MW00787210

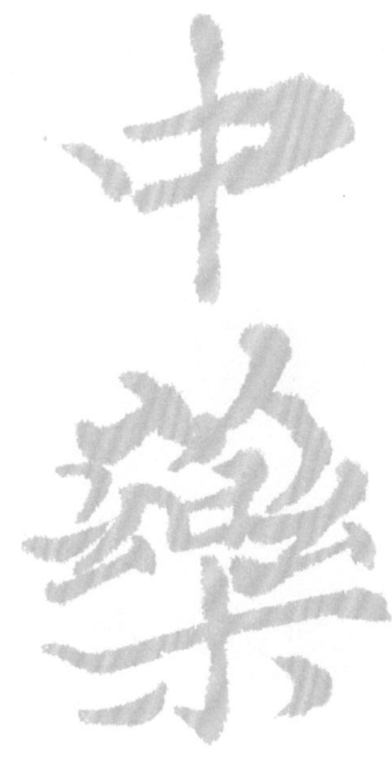

Chinese Medical Herbology and Pharmacology

John K. Chen • Tina T. Chen

with Laraine Crampton

中藥藥理學

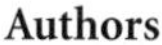

Chinese Medical Herbology and Pharmacology

John K. Chen • Tina T. Chen

with Laraine Crampton

Authors
John K. Chen, PhD, PharmD, OMD, LAc
Tina T. Chen, MS, LAc
with Laraine Crampton, MPW, MATCM, LAc

Editor
Laraine Crampton, MPW, MATCM, LAc

Associate Editors
Colleen Burke, DOM, LAc
Vanessa G Au, LAc, DC

Contributing Editors
Christian DellaCorte, PhD
Joerg Fritschi, MD
Steve Given, LAc, Dipl Ac
Glenn Grossman, MS, LAc, Dipl Ac & CH
Steve Jarsky, LAc
Anita Chen Marshall, PharmD, MS, Dipl Ac, LAc
Cathy McNease, Dipl CH
Larry Miller, LAc
William R. Morris, DOM, LAc
Daoshing Ni, LAc, DOM, PhD
Ray Rubio, LAc

Peer Review Committee
Subhuti Dharmanada, PhD
Susan Diva, RN
Jake Paul Fratkin, OMD, LAc
Jing-Lih Lily Ko, LAc
David Karaba, LAc
Richard Ko, PharmD, PhD
Cheri Levine, LAc, RN, CEN
Frederick Obey, LAc
Kevin Park, PharmD
Eric Rhim, PharmD
Marc Ryan, LAc
Tierney Tully, MSOM, Dipl Ac
Roy Upton, Herbalist
Ronda Wimmer, LAc

Copy Editors
Lily Huang, LAc
Delicia Liu, LAc
Minh Thanh Nguyen, LAc

Research Associates
Meng-Chau (Victor) Jang, LAc
Delicia Liu, LAc

Art of Medicine Press, Inc.
City of Industry, CA USA

ISBN: 0-9740635-0-9
Standard Address Number: 255-3376
Library of Congress Number: 2003105436

Art of Medicine Press, Inc.
P.O. Box 90878
City of Industry, CA 91715-0878

Website: www.aompress.com
Email: editor@aompress.com

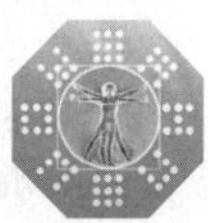

Preface to the Second Print

Chinese Medical Herbology and Pharmacology is intended to be used with *Chinese Herbal Formulas and Applications*. The former text provides indepth understanding of how each individual herb functions within Chinese herbal formulas, while the latter text provides insight on how these formulas are used specifically in clinical practice.

In referencing between these two texts, it is important to note that the nomenclature for some herbs has been changed since the publication of *Chinese Medical Herbology and Pharmacology* in 2004. Most changes correspond to the 2005 edition of 中华人民共和国药典 *Zhong Hua Ren Min Gong He Guo Yao Dian* (Pharmacopoeia of the People's Republic of China), which is the official pharmacopoeia in China, as well as our primary reference. Therefore, in the second print of *Chinese Medical Herbology and Pharmacology*, changes have been made to:

- correctly pronounce the *pinyin* name, from *Huang Bai* (Cortex Phellodendri) to *Huang Bo* (Cortex Phellodendri Chinensis)
- precisely describe the processing method, from *Zhi Gan Cao* (Radix Glycyrrhizae Praeparata) to *Zhi Gan Cao* (Radix et Rhizoma Glycyrrhizae Praeparata cum Melle)
- be more specific: *Kun Bu* (Thallus Laminariae seu Eckloniae) is separated into *Hai Dai* (Thallus Laminariae) and *Kun Bu* (Thallus Eckloniae)
- be more inclusive: from *Shan Ci Gu* (Pseudobulbus Cremastrae) to *Shan Ci Gu* (Pseudobulbus Cremastrae seu Pleiones)
- adapt to the current rules and regulations, from *Xi Xin* (Herba Asari) to *Xi Xin* (Radix et Rhizoma Asari). Note: The aerial parts of asarum contain aristolochic acid, and have been banned by many countries around the world. As a result, the root and rhizome of asarum are now used, as they are believed to have little or no aristolochic acid.[1]
- and lastly, to humbly correct our previous errors, such as replacing the incorrect *Mu Fang Ji* (Radix Couulus Trilobus) with *Mu Fang Ji* (Radix Cocculi Trilobi).

Chinese Medical Herbology and Pharmacology, first print in 2004	*Chinese Medical Herbology and Pharmacology, second print in 2012*
Ba Yue Zha (Fructus Akebiae)	*Yu Zhi Zi* (Fructus Akebiae)
Bai Dou Kou (Fructus Amomi Rotundus)	*Dou Kou* (Fructus Amomi Rotundus)
Bai Dou Kou Ke (Pericarpium Amomi Rotundus)	*Dou Kou Ke* (Pericarpium Amomi Rotundus)
Bai Hua She (Bungarus Parvus)	*Jin Qian Bai Hua She* (Bungarus Parvus)
Bai Hua She She Cao (Herba Oldenlandia)	*Bai Hua She She Cao* (Herba Hedyotis)
Bai Ji Li (Fructus Tribuli)	*Ji Li* (Fructus Tribuli)
Bai Qian (Rhizoma Cynanchi Stauntonii)	*Bai Qian* (Rhizoma et Radix Cynanchi Stauntonii)
Bai Wei (Radix Cynanchi Atrati)	*Bai Wei* (Radix et Rhizoma Cynanchi Atrati)
Bei Mu (Bulbus Fritillaria)	*Bei Mu* (Bulbus Fritillariae)
Bei Wu Jia Pi (Cortex Periploca Sepium Radicis)	*Xiang Jia Pi* (Cortex Periplocae)
Bi Ba (Fructus Piperis Longi)	*Bi Bo* (Fructus Piperis Longi)
Bi Xie (Rhizoma Dioscoreae Hypoglaucae)	*Fen Bi Xie* (Rhizoma Dioscoreae Hypoglaucae)
Bian Dou (Semen Lablab Album)	*Bai Bian Dou* (Semen Lablab Album)
Can Sha (Excrementum Bombycis Mori)	*Can Sha* (Faeces Bombycis)
Chi Fu Ling (Poria Rubrae)	*Chi Fu Ling* (Poria Rubra)
Chi Shao (Radix Paeoniae Rubrae)	*Chi Shao* (Radix Paeoniae Rubra)
Chong Wei Zi (Semen Leonuri)	*Chong Wei Zi* (Fructus Leonuri)
Chuan Xiong (Rhizoma Ligustici Chuanxiong)	*Chuan Xiong* (Rhizoma Chuanxiong)
Chun Gen Pi (Cortex Ailanthi)	*Chun Pi* (Cortex Ailanthi)
Ci Wu Jia (Radix et Caulis Acanthopanacis Senticosi)	*Ci Wu Jia* (Radix et Rhizoma seu Caulis Acanthopanacis Senticosi)
Da Hui Xiang (Fructus Anisi Stellati)	*Ba Jiao Hui Xiang* (Fructus Anisi Stellati)

Preface to the Second Print

Chinese Medical Herbology and Pharmacology, first print in 2004	*Chinese Medical Herbology and Pharmacology, second print in 2012*
Da Ji (Herba seu Radix Cirsii Japonici)	*Da Ji* (Herba Cirsii Japonici)
Dai Zhe Shi (Haematitum)	*Zhe Shi* (Haematitum)
Dan Shen (Radix Salviae Miltiorrhizae)	*Dan Shen* (Radix et Rhizoma Salviae Miltiorrhizae)
Dang Gui (Radicis Angelicae Sinensis)	*Dang Gui* (Radix Angelicae Sinensis)
Dang Gui Shen (Corpus Radicis Angelicae Sinensis)	*Dang Gui Shen* (Corpus Radix Angelicae Sinensis)
Dang Gui Tou (Caput Radicis Angelicae Sinensis)	*Dang Gui Tou* (Caput Radix Angelicae Sinensis)
Dang Gui Wei (Extremitas Radicis Angelicae Sinensis)	*Dang Gui Wei* (Extremitas Radix Angelicae Sinensis)
Di Bie Chong (Eupolyphaga)	*Tu Bie Chong* (Eupolyphaga seu Steleophaga)
Duan Shi Gao (Gypsum Fibrosum Preparata)	*Duan Shi Gao* (Gypsum Fibrosum Praeparatum)
Fen Fang Ji (Radix Stephaniae Tetandrae)	*Fang Ji* (Radix Stephaniae Tetrandrae)
Fu Xiao Mai (Semen Tritici Aestivi Levis)	*Fu Xiao Mai* (Fructus Tritici Levis)
Gan Cao (Radix Glycyrrhizae)	*Gan Cao* (Radix et Rhizoma Glycyrrhizae)
Gan Song (Radix seu Rhizoma Nardostachys)	*Gan Song* (Radix et Rhizoma Nardostachydis)
Gan Sui (Radix Euphorbiae Kansui)	*Gan Sui* (Radix Kansui)
Gao Ben (Rhizoma Ligustici)	*Gao Ben* (Rhizoma et Radix Ligustici)
Ge Gen (Radix Puerariae)	*Ge Gen* (Radix Puerariae Lobatae)
Gu Zhi Hua (Semen Oroxyli)	*Mu Hu Die* (Semen Oroxyli)
Gua Lou Ren (Semen Trichosanthis)	*Gua Lou Zi* (Semen Trichosanthis)
Gua Lou Shi (Fructus Trichosanthis)	*Gua Lou* (Fructus Trichosanthis)
Guan Bai Fu (Rhizoma Aconitum Coreanum)	*Guan Bai Fu* (Radix Aconiti Coreani)
Guan Ye Lian Qiao (Herba Hypericum)	*Guan Ye Jin Si Tao* (Herba Hyperici Perforati)
Guan Zhong (Rhizoma Dryopteridis)	*Mian Ma Guan Zhong* (Rhizoma Dryopteridis Crassirhizomatis)
Hai Ge Fen (Concha Meretricis seu Cyclinae)	*Ge Qiao* (Concha Meretricis seu Cyclinae)
Hai Jin Sha (Herba Lygodii)	*Hai Jin Sha* (Spora Lygodii)
Han Fang Ji (Radix Stephaniae Tetandrae)	*Fang Ji* (Radix Stephaniae Tetrandrae)
Han Lian Cao (Herba Ecliptae)	*Mo Han Lian* (Herba Ecliptae)
Hei Cha (Folium Camelliae Nigrum)	*Hei Cha* (Folium Camelliae Nigrum)
Hei Dou (Semen Glycine Max)	*Hei Dou* (Semen Sojae)
Hong Dou Kou (Fructus Alphiniae Galangae)	*Hong Dou Kou* (Fructus Galangae)
Hong Teng (Caulis Sargentodoxae)	*Da Xue Teng* (Caulis Sargentodoxae)
Hu Jiao (Fructus Piper)	*Hu Jiao* (Fructus Piperis)
Hu Zhang (Rhizoma Polygoni Cuspidati)	*Hu Zhang* (Rhizoma et Radix Polygoni Cuspidati)
Huai Niu Xi (Radix Achyranthis Bidentatae)	*Niu Xi* (Radix Achyranthis Bidentatae)
Huang Bai (Cortex Phellodendri)	*Huang Bo* (Cortex Phellodendri Chinensis)
Huang Teng (Caulis Fibraurea)	*Huang Teng* (Caulis Fibraureae)
Huo Xiang (Herba Agastache)	*Huo Xiang* (Herba Agastaches)
Huo Xiang Ye (Folium Agastache)	*Huo Xiang Ye* (Folium Agastaches)
Jin Bo (Native Gold)	*Jin Bo* (gold foil)
Jin Yin Hua (Flos Lonicerae)	*Jin Yin Hua* (Flos Lonicerae Japonicae)
Jing Jie Sui (Flos Schizonepetae)	*Jing Jie Sui* (Spica Schizonepetae)
Jing Sui (Flos Schizonepetae)	*Jing Jie Sui* (Spica Schizonepetae)
Ju He (Semen Citri Rubrum)	*Ju He* (Semen Citri Reticulatae)

Preface to the Second Print

Chinese Medical Herbology and Pharmacology, first print in 2004	*Chinese Medical Herbology and Pharmacology, second print in 2012*
Ju Luo (Fibra Citri Rubrum)	*Ju Luo* (Vascular Citri Reticulatae)
Ju Ye (Folium Citri Rubrum)	*Ju Ye* (Folium Citri Reticulatae)
Ku Shen Gen (Radix Sophorae Flavescentis)	*Ku Shen* (Radix Sophorae Flavescentis)
Kun Bu (Thallus Laminariae seu Eckloniae)	*Kun Bu* (Thallus Eckloniae)
Long Dan Cao (Radix Gentianae)	*Long Dan* (Radix et Rhizoma Gentianae)
Lu Cha (Folium Camellia Sinensis)	*Cha Ye* (Folium Camelliae)
Lu Feng Fang (Nidus Vespae)	*Feng Fang* (Nidus Vespae)
Lu Han Cao (Herba Pyrolae)	*Lu Xian Cao* (Herba Pyrolae)
Lu Jiao Jiao (Gelatinum Cornu Cervi)	*Lu Jiao Jiao* (Colla Cornus Cervi)
Lu Jiao Shuang (Cornu Cervi Degelatinatium)	*Lu Jiao Shuang* (Cornu Cervi Degelatinatum)
Ma Huang Gen (Radix Ephedrae)	*Ma Huang Gen* (Radix et Rhizoma Ephedrae)
Mai Men Dong (Radix Ophiopogonis)	*Mai Dong* (Radix Ophiopogonis)
Mi Jiao (Cornu Elapnurus)	*Mi Lu Jiao* (Cornu Elaphuri)
Mi Rong (Cornu Elapnurus Parvum)	*Mi Lu Rong* (Cornu Elaphuri Pantotrichum)
Ming Fan (Alumen)	*Bai Fan* (Alumen)
Mu Fang Ji (Radix Couulus Trilobus)	*Mu Fang Ji* (Radix Cocculi Trilobi)
Niu Xi (Radix Cyathulae seu Achyranthis)	*Niu Xi* (Radix Achyranthis Bidentatae)
Pao Jiang (Rhizoma Zingiberis Preparatum)	*Pao Jiang* (Rhizoma Zingiberis Praeparatum)
Qian Cao (Radix Rubiae)	*Qian Cao* (Radix et Rhizoma Rubiae)
Qian Jin Zi (Semen Euphorbiae Lathyridis)	*Qian Jin Zi* (Semen Euphorbiae)
Ren Dong Cao (Herba Lonicerae)	*Ren Dong Cao* (Herba Lonicerae Japonicae)
Ren Dong Teng (Caulis Lonicerae)	*Ren Dong Teng* (Caulis Lonicerae Japonicae)
Ren Gong Niu Huang (Calculus Bovis Syntheticum)	*Ren Gong Niu Huang* (Calculus Bovis Artifactus)
Ren Shen (Radix Ginseng)	*Ren Shen* (Radix et Rhizoma Ginseng)
Rui Ren (Semen Prinsepiae)	*Rui Ren* (Nux Prinsepiae)
San Qi (Radix Notoginseng)	*San Qi* (Radix et Rhizoma Notoginseng)
Sang Shen Zi (Fructus Mori)	*Sang Shen* (Fructus Mori)
Shan Ci Gu (Pseudobulbus Cremastrae)	*Shan Ci Gu* (Pseudobulbus Cremastrae seu Pleiones)
Shan Dou Gen (Radix Sophorae Tonkinensis)	*Shan Dou Gen* (Radix et Rhizoma Sophorae Tonkinensis)
Sheng Di Huang (Radix Rehmanniae)	*Di Huang* (Radix Rehmanniae)
Shi Chang Pu (Rhizoma Acori)	*Shi Chang Pu* (Rhizoma Acori Tatarinowii)
Shi Hu (Herba Dendrobii)	*Shi Hu* (Caulis Dendrobii)
Shu Di Huang (Radix Rehmanniae Preparata)	*Shu Di Huang* (Radix Rehmanniae Praeparata)
Shui Chang Pu (Rhizoma Acori Calami)	*Zang Chang Pu* (Rhizoma Acori Calami)
Su Geng (Caulis Perillae)	*Zi Su Geng* (Caulis Perillae)
Su Ye (Folium Perillae)	*Zi Su Ye* (Folium Perillae)
Su Zi (Fructus Perillae)	*Zi Su Zi* (Fructus Perillae)
Suan Zao Ren (Semen Zizyphi Spinosae)	*Suan Zao Ren* (Semen Ziziphi Spinosae)
Tian Men Dong (Radix Asparagi)	*Tian Dong* (Radix Asparagi)
Tu Bei Mu (Bulbus Bolbostemma Paniculatum)	*Tu Bei Mu* (Rhizoma Bolbostematis)
Tu Niu Xi (Radix Achyranthes Longifolia)	*Tu Niu Xi* (Radix Achyranthis Longifoliae)
Wan Nian Song (Herba Selaginellae)	*Juan Bai* (Herba Selaginellae)
Wei Ling Xian (Radix Clematidis)	*Wei Ling Xian* (Radix et Rhizoma Clematidis)

Preface to the Second Print

Chinese Medical Herbology and Pharmacology, first print in 2004	*Chinese Medical Herbology and Pharmacology, second print in 2012*
Wu Ling Zhi (Excrementum Trogopteri seu Pteromi)	*Wu Ling Zhi* (Faeces Trogopteri)
Wu Long Cha (Folium Camellia Sinensis Fermentata)	*Wu Long Cha* (Folium Camelliae Fermentata)
Xi Xin (Herba Asari)	*Xi Xin* (Radix et Rhizoma Asari)
Xiang Ru (Herba Elsholtziae seu Moslae)	*Xiang Ru* (Herba Moslae)
Xiao Ji (Herba Cirisii)	*Xiao Ji* (Herba Cirsii)
Xing Ren (Semen Armeniacae Amarum)	*Ku Xing Ren* (Semen Armeniacae Amarum)
Xu Chang Qing (Radix Cynanchi Paniculati)	*Xu Chang Qing* (Radix et Rhizoma Cynanchi Paniculati)
Xuan Ming Fen (Matrii Sulfas Exsiccatus)	*Xuan Ming Fen* (Natrii Sulfas Exsiccatus)
Ye Jiao Teng (Caulis Polygoni Multiflori)	*Shou Wu Teng* (Caulis Polygoni Multiflori)
Ye Ming Sha (Excrementum Vespertilionis Murini)	*Ye Ming Sha* (Faeces Vespertilionis Murini)
Yi Tang (Saccharum Granorum)	*Yi Tang* (Maltosum)
Yi Zhi Ren (Fructus Alpiniae Oxyphyllae)	*Yi Zhi* (Fructus Alpiniae Oxyphyllae)
Yin Chen Hao (Herba Artemisiae Scopariae)	*Yin Chen* (Herba Artemisiae Scopariae)
Yin Guo Ye (Folium Ginkgo)	*Yin Xing Ye* (Folium Ginkgo)
Yuan Ming Fen (Matrii Sulfas Exsiccatus)	*Xuan Ming Fen* (Natrii Sulfas Exsiccatus)
Zang Hong Hua (Flos Crocus Sativus)	*Xi Hong Hua* (Stigma Croci)
Zhen Zhu Mu (Concha Margaritaferae)	*Zhen Zhu Mu* (Concha Margaritiferae)
Zhi Gan Cao (Radix Glycyrrhizae Preparata)	*Zhi Gan Cao* (Radix et Rhizoma Glycyrrhizae Praeparata cum Melle)
Zhi Ke (Fructus Aurantii)	*Zhi Qiao* (Fructus Aurantii)
Zhi Mu (Radix Anemarrhenae)	*Zhi Mu* (Rhizoma Anemarrhenae)
Zi Cao Gen (Radix Lithospermi)	*Zi Cao* (Radix Arnebiae)
Zi Wan (Radix Asteris)	*Zi Wan* (Radix et Rhizoma Asteris)
Zong Lu Pi (Fibra Stipulae Trachycarpi)	*Zong Lu* (Petiolus Trachycarpi)

[1] Wu KM, Farrelly JG, Upton R, Chen J. Complexities of the herbal nomenclature system in traditional Chinese medicine (TCM): Lessons learned from the misuse of Aristolochia-related species and the importance of the pharmaceutical name during botanical drug product development. Phytomedicine 2007;14:273-279.

Abbreviated Table of Contents

Table of Contents

Table of Contents

Table of Contents

Table of Contents

Table of Contents

Table of Contents

Table of Contents

Table of Contents

Preface

As an herbalist and a pharmacist, it has always been my goal to produce an herbal medicine textbook that appropriately merges the concepts of traditional Chinese medicine with those of western medicine. Throughout my years of practice, I have often been asked about integration and interpretation of both paradigms of medicine. Practitioners of herbal medicine often ask whether certain herbs can be prescribed for particular patients because of potential herb-drug interactions. On the other hand, practitioners of western pharmaceutical-based medicine are often skeptical of herbs as authentic medicine because they have not gained understanding of "how or if herbs really work." While helpful answers have not always been promptly available, the question is crystal clear. There is a dire need for resources that integrate the two systems of medicine.

The objective for the compilation of *Chinese Medical Herbology and Pharmacology* is to create an informative and useful text on Chinese herbal medicine accessible to all healthcare practitioners. For herbal medicine practitioners, it offers comprehensive information on the traditional uses and applications of herbs. For other healthcare professionals, this text offers detailed discussion of the pharmacology and clinical applications of herbs. Those who practice in integrative settings will benefit from the understanding of contemporary frontiers of herb/drug interaction and toxicology information. This book is written for practitioners and students of medicine, and the contents are best understood by readers who have a basic understanding of both traditional Chinese and western medicines.

Chinese Medical Herbology and Pharmacology is dedicated to all who believe in the healing power of herbs, and believe that the next cure may be found in nature.

John K. Chen, Ph.D., Pharm.D., O.M.D, L.Ac.
Tina T. Chen, M.S., L.Ac.
June 2003

Writing any textbook requires commitment and self-sacrifice. Writing, translating, and compiling a highly-technical and detailed book is undertaken only by seriously-determined individuals with a lot of energy and broad knowledge, willing to invest many hours of disciplined effort and patience in organizing myriad details and establishing consistency throughout many hundreds of pages and dozens of pre-publication editions. Insuring that the whole of that material is accessible and clear for a widely-diverse audience of professionals in multiple disciplines requires a stubborn perfectionism that calls for even more patience.

I have been enormously fortunate to have been invited into the process of completing *Chinese Medical Herbology and Pharmacology* by John Chen and Tina Chen. They exhibited not only the qualities mentioned above, but have shown great tolerance for my fierce editing, and generous openness to my ideas. John in particular has exercised forbearance with my persistent communication about thousands of details. I join John and Tina in hoping that the years invested in this work will be transformed through publication into genuine benefit to our profession and to ever-improving healthcare services for all individuals seeking to regain vitality and well-being.

Laraine Crampton, MPW, MATCM, L.Ac.
June 2003

Acknowledgements

We would like to thank all our teachers, who have taught us everything we know, especially Drs. Jimmy Wei-Yen Chang, Jiao Shu-De, Sam Liang, Richard Teh-Fu Tan, Liu Zhi-Tong, Tsai Wen-Qi, and Zhang Xiao-Ping.

We would like to thank Laraine for her unyielding pursuit of perfection. We truly appreciate everything you have done, and all the sacrifices you have made. You complete and compliment our strengths and weaknesses.

Our thanks to Dan Bensky, Randall Barolet, Andrew Gamble, Giovanni Maciocia, Subhuti Dharmanada, Him-che Yeung, Nigel Wiseman and Feng Ye for their contributions to Chinese herbal medicine.

The contributing editors and Peer Review committee have offered inestimable improvements for the material through their review, suggestions and contributions.

Jake Paul Fratkin, Felice Dunas, Giovanni Maciocia and Bob Felt, thank you for your wisdom on writing and publishing.

To our dear friend and colleague, who wishes to stay anonymous, our sincere thanks for his wisdom and support.

Most importantly, we would like to thank our family: our father, for his vision and inspiration; our mom, for her endless love and support; and our family for reminding us to stop and smell the herbs throughout this eight-year journey.

The publication of *Chinese Medical Herbology and Pharmacology* would not have been possible without the help of everyone who has contributed. This book belongs to all of us.

John K. Chen
Tina T. Chen

I would never have worked on this book if Dr. Maoshing Ni had not given me a life-changing introduction to Chinese medicine.

It has been a great privilege, and often fun, to work with and learn from John and Tina: you have broadened my understanding of our field and its potential. Your patience has been huge, hyphens and all.

My thanks to always-inspiring Cathy McNease and Denise Neumark-Reimer for patience and kindness as I learned herbology, and to my other teachers, not least Steve Given and Daoshing Ni, for emphasizing the critical importance of these potent medicines. Thanks to my patients, who inspire me to keep learning.

Colleen and Richard, I would have been lost without your generous hard work. Vanessa, Lily, Delicia, Nina, and recently, Minh, Larry and David: there is no way to quantify the value of your efforts. Rick and Charles, your creativity, brilliance and perseverance are the visual beauty of this book.

To Jeffrey Clark, Sollace Mitchell, and Brad Schreiber, my warmest thanks for graciously answering my calls and e-mails about arcane details of language. David G., thanks for great resources. Kathy and Mark, your meals and encouragement kept me going when the task grew long. Mom, you never complained when I had to postpone visits because of the book. Thanks always for your love and generosity of spirit.

Laraine Crampton

Contributors

Authors
John K. Chen, PhD, PharmD, OMD, LAc
Tina T. Chen, MS, LAc
with Laraine Crampton, MPW, MATCM, LAc

Editor
Laraine Crampton, MPW, MATCM, LAc

Associate Editors
Colleen Burke, DOM, LAc
Vanessa G Au, LAc, DC

Contributing Editors
Christian DellaCorte, PhD
Joerg Fritschi, MD
Steve Given, LAc, Dipl Ac
Glenn Grossman, MS, LAc, Dipl Ac & CH
Steve Jarsky, LAc
Jing-Lih Lily Ko, LAc
Anita Chen Marshall, PharmD, MS, Dipl Ac, LAc
Cathy McNease, Dipl CH
Larry Miller, LAc
William R. Morris, DOM, LAc
Daoshing Ni, LAc, DOM, PhD
Ray Rubio, LAc

Copy Editors
Lily Huang, LAc
Delicia Liu, LAc
Minh Thanh Nguyen, LAc

Research Associates
Meng-Chau (Victor) Jang, LAc
Delicia Liu, LAc

Peer Review Committee
Subhuti Dharmananda, PhD
Susan Diva, RN
Jake Paul Fratkin, OMD, LAc
David Karaba, LAc
Richard Ko, PharmD, PhD
Cheri Levine, LAc, RN, CEN
Frederick Obey, LAc
Kevin Park, PharmD
Eric Rhim, PharmD
Marc Ryan, LAc
Tierney Tully, MSOM, Dipl Ac
Roy Upton, Herbalist
Ronda Wimmer, LAc

Book Design
Rick Friesen — birdbrainArts

Contributors

Cover Design and Photography
Charles Funk

Text Herb Illustrations
Rick Friesen — birdbrainArts
Charles Funk

Calligraphy
Tu Chin-Sheng

Typists
Richard Kearns
Nina Luu

Legal Advisor
Eric K. Chen, PhD, OMD, LAc, JD

Proofreaders
James Chi-Wei Chen
Gil Cruz
David Fiden
Donna Greenberg
Steven Davis Kanovitz
Debbie Kim
Aram Nalbandyan
Sara Pettitt
Kiumars Pharrahpur
Sami Rank
Gail Ritzer
Maureen Santucci
Star Urmston
Nathalie Valkov
Shawn Welch
Dena Zachara

Chemical Structure Illustrations
Chemical structure diagrams were used with permission from:
The Merck Index 12th edition, Chapman & Hall/CRCnetBASE/Merck, 2000
Traditional Chinese Medicines Molecular Structures, Natural Sources and Applications; Yan X, Zhou J, and Xie G, Ashgate, 1999; 2598

Herb Samples
Mayway Corp.
NuHerb
Sheng Foong Pharmaceutical Company
Robert Chu, LAc
South Baylo University Clinic
Spring Wind Herbs

Contributing Authors:
Chang Jie-An, Director and Vice-President of Wuhan TCM Hospital, Wuhan, China
Chang Wei-Yen (Jimmy), Jian Tai Clinic, Hacienda Heights, CA, USA
Chen Ke-Fen, Professor of Tianjin TCM Hospital, Tianjin, China

Contributors

Chen Shu-Sheng, Consultant for the First Tuberculosis Research Hospital of Shanghai, Shanghai, China
Chen Yuan-Da, Chen's Clinic, La Puente, CA, USA
Cheng Chun-Fu, Professor of Hubei TCM University, Hubei, China
Ding Guang-Di, Professor of Nanjing TCM University, Nanjing, China
Gan Zhu-Wang, Professor of TCM University of Nanjing, Director of Nanjing TCM Hospital, Nanjing, China
He Shi-Xi, Shanghai TCM Hospital, Shanghai, China
He Zi-Jun, Director of Hangzhou TCM Hospital, Hangzhou, China
Hu Qing-Shan, Heilongjiang TCM Hospital, Heilongjiang, China
Jang Meng-Chau, Rosemead, CA, USA
Jiao Shu-De, Profession of Beijing TCM University, Beijing, China
Li Shou-Shan, Consultant and Professor of TCM Hospital of Dalian, Dalian, China
Li Tong-Sheng, President of the Hubei TCM Research Center, Hubei, China
Li Zi-Zi, Director of TCM University in Gansu Province, Gansu, China
Liang, Sam, Golden Needle, El Toro, CA, USA
Liu Feng-Wu, Director of Gynecology Department Beijing TCM Hospital, Beijing, China
Liu Hong-Xiang, Director of Taian City Hospital, Weifang, China
Liu Shao-An, Director of Internal Medicine, People's First TCM Hospital of Guiyang, Guiyang, China
Liu Zhi-Tong, Tianjin Military Hospital, Tianjin, China
Long Pang-Chi, Professor of Shanghai TCM University, Director of Gynecology Department Shuguang Hospital, Shanghai, China
Shen Yen-Nan, Professor of Guangzhou TCM University, Guangzhou, China
Shu Run-San, Director of Gynecology Department, Beijing Sino-Japanese Hospital, Beijing, China
Tan Teh-Fu (Richard), San Diego, CA, USA
Tsai Wen-Qi, Alhambra, CA, USA
Wei Jia, Director of Jiangxi TCM Hospital, Professor of Jiangxi University of TCM, Jiangxi, China
Xu Fu-He, Professor of TCM University of Nanjing, Director of Nanjing TCM Hospital, Nanjing, China
Yin Hui-He, Director of Sino-Japanese Hospital of Beijing, Beijing, China
Zhang Xiao-Ping, Director of Anhui TCM Hospital, Professor of Anhui TCM University, Anhui, China
Zhang Xue-Wen, Director and Professor of Shanxi TCM University, Shanxi, China
Zhu Fang-Shou, Professor of Nanjing TCM Hospital and Director of Sujiang Province TCM Hospital, Sujiang, China
Zhu Lang-Chun, Director of Nantong TCM Hospital, Nantong, China
Zhu Shen-Yu, Director of TCM Department, TCM Science Hospital, Beijing, China

Using this Book

Chinese Medical Herbology and Pharmacology has been designed for use in the clinic, in the classroom, in research, and to preserve and convey valuable historical information that may yet prove crucial in our future. Written to empower practitioner readers to become better clinicians, it offers detailed discussion on traditional applications, dosages and preparation of herbs, cautions and/or contraindications, overdosage and its treatment, and a contemporary expansion of clinician training: potential herb-drug interactions. All of these features simultaneously serve students and faculty in academic settings. Research professionals will find chemical structures and components, *in vitro* information on pharmacological effects and toxicology, and *in vivo* information from clinical studies. Some rare or potentially lethal medicinal substances that are *not* in contemporary use are included and discussed strictly to illustrate important concepts or historical value in traditional Chinese medicine. Among these are endangered species [such as *Hu Gu* (Os Tigris) and *Xi Jiao* (Cornu Rhinoceri)] and dangerous heavy metals [such as *Shui Yin* (Hydrargyrum) and *Qian Dan* (Minium)]. Their inclusion in no way advocates resumption of use or further destruction of species or resources.

Although pertinent to the history, practice, and research of Chinese herbal medicine, not all herbs discussed herein are commercially available. Some are prohibited as illegal substances (such as *Ying Su Ke* (Pericarpium Papaveris)), some, as mentioned above, carry excessive potential for toxicity (such as *Zhu Sha* (Cinnabaris)) or are restricted due to endangered status (such as *Xi Jiao* (Cornu Rhinoceri)). These substances are included only to offer the accurate history of their critically important usage in traditional herbal medicine, and to serve as models for appropriate usage of effective *substitute* substances. The readers are strongly encouraged to know and respect the rules and regulations for use of these substances in their own states and/or countries.

ILLUSTRATIONS

- Black-and-white photographs of substances are displayed in actual size, unless noted otherwise. Because most users of this text will not be gathering herbs direct from nature, we have chosen to provide illustrations of the harvested, processed, manicured substances as our readers would encounter them in realistic purchasing and clinical situations.
- Herb samples available at the time of publication are displayed in a full-color section, in alphabetical order by pinyin name. Matching black-and-white photographs accompany the primary herb entries throughout the text. We encourage the readers to always refer to the color pictures when seeking more complete and life-like illustration of herb samples.

NOMENCLATURE

- Traditional and simplified **Chinese Characters** lead each herb monograph to provide the most accurate Chinese name and to facilitate understanding of the herb under discussion. Simplified characters serve as the default in cases in which the traditional and simplified are identical.
- **Herbs and Formulas:** It is our goal to be as comprehensive and precise as possible. Traditional nomenclature of herbs is often vague: one herb may have several alternate names, and may be replaced by substitute plants from varied sources, species or genus. Thus, we have listed in the monographs Chinese characters, pinyin name, alternate pinyin name(s), literal name(s), common English name(s), botanical/zoological name(s) and pharmaceutical name(s). When an herb is commonly obtained from more than one natural source, identification is made of all pinyin, pharmaceutical and botanical names. Because differences in therapeutic effect are often distinguished by names, these distinctions are made clear. For example, *Sha Shen* (Radix Glehniae seu Adenophorae) is stated as *Nan Sha Shen* (Radix Adenophorae) or *Bei Sha Shen* (Radix Glehniae) whenever possible because of the unique clinical applications of each. "*Mu Tong*" has been separated appropriately into *Chuan Mu Tong* (Caulis Clematidis Armandii), *Guan Mu Tong* (Caulis Aristolochiae Manshuriensis), *San Ye Mu Tong* (Caulis Akebia Trifoliata), *Wu Ye Mu Tong* (Caulis Akebia Quinata), and *Bai Mu Tong* (Caulis Akebia Trifoliata Australis), since these plants are not only from different genus and species, but also have different therapeutic effects and safety profiles.

Using this Book

The following are the primary sources the authors relied upon for nomenclature of herbs and formulas:

Zhong Hua Ren Min Gong He Guo Yao Dian (Chinese Herbal Pharmacopoeia by People's Republic of China), People's Republic of China, 2000. Our standard reference for nomenclature of pinyin and pharmaceutical names, this text offers the most precise, accurate and current information on the identification of Chinese herbs and other medicinal substances.

Xian Dai Zhong Yao Yao Li Xue (Contemporary Pharmacology of Chinese Herbs) by Wang Ben-Yang, Tianjing Science and Technology Press, 1999.

Chinese Herbal Medicine Materia Medica, by Dan Bensky and Andrew Gamble, Eastland Press, 1993.

Chinese Herbal Medicine Formulas & Strategies, by Dan Bensky and Randall Barolet, Eastland Press, 1990.

A Practical Dictionary of Chinese Medicine 2nd Edition, by Nigel Wiseman and Feng Ye, Paradigm Publications, 1998.

CHINESE THERAPEUTIC ACTIONS

- **Traditional Chinese Medicine (TCM) terminology**. Because traditional Chinese medicine and western medicine have distinct cultural and philosophical influences, it is challenging to accurately convey some TCM terms and concepts by using English or allopathic clinical language. We have made sincere efforts to provide consistent standards for terms and concepts to bridge the gap, as follows:

  Terms that have become an accepted part of English language discourse and are well understood by the general public, such as qi, yin and yang, are not italicized nor capitalized.

  Terms unique to the profession, understood primarily by TCM practitioners, are given in pinyin, italicized and translated but not capitalized; such as *bi zheng* (painful obstruction syndrome), *xiao ke* (wasting and thirsting) syndrome, and *lin zheng* (dysuria syndrome).

  Nouns distinct to herbal medicine are italicized, capitalized and translated, such as *Ren Shen* (Radix Ginseng) and *Bu Zhong Yi Qi Tang* (Tonify the Middle and Augment the Qi Decoction).

  Translations are omitted after the first full use of the term in one monograph or segment of a monograph, unless repetition is necessary to insure clarity and safety in discriminating between substances or concepts.

  To avoid confusion, herbs other than the principle herb under consideration in a given monograph will be listed with their full pinyin and pharmaceutical names at each use, unless mentioned multiple times within a given paragraph.

  It is important to note that anatomical organ names in TCM imply functions distinct from their common understanding in western medicine. Therefore, organ names are capitalized when discussed within the context of traditional Chinese medicine but not when referring exclusively to anatomical function. For example, *Huang Qin* (Radix Scutellariae) is commonly used to clear **Lung** heat because the herb has shown antibiotic effectiveness to treat infection of the **lungs**.

  In some few instances, the authors felt that rendering a highly precise translation of a Chinese word misses the common professional meaning/usage of the term. In these cases, the common usage has been chosen for the body of the text, while precise translation is offered in the glossary.

  The Glossary provides additional information on individual terms and definitions. A cross-reference with the terminology chosen by **Wiseman** and **Ye** is also listed.

- **Formulas and Compositions:** Examples of Chinese herbal formulas are mentioned throughout this text, to enhance understanding of the qualities of an individual herb, and its applications. Herbal formula names are cross-referenced in Appendix 5, Cross-Reference of Herbal Formula Names. Further discussion, including the full composition of each formula in a thorough monograph, will be available in our next book.

Note: A keen reader may notice that the ingredients listed in some exemplar formulas here may differ slightly from standard classic formulas. We name the classic formula to demonstrate the

Using this Book

intent and basic strategy of the formulation in clinical application, but *not* to list the exact composition of the ingredients. Thus, in any given exemplar formula, additional herbs may be listed (as modifications) to optimize treatment in the particular contextual situation.

DOSAGE

- **Standard dosage:** Listed in this text is the standard dosage of ***dried*** herb to be used ***in decoction*** for an ***average adult***, unless otherwise specified. Adjustments are needed if the herbs are to be used in other forms: higher dosage (generally double) for the fresh herb, and lower dosage for herbs ingested in powder or pill forms. The average adult is defined as being between 18 and 60 years of age, weighing approximately 150 pounds. Thus, dosage must be adjusted more precisely depending on individual attributes. Additional information and guidelines for dosage adjustment can be found in Appendix 8, Dosing Guidelines.
- **Weights and Measurement:** Units of measurement have been converted from the traditional Chinese system to the metric system. Additional information on comparison and conversions can be found in Appendix 9, Weights and Measures: Chinese, British and Metric Systems.
- **Herb status:** Herbs in many forms are mentioned, accurately reflecting the marketplace and the clinic.

  Fresh herbs are those that are recently harvested. Fresh herbs are the most potent because the active components are completely or largely intact and available. Paradoxically, the dosage for fresh herbs is generally higher, as they still naturally contain a large amount of water.

  Dried herbs are those from which the water has been removed, usually by drying under the sun. Drying is an essential process that makes it possible to store herbs for longer periods of time without their becoming spoiled. Dried herbs are nonetheless frequently referred to as "raw herbs," not to be confused with fresh herbs. Most herbs sold in herb stores are dried.

  Unprocessed herbs have not been treated to alter their properties. Herbs are assumed to be unprocessed unless stated otherwise. "Unprocessed" is used in this text specifically to contrast differences in function and property with those of "processed" herbs.

  Processed herbs have been treated to alter or enhance certain properties and functions. There are numerous ways to "process" an herb, including dry-frying, charring to ash, calcining, roasting, boiling, steaming, quenching, and simmering, among others.

  The most common way in which herbs are stored and sold is dried and unprocessed. Therefore, most herbs in this text are assumed for purposes of discussion to be dried and unprocessed unless stated otherwise. Fresh herbs must be indicated specifically in contrast with dried herbs. If processed, the exact mechanism of processing must be indicated to differentiate the product from unprocessed substances.
- **Preparation and Processing of Herbs:** Processing enhances or alters therapeutic actions of herbs, and reduces side effects and/or toxicity. A general description of preparation and processing strategies and modalities is offered in Part I of this text, Chapter 5, Preparation and Processing of Chinese Herbs. The purposes and final effects of preparation and processing for each herb are listed in the Dosage section of the individual herb monographs.

CAUTIONS / CONTRAINDICATIONS

While it may be self-evident to experienced practitioners, new students and researchers or healthcare professionals from other fields will want to particularly note the cautions or contraindications mentioned for use of each substance under consideration. (If there are none reported, none will be mentioned.) In some cases these follow from observations made by practitioners hundreds or even thousands of years in the past, and the careful and accurate transmission of these key pieces of information from one generation of herbal practitioners to the next is one of the factors contributing to the long tradition of safe and effective practice of Chinese herbal medicine with a minimum of unwanted side effects.

OVERDOSAGE & TREATMENT

When used properly by trained practitioners, herbal medicines are generally considered safe and effective. Many examples of overdosage listed in this text are based on accidental ingestion, and ***not*** the intentional use of herbs by practitioners. Nonetheless, dosage is often the critical dividing line between a "medicine" and a "poison." The information on overdosage and its treatment is cited from numerous references. It is important to keep in mind that, while most cases of overdosage can be treated with the traditional methods listed, acute and life-threatening situations may require emergency medical intervention, as traditional methods may be inadequate in some contemporary clinics, because of the time and/or methods required for processing or preparation of remedies.

CHEMICAL COMPOSITION

- The chemical composition of herbs is extremely complex. The authors have accessed many resources for the compilation of this section in each monograph. For herbs in common use, the main active constituents have been studied extensively and are well understood. However, for herbs that have not been used as frequently, much research is still needed for complete understanding.
- The chemical structures of the main constituents are diagramed in the herb monographs, whenever relevant and available. The diagrams of chemical structures are provided with permission from *The Merck Index* 12th edition by Chapman & Hall/CRCnetBASE/Merck, and from *Traditional Chinese Medicines Molecular Structures, Natural Sources and Applications* by Yan X, Zhou J, and Xie G.

WESTERN SCIENCES

- **References:** It has been our intention to cite from original and credible sources whenever possible. Selection of references was based on relevance, strong study design, English language, use of human subjects whenever and wherever possible, with preference given to randomized, blinded, controlled studies over observational reports. However, not all references meet our selection criteria, mostly because studies on Chinese herbs were done predominately in China, in Chinese. Therefore, instead of restricting ourselves and the readers to the limited amount of information that fit these strict criteria, we decided to use our best judgment in including relevant information from credible sources. Another limitation we encountered during the compilation of this text is the inaccessibility of some original articles, texts, and references: some are out of press, others simply cannot be located. Although it is not always as complete, detailed or current as the authors would prefer, we have made our best effort in all cases to convey as much information on the original source as possible, judging even limited information to be of some value.
- **Scientific and Medical Terminology:** For the occasional allopathic term that readers might find puzzling, we recommend accessing any standard allopathic medical dictionary (see next entry for example). Since there is no need for translation or interpretation of these terms, we concluded that it was unnecessary and cumbersome to include such terms in the glossary for this text.
- **Medical Abbreviations and Symbols** are used in accordance with *Dorland's Illustrated Medical Dictionary*, 28th Edition, by Saunders.
- **Drug Names** are designated in this text by generic names only, or the combination of generic (proprietary) names. The generic (proprietary) names are referenced according to *Drug Facts and Comparisons*, updated monthly by Facts and Comparisons, a Wolters Kluwer Company.
- **Pharmacological Effects:** Most pharmacological studies focus on the anatomical and physiological influences of the herbs 1) on the body or 2) against pathogens. For example, many herbs are described as having antihypertensive effects, as the administration of the herbs leads directly to a decrease in blood pressure. Others are said to have antibacterial effects, as the introduction of the herb leads to the inhibition or death of bacteria. However, the exact mechanisms of action for many herbs are still not well understood at this time.
- **Clinical Studies and Research**. Chinese herbs are used in multiple-herb formulas to treat patients. Thus, most clinical studies and research cited include use of many herbs, not solely a single sub-

Using this Book

stance under consideration. Though this increases the number of variables influencing outcome, this nonetheless reflects the actual practice of Chinese herbal medicine and the basis on which centuries of refinement have been effectively carried forward.

HERB-DRUG INTERACTION

Herb-Drug Interaction is a critically important subject, yet there is little extensively definitive information available. Basic understandings of this topic are detailed in Part I, Chapter 8, Concurrent Use of Herbal Medicines and Pharmaceuticals. Documented and potential interactions (based on our best understanding of herbs and drugs) are discussed in each herb monograph when relevant. Herb monographs that do not contain herb-drug interaction information imply that there was no known or documented interaction at the time of publication. However, readers are strongly encouraged to stay updated, as new information on herb-drug complementarities and conflicts is regularly being published.

TOXICOLOGY

The toxicology of individual herbs or of their constituents is reported based on *in vitro* studies. Readers are urged to examine and understand these reports with the same attention to context, proportion and clinical application as would be the case in reviewing toxicology and/or *in vitro* studies for any medicine or supplement.

SUPPLEMENT

Frequently, additional herbs have names and/or functions similar to the primary substance under discussion in a particular monograph. These are brought for consideration in the Supplement section, particularly when they might serve as substitutes or be inappropriate substitutes. Many herbs included in this section are derived from the same botanical sources as the main herb in the monograph, and are mentioned for quick comparison purposes.

AUTHORS' COMMENTS

When there is relevant clinical information that does not sensibly fall under other categories, or when the authors wish to provide additional insights on a particular herb or its uses or a related topic, or to offer clinical experience volunteered by their teachers, this information is discussed in this closing segment of the monographs.

REFERENCES

Reference material is embedded in the text for ease of access via endnotes in each monograph. The key information from all of these notes has been carefully consolidated into two thorough bibliographic resources.

- The complete names of historical books (given in Chinese characters, pinyin names, and English names) are listed in the Bibliography of Historical Texts.
- The complete names for recent journals, articles and books are listed in the Bibliography of Contemporary References.

ADDITIONAL RESOURCES

In a text involving so many hundreds of pieces of information as *Chinese Medical Herbology and Pharmacology*, it is inevitable that on any given page a reader might find information that inspires curiosity about specific details that are not included in that particular monograph. The authors want both to provide as much information as possible and to avoid overwhelming students and practitioners with excessive repetition and complexity that obscures key concepts and bogs down progress through the general text.

For this reason, the reader will find in Part III that there are no less than ten specialty appendices to provide intensive bodies of information at the close of the text, followed by a thorough glossary and the two bibliographies mentioned above. Each of these is self-contained and self-explanatory.

The authors are proud and grateful to have had an excellent gathering of committed and experienced professionals contributing to and evaluating the content of this textbook. We invite the reader to appreciate the wealth of training and experience these contributors have brought to bear on behalf of *Chinese Medical Herbology and Pharmacology*, as listed in the section titled "About the Authors and Contributors."

There is, last but not least, an extensive index at the close of Part III, linking terminology and topics throughout the text for the convenience of students, practitioners and researchers.

It is our hope that these features will contribute to the greatest accessibility and convenience in your use of this volume.

DISCLAIMER

Great care has been taken by the authors, editors, and other contributors to maintain the accuracy of the information contained in *Chinese Medical Herbology and Pharmacology*. All information has been evaluated, double-checked and cross-verified. However, in view of the potential for human, electronic, or mechanical error, neither the authors nor the publisher nor any other contributors involved in the preparation or publication of this text warrant that the information contained herein is in every aspect accurate, and they are not responsible for any errors or omissions nor for the results obtained from the use of said information.

Chinese Medical Herbology and Pharmacology is intended as an educational guide for healthcare practitioners, as professional training and expertise are essential to the safe practice of herbal medicine in recommendation of and effective guidance for use of herbs. We cannot anticipate all conditions under which this information may be used. In view of ongoing research, changes in governmental regulation, and the constant flow of information relating to Chinese and western medicine, the reader is urged to check with other sources for all up-to-date information. In recognition that practitioners accessing information in this text will have varying levels of training and expertise, we accept no responsibility for the results obtained by the application of the information within this text. Neither the publisher, authors, editors, nor other contributors can be held responsible for errors of fact or omission, or for any consequences arising from the use or misuse of the information herein.

It is our intention to continually update and improve this text to maintain and enhance its usefulness. We welcome and encourage your comments and suggestions.

— Herb Indentification Guide (Color Photographs)

中药图鉴

Herb Indentification Guide

Full-color photographs are displayed in alphabetical order by pinyin name in this section, to assist in accurate recognition of individual herbs. Because of limitations of space, many of these images are not reproduced in life-size scale.

However, the black-and-white images matched to corresponding herb monographs throughout the text are life-size unless otherwise noted.

Because most users of this text will not be gathering herbs directly from nature, we have chosen to provide illustrations of the harvested, processed, manicured substances as our readers would encounter them in realistic purchasing and clinical situations.

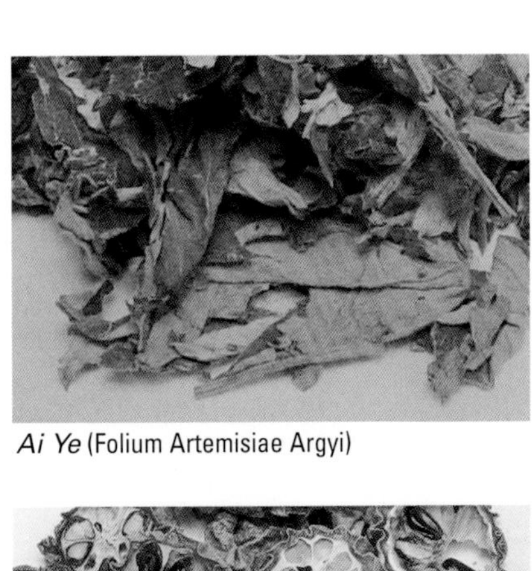

Ai Ye (Folium Artemisiae Argyi)

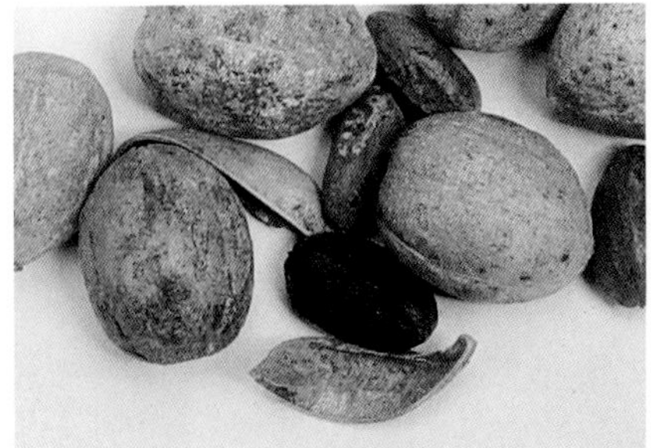

Ba Dou (Fructus Crotonis)

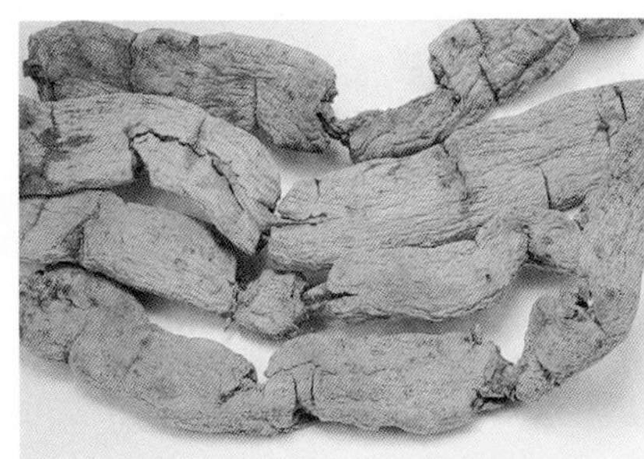

Ba Ji Tian (Radix Morindae Officinalis)

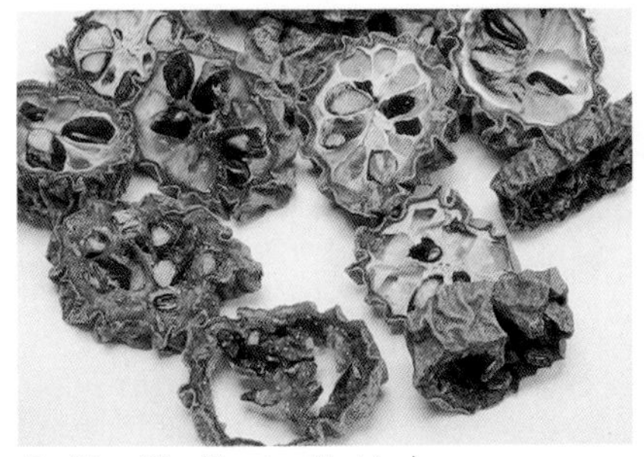

Ba Yue Zha (Fructus Akebiae)

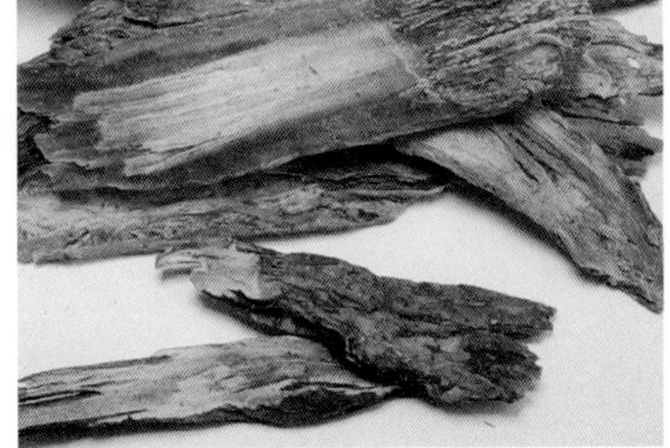

Bai Bu (Radix Stemonae)

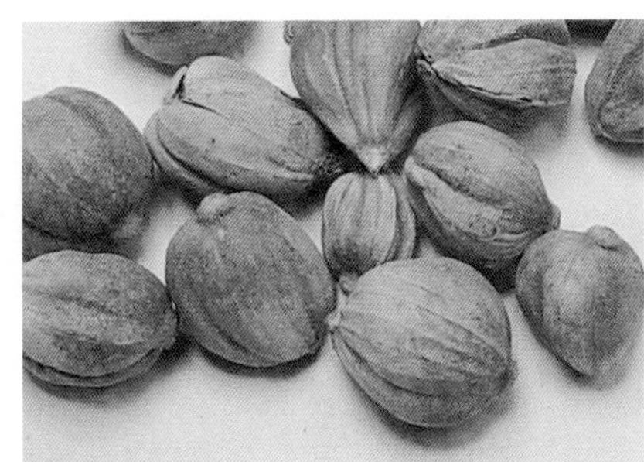

Bai Dou Kou (Fructus Amomi Rotundus)

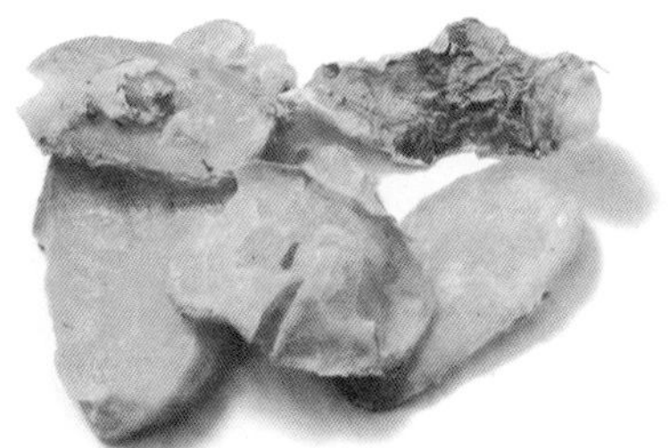

Bai Fu Zi (Rhizoma Typhonii)

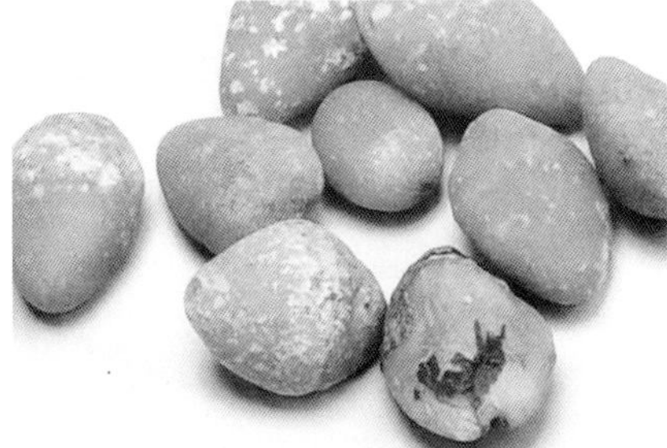

Bai Guo (Semen Ginkgo)

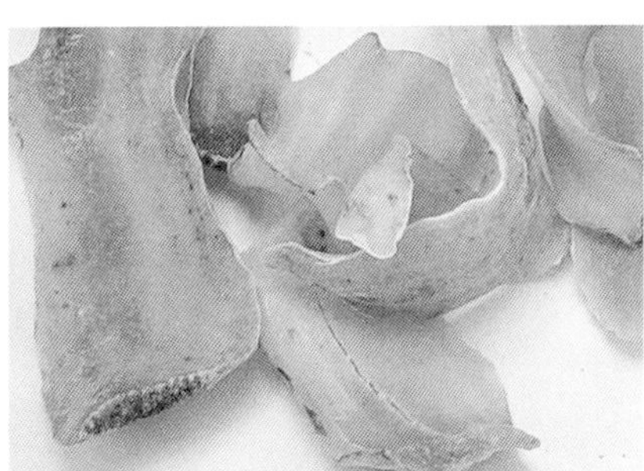

Bai He (Bulbus Lilii)

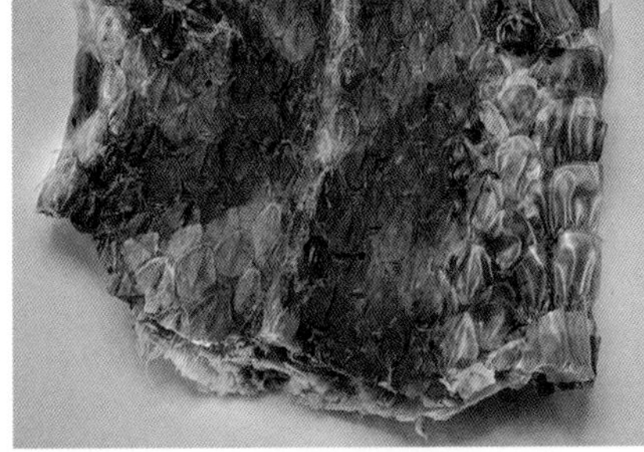

Bai Hua She (Bungarus Parvus)

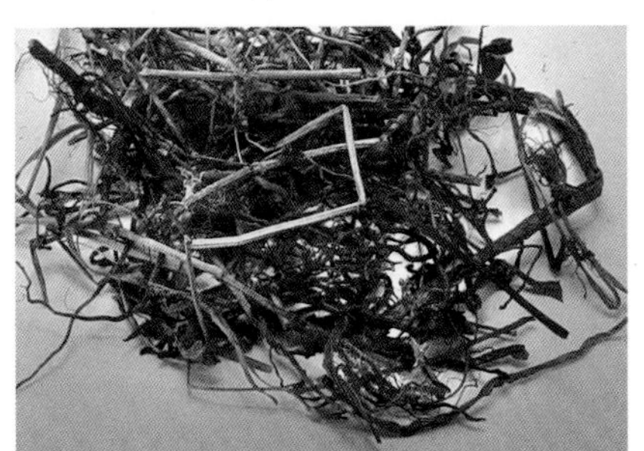

Bai Hua She She Cao (Herba Oldenlandia)

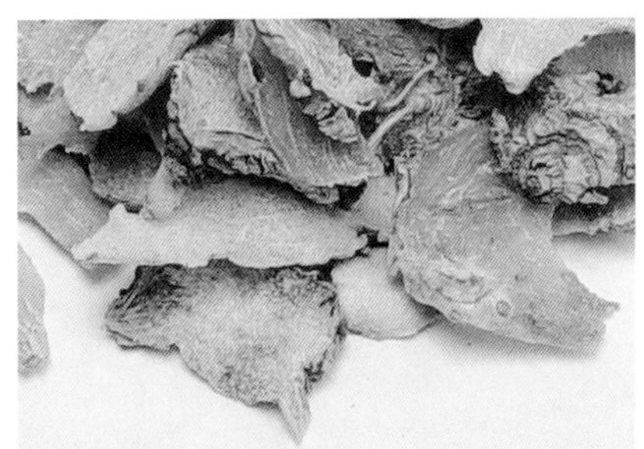

Bai Ji (Rhizoma Bletillae)

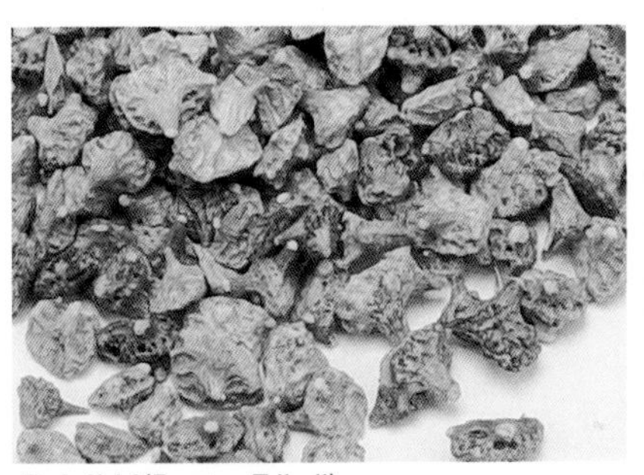

Bai Ji Li (Fructus Tribuli)

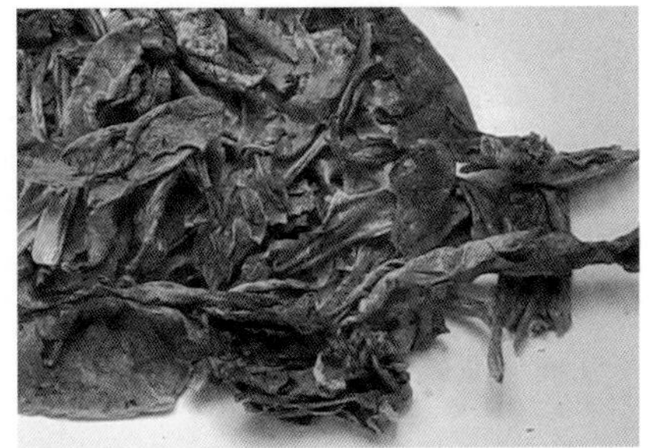

Bai Jiang Cao (Herba cum Radice Patriniae)

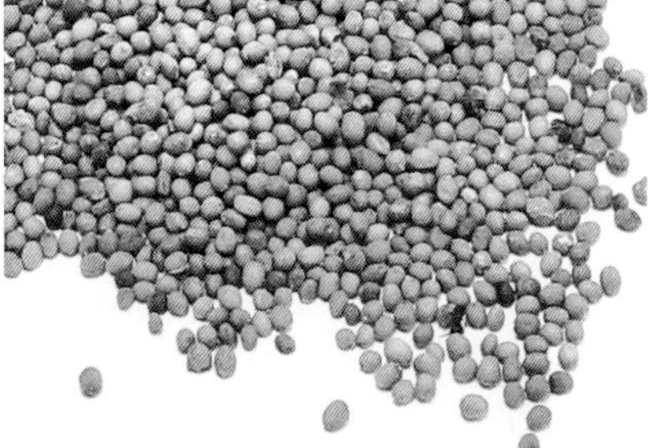

Bai Jie Zi (Semen Sinapis)

Herb Indentification Guide

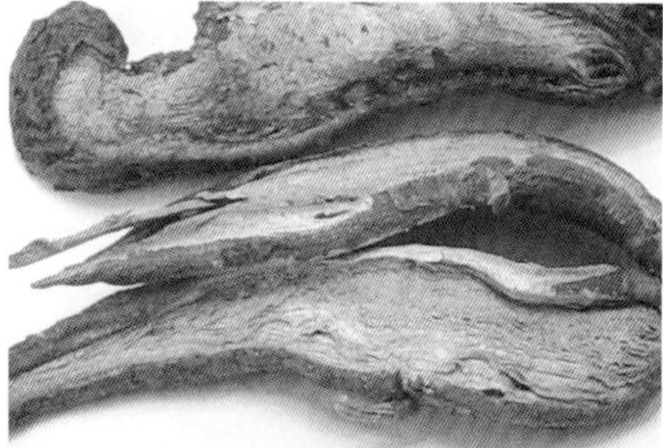

Bai Lian (Radix Ampelopsis)

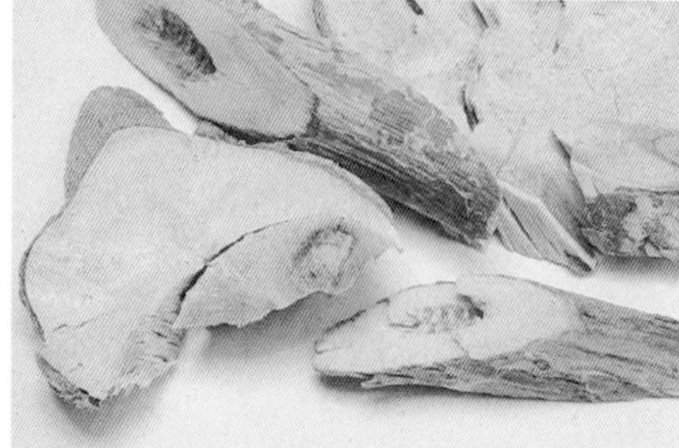

Bai Long Chuan Hua Tou (Radix Clerodendron Paniculatum)

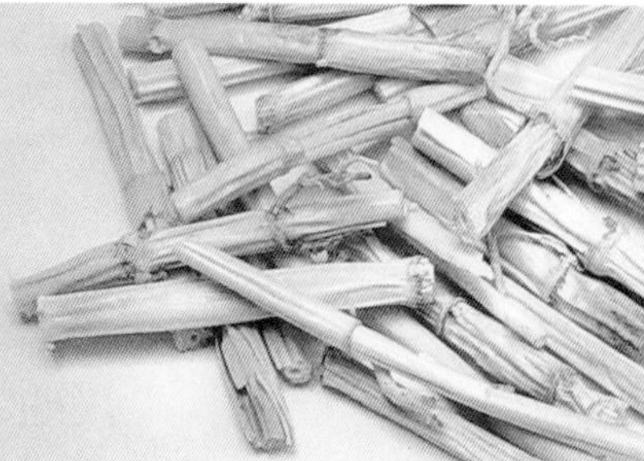

Bai Mao Gen (Rhizoma Imperatae)

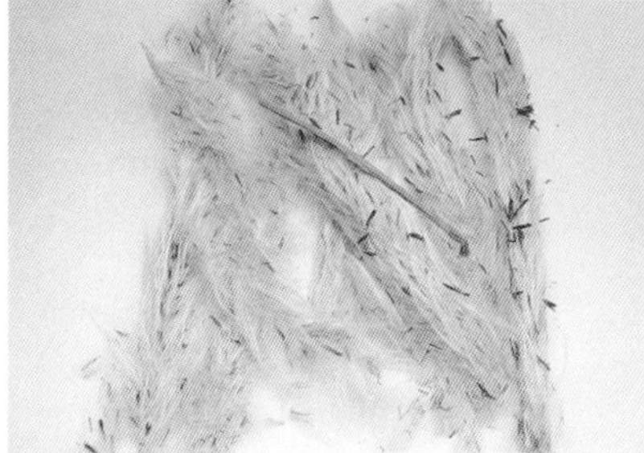

Bai Mao Hua (Flos Imperatae)

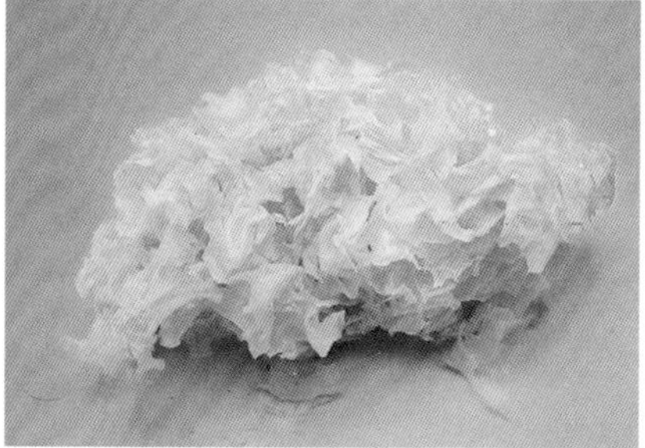

Bai Mu Er (Fructificatio Tremellae Fuciformis)

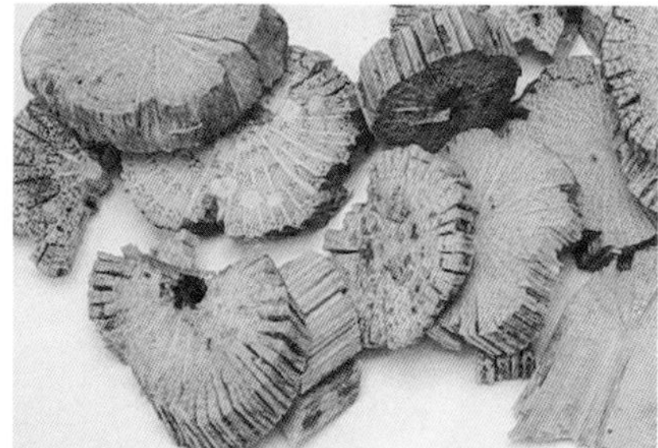

Bai Mu Tong (Caulis Akebia Trifoliata Australis)

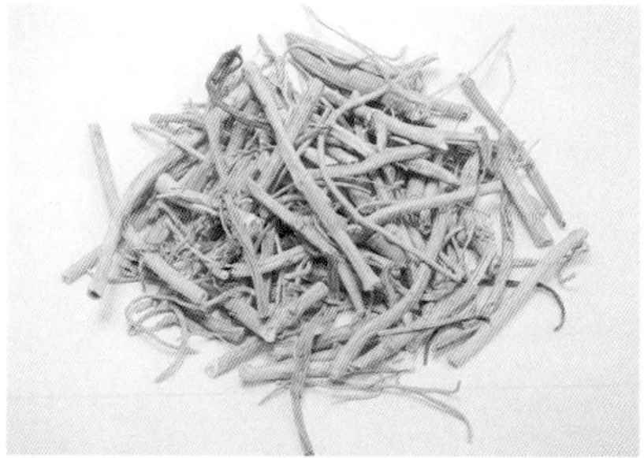

Bai Qian (Rhizoma Cynanchi Stauntonii)

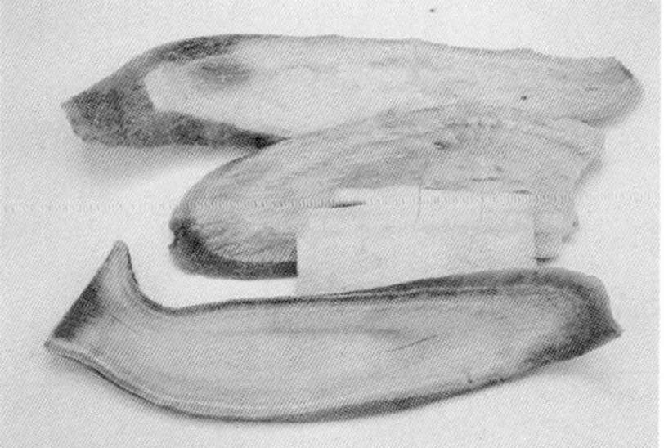

Bai Shao (Radix Paeoniae Alba)

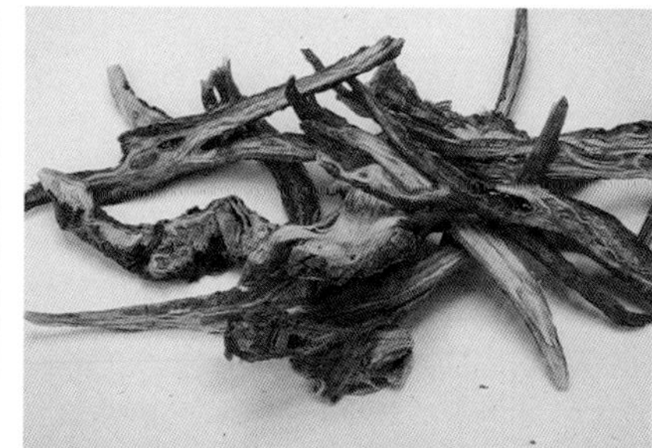

Bai Tou Weng (Radix Pulsatillae)

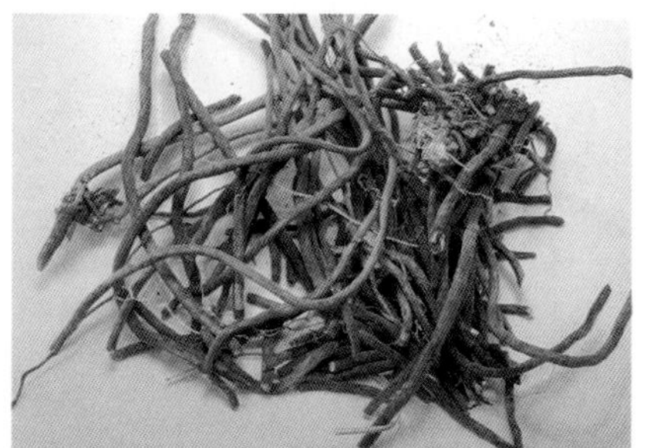

Bai Wei (Radix Cynanchi Atrati)

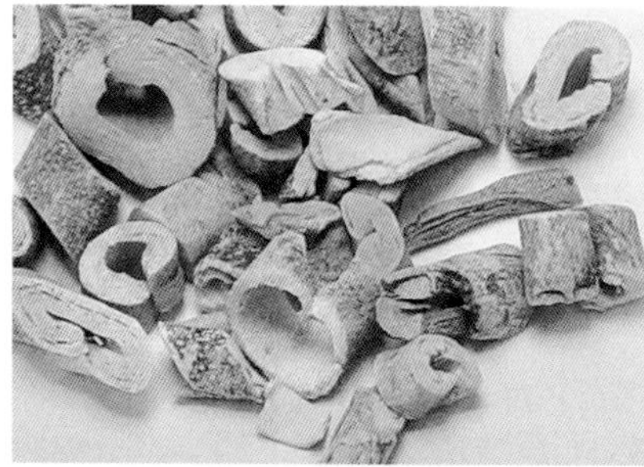

Bai Xian Pi (Cortex Dictamni)

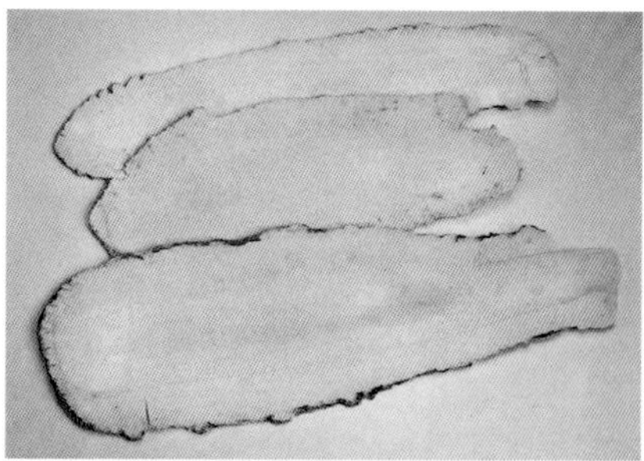

Bai Zhi (Radix Angelicae Dahuricae)

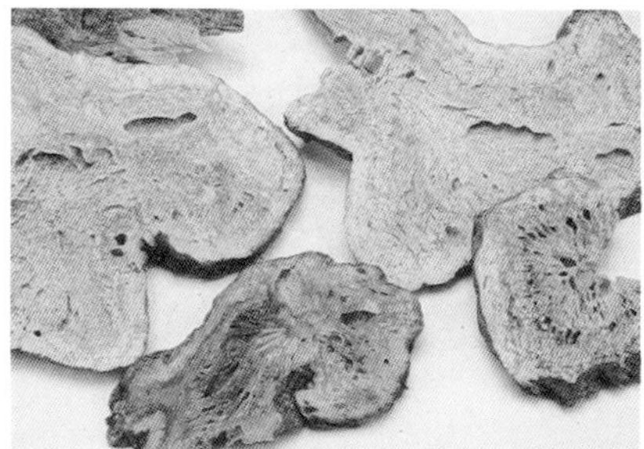

Bai Zhu (Rhizoma Atractylodis Macrocephalae)

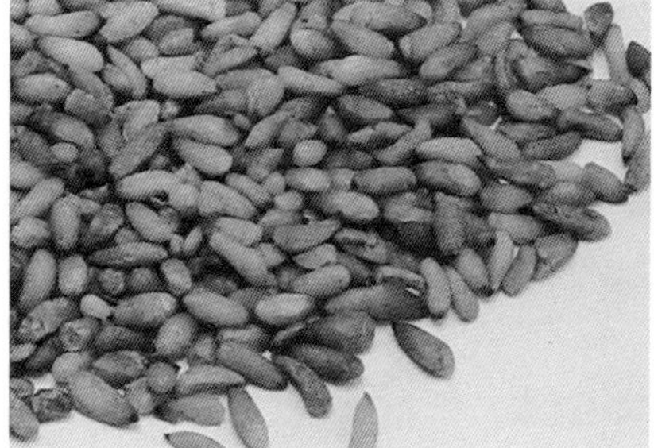

Bai Zi Ren (Semen Platycladi)

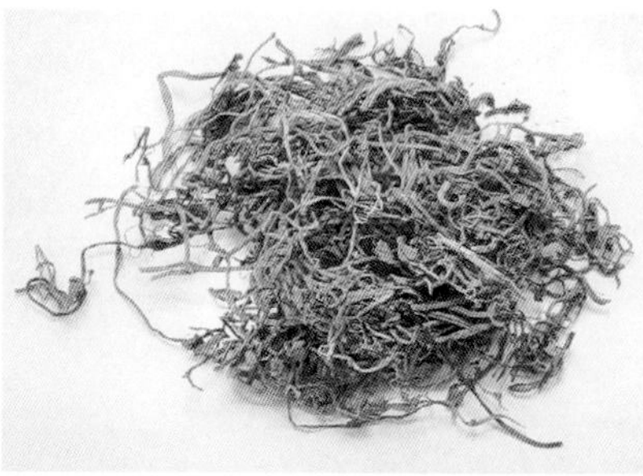

Ban Bian Lian (Herba Lobeliae Chinensis)

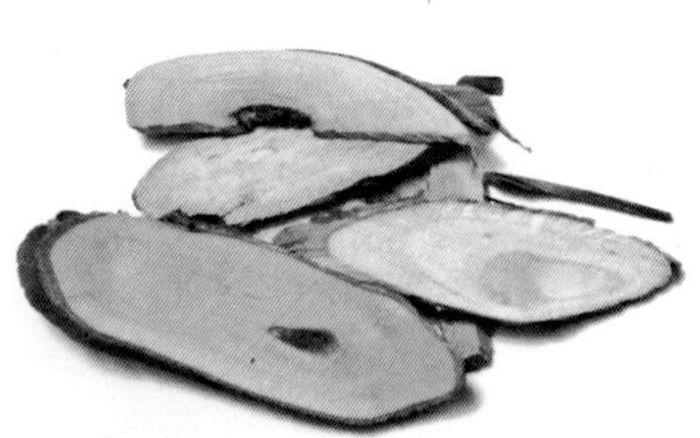
Ban Lan Gen (Radix Isatidis)

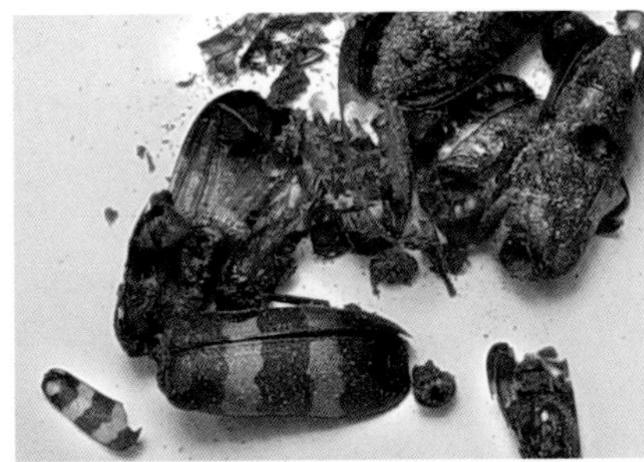
Ban Mao (Mylabris)

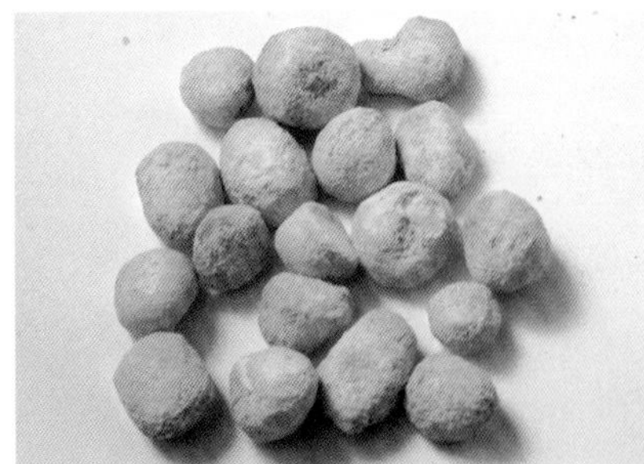
Ban Xia (Rhizoma Pinelliae)

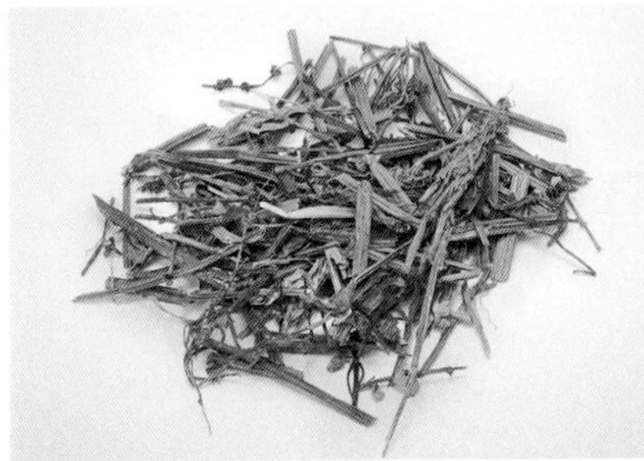
Ban Zhi Lian (Herba Scutellariae Barbatae)

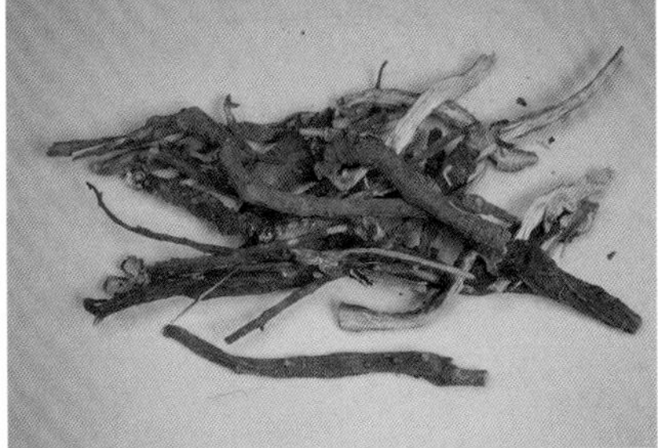
Bei Chai Hu (Radix Bupleurum Chinensis)

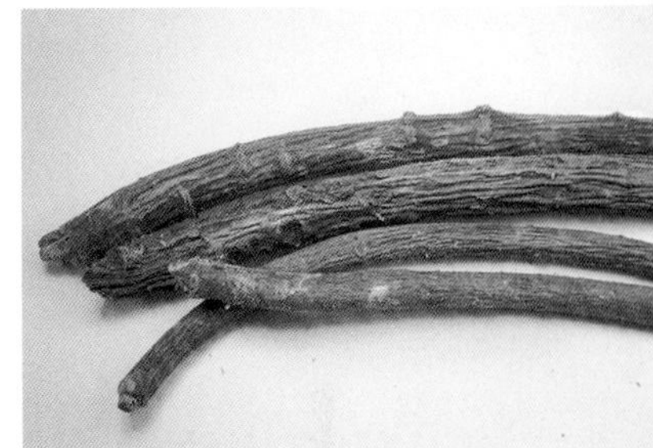
Bei Dou Gen (Rhizoma Menispermi)

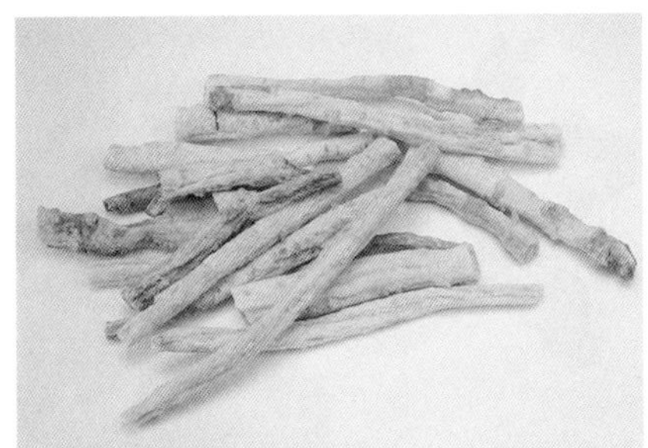
Bei Sha Shen (Radix Glehniae)

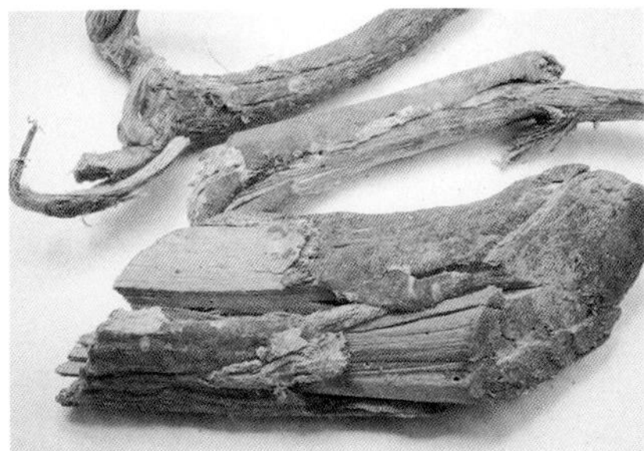
Bei Wu Jia Pi (Cortex Periploca Sepium Radicis)

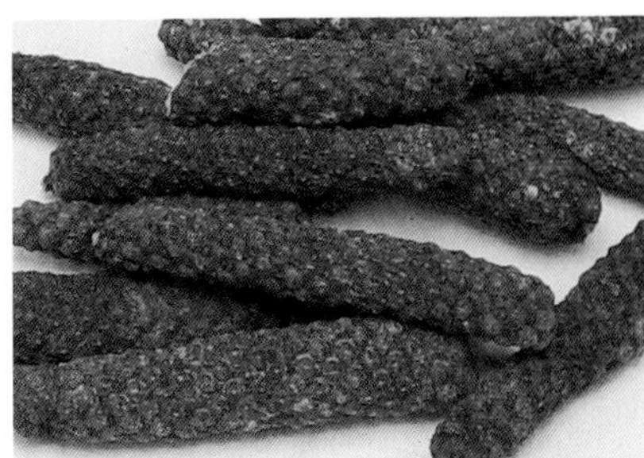
Bi Ba (Fructus Piperis Longi)

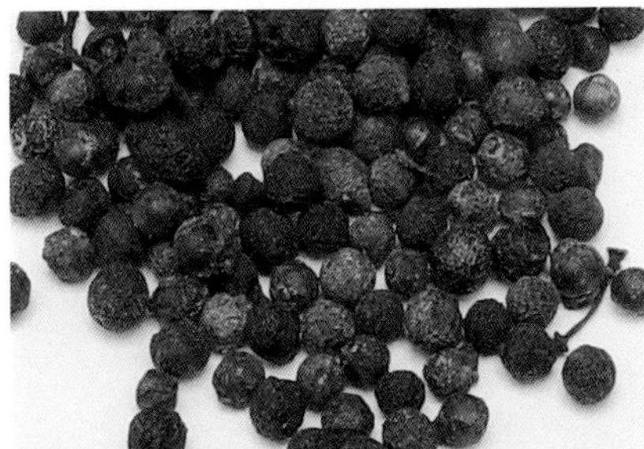
Bi Cheng Qie (Fructus Litseae)

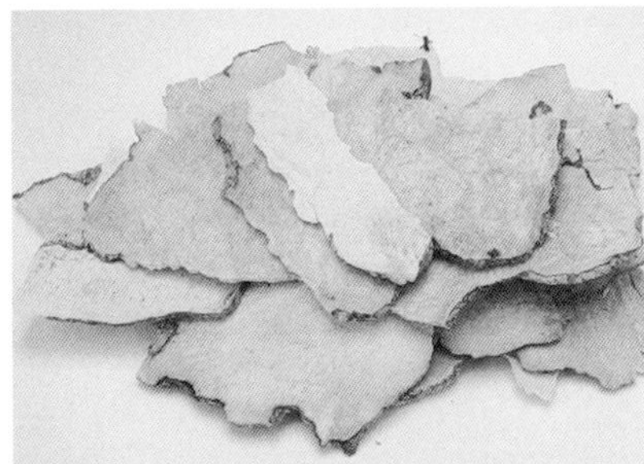
Bi Xie (Rhizoma Dioscoreae Hypoglaucae)

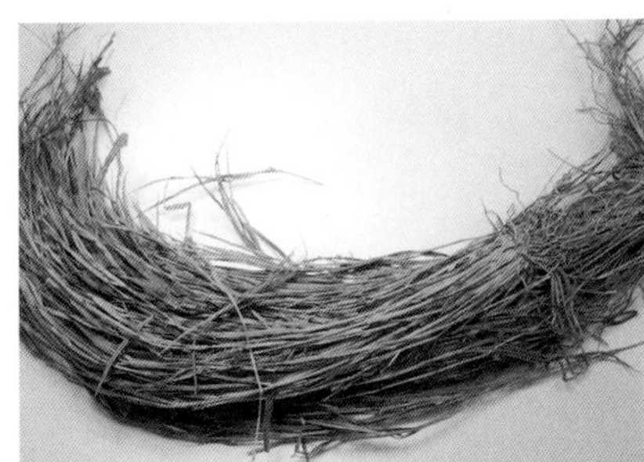
Bi Zi Cao (Herba Pogonantheri Criniti)

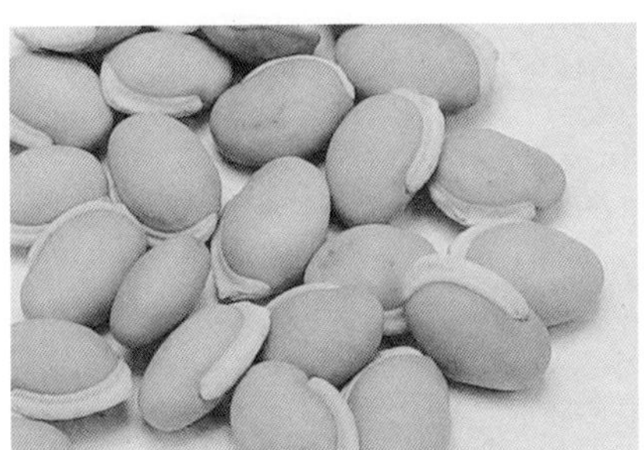
Bian Dou (Semen Lablab Album)

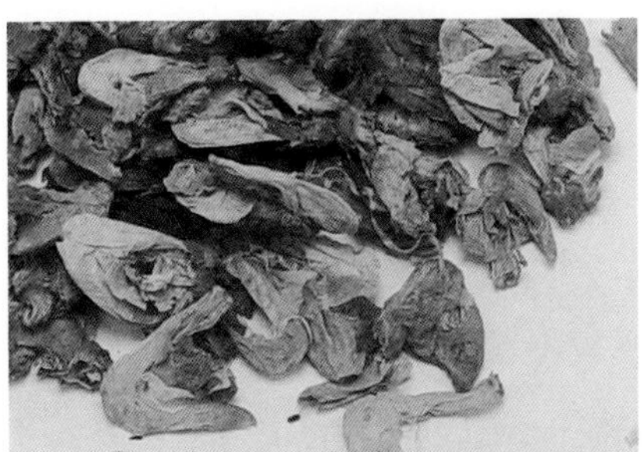
Bian Dou Hua (Flos Lablab Album)

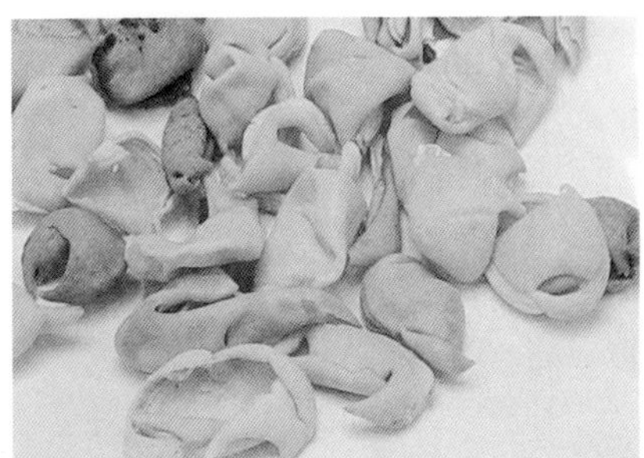
Bian Dou Yi (Pericarpium Lablab Album)

Herb Indentification Guide

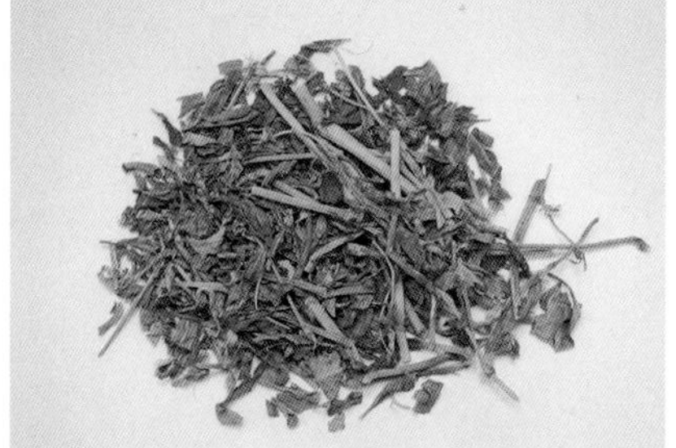
Bian Xu (Herba Polygoni Avicularis)

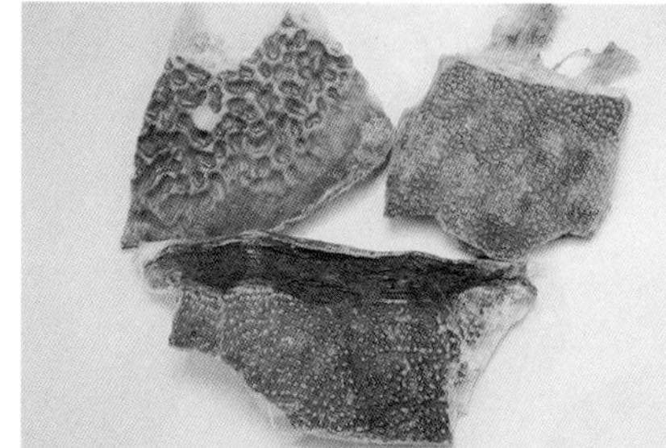
Bie Jia (Carapax Trionycis)

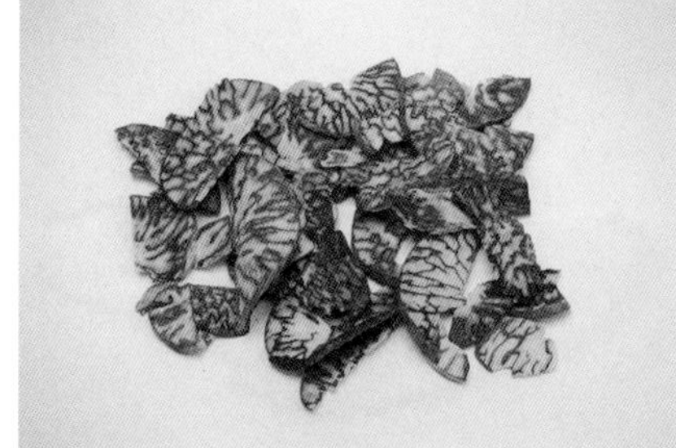
Bing Lang (Semen Arecae)

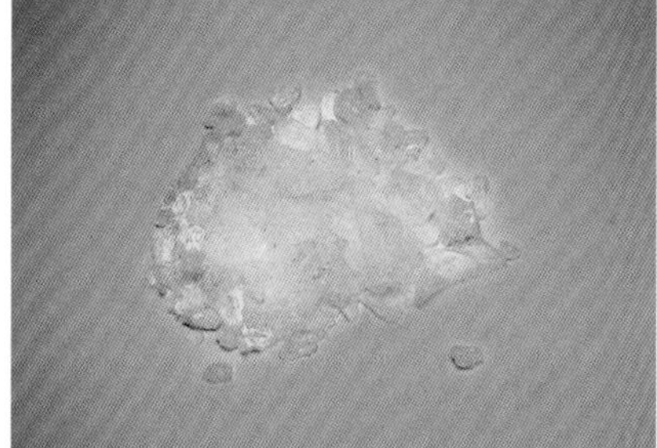
Bing Pian (Borneolum Syntheticum)

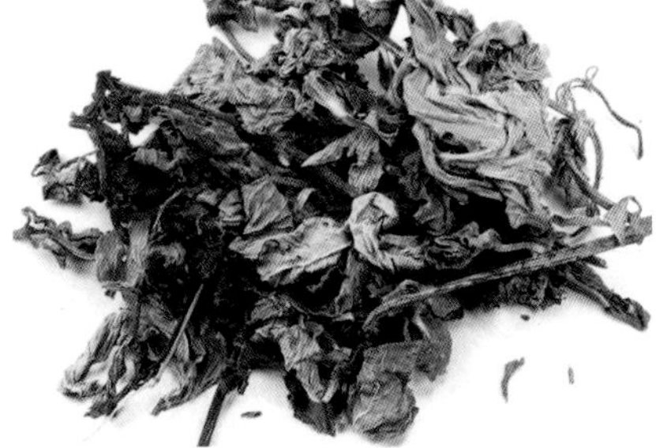
Bo He (Herba Menthae)

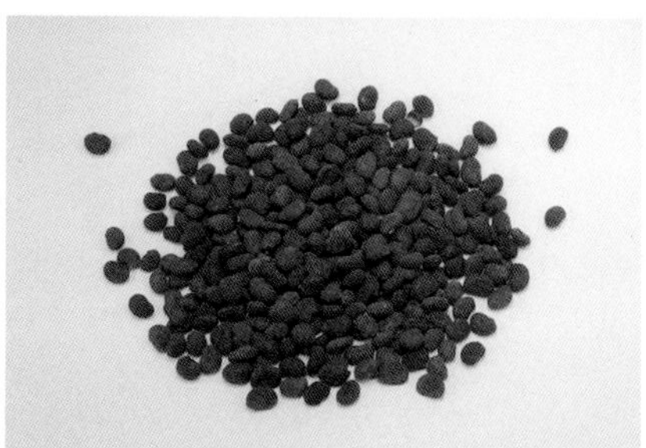
Bu Gu Zhi (Fructus Psoraleae)

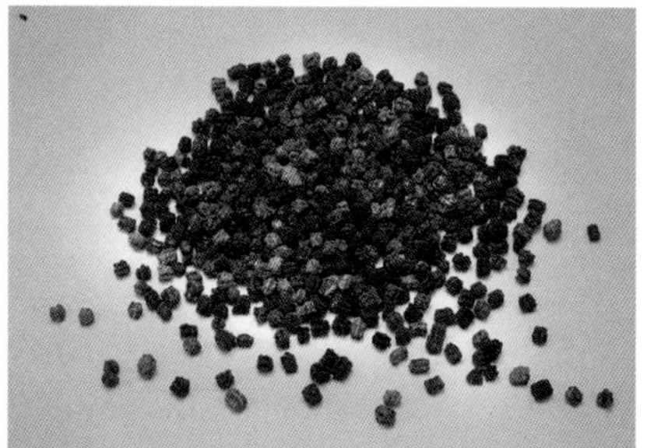
Can Sha (Excrementum Bombycis Mori)

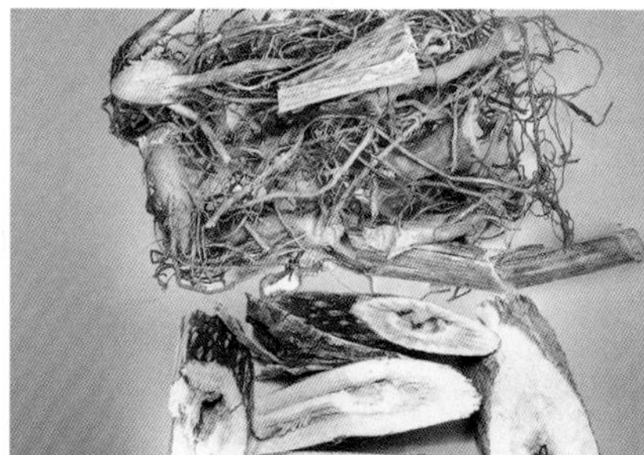
Cang Er Gen (Radix Xanthii)

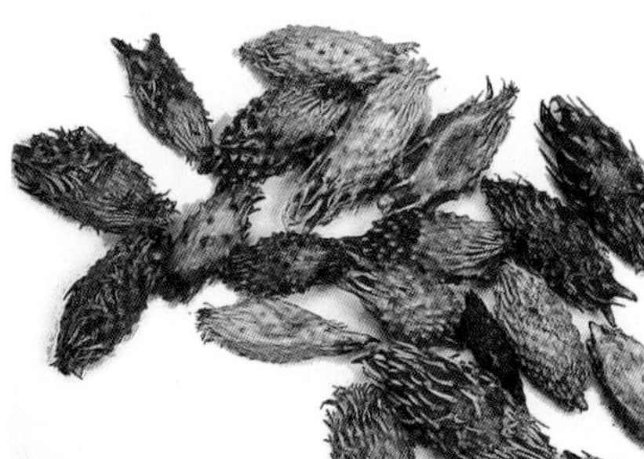
Cang Er Zi (Fructus Xanthii)

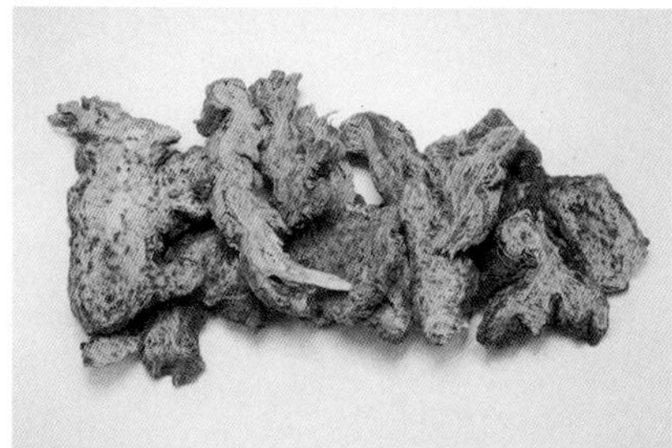
Cang Zhu (Rhizoma Atractylodis)

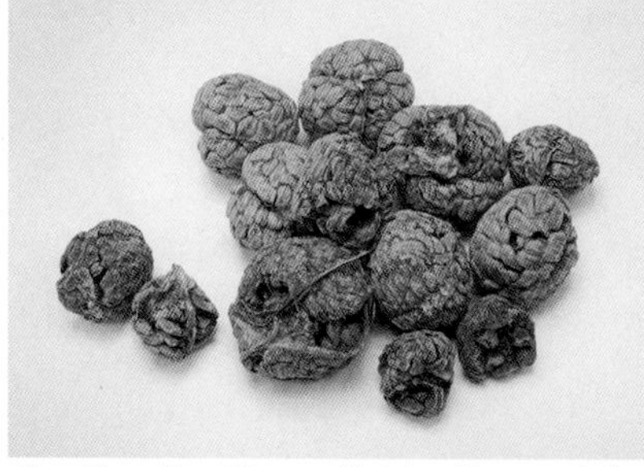
Cao Dou Kou (Semen Alpiniae Katsumadai)

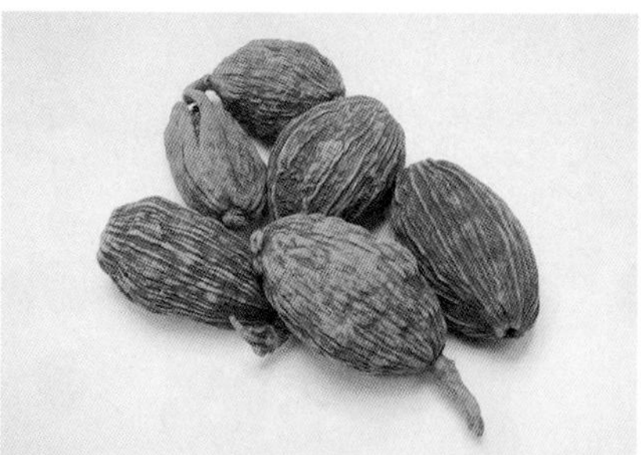
Cao Guo (Fructus Tsaoko)

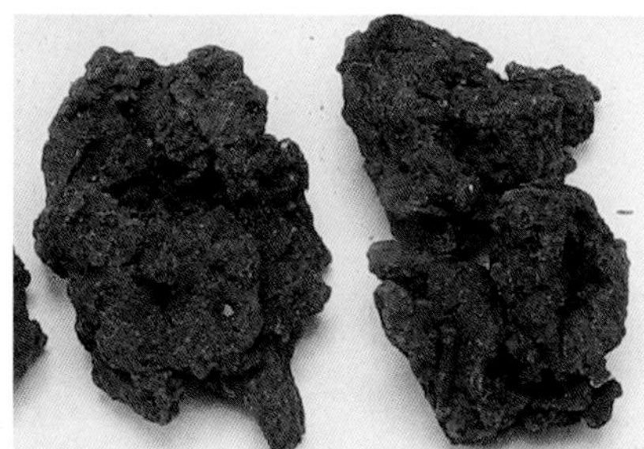
Cao Wu (Radix Aconiti Kusnezoffii)

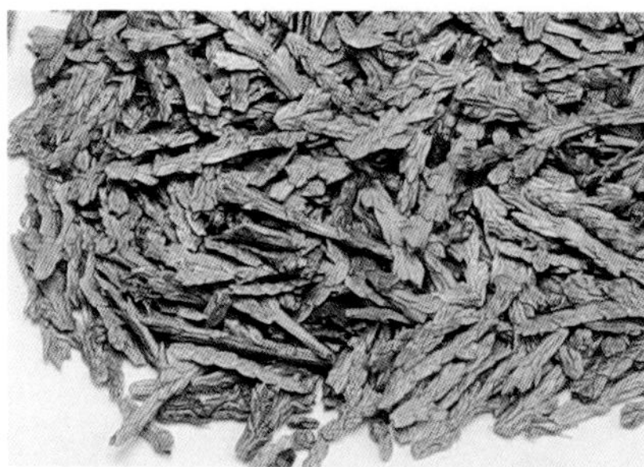
Ce Bai Ye (Cacumen Platycladi)

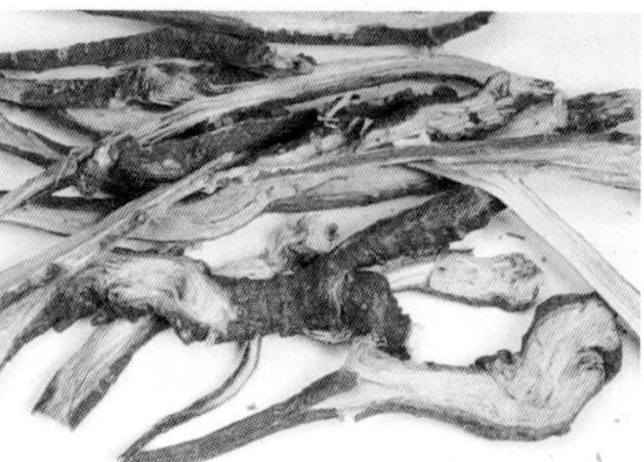
Chai Hu (Radix Bupleuri)

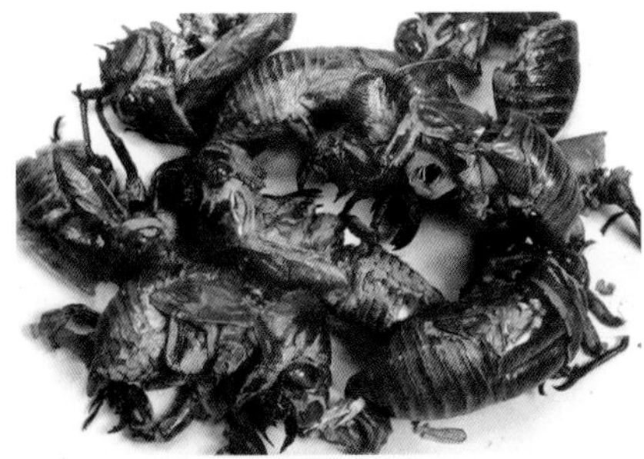
Chan Tui (Periostracum Cicadae)

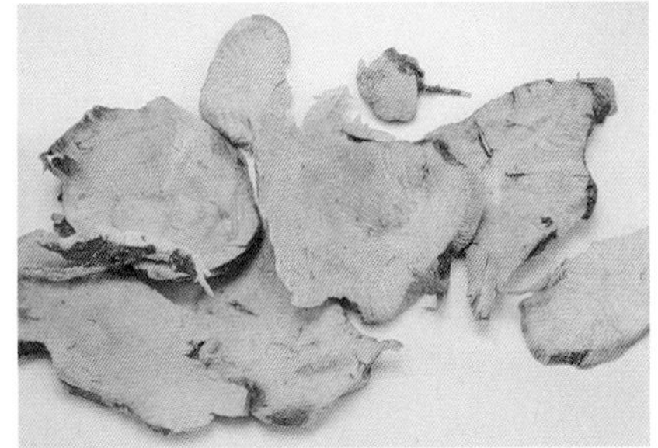
Chang Shan (Radix Dichroae)

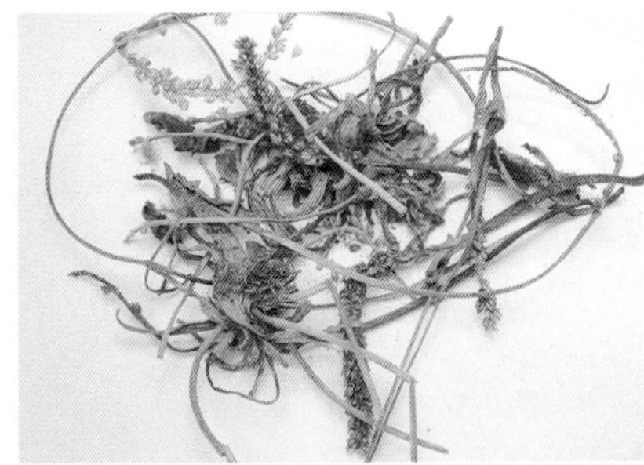
Che Qian Cao (Herba Plantaginis)

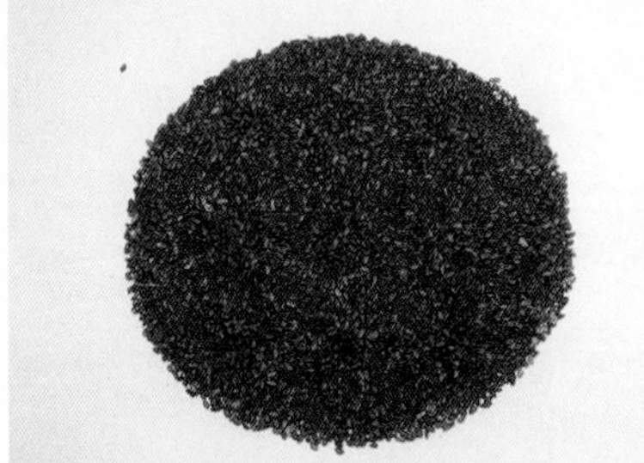
Che Qian Zi (Semen Plantaginis)

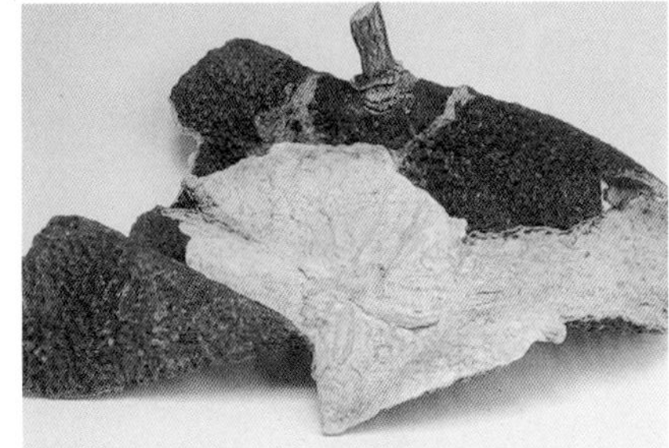
Chen Pi (Pericarpium Citri Reticulatae)

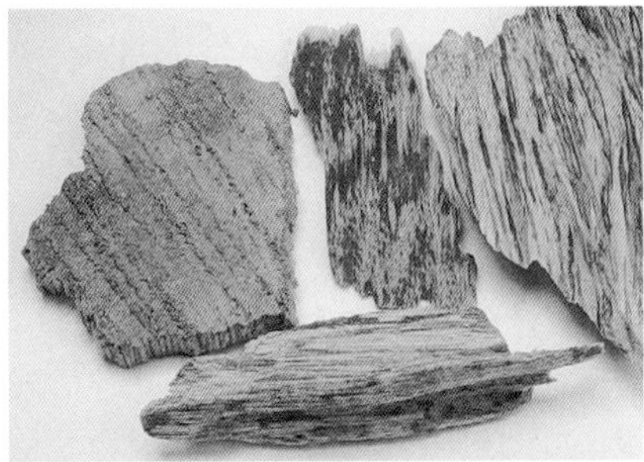
Chen Xiang (Lignum Aquilariae Resinatum)

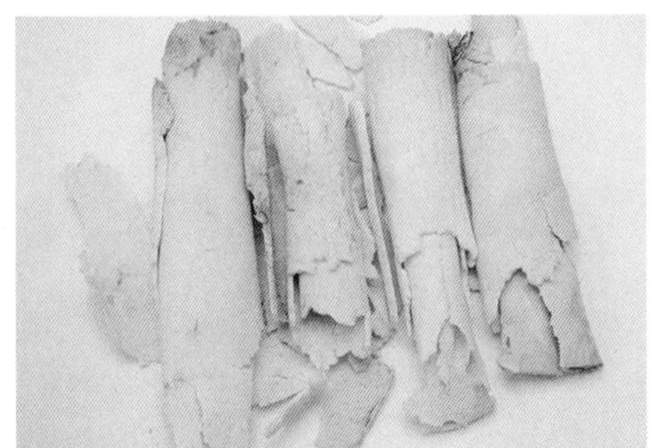
Chi Fu Ling (Poria Rubrae)

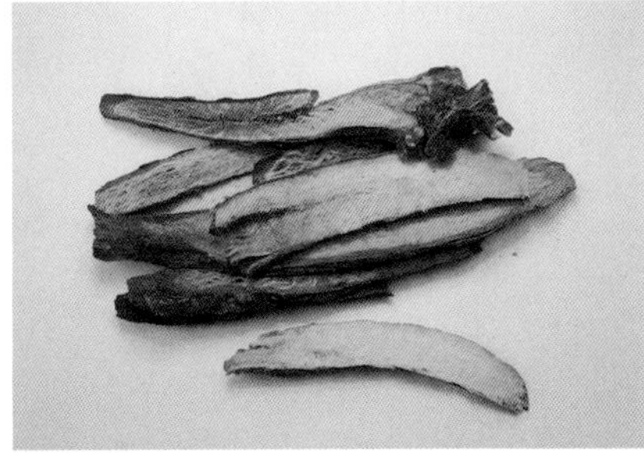
Chi Shao (Radix Paeoniae Rubrae)

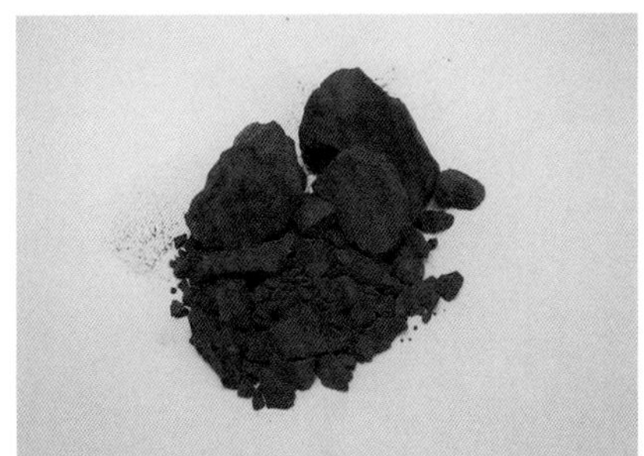
Chi Shi Zhi (Halloysitum Rubrum)

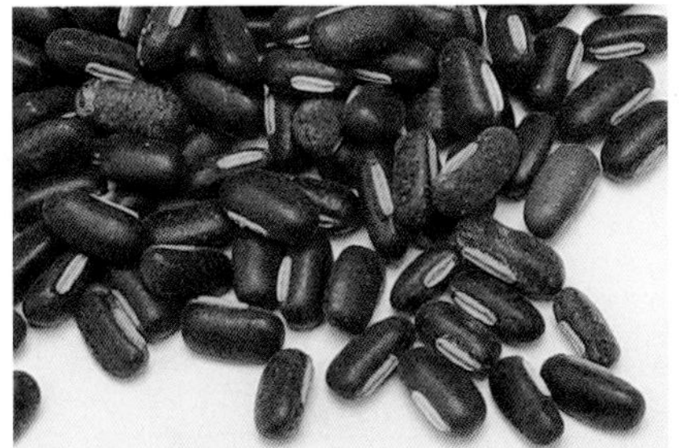
Chi Xiao Dou (Semen Phaseoli)

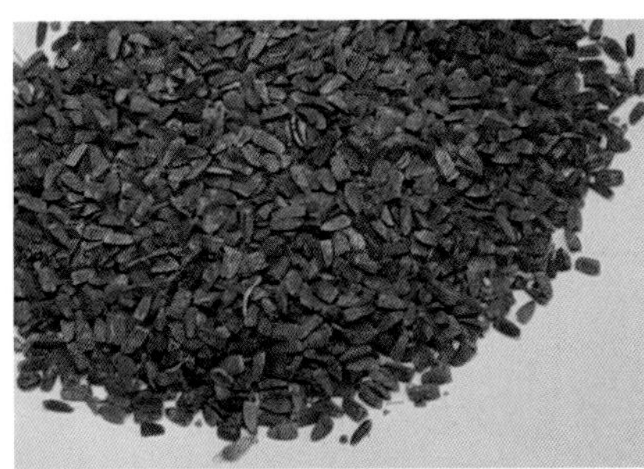
Chong Wei Zi (Semen Leonuri)

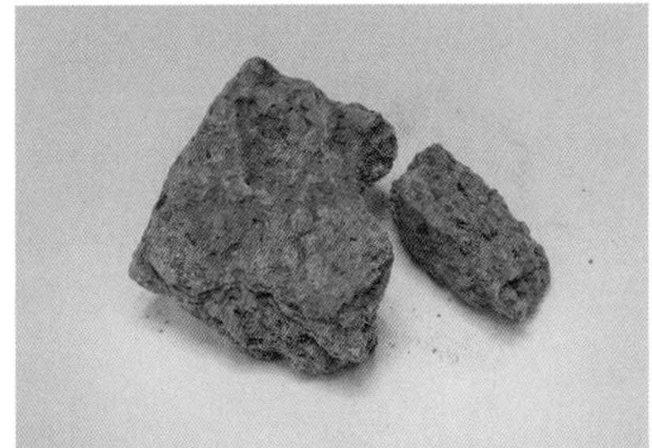
Chou Wu Tong (Folium Clerodendri Trichotomi)

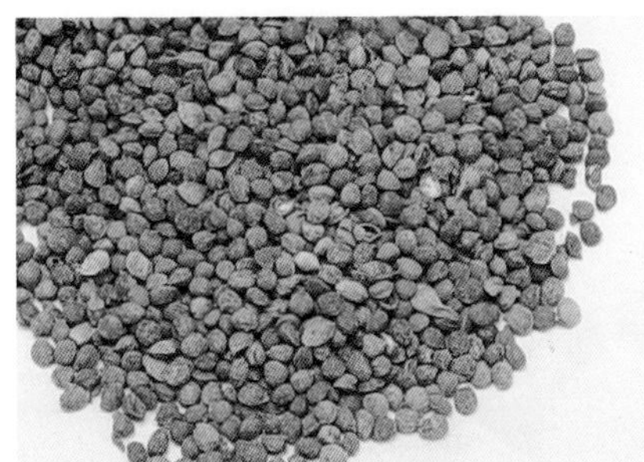
Chu Shi Zi (Fructus Broussonetiae)

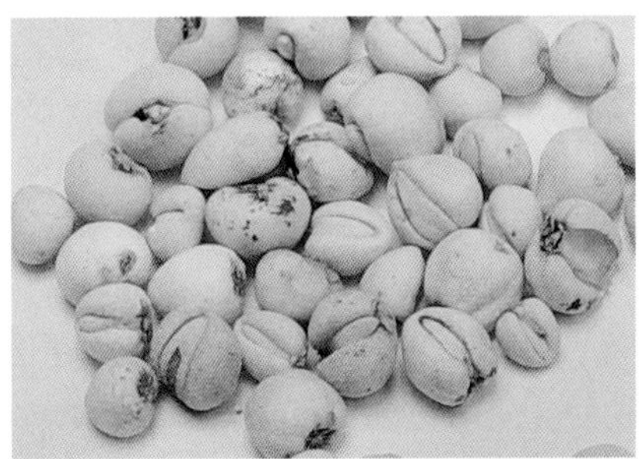
Chuan Bei Mu (Bulbus Fritillariae Cirrhosae)

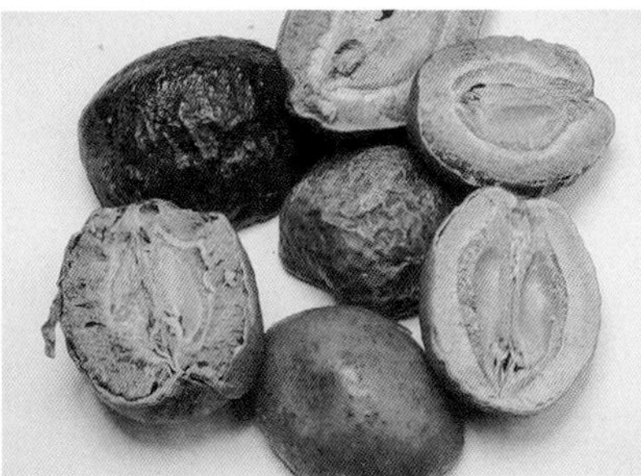
Chuan Lian Zi (Fructus Toosendan)

Herb Indentification Guide

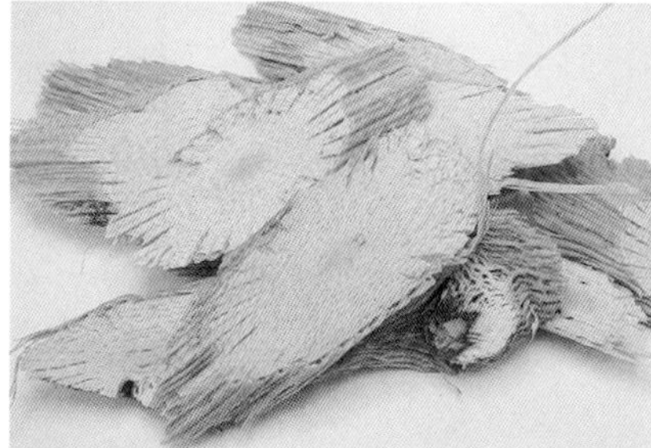
Chuan Mu Tong (Caulis Clematidis Armandii)

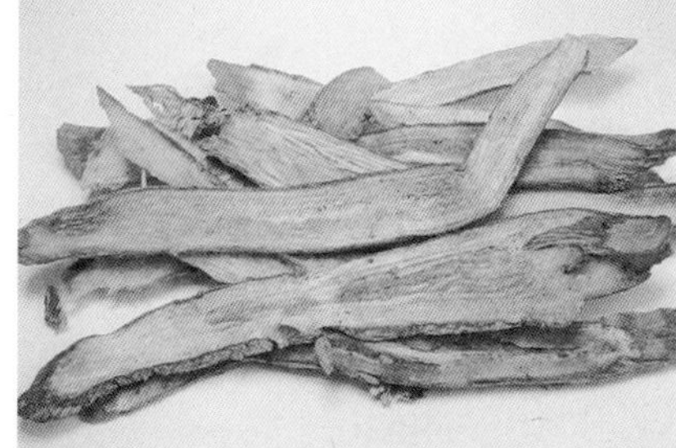
Chuan Niu Xi (Radix Cyathulae)

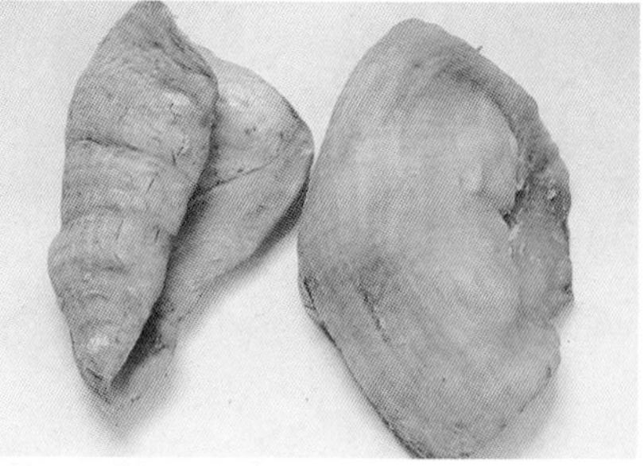
Chuan Shan Jia (Squama Manis)

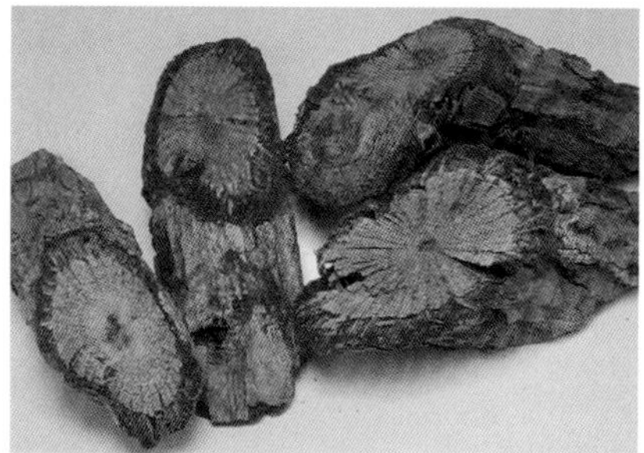
Chuan Shan Long
(Rhizoma Dioscoreae Nipponicae)

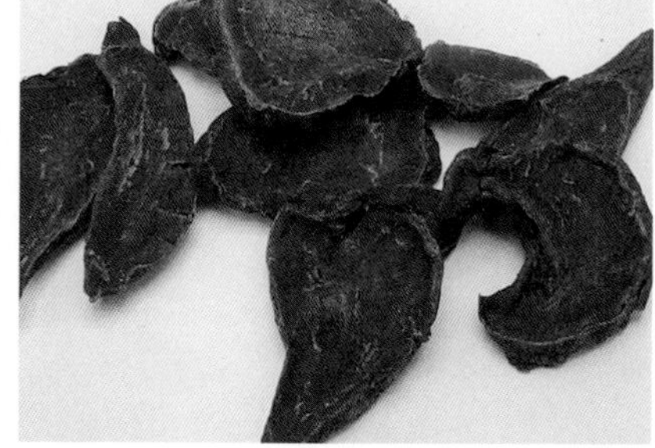
Chuan Wu (Radix Aconiti Preparata)

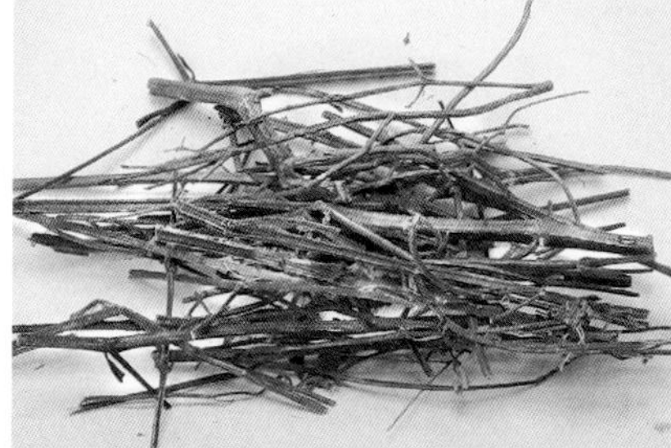
Chuan Xin Lian (Herba Andrographis)

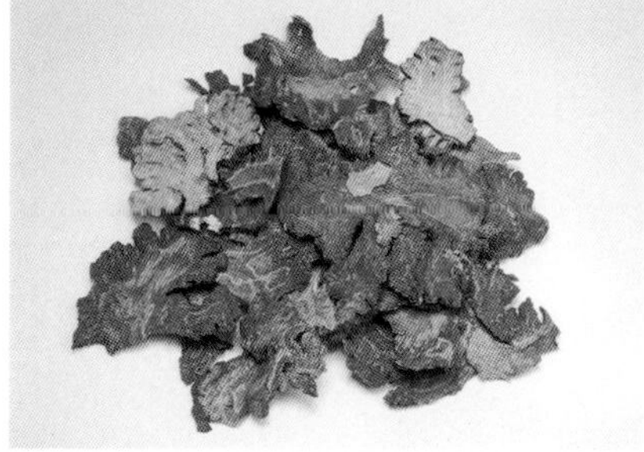
Chuan Xiong (Rhizoma Ligustici Chuanxiong)

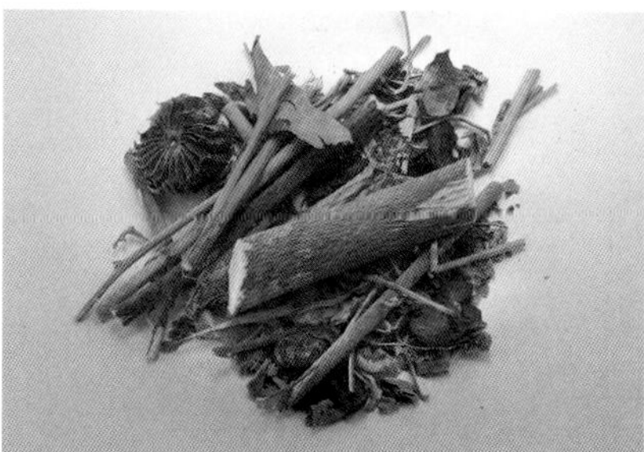
Chui Pen Cao (Herba Sedi)

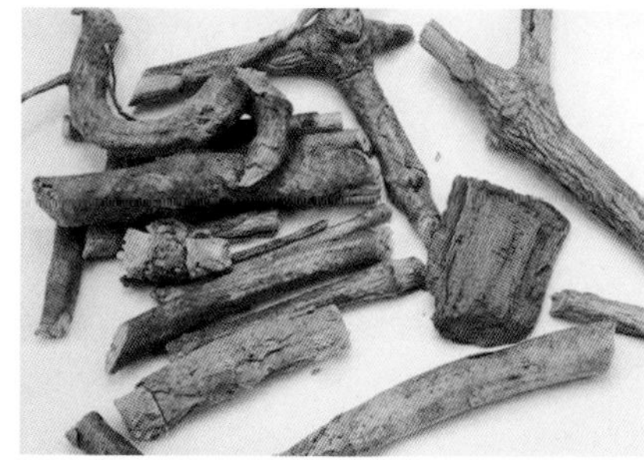
Chun Gen (Radix Ailanthi)

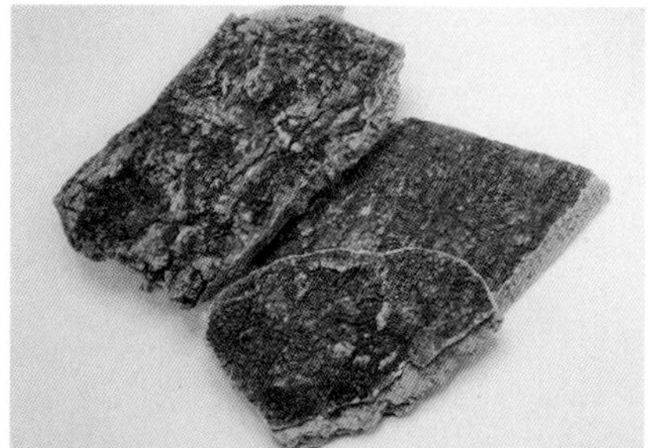
Chun Gen Pi (Cortex Ailanthi)

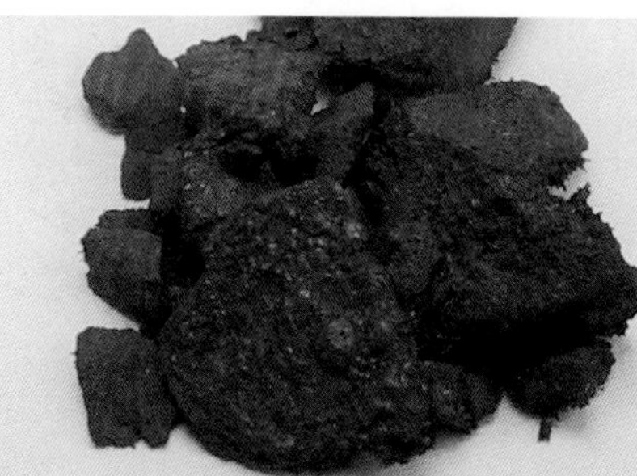
Ci Shi (Magnetitum)

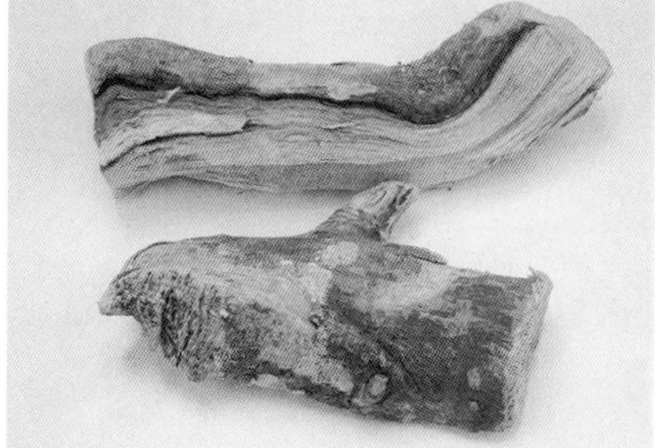
Ci Wu Jia
(Radix et Caulis Acanthopanacis Senticosi)

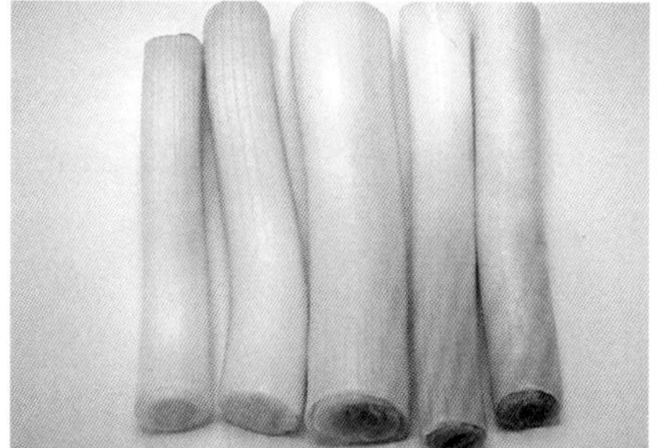
Cong Bai (Bulbus Allii Fistulosi)

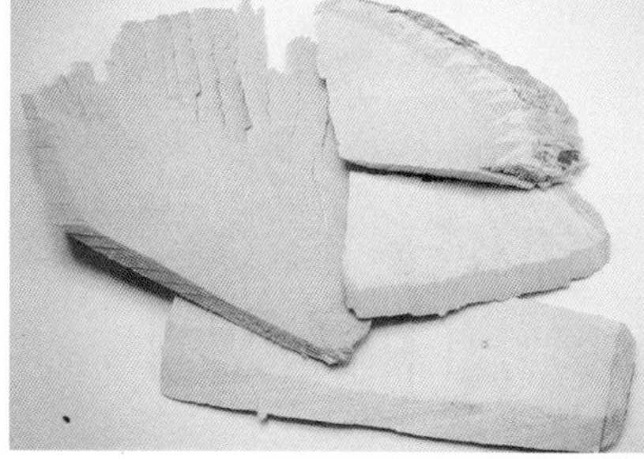
Da Ding Huang (Caulis Euonymi)

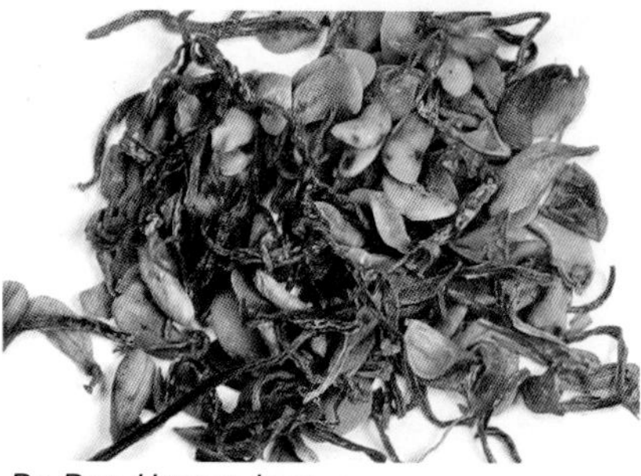
Da Dou Huang Juan
(Semen Glycines Germinatum)

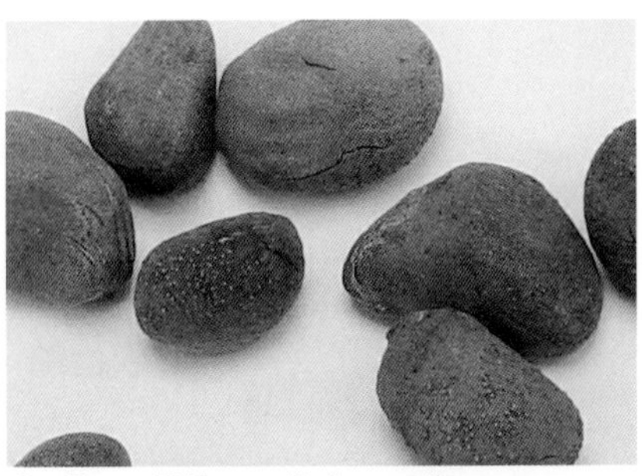
Da Feng Zi (Semen Hydnocarpi)

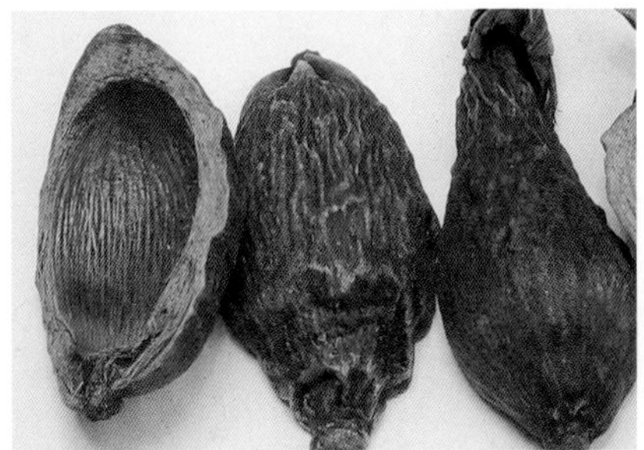
Da Fu Pi (Pericarpium Arecae)

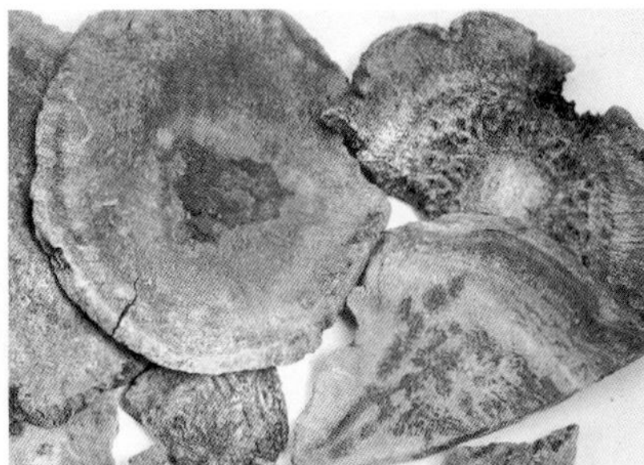
Da Huang (Radix et Rhizoma Rhei)

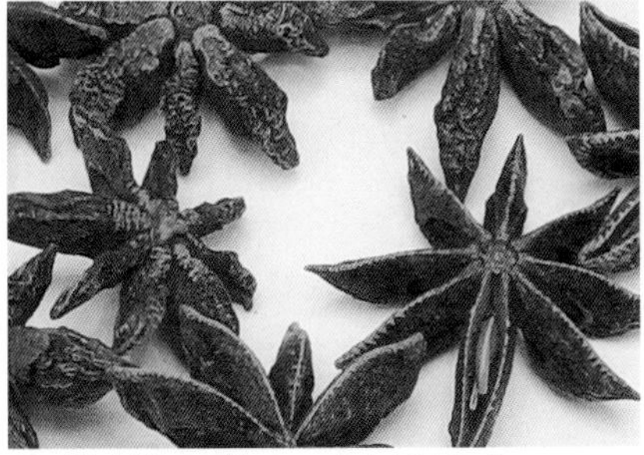
Da Hui Xiang (Fructus Anisi Stellati)

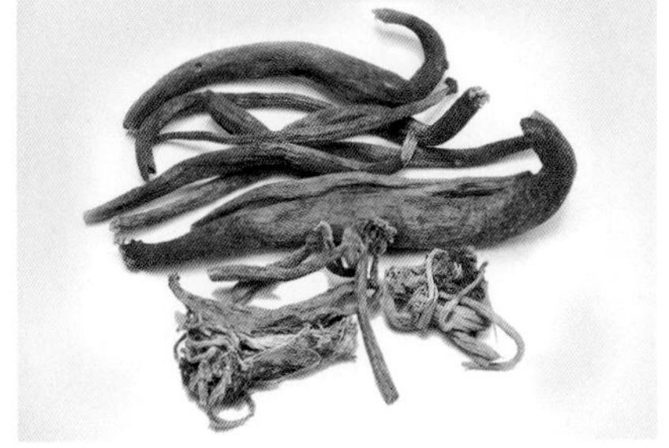
Da Ji (Herba seu Radix Cirsii Japonici)

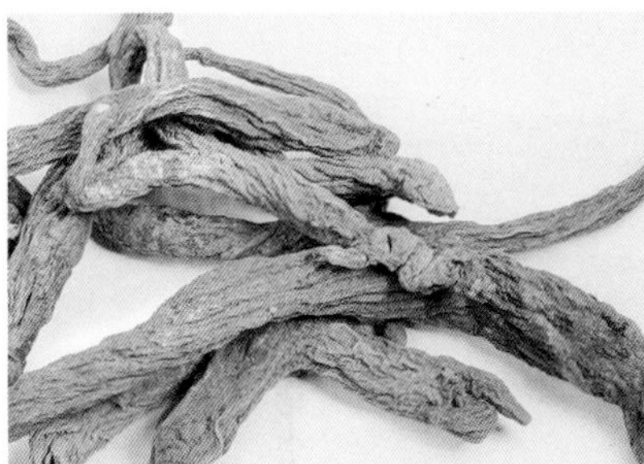
Da Ji (Radix Euphorbiae seu Knoxiae)

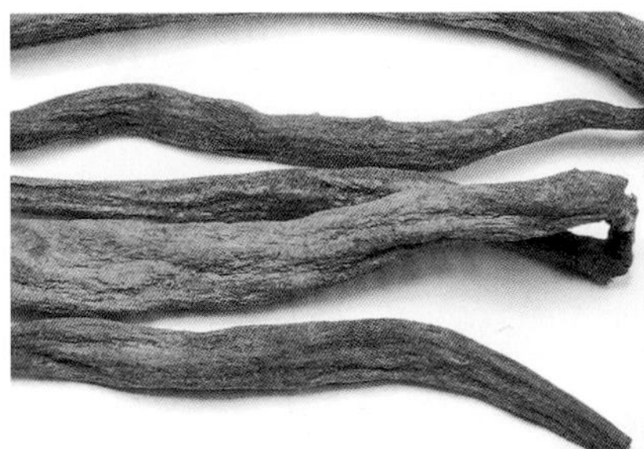
Da Ji Gen (Radix Cirsii Japonici)

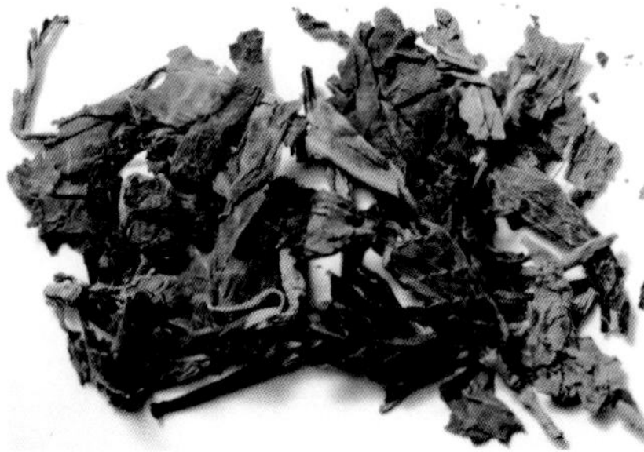
Da Qing Ye (Folium Isatidis)

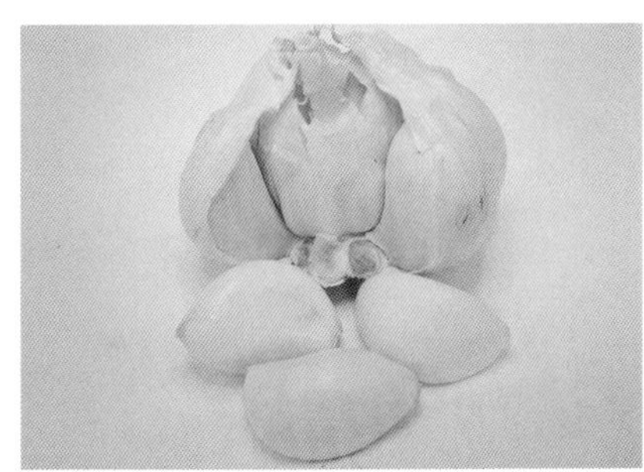
Da Suan (Bulbus Alli Sativi)

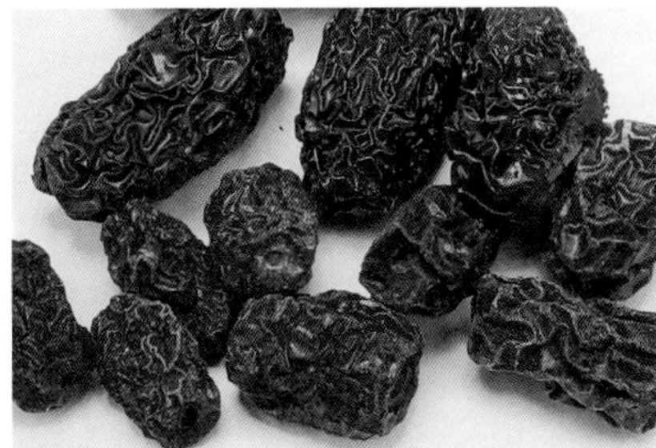
Da Zao (Fructus Jujubae)

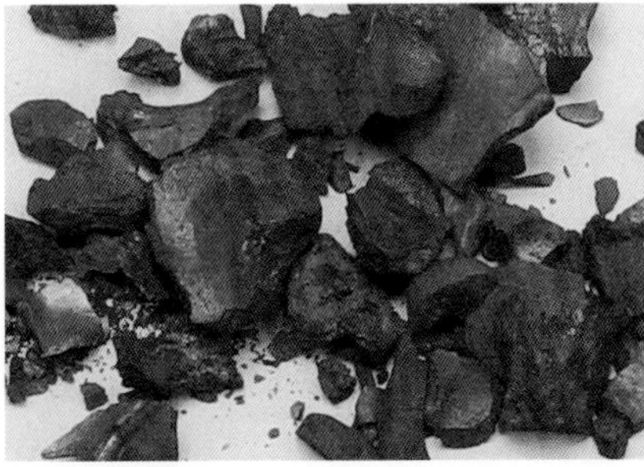
Dai Zhe Shi (Haematitum)

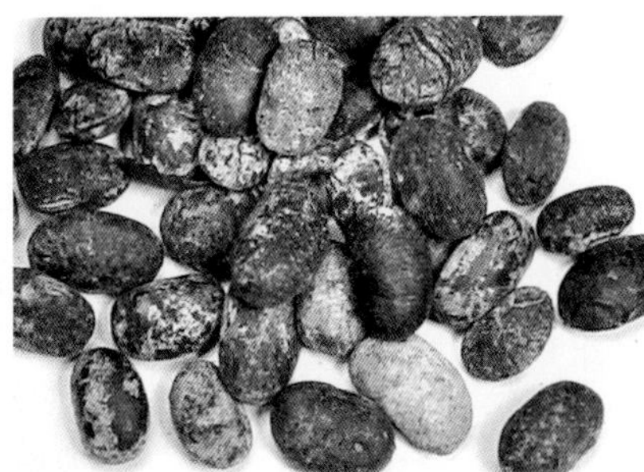
Dan Dou Chi (Semen Sojae Praeparatum)

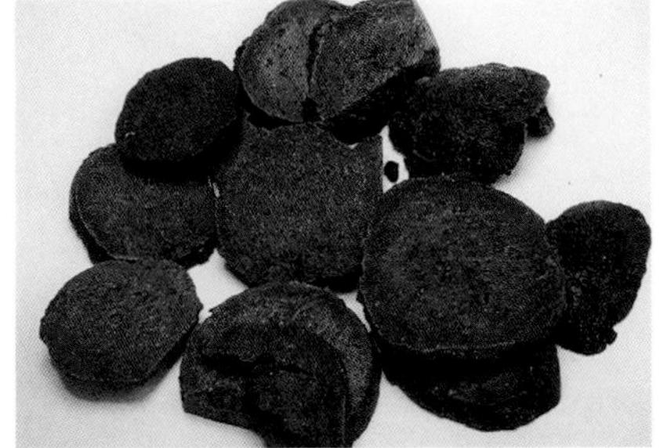
Dan Nan Xing (Arisaema cum Bile)

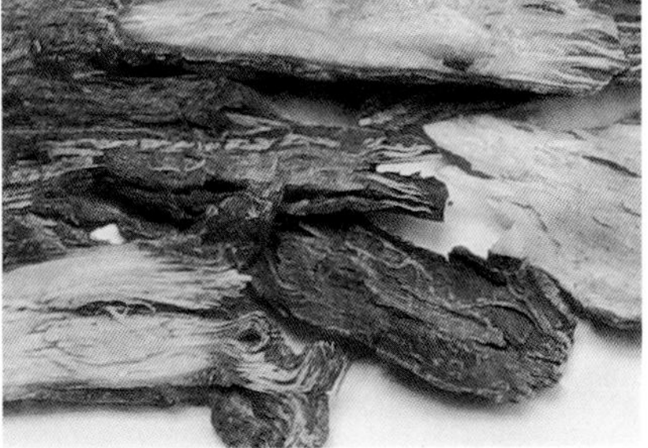
Dan Shen (Radix Salviae Miltiorrhizae)

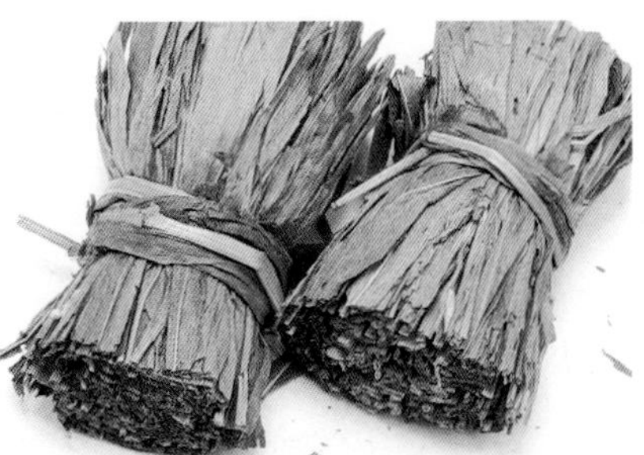
Dan Zhu Ye (Herba Lophatheri)

Herb Indentification Guide

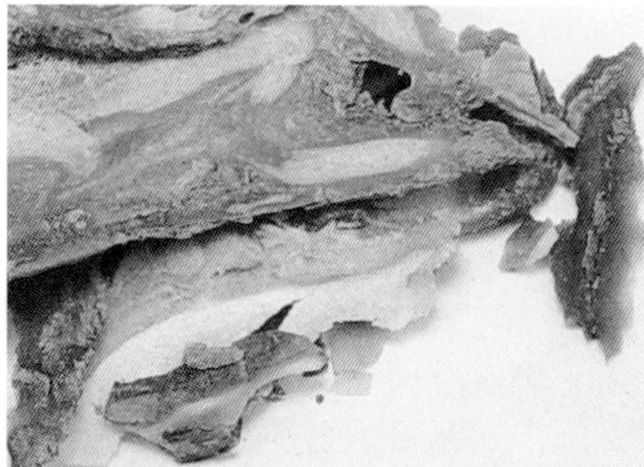

Dang Gui Shen (Corpus Radicis Angelicae Sinensis)

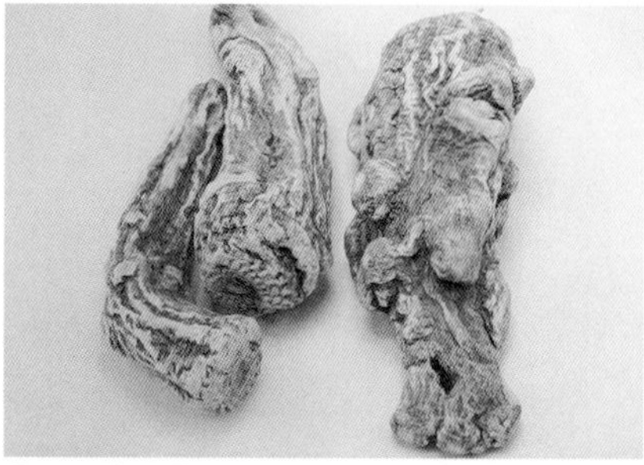

Dang Gui Tou (Caput Radicis Angelicae Sinensis)

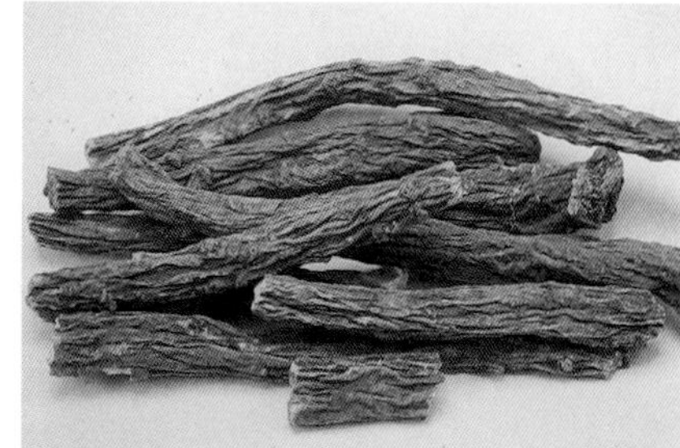

Dang Gui Wei (Extremitas Radicis Angelicae Sinensis)

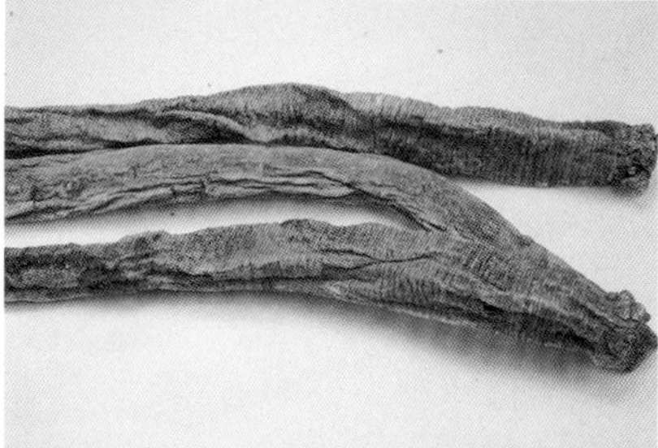

Dang Shen (Radix Codonopsis)

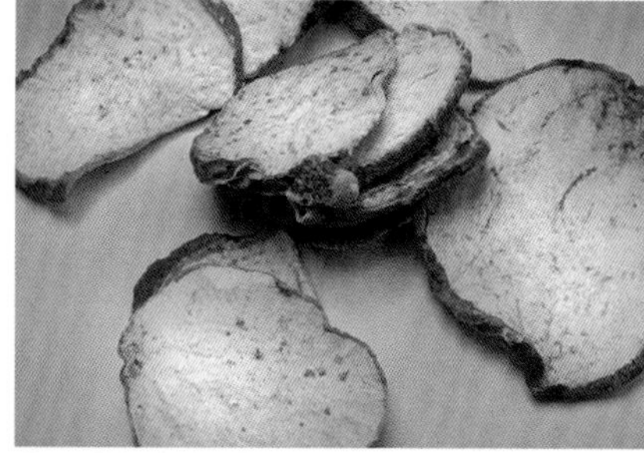

Dao Diao Jin Zhong (Melothria Maderospatana)

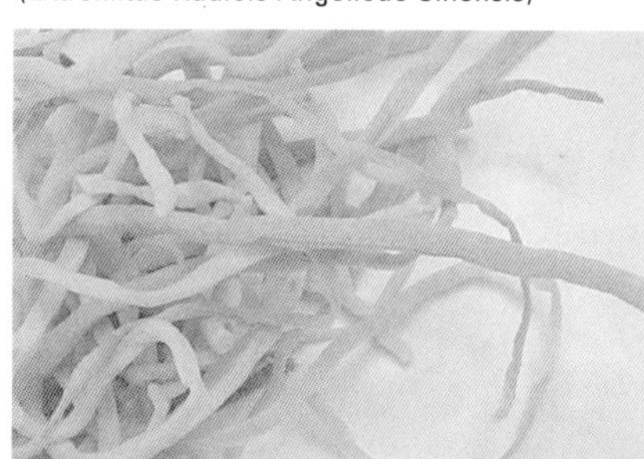

Deng Xin Cao (Medulla Junci)

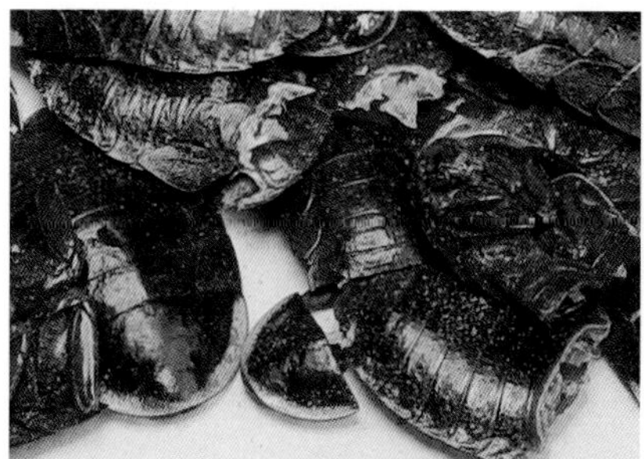

Di Bie Chong (Eupolyphaga)

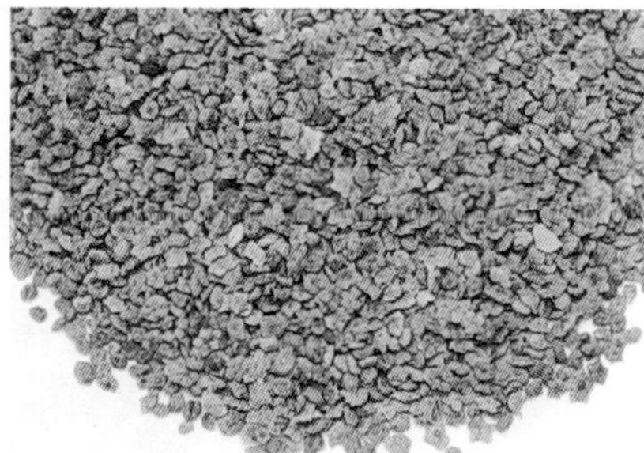

Di Fu Zi (Fructus Kochiae)

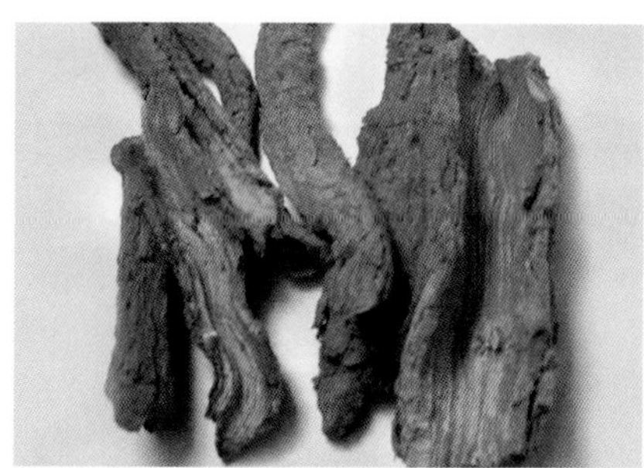

Di Gu Pi (Cortex Lycii)

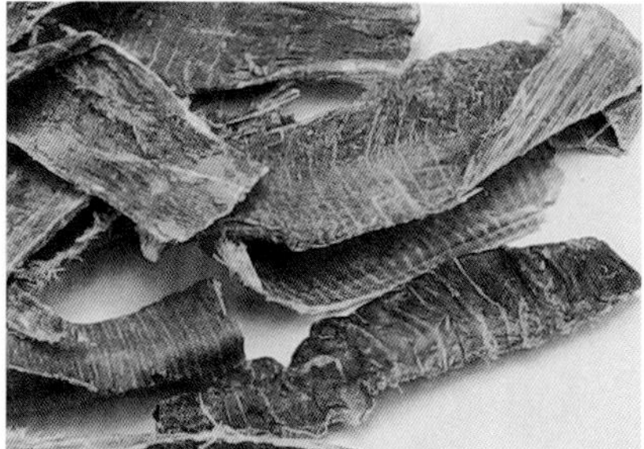

Di Long (Pheretima)

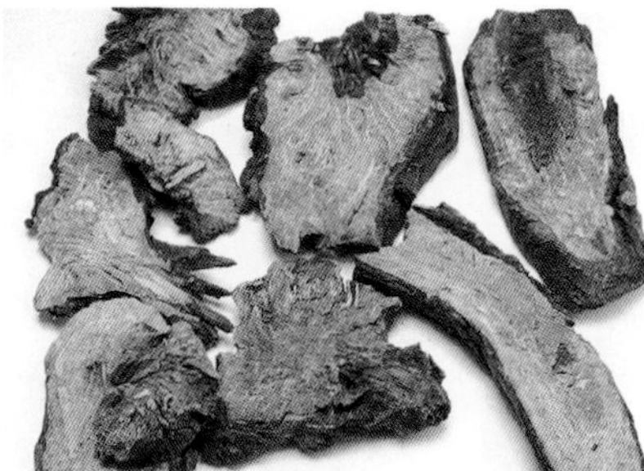

Di Yu (Radix Sanguisorbae)

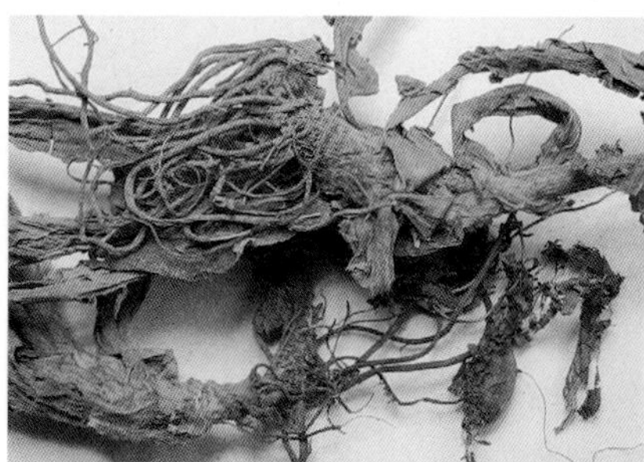

Ding Shu Xiu (Herba Elephantopus Scaber)

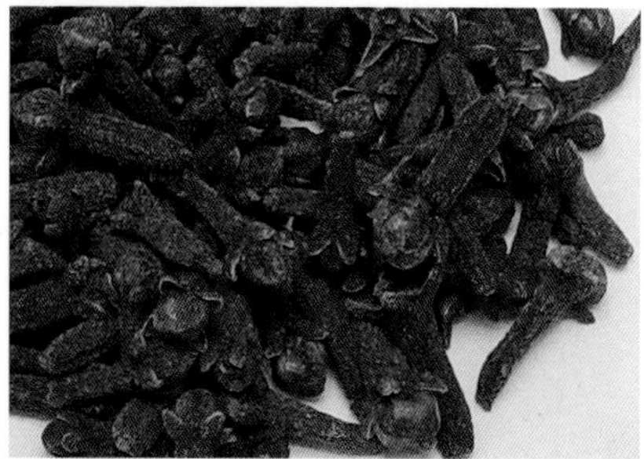

Ding Xiang (Flos Caryophylli)

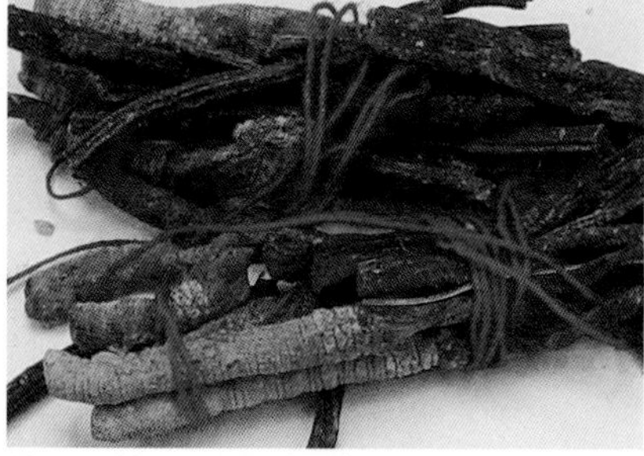

Dong Chong Xia Cao (Cordyceps)

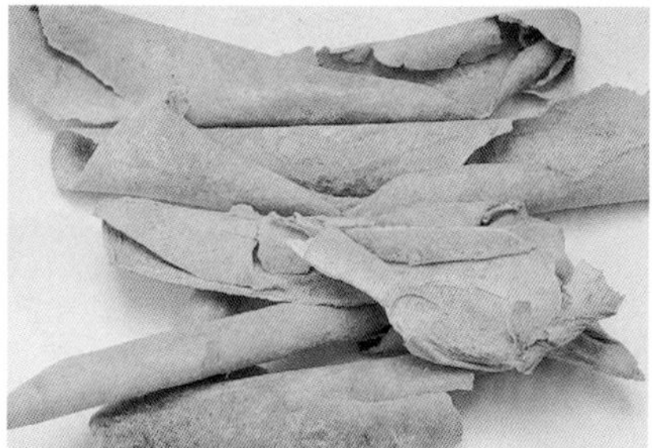

Dong Gua Pi (Exocarpium Benincasae)

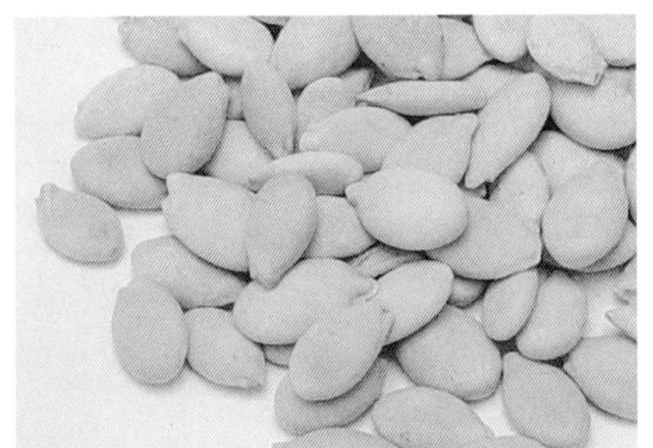
Dong Gua Zi (Semen Benincasae)

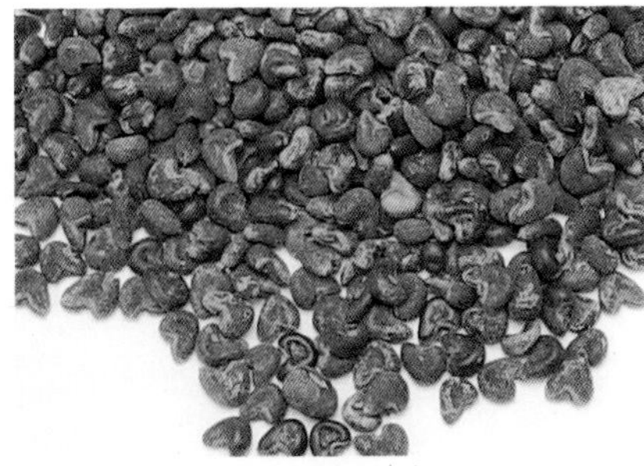
Dong Kui Zi (Semen Malvae)

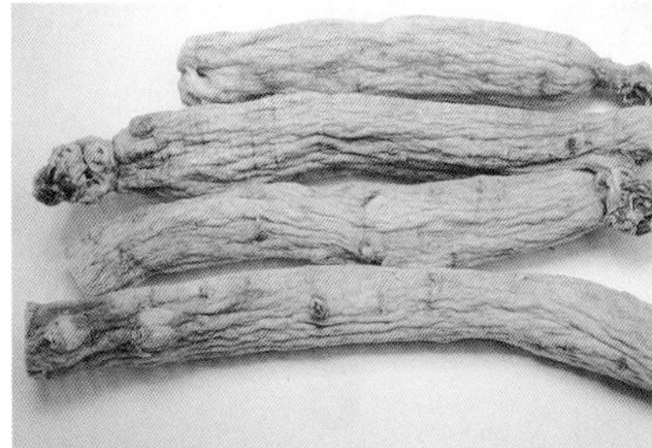
Dong Yang Shen (Radix Ginseng Japonica)

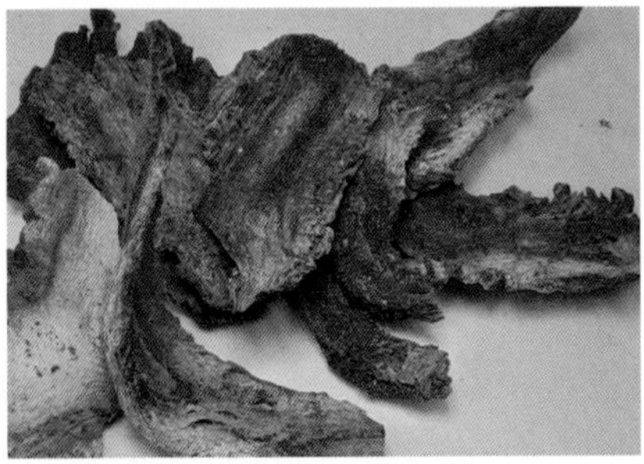
Du Huo (Radix Angelicae Pubescentis)

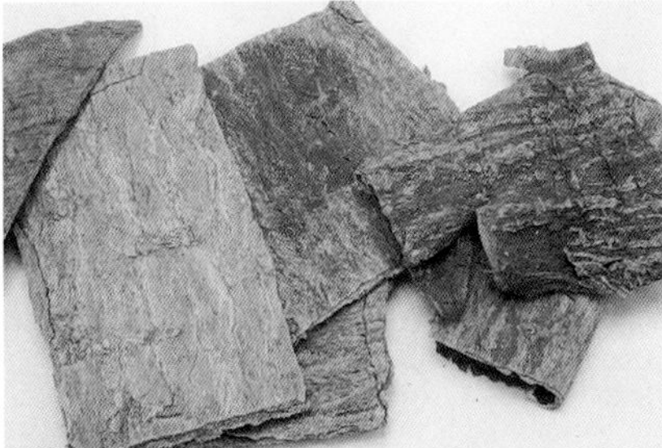
Du Zhong (Cortex Eucommiae)

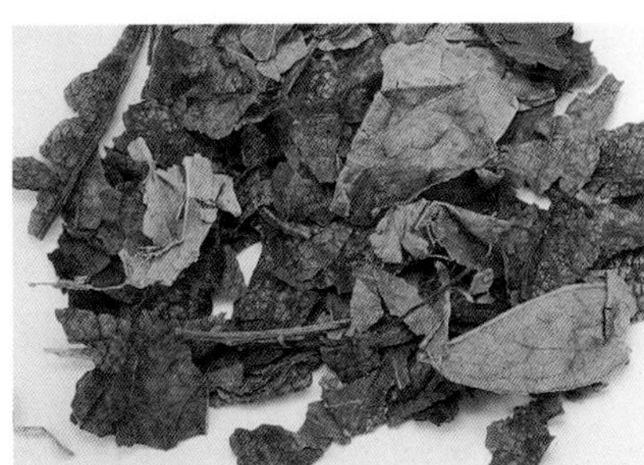
Du Zhong Ye (Folium Eucommiae)

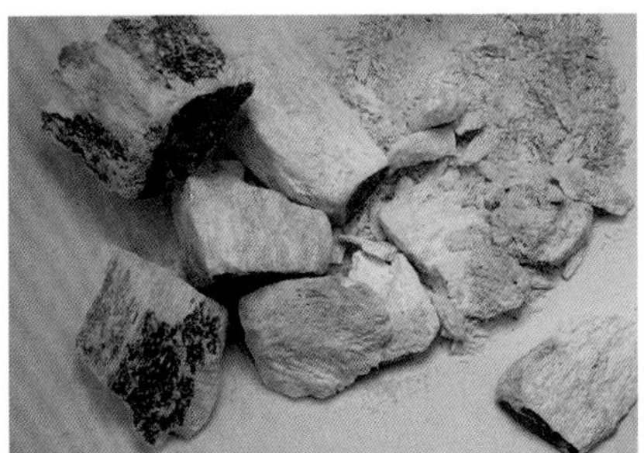
Duan Shi Gao (Gypsum Fibrosum Preparata)

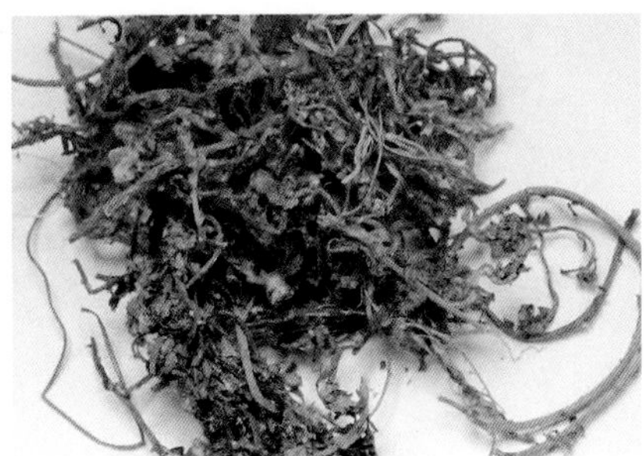
E Bu Shi Cao (Herba Centipedae)

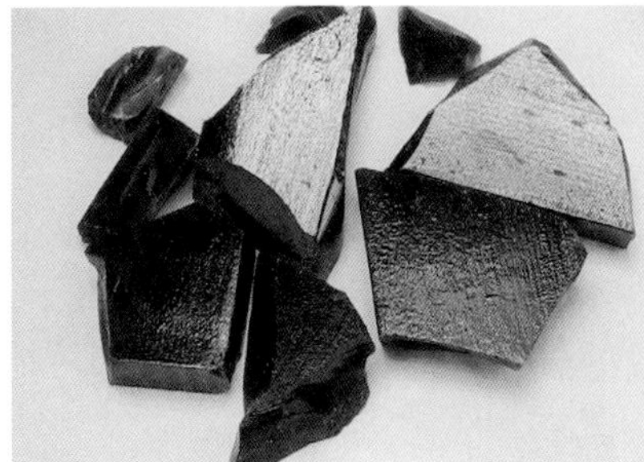
E Jiao (Colla Corii Asini)

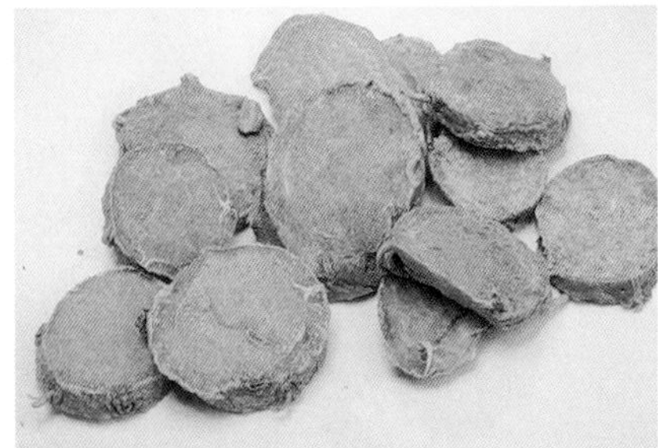
E Zhu (Rhizoma Curcumae)

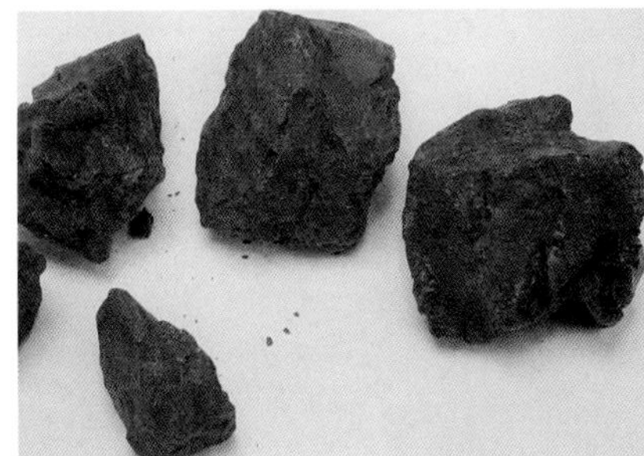
Er Cha (Catechu)

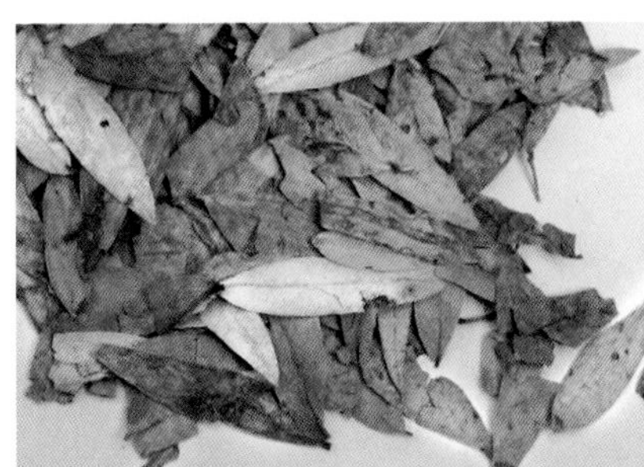
Fan Xie Ye (Folium Sennae)

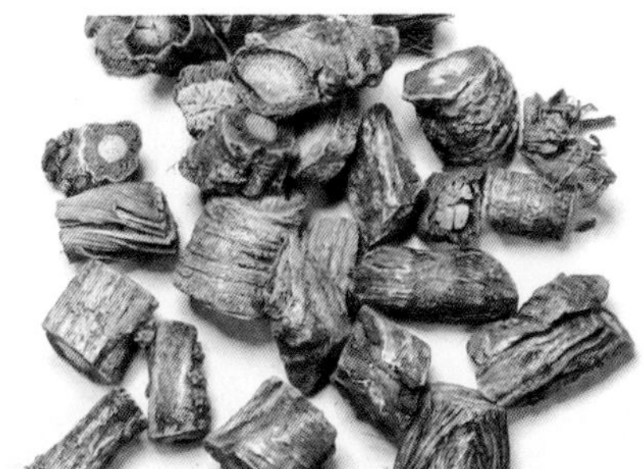
Fang Feng (Radix Saposhnikoviae)

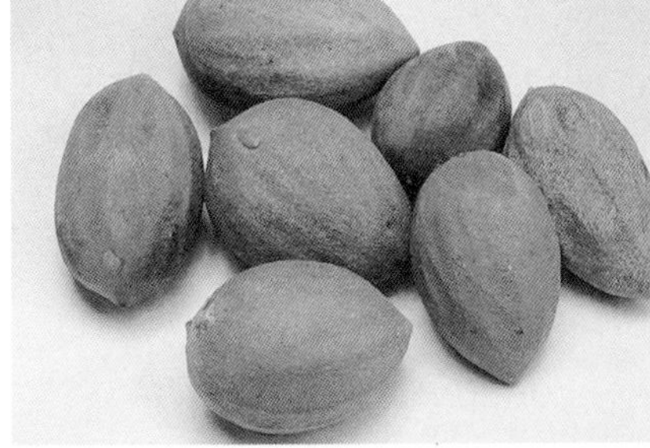
Fei Zi (Semen Torreyae)

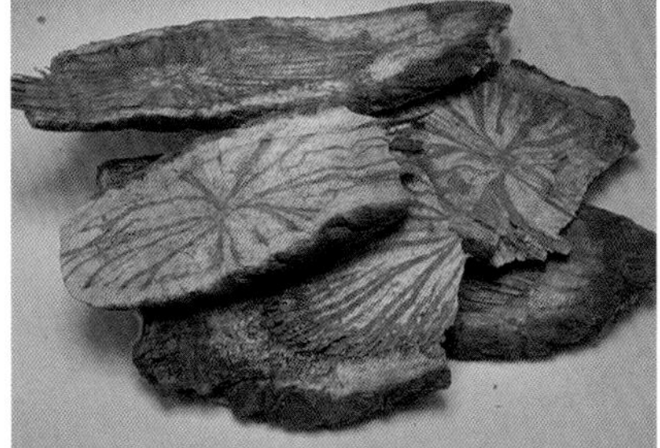
Fen Fang Ji (Radix Stephaniae Tetandrae)

Herb Indentification Guide

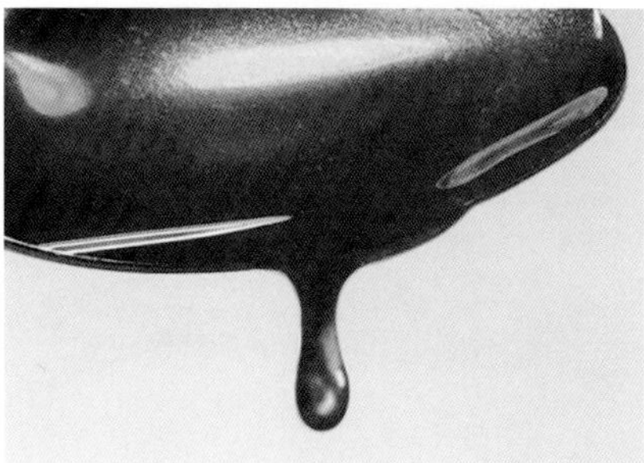
Feng Mi (Mel)

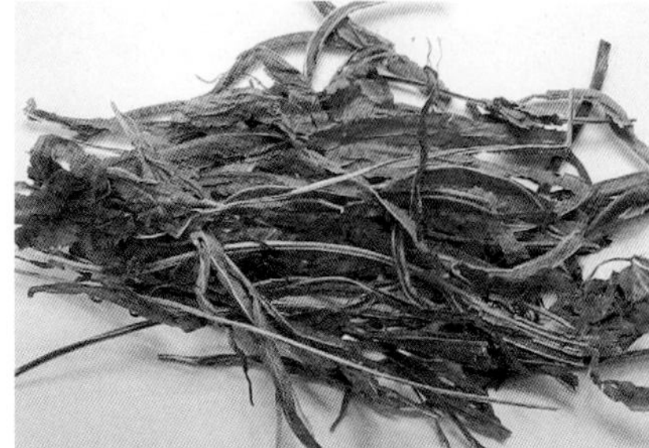
Feng Wei Cao (Herba Pteris)

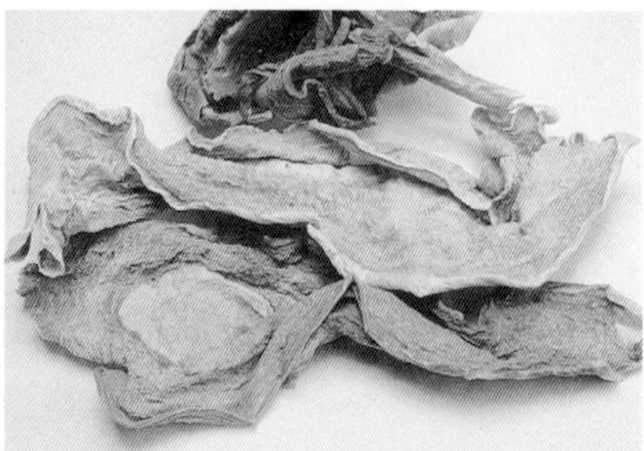
Fo Shou (Fructus Citri Sarcodactylis)

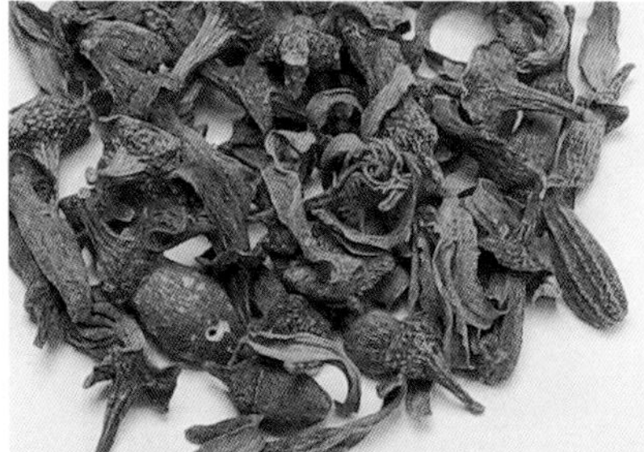
Fo Shou Hua (Flos Citri Sarcodactylis)

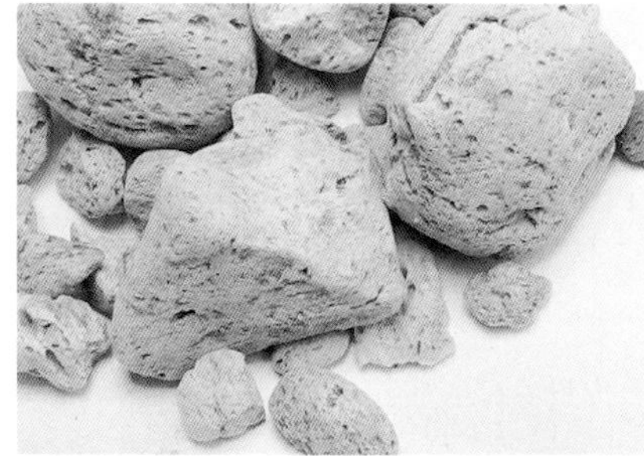
Fu Hai Shi (Pumice)

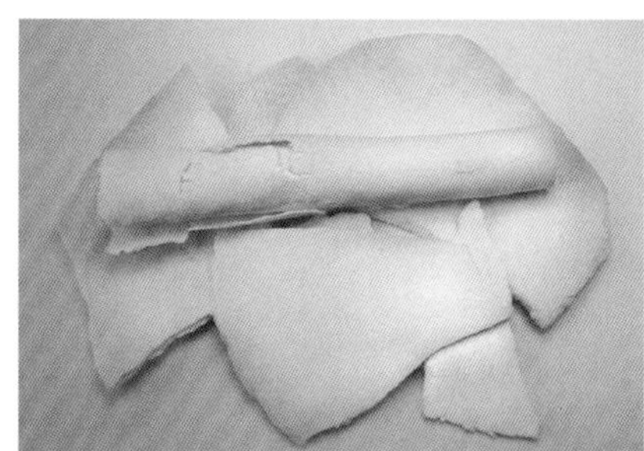
Fu Ling (Poria)

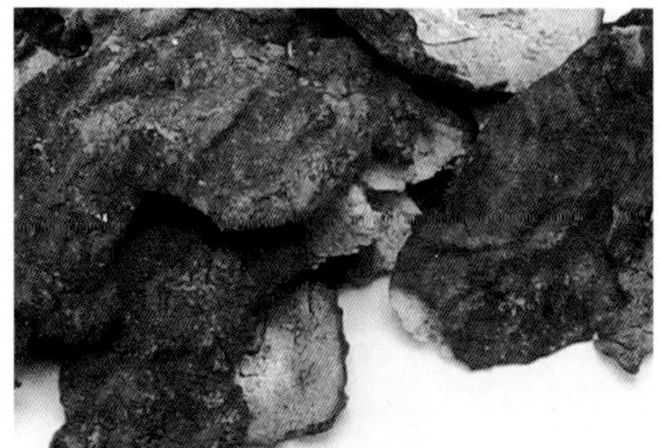
Fu Ling Pi (Cortex Poria)

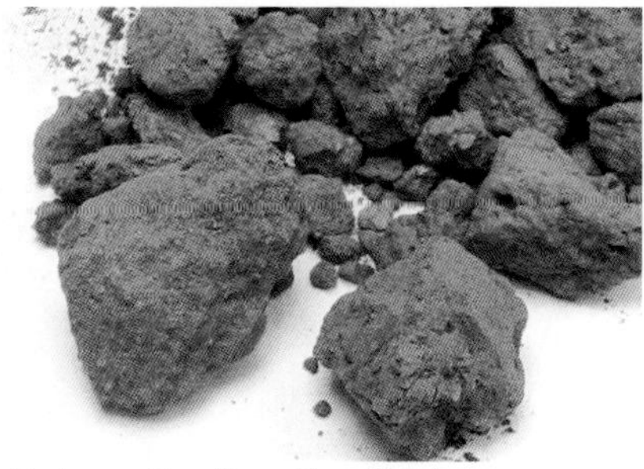
Fu Long Gan (Terra Flava Usta)

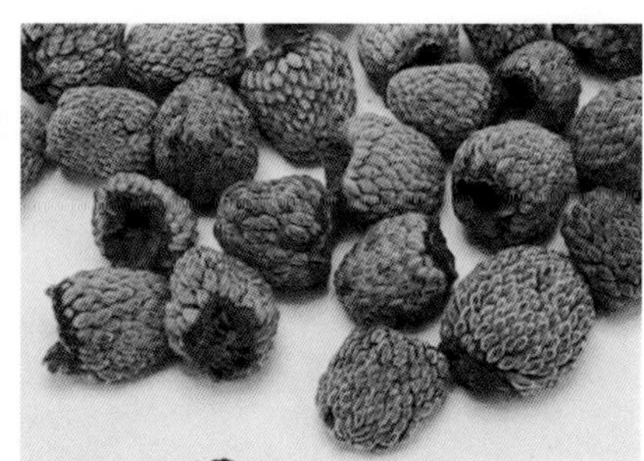
Fu Pen Zi (Fructus Rubi)

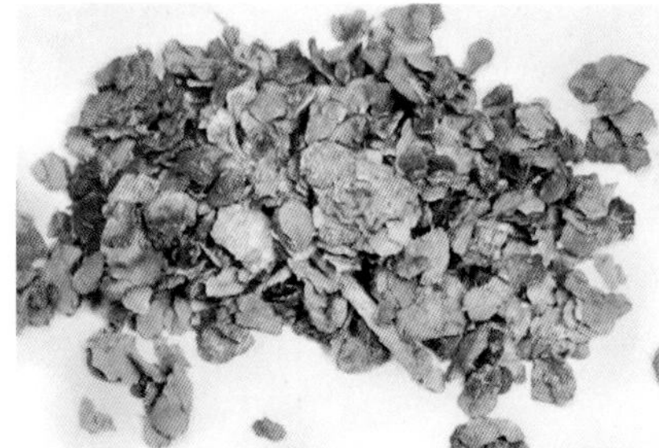
Fu Ping (Herba Spirodelae)

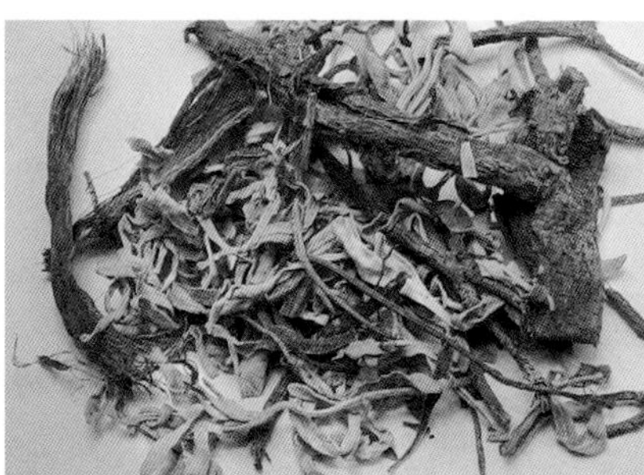
Fu Rong (Radix Hibisci)

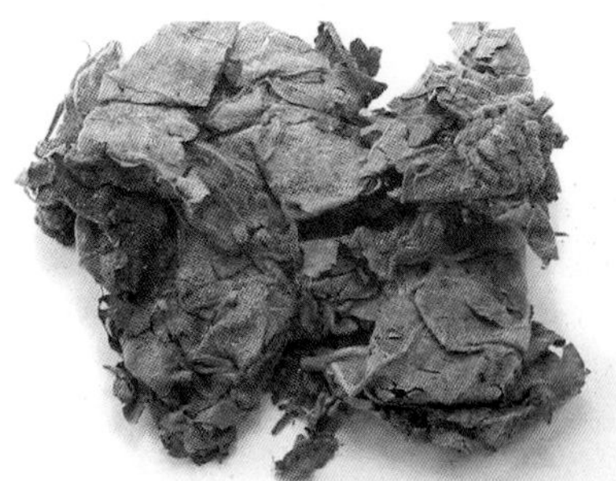
Fu Rong Ye (Folium Hibisci)

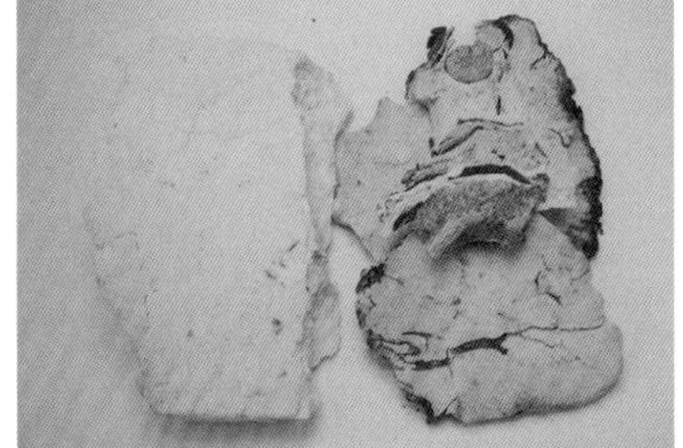
Fu Shen (Poria Paradicis)

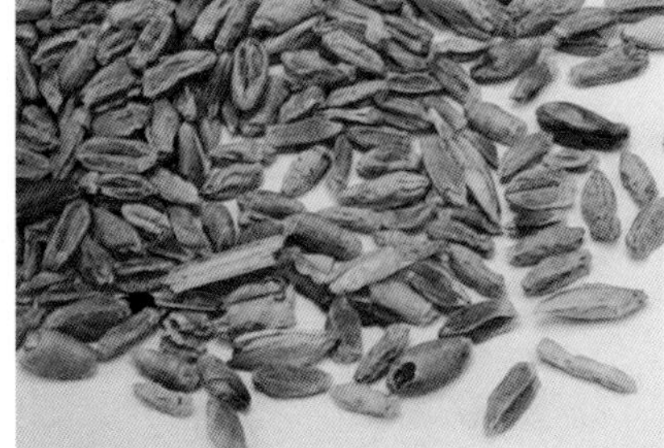
Fu Xiao Mai (Semen Tritici Aestivi Levis)

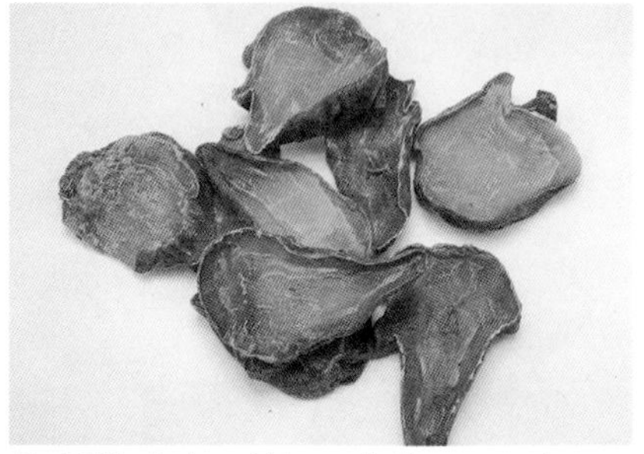
Fu Zi (Radix Aconiti Lateralis Praeparata)

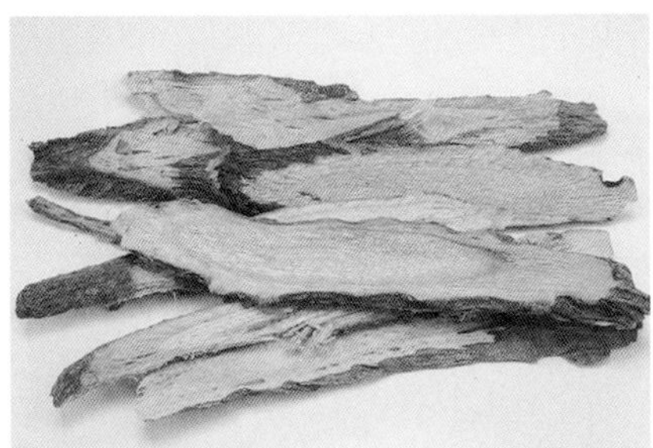
Gan Cao (Radix Glycyrrhizae)

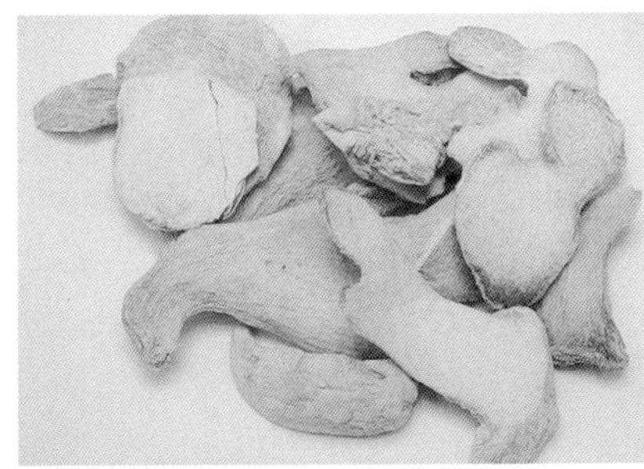
Gan Jiang (Rhizoma Zingiberis)

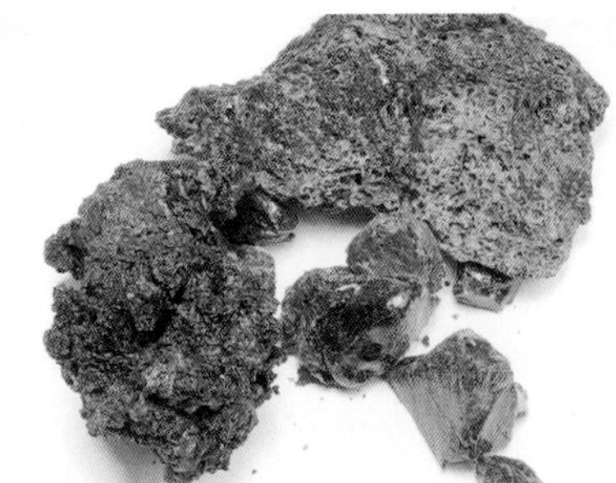
Gan Qi (Resina Toxicodendri)

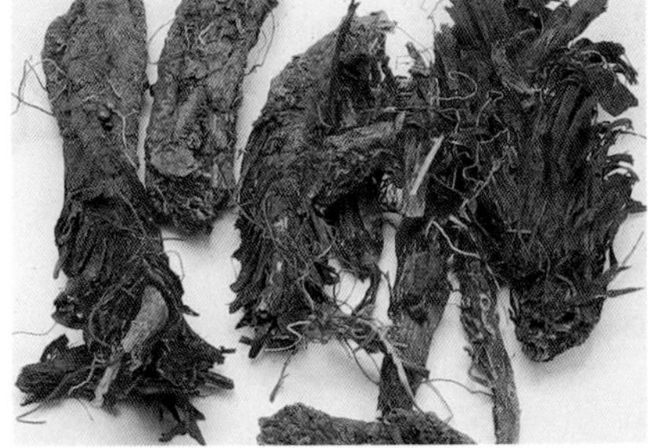
Gan Song (Radix seu Rhizoma Nardostachys)

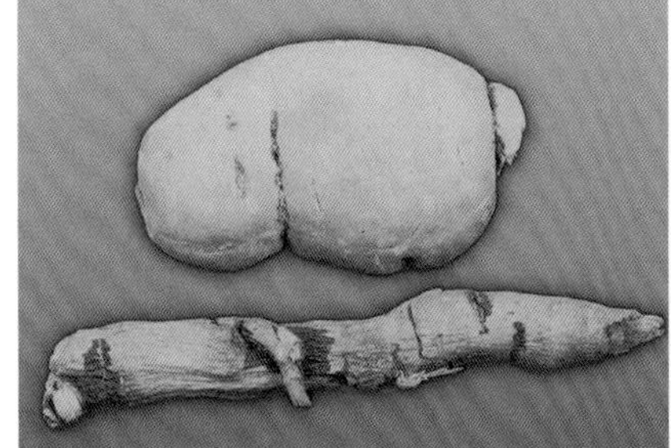
Gan Sui (Radix Euphorbiae Kansui)

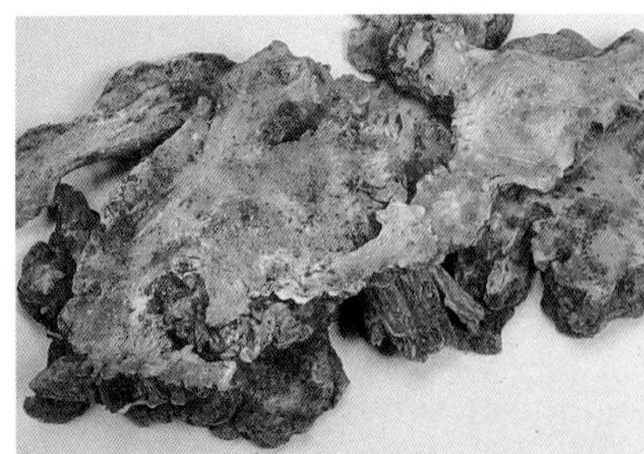
Gao Ben (Rhizoma Ligustici)

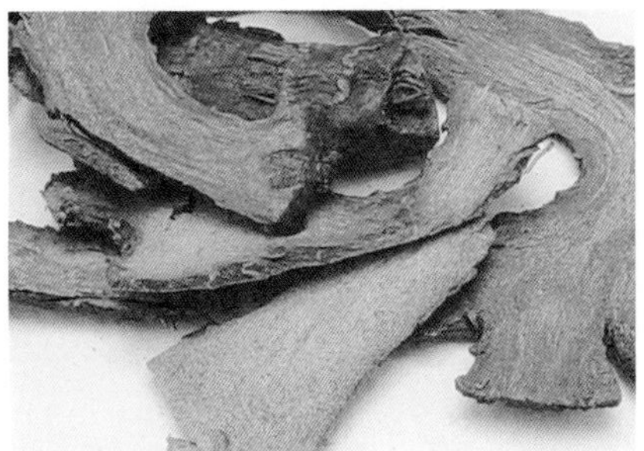
Gao Liang Jiang
(Rhizoma Alpiniae Officinarum)

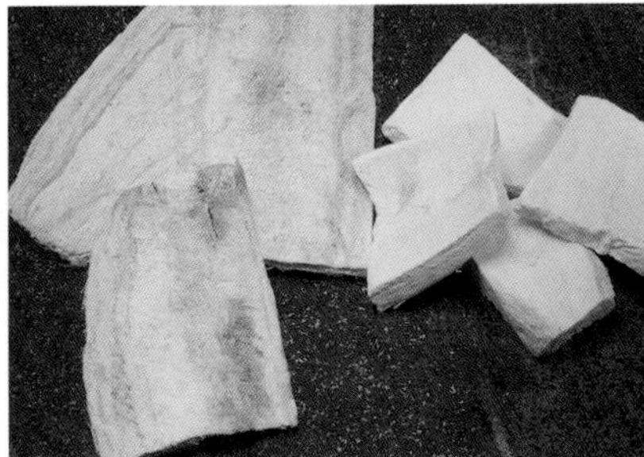
Ge Gen (Radix Puerariae)

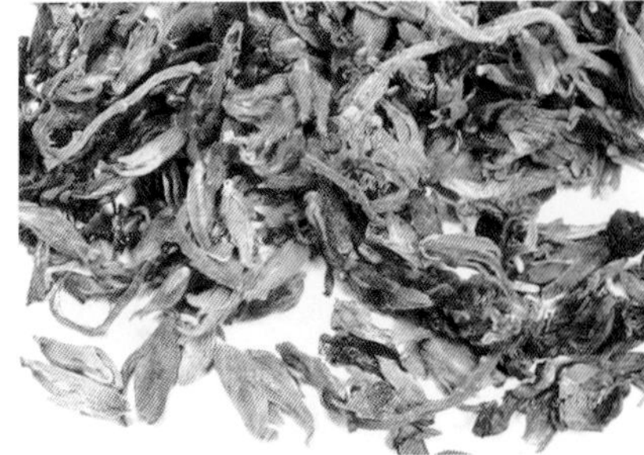
Ge Hua (Flos Puerariae)

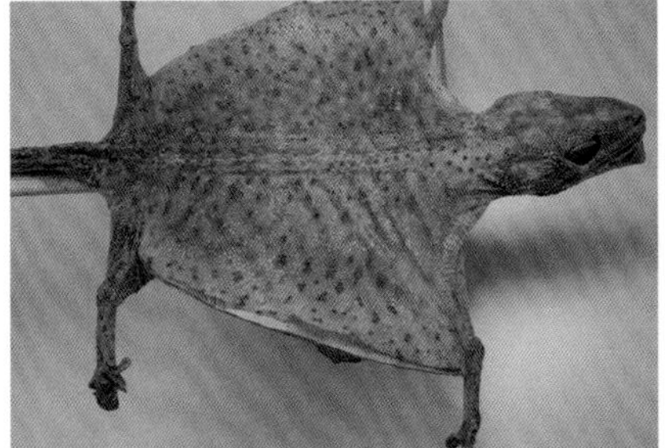
Ge Jie (Gecko)

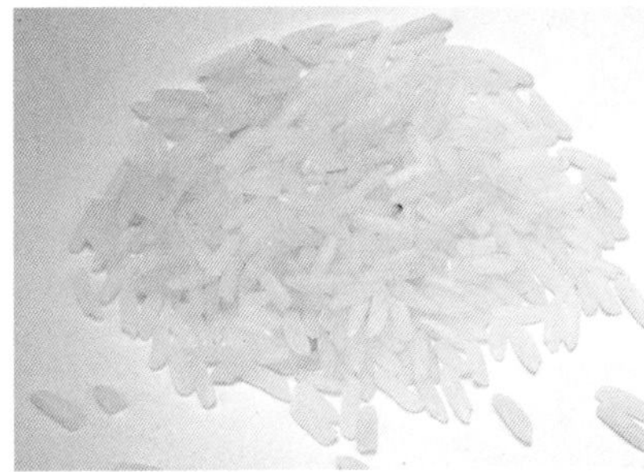
Geng Mi (Semen Oryzae)

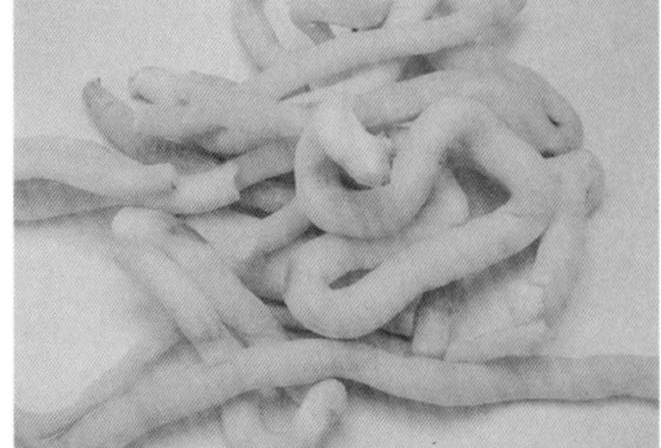
Geng Tong Cao
(Ramulus Aeschynomene Indica)

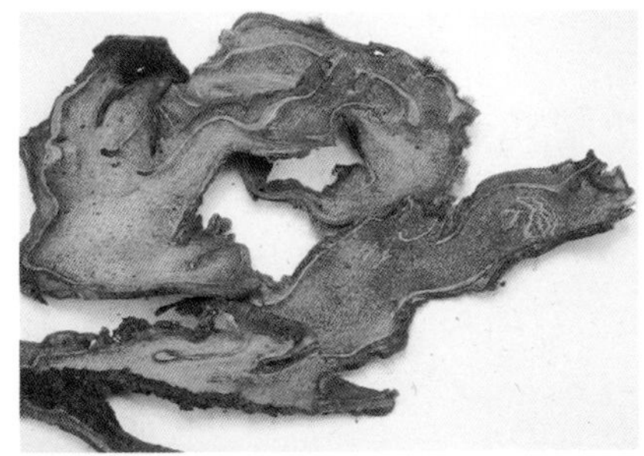
Gou Ji (Rhizoma Cibotii)

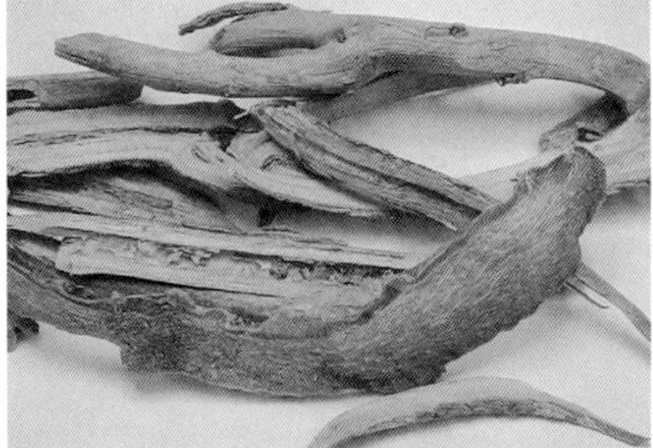
Gou Qi Gen (Radix Lycii)

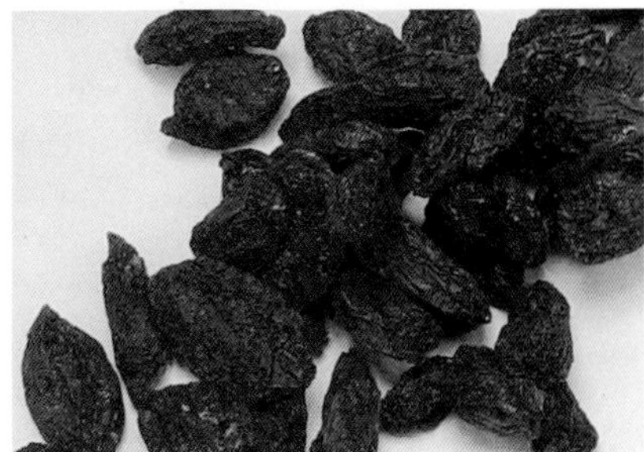
Gou Qi Zi (Fructus Lycii)

Herb Indentification Guide

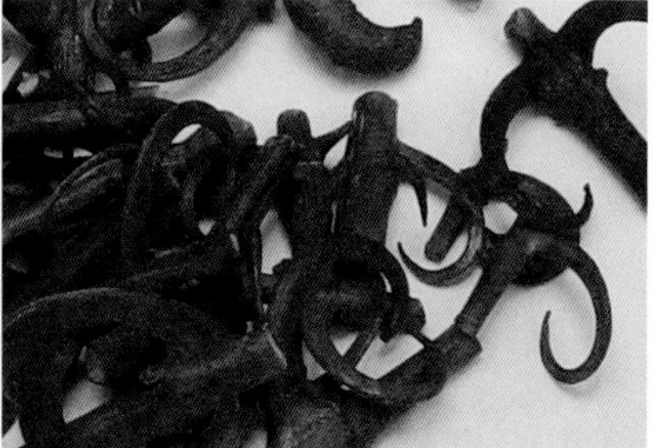
Gou Teng (Ramulus Uncariae cum Uncis)

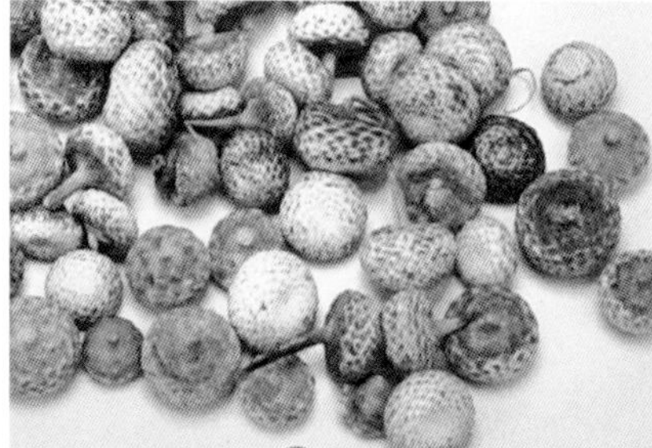
Gu Jing Cao (Flos Eriocauli)

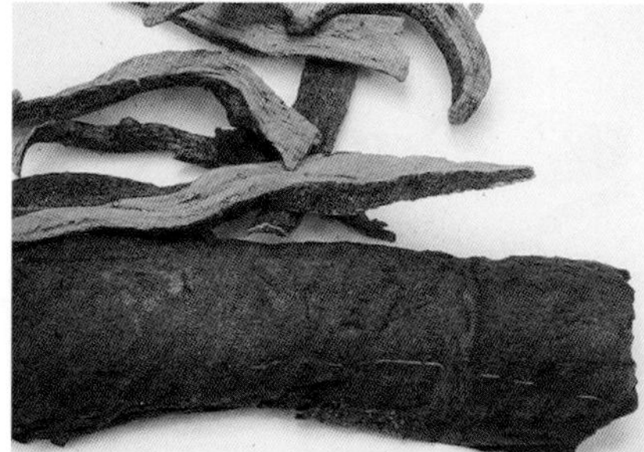
Gu Sui Bu (Rhizoma Drynariae)

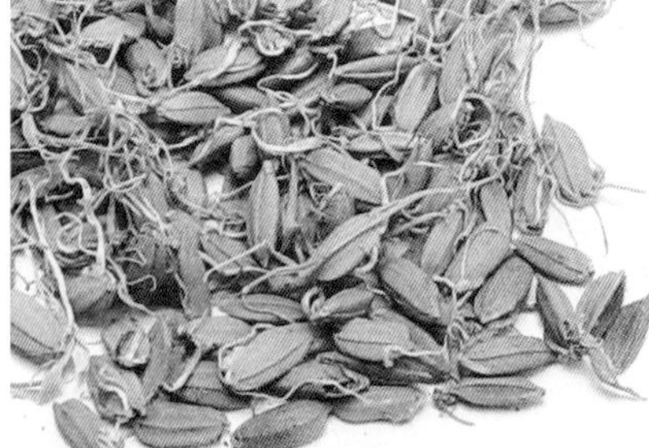
Gu Ya (Fructus Setariae Germinatus)

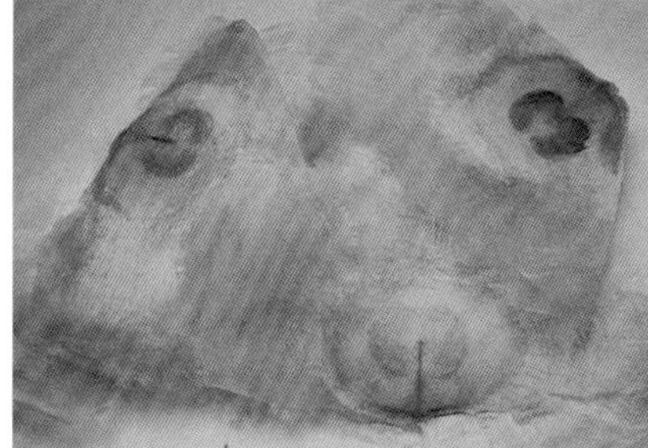
Gu Zhi Hua (Semen Oroxyli)

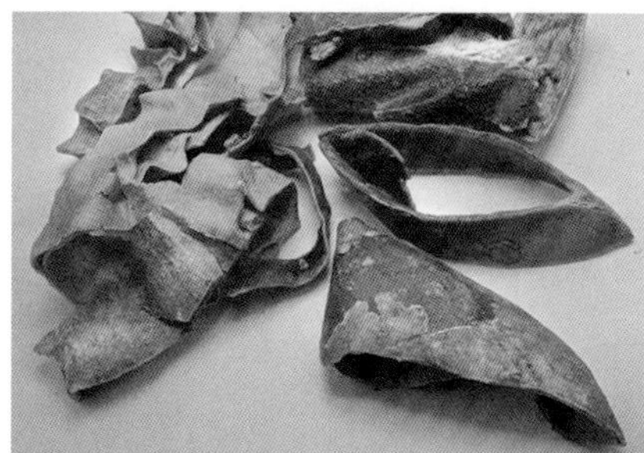
Gua Lou Pi (Pericarpium Trichosanthis)

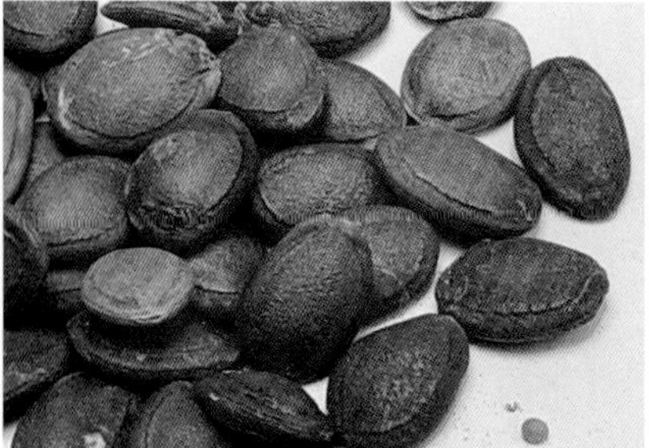
Gua Lou Ren (Semen Trichosanthis)

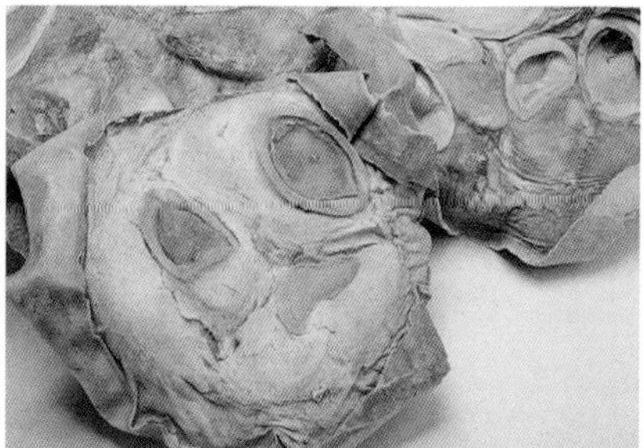
Gua Lou Shi (Fructus Trichosanthis)

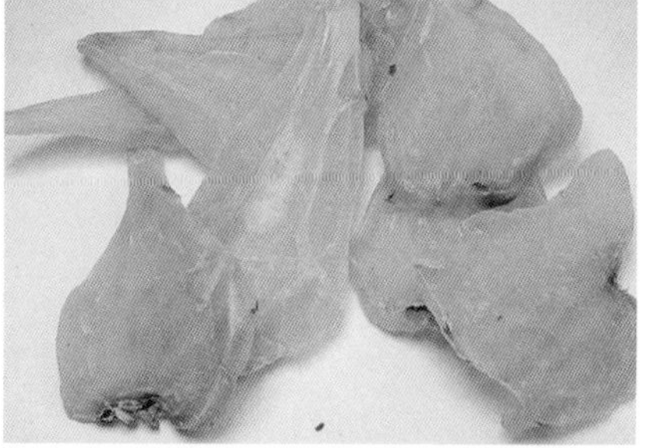
Guan Bai Fu (Rhizoma Aconitum Coreanum)

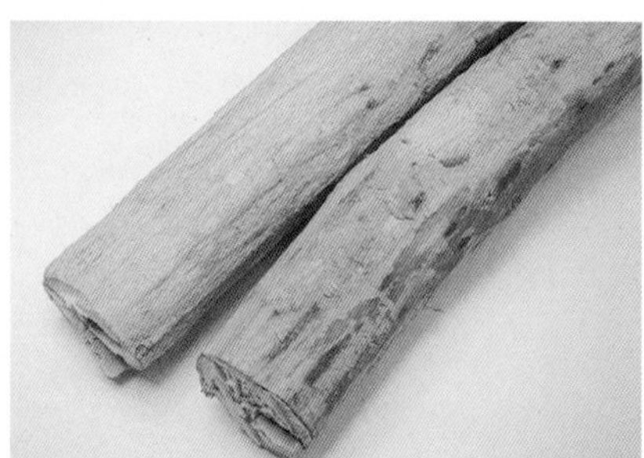
Guan Mu Tong
(Caulis Aristolochiae Manshuriensis)

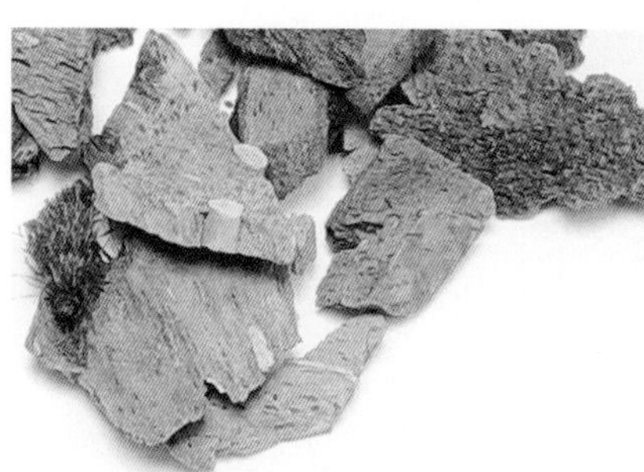
Guan Zhong (Rhizoma Dryopteridis)

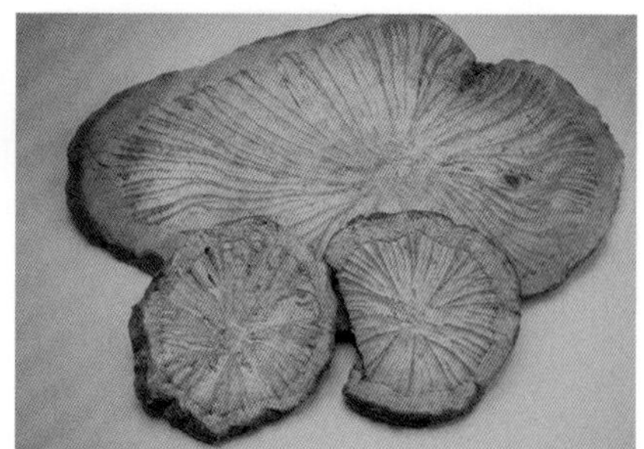
Guang Fang Ji (Radix Aristolochiae Fangchi)

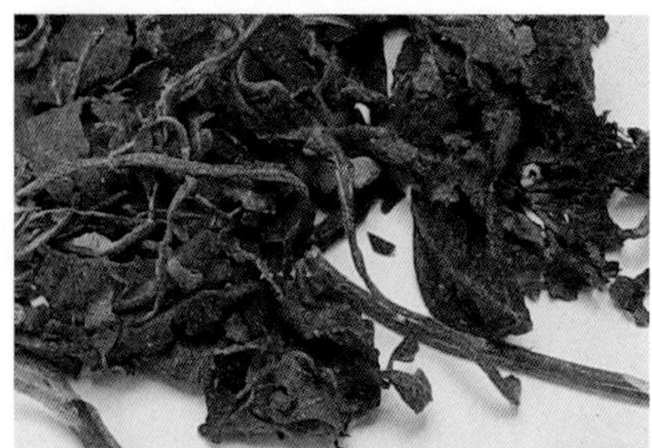
Guang Huo Xiang (Herba Pogostemonis)

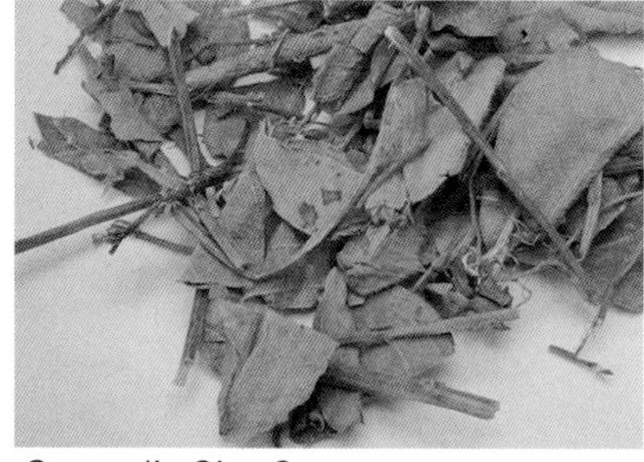
Guang Jin Qian Cao
(Herba Desmodii Styracifolii)

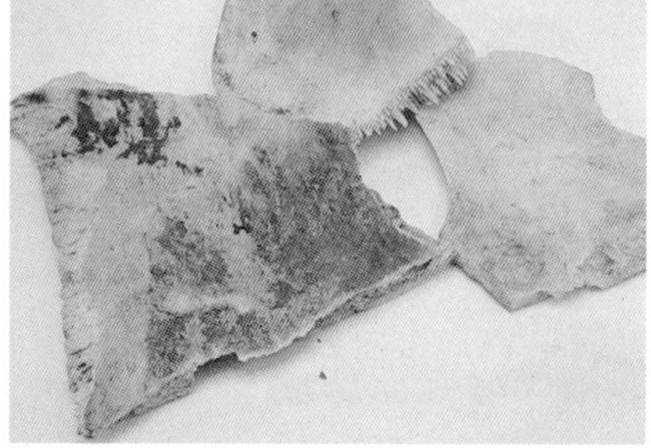
Gui Ban (Plastrum Testudinis)

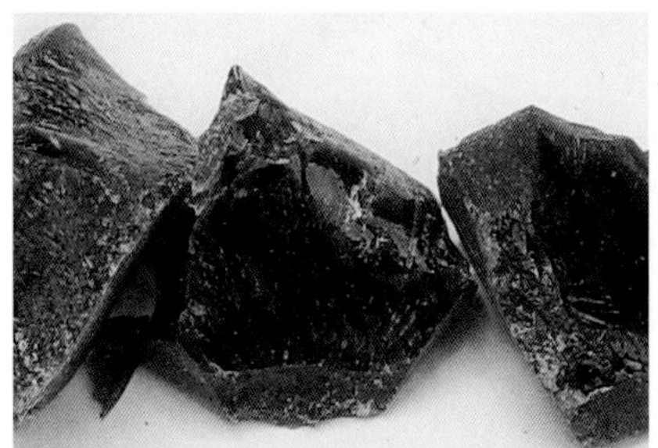
Gui Ban Jiao (Gelatinum Plastrum Testudinis)

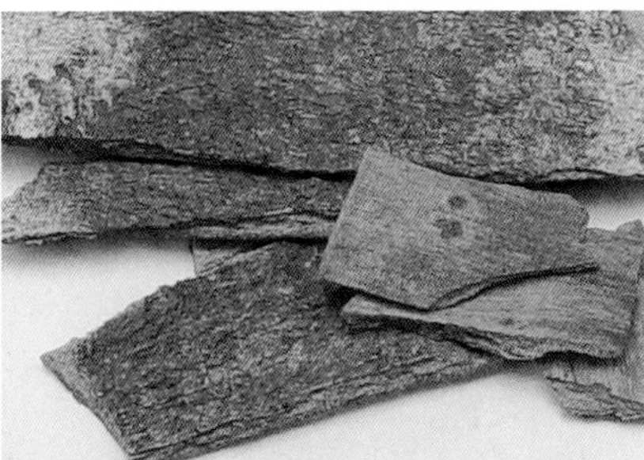
Gui Xin (Cortex Rasus Cinnamomi)

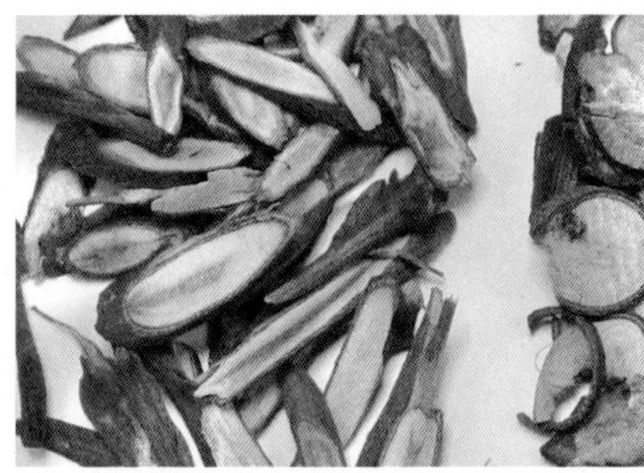
Gui Zhi (Ramulus Cinnamomi)

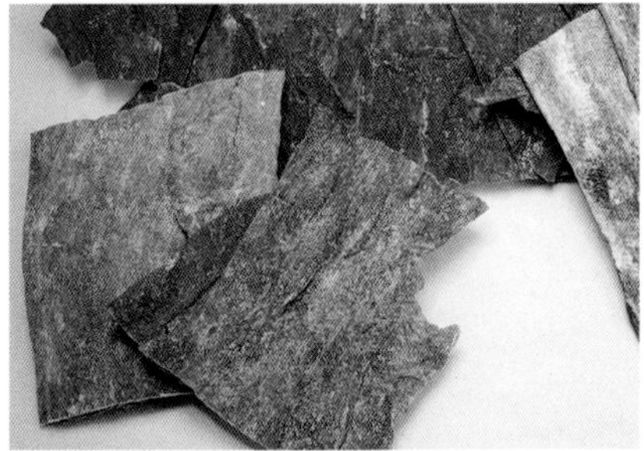
Hai Dai (Thallus Laminariae)

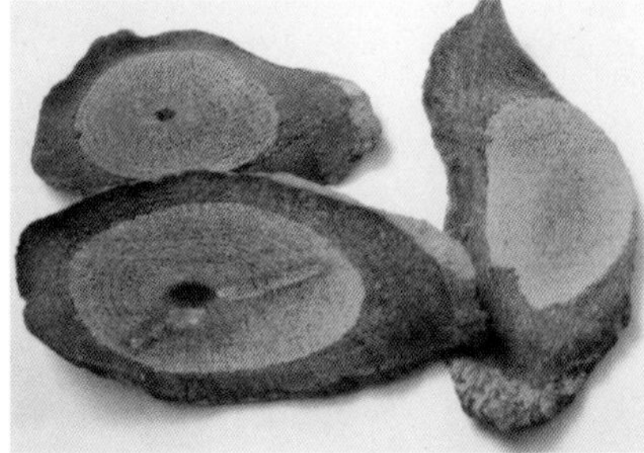
Hai Feng Teng (Caulis Piperis Kadsurae)

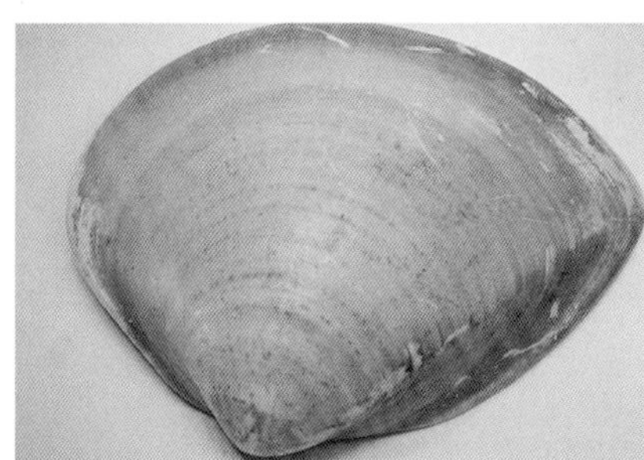
Hai Ge Fen (Concha Meretricis seu Cyclinae)

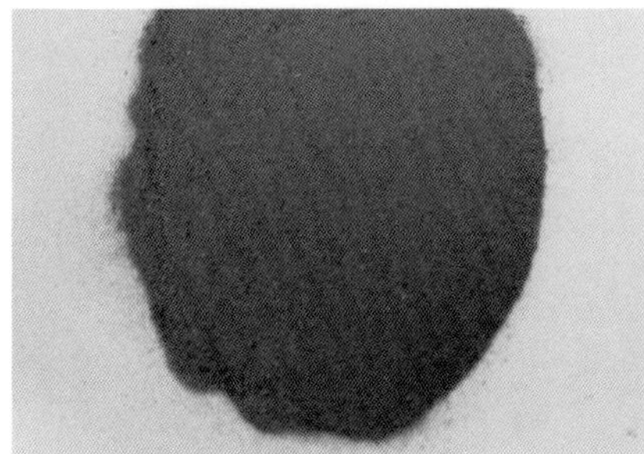
Hai Jin Sha (Herba Lygodii)

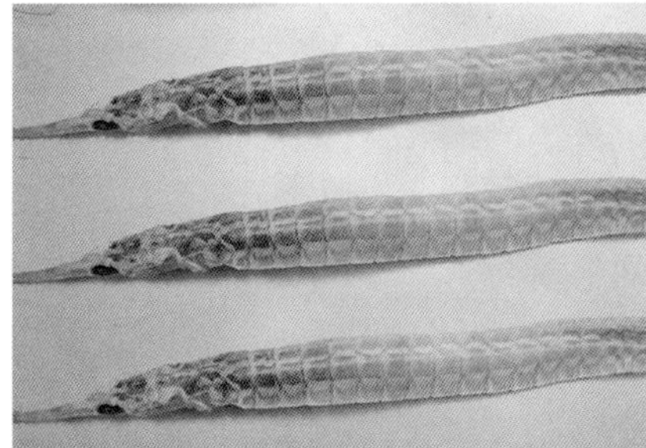
Hai Long (Syngnathus)

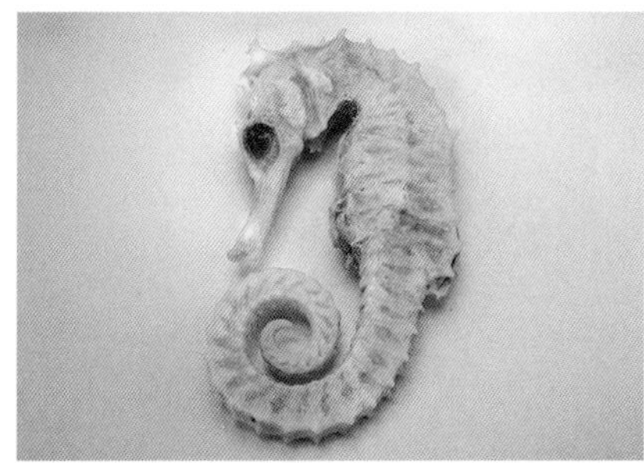
Hai Ma (Hippocampus)

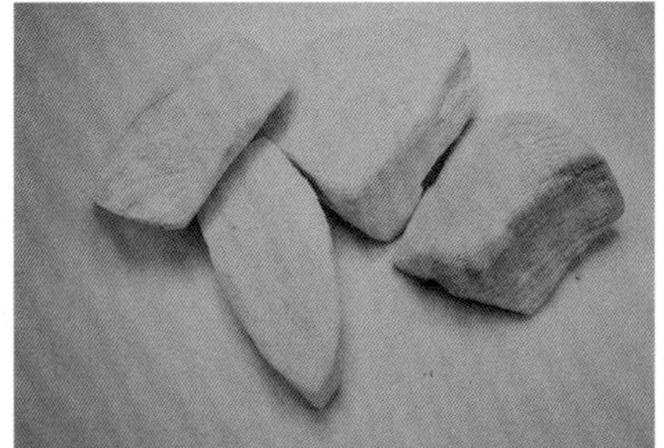
Hai Piao Xiao (Endoconcha Sepiae)

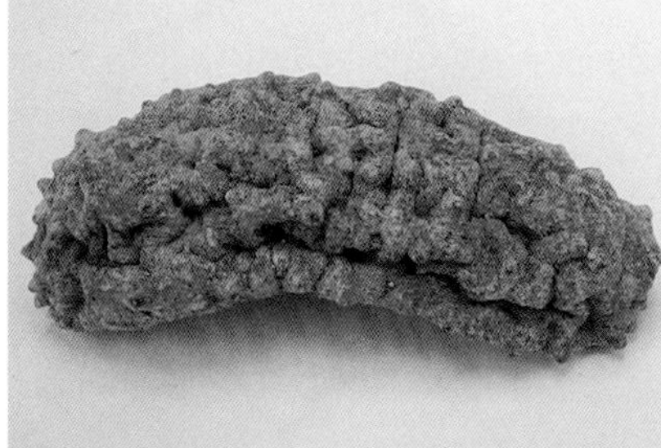
Hai Shen (Strichopus Japonicus)

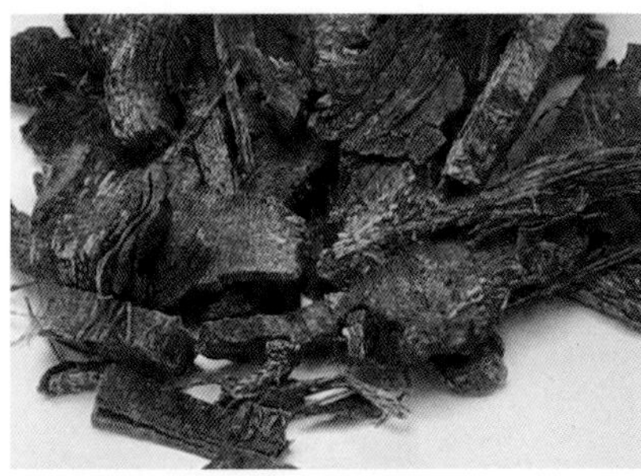
Hai Tong Pi (Cortex Erythrinae)

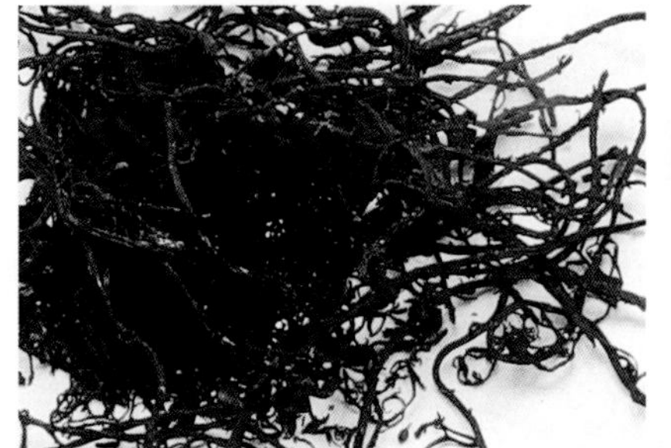
Hai Zao (Sargassum)

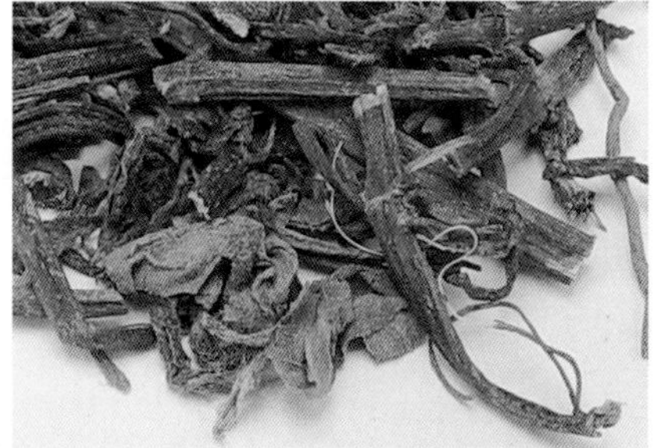
Han Lian Cao (Herba Ecliptae)

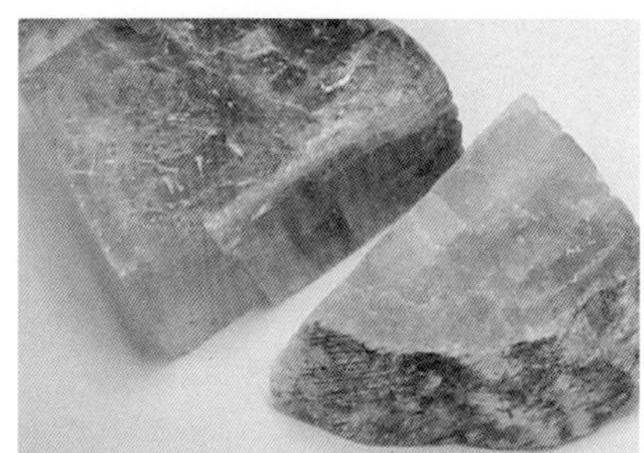
Han Shui Shi (Mirabilite)

Herb Indentification Guide

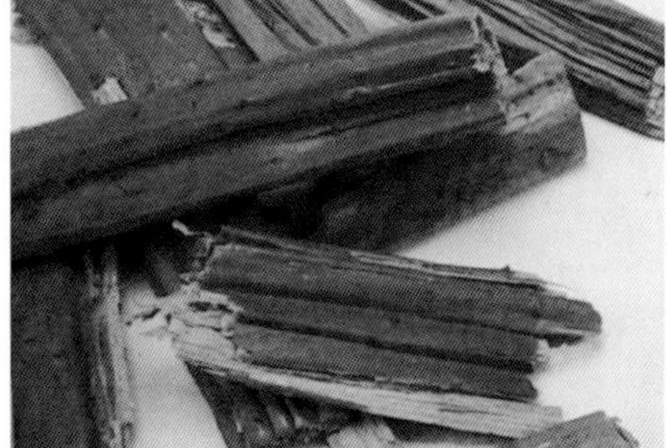
He Geng (Caulis Nelumbinis)

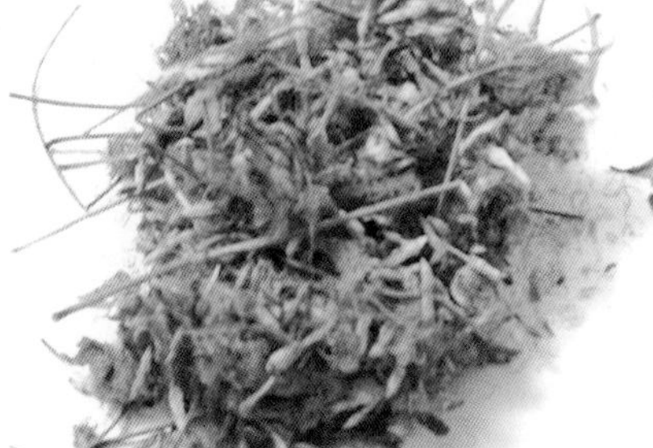
He Huan Hua (Flos Albiziae)

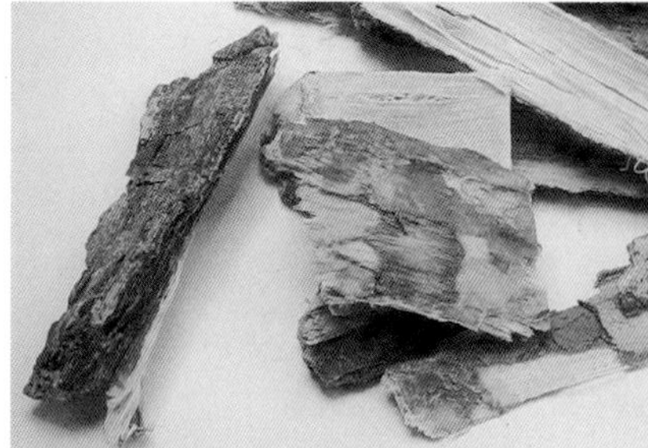
He Huan Pi (Cortex Albiziae)

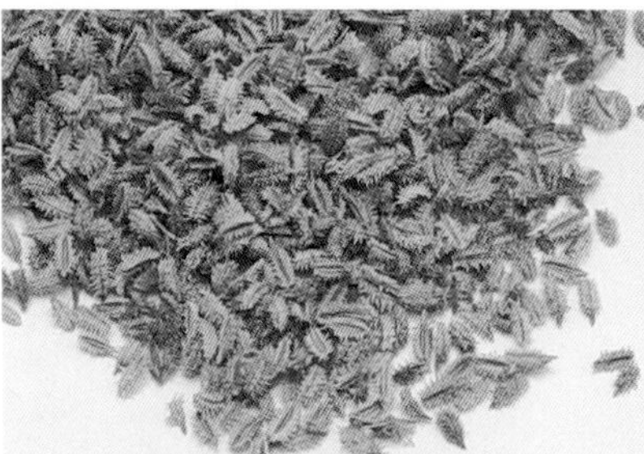
He Shi (Fructus Carpesii)

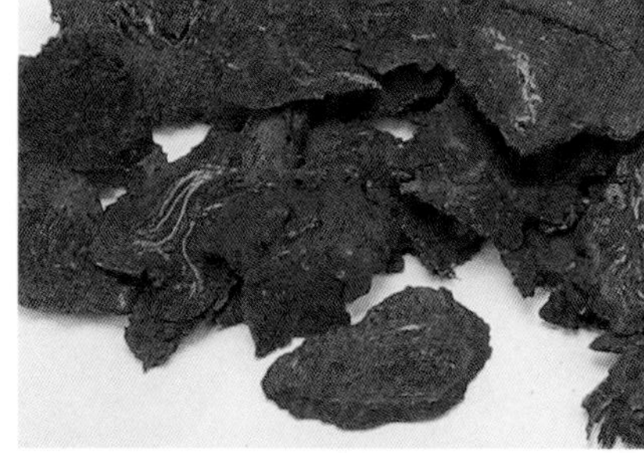
He Shou Wu (Radix Polygoni Multiflori)

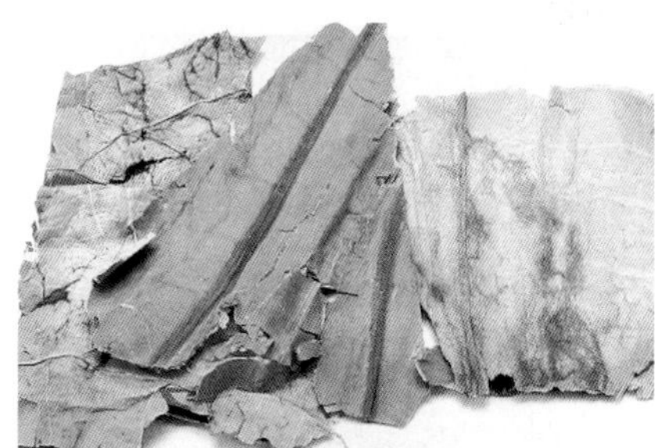
He Ye (Folium Nelumbinis)

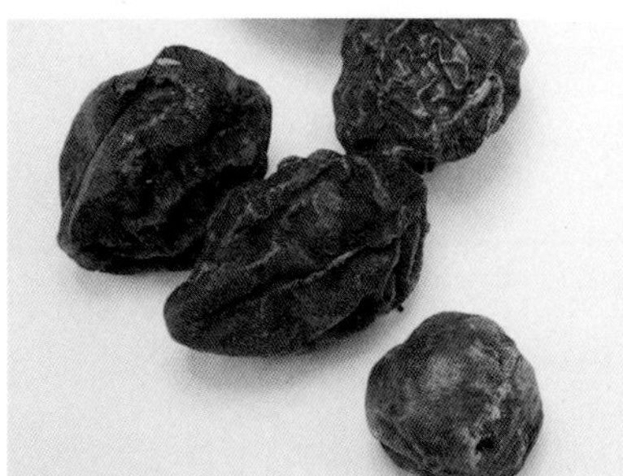
He Zi (Fructus Chebulae)

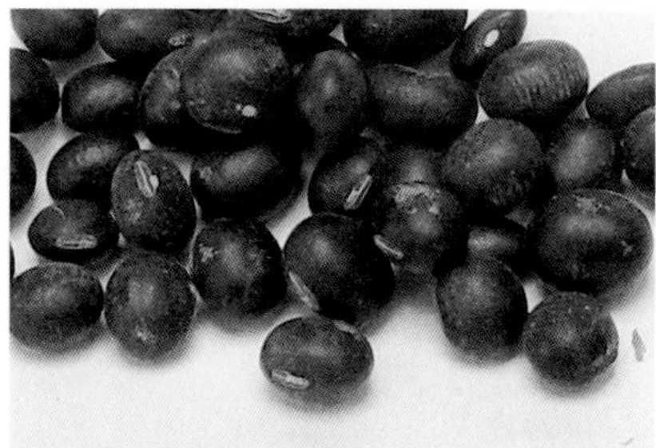
Hei Dou (Semen Glycine Max)

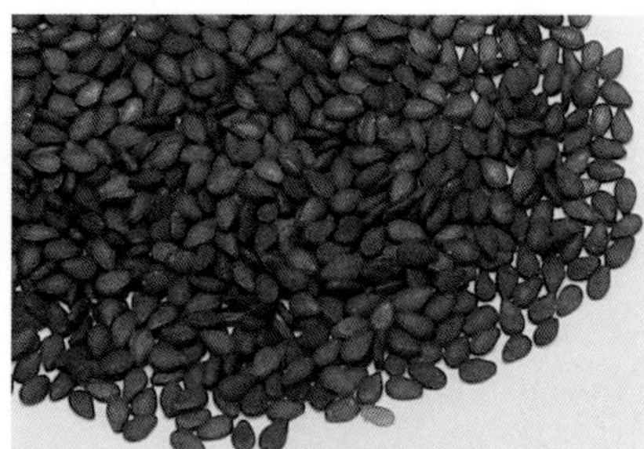
Hei Zhi Ma (Semen Sesami Nigrum)

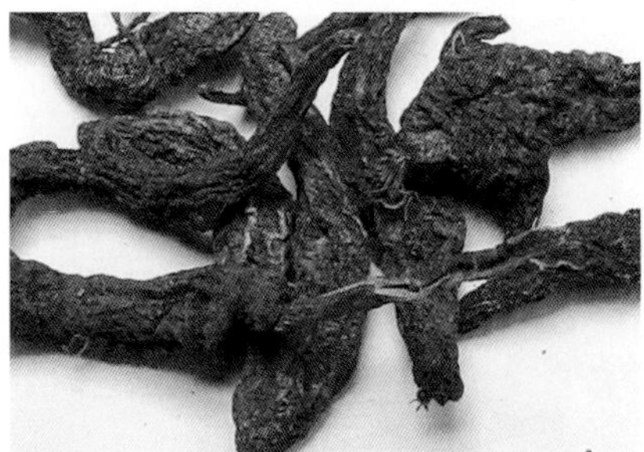
Hong Da Ji (Radix Knoxiae)

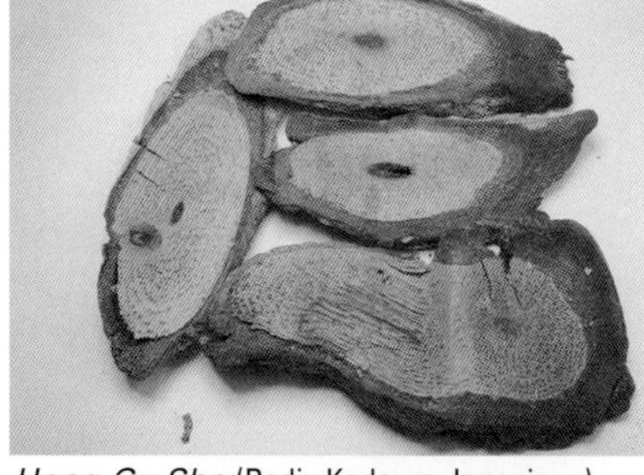
Hong Gu She (Radix Kadsura Japonicae)

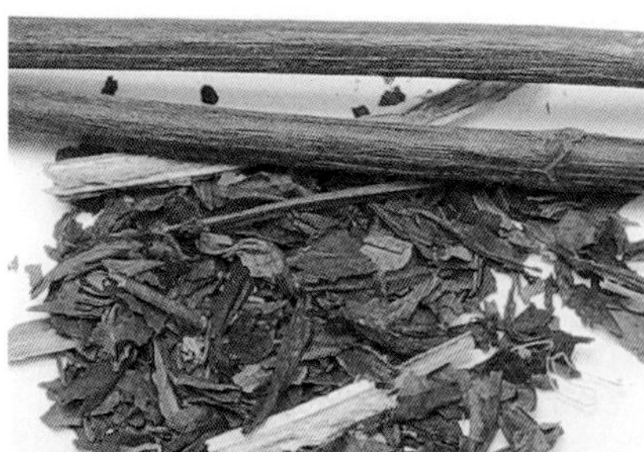
Hong Han Lian (Herba Hypericum Ascyron)

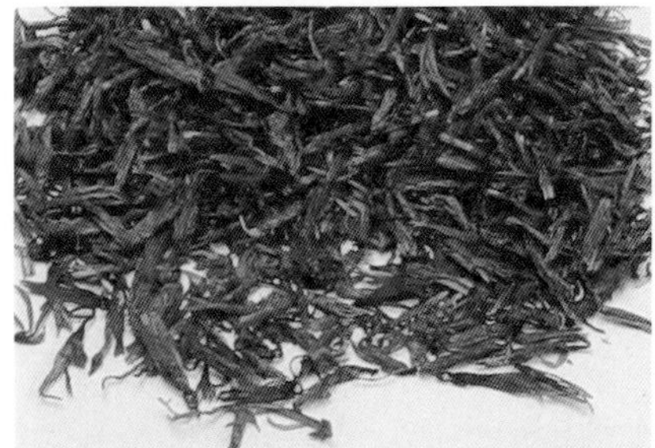
Hong Hua (Flos Carthami)

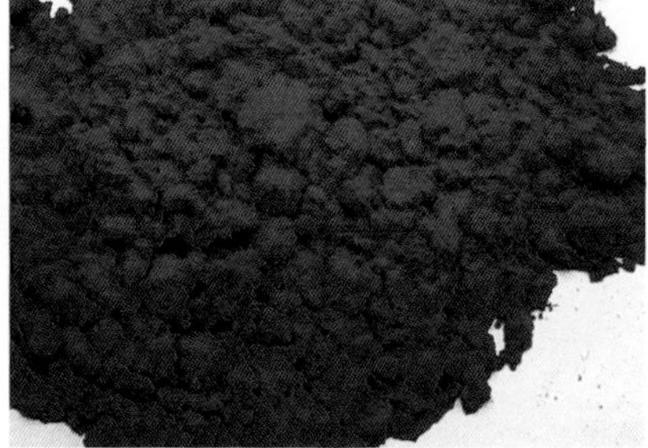
Hong Qu (Monascus)

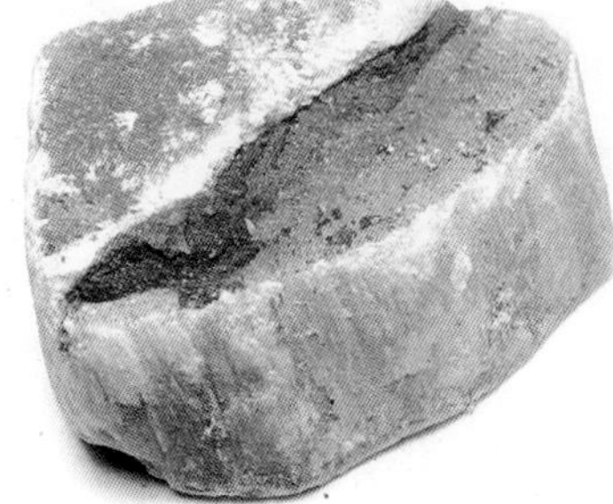
Hong Shi Gao (Gypsum Rubrae)

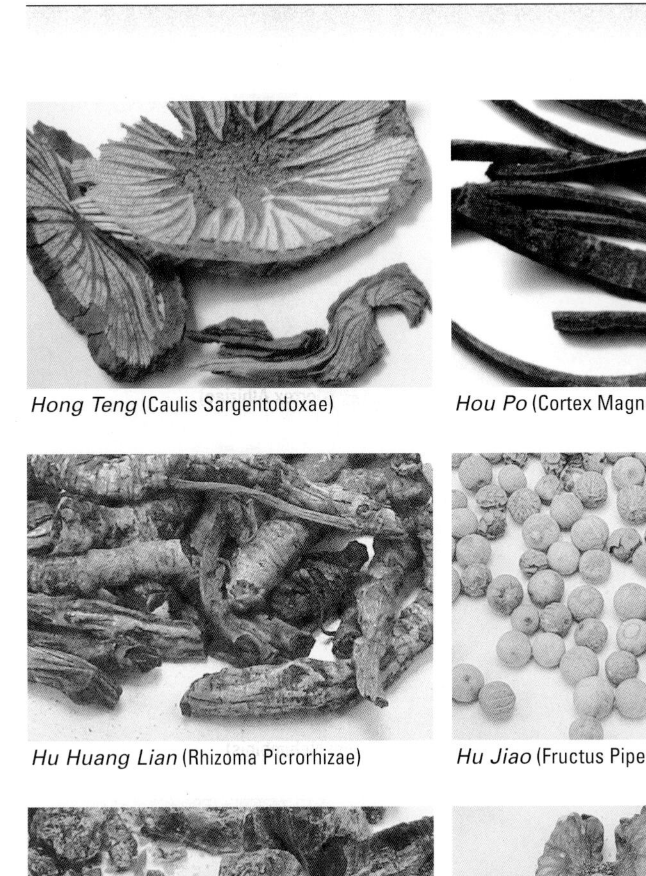

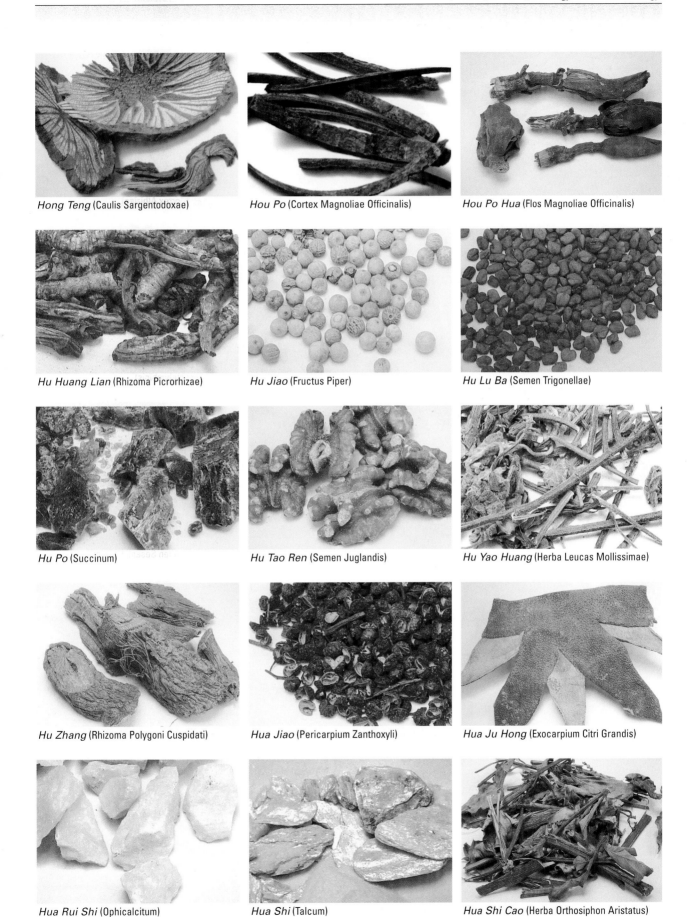

Hong Teng (Caulis Sargentodoxae)

Hou Po (Cortex Magnoliae Officinalis)

Hou Po Hua (Flos Magnoliae Officinalis)

Hu Huang Lian (Rhizoma Picrorhizae)

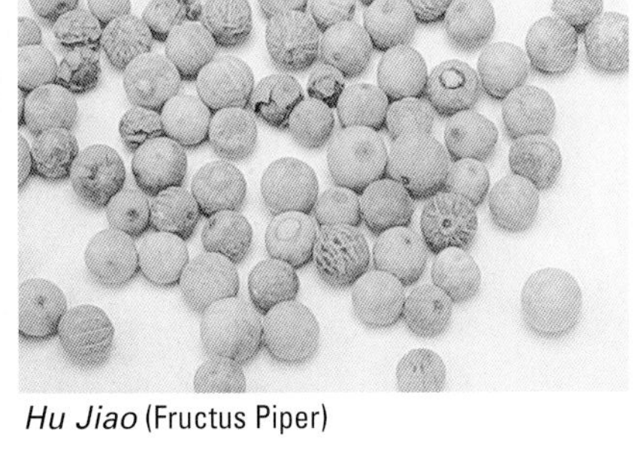

Hu Jiao (Fructus Piper)

Hu Lu Ba (Semen Trigonellae)

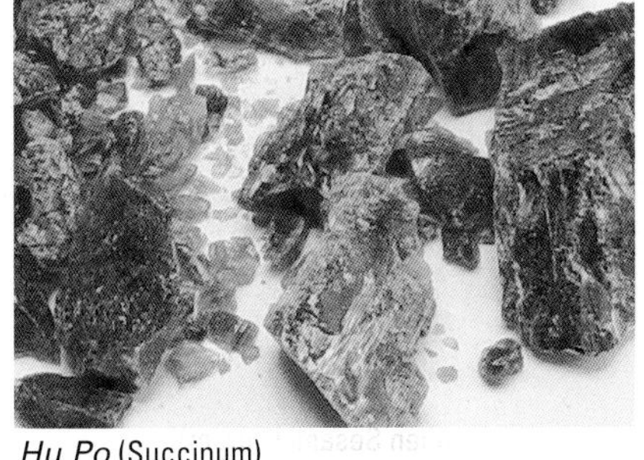

Hu Po (Succinum)

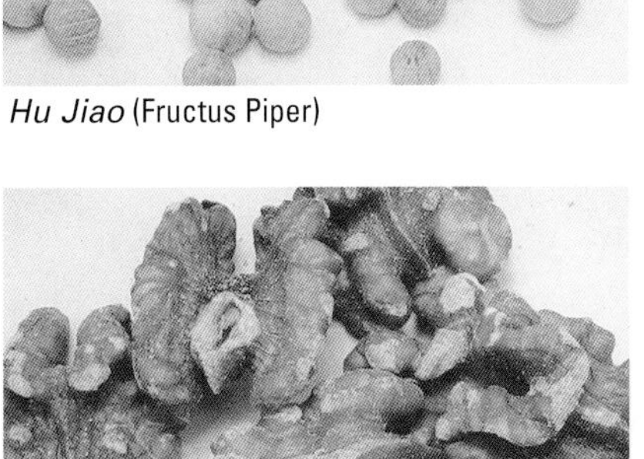

Hu Tao Ren (Semen Juglandis)

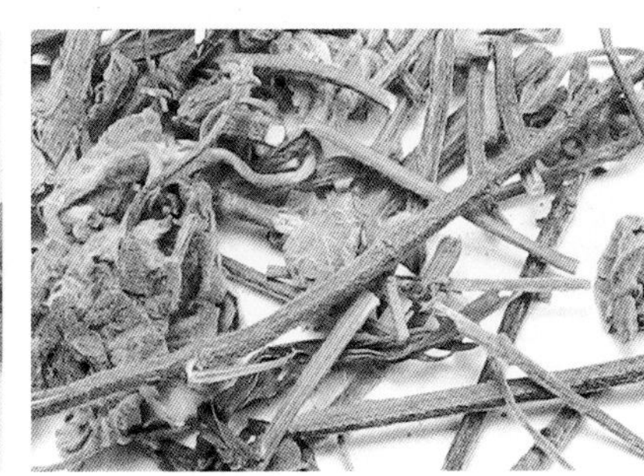

Hu Yao Huang (Herba Leucas Mollissimae)

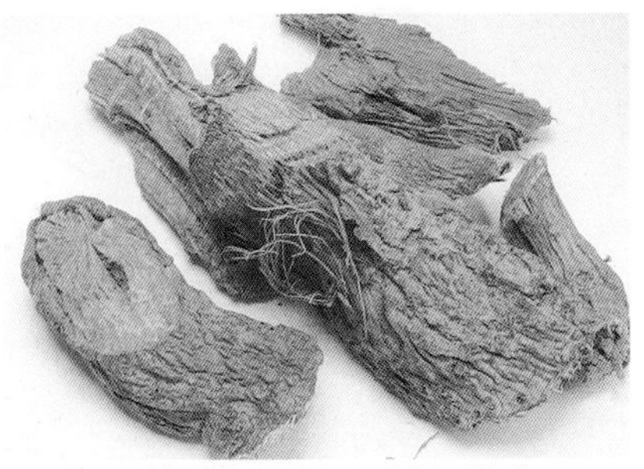

Hu Zhang (Rhizoma Polygoni Cuspidati)

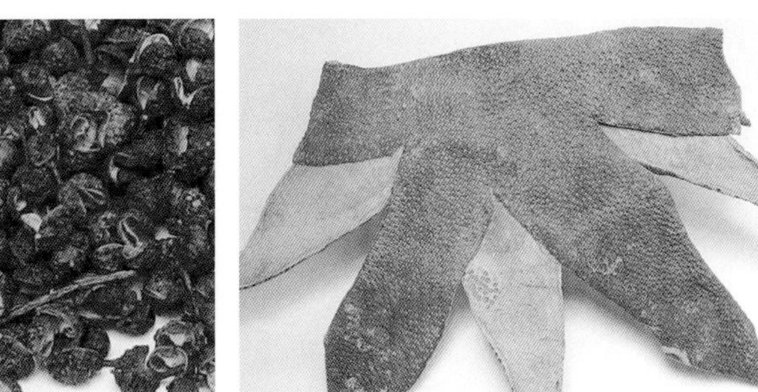

Hua Jiao (Pericarpium Zanthoxyli)

Hua Ju Hong (Exocarpium Citri Grandis)

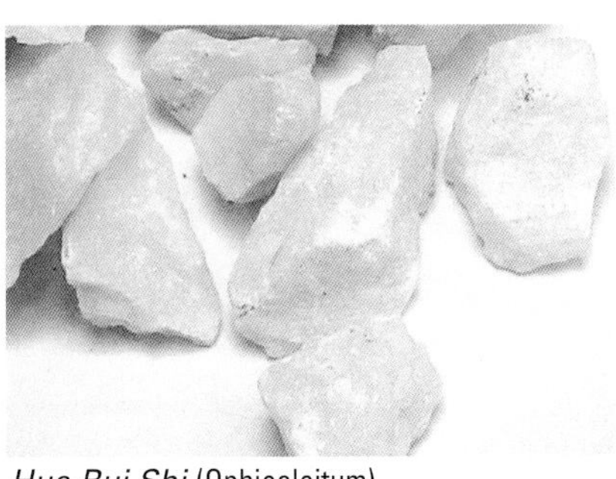

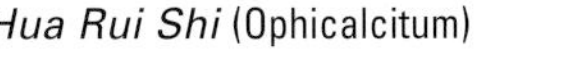

Hua Rui Shi (Ophicalcitum)

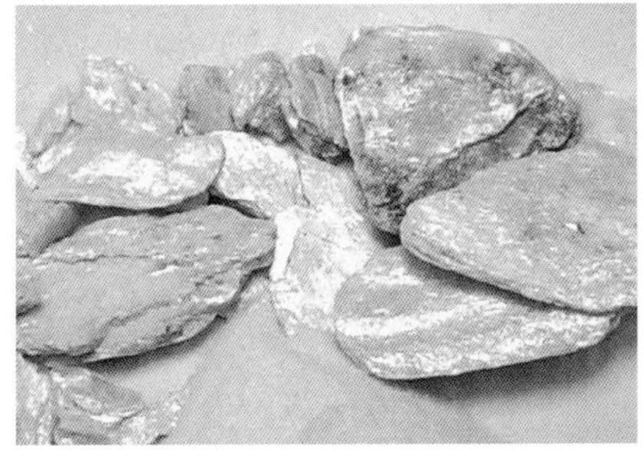

Hua Shi (Talcum)

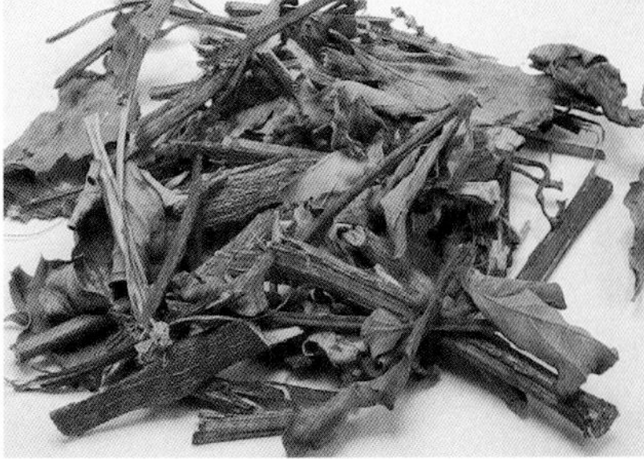

Hua Shi Cao (Herba Orthosiphon Aristatus)

Herb Indentification Guide

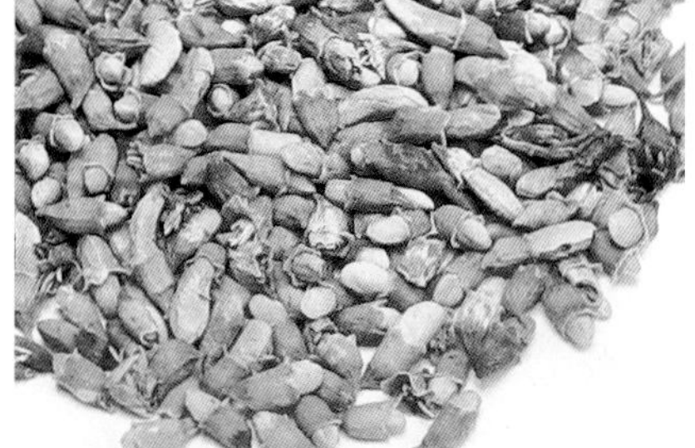
Huai Hua (Flos Sophorae)

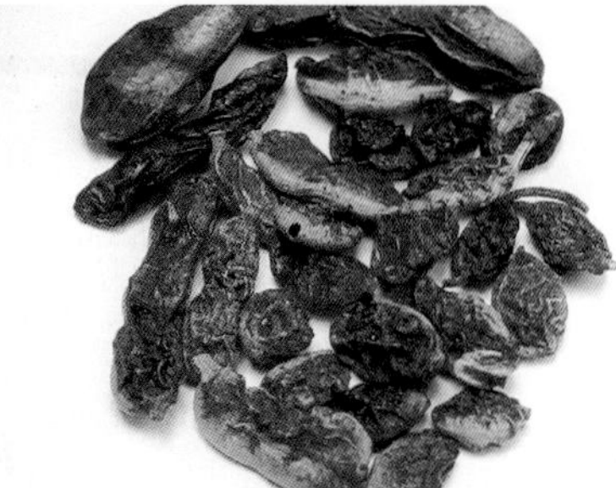
Huai Jiao (Fructus Sophorae)

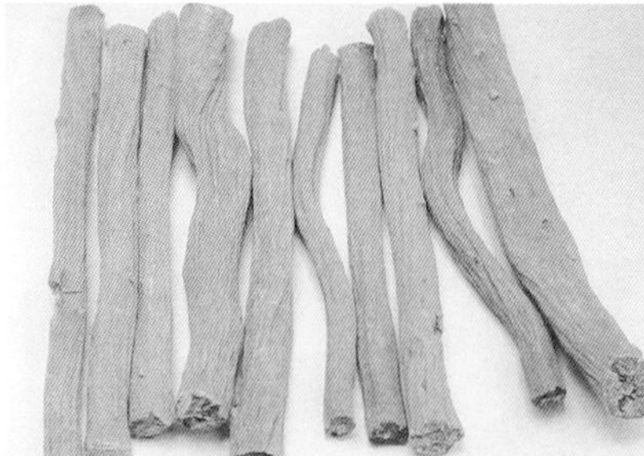
Huai Niu Xi (Radix Achyranthis Bidentatae)

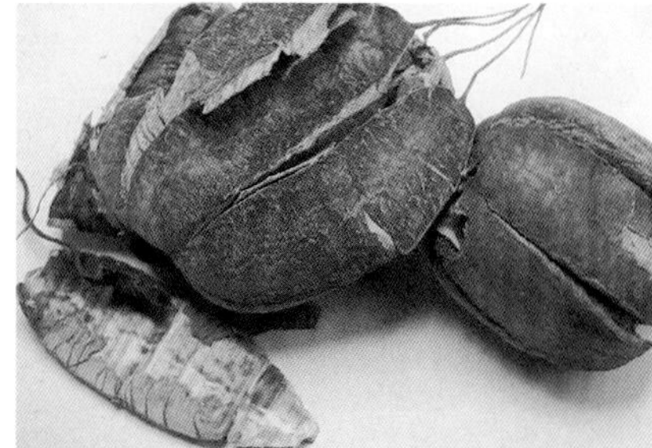
Huai Tong Ma Dou Ling (Caulis Aristolochiae Moupinensis)

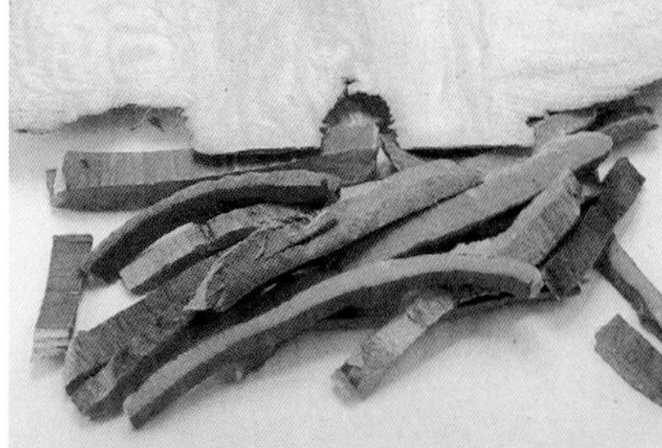
Huang Bai (Cortex Phellodendri)

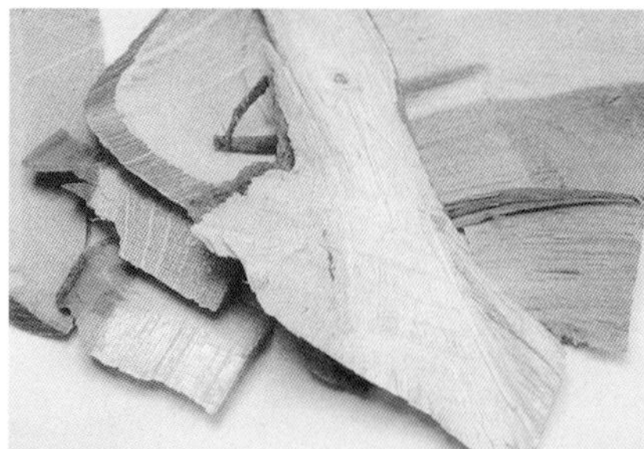
Huang Jin Gui (Caulis Vanieriae)

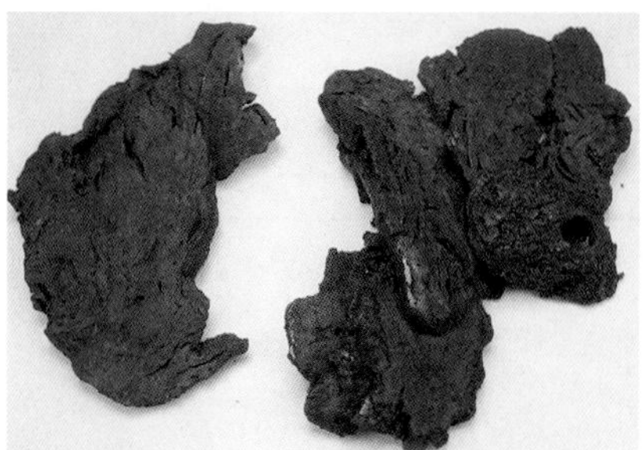
Huang Jing (Rhizoma Polygonati)

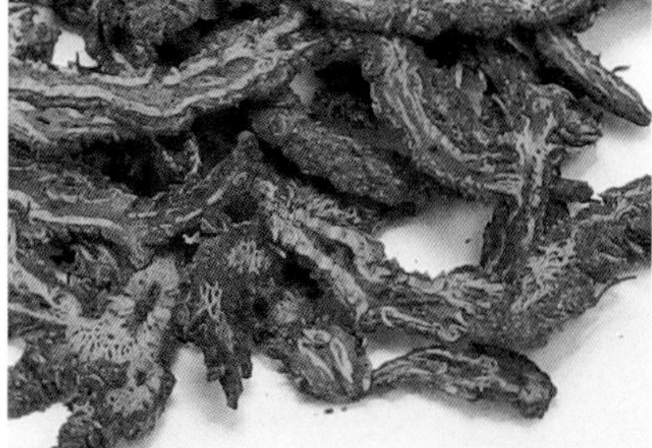
Huang Lian (Rhizoma Coptidis)

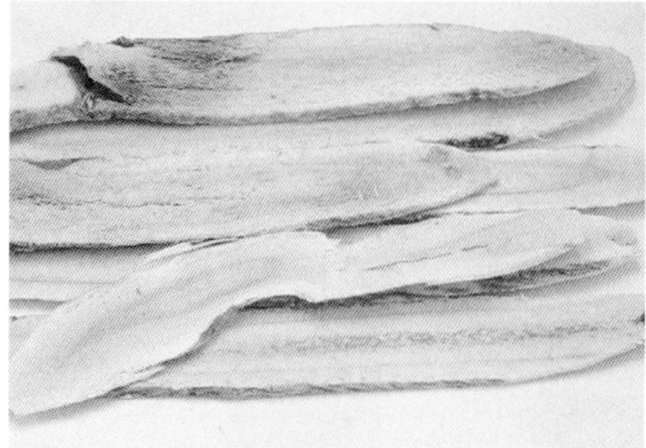
Huang Qi (Radix Astragali)

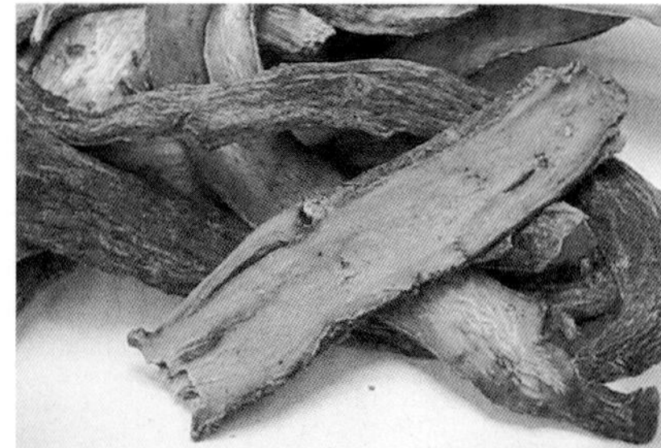
Huang Qin (Radix Scutellariae)

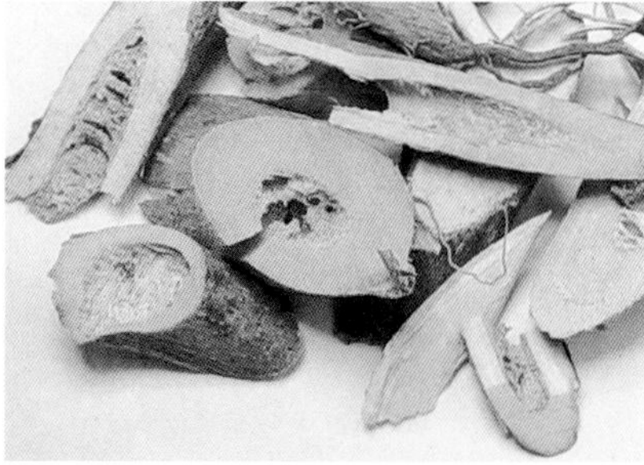
Huang Shui Qie (Herba Solani)

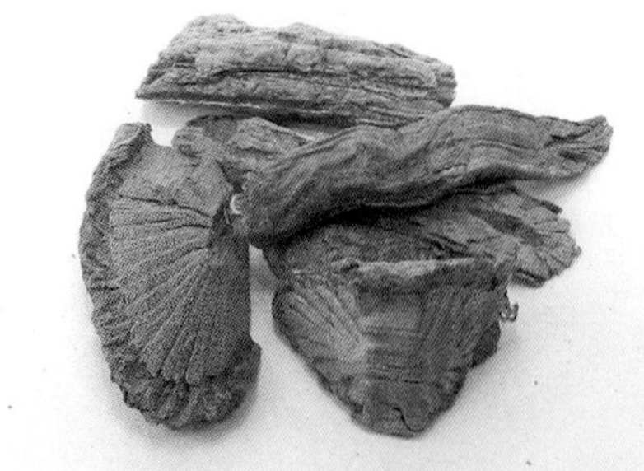
Huang Teng (Caulis Fibraurea)

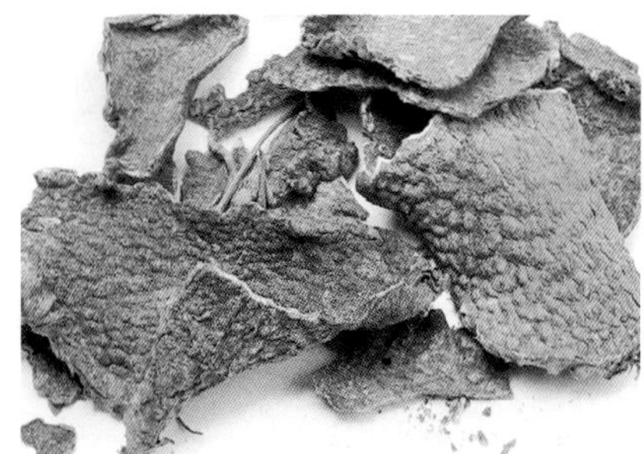
Huang Yao Zi (Herba Dioscoreae Bulbiferae)

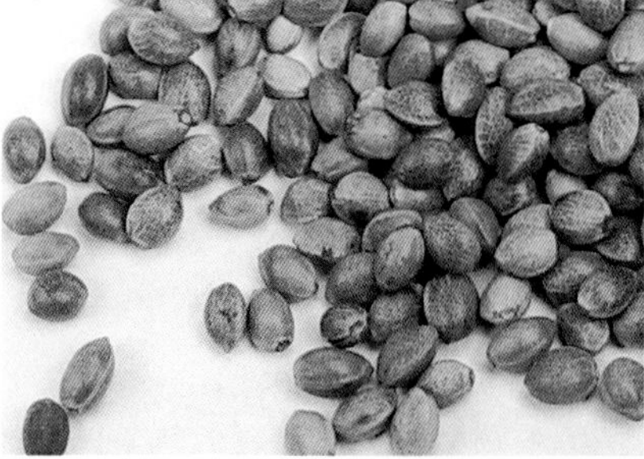
Huo Ma Ren (Fructus Cannabis)

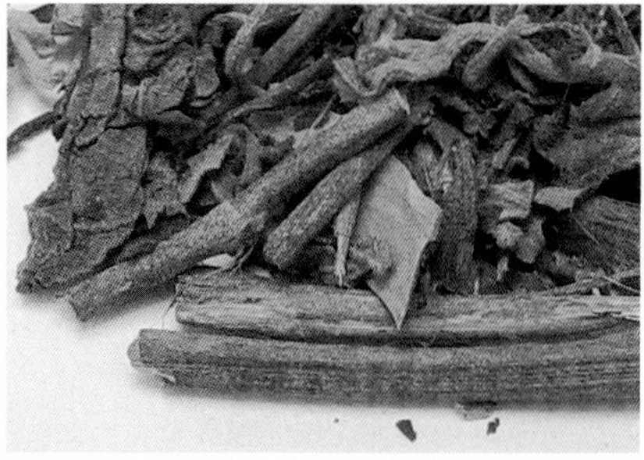
Huo Xiang (Herba Agastache)

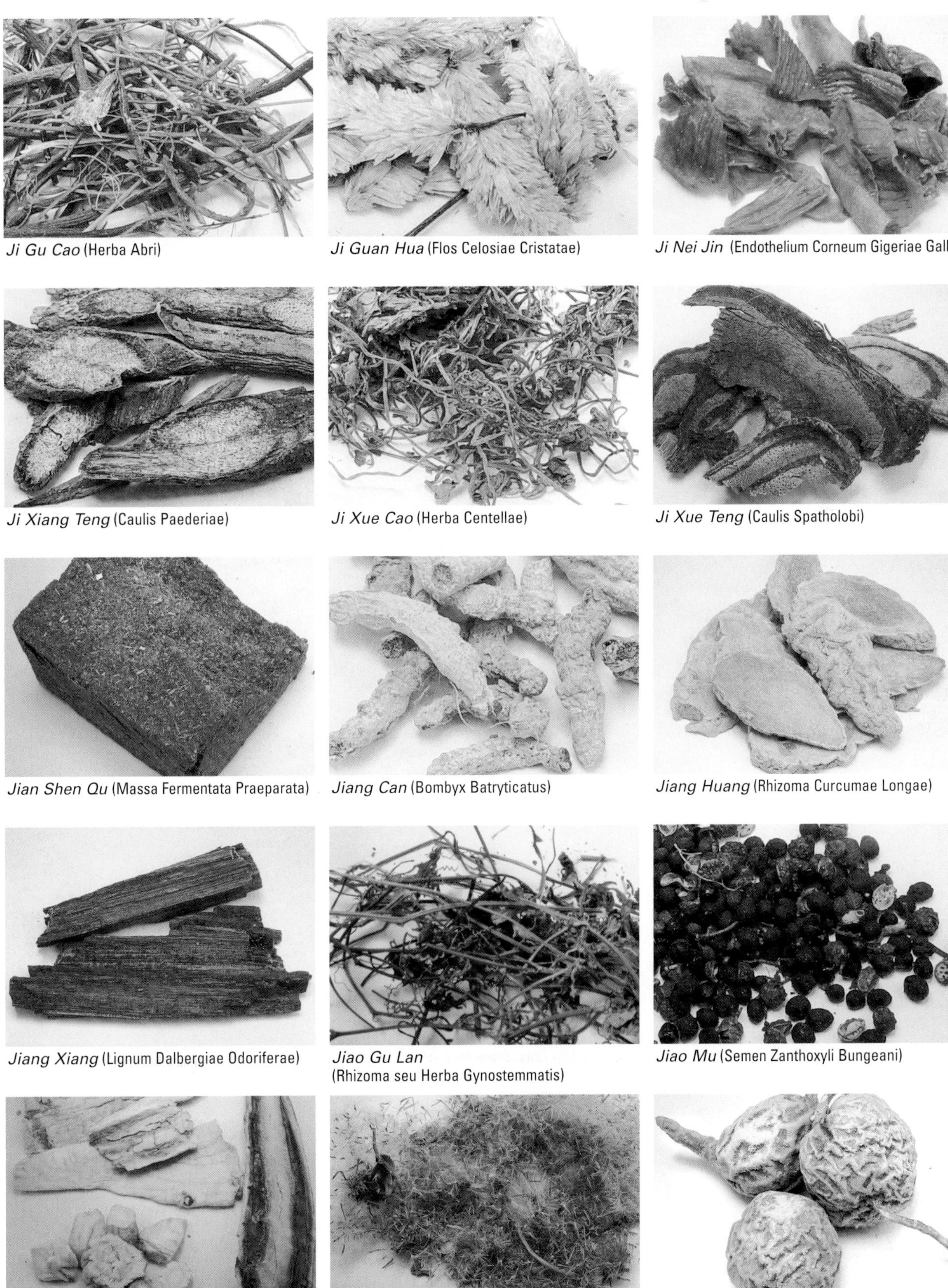

Ji Gu Cao (Herba Abri)

Ji Guan Hua (Flos Celosiae Cristatae)

Ji Nei Jin (Endothelium Corneum Gigeriae Galli)

Ji Xiang Teng (Caulis Paederiae)

Ji Xue Cao (Herba Centellae)

Ji Xue Teng (Caulis Spatholobi)

Jian Shen Qu (Massa Fermentata Praeparata)

Jiang Can (Bombyx Batryticatus)

Jiang Huang (Rhizoma Curcumae Longae)

Jiang Xiang (Lignum Dalbergiae Odoriferae)

Jiao Gu Lan (Rhizoma seu Herba Gynostemmatis)

Jiao Mu (Semen Zanthoxyli Bungeani)

Jie Geng (Radix Platycodonis)

Jin Fei Cao (Herba Inulae)

Jin Guo Lan (Radix Tinosporae)

Herb Indentification Guide

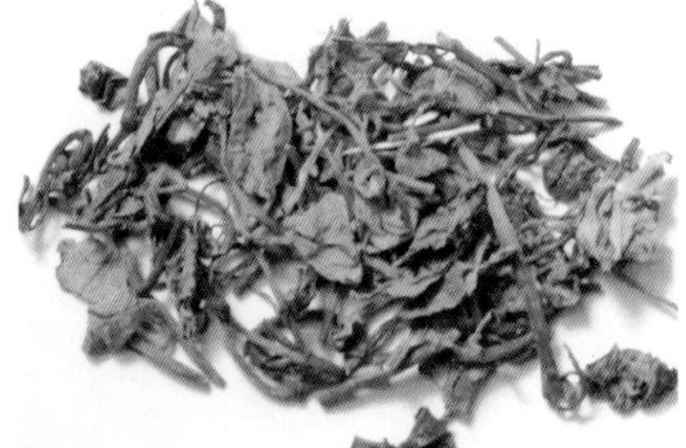
Jin Qian Cao (Herba Lysimachiae)

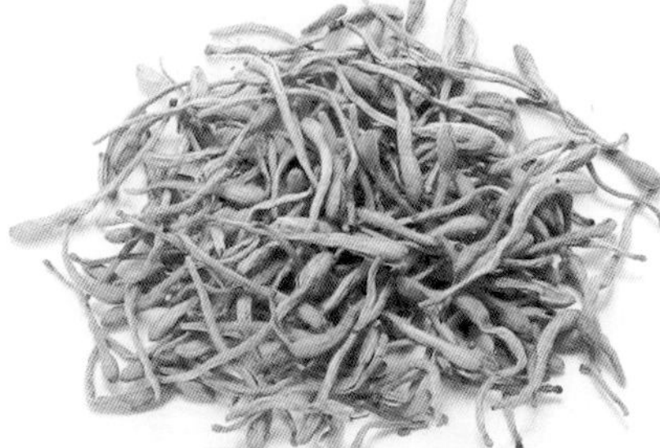
Jin Yin Hua (Flos Lonicerae)

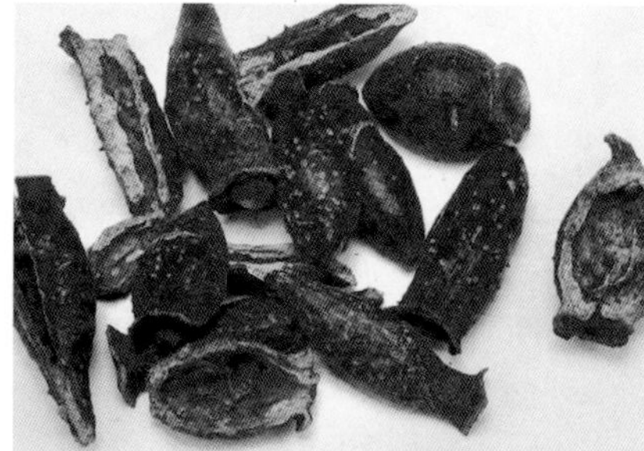
Jin Ying Zi (Fructus Rosae Laevigatae)

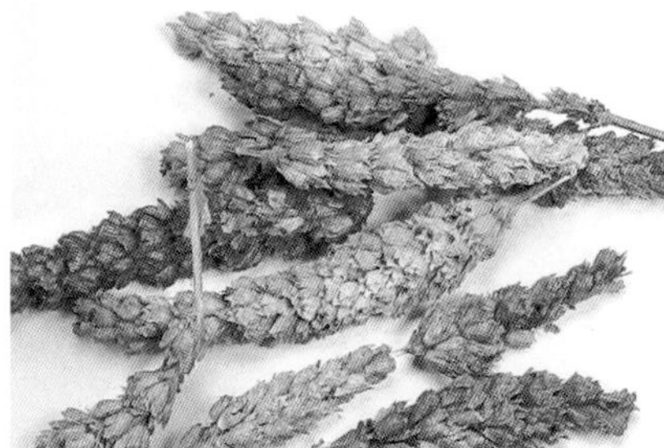
Jing Jie (Herba Schizonepetae)

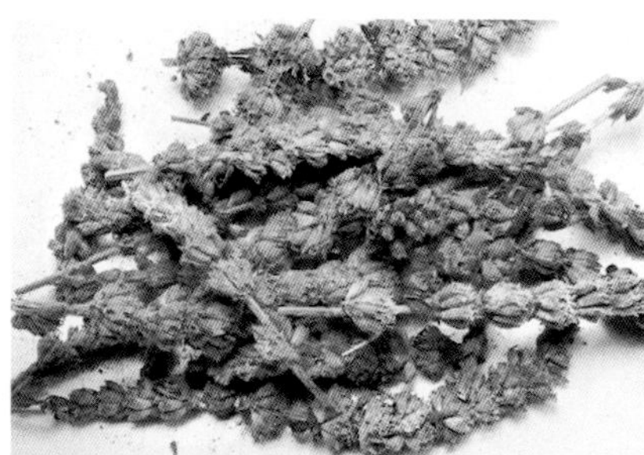
Jing Sui (Flos Schizonepetae)

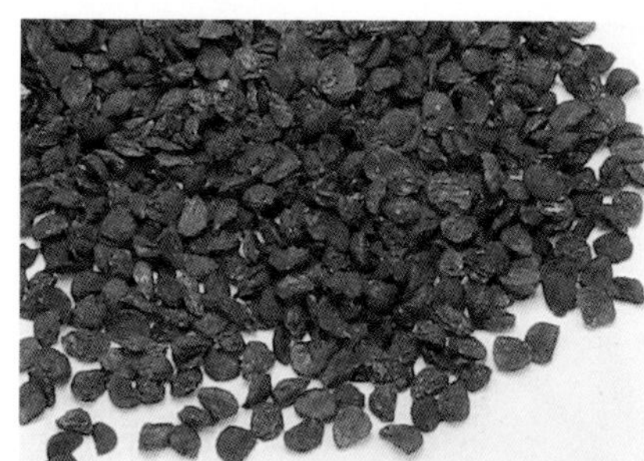
Jiu Cai Zi (Semen Allii Tuberosi)

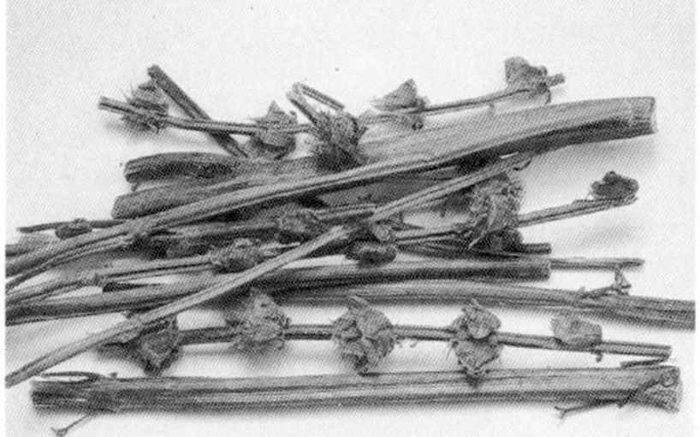
Jiu Ceng Ta (Herba Ocimi Basilici)

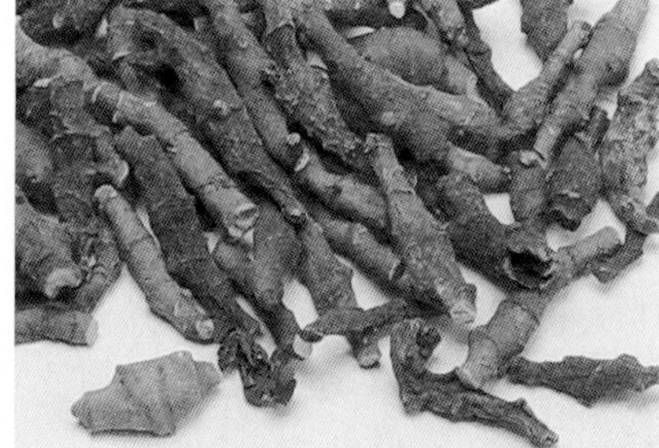
Jiu Jie Chang Pu (Rhizoma Anemones Altaicae)

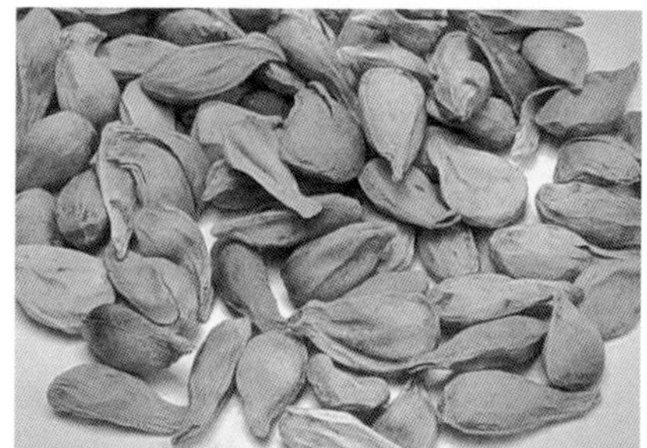
Ju He (Semen Citri Rubrum)

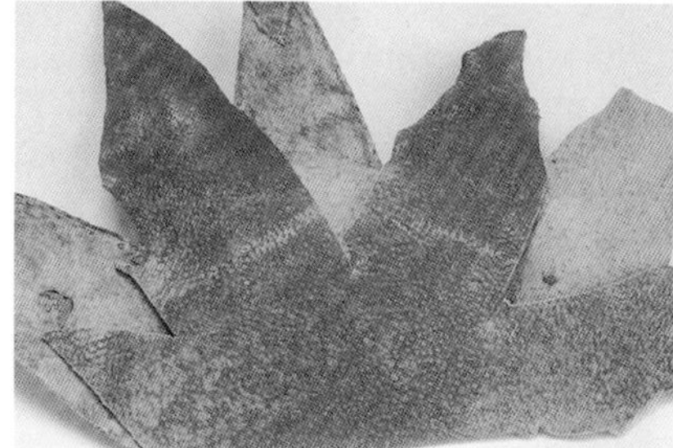
Ju Hong (Exocarpium Citri Rubrum)

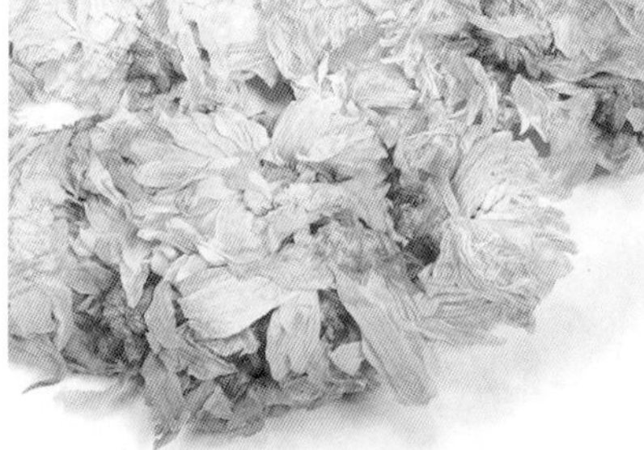
Ju Hua (Flos Chrysanthemi)

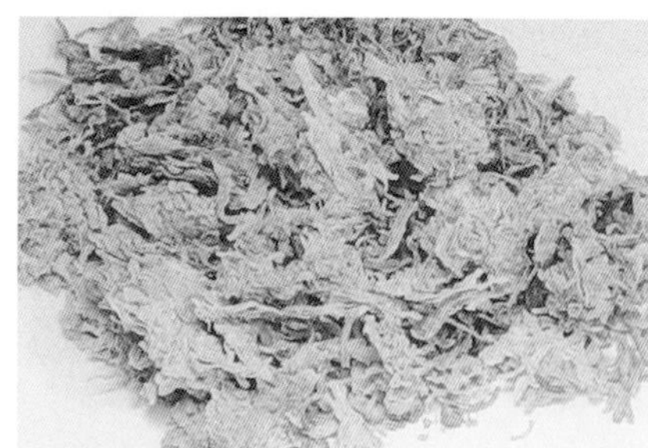
Ju Luo (Fibra Citri Rubrum)

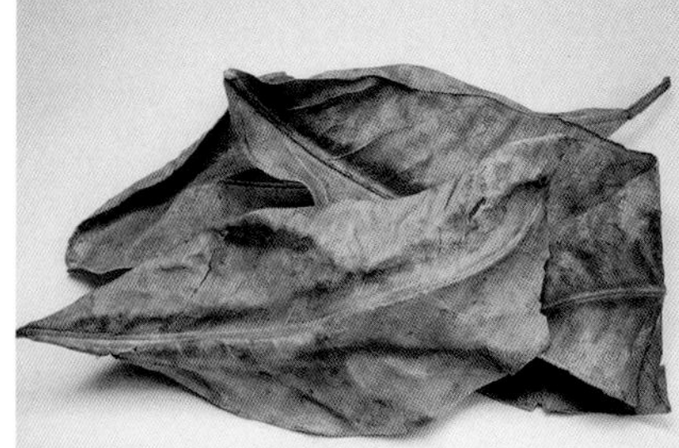
Ju Ye (Folium Citri Rubrum)

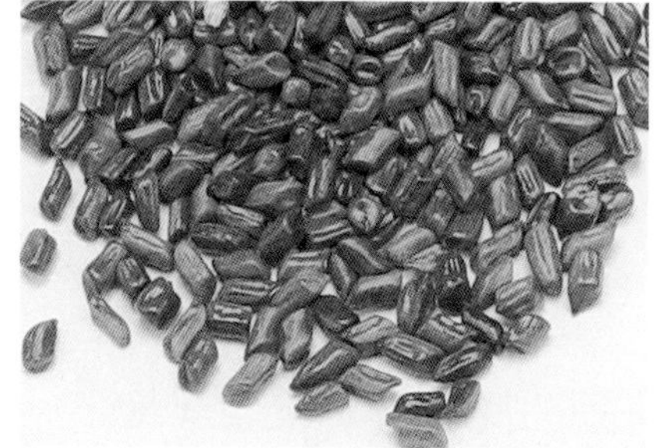
Jue Ming Zi (Semen Cassiae)

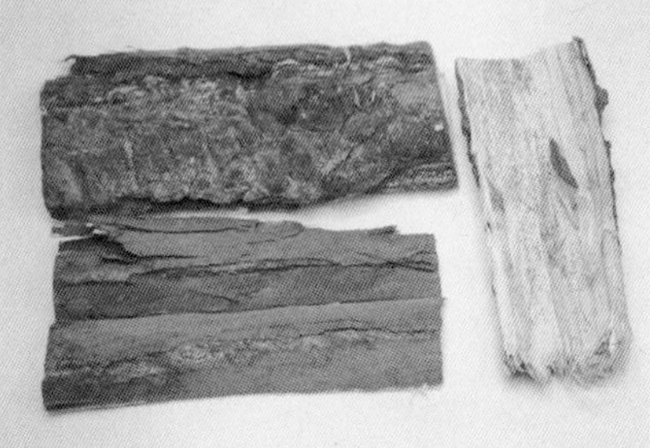
Ku Lian Pi (Cortex Meliae)

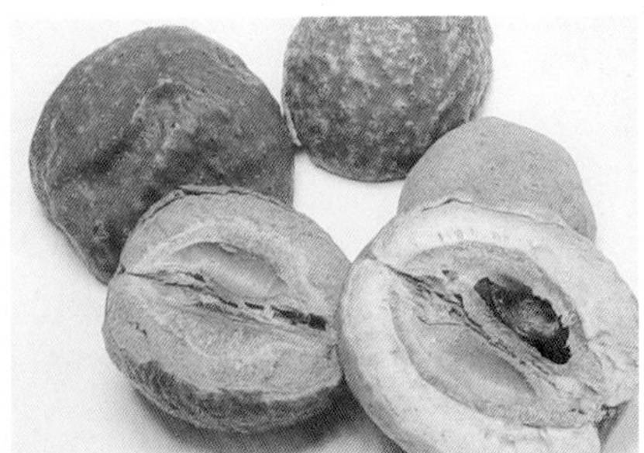
Ku Lian Zi (Fructus Meliae)

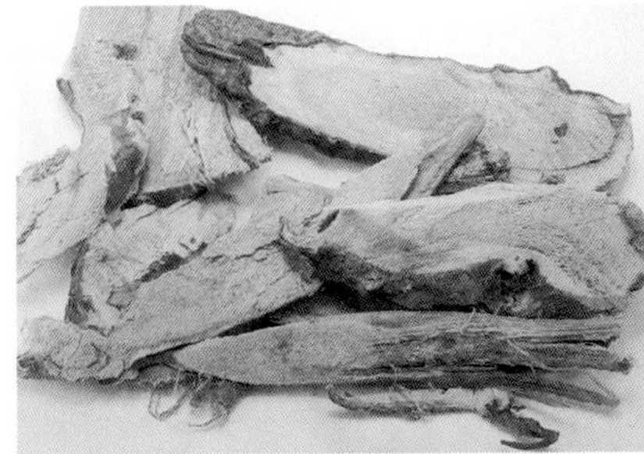
Ku Shen Gen (Radix Sophorae Flavescentis)

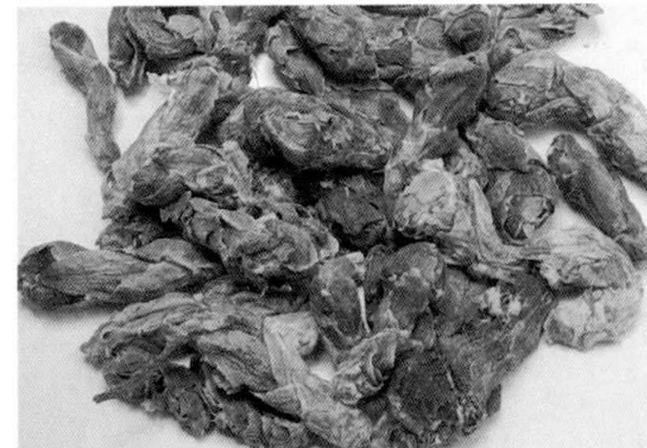
Kuan Dong Hua (Flos Farfarae)

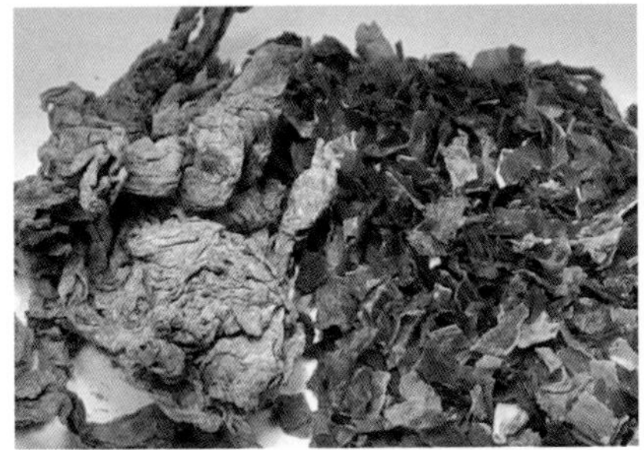
Kun Bu (Thallus Laminariae seu Eckloniae)

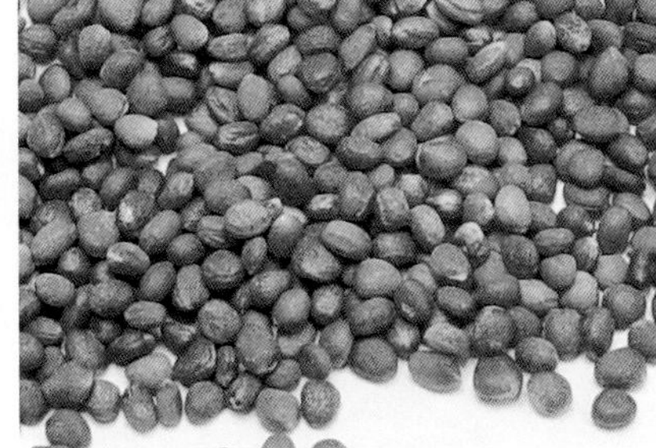
Lai Fu Zi (Semen Raphani)

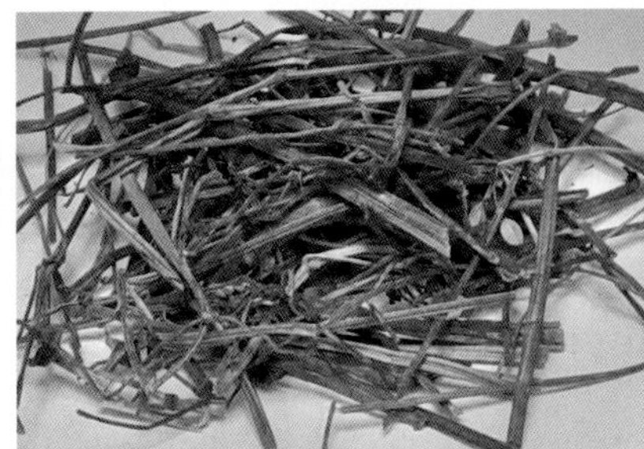
Lao Guan Cao (Herba Erodii seu Geranii)

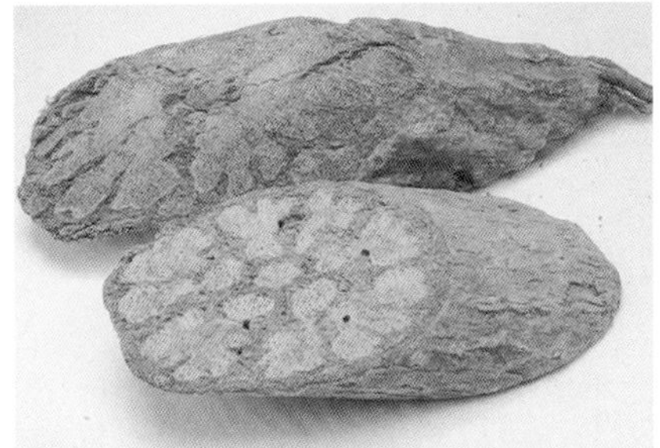
Lei Gong Teng (Radix Tripterygii Wilfordii)

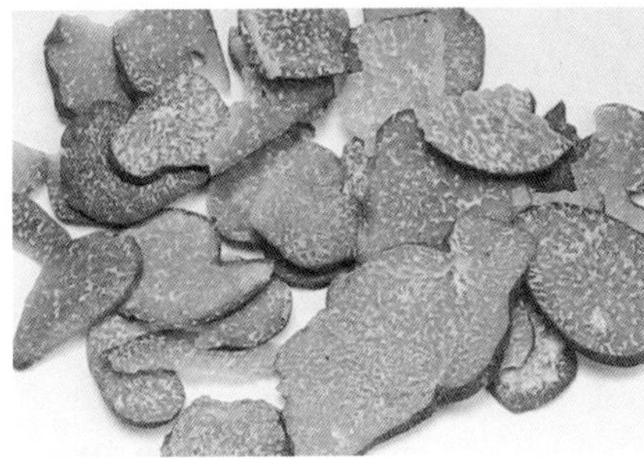
Lei Wan (Omphalia)

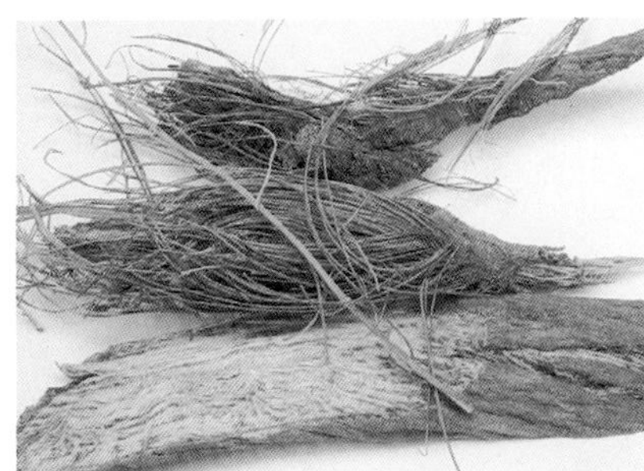
Li Lu (Radix et Rhizoma Veratri)

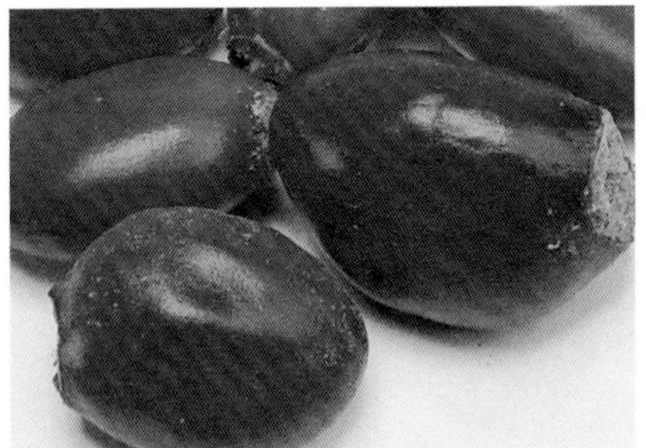
Li Zhi He (Semen Litchi)

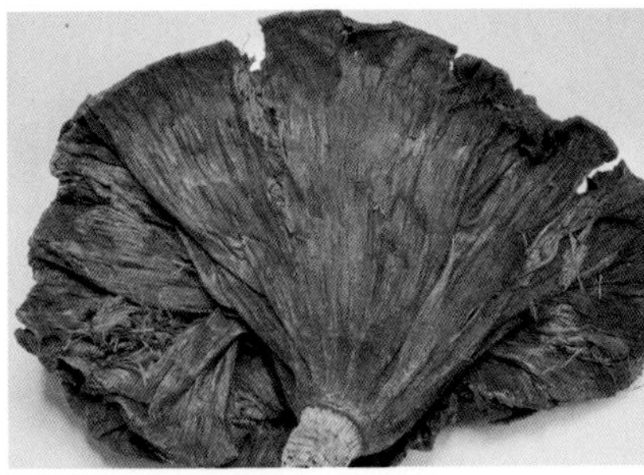
Lian Fang (Receptaculum Nelumbinis)

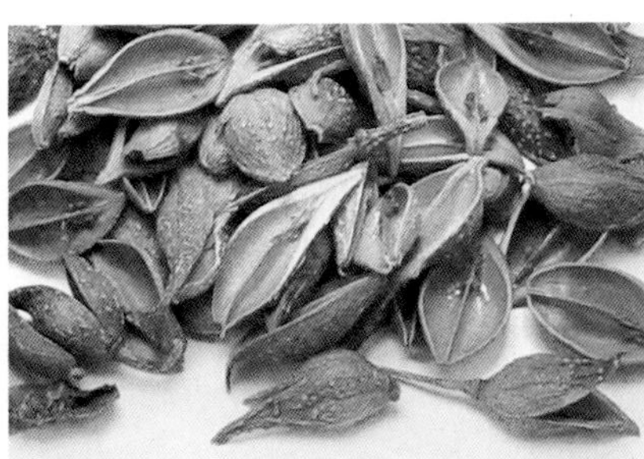
Lian Qiao (Fructus Forsythiae)

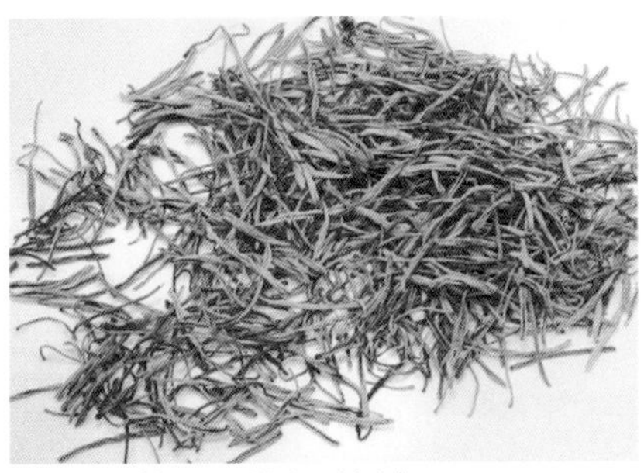
Lian Xu (Stamen Nelumbinis)

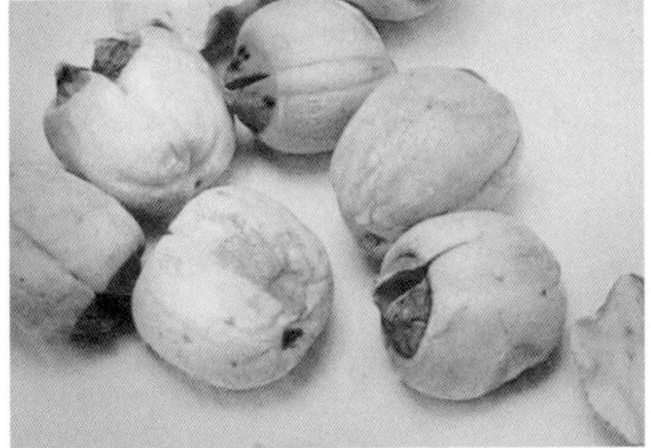
Lian Zi (Semen Nelumbinis)

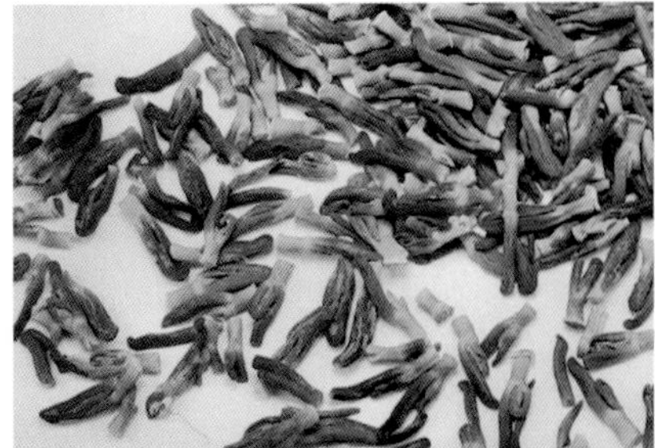
Lian Zi Xin (Plumula Nelumbinis)

Herb Indentification Guide

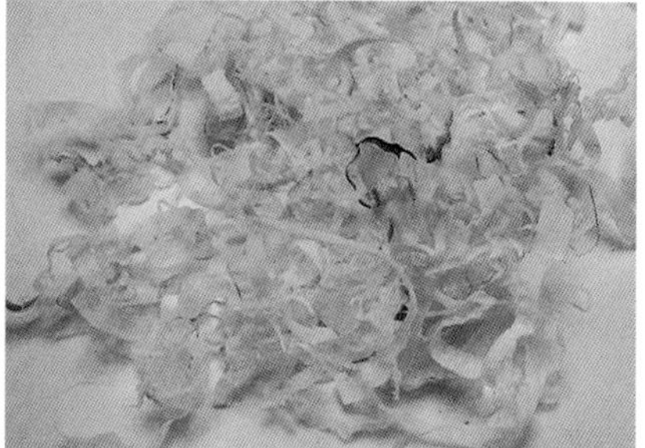
Ling Yang Jiao (Cornu Saigae Tataricae)

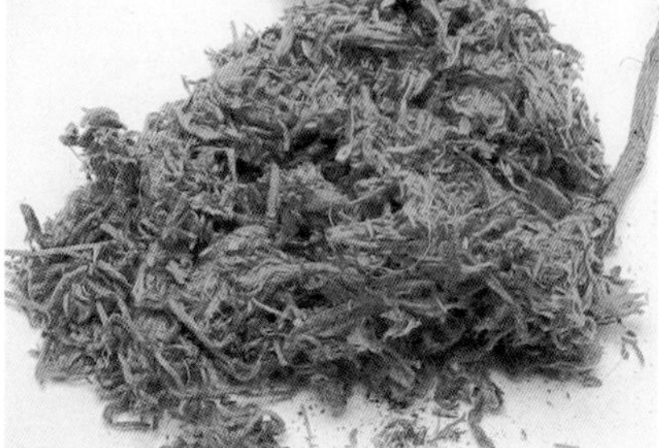
Ling Yin Chen (Herba Siphonostegia Chinensis)

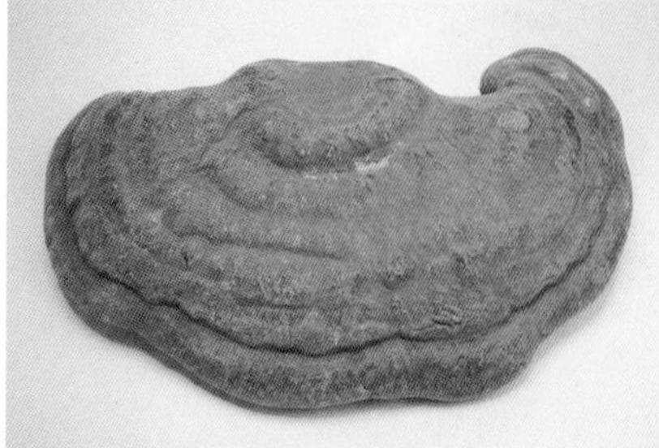
Ling Zhi (Ganoderma)

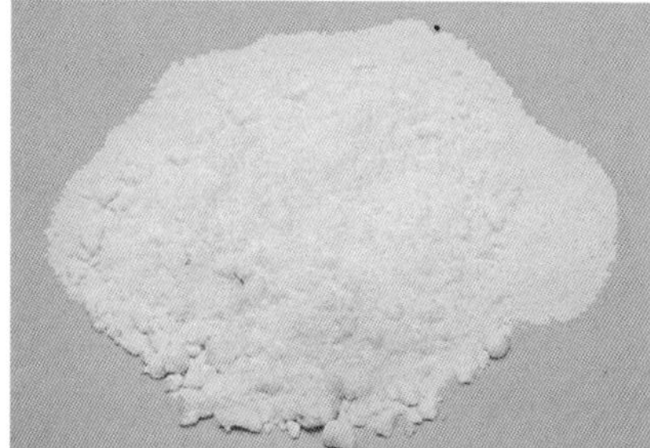
Liu Huang (Sulfur)

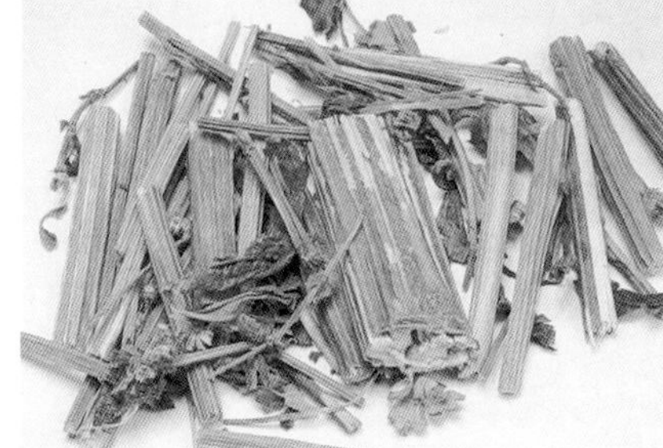
Liu Ji Nu (Herba Artemisiae Anomalae)

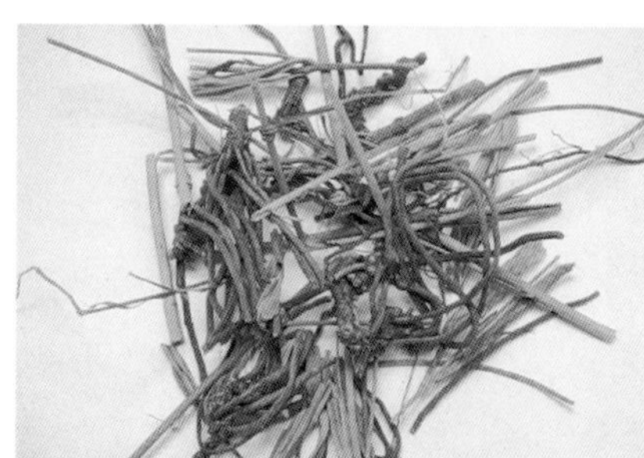
Liu Zhi Huang (Herba Solidaginis)

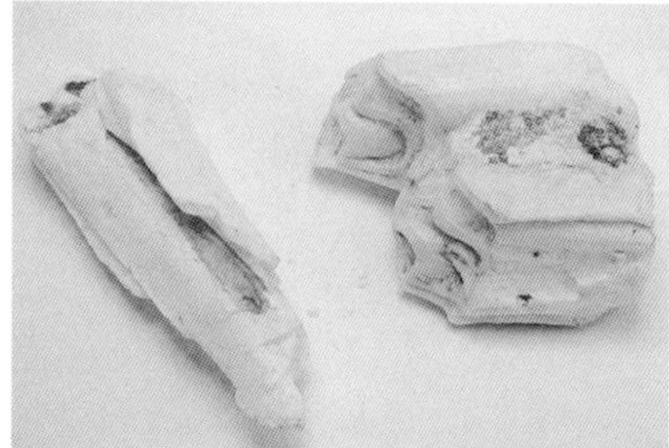
Long Chi (Dens Draconis)

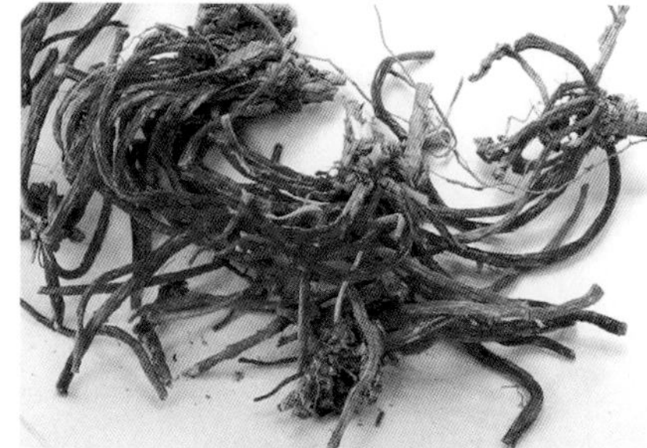
Long Dan Cao (Radix Gentianae)

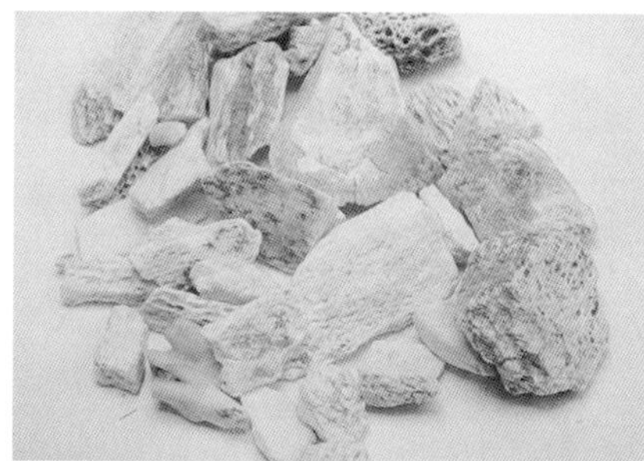
Long Gu (Os Draconis)

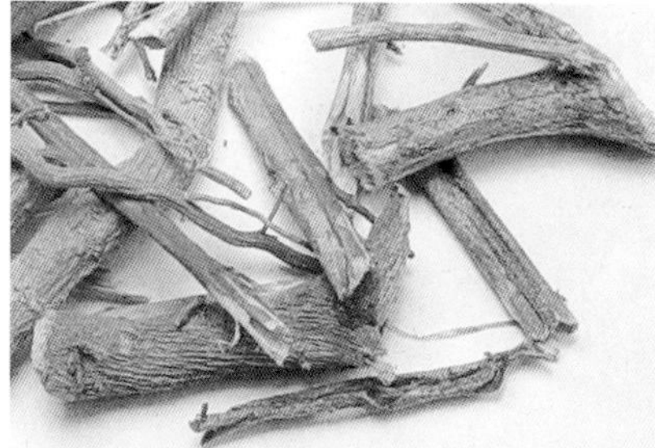
Long Kui (Herba Solanum Nigrum)

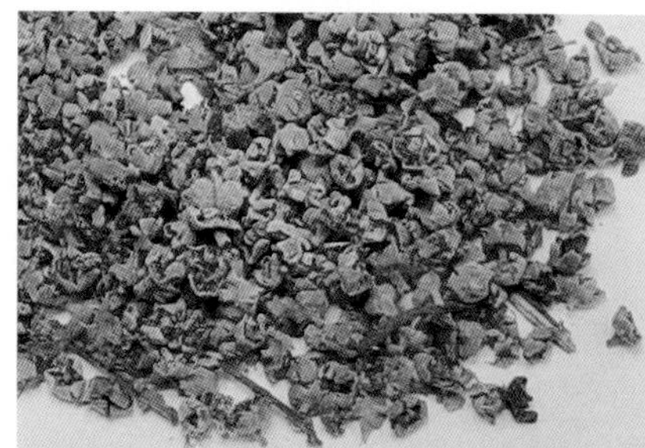
Long Yan Hua (Flos Longan)

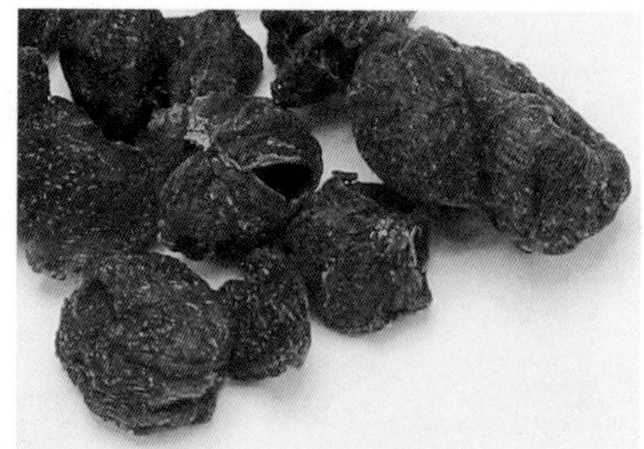
Long Yan Rou (Arillus Longan)

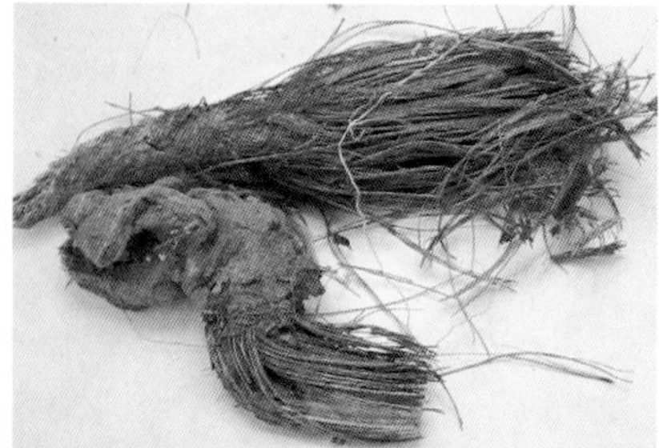
Lou Lu (Radix Rhapontici)

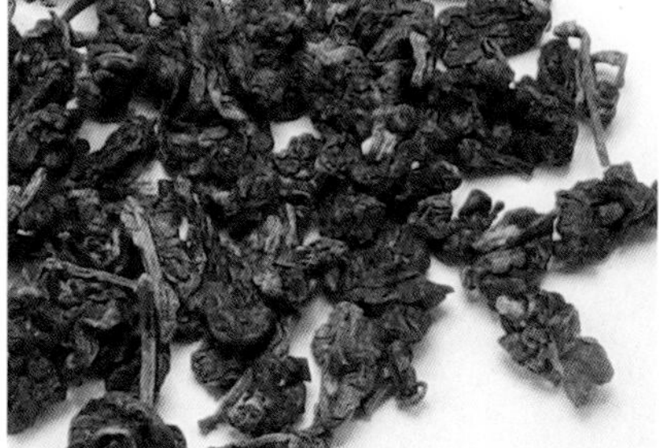
Lu Cha (Folium Camellia Sinensis)

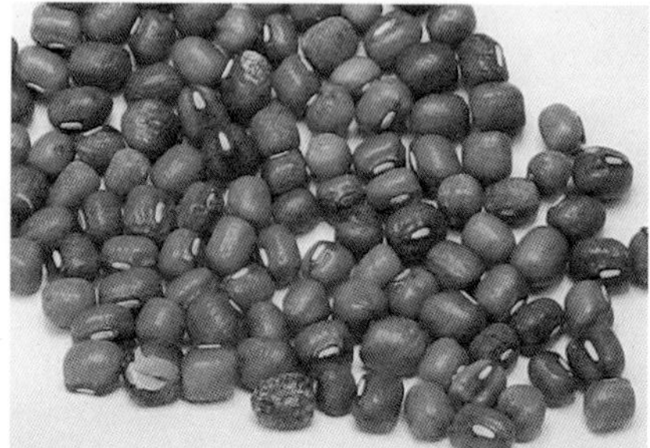
Lu Dou (Semen Phaseoli Radiati)

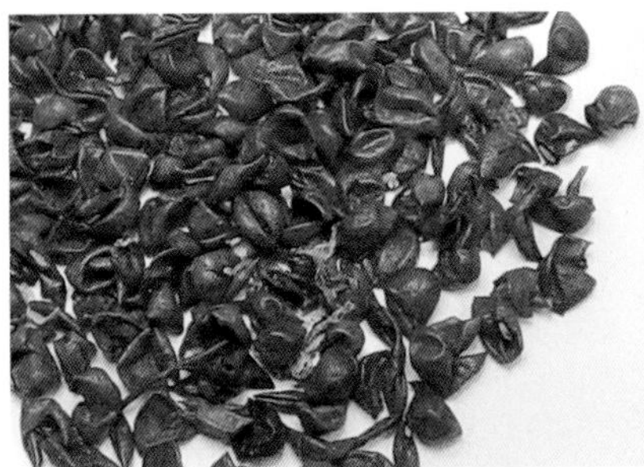
Lu Dou Yi (Pericarpium Phaseoli Radiati)

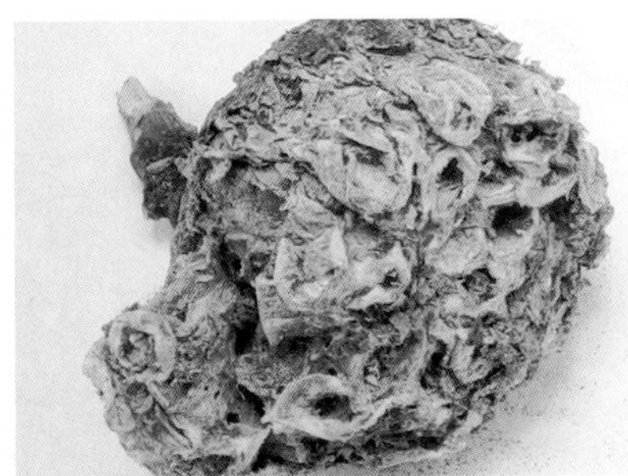
Lu Feng Fang (Nidus Vespae)

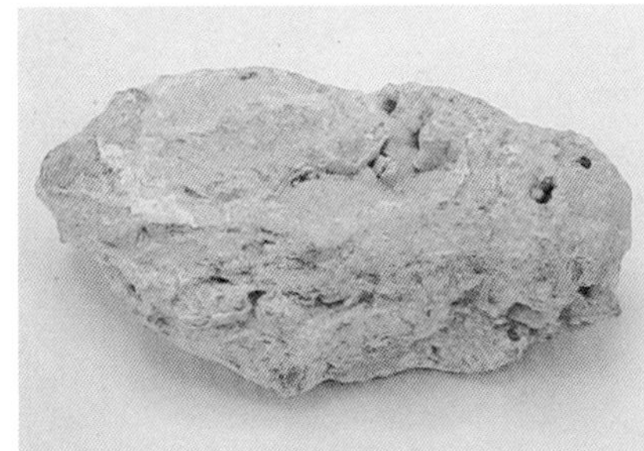
Lu Gan Shi (Galamina)

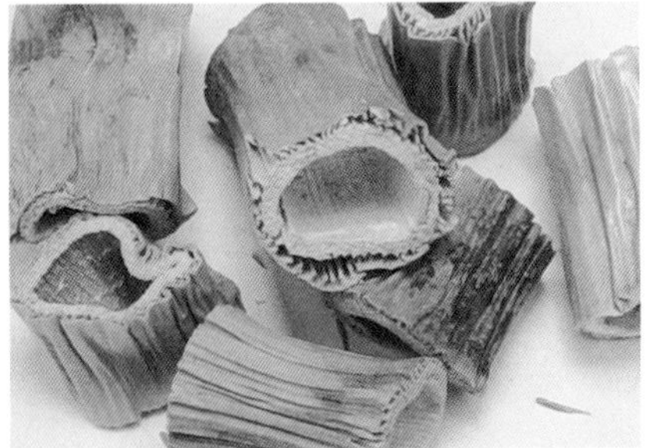
Lu Gen (Rhizoma Phragmitis)

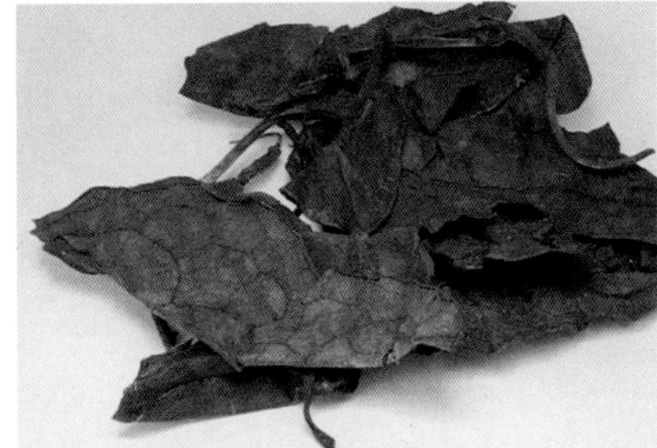
Lu Han Cao (Herba Pyrolae)

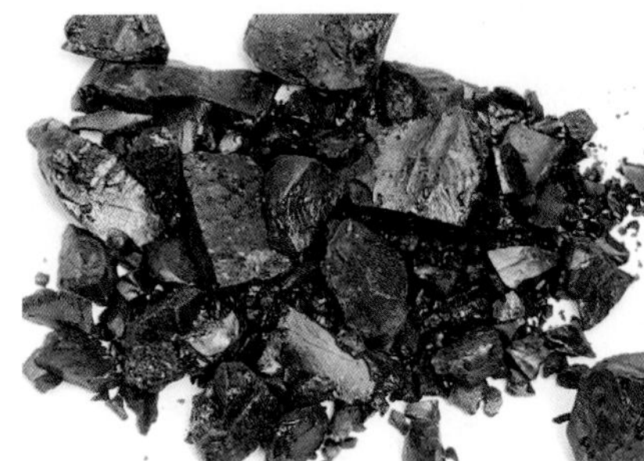
Lu Hui (Aloe)

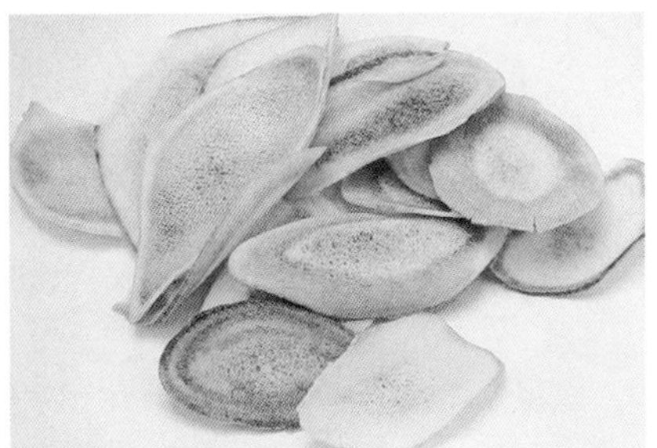
Lu Jiao (Cornu Cervi)

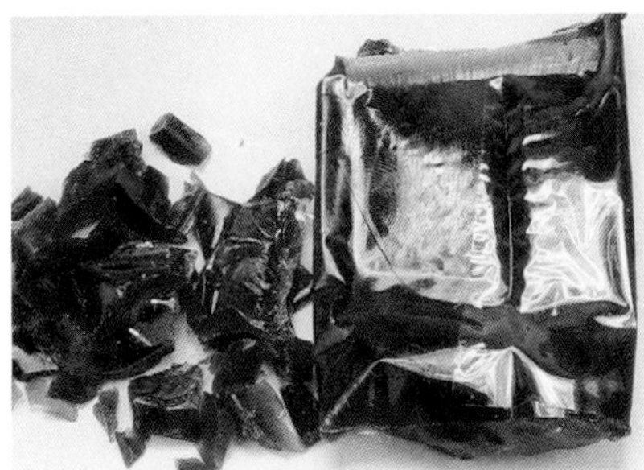
Lu Jiao Jiao (Gelatinum Cornu Cervi)

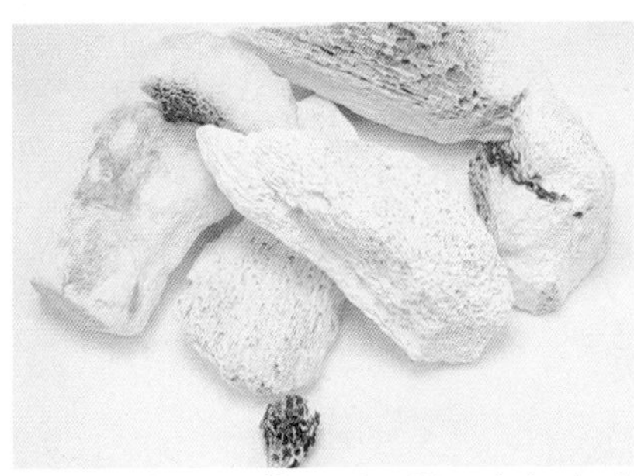
Lu Jiao Shuang (Cornu Cervi Degelatinatium)

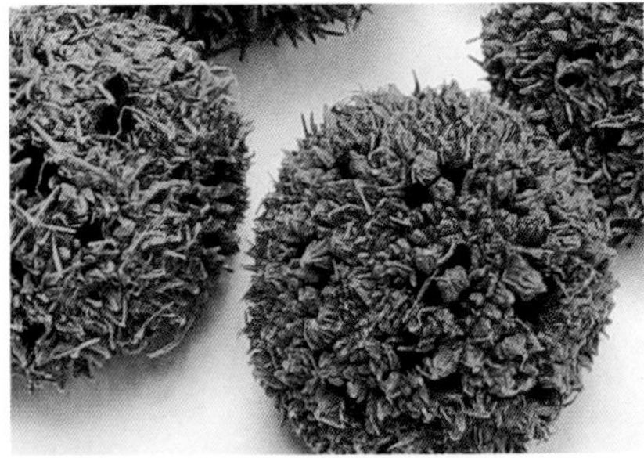
Lu Lu Tong (Fructus Liquidambaris)

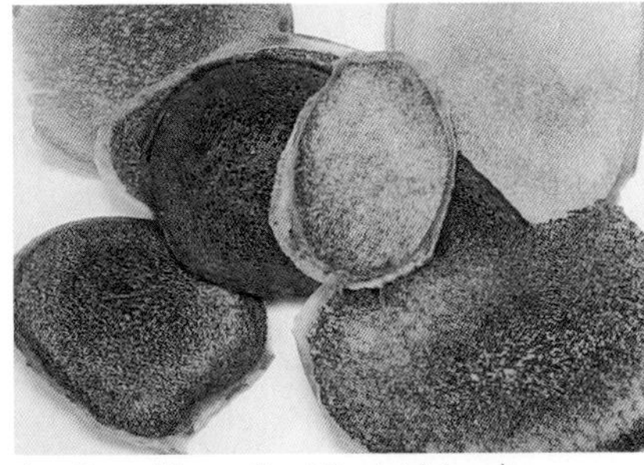
Lu Rong (Cornu Cervi Pantotrichum)

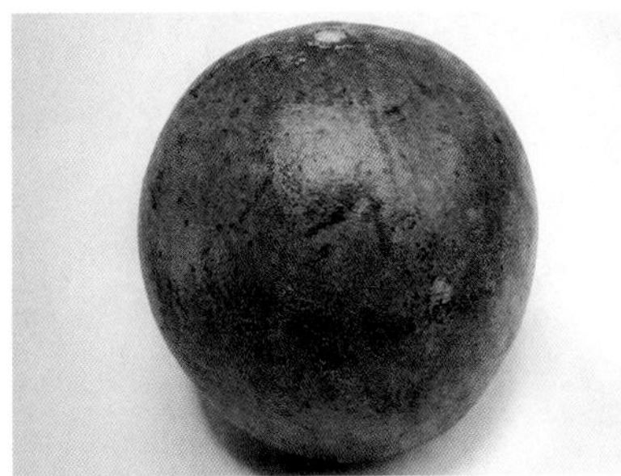
Luo Han Guo (Fructus Momordicae)

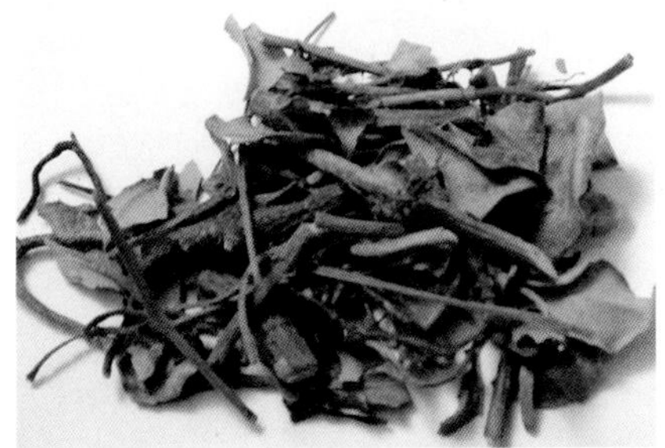
Luo Shi Teng (Caulis Trachelospermi)

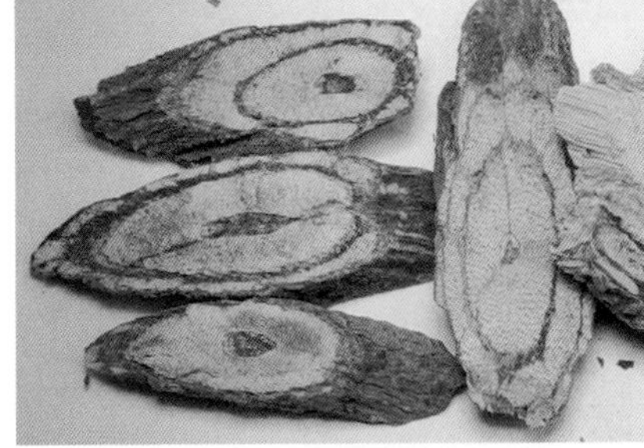
Ma An Teng (Herba Ipomoea Pes-caprae)

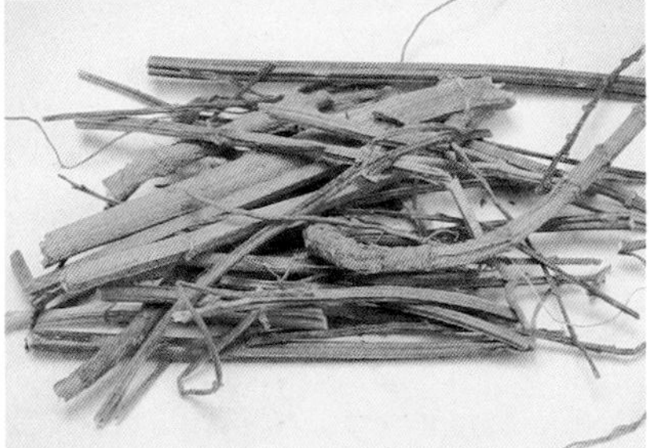
Ma Bian Cao (Herba Verbenae)

Herb Indentification Guide

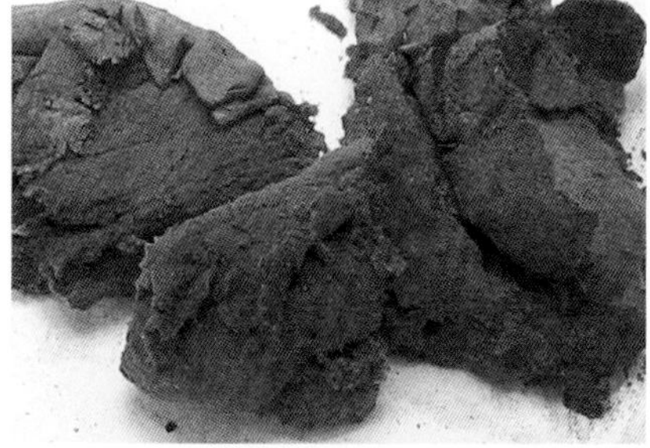
Ma Bo (Lasiosphaera seu Calvatia)

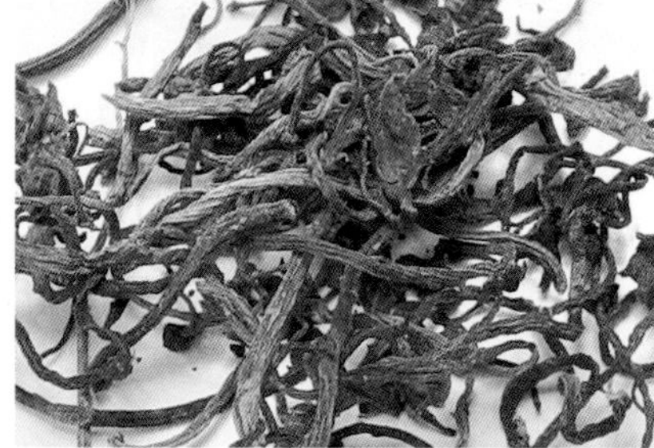
Ma Chi Xian (Herba Portulacae)

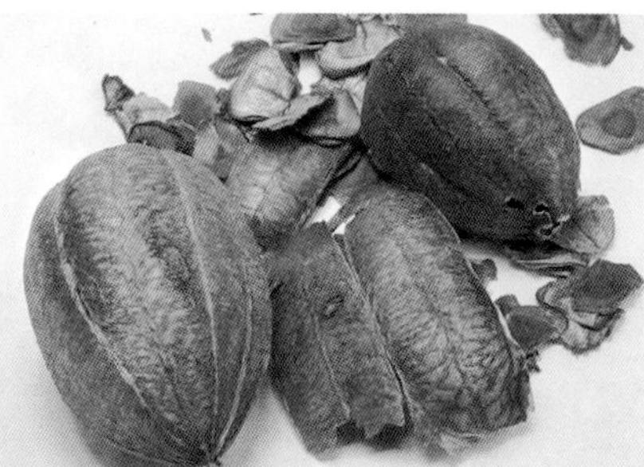
Ma Dou Ling (Fructus Aristolochiae)

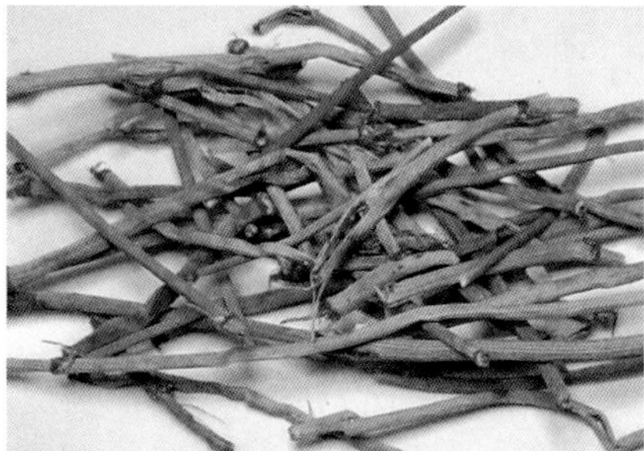
Ma Huang (Herba Ephedrae)

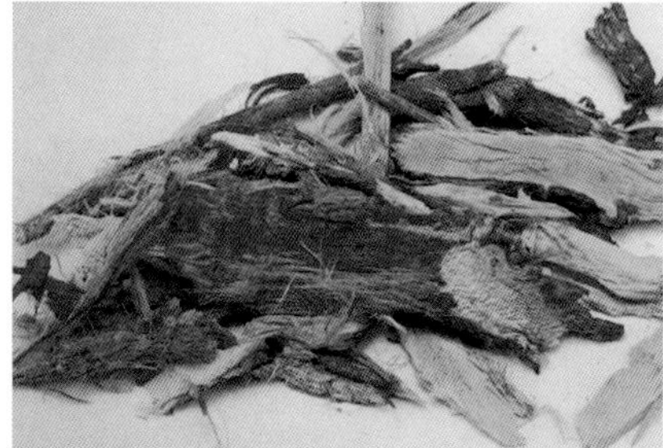
Ma Huang Gen (Radix Ephedrae)

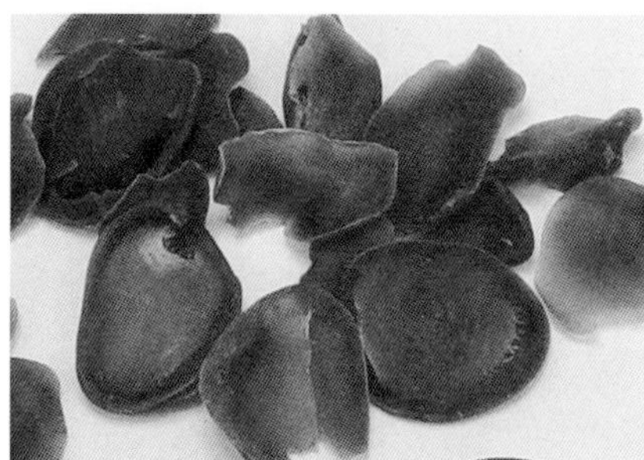
Ma Qian Zi (Semen Strychni)

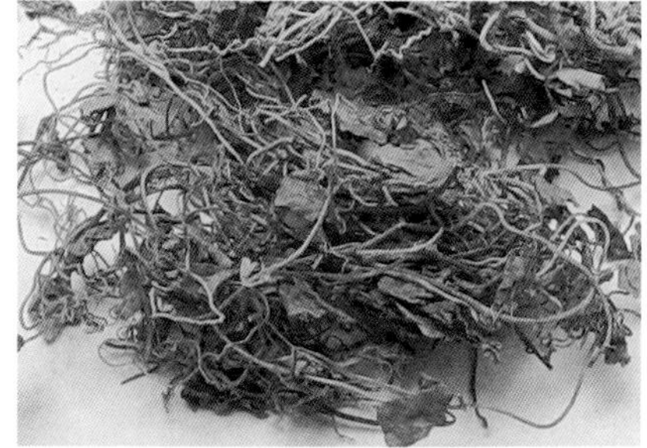
Ma Ti Jin (Herba Dichondrae Repentis)

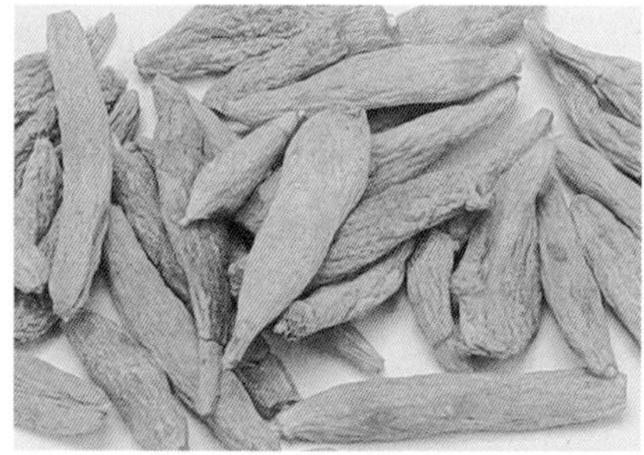
Mai Men Dong (Radix Ophiopogonis)

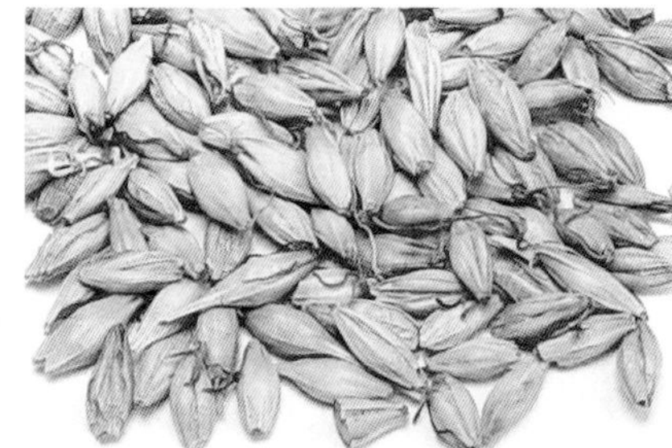
Mai Ya (Fructus Hordei Germinatus)

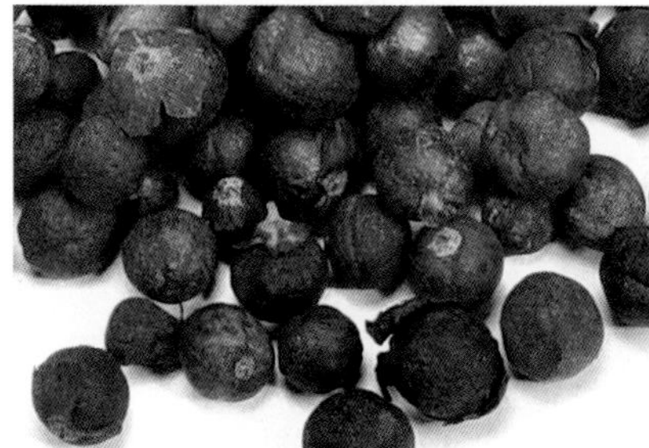
Man Jing Zi (Fructus Viticis)

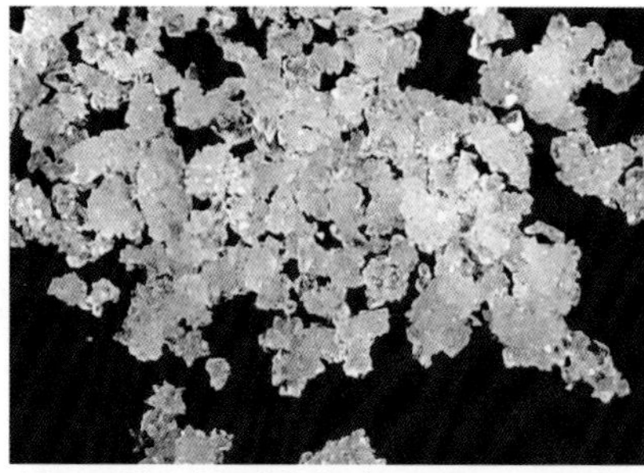
Mang Xiao (Natrii Sulfas)

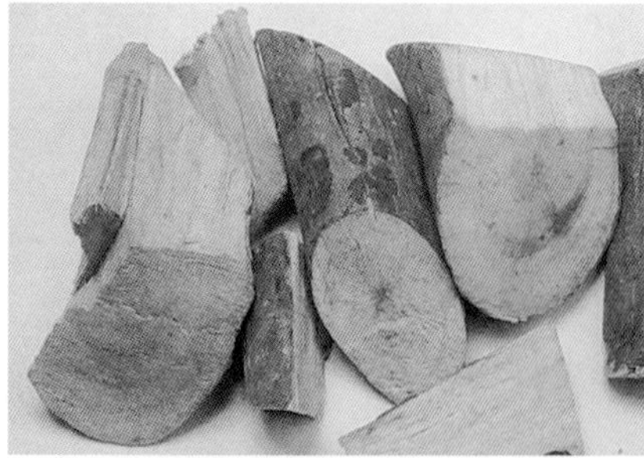
Mao Dong Qing (Radix Ilicis Pubescentis)

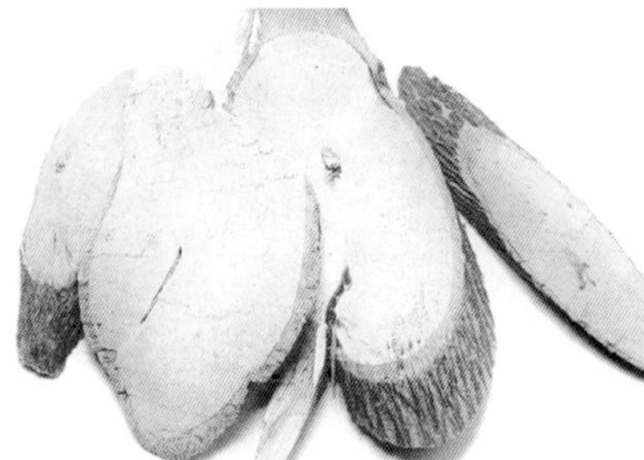
Mao Zi Dun Tou (Herba Abutilon Indicum)

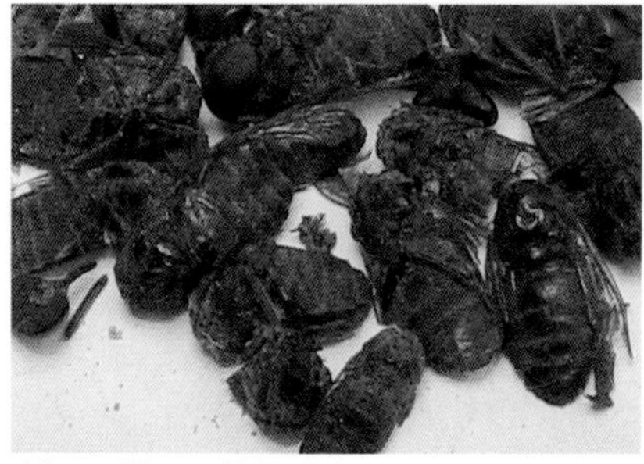
Meng Chong (Tabanus)

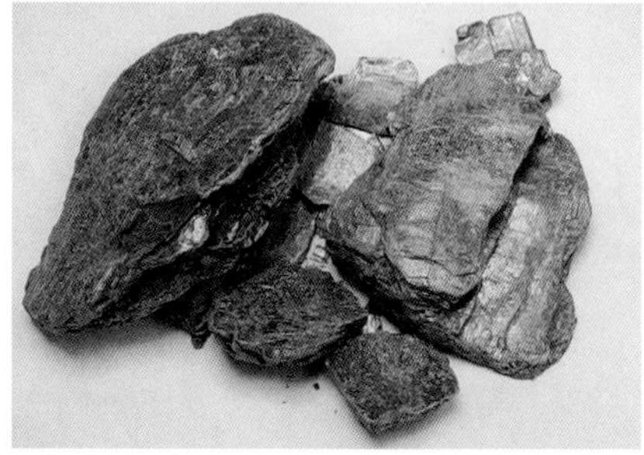
Meng Shi (Lapis Micae seu Chloriti)

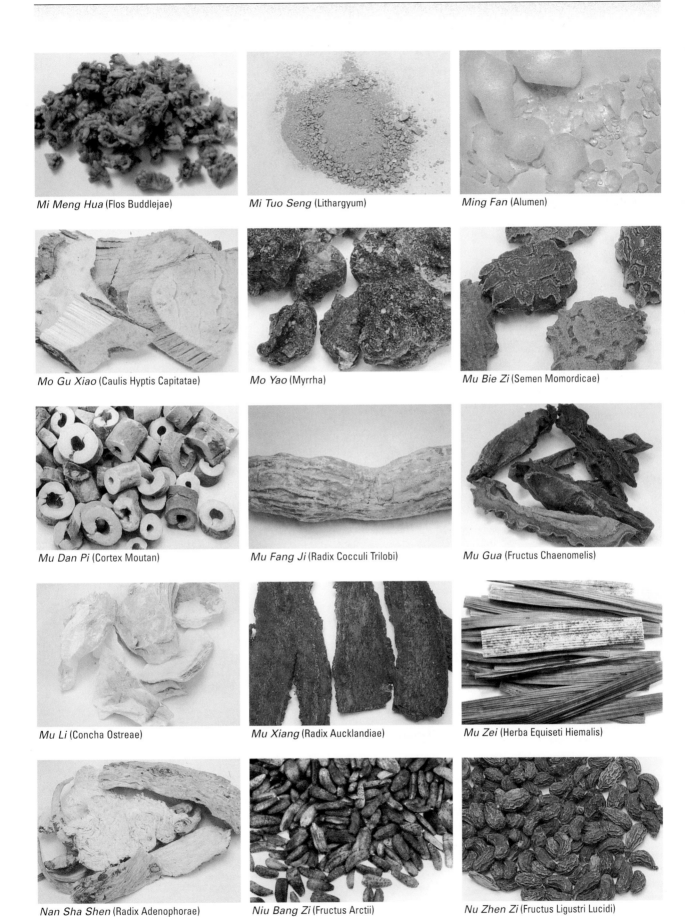

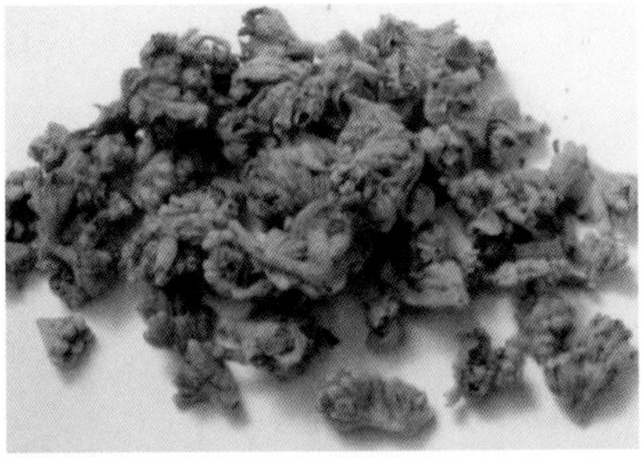

Mi Meng Hua (Flos Buddlejae)

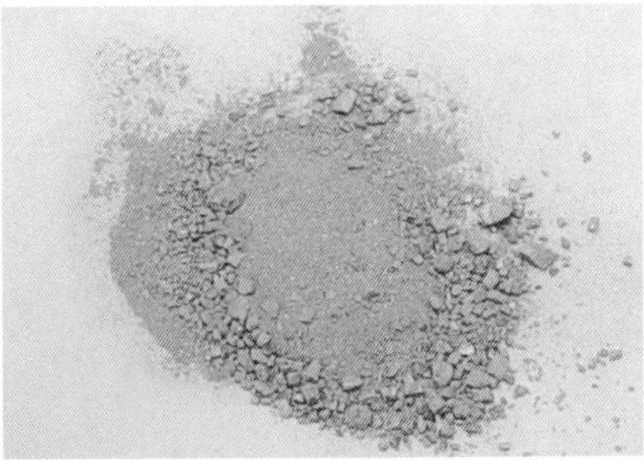

Mi Tuo Seng (Lithargyum)

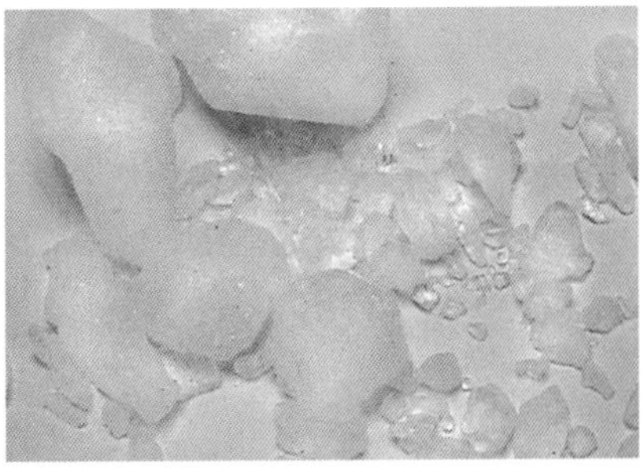

Ming Fan (Alumen)

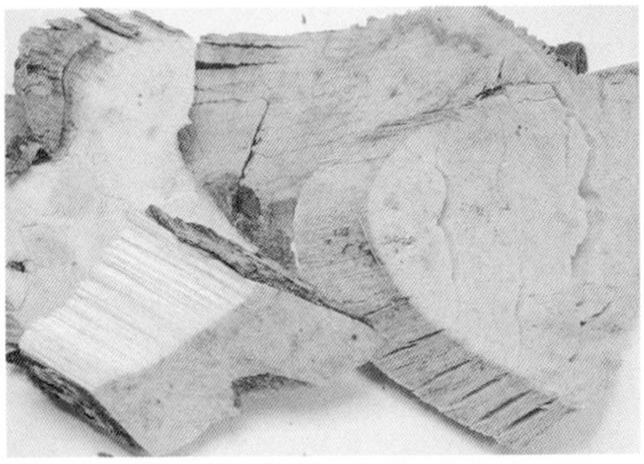

Mo Gu Xiao (Caulis Hyptis Capitatae)

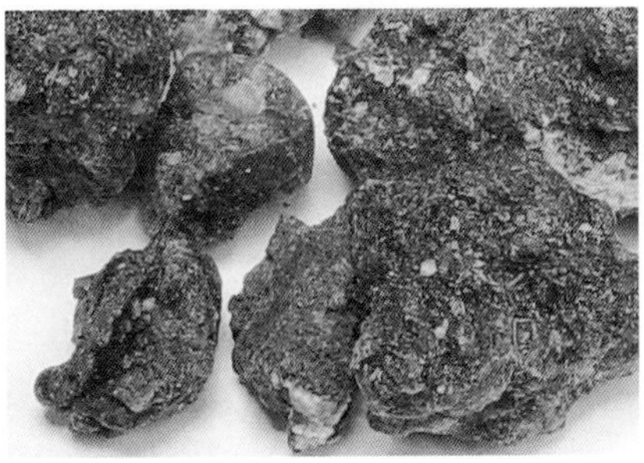

Mo Yao (Myrrha)

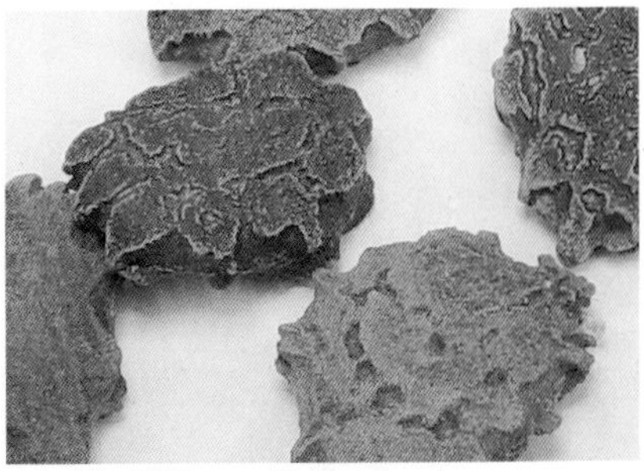

Mu Bie Zi (Semen Momordicae)

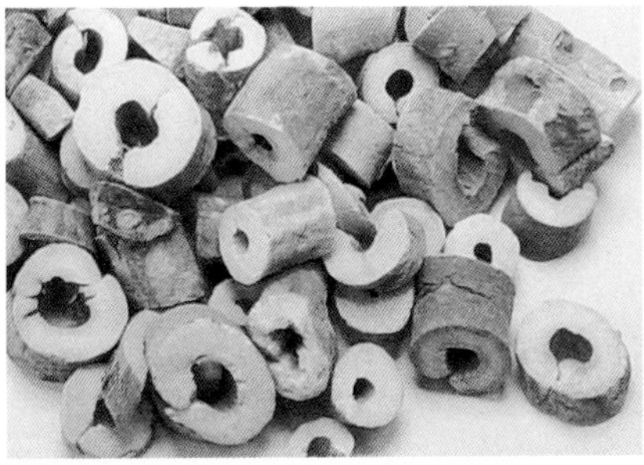

Mu Dan Pi (Cortex Moutan)

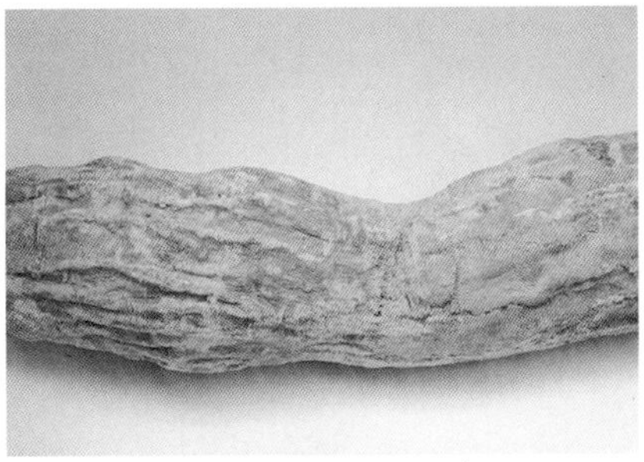

Mu Fang Ji (Radix Cocculi Trilobi)

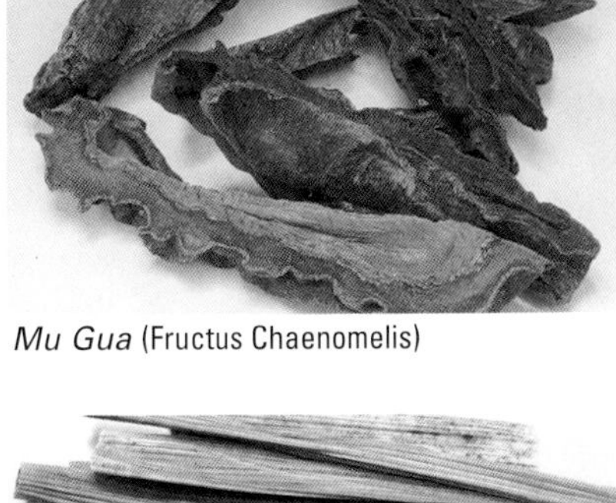

Mu Gua (Fructus Chaenomelis)

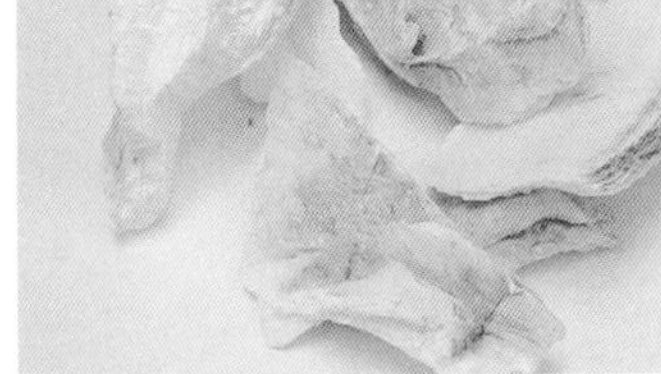

Mu Li (Concha Ostreae)

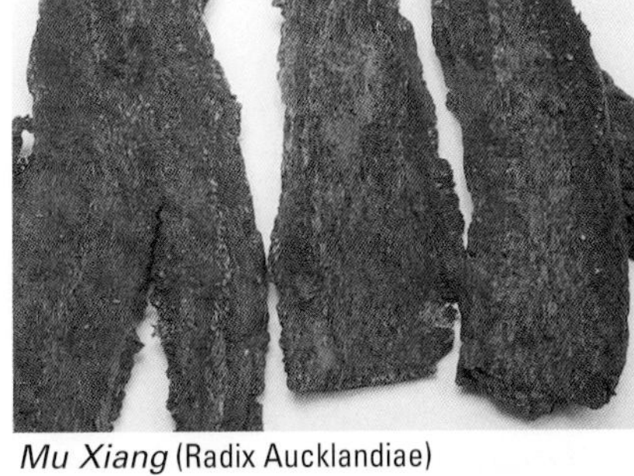

Mu Xiang (Radix Aucklandiae)

Mu Zei (Herba Equiseti Hiemalis)

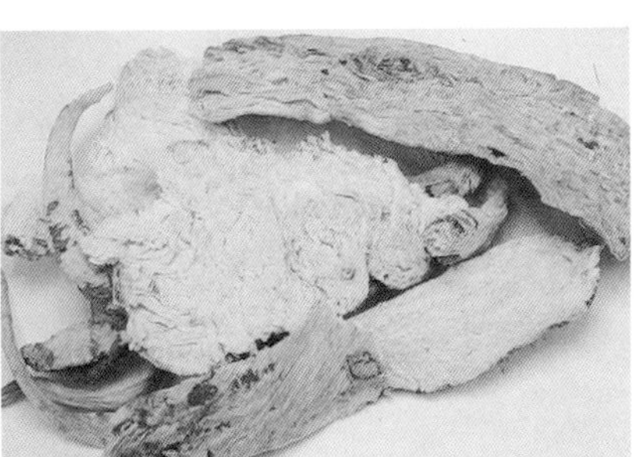

Nan Sha Shen (Radix Adenophorae)

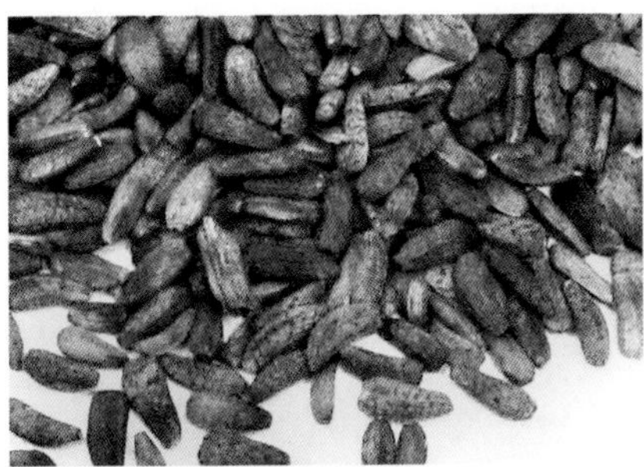

Niu Bang Zi (Fructus Arctii)

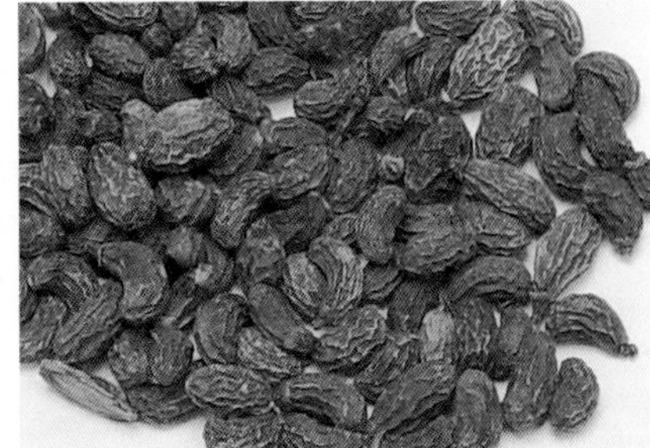

Nu Zhen Zi (Fructus Ligustri Lucidi)

Herb Indentification Guide

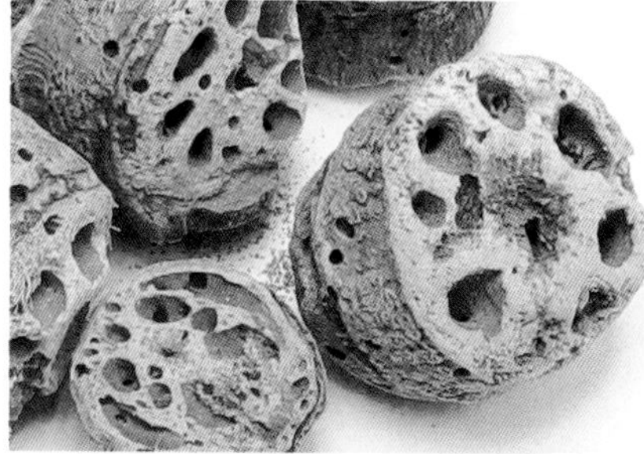
Ou Jie (Nodus Nelumbinis Rhizomatis)

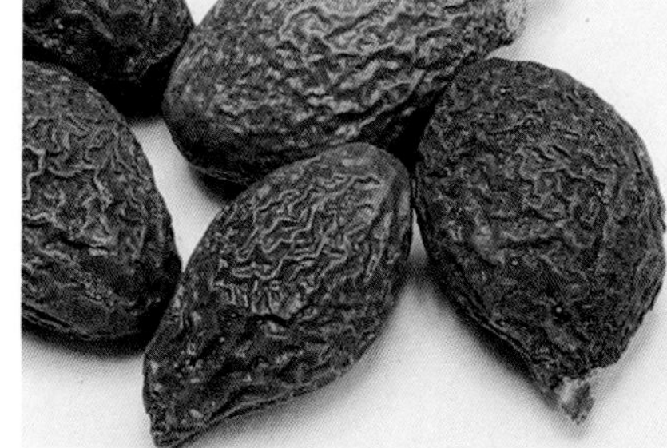
Pang Da Hai (Semen Sterculiae Lychnophorae)

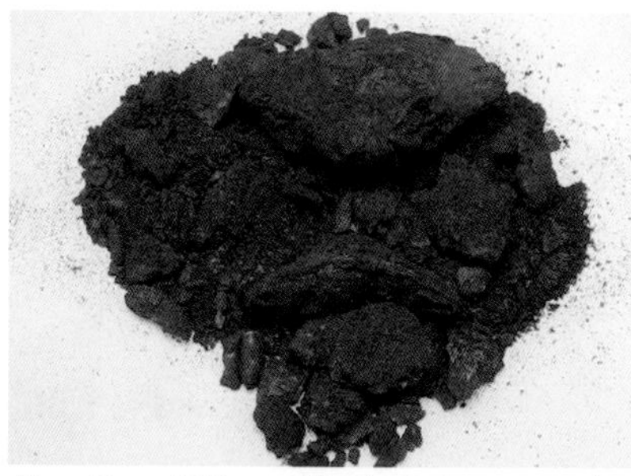
Pao Jiang (Rhizoma Zingiberis Preparatum)

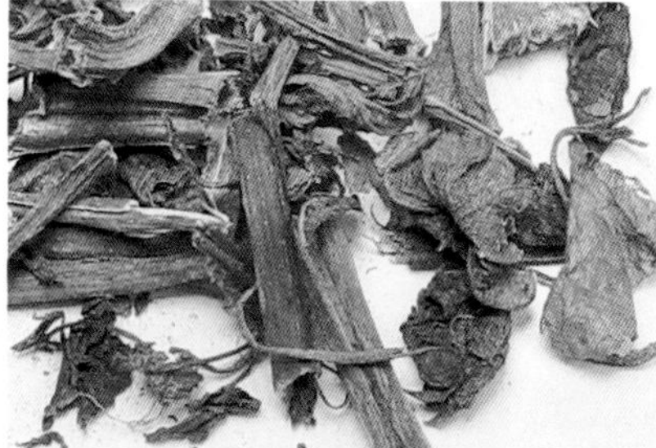
Pao Zai Cao (Herba Physalis Angulatae)

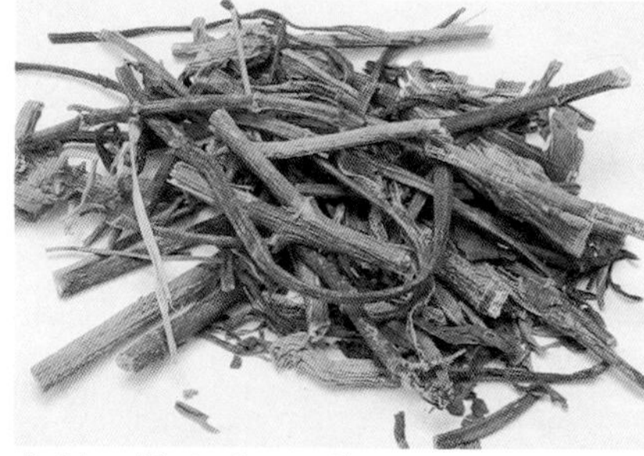
Pei Lan (Herba Eupatorii)

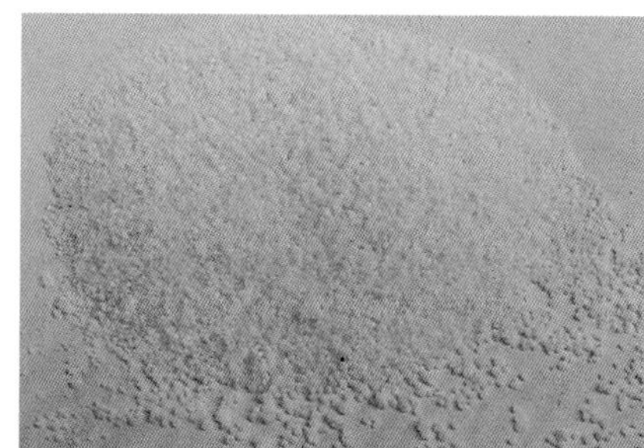
Peng Sha (Borax)

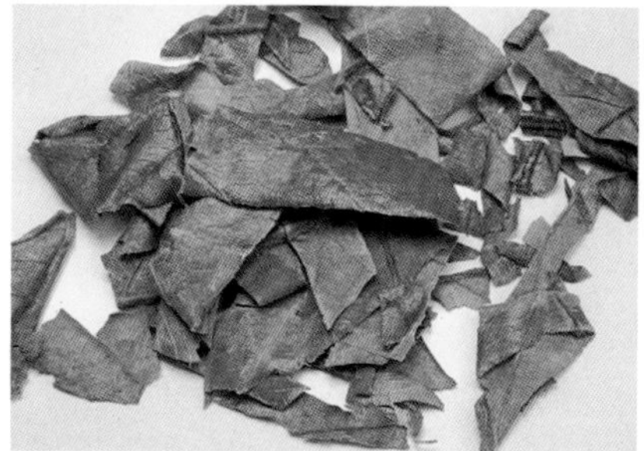
Pi Pa Ye (Folium Eriobotryae)

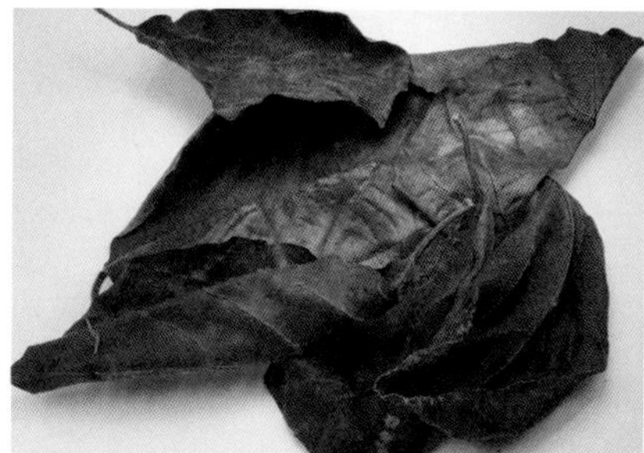
Po Bu Zi Ye (Folium Cordia Dichotoma)

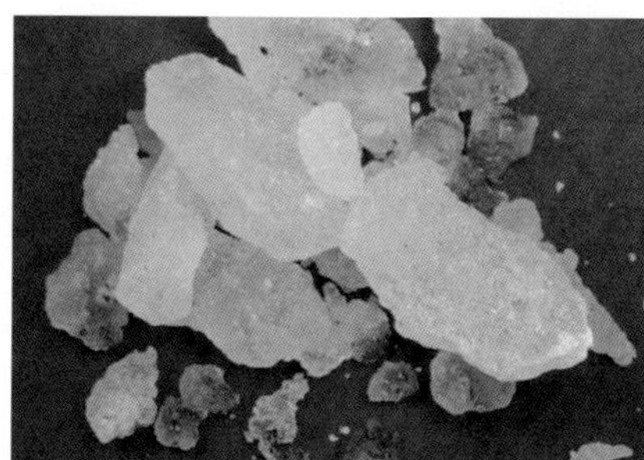
Po Xiao (Sal Glauberis)

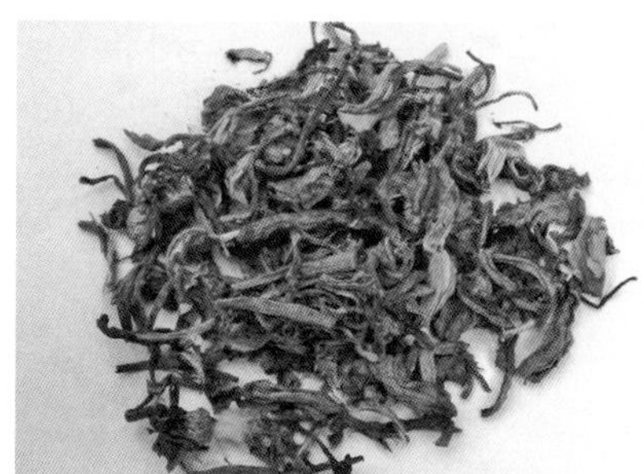
Pu Gong Ying (Herba Taraxaci)

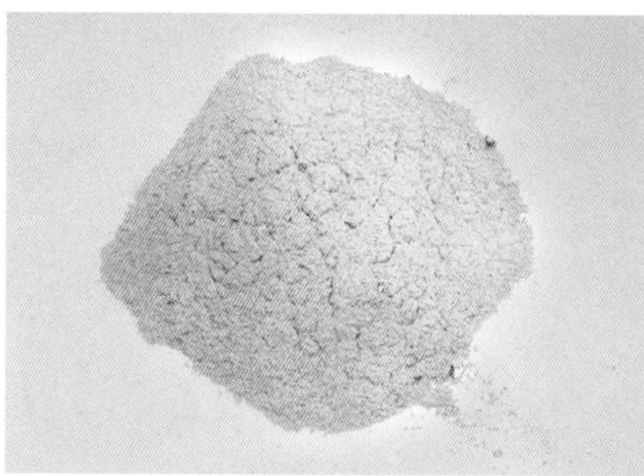
Pu Huang (Pollen Typhae)

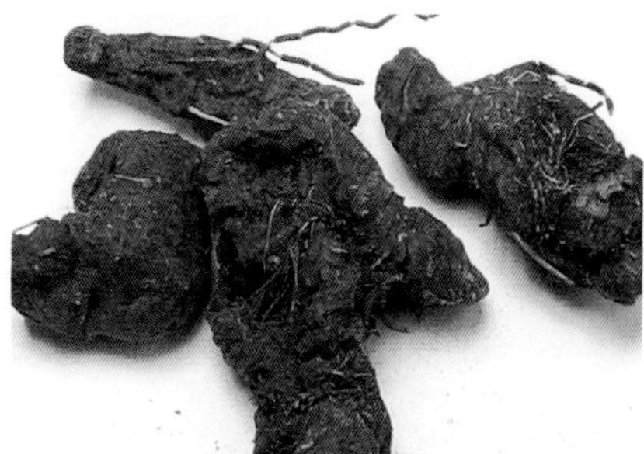
Qi Ye Lian (Radix Schefflerae)

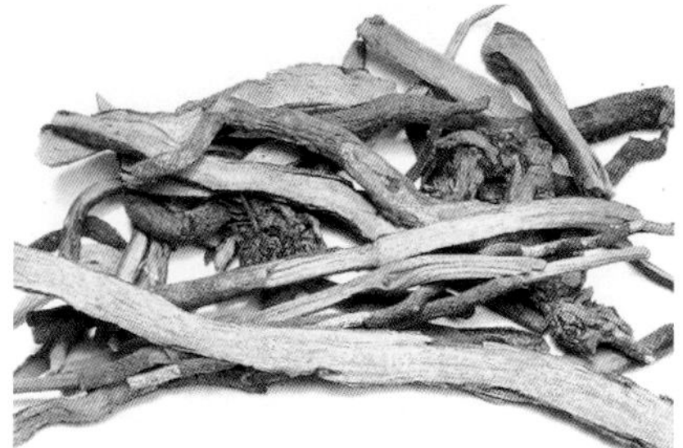
Qian Cao (Radix Rubiae)

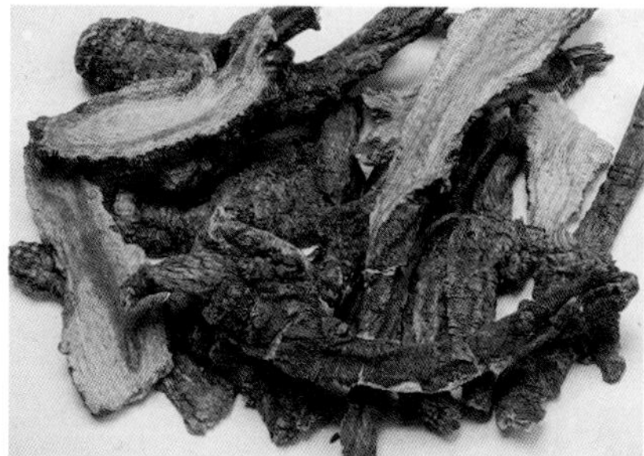
Qian Hu (Radix Peucedani)

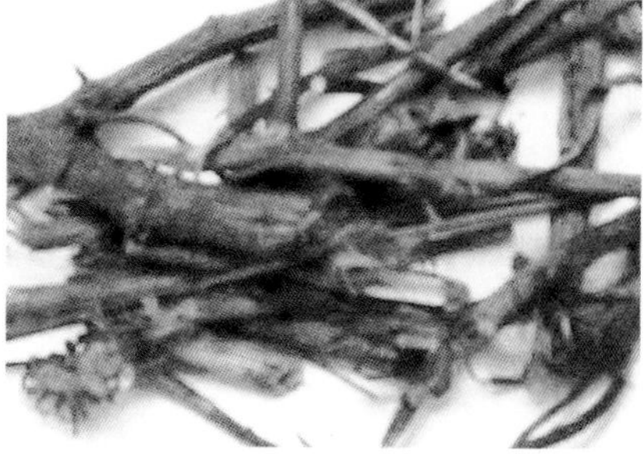
Qian Li Guang (Herba Senecionis Scandens)

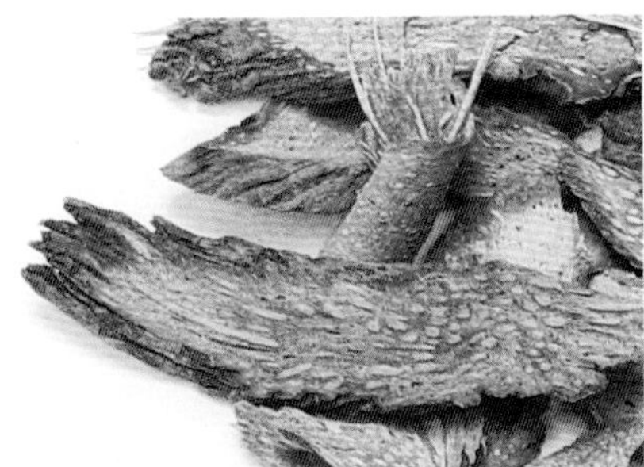
Qian Nian Jian (Rhizoma Homalomenae)

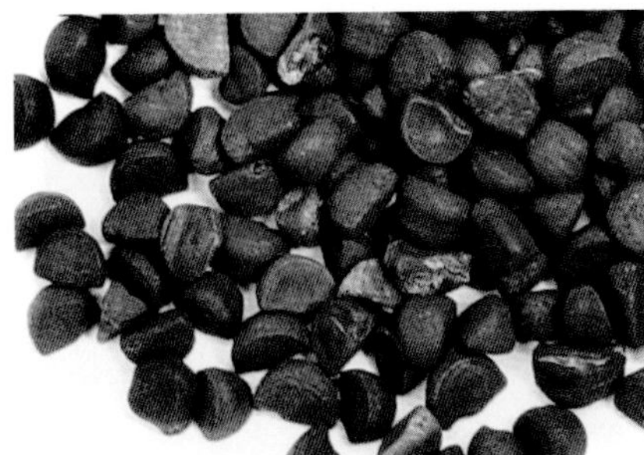
Qian Niu Zi (Semen Pharbitidis)

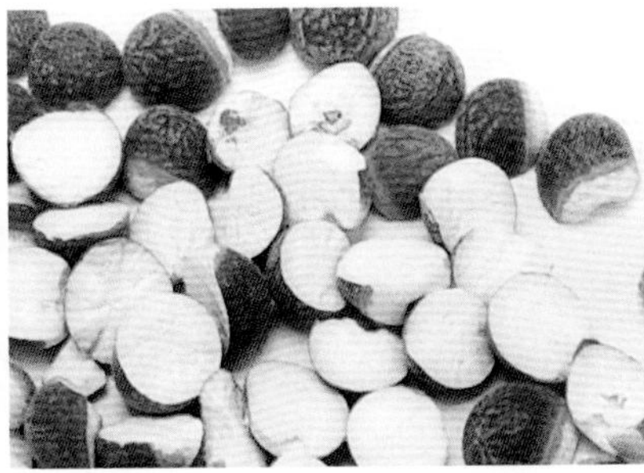
Qian Shi (Semen Euryales)

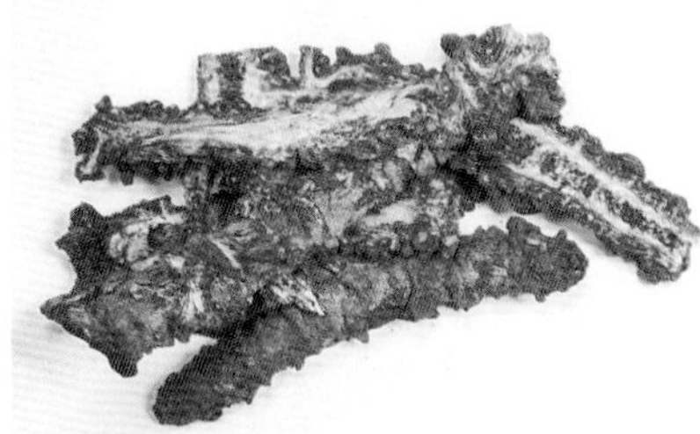
Qiang Huo (Rhizoma et Radix Notopterygii)

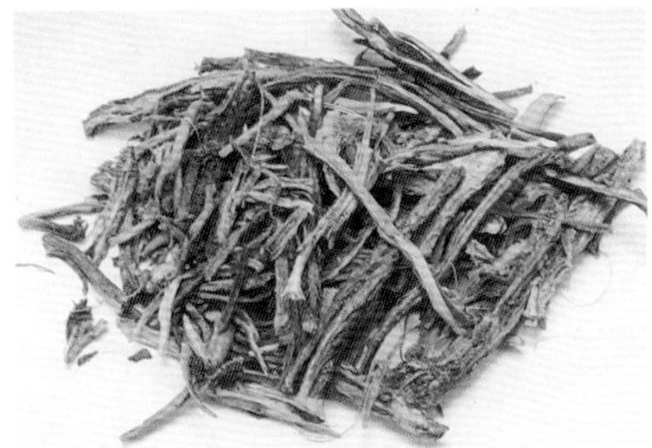
Qin Jiao (Radix Gentianae Macrophyllae)

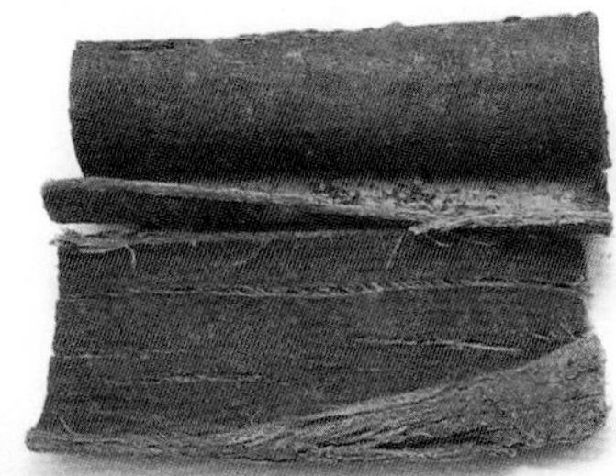
Qin Pi (Cortex Fraxini)

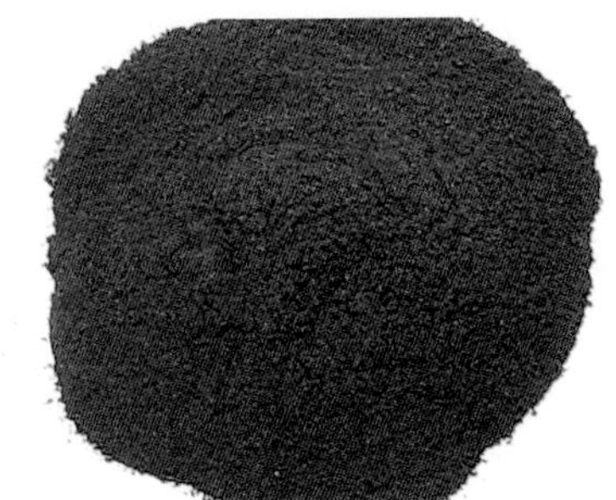
Qing Dai (Indigo Naturalis)

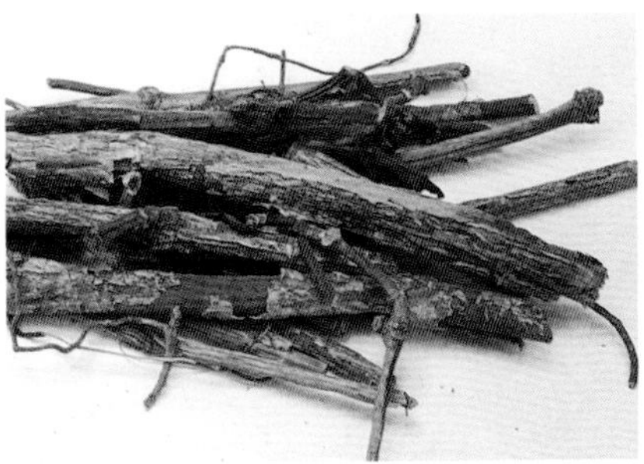
Qing Feng Teng (Caulis Sinomenii)

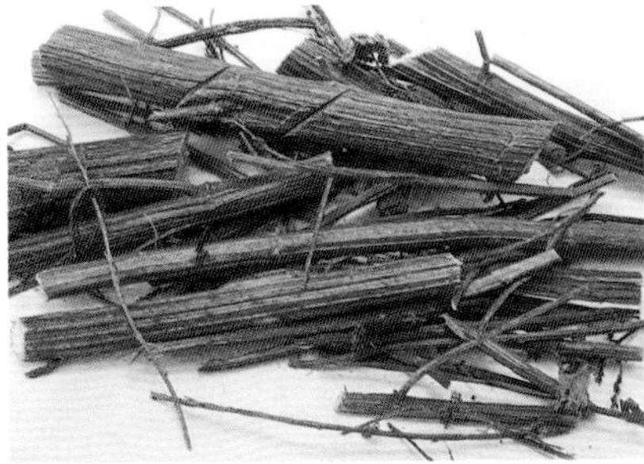
Qing Hao (Herba Artemisiae Annuae)

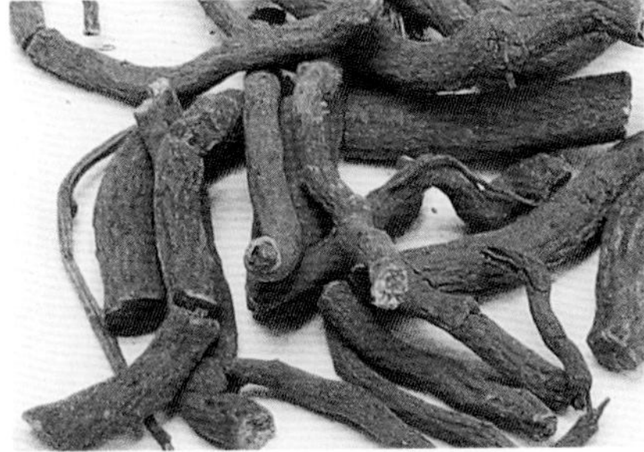
Qing Mu Xiang (Radix Aristolochiae)

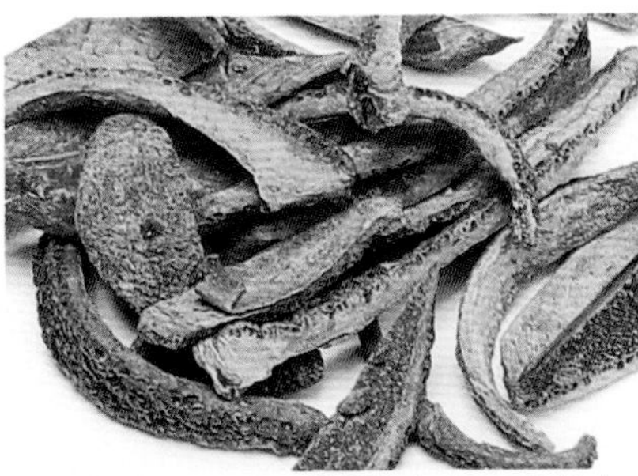
Qing Pi (Pericarpium Citri Reticulatae Viride)

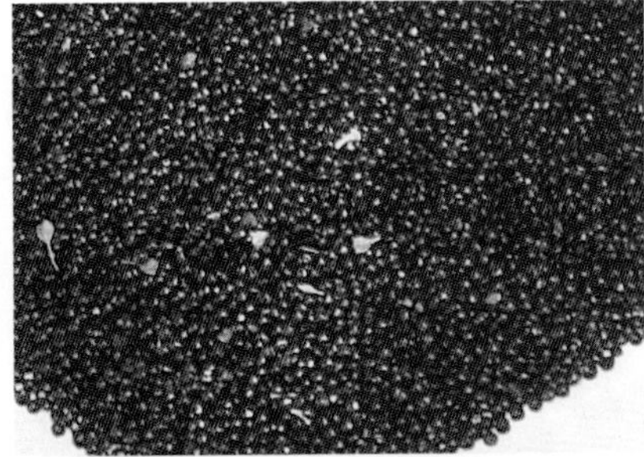
Qing Xiang Zi (Semen Celosiae)

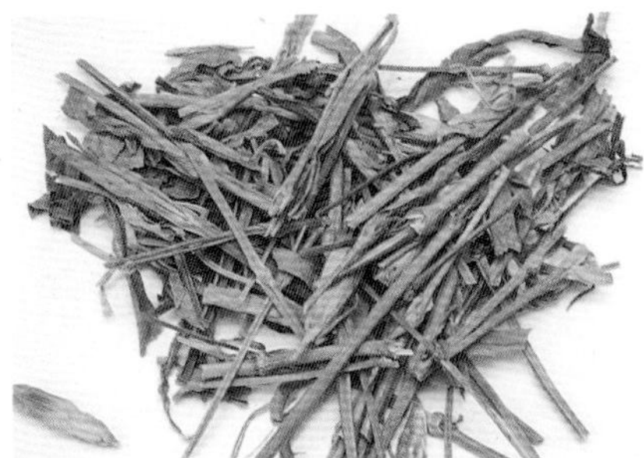
Qu Mai (Herba Dianthi)

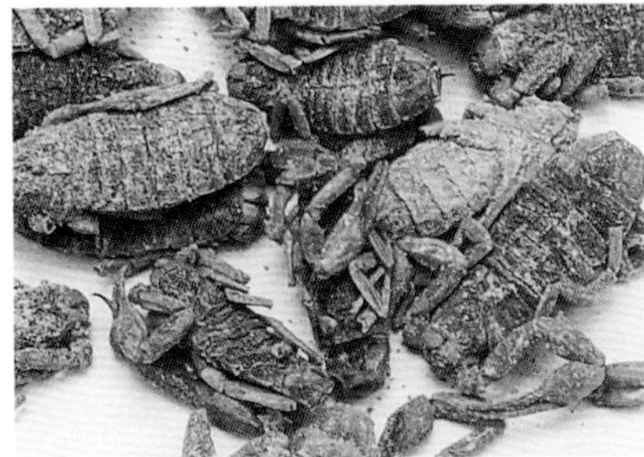
Quan Xie (Scorpio)

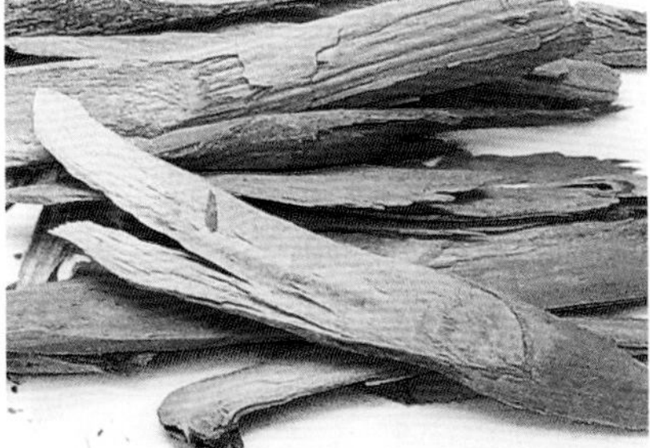
Ren Dong Teng (Caulis Lonicerae)

Herb Indentification Guide

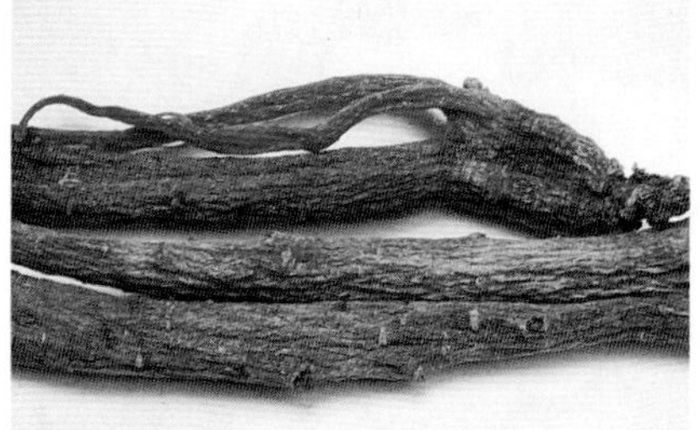
Ren Shen (Radix Ginseng)

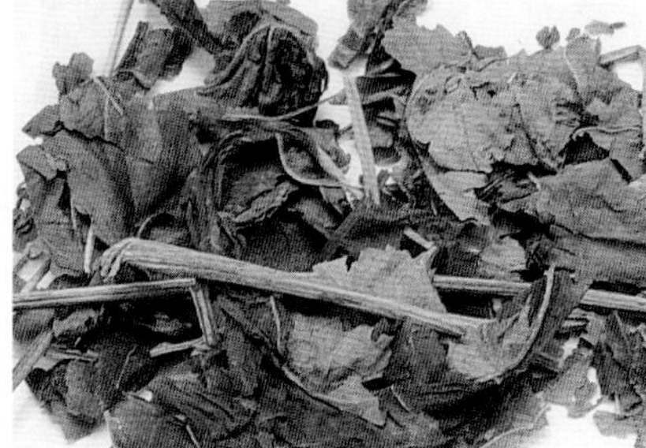
Ren Shen Ye (Folium Ginseng)

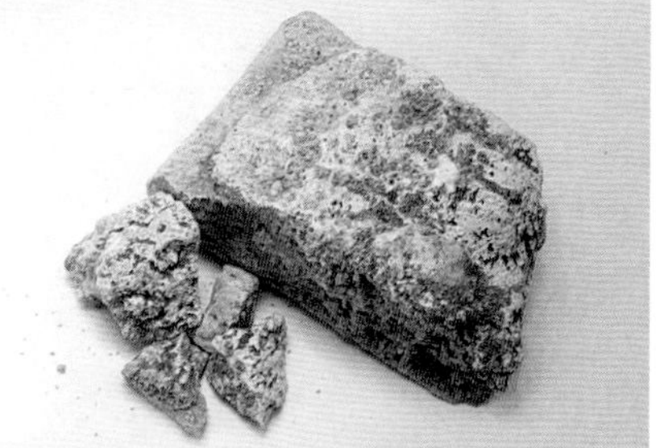
Ren Zhong Bai (Urinae Hominis Sedimen)

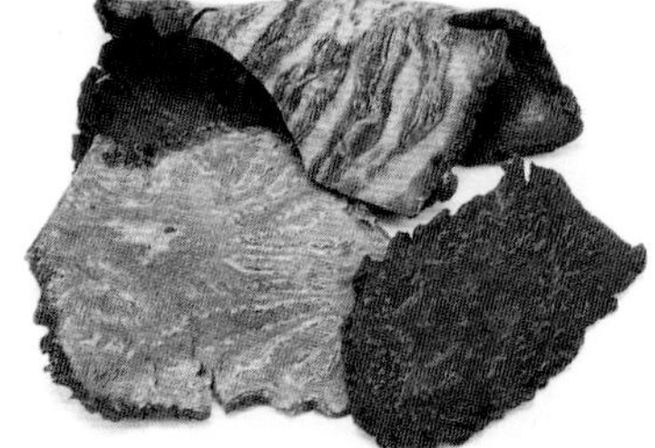
Rou Cong Rong (Herba Cistanches)

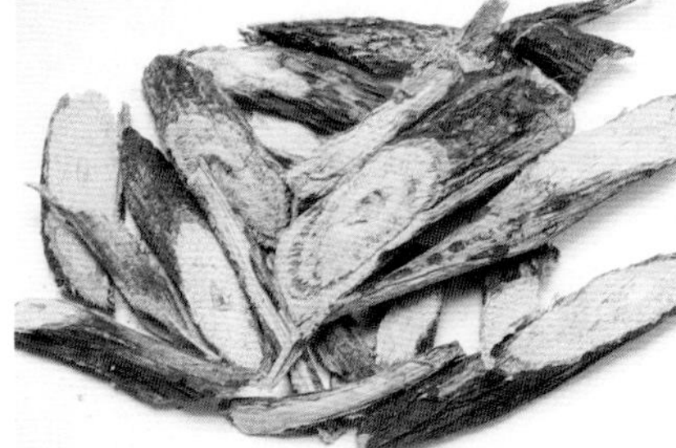
Rou Dou Gen (Radix Myristicae)

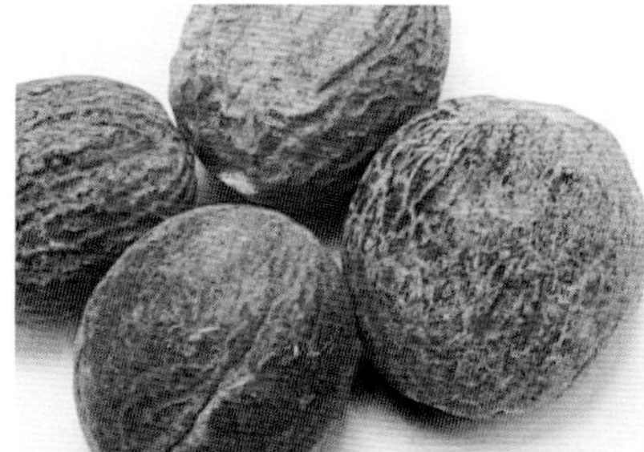
Rou Dou Kou (Semen Myristicae)

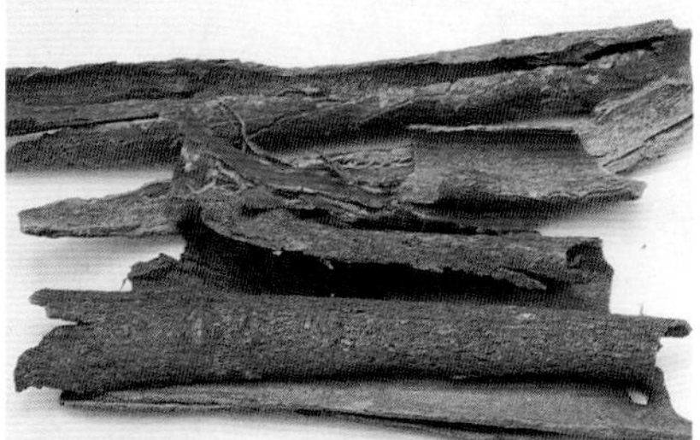
Rou Gui (Cortex Cinnamomi)

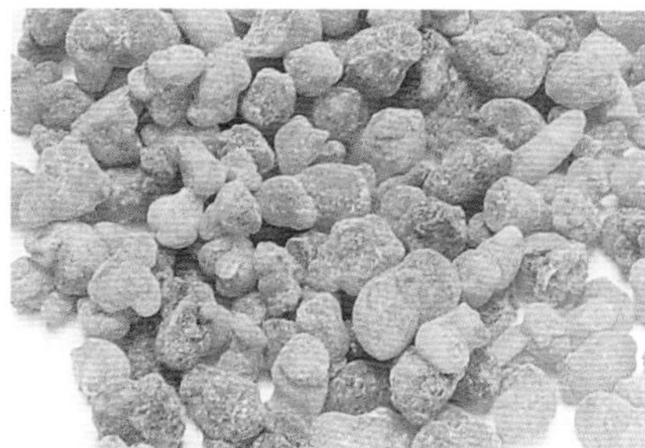
Ru Xiang (Gummi Olibanum)

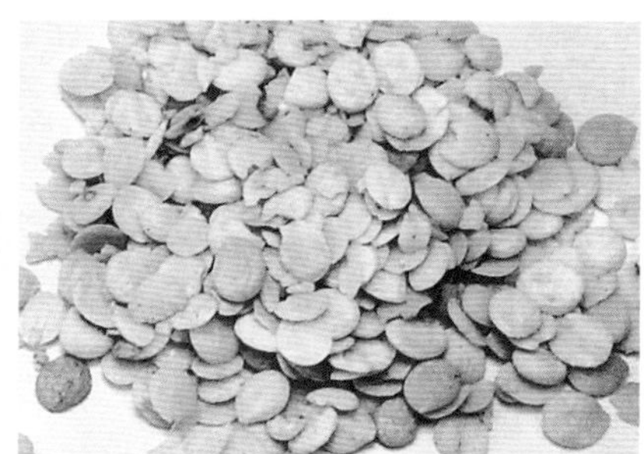
Rui Ren (Semen Prinsepiae)

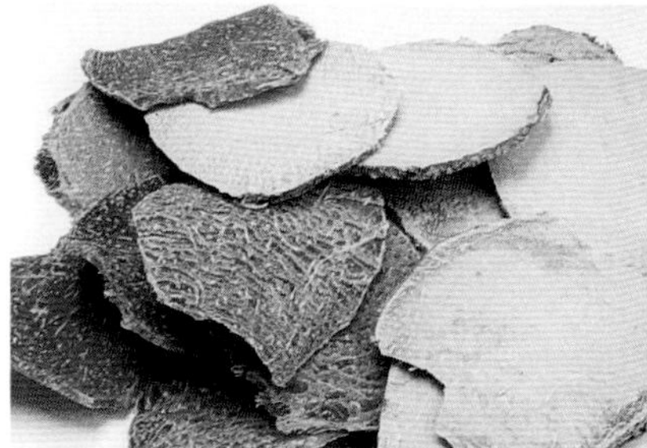
San Leng (Rhizoma Sparganii)

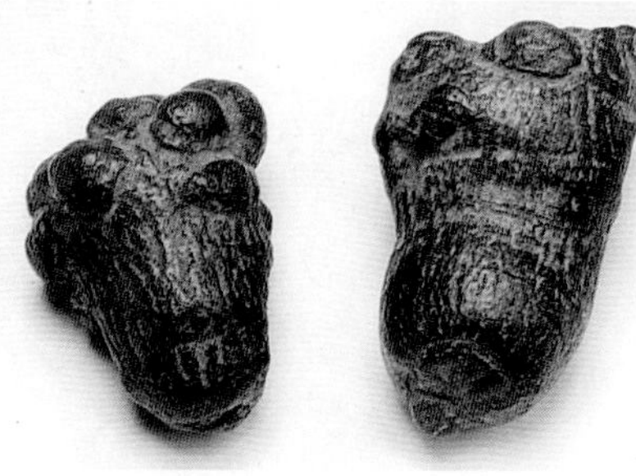
San Qi (Radix Notoginseng)

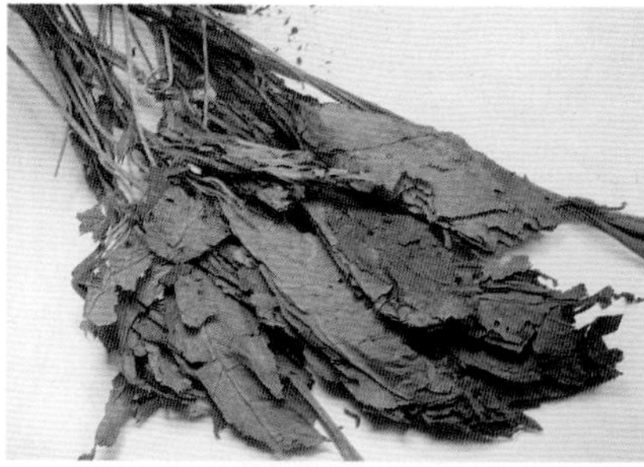
San Qi Ye (Folium Notoginseng)

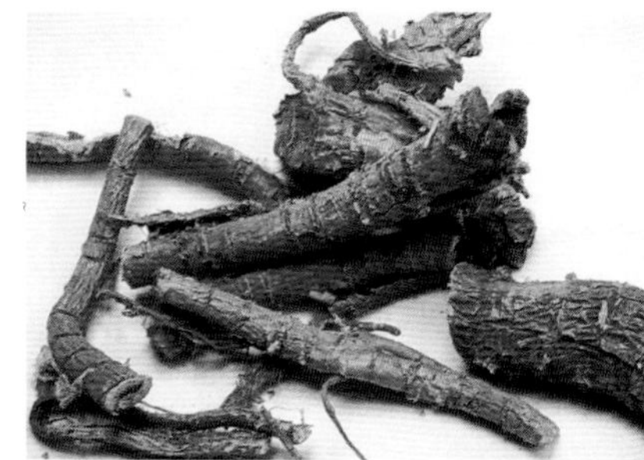
Sang Bai Pi (Cortex Mori)

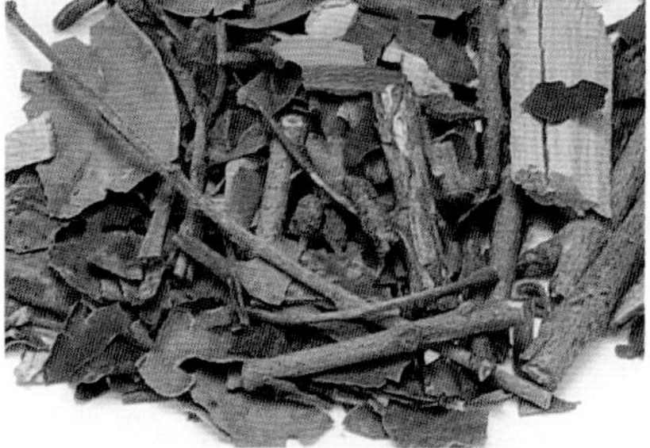
Sang Ji Sheng (Herba Taxilli)

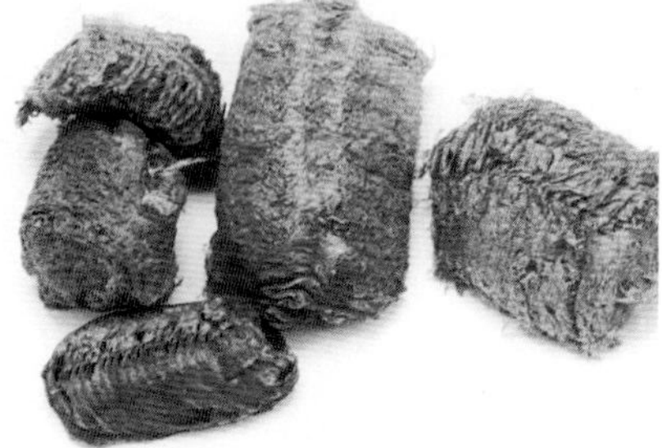
Sang Piao Xiao (Ootheca Mantidis)

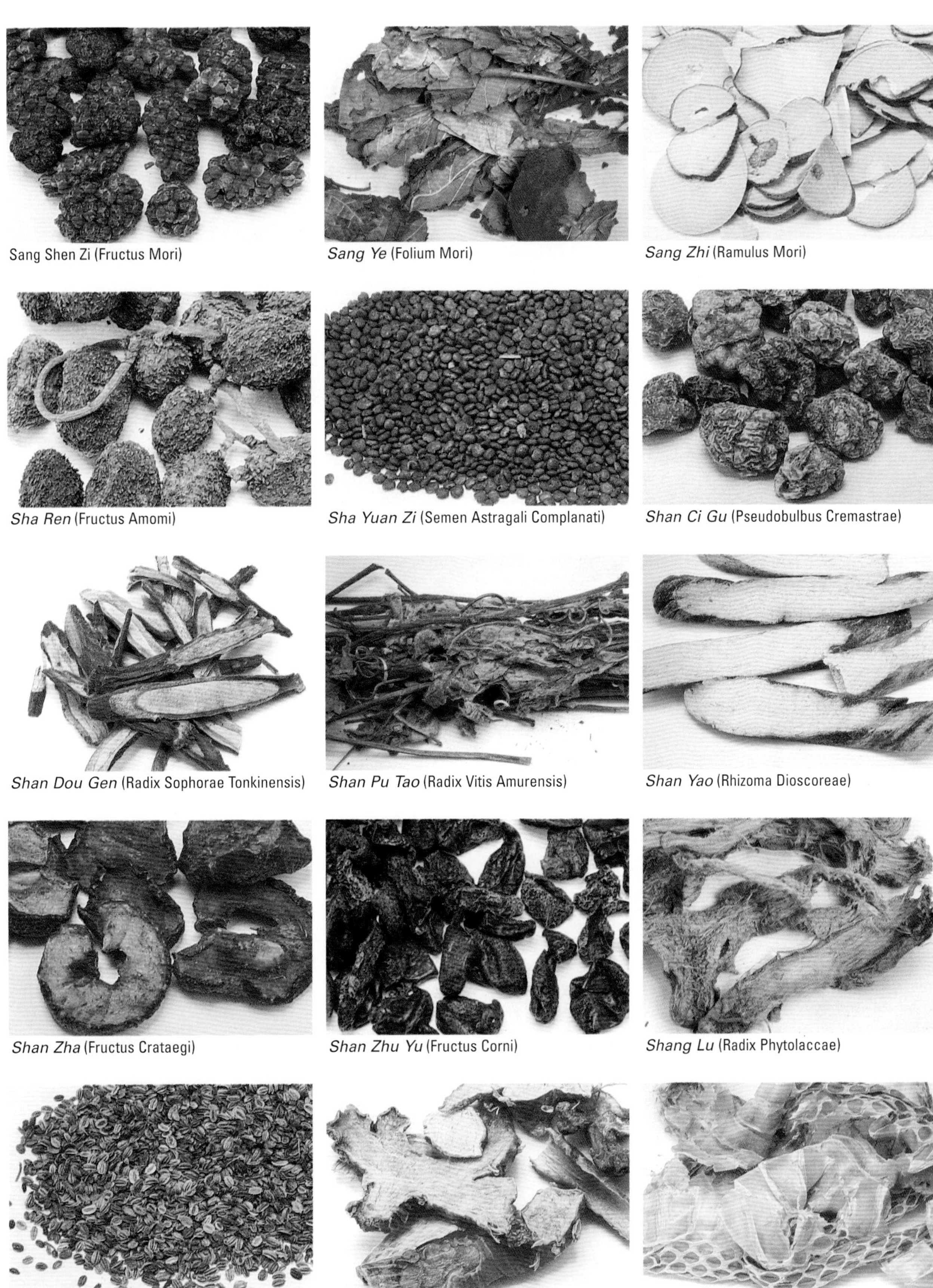

Sang Shen Zi (Fructus Mori)

Sang Ye (Folium Mori)

Sang Zhi (Ramulus Mori)

Sha Ren (Fructus Amomi)

Sha Yuan Zi (Semen Astragali Complanati)

Shan Ci Gu (Pseudobulbus Cremastrae)

Shan Dou Gen (Radix Sophorae Tonkinensis)

Shan Pu Tao (Radix Vitis Amurensis)

Shan Yao (Rhizoma Dioscoreae)

Shan Zha (Fructus Crataegi)

Shan Zhu Yu (Fructus Corni)

Shang Lu (Radix Phytolaccae)

She Chuang Zi (Fructus Cnidii)

She Gan (Rhizoma Belamcandae)

She Tui (Periostracum Serpentis)

Herb Indentification Guide

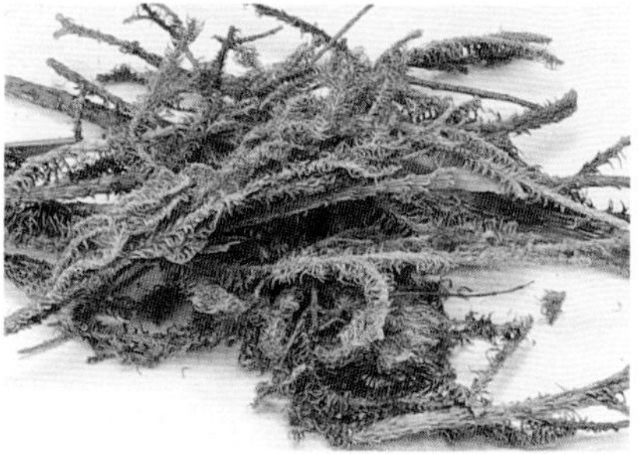

Shen Jin Cao (Herba Lycopodii)

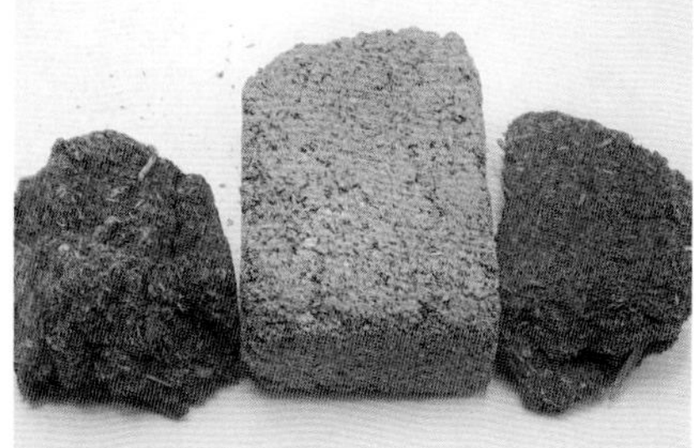

Shen Qu (Massa Fermentata)

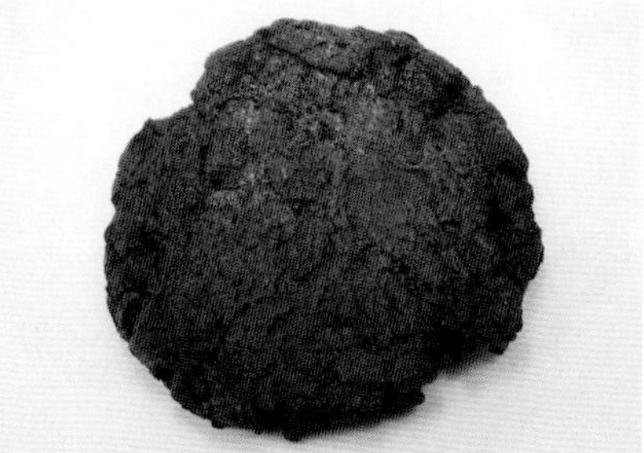

Sheng Di Huang (Radix Rehmanniae)

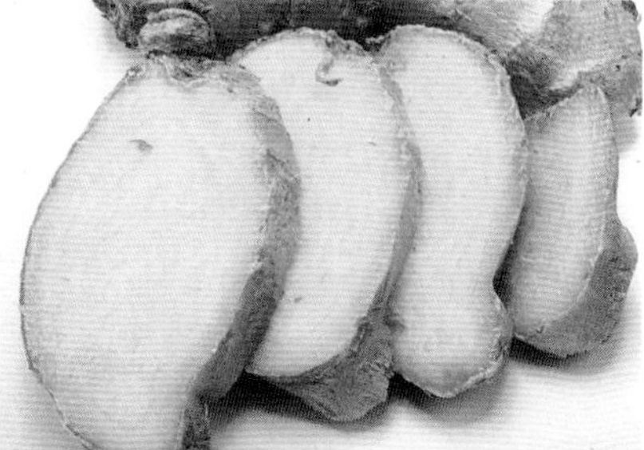

Sheng Jiang (Rhizoma Zingiberis Recens)

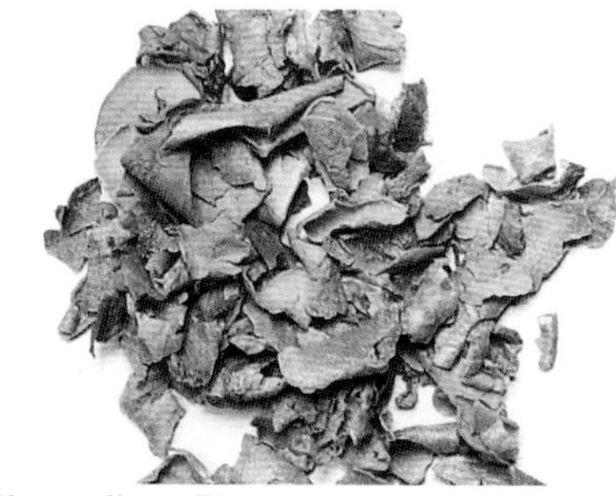

Sheng Jiang Pi (Pericarpium Zingiberis Recens)

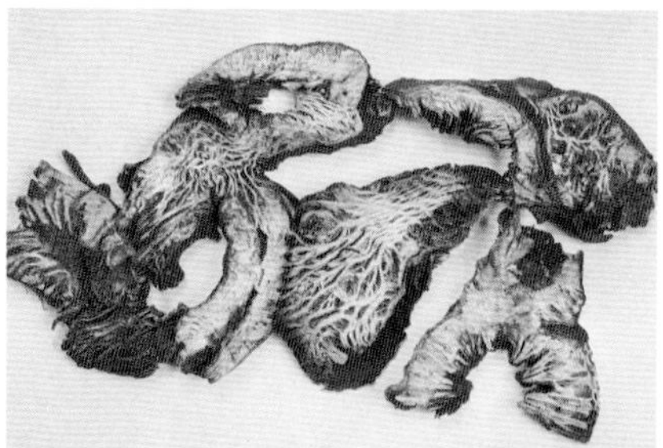

Sheng Ma (Rhizoma Cimicifugae)

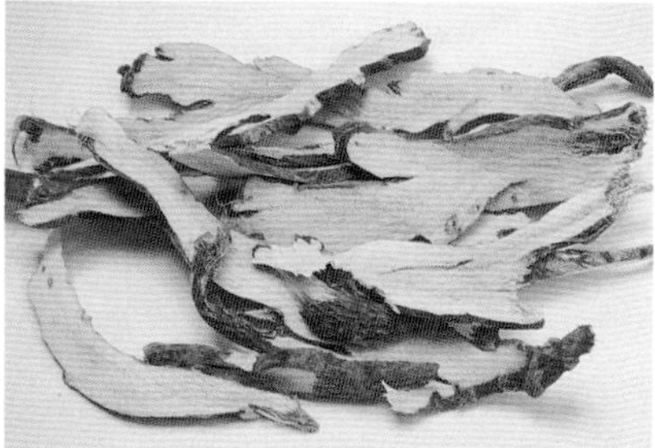

Shi Chang Pu (Rhizoma Acori)

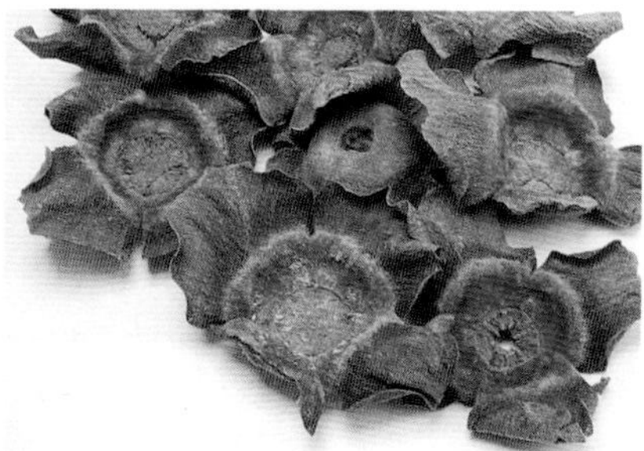

Shi Di (Calyx Kaki)

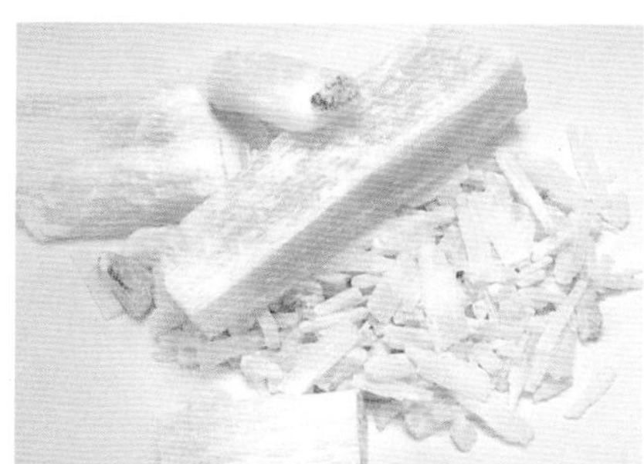

Shi Gao (Gypsum Fibrosum)

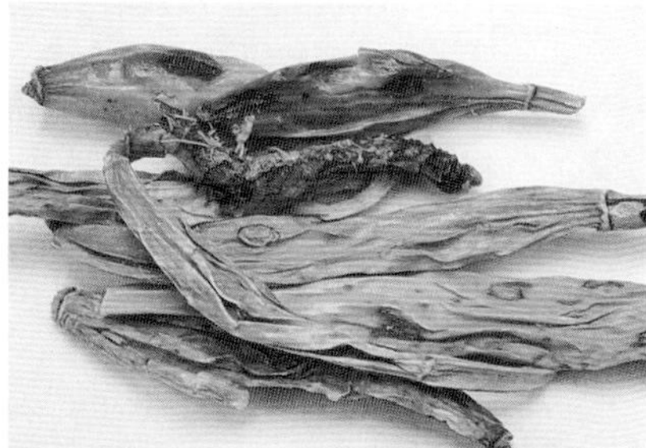

Shi Hu (Herba Dendrobii)

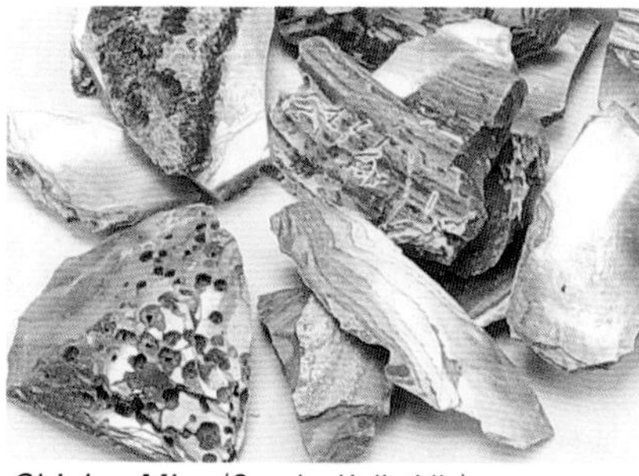

Shi Jue Ming (Concha Haliotidis)

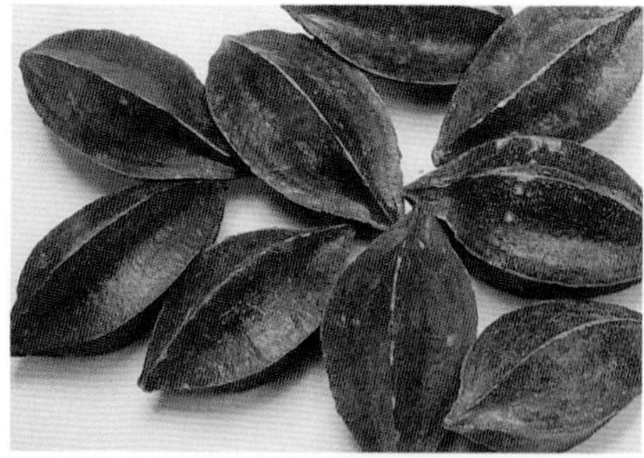

Shi Jun Zi (Fructus Quisqualis)

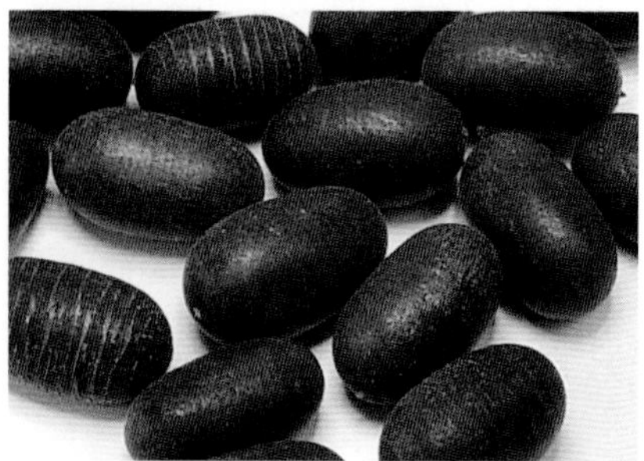

Shi Lian Zi (Herba Sinocrassulae Indicae)

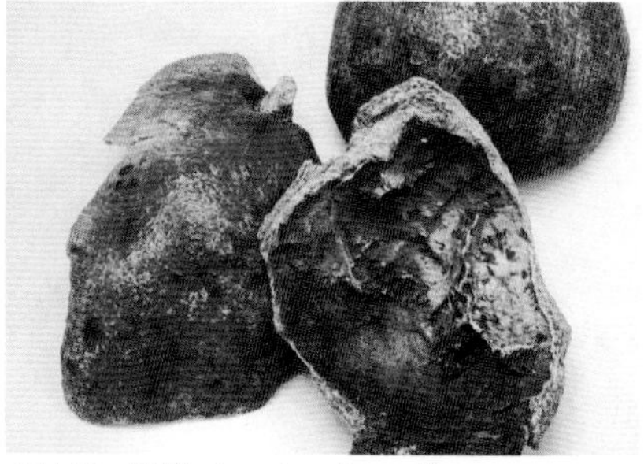

Shi Liu Pi (Pericarpium Granati)

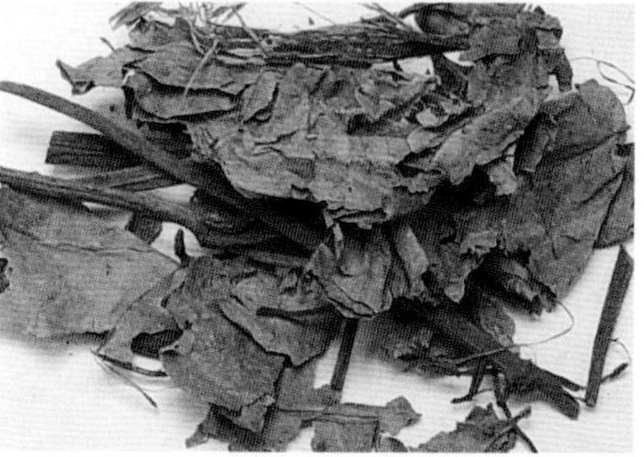

Shi Nan Teng (Ramulus Piper)

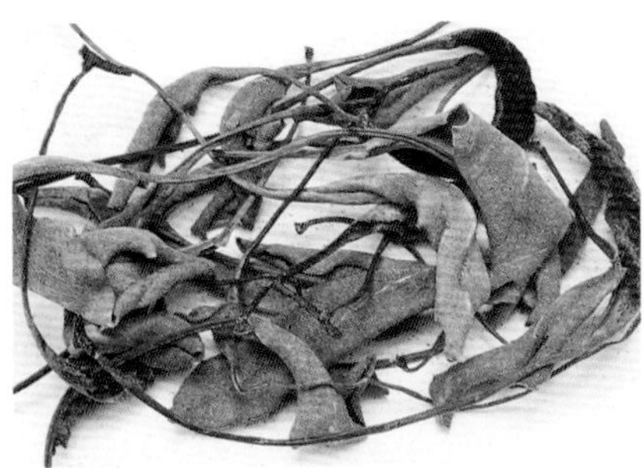
Shi Wei (Folium Pyrrosiae)

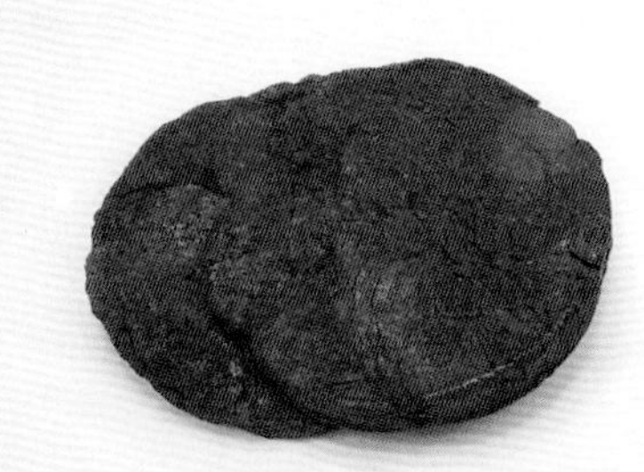
Shu Di Huang (Radix Rehmanniae Preparata)

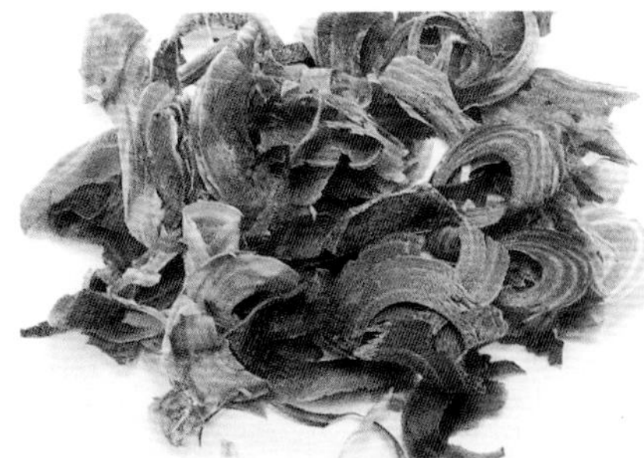
Shui Niu Jiao (Cornu Bubali)

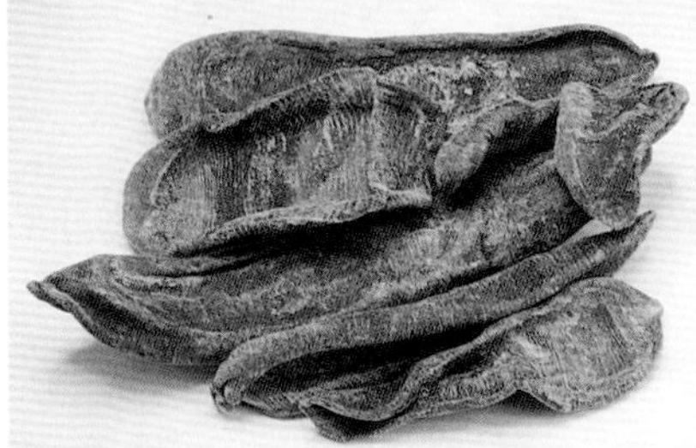
Shui Zhi (Hirudo)

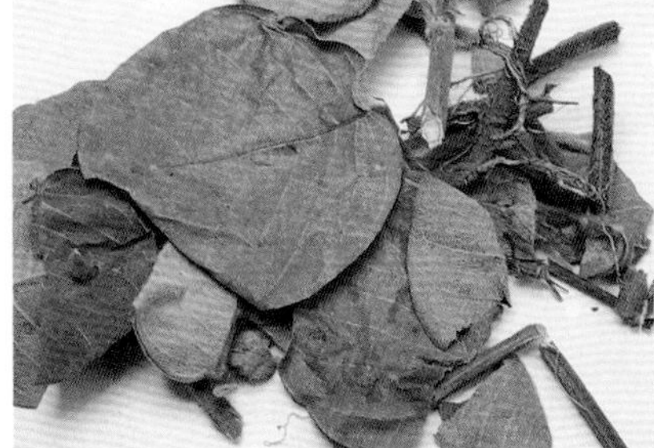
Si Chuan Da Jin Qian Cao (Herba Lysimachia Christinae)

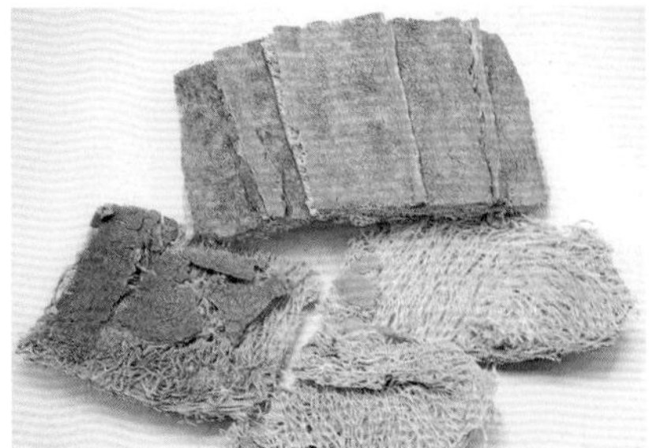
Si Gua Luo (Retinervus Luffae Fructus)

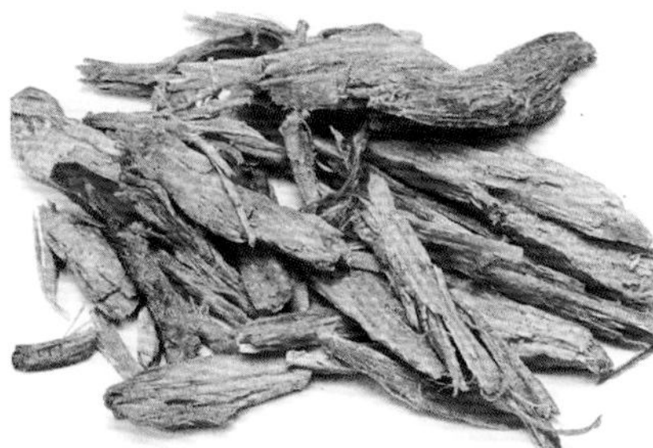
Song Jie (Lignum Pini Nodi)

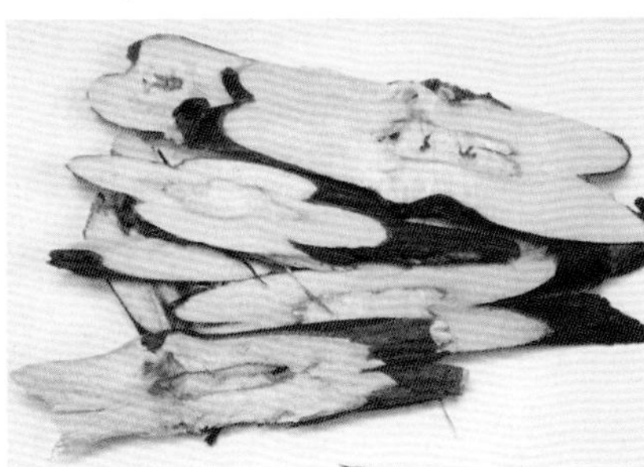
Su Geng (Caulis Perillae)

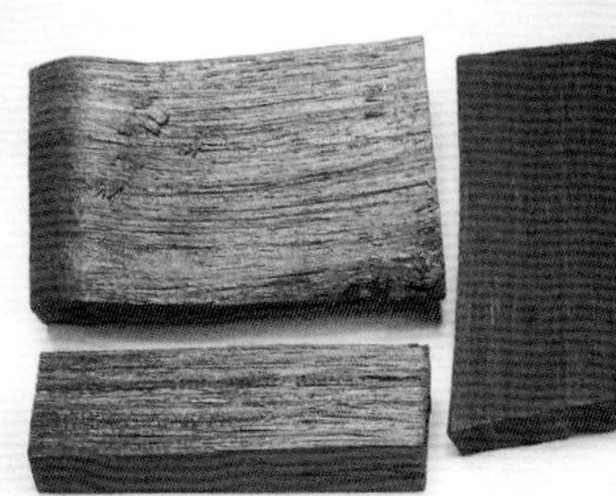
Su Mu (Lignum Sappan)

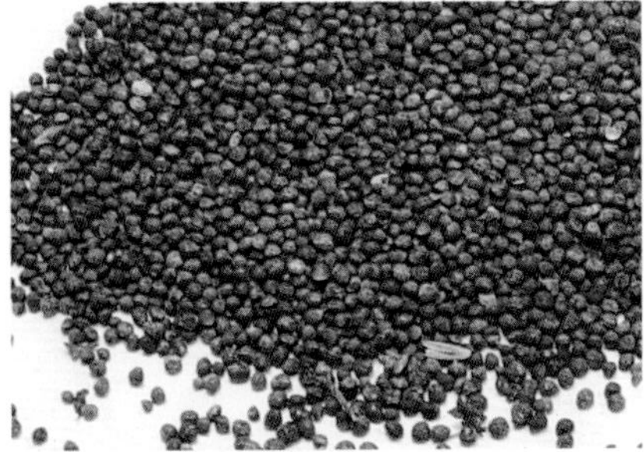
Su Zi (Fructus Perillae)

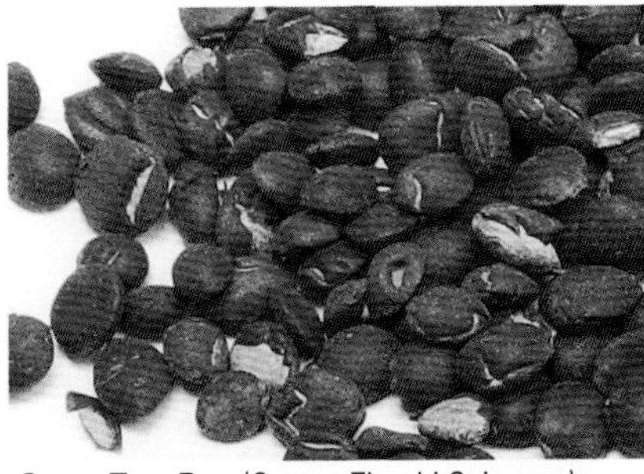
Suan Zao Ren (Semen Zizyphi Spinosae)

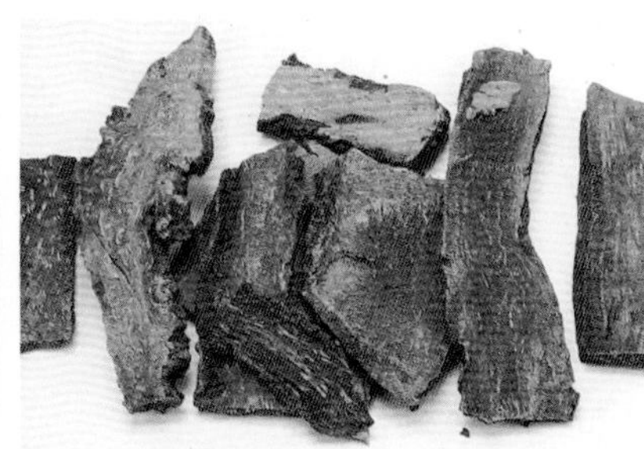
Suo Yang (Herba Cynomorii)

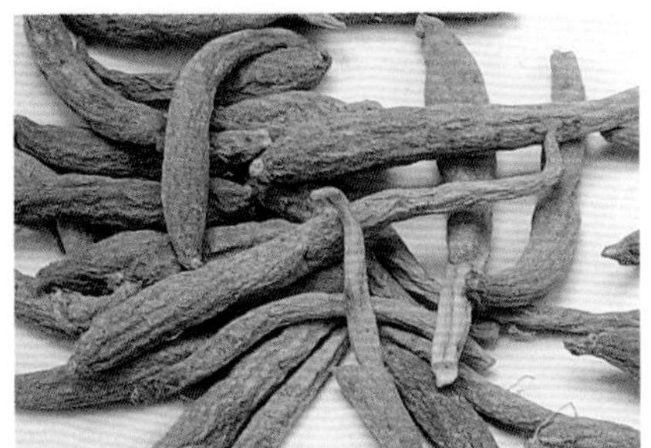
Tai Zi Shen (Radix Pseudostellariae)

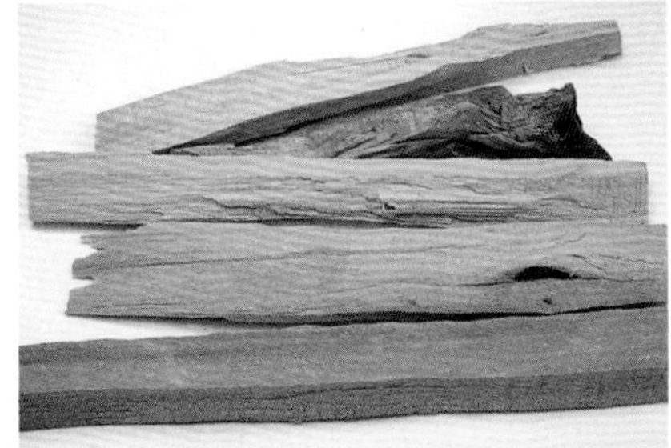
Tan Xiang (Lignum Santali Albi)

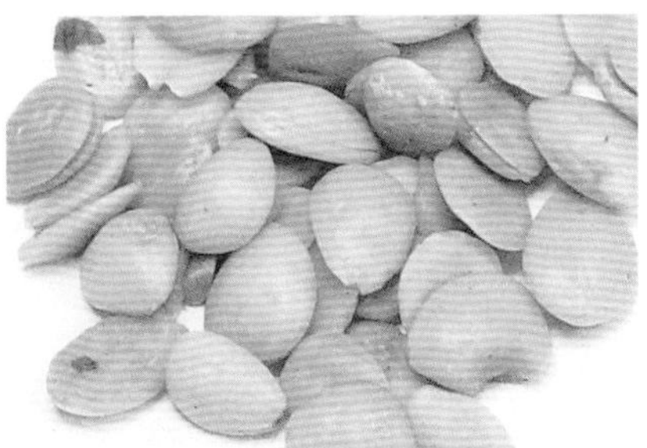
Tao Ren (Semen Persicae)

Herb Indentification Guide

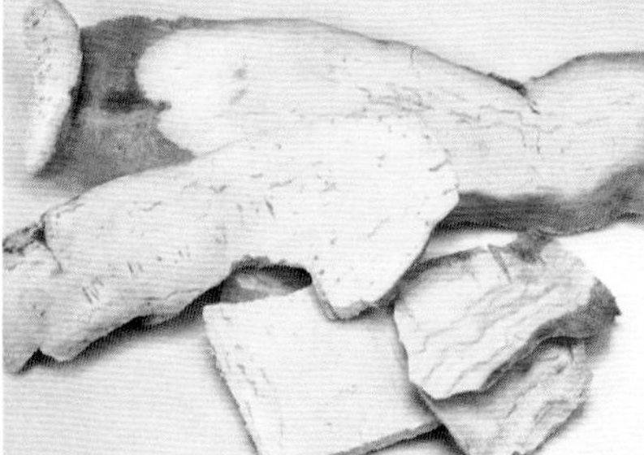
Tian Hua Fen (Radix Trichosanthis)

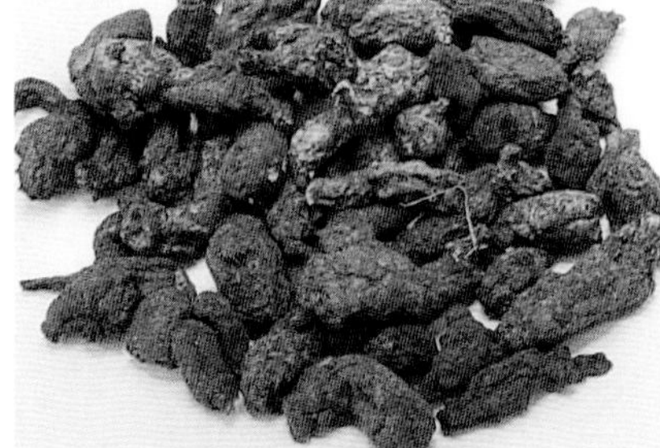
Tian Kui Zi (Radix Semiaquilegiae)

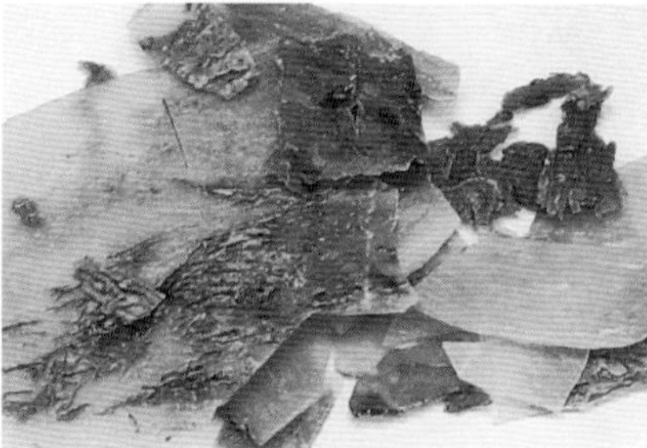
Tian Ma (Rhizoma Gastrodiae)

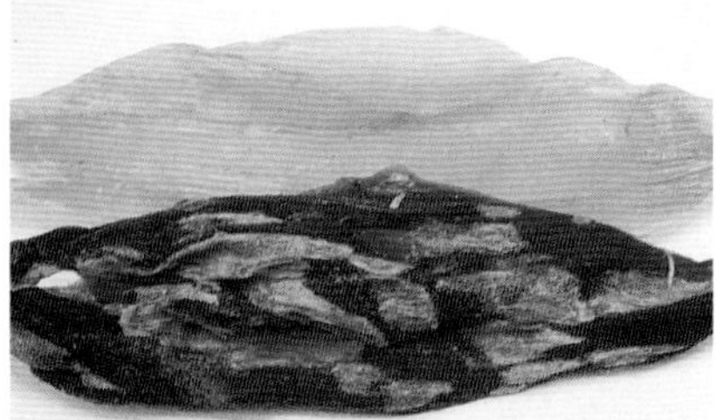
Tian Men Dong (Radix Asparagi)

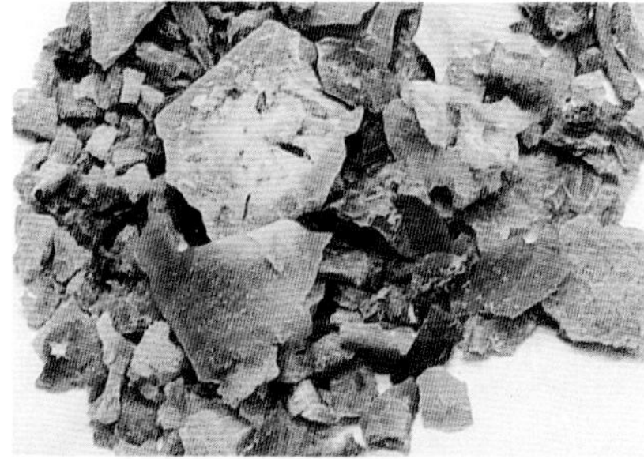
Tian Nan Xing (Rhizoma Arisaematis)

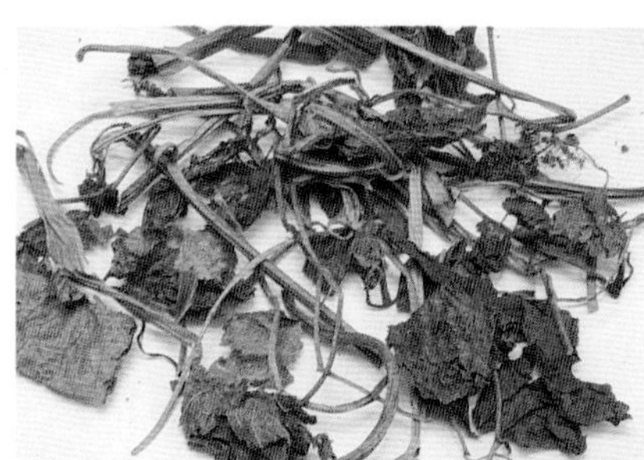
Tian Xian Teng (Herba Aristolochiae)

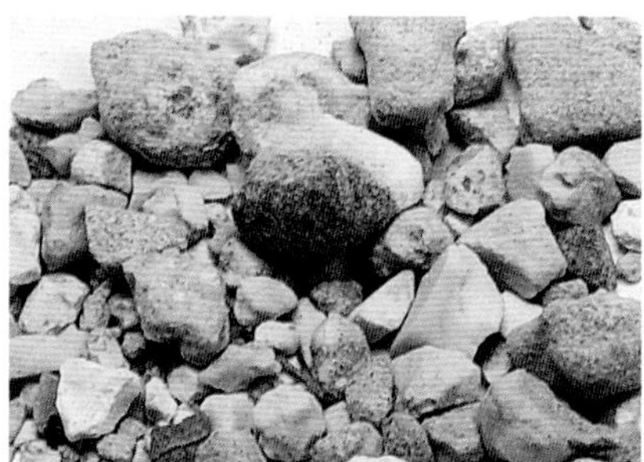
Tian Zhu Huang (Concretio Silicea Bambusae)

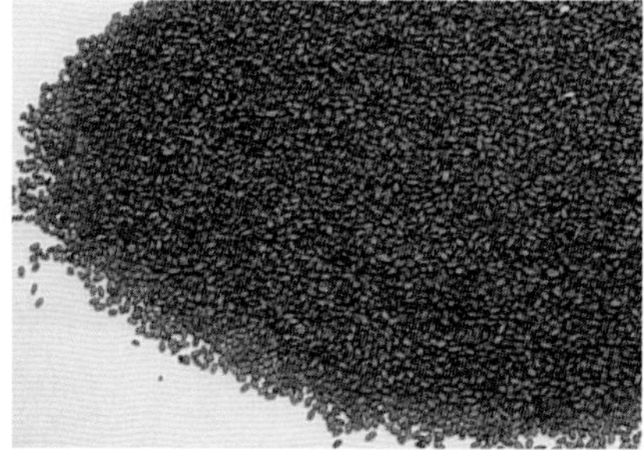
Ting Li Zi (Semen Descurainiae seu Lepidii)

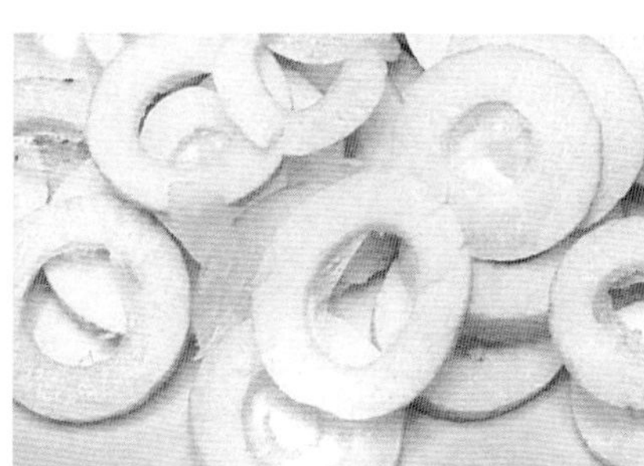
Tong Cao (Medulla Tetrapanacis)

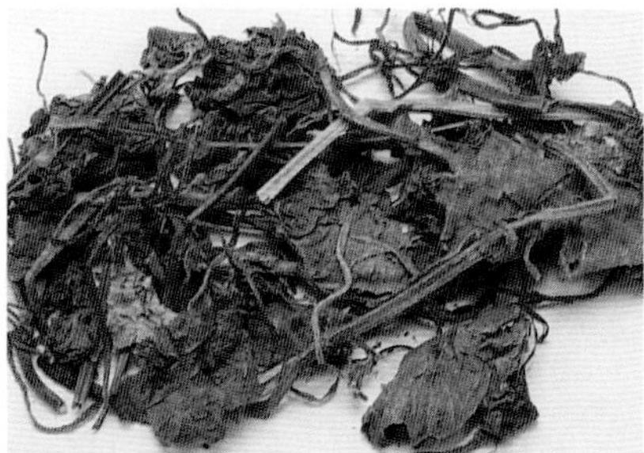
Tou Gu Cao (Caulis Impatientis)

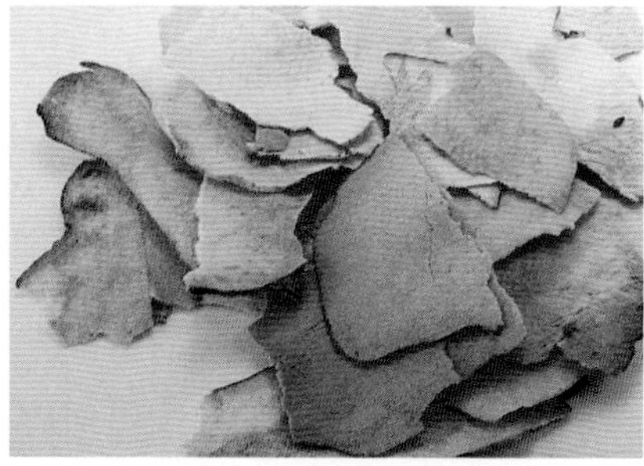
Tu Fu Ling (Rhizoma Smilacis Glabrae)

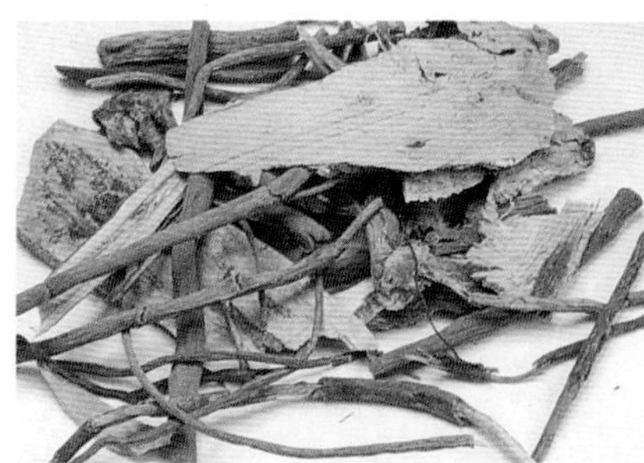
Tu Niu Xi (Radix Achyranthes Longifolia)

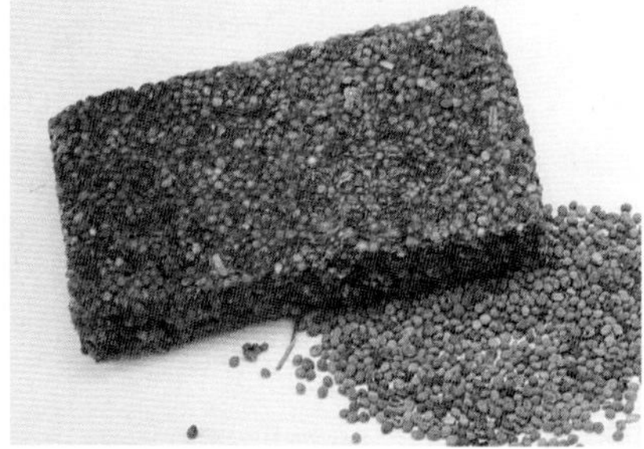
Tu Si Zi (Semen Cuscutae)

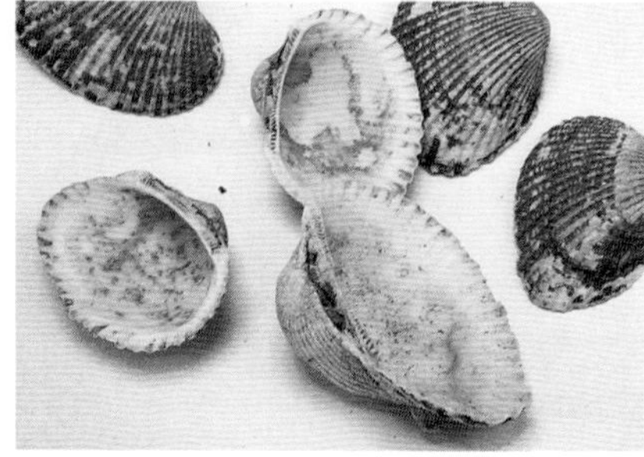
Wa Leng Zi (Concha Arcae)

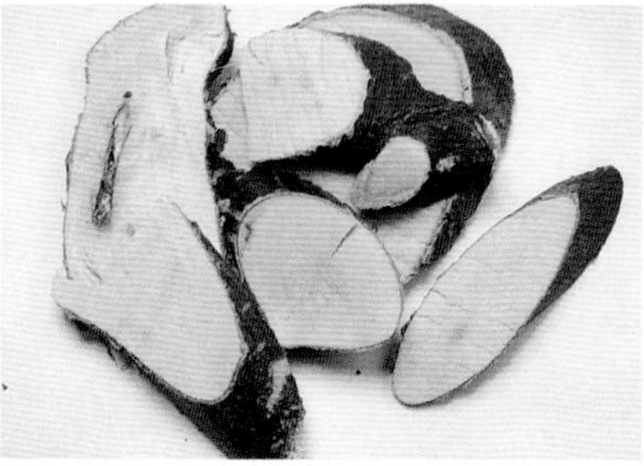
Wan Dian Jin (Radix Ilicis Asprellae)

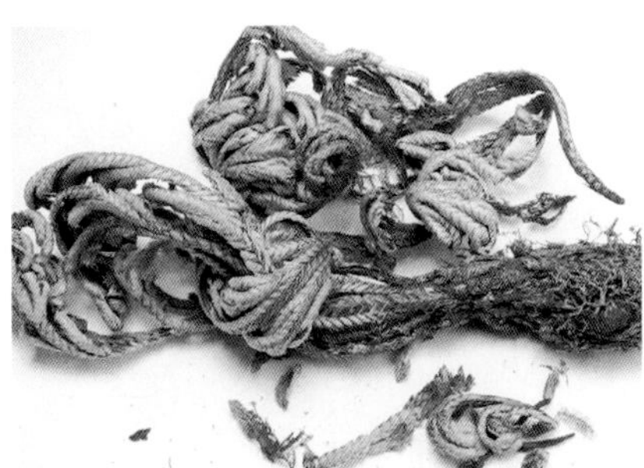
Wan Nian Song (Herba Selaginellae)

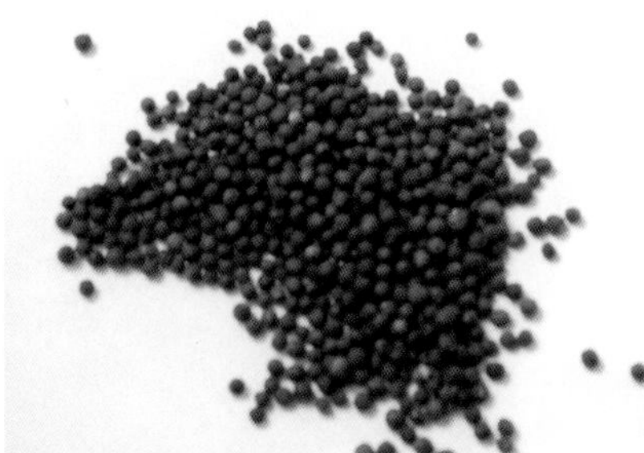
Wang Bu Liu Xing (Semen Vaccariae)

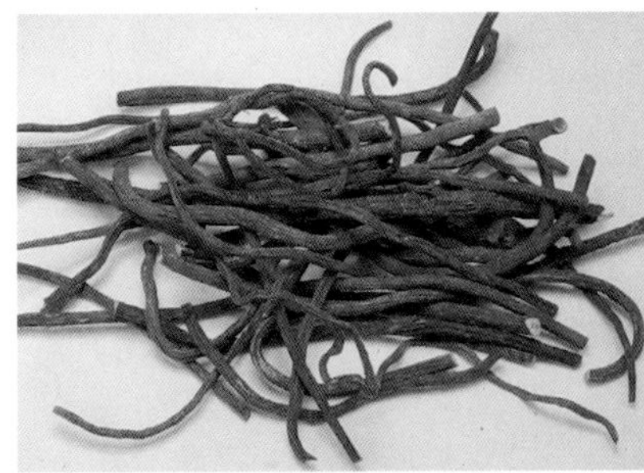
Wei Ling Xian (Radix Clematidis)

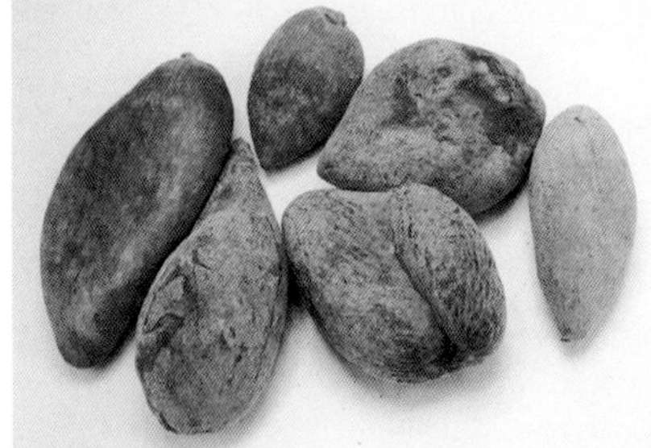
Wu Bei Zi (Galla Chinensis)

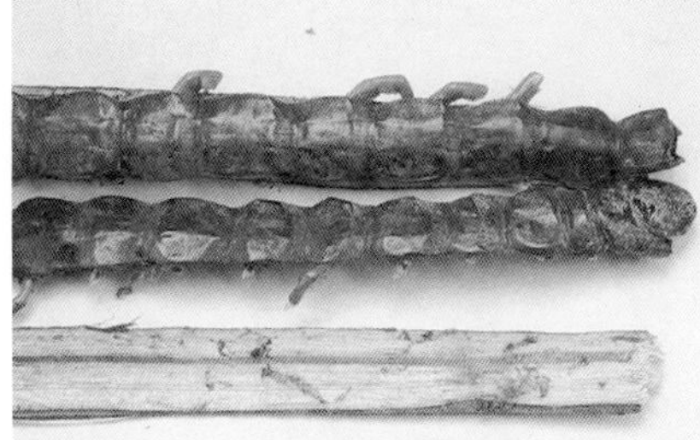
Wu Gong (Scolopendra)

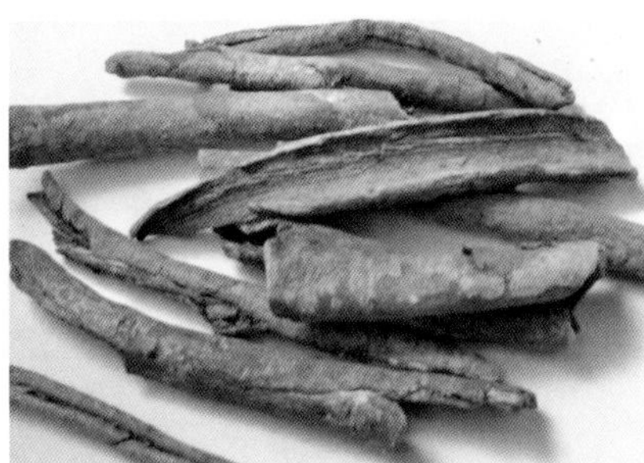
Wu Jia Pi (Cortex Acanthopanacis)

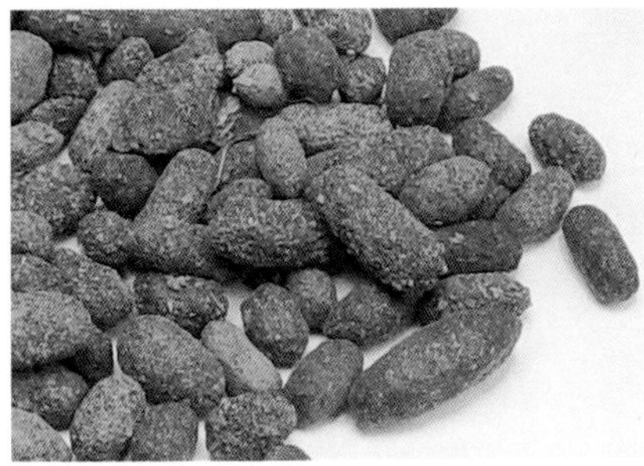
Wu Ling Zhi
(Excrementum Trogopteri seu Pteromi)

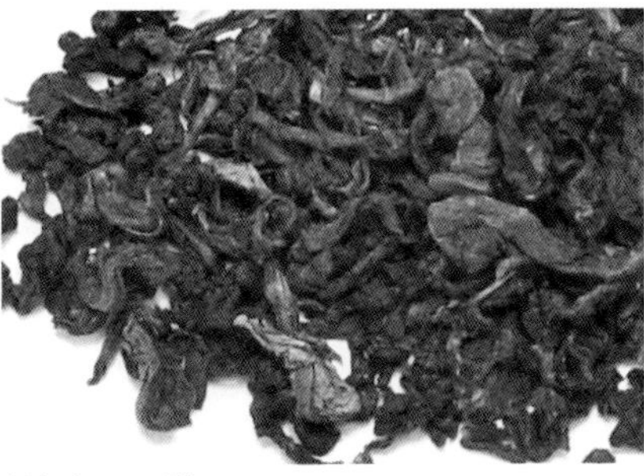
Wu Long Cha
(Folium Camellia Sinensis Fermentata)

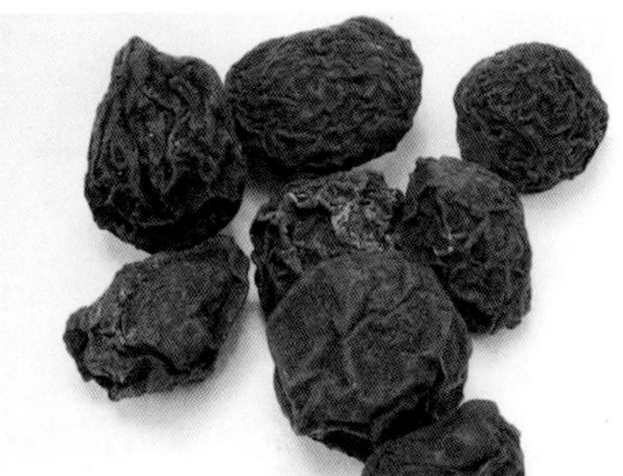
Wu Mei (Fructus Mume)

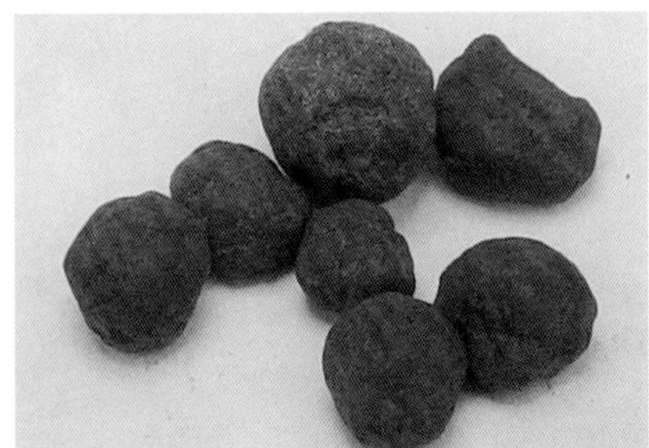
Wu Ming Yi (Pyrolusitum)

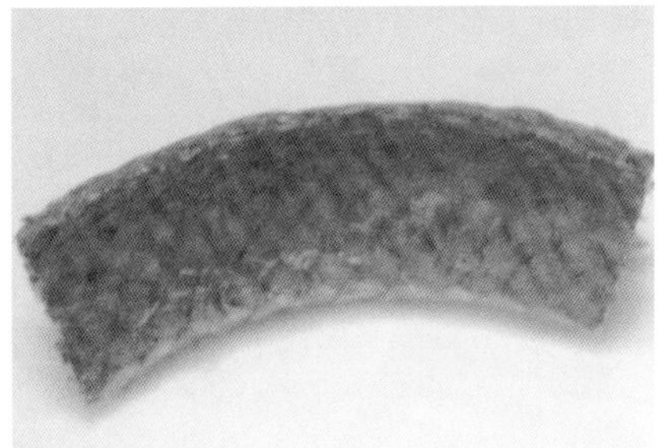
Wu Shao She (Zaocys)

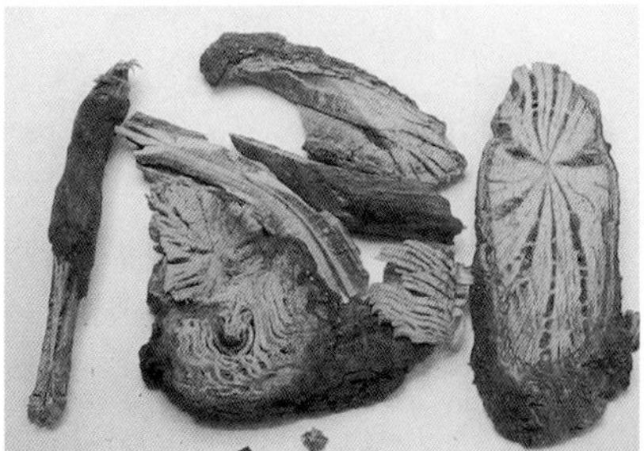
Wu Teng (Ramulus Linderae Strychnifolia)

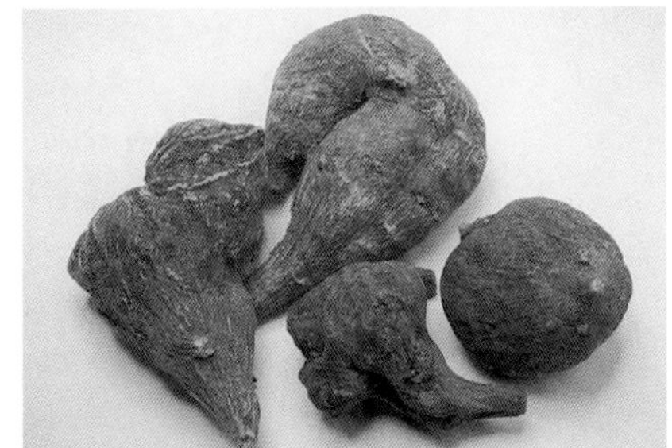
Wu Tou (Radix Aconiti)

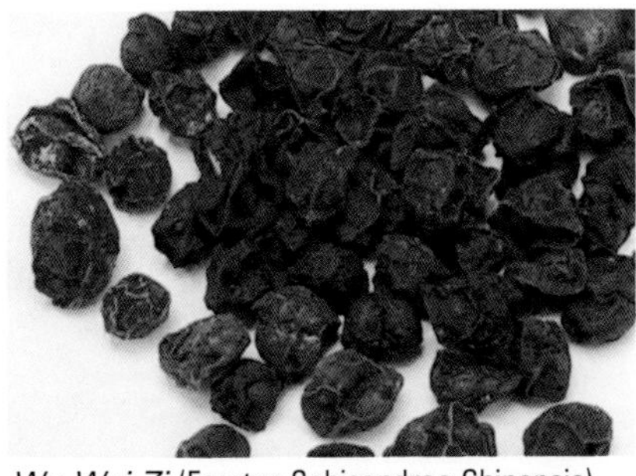
Wu Wei Zi (Fructus Schisandrae Chinensis)

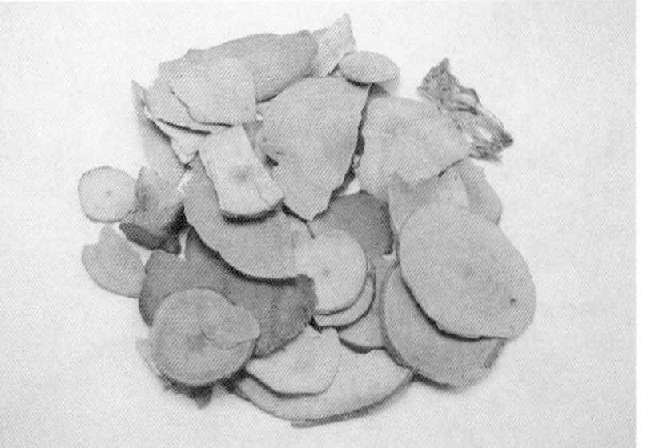
Wu Yao (Radix Linderae)

Herb Indentification Guide

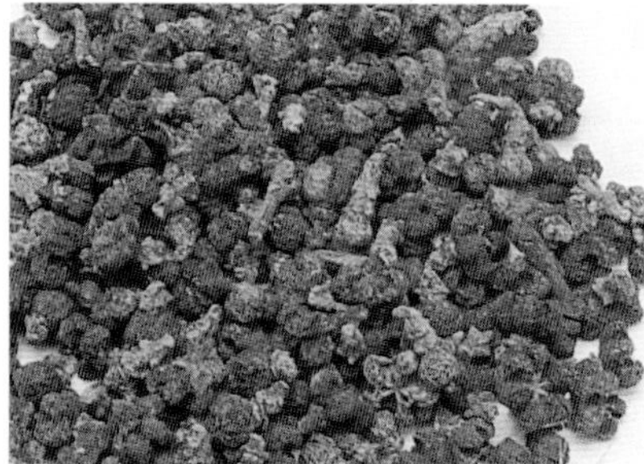
Wu Zhu Yu (Fructus Evodiae)

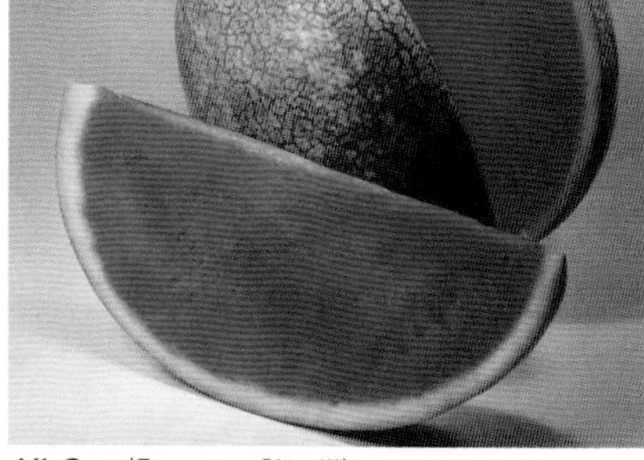
Xi Gua (Frucutus Citrulli)

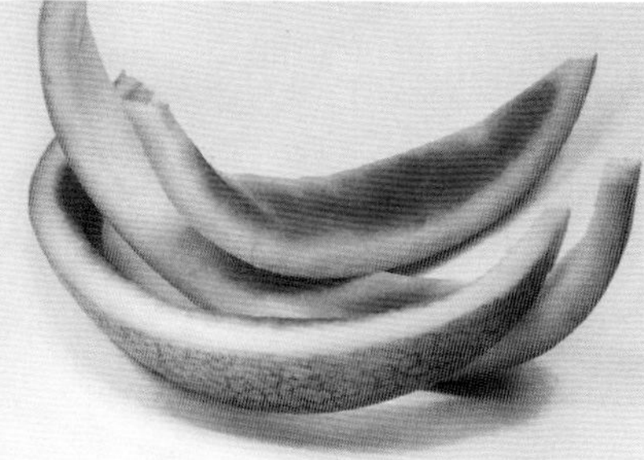
Xi Gua Pi (Pericarpium Citrulli)

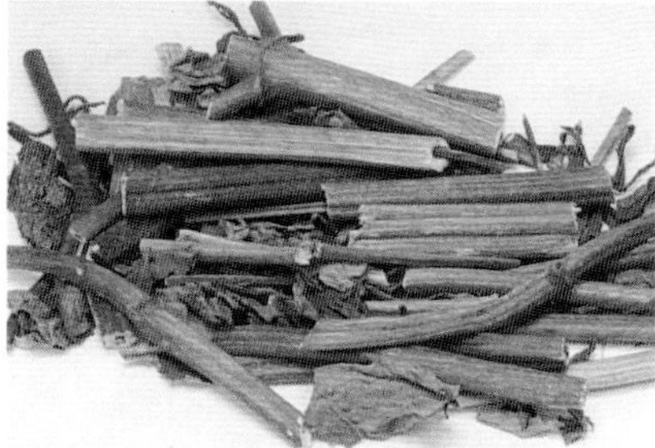
Xi Xian Cao (Herba Siegesbeckiae)

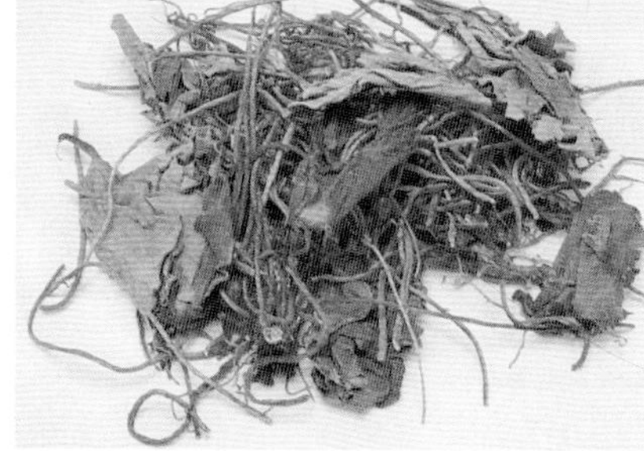
Xi Xin (Herba Asari)

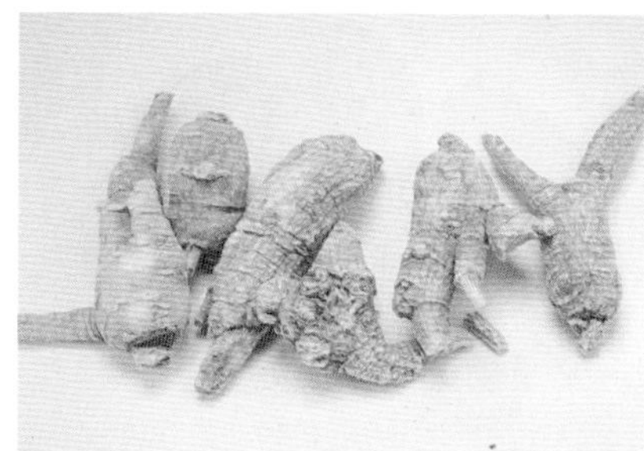
Xi Yang Shen (Radix Panacis Quinquefolii)

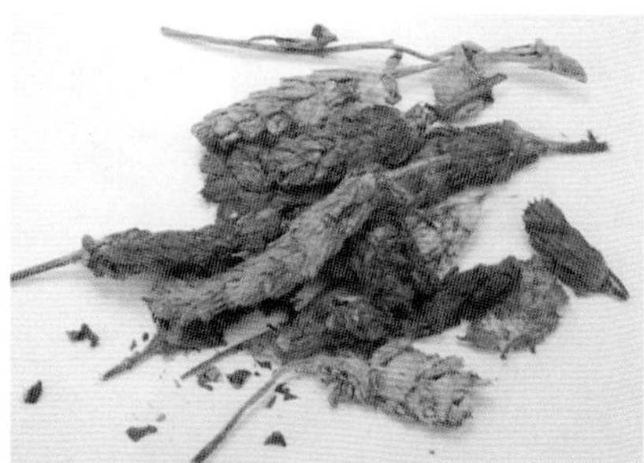
Xia Ku Cao (Spica Prunellae)

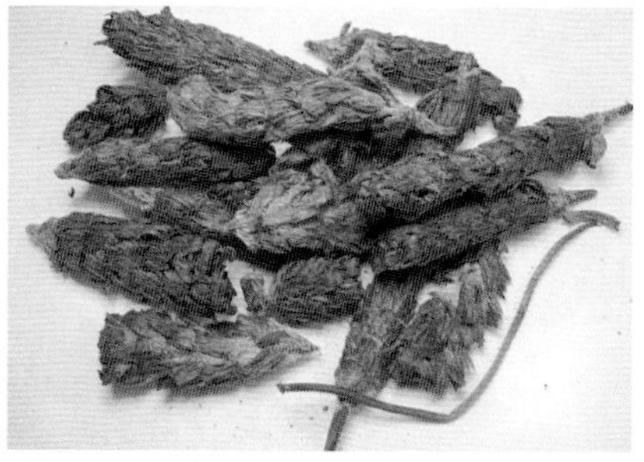
Xia Ku Hua (Flos Prunellae)

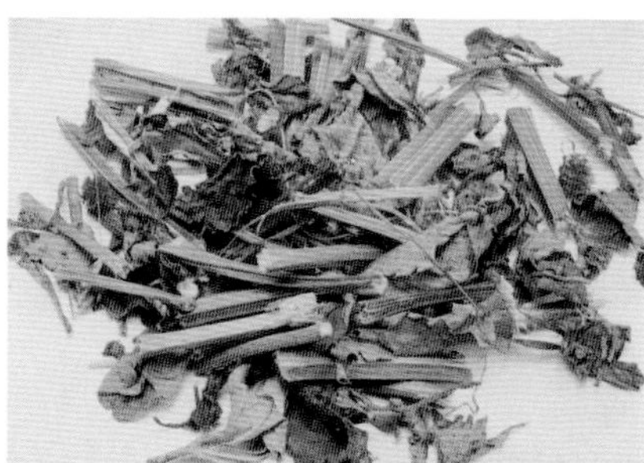
Xian Feng Cao (Herba Bidentis)

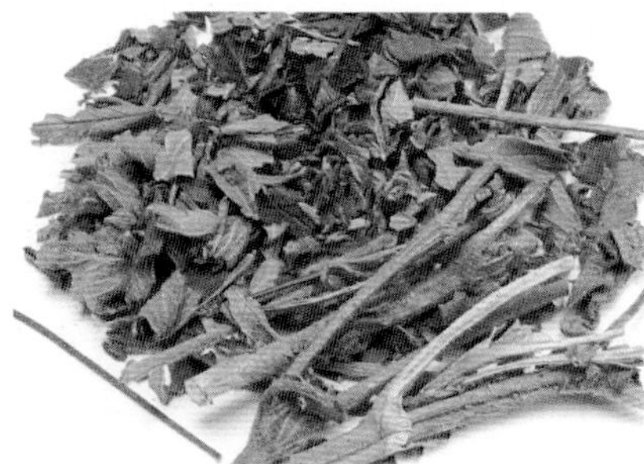
Xian He Cao (Herba Agrimoniae)

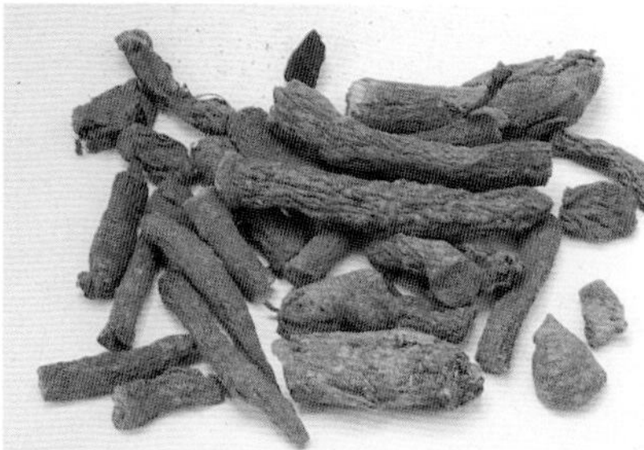
Xian Mao (Rhizoma Curculiginis)

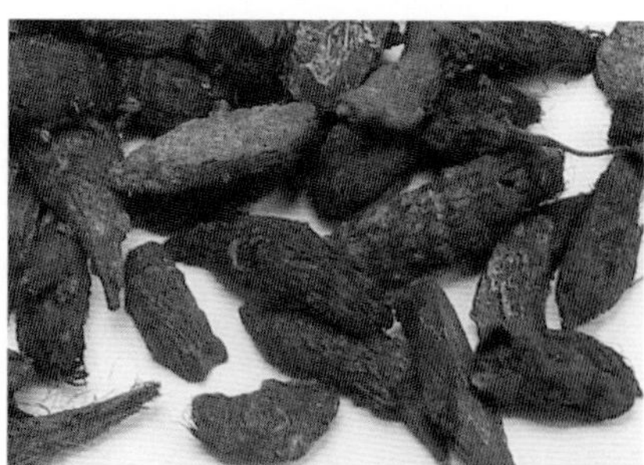
Xiang Fu (Rhizoma Cyperi)

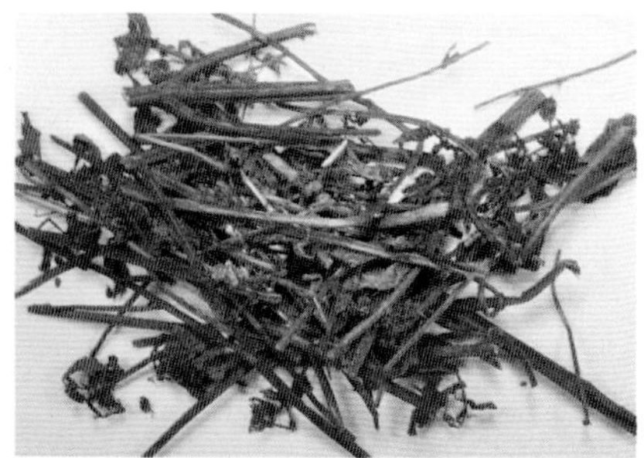
Xiang Ru (Herba Elsholtziae seu Moslae)

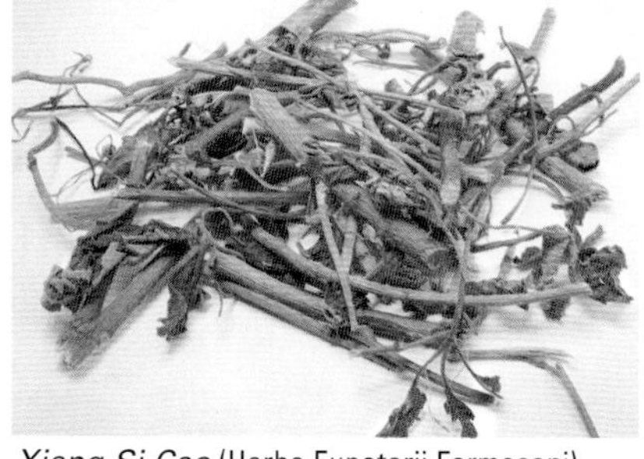
Xiang Si Cao (Herba Eupatorii Formosani)

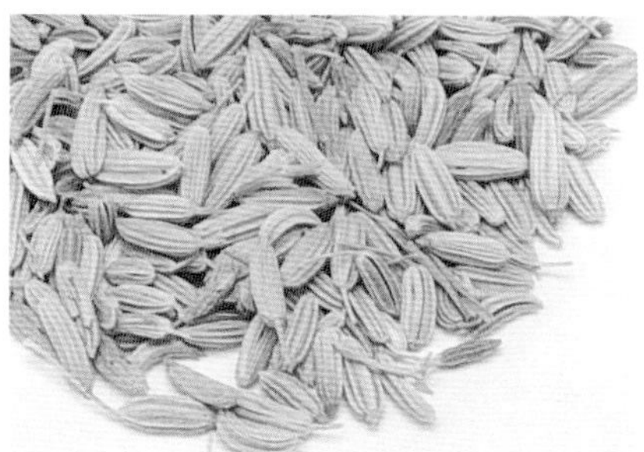
Xiao Hui Xiang (Fructus Foeniculi)

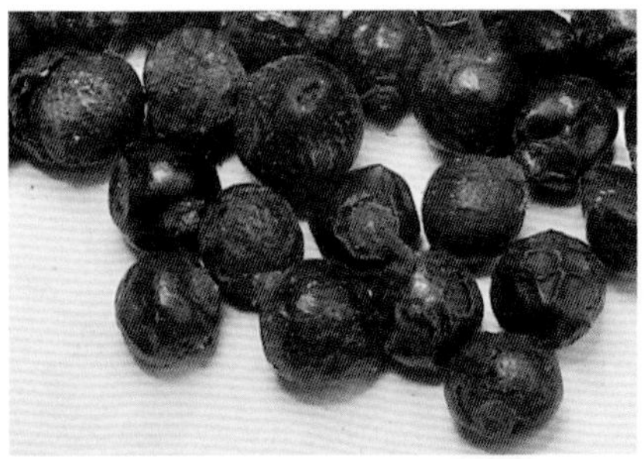
Xiao Jin Ying (Fructus Rosae Cymosae)

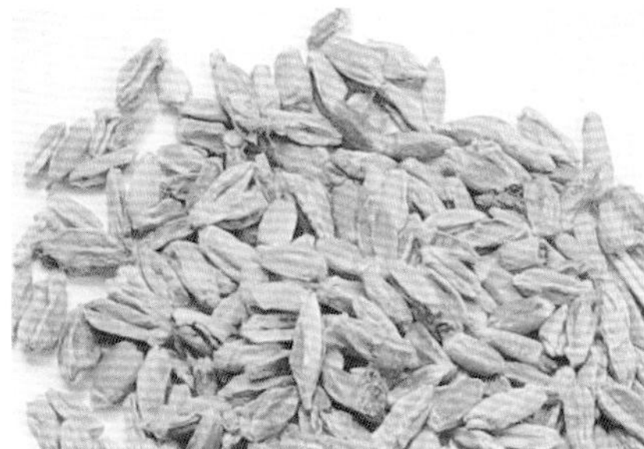
Xiao Mai (Fructus Tritici)

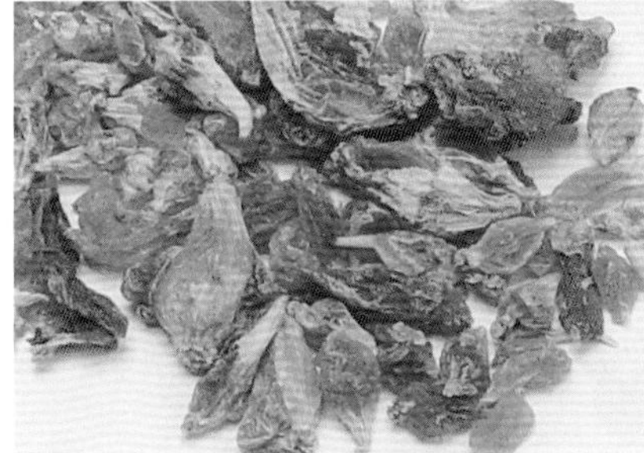
Xie Bai (Bulbus Allii Macrostemonis)

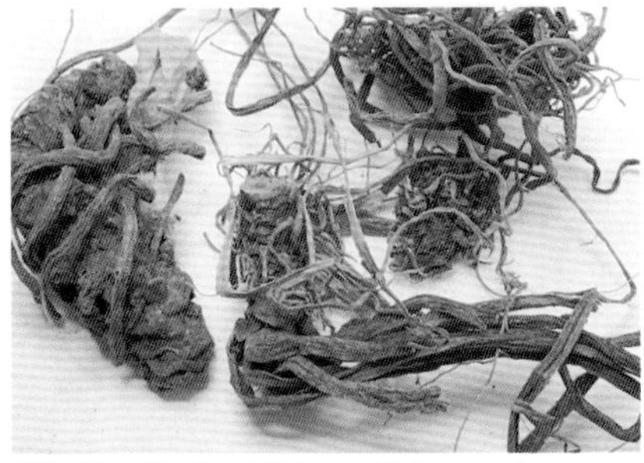
Xie Cao (Radix et Rhizoma Valerianae)

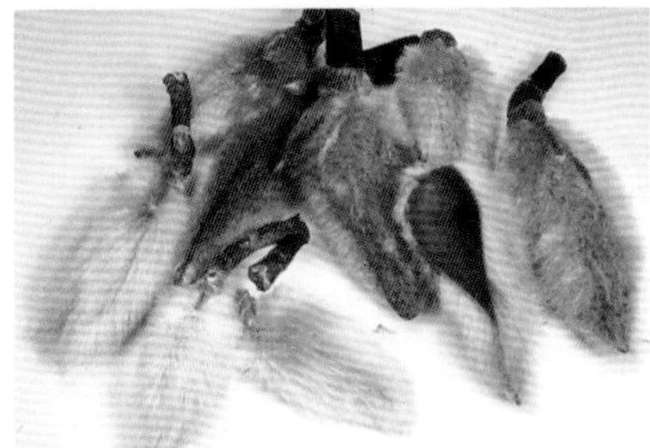
Xin Yi Hua (Flos Magnoliae)

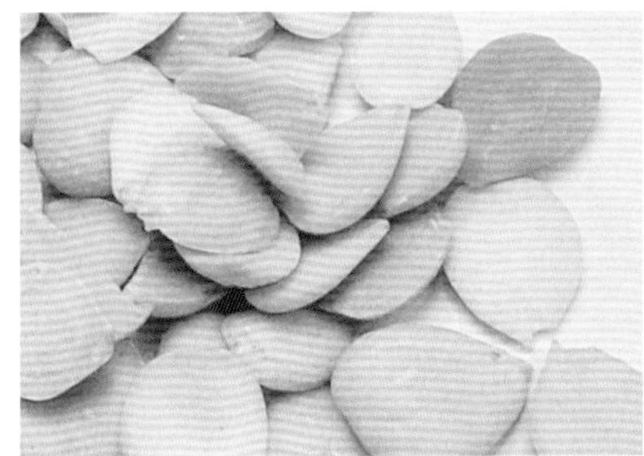
Xing Ren (Semen Armeniacae Amarum)

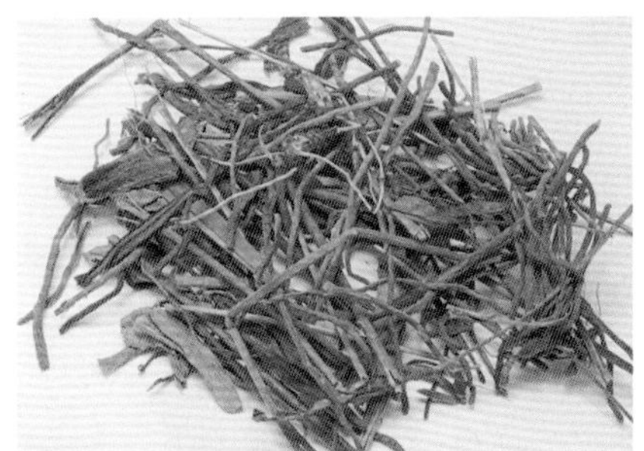
Xu Chang Qing (Radix Cynanchi Paniculati)

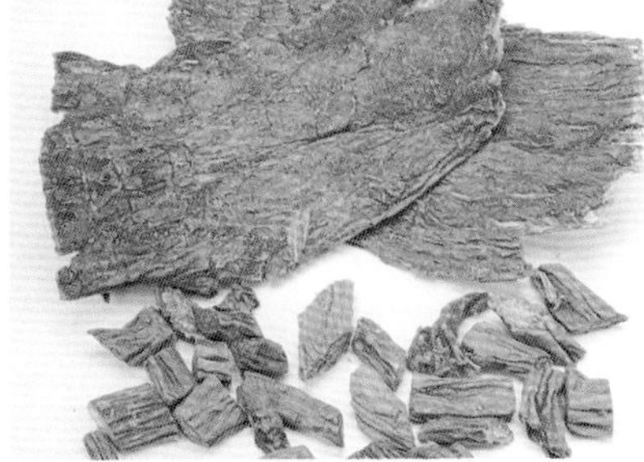
Xu Duan (Radix Dipsaci)

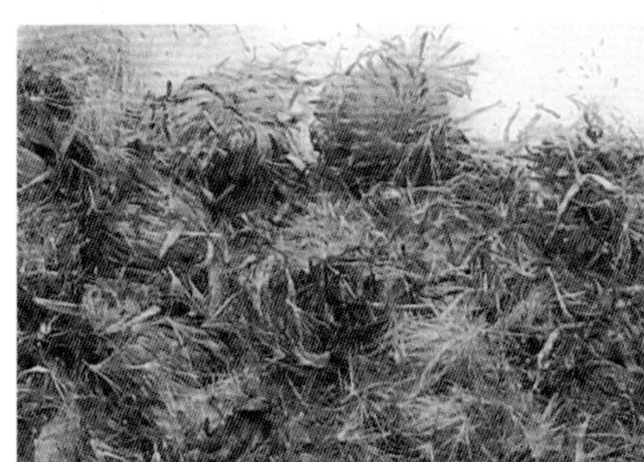
Xuan Fu Hua (Flos Inulae)

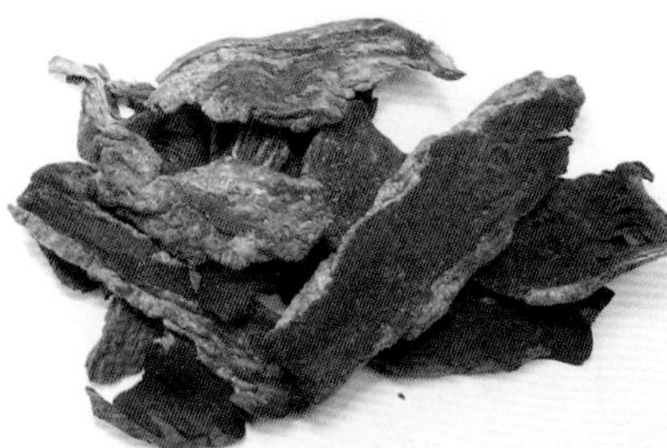
Xuan Shen (Radix Scrophulariae)

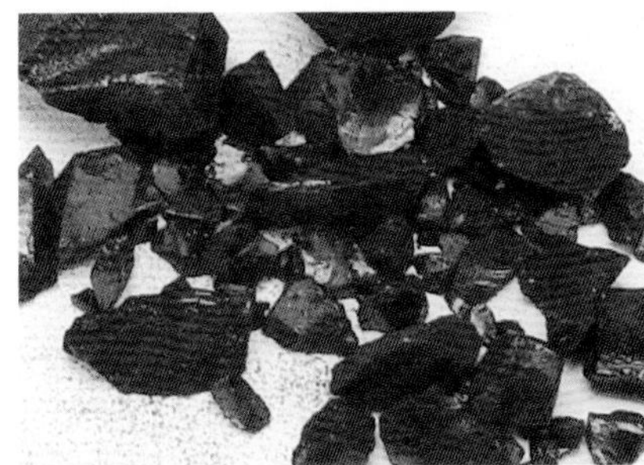
Xue Jie (Sanguis Draconis)

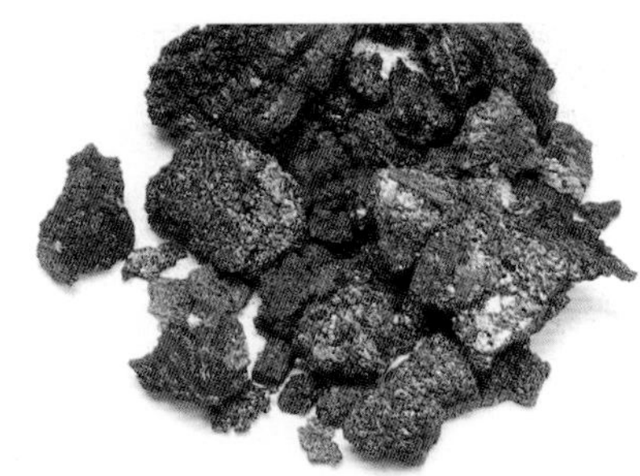
Xue Yu Tan (Crinis Carbonisatus)

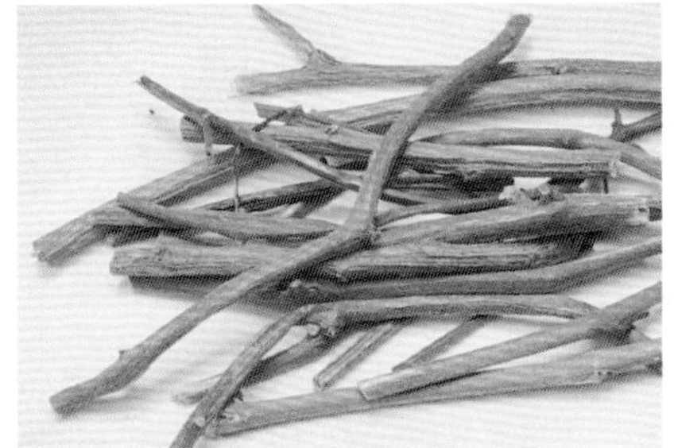
Xun Gu Feng
(Herba Aristolochiae Mollissimae)

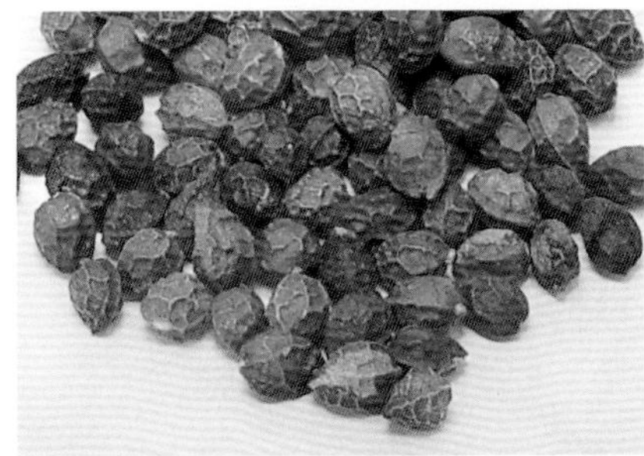
Ya Dan Zi (Fructus Bruceae)

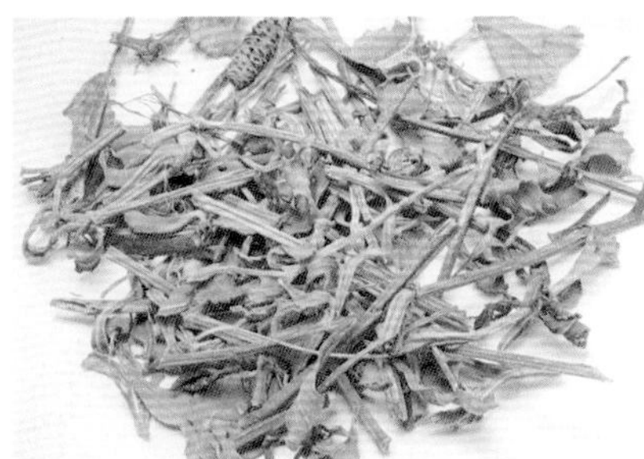
Ya She Huang (Herba Lippiae)

Herb Indentification Guide

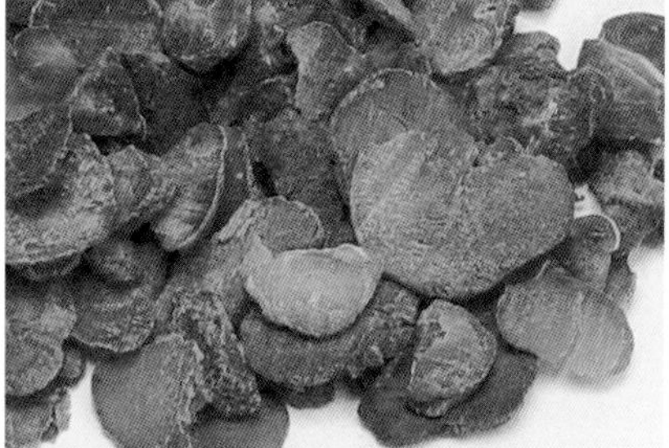
Yan Hu Suo (Rhizoma Corydalis)

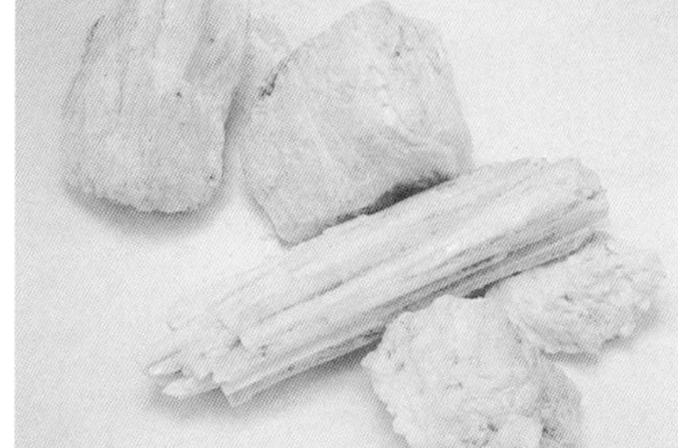
Yang Qi Shi (Actinolitum)

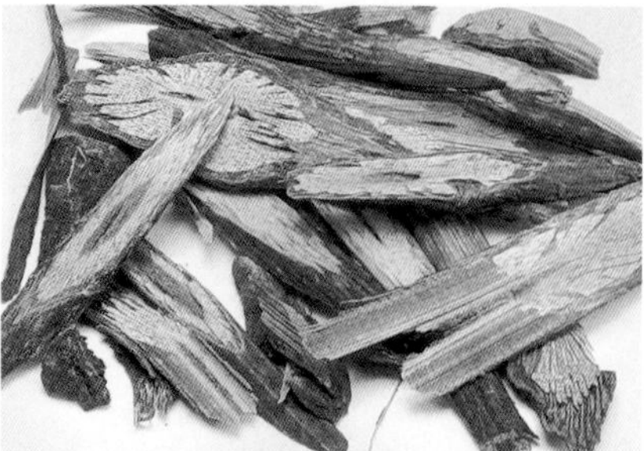
Ye Jiao Teng (Caulis Polygoni Multiflori)

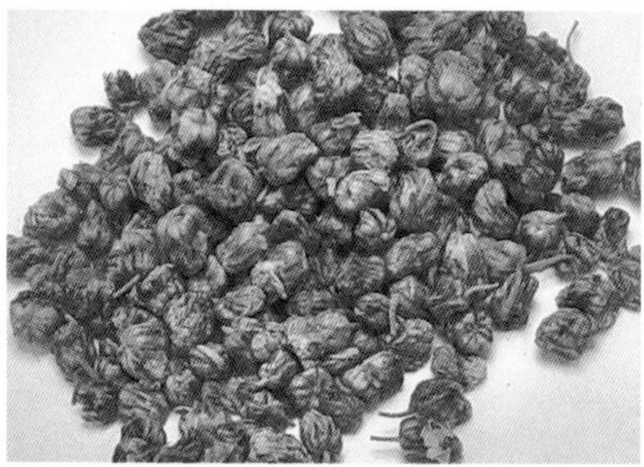
Ye Ju Hua (Flos Chrysanthemi Indici)

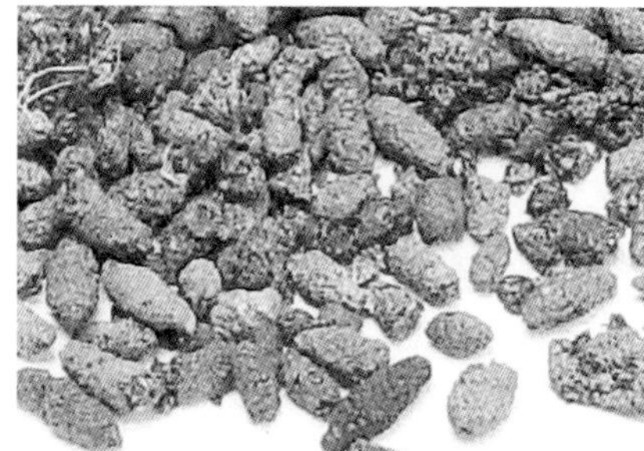
Ye Ming Sha (Excrementum Vespertilionis Murini)

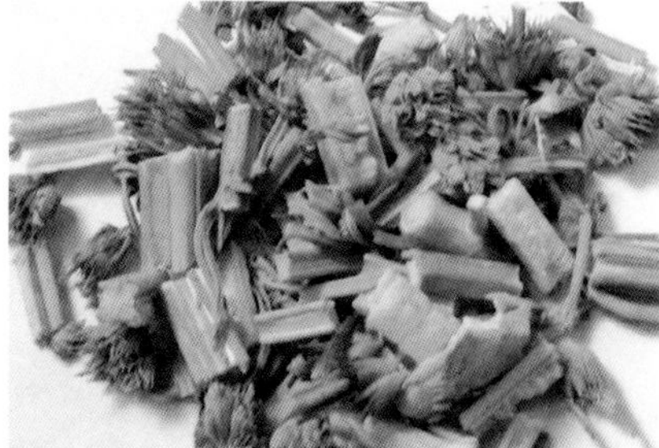
Yi Mu Cao (Herba Leonuri)

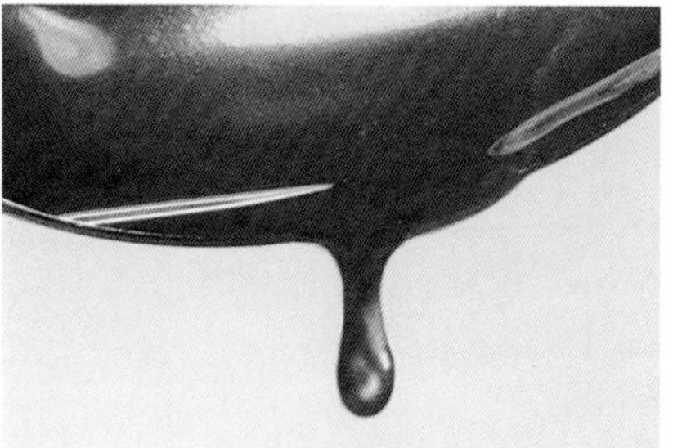
Yi Tang (Saccharum Granorum)

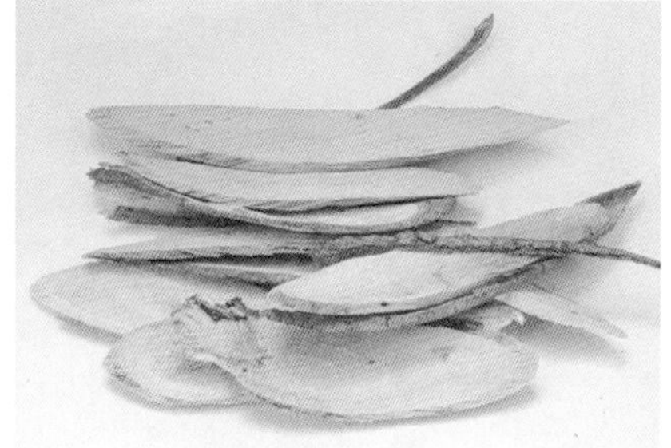
Yi Tiao Gen (Radix Moghaniae)

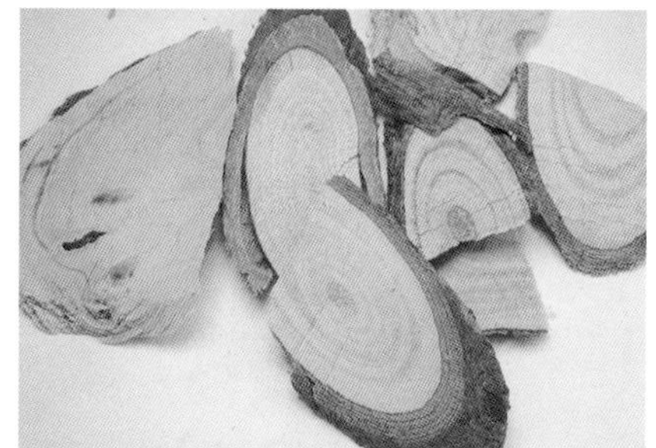
Yi Wu Gen (Radix Elaeagni)

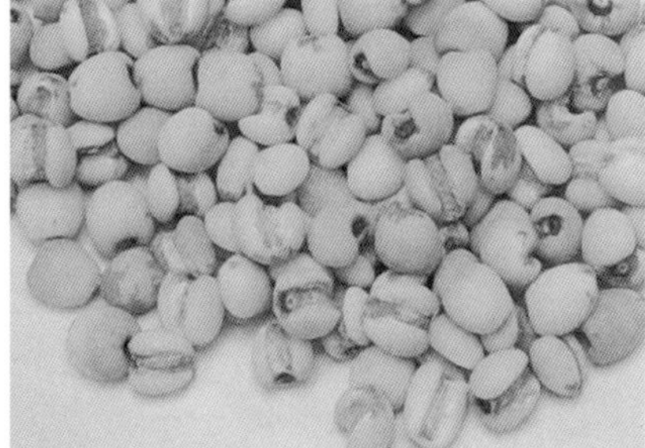
Yi Yi Ren (Semen Coicis)

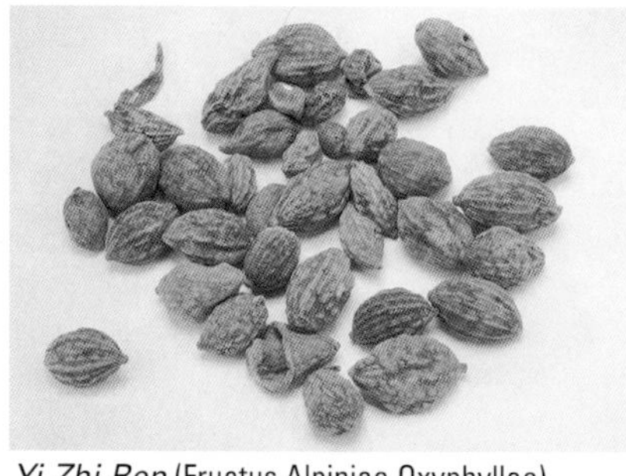
Yi Zhi Ren (Fructus Alpiniae Oxyphyllae)

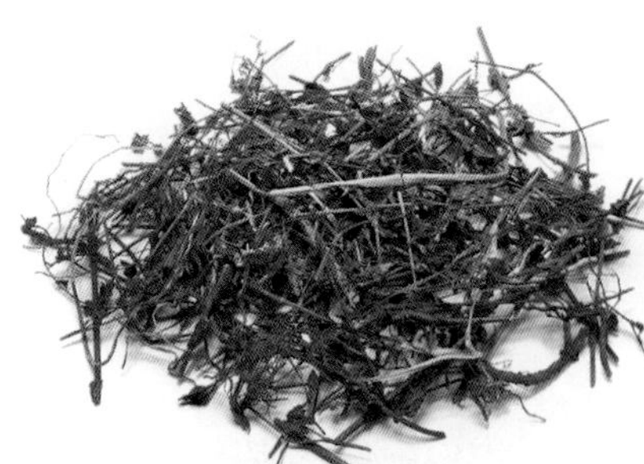
Yi Zhi Xiang (Herba Vernoniae Cinereae)

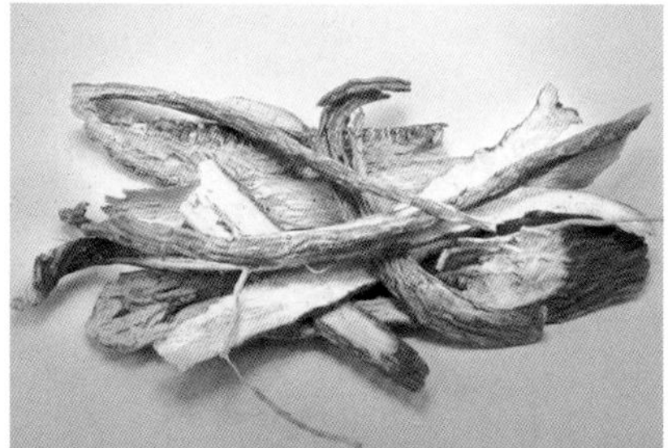
Yin Chai Hu (Radix Stellariae)

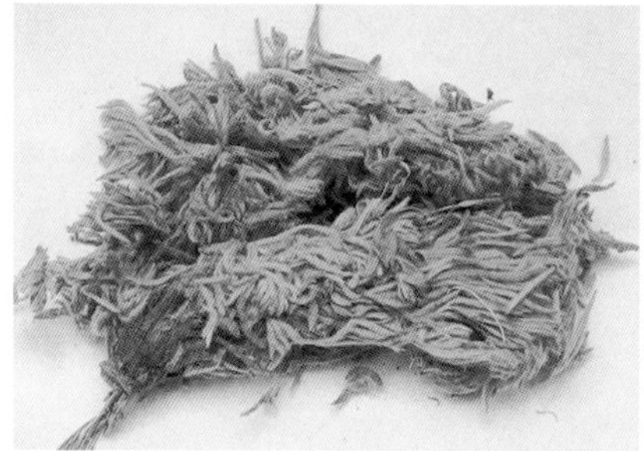
Yin Chen Hao (Herba Artemisiae Scopariae)

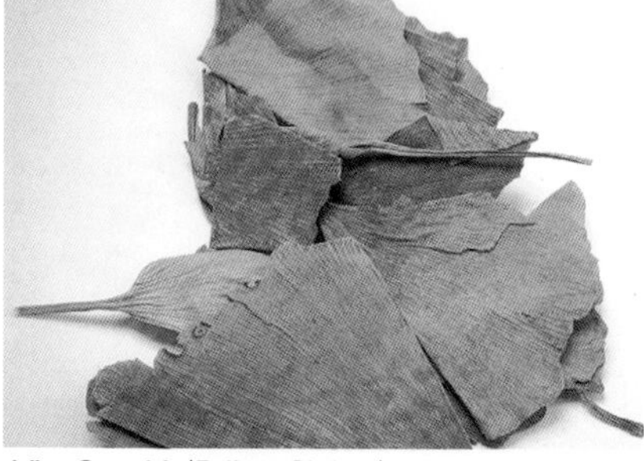
Yin Guo Ye (Folium Ginkgo)

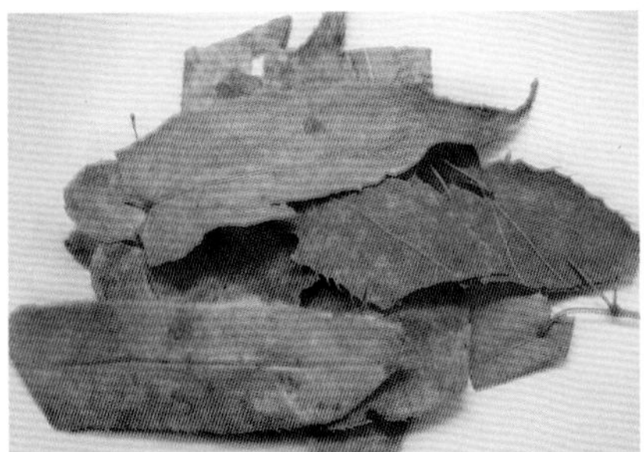
Yin Yang Huo (Herba Epimedii)

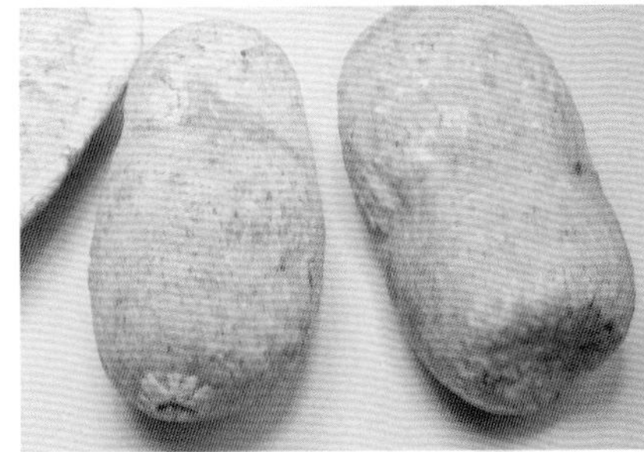
Yu Bai Fu (Rhizoma Typhonium Giganteum)

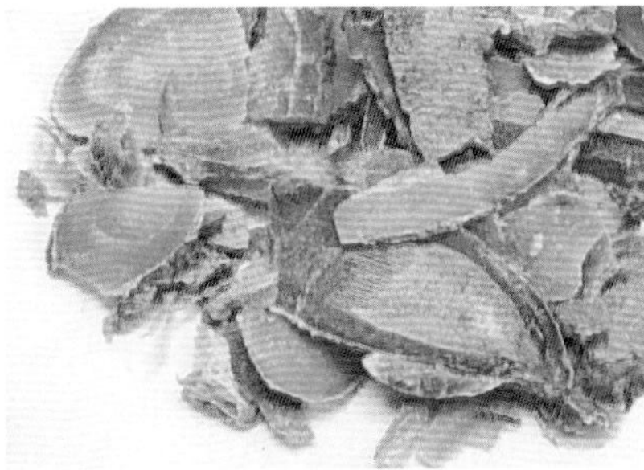
Yu Jin (Radix Curcumae)

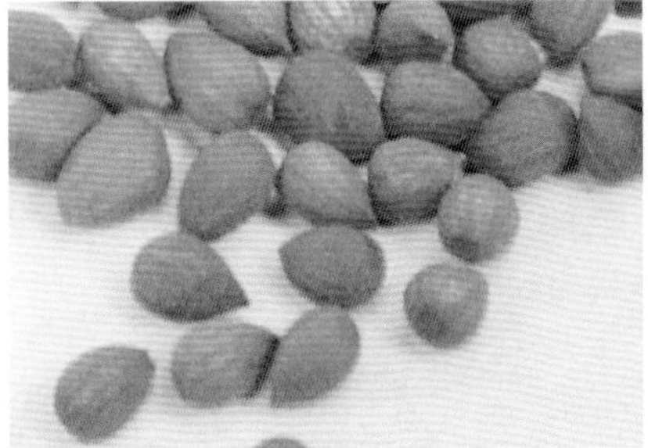
Yu Li Ren (Semen Pruni)

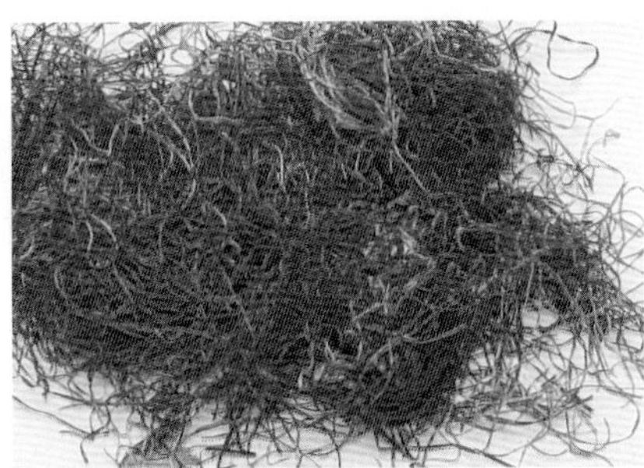
Yu Mi Xu (Stigma Maydis)

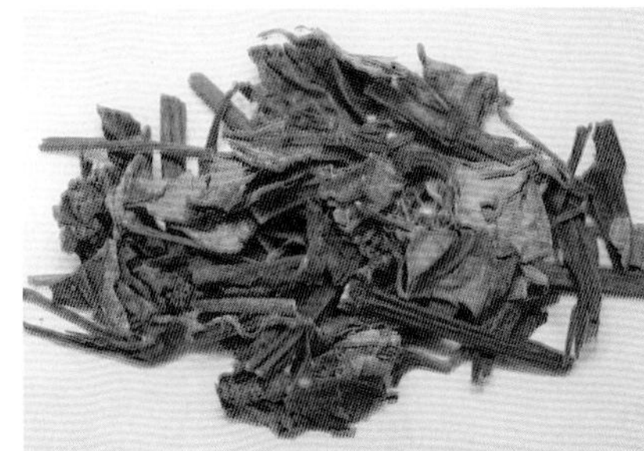
Yu Xing Cao (Herba Houttoyniae)

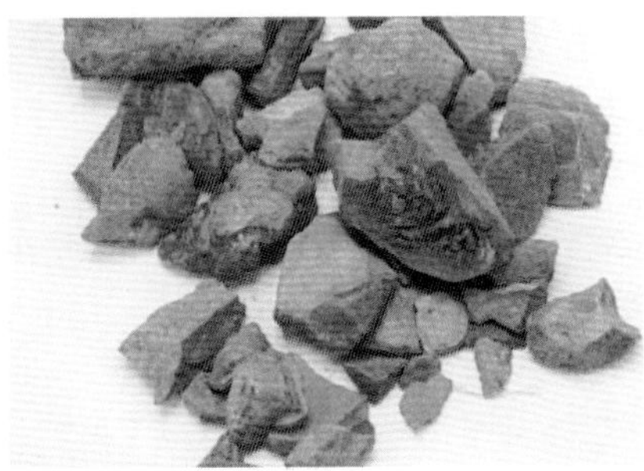
Yu Yu Liang (Limonitum)

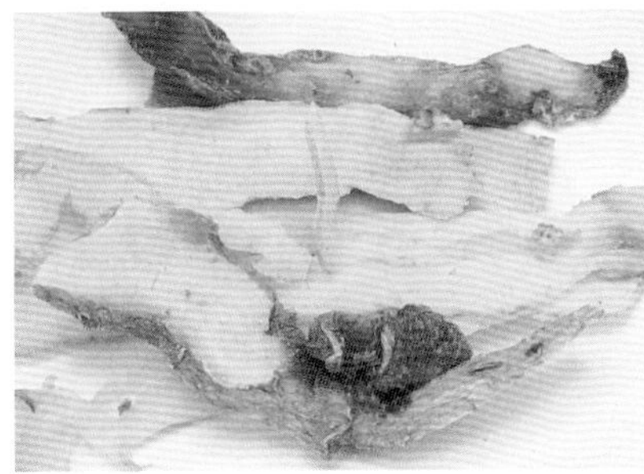
Yu Zhu (Rhizoma Polygonati Odorati)

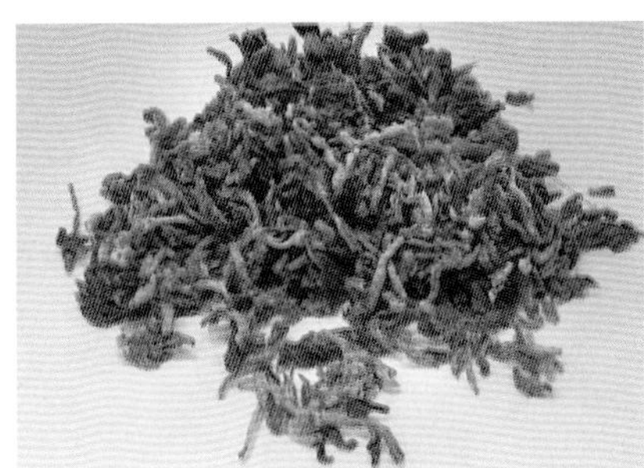
Yuan Hua (Flos Genkwa)

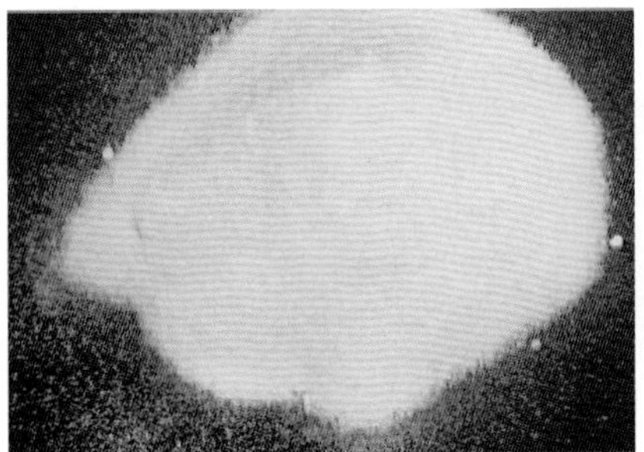
Yuan Ming Fen (Matrii Sulfas Exsiccatus)

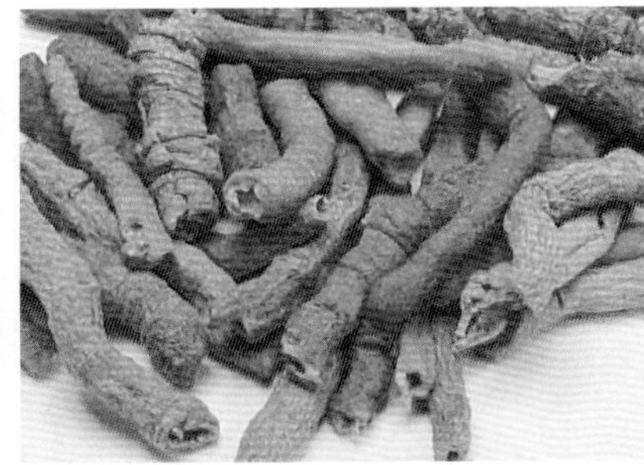
Yuan Zhi (Radix Polygalae)

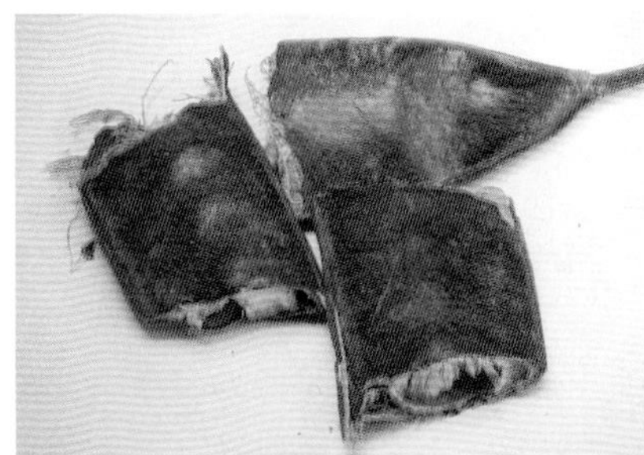
Zao Jiao (Fructus Gleditsiae)

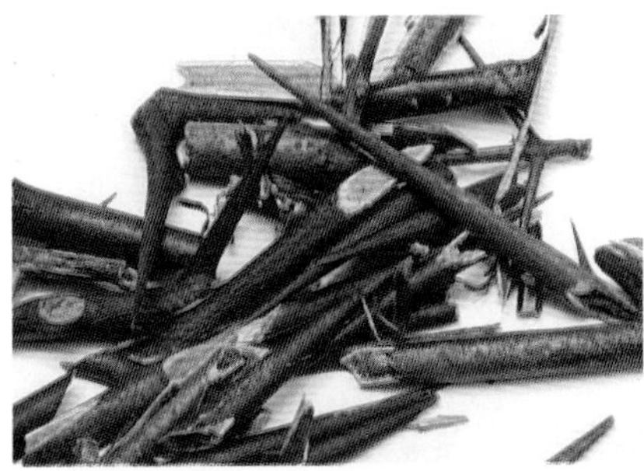
Zao Jiao Ci (Spina Gleditsiae)

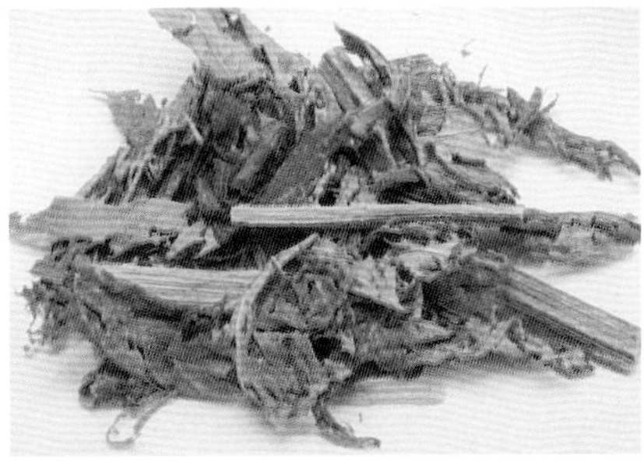
Ze Lan (Herba Lycopi)

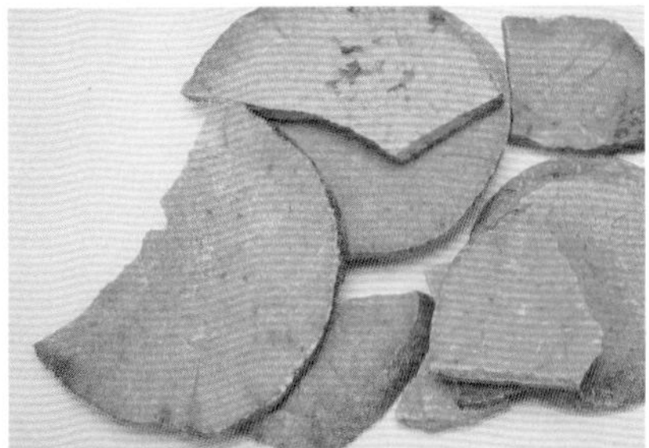
Ze Xie (Rhizoma Alismatis)

Herb Indentification Guide

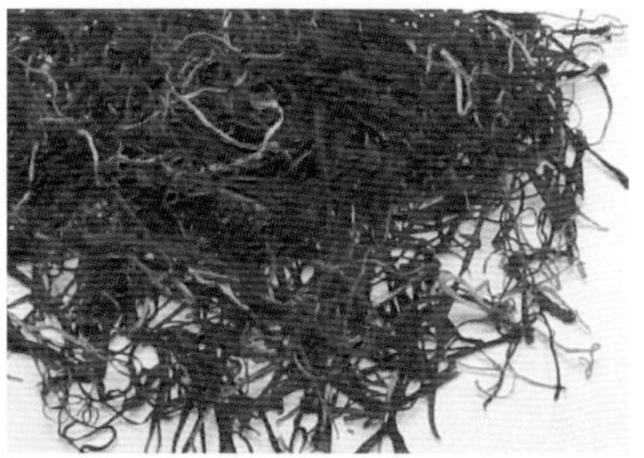
Zhang Hong Hua (Flos Crocus Sativus)

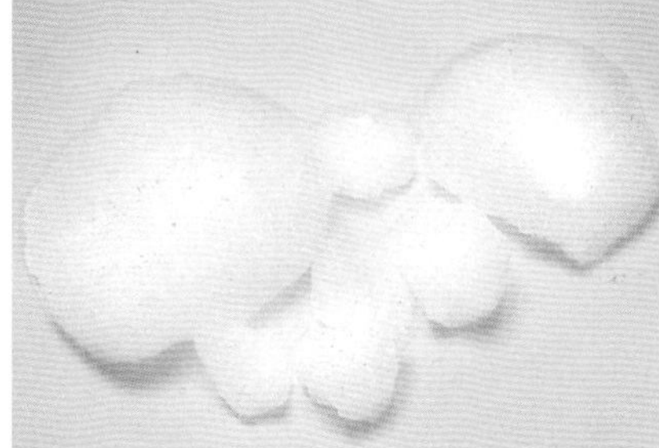
Zhang Nao (Camphora)

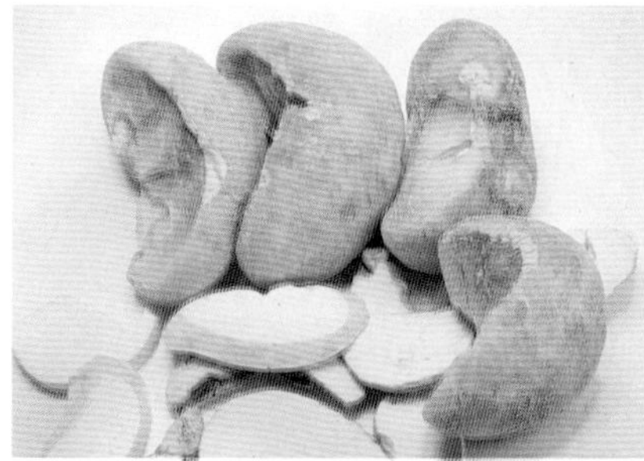
Zhe Bei Mu (Bulbus Fritillariae Thunbergii)

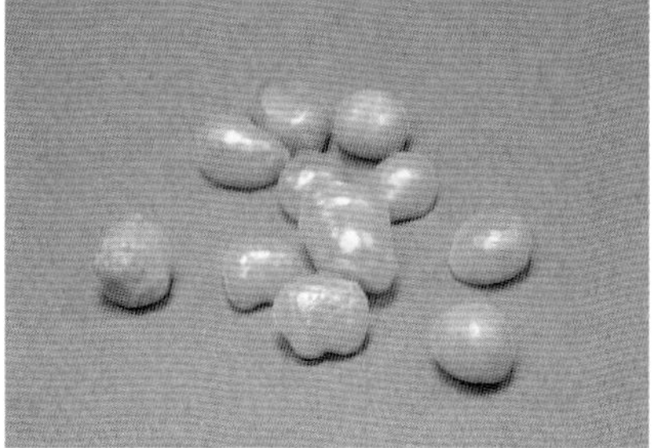
Zhen Zhu (Margarita)

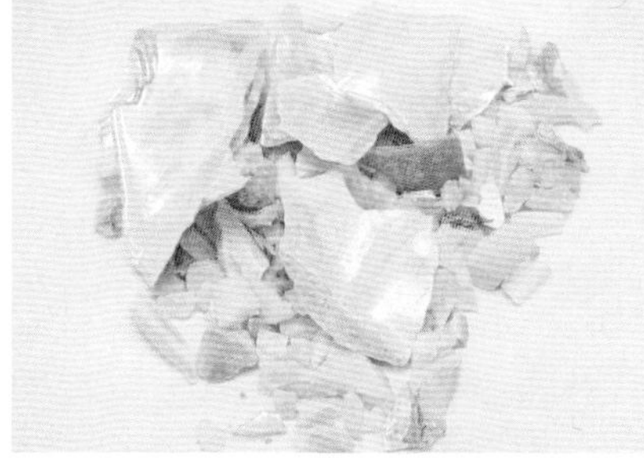
Zhen Zhu Mu (Concha Margaritaferae)

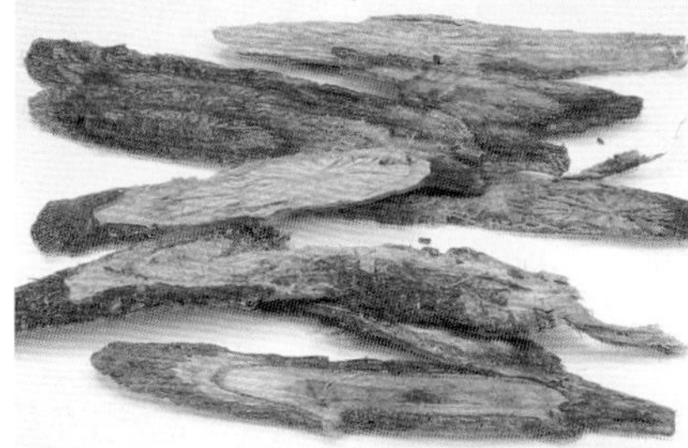
Zhi Gan Cao (Radix Glycyrrhizae Preparata)

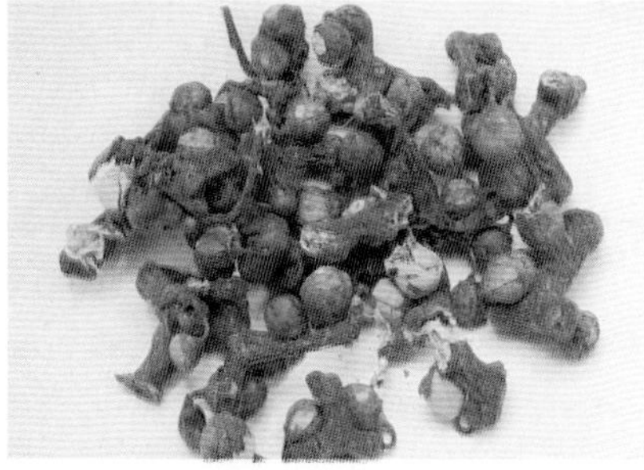
Zhi Ju Zi (Fructus Hoveniae)

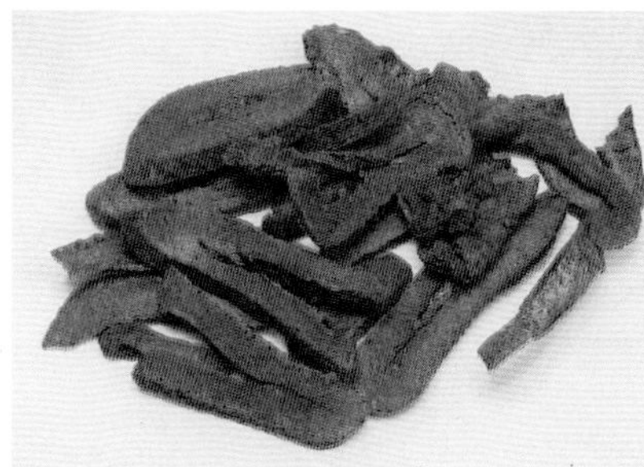
Zhi Ke (Fructus Aurantii)

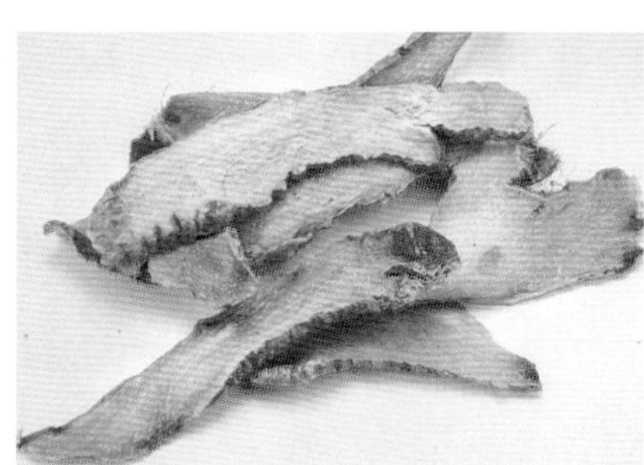
Zhi Mu (Radix Anemarrhenae)

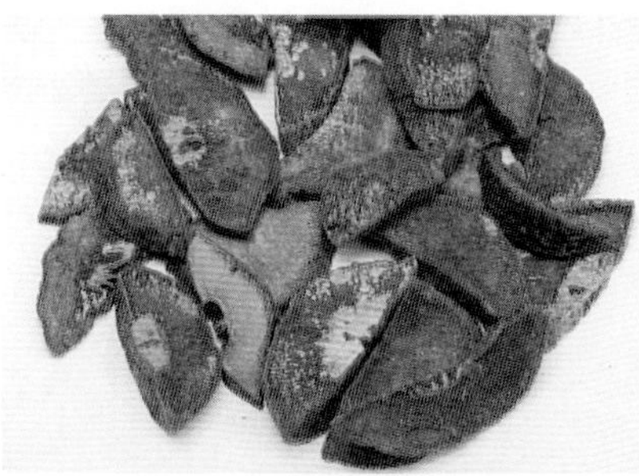
Zhi Shi (Fructus Aurantii Immaturus)

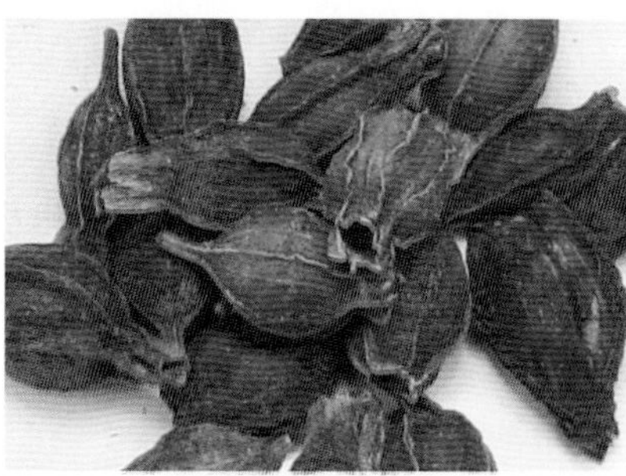
Zhi Zi (Fructus Gardeniae)

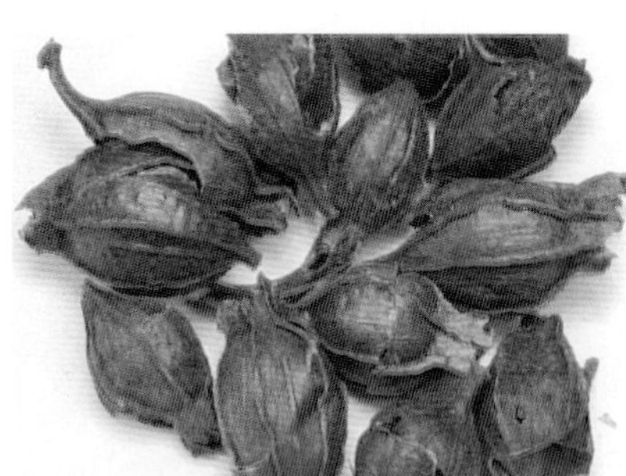
Zhi Zi Pi (Pericarpium Gardeniae)

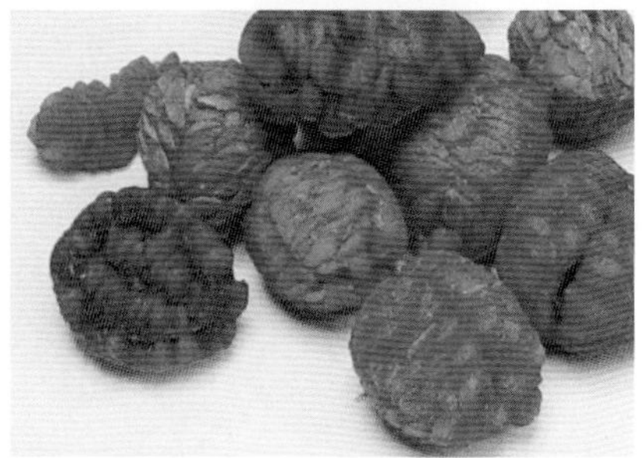
Zhi Zi Ren (Semen Gardeniae)

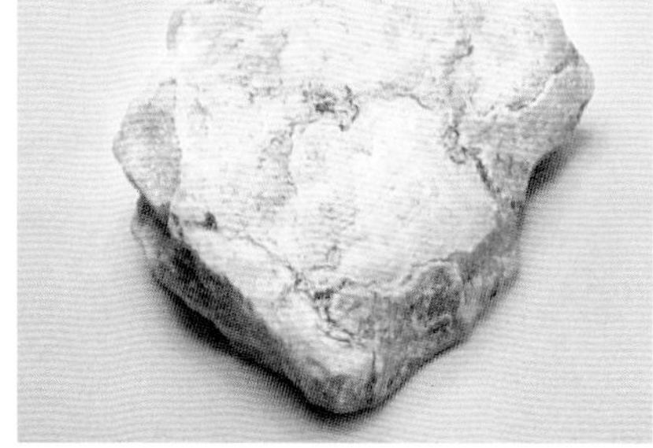
Zhong Ru Shi (Stalactitum)

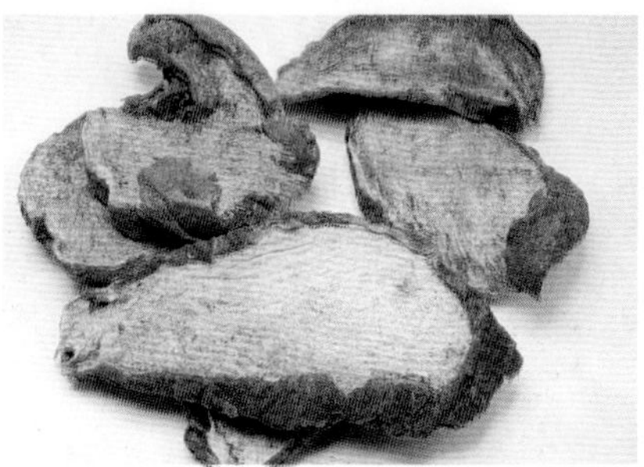
Zhu Fan Hua Tou (Rhizoma Mirabilidis)

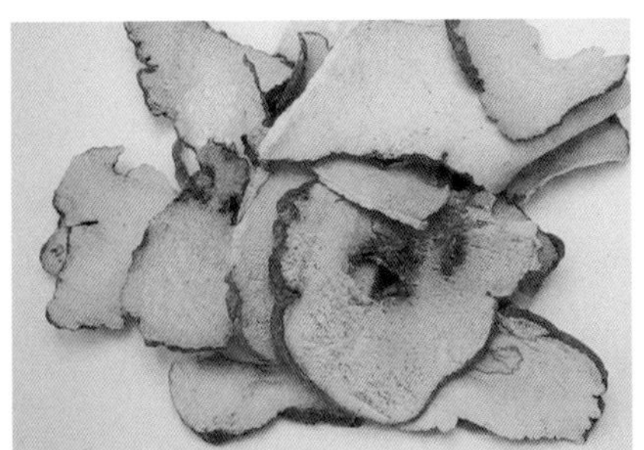
Zhu Ling (Polyporus)

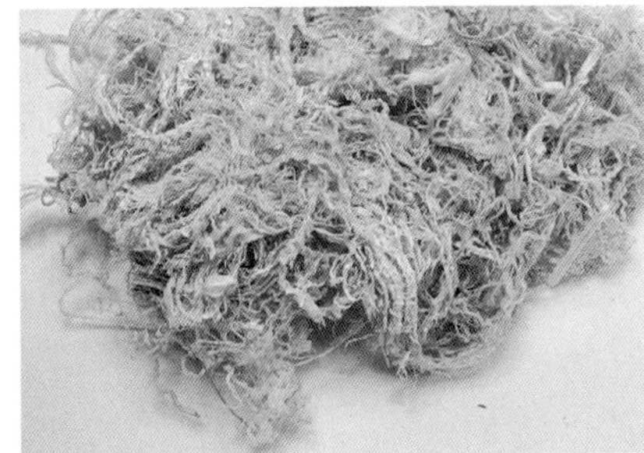
Zhu Ru (Caulis Bambusae in Taenia)

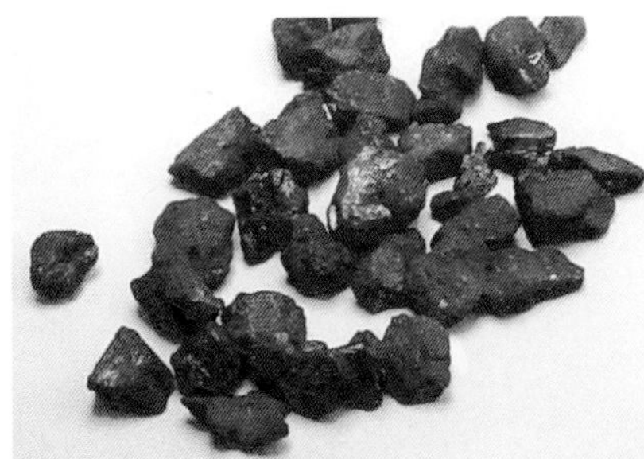
Zhu Sha (Cinnabaris)

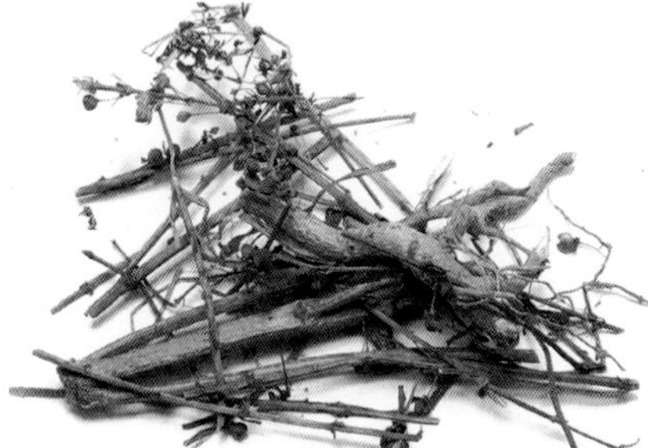
Zhu Zi Cao (Herba Euphorbiae Thymifoliae)

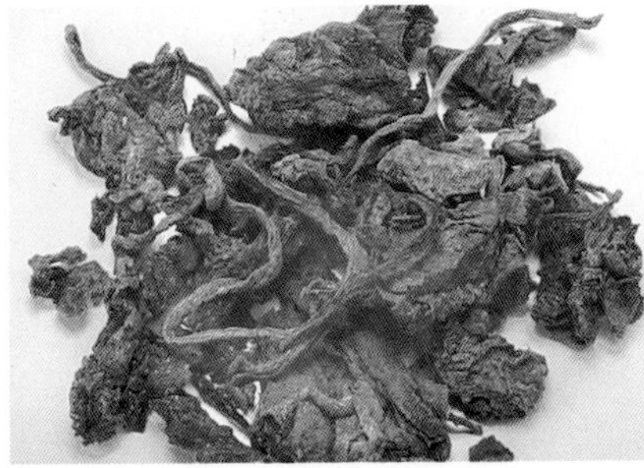
Zi Bei Tian Kui (Herba Semiaquilegiae)

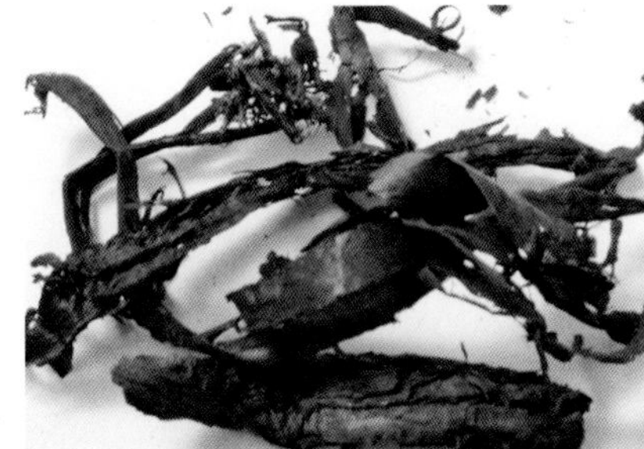
Zi Cao Gen (Radix Lithospermi)

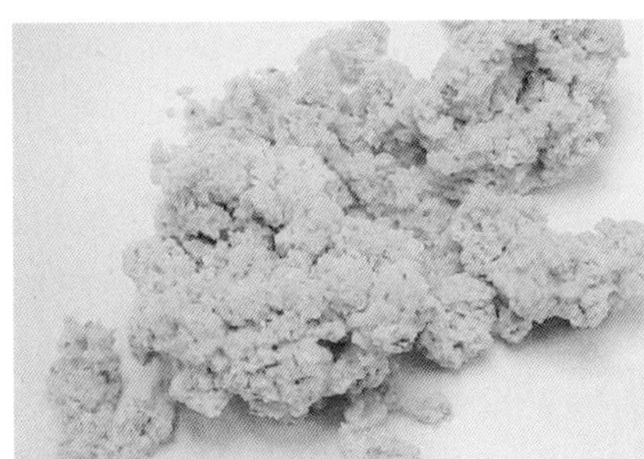
Zi He Che (Placenta Hominis)

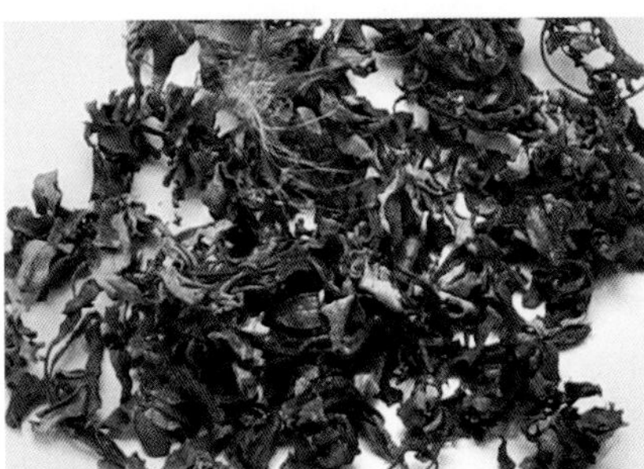
Zi Hua Di Ding (Herba Violae)

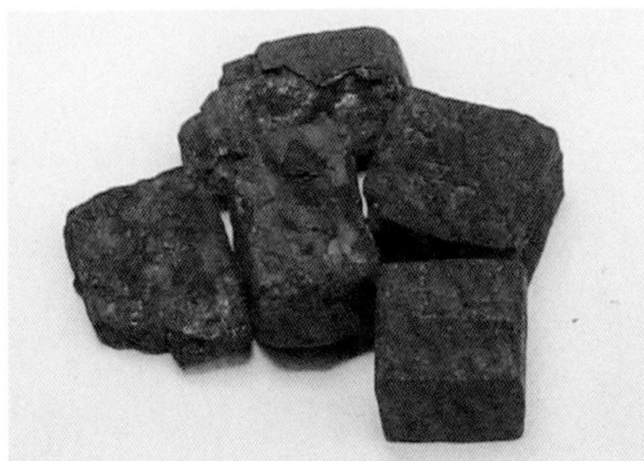
Zi Ran Tong (Pyritum)

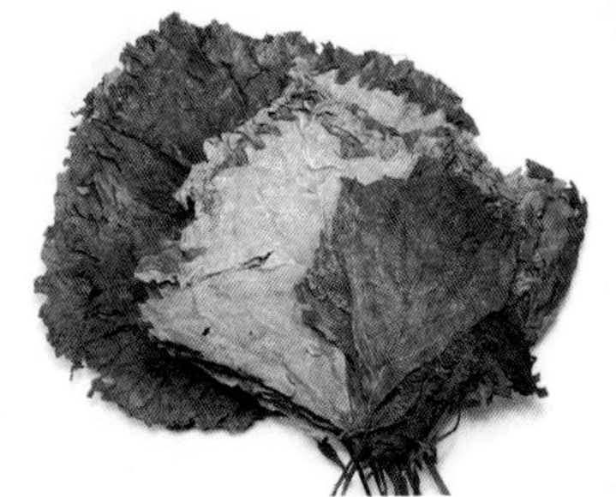
Zi Su Ye (Folium Perillae)

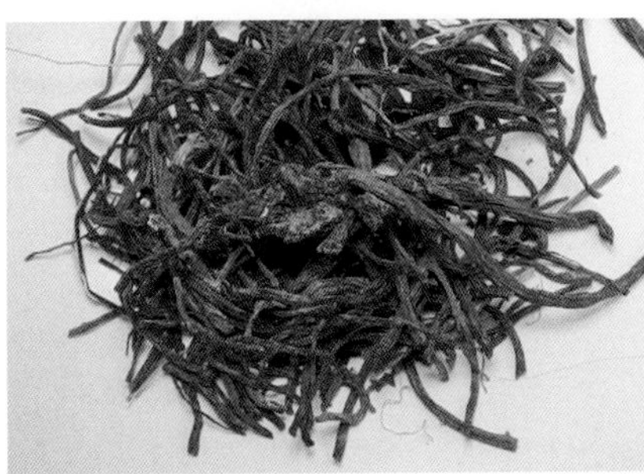
Zi Wan (Radix Asteris)

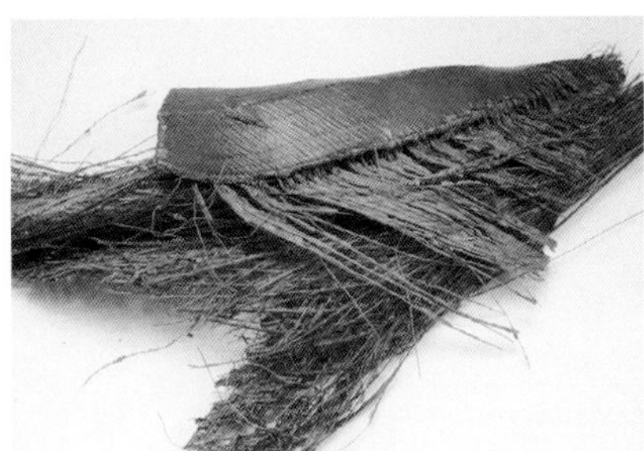
Zong Lu Pi (Fibra Stipulae Trachycarpi)

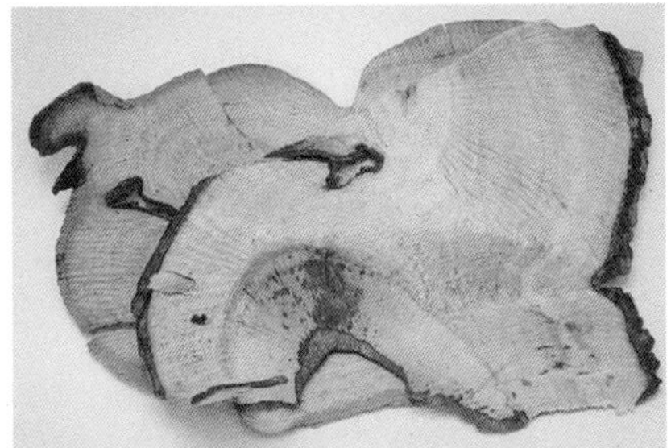
Zou Ma Tai (Rhizoma Ardisiae)

Part I — Overview

总

论

Chapter 1

历史 — The History of Chinese Herbal Medicine

Chinese Herbal Medicine is a system of medicine based on a long history of empirical observation and on centuries of clinical trial and error. Whether addressing illness or enhancing health, healers and common folk alike have tested myriad herbs throughout time, and observed their effects on the human body. Through countless years of intentional and unintentional uses, the experience and knowledge of herbs gradually have been recorded and passed along, leading to Chinese Herbal Medicine as it is practiced today.

Table 1. Summary of Important Historical Texts on Chinese Herbs

Name	Author	Time	Description
Unknown	Unknown	1066-221 B.C.	Scattered listings of medicinal substances, case studies, and toxicity information
Shen Nong Ben Cao Jing (Divine Husbandman's Classic of the Materia Medica)	numerous authors	2nd century, A.D.	Detailed descriptions of 365 herbs
Ben Cao Jing Ji Zhu (Collection of Commentaries on the Classic of the Materia Medica)	Tao Hong-Jing	480-498 A.D.	Detailed descriptions of 730 herbs, with additional information such as methods of preparation and correct identification of the herbs
Tang Ben Cao (Tang Materia Medica)	Su Jing and 23 others	657-659 A.D.	Detailed descriptions and illustrations of 850 medicinal substances
Ben Cao Shi Yi (Omissions from the [Classic of the] Materia Medica)	Chen Cang-Qi	741 A.D.	Discussed single herbs and herbal formulas
Yao Xing Ben Cao (Materia Medica of Medicinal Properties)	Zhen Quan	600 A.D.	Focused on theory and functions of herbs
Shi Liao Ben Cao (Materia Medica of Diet Therapy)	Meng Shan	7th century	Emphasized the importance of diet and the use of 227 herbs as therapeutic agents
Hai Yao Ben Cao (Materia Medica of Herbs from [Across the] Seas)	Li Xun	7th century	Discussed aromatic herbs and herbs grown overseas
Kai Bao Ben Cao (Materia Medica of the Kai Bao Era)	Ma Zhi	973-974 A.D.	Contained descriptions of 983 herbs
Jia You Ben Cao (Materia Medica of the Jia You Era)	Zhang Yu-Xi and Su Song	1057-1060 A.D.	Listed profiles of 1082 herbs
Jing Shi Zheng Lei Bei Ji Ben Cao (Differentiation and Application of Materia Medica)	Tang Shen-Wei	1082 A.D.	Included compilation of 1558 herbs
Ben Cao Gang Mu (Materia Medica)	Li Shi-Zhen	1578 A.D.	Detailed descriptions and illustrations of 1,892 individual herbs (374 herbs not previously documented) and 11,000 herbal formulas
Ben Cao Gang Mu Shi Yi (Omissions from the Grand Materia Medica)	Zhao Xue-Min	1765 A.D.	Included 716 substances described for the first time.

Written records documenting Chinese herbal medicine extend over three thousand years into the past. Artifacts made between 1066-221 B.C. have been discovered, listing botanical and animal medicinal substances, giving case studies, and focusing on topics such as toxicity. Unfortunately, most of those early documents were incomplete when discovered, as they were damaged, or in

Chapter 1 — The History of Chinese Herbal Medicine

some cases, almost destroyed. The first authoritative documentation of Chinese herbal medicine extant in its complete form today is *Shen Nong Ben Cao Jing* (Divine Husbandman's Classic of the Materia Medica), compiled by numerous authors by the second century, A.D. It contains information on 365 herbs, including details such as the thermal property, taste and toxicity of each herb, also dosages, dosage forms, and similar data. Many treatment protocols listed in that text are still in use today, such as the means of using *Ma Huang* (Herba Ephedrae) to relieve asthma, *Dang Gui* (Radicis Angelicae Sinensis) to regulate menstruation, and *Huang Lian* (Rhizoma Coptidis) to treat diarrhea.

As commerce between countries became more common, many herbs from neighboring countries were introduced to China. These herbs gradually gained acceptance in medicinal use and were documented accordingly. *Ben Cao Jing Ji Zhu* (Collection of Commentaries on the Classic of the Materia Medica), compiled by Tao Hong-Jing in 480-498 A.D., is the second oldest major text of Chinese herbal medicine known today. It describes 730 herbs and offers additional information such as methods of preparation and how to correctly identify the herbs.

The Tang dynasty (618 A.D. to 907 A.D.) was one of the more significant periods in the history of China, as the civilization experienced tremendous progress in medicine and culture. Numerous important classics were written during that time. *Tang Ben Cao* (Tang Materia Medica), also known as the *Xin Xiu Ben Cao* (Newly Revised Materia Medica) was compiled in 657-659 A.D. by Su Jing and 23 others. The book included detailed descriptions and illustrations of 850 medicinal substances, and even offered a description of the use of goat liver to improve vision and treat night blindness.

Also during the Tang dynasty, *Ben Cao Shi Yi* (Omissions from the [Classic of the] Materia Medica), compiled by Chen Cang-Qi in 741 A.D., described folklore uses of herbal medicines and formulas. It included the use of *Zi He Che* (Placenta Hominis) to improve immunity.

In 600 A.D., another Tang dynasty text, Zhen Quan's *Yao Xing Ben Cao* (Materia Medica of Medicinal Properties) focused on the theory and functions of herbs. It provided uses for and accurate descriptions of fermented herbs, such as *Shen Qu* (Massa Fermentata).

Meng Shan's *Shi Liao Ben Cao* (Materia Medica of Diet Therapy), written in the seventh century, emphasized the importance of diet in health and the use of 227 herbs as therapeutic agents. In *Hai Yao Ben Cao* (Materia Medica of Herbs from [Across the] Seas), Li Xun expanded the scope of herbal medicine by focusing on 124 herbs that were either aromatic or derived from herbs grown overseas.

During the Song Dynasty, *Kai Bao Ben Cao* (Materia Medica of the Kai Bao Era), written by Ma Zhi in 973-974 A.D., was the most comprehensive source of information about herbal medicine of its time, providing descriptions of 983 herbs.

In 1057-1060 A.D., *Jia You Ben Cao* (Materia Medica of the Jia You Era), compiled by Zhang Yu-Xi and Su Song, detailed profiles of 1082 herbs.

Jing Shi Zheng Lei Bei Ji Ben Cao (Differentiation and Application of Materia Medica), by Tang Shen-Wei in 1082 A.D., combined references from many texts, and boosted the overall compilation to 1,558 herbs.

In 1578 A.D., during the Ming Dynasty, Li Shi-Zhen wrote one of the most important texts of Chinese herbal medicine, the *Ben Cao Gang Mu* (Materia Medica). Li Shi-Zhen spent his entire life studying herbal medicine, and invested over 27 years in compiling this text. Many herbalists/scholars consider this to be the most comprehensive and historically significant text in the field. It contains detailed descriptions and illustrations of 1,892 individual herbs (374 herbs not previously documented) and 11,000 herbal formulas. The *Ben Cao Gang Mu* corrected many errors found in previous texts. The text encompassed a wide variety of medicinal substances, ranging from plants, animals, and insects to minerals.

More recently, *Ben Cao Gang Mu Shi Yi* (Omissions from the Grand Materia Medica) by Zhao Xue-Min in 1765 A.D., brought to attention many herbs used in folk medicine but not previously formally documented in texts. Though it only contained descriptions of 920 herbs, over three-quarters, that is 716, were described for the first time in this herbal text.

The texts mentioned above highlight only some of the landmarks of accomplishment throughout the history of the profession. As this text is being prepared for publication, the total number of herbs that have been documented thus far is 11,146. The complete list of historical references used to obtain the above information can be found in the Bibliography of Historical Texts.

Chapter 2 — Nomenclature of Chinese Herbs

命名

Chinese herbal medicine draws upon a wide variety of sources for medicinal substances, including plants, animals, insects, and minerals. Though not all of these are, strictly speaking, 'botanical substances,' they are generally referred to as a whole as 'Chinese Herbal Medicine.' Because of this wide variety of sources and unique individual characteristics, the functions of and indications for use of each of the herbs are significantly different. Often, the original name of the herb and the botanical or scientific category(ies) in which it is placed offer clues to these characteristics. Therefore, understanding the naming traditions or strategies (nomenclature) and the classification criterion (discussed in Chapter 3) for the substances provides an advantage for those who wish to pursue the study of Chinese herbal medicine.

For those unfamiliar with the *pinyin* transliteration of Chinese words: the pronunciation differences made possible by the Chinese tonal system are not immediately apparent in printed *pinyin* (particularly in the absence of diacritical marks). Thus, it may appear that one word has many meanings. Additionally, the context in which a Chinese word appears often defines the word. For example, the word '*jiao*' might mean 'horn' in one name while meaning 'gelatin' in another, because of the verbal context surrounding '*jiao*.' Reference to the Chinese characters provided at the heading **Chinese Name** in each herb profile will confirm the precise original name.

Context often defines Chinese words: '*jiao*' means 'horn' in one context, 'gelatin' in another. The Chinese characters provide the precise original word.

NOMENCLATURE BASED ON SHAPE

Many herbs earn their names from their unique physical appearance. Examples of such naming practices include:

- *Ru Xiang* (Gummi Olibanum), literally 'breast fragrant,' derives its name from both the breast-like shape the gel forms as it seeps from the tree, and its fragrance.
- *Bai Mu Er* (Fructificatio Tremellae Fuciformis), 'white wood ear,' is white and resembles an ear.
- *Niu Xi* (Radix Cyathulae seu Achyranthis), 'cow's knees,' has big joints that might look like cow knees.
- *Gou Teng* (Ramulus Uncariae cum Uncis), 'hook vine,' identifies vines that have hook-like tendril attachments.
- *Long Yan Rou* (Arillus Longan), 'dragon eye meat,' refers to the meaty part of the Longan fruit that looks like the eyes of a dragon.
- *Gou Ji* (Rhizoma Cibotii), 'dog spine,' resembles the spine of a dog.

Additional examples appear under the **Literal Name** heading within individual herb profiles.

Chapter 2 — Nomenclature of Chinese Herbs

NOMENCLATURE BASED ON COLOR

Color is not only a valuable means of identifying herbs for purchasing or pharmacy use, but in many cases also provides information about the therapeutic attributes of the herb. Thus, color is an essential element of nomenclature in this herbal tradition.

Red herbs are labeled *hong* (red), *chi* (bright red), or *zhu* (dull red). For example, *Hong Hua* (Flos Carthami) means 'red flower,' *Chi Shao* (Radix Paeoniae Rubrae) is 'bright red peony,' and *Zhu Sha* (Cinnabaris), 'dull red sand.'

Yellow herbs are referred to as *huang* (yellow) or *jin* (gold). *Huang Bai* (Cortex Phellodendri) means 'yellow fir,' *Da Huang* (Radix et Rhizoma Rhei) is known as 'big yellow,' and *Jin Yin Hua* (Flos Lonicerae) has the label 'golden silver flower.'

Herbs that are white may be called *bai* (white) or *yin* (silver). *Bai Shao* (Radix Paeoniae Alba) translates to 'white peony,' and *Yin Guo Ye* (Folium Ginkgo) is 'silver fruit leaf.'

Qing designates blue-green herbs. *Qing Pi* (Pericarpium Citri Reticulatae Viride) is 'blue-green peel' and *Da Qing Ye* (Folium Isatidis) means 'big blue-green leaf.'

Those herbs that are simply green are referred to as *lu*. Among green herbs: *Lu Dou* (Semen Phaseoli Radiati) 'green bean' and *Lu Cha* (Folium Camellia Sinensis) 'green tea.'

Black-colored herbs incorporate *hei* or *wu* in their names, such as *Hei Dou* (Semen Glycine Max) 'black bean,' *Hei Zao* (Fructus Jujubae) 'black jujube,' and *Wu Yao* (Radix Linderae) 'black medicine.'

Purple herbs are tagged with *zi*: *Zi Cao Gen* (Radix Lithospermi) 'purple herb root' and *Zi Hua Di Ding* (Herba Violae) 'purple flower earth herb.'

Similar instances throughout the text are specified in the **Literal Name** heading in each herb profile.

Table 2. Nomenclature Based on Color

Pinyin	Meaning	Pinyin Name	Literal Name	Pharmaceutical Name
Hong	Red	*Hong Hua*	Red flower	Flos Carthami
Chi	Bright red	*Chi Shao*	Bright red peony	Radix Paeoniae Rubrae
Zhu	Dull red	*Zhu Sha*	Dull red sand	Cinnabaris
Huang	Yellow	*Da Huang*	Big yellow	Radix et Rhizoma Rhei
Jin	Gold	*Jin Yin Hua*	Golden silver flower	Flos Lonicerae
Bai	White	*Bai Shao*	White peony	Radix Paeoniae Alba
Yin	Silver	*Yin Guo Ye*	Silver fruit leaf	Folium Ginkgo
Qing	Blue-green	*Qing Pi*	Blue-green peel	Pericarpium Citri Reticulatae Viride
Lu	Green	*Lu Dou*	Green beans	Semen Phaseoli Radiati
Hei	Black	*Hei Dou*	Black beans	Semen Glycine Max
Zi	Purple	*Zi Cao Gen*	Purple herb root	Radix Lithospermi

NOMENCLATURE BASED ON SMELL AND TASTE

A unique fragrance or odor determines part of the identifying name for some herbs. *Xiang* 'fragrant' describes herbs that are fragrant. For example, *Mu Xiang* (Radix Aucklandiae) means 'fragrant wood,' and *Jiang Xiang* (Lignum Dalbergiae Odoriferae), 'descending fragrance.' *Yu Xing Cao* (Herba Houttuyniae) 'fish smell herb' has a unique fishy odor. *Bai Jiang Cao* (Herba cum Radice Patriniae) 'rotten paste herb' smells similar to rotten paste.

Unique flavors define specific names for some substances. *Gan* means 'sweet,' so *Gan Cao* (Radix Glycyrrhizae) is 'sweet herb.' *Ku* is 'bitter,' thus *Ku Shen Gen* (Radix Sophorae Flavescentis) translates as 'bitter herb root.' *Suan* is 'sour,' thus *Suan Zao Ren* (Semen Zizyphi Spinosae) describes 'sour date seed.' *Xin* is 'acrid,' as used in *Xi Xin* (Herba Asari) 'thin acrid.' *Dan* is 'bland,' so *Dan Zhu Ye* (Herba Lophatheri) means 'bland bamboo leaves.' Lastly, *Wu Wei Zi* (Fructus Schisandrae Chinensis) means 'five-flavored seed,' referring to its five (*wu*) distinct flavors, namely sour, sweet, bitter, acrid, and salty. Related examples are offered throughout the text.

Chapter 2 — Nomenclature of Chinese Herbs

Table 3. Nomenclature Based on Smell and Taste

Pinyin	Meaning	Pinyin Name	Literal Name	Pharmaceutical Name
Xiang	Fragrant	*Mu Xiang*	Fragrant wood	Radix Aucklandiae
Gan	Sweet	*Gan Cao*	Sweet herb	Radix Glycyrrhizae
Ku	Bitter	*Ku Shen Gen*	Bitter herb root	Radix Sophorae Flavescentis
Suan	Sour	*Suan Zao Ren*	Sour date seed	Semen Zizyphi Spinosae
Xin	Acrid	*Xi Xin*	Thin acrid	Herba Asari
Dan	Bland	*Dan Zhu Ye*	Bland bamboo leaf	Herba Lophatheri

NOMENCLATURE BASED ON GEOGRAPHIC LOCATION

The geographic locations or provinces in which herbs are grown often figure into herb names.

Compass references: *bei* refers to north, *nan* to south, *dong* to east, and *xi* to west. *Bei Sha Shen* (Radix Glehniae) is grown and harvested in northern China. *Nan Sha Shen* (Radix Adenophorae) originated in southern China. *Dong Yang Shen* (Radix Ginseng Japonica) describes 'eastern' ginseng from Japan. *Xi Yang Shen* (Radix Panacis Quinquefolii) indicates 'western' ginseng from the American continent.

Province references: *Chuan* indicates Sichuan province, with examples like *Chuan Bei Mu* (Bulbus Fritillariae Cirrhosae) and *Chuan Niu Xi* (Radix Cyathulae). *Zhe* refers to Zhejiang Province, as in *Zhe Bei Mu* (Bulbus Fritillariae Thunbergii). *Huai* refers to a place in Henan Province called Huaiqingfu, pinpointing the geographic origin of *Huai Niu Xi* (Radix Achyranthis Bidentatae).

Zhang refers to Tibet, thus *Zhang Hong Hua* (Flos Crocus Sativus) indicates the variety of *Hong Hua* (Flos Carthami) that comes from Tibet. *Fan*, 'barbarians,' identifies herbs imported to China, such as *Fan Xie Ye* (Folium Sennae).

NOMENCLATURE BASED ON PLANT LIFE CYCLES

The life and growth cycles of herbs provide useful input for names. *Xia Ku Cao* (Spica Prunellae), 'summer dry herb,' becomes withered and dry in summer. *Ren Dong Teng* (Caulis Lonicerae), 'tolerate winter vine,' continues to grow through the winter. *Dong Chong Xia Cao* (Cordyceps), 'winter bug summer herb,' is a fungal herb that grows in winter and is dormant in summer.

NOMENCLATURE BASED ON SPECIFIC PARTS

Specific plant and animal parts figure prominently in herb names. The most common examples are described below; other examples appear under the **Literal Name** headings in the main text.

Gen 'root' indicates the root as being the medicinal part of a particular herb. *Lu Gen* (Rhizoma Phragmitis) specifies phragmites root, and *Ma Huang Gen* (Radix Ephedrae), ephedra root.

Geng means 'branches,' and *zhi* means 'twigs,' referring to the branches/twigs as the medicinal component of the herb. *Su Geng* (Caulis Perillae) points to perilla branches, and *Gui Zhi* (Ramulus Cinnamomi), cinnamon twigs.

Ye 'leaves' selects leaves as the desired plant part. *Sang Ye* (Folium Mori) 'mulberry leaves,' and *Zhu Ye* (Herba Phyllostachys) 'bamboo leaves' are two common examples.

Hua 'flower' directs the herbalist to choose the flower as the medicinal portion of the herb. *Hong Hua* (Flos Carthami) specifies red flower, and *Ju Hua* (Flos Chrysanthemi) denotes the chrysanthemum flower.

Guo, literally meaning 'fruit,' designates the fruit. *Cao Guo* (Fructus Tsaoko) is 'herb fruit.'

Pi 'peel' identifies the peels or skins as the chosen medicinal component. *Qing Pi* (Pericarpium Citri Reticulatae Viride) means 'blue-green peel,' and *Chen Pi* (Pericarpium Citri Reticulatae) identifies 'aged peels.'

Zi or *ren* both indicate 'seeds' to be the medicinal element. *Dong Gua Zi* (Semen Benincasae) is 'wintermelon seed,' and *Tao Ren* (Semen Persicae), 'persica seed.'

Jiao 'horn' designates animal horn. *Lu Jiao* (Cornu Cervi) identifies deer horn, while *Shui Niu Jiao* (Cornu Bubali) is 'water buffalo horn.'

Chapter 2 — Nomenclature of Chinese Herbs

Dan 'gallbladder' specifies animal gallbladder for therapeutic use. For example, *Zhu Dan* (Fel Porcus) means 'pig gallbladder.'

Table 4. Nomenclature Based on Specific Parts

Chinese	English	Latin	Examples	Common Name
Cao	Herb	Herba	*Che Qian Cao* (Herba Plantaginis)	Plantain herb
Dan	Gallbladder	Fel	*Zhu Dan* (Fel Porcus)	Pig gallbladder
Dou	Seed	Semen	*Lu Dou* (Semen Phaseoli Radiati)	Mung bean
Gen	Root	Radix	*Ban Lan Gen* (Radix Isatidis)	Isatis root
Gen	Rhizome	Rhizoma	*Bai Mao Gen* (Rhizoma Imperatae)	Imperata root
Geng	Branch/stem	Caulis	*Su Geng* (Caulis Perillae)	Perilla branch
Gua	Fruit	Fructus	*Mu Gua* (Fructus Chaenomelis)	Papaya fruit
Hua	Flower	Flos	*Hong Hua* (Flos Carthami)	Safflower
Jiao	Horn	Cornu	*Lu Jiao* (Cornu Cervi)	Deer horn
Jiao	Gelatin	Gelatinum	*Gui Ban Jiao* (Gelatinum Plastrum Testudinis)	Tortoise shell gelatin
Ke	Shell	Concha	*Shi Jue Ming* (Concha Haliotidis)	Abalone shell
Mu	Wood	Lignum	*Su Mu* (Lignum Sappan)	Sappan wood
Pi	Bark	Cortex	*He Huan Pi* (Cortex Albiziae)	Albizia bark
Pi	Outer skin	Exocarpium	*Dong Gua Pi* (Exocarpium Benincasae)	Wintermelon peel
Pi	Peel/skin	Pericarpium	*Chen Pi* (Pericarpium Citri Reticulatae)	Orange peel
Ren	Fruit	Fructus	*Huo Ma Ren* (Fructus Cannabis)	Cannabis seed
Ren	Seed	Semen	*Xing Ren* (Semen Armeniacae Amarum)	Bitter almond seed
Shi	Stone	Calculus	*Niu Huang* (Calculus Bovis)	Cattle gallstone
Teng	Vine	Caulis	*Ren Dong Teng* (Caulis Lonicerae)	Honeysuckle vine
Ye	Leaf	Folium	*Yin Guo Ye* (Folium Ginkgo)	Ginkgo leaf
Zhi	Branch/twig	Ramulus	*Gui Zhi* (Ramulus Cinnamomi)	Cinnamon twig
Zi	Seed	Semen	*Lian Zi* (Semen Nelumbinis)	Lotus seed

NOMENCLATURE BASED ON FUNCTION

Herb names also arise from unique individual functions. For example, *Fang Feng* (Radix Saposhnikoviae), literally 'prevent wind,' prevents or treats wind-related illnesses. *Yi Mu Cao* (Herba Leonuri), literally 'benefit mother herb,' is often used in gynecology. *Xu Duan* (Radix Dipsaci), literally 'restore the broken,' effectively treats torn soft tissues and broken bones. *Yin Yang Huo* (Herba Epimedii), literally 'horny goat wort (or grass),' increases sexual desire and performance. *Yang Qi Shi* (Actinolitum), literally 'yang lifting the rock,' tonifies yang, and is said to do this so effectively that the male penis is strong enough to lift rocks.

NOMENCLATURE BASED ON HUMANS OR THE HUMAN ACTION INVOLVED

Some herbs are named after the individuals who discovered them. *Liu Ji Nu* (Herba Artemisiae Anomalae), 'live-in slave Liu,' identifies the first individual credited with finding or using the herb. *He Shou Wu* (Radix Polygoni Multiflori) credits 'dark-haired Mr. He's' continuous use of the herb to maintain black hair. *Qian Niu Zi* (Semen Pharbitidis), 'walk cow seed,' refers to how an old man found the herb while walking his cows.

NOMENCLATURE BASED ON COUNTRY OF ORIGIN

Through international commerce, many herbs indigenous to other countries have been incorporated into the Chinese materia medica. *Xi Yang Shen* (Radix Panacis Quinquefolii), imported from North American crops, translates as 'western ginseng,' while *Dong Yang Shen* (Radix Ginseng Japonica), grown in and imported from North Asian countries, is 'eastern ginseng.' Similar examples are noted in the text whenever geography matters in herb selection.

OTHER NAME DIFFERENTIATIONS

In addition to the methods above, there are more approaches to herbal nomenclature. For example, there are three types of *Di Huang* (Rehmannia): *Xian Di Huang* (Radix Rehmanniae Recens) is the fresh root, *Sheng Di Huang* (Radix Rehmanniae) is dried, and *Shu Di Huang* (Radix Rehmanniae Preparata) is prepared (steamed).

Chapter 3 分类 — Classification of Chinese Herbs

The organization of Chinese herbal medicines into specific classes (of action, source, therapeutic function, or other criteria) has long been a challenging task. While the *Shen Nong Ben Cao Jing* (Divine Husbandman's Classic of the Materia Medica), one of the earliest texts, listed only 365 herbs, *Zhong Yao Da Ci Dien* (The Dictionary of Chinese Herbs), one of the latest contemporary references, covers 9,000 herbs. Reasonably, herbal medicine practitioners need systematic approaches to finding their way around this huge pharmacopoeia. Based on the vast number of herbs to be assessed, several approaches to classification have been incorporated over the years.

CLASSIFICATION BY THERAPEUTIC ACTIONS AND SIDE EFFECTS

Some texts classify herbs as superior-, medium- and inferior-grade, based on their therapeutic effectiveness and possible side effects.

Herbs of **superior** status have excellent therapeutic action, few or no side effects, and may safely be taken for a long period of time. Superior herbs include *Ren Shen* (Radix Ginseng), *Gan Cao* (Radix Glycyrrhizae), *Di Huang* (Radix Rehmanniae), *Shi Hu* (Herba Dendrobii), *Ba Ji Tian* (Radix Morindae Officinalis), *Huang Qi* (Radix Astragali), *Gou Qi Zi* (Fructus Lycii), and others. These herbs are safe not only as medicine but also as food.

Herbs given **medium** status have both therapeutic benefit and possible side effects, requiring professional supervision for medicinal usage. Medium-status herbs include *Gan Jiang* (Rhizoma Zingiberis), *Ma Huang* (Herba Ephedrae), *Dang Gui* (Radicis Angelicae Sinensis), *Bai Shao* (Radix Paeoniae Alba), *Wu Zhu Yu* (Fructus Evodiae), and *Hou Po* (Cortex Magnoliae Officinalis), among others.

Herbs assigned **inferior** status may have more side effects and/or toxicities than therapeutic benefits (especially if not properly processed or administered). Such herbs are used only when the key benefits outweigh the risks, and only under professional supervision. Examples of inferior herbs include *Fu Zi* (Radix Aconiti Lateralis Praeparata), *Ban Xia* (Rhizoma Pinelliae), *Da Huang* (Radix et Rhizoma Rhei), *Gan Sui* (Radix Euphorbiae Kansui), *Ba Dou* (Fructus Crotonis), and *Wu Gong* (Scolopendra), to name a few. This designation does not mean that these herbs have lesser value in clinical practice.

Chapter 3 — Classification of Chinese Herbs

CLASSIFICATION BY THE SOURCE OF THE HERBS

Other texts classify substances based on the original source of the substance. While the majority of medicinal substances are herbs, many are derived from and thus categorized by other sources:

- Plants
  Leaves, Branches, Stems, Fruits, Seeds, Roots, Barks, Twigs
- Animals
- Fish
- Shellfish
- Insects
- Minerals

CLASSIFICATION BY THERAPEUTIC FUNCTION

Most texts classify herbs based on the therapeutic function of each substance. The following terms are used to describe the effects various herbs have on qi, blood, *shen* (spirit), yin, yang, body fluids or pathogens:

- disperse
- astringe
- tonify
- sedate
- warm
- cool
- moisten
- dry
- eliminate toxins
- move

CLASSIFICATION BASED ON INTERNAL ORGANS

Some texts primarily classify herbs based on the affected *zang* (solid) and *fu* (hollow) organs. *Zang* organs include Kidney, Liver, Heart, Pericardium, Spleen, and Lung. *Fu* organs include Urinary Bladder, Gallbladder, Small Intestine, *San Jiao*, Stomach and Large Intestine. Details are also given as to how the herbs affect the organs: tonify, harmonize, attack, disperse, cool, or warm. A specific herb, for example, might 'tonify Liver yin,' boosting and nourishing the yin energy of the Liver.

OTHER STRATEGIES

Chinese medicine texts are published in several languages for varied professional audiences. In addition to the approaches mentioned above, there are specialty texts that classify the herbs based on details such as:

- the number of strokes required to create the Chinese characters of each herb name
- presenting the herb *pinyin* names in alphabetical order
- the general disease syndromes under consideration, or other such choices.

Chapter 4

採集 — Growing and Harvesting Chinese Herbs

Herbs are products of nature: through millions of years of natural selection they have adapted to the environments most favorable for their growth and survival. Climate, geography and timing of harvest are significant factors influencing the quality of the herbs and thus, their individual usefulness in treating specific conditions. Herbalists through the centuries have recorded and passed on information about these details; contemporary scientists are bringing sophisticated laboratory analysis to study these facts.

Some herbs reach optimum quality if grown on the east coast of China in the humid ocean climate; some are best gathered on the dry West coast desert; some thrive only in the north, with long, cold winters; and others do best in the long summers and hot climate of the South.

Increasing use of Chinese herbs worldwide may result in over-harvesting in China and endanger indigenous herb supplies, unless international efforts are made to protect and cultivate these herbs elsewhere.

GEOGRAPHIC CLIMATE

Although a specific herb may be cultivated successfully in several regions of China, some herbs are named after a specific province to emphasize the impact of geographic climate on quality. This traditional emphasis on geographic location has been validated in several cases by modern science. In one laboratory study, it was found that samples of *Dan Shen* (Radix Salviae Miltiorrhizae) obtained from different provinces had significantly different contents of an element called tanshinone II A, with variations of up to several levels of concentration.[1] Similarly, essential oil content of *Bo He* (Herba Menthae) from various regions can fluctuate up to 10 times in concentration.[2]

Specific examples of herbs and their association with geographic climate include modifiers to herb names derived from such provinces as Sichuan, Zhejiang, Henan, and Guangdong.

Sichuan province is commonly abbreviated as *chuan. Chuan Xiong* (Rhizoma Ligustici Chuanxiong), *Chuan Wu* (Radix Aconiti Preparata), *Chuan Niu Xi* (Radix Cyathulae), *Chuan Lian Zi* (Fructus Toosendan), and *Chuan Bei Mu* (Bulbus Fritillariae Cirrhosae) are most effective if grown and harvested in Sichuan.

Zhejiang province is commonly abbreviated as *zhe* or *hang*, with such examples as *Zhe Bei Mu* (Bulbus Fritillariae Thunbergii) and *Hang Ju Hua* (Flos Chrysanthemi).

The common derivation of Henan province is *huai*, with examples like *Huai Niu Xi* (Radix Achyranthis Bidentatae), *Huai Shan Yao* (Rhizoma Dioscoreae), and *Huai Ju Hua* (Flos Chrysanthemi).

Guangdong province is commonly abbreviated *guang*, as in *Guang Chen Pi* (Pericarpium Citri Reticulatae).

However, due to an increase in the use of Chinese herbs worldwide, harvesting herbs from the wild in the ideal provinces indicated by their names will not always meet the demand. This may result in over-harvesting local resources and even endangering the original supply of indigenous herbs. Therefore, many herbs are now cultivated rather than gathered wild; grown, if not in the ideal province, at least in a similar climate, to ensure maximum effectiveness.

TIME OF HARVEST

The timing of harvest significantly affects the potency of herbs as the plants go through seasonal changes of growth, maturation, blossoming, bearing fruit, withering, and dormancy. Different plant parts are harvested at specific seasons or stages to ensure maximum potency for desired actions.

In collecting Chinese herbs that make use of the entire plant, such as *Yi Mu Cao* (Herba Leonuri) and *Xian He Cao* (Herba Agrimoniae), it is best to harvest immediately prior to the blossoming of the flowers.

Chapter 4 — Growing and Harvesting Chinese Herbs

When leaves are the primary medicinal component, as is the case with *Da Qing Ye* (Folium Isatidis), *He Ye* (Folium Nelumbinis), and *Ai Ye* (Folium Artemisiae Argyi), the leaves are ideally harvested immediately before or during the blooming of flowers, when the leaves contain the highest levels of active ingredients and aroma.

When flowers are the key herbal component desired, such as *Ju Hua* (Flos Chrysanthemi), *Xuan Fu Hua* (Flos Inulae), and *Huai Hua* (Flos Sophorae), they are harvested while in bloom. Some herbs like *Ju Hua* (Flos Chrysanthemi) require multiple harvests, as flowers often blossom repeatedly or plants mature at different rates because of differences in exposure, water or other factors. Others, like *Jin Yin Hua* (Flos Lonicerae) and *Xin Yi Hua* (Flos Magnoliae), should be gathered while the flower is still within the bud, immediately before blossoming. Still others, like *Hong Hua* (Flos Carthami), are best harvested as the flowers begin to change color (in this case, from yellow to red), yielding maximum fragrance and potency.

Seed and fruit substances, such as *Gua Lou Shi* (Fructus Trichosanthis), *Xing Ren* (Semen Armeniacae Amarum), and *Wu Wei Zi* (Fructus Schisandrae Chinensis), ought to be collected in the early to middle stages of fruit formation. Fully-mature fruit may bruise or burst during drying and transport, creating difficulties with distribution. Some herbs specifically must be immature fruit, such as *Qing Pi* (Pericarpium Citri Reticulatae Viride), *Zhi Shi* (Fructus Aurantii Immaturus), and *Wu Mei* (Fructus Mume), and therefore must be harvested prior to reaching maturity.

Chinese herbs that are barks, such as *Huang Bai* (Cortex Phellodendri), *Hou Po* (Cortex Magnoliae Officinalis), *Du Zhong* (Cortex Eucommiae), and *Qin Pi* (Cortex Fraxini), should be collected in spring and summer, when plant growth insures that a maximum level of nutrients is circulating in the bark. To ensure a continuous supply of these herbs both in the short- and long-range future, the plants should <u>not</u> be cut down to facilitate harvesting, and the bark should be removed in sections without stripping the entire circumference of the tree or shrub. Such stripping may harm or kill the plant.

When roots are the medicinal substance, as is the case with *Tian Ma* (Rhizoma Gastrodiae), *Cang Zhu* (Rhizoma Atractylodis), *Ge Gen* (Radix Puerariae), *Jie Geng* (Radix Platycodonis), *Da Huang* (Radix et Rhizoma Rhei), *Dan Shen* (Radix Salviae Miltiorrhizae), and *Tian Nan Xing* (Rhizoma Arisaematis), the roots must be harvested during the dormant phase of the plant, in late winter or early spring, while all the nutrients are stored in the roots.

Organic medicinal substances other than flora should be harvested following a similar rationale. Insects should be collected in spring and summer to ensure maximum potency. Animals are generally farmed and animal products harvested at appropriate seasons specifically for medicinal purposes. Ideally, farming ensures that the animals will not be treated cruelly, and that wild populations will not be depleted. On the other hand, minerals, not subject to seasonal variation, may be gathered year round.

Harvest timing has a significant impact on herb potency, as documented by numerous studies. For example, in one laboratory study, samples of *Qing Hao* (Herba Artemisiae Annuae) were collected at various stages of growth, to analyze the content of arteannuin—an active constituent in *Qing Hao* that plays a key role in treatment of malaria. It was concluded that the sample taken immediately prior to the blooming of the flowers contained the highest concentration of arteannuin.[3]

Another study reported that winter-harvested *Dan Shen* (Radix Salviae Miltiorrhizae) contained two to three times the amount of the component tanshinone than samples harvested during other seasons.[4]

Lastly, an investigation determined that samples of *Shi Chang Pu* (Rhizoma Acori) harvested in winter exhibited a higher content of essential oil than samples gathered in spring and summer.[5]

Chapter 5

炮制

– Preparation and Processing of Chinese Herbs

The preparation and processing of herbs are essential activities of Chinese herbal medicine. While some herbs are used in their fresh or original forms, most must be prepared or processed before use, to achieve maximum availability of their constituents. Each method of preparation or processing has a specific purpose or function that influences the final product and its therapeutic impact.

PURPOSES OF PREPARATION AND PROCESSING

There are seven main purposes for the preparation and subsequent processing of herbal substances:

- to enhance or alter therapeutic actions
- to minimize loss of active components
- to maximize extraction of constituents
- to reduce side effects and/or toxicity
- to increase surface area and facilitate extraction
- to prevent spoilage and prolong shelf life
- to clean herbs prior to ingestion

To **enhance or alter therapeutic actions**, herbs may be processed (with honey, vinegar or grain-based liquor), steamed, baked, roasted, or charred to ashes, or cooked for greater or lesser periods of time. Processing *Kuan Dong Hua* (Flos Farfarae) with honey enhances its action to moisten the Lung and relieve coughing. Processing *Huang Qin* (Radix Scutellariae) with grain-based liquor strengthens its ability to clear heat from the upper *jiao*. Vinegar-processing *Chai Hu* (Radix Bupleuri) or *Xiang Fu* (Rhizoma Cyperi) facilitates entrance to the Liver for treatment of liver-related disorders.

To **alter therapeutic action**, *Sheng Di Huang* (Radix Rehmanniae), a cold substance that cools heat in the blood, is steamed to yield *Shu Di Huang* (Radix Rehmanniae Preparata), a warm herb used to tonify blood. Roasting the exterior-relieving *Sheng Jiang* (Rhizoma Zingiberis Recens) yields interior-warming *Pao Jiang* (Rhizoma Zingiberis Preparatum). Charring *Ai Ye* (Artemisiae Argyi) to ash enhances its capacity to stop bleeding.

To **minimize loss of active components**, some herbs are cooked only for a short period of time, such as volatile mint leaves, *Bo He* (Herba Menthae), and agastache, *Huo Xiang* (Herba Agastache). This method is known as post-decoction.

To **maximize extraction of active constituents**, some herbs are cooked for a prolonged period of time. *Ren Shen* (Radix Ginseng), is often cooked by itself for a relatively long time for single use, or cooked separately prior to being added to other herbs for further cooking in a formula. Both the relatively high cost of ginseng and the relatively high potency of this herb make the longer cooking time quite appropriate. This process is called pre-decoction.

To **reduce side effects and/or toxicity**, certain raw materials are pre-processed. Both *Chuan Wu* (Radix Aconiti Preparata) and *Cao Wu* (Radix Aconiti Kusnezoffii) are examples of herbs that are toxic when raw and should be processed with *Gan Cao* (Radix Glycyrrhizae) and *Hei Dou* (Semen Glycine Max) to decrease toxicity and minimize side effects. Processing *Chang Shan* (Radix Dichroae) with grain-based liquor reduces its tendency to cause nausea and vomiting. *Ban Xia* (Rhizoma Pinelliae) and *Tian Nan Xing* (Rhizoma Arisaematis) require additional preparation and processing to reduce toxicity.

To **increase available herb surface area and facilitate extraction**, minerals, seeds, and shells must be ground or crushed to increase the surface area interacting with the surrounding solution, to ensure maximum extraction of active components. Specific examples include *Zi Ran Tong*

Chapter 5 — Preparation and Processing of Chinese Herbs

(Pyritum), *Ci Shi* (Magnetitum), *Chuan Shan Jia* (Squama Manis), *Zhen Zhu Mu* (Concha Margaritaferae), *Gui Ban* (Plastrum Testudinis), and *Bie Jia* (Carapax Trionycis).

To **prevent spoilage and prolong shelf life,** most plant-based herbs or moisture-sensitive substances must be dried completely prior to storage, to prolong shelf life and avoid spoilage. In addition, many tonic herbs are soaked in grain-based liquor to make herbal wine. The alcohol acts as an effective solvent to extract active constituents, and as a preservative to prevent degradation and spoilage of the herbs.

Cleaning herbs prior to ingestion is an important aspect of the preparation of herbal substances. This purifying involves removing dirt, contamination, odors, and inactive components. Herbs of botanic origin require thorough washing to remove dirt and debris. Other plants or weeds must be removed. Strongly odorous substances may be washed, processed with grain-based liquor or vinegar, or dry-fried until they turn a yellowish color, to release the objectionable odors. Inactive or irrelevant parts of the medicinal substance, such as the head and legs of the cicada *Chan Tui* (Periostracum Cicadae), should be removed prior to final processing and ingestion.

METHODS OF PREPARATION AND PROCESSING

The many substances of Chinese herbal medicine require various methods of preparation to make them available for human use: mechanical processing, water techniques, the use of heat, combined water and heat applications, and more.

Mechanical processing methods are sub-divided into cleaning, pulverizing and slicing:

- Cleaning removes the non-medicinal parts of the material through sorting, sifting and peeling techniques. Examples of cleaning include removal of leaves and branches from *He Huan Hua* (Flos Albiziae), or removal of hair from *Pi Pa Ye* (Folium Eriobotryae).
- Pulverizing works to increase the surface area of substances and facilitate ingestion through grinding, pounding, and crushing techniques. Examples of pulverizing include pounding *Long Gu* (Os Draconis) and *Mu Li* (Concha Ostreae) into small pieces prior to cooking, or grinding *Ling Yang Jiao* (Cornu Saigae Tataricae) into fine powder to allow effective ingestion.
- Slicing is another method of increasing the available surface area of herbs, as well as allowing the herbalist to create standard portion weights and sizes, facilitate drying, and prolong shelf life.

Water processing techniques are sub-divided into moistening, washing, and *shui fei* (refining with water):

- Moistening requires soaking the herbs in water to soften the substances prior to slicing, or to ensure complete extraction prior to cooking in decoctions.
- Washing requires repeated soaking of herbs and removal of the soak water to eliminate undesired odor and components. For example, *Zi He Che* (Placenta Hominis) is washed to remove odor, and *Hai Zao* (Sargassum) and *Kun Bu* (Thallus Laminariae seu Eckloniae) are washed to remove excess salt.
- *Shui fei* (refining with water) technique literally means "flying in water." This technique begins with placing the herbs in a large container with water. The herbs are then crushed and ground, leaving large and heavy particles to settle to the bottom, while small and light particles remain suspended, "flying in water." The small and light particles are poured with the water into another container, and the heavier, sedimentary, particles are ground again. The process of grinding and pouring is repeated several times until only the smallest, lightest particles remain. This is a relatively lengthy, complex method, generally reserved for minerals, shells, and other medicinal substances normally insoluble in water. The purpose of this technique is to extract only the smallest and lightest particles that remain suspended in water. Herbs used for ophthalmic preparations are often processed by *shui fei*.

Methods using heat are subdivided into *chao* (dry-frying), *tan* (charring to ash), *zhi* (frying with liquid), *duan* (calcining), and *wei* (roasting):

- *Chao* (dry-frying) requires stir-frying herbs, without adding liquid, until the herbs turn yellow or black, or turn to ash. This increases the warmth of the herb, harmonizes and moderates therapeutic effects, and facilitates extraction of active constituents.

- *Tan* (charring to ash), burning the herbs to ash, harmonizes and moderates therapeutic effects, reduces side effects, and potentiates the 'stop bleeding' properties of specific substances.
- *Zhi* (frying with liquid) changes the properties of herbs by introducing a new component while heating. This is done to enhance therapeutic effectiveness and reduce side effects. Liquids used for frying include honey, grain-based liquor, vinegar, ginger juice, and salt water.
  Honey enhances the moisturizing effect.
  Grain-based liquor enhances the invigorating function to move qi and blood.
  Vinegar facilitates entrance to the Liver and treatment of Liver disorders.
  Ginger juice increases warmth and relieves nausea and vomiting.
  Salt facilitates entrance to the Kidney and treatment of Kidney disorders.
- *Duan* (calcining) places an herb directly or indirectly into flames until the substance turns red and brittle. This method is often reserved for minerals or shell-like substances, to facilitate pulverization.
- *Wei* (roasting) is a technique that reduces toxicity or moderates the drastic actions of some herbs. Roasting involves wrapping the herbs in wet cloth, paper, or mud, and heating this bundle in hot cinders until the coating has turned black or burned away.

Methods using both water and heat are sub-divided into *zhu* (boiling), *zheng* (steaming), *cui* (quenching), and *ao* (simmering):

- *Zhu* (boiling): Cooking certain herbs in boiling water or another medium enhances the therapeutic effect or reduces toxicity. For example, boiling *Da Ji* (Radix Euphorbiae seu Knoxiae) in vinegar reduces its toxicity.
- *Zheng* (steaming): This method indirectly introduces heat and water to the herbs, again altering the therapeutic effect or reducing toxicity. Steaming *Da Huang* (Radix et Rhizoma Rhei) with grain-based liquor moderates its purgative and laxative properties. Repeated steaming and drying of *He Shou Wu* (Radix Polygoni Multiflori) enhances its tonic strength and reduces its laxative effect.
- *Cui* (quenching): This procedure involves calcining the herbs until they turn red, followed by dipping the calcined product in cold water, making the substance brittle, to facilitate pulverization of the herbs.
- *Ao* (simmering): This process slowly cooks the herbs, extracts active constituents, and removes excess water. Gels, pastes, and extracts are made using this method.

Chapter 6

性能 — Characteristics of Chinese Herbal Medicines

One of the great strengths of Chinese herbal medicine is the high degree of effectiveness obtained by precise differentiation of *both* the symptom pattern *and* the nature and properties of individual herbs. This allows unique prescription of a formula that incorporates herbs selected for the specific characteristics and functions that address the particular symptom pattern that has been identified.

The characteristics of herbs are highly interdependent with herb functions, and vice-versa. The term 'characteristics' refers to a set of values that describe the thermal property, taste, direction, channel affiliations, and toxicity (if any) of each substance. Herb 'functions' describe therapeutic effects (and possible side effects). Throughout the history of traditional Chinese medicine, there has been continuous observation and evaluation of the therapeutic behaviors of herbs. After countless years of recorded experience, the overall effects of herbs are clearly understood, their characteristics well established. While knowing the characteristics of each herb enables the herbalist to interpret its functions, a clear understanding of the herb functions allows one to establish its characteristics.

Most authorities agree on fundamental characteristics and functions of herbs, but there are occasional differences in detail from one text to another.

Most authorities agree on the fundamental characteristics and functions of the majority of herb substances. However, because the interpretation of taste, thermal property, channels affiliations and therapeutic effects are somewhat subjective, there are occasional differences from one text to another.

TASTE

Each herb has a specific taste attribute within the following array: **acrid, sweet, sour, bitter, salty, bland**, and **astringent**. The first five distinctions comprise the five fundamental tastes used in classical herbal medicine. Detailed functions and specific examples of each taste are as follows:

Acrid (pungent): Acrid-tasting herbs often have dispersing and moving properties. For example, herbs that release the exterior, such as *Ma Huang* (Herba Ephedrae), *Gui Zhi* (Ramulus Cinnamomi), *Jing Jie* (Herba Schizonepetae), and *Bo He* (Herba Menthae), are acrid. These herbs function to disperse outward, induce diaphoresis, and dispel exterior pathogenic factors. Herbs that invigorate the circulation of qi and blood, such as *Chen Pi* (Pericarpium Citri Reticulatae), *Mu Xiang* (Radix Aucklandiae), *Chuang Xiong* (Rhizoma Ligustici Chuanxiong), and *Hong Hua* (Flos Carthami), are also acrid: they disperse and move qi and blood. Since acrid herbs are both dispersing and drying, they should be used with caution in patients with deficiency of qi, yin, or body fluids, and in cases of spontaneous perspiration.

Sweet: Sweet herbs often have tonifying and harmonizing properties. *Ren Shen* (Radix Ginseng) and *Huang Qi* (Radix Astragali), both sweet, are key herbs to tonify qi. In addition, many herbs that have harmonizing and moderating properties are also sweet. *Gan Cao* (Radix Glycyrrhizae) and *Da Zao* (Fructus Jujubae) are sweet herbs that provide excellent catalysts to harmonize an herbal formula, moderate the drastic effects of some herbs, and relieve pain. Since sweet herbs are often rich or cloying and hard to digest, thus, may cause stagnation, they should be used with caution in patients who have Spleen deficiency with accumulated dampness.

Sour: Herbs that are said to taste sour often function to stabilize and bind, thereby reducing or preventing the loss of body fluids through perspiration, diarrhea, bleeding, leukorrhea, urinary incontinence, enuresis, spermatorrhea, and nocturnal emissions. For example, *Wu Wei Zi* (Fructus Schisandrae Chinensis) and *Wu Bei Zi* (Galla Chinensis) function to stop perspiration; *Xian He Cao* (Herba Agrimoniae) and *Bai Ji* (Rhizoma Bletillae) stop bleeding; *Chi Shi Zhi* (Halloysitum Rubrum) and *Shi Liu Pi* (Pericarpium Granati) stop diarrhea; and *Jin Ying Zi* (Fructus Rosae Laevigatae) and *Sang Piao Xiao* (Ootheca Mantidis) halt spermatorrhea and nocturnal emissions.

Chapter 6 — Characteristics of Chinese Herbal Medicines

In addition, sour herbs nourish Stomach yin and improve appetite, as is true of *Wu Mei* (Fructus Mume) and *Wu Wei Zi* (Fructus Schisandrae Chinensis); others, such as *Mu Gua* (Fructus Chaenomelis) and *Bai Shao* (Radix Paeoniae Alba) treat muscle spasms and cramps caused by damage to body fluids. *Wu Mei* (Fructus Mume) is one example of several sour herbs that calm intestinal parasites and relieve pain.

Bitter: Bitter-tasting herbs function to sedate, to purge, and/or to dry dampness. The sedating and purging functions refer to the elimination of heat and other excess factors via the downward movement of the herbs. For example, *Da Huang* (Radix et Rhizoma Rhei), a bitter herb, drains heat and fire downwards to relieve constipation; *Xing Ren* (Semen Armeniacae Amarum), also a bitter herb, sends inappropriately rising Lung qi back downwards to relieve wheezing and dyspnea; and *Zhi Zi* (Fructus Gardeniae) purges fire to treat various infections accompanied by elevated body temperature.

Furthermore, bitter-tasting herbs function to dry dampness. Bitter and cold herbs, such as *Huang Lian* (Rhizoma Coptidis), treat syndromes characterized by dampness and heat. Bitter and warm herbs, such as *Cang Zhu* (Rhizoma Atractylodis), address syndromes characterized by dampness and cold.

Herbs distinguished by the bitter taste have been found to stimulate the nervous system and increase production of gastric acid. Therefore, a small quantity of bitter herbs taken before meals will increase appetite and improve digestion. A large quantity, however, may have the opposite effect, inducing nausea and vomiting. Since bitter herbs are drying in nature, they should be used with caution in cases of deficiency of yin and body fluids.

Salty: The functions of the salty-tasting herbs are to purge excess, soften hardness, and facilitate entrance to the Kidney and/or Kidney channel. For example, *Mang Xiao* (Natrii Sulfas) has purgative action to treat constipation; *Mu Li* (Concha Ostreae) softens hardness to treat scrofula, enlarged thyroid, and nodules. In addition, herbs that are salty or have been processed with salt, such as *Lu Rong* (Cornu Cervi Pantotrichum) and *Ge Jie* (Gecko), enter the Kidney and treat Kidney-related disorders.

Bland: Not surprisingly, bland-tasting herbs have little or no taste. They generally exert diuretic influence, and are commonly used to treat edema and dysuria. *Fu Ling* (Poria) and *Zhu Ling* (Polyporus) are common examples.

Astringent: Herbs designated as having an astringent property are basically the same as sour-tasting herbs, functioning to retain and bind, that is, draw or bind together and preserve or prevent leakage of bodily substances. For example, *Wu Wei Zi* (Fructus Schisandrae Chinensis) contains the leakage of Lung qi to treat cough, *Chi Shi Zhi* (Halloysitum Rubrum) binds the intestines to stop diarrhea, and *Fu Xiao Mai* (Semen Tritici Aestivi Levis) stops spontaneous sweating.

It is important to note that tastes and functions do not always correspond to each other. Foods that have the flavors described above may not have any identified medicinal properties; herbs with specific therapeutic effects may not always have the usual corresponding taste. For example, *Ge Gen* (Radix Puerariae) acts to dispel heat and release the exterior, yet does not taste acrid. Another example, *Ying Su Ke* (Pericarpium Papaveris) stabilizes and binds the intestines to treat diarrhea, yet does not have either sour or astringent tastes.

Table 6. Relationship of Taste and Function

Taste	Function
Acrid	Release the exterior, disperse outwards, move qi and blood
Sweet	Tonify deficiencies, harmonize herbs within a formula
Sour	Stabilize and bind, reduce and prevent the loss of body fluids
Bitter	Sedate heat, purge fire, drain downwards, dry dampness
Salty	Purge excess, soften hardness, facilitate entrance to the Kidney
Bland	Promote urination
Astringent	Stabilize and bind, reduce and prevent the loss of body fluids

Chapter 6 — Characteristics of Chinese Herbal Medicines

THERMAL PROPERTY

Thermal property describes the 'temperature' of the herbs, expressed as a progressive range: cold, cool, neutral, warm, hot. Describing a traditional approach to treatment, many classic texts state: "Cold diseases must be warmed, and hot diseases must be cooled." Therefore, cold or cool herbs, such as *Huang Qin* (Radix Scutellariae) and *Ban Lan Gen* (Radix Isatidis), are commonly used to treat disorders characterized by heat, such as fever and sore throat. Warm and hot herbs, such as *Gan Jiang* (Rhizoma Zingiberis) and *Fu Zi* (Radix Aconiti Lateralis Praeparata), treat disorders characterized by cold, such as abdominal cold and pain, and cold extremities. Neutral herbs, such as *Fu Ling* (Poria), may be used for conditions on either side of the temperature range. Accurate diagnosis of the temperature of the health imbalance, followed by a correct corresponding prescription, promotes successful treatment of the illness.

DIRECTION

The concept of **direction** refers to the dynamic or developmental movement of the disease and to the directional affinity of the herbs. There are disorders that move *upwards* (such as cough and vomiting), *downwards* (diarrhea, dysentery, prolapse of rectum), *inward* (transformation from a common cold to pneumonia), and *outward* (spontaneous or night perspiration). Similarly, each herb has its own directional characteristics, some more pronounced than others. Flowers or rapidly-growing plants tend to carry lighter, upward-moving qi, while substances found deeper in the earth, such as roots or minerals, often possess heavier, or downward-bearing energy.

Therefore, disorders typified by a distinct directional flow may be countered by the use of herbs that influence movement in the opposite direction. For example, a cough (Lung qi moving up) may be relieved by herbs that cause qi to descend; prolapse of the rectum may be treated with herbs that lift qi (raise or cause it to ascend); the inward invasion of a common cold may be treated by the use of herbs that disperse and dispel the exterior pathogenic factor; and spontaneous perspiration may be treated with herbs that retain fluids and/or bind substances to prevent loss.

Herbs with particular directional affinities may also be useful as 'guide herbs' to direct the therapeutic effect of the treatment to the affected area. For example, *Qiang Huo* (Rhizoma et Radix Notopterygii) moves upwards, thus it treats musculoskeletal disorders of the upper body (and guides other herbs in a formula to the upper body). Conversely, *Du Huo* (Radix Angelicae Pubescentis) moves downwards and thus treats (and/or guides other herbs to treat) musculoskeletal disorders of the lower body.

CHANNELS AFFILIATIONS

The appointment of one or more of the 14 classic energetic channels of the body to each herb is done gradually via the accumulated understanding of the functions of and indications for each herb. The criteria this assignment is based upon include **direct effect, indirect effect**, and **specific effect**.

The system of assigning channels by **direct effect** refers to the specific function and indications of the herb. For example, *Xing Ren* (Semen Armeniacae Amarum) is said to enter the Lung channel because it treats cough and wheezing; classic texts list *Ban Xia* (Rhizoma Pinelliae) as entering the Stomach channel because it relieves nausea and vomiting; and tradition holds that *Zhu Ling* (Polyporus) goes to the Urinary Bladder channel because it promotes urination.

Channels are also appointed to the herb **indirectly** via the interpretation of its function. For example, *Bu Gu Zhi* (Fructus Psoraleae) warms the Spleen and Kidney to (indirectly) relieve chronic diarrhea, so is said to enter the Spleen and Kidney channels; and *Fu Pen Zi* (Fructus Rubi) treats frequent urination by tonifying Kidney qi, thus is identified as influencing the Kidney channel. *Xu Duan* (Radix Dipsaci) nourishes bones and tendons, effectively treating bone fractures and soft tissue injuries. Since tendons are controlled by the Liver and bones by the Kidney, *Xu Duan* is said to enter the Liver and Kidney channels.

Furthermore, there are some herbs that have **specific effects** for treating certain organs and particular kinds of headache, and are appointed channels based on observation of those affinities. For example, *Yin Chen Hao* (Herba Artemisiae Scopariae) is one of the most effective herbs for

Chapter 6 — Characteristics of Chinese Herbal Medicines

treatment of jaundice, and thus is assigned to enter the Liver and Gallbladder channels.

A classic example of how this differentiation is applied in clinical practice is the use of herbs for headache: *Qiang Huo* (Rhizoma et Radix Notopterygii) is most effective in treating *taiyang* headaches; *Chai Hu* (Radix Bupleuri) most directly addresses *shaoyang* headaches; and *Bai Zhi* (Radix Angelicae Dahuricae) excels at treating *yangming* headaches. *Taiyin* headaches should be treated with *Cang Zhu* (Rhizoma Atractylodis), *shaoyin* headaches are best treated with *Xi Xin* (Herba Asari), and *jueyin* headaches can be dealt with by adding *Wu Zhu Yu* (Fructus Evodiae). Thus, each of these herbs are assigned to the corresponding channels.

SUMMARY

It is important to keep in mind that while thermal property, taste, direction and channels are four separate evaluative criteria, each of them must be taken into account when treating patients. Choosing the correct taste but the wrong temperature, or the appropriate temperature but the wrong channels will result in inappropriate treatment.

For example, just because *Huang Lian* (Rhizoma Coptidis), *Huang Qin* (Radix Scutellariae), and *Long Dan Cao* (Radix Gentianae) are all cold does not mean they have the same function and indications. *Huang Lian* clears Heart fire, *Huang Qin* clears Lung fire, and *Long Dan Cao* clears Liver fire.

In addition, just because *Huang Qin* (Radix Scutellariae), *Gan Jiang* (Rhizoma Zingiberis), *Bai He* (Bulbus Lilii) and *Ting Li Zi* (Semen Descurainiae seu Lepidii) all enter the Lung channel does not mean they can be used indiscriminately for Lung disorders. *Huang Qin* clears Lung fire, *Gan Jiang* warms the Lung, *Bai He* tonifies Lung yin, and *Ting Li Zi* sedates excess Lung energy.

To obtain maximum impact for the efforts put into integrating temperature, taste, direction and channels, it is important to correctly diagnose the disorder. For example, when treating patients with wheezing and dyspnea, it is important to know whether the disorder is caused by the Lung or the Kidney. Wheezing and dyspnea caused by a Lung disorder should be treated with *Ma Huang* (Herba Ephedrae) and *Xing Ren* (Semen Armeniacae Amarum) to disperse and descend qi; while wheezing and dyspnea caused by Kidney deficiency should be treated with *Ge Jie* (Gecko) and *Bu Gu Zhi* (Fructus Psoraleae) to tonify the Lung and help Kidney energy to grasp the qi and draw it down.

Following precise diagnostic protocols will similarly allow the practitioner to select appropriate herbs for such regional issues as headaches, as discussed above, and *bi zheng* (painful obstruction syndrome), that have unique causes and locations.

TOXICITY

Toxicity refers to the potential for an herb to cause side effects and adverse reactions. While the majority of herbs are safe when used correctly and within the suggested dosage range, there are some that may cause undesired effects even within normal dosage ranges. Such herbs are designated as having toxic properties. These herbs have a narrow safety index and must be used only when the benefits of usage outweigh the risks.

From over 7,000 species of medicinal plants in China, not more than 10 species are considered toxic.

The impact of toxicity is often dose-related. Smaller doses are associated with less toxic reactions, while larger doses are associated with more toxic impact. From over 7,000 species of medicinal plants in China, not more than 10 species are considered toxic. Examples of toxic herbs from these species include various aconite roots and datura species, a tiny group of substances that account for up to 76% of all serious reactions that require urgent medical treatment.[6]

Some of these herbs are inherently toxic and their uses must be monitored carefully. *Huang Yao Zi* (Herba Dioscoreae Bulbiferae) is very effective for treatment of hyperthyroid conditions. However, its use has been associated with liver damage in rare cases. Therefore, *Huang Yao Zi* must be prescribed in small dosages, monitored carefully, and discontinued if symptoms and signs of potential liver damage occur.

Proper combining with other herbs is also an effective solution to reduce noxious impact. For example, concurrent use of *Gan Cao* (Radix Glycyrrhizae) reduces the toxicity of *Fu Zi* (Radix

Chapter 6 — Characteristics of Chinese Herbal Medicines

Aconiti Lateralis Praeparata); use of *Sheng Jiang* (Rhizoma Zingiberis Recens) decreases the toxicity of *Ban Xia* (Rhizoma Pinelliae); and use of *Bing Lang* (Semen Arecae) relieves nausea caused by *Chang Shan* (Radix Dichroae).

Reducing dosage while increasing frequency of intake is another approach to reducing the negative impact of a toxic herb. This method reduces the peak blood concentration associated with a large dosage, and stabilizes the blood concentration by more frequent dosing. This is especially effective for patients who suffer side effects or adverse reactions immediately after ingesting herbs.

Toxicity is sometimes caused by adulteration and contamination of herbs. While most herbal products are safe and effective, there are some products that may contain pharmaceutical drugs, herbicides, pesticides, sulfur, heavy metals, bacteria and fungus. Adverse reactions due to adulteration and contamination of herbs are problems associated with lack of quality control during the manufacturing procedure. Such instances are to be evaluated as manufacturing errors, not as inherent toxicity of the herbs.

It is important to note that allergic reactions are <u>not</u> toxic reactions. An *allergy* is a hypersensitive reaction that is specific and may differ in every individual. Allergic reactions occur with exposure to the offending agent. A mild allergy is characterized by skin rash and itching, while a severe allergic reaction may cause dyspnea and shortness of breath. Unfortunately, it is difficult, if not impossible, to predict which herb may cause allergy to what degree of severity in which individual.

Inappropriate Use

Correct diagnosis and appropriate usage of herbs contribute a great deal to prevention of unwanted results. For example, a patient suffering from a deficiency needs to have that deficiency tonified. However, if yang tonics are incorrectly prescribed to treat yin deficiency, not only will the treatment be ineffective, but the condition will also deteriorate further, since warm, yang-building herbs will further deplete stores of yin.

Gan Cao (Radix Glycyrrhizae) is an example of an herb that is generally safe and effective in a variety of uses and combinations. However, if used incorrectly in large dosages over a prolonged period of time, it will undoubtedly cause edema and an unwanted increase in blood pressure.

The toxicity of the few suspect herbs can be reduced and/or minimized when the herbs are processed correctly. For example, while unprocessed aconite roots are considered toxic, cooking them in boiling water for 30 to 60 minutes will reduce the toxicity to 1/2000 to 1/4000th of the toxicity of the unprocessed herb, making the resultant product safe for further incorporation in preparing a combination formula. While unprocessed *Ba Dou* (Fructus Crotonis) is extremely toxic, removal of all of its essential oils will eliminate most of its toxic component, leaving only laxative influence.

Chapter 7

– Clinical Applications of Chinese Herbal Medicine

Chinese herbal medicine is a combination of both the art and the science of medicine. While traditional Chinese medicine offers many approaches to the treatment of any one illness, there are also strict guidelines that every practitioner must follow. Optimal therapeutic effects can only be achieved through clear understanding of the disorder being treated, correct differential diagnosis, and precise formulation of herbs. When creating an herbal formula, it is important to consider the herbs selected (formulation), any accompanying cautions or contraindications, appropriate dosage, and the most advantageous preparation methods.

FORMULATION

Chinese herbs may be prescribed either as single herbs or, most commonly, as combined herbal formulations. Single herbs are used in treatment when the illness has a clear diagnosis with no complications. For example, *Ren Shen* (Radix Ginseng) is sometimes used alone to restore collapsed qi. However, using one herb individually is generally not sufficient for treatment: most disease conditions are complex and require the administration of multiple herbs. Furthermore, using a large dosage of a single herb exposes the patient to higher risk of side effects and adverse reactions. Therefore, multiple herbs are generally combined as an herbal formula to achieve maximum benefit with minimal side effects.

As the prescription of herbal formulas is naturally more complicated than the use of single herbs, rules and guidelines for proper formulation must be followed closely. While combinations of certain herbs will boost the overall therapeutic effect of a formula, the combination of others might lead to reduced effectiveness or even undesired effects. There are six major categories of herb-to-herb interaction that serve as reliable guidelines for the practitioner seeking maximum effectiveness. The examples below are classic examples found in standard textbooks of *Zhong Yao Xue* (Chinese Herbology).

- *Xiang xu* (mutual accentuation): Herbs with similar functions combine to amplify the overall therapeutic effect. For example, *Shi Gao* (Gypsum Fibrosum) and *Zhi Mu* (Radix Anemarrhenae) are combined to accentuate their individual abilities to clear heat and purge fire; *Da Huang* (Radix et Rhizoma Rhei) and *Mang Xiao* (Natrii Sulfas) are put together to potentiate purgative and laxative actions.
- *Xiang shi* (mutual enhancement): Herbs with different functions combine such that one herb enhances the properties of another. For example, *Fu Ling* (Poria) amplifies the nature of *Huang Qi* (Radix Astragali) to tonify qi and regulate water circulation; and *Da Huang* (Radix et Rhizoma Rhei) serves as a catalyst for the ability of *Huang Qin* (Radix Scutellariae) to clear heat and purge fire.
- *Xiang wei* (mutual counteraction): One herb minimizes or neutralizes a toxic aspect of another. For example, the toxicity of *Ban Xia* (Rhizoma Pinelliae) can be reduced by adding *Sheng Jiang* (Rhizoma Zingiberis Recens). [Note: The concept of "mutual" may not seem at first to apply to *xiang wei* and *xiang sha* (below), confusing readers. It may be helpful to think of counteraction and suppression as the need for the toxic or side-effect laden herb and its partners to work together to provide safe and comfortable effectiveness.]
- *Xiang sha* (mutual suppression): Addition of an herb to suppress or reduce unwanted side effects from another. For example, the addition of *Sheng Jiang* (Rhizoma Zingiberis Recens) reduces the side effects that may accompany *Tian Nan Xing* (Rhizoma Arisaematis). *Xiang wei* (mutual counteraction) and *xiang sha* (mutual suppression) are essentially the same: both achieve the same goal. The only difference is the emphasis. *Xiang wei* (mutual counteraction) emphasizes that a toxic effect <u>must</u> be reduced by adding other herbs, while *xiang sha* (mutual suppression) empha-

sizes that addition of certain herbs suppresses unwanted actions of certain other herbs.

- *Xiang wu* (mutual antagonism): A combination in which the desired therapeutic effect of an herb is reduced by the addition of another. For example, the qi-tonifying attributes of *Ren Shen* (Radix Ginseng) are reduced if *Lai Fu Zi* (Semen Raphani) is added to the formula.
- *Xiang fan* (mutual incompatibility): The combination of two specific herbs will lead to undesirable side effects and/or adverse reactions. This is an illustration of adverse herb-herb interactions (discussed further in chapter 8). Examples of *xiang fan* (mutual incompatibility) include *Shi Ba Fan* (Eighteen Incompatibles) and *Shi Jiu Wei* (Nineteen Counteractions). More details are listed in the section below.

CAUTIONS AND CONTRAINDICATIONS IN CLINICAL PRACTICE

There are two levels of further instruction that herbalists have communicated over the centuries to insure safe and effective treatment: cautions or contraindications, 1) related to the interaction of the nature of the herbs with the specific symptoms of the patient, and 2) similar guidelines related to the interaction of the herbs with other herbs.

In the first category, an herb with diuretic functions might be labeled for use with caution in patients who are experiencing deficiency of yin or body fluids, while an herb that has a strong upward-moving characteristic might be identified as contraindicated for treatment of a patient at risk for stroke.

The second category refers to examples of herb-to-herb interactions. While most herbs are believed to be safe when used individually or together with other herbs, certain combinations have proven to create undesirable side effects and adverse reactions. For centuries, there have been listings of exactly which herbs are not to be combined. The *Shi Ba Fan* (Eighteen Incompatibles) is a classic list of eighteen herb-to-herb interactions. The *Shi Jiu Wei* (Nineteen Counteractions) is a classic list of nineteen herbal combinations in which the herbs counteract each other. Combinations of such herbs will likely lead to adverse side effects and/or toxic reactions. It should be noted here: these are not exhaustive lists. The observant reader will find other examples of incompatibilities noted specifically in the individual herb monographs.

***Shi Ba Fan* (Eighteen Incompatibles)** is a list of herbs that are incompatible when combined. The original list contained only 18 herbs, but the list has since been expanded.

- *Gan Cao* (Radix Glycyrrhizae) is incompatible with:
  Gan Sui (Radix Euphorbiae Kansui)
  Jing Da Ji (Radix Euphorbiae Pekinensis)
  Hong Da Ji (Radix Knoxiae)
  Yuan Hua (Flos Genkwa)
  Hai Zao (Sargassum)

- *Fu Zi* (Radix Aconiti Lateralis Praeparata), *Chuan Wu* (Radix Aconiti Preparata) and *Cao Wu* (Radix Aconiti Kusnezoffii) are incompatible with:
  Ban Xia (Rhizoma Pinelliae)
  Chuan Bei Mu (Bulbus Fritillariae Cirrhosae)
  Zhe Bei Mu (Bulbus Fritillariae Thunbergii)
  Gua Lou Shi (Fructus Trichosanthis)
  Gua Lou Ren (Semen Trichosanthis)
  Gua Lou Pi (Pericarpium Trichosanthis)
  Tian Hua Fen (Radix Trichosanthis)
  Bai Ji (Rhizoma Bletillae)
  Bai Lian (Radix Ampelopsis)

- *Li Lu* (Radix et Rhizoma Veratri) is incompatible with:
  Ren Shen (Radix Ginseng)
  Dang Shen (Radix Codonopsis)
  Nan Sha Shen (Radix Adenophorae)
  Bei Sha Shen (Radix Glehniae)
  Dan Shen (Radix Salviae Miltiorrhizae)
  Xuan Shen (Radix Scrophulariae)
  Ku Shen Gen (Radix Sophorae Flavescentis)
  Chi Shao (Radix Paeoniae Rubrae)
  Bai Shao (Radix Paeoniae Alba)
  Xi Xin (Herba Asari)

***Shi Jiu Wei* (Nineteen Counteractions)** consists of nineteen herbs combined as ten pairs that antagonize each other:

Liu Huang (Sulfur) and *Po Xiao* (Sal Glauberis)
Shui Yin (Hydrargyum) and *Pi Shuang* (Arsenolite)
Lang Du (Radix Euphorbiae Fischerianae) and *Mi Tuo Seng* (Lithargyrum)
Ba Dou (Fructus Crotonis) and *Qian Niu Zi* (Semen Pharbitidis)
Ding Xiang (Flos Caryophylli) and *Yu Jin* (Radix Curcumae)
Ya Xiao (Nitrum) and *San Leng* (Rhizoma Sparganii)
Xi Jiao (Cornu Rhinoceri) and *Cao Wu* (Radix Aconiti Kusnezoffii)
Xi Jiao (Cornu Rhinoceri) and *Chuan Wu* (Radix Aconiti Preparata)
Ren Shen (Radix Ginseng) and *Wu Ling Zhi* (Excrementum Trogopteri seu Pteromi)
Rou Gui (Cortex Cinnamomi) and *Chi Shi Zhi* (Halloysitum Rubrum)

DIETARY CONSIDERATIONS

There are historically documented interactions between certain foods and particular herbs. The wise practitioner informs patients about factors that diminish digestive effectiveness or compete with the digestion of herbs. In general, foods that are cold, raw, greasy, rotten or spoiled, and other foods that are difficult to digest, should be avoided when taking herbal medicines.

During herbal therapy, avoiding specific foods will prevent unwanted reactions. For example, onions should not be eaten when ingesting an herbal formula including *Chang Shan* (Radix Dichroae); onions and garlic should not be taken with *Sheng Di Huang* (Radix Rehmanniae), *Shu Di Huang* (Radix Rehmanniae Preparata), and *He Shou Wu* (Radix Polygoni Multiflori); vinegar should not be used by a patient being treated with *Fu Ling* (Poria); and raw onion should not be taken with *Feng Mi* (Mel).

Foods that are cold, raw, greasy, rotten or spoiled, and other foods that are difficult to digest, should be avoided when taking herbal medicines.

USE OF HERBS DURING PREGNANCY

Certain herbs have a recognized potential to endanger or cause harm to a fetus during pregnancy, thus possibly causing birth defects or miscarriage. As a general rule, herbs with potent effects to regulate qi, move blood, or drain downwards should be avoided during pregnancy. These herbs are classified as **contraindicated** or for **use with caution** in treatment of pregnant women. Please note that these are not comprehensive lists—additional information is listed in each individual herb monograph. On the other hand, there are many herbs that are specifically used during pregnancy to **stabilize pregnancy** and prevent miscarriage.

Herbs that are **contraindicated** during pregnancy are generally toxic, or have potent effect to break stagnation or drain downwards.

Ba Dou (Semen Crotonis)
Ban Mao (Mylabris)
Da Huang (Radix et Rhizoma Rhei)

Da Ji (Radix Euphorbiae seu Knoxiae)
E Zhu (Rhizoma Curcumae)
Mang Xiao (Natrii Sulfas)
Meng Chong (Tabanus Bivttatus Matsumura)
Qian Niu Zi (Semen Pharbitidis)
San Leng (Rhizoma Sparganii)
Shang Lu (Radix Phytolaccae)
She Xiang (Moschus)
Shui Zhi (Hirudo)

Herbs that must be **used with caution** during pregnancy are usually pungent and warm in nature. These substances activate qi, activate blood circulation, and remove blood stasis. They are very potent and should be avoided, or used only in later stages of pregnancy *if* the benefits of using the herbs outweigh the risks.
Fu Zi (Radix Aconiti Lateralis Praeparata)
Gan Jiang (Rhizoma Zingiberis)
Hong Hua (Flos Carthami)
Rou Gui (Cortex Cinnamomi)
Tao Ren (Semen Persicae)
Zhi Shi (Fructus Aurantii Immaturus)

Herbs that **stabilize pregnancy** can be used if needed to prevent miscarriage.
Bai Zhu (Rhizoma Atractylodis Macrocephalae)
Du Zhong (Cortex Eucommiae)
Huang Qin (Radix Scutellariae)
Sha Ren (Fructus Amomi)
Zi Su Ye (Folium Perillae)

USE OF HERBS DURING NURSING

Little information has been noted historically regarding the safety of nursing mothers ingesting herbs. It is best not to assume that herbs ingested by the mother will not become evident in her breast milk. Therefore, it is prudent to advise nursing mothers to temporarily avoid using herbs.

However, if herbal medicine should become necessary for a nursing mother, the prescribing practitioner must follow simple safety guidelines concerning both the physical nature of the herbs and their possible influence. More lipophilic materials, such as animal and insect substances, and seeds, are more likely to be transmitted in breast milk; herbs that are more hydrophilic, certain minerals, leaves, and roots, are less apt to show up in breast milk. Gauging the desired action of the herbs for the mother, the practitioner can anticipate what effect the herbs may have on the infant, and take precautionary steps if necessary.

There are herbs used specifically to promote lactation during nursing. Such herbs dispel stagnation and promote the generation of breast milk. Examples include:
Chuan Mu Tong (Caulis Clematidis Armandii)
Chuan Shan Jia (Squama Manis)
Dong Kui Zi (Semen Malvae)
Lou Lu (Radix Rhapontici)
Nan Gua Zi (Semen Cucurbitae Moschatae)
Si Gua Luo (Retinervus Luffae Fructus)
Tong Cao (Medulla Tetrapanacis)
Wang Bu Liu Xing (Semen Vaccariae)
Zi He Che (Placenta Hominis)

Chapter 7 — Clinical Applications of Chinese Herbal Medicine

There are herbs to inhibit lactation when necessary:

Mang Xiao (Natrii Sulfas)
Shen Qu (Massa Fermentata)
Mai Ya (Fructus Hordei Germinatus)
Hua Jiao (Pericarpium Zanthoxyli)

WEIGHTS AND MEASURES

The traditional system of measurement in China is significantly different from the British and metric systems. Listed below are conversions between the traditional Chinese system and the metric system:

1 *liang* = 30 grams
1 *qian* = 3 grams
1 *fen* = 0.3 gram
1 *li* = 0.03 gram

DOSING

The dosages listed in this text refer to the daily dose for an adult of average height and weight, when using dehydrated herbs. However, the actual prescribed dosage will vary significantly, based not only on the characteristics of the illness and overall condition of the patient, but also on his or her size and age. Generally speaking, single herbs used individually require higher dosages, while herbs used as part of an herbal formula are chosen in smaller amounts. Treatment of an acute condition necessitates higher dosages, and treatment of a mild condition, smaller dosages. One must also consider the constitution of the patient. Those who are basically healthy and strong may tolerate larger doses, while weak and/or deficient patients will need a smaller dose.

Recommended ingestion levels must be adjusted to reflect variations in age and body weight. The principle behind the *Age-to-Dose Guideline* is based on assessment of the maturity of the internal organs and their capacity to metabolize, utilize and eliminate herbs. This highly-detailed chart is especially useful for infants and younger children. The recommendations are taken from *Zhong Cao Yao* (Chinese Herbal Medicine), published by the Nanjing College of Traditional Chinese Medicine.

The principle behind the *Weight-to-Dose Guideline* is based on the effective concentration of the herbal medicine once it is distributed throughout different areas of the body. This dosing strategy is especially useful for patients whose body weight falls outside of the normal range. All calculations are based on Clark's Rule in "*Pharmaceutical Calculations*," written by Mitchell Stoklosa and Howard Ansel.

These charts provide herbal practitioners a handy reference for dosing those patients who fall outside the definition of an average adult. It is important to remember, however, that the charts serve only as guidelines—not as absolute rules. One must always remember to treat each patient as a unique individual, not as a statistic on a chart!

Table 7. Age-to-Dose Dosing Guideline

Age	Recommended Daily Dosage
0 – 1 month	1/18 – 1/14 of adult dose
1 – 6 month	1/14 – 1/7 of adult dose
6 – 12 month	1/7 – 1/5 of adult dose
1 – 2 years	1/5 – 1/4 of adult dose
2 – 4 years	1/4 – 1/3 of adult dose
4 – 6 years	1/3 – 2/5 of adult dose
6 – 9 years	2/5 – 1/2 of adult dose
9 – 14 years	1/2 – 2/3 of adult dose
14 – 18 years	2/3 – full adult dose
18 – 60 years	**adult dose**
60 years and over	3/4 or less of adult dose

Chapter 7 — Clinical Applications of Chinese Herbal Medicine

Table 8. Weight-to-Dose Dosing Guideline

Weight	Recommended Daily Dosage
30 – 40 lbs	20% – 27% of adult dose
40 – 50 lbs	27% – 33% of adult dose
50 – 60 lbs	33% – 40% of adult dose
60 – 70 lbs	40% – 47% of adult dose
70 – 80 lbs	47% – 53% of adult dose
80 – 100 lbs	53% – 67% of adult dose
100 – 120 lbs	67% – 80% of adult dose
120 – 150 lbs	80% – 100% of adult dose
150 lbs	**adult dose**
150 – 200 lbs	100% – 133% of adult dose
200 – 250 lbs	133% – 167% of adult dose
250 – 300 lbs	167% – 200% of adult dose

PREPARATION OF HERBS

The decoction is the most common dosage form for herbs in China. While the exact preparation of decoctions varies with the herbs prescribed, the general rules remain the same. The herbs must first be soaked for some period of time (determined by the nature of the herbs and the purpose for which they are being prepared), in enough water to completely cover the herbs. The herbs are then cooked until the water boils, at which point the decoction is simmered for some period of time (again, dependent upon the particular blend of herbs in the decoction) before the resultant 'tea' (or, decoction) is poured off for consumption. The cooked herb dregs may be cooked a second time, discarded, or even (in some cases) added to foods for the patient.

PREPARATION METHODS

Cooking processes vary depending on the herbs used, to maximize the therapeutic effects and minimize side effects.

Pre-decoction is a process by which herbs are cooked for an extended period of time. Tonic or rich herbs must be pre-decocted by cooking them for a longer period of time to ensure extraction of active components. Mineral substances are cooked for even longer, as many constituents have low water solubility and are hard to extract. On the other hand, some herbs, such as *Fu Zi* (Radix Aconiti Lateralis Praeparata), are cooked for an extended period of time to minimize toxicity.

Post-decoction is a specific instruction to add the herbs at the end of the decoction process and cook them for only a short period of time (about 5 to 10 minutes). Acrid or aromatic herbs, such as *Bo He* (Herba Menthae) and *Huo Xiang* (Herba Agastache), contain essential oils which easily evaporate if cooked at high temperatures for a prolonged period of time. Herbs that contain constituents that are easily deactivated by heat, such as *Da Huang* (Radix et Rhizoma Rhei) and *Fan Xie Ye* (Folium Sennae), are also added at the end of the cooking process to preserve the integrity of the active components.

Other specifics:

Some herbs, such as *Xin Yi Hua* (Flos Magnoliae), should be wrapped in cheesecloth during the cooking process, because their fibers are irritating to the throat when ingested.

Some herbs are added to the decoction after the preparation process, immediately prior to ingestion, such as *Mang Xiao* (Natrii Sulfas). Juices from fresh herbs, like *Zhu Li* (Succus Bambusae) and *Sheng Jiang* (Rhizoma Zingiberis Recens), are also added at the end of preparation, prior to ingestion.

Herbs that are more expensive, such as *Ren Shen* (Radix Ginseng) and *San Qi* (Radix Notoginseng), are commonly taken as powder without cooking, or are cooked separately to ensure maximal use of the herb and maximal therapeutic effectiveness.

INGESTION STRATEGIES

Generally speaking, decoctions should be warm when ingested. More specifically, exterior wind-cold conditions should be treated with warm decoctions and the patient's body covered with blankets to induce perspiration. Cases of vomiting should be treated with small doses of decoctions taken more frequently, in order to minimize irritation. Herbs in solid dosage forms, such as capsules, tablets, and pills, are best taken with warm water to facilitate absorption. Taking the herbs with tea or soda may decrease the absorption of the herbs or create unwanted gastrointestinal side effects.

TIMING OF DOSING

Tonic herbs are often taken *after* meals to improve the tonic effect. Antiparasitic herbs and laxative herbs are taken *on an empty stomach* one hour before or two hours after meals. Herbs that strengthen the Spleen and Stomach, or herbs that are irritating to the gastrointestinal tract, are taken *after meals,* while food is present to cushion the effect of the herbal substances. Herbs that induce sleep are taken *before bedtime.*

FREQUENCY

Herbs are generally taken three times daily. However, acute or severe conditions may require dosing up to every four hours, while chronic or mild conditions may only need two daily doses. Furthermore, aggressive treatment, such as releasing the exterior or draining the bowels, should be used only when necessary and discontinued as soon as the desired effect is achieved, to avoid unnecessary adverse effects.

Chapter 8 — Concurrent Use of Herbal Medicines and Pharmaceuticals

中西药

The practice of medicine is now at a crossroads: countless patients are being treated simultaneously with both Western and Oriental medicine. It is quite common for a patient to seek herbal treatment while taking several prescription medications. According to JAMA, an estimated 15 million adults in the United States (representing 18.4% of all prescription pharmaceutical users) took prescription drugs concurrently with herbal remedies and/or vitamins in 1997.[7]

As the general public grows increasingly open to the use of herbs and supplements, both patients and the health professionals who care for them are becoming more alert to the potential for occasional adverse herb-drug interactions. Safety has become a major topic of discussion. Even though herbal remedies are classified as dietary supplements, it must be noted that if used incorrectly, herbs, like any substance, may affect patients adversely. The safest route of access to herbal therapy is through a well-qualified herbalist.

Although Chinese herbal medicine has been prescribed safely by professionals in the West for many years now and a great deal of research has been amassed in China, there are still few formal studies published in English to document the safety and efficacy of combining herbs with prescription drugs. Some questions posed by Western healthcare professionals or patients are difficult to answer quickly with documented specifics. However, with some general insights into pharmacology, one can foresee possible interactions and take appropriate precautions to prevent incompatible combinations.

The concept of 'interaction' refers to the possibility that, when two (or more) substances are given concurrently, one substance may interact with another, or alter its bioavailability or clinical action. The net result may be an increase or a decrease in the effectiveness of one or both substances. It is important to note that interactions may yield positive effects (achieving better therapeutic effects at lower dosage) or negative results (creating unwanted side effects or adverse reactions). Most of the possible interactions may be classified in two major categories: pharmacokinetic and pharmacodynamic.[8, 9]

PHARMACOKINETIC INTERACTIONS

'Pharmacokinetic interaction' refers to the fluctuation in bioavailability of herb/drug molecules in the body as a result of changes in absorption, distribution, metabolism and elimination.[8, 9]

Absorption

Absorption is the term that describes the process of the physical passage of herbs or drugs from the outside to the inside of the body. The majority of all absorption occurs in the intestines, where herbs or drugs must pass through the intestinal wall to enter the bloodstream. Several mechanisms may interfere with the absorption of drugs through the intestines.[10, 11]

The absorption of herbs may be adversely affected if herbs are administered with drugs that may promote binding in the gastrointestinal (G.I.) tract. Drugs such as cholestyramine (Questran), colestipol (Colestid) and sucralfate (Carafate) may bind to certain herbs, forming an insoluble complex that decreases absorption of both substances. Because of the large size of the insoluble complex, few or no molecules of either substance pass through the intestinal wall.[10, 11, 12]

Herb absorption may be adversely affected in the presence of drugs that change the pH of the stomach. Antacids, cimetidine (Tagamet), famotidine (Pepcid), nizatidine (Axid), ranitidine (Zantac) and omeprazole (Prilosec) may neutralize, decrease or inhibit the secretion of stomach acids.[10,11] With this subsequent decrease in stomach acidity, herbs may not be broken down properly in the stomach, leading to poor absorption in the intestines. To minimize this interaction, herbs are best taken separately from these drugs by approximately two hours.

Drugs that affect gastrointestinal motility may also affect the absorption of herbs. G.I. motility is the rate at which the intestines contract to push food products from the stomach to the rectum. Slower G.I. motility means that the herbs stay in the intestines for a longer period of time, thereby increasing the potential absorption. Conversely, more rapid G.I. motility means that the herbs stay in the intestines for a shorter time, which may decrease absorption. Drugs such as haloperidol (Haldol) decrease G.I. motility and may increase herb absorption; while drugs such as metoclopramide (Reglan) increase G.I. motility and possibly decrease herb absorption.

Therefore, it may be necessary to decrease the dosage of herbs when the patient is taking a drug that decreases G.I. motility and increases overall absorption. Likewise, it is probably helpful to increase the dosage of herbs when the patient is taking a drug that increases G.I. motility and thus decreases overall absorption.

Distribution

After absorption, herbs or drugs must be delivered to the targeted area in order to exert their influence. 'Distribution' refers to the processes by which herbs or drugs (once absorbed) are carried and released to different parts of the body. Currently, it appears that the majority of herbs and drugs do not have any clinically-significant interactions affecting distribution and thus can safely be taken together. The exception seems to be if a drug has a narrow range-of-safety index, and is highly protein-bound, in which case interaction with other substances might occur during the distribution phase. Examples of drugs that have both a narrow range-of-safety index and a highly protein-bound ratio include warfarin (Coumadin) and phenytoin (Dilantin). Unfortunately, it is very difficult to predict whether an individual herb will interact with either one of these drugs because there are no known tests or experiments documenting such interactions.[10,11]

Metabolism

Once metabolized by the liver, most herbs and drugs become inactive derivatives. The rate at which the liver metabolizes a substance determines the length of time it stays active in the body. If the liver were induced to speed up its metabolic rate, herbs and drugs would be deactivated at a more rapid pace, and the overall effectiveness of ingested substances would be lower. On the other hand, if the liver were made to slow its metabolism, herbs and drugs would be deactivated at a slower pace and the overall impact of the substances would be greater.

Drugs that induce greater liver metabolism do not exert an immediate effect; while drugs that inhibit liver metabolism have immediate onset of action.

In general, drugs that induce greater liver metabolism do not exert an immediate effect. The metabolism rate of the liver changes slowly, over several weeks. Therefore, the effect of accelerated liver metabolism is not seen until weeks after the initiation of drug therapy. Some examples of pharmaceuticals that speed hepatic metabolism are: phenytoin (Dilantin), carbamazepine (Tegretol), phenobarbitals and rifampin (Rifadin).[10,11] Therefore, herbs given in the presence of one of these products may be deactivated more rapidly, and their overall effectiveness lowered. Under these circumstances, a higher dose of herbs may be required to achieve the desired effect.

In great contrast, drugs that inhibit liver metabolism have an immediate onset of action. The rate of liver metabolism may be greatly impaired within a few days. Pharmaceuticals that slow or inhibit liver metabolism include: cimetidine (Tagamet), erythromycin, ethanol, fluconazole (Diflucan), itraconazole (Sporanox) and ketoconazole (Nizoral), among others.[10,11] When a patient takes these drugs concurrently with herbs, there is a higher risk of herbal components accumulating in the body, as the ability of the liver to neutralize them is compromised. If the herbs are metabolized more slowly, their overall effectiveness may be prolonged. In this case, one may need to lower the dosage of herbs to avoid unwanted side effects.

Depending on the half-life in the body of drugs that influence liver metabolism, it may be necessary to increase or decrease the dosages of herbs for weeks or even months after discontinuation of the pharmaceutical substance, along with consistent monitoring.

Elimination

While the liver neutralizes incoming drugs and herbs, the kidneys are responsible for eliminating the substances and their metabolites from the body. If the kidneys are damaged, then the rate of elimination is slowed, leading to an accumulation of active substances in the body. Important examples of drugs that damage the kidneys include amphotericin B, methotrexate, tobramycin and gentamicin.[10,11] As a safety precaution, when prescribing herbs for a patient who is currently taking or has recently taken one of these drugs, it may be wise to lower the dose of herbs to avoid unnecessary and unwanted side effects.

Summary of Pharmacokinetic Interactions

The pharmacokinetic interactions listed above include both theoretical and actual interactions. Though such interactions are possible, the extent and severity of each interaction will vary depending on the specific circumstances, such as the dosages of all substances, the inherent sensitivity of each patient, individual body weight, and metabolic rate.

PHARMACODYNAMIC INTERACTIONS

The study of pharmacodynamics provides insight into the dynamic behavior of drugs inside the human body. The phrase 'pharmacodynamic interactions' in our context refers to fluctuations in the bioavailability of ingested substances as a result of synergistic or antagonistic interactions between herb and drug molecules. Pharmacodynamic interactions are generally more difficult to predict and prevent than pharmacokinetic interactions. Most of the currently-known pharmaco-

Chapter 8 – Concurrent Use of Herbal Medicines and Pharmaceuticals

dynamic interactions have been documented through actual cases, not by laboratory experiments. The best way to prevent pharmacodynamic interactions is to follow the patient closely and monitor all clinical signs and symptoms, and particularly any abnormal reactions.

A ***synergistic*** interaction occurs when two drugs with similar properties show an additive or even exponential increase in clinical impact when given together. An ***antagonistic*** interaction occurs when two drugs with similar properties are administered simultaneously and show lessened or no clinical effectiveness.[13]

Synergistic or antagonistic interactions may occur with any concurrent use of medicinal substances, regardless of whether they are herbs, drugs, or both.

Herb-to-Herb Interactions

Oriental Medicine has tracked cases of herb-to-herb pharmacodynamic interactions for centuries. As discussed more thoroughly in part 1, chapter 7, "Clinical Applications of Chinese Herbal Medicine," the additive effect is generally referred to as *xiang xu* (mutual accentuation) or *xiang shi* (mutual enhancement), such as takes place in the combination of *Shi Gao* (Gypsum Fibrosum) and *Zhi Mu* (Radix Anemarrhenae) to clear heat and purge fire. The antagonistic effect is generally referred to as *xiang wei* (mutual counteraction), *xiang sha* (mutual suppression) or *xiang wu* (mutual antagonism), such as happens in the combination of *Lai Fu Zi* (Semen Raphani) and *Ren Shen* (Radix Ginseng), in which the therapeutic action of the latter herb is decreased by the addition of *Lai Fu Zi*.

Classic Chinese texts describe numerous other herb-to-herb interactions, such as the *Shi Ba Fan* (Eighteen Incompatibles) and *Shi Jiu Wei* (Nineteen Counteractions), discussed in greater detail earlier in this text. Ill-advised combinations of these herbs will likely lead to adverse side effects and/or toxic reactions.

Herb-to-Drug Interactions

Pharmacodynamic herb-to-drug interactions are best identified by analyzing the therapeutic profile of the herbs as well as that of the drugs. Concurrent use of herbs and drugs with similar therapeutic actions poses potential for herb-drug interactions. In these cases, the increased potency of treatment may interfere with optimal outcome, as the desired effect becomes less predictable and harder to obtain with precision. The highest risk of clinically-significant interactions occurs between herbs and drugs that have **sympathomimetic, anticoagulant, antiplatelet, diuretic** and **antidiabetic** effects.[14]

Herbs that exert **sympathomimetic** effects may interfere with antihypertensive and antiseizure drugs. The classic example of this type of herb is *Ma Huang* (Herba Ephedrae), containing ephedrine, pseudoephedrine, norephedrine and other ephedrine alkaloids. *Ma Huang* may interact with other drugs and disease conditions and should always be used with caution in patients vulnerable to hypertension, seizures, diabetes, thyroid conditions, and similar regulatory imbalances.[14]

Herbs with **anticoagulant** and **antiplatelet** effects include herbs that have blood-activating and blood-stasis-removing functions, such as *Dan Shen* (Radix Salviae Miltiorrhizae), *Dang Gui* (Radix Angelicae Sinensis), *Chuan Xiong* (Rhizoma Ligustici Chuanxiong), *Tao Ren* (Semen Persicae), *Hong Hua* (Flos Carthami) and *Shui Zhi* (Hirudo). These herbs may interfere with anticoagulant and antiplatelet drugs, including warfarin (Coumadin), enoxaparin (Lovenox), aspirin, dipyridamole (Persantine), and clopidogrel (Plavix). Without proper supervision, concurrent use of these herbs and drugs may lead to prolonged and excessive bleeding. Thus, individuals taking anticoagulant or antiplatelet drugs must be very cautious about concurrently using herbs, and would be wise to so only under the supervision of well-trained healthcare professionals.[14]

Concomitant use of **diuretic** herbs and diuretic drugs may create additive or synergistic effects, making hypertension more difficult to control, or hypotensive episodes more likely.[14] The dosage of herbs and/or drugs must be adjusted to achieve optimal treatment outcome. Commonly-used diuretic herbs include *Fu Ling* (Poria), *Zhu Ling* (Polyporus), *Che Qian Zi* (Semen Plantaginis), and *Ze Xie* (Rhizoma Alismatis).

Chapter 8 – Concurrent Use of Herbal Medicines and Pharmaceuticals

Antidiabetic herbs may interfere with antidiabetic drugs by accentuating the decrease of plasma glucose levels. The dosage of these herbs and drugs must be balanced carefully to effectively control blood glucose levels without causing hyper- or hypo-glycemia.[14] Herbs with definite antidiabetic effects include the following pairs of herbs: *Zhi Mu* (Radix Anemarrhenae) and *Shi Gao* (Gypsum Fibrosum); *Xuan Shen* (Radix Scrophulariae) and *Cang Zhu* (Rhizoma Atractylodis); and *Shan Yao* (Rhizoma Dioscoreae) and *Huang Qi* (Radix Astragali).

Summary of Pharmacodynamic Interactions

Understanding synergistic and antagonistic interactions from both an Oriental medicine perspective and the realm of pharmaceutical medicines helps practitioners to anticipate, prevent, and/or monitor for unwanted interactions in patients who need or elect to rely on multiple therapeutic substances.

SUMMARY: CONCURRENT USE OF HERBAL MEDICINES AND PHARMACEUTICALS

Historically, herbs and drugs have been presumed to be very different treatment modalities, that have rarely, if ever, been used together. The line that separates use of herbs and drugs, however, has blurred in recent decades as the lay public gains increased accessibility to multiple treatment modalities. It is not uncommon for one patient to seek care from several health professionals for an ailment. As a result, a patient may easily be taking multiple drugs, herbs, supplements, and vitamins concurrently. It becomes difficult to predict whether the combination of all these substances will lead to unwanted side effects and/or interactions. It is imprudent to assume that there will be no interactions. On the other hand, it is just as unwise to abandon treatment simply for fear of possible interactions. The solution to this situation is in the understanding of pharmacokinetic and pharmacodynamic herb-drug interactions. By understanding these mechanisms, one can recognize potential interactions and take proper actions to prevent their occurrence.

References

1. *Zhong Cao Yao* (Chinese Herbal Medicine), 1980; 11(6):276
2. *Zhong Cheng Yao Yan Jiu* (Research of Chinese Patent Medicine), 1983; 1:12
3. *Zhong Cao Yao Tong Xun* (Journal of Chinese Herbal Medicine), 1979; 1:6
4. *Zhong Cao Yao* (Chinese Herbal Medicine), 1980; 6:276
5. *Yao Xue Tong Bao* (Report of Herbology), 1981; 4:15
6. Thomas Chan, Anticholinergic poisoning due to Chinese Herbal Medicine, *Vet Human Toxicol* 37 (2) April 1995
7. David M. Eisenberg, et al. *Trends in Alternative Medicine Use in the United States,* 1990-1997. JAMA. November 11, 1998
8. Robert Berkow and Andrew J. Fletcher: *The Merck Manual of Diagnosis and Therapy 16th Edition.* Merck Research Laboratories, 1992
9. Anthony S. Fauci, et al: *Harrison's Principles of Internal Medicine 14th Edition.* McGraw-Hill Health Professions Division, 1998
10. Philip D. Hansten: *Understanding Drug-Drug Interactions. Science and Medicine* 16-25. January-February 1998
11. Philip D. Hansten: *Chapter Three Drug Interactions. Applied Therapeutics.* Applied Therapeutics, Inc. 1993
12. Sophia Segal and Susan Kaminski: *Drug-Nutrient Interactions.* American Druggist 42-49. July 1996
13. Harold Kalant and Walter H.E. Roschlau: *Principles of Medical Pharmacology Sixth Edition.* Oxford University Press, 1998
14. P.F.D'Arcy: Adverse Reactions and Interactions With Herbal Medicine. Part 2 – Drug Interactions. *Adverse Drug React. Toxicol.* Rev. 1993, 12(3) 147-162 Oxford University Press

Part II — Herb Monographs

各论

Chapter 1

— Exterior-Releasing Herbs

解表药

Chapter 1 — Exterior-Releasing Herbs

Section 1 Wind-Cold Releasing Herbs

Section 2 Wind-Heat Releasing Herbs

Chapter 1 — Exterior-Releasing Herbs

解表药

Definition: Substances that 'release the exterior' act to dispel pathogenic factors from the external and superficial parts of the body.

The term 'pathogenic factors' describes normally benign environmental factors, such as wind, cold or heat, that have combined to disrupt normal physiological functioning and express themselves in the form of wind-cold and wind-heat. With drastic or sudden changes in the weather, or with a decline in health or immunity, these factors commonly attack the exterior or superficial parts of the body, that is, the skin and muscle layers. Therefore, an 'exterior syndrome' refers to a condition characterized by wind-cold or wind-heat attacking (or 'invading') the skin and muscle layers of the body, causing symptoms and signs such as aversion to cold, chills, fever, headache, muscle aches and pain, the inappropriate presence or absence of perspiration, and a superficial pulse.

The herbs in this category stimulate immune response, alleviate pain, regulate body temperature, and induce perspiration. They are most often used to treat common colds, influenza, and complications of complex internal disorders.

Exterior-releasing herbs stimulate immune response, alleviate pain, regulate body temperature, and induce perspiration, treating common colds, influenza and complications of complex internal disorders.

SUBCATEGORIES OF ACTION

Clinically, exterior-releasing herbs fall into two categories to address the problems of exterior wind-cold or exterior wind-heat syndromes.

1. ***Dispel wind-cold***: These herbs are generally acrid and warm in thermal property. They induce perspiration, dispel wind-cold from the exterior, and promote warming and relaxation of the skin and muscle layers.
2. ***Dispel wind-heat***: These herbs are commonly acrid and cold in thermal property. They dispel wind-heat to relieve fever and pain or inflammation in the throat, eyes and skin.

Herbs from both categories are generally used in the treatment of common colds, influenza, bacterial infections, asthma, coughing, wheezing, measles, chest congestion, nausea, vomiting, edema, arthritis, and eye disorders. Herbs that release the exterior may also serve multiple purposes: to regulate qi circulation to relieve pain, relieve wheezing and dyspnea, dissolve phlegm, promote the eruption of measles, relieve nausea and vomiting, regulate water circulation and eliminate dampness, and brighten the eyes.

Ma Huang (Herba Ephedrae)
Ben Cao Gang Mu (Materia Medica),
by Li Shi-Zhen, 1578 A.D.

DIFFERENTIAL DIAGNOSIS AND TREATMENT

Accurate differential diagnosis of the external pathogen and the degree to which it has penetrated is of vital importance: treatment of wind-cold and wind-heat can be significantly different. Furthermore, it is important to determine the basic underlying condition of the patient prior to prescribing any herbal formula.

Pre-existing constitutional deficiency or chronic illness may require the addition of tonics to enhance the overall therapeutic effect. However, tonics must <u>not</u> be used alone or casually in the presence of an exterior condition, as this will only send the pathogenic factors deeper into the interior of the body, thus complicating the illness.

Chapter 1 — Exterior-Releasing Herbs

Differential Diagnosis of Wind-Cold and Wind-Heat

Diagnosis	Symptoms	Tongue	Pulse
Wind-cold	aversion to cold, fever, lack of perspiration, headache, body aches and pain	thin and white tongue coat	superficial, tight pulse
Wind-heat	fever, mild aversion to wind and cold, dry or sore throat, thirst	thin and yellow tongue coat	superficial, rapid pulse

CAUTIONS/CONTRAINDICATIONS

~

As soon as desired therapeutic results are achieved, intake of exterior-releasing herbs should immediately be discontinued.

~

- Many herbs that release the exterior do so via inducing perspiration. Overdose, prolonged use, or inappropriate use of these herbs will consume qi and body fluids, resulting in qi deficiency, dryness and/or yin deficiency. Therefore, they should be used only when necessary. Furthermore, intake of these herbs should be discontinued immediately, when the desired therapeutic results are achieved.
- Herbs that release the exterior should be prescribed with caution for individuals who have a deficiency of qi, yin, blood or body fluids.
- Exterior-releasing herbs should be used with caution in patients with an exterior condition accompanied by sores and abscess, *lin zheng* (dysuria syndrome), or bleeding.

PROCESSING

Many herbs that release the exterior are aromatic and contain volatile essential oils. Cooking these herbs for a prolonged period of time causes evaporation and destruction of many active constituents. Therefore, these more volatile herbs (often leaves and flowers) should be added at the end of the cooking time for the main formula, so that they are only decocted briefly, simmering for no more than 5 minutes, long enough to release their potent influence without diminishing their actions. The practice of adding the herb at the end of the cooking process is referred to in this text as "post-decoction."

PHARMACOLOGICAL EFFECTS

- **Diaphoretic**: Many herbs in this category induce perspiration. Of these herbs, *Ma Huang* (Herba Ephedrae) exerts the strongest diaphoretic function by directly stimulating the sweat glands, as verified by *in vivo* and *in vitro* studies. The effect of *Ma Huang* may be potentiated by the addition of *Gui Zhi* (Ramulus Cinnamomi), which dilates peripheral blood vessels and increases blood circulation to the superficial parts of the body. Among other herbs that have both diaphoretic and antipyretic influences are *Sheng Jiang* (Rhizoma Zingiberis Recens) and *Bo He* (Herba Menthae).
- **Antipyretic**: Many exterior-releasing herbs reduce body temperature in subjects experiencing either elevated or normal body temperature (in the case of normal temperature, these substances may bring body temperature below normal levels). The mechanisms of antipyretic action vary depending on the herb. *Ma Huang* (Herba Ephedrae), *Gui Zhi* (Ramulus Cinnamomi) and *Bo He* (Herba Menthae) act on the central nervous system and disperse heat via diaphoresis. *Gui Zhi* (Ramulus Cinnamomi), *Sheng Jiang* (Rhizoma Zingiberis Recens) and *Bo He* (Herba Menthae) reduce body temperature by promoting blood circulation to superficial parts of the body, dilating blood vessels, and opening skin pores to release heat. In addition, these three herbs have anti-inflammatory, antibacterial and antiviral actions that contribute to reducing body temperature. Other herbs with antipyretic effects include *Zi Su Ye* (Folium Perillae), *Jing Jie* (Herba Schizonepetae), *Fang Feng* (Radix Saposhnikoviae), and *Bai Zhi* (Radix Angelicae Dahuricae).
- **Sedative**: Some herbs that relieve the exterior also exert a sedative influence, such as *Gui Zhi* (Ramulus Cinnamomi), *Sheng Jiang* (Rhizoma Zingiberis Recens), *Chai Hu* (Radix Bupleuri), *Jing Jie* (Herba Schizonepetae), and *Fang Feng* (Radix Saposhnikoviae). Administering these herbs reduces spontaneous physical activities (such as restlessness, spasms and twitches), and potentiates the effect of barbiturates.

Chapter 1 — Exterior-Releasing Herbs

- **Antibiotic**: Both antibacterial and antiviral properties are integral to certain exterior-releasing herbs, such as *Ma Huang* (Herba Ephedrae), *Gui Zhi* (Ramulus Cinnamomi), *Zi Su Ye* (Folium Perillae), *Chai Hu* (Radix Bupleuri), *Fang Feng* (Radix Saposhnikoviae), *Bo He* (Herba Menthae), *Gao Ben* (Rhizoma Ligustici), *Xiang Ru* (Herba Elsholtziae seu Moslae), *Xin Yi Hua* (Flos Magnoliae) and *Man Jing Zi* (Fructus Viticis). Others may have only antibacterial or antiviral effects.
- **Metabolic**: Many exterior-releasing herbs act to lower blood glucose levels, as is the case with *Sang Ye* (Folium Mori) and *Ge Gen* (Radix Puerariae). Others, like *Ma Huang* (Herba Ephedrae), stimulate the basal metabolic rate.
- **Diuretic**: Some herbs in this category promote diuresis to eliminate excess water accumulation, including: *Ma Huang* (Herba Ephedrae), *Fu Ping* (Herba Spirodelae), *Niu Bang Zi* (Fructus Arctii), *Mu Zei* (Herba Equiseti Hiemalis) and *Xiang Ru* (Herba Elsholtziae seu Moslae).
- **Cardiovascular**: Herbs such as *Ge Gen* (Radix Puerariae) and *Ju Hua* (Flos Chrysanthemi) increase perfusion of blood to the coronary arteries.
- **Antispasmodic**: *Jing Jie* (Herba Schizonepetae), *Ma Huang* (Herba Ephedrae), *Ge Gen* (Radix Puerariae), and others relax the smooth muscles to prevent spasms and cramps.
- **Analgesic**: *In vitro* and *in vivo* studies confirm that many herbs simultaneously relieve pain and release pathogens at the exterior levels. *Fang Feng* (Radix Saposhnikoviae) relieves pain via its effect on the central nervous system. *Sheng Jiang* (Rhizoma Zingiberis Recens) reduces inflammation and pain via its effect on the peripheral nervous system. Other analgesic herbs include *Jing Jie* (Herba Schizonepetae), *Qiang Huo* (Rhizoma et Radix Notopterygii), *Man Jing Zi* (Fructus Viticis), *Gao Ben* (Rhizoma Ligustici), and *Xin Yi Hua* (Flos Magnoliae), but the mechanisms of their actions are not well understood at this time.
- **Anti-inflammatory**: *Chai Hu* (Radix Bupleuri) reduces inflammation by stimulating the release of hormones from the adrenal cortex. *Qiang Huo* (Rhizoma et Radix Notopterygii) reduces inflammation by stimulating the endocrine system, particularly the pituitary gland and adrenal cortex. *Sheng Jiang* (Rhizoma Zingiberis Recens) and *Ma Huang* (Herba Ephedrae) exert their anti-inflammatory effect by inhibiting prostaglandin synthesis in the periphery.
- **Antivenin**: Some exterior-relieving herbs are useful as antidotes for snake bites, such as *Bai Zhi* (Radix Angelicae Dahuricae).

POTENTIAL HERB-DRUG INTERACTIONS

Exterior-releasing herbs are characterized by diaphoretic action, inducing perspiration. Some achieve this by stimulating sweat glands, others by dilating peripheral blood vessels. Herbal diaphoretic activity is generally not associated with reported or potential herb-drug interactions.

- **Sedatives**: Herbs that release the exterior have many other pharmacological effects, as described above, and therefore may interact with other medicinal agents. For example, the sedative influence may be potentiated when one takes both herbs and drugs with sedative properties. The sedative effect of the herbs may also be potentiated by intake of alcohol. Excessive sedation interferes with alertness, increasing the risk of injury if one drives an automobile or operates heavy machinery.
- **Antibiotics**: Antibiotic activity may be potentiated by concurrent use of herbs and drugs.
- **Diuretics**: Some exterior-releasing herbs promote diuresis. Therefore, it is prudent to avoid combining those herbs with drugs that exert diuretic effects, as there may be additive or synergistic results. Inappropriate combination therapy may lead to excessive loss of fluids and electrolytes.

Section 1

— Wind-Cold Releasing Herbs

Ma Huang (Herba Ephedrae)

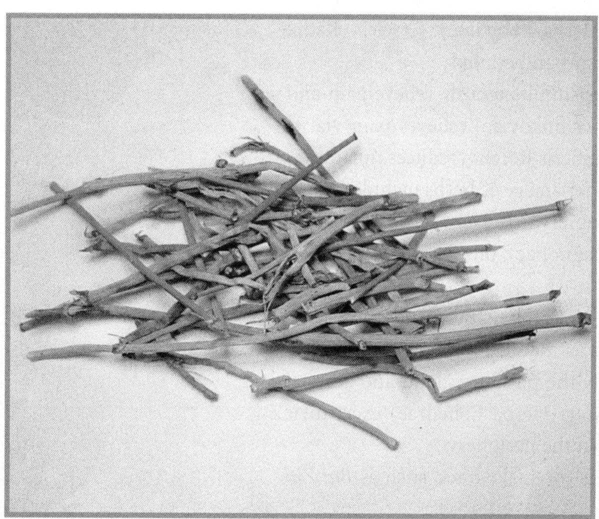

麻黄

Pinyin Name: *Ma Huang*
Literal Name: "hemp yellow," "numb yellow herb"
Alternate Chinese Names: *Jing Ma Huang, Ma Huang Rong*
Original Source: *Shen Nong Ben Cao Jing* (Divine Husbandman's Classic of the Materia Medica) in the second century
English Name: ephedra
Botanical Name: *Ephedra sinica* Stapf. (*Mu Cao Ma Huang*); *Ephedra equisetina* Bunge. (*Mu Zei Ma Huang*)
Pharmaceutical Name: Herba Ephedrae
Properties: acrid, bitter, warm
Channels Entered: Lung, Urinary Bladder

CHINESE THERAPEUTIC ACTIONS

1. Releases the Exterior through Diaphoresis

Exterior-excess, wind-cold condition: Acrid and warm, *Ma Huang* (Herba Ephedrae) ventilates the Lung and is commonly used to treat exterior-excess, wind-cold syndrome characterized by symptoms such as chills, aversion to cold, fever, absence of perspiration, headache, body aches and pain, nasal obstruction, and a superficial, tight pulse. Its dispersing function also opens peripheral channels and collaterals.

- Exterior-excess, wind-cold syndrome: use it with *Gui Zhi* (Ramulus Cinnamomi) to enhance the diaphoretic action. **Exemplar Formula:** *Ma Huang Tang* (Ephedra Decoction).

2. Relieves Wheezing and Dyspnea, Stops Cough

Wind-cold constriction of the Lung leading to Lung qi reversal: *Ma Huang* ventilates Lung qi and is useful in treatment of wheezing, dyspnea and cough characterized by wind-cold attacking the exterior that leads to abnormal rising of Lung qi.

- Cough from wind-cold attacking the exterior and constricting Lung qi: use it with *Xing Ren* (Semen Armeniacae Amarum). *Ma Huang* and *Xing Ren* work synergistically to treat cough, as the former herb disperses Lung qi and relieves stagnation while the latter herb sends qi downward.
- Wheezing or cough caused by Lung heat: combine it with *Shi Gao* (Gypsum Fibrosum) and *Xing Ren* (Semen Armeniacae Amarum). *Ma Huang* and *Xing Ren* have synergistic functions in treating wheezing and dyspnea. *Shi Gao* clears Lung heat and neutralizes the warm property of *Ma Huang* to prevent the possible side effect of excess perspiration. **Exemplar Formula**: *Ma Xing Gan Shi Tang* (Ephedra, Apricot Kernel, Licorice, and Gypsum Decoction).
- Wheezing or cough from wind-cold attack at the exterior and cold stagnation in the interior: add it to *Gan Jiang* (Rhizoma Zingiberis), *Xi Xin* (Herba Asari) and *Ban Xia* (Rhizoma Pinelliae). **Exemplar Formula**: *Xiao Qing*

Ma Huang (Herba Ephedrae)

Long Tang (Minor Bluegreen Dragon Decoction).

- Wheezing and dyspnea caused by stagnation of qi and phlegm: combine it with *Xing Ren* (Semen Armeniacae Amarum), *Chen Pi* (Pericarpium Citri Reticulatae) and *Hou Po* (Cortex Magnoliae Officinalis). **Exemplar Formula:** *Shen Mi Tang* (Mysterious Decoction).

3. Regulates Water Circulation and Relieves Edema

Edema with exterior syndrome: *Ma Huang* enters the Lung and Urinary Bladder channels to regulate water circulation and eliminate edema. Excess water is generally eliminated through perspiration, increased urination, or both.

- Edema with exterior wind-cold signs or symptoms: use *Ma Huang* with *Sheng Jiang* (Rhizoma Zingiberis Recens), *Bai Zhu* (Rhizoma Atractylodis Macrocephalae) and *Gan Cao* (Radix Glycyrrhizae) to dispel the exterior condition and eliminate water accumulation. **Exemplar Formula:** *Yue Bi Jia Zhu Tang* (Maidservant from Yue Decoction plus Atractylodes).

4. Disperses Cold

***Bi zheng* (painful obstruction syndrome)**: Warm and dispersing in nature, *Ma Huang* disperses and eliminates cold and damp from the exterior parts of the body.

- *Bi zheng* caused by wind-damp: use it with *Yi Yi Ren* (Semen Coicis), *Xing Ren* (Semen Armeniacae Amarum) and *Gan Cao* (Radix Glycyrrhizae) to treat muscle aches and pain of the extremities caused by wind-damp.

Yin sores: This condition is characterized by localized, painful swellings without heads, that blend into the surrounding tissues. They often appear to be the same color as the skin and are not hot to the touch. The underlying cause of this problem is blood deficiency with stagnation of cold and phlegm.

- Yin sores: use *Ma Huang* with *Shu Di Huang* (Radix Rehmanniae Preparata), *Bai Jie Zi* (Semen Sinapis) or *Lu Jiao Jiao* (Gelatinum Cornu Cervi).
- Arteritis obliterans, obliterating phlebitis or Raynaud's disease: use it with *Shu Di Huang* (Radix Rehmanniae Preparata), *Bai Jie Zi* (Semen Sinapis), *Lu Jiao Jiao* (Gelatinum Cornu Cervi), *Rou Gui* (Cortex Cinnamomi) and *Gan Cao* (Radix Glycyrrhizae).

DOSAGE

1.5 to 10 grams in decoction. The maximum dosage of *Ma Huang* is 20 to 25 grams. Use of *Ma Huang* in treating edema requires dosage between 10 and 15 grams.

The proper method for preparing *Ma Huang* is to predecoct it and remove the resultant foam from the solution prior to the addition of other herbs. Classic texts state that the foam is the component more likely to cause irritability. To minimize diaphoresis and neutralize the warm nature of *Ma Huang, Shi Gao* (Gypsum Fibrosum) is frequently used with *Ma Huang* in a three-to-one ratio (*Shi Gao* 3 : *Ma Huang* 1).

Different types of *Ma Huang* have slightly different therapeutic functions: unprocessed *Ma Huang* has a stronger function to induce perspiration and is commonly used to treat wind-cold conditions; honey-fried *Ma Huang* is weaker in inducing perspiration but more strongly moistens the Lung and relieves wheezing, dyspnea and cough; and crushed *Ma Huang Rong* is milder in inducing perspiration and is generally used in pediatric medicine to relieve exterior syndromes.

CAUTIONS / CONTRAINDICATIONS

- Because *Ma Huang* strongly functions to induce diaphoresis and ventilate the lungs, inappropriate use may damage qi, yin and body fluids. It should be used with caution in patients with weak constitutions, spontaneous perspiration arising from qi deficiency, night perspiration due to yin deficiency, wheezing or dyspnea caused by Kidney deficiency (manifesting in long exhalation and short inhalation), or edema due to Spleen deficiency.
- Chronic or repetitive use of *Ma Huang* to treat wheezing/dyspnea is not recommended, as it may damage Lung qi and lead to further complications. Other herbs must be added to harmonize its strong effects.
- Ingesting *Ma Huang* is not recommended in patients with Liver yang rising or yin-deficient fire, as its use may lead to vertigo, epistaxis, or hematemesis.
- *Ma Huang* has a stimulating effect on the sympathetic nervous system. Thus, it should be used with caution in patients with such medical conditions as convulsions, epilepsy and seizure disorders, diabetes mellitus, hypertension, hyperthyroidism and prostatic enlargement.
- Use *Ma Huang* with caution during pregnancy because of its stimulating effect on the uterus.[1]

OVERDOSAGE

Overdose of *Ma Huang* is characterized by stimulation of the sympathetic nervous system by the numerous ephedrine alkaloids in the herb. Symptoms include excitation, irritability, restlessness, hypersensitivity, tinnitus, insomnia, nausea, vomiting, red face, upper abdominal discomfort, poor appetite, thirst, perspiration, increased blood pressure, dizziness, elevated blood glucose levels, chest pain, and tremor. In severe cases, there may be cardiac arrhythmia, increased blood pressure, and possibly epilepsy and convulsions. Adverse reactions generally occur between one-half and two hours following ingestion of an excessive quantity of the herb.[2]

Ma Huang (Herba Ephedrae)

TREATMENT OF OVERDOSAGE

Overdose of *Ma Huang* may be treated with either of two herbal formulas:

- Formula one contains *Da Huang* (Radix et Rhizoma Rhei) 9g, *Hou Po* (Cortex Magnoliae Officinalis) 9g, *Mu Xiang* (Radix Aucklandiae) 9g, *Mang Xiao* (Natrii Sulfas) 15g, and *Gan Cao* (Radix Glycyrrhizae) 6g. The decoction is to be taken once every four hours until toxic symptoms are alleviated.
- Formula two contains *Lu Dou* (Semen Phaseoli Radiati) 15g and *Gan Cao* (Radix Glycyrrhizae) 30g cooked in water to yield 300 ml of decoction. Patients are instructed to take 150 ml per dose, every two hours, for 3 to 5 doses.[2,3]

CHEMICAL COMPOSITION

Ephedrine alkaloids 0.481-2.47% (l-ephedrine, d-pseudoephedrine, l-norephedrine, d-norpseudoephedrine, l-methylephedrine, d-methylpseudoephedrine), ephedroxane, 2,3,4-trimethyl-5-phenyloxazolidine benzylmethylamine, 2,3,5,6-tetramethylpyrazine, essential oil 0.25% (l-α-terpineol).[4,5]

OH H N CH_3 CH_3

Ephedrine

PHARMACOLOGICAL EFFECTS

- **Diaphoresis**: In humans, administration of ephedrine alkaloids is associated with increased perspiration, but only in subjects with elevated body temperature.[6]
- **Antipyretic**: Essential oil of *Ma Huang* is associated with antipyretic action in rabbits with artificially-induced fever. It also reduces temperature in mice with normal body temperature. However, it has no effect on cats with normal body temperature.[7]
- **Respiratory**: Both ephedrine and pseudoephedrine have mild, prolonged bronchodilating effects. Ephedrine has a more rapid onset of action, but its effectiveness may decrease if it is used repeatedly in a short period of time.[8] Water extract of *Ma Huang* administered via oral or intraperitoneal injection is also associated with an antitussive effect.[9]
- **Diuresis**: Pseudoephedrine has a diuretic function.[10]
- **Cardiovascular**: Use of *Ma Huang* is associated with an increase in both systolic and diastolic blood pressures. Ephedrine has a mild but prolonged effect to constrict blood vessels and raise blood pressure.[11]
- **CNS stimulant**: Ephedrine has a marked stimulating influence on the central nervous system (CNS), cardiovascular system, and respiratory system. It may cause such side effects as irritability, insomnia, restlessness and tremor.[12,13]
- **Antibiotic**: Decoction of *Ma Huang* has varying degrees of inhibitory effect *in vitro* against *Staphylococcus aureus*, α-streptococcus, β-streptococcus, *Bacillus anthracis*, *Corynebacterium diphtheriae*, *Pseudomonas aeruginosa*, *Bacillus dysenteriae*, and *Salmonella typhi*.[14] The essential oil of *Ma Huang* has an inhibitory effect against *E. coli*, *Candida albicans*, and various types of influenza virus.[15]

CLINICAL STUDIES AND RESEARCH

- **Infantile diarrhea**: According to one report, 138 patients with infantile diarrhea were treated with *Ma Huang* (2 to 4 grams) and *Qian Hu* (Radix Peucedani) (4 to 8 grams). The herbs were given once daily as an herbal decoction with the addition of a small amount of sugar. Out of 138 patients, 126 (91.3%) showed significant improvement, and 124 (90%) responded within 1 to 2 doses. This study demonstrates the *zang fu* relationship between the Lung and Large Intestine, in that ventilation of the Lung helps with water retention of the Large Intestine.[16]
- **Coughing and wheezing**: In a clinical trial, 260 patients with coughing, wheezing and asthma from various causes were treated with Chinese herbal formulas, with complete recovery in 148 patients, marked improvement in 107 patients, and no response in 5 patients. The formulas were given as decoctions, six to eight times daily for children, and three times daily for adults. The fundamental formula included *Ma Huang* 10g, *Pi Pa Ye* (Folium Eriobotryae) 10g, *Zi Wan* (Radix Asteris) 15g, *Kuan Dong Hua* (Flos Farfarae) 15g, *Bai Qian* (Rhizoma Cynanchi Stauntonii) 15g, *Sang Bai Pi* (Cortex Mori) 15g, *Ting Li Zi* (Semen Descurainiae seu Lepidii) 10g, *Bai Jie Zi* (Semen Sinapis) 10g, *Su Zi* (Fructus Perillae) 10g, *Lai Fu Zi* (Semen Raphani) 10g, *Wu Wei Zi* (Fructus Schisandrae Chinensis) 10g, *Tu Si Zi* (Semen Cuscutae) 10g, *Bei Mu* (Bulbus Fritillaria) 10g, *Ban Xia* (Rhizoma Pinelliae) 10g, *Chen Pi* (Pericarpium Citri Reticulatae) 10g, *Xing Ren* (Semen Armeniacae Amarum) 15g, and *Jie Geng* (Radix Platycodonis) 15g. Modifications to the fundamental formula included *Gan Jiang* (Rhizoma Zingiberis) for cold; *Huang Qin* (Radix Scutellariae) and *Huang Lian* (Rhizoma Coptidis) for heat; *Dang Shen* (Radix Codonopsis) and *Huang Qi* (Radix Astragali) for deficiency; and *Da Huang* (Radix et Rhizoma Rhei) and *Mang Xiao* (Natrii Sulfas) for excess.[17]
- **Asthma**: An herbal formula containing *Ma Huang*, *Di Long* (Pheretima), *Chuan Bei Mu* (Bulbus Fritillariae Cirrhosae), *Chan Tui* (Periostracum Cicadae) and *Gan Cao* (Radix Glycyrrhizae) was used to treat asthma patients. Minor modifications to the formula were made, depending on the condition of each individual patient, if deemed necessary by the doctors. Out of 55 patients, 28

Ma Huang (Herba Ephedrae)

showed marked improvement, 15 showed moderate improvement, and 2 showed no response.[18]

HERB-DRUG INTERACTION

- **General effect:** *Ma Huang* contains ephedrine alkaloids that stimulate the central nervous system and the cardiovascular system. Combining *Ma Huang* with cardiac glycosides may lead to cardiac arrhythmia. *Ma Huang* should not be combined with other sympathomimetic drugs, such as ephedrine, pseudoephedrine, theophylline, caffeine, monoamine oxidase inhibitors (MAOI), or substances with similar properties.[19]
- **Beta blockers:** The effect of beta blockers may be reduced when combined with *Ma Huang* because of increased levels of norepinephrine caused by the herb.[20] [Note: Examples of beta blockers include atenolol (Tenormin), metoprolol (Lopressor/Toprol), sotalol (Betapace), propranolol (Inderal), and labetalol (Normodyne/Trandate).]
- **Diuretics:** *Ma Huang* has a diuretic effect. Though this potential interaction has not been documented, concurrent use with diuretic drugs may lead to increased elimination of water and/or electrolytes.[21] [Note: Examples of diuretics include chlorothiazide, hydrochlorothiazide, furosemide (Lasix), bumetanide (Bumex), and torsemide (Demadex).]

TOXICOLOGY

Ephedrine and pseudoephedrine are well-absorbed. Peak plasma concentration is reached 1 to 2 hours after oral ingestion of the herb. Ephedrine and pseudoephedrine are distributed throughout the body, with higher concentrations found in the liver and kidneys, followed by the brain, spleen, fatty tissues, and saliva. The half-lives of these compounds range from 4.73 to 7.1 or 13.4 hours (when the urinary pH is 5.2, 6, and 7, respectively). Up to 75% of these compounds can be recovered unchanged in the urine.[4]

The LD_{50} for water-extracted *Ma Huang* in mice via intraperitoneal injection is 650 mg/kg. The LD_{50} for essential oil of *Ma Huang* in mice is 1.35 ml/kg via intraperitoneal injection, and 2.79 ml/kg via oral ingestion.[22]

AUTHORS' COMMENTS

Ma Huang is one of the most extensively studied Chinese herbs. Several ephedrine alkaloids, such as ephedrine and pseudoephedrine, have been isolated and used as pharmaceutical drugs. Though the herb is not as potent as its drug counterpart, the herb still possesses strong medicinal properties and stimulates both the central nervous system and the cardiovascular system.

Ma Huang must be prescribed carefully and its use supervised. Respectful attention to dosages and the clear guidelines for use of this herb will result in safe applications in the majority of cases. Inappropriate or prolonged use, or high dosages, may lead to adverse reactions and unwanted side effects. While taking this herb, patient symptoms and progress must be closely monitored, as adverse reactions and side effects may occur in individuals with pre-existing medical conditions.

Traditionally, *Ma Huang* is pre-decocted and the resultant foam removed, prior to addition of the other herbs. Various sources offer several reasons for this. Some indicate that the foam may cause irritability. Others state that the foam is representative of the diaphoretic function of *Ma Huang* and is strongest in inducing perspiration. Therefore, the foam is best removed to prevent irritability and excessive diaphoresis.

Patients with initial wind-cold invasion may require the use of unprocessed *Ma Huang,* as it is strongest in inducing perspiration and driving out external pathogenic factors lingering in the *wei* (defense) level. However, if the patient has overcome the exterior condition but still is experiencing coughing, dyspnea or wheezing, then it is best to choose honey-fried *Ma Huang,* as it has a weaker diaphoretic function but is stronger to relieve rebellious Lung qi. Honey-fried *Ma Huang* should be used instead of unprocessed *Ma Huang* when treating respiratory disorders not caused by exterior wind-cold invasion manifesting in cough, dyspnea or wheezing.

According to the clinical experience of Dr. Chen Shu-Sheng, *Ma Huang* constricts blood vessels and should be used with caution for hypertensive patients. The strong diaphoretic effect contraindicates its use for weak patients or those experiencing excessive sweating. However, *Ma Huang Gen* (Radix Ephedrae) has the exact opposite effect. It dilates the blood vessels to lower blood pressure and consolidates the *wei* (defensive) level and stops perspiration. When used together, the herb and root regulate respiration and increase the physiological efficiency of the lung without causing the side effects of hyperactivity or increased blood pressure.

References

1. Brinker, Francis. *The Toxicology of Botanical Medicines,* rev. 2nd ed., 1996
2. *Zhong Yao Bu Liang Fan Ying Yu Zhi Liao* (Adverse Reactions and Treatment of Chinese Herbal Medicine), 1996; 158:159
3. Ibid.
4. *Xian Dai Zhong Yao Yao Li Xue* (Contemporary Pharmacology of Chinese Herbs), 1997; 32-33
5. *The Merck Index* 12th edition, Chapman & Hall/CRCnetBASE/Merck, 2000
6. *Zhong Xi Yi Jie He Za Zhi* (Journal of Integrated Chinese and Western Medicine), 1989; 9(4):255
7. *Zhong Yao Yao Li Yu Ying Yong* (Pharmacology and Applications of Chinese Herbs), 1983; 1082

Ma Huang (Herba Ephedrae)

8. *Zhong Yao Xue* (Chinese Herbology), 1998; 63:65
9. *Yao Xue Tong Bao* (Report of Herbology), 1986; 21(4):235
10. *Zhong Yao Xue* (Chinese Herbology), 1998; 63:65
11. *Zhong Yao Yao Li Yu Ying Yong* (Pharmacology and Applications of Chinese Herbs), 1983: 1082
12. Ibid.
13. *Neuropharmacology*, 1984; 23:1241
14. *Zhong Yao Yao Li Yu Ying Yong* (Pharmacology and Applications of Chinese Herbs), 1983; 1082
15. *Zhong Xi Yi Jie He Za Zhi* (Journal of Integrated Chinese and Western Medicine), 1989; 9(4):255
16. Ibid., 1988; 6:351
17. *Shan Xi Zhong Yi* (Shanxi Chinese Medicine), 1991; 12(7):320
18. *Hu Bei Zhong Yi Za Zhi* (Hubei Journal of Chinese Medicine), 1990; (4):43
19. Brinker, Francis. *Herb Contraindications and Drug Interactions*, 1997; 63
20. *The IBIS Guide to Drug-Herb and Drug-Nutrient Interactions*, 1999
21. Chen, J. Recognition & prevention of Herb-drug interactions, *Medical Acupuncture*, Fall/Winter 1998/1999; volume 10/number 2; 9-13
22. *Zhong Yao Yao Li Yu Ying Yong* (Pharmacology and Applications of Chinese Herbs), 1983; 1082

Gui Zhi (Ramulus Cinnamomi)

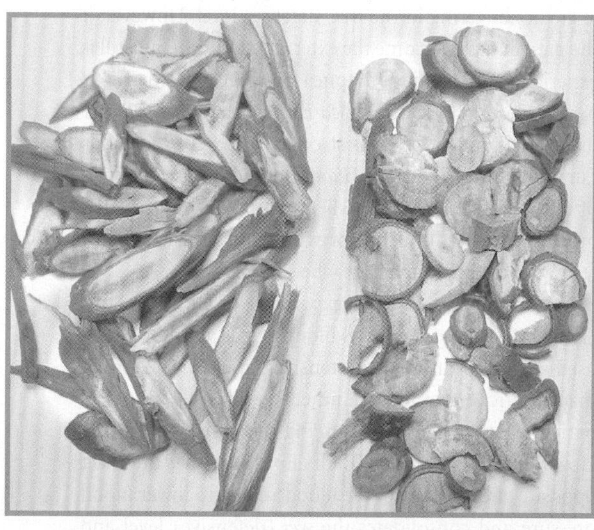

桂枝

Pinyin Name: *Gui Zhi*
Literal Name: "cinnamon twigs"
Alternate Chinese Names: *Liu Gui*
Original Source: *Shen Nong Ben Cao Jing* (Divine Husbandman's Classic of the Materia Medica) in the second century
English Name: cinnamon twigs, cassia twigs
Botanical Name: *Cinnamomum cassia* Presl.
Pharmaceutical Name: Ramulus Cinnamomi
Properties: acrid, sweet, warm
Channels Entered: Heart, Lung, Urinary Bladder

CHINESE THERAPEUTIC ACTIONS

1. Releases the Exterior through Diaphoresis

Exterior-excess, wind-cold condition: Acrid, sweet and warm, *Gui Zhi* (Ramulus Cinnamomi) exerts a diaphoretic function to release the exterior. It induces perspiration, relieves the exterior and warms the yang. *Gui Zhi* is used for exterior-excess conditions in which there is an absence of perspiration due to wind-cold constricting the pores and not allowing perspiration to occur. This herb can also be used for exterior-deficiency conditions, in which perspiration results from *wei* (defensive) *qi* deficiency in controlling the opening and closing of pores.

- Exterior-excess, wind-cold conditions in the absence of perspiration: use *Gui Zhi* with *Ma Huang* (Herba Ephedrae). **Exemplar Formula:** *Ma Huang Tang* (Ephedra Decoction).
- Wind-cold, exterior-deficient conditions with perspiration and aversion to wind: combine it with *Bai Shao* (Radix Paeoniae Alba). **Exemplar Formula:** *Gui Zhi Tang* (Cinnamon Twig Decoction).

2. Warms and Opens the Channels and Collaterals

***Bi zheng* (painful obstruction syndrome):** *Gui Zhi* is acrid and warm and is commonly used to treat *bi zheng* caused by stagnation of wind, cold and dampness. *Gui Zhi* travels to the superficial layers of the body, warms the muscles, and opens the channels and collaterals, thus relieving pain. It may be used as a guiding herb, and to treat pain.

- *Bi zheng:* use it with *Chuan Wu* (Radix Aconiti Preparata) and *Cao Wu* (Radix Aconiti Kusnezoffii) to

Gui Zhi (Ramulus Cinnamomi)

dispel cold and dampness, open the channels and collaterals, and relieve pain.

- *Bi zheng* in the upper body, especially the shoulders: add *Jiang Huang* (Rhizoma Curcumae Longae) and *Fang Feng* (Radix Saposhnikoviae).
- Rheumatoid arthritis: combine with *Qiang Huo* (Rhizoma et Radix Notopterygii), *Du Huo* (Radix Angelicae Pubescentis), *Fang Feng* (Radix Saposhnikoviae), and *Wei Ling Xian* (Radix Clematidis).

3. Warms Yang to Eliminate Water or Phlegm Stagnation

Edema and dysuria: Yang deficiency interferes with normal transportation and transformation of fluids in the body. Such interference leads to abnormal water circulation and water accumulation, characterized by symptoms such as edema and dysuria.

- Edema and dysuria due to yang deficiency: use *Gui Zhi* with *Fu Ling* (Poria), *Zhu Ling* (Polyporus), *Ze Xie* (Rhizoma Alismatis) and *Bai Zhu* (Rhizoma Atractylodis Macrocephalae). **Exemplar Formula:** *Wu Ling San* (Five-Ingredient Powder with Poria).

***Tan yin* (phlegm retention):** *Gui Zhi* treats yang-deficiency accumulation of phlegm with presentations such as fullness of the chest and hypochondrium, dizziness, vertigo and palpitations. Excess accumulation in the upper *jiao* interferes with normal functioning of transportation and transformation.

- Phlegm accumulation with fullness in the chest and hypochondrium, dizziness, vertigo, and palpitations: combine *Gui Zhi* with *Fu Ling* (Poria), *Bai Zhu* (Rhizoma Atractylodis Macrocephalae) and *Gan Cao* (Radix Glycyrrhizae) to tonify yang and resolve phlegm stagnation. **Exemplar Formula:** *Ling Gui Zhu Gan Tang* (Poria, Cinnamon Twig, Atractylodes Macrocephala, and Licorice Decoction).

4. Warms Yang in the Chest

***Xiong bi* (painful obstruction of the chest):** *Gui Zhi* warms yang energy in the chest and eliminates cold or phlegm stagnation. With yang deficiency, cold and phlegm may invade the chest, leading to symptoms such as *xiong bi*, cough, chest pain that may radiate to the scapulae, shortness of breath, and related discomforts. *Gui Zhi* is commonly used today to treat myocardial infarction, angina pectoris and cardiac insufficiency caused by yang deficiency, when no signs of heat are present.

- *Xiong bi* due to yang deficiency: use *Gui Zhi* with *Gua Lou Shi* (Fructus Trichosanthis) and *Xie Bai* (Bulbus Allii Macrostemonis) to warm yang in the chest, activate qi circulation, and remove stagnation.
- Palpitations and intermittent pulse because of Heart yin and yang deficiencies: combine it with *Zhi Gan Cao* (Radix Glycyrrhizae Preparata), *Ren Shen* (Radix Ginseng) and *E Jiao* (Colla Corii Asini) to tonify Heart yin and yang and restore normal pulse. **Exemplar Formula:** *Zhi Gan Cao Tang* (Honey-Fried Licorice Decoction).

5. Warms Yang in the *Chong* (Thoroughfare) and *Ren* (Conception) Channels to Restore Normal Menstruation

In traditional Chinese medicine, the *chong* channel is the sea of blood and the *ren* channel governs the uterus. Yang deficiency of the *chong* and *ren* channels, combined with qi stagnation, leads to abnormal blood flow, manifesting in symptoms such as irregular menstruation, dysmenorrhea, amenorrhea and other gynecological disorders. *Gui Zhi* warms the *chong* and *ren* channels and disperses stagnation by facilitating the flow of blood in the vessels.

- Irregular menstruation due to yang deficiency and cold stagnation: use it with *Dang Gui* (Radicis Angelicae Sinensis) and *Chuan Xiong* (Rhizoma Ligustici Chuanxiong) to warm the channels, eliminate cold stagnation, and nourish blood. **Exemplar Formula:** *Wen Jing Tang* (Warm the Menses Decoction).
- Blood stagnation and masses in the lower abdomen: combine this herb with *Mu Dan Pi* (Cortex Moutan) and *Tao Ren* (Semen Persicae) to disperse blood stasis. **Exemplar Formula:** *Gui Zhi Fu Ling Wan* (Cinnamon Twig and Poria Pill).

DOSAGE

5 to 10 grams. Maximum dosage for *Gui Zhi* is 30 grams. It may be used in decoction, pills, or powder.

CAUTIONS / CONTRAINDICATIONS

- Because *Gui Zhi* stimulates blood circulation, it should be used with caution in patients with high risk of bleeding, pregnant women, or women with hypermenorrhea.
- *Gui Zhi* is acrid and warm and may damage yin if used inappropriately. Therefore, it is contraindicated in patients with febrile disorders, yang excess related to yin deficiency, heat in the blood, or other heat-dominant disorders.

CHEMICAL COMPOSITION

Essential oils 0.43-1.35% (cinnamaldehyde, benzyl benzoate, cinnamyl acetate, calamenene, β-cadinene, terpinon-4-ol), trans-cinnamic acid, coumarin, protocatechuic acid.[1]

PHARMACOLOGICAL EFFECTS

- **Antibiotic**: *Gui Zhi* has both antibacterial and antiviral effects. It exerts an inhibitory effect against *Staphylococcus*

Gui Zhi (Ramulus Cinnamomi)

aureus, Salmonella typhi, some dermatophytes, and influenza viruses.[2]

- **Diuretic**: The essential oil of *Gui Zhi* has a mild diuretic effect to reduce edema.[3]
- **Diaphoretic and antipyretic**: The essential oil of *Gui Zhi* induces perspiration and lowers body temperature through dilation of blood vessels at the peripheral regions of the body.[4]
- **Analgesic**: It exerts analgesic action.[5]
- **Circulatory**: *Gui Zhi* dilates blood vessels and promotes blood circulation to the uterus.[6]
- **Other**: *Gui Zhi* has cardiotonic, sedative and hypnotic, and antitussive effects.[7]

CLINICAL STUDIES AND RESEARCH

- **Frostbite**: According to one report, 6 patients with frostbite were treated with an herbal decoction twice daily for 5 to 10 days with satisfactory results. The formula contained *Gui Zhi, Chi Shao* (Radix Paeoniae Rubrae), *Dang Gui* (Radicis Angelicae Sinensis), *Gan Cao* (Radix Glycyrrhizae), *Sheng Jiang* (Rhizoma Zingiberis Recens) and *Da Zao* (Fructus Jujubae).[8]

  In another study, *Gui Zhi* was used topically to treat frostbite with excellent results. The herbal decoction was prepared by cooking 60 grams of *Gui Zhi* in 1,000 ml of water for 10 minutes. The herbal decoction was applied topically to the affected area for 10 to 15 minutes twice daily. Treatment duration ranged between 1 and 6 topical applications.[9]
- **Facial numbness**: In a clinical study, 30 patients with facial numbness were treated by topical application of herbs, with complete recovery in 26 patients, moderate improvement in 3 patients, and no response in 1 patient. The duration of treatment ranged from 6 to 15 days. The herbal formula included *Gui Zhi* 30g, *Fang Feng* (Radix Saposhnikoviae) 20g, and *Chi Shao* (Radix Paeoniae Rubrae) 15g. The treatment protocol was to cook the herbs in decoction, and apply the decoction to the affected area with gentle massage for 20 minutes, twice daily. There should be mild warmth and redness in the area after each treatment session.[10]
- **Hypotension**: In one report, 117 patients with low blood pressure were treated with an herbal formula, with marked effectiveness in all patients within 2 to 3 days. The herbal formula consisted of *Gui Zhi* 40g, *Rou Gui* (Cortex Cinnamomi) 40g, and *Gan Cao* (Radix Glycyrrhizae) 20g, cooked in decoction and administered in three equally-divided doses daily.[11]
- **Arthritis**: In one report, 30 arthritic patients were treated with herbal formulas, with complete recovery in 15 patients, marked improvement in 6 patients, moderate effectiveness in 5 patients, and no response in 4 patients. The patients were given the herbs as decoction once daily. Duration of treatment was not specified. The herbal formula included *Gui Zhi* 15g, *Bai Shao* (Radix Paeoniae Alba) 15g, *Gan Cao* (Radix Glycyrrhizae) 6g, *Ma Huang* (Herba Ephedrae) 6g, *Bai Zhu* (Rhizoma Atractylodis Macrocephalae) 12g, *Zhi Mu* (Radix Anemarrhenae) 10g, *Fang Feng* (Radix Saposhnikoviae) 10g, *Fu Zi* (Radix Aconiti Lateralis Praeparata) 30 to 60g, and *Sheng Jiang* (Rhizoma Zingiberis Recens) 5g. For patients with chronic and stubborn arthritis, *Quan Xie* (Scorpio) 10g, *Wu Gong* (Scolopendra) 10g, *Wu Shao She* (Zaocys) 10g, and *Chuan Shan Jia* (Squama Manis) 10g were added to the formula.[12]

HERB-DRUG INTERACTION

Diuretics: *Gui Zhi* has a mild diuretic effect. Though this potential interaction has not been documented, concurrent use with diuretic drugs may lead to increased elimination of water and/or electrolytes.[13] [Note: Examples of diuretics include chlorothiazide, hydrochlorothiazide, furosemide (Lasix), bumetanide (Bumex), and torsemide (Demadex).]

TOXICOLOGY

The LD_{50} for cinnamic aldehyde in mice was 132 mg/kg via intravenous injection, 610 mg/kg via intraperitoneal injection, and 2,225 mg/kg via oral ingestion. Interestingly, there were more adverse toxicities and fatalities in the daytime than at night.[14]

References

1. *Xian Dai Zhong Yao Yao Li Xue* (Contemporary Pharmacology of Chinese Herbs), 1997; 46
2. *Zhong Yao Xue* (Chinese Herbology), 1998; 65:67
3. Ibid.
4. Ibid.
5. Ibid.
6. Ibid.
7. Ibid.
8. *Zhong Hua Yi Xue Za Zhi* (Chinese Journal of Medicine), 1956; 10:978
9. *Xin Zhong Yi* (New Chinese Medicine), 1980; 16
10. *Hu Nan Zhong Yi Za Zhi* (Hunan Journal of Chinese Medicine), 1987; 8(2):4
11. *Zhong Guo Nong Cun Yi Xue* (Chinese Agricultural Medicine), 1985; (5):11
12. *Shi Zhen Guo Yao Yan Jiu* (Research of Shizhen Herbs), 1991; 5(4):36
13. Chen, J. Recognition & prevention of herb-drug interactions, *Medical Acupuncture*, Fall/Winter 1998/1999; volume 10/number 2; 9-13
14. *Chang Yong Zhong Yao Xian Dai Yan Jiu Yu Lin Chuan* (Recent Study & Clinical Application of Common Traditional Chinese Medicine), 1995; 6:8

Zi Su Ye (Folium Perillae)

紫蘇葉 紫苏叶

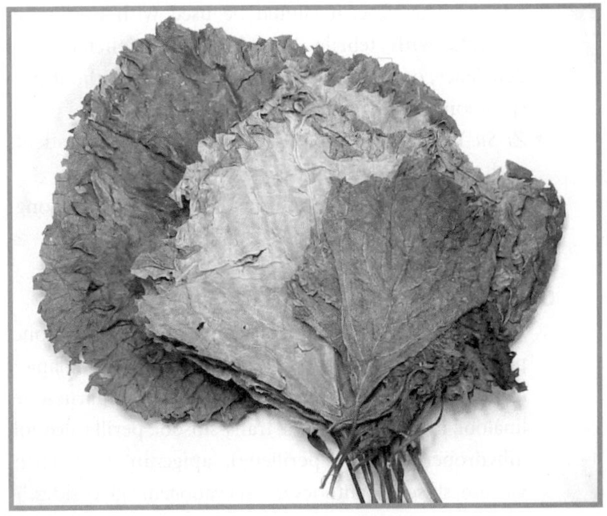

Pinyin Name: *Zi Su Ye*
Literal Name: "purple perilla leaf"
Alternate Chinese Names: *Su Ye, Zi Su*
Original Source: *Ben Cao Jing Ji Zhu* (Collection of Commentaries on the Classic of the Materia Medica) by Tao Hong-Jing in 480-498 A.D.
English Name: perilla, perilla leaf
Botanical Name: *Perilla frutescens* (L.) Britt. var. *crispa* (Thunb.) Hand. – Mazz.
Pharmaceutical Name: Folium Perillae
Properties: acrid, warm
Channels Entered: Lung, Spleen

CHINESE THERAPEUTIC ACTIONS

1. Releases the Exterior and Dispels Cold

Exterior wind-cold syndrome: Acrid and warm in nature, *Zi Su Ye* (Folium Perillae) releases the exterior, dispels wind and cold, and ventilates Lung qi. It is commonly used to treat exterior wind-cold syndrome.

- Exterior wind-cold syndrome with aversion to cold, fever, headache, nasal obstruction, absence of perspiration, and cough: use *Zi Su Ye* with *Qian Hu* (Radix Peucedani), *Xing Ren* (Semen Armeniacae Amarum) and *Jie Geng* (Radix Platycodonis). **Exemplar Formula:** *Xing Su San* (Apricot Kernel and Perilla Leaf Powder).
- Exterior wind-cold syndrome with qi stagnation and chest congestion: combine it with *Chen Pi* (Pericarpium Citri Reticulatae) and *Xiang Fu* (Rhizoma Cyperi) to activate and regulate qi circulation.

2. Regulates Qi and Expands the Chest, Harmonizes the Middle Jiao, Alleviates Nausea and Vomiting

Nausea and vomiting: *Zi Su Ye* is commonly used to treat chest fullness and congestion, nausea and vomiting secondary to qi stagnation of the Spleen and Stomach.

- Stomach flu, acute enteritis due to qi stagnation of the Spleen and Stomach, manifesting as abdominal pain, vomiting and diarrhea: use this herb with *Chen Pi* (Pericarpium Citri Reticulatae), *Ban Xia* (Rhizoma Pinelliae) and *Huo Xiang* (Herba Agastache). **Exemplar Formula:** *Huo Xiang Zheng Qi San* (Agastache Powder to Rectify the Qi).
- Qi stagnation of the Spleen and Stomach with heat: combine it with *Huang Lian* (Rhizoma Coptidis).
- Qi stagnation of the Spleen and Stomach with phlegm stagnation: add *Ban Xia* (Rhizoma Pinelliae) and *Hou Po* (Cortex Magnoliae Officinalis).

3. Calms the Fetus

Morning sickness or restless fetus: In pregnant women, upward reversal of fetal qi may lead to nausea and morning sickness. Abnormal descending of fetal qi may lead to restless fetus or threatened abortion. *Zi Su Ye* can be used during pregnancy to regulate qi circulation to relieve nausea and morning sickness, and stabilize the fetus.

- Morning sickness, restless fetus or threatened abortion: use this herb with *Chen Pi* (Pericarpium Citri Reticulatae), *Mu Xiang* (Radix Aucklandiae) and *Sha Ren* (Fructus Amomi) to regulate qi and stabilize pregnancy.

4. Alleviates Seafood Poisoning

Seafood poisoning: *Zi Su Ye* is commonly used to treat seafood poisoning characterized by nausea, vomiting, diarrhea and abdominal pain. It is most effective for poisoning from ingesting fish and crabs.

- Seafood poisoning: decoct *Zi Su Ye* by itself or in combination with *Sheng Jiang* (Rhizoma Zingiberis Recens).
- Rash or itching because of allergy: combine it with *Chan Tui* (Periostracum Cicadae) and *Fang Feng* (Radix Saposhnikoviae).

DOSAGE

5 to 10 grams. The herbal decoction may be taken orally or applied topically. When cooking the decoction, *Zi Su Ye* should be added last and cooked for only a few minutes.

CAUTIONS / CONTRAINDICATIONS

- Since *Zi Su Ye* is acrid and warm, it can easily damage yin

Zi Su Ye (Folium Perillae)

and qi. Therefore, it should be used with caution in patients with febrile disorders, yin deficiency, qi deficiency, or exterior-deficient syndromes without perspiration.

- *Zi Su Ye* should also be used with caution for patients with nausea caused by heat.
- *Zi Su Ye* should be used only on a short-term basis. Long-term use may lead to qi deficiency.

CHEMICAL COMPOSITION

Essential oils 0.2-0.9% (perillaldehyde, elsholtziaketone, perilla ketone, naginataketone, isoegomaketone, dillapiol, elemicin, wyristicin, citral, caryophellene, farnesene, linalool, methene, menthol, trans-shisool, perilla alcohol, dihydroperillalcohol, perillene), apigenin, scutellarin, vicenin, shisonin, anthocyanins, cyanogenic glycosides.[1,2]

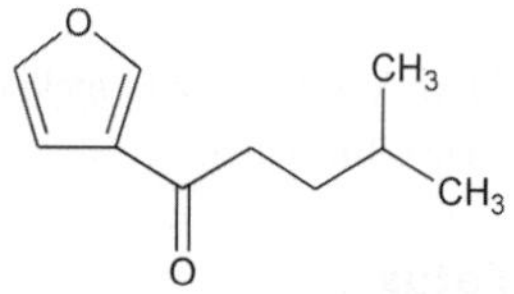

CH_3 CH_3 O O

Perilla Ketone

PHARMACOLOGICAL EFFECTS

- **Antipyretic and diaphoretic**: Decoction of *Zi Su Ye* dilates peripheral blood vessels and stimulates perspiration. At 2 g/kg via oral ingestion, it has a mild antipyretic effect in rabbits.[3]
- **Respiratory**: *Zi Su Ye* has been shown to promote bronchodilation and relieve bronchospasm. It also reduces secretion from the bronchioli.[4]
- **Antibiotic**: *Zi Su Ye* has been shown to inhibit the activity of *Staphylococcus aureus*. The minimum inhibitory concentration (MIC) of *Zi Su Ye* extract is 200 to 1,600 mg/ml.[5]
- **Gastrointestinal**: The perilla ketone of *Zi Su Ye* stimulates the gastrointestinal tract by increasing stomach acid secretion and intestinal peristalsis in rats.[6]
- **Hyperglycemic**: Essential oils of *Zi Su Ye* at 0.35 ml/kg given via oral ingestion in rabbits increase blood glucose levels.[7]

CLINICAL STUDIES AND RESEARCH

- **Common warts**: In one study, patients with common warts were treated by topical application of herbs with satisfactory results. *Zi Su Ye* ground into paste was applied topically for 10 to 15 minutes once daily, to treat common warts. Observation of 20 patients treated with this method revealed satisfactory results, with treatment duration ranging from 2 to 6 treatments.[8]
- **Cervical bleeding**: *Zi Su Ye* was extracted to yield a final solution with concentration of 2 grams of the herb in 1 ml of final solution. The solution was sterilized and applied topically to the affected area to stop bleeding. Of 108 patients, 86 (79.63%) reported satisfactory responses.[9]

TOXICOLOGY

Administration of *Zi Su Ye* is occasionally associated with adverse reactions, over stimulation, and allergic reactions.[10]

SUPPLEMENT

- 蘇梗 / 苏梗 *Su Geng* (Caulis Perillae), first cited in *Ming Yi Za Zhu* (Miscellaneous Records of Famous Physicians) by Tao Hong-Jing in 500 A.D., is derived from branches of the same plant as *Zi Su Ye*. It is acrid, sweet, and slightly warm and enters the Lung, Spleen and Stomach. Its main functions are to expand the chest and hypochondrium, regulate qi and calm the fetus. Because of its mild nature, *Su Geng* is most suitable for deficient patients with qi stagnation in the middle *jiao*. Its diaphoretic function is weaker than that of *Zi Su Ye*. The usual dosage is 5 to 10 grams. *Su Geng* should be added to the decoction last, and cooked for only a short time.

AUTHORS' COMMENTS

Please refer to *Su Zi* (Fructus Perillae) for comparison and contrast of *Zi Su Ye* (Folium Perillae), *Su Zi* (Fructus Perillae), and *Su Geng* (Caulis Perillae).

Zi Su Ye, *Shi Chang Pu* (Rhizoma Acori), *Ze Xie* (Rhizoma Alismatis) and *Shan Zha* (Fructus Crataegi) taken as tea on a daily basis is effective to reduce body weight and lower cholesterol.

References

1. *Xian Dai Zhong Yao Yao Li Xue* (Contemporary Pharmacology of Chinese Herbs), 1997; 72-73
2. *The Merck Index* 12th edition, Chapman & Hall/CRCnetBASE/Merck, 2000
3. *Planata Med*, 1985; (6):4
4. *Zhong Yao Xue* (Chinese Herbology), 1998; 67:68
5. *Zhong Guo Zhong Yao Za Zhi* (People's Republic of China Journal of Chinese Herbology), 1990; 25(2):31
6. *Planata Med*, 1985; (6):4
7. *Zhong Yao Xue* (Chinese Herbology), 1988: 665
8. *Zhong Hua Pi Fu Ke Xue Za Zhi* (Chinese Journal of Dermatology), 1965; 6:391
9. *Zhong Yi Za Zhi* (Journal of Chinese Medicine), 1988; 8:49
10. *Food Toxicol*, 1981; 19(2):253

Sheng Jiang (Rhizoma Zingiberis Recens)

生薑 生姜

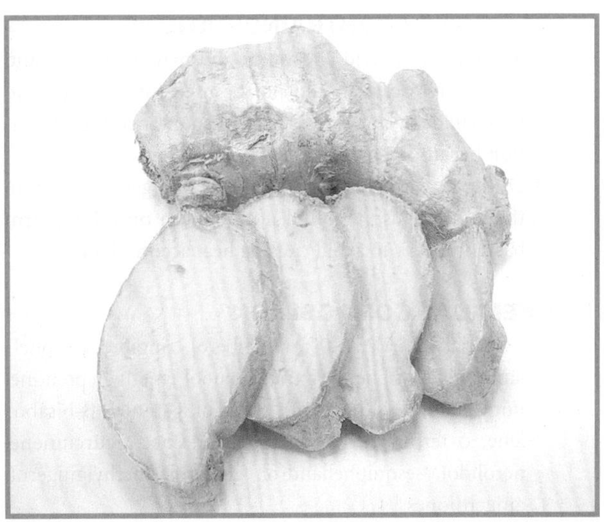

Pinyin Name: *Sheng Jiang*
Literal Name: "fresh ginger"
Original Source: *Ming Yi Za Zhu* (Miscellaneous Records of Famous Physicians) by Tao Hong-Jing in 500 A.D.
English Name: fresh ginger
Botanical Name: *Zingiber officinale* Rosc.
Pharmaceutical Name: Rhizoma Zingiberis Recens
Properties: acrid, slightly warm
Channels Entered: Lung, Spleen, Stomach

CHINESE THERAPEUTIC ACTIONS

1. Releases the Exterior and Induces Perspiration

Exterior wind-cold syndrome: *Sheng Jiang* (Rhizoma Zingiberis Recens), used as food on many occasions, has a mild function to release the exterior and induce perspiration. It is commonly used to treat mild or early stages of wind-cold syndrome. Because it is relatively mild, it must be used with stronger diaphoretic herbs in order to induce perspiration for releasing exterior syndromes.

- Early stage of common colds or influenza: use *Sheng Jiang* alone, or with *Gui Zhi* (Ramulus Cinnamomi) to dispel wind-cold or induce diaphoresis. **Exemplar Formula:** *Gui Zhi Tang* (Cinnamon Twig Decoction).
- To prevent catching a cold during cold or rainy weather: cook 15 to 20 slices *Sheng Jiang* for 10 minutes as a decoction in about two bowls of water, with brown sugar added at the end. Serve the decoction while it is still warm to alleviate minor wind-cold signs and symptoms.

2. Warms the Middle Jiao and Alleviates Vomiting

Vomiting caused by Stomach cold: *Sheng Jiang* warms the Stomach, harmonizes the middle *jiao* and is commonly used to relieve nausea and vomiting.

- Nausea and vomiting: use it alone or with *Da Zao* (Fructus Jujubae).
- Nausea and vomiting due to Stomach cold: combine *Sheng Jiang* with *Ban Xia* (Rhizoma Pinelliae).
- Nausea and vomiting due to Stomach heat: use it with *Zhu Ru* (Caulis Bambusae in Taenia), *Pi Pa Ye* (Folium Eriobotryae) and *Huang Lian* (Rhizoma Coptidis). **Exemplar Formula:** *Ju Pi Zhu Ru Tang* (Tangerine Peel and Bamboo Shaving Decoction).

3. Warms the Lung and Stops Coughing

Cough with profuse sputum caused by wind-cold: Wind-cold constricts Lung qi and may lead to coughing and formation of phlegm. *Sheng Jiang* warms the Lung, dispels cold, and stops coughing.

- Cough: use it with *Zi Su Ye* (Folium Perillae), *Xing Ren* (Semen Armeniacae Amarum), *Zi Wan* (Radix Asteris) and *Chen Pi* (Pericarpium Citri Reticulatae). **Exemplar Formula:** *Xing Su San* (Apricot Kernel and Perilla Leaf Powder).

4. Eliminates Toxins

Seafood poisoning: *Sheng Jiang* eliminates toxins and treats food poisoning characterized by vomiting and diarrhea. It works best for food poisoning commonly associated with seafood such as shrimp and crabs.

- Seafood poisoning: use *Sheng Jiang* individually or with *Zi Su Ye* (Folium Perillae).

Toxicity of herbs: *Sheng Jiang* is commonly used to neutralize or eliminate the toxicity of other herbs, often by either simultaneous use or by using *Sheng Jiang* as a preprocessing agent.

- Detoxification: *Tian Nan Xing* (Rhizoma Arisaematis) and *Ban Xia* (Rhizoma Pinelliae) should be preprocessed with *Sheng Jiang* to reduce unwanted toxic side effects. If numbness and swelling of the tongue or throat occur, drink *Sheng Jiang* decoction immediately to neutralize the toxins.

DOSAGE

3 to 10 grams for fresh herb in decoction. Maximum dosage for *Sheng Jiang* is 30 grams. Fresh *Sheng Jiang* may be ground into paste for topical application.

Sheng Jiang (Rhizoma Zingiberis Recens)

CAUTIONS / CONTRAINDICATIONS

- *Sheng Jiang* is acrid and warm and may damage qi and yin. Therefore, it should not be used for patients who have yin deficiency, excess heat, or spontaneous perspiration because of qi deficiency.
- Due to its warm nature, *Sheng Jiang* may generate heat in the body. Thus, it should not be given on a long-term basis, in order to avoid causing heat accumulation.

CHEMICAL COMPOSITION

Essential oils 0.25-3.0% (zingiberol, zingiberene, phellandrene, camphene, citral, linalool, methyheptenone, nonyladehyde, d-borneol), geraniol, geranial, β-bisabolene, α-terpineol, β-sesquiphellandrene, arcurcumene, nerolidol, sesquiphellandrol, gingerol, methylgingerol, gingerdiones.[1]

PHARMACOLOGICAL EFFECTS

- **Gastrointestinal:** Oral administration of *Sheng Jiang* in rats has demonstrated a marked influence on the gastrointestinal system. It exerts protective effects on the gastrointestinal system by stimulating the production of stomach mucous membranes. It also increases stomach acid secretion and intestinal motility.[2]
- **Cardiovascular:** The use of *Sheng Jiang* has been associated with an increase in heart rate, respiration rate, and blood pressure.[3]
- **Antibiotic:** *Sheng Jiang* has been shown to have an inhibitory effect on *Salmonella typhi*, *Vibrio cholerae* and *Trichomonas vaginalis*.[4]

CLINICAL STUDIES AND RESEARCH

- **Arthritis and low back pain:** Injections of a *Sheng Jiang* preparation were given to 113 patients to evaluate its effect on arthritis and low back pain. The injections were administered to pressure points daily or every other day, for 3 to 5 treatments per course. The rate of effectiveness was 83%.[5]
- **Arthritis:** Injections of a *Sheng Jiang* preparation were given to 125 patients to evaluate its effectiveness in treating arthritis. The injections were administered to various pressure points in the upper and lower limbs daily or every other day. Each course of treatment consisted of 7 injections, with 4 to 7 days of rest in between courses of treatment. Of 125 patients, 113 showed improvement.[6]
- **Intestinal obstruction due to parasites:** In one report, 541 patients with intestinal obstruction caused by parasites were given an herbal preparation (30 grams of *Sheng Jiang* and 60 grams of honey). This was given three times daily at varying dosages depending on the age of the patients, that ranged from 1 to 15 years of age. The patients also received supportive treatment with allopathic medicine when necessary. Of 541 patients, 87.6% reported improvement.[7]
- **Nausea and vomiting:** A slice of *Sheng Jiang* placed topically on point *Neiguan* (PC 6) showed marked effectiveness in relieving nausea and vomiting in 10 patients.[8]
- **Severe nausea and vomiting:** Administration of *Sheng Jiang* via simple tea or decoction effectively reduced the severity of nausea and vomiting associated with chemotherapy and radiation treatments.[9]
- **Motion sickness:** In one report, patients with frequent history of motion sickness were treated with *Sheng Jiang* placed topically on *Neiguan* (PC 6), on the right hand for females and left hand for males. Of 39 patients treated, following a motorcycle ride only one experienced motion sickness.[10]
- **Vitiligo:** *Sheng Jiang* was reported to be effective in treating vitiligo when it was used to rub the affected area of the skin three to four times daily for 2 to 3 months.[11]
- **Burn:** Topical application of fresh *Sheng Jiang* juice with a cotton ball showed marked effectiveness in treating burns, whether blistered or not, in 400 to 500 patients, without unwanted side effects.[12]

TOXICOLOGY

No fatalities were noted following intramuscular injection of *Sheng Jiang* in mice at a dose 625 times the normal adult dose in humans.[13]

SUPPLEMENT

- 生薑皮 / 生姜皮 *Sheng Jiang Pi* (Pericarpium Zingiberis Recens), first cited in *Tu Jing Ben Cao* (Illustrated Classic of the Materia Medica) by Su Song in 1061, is derived from the skin of the ginger root. It is acrid and cool, and functions to harmonize the middle *jiao*, dispel water and reduce edema. It is often used in patients with edema and urinary dysfunction. *Sheng Jiang Pi*, *Da Fu Pi* (Pericarpium Arecae), *Sang Bai Pi* (Cortex Mori), *Fu Ling Pi* (Cortex Poria) and *Chen Pi* (Pericarpium Citri Reticulatae) are five herbs often combined together to relieve edema, such as in *Wu Pi Yin* (Five-Peel Decoction). The dosage for *Sheng Jiang Pi* is 3 to 10 grams.

AUTHORS' COMMENTS

Sheng Jiang (Rhizoma Zingiberis Recens) and *Gan Jiang* (Rhizoma Zingiberis) are two herbs with similar yet different functions. *Sheng Jiang* is acrid and warm, and is best at dispelling exterior wind-cold. *Gan Jiang* is acrid and hot, and is most effective to warm the interior.

References

1. *Xian Dai Zhong Yao Yao Li Xue* (Contemporary Pharmacology of Chinese Herbs), 1997; 64

Sheng Jiang (Rhizoma Zingiberis Recens)

2. Ibid., 66
3. *Zhong Yao Xue* (Chinese Herbology), 1998; 69:72
4. Ibid.
5. *He Bei Xin Yi Yao* (Hebei New Medicine and Herbology), 1972; 3:31
6. *Chi Jiao Yi Shi Za Zhi* (Journal of Barefoot Doctors), 1077; 11:13
7. *Zhong Xi Yi Jie He Za Zhi* (Journal of Integrated Chinese and Western Medicine), 1986; 2:114
8. *Xin Zhong Yi* (New Chinese Medicine), 1986; 12:24
9. *Dissertation Abstr Interant*, 1987, 8:3297
10. *Da Zhong Yi Xue* (Public Medicine), 1980; 9:7
11. *Zhe Jiang Zhong Yi Za Zhi* (Zhejiang Journal of Chinese Medicine) 1966; 3:97
12. *Xin Zhong Yi* (New Chinese Medicine), 1984; 2:22
13. *Chang Yong Zhong Yao Xian Dai Yan Jiu Yu Lin Chuan* (Recent Study & Clinical Application of Common Traditional Chinese Medicine), 1995; 10:13

Xiang Ru (Herba Elsholtziae seu Moslae)

香薷 香薷

Pinyin Name: *Xiang Ru*
Alternate Chinese Names: *Xi Xiang Ru*
Original Source: *Ming Yi Za Zhu* (Miscellaneous Records of Famous Physicians) by Tao Hong-Jing in 500 A.D.
English Name: elsholtzia
Botanical Name: *Elsholtzia splendens* Nakai ex F. Maekawa (*Xiang Ru*); *Mosla chinensis* Maxim. (*Shi Xiang Ru*)
Pharmaceutical Name: Herba Elsholtziae seu Moslae
Properties: acrid, slightly warm
Channels Entered: Lung, Stomach

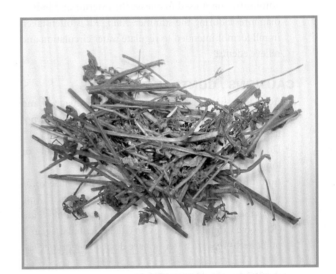

CHINESE THERAPEUTIC ACTIONS

1. Releases the Exterior and Induces Diaphoresis

Wind-cold with dampness: *Xiang Ru* (Herba Elsholtziae seu Moslae) is best for patients who catch common colds while outdoors trying to cool off on hot summer nights. As the weather is humid in Asia, this acrid and slightly warm herb is used to dispel wind-cold and the dampness factor that is present during the summer. It is used less often in environments where the weather is predominantly dry.

- Exterior wind-cold syndrome in summer with fever, aversion to cold, headache, chest fullness and congestion, but no perspiration: use this herb with *Hou Po* (Cortex Magnoliae Officinalis) and *Bian Dou* (Semen Lablab Album) to dispel wind-cold. **Exemplar Formula:** *Xiang Ru Yin* (Elsholtzia Combination).
- Exterior wind-cold syndrome in summer with fever, chills, thirst, and no perspiration: combine it with *Jin Yin Hua* (Flos Lonicerae), *Lian Qiao* (Fructus Forsythiae) and *Bo He* (Herba Menthae).

2. Eliminates Dampness and Harmonizes the Middle Jiao

Gastrointestinal disorders in summer: *Xiang Ru* is commonly used to treat gastrointestinal disorders, such as nausea, vomiting and diarrhea, caused by excessive intake of cold or contaminated beverages or foods in the summer. These conditions are characterized by dampness attacking the middle *jiao,* impeding the Spleen's normal transformation and transportation functions. Again, *Xiang Ru* is not often used for this purpose in developed countries where sanitation is not a problem, or in areas with predominantly dry weather patterns.

- Nausea and vomiting: use it with *Hou Po* (Cortex Magnoliae Officinalis) and *Sheng Jiang* (Rhizoma Zingiberis Recens).
- Diarrhea: combine it with *Bian Dou* (Semen Lablab

Xiang Ru (Herba Elsholtziae seu Moslae)

Album), *Huang Qin* (Radix Scutellariae), *Hou Po* (Cortex Magnoliae Officinalis) and *Fu Ling* (Poria).

3. Promotes Urination and Relieves Edema

Edema and dysuria: *Xiang Ru* raises yang qi, strengthens the Spleen, dispels dampness, and promotes circulation of water. It treats edema and dysuria, such as those seen in acute nephritis.

- Edema and dysuria: use *Xiang Ru* with *Bai Zhu* (Rhizoma Atractylodis Macrocephalae).

DOSAGE

3 to 10 grams. Maximum dosage is 30 grams. The decoction should be cooled to room temperature prior to administration if used to release the exterior and induce diaphoresis during the summer. *Xiang Ru* is often taken in pill form if intended to regulate water circulation and relieve edema.

CAUTIONS / CONTRAINDICATIONS

- Acrid and slightly warm, *Xiang Ru* may damage qi and yin. Thus, patients with qi or yin deficiency should not take this herb.
- Do not use *Xiang Ru* as tea for drinking on a daily or long-term basis.
- Administration of the warm decoction may cause vomiting, which may be alleviated by the addition of *Xing Ren* (Semen Armeniacae Amarum), *Huang Lian* (Rhizoma Coptidis), *Huang Qin* (Radix Scutellariae) and other herbs that are bitter or have descending properties.

CHEMICAL COMPOSITION

Essential oils 0.1-0.9% (carvacrol, m-cymene, p-cymene, o-cymene, r-terpinene, humulene, α-phellandrene, β-ionone, α-terpineol, eugenol, cedrol), quercetin, apigenin, 2-methylbaicalein, ursolic acid, syringic acid, caffeic acid.[1]

PHARMACOLOGICAL EFFECTS

- **Antipyretic:** The essential oil of *Xiang Ru* has diaphoretic and antipyretic effects.[2]
- **Gastrointestinal:** *Xiang Ru* stimulates the secretion of gastric acid, but inhibits intestinal peristalsis in mice, rats and guinea pigs.[3]
- **Antibiotic:** It has inhibitory activity against *E. coli*, *Staphylococcus aureus*, β-hemolytic streptococcus, and some dermatomyces.[4]
- **Others:** Some studies report expectorant and diuretic effects.[5]

CLINICAL STUDIES AND RESEARCH

- **Common cold:** According to one report, 200 patients suffering from common colds were treated topically with an herbal formula, with complete recovery in 196 cases and no effect in 4 cases. Out of 196 that responded, 164 reported positive improvement after one dose and 32 reported positive effects after two doses. The herbal formula contained in fine powder: *Xiang Ru* 15g, *Ma Huang* (Herba Ephedrae) 15g, *Ban Lan Gen* (Radix Isatidis) 10g, *Pu Gong Ying* (Herba Taraxaci) 10g and *Jie Geng* (Radix Platycodonis) 12g. The herbal powder was placed topically on the umbilicus and held in place with gauze. The dosage was 3.5g for adults and 1.0g for pediatric patients.[6]
- **Diarrhea in the summer time:** An herbal decoction given three times daily was effective in 89 of 90 patients with diarrhea. The herbal decoction contained *Xiang Ru* 10g, *Qin Pi* (Cortex Fraxini) 10g, *Bian Dou* (Semen Lablab Album) 10g, *Liu Yi San* (Six-to-One Powder) 10g, *Hou Po* (Cortex Magnoliae Officinalis) 10g, *Huo Xiang* (Herba Agastache) 10g, *Bai Zhu* (Rhizoma Atractylodis Macrocephalae) 10g, *Ban Xia* (Rhizoma Pinelliae) 10g, *Mu Xiang* (Radix Aucklandiae) 10g, *Huang Lian* (Rhizoma Coptidis) 5g, and *Fu Ling* (Poria) 15g. If there were symptoms of food stagnation, *Shan Zha* (Fructus Crataegi) 10g, *Shen Qu* (Massa Fermentata) 10g, and *Mai Ya* (Fructus Hordei Germinatus) 10g were added.[7]

AUTHORS' COMMENTS

It is generally accepted that the herb of choice to dispel wind-cold from the exterior is *Ma Huang* (Herba Ephedrae) in winter and *Xiang Ru* in summer. Use of *Ma Huang* in summer is not appropriate, as it may be too strong and damage body fluids. Similarly, use of *Xiang Ru* in winter is not sufficient, as it is not powerful enough to dispel wind-cold under winter conditions.

References

1. *Xian Dai Zhong Yao Yao Li Xue* (Contemporary Pharmacology of Chinese Herbs), 1997; 90
2. *Zhong Yao Xue* (Chinese Herbology), 1998; 72:73
3. *Zhong Yao Yao Li Yu Ying Yong* (Pharmacology and Applications of Chinese Herbs), 1988; 4(2):30
4. *Zhong Cao Yao Tong Xun* (Journal of Chinese Herbal Medicine), 1973; (1):44
5. *Zhong Yao Xue* (Chinese Herbology), 1998; 72:73
6. *An Hui Zhong Yi Xue Yuan Xue Bao* (Journal of Anhui University School of Medicine), 1989; (2):28
7. *He Bei Zhong Yi* (Hebei Chinese Medicine), 1991; 13(1):5

Jing Jie (Herba Schizonepetae)

荆芥 荊芥

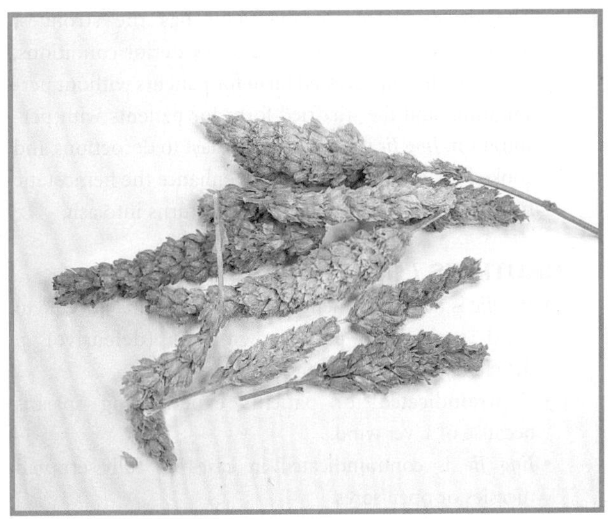

Pinyin Name: *Jing Jie*
Alternate Chinese Names: *Jing Jie Sui*
Original Source: *Shen Nong Ben Cao Jing* (Divine Husbandman's Classic of the Materia Medica) in the second century
English Name: schizonepeta, fine-leaf schizonepeta
Botanical Name: *Schizonepeta tenuifolia* Briq.
Pharmaceutical Name: Herba Schizonepetae
Properties: acrid, slightly warm
Channels Entered: Lung, Liver

CHINESE THERAPEUTIC ACTIONS

1. Releases the Exterior and Dispels Wind

Wind-heat or wind-cold: *Jing Jie* (Herba Schizonepetae) is rather mild in action. It is acrid, yet not damaging to the yin; it is warm but not drying. It is commonly used to dispel wind-cold or wind-heat from the exterior.

- Exterior wind-cold with aversion to cold, fever, headache and no perspiration: use *Jing Jie* with *Fang Feng* (Radix Saposhnikoviae) and *Qiang Huo* (Rhizoma et Radix Notopterygii) to dispel wind-cold and release the exterior. **Exemplar Formula:** *Jing Fang Bai Du San* (Schizonepeta and Saposhnikovia Powder to Overcome Pathogenic Influences).
- Exterior wind-heat with fever, headache, sore throat and red eyes: combine *Jing Jie* with *Bo He* (Herba Menthae), *Lian Qiao* (Fructus Forsythiae) and *Jin Yin Hua* (Flos Lonicerae) to dispel wind-heat. **Exemplar Formula:** *Yin Qiao San* (Honeysuckle and Forsythia Powder).

2. Dispels Wind and Relieves Muscle Spasms

- Postpartum spasms and trismus: *Jing Jie* is useful to relieve these problems caused by exposure to wind.
- Muscle cramps and spasms caused by wind exposure: use this herb by itself as powder, or in combination with other herbs that arrest wind and stop tremors.

3. Dispels Wind, Vents Rashes and Alleviates Itching

Dermatological disorders are often the direct manifestation of wind attacking the exterior of the body. *Jing Jie* dispels this wind and is commonly used to treat measles, rashes, eczema, pruritic itching, carbuncles, furuncles, abscesses, and similar eruptions or sores.

- Measles: use it with *Chan Tui* (Periostracum Cicadae), *Niu Bang Zi* (Fructus Arctii), *Bo He* (Herba Menthae), and *Jin Yin Hua* (Flos Lonicerae) to dispel wind and promote the eruption of measles.
- Pruritic itching: combine it with *Fang Feng* (Radix Saposhnikoviae) to dispel wind and relieve itching.
- Early-stage carbuncles, furuncles, and abscesses with heat: use *Jing Jie* with *Lian Qiao* (Fructus Forsythiae), *Bo He* (Herba Menthae), *Niu Bang Zi* (Fructus Arctii), *Mu Dan Pi* (Cortex Moutan) and *Zhi Zi* (Fructus Gardeniae).
- Early-stage carbuncles, furuncles and abscesses with exterior signs and symptoms: use it with *Fang Feng* (Radix Saposhnikoviae), *Jin Yin Hua* (Flos Lonicerae) and *Lian Qiao* (Fructus Forsythiae).

4. Stops Bleeding

Bleeding from various causes: *Jing Jie* has excellent effects to stop bleeding, if the charred form is used.

- Epistaxis, hemoptysis and hematemesis: use it with fresh juice of *Sheng Di Huang* (Radix Rehmanniae).
- Hematochezia or bleeding hemorrhoids: add it to *Huai Hua* (Flos Sophorae), *Ce Bai Ye* (Cacumen Platycladi), and *Zhi Ke* (Fructus Aurantii). **Exemplar Formula:** *Huai Hua San* (Sophora Japonica Flower Powder).
- Hematuria: combine *Jing Jie* with *Xiao Ji* (Herba Cirisii), *Sheng Di Huang* (Radix Rehmanniae), *Ou Jie* (Nodus Nelumbinis Rhizomatis), *Hua Shi* (Talcum), *Tong Cao* (Medulla Tetrapanacis), and *Pu Huang* (Pollen Typhae).
- For hypermenorrhea, abnormal uterine bleeding or postpartum bleeding: use it with *E Jiao* (Colla Corii Asini), *Ai Ye* (Folium Artemisiae Argyi), and *Gan Cao* (Radix Glycyrrhizae).

DOSAGE

5 to 10 grams. Maximum dosage of *Jing Jie* is 30 grams.

Jing Jie (Herba Schizonepetae)

The tip or flower of the plant has the strongest diaphoretic effect. For treatment of exterior conditions, prescribe the unprocessed form for patients without perspiration, and the stir-fried form for patients with perspiration. *Jing Jie* should be added last to decoctions and cooked for only a short time. To enhance the hemostatic function, the herb is charred until it turns into ash.

CAUTIONS / CONTRAINDICATIONS

- *Jing Jie* is not recommended if perspiration is not due to wind, such as in patients with *wei* (defensive) *qi* deficiency or yin-deficient heat.
- Contraindicated for patients experiencing spasms because of Liver wind.
- *Jing Jie* is contraindicated in cases of fully erupted measles or open sores.
- While taking *Jing Jie*, patients should avoid foods such as fish, crab, goose or duck, as consumption of these foods may increase itching of the skin.

CHEMICAL COMPOSITION

Essential oils 0.43-2.05% (menthone, pulegone, isomenthone, isopulegone, limonene), schizomodiol, schizonepetoside A-E. Charred *Jing Jie* has a significantly lower content of essential oils (0.06%).[1]

PHARMACOLOGICAL EFFECTS

- **Antipyretic and diaphoretic**: Water and alcohol extracts of *Jing Jie* given orally at 2 g/kg are associated with mild antipyretic effects in rabbits with artificially-induced fevers.[2]
- **Antibiotic**: Decoction of *Jing Jie* has shown antimicrobial effectiveness against *Staphylococcus aureus, Corynebacterium diphtheriae, Bacillus anthracis,* β-streptococcus, *Salmonella typhi, Bacillus dysenteriae, Pseudomonas aeruginosa,* and *Bacillus tuberculi*.[3]
- **Hemostatic**: In one laboratory study, the hemostatic effects of unprocessed *Jing Jie* and charred *Jing Jie* were evaluated in mice and rabbits. The study reported that unprocessed *Jing Jie* shortened coagulation time by 30%, while charred *Jing Jie* did so by 77.7%. The study concluded that charred *Jing Jie* is more effective than unprocessed *Jing Jie* as a hemostatic agent.[4]
- **Analgesic**: Decoction of *Jing Jie* demonstrated analgesic influence.[5]
- **Respiratory**: Essential oil of *Jing Jie* exerts bronchodilating action to relieve bronchospasm, treating wheezing and dyspnea.[6]

CLINICAL STUDIES AND RESEARCH

- **Dermatological disorders**: *Jing Jie* powder can be applied topically for various dermatological disorders, such as measles, pruritic rash and itching. Apply the powder to the affected area and gently rub it against the skin until there is a sensation of mild warmth. Mild dermatological conditions require 1 or 2 treatments, while severe conditions require 2 to 4 treatments.[7]

TOXICOLOGY

The LD_{50} for decoction of *Jing Jie* via intraperitoneal injection in mice is 30,046 mg/kg.[8]

SUPPLEMENT

- 荊穗 / 荆穗 *Jing Sui* (Flos Schizonepetae), the flower, treats wind invasion affecting the head. By comparison, *Jing Jie* (Herba Schizonepetae), the aerial part of the plant, treats wind invasion throughout the body.

References

1. *Xian Dai Zhong Yao Yao Li Xue* (Contemporary Pharmacology of Chinese Herbs), 1997; 53
2. *Zhong Yao Yao Li Yu Ying Yong* (Pharmacology and Applications of Chinese Herbs), 1983; 744
3. Ibid.
4. *Zhong Yao Cai* (Study of Chinese Herbal Material), 1989; 12(6):37
5. Ibid.
6. *Zhong Yao Xue* (Chinese Herbology), 1998; 73:75
7. *Zhong Yi Za Zhi* (Journal of Chinese Medicine), 12:18
8. *Zhong Yao Cai* (Study of Chinese Herbal Material), 1989; 12(6):37

Fang Feng (Radix Saposhnikoviae)

防風 防风

Pinyin Name: *Fang Feng*
Literal Name: "guard against wind," "wind-preventing herb"
Alternate Chinese Names: *Qing Fang Feng, Cao Fang Feng*
Original Source: *Shen Nong Ben Cao Jing* (Divine Husbandman's Classic of the Materia Medica) in the second century
English Name: siler
Botanical Name: *Saposhnikovia divaricata* (Turcz.) Schischk; *Ledebouriella divaricata* (Turcz.) Hiroe
Pharmaceutical Name: Radix Saposhnikoviae
Properties: acrid, sweet, slightly warm
Channels Entered: Urinary Bladder, Liver, Spleen

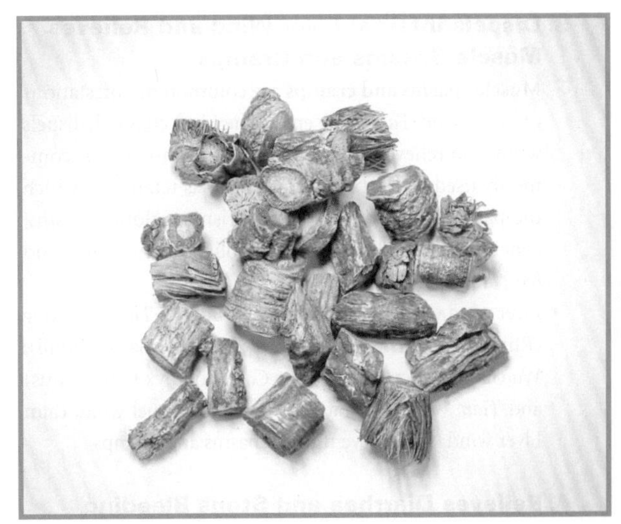

CHINESE THERAPEUTIC ACTIONS

1. Dispels Wind and Releases the Exterior

Exterior wind-heat or wind-cold syndrome: Due to its acrid and sweet properties, *Fang Feng* (Radix Saposhnikoviae) is one of the most effective herbs for dispelling wind without causing dryness. Because the function of *Fang Feng* in dispelling wind is stronger than the influence of its warming property, it can be used for both wind-cold and wind-heat conditions. *Fang Feng* is the herb of choice when body aches and pain are the chief complaints in an exterior syndrome.

- Exterior wind-cold syndrome with aversion to cold, fever, and headache: use this herb with *Zi Su Ye* (Folium Perillae), *Jing Jie* (Herba Schizonepetae), and *Bai Zhi* (Radix Angelicae Dahuricae).
- Exterior wind-cold syndrome with aversion to cold, headache, muscle aches and pain: combine it with *Jing Jie* (Herba Schizonepetae), *Qiang Huo* (Rhizoma et Radix Notopterygii) and *Qian Hu* (Radix Peucedani).
- Exterior wind-heat syndrome with red eyes and sore throat: combine it with *Jing Jie* (Herba Schizonepetae), *Lian Qiao* (Fructus Forsythiae) and *Bo He* (Herba Menthae).
- To strengthen *wei* (defensive) *qi*: add *Huang Qi* (Radix Astragali).
- Exterior wind-heat syndrome with accumulation of interior heat: use with *Ma Huang* (Herba Ephedrae) and *Jing Jie* (Herba Schizonepetae) to dispel wind-heat from the exterior, and with *Huang Qin* (Radix Scutellariae) and *Zhi Zi* (Fructus Gardeniae) to clear heat from the interior. **Exemplar Formula:** *Jing Fang Bai Du San* (Schizonepeta and Saposhnikovia Powder to Overcome Pathogenic Influences).

Dermatological disorders with itching: Wind is the predominant factor in dermatological disorders such as rashes, eczema, boils, rubella and urticaria. *Fang Feng* dispels wind and relieves itching.

- Dermatological disorders with itching, rash, and irritation: use it with *Jing Jie* (Herba Schizonepetae) and *Chan Tui* (Periostracum Cicadae). **Exemplar Formula:** *Xiao Feng San* (Eliminate Wind Powder).
- Acne due to wind-heat attacking the upper body: use it with *Bo He* (Herba Menthae), *Lian Qiao* (Fructus Forsythiae), *Huang Qin* (Radix Scutellariae), and *Huang Lian* (Rhizoma Coptidis). **Exemplar Formula:** *Qing Shang Fang Feng Tang* (Clear the Upper and Guard the Wind Decoction).

2. Dispels Wind, Cold, and Dampness and Relieves Pain

***Bi zheng* (painful obstruction syndrome):** Wind, cold and dampness are factors that commonly attack the muscles and joints, leading to arthritis, also known as *bi zheng*. These pathogens obstruct the normal circulation of qi and blood, leading to joint pain and muscle spasms. This type of pain is usually aggravated in cold or rainy seasons.

- *Bi zheng* arising from wind, cold, and dampness: use *Fang Feng* with *Qiang Huo* (Rhizoma et Radix Notopterygii), *Dang Gui* (Radicis Angelicae Sinensis), *Jiang Huang* (Rhizoma Curcumae Longae), *Chi Shao* (Radix Paeoniae Rubrae), *Huang Qi* (Radix Astragali), and *Gan Cao* (Radix Glycyrrhizae) to eliminate pathogenic factors and relieve pain. **Exemplar Formula:** *Juan Bi Tang* (Remove Painful Obstruction Decoction).

Fang Feng (Radix Saposhnikoviae)

3. Dispels Internal Liver Wind and Relieves Muscle Spasms and Cramps

Muscle spasms and cramps are common manifestations of Liver wind. *Fang Feng* enters the Liver channel, dispels wind, and relieves muscle spasms and cramps. It is commonly used to treat conditions such as tetanus in which the patients have hyperreflexia, trismus, glottal spasms, generalized muscle spasms, trembling of the hands and feet, and seizures.

- Liver wind with spasms: use *Fang Feng* with *Tian Nan Xing* (Rhizoma Arisaematis), *Bai Fu Zi* (Rhizoma Typhonii), *Wu Gong* (Scolopendra), *Jiang Can* (Bombyx Batryticatus) and *Tian Ma* (Rhizoma Gastrodiae) to dispel wind, calm Liver wind, and relieve muscle spasms and cramps.

4. Relieves Diarrhea and Stops Bleeding

Liver and Spleen disharmony: Clinical manifestations include recurrent, painful diarrhea with borborygmus and abdominal pain that may or may not be relieved by evacuation. Bright red blood may also be present in the stool. *Fang Feng* can be used in combination with other herbs to treat diarrhea caused by Liver and Spleen disharmony.

- Diarrhea with abdominal pain: use *Fang Feng* with *Chen Pi* (Pericarpium Citri Reticulatae), *Bai Zhu* (Rhizoma Atractylodis Macrocephalae) and *Bai Shao* (Radix Paeoniae Alba) to stop diarrhea and relieve abdominal pain. **Exemplar Formula:** *Tong Xie Yao Fang* (Important Formula for Painful Diarrhea).
- Chronic, recurrent diarrhea with blood caused by *chang feng* (intestinal wind): use this herb with charred *Di Yu* (Radix Sanguisorbae), charred *Huai Jiao* (Fructus Sophorae), and *Huai Hua* (Flos Sophorae).

5. Hemostatic

When charred to ashes, *Fang Feng* stops bleeding.

- Excessive menstrual bleeding: stir-fry *Fang Feng* until it turns to ash, then administer 6 grams orally, with water.

DOSAGE

3 to 10 grams. Maximum dosage of *Fang Feng* is 30 grams. Use the unprocessed form for the strongest exterior-releasing action; use the charred herb for maximum hemostatic effect.

CAUTIONS / CONTRAINDICATIONS

- Acrid and slightly warm, *Fang Feng* may consume qi, yin and body fluids. Therefore, it is contraindicated for patients who have yin-deficient fire, muscle cramps and spasms because of blood deficiency, or who have conditions that do not include the presence of wind, cold, or dampness.
- Since *Fang Feng* is ascending in nature, it should not be used in patients with headaches or dizziness due to Liver yang or Liver wind rising.

CHEMICAL COMPOSITION

Essential oil 0.3-0.6%, saccharides (saposhnikovan A, B, C), imperatorin, phellopterin, hamaudol, 3-o-angeloylhamaudol, ledebouriellol, sec-o-glycosylhamaudol, 5-o-methylvisamminol, cimifugin, prim-o-glycosylcimifugin, anomalin, xanthotoxin, scopoletin, falcarindiol.[1]

PHARMACOLOGICAL EFFECTS

- **Antipyretic:** Decoction of *Fang Feng* at 2 g/kg has a mild antipyretic effect in subjects with artificially-induced fever. The peak effect was observed within 1 to 2 hours after ingestion.[2]
- **Antibiotic:** *Fang Feng* has been shown to have antibacterial effect against *Shigella* spp., *Pseudomonas aeruginosa,* and *Staphylococcus aureus*. *Fang Feng* was also shown to exert antiviral action against influenza viruses.[3]

CLINICAL STUDIES AND RESEARCH

- **Antidote for arsenic poisoning:** In one study, 278 patients were treated for arsenic poisoning with an herbal decoction consisting of *Fang Feng* 12g, *Lu Dou* (Semen Phaseoli Radiati) 9g, *Gan Cao* (Radix Glycyrrhizae) 3g, and sugar 9g. The herbal decoction was given twice daily for 14 days per course of treatment, for a total of 2 courses. At the end of the treatment, 155 (55.76%) patients reported significant improvement in subjective signs and symptoms with normal levels of arsenic found through urinalysis.[4]
- **Chronic low back pain:** In one report, 336 patients were treated for chronic low back pain using an injected herbal formulation consisting of *Fang Feng, Niu Xi* (Radix Cyathulae seu Achyranthis), and *Gui Zhi* (Ramulus Cinnamomi). The treatment protocol was to inject 0.5 to 1.0 ml of the solution into tender points in the lower back once daily for 5 to 7 days. Out of 336 patients, the study reported an overall effective rate of 96% with 40% showing marked improvement.[5]

TOXICOLOGY

The LD_{50} for oral ingestion of *Fang Feng* in mice is 213.8 g/kg.[6]

AUTHORS' COMMENTS

Saposhnikovia divaricata is the standard source of *Fang Feng*.[7] *Ledebouriella divaricata* is considered to be the substitute.

Fang Feng can be used to detoxify the body from many substances, such as heavy metal (arsenic) and overdose of herbs such as *Fu Zi* (Radix Aconiti Lateralis Praeparata).

Fang Feng (Radix Saposhnikoviae)

References

1. *Xian Dai Zhong Yao Yao Li Xue* (Contemporary Pharmacology of Chinese Herbs), 1997; 58
2. *Zhong Yi Yao Xin Xi* (Information on Chinese Medicine and Herbology), 1990; (4):39
3. *Zhong Yao Tong Bao* (Journal of Chinese Herbology), 1988; 13(6):364
4. *Xin Yi Xue* (New Medicine), 1973; 7:6
5. *Shanxi Traditional Chinese Medicine*, 1988; 10:461
6. *Zhong Yao Tong Bao* (Journal of Chinese Herbology), 1988; 13(6):364
7. *Zhong Hua Ren Min Gong He Guo Yao Dian* (Chinese Herbal Pharmacopoeia by People's Republic of China), 2000

Qiang Huo (Rhizoma et Radix Notopterygii)

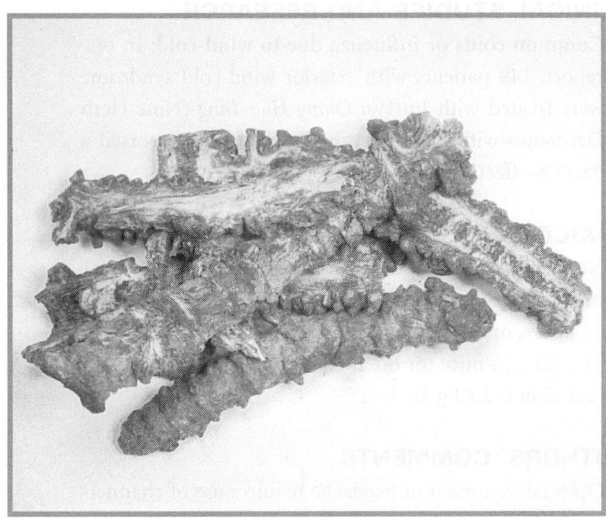

羌活

Pinyin Name: *Qiang Huo*

Alternate Chinese Names: *Chuan Qiang Huo, Xi Qiang Huo*

Original Source: *Shen Nong Ben Cao Jing* (Divine Husbandman's Classic of the Materia Medica) in the second century

English Name: notopterygium, incised notopterygium rhizome or root, forbes notopterygium rhizome or root

Botanical Name: *Notopterygium incisum* Ting. (*Qiang Huo*); *Notopterygium forbesii* Boiss. (*Quan Ye Qiang Huo*); *Notopterygium franchetii* Boiss. (*Chuan Qiang Huo*)

Pharmaceutical Name: Rhizoma et Radix Notopterygii

Properties: acrid, bitter, warm

Channels Entered: Urinary Bladder, Kidney

CHINESE THERAPEUTIC ACTIONS

1. Releases the Exterior and Dispels Cold

Pain due to wind-cold: Ascending and dispersing in nature, *Qiang Huo* (Rhizoma et Radix Notopterygii) strongly functions to release the exterior by dispelling cold and dampness in the channels at the superficial level. It is best for occipital headache or pain associated with feelings of heaviness, sleepiness or the lack of desire to move, all of which may be caused by dampness. It is often used as a channel guiding herb to the *taiyang* and *du* (governing) channels, where it exerts its best influence to relieve pain.

- Exterior wind-cold syndrome with aversion to cold, fever, headache and muscle aches: use *Qiang Huo* with *Bai Zhi* (Radix Angelicae Dahuricae), *Fang Feng* (Radix Saposhnikoviae), *Xi Xin* (Herba Asari) and *Chuan Xiong* (Rhizoma Ligustici Chuanxiong). **Exemplar Formula:** *Jiu Wei Qiang Huo Tang* (Nine-Herb Decoction with Notopterygium).
- Occipital headache from wind-cold, without perspiration: use this herb with *Jing Jie* (Herba Schizonepetae) and *Fang Feng* (Radix Saposhnikoviae).
- Heavy-headed sensations: combine it with *Cang Zhu* (Rhizoma Atractylodis).
- Red eyes from wind-heat attacking the head: use *Qiang Huo* with *Long Dan Cao* (Radix Gentianae), *Huang Lian* (Rhizoma Coptidis), *Chan Tui* (Periostracum Cicadae) and *Bai Ji Li* (Fructus Tribuli).

2. Eliminates Wind, Cold and Dampness to Relieve Pain

***Bi zheng* (painful obstruction syndrome) due to wind, cold and dampness:** Wind, cold and dampness are three external factors that commonly attack the muscles and joints, leading to arthritis, which is also known as *bi zheng*. The exterior pathogens obstruct the normal circulation of qi and blood, leading to pain and spasms of the affected area. *Qiang Huo* is most effective to eliminate

Qiang Huo (Rhizoma et Radix Notopterygii)

wind, cold and dampness from the upper body and is commonly used to treat conditions such as occipital headache, neck and shoulder muscle aches and pains, and joint pain in the upper body.

- Muscle aches and joint pain caused by wind, cold and dampness: combine *Qiang Huo* with *Fang Feng* (Radix Saposhnikoviae), *Jiang Huang* (Rhizoma Curcumae Longae), *Dang Gui* (Radicis Angelicae Sinensis), *Chi Shao* (Radix Paeoniae Rubrae) and *Gan Cao* (Radix Glycyrrhizae). **Exemplar Formula:** *Juan Bi Tang* (Remove Painful Obstruction Decoction).
- Arthritis of the upper body or limbs: use this herb with *Jiang Huang* (Rhizoma Curcumae Longae) and *Gui Zhi* (Ramulus Cinnamomi).
- Wind-damp headache: add it to *Fang Feng* (Radix Saposhnikoviae), *Gao Ben* (Rhizoma Ligustici), and *Chuan Xiong* (Rhizoma Ligustici Chuanxiong) to dispel wind and relieve pain. **Exemplar Formula:** *Qiang Huo Sheng Shi Tang* (Notopterygium Decoction to Overcome Dampness).
- General arthritis: use it with *Du Huo* (Radix Angelicae Pubescentis), *Gui Zhi* (Ramulus Cinnamomi), *Chi Shao* (Radix Paeoniae Rubrae), *Hong Hua* (Flos Carthami) and *Wei Ling Xian* (Radix Clematidis).

DOSAGE

3 to 10 grams. Maximum dosage of *Qiang Huo* is 30 grams.

CAUTIONS / CONTRAINDICATIONS

- Use of *Qiang Huo* is contraindicated for patients having febrile disorders, yin deficiency, or muscle aches and pain because of blood deficiency.
- It is also contraindicated for patients with *bi zheng* (painful obstruction syndrome) who have red tongues with little or no tongue coating.

OVERDOSAGE

Overdose of *Qiang Huo* may injure the Stomach and cause nausea and vomiting. This may be alleviated by decreasing the dosage or by taking it with herbs that harmonize the Stomach, such as *Da Zao* (Fructus Jujubae) and *Sheng Jiang* (Rhizoma Zingiberis Recens).

CHEMICAL COMPOSITION

Essential oil 0.16-2.70% (α-pinene, β-pinene, limonene, α-phellandrene), coumarins (nodakenin, notopterol, 6-O-transferuloynodakenin, isoimperatorin, cnidilin, nodakenetin, bergaptin, bergapten, bergaptol, demethylfuropinnarin, phellopterin, osthenol, notoptol, anhydronotoptol, karatavicin, marmesin, imperatorin, columbianetin), p-hydroxyphenethyl anisate, ferulic acid, phenethyl ferulate.[1,2]

PHARMACOLOGICAL EFFECTS

- **Antipyretic**: Essential oil of *Qiang Huo* administered via intraperitoneal injection and oral ingestion has been shown to lower body temperature in rats.[3]
- **Analgesic**: Essential oil of *Qiang Huo* administered via intraperitoneal injection for three days showed marked usefulness to relieve muscle aches and pain in mice.[4]
- **Cardiovascular**: The essential oil of *Qiang Huo* has been shown to increase blood circulation to the coronary artery in mice. *Qiang Huo* has also demonstrated good effects in treating arrhythmia in mice, especially if the arrhythmia is associated with overdose of aconitine.[5,6]

CLINICAL STUDIES AND RESEARCH

- **Common colds or influenza due to wind-cold**: In one report, 149 patients with exterior wind-cold syndrome were treated with *Jiu Wei Qiang Huo Tang* (Nine-Herb Decoction with Notopterygium). The study reported a 93.33% effective rate.[7]

TOXICOLOGY

No fatalities were observed in mice following either oral ingestion of water extract of *Qiang Huo* at 12 g/kg for 72 hours, or essential oil of *Qiang Huo* at 0.75 g/kg.[8] The LD_{50} in mice for essential oil of *Qiang Huo* via oral ingestion is 2.83 g/kg.[9]

AUTHORS' COMMENTS

Optimal treatment of headache requires use of channel-guiding herbs to deliver the therapeutic effect of the herbs to the affected area. The following is a list of the commonly used channel-guiding herbs:

- *Taiyang* channels: *Qiang Huo* (Rhizoma et Radix Notopterygii)
- *Shaoyang* channels: *Chai Hu* (Radix Bupleuri)
- *Yangming* channels: *Bai Zhi* (Radix Angelicae Dahuricae)
- *Taiyin* channels: *Cang Zhu* (Rhizoma Atractylodis)
- *Shaoyin* channels: *Xi Xin* (Herba Asari)
- *Jueyin* channels: *Wu Zhu Yu* (Fructus Evodiae)

Qiang Huo (Rhizoma et Radix Notopterygii), *Chuan Xiong* (Rhizoma Ligustici Chuanxiong), *Bai Zhi* (Radix Angelicae Dahuricae), *Chai Hu* (Radix Bupleuri) and *Gao Ben* (Rhizoma Ligustici) all treat headaches. According to Dr. Li Shou-Shan, the differences between these herbs are as follows:

- *Qiang Huo* is more specific to occipital headaches.
- *Chuan Xiong* is most effective for headaches related to menstruation.
- *Bai Zhi* focuses on frontal headaches.
- *Chai Hu* treats temporal headaches.
- *Gao Ben* is best for vertex headaches.

Qiang Huo (Rhizoma et Radix Notopterygii)

References

1. *Xian Dai Zhong Yao Yao Li Xue* (Contemporary Pharmacology of Chinese Herbs), 1997; 86
2. *The Merck Index* 12th edition, Chapman & Hall/CRCnetBASE/Merck, 2000
3. *Zhong Cao Yao* (Chinese Herbal Medicine), 1991; 22(1):28
4. Ibid.
5. *Zhong Yao Tong Bao* (Journal of Chinese Herbology), 1982; (1):31
6. Ibid., 12(12):45
7. *Fu Jian Zhong Yi Yao* (Fujian Chinese Medicine and Herbology), 1964; 5:13
8. *Zhong Yao Tong Bao* (Journal of Chinese Herbology), 1982; (1):31
9. *Zhong Cheng Yao Yan Jiu* (Research of Chinese Patent Medicine), 1981; (12):41

Gao Ben (Rhizoma Ligustici)

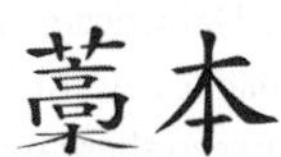

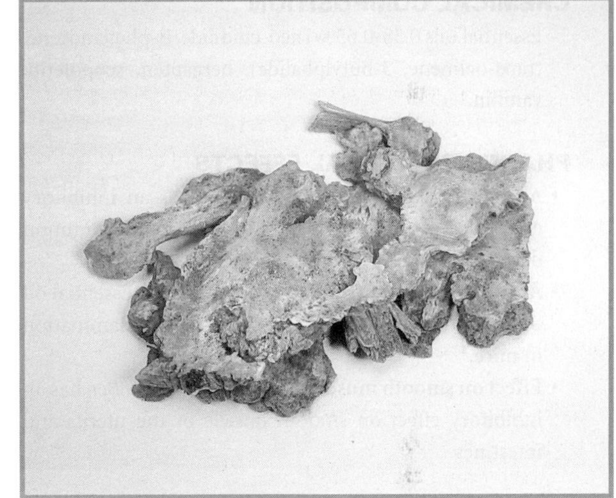

Pinyin Name: *Gao Ben*
Alternate Chinese Names: *Gao Ban*
Original Source: *Shen Nong Ben Cao Jing* (Divine Husbandman's Classic of the Materia Medica) in the second century
English Name: ligusticum, chinese ligusticum rhizome, jehol ligusticum rhizome, Chinese lovage root
Botanical Name: *Ligusticum sinense* Oliv. (*Gao Ben*); *Ligusticum jeholense* Nakai et Kitag. (*Liaoning Gao Ben*)
Pharmaceutical Name: Rhizoma Ligustici
Properties: acrid, warm
Channels Entered: Urinary Bladder

CHINESE THERAPEUTIC ACTIONS

1. Releases the Exterior and Dispels Cold

Headache due to wind-cold: Acrid and warm, *Gao Ben* (Rhizoma Ligustici) releases the exterior and dispels wind-cold. It is an essential herb in treating pain caused by wind or cold and is often used as a channel-guiding herb to lead the effects of other herbs to the head.

- Exterior wind-cold syndrome with aversion to cold, fever, headache, muscle aches and pain: use this herb with *Jing Jie* (Herba Schizonepetae), *Fang Feng* (Radix Saposhnikoviae), *Cang Zhu* (Rhizoma Atractylodis) and *Chen Pi* (Pericarpium Citri Reticulatae).
- Exterior wind-cold syndrome with dampness: add to *Qiang Huo* (Rhizoma et Radix Notopterygii) and *Fang Feng* (Radix Saposhnikoviae).

Vertex headache or lower back pain: *Gao Ben* enters the *du* (governing) channel. Thus, it can be used to treat pain at both ends of the *du* channel caused by wind-cold invasion.

2. Dispels Wind, Cold, and Damp and Relieves Pain

***Bi zheng* (painful obstruction syndrome):** Wind, cold and dampness are three exterior factors that commonly attack the muscles and joints, leading to *bi zheng*. Wind, cold and dampness obstruct the normal circulation of qi and blood, causing pain in the affected area. Warm and acrid, *Gao Ben* opens the channels and disperses stagnation. This herb is most effective in treating headaches caused by wind-cold.

- *Bi zheng* caused by wind, cold and dampness: add *Qiang Huo* (Rhizoma et Radix Notopterygii), *Fang Feng* (Radix Saposhnikoviae), and *Wei Ling Xian* (Radix Clematidis).
- Headache due to cold and dampness: use this herb with *Chuan Xiong* (Rhizoma Ligustici Chuanxiong) and *Xi Xin* (Herba Asari).
- Frontal and migraine headaches: combine it with *Xi Xin* (Herba Asari), *Shi Gao* (Gypsum Fibrosum) and *Bai Zhi* (Radix Angelicae Dahuricae).

Gao Ben (Rhizoma Ligustici)

- Abdominal pain due to cold and dampness: use it with *Cang Zhu* (Rhizoma Atractylodis).

DOSAGE

3 to 10 grams. The maximum dosage of *Gao Ben* is 20 grams.

CAUTIONS / CONTRAINDICATIONS

- Use of *Gao Ben* is contraindicated in patients with heat symptoms, or headache caused by blood deficiency or Liver yang rising.
- *Gao Ben* is acrid and warm and may damage the yin. Yin-deficient patients should use this herb with caution.
- Long-term use of *Gao Ben* is not recommended.

CHEMICAL COMPOSITION

Essential oils 0.38-0.65% (neo-cnidilide, β-phellandrene, trans-ocimene, 3-butylphalide), bergapten, scopoletin, vanillin.[1]

PHARMACOLOGICAL EFFECTS

- **Antibiotic**: Essential oil of *Gao Ben* has an inhibitory effect against influenza viruses and many common dermatomycoses.[2,3]
- **Antipyretic and anti-inflammatory effects**: Essential oil of *Gao Ben* reduced body temperature and inflammation in mice.[4]
- **Effect on smooth muscle:** Essential oil of *Gao Ben* has an inhibitory effect on smooth muscle of the uterus and intestines.[5]

CLINICAL STUDIES AND RESEARCH

- **Headache**: In one study, 97 patients with headaches from various causes were treated with an herbal formula with up to 93.8% effectiveness. The herbal formula was given in decoction, and contained *Gao Ben* 15g, *Dang Gui* (Radicis Angelicae Sinensis) 15g, *Tao Ren* (Semen Persicae) 15g, *Hong Hua* (Flos Carthami) 15g, *Chuan Xiong* (Rhizoma Ligustici Chuanxiong) 15g, *Huang Qi* (Radix Astragali) 15g, *Sheng Di Huang* (Radix Rehmanniae) 15g, *Dan Shen* (Radix Salviae Miltiorrhizae) 25g, *Long Gu* (Os Draconis) 25g, *Mu Li* (Concha Ostreae) 25g, *Xi Xin* (Herba Asari) 5g, *Gan Cao* (Radix Glycyrrhizae) 10g, and *Wu Gong* (Scolopendra) 3 pieces.[6]

TOXICOLOGY

The LD_{50} in mice for essential oil of *Gao Ben* given via oral ingestion was 70.17 g/kg (based on the use of dried herb).[7]

AUTHORS' COMMENTS

Gao Ben (Rhizoma Ligustici), *Chuan Xiong* (Rhizoma Ligustici Chuanxiong), *Qiang Huo* (Rhizoma et Radix Notopterygii), *Bai Zhi* (Radix Angelicae Dahuricae), and *Chai Hu* (Radix Bupleuri) all treat headaches. According to Dr. Li Shou-Shan, the differences between these herbs are as follows:

- *Gao Ben* is best for vertex headaches.
- *Chuan Xiong* is most effective for headaches related to menstruation.
- *Qiang Huo* is more specific to occipital headaches.
- *Bai Zhi* focuses on frontal headaches.
- *Chai Hu* treats temporal headaches.

References

1. *Xian Dai Zhong Yao Yao Li Xue* (Contemporary Pharmacology of Chinese Herbs), 1997; 84
2. *Zhong Cao Yao Xue* (Study of Chinese Herbal Medicine), 1976:779
3. *Zhong Yao Xue* (Chinese Herbology), 1998; 80:81
4. *Zhong Xi Yi Jie He Za Zhi* (Journal of Integrated Chinese and Western Medicine), 1987; 7(12):738
5. *Zhong Yao Tong Bao* (Journal of Chinese Herbology), 1987; 12(4):48
6. *Ji Lin Zhong Yi Yao* (Jilin Chinese Medicine and Herbology), 1991; (5):14
7. *Chang Yong Zhong Yao Cheng Fen Yu Yao Li Shou Ce* (A Handbook of the Composition and Pharmacology of Common Chinese Drugs), 1994; 1834:1841

Ji Xiang Teng (Caulis Paederiae)

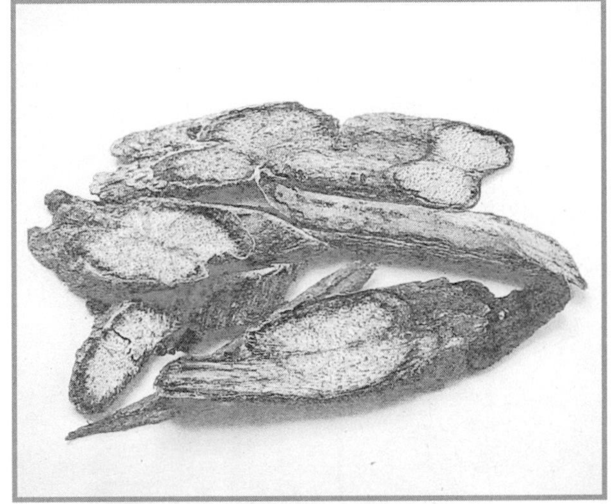

雞香藤 鸡香藤

Pinyin Name: *Ji Xiang Teng*
Alternate Chinese Names: *Ji Shi Teng, Wu De Teng, Chou Xing Teng, Niu Pi Dong*
English Name: paederia
Botanical Name: *Paederia scandens* (Lour.) Merr.
Pharmaceutical Name: Caulis Paederiae
Properties: sweet, neutral to slightly warm
Channels Entered: Lung, Liver

CHINESE THERAPEUTIC ACTIONS

1. Dispels Wind-Cold

Body aches associated with an exterior condition: The chief characteristic of *Ji Xiang Teng* (Caulis Paederiae) is that it helps relieve body aches and joint pain caused by wind-cold invasion. This is the herb of choice for pain associated with a common cold. It can be used by itself to relieve pain, or combined with other warm diaphoretic herbs. Other clinical manifestations include clear nasal discharge, sputum and aversion to cold.

- Joint pain and body aches of the entire body from wind-cold: use *Ji Xiang Teng* with *Fang Feng* (Radix Saposhnikoviae), *Hong Gu She* (Radix Kadsura Japonicae) and *Dao Di Wu Gong* (Rhizoma Heliminthostachytis).
- Cough with profuse sputum: combine it with *Wu Tian* (Radix et Folium Viticis Quinatae) and *Fu Rong* (Radix Hibisci).

2. Dispels Cold and Dampness

***Bi zheng* (painful obstruction syndrome) caused by cold and dampness:** *Ji Xiang Teng* relieves pain by dispelling wind, cold and dampness. It treats *bi zheng* caused by cold and dampness, with pain in a fixed location, that worsens with exposure to cold.

- *Bi zheng:* use this herb with *Yi Tiao Gen* (Radix Moghaniae), *Chuan Shan Long* (Rhizoma Dioscoreae Nipponicae) and *Du Huo* (Radix Angelicae Pubescentis).

3. Eliminates Toxins

- Neurodermatitis: apply *Ji Xiang Teng* topically.
- Organophosphorus pesticide poisoning: combine this herb with *Lu Dou* (Semen Phaseoli Radiati). After ingestion of the herbs, vomiting or diarrhea may occur as signs of detoxification in progress.

DOSAGE

5 to 30 grams in decoction.

Cong Bai (Bulbus Allii Fistulosi)

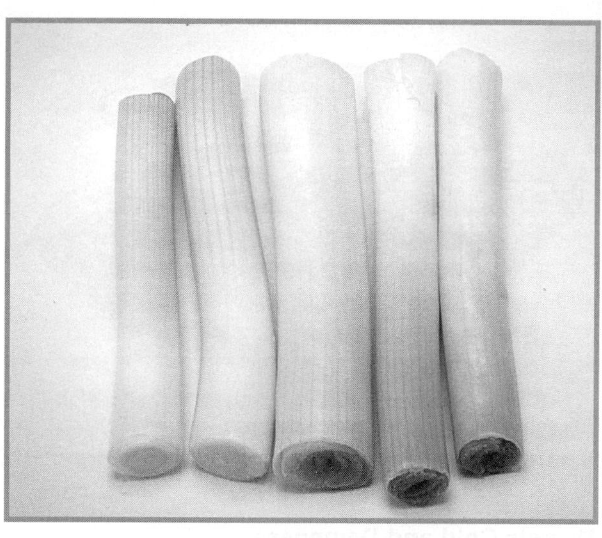

蔥白 葱白

Pinyin Name: *Cong Bai*
Literal Name: "white allium"
Alternate Chinese Names: *Cong Jing Bai, Cong Bai Tou*
Original Source: *Shen Nong Ben Cao Jing* (Divine Husbandman's Classic of the Materia Medica) in the second century
English Name: allium, scallion, green onion
Botanical Name: *Allium fistulosum* L.
Pharmaceutical Name: Bulbus Allii Fistulosi
Properties: acrid, warm
Channels Entered: Lung, Stomach

CHINESE THERAPEUTIC ACTIONS

1. Releases the Exterior and Induces Perspiration

Mild cases of wind-cold invasion: Acrid and warm, *Cong Bai* (Bulbus Allii Fistulosi) releases the exterior and induces perspiration. Its diaphoretic function, however, is rather weak, thus *Cong Bai* should only be used in treating early or mild cases of wind-cold syndrome.

- Wind-cold syndrome: use *Cong Bai* with *Dan Dou Chi* (Semen Sojae Praeparatum) to dispel wind-cold.
- Wind-cold syndrome without perspiration: combine it with *Ma Huang* (Herba Ephedrae) and *Ge Gen* (Radix Puerariae).
- Presence of exterior wind-cold with interior heat: combine it with *Zhi Zi* (Fructus Gardeniae), *Lian Qiao* (Fructus Forsythiae), *Bo He* (Herba Menthae) and *Dan Dou Chi* (Semen Sojae Praeparatum).

2. Disperses Cold and Unblocks Yang

Abdominal pain: *Cong Bai* treats abdominal pain characterized by cold stagnation in the interior, leading to inability of yang energy to circulate and warm the interior of the body. This inability of yang to enter and warm the interior subsequently leads to abdominal pain, clear and watery diarrhea, extreme cold of the body and extremities, and a weak and forceless pulse. Warm in nature, *Cong Bai* disperses cold and warms yang.

- Interior cold stagnation blocking the yang: use it with *Fu Zi* (Radix Aconiti Lateralis Praeparata) and *Gan Jiang* (Rhizoma Zingiberis).
- Interior cold stagnation with abdominal coldness, pain and dysuria: place *Cong Bai* directly on the navel to disperse cold and to warm yang.

Dysuria and constipation: *Cong Bai* treats these conditions by unblocking yang qi.

- Dysuria: *Cong Bai* should be stir-fried and applied while warm as a topical on the lower abdomen.
- Constipation: use it with *E Jiao* (Colla Corii Asini).

3. Eliminates Toxins and Disperses Clumps

Sores and abscesses: Topical application of *Cong Bai* relieves toxicity and disperses clumps. Use the herb alone as a poultice.

4. Kills Parasites

Abdominal pain caused by intestinal parasites: The juice of *Cong Bai* kills intestinal parasites and relieves pain.

DOSAGE

3 to 10 grams for the fresh herb (or 2 to 5 scallions, using the white part and the root). The maximum dosage of fresh *Cong Bai* is 100 grams. For topical application, *Cong Bai* can be crushed into paste, made into a poultice or stir-fried.

CAUTIONS / CONTRAINDICATIONS

- *Cong Bai* should be used with caution in patients with yin deficiency and yang excess, and in patients with spontaneous perspiration arising from qi deficiency.
- *Cong Bai* is incompatible with honey (when used internally) and with *Chang Shan* (Radix Dichroae).

CHEMICAL COMPOSITION

Essential oils (allicin, disulfides, polysulfides, dipropyldisulfide, dipropyltrisulfide, allylpropyl disulfide, s-methylpropane trisulfonate), thiaheterocycles, s-allylmercaptocysteine, s-methylmercaptocysteine, s-propenyl-L-cysteine sulfoxide, cycloalliin.[1]

Cong Bai (Bulbus Allii Fistulosi)

PHARMACOLOGICAL EFFECTS

- **Antibiotic:** *Cong Bai* has an inhibitory influence *in vitro* against *Corynebacterium diphtheriae, Staphylococcus* spp., *Streptococcus* spp., and *Shigella* spp., and dermatomyces.[2]
- **Others:** It has antipyretic, diuretic, and expectorant effects.[3]

CLINICAL STUDIES AND RESEARCH

- **Common cold:** Topical herbal paste (*Cong Bai, Sheng Jiang* (Rhizoma Zingiberis Recens) and salt) was applied to the center of the chest, back, soles, palms, popliteal fossa, and cubital fossa for 1 to 2 days in 107 patients, resulting in marked improvement.[4]
- **Acute abdominal pain caused by intestinal parasites:** According to one report, 25 children with acute abdominal pain caused by intestinal parasites were treated with an herbal solution (30 grams each of *Cong Bai* juice and sesame oil), taken on an empty stomach. Most patients reported pain relief after 1 to 2 doses.[5]
- **Intestinal obstruction caused by parasites:** In one report, parasitic intestinal obstruction in 24 patients was treated with an herbal solution (equal portions of *Cong Bai* and nut oil), with good results.[6]
- **Abscesses and inflammation of the skin:** An herbal paste (2 parts *Cong Bai* and 1 part honey) was applied topically, treating 100 patients with skin abscesses and inflammation with satisfactory results. The herbal paste was changed and re-applied once daily or every other day.[7]
- **Urticaria:** According to one study, 100 patients with urticaria were treated with Chinese herbs. Urticaria from wind-cold was treated with 15 bulbs of *Cong Bai*, 10 grams of *Jing Jie* (Herba Schizonepetae) and 3 grams of *Gan Cao* (Radix Glycyrrhizae). Urticaria from wind-heat was treated with 15 bulbs of *Cong Bai*, 15 grams of *Da Qing Ye* (Folium Isatidis), and 15 grams of *Lian Qiao* (Fructus Forsythiae). The herbal decoctions were given once daily. In addition, 20 bulbs of *Cong Bai* were cooked to prepare a topical solution that was applied to the affected area once daily. All 100 patients showed marked improvement within 1 to 8 days.[8]

References

1. *Xian Dai Zhong Yao Yao Li Xue* (Contemporary Pharmacology of Chinese Herbs), 1997; 108
2. *Zhong Yao Xue* (Chinese Herbology), 1998; 85:88
3. Ibid.
4. *Zhong Ji Yi Kan* (Medium Medical Journal), 19635; 9:580
5. *Zhe Jiang Zhong Yi Za Zhi* (Zhejiang Journal of Chinese Medicine), 1966, 4:13
6. *Xin Yi Xue* (New Medicine), 1972; 8:37
7. *Ji Lin Wei Shen* (Jilin Public Health), 1960; 1:40
8. *Zhe Jiang Zhong Yi Za Zhi* (Zhejiang Journal of Chinese Medicine), 1987; 1:16

Bai Zhi (Radix Angelicae Dahuricae)

白芷 白芷

Pinyin Name: *Bai Zhi*
Literal Name: "white rootlet"
Alternate Chinese Names: *Xiang Bai Zhi*
Original Source: *Shen Nong Ben Cao Jing* (Divine Husbandman's Classic of the Materia Medica) in the second century
English Name: angelica, dahurican angelica root, Taiwan angelica root
Botanical Name: *Angelica dahurica* (Fisch ex Hoffm.) Benth. et Hook. f. (*Bai Zhi*); *Angelica dahurica* (Fisch. ex Hoffm.) Benth. et Hook. var. *formosana* (Boiss.) Shan et Yuan (*Hang Bai Zhi*)
Pharmaceutical Name: Radix Angelicae Dahuricae
Properties: acrid, warm
Channels Entered: Lung, Stomach, Spleen

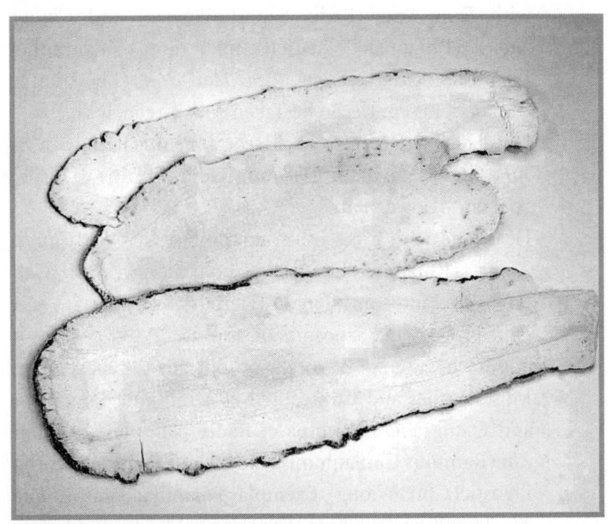

Bai Zhi (Radix Angelicae Dahuricae)

CHINESE THERAPEUTIC ACTIONS

1. Releases the Exterior, Dispels Wind and Opens Orifices

Wind-cold: Acrid and warm, *Bai Zhi* (Radix Angelicae Dahuricae) releases the exterior and dispels wind. It opens orifices to relieve nasal obstruction.

- Wind-cold with headache, muscle aches, nasal obstruction and clear nasal discharge: use *Bai Zhi* with *Sheng Jiang* (Rhizoma Zingiberis Recens) and *Dan Dou Chi* (Semen Sojae Praeparatum).
- Sinusitis and rhinitis with turbid white nasal discharge or nasal obstruction due to cold: use it with *Cang Er Zi* (Fructus Xanthii) and *Xin Yi Hua* (Flos Magnoliae) to dispel wind and open nasal passages. **Exemplar Formula:** *Cang Er San* (Xanthium Powder).
- Sinusitis and rhinitis with turbid yellow nasal discharge or nasal obstruction caused by heat: combine it with *Shi Gao* (Gypsum Fibrosum), *Huang Qin* (Radix Scutellariae) and *Pu Gong Ying* (Herba Taraxaci).

2. Dispels Cold and Relieves Pain

Pain along the Stomach channel: Acrid and warm, *Bai Zhi* releases the exterior and dispels wind and dampness from the Lung, Stomach and Large Intestine channels. It is most effective in treating disorders along the Stomach channel and is commonly used for frontal headaches, pain around the eyes, toothache, nasal obstruction and nasal discharge.

- Headache and nasal obstruction from wind-cold: use *Bai Zhi* with *Qiang Huo* (Rhizoma et Radix Notopterygii) and *Fang Feng* (Radix Saposhnikoviae) to dispel wind-cold. **Exemplar Formula:** *Jiu Wei Qiang Huo Tang* (Nine-Herb Decoction with Notopterygium).
- *Yangming* channel headache with pain around the eyes, frontal headache, and toothache: use *Bai Zhi* alone, or with *Fang Feng* (Radix Saposhnikoviae) and *Chuan Xiong* (Rhizoma Ligustici Chuanxiong). **Exemplar Formula:** *Chuan Xiong Cha Tiao San* (Ligusticum Chuanxiong Powder to be Taken with Green Tea).
- Headache with excessive cold: combine this herb with *Xi Xin* (Herba Asari) and *Wu Tou* (Radix Aconiti) to dispel cold and relieve pain.
- Headache with excessive heat: combine it with *Chuan Xiong* (Rhizoma Ligustici Chuanxiong), *Shi Gao* (Gypsum Fibrosum), *Jing Jie* (Herba Schizonepetae) and *Fang Feng* (Radix Saposhnikoviae).
- Toothache: use *Bai Zhi* orally or topically to relieve pain.
- Muscle aches and pain caused by wind and dampness: add *Qiang Huo* (Rhizoma et Radix Notopterygii), *Gui Zhi* (Ramulus Cinnamomi), and *Chuan Xiong* (Rhizoma Ligustici Chuanxiong). **Exemplar Formula:** *Shang Zhong Xia Tong Yong Tong Feng Wan* (Upper Middle and Lower General-Use Pills for Wind-Pain).

3. Reduces Swelling, Expels Pus and Eliminates Toxins

Sores, carbuncles or furuncles with pus and swelling: *Bai Zhi* eliminates the accumulation of wind and dampness that commonly causes muscle aches and itching. But accumulation of dampness in the skin can also result in sores and carbuncles. This herb helps to reduce swelling, discharge pus and regenerate tissue.

- Rashes and itching caused by wind and dampness: combine *Bai Zhi* with *Qin Jiao* (Radix Gentianae Macrophyllae), *Jing Jie* (Herba Schizonepetae), and *Xi Xian Cao* (Herba Siegesbeckiae).
- Dermatological disorders with abscesses and swelling: use it with *Jin Yin Hua* (Flos Lonicerae), *Chuan Shan Jia* (Squama Manis), and *Tian Hua Fen* (Radix Trichosanthis).
- Formation of pus without ulceration: use it with *Niu Bang Zi* (Fructus Arctii), *Jin Yin Hua* (Flos Lonicerae), *Chuan Shan Jia* (Squama Manis) and *Zao Jiao Ci* (Spina Gleditsiae).
- Formation of pus with ulceration or prolonged delay in healing: combine it with *Dang Shen* (Radix Codonopsis), *Huang Qi* (Radix Astragali), *Jin Yin Hua* (Flos Lonicerae) and *Gan Cao* (Radix Glycyrrhizae).
- Acute appendicitis or intestinal abscess: combine it with *Mu Dan Pi* (Cortex Moutan), *Dong Gua Zi* (Semen Benincasae), *Bai Jiang Cao* (Herba cum Radice Patriniae), *Hong Teng* (Caulis Sargentodoxae) and *Da Huang* (Radix et Rhizoma Rhei).
- Breast abscesses: use *Bai Zhi* with *Chi Shao* (Radix Paeoniae Rubrae), *Hong Hua* (Flos Carthami), *Pu Gong Ying* (Herba Taraxaci), *Zi Hua Di Ding* (Herba Violae), *Ye Ju Hua* (Flos Chrysanthemi Indici) and *Jin Yin Hua* (Flos Lonicerae).

4. Dispels Dampness and Treats Leukorrhea and Diarrhea

Leukorrhea: *Bai Zhi* dispels accumulated damp in the lower *jiao* that causes leukorrhea.

- White, turbid leukorrhea due to cold and dampness: use *Bai Zhi* with *Hai Piao Xiao* (Endoconcha Sepiae), *Bai Zhu* (Rhizoma Atractylodis Macrocephalae), *Fu Ling* (Poria) and *Ji Guan Hua* (Flos Celosiae Cristatae).
- Yellow, turbid leukorrhea caused by heat and dampness: combine it with *Huang Bai* (Cortex Phellodendri) and *Che Qian Zi* (Semen Plantaginis).

Diarrhea: *Bai Zhi* dispels accumulation of dampness in the lower *jiao* that causes diarrhea.

- Chronic diarrhea due to Spleen deficiency and damp accumulation: combine this herb with *Rou Dou Kou* (Semen Myristicae), *He Zi* (Fructus Chebulae), *Fu Ling* (Poria) and *Qian Shi* (Semen Euryales).

Bai Zhi (Radix Angelicae Dahuricae)

DOSAGE

3 to 10 grams. The maximum dosage of *Bai Zhi* is 30 grams. It can be taken internally, or applied topically in powdered form. When treating dermatological disorders, the dosage should be decreased as the sores heal.

CAUTIONS / CONTRAINDICATIONS

- Acrid and warm, *Bai Zhi* may damage yin and should be used with caution for patients who have yin-deficient fire, Liver yang rising, or Liver or Kidney yin deficiency.
- This herb is contraindicated for patients with febrile disorders.
- Overdose of *Bai Zhi* may cause nausea, vomiting, numbness of the limbs, epilepsy and convulsions.

CHEMICAL COMPOSITION

Coumarins (oxypeucedanin, imperatorin, isoimperatorin), byak-angelicin, byak-angelicol, anhydrobyakangelicin, neobyakangelicol, oxypeucedanin hydrate, phellopterin, xanthotoxin, scopoletin, byakangelicin hydrate, xanthotoxol, isooxypeucedanin, cnidilin, pabulenol, essential oil 0.24% (methylcyclodecanc, l-tetradecene).[1,2]

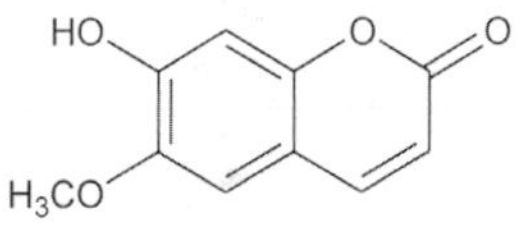

HO, O, O, H_3CO

Scopoletin

PHARMACOLOGICAL EFFECTS

- **Antibiotic**: Decoction of *Bai Zhi* has an inhibitory effect against *E. coli, Bacillus dysenteriae, Bacillus proteus, Salmonella typhi, Pseudomonas aeruginosa, Vibrio cholerae, Mycobacterium tuberculosis hominis*, and *Shigella* spp.[3]
- **Anti-inflammatory**: Decoctions of *Bai Zhi* have demonstrated marked anti-inflammatory effects in mice. Administration of 4g/kg of *Bai Zhi* was effective in treating otitis media in mice.[4]
- **Analgesic and antipyretic**: Decoctions of *Bai Zhi* at a dosage of 15 g/kg have demonstrated significant analgesic and antipyretic actions in mice. The dosage of 8 g/kg was slightly less effective than the dosage of 15 g/kg.[5]
- **Antispasmodic**: Various components of *Bai Zhi* have demonstrated marked muscle-relaxant qualities to treat muscle spasms and cramps. Scopoletin showed marked antispasmodic effect on the uterus in mice with ED_{50} of 0.09 mg/kg.[6,7]
- **Other**: In laboratory animals, *Bai Zhi* affects the cardiovascular system by lowering heart rate and decreasing blood pressure, excites the respiratory system to increase the depth of breathing, and also stimulates the nervous system. In addition, it has a mild hemostatic effect.[8]

CLINICAL STUDIES AND RESEARCH

- **Headache**: According to one report, patients with occipital headaches were treated twice daily with 30 grams of *Bai Zhi* in decoction. Out of 73 patients, 69 showed significant improvement, 3 showed slight improvement, and 1 showed no response.[9]

  In another study, a 5% solution of *Bai Zhi* was given to 62 patients with headaches. One course of treatment ranged from 10 to 15 days, and patients received 1 to 2 courses of treatment. Of 62 patients, 54 showed significant improvement.[10]
- **Vitiligo**: Topical preparations of *Bai Zhi* were used to treat 321 patients with vitiligo. After topical application, the affected area was exposed to sunlight for periods of 5, 10 or 30 minutes. Of 321 patients, 61.5% showed significant improvement.[11]
- **Psoriasis**: In one study, 159 patients with psoriasis were treated with *Bai Zhi* in various preparations. The dosage forms included capsules for oral administration, and herbal decoction. All patients received treatment daily or every other day. The overall effective rate was 94.4%.[12]

HERB-DRUG INTERACTION

- **Liver metabolism**: Administration of *Bai Zhi* extract in rats is associated with an inhibitory effect on liver microsomal cytochrome P-450. Because of inhibited metabolism, concurrent use of the herb may lead to increased plasma concentration of other drugs, such as testosterone, tolbutamide, nifedipine, bufuralol and diazepam.[13]

TOXICOLOGY

The LD_{50} for decoction of *Bai Zhi* in mice via oral ingestion is 53.82 g/kg. Possible adverse reactions to *Bai Zhi* include increased blood pressure, slowed heart rate, increased depth of respiration, vomiting, and in severe cases of gross overdose, seizures and convulsions.[14,15,16,17,18]

AUTHORS' COMMENTS

Optimal treatment of headache requires use of channel-guiding herbs to deliver the therapeutic effect of the herbs to the affected area. The following is a list of the commonly used channel-guiding herbs:

- *Taiyang* channels: *Qiang Huo* (Rhizoma et Radix Notopterygii)
- *Shaoyang* channels: *Chai Hu* (Radix Bupleuri)
- *Yangming* channels: *Bai Zhi* (Radix Angelicae Dahuricae)
- *Taiyin* channels: *Cang Zhu* (Rhizoma Atractylodis)
- *Shaoyin* channels: *Xi Xin* (Herba Asari)
- *Jueyin* channels: *Wu Zhu Yu* (Fructus Evodiae)

Bai Zhi (Radix Angelicae Dahuricae), *Chuan Xiong* (Rhizoma Ligustici Chuanxiong), *Qiang Huo* (Rhizoma

Bai Zhi (Radix Angelicae Dahuricae)

et Radix Notopterygii), *Chai Hu* (Radix Bupleuri) and *Gao Ben* (Rhizoma Ligustici) all treat headaches. According to Dr. Li Shou-Shan, the differences between these herbs are as follows:

- *Bai Zhi* focuses on frontal headaches.
- *Chuan Xiong* is most effective for menstrual headaches.
- *Qiang Huo* is more specific to occipital headaches.
- *Chai Hu* treats temporal headaches.
- *Gao Ben* is best for vertex headaches.

Bai Zhi is traditionally used as a component of cosmetic foundations. It whitens and softens the skin, and invigorates blood circulation.

References

1. *Xian Dai Zhong Yao Yao Li Xue* (Contemporary Pharmacology of Chinese Herbs), 1997; 77
2. *The Merck Index* 12th edition, Chapman & Hall/CRCnetBASE/Merck, 2000
3. *Zhong Yao Yao Li Yu Ying Yong* (Pharmacology and Applications of Chinese Herbs), 1983:796
4. *Zhong Guo Zhong Yao Za Zhi* (People's Republic of China Journal of Chinese Herbology), 1991; 16(9):560
5. Ibid.
6. *Zhong Yao Yao Li Yu Ying Yong* (Pharmacology and Applications of Chinese Herbs), 1983:796
7. *Zhi Wu Yao You Xiao Cheng Fen Shou Ce* (Manual of Plant Medicinals and Their Active Constituents), 1986: 624,603,197
8. *Zhong Yao Xue* (Chinese Herbology), 1998; 78:80
9. *Xin Yi Xue* (New Medicine), 1976; 1:8
10. *Xin Yi Yao Xue Za Zhi* (New Journal of Medicine and Herbology), 1976; 8:35
11. *Pi Fu Bing Fang Zhi Yan Jiu Tong Xun* (Research Journal on Prevention and Treatment of Dermatological Disorders), 1980; 1:8
12. *Zhong Hua Pi Fu Ke Xue Za Zhi* (Chinese Journal of Dermatology), 1981; 3:129
13. Ishihara K, et al. Interaction of drugs and Chinese herbs: pharmacokinetic changes of tolbutamide and diazepam caused by extract of Angelica dahurica. *Journal of Pharmacy & Pharmacology*, 52(8):1023-9; 2000 Aug
14. *Hua Xi Yao Xue Za Zhi* (Huaxi Herbal Journal), 1990; 5(1):22
15. *Zhong Yao Yao Li Yu Ying Yong* (Pharmacology and Applications of Chinese Herbs), 1983:796
16. *Hua Xi Yao Xue Za Zhi* (Huaxi Herbal Journal), 1991; 6(1):16
17. *Zhong Cao Yao* (Chinese Herbal Medicine), 1988; 19(11):23
18. Ibid., 19(10):22

Cang Er Zi (Fructus Xanthii)

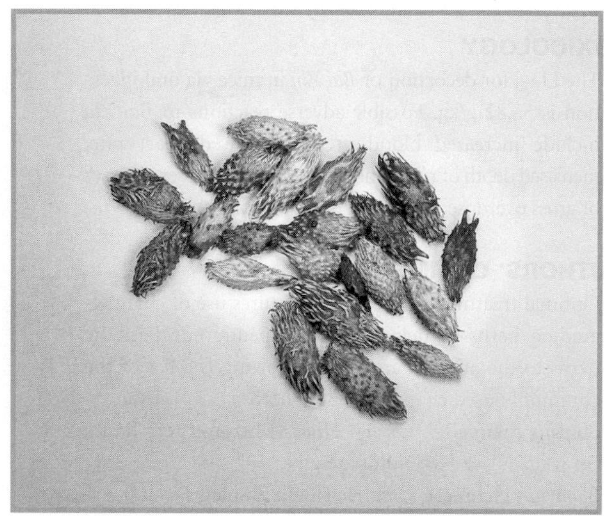

蒼耳子 苍耳子

Pinyin Name: *Cang Er Zi*
Literal Name: "deep green ear seeds"
Alternate Chinese Names: *Cang Zi, Cang Er Ji Li*
Original Source: *Shen Nong Ben Cao Jing* (Divine Husbandman's Classic of the Materia Medica) in the second century
English Name: xanthium fruit, Siberian cocklebur fruit
Botanical Name: *Xanthium sibiricum* Patr. et Widd.; *Xanthium strumarium* L.
Pharmaceutical Name: Fructus Xanthii
Properties: bitter, acrid, warm
Channels Entered: Lung, Liver
Safety Index: toxic

CHINESE THERAPEUTIC ACTIONS

1. Opens Nasal Passages and Relieves Pain

Sinus disorders with headache: Acrid in nature, *Cang Er Zi* (Fructus Xanthii) is commonly used for sinusitis, rhinitis, sinus headaches, nasal blockage, turbid nasal discharge or loss of smell.

- Sinusitis or rhinitis with nasal obstruction, loss of smell, and nasal discharge: combine this herb with *Bai Zhi* (Radix Angelicae Dahuricae) and *Xin Yi Hua* (Flos Magnoliae).

Exemplar Formula: *Cang Er San* (Xanthium Powder).

Cang Er Zi (Fructus Xanthii)

- Sinus headache caused by wind-cold: use it with *Fang Feng* (Radix Saposhnikoviae), *Bai Zhi* (Radix Angelicae Dahuricae) and *Gao Ben* (Rhizoma Ligustici).

2. Dispels Wind and Dampness

Bi zheng **(painful obstruction syndrome):** *Cang Er Zi* dispels wind and dampness from the muscles to relieve pain. Its clinical applications include *bi zheng* caused by wind and dampness, as well as muscle spasms and cramps.

- *Bi zheng*: use *Cang Er Zi* individually, or with *Wei Ling Xian* (Radix Clematidis), *Chuan Xiong* (Rhizoma Ligustici Chuanxiong) and *Cang Zhu* (Rhizoma Atractylodis).

Dermatological disorders: *Cang Er Zi* also dispels wind and dampness from the skin to relieve itching and rash.

- Itching and rash: use it with *Bai Ji Li* (Fructus Tribuli), *Di Fu Zi* (Fructus Kochiae), *Chan Tui* (Periostracum Cicadae), *Bai Xian Pi* (Cortex Dictamni) and *Jing Jie* (Herba Schizonepetae).

DOSAGE

3 to 10 grams. *Cang Er Zi* should be dry-fried to minimize toxicity and maximize extraction of active components. The general guideline is to dry-fry the seeds until the outside 'spikes' are blunted and loose their sharpness. The fresh, unprocessed herb is generally not used due to its significantly higher risk of toxicity.

CAUTIONS / CONTRAINDICATIONS

Due to its drying nature, *Cang Er Zi* consumes qi and blood, and should be used with caution in patients having these deficiencies. It should also be used with caution during pregnancy.

OVERDOSAGE

Overdose of *Cang Er Zi* may lead to nausea, vomiting, abdominal pain, diarrhea or constipation, headache, dizziness, lethargy, and poor appetite. Gross overdose of *Cang Er Zi* is divided into early or late stage. Early stage overdose is characterized by jaundice and hypochondriac pain. The late stage is characterized by jaundice, severe hypochondriac pain, tonic-clonic convulsions, and possibly death. In adults, adverse reactions may occur following ingestion of 30 pieces of the fresh, unprocessed seeds. Hepatitis and nephritis may occur following ingestion of 50 seeds, and death following 100 seeds.[1] [Note: Fresh, unprocessed seeds are significantly more toxic than dry-fried seeds.]

The entire xanthium plant is toxic. The fruit is more toxic than the leaves, and fresh leaves are more toxic than the dried ones. The toxic components of the herb are soluble in water. Toxic signs and symptoms include liver damage, unconsciousness, shock, and respiratory and renal suppression.

TREATMENT OF OVERDOSAGE

Overdose of *Cang Er Zi* may be treated by the following general methods:

- An herbal decoction using *Gan Cao* (Radix Glycyrrhizae) 30g and *Lu Dou* (Semen Phaseoli Radiati) 120g.
- An herbal decoction using *Ban Lan Gen* (Radix Isatidis) 120g.
- An herbal decoction using *Lu Gen* (Rhizoma Phragmitis) 60g, *Lu Dou* (Semen Phaseoli Radiati) 30g, *Jin Yin Hua* (Flos Lonicerae) 15g, *Ge Gen* (Radix Puerariae) 9g, and *Gan Cao* (Radix Glycyrrhizae) 9g.

For gastrointestinal bleeding caused by overdose of *Cang Er Zi*, treat with a decoction containing *Gan Cao* (Radix Glycyrrhizae) 30g, *Yuan Zhi* (Radix Polygalae) 9g, *Sha Shen* (Radix Glehniae seu Adenophorae) 9g, *Xue Yu Tan* (Crinis Carbonisatus) 9g, and *San Qi* (Radix Notoginseng) 1.5g. Take the decoction every 4 hours for 2 to 6 doses.[2]

CHEMICAL COMPOSITION

Xanthostrumarin 1.27%, resin 3.3%, oil 39%, essential oil, alkaloid, vitamin C, carbohydrates.[3]

PHARMACOLOGICAL EFFECTS

- **Antidiabetic**: Intraperitoneal injection of xanthostrumarin at 10 mg/kg may lower plasma glucose levels in rats for up to 2 hours.[4]
- **Antitussive:** Decoction of *Cang Er Zi* has been shown to suppress coughing.[5]

CLINICAL STUDIES AND RESEARCH

- **Chronic sinusitis:** Two-hundred and seven patients with chronic sinusitis were treated by topical application of *Cang Er Zi* with satisfactory results. The topical solution was prepared by crushing 30 to 40 pieces of the herb, cooking it with 30 ml sesame oil, then filtering out the herb. The herbal solution was applied to the nasal cavity via a cotton swab two to three times daily for 2 weeks per course of treatment.[6] In another study, 1,576 patients with chronic sinusitis were treated with 86.9% effective rate using topical application of an herbal formula. The herbal solution was instilled into the nose three to four times daily for 7 to 30 days per course of treatment, for a total of 2 to 3 courses total. The herbal solution was prepared by soaking *Cang Er Zi* 160g and *Xin Yi Hua* (Flos Magnoliae) 16g in 1,000 ml of sesame oil for 24 hours, then cooked and filtered to yield 800 ml of the final solution.[7]
- **Chronic tracheitis:** One report says 275 patients with chronic tracheitis were treated with a preparation of

Cang Er Zi (Fructus Xanthii)

Cang Er Zi with a 97.5% rate of effectiveness. Patients were given the herb three times daily for 10 days for each course of treatment.[8]

- **Pain in the low back and legs:** Trigger point injection of *Cang Er Zi* every other day for 10 days was 89% effective in treating 163 patients with pain in the lower back and legs from various causes.[9]
- **Acute bacterial dysentery:** Decoction of 120 to 150 grams of *Cang Er Zi* given three to four times daily was effective in treating 109 out of 110 patients with acute bacterial dysentery. Most patients responded within 2 to 8 days.[10]
- **Acute localized inflammation**: An herbal paste made from water extract of *Cang Er Zi* and vinegar was used to treat 152 patients with acute localized inflammations. The herbal paste was applied to the affected area for 1 to 2 days before removal and application of a new dose. The study determined that the treatment outcome was satisfactory.[11]

HERB-DRUG INTERACTION

- **Antidiabetics:** Herbs that lower plasma glucose levels, such as *Cang Er Zi,* should be used with caution with insulin, sulfonylureas, and other antidiabetic medications as the combination may have a synergistic effect, leading to hypoglycemia.[12] [Note: Examples of antidiabetic drugs include insulin, tolbutamide (Orinase), glipizide (Glucotrol), and glyburide (Diabeta/Micronase).]

TOXICOLOGY

The LD_{50} for intraperitoneal injection of *Cang Er Zi* is 0.93 g/kg in mice.[13]

SUPPLEMENT

- 蒼耳根 / 苍耳根 *Cang Er Gen* (Radix Xanthii), the root, is bitter, cool and slightly toxic. It enters the Lung and clears heat, eliminates toxins, and treats common colds caused by wind-heat invasions, as well as reducing scrofulae or other toxic swellings such as tonsillitis. Because *Cang Er Gen* is slightly toxic, it is should be used with caution during pregnancy, and in cases of deficiency. The dose for *Cang Er Gen* is 3 to 12 grams.
- 蒼耳草 / 苍耳草 *Cang Er Cao* (Herba Xanthii), the entire plant, is acrid, bitter, cool, and slightly toxic. Its main functions include: dispelling wind, and clearing heat and toxins. Chief applications include: *bi zheng* (painful obstruction syndrome), spasms and cramps. It can be used for dermatological disorders, yin sores, rashes or pruritus. Because it is toxic, this herb should not be taken at a high dose when taken internally, nor should it be used by deficient patients or taken for a long period of time, as it may drain qi and blood. The recommended dose of *Cang Er Cao* is 6 to 15 grams.

AUTHORS' COMMENTS

Cang Er Zi has two main functions that are equally important: it dispels wind and dampness, and opens nasal passages. Thus, this herb is commonly classified as either an exterior-releasing herb or a wind-damp dispelling herb.

Cang Er Zi and *Tian Ma* (Rhizoma Gastrodiae) both treat wind. *Cang Er Zi* dispels external wind, and treats headaches and dizziness. *Tian Ma* extinguishes internal wind, and relieves headaches, dizziness and vertigo.

According to Dr. Gan Zhu-Wang, *Cang Er Zi, Bo He* (Herba Menthae), *Bai Zhi* (Radix Angelicae Dahuricae), and *Xin Yi Hua* (Flos Magnoliae) treat acute allergic rhinitis, while *He Zi* (Fructus Chebulae) and *Shi Liu Pi* (Pericarpium Granati) resolve clear white nasal discharge.

References

1. *Zhong Yao Bu Liang Fan Ying Yu Zhi Liao* (Adverse Reactions and Treatment of Chinese Herbal Medicine), 1996; 195:197
2. Ibid.
3. *Xian Dai Zhong Yao Yao Li Xue* (Contemporary Pharmacology of Chinese Herbs), 1997; 98-99
4. *Zhong Yao Xue* (Chinese Herbology), 1998; 81:83
5. Ibid.
6. *Xin Yi Xue* (New Medicine), 1972; 10:51
7. *Zhong Xi Yi Jie He Za Zhi* (Journal of Integrated Chinese and Western Medicine), 1984; 4:211
8. *He Bei Xin Yi Yao* (Hebei New Medicine and Herbology), 1974; 5:12
9. *Zhong Cao Yao Tong Xun* (Journal of Chinese Herbal Medicine), 1972; 2:50
10. *Xin Zhong Yi* (New Chinese Medicine), 1984; 9:18
11. *Jiang Su Yi Yao* (Jiangsu Journal of Medicine and Herbology), 1977; 5:36
12. Chen, J. Recognition & prevention of herb-drug interactions, *Medical Acupuncture*, Fall/Winter 1998/1999; volume 10/number 2; 9-13
13. *Zhong Yao Xue* (Chinese Herbology), 1998; 81:83

Xin Yi Hua (Flos Magnoliae)

辛夷花 辛夷花

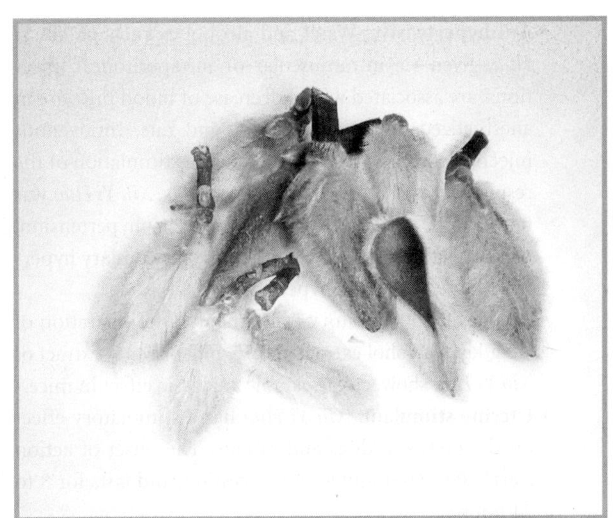

Pinyin Name: *Xin Yi Hua*

Literal Name: "lily-flowered magnolia," "pungent magnolia flower"

Alternate Chinese Names: *Xin Yi*

Original Source: *Shen Nong Ben Cao Jing* (Divine Husbandman's Classic of the Materia Medica) in the second century

English Name: magnolia flower, biond magnolia flower bud, sprenger magnolia flower bud, yulan magnolia flower bud

Botanical Name: *Magnolia biondii* Pamp. (*Qiao Mu Wang Chun Hua*); *Magnolia sprengeri* Pamp. (*Wu Dang Yu Lan*); *Magnolia denudata* Desr. (*Yu Lan*)

Pharmaceutical Name: Flos Magnoliae

Properties: acrid, warm

Channels Entered: Lung, Stomach

CHINESE THERAPEUTIC ACTIONS

1. Dispels Wind-Cold

Nasal obstruction due to wind-cold: *Xin Yi Hua* (Flos Magnoliae) has a rather mild function of dispelling exterior wind-cold. It is most effective for opening nasal obstruction and draining nasal discharge caused by wind-cold.

- Nasal obstruction and clear nasal discharge from wind-cold: use *Xin Yi Hua* with *Bai Zhi* (Radix Angelicae Dahuricae) and *Fang Feng* (Radix Saposhnikoviae). **Exemplar Formula:** *Xin Yi San* (Magnolia Flower Powder).
- Wind-cold attacking the Lung and Stomach with continuous, clear, watery nasal discharge: combine it with *Xi Xin* (Herba Asari), *Gan Jiang* (Rhizoma Zingiberis) and *Fu Zi* (Radix Aconiti Lateralis Praeparata) to dispel cold.

2. Opens Nasal Orifices

Xin Yi Hua has an excellent dispersing function to open sensory orifices and unblock nasal obstruction.

- Sinusitis and rhinitis with loss of smell: use it with *Cang Er Zi* (Fructus Xanthii). **Exemplar Formula:** *Cang Er San* (Xanthium Powder).
- Sinusitis or rhinitis due to cold: combine it with *Qiang Huo* (Rhizoma et Radix Notopterygii), *Fang Feng* (Radix Saposhnikoviae), and *Xi Xin* (Herba Asari). **Exemplar Formula:** *Xin Yi San* (Magnolia Flower Powder).
- Chronic sinusitis or rhinitis caused by damp-heat: use this herb with *Shi Gao* (Gypsum Fibrosum) and *Da Huang* (Radix et Rhizoma Rhei). **Exemplar Formula:** *Qing Bi Tang* (Clear the Nose Decoction).
- Sinusitis or rhinitis caused by heat: use it with *Zhi Zi* (Fructus Gardeniae), *Xuan Shen* (Radix Scrophulariae), *Chuan Bei Mu* (Bulbus Fritillariae Cirrhosae) and *Chai Hu* (Radix Bupleuri).
- Sinusitis or rhinitis with Lung heat: use it with *Zhi Zi* (Fructus Gardeniae), *Huang Qin* (Radix Scutellariae), *Shi Gao* (Gypsum Fibrosum) and *Sheng Ma* (Rhizoma Cimicifugae). **Exemplar Formula:** *Xin Yi Qing Fei Yin* (Magnolia and Gypsum Fibrosum Combination).

DOSAGE

3 to 10 grams. The maximum dosage of *Xin Yi Hua* is 20 grams. It may be given orally or applied topically. For oral administration, *Xin Yi Hua* should be enclosed in cheesecloth during cooking, as fibers from the flowers may be irritating to the throat. Topical applications use either the powdered form or the essential oil of the herb.

CAUTIONS / CONTRAINDICATIONS

Xin Yi Hua should be used with caution in patients with yin-deficient fire or Liver yang rising.

CHEMICAL COMPOSITION

Essential oils 2.68-5.0% (camphor, 1,8-cineole, β-pinene, sabinene, myrcene), lignans, pinoresinol bimethyl ether, lirioresinol bimethyl ether, magnolin, fargesin, sesamin, eudesmin, d-coclaurine, d-reticuline, yuzirine, rutin.[1]

PHARMACOLOGICAL EFFECTS

- **Effect on nasal mucosa:** Topical application of essential oil of *Xin Yi Hua* has been associated with reduction of mucous secretion, reduction of inflammation, and relief of nasal obstruction.[2]

Xin Yi Hua (Flos Magnoliae)

- **Antihypertensive**: Water and alcohol extracts of *Xin Yi Hua*, given via intramuscular or intraperitoneal injections, are associated with a decrease of blood pressure in anesthetized dogs, cats, rabbits, and rats. Intravenous injection is sometimes associated with stimulation of the respiratory system. In other experiments, *Xin Yi Hua* was found to be effective in cases of primary hypertension, but not necessarily effective in cases of secondary hypertension, such as renal hypertension.[3]
- **Analgesic**: In laboratory experiments, administration of 6.5 g/kg of alcohol extract and 15 g/kg of water extract of *Xin Yi Hua* showed comparable analgesic effect in mice.[4]
- **Uterine stimulant**: *Xin Yi Hua* has a stimulatory effect on the uterus in dogs and rabbits. The onset of action starts 20 to 60 minutes after ingestion, and lasts for 8 to 24 hours.[5]
- **Antibiotic**: Decoction of *Xin Yi Hua* has an inhibitory effect on dermatomycoses, and some species of streptococcus and staphylococcus.[6]

CLINICAL STUDIES AND RESEARCH

- **Sinusitis**: In one study, 46 patients with chronic sinusitis were treated with an herbal formula with marked effectiveness in 35 cases, moderate improvement in 8 cases, and no response in 3 cases. The herbal formula was given in decoction, once daily, for 7 days per course of treatment. The herbal formula contained *Xin Yi Hua* 12g, *Cang Er Zi* (Fructus Xanthii) 12g, *Gao Ben* (Rhizoma Ligustici) 9g, *Sheng Ma* (Rhizoma Cimicifugae) 9g, *Huang Qin* (Radix Scutellariae) 9g, *Fang Feng* (Radix Saposhnikoviae) 9g, *Jing Jie* (Herba Schizonepetae) 9g, *Niu Bang Zi* (Fructus Arctii) 9g, *Chan Tui* (Periostracum Cicadae) 9g, *Lian Qiao* (Fructus Forsythiae) 10g, *Chuan Xiong* (Rhizoma Ligustici Chuanxiong) 10g, and *Bai Zhi* (Radix Angelicae Dahuricae) 15g. Modifications were made if deemed necessary.[7]
- **Sinusitis and rhinitis**: In one study, patients with sinusitis or rhinitis were treated with Chinese herbs once or twice daily. All patients were prescribed 3 grams of *Xin Yi Hua*. Those diagnosed with wind-cold also received 10 grams of *Huo Xiang* (Herba Agastache), and those with wind-heat also received 10 grams of *Huai Hua* (Flos Sophorae). Out of 120 patients, the effective rate was 95%.[8]
- **Sinusitis and rhinitis**: In one study, 2,450 patients with sinusitis or rhinitis were treated with intranasal instillation and intramuscular injection of *Xin Yi Hua* preparations. The patients in this study received varied doses according to their age. The study reported 17.3% had marked improvement, 28.5% had moderate improvement, 46.7% had slight improvement, and 7.5% showed no response.[9]

TOXICOLOGY

Xin Yi Hua has very low toxicity. No fatalities were reported following intravenous injection at 1 g/kg in dogs and 4.75 g/kg in rabbits. Furthermore, no abnormalities were noted following oral ingestion of alcohol extract at 18 g/kg and water extract at 30 g/kg in rats for 1 month.[10]

References

1. *Xian Dai Zhong Yao Yao Li Xue* (Contemporary Pharmacology of Chinese Herbs), 1997; 93-94
2. *Zhong Yao Cai* (Study of Chinese Herbal Material), 1990; 13(9):33
3. *Zhong Yao Yao Li Yu Ying Yong* (Pharmacology and Applications of Chinese Herbs), 1983:541
4. *Zhong Yao Cai* (Study of Chinese Herbal Material), 1990; 13(9):33
5. *Zhong Yao Yao Li Yu Ying Yong* (Pharmacology and Applications of Chinese Herbs), 1983:541
6. *Zhong Yao Xue* (Chinese Herbology), 1998; 84:85
7. *Shan Xi Zhong Yi* (Shanxi Chinese Medicine), 1991; 12(4):177
8. *Zhong Yao Tong Bao* (Journal of Chinese Herbology), 1985; 5:45
9. *Xin Yi Xue* (New Medicine), 1981; 1:12
10. *Zhong Yao Cai* (Study of Chinese Herbal Material), 1990; 13(9):33

E Bu Shi Cao (Herba Centipedae)

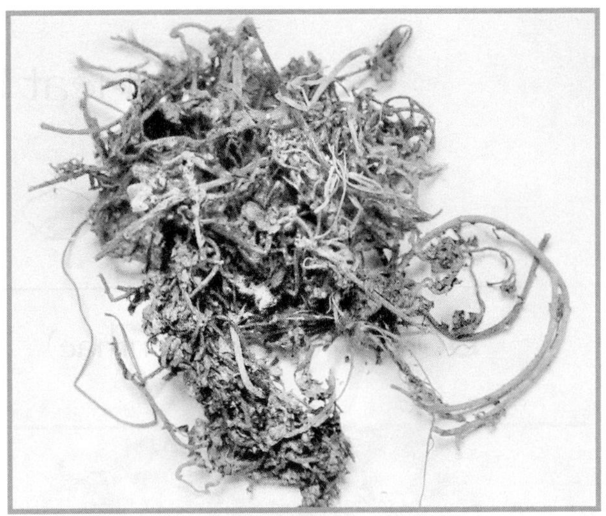

鵝不食草
鹅不食草

Pinyin Name: *E Bu Shi Cao*
Alternate Chinese Names: *Shi Hu Wei, Die Zai Cao, Man Tian Xing*
English Name: centipeda herb, small centipeda herb
Botanical Name: *Centipeda minima* (L.) A.
Pharmaceutical Name: Herba Centipedae
Properties: acrid, warm
Channels Entered: Lung, Liver

CHINESE THERAPEUTIC ACTIONS

1. Opens the Nasal Orifices, Removes Superficial Visual Obstruction

Hypertrophic rhinitis, sinus polyps, nasal obstruction: *E Bu Shi Cao* (Herba Centipedae) opens the nasal orifices to treat symptoms related to nasal disorders.

- Nasal disorders: use *E Bu Shi Cao* with *Fu Rong* (Radix Hibisci) and *Xin Yi Hua* (Flos Magnoliae) in herbal decoction. The fresh juice of *E Bu Shi Cao* can also be applied topically as nose drops.

Cataract: *E Bu Shi Cao* removes superficial visual obstruction and treats cataracts.

- Cataracts: combine it with *Qian Li Guang* (Herba Senecionis Scandens).

2. Dispels Wind and Dampness and Benefits the Joints

Traumatic injuries, arthritis: *E Bu Shi Cao* treats arthritic pain caused by wind and dampness lodged in the joints after traumatic injuries.

- Pain: combine it with *Yi Tiao Gen* (Radix Moghaniae), *Jin Bu Huan* (Herba Lycopodii Serrati), *Mo Gu Xiao* (Caulis Hyptis Capitatae), *Huang Jin Gui* (Caulis Vanieriae) and *Liu Zhi Huang* (Herba Solidaginis).

DOSAGE

3 to 9 grams in decoction.

CAUTIONS / CONTRAINDICATIONS

- Use *E Bu Shi Cao* with caution for patients with weak digestive systems.
- *E Bu Shi Cao* is contraindicated in patients with gastritis or duodenal ulcers.

AUTHORS' COMMENTS

Use of *E Bu Shi Cao* is sometimes associated with irritation to the stomach lining, which is why it should be used with caution in patients with sensitive stomachs. This side effect can be minimized by adding herbs that protect the stomach, such as such as *Bai Ji* (Rhizoma Bletillae), *Wu Bei Zi* (Galla Chinensis), *Hai Piao Xiao* (Endoconcha Sepiae) and *Chuan Bei Mu* (Bulbus Fritillariae Cirrhosae).

Section 2

— Wind-Heat Releasing Herbs

Bo He (Herba Menthae)

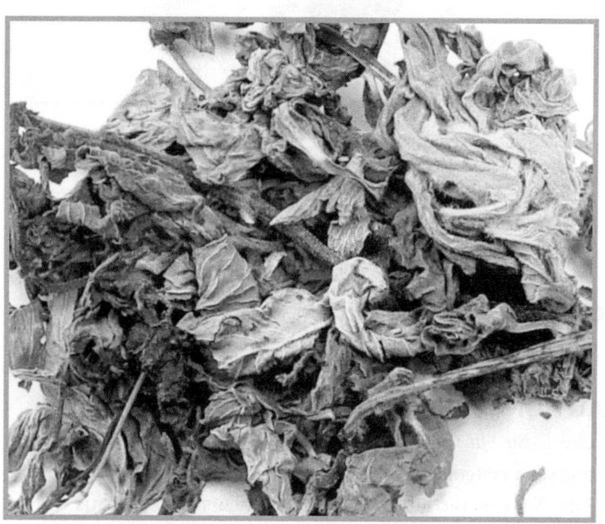

薄荷 薄荷

Pinyin Name: *Bo He*

Alternate Chinese Names: *Bo He Ye, Bo He Geng, Su Bo He*

Original Source: *Yao Xing Ben Cao* (Materia Medica of Medicinal Properties) by Zhen Quan in 600 A.D.

English Name: mint, wild mint

Botanical Name: *Mentha haplocalyx* Briq.

Pharmaceutical Name: Herba Menthae

Properties: acrid, cool

Channels Entered: Lung, Liver

CHINESE THERAPEUTIC ACTIONS

1. Releases the Exterior and Dispels Wind-Heat

Wind-heat: *Bo He* (Herba Menthae) is commonly used to treat the initial stages of febrile disorders, or wind-heat syndrome, characterized by symptoms such as headache, fever, the absence of perspiration, dry mouth and/or sore throat, yellow tongue coat, and superficial, rapid pulse. Because its acrid taste can overcome its cold nature, *Bo He* can also be used to treat wind-cold syndrome, if combined with acrid, warm herbs.

- Wind-heat syndrome: use this herb with *Jing Jie* (Herba Schizonepetae), *Jie Geng* (Radix Platycodonis), *Sang Ye* (Folium Mori), *Ju Hua* (Flos Chrysanthemi) and *Niu Bang Zi* (Fructus Arctii) to dispel wind-heat and remove toxins. **Exemplar Formulas:** *Sang Ju Yin* (Mulberry Leaf and Chrysanthemum Decoction) and *Yin Qiao San* (Honeysuckle and Forsythia Powder).
- Early-stage febrile disorders: combine it with *Chan Tui* (Periostracum Cicadae), *Shi Gao* (Gypsum Fibrosum) and *Gan Cao* (Radix Glycyrrhizae).
- Wind-cold syndrome: use it with *Zi Su Ye* (Folium Perillae), *Fang Feng* (Radix Saposhnikoviae), and *Qiang Huo* (Rhizoma et Radix Notopterygii).

2. Clears the Head, Brightens the Eyes and Benefits the Throat

Headache, sore throat, and red eyes: *Bo He* is commonly said to have light, floating or ascending properties. Thus, it is most effective in treating wind-heat in the upper body, such as disorders of the throat and head. The most suitable clinical applications include headache, sore throat, and red eyes.

- Sore throat from wind-heat: use this herb with *Niu Bang Zi* (Fructus Arctii), *Ban Lan Gen* (Radix Isatidis) and *She Gan* (Rhizoma Belamcandae).
- Sore throat with loss of voice: combine it with *Lian Qiao* (Fructus Forsythiae), *Jie Geng* (Radix Platycodonis) and *Gu Zhi Hua* (Semen Oroxyli).
- Red eyes from wind-heat: use it with *Ju Hua* (Flos Chrysanthemi), *Niu Bang Zi* (Fructus Arctii) and *Gan Cao* (Radix Glycyrrhizae).

Bo He (Herba Menthae)

3. Vents Rashes

Dermatological disorders: Dispersing by nature, *Bo He* is commonly used to treat wind-heat attacking the skin, characterized by disorders such as rashes, measles, and other dermatological diseases. It promotes a more rapid recovery by shortening the duration of illness.

- Measles: combine it with *Jing Jie* (Herba Schizonepetae), *Niu Bang Zi* (Fructus Arctii) and *Lian Qiao* (Fructus Forsythiae) to promote the eruption of measles.
- Rash, eczema and general itching: use it with *Chan Tui* (Periostracum Cicadae), *Jing Jie* (Herba Schizonepetae), *Di Fu Zi* (Fructus Kochiae) and *Niu Bang Zi* (Fructus Arctii).

4. Soothes and Relieves Liver Qi Stagnation

Liver qi stagnation: *Bo He* enters the Liver channel and is commonly used to treat Liver qi stagnation characterized by feelings of discomfort, distention, and pain in the chest and hypochondrium.

- Liver qi stagnation: use it with *Chai Hu* (Radix Bupleuri), *Bai Shao* (Radix Paeoniae Alba), and *Dang Gui* (Radicis Angelicae Sinensis). **Exemplar Formula:** *Xiao Yao San* (Rambling Powder).
- Red eyes, blurred vision and headache in hypertension caused by Liver yang rising: add *Ju Hua* (Flos Chrysanthemi) and *Sang Ye* (Folium Mori).

5. Disperses Turbid Qi from the Abdomen

Damp-heat accumulation in the abdomen: In the summer, an inappropriate diet of uncooked or unsanitary food may introduce heat and dampness to the abdomen. With the accumulation of heat and dampness, patients will experience abdominal pain, vomiting, diarrhea, and other gastrointestinal disturbances. In combination with other herbs, *Bo He* can effectively treat this type of gastrointestinal disorder.

- Vomiting and diarrhea due to summer-heat and dampness: use it with *Huo Xiang* (Herba Agastache), *Lian Qiao* (Fructus Forsythiae), and *Bai Dou Kou* (Fructus Amomi Rotundus). **Exemplar Formula:** *Gan Lu Xiao Du Dan* (Sweet Dew Special Pill to Eliminate Toxin).

DOSAGE

2 to 10 grams. The maximum dosage of *Bo He* is 20 grams. *Bo He* should be added last to the decoction, and cooked only for a short period of time, no more than 5 to 10 minutes. The leaves have stronger diaphoretic action, while the stems have stronger qi-regulating action.

CAUTIONS / CONTRAINDICATIONS

- Aromatic and acrid, *Bo He* has a dispersing nature and may consume qi and yin. Therefore, it should be used with caution in patients with yin deficiency, yin-deficient heat, *xiao ke* (wasting and thirsting) syndrome, perspiration from qi deficiency, Liver yang excess, and those patients who are recovering from chronic illnesses or have deficiency symptoms.
- Chronic, repetitive use may lead to depletion of qi and yang reserves.

CHEMICAL COMPOSITION

Essential oils 1-3% (menthol, menthone, isomenthol, pulegone, menthenone, neomenthol), lipophilic flavones, coumarins.[1,2]

Menthone

PHARMACOLOGICAL EFFECTS

- **Dermatologic**: Topical application of *Bo He* increases local blood circulation. It produces a cool sensation initially, followed by a warm sensation. It is commonly used to relieve itching and pain.[3]
- **Others**: *Bo He* has antipyretic, diaphoretic and anti-inflammatory effects.[4]

CLINICAL STUDIES AND RESEARCH

- **Fever**: In one report, 73 patients with high fevers due to infection were treated successfully with an herbal formula. The overall effective rate was 92.76%, with 13 patients showing complete recovery within 24 hours. The herbal formula included 10 grams each of *Bo He*, *Jing Jie* (Herba Schizonepetae), *Jin Yin Hua* (Flos Lonicerae), *Xing Ren* (Semen Armeniacae Amarum), *Shi Gao* (Gypsum Fibrosum), *Qian Hu* (Radix Peucedani), *Huang Qin* (Radix Scutellariae), *Zhu Ye* (Herba Phyllostachys), *Chai Hu* (Radix Bupleuri), *Gan Cao* (Radix Glycyrrhizae), and *Ban Lan Gen* (Radix Isatidis), and 15 grams of *Lian Qiao* (Fructus Forsythiae). The herbal decoction was given four to eight times daily as needed to control fever.[5]
- **Acute mastitis**: In one report, topical application of an herbal solution to the affected area twice daily showed satisfactory results in 40 cases of acute mastitis. The herbal solution was made by cooking 60 grams each of *Bo He* and *Jie Geng* (Radix Platycodonis) with the herb residue filtered out to yield the topical solution.[6]

TOXICOLOGY

The LD_{50} for menthone in rats is 2.0 g/kg via subcutaneous injection.[7]

Bo He (Herba Menthae)

References
1. *Xian Dai Zhong Yao Yao Li Xue* (Contemporary Pharmacology of Chinese Herbs), 1997; 165
2. Yan X, Zhou J, Xie G, *Traditional Chinese Medicines Molecular Structures, Natural Sources and Applications*; Ashgate, 1999; 4168
3. *Zhong Cao Yao Xue* (Study of Chinese Herbal Medicine), 1980; 932
4. *Zhong Yao Xue* (Chinese Herbology), 1998; 89:91
5. *Zhong Yi Za Zhi* (Journal of Chinese Medicine), 1991; 32(3):52
6. *Guang Xi Chi Jiao Yi Shen* (Guangxi Barefoot Doctor), 1977; (1):43
7. *Zhong Cao Yao Xue* (Study of Chinese Herbal Medicine), 1980; 932

Níu Bang Zi (Fructus Arctii)

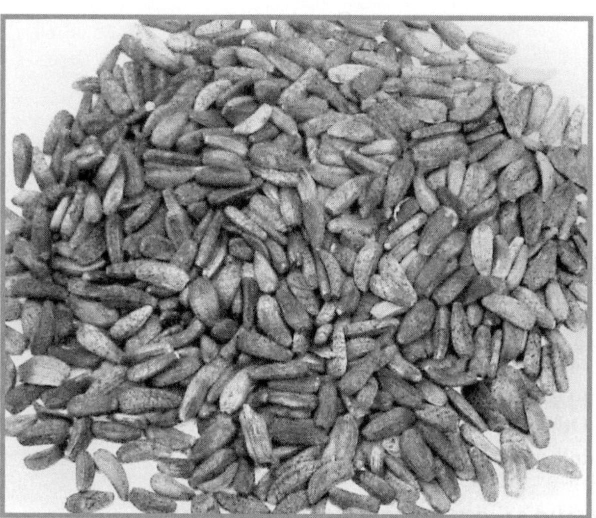

牛蒡子 牛蒡子

Pinyin Name: *Niu Bang Zi*
Alternate Chinese Names: *Su Nien Zi, Da Li Zi, E Shi*
Original Source: *Ming Yi Za Zhu* (Miscellaneous Records of Famous Physicians) by Tao Hong-Jing in 500 A.D.
English Name: arctium, achene of great burdock, burdock fruit
Botanical Name: *Arctium lappa* L.
Pharmaceutical Name: Fructus Arctii
Properties: acrid, bitter, cold
Channels Entered: Lung, Stomach

CHINESE THERAPEUTIC ACTIONS

1. Dispels Wind and Clears Heat

Wind-heat: Due to its cold nature, *Niu Bang Zi* (Fructus Arctii) effectively dispels wind-heat and toxins or wind-heat at the early stage of a febrile disorder. It is commonly used to treat wind-heat affecting the Lung, accompanied by headache, fever, sore throat with swelling and pain, cough, and yellow sputum.

- Sore throat caused by febrile disorder or wind-heat syndrome: use *Niu Bang Zi* with *Jin Yin Hua* (Flos Lonicerae), *Bo He* (Herba Menthae), *Jie Geng* (Radix Platycodonis), and *Lian Qiao* (Fructus Forsythiae). **Exemplar Formula:** *Yin Qiao San* (Honeysuckle and Forsythia Powder).
- Severe sore throat or swollen tonsils due to wind-heat with excessive heat and toxins: use this herb with *Ma Bo* (Lasiosphaera seu Calvatia), *Huang Qin* (Radix Scutellariae), *Shan Dou Gen* (Radix Sophorae Tonkinensis) or *Da Huang* (Radix et Rhizoma Rhei).
- Cough and phlegm due to wind-heat invading the Lung: add it to *Jie Geng* (Radix Platycodonis), *Sang Ye* (Folium Mori), *Bei Mu* (Bulbus Fritillaria) and *Gan Cao* (Radix Glycyrrhizae), to dispel wind-heat and clear Lung heat.

2. Eliminates Toxins and Vents Rashes

Dermatological disorders: *Niu Bang Zi* dispels wind-heat and eliminates toxic heat from the skin. It is commonly used to treat various dermatological disorders, such as red swellings, rashes, eczema, carbuncles, erythemas, mumps, acute febrile maculopapular rashes, and measles in cases of incomplete eruption or expression. *Niu Bang Zi* vents rashes, promotes their eruption and clears toxins from the body.

- Dermatological disorders caused by wind-heat (in which there is more itching but the basic condition is less severe): use *Niu Bang Zi* with *Chan Tui* (Periostracum Cicadae), *Bo He* (Herba Menthae), *Jing Jie* (Herba Schizonepetae) and *Ge Gen* (Radix Puerariae).
- Dermatological disorders from the accumulation of heat and toxins (there is more redness or pain, and the condition is more severe): use it with *Da Qing Ye* (Folium Isatidis), *Zi Cao Gen* (Radix Lithospermi) and *Sheng Ma* (Rhizoma Cimicifugae).

Níu Bang Zi (Fructus Arctii)

- Sores, carbuncles or fixed swellings with redness and pain: combine it with *Jin Yin Hua* (Flos Lonicerae), *Lian Qiao* (Fructus Forsythiae), *Ku Shen Gen* (Radix Sophorae Flavescentis), *Dang Gui Wei* (Extremitas Radicis Angelicae Sinensis) and *Chi Shao* (Radix Paeoniae Rubrae).

3. Clears Heat and Eliminates Toxins from the Throat

Sore throat: *Niu Bang Zi* dispels wind-heat, eliminates toxins and is very effective in treating sore throat with severe pain and swelling, such as acute tonsillitis, pharyngitis and laryngitis.

- Sore throat: use it with *Ma Bo* (Lasiosphaera seu Calvatia), *Ban Lan Gen* (Radix Isatidis), *Xuan Shen* (Radix Scrophulariae), *Jie Geng* (Radix Platycodonis), and *Lian Qiao* (Fructus Forsythiae) to clear heat and eliminate toxins. **Exemplar Formula:** *Pu Ji Xiao Du Yin* (Universal Benefit Decoction to Eliminate Toxin).

DOSAGE

3 to 10 grams. The maximum dosage for *Niu Bang Zi* is 30 grams. The seeds should be crushed prior to cooking to maximize the available surface area and ensure complete extraction of the active constituents. Due to the cold thermal property of the herb, consumption of the unprocessed form is sometimes associated with diarrhea. Therefore, dry-frying the herb to increase its warmth will reduce the possibility of diarrhea.

CAUTIONS / CONTRAINDICATIONS

- Due to its cold nature, *Niu Bang Zi* should be used only for patients with heat or excess syndromes.
- Use of *Niu Bang Zi* is contraindicated in patients with Spleen qi deficiency with loose stools.

CHEMICAL COMPOSITION

Arctiin, arcti-genin, isoarctigenin, essential oil 25-30%, gobosterin, lappaol A,B,C,D,E,F,H.[1]

PHARMACOLOGICAL EFFECTS

- **Antibiotic**: *Niu Bang Zi* has been shown to inhibit *Streptococcus pneumoniae* and some pathogenic fungi.[2]
- **Antidiabetic**: Extract of *Niu Bang Zi* has been shown to decrease blood glucose levels, with a prolonged duration of effect, in rats.[3]
- **Renal**: Intraperitoneal injection of arctiin at 10 mg/kg daily for 10 days showed promising results in treating kidney diseases by reducing the amount of protein present in the urine.[4]
- **Others**: *Niu Bang Zi* has anti-inflammatory, antipyretic and diuretic effects.[5]

CLINICAL STUDIES AND RESEARCH

- **Migraine**: *Niu Bang Zi* was used to treat migraine headache in 40 patients. Each patient received 9 grams of powdered *Niu Bang Zi*, taken with grain-based liquor, once daily. Patients were covered with blankets after administration of the herbs to enhance diaphoresis. Out of 40 patients, 34 reported significant improvement.[6]
- **Facial paralysis**: According to one report, 47 patients with facial paralysis were treated with an herbal decoction twice daily with all patients reporting at least slight improvement in their condition. The herbal formula contained *Niu Bang Zi* 30g, *Bai Zhi* (Radix Angelicae Dahuricae) 10g, *Nu Zhen Zi* (Fructus Ligustri Lucidi) 12g, and *Han Lian Cao* (Herba Ecliptae) 12g.[7]

HERB-DRUG INTERACTION

- **Antidiabetics:** Herbs that lower the plasma glucose levels, such as *Niu Bang Zi,* should be used with caution with insulin, sulfonylureas, and other antidiabetic medications as the combination may have a synergistic effect, leading to hypoglycemia.[8] [Note: Examples of antidiabetic drugs include insulin, tolbutamide (Orinase), glipizide (Glucotrol), and glyburide (DiaBeta/Micronase).]
- **Acetaminophen**: It has been shown that *Niu Bang Gen* (Radix Arctii) has marked hepatoprotective effects. *Niu Bang Gen* suppressed the elevated SGOT and SGPT levels induced by carbon tetrachloride or acetaminophen in a dose-dependent manner. It also alleviated the severity of liver damage based on histopathological observations. The mechanism of this hepatoprotective action is based on the antioxidative effect of *Niu Bang Gen* on hepatocytes, hence eliminating the deleterious effects of toxic metabolites from carbon tetrachloride or acetaminophen.[9]

SUPPLEMENT

- 牛蒡根 / 牛蒡根 *Niu Bang Gen* (Radix Arctii) is derived from the root of the same plant as *Niu Bang Zi.* Historically, *Niu Bang Gen* has rarely been used. However, its use has increased in light of its beneficial action to protect the liver from chemically-induced damage, such as caused by use of acetaminophen or carbon tetrachloride.

References

1. *Xian Dai Zhong Yao Yao Li Xue* (Contemporary Pharmacology of Chinese Herbs), 1997; 172
2. *Zhong Yao Zhi* (Chinese Herbology Journal), 1984; 250
3. Ibid.
4. *Guo Wai Yi Xue Zhong Yi Zhong Yao Fen Ce* (Monograph of Chinese Herbology from Foreign Medicine), 1990; 12(6):47
5. *Zhong Yao Xue* (Chinese Herbology), 1998; 91:92
6. *Liao Ning Zhong Yi Za Zhi* (Liaoning Journal of Chinese Medicine), 1959; 2:5
7. *Shi Yong Zhong Yi Nei Ke Za Zhi* (Journal of Practical Chinese Internal Medicine), 1988; 3:128

Níu Bang Zi (Fructus Arctii)

8. Chen, J. Recognition & prevention of herb-drug interactions, *Medical Acupuncture*, Fall/Winter 1998/1999; volume 10/number 2; 9-13
9. Lin SC. Chung TC. Lin CC. Ueng TH. Lin YH. Lin SY. Wang LY., Hepatoprotective effects of Arctium lappa on carbon tetrachloride- and acetaminophen-induced liver damage. *American Journal of Chinese Medicine*. 28(2):163-73, 2000

Chan Tui (Periostracum Cicadae)

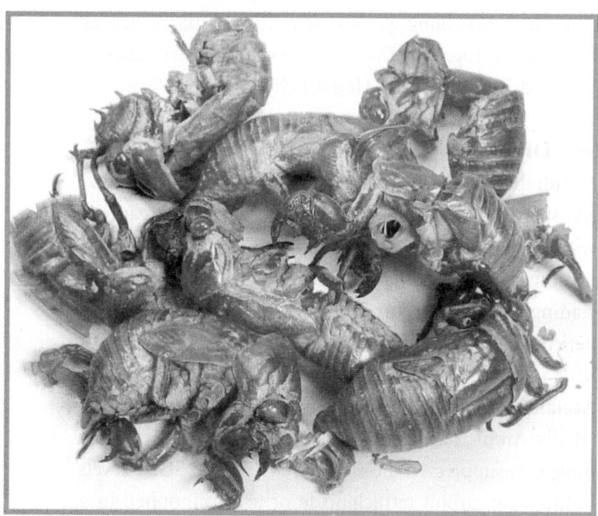

蟬蛻 蝉蜕

Pinyin Name: *Chan Tui*
Literal Name: "slough of cicada"
Alternate Chinese Names: *Chan Yi*, *Chan Ke*
Original Source: *Ming Yi Za Zhu* (Miscellaneous Records of Famous Physicians) by Tao Hong-Jing in 500 A.D.
English Name: cicada moulting
Zoological Name: *Cryptotympana atrata* Fabr.; *Cryptotympana pustulata* Fabr.
Pharmaceutical Name: Periostracum Cicadae
Properties: sweet, cold
Channels Entered: Liver, Lung

CHINESE THERAPEUTIC ACTIONS

1. Dispels Wind-Heat

Wind-heat: *Chan Tui* (Periostracum Cicadae) dispels wind-heat, especially from the head or eyes. It is commonly used to treat early-stage febrile disorders or wind-heat syndrome affecting the throat. Representative symptoms include loss or hoarseness of voice, sore throat, headache and fever.

- Early-stage febrile disorders or wind-heat syndrome: combine *Chan Tui* with *Ju Hua* (Flos Chrysanthemi), *Bo He* (Herba Menthae), and *Lian Qiao* (Fructus Forsythiae). **Exemplar Formula:** *Sang Ju Yin* (Mulberry Leaf and Chrysanthemum Decoction).
- Loss of voice: combine it with *Pang Da Hai* (Semen Sterculiae Lychnophorae), *Niu Bang Zi* (Fructus Arctii), and *Jie Geng* (Radix Platycodonis).

2. Vents Rashes and Relieves Itching

Incomplete expression of rashes, and itching: *Chan Tui* dispels heat from the skin and is commonly used to treat various dermatological disorders, including but not limited to urticaria, rash, eczema, measles, chickenpox and itching. *Chan Tui* promotes a more rapid recovery by shortening the duration of illness.

- To promote the eruption of dermatological disorders: use it with *Niu Bang Zi* (Fructus Arctii), *Ge Gen* (Radix Puerariae) and *Bo He* (Herba Menthae).
- Itching: add to *Jing Jie* (Herba Schizonepetae), *Bai Ji Li* (Fructus Tribuli), and *Fang Feng* (Radix Saposhnikoviae).

3. Brightens the Eyes

Superficial visual obstruction: As the Liver opens to the eyes - either wind or wind-heat affecting the Liver will lead to superficial visual obstruction, blurred vision, red eyes and excessive secretion of tears.

- Red eyes: use *Chan Tui* with *Ju Hua* (Flos Chrysanthemi) and *Mu Zei* (Herba Equiseti Hiemalis).

4. Extinguishes Liver Wind and Relieves Spasms

Tetanus: *Chan Tui* enters the Liver channel and extinguishes Liver wind. It treats muscle spasms, twitching, convulsions with high fever, facial paralysis, post-stroke speech impairment, tetanus, and constant crying in infants, or infantile seizures.

- Muscle spasms and twitching: combine it with *Quan Xie*

Chan Tui (Periostracum Cicadae)

(Scorpio), *Jiang Can* (Bombyx Batryticatus), and *Gou Teng* (Ramulus Uncariae cum Uncis).

- Mild tetanus: use *Chan Tui* alone in powder and serve with rice-based liquor.
- Severe tetanus: *Chan Tui* is most useful in combination with *Tian Nan Xing* (Rhizoma Arisaematis), *Tian Ma* (Rhizoma Gastrodiae), *Jiang Can* (Bombyx Batryticatus), and *Quan Xie* (Scorpio).
- Constant crying in infants due to fear or fright: use this herb with *Gou Teng* (Ramulus Uncariae cum Uncis) and *Bo He* (Herba Menthae).

DOSAGE

3 to 10 grams. The maximum dosage of *Chan Tui* is 30 grams. It can also be used alone as powder or pills.

CAUTIONS / CONTRAINDICATIONS

- *Chan Tui* should be used with caution in pregnant women, as it may impair labor and cause difficulty in delivery.
- Chronic or repetitive use of *Chan Tui* may consume qi and yin. Therefore, use with caution in patients with these deficiencies.
- Use of *Chan Tui* may be associated with possible drowsiness and sedation. Therefore, individuals who take this herb should exercise caution in driving or operating heavy machinery.

CHEMICAL COMPOSITION

Protein, amino acid, organic acid, carbohydrates, lipids, essential oil.[1]

PHARMACOLOGICAL EFFECTS

- **CNS suppressant:** *Chan Tui* has demonstrated an inhibitory influence on the central nervous system (CNS). Laboratory experiments show that it prevents and treats seizures, treats tetanus, prolongs sleeping time induced by barbiturates, reduces spontaneous activity and counters excitation induced by caffeine in mice.[2,3]

CLINICAL STUDIES AND RESEARCH

- **Tetanus:** According to one report, 8 patients with tetanus were treated with *Chan Tui*. Adults received 45 to 60 grams of *Chan Tui* powder twice daily with 90 to 120 ml of grain-based liquor. The dosage for the children was adjusted according to their age and body weight. All patients received concurrent supportive treatment and antibiotic therapy. All patients recovered within 7 to 17 days.[4]
- **Chronic urticaria:** In one study, chronic urticaria was treated with 9 grams of an herbal formula, in pills, two to three times daily. The pills consisted of 2 parts *Chan Tui*, 1 part *Bai Ji Li* (Fructus Tribuli), and honey. Out of 30 patients, 7 reported significant improvement, 15 reported moderate improvement, and 5 reported slight improvement.[5]
- **Prolapse of rectum:** *Chan Tui* powder was used topically to treat rectal prolapse. Satisfactory results were reported in 15 patients who applied the herb topically after one to five applications.[6]

HERB-DRUG INTERACTION

- **Sedatives:** *Chan Tui* has an inhibitory influence on the central nervous system. It potentiates the sedative effect of barbiturates, and reduces the stimulant effect of caffeine.[7] [Note: Many categories of drugs induce sedation, such as antihistamines, narcotic analgesics, barbiturates, benzodiazepines and others.]

TOXICOLOGY

No fatalities were reported following oral administration of alcohol extract of *Chan Tui* at 8,000 mg/kg in mice.[8,9]

AUTHORS' COMMENTS

According to the *Ben Cao Gang Mu* (Materia Medica) by Li Shi-Zhen in 1578, cicada treats all symptoms related to wind-heat. The entire insect is more effective for the treatment of diseases of the internal organs, such as to calm Liver wind and relieve muscle spasms. The moulted casing is more appropriate to treat exterior disorders, such as dermatological disorders caused by wind-heat.

References

1. *Xian Dai Zhong Yao Yao Li Xue* (Contemporary Pharmacology of Chinese Herbs), 1997; 175
2. *Zhong Yao Cai* (Study of Chinese Herbal Material), 1985; 3:39
3. *Zhong Cao Yao* (Chinese Herbal Medicine), 1986; 17(11):21
4. *Shan Xi Zhong Yi* (Shanxi Chinese Medicine), 1985; 7:322
5. *Pi Fu Bing Fang Zhi Yan Jiu Tong Xun* (Research Journal on Prevention and Treatment of Dermatological Disorders), 1972; 3:215
6. *Xin Zhong Yi* (New Chinese Medicine), 1980; 2:49
7. *Zhong Yao Cai* (Study of Chinese Herbal Material), 1985; 3:39
8. *Zhong Cao Yao* (Chinese Herbal Medicine), 1986; 17(11):21
9. *Zhong Guo Yi Yuan Yao Xue Za Zhi* (Chinese Hospital Journal of Herbology), 1988; 8(3):8

Sang Ye (Folium Mori)

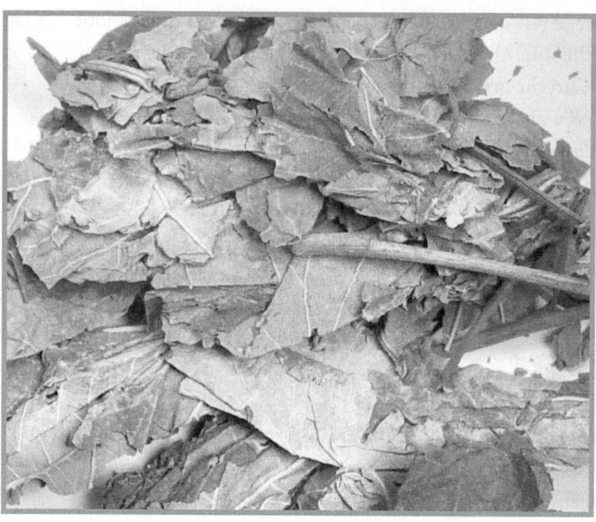

桑葉 桑叶

Pinyin Name: *Sang Ye*
Literal Name: "mulberry leaves"
Alternate Chinese Names: *Dong Sang Ye, Shuang Sang Ye*
Original Source: *Shen Nong Ben Cao Jing* (Divine Husbandman's Classic of the Materia Medica) in the second century
English Name: mulberry leaf
Botanical Name: *Morus alba* L.
Pharmaceutical Name: Folium Mori
Properties: bitter, sweet, cold
Channels Entered: Lung, Liver

CHINESE THERAPEUTIC ACTIONS

1. Dispels Wind-Heat

Wind-heat: *Sang Ye* (Folium Mori) is one of the most commonly used herbs to treat wind-heat syndrome, characterized by cough, fever, headache and sore throat.

- Wind-heat with cough: use *Sang Ye* with *Ju Hua* (Flos Chrysanthemi), *Bo He* (Herba Menthae), *Lian Qiao* (Fructus Forsythiae), and *Jie Geng* (Radix Platycodonis).

2. Clears Lung Heat and Moistens Dryness

Heat and dryness injuring the Lung: Key symptoms include cough, scanty or no sputum, difficult-to-expectorate sputum, and dry mouth and throat caused by heat and dryness damaging the Lung.

- Lung heat and dryness: use *Sang Ye* with *Xing Ren* (Semen Armeniacae Amarum), *Chuan Bei Mu* (Bulbus Fritillariae Cirrhosae), *Mai Men Dong* (Radix Ophiopogonis) and *Sha Shen* (Radix Glehniae seu Adenophorae). **Exemplar Formula:** *Sang Xing Tang* (Mulberry Leaf and Apricot Kernel Decoction).
- Coughing with blood: combine this herb with *Sheng Di Huang* (Radix Rehmanniae), *E Jiao* (Colla Corii Asini), *Shi Gao* (Gypsum Fibrosum) and *Pi Pa Ye* (Folium Eriobotryae).

3. Calms the Liver and Brightens the Eyes

Liver yang rising: *Sang Ye* enters the Liver channel to treat Liver yang rising, Liver fire and Liver yin deficiency. Liver yang rising is characterized by dizziness, vertigo and headache. Liver fire is characterized by redness, swelling and painful eyes. Liver yin deficiency is characterized by dizziness and blurred vision.

- Liver yang rising: use *Sang Ye* with *Ju Hua* (Flos Chrysanthemi), *Shi Jue Ming* (Concha Haliotidis), and *Bai Shao* (Radix Paeoniae Alba).
- Liver fire: combine it with *Ju Hua* (Flos Chrysanthemi), *Jue Ming Zi* (Semen Cassiae) and *Che Qian Zi* (Semen Plantaginis). *Sang Ye* is sometimes used as an external wash to relieve eye disorders caused by Liver fire.
- Liver yin deficiency: use it with *Hei Zhi Ma* (Semen Sesami Nigrum) and *Gou Qi Zi* (Fructus Lycii).

Eye disorders due to wind-heat: Key symptoms include itching and redness of the eyes.

- Itching and redness of the eyes: combine *Sang Ye* with *Chan Tui* (Periostracum Cicadae).

4. Cools the Blood and Stops Bleeding

Hematemesis due to heat: Excess heat in the Stomach forces blood out of its channels and thus causes vomiting of blood. *Sang Ye* can both cool the blood and stop bleeding.

- Hematemesis: use *Sang Ye* with blood-cooling herbs, such as *Xiao Ji* (Herba Cirisii).

DOSAGE

5 to 10 grams for dried *Sang Ye*, with a maximum dosage of 50 grams. Double the dosage up to 100 grams if fresh *Sang Ye* is used. *Sang Ye* may be taken internally as a decoction or applied topically as an herbal paste. For decoctions, *Sang Ye* processed with honey has a stronger function to moisten the Lung and relieve cough. For topical applications, it should be crushed into paste prior to use.

CAUTIONS / CONTRAINDICATIONS

- Due to its cold nature, *Sang Ye* should be used with caution for patients who have constitutional deficiencies or cold.

Sang Ye (Folium Mori)

CHEMICAL COMPOSITION

Flavonoids (rutin 1.38-3.06%, quercetin, isoquercitrin), moracetin, campesterol, lupeol, myoinsitol, inokosterone, ecdysterone, hemolysin, moracelin, scopoletin, scoplin, phenolics hydroxycinnamic acid, 8-cyclohexenyflavones, cyclomorusin, oxydihydromorusin, astragalin, morusenin A, B; hydroxycoumarin, essential oils (linalool, eugenol).[1]

PHARMACOLOGICAL EFFECTS

- **Antibiotic**: *Sang Ye* has bactericidal action against *Staphylococcus aureus*, β-hemolytic streptococcus, *Bacillus diphtheriae, E. coli, Pseudomonas aeruginosa,* and leptospirosis.[2]
- **Metabolic**: The use of *Sang Ye* has been associated with decreased blood glucose and serum cholesterol levels in rats.[3]

CLINICAL STUDIES AND RESEARCH

- **Elephantiasis**: In one study, 1,638 patients with elephantiasis were treated with injections of 4 ml of 25 to 50% solution of *Sang Ye* one or two times daily. These patients also received herbs to reduce swelling and promote diuresis. The lower limbs of these patients were wrapped. The treatment duration ranged between 15 and 20 days per treatment course, totaling three courses of treatment per patient. The overall effective rate was reported to be approximately 99%.[4]
- **Psoriasis**: Intramuscular injections of *Sang Ye* were evaluated in the treatment of psoriasis in 31 patients. The treatment protocol was to administer 4 ml of *Sang Ye* via injection twice daily, for 7 days per treatment course. The study reported significant improvement in 81% of the patients.[5]

TOXICOLOGY

No fatalities were reported following a bolus intraperitoneal injection of 10% *Sang Ye* in mice at a dosage 250 times the normal adult human dose. In a follow-up study, daily intraperitoneal injection with 10% *Sang Ye* for 21 days did not cause any damage to internal organs, such as the liver, kidneys, and lungs.[6]

AUTHORS' COMMENTS

According to the *Ben Cao Gang Mu* (Materia Medica) by Li Shi-Zhen in 1578, *Sang Ye* also stimulates hair growth.

References

1. *Xian Dai Zhong Yao Yao Li Xue* (Contemporary Pharmacology of Chinese Herbs), 1997; 168-169
2. *Zhong Yao Yao Li Yu Ying Yong* (Pharmacology and Applications of Chinese Herbs), 1983
3. Ibid.
4. *Zhe Jiang Zhong Yi Yao* (Zhejiang Chinese Medicine and Herbology), 1979; 8:278
5. *Zhong Guo Nong Cun Yi Xue* (Chinese Agricultural Medicine), 1983; 3:24
6. *Zhong Yao Yao Li Yu Ying Yong* (Pharmacology and Applications of Chinese Herbs), 1983

Ju Hua (Flos Chrysanthemi)

菊花 菊花

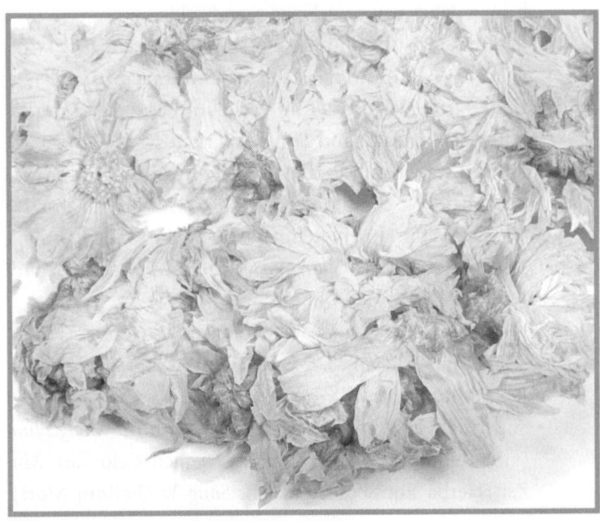

Pinyin Name: *Ju Hua*
Literal Name: "chrysanthemum flower"
Alternate Chinese Names: *Hang Ju, Bai Ju Hua, Huang Ju Hua, Hang Ju Hua*
Original Source: *Shen Nong Ben Cao Jing* (Divine Husbandman's Classic of the Materia Medica) in the second century
English Name: chrysanthemum flower
Botanical Name: *Chrysanthemum morifolium* Ramat.
Pharmaceutical Name: Flos Chrysanthemi
Properties: acrid, sweet, bitter, cool
Channels Entered: Lung, Liver

Ju Hua (Flos Chrysanthemi)

CHINESE THERAPEUTIC ACTIONS

1. Dispels Wind-Heat

Wind-heat: *Ju Hua* (Flos Chrysanthemi) is commonly used to dispel wind-heat and treat early-stage febrile disorders and wind-heat syndromes characterized by headache, fever, red and painful eyes, dizziness, dry mouth and throat, and a yellow tongue coat.

- Febrile disorders and wind-heat syndrome: use *Ju Hua* with *Sang Ye* (Folium Mori), *Bo He* (Herba Menthae), *Lu Gen* (Rhizoma Phragmitis), and *Lian Qiao* (Fructus Forsythiae). **Exemplar Formula:** *Sang Ju Yin* (Mulberry Leaf and Chrysanthemum Decoction).
- Headache: add *Qiang Huo* (Rhizoma et Radix Notopterygii), *Fang Feng* (Radix Saposhnikoviae), *Bai Zhi* (Radix Angelicae Dahuricae) and *Xi Xin* (Herba Asari) to relieve occipital or frontal headache, caused either by wind-heat or wind-cold.
- Headache from wind-heat: add it to *Chuan Xiong* (Rhizoma Ligustici Chuanxiong) and *Shi Gao* (Gypsum Fibrosum).
- Headache due to Liver wind and yin-deficient fire: use this herb with *Gou Teng* (Ramulus Uncariae cum Uncis), *Sheng Di Huang* (Radix Rehmanniae) and *Bai Shao* (Radix Paeoniae Alba).
- Wind-heat with sore throat: combine it with *Ban Lan Gen* (Radix Isatidis) or *Shan Dou Gen* (Radix Sophorae Tonkinensis).

2. Clears the Liver and Benefits the Eyes

Disorders of the eyes: *Ju Hua* is one of the most commonly used herbs in treatment of eye disorders. It treats eye disorders caused by wind-heat attacking the Liver channel, or Liver fire rising, with symptoms such as redness, swelling and pain in the eyes, superficial visual obstruction, and increased production of tears on exposure to wind. It treats blurred vision and dizziness from Liver and Kidney yin deficiencies. It is, however, contraindicated if the diagnosis is yang deficiency, or deficiency and cold.

- Redness, swelling and pain in the eyes: use *Ju Hua* with *Sang Ye* (Folium Mori), *Xia Ku Cao* (Spica Prunellae), *Chan Tui* (Periostracum Cicadae), *Mu Zei* (Herba Equiseti Hiemalis) and *Bai Ji Li* (Fructus Tribuli).
- Blurred vision and dizziness caused by Liver and Kidney yin deficiency: combine it with *Gou Qi Zi* (Fructus Lycii), *Shu Di Huang* (Radix Rehmanniae Preparata), *Shan Zhu Yu* (Fructus Corni), *Shan Yao* (Rhizoma Dioscoreae) and *Mu Dan Pi* (Cortex Moutan).
- Near-sightedness: add it to *Sheng Di Huang* (Radix Rehmanniae), *Tian Men Dong* (Radix Asparagi) and *Zhi Ke* (Fructus Aurantii).
- Superficial visual obstruction: use it with *Mi Meng Hua* (Flos Buddlejae), *Qing Xiang Zi* (Semen Celosiae), *Mu Zei* (Herba Equiseti Hiemalis), *Sang Ye* (Folium Mori) and *Chan Tui* (Periostracum Cicadae).
- Visual disturbances with dizziness and headache due to Liver yang rising: use *Ju Hua* with *Bai Ji Li* (Fructus Tribuli), *Jue Ming Zi* (Semen Cassiae), *Bai Shao* (Radix Paeoniae Alba) and *Man Jing Zi* (Fructus Viticis).

3. Calms Liver Yang

Hypertension: *Ju Hua* enters the Liver channel and calms rising Liver yang. It is commonly used to treat hypertension, dizziness, vertigo, and swelling and pain in the head associated with Liver yang rising.

- Liver yang rising: use it with *Shi Jue Ming* (Concha Haliotidis), *Bai Shao* (Radix Paeoniae Alba) and *Gou Teng* (Ramulus Uncariae cum Uncis).

4. Clears Heat and Eliminates Toxins

Dermatological disorders: *Ju Hua* clears heat and eliminates toxins from the exterior of the body and treats various dermatological disorders with abscesses and ulcerations.

- Sores, carbuncles and abscesses of the skin: use it with *Gan Cao* (Radix Glycyrrhizae), *Jin Yin Hua* (Flos Lonicerae) and *Pu Gong Ying* (Herba Taraxaci), and apply topically.

DOSAGE

10 to 15 grams. The maximum dosage of *Ju Hua* is 100 grams. *Ju Hua* can be used orally or topically. For oral administration, use in herbal decoction. For topical administration, the herb should be crushed into paste prior to application. It can also be taken as herbal tea on a daily basis to prevent buildup of heat.

CAUTIONS / CONTRAINDICATIONS

- Since *Ju Hua* is cool, it should be used with caution in patients with qi deficiency or cold in the Stomach, characterized by diarrhea, lack of appetite, or decreased food intake.
- *Ju Hua* is contraindicated for use in the presence of yang deficiency, or deficiency and cold.

CHEMICAL COMPOSITION

Essential oils 0.2-0.85% (borneol, bornyl acetate, chrysanthenone, camphor), flavone (luteolin, apigenin, acacetin), chrysanthemin A, B; chlorochrymorin, chrysandiol.[1]

PHARMACOLOGICAL EFFECTS

- **Vasodilative:** *Ju Hua* has been shown to dilate blood vessels. It increases blood perfusion to the coronary arteries, lowers blood pressure, and decreases body temperature.[2]
- **Antibiotic:** *Ju Hua* has been shown to inhibit *Staphylococcus aureus*, β-hemolytic streptococcus, and *Shigella sonnei*. It also has an inhibitory effect against leptospira at high doses.[3]

Ju Hua (Flos Chrysanthemi)

CLINICAL STUDIES AND RESEARCH

- **Coronary artery disease:** According to one study, 164 patients with coronary artery disease were treated with a preparation of *Ju Hua* (containing the equivalent of 50 grams of dried herb) for 2 months per treatment course, with a total treatment duration ranging between 1 and 2 courses. The study reported improvement based on symptom evaluation in 86.5% of patients, and improvement based on EKG evaluation in 45.3% of patients.[4]
- **Hypertension:** According to one report, 46 patients with hypertension were treated with herbs, with good results. The herbal formulation consisted of 24 to 30 grams each of *Ju Hua* and *Jin Yin Hua* (Flos Lonicerae) as the base formula. Furthermore, 12 grams of *Sang Ye* (Folium Mori) were added to address dizziness, and 12 to 24 grams of *Shan Zha* (Fructus Crataegi) to treat high cholesterol. After herbal treatment for 3 to 7 days, the study reported that 35 of 46 patients showed reduction of blood pressure, dizziness and insomnia.[5]

AUTHORS' COMMENTS

There are three different types of "*Ju Hua*" that are used medicinally:

- *Ye Ju Hua*, wild chrysanthemum flower, is strongest in clearing heat, eliminating toxins and treating sore throat, sores and carbuncles, and swollen, painful eyes.
- *Huang Ju Hua*, yellow chrysanthemum flower, is the strongest in dispelling wind-heat.
- *Bai Ju Hua*, white chrysanthemum flower, is strongest in sedating Liver fire, brightening the eyes and treating redness and pain in the eyes.

References

1. *Xian Dai Zhong Yao Yao Li Xue* (Contemporary Pharmacology of Chinese Herbs), 1997; 160-161
2. *Zhong Yao Xue* (Chinese Herbology), 1998; 97:99
3. *Yi Xue Ji Shu Zi Liao* (Resource of Medical Techniques), 1974; (1:2):113
4. *Zhe Jiang Yi Ke Da Xue Xue Bao* (Journal of Zhejiang Province School of Medicine), 1978; 4:9
5. *Xin Yi Yao Xue Za Zhi* (New Journal of Medicine and Herbology), 1972; 2:32

Man Jing Zi (Fructus Viticis)

蔓荆子 蔓荊子

Pinyin Name: *Man Jing Zi*
Alternate Chinese Names: *Man Jing Shi, Jing Zi*
Original Source: *Shen Nong Ben Cao Jing* (Divine Husbandman's Classic of the Materia Medica) in the second century
English Name: vitex, chastetree fruit, three-leaf chastetree fruit
Botanical Name: *Vitex rotundifolia* L. (*Dan Ye Mang Jing*); *Vitex trifolia* L. (*Mang Jing*)
Pharmaceutical Name: Fructus Viticis
Properties: acrid, bitter, cool
Channels Entered: Liver, Stomach, Urinary Bladder

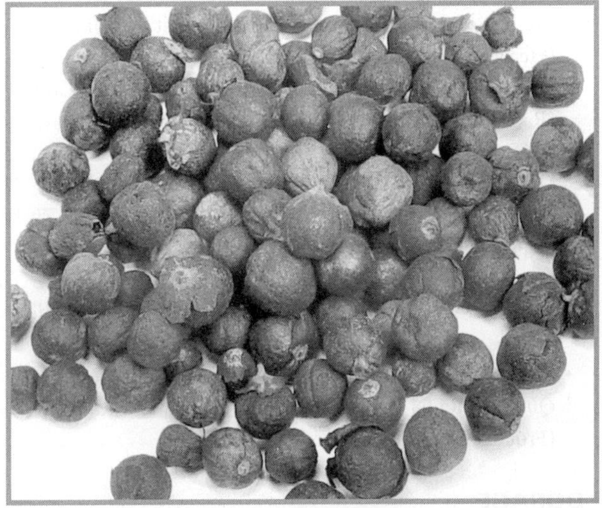

CHINESE THERAPEUTIC ACTIONS

1. Dispels Wind-Heat

Wind-heat: With its ascending and dispersing properties, *Man Jing Zi* (Fructus Viticis) is a strategic choice for dispelling wind-heat from the head and face. Clinical applications include dizziness, headache, and swelling and pain in the gums. It is especially useful when treating temporal headaches.

- Headache due to wind-heat: combine *Man Jing Zi* with *Fang Feng* (Radix Saposhnikoviae), *Ju Hua* (Flos

Man Jing Zi (Fructus Viticis)

Chrysanthemi), *Chuan Xiong* (Rhizoma Ligustici Chuanxiong) and *Shi Gao* (Gypsum Fibrosum).

- Headache, facial swelling and pain caused by wind-heat: add it to *Bo He* (Herba Menthae), *Jing Jie* (Herba Schizonepetae) and *Ju Hua* (Flos Chrysanthemi).
- Frontal or migraine headache: use *Man Jing Zi* individually, or in combination with *Ju Hua* (Flos Chrysanthemi), *Jing Jie* (Herba Schizonepetae) and *Tian Ma* (Rhizoma Gastrodiae).
- Temporal headache from wind-heat: use it with *Jing Jie* (Herba Schizonepetae), *Fang Feng* (Radix Saposhnikoviae), *Ju Hua* (Flos Chrysanthemi) and *Bai Ji Li* (Fructus Tribuli).
- Headache from internal wind resulting from blood deficiency: combine it with *Qiang Huo* (Rhizoma et Radix Notopterygii), *Fang Feng* (Radix Saposhnikoviae) and *Si Wu Tang* (Four-Substance Decoction).

2. Dispels Wind-Heat in the Liver Channel, Brightens the Eyes

Eye disorders: *Man Jing Zi* dispels wind-heat attacking the Liver channel. As wind-heat travels upwards along the Liver channel, it causes dizziness, redness and swelling of the eyes, and excessive tears. *Man Jing Zi* is also used for other eye disorders if combined with appropriate herbs.

- Eye disorders due to wind-heat attacking the Liver channel: use this herb with *Ju Hua* (Flos Chrysanthemi), *Chan Tui* (Periostracum Cicadae) and *Bai Ji Li* (Fructus Tribuli).
- Eye disorders due to wind-cold: combine it with *Jing Jie* (Herba Schizonepetae), *Fang Feng* (Radix Saposhnikoviae), *Bai Ji Li* (Fructus Tribuli), and *Gan Cao* (Radix Glycyrrhizae).

3. Dispels Wind and Relieves Pain

***Bi zheng* (painful obstruction syndrome):** *Man Jing Zi* dispels wind and dampness that has attacked the muscles, to relieve various aches and pains. It is commonly used to treat arthritis or painful joints with spasms and cramps caused by wind and dampness.

- *Bi zheng:* use it with *Fang Feng* (Radix Saposhnikoviae), *Qin Jiao* (Radix Gentianae Macrophyllae), and *Mu Gua* (Fructus Chaenomelis).

DOSAGE

6 to 12 grams. The maximum dosage of *Man Jing Zi* is 30 grams. This herb should be dry-fried and crushed to facilitate extraction of the active constituents.

CAUTIONS / CONTRAINDICATIONS

- *Man Jing Zi* should be used with caution for patients who have Spleen and Stomach deficiencies, or yin-deficient fire.
- *Man Jing Zi* should be used with caution in patients who have dizziness or headaches because of blood deficiency. In this case, blood tonics should be used.

CHEMICAL COMPOSITION

Vitexicarpin, vitexilactone, previtexilactone, luteolin, p-hydroxybenzoic acid, vanillic acid, camphene, pinene, vitamin A.[1,2]

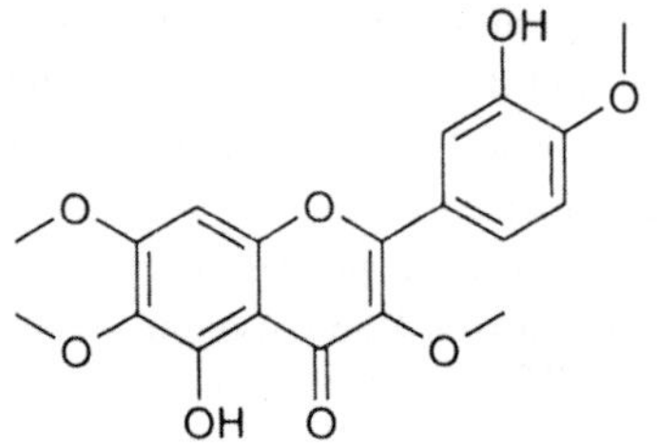

Vitexicarpin

PHARMACOLOGICAL EFFECTS

- **Antibiotic**: Vitexicarpin has an inhibitory effect against *Staphylococcus aureus*, *Bacillus cereus*, and *Bacillus megaterium*.[3]
- **Others**: It has antipyretic, analgesic and sedative effects.[4]

CLINICAL STUDIES AND RESEARCH

- **Allergic sinusitis:** According to one report, 35 patients with allergic sinusitis were treated with a topical solution consisting of 20% *Man Jing Ye* (Folium Viticis). The treatment protocol was to instill 3 to 5 drops of the solution directly into the nostrils three to five times daily for 2 days. This short-term treatment was effective for most patients.[5]

AUTHORS' COMMENTS

Man Jing Zi and *Tian Ma* (Rhizoma Gastrodiae) both treat headache due to wind. *Man Jing Zi* is used for headaches caused by exterior wind-heat, while *Tian Ma* is used for headaches and vertigo due to internal Liver wind.

References

1. *Xian Dai Zhong Yao Yao Li Xue* (Contemporary Pharmacology of Chinese Herbs), 1997; 183
2. Yan X, Zhou J, Xie G, *Traditional Chinese Medicines Molecular Structures, Natural Sources and Applications*; Ashgate, 1999; 6672
3. *Zhong Cao Yao Xue* (Study of Chinese Herbal Medicine), 1980; 915
4. *Zhong Yao Xue* (Chinese Herbology), 1998; 99:100
5. *Guang Xi Wei Sheng* (Guangxi Province Public Health), 1976; 1:32

Mu Zeí (Herba Equiseti Hiemalis)

木賊 木贼

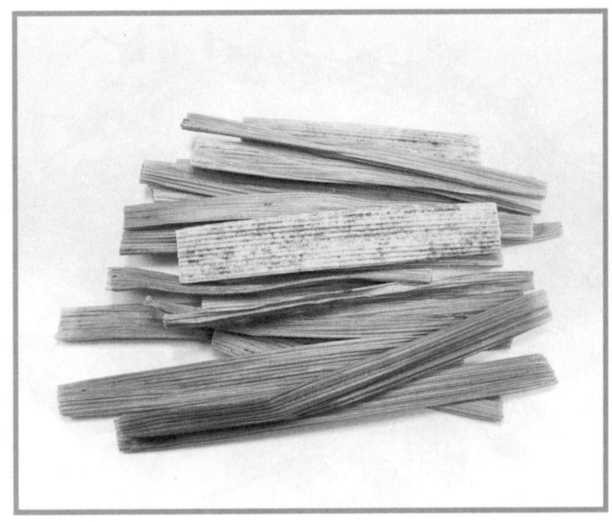

Pinyin Name: *Mu Zei*
Literal Name: "wood thief"
Alternate Chinese Names: *Mu Zei Cao, Jie Jie Cao*
Original Source: *Jia You Ben Cao* (Materia Medica of the Jia You Era) by Zhang Yu-Xi and Su Song in 1057-1060
English Name: equisetum, common scouring rush, Dutch rushes, rough horsetail
Botanical Name: *Equisetum hiemale* L.
Pharmaceutical Name: Herba Equiseti Hiemalis
Properties: sweet, bitter, neutral
Channels Entered: Lung, Liver, Gallbladder

CHINESE THERAPEUTIC ACTIONS

1. Dispels Wind-Heat, Brightens the Eyes and Removes Superficial Visual Obstruction

Eye disorders accompanying wind-heat invasion: *Mu Zei* (Herba Equiseti Hiemalis) dispels wind-heat affecting the Lung, Liver and Gallbladder channels. It is commonly used to treat red eyes, excessive tearing, blurred vision, and pterygium caused by wind-heat.

- Blurred vision and excessive tearing: use *Mu Zei* with *Cang Zhu* (Rhizoma Atractylodis).
- Redness, swelling and pain in the eyes, pterygium: combine it with *Ju Hua* (Flos Chrysanthemi).
- Red eyes: use *Mu Zei* with *Shi Jue Ming* (Concha Haliotidis).
- Night blindness due to Liver blood deficiency: combine this herb with *Ye Ming Sha* (Excrementum Vespertilionis Murini), *Dang Gui* (Radicis Angelicae Sinensis), *Chan Tui* (Periostracum Cicadae) and goat liver to tonify the Liver and nourish the blood.

2. Stops Bleeding

Hematochezia or hemorrhoids: *Mu Zei* has hemostatic action, and is commonly used to treat gastrointestinal bleeding and hemorrhoids.

- Hematochezia or hemorrhoids: use this herb with *Di Yu* (Radix Sanguisorbae) and *Huai Jiao* (Fructus Sophorae) to clear heat and stop bleeding.
- Bloody dysentery: use 15 or 30 grams of *Mu Zei* individually.

DOSAGE

3 to 10 grams. The maximum dosage of *Mu Zei* is 30 grams.

CAUTIONS / CONTRAINDICATIONS

- Use *Mu Zei* with caution for patients with deficiency of qi, blood, yin or yang.
- Use *Mu Zei* with caution for pregnant women.
- *Mu Zei* is not recommended for patients with red eyes caused by Liver yang rising.
- Long-term usage of this herb is not recommended.

CHEMICAL COMPOSITION

Flavones 0.10% (kaempferol, kaempferol-3,7-diglucoside, kaempferol-3-diglucoside, hippochaete, herbacetrin, gossypitrin), succinic acid, ferulic acid, caffic acid, vanillin, palustrine, dimethyl sulfone, thymine.[1]

PHARMACOLOGICAL EFFECTS

- **Antihypertensive**: Intraperitoneal injection of alcohol extract of *Mu Zei* has a prolonged influence in reducing blood pressure in anesthetized cats. The antihypertensive effect of *Mu Zei* has a positive dose-to-effect relationship.[2]
- **Others**: It has mild anti-inflammatory, diuretic, sedative, and antiplatelet actions.[3,4]

References

1. *Xian Dai Zhong Yao Yao Li Xue* (Contemporary Pharmacology of Chinese Herbs), 1997; 180
2. *Hu Bei Zhong Yi Za Zhi* (Hubei Journal of Chinese Medicine), 1980; (5):52
3. *Zhong Yao Xue* (Chinese Herbology), 1998; 109:110
4. *Yi Xue Xue Bao* (Report of Medicine), 1980; 15(6):321

Yi Zhi Xiang (Herba Vernoniae Cinereae)

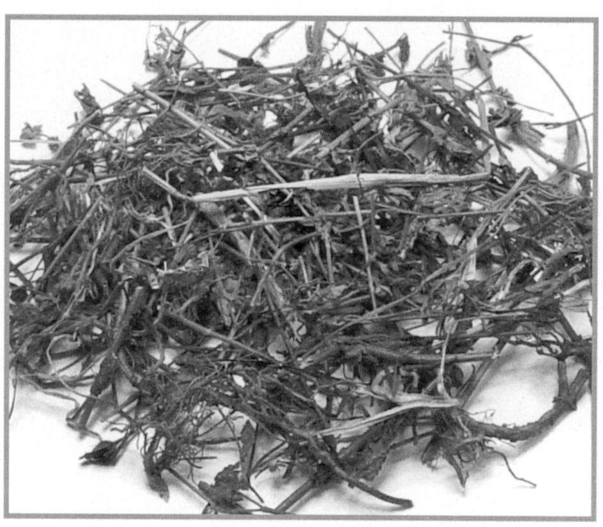

一枝香

Pinyin Name: *Yi Zhi Xiang*
Literal Name: "individual fragrance"
Alternate Chinese Names: *Shang Han Cao, Ye Zai Cao, Sheng Zhi Xiang*
English Name: vernonia
Botanical Name: *Vernonia cinerea* Less
Pharmaceutical Name: Herba Vernoniae Cinereae
Properties: acrid, bitter, cool
Channels Entered: Lung, Liver

CHINESE THERAPEUTIC ACTIONS

1. Dispels Wind-Heat and Clears Lung Heat

Lung heat or wind-heat: *Yi Zhi Xiang* (Herba Vernoniae Cinereae) is excellent for treating invasion of wind-heat that is turning into Lung heat with sore throat, cough, yellow phlegm and possibly fever.

- Sore throat caused by wind-heat: use *Yi Zhi Xiang* with *Ban Lan Gen* (Radix Isatidis), *Zao Xiu* (Rhizoma Paridis) and *Da Qing Ye* (Folium Isatidis).
- Inflammation of the throat, bronchitis: combine it with *Zhu Zi Cao* (Herba Euphorbiae Thymifoliae), *Ya She Huang* (Herba Lippiae), *Pao Zai Cao* (Herba Physalis Angulatae) and *Ban Bian Lian* (Herba Lobeliae Chinensis).

2. Sedates Liver Fire

Yi Zhi Xiang disperses qi stagnation, reduces inflammation and eliminates toxins in cases of Liver fire.

- Conjunctivitis: use it with *Shan Pu Tao* (Radix Vitis Amurensis), *Qian Li Guang* (Herba Senecionis Scandens) and *Long Dan Xie Gan Tang* (Gentiana Decoction to Drain the Liver).
- Bloody dysentery, abdominal bloating: combine this herb with *Feng Wei Cao* (Herba Pteris), *Bai Tou Weng* (Radix Pulsatillae), *Qin Pi* (Cortex Fraxini), *Huang Lian* (Rhizoma Coptidis), *Huang Bai* (Cortex Phellodendri), *Huai Hua* (Flos Sophorae) and charred *Di Yu* (Radix Sanguisorbae).

DOSAGE

6 to 30 grams in decoction.

CAUTIONS / CONTRAINDICATIONS

- Use *Yi Zhi Xiang* with caution in patients with deficiency and cold of the Spleen and Stomach.

Ge Gen (Radix Puerariae)

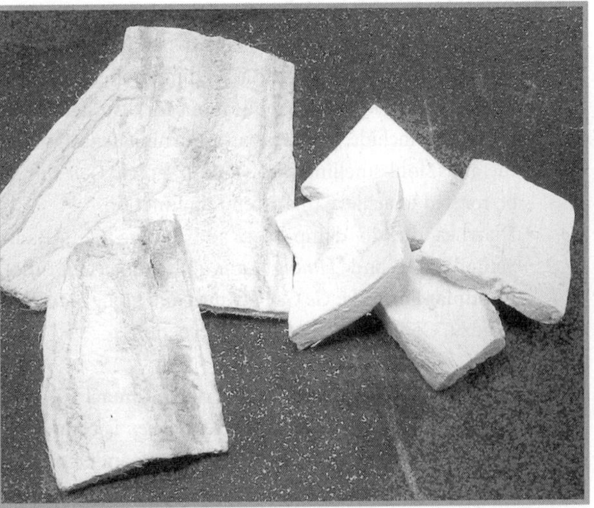

葛根 葛根

Pinyin Name: *Ge Gen*
Literal Name: "Ge's root"
Alternate Chinese Names: *Gan Ge, Fen Ge*
Original Source: *Shen Nong Ben Cao Jing* (Divine Husbandman's Classic of the Materia Medica) in the second century
English Name: pueraria root, kudzu, lobed kudzuvine root, thomson kudzuvine root
Botanical Name: *Pueraria lobata* (*Wild.*) Ohwi. (*Ye Ge*); *Pueraria thomsonii* Benth. (*Gan Ge*)
Pharmaceutical Name: Radix Puerariae
Properties: sweet, acrid, cool
Channels Entered: Spleen, Stomach

CHINESE THERAPEUTIC ACTIONS

1. Dispels Wind from the Exterior and Releases Muscles

Wind-heat: *Ge Gen* (Radix Puerariae) is excellent for relieving wind-heat that manifests in headache, fever, stiffness and pain in the neck and shoulders. This herb enters the Spleen, which controls the muscles. *Ge Gen* is acrid and cool, and thus dispels pathogenic factors from the muscle layer and relieves pain. When combined with other herbs, it can treat both wind-cold and wind-heat syndromes. The unprocessed form is stronger for this application.

- Wind-cold syndrome without perspiration: use *Ge Gen* with *Gui Zhi* (Ramulus Cinnamomi) and *Ma Huang* (Herba Ephedrae) to promote diaphoresis and dispel wind-cold. **Exemplar Formula:** *Ge Gen Tang* (Kudzu Decoction).
- Wind-heat: use it with *Chai Hu* (Radix Bupleuri), *Huang Qin* (Radix Scutellariae) and *Shi Gao* (Gypsum Fibrosum). **Exemplar Formula:** *Chai Ge Jie Ji Tang* (Bupleurum and Kudzu Decoction to Release the Muscle Layer).
- Wind-cold syndrome with perspiration: add this herb to *Gui Zhi* (Ramulus Cinnamomi) and *Bai Shao* (Radix Paeoniae Alba) to dispel wind-cold and harmonize *wei* (defense) and *ying* (nutritive) levels. **Exemplar Formula:** *Gui Zhi Jia Ge Gen Tang* (Cinnamon Twig Decoction plus Kudzu).
- Half-exterior and half-interior syndrome: combine it with *Qiang Huo* (Rhizoma et Radix Notopterygii), *Chai Hu* (Radix Bupleuri), *Huang Qin* (Radix Scutellariae) and *Shi Gao* (Gypsum Fibrosum) to harmonize the exterior and the interior, and to relieve symptoms such as fever, aversion to heat, thirst, and inappropriate absence of perspiration.

2. Promotes the Eruption of Measles

Incomplete expression of measles: *Ge Gen* releases pathogenic factors from the skin and muscles, and is commonly used to promote eruption of measles.

- Measles: use *Ge Gen* with *Sheng Ma* (Rhizoma Cimicifugae), *Bai Shao* (Radix Paeoniae Alba) and *Gan Cao* (Radix Glycyrrhizae).

3. Clears Heat, Generates Fluids

Febrile disorders: *Ge Gen* has a dual action of clearing heat and generating body fluids simultaneously. It is commonly used for patients in whom internal heat is drying body fluids (especially those of the Stomach), leading to thirst, dry mouth, increased intake of water, and possibly fidgeting and irritability. It is one of the key herbs in clearing *yangming* stage heat where thirst is one of the predominant signs. Patients manifesting such symptoms might have febrile disorders or *xiao ke* (wasting and thirsting) syndrome.

- Internal heat with fluid deficiency: use *Ge Gen* with *Tian Hua Fen* (Radix Trichosanthis), *Huang Qi* (Radix Astragali), and *Mai Men Dong* (Radix Ophiopogonis). **Exemplar Formula:** *Yu Quan Wan* (Jade Spring Pills).
- *Xiao ke* (wasting and thirsting) syndrome: combine it with *Tian Hua Fen* (Radix Trichosanthis), *Sheng Di Huang* (Radix Rehmanniae), *Mai Men Dong* (Radix Ophiopogonis), *Shi Gao* (Gypsum Fibrosum) and *Zhi Mu* (Radix Anemarrhenae) to sedate heat, moisten dryness, and promote secretion of body fluids.
- Irritability: combine *Ge Gen* with *Zhi Zi* (Fructus Gardeniae).

Ge Gen (Radix Puerariae)

4. Lifts Yang Qi and Stops Diarrhea

Diarrhea due to damp-heat: *Ge Gen* separates the clear from the turbid, and with its ascending property, it helps to stop diarrhea. Clinical applications for disorders in the lower *jiao* include diarrhea with burning sensations of the anus, foul-smelling stools and fever. *Ge Gen* should be roasted to achieve this ascending function.

- Diarrhea due to damp-heat: add *Huang Qin* (Radix Scutellariae) and *Huang Lian* (Rhizoma Coptidis). **Exemplar Formula:** *Ge Gen Huang Qin Huang Lian Tang* (Kudzu, Coptis, and Scutellaria Decoction).

Chronic diarrhea from Spleen and Stomach qi prolapse: Due to its ascending nature, *Ge Gen* is commonly used to raise the yang qi of the Spleen and Stomach. Patients suffering from this condition will show fatigue, poor appetite and chronic diarrhea. The roasted form of *Ge Gen* should be used here to protect the middle *jiao*.

- Chronic diarrhea due to Spleen qi deficiency: use it with *Ren Shen* (Radix Ginseng), *Bai Zhu* (Rhizoma Atractylodis Macrocephalae), *Fu Ling* (Poria), and *Mu Xiang* (Radix Aucklandiae).

5. Treats Hypertension

Hypertension: *Ge Gen* has recently been used to successfully treat hypertension, headache, stiff neck, tinnitus and dizziness. It is also useful for coronary heart disease, angina pectoris and sudden deafness.

DOSAGE

10 to 20 grams. The maximum dosage of *Ge Gen* is 60 grams. The unprocessed herb has a stronger function to release pathogenic factors from the muscle layer and reduce fever. Roasting increases the warmth of any herb; therefore, roasted *Ge Gen* has a stronger effect to treat diarrhea, but is weaker for releasing the exterior than it would be in its unprocessed form.

CAUTIONS / CONTRAINDICATIONS

- Use of *Ge Gen* may be associated with nausea and vomiting because of its cool nature. Patients with cold in the Stomach, or yang deficiency, should use this herb with caution.
- *Ge Gen* also should be used with caution during the summer, when excess perspiration accompanies wind-heat invasion.

CHEMICAL COMPOSITION

Isoflavonoids 1.43 to 12.30% (puerarin, daidzin, daidzein, daidzein 4,7-diglucoside, formononetin, genistein), triterpenoid sapogenols.[1,2]

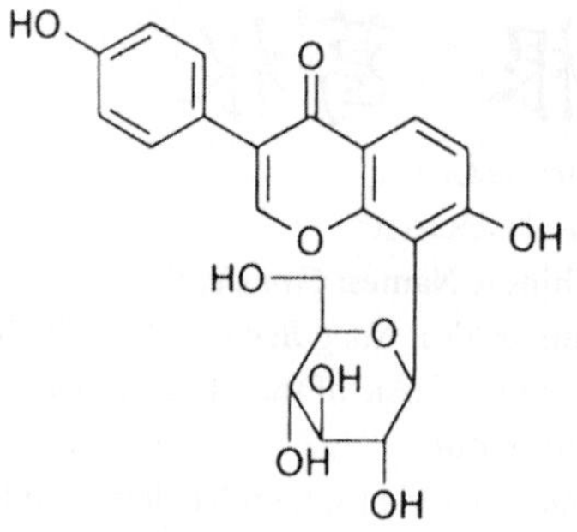

HO, O, OH, HO, O, OH, OH, OH

Puerarin

PHARMACOLOGICAL EFFECTS

- **Cardiovascular:** *Ge Gen* has marked effectiveness in dilating coronary blood vessels, relieving spasms of these vessels, and reducing the oxygen requirement of the cardiac muscles. In one laboratory study, administration of water or alcohol extracts of *Ge Gen* via intraperitoneal or subcutaneous injection was effective in treating rats with acute myocardial ischemia. *Ge Gen* also dilates the blood vessels of the brain and increases local perfusion.[3,4]
- **Antiplatelet:** Puerarin has been shown to inhibit platelet aggregation in mice.[5]
- **Antihypertensive:** Both water and alcohol extracts of *Ge Gen* have shown marked effectiveness in lowering blood pressure.[6]
- **Antipyretic:** *Ge Gen* has mild antipyretic action through vessel dilation.[7]
- **Antidiabetic:** Oral administration of *Ge Gen* in herbal decoction has been shown to have mild influence in lowering blood glucose levels.[8]
- **Antispasmodic:** *Ge Gen* has been shown to relieve intestinal muscle spasms and cramps.[9]
- **Antialcoholic:** Administration of isoflavonoids of *Ge Gen*, namely daidzin and daidzein, have been associated with marked antialcoholic effects in hamsters that were trained or genetically bred to prefer and consume large amounts of ethanol.[10]

CLINICAL STUDIES AND RESEARCH

- **Coronary artery disorder:** Intravenous injection of puerarin was evaluated for the treatment of coronary artery disorder. Thirty patients received this treatment for 6 days. The study authors reported a decrease of oxygen consumption requirement by cardiac muscle. The study concluded that puerarin injections may be useful in the treatment of coronary artery disease.[11]
- **Hypertension:** In one study, 222 patients with hypertension accompanied by neck stiffness and pain were treated with *Ge Gen*, with a rate of effectiveness between 78 and 90%.[12]

Ge Gen (Radix Puerariae)

- **Sudden deafness**: According to one report, 100 patients with sudden deafness were treated with *Ge Gen* pills and injectables. *Ge Gen* pills (1.5 to 4.5 grams of dried herb per dose) were administered orally three times daily and the injectables (100 mg of daidzein) were administered twice daily. The treatment duration ranged between 1 to 2 months, with an overall 76% rate of effectiveness.[13]
- **Migraine headache**: In one study, 53 patients with migraine headaches were given *Ge Gen* pills, containing 100 mg of puerarin, three times daily, for 2 to 22 days. The overall rate of effectiveness reported was 83%.[14]

HERB-DRUG INTERACTION

- **Antidiabetics:** It is prudent to use *Ge Gen* with caution with insulin, sulfonylureas, and other antidiabetic medications as the combination may have a synergistic effect, leading to hypoglycemia.[15] [Note: Examples of antidiabetic drugs include insulin, tolbutamide (Orinase), glipizide (Glucotrol), and glyburide (DiaBeta/Micronase).]
- **Anticoagulant or antiplatelet drugs:** *Ge Gen* has an antiplatelet effect, and should be used with caution in patients who take anticoagulant or antiplatelet medications. Though this potential interaction has not been documented, this herb may potentiate the effect of drugs such as warfarin.[16] [Note: Examples of anticoagulants include heparin, warfarin (Coumadin) and enoxaparin (Lovenox); and examples of antiplatelets include aspirin, dipyridamole (Persantine), and clopidogrel (Plavix).]

TOXICOLOGY

No toxic reaction was observed following oral administration of *Ge Gen* powder at 10 to 20 g/kg for 3 days. The LD_{50} for intravenous injection of alcohol extract of *Ge Gen* is 2.1 +/- 0.12 g/kg in mice.[17]

SUPPLEMENT

- 葛花 / 葛花 *Ge Hua* (Flos Puerariae), the flower derived from the same plant as *Ge Gen*, is usually harvested as a bud, or before it completely blossoms. It was first cited in the *Shen Nong Ben Cao Jing* (Divine Husbandman's Classic of the Materia Medica) in the second century. It is sweet, neutral and enters the Stomach channel. It increases the metabolism of alcohol, relieves hangover and promotes the process of regaining sobriety. Common clinical applications include: excessive intake of alcohol, headache, fever, irritability, thirst, chest and abdominal fullness and distention, lack of appetite, vomiting of sour fluids. Both the root and the flower are believed to have the same property for treatment of alcoholism, hangover, and liver-related disorders caused by alcohol. *Ge Hua* is often combined with *Ren Shen* (Radix Ginseng), *Bai Dou Kou* (Fructus Amomi Rotundus) and *Chen Pi* (Pericarpium Citri Reticulatae) to relieve hangover, such as the combination *Ge Hua Jie Cheng San* (Pueraria Flower Powder for Detoxification and Awakening). Common dosage for *Ge Hua* is 3 to 12 grams in decoctions or in pills. *Ge Hua* is contraindicated in patients who are not experiencing hangover, as it may injure the yin with its strong dispersing property.

AUTHORS' COMMENTS

According to Dr. Chen Yuan-Da, *Ge Gen* is one of the best and most effective herbs for the treatment of acute neck and shoulder injuries. Immediate pain relief and increased range of motion can be achieved immediately when a large dose of *Ge Gen* is used in conjunction with *Bai Shao* (Radix Paeoniae Alba) and *Gan Cao* (Radix Glycyrrhizae).

References

1. *Xian Dai Zhong Yao Yao Li Xue* (Contemporary Pharmacology of Chinese Herbs), 1997; 145-146
2. Yan X, Zhou J, Xie G, *Traditional Chinese Medicines Molecular Structures, Natural Sources and Applications*; Ashgate, 1999; 5397
3. *Yi Xue Yan Jiu Tong Xun* (Report of Medical Studies), 1972; (2):14
4. *Zhong Hua Yi Xue Za Zhi* (Chinese Journal of Medicine), 1979; 59(8):479
5. *Xin Zhang Xue Guan Ji Bing* (Cardiovascular Diseases), 1979; (12):1
6. *Zhong Yao Xue* (Chinese Herbology), 1998; 101:103
7. Ibid.
8. Ibid.
9. Ibid.
10. *Phytochemistry.* 47(4):499-506, 1998 Feb.
11. *Zhong Hua Xin Xue Guan Bing Za Zhi* (Chinese Journal of Cardiology), 1985; 3:175
12. *Zhong Cao Yao Tong Xun* (Journal of Chinese Herbal Medicine), 1975; 2:34
13. *Zhong Hua Yi Xue Za Zhi* (Chinese Journal of Medicine), 1973, 10:591
14. *Zhong Hua Nei Ke Za Zhi* (Chinese Journal of Internal Medicine), 1977; 6:326
15. Chen, J. Recognition & prevention of herb-drug interactions, *Medical Acupuncture*, Fall/Winter 1998/1999; volume 10/number 2; 9-13
16. Ibid.
17. *Zhong Guo Yao Li Xue Yu Du Li Xue Za Zhi* (Journal of Herbology and Toxicology), 1992; 8(3):233

Chai Hu (Radix Bupleuri)

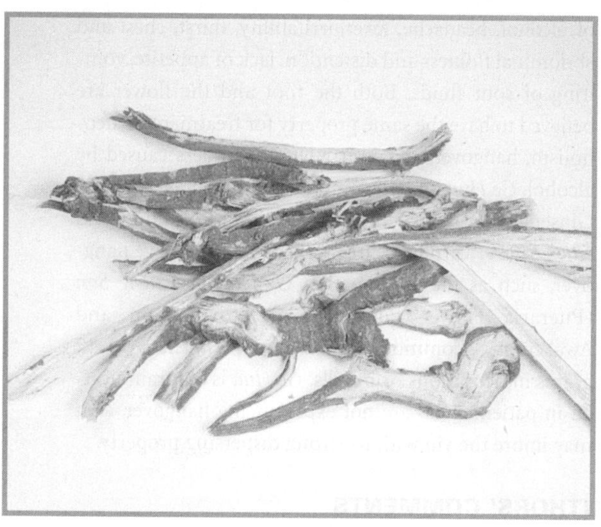

柴胡

Pinyin Name: *Chai Hu*
Literal Name: "kindling of the barbarians"
Original Source: *Shen Nong Ben Cao Jing* (Divine Husbandman's Classic of the Materia Medica) in the second century
English Name: bupleurum, hare's ear, Chinese thorowax root, red thorowax root
Botanical Name: *Bupleurum chinense* DC. (*Bei Chai Hu*); *Bupleurum scorzoneraefolium* Willd. (*Nan Chai Hu*)
Pharmaceutical Name: Radix Bupleuri
Properties: bitter, acrid, cool
Channels Entered: Liver, Gallbladder

CHINESE THERAPEUTIC ACTIONS

1. Harmonizes the Exterior and the Interior

***Shaoyang* syndrome:** *Chai Hu* (Radix Bupleuri), with its ascending and dispersing functions, is the key herb in treating *shaoyang* syndrome, a disorder in which the pathogenic factor is trapped halfway between the exterior and the interior. Due to the complexity of this condition, patients will exhibit both exterior and interior symptoms and signs, such as alternate spells of chills and fever, fullness and distention of the chest and hypochondriac region, a bitter taste in the mouth, dry throat, poor appetite, nausea and vertigo, irritability, and a wiry pulse. *Chai Hu* harmonizes *shaoyang* conditions, meaning that it will guide the trapped pathogenic factors outwards.

- *Shaoyang* syndrome: use *Chai Hu* with *Huang Qin* (Radix Scutellariae). *Chai Hu* eliminates the pathogenic factor from the exterior and *Huang Qin* clears heat from the interior. The combination of these two herbs eliminates pathogenic factors from both the exterior and the interior, and harmonizes half-exterior half-interior conditions. **Exemplar Formula:** *Xiao Chai Hu Tang* (Minor Bupleurum Decoction).
- *Shaoyang* and *yangming* syndromes together: use this herb with *Huang Qin* (Radix Scutellariae), *Bai Shao* (Radix Paeoniae Alba), *Zhi Zi* (Fructus Gardeniae) and *Da Huang* (Radix et Rhizoma Rhei). **Exemplar Formula:** *Da Chai Hu Tang* (Major Bupleurum Decoction).
- Lingering exterior conditions with the pathogenic factor entering the *shaoyang* stage, with fever: combine *Chai Hu* with *Ge Gen* (Radix Puerariae) and *Huang Qin* (Radix Scutellariae). **Exemplar Formula:** *Chai Ge Jie Ji Tang* (Bupleurum and Pueraria Combination).

Malaria is considered a *shaoyang* disorder, as patients often have alternating spells of chills and fever. *Chai Hu* is used for its ability to dispel the pathogenic factor and harmonize the interior and exterior.

- Malaria: use *Chai Hu* with *Qing Hao* (Herba Artemisiae Annuae), *Bing Lang* (Semen Arecae), *Chang Shan* (Radix Dichroae) and *Cao Guo* (Fructus Tsaoko).

2. Spreads the Liver and Relieves Liver Qi Stagnation

Liver qi stagnation: Acrid and aromatic, *Chai Hu* has ascending and dispersing characteristics. It is commonly used to unblock Liver qi stagnation and spread Liver qi. Clinical manifestations of Liver qi stagnation include emotional distress, fullness and distention of the chest and hypochondrium, irritability, headache, eye disorders, breast swelling and pain, irregular menstruation, amenorrhea or menstrual cramps, and jaundice.

- Liver qi stagnation with stress and emotional distress: combine *Chai Hu* with *Bai Shao* (Radix Paeoniae Alba), *Dang Gui* (Radicis Angelicae Sinensis), and *Bo He* (Herba Menthae). **Exemplar Formula:** *Xiao Yao San* (Rambling Powder).
- Liver qi stagnation causing hypochondriac fullness and pain: use this herb with *Bai Shao* (Radix Paeoniae Alba), *Chuan Xiong* (Rhizoma Ligustici Chuanxiong) and *Zhi Ke* (Fructus Aurantii). **Exemplar Formula:** *Chai Hu Shu Gan Tang* (Bupleurum Powder to Spread the Liver).
- Liver qi stagnation with cold extremities: add *Xiang Fu* (Rhizoma Cyperi), *Zhi Shi* (Fructus Aurantii Immaturus) and *Bai Shao* (Radix Paeoniae Alba). **Exemplar Formula:** *Si Ni San* (Frigid Extremities Powder).
- Migraine headache: combine *Chai Hu* with *Chuan Xiong* (Rhizoma Ligustici Chuanxiong), *Xiang Fu*

Chai Hu (Radix Bupleuri)

(Rhizoma Cyperi) and *Bai Shao* (Radix Paeoniae Alba) to treat migraine headache caused by *shaoyang* fire attacking the head.

- Eye disorders: use it with *Huang Qin* (Radix Scutellariae), *Zhi Zi* (Fructus Gardeniae), *Fang Feng* (Radix Saposhnikoviae) and *Jue Ming Zi* (Semen Cassiae) to treat eye disorders due to Liver fire rising, characterized by eye redness, swelling and pain.
- Irregular menstruation with pain and cramps: use *Chai Hu* with *Dang Gui* (Radicis Angelicae Sinensis), *Bai Shao* (Radix Paeoniae Alba), *Xiang Fu* (Rhizoma Cyperi) and *Mu Dan Pi* (Cortex Moutan) to nourish blood and regulate menstruation.
- Jaundice: add *Yin Chen Hao* (Herba Artemisiae Scopariae), *Da Huang* (Radix et Rhizoma Rhei), and *Zhi Zi* (Fructus Gardeniae) to clear damp-heat attacking both Liver and Gallbladder (leading to stasis of bile).

3. Lifts Yang Qi

Prolapsed organs: Because of its ascending nature, *Chai Hu* is commonly used to treat prolapse of internal organs caused by yang or qi deficiency. Clinical applications include prolapse of the rectum and uterus with shortness of breath, fatigue, hypermenorrhea, polyuria and other symptoms of yang and qi deficiency.

- Prolapse of internal organs: use *Chai Hu* with *Sheng Ma* (Rhizoma Cimicifugae) and *Huang Qi* (Radix Astragali) to raise yang and tonify qi. **Exemplar Formula:** *Bu Zhong Yi Qi Tang* (Tonify the Middle and Augment the Qi Decoction).

DOSAGE

3 to 10 grams. The maximum dosage of *Chai Hu* is 60 grams. Treatment of organ prolapse relies on only a small dosage (3 grams) to raise yang qi. Treatment of malaria, however, requires a larger dose (10 to 15 grams). Unprocessed *Chai Hu* has a stronger effect to ascend and disperse, and is commonly used to release the exterior and reduce fever. The vinegar-fried herb more effectively regulates Liver qi, and is commonly used to relieve hypochondriac pain, abdominal pain, and menstrual cramps.

CAUTIONS / CONTRAINDICATIONS

- *Chai Hu* has ascending and dispersing functions, so prolonged use or overdose may consume yin. Therefore, this herb should be used with caution in yin-deficient patients, those with yin-deficient fire, Liver yang rising, or Liver wind rising.
- *Chai Hu* should not be used for an individual having only an exterior syndrome but no interior symptoms or condition. Use of *Chai Hu* under these circumstances may lead the pathogenic factor inward, making the disease more difficult to treat.

CHEMICAL COMPOSITION

Triterpenoids (saikosaponin A, B, C, D, E; saikogenin F, G, E; saikoside), essential oils 0.06-0.16% (r-heptalactone, r-decalactone), carbohydrates, flavone, coumarin, organic acid.[1,2]

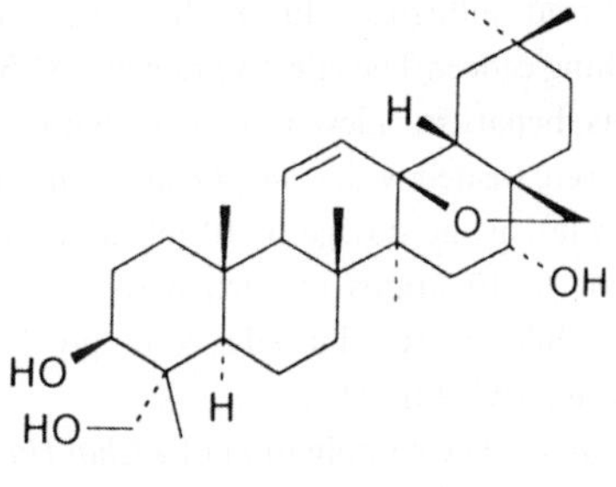

Saikosaponin

PHARMACOLOGICAL EFFECTS

- **Analgesic and antipyretic**: According to laboratory studies, essential oil, saikosaponin, and decoction of *Chai Hu* all have demonstrated marked analgesic and antipyretic effects. The analgesic effect was partially blocked with oral ingestion of atropine at 25 mg/kg or subcutaneous injection of naloxone at 0.26 mg/kg.[3]
- **Sedative**: *Chai Hu* and saikosaponin have both demonstrated a sedative effect. Oral ingestion of saikosaponin at 200 to 800 mg/kg has a marked sedative effect in mice. At 500 mg/kg, saikosaponin prolonged sleeping time induced by barbiturates.[4]
- **Anti-inflammatory**: *Chai Hu* reduces inflammation by decreasing capillary permeability caused by histamine and 5-hydroxy-tryptamine.[5]
- **Hepatoprotective**: *Chai Hu* has demonstrated hepatoprotective activity in laboratory animals, especially against carbon tetrachloride-induced liver damage.[6]
- **Cholagogic**: *Chai Hu* has a marked cholagogic effect, achieved by increased production and excretion of bile.[7]
- **Antihyperlipidemic**: Saikosaponin A and D have demonstrated marked effectiveness in reducing triglycerides and moderate influence in reducing cholesterol.[8]
- **Immunostimulant**: *Chai Hu* stimulates both humoral and cellular immunity in mice.[9]
- **Antibiotic**: *Chai Hu* has demonstrated an inhibitory effect against β-hemolytic streptococcus, *Vibrio cholerae*, *Mycobacterium tuberculosis*, leptospira, some influenza viruses, poliomyelitis viruses, and hepatitis viruses.[10]

CLINICAL STUDIES AND RESEARCH

- **Common cold**: According to one study, 666 patients with common colds were treated with an herbal formulation consisting of *Chai Hu*, *Fang Feng* (Radix Saposhnikoviae), *Chen Pi* (Pericarpium Citri Reticulatae), *Bai Shao* (Radix Paeoniae Alba), *Gan Cao* (Radix Glycyrrhizae), and *Sheng*

Chai Hu (Radix Bupleuri)

Jiang (Rhizoma Zingiberis Recens). The patients received 12 grams of the herbal formulation three times daily. The rate of effectiveness was 79%.[11]

- **Cough**: In one study, 1,005 patients were treated with a preparation of *Chai Hu*. The etiology of cough included common cold, influenza, chronic bronchitis, pneumonia, and lung cancer. The effective rate was 85.5%.[12]
- **Infectious hepatitis**: Eleven patients with infectious hepatitis were treated with *Chai Hu* and *Gan Cao* (Radix Glycyrrhizae), at the dosage of 10 ml three times daily (equivalent to 15 grams of each herb per day). The dosage for children was adjusted accordingly. The overall results were satisfactory.[13]
- **Liver cirrhosis**: The combination of a *Chai Hu* and *Gan Cao* (Radix Glycyrrhizae) preparation has demonstrated preventative influence against liver cirrhosis in laboratory mice.[14]
- **Hyperlipidemia**: In one study, 86 patients with hyperlipidemia were treated with an herbal formula (3 grams of *Chai Hu* with *Luo Han Guo* (Fructus Momordicae) added as a flavoring agent) three times daily for 3 weeks per course of treatment. The study reported marked effectiveness in reduction of triglycerides.[15]
- **Erythema**: Thirteen patients with erythema were treated with 2 ml of *Chai Hu* injectable (equivalent to 4 grams of herb) twice daily for 10 days. The study reported good results in all patients.[16]
- **Globus hystericus**: According to one report, 25 patients with globus hystericus were treated with 2 ml of a *Chai Hu* preparation injected into *Tiantu* (CV 22) daily or every other day. After 4 treatments, 15 patients reported marked improvement, 6 reported moderate improvement, and 4 reported no response.[17]

HERB-DRUG INTERACTION

The following cases of herb-drug interaction are based on *Xiao Chai Hu Tang* (Minor Bupleurum Decoction), an herbal formula that contains *Chai Hu* as the main ingredient. Additional information is not available at this time whether *Chai Hu*, as a single herb, is associated with the same risk of not.

- **Tolbutamide:** It was demonstrated in one study that the formula *Xiao Chai Hu Tang* (Minor Bupleurum Decoction) reduced the bioavailability of tolbutamide after oral administration in rats. *Xiao Chai Hu Tang* was found to accelerate the initial absorption rate, reduce the area under the plasma concentration-time curve, and decrease the overall bioavailability of tolbutamide. The mechanism of interaction was not related to hepatic metabolism.[18]
- **Ofloxacin:** In an open, random-crossover investigation study with seven volunteers, a single dose of ofloxacin and a one-week dose of *Xiao Chai Hu Tang* (Minor Bupleurum Decoction) were given concurrently. Using high-performance liquid chromatography to evaluate the bioavailability of ofloxacin, it was determined that there is no significant effect on the rate or extent of bioavailability of ofloxacin when given concurrently with *Xiao Chai Hu Tang*.[19]
- **Interferon:** It has been reported that increased risk of acute pneumonitis may be associated with use of interferon, Sho-saiko-to [*Xiao Chai Hu Tang* (Minor Bupleurum Decoction)], or both in combination. Among patients with chronic hepatitis or liver cirrhosis, the frequency of drug-induced pneumonitis was 0.5% in those given only interferon-alpha, 0.7% in those given only Sho-saiko-to, and 4.0% in those given both interferon-alpha and Sho-saiko-to. The herbs have not been shown to injure the lung tissues, but may over stimulate the neutrophils to release granulocytes elastase and oxygen radicals, which subsequently damage lung tissue. The fibroblasts that repair the damaged tissue may increase the risk of pulmonary fibrosis.[20,21]

TOXICOLOGY

Chai Hu has very low toxicity. The LD_{50} in mice is 1.19 g/kg via intraperitoneal injection for essential oil of *Chai Hu*, and 1.906 g/kg for saikosaponin.[22]

SUPPLEMENT

There are two types of *Chai Hu*:

- 北柴胡 *Bei Chai Hu* (Radix Bupleurum Chinensis), harvested in northern China, is generally used as the standard source for *Chai Hu*. It has an excellent ability to disperse stagnation and treat Liver qi stagnation accompanied by heat.
- 南柴胡 *Nan Chai Hu* (Radix Bupleurum Scorzoneraefolium), harvested in southern China, has a milder overall function.

AUTHORS' COMMENTS

Optimal treatment of headache requires use of channel-guiding herbs to deliver the therapeutic effect of the herbs to the affected area. The following is a list of the commonly used channel-guiding herbs:

- *Taiyang* channels: *Qiang Huo* (Rhizoma et Radix Notopterygii)
- *Shaoyang* channels: *Chai Hu* (Radix Bupleuri)
- *Yangming* channels: *Bai Zhi* (Radix Angelicae Dahuricae)
- *Taiyin* channels: *Cang Zhu* (Rhizoma Atractylodis)
- *Shaoyin* channels: *Xi Xin* (Herba Asari)
- *Jueyin* channels: *Wu Zhu Yu* (Fructus Evodiae)

Chai Hu (Radix Bupleuri), *Chuan Xiong* (Rhizoma Ligustici Chuanxiong), *Qiang Huo* (Rhizoma et Radix

Chai Hu (Radix Bupleuri)

Notopterygii), *Bai Zhi* (Radix Angelicae Dahuricae), and *Gao Ben* (Rhizoma Ligustici) all treat headaches. According to Dr. Li Shou-Shan, the differences between these herbs are as follows:

- *Chai Hu* treats temporal headaches.
- *Chuan Xiong* is most effective for headaches related to menstruation.
- *Qiang Huo* is more specific to occipital headaches.
- *Bai Zhi* focuses on frontal headaches.
- *Gao Ben* is best for vertex headaches.

References

1. *Xian Dai Zhong Yao Yao Li Xue* (Contemporary Pharmacology of Chinese Herbs), 1997; 126-127
2. Yan X, Zhou J, Xie G, *Traditional Chinese Medicines Molecular Structures, Natural Sources and Applications*; Ashgate, 1999; 5660
3. *Shen Yang Yi Xue Yuan Xue Bao* (Journal of Shenyang University of Medicine), 1984; 1(3):214
4. *Zhong Yao Yao Li Yu Ying Yong* (Pharmacology and Applications of Chinese Herbs), 1983; 888
5. Ibid.
6. Ibid.
7. *Zhong Yi Yao Xue Bao* (Report of Chinese Medicine and Herbology), 1988; (1):45
8. *Zhong Yao Xue* (Chinese Herbology), 1998; 103:106
9. *Shang Hai Yi Ke Da Xue Xue Bao* (Journal of Shanghai University of Medicine), 1986; 13(1):20
10. *Zhong Yao Xue* (Chinese Herbology), 1998; 103:106
11. *Zhong Yi Za Zhi* (Journal of Chinese Medicine), 1985; 12:13
12. *Zhong Yao Xue* (Chinese Herbology), 1998; 105
13. *Xin Yi Yao Xue Za Zhi* (New Journal of Medicine and Herbology), 1974; 2:18
14. Ibid., 2:28
15. *Zhong Yi Za Zhi* (Journal of Chinese Medicine), 1988; 2:62
16. *Pi Fu Bing Fang Zhi Yan Jiu Tong Xun* (Research Journal on Prevention and Treatment of Dermatological Disorders), 1979; 2:110
17. *Zhe Jiang Zhong Yi Xue Yuan Xue Bao* (Journal of Zhejiang University of Chinese Medicine), 1987; 6:52
18. *American Journal of Chinese Medicine.* 27(3-4):355-63, 1999
19. *International Journal of Clinical Pharmacology and Therapeutics.* 32(2):57-61, 1994 Feb.
20. Nakagawa A et al. Five cases of drug-induced pneumonitis due to Sho-saiko-to or interferon-alpha or both. *Nihon Kyobu Shikkan Gakkai Zasshi.* 1995 Dec;33(12):1361-1366
21. Murakami K et al. A possible mechanism of interstitial pneumonia during interferon therapy with sho-saiko-to. *Nihon Kyobu Shikkan Gakkai Zasshi.* 1995 Apr;33(4):389-94
22. *Yao Xue Tong Bao* (Report of Herbology), 1979; 14(6):252

Sheng Ma (Rhizoma Cimicifugae)

升麻

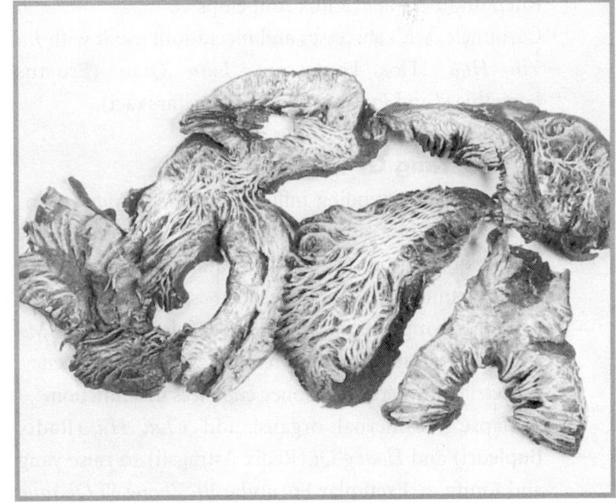

Pinyin Name: *Sheng Ma*
Literal Name: "ascending hemp"
Original Source: *Shen Nong Ben Cao Jing* (Divine Husbandman's Classic of the Materia Medica) in the second century
English Name: cimicifuga, large trifoliolious bugbane rhizome, dahurian bugbane rhizome, skunk bugbane rhizome
Botanical Name: *Cimicifuga heracleifolia* Kom. (*Da San Ye Sheng Ma*); *Cimicifuga dahurica* (Turcz.) Maxim. (*Xing An Sheng Ma*); *Cimicifuga foetida* L. (*Sheng Ma*)
Pharmaceutical Name: Rhizoma Cimicifugae
Properties: acrid, sweet, cool
Channels Entered: Lung, Spleen, Large Intestine, Stomach

CHINESE THERAPEUTIC ACTIONS

1. Releases the Exterior and Vents Measles

Dermatological disorders: The ascending and dispersing influences of *Sheng Ma* (Rhizoma Cimicifugae) are commonly used to dispel wind-heat. Clinical applications include headache, fever, rash, itching, the initial stages of measles, or measles with incomplete eruptions.

- Measles: use *Sheng Ma* with *Ge Gen* (Radix Puerariae),

Sheng Ma (Rhizoma Cimicifugae)

Niu Bang Zi (Fructus Arctii), *Huang Qin* (Radix Scutellariae) and *Bo He* (Herba Menthae).

- Incomplete expression of measles: combine it with *Ge Gen* (Radix Puerariae), *Bai Shao* (Radix Paeoniae Alba) and *Gan Cao* (Radix Glycyrrhizae). **Exemplar Formula:** *Sheng Ma Ge Gen Tang* (Cimicifuga and Kudzu Decoction).
- Facial skin disorders: add *He Ye* (Folium Nelumbinis), *Cang Zhu* (Rhizoma Atractylodis) and *Gan Cao* (Radix Glycyrrhizae).

2. Clears Heat and Eliminates Toxins

Various heat-toxin disorders: The disorder in which heat-toxins attack the *yangming* channel is characterized by headache, swelling and pain of the gums, and mouth and tongue ulceration. The attack of heat toxins in the throat is characterized by throat pain and soreness.

- Swollen, painful gums or oral ulcers: use *Sheng Ma* with *Huang Lian* (Rhizoma Coptidis), *Sheng Di Huang* (Radix Rehmanniae) and *Mu Dan Pi* (Cortex Moutan). **Exemplar Formula:** *Qing Wei San* (Clear the Stomach Powder).
- Throat pain and soreness: combine it with *Jie Geng* (Radix Platycodonis) and *Xuan Shen* (Radix Scrophulariae).
- Febrile diseases with maculae: add *Shi Gao* (Gypsum Fibrosum) and *Da Qing Ye* (Folium Isatidis).
- Toothache: use it with *Huang Lian* (Rhizoma Coptidis), *Shi Gao* (Gypsum Fibrosum) and *Sheng Di Huang* (Radix Rehmanniae).
- Carbuncles without abscess: combine this herb with *Lian Qiao* (Fructus Forsythiae), *Da Huang* (Radix et Rhizoma Rhei) and *Bai Lian* (Radix Ampelopsis).
- Carbuncles with abscesses and ulceration: use it with *Jin Yin Hua* (Flos Lonicerae), *Lian Qiao* (Fructus Forsythiae) and *Pu Gong Ying* (Herba Taraxaci).

3. Raises Yang Qi

Prolapse: The ascending influence of *Sheng Ma* is commonly used to treat prolapse of internal organs caused by yang or qi deficiency. Clinical applications include prolapse of the rectum and uterus with shortness of breath, fatigue, and other symptoms of yang and qi deficiencies. *Sheng Ma* also treats profuse bleeding resulting from qi deficiency. Processing the herb with honey enhances this function.

- Prolapse of internal organs: add *Chai Hu* (Radix Bupleuri) and *Huang Qi* (Radix Astragali) to raise yang and tonify qi. **Exemplar Formula:** *Bu Zhong Yi Qi Tang* (Tonify the Middle and Augment the Qi Decoction).

DOSAGE

3 to 10 grams. The maximum dosage of *Sheng Ma* is 15 grams. Use smaller doses to raise yang qi. Use larger dosages to clear heat and eliminate toxins. Honey-processed *Sheng Ma* more effectively lifts yang qi.

CAUTIONS / CONTRAINDICATIONS

- Due to its ascending and floating nature, *Sheng Ma* should be used with caution in patients who have yin deficiency, bleeding in the upper body, Liver yang rising, heat signs, complete eruption of measles, nausea due to reversed Stomach qi, or dyspnea due to reversed Lung qi.

OVERDOSAGE

Overdose of *Sheng Ma* is associated with adverse reactions such as nausea, vomiting, headache, muscle stiffness, convulsions, and delirium.[1]

CHEMICAL COMPOSITION

Triterpenoids 4.17% (cimigenol, cimigenol xyloside, dahurinol, 12-hydroxycimigenol arabinoside), visnagin, visamminol, norvisnagin, cimifugin, isoferulic acid, ferulic acid, caffeic acid, cimicifugoside, cimicifogine.[2]

PHARMACOLOGICAL EFFECTS

- **Cardiovascular:** *Sheng Ma* has an inhibitory effect on the cardiovascular system to lower blood pressure and heart rate.[3]
- **Antibiotic:** It has an inhibitory effect against *Mycobacterium tuberculosis,* dermatomyces, and many pathogenic fungi.[4]
- **Antipyretic:** Oral ingestion of *Sheng Ma* extract at 1 to 2 g/kg lowered body temperature in rats with artificially-induced fever.[5]
- **Others:** *Sheng Ma* has mild anti-inflammatory and analgesic effects.[6]

CLINICAL STUDIES AND RESEARCH

- **Gastric prolapse:** Intramuscular injection of an herbal preparation was evaluated for its effect in treating gastric prolapse. The herbal injectables contained *Sheng Ma* and *Huang Qi* (Radix Astragali). Acupuncture points included *Zusanli* (ST 36), *Weishu* (BL 21), and *Pishu* (BL 20), used in rotation in each treatment. The treatment protocol was to inject 3 ml of the preparation to each point one time daily for 6 days, followed by 1 day of rest. The patients were also advised to exercise. The length of treatment was between 1 and 3 months. Out of 146 patients, the effective rate was 96.7%.[7]
- **Severe rectal prolapse:** According to one report, 32 patients with severe rectal prolapse underwent an intensive herbal treatment that included administration of topical and oral herbs. The topical solution was prepared by adding 30 grams of *Mang Xiao* (Natrii Sulfas) and 9 grams of *Gan Cao* (Radix Glycyrrhizae) to 2,500 to 3,000 ml of boiling water, for 5 minutes. The oral herbal decoction consisted of 30 grams of *Dang Shen* (Radix Codonopsis), 9 grams of *Sheng Ma* and 6 grams of *Gan Cao* (Radix Glycyrrhizae). Patients

Sheng Ma (Rhizoma Cimicifugae)

were advised to sit and soak in the herbal solution twice daily, and take the herbal decoction two to four times daily. Of the 32 patients, 28 reported marked improvement and 4 reported moderate improvement.[8]

AUTHORS' COMMENTS

Sheng Ma, *Chai Hu* (Radix Bupleuri), and *Ge Gen* (Radix Puerariae) are three herbs with excellent ascending functions. They are commonly used to treat prolapse of internal organs, such as the stomach, uterus, and rectum.

References

1. *Zhong Yao Da Ci Dien* (Dictionary of Chinese Herbs), 1975; 451
2. *Xian Dai Zhong Yao Yao Li Xue* (Contemporary Pharmacology of Chinese Herbs), 1997; 155-156
3. *Zhong Yao Da Ci Dien* (Dictionary of Chinese Herbs), 1975; 451
4. *Zhong Yao Xue* (Chinese Herbology), 1998; 106:108
5. *Yao Xue Za Zhi* (Journal of Medicinals), 1975; 95:539
6. *Zhong Yao Xue* (Chinese Herbology), 1998; 106:108
7. *Hu Bei Zhong Yi Za Zhi* (Hubei Journal of Chinese Medicine), 1985; 2:44
8. *Zhong Yi Za Zhi* (Journal of Chinese Medicine), 1963; 6:16

Dan Dou Chi (Semen Sojae Praeparatum)

淡豆鼓

Pinyin Name: *Dan Dou Chi*
Alternate Chinese Names: *Xiang Dou Chi*
Original Source: *Ming Yi Za Zhu* (Miscellaneous Records of Famous Physicians) by Tao Hong-Jing in 500 A.D.
English Name: soja, soybean, fermented soybean
Botanical Name: *Glycine max* (L.) Merr.
Pharmaceutical Name: Semen Sojae Praeparatum
Properties: acrid, sweet, slightly bitter, cold
Channels Entered: Lung, Stomach

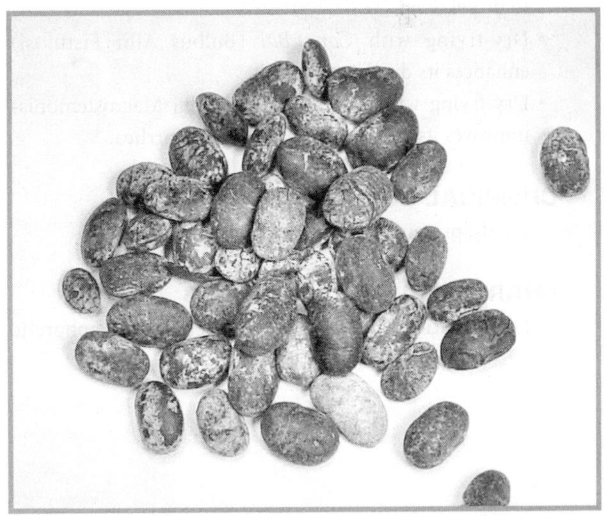

CHINESE THERAPEUTIC ACTIONS

1. Releases the Exterior

Exterior syndromes: *Dan Dou Chi* (Semen Sojae Praeparatum) is relatively mild and is often used as a spice or food. The gentle action of this herb to dispel exterior pathogenic factors makes it suitable for irritability or exterior syndromes in chronic, deficiency or elderly patients. It can be used for both wind-cold and wind-heat syndromes.

- Wind-cold syndromes in the early stage: combine *Dan Dou Chi* with *Cong Bai* (Bulbus Allii Fistulosi) and *Sheng Jiang* (Rhizoma Zingiberis Recens).
- Wind-cold syndrome with tight pulse and no perspiration: use it with *Ma Huang* (Herba Ephedrae), and *Ge Gen* (Radix Puerariae).
- Wind-heat syndromes: add *Bo He* (Herba Menthae), *Jin Yin Hua* (Flos Lonicerae) and *Lian Qiao* (Fructus Forsythiae). **Exemplar Formula:** *Yin Qiao San* (Honeysuckle and Forsythia Powder).

2. Eliminates Irritability and Harmonizes the Middle *Jiao*

Irritability and feelings of chest oppression: With its dispersing activity, *Dan Dou Chi* clears heat and relieves irritability and feelings of oppression in the chest. Furthermore, it clears heat in the Stomach to eliminate food stagnation from the gastrointestinal tract.

- Heat in the chest with irritability and insomnia: use *Dan Dou Chi* with *Zhi Zi* (Fructus Gardeniae). **Exemplar Formula:** *Zhi Zi Chi Tang* (Gardenia and Soja Decoction).
- Diarrhea from damp-heat in the middle *jiao*: add *Huang Lian* (Rhizoma Coptidis) and *Xie Bai* (Bulbus Allii Macrostemonis).

Dan Dou Chi (Semen Sojae Praeparatum)

- Lack of appetite because of Spleen deficiency or food stagnation: use *Dan Dou Chi* individually in decoction.

DOSAGE

10 to 15 grams. The maximum dosage of *Dan Dou Chi* is 50 grams. *Dan Dou Chi* has different properties and functions depending on the processing methods chosen. To maximize heat-clearing effect, *Dan Dou Chi* should be cooked prior to the addition of other herbs. To maximize the exterior-releasing function, this herb should be added to the decoction last and cooked only for a short time.

- Dry-frying increases its function to stop perspiration.
- Dry-frying with black beans changes the thermal property to neutral-to-warm.
- Dry-frying with salt enhances its emetic effect.
- Dry-frying with garlic helps to stop bleeding.
- Dry-frying with grain-based liquor enhances its ability to dispel wind.
- Dry-frying with *Cong Bai* (Bulbus Allii Fistulosi) enhances its diaphoretic effect.
- Dry-frying with *Xie Bai* (Bulbus Allii Macrostemonis) improves its effectiveness in treating diarrhea.

CHEMICAL COMPOSITION

Lipids, protein, carbohydrates, vitamin B_1, B_2.

PHARMACOLOGICAL EFFECTS

Diaphoretic: *Dan Dou Chi* has a very mild diaphoretic effect.[1]

SUPPLEMENT

- 大豆黄卷 *Da Dou Huang Juan* (Semen Glycines Germinatum), first cited in *Shen Nong Ben Cao Jing* (Divine Husbandman's Classic of the Materia Medica) in the second century, is the germinated form of unprocessed *Dan Dou Chi. Da Dou Huang Juan* is normally processed with *Ma Huang* (Herba Ephedrae) to enhance its diaphoretic effect. *Da Dou Huang Juan* is neutral, sweet and enters the Stomach channel. Its functions include releasing the exterior through diaphoresis, clearing damp-heat, raising yang qi and opening channels and collaterals. It is used for summer-heat or damp-heat combined with exterior patterns. It can also be used to treat spasms caused by *bi zheng* (painful obstruction syndrome). The normal dosage of *Da Dou Huang Juan* is 10 to 15 grams.

AUTHORS' COMMENTS

Dan Dou Chi can be either warm or cold depending on the herb with which it is processed. It is cold in nature and if processed with *Sang Ye* (Folium Mori) and *Qing Hao* (Herba Artemisiae Annuae). On the other hand, it is warm in thermal property if it is processed with *Zi Su Ye* (Folium Perillae) and *Ma Huang* (Herba Ephedrae). When using *Dan Dou Chi,* it is important to determine how it has been processed, so that it can be used appropriately.

References

1. *Zhong Yao Xue* (Chinese Herbology), 1998; 94:95

Wu Tian (Radix et Folium Viticis Quinatae)

烏甜 乌甜

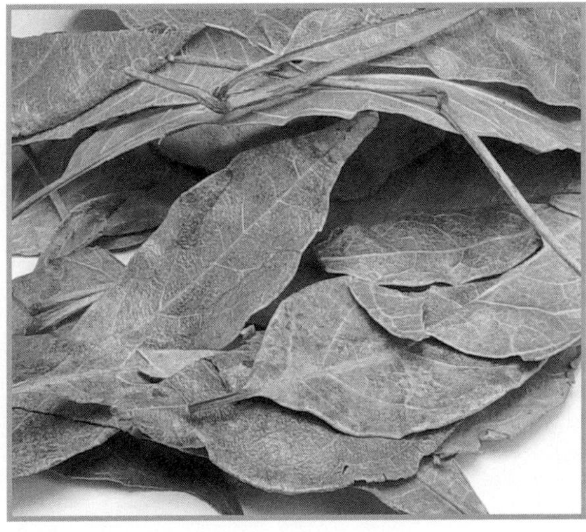

Pinyin Name: *Wu Tian*
Literal Name: "black sweet"
Alternate Chinese Names: *Wu Tian Ye, Pu Jiang Mu, Shan Pu Jiang, Mu Jing, Shan Mu Jing*
English Name: vitex root and leaves
Botanical Name: *Vitex quinata*
Pharmaceutical Name: Radix et Folium Viticis Quinatae
Properties: sweet, acrid, bland, cold
Channels Entered: Lung

CHINESE THERAPEUTIC ACTIONS

1. Clears Lung Heat, Cools Blood and Arrests Cough

Lung heat: *Wu Tian* (Radix et Folium Viticis Quinatae) treats various symptoms of Lung heat such as cough and hemoptysis.

- Cough caused by yin-deficient heat: use *Wu Tian* with *Bai He* (Bulbus Lilii), *Shi Hu* (Herba Dendrobii) and *Sang Bai Pi* (Cortex Mori).
- Dry cough: combine it with *Chuan Bei Mu* (Bulbus Fritillariae Cirrhosae), *E Jiao* (Colla Corii Asini) and *Pi Pa Ye* (Folium Eriobotryae).
- Epistaxis or hematemesis: use it with *Bai He* (Bulbus Lilii), *Mai Men Dong* (Radix Ophiopogonis), charred *Ai Ye* (Folium Artemisiae Argyi) and charred *Ce Bai Ye* (Cacumen Platycladi).
- Hemoptysis: add *Sang Ye* (Folium Mori), *Ce Bai Ye* (Cacumen Platycladi), *Zhu Ye* (Herba Phyllostachys) and *Ji Xue Teng* (Caulis Spatholobi).
- Chest congestion: use *Wu Tian* with *Chai Hu* (Radix Bupleuri), *Pi Pa Ye* (Folium Eriobotryae), *Ze Lan* (Herba Lycopi), *Ou Jie* (Nodus Nelumbinis Rhizomatis), *Zhi Ke* (Fructus Aurantii) and *Jie Geng* (Radix Platycodonis).
- Cough with profuse sputum: add *Jie Geng* (Radix Platycodonis) and *Gua Lou Shi* (Fructus Trichosanthis).

DOSAGE

3 to 12 grams in decoction.

AUTHORS' COMMENTS

Both *Wu Tian* and *Fu Rong* (Radix Hibisci) enter the Lung and treat Lung heat. However, *Wu Tian* treats Lung heat manifesting in cough or hemoptysis, while *Fu Rong* treats nasal disorders such as sinusitis.

Fu Ping (Herba Spirodelae)

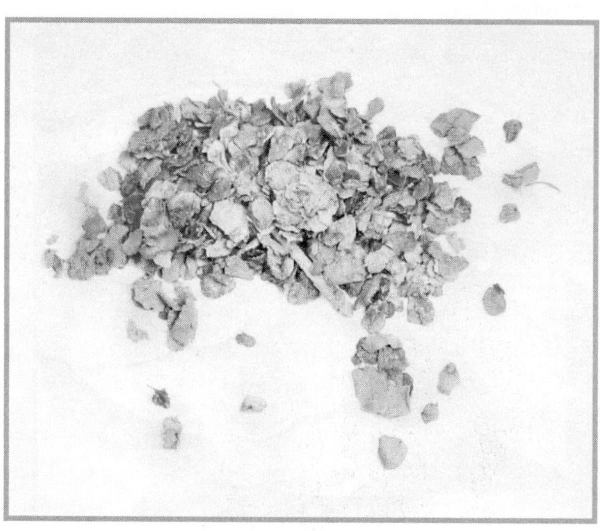

浮萍 浮萍

Pinyin Name: *Fu Ping*
Literal Name: "floating spirodela"
Alternate Chinese Names: *Sui Ping, Tian Ping*
Original Source: *Shen Nong Ben Cao Jing* (Divine Husbandman's Classic of the Materia Medica) in the second century
English Name: spirodela, common duckweed
Botanical Name: *Spirodela polyrrhiza* (L.) Schleid.
Pharmaceutical Name: Herba Spirodelae
Properties: acrid, cold
Channels Entered: Lung, Urinary Bladder

CHINESE THERAPEUTIC ACTIONS

1. Releases the Exterior and Induces Diaphoresis

Wind-heat: Acrid and cold, *Fu Ping* (Herba Spirodelae) has ascending and dispersing properties. It is commonly used to dispel wind-heat through diaphoresis. Common symptoms include fever, headache, absence of perspiration, thirst, sore throat, and a superficial, rapid pulse.

- Wind-heat syndrome: combine *Fu Ping* with *Jing Jie* (Herba Schizonepetae), *Bo He* (Herba Menthae), and *Lian Qiao* (Fructus Forsythiae).
- Wind-heat syndrome with thirst: use it with *Tian Hua Fen* (Radix Trichosanthis).

2. Vents Rashes and Stops Itching

Incomplete eruption of measles or rashes with itching: *Fu Ping* is commonly used for symptoms of wind attacking the skin, manifesting as measles, urticaria, rash and itching.

- Incomplete expression of measles: add this herb to *Bo He* (Herba Menthae), *Niu Bang Zi* (Fructus Arctii), and *Chan Tui* (Periostracum Cicadae).
- Itching: use it with *Niu Bang Zi* (Fructus Arctii) and *Bo He* (Herba Menthae).

3. Eliminates Water and Reduces Swelling and Edema

- **Exterior syndrome with edema and fever:** *Fu Ping* regulates water circulation and eliminates water accumulation. It is commonly used for patients with exterior syndromes accompanied by edema.

DOSAGE

3 to 10 grams. The maximum dosage of *Fu Ping* is 30 grams. Generally, this herb is added only in the last 5 to 10 minutes of cooking a decoction, to preserve its potency. *Fu Ping* may be used individually or in combination with other herbs, as a decoction or topical substance.

CAUTIONS / CONTRAINDICATIONS

- *Fu Ping* should be used with caution in patients who have spontaneous perspiration from qi deficiency, night sweating and/or thirst and dry mouth caused by yin deficiency.
- *Fu Ping* should also be used with caution in cases of edema caused by yang deficiency.

CHEMICAL COMPOSITION

Flavones (orientin, vitexin, isoorientin, isovitexin, rutin, luteolin-7-O-glucoside), stigmasterol, campesterol, β-sitosterol, protein 18-25% (albumins, glutelins), lycopersene.[1]

PHARMACOLOGICAL EFFECTS

- *Fu Ping* has mild cardiotonic, diuretic and antipyretic effects.[2]

References

1. *Xian Dai Zhong Yao Yao Li Xue* (Contemporary Pharmacology of Chinese Herbs), 1997; 178-179
2. *Zhong Yao Xue* (Chinese Herbology), 1998; 108:109

Shuang Liu Huang (Herba Vernoniae Patulae)

雙柳黃 双柳黄

Pinyin Name: *Shuang Liu Huang*
Literal Name: "double willow yellow"
Alternate Chinese Names: *Xian Xia Hua, Gou Zi Hua, Gou Zi Cai*
English Name: half-spreading ironweed
Botanical Name: *Vernonia patula* (Ait.) Merr.
Pharmaceutical Name: Herba Vernoniae Patulae
Properties: bitter, neutral
Channels Entered: Lung, Large Intestine

CHINESE THERAPEUTIC ACTIONS

1. Dispels Wind-Heat

Shuang Liu Huang (Herba Vernoniae Patulae) may be used alone to treat common colds or influenza characterized by wind-heat. It also relieves headache.

- Exterior wind-heat: use 3 grams of *Shuang Liu Huang*.
- Headache: use 10 grams of *Shuang Liu Huang*.

2. Clears Heat, Stops Diarrhea

Shuang Liu Huang clears heat, stops diarrhea, and is often incorporated in herbal formulas to treat traveler's diarrhea or dysentery.

DOSAGE

3 to 10 grams in decoction.

CHEMICAL COMPOSITION

Flavonoids, terpenoids, essential oil, amino acids, organic acids.[1]

References

1. *Zhong Yao Da Ci Dien* (Dictionary of Chinese Herbs), 2799

Mao Zi Dun Tou (Herba Abutilon Indicum)

帽仔盾頭
帽仔盾头

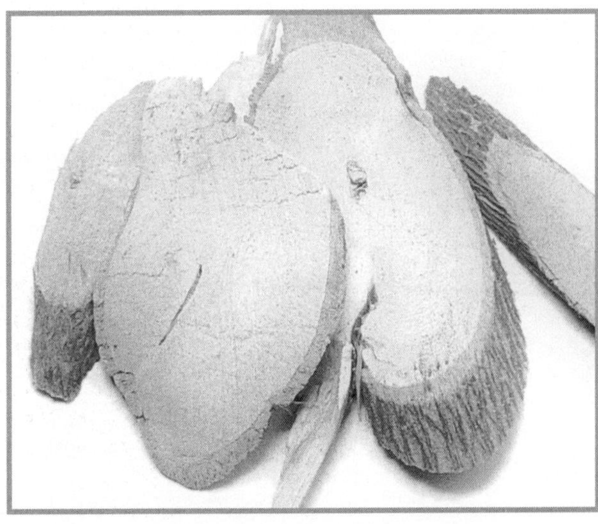

Pinyin Name: *Mao Zi Dun Tou*
Alternate Chinese Names: *Mo Pan Cao, Mi Lan Cao, Si Mu Cao, Er Xiang Cao, Jin Hua Cao*
English Name: Indian abutilon
Botanical Name: *Abutilon indicum* (L.) Sweet.
Pharmaceutical Name: Herba Abutilon Indicum
Properties: sweet, neutral
Channels Entered: Lung, Liver, Gallbladder, Spleen
Safety Index: slightly toxic

Mao Zi Dun Tou (Herba Abutilon Indicum)

CHINESE THERAPEUTIC ACTIONS

1. Dispels Wind-Heat

Wind-heat: *Mao Zi Dun Tou* (Herba Abutilon Indicum) may be used to dispel wind-heat from the exterior with symptoms of sore throat, fever, cough with yellow sputum, or yellow nasal discharge.

- Wind-heat: use this herb with *Jin Yin Hua* (Flos Lonicerae), *Huang Qin* (Radix Scutellariae), *Pu Gong Ying* (Herba Taraxaci), *Feng Wei Cao* (Herba Pteris) and *Ban Lan Gen* (Radix Isatidis).

2. Separates Turbidity, Opens Orifices, Invigorates Blood, and Reduces Swellings and Abscesses

Mao Zi Dun Tou is commonly used to treat deafness, tinnitus and ear pain. It has also been used to treat abscesses, swelling and splenomegaly.

- Deafness, tinnitus and ear pain arising from fire in the Liver and Gallbladder channels: use this herb with *Long Dan Cao* (Radix Gentianae), *Hu Zhang* (Rhizoma Polygoni Cuspidati), *Hu Yao Huang* (Herba Leucas Mollissimae), *Ma Bian Cao* (Herba Verbenae) and *Qian Li Guang* (Herba Senecionis Scandens).
- Abscess and swelling: combine it with *San Leng* (Rhizoma Sparganii), *E Zhu* (Rhizoma Curcumae), *Hong Hua* (Flos Carthami), *Tao Ren* (Semen Persicae), *Tian Hua Fen* (Radix Trichosanthis), *Xia Ku Cao* (Spica Prunellae), *Mu Li* (Concha Ostreae) and *Zao Jiao Ci* (Spina Gleditsiae).
- Splenomegaly: use *Mao Zi Dun Tou* with *Hu Zhang* (Rhizoma Polygoni Cuspidati), *Mu Li* (Concha Ostreae), *Bie Jia* (Carapax Trionycis), *San Leng* (Rhizoma Sparganii), *E Zhu* (Rhizoma Curcumae) and *Tian Hua Fen* (Radix Trichosanthis).

3. Strengthens the Spleen and Promotes Digestion

Mao Zi Dun Tou treats chronic indigestion or weak digestion in children.

- Indigestion: combine it with *Dang Shen* (Radix Codonopsis), *Bai Zhu* (Rhizoma Atractylodis Macrocephalae), *Fu Ling* (Poria), *Gan Cao* (Radix Glycyrrhizae), *Shan Zha* (Fructus Crataegi), *Mai Ya* (Fructus Hordei Germinatus) and *Shen Qu* (Massa Fermentata).

DOSAGE

1 to 3 grams.

CAUTIONS / CONTRAINDICATIONS

- *Mao Zi Dun Tou* is slightly toxic. Therefore, it should not be prescribed in excess of 5 (five) grams.

AUTHORS' COMMENTS

Mao Zi Dun Tou has long been used as a medicinal herb in various countries. It has been used in the Philippines, to treat constipation by lubricating the bowels; in India, to relieve cystitis by promoting urination; and in Malaysia, to relieve toothache and ear pain via topical application. Other historical applications indicate sedative, aphrodisiac, antitussive and anti-inflammatory uses.

Chapter 1 summary

— Exterior-Releasing Herbs

SECTION 1: WIND-COLD RELEASING HERBS

Name	Similarities	Differences
Ma Huang (Herba Ephedrae)	Induce perspiration, disperse cold	Dilates the Lung, relieves wheezing, regulates water, relieves edema
Gui Zhi (Ramulus Cinnamomi)		Warms the channels, unblocks the yang, relieves pain in the upper extremities
Zi Su Ye (Folium Perillae)	Dispel wind-cold, harmonize Spleen and Stomach	Regulates Spleen and Stomach qi, calms fetus and detoxifies
Sheng Jiang (Rhizoma Zingiberis Recens)		Warms the Stomach, relieves vomiting, detoxifies
Xiang Ru (Herba Elsholtziae seu Moslae)		Relieves summer-dampness, regulates water, relieves edema
Jing Jie (Herba Schizonepetae)	Dispel wind, release the exterior	Vents rashes, stops bleeding (the charred 'ash' form)
Fang Feng (Radix Saposhnikoviae)		Dispels both external and internal wind
Qiang Huo (Rhizoma et Radix Notopterygii)		Disperses cold, dries dampness, relieves upper body pain, treats occipital headache
Gao Ben (Rhizoma Ligustici)		Treats vertex headache
Ji Xiang Teng (Caulis Paederiae)		Relieves pain, clears toxins
Cong Bai (Bulbus Allii Fistulosi)		Disperses coldness, eliminates toxins to treat sores topically
Bai Zhi (Radix Angelicae Dahuricae)	Disperse wind-cold, open nasal passages	Treats frontal headache, clears turbid nasal discharge
Cang Er Zi (Fructus Xanthii)		Relieves continuous nasal discharge, treats headache
Xin Yi Hua (Flos Magnoliae)		Restores sense of smell, treats clear, watery nasal discharge
E Bu Shi Cao (Herba Centipedae)		Clears nose and removes visual obstruction

General Characteristics of Wind-Cold Releasing Herbs:

Taste: acrid
Thermal property: warm
Channels entered: Lung
Therapeutic actions: dispel wind-cold, release the exterior, induce diaphoresis

These herbs treat wind-cold, a condition characterized by aversion to wind and cold, chills more prominent than fever, body aches, the absence of perspiration, a thin, white tongue coating and superficial, tight pulse. Additional uses include treatment of dyspnea, cough, wheezing, edema, *bi zheng* (painful obstruction syndrome), arthritis, and dermatological disorders including but not limited to sores and abscesses.

Ma Huang (Herba Ephedrae) and ***Gui Zhi*** (Ramulus Cinnamomi) disperse wind-cold in the *taiyang* channels.

Ma Huang is the stronger of the two to induce perspiration and release the exterior. Therefore, it is more suitable for exterior excess conditions. In addition, *Ma Huang* dilates the Lung to relieve dyspnea and wheezing, and increases urine output to reduce edema.

Gui Zhi, moderate in potency, treats both excess and deficiency cases of wind-cold invasion. *Gui Zhi* warms the channels, the chest and the *chong* (thoroughfare) channel to treat *bi zheng* (painful obstruction syndrome), arthritis, chest pain and palpitations caused by cold and phlegm accumulation, and irregular menstruation or lower abdominal pain and coldness.

Chapter 1 summary

Zi Su Ye (Folium Perillae) disperses wind-cold, and regulates Spleen and Stomach qi. It expands the chest to relieve congestion, relieves nausea and vomiting, stabilizes the fetus during pregnancy, and relieves abdominal pain and diarrhea associated with seafood poisoning, all of which are problems caused by qi stagnation in the middle *jiao*. *Zi Su Ye*'s function of diaphoresis is not as strong as that of *Ma Huang* or *Gui Zhi*; it is therefore more suitable for clearing mild wind-cold invasions.

Sheng Jiang (Rhizoma Zingiberis Recens), gentle in nature, is used more frequently for milder cases of wind-cold invasion. With its excellent influence of harmonizing the middle *jiao*, *Sheng Jiang* increases the appetite, and relieves abdominal pain, diarrhea, nausea, and vomiting. It counteracts the toxicity of herbs such as *Ban Xia* (Rhizoma Pinelliae) and *Tian Nan Xing* (Rhizoma Arisaematis).

Xiang Ru (Herba Elsholtziae seu Moslae) is a key herb for treating summer night invasions of wind-cold-dampness manifesting in aversion to cold, fever, headache, abdominal pain, vomiting, diarrhea, and the absence of perspiration. It harmonizes the middle *jiao*, transforms dampness, and treats edema accompanied by dysuria.

Jing Jie (Herba Schizonepetae) and ***Fang Feng*** (Radix Saposhnikoviae) are both excellent herbs to disperse wind.

Jing Jie has a stronger diaphoretic function than *Fang Feng*. *Jing Jie* is acrid but mild, slightly warm but not drying, and depending on with what other herbs it is prescribed, disperses either wind-cold or wind-heat. Because the strength of *Jing Jie* is in dispelling wind, it treats various itching and dermatological disorders in which *wind* is the underlying cause. Charred *Jing Jie* stops bleeding.

Fang Feng dispels wind, cold and dampness. It relieves pain in the head, eyes, throat, body, and joints. It relieves arthritis caused by *bi zheng* (painful obstruction syndrome), or spasms, cramps or tetany from internal Liver wind.

Qiang Huo (Rhizoma et Radix Notopterygii) and ***Gao Ben*** (Rhizoma Ligustici) relieve arthritic pain, especially in the upper body.

Qiang Huo relieves pain of the *taiyang* Urinary Bladder channel, when there is neck and occipital stiffness and pain.

Gao Ben is best for vertex headaches.

Ji Xiang Teng (Caulis Paederiae) dispels wind, relieves pain, and clears toxins.

Cong Bai (Bulbus Allii Fistulosi) is relatively weak, and relieves mild cases of exterior wind-cold. It also warms the body to treat yang deficiency. Applied topically, *Cong Bai* alleviates carbuncles.

Bai Zhi (Radix Angelicae Dahuricae), acrid and aromatic, addresses wind-cold characterized by frontal headaches, supra-orbital pain, toothache and nasal obstruction. Because it also dries dampness, *Bai Zhi* treats *bi zheng* (painful obstruction syndrome), dermatological disorders that involve swelling and pus, and lower abdominal coldness and pain with leukorrhea.

Cang Er Zi (Fructus Xanthii) disperses wind, dispels dampness and induces perspiration. It is primarily used for headaches, yellow nasal discharge, itching rashes, *bi zheng* (painful obstruction syndrome) and spasms and cramps. However, it is slightly toxic and should be used with caution.

Xin Yi Hua (Flos Magnoliae) disperses wind-cold, opens nasal passages and relieves headache. It is best for sinusitis or to aid wind-cold sufferers who have lost their sense of smell because of nasal obstruction.

E Bu Shi Cao (Herba Centipedae) releases wind-cold to open nasal passages and clear visual obstruction. It also dispels wind-damp to benefit the joints.

Chapter 1 summary

SECTION 2: WIND-HEAT RELEASING HERBS

Name	Similarities	Differences
Bo He (Herba Menthae)	Disperse wind-heat, benefit the throat, vent rashes	Clears the head, weaker in dispersing wind-heat
Niu Bang Zi (Fructus Arctii)		Soothes sore throat, clears heat and eliminates toxins
Chan Tui (Periostracum Cicadae)		Benefits voice, relieves spasms, itching, superficial visual obstruction
Sang Ye (Folium Mori)	Disperse wind-heat, clear heat in the Liver, brighten the eyes	Clears the Lung, stops coughing, stops bleeding
Ju Hua (Flos Chrysanthemi)		Stronger in clearing heat in the Liver, clears toxins
Man Jing Zi (Fructus Viticis)		Relieves headache
Mu Zei (Herba Equiseti Hiemalis)		Stops bleeding
Yi Zhi Xiang (Herba Vernoniae Cinereae)		Clears Lung and Liver heat, clears toxins
Ge Gen (Radix Puerariae)	Relieve wind-heat, raise the yang	Relieves stiff neck, generates fluids, vents rashes
Chai Hu (Radix Bupleuri)		Harmonizes *shaoyang* channels, disperses Liver qi stagnation
Sheng Ma (Rhizoma Cimicifugae)		Vents rashes, clears heat and eliminates toxins
Dan Dou Chi (Semen Sojae Praeparatum)	Disperse wind-heat	Relieves irritability
Wu Tian (Radix et Folium Viticis Quinatae)		Cools blood, relieves cough
Fu Ping (Herba Spirodelae)		Dispels dampness
Shuang Liu Huang (Herba Vernoniae Patulae)		Clears heat and relieves diarrhea
Mao Zi Dun Tou (Herba Abutilon Indicum)		Opens sensory orifices, reduces swellings and abscesses

General Characteristics of Wind-Heat Releasing Herbs:

Taste: acrid
Thermal property: cool, cold
Channels entered: Lung, Liver
Therapeutic actions: dispel wind-heat, release the exterior, reduce swelling and inflammation

These herbs treat wind-heat, a condition characterized by sore throat, aversion to wind and cold, fever, dry throat, thirst, thin white or thin yellow tongue coating, and superficial, rapid pulse. They also address headache, red eyes, cough, rashes, and Liver qi stagnation.

Bo He (Herba Menthae), cool and acrid, induces perspiration. It clears wind-heat from the head, vents rashes and treats initial stages of warm febrile disorders in the absence of perspiration; it relieves headache, red eyes and sore throat, alleviates canker sores, and addresses itching of the skin with rashes that have not erupted. It is slightly aromatic and relieves chest and hypochondriac fullness and distention caused by Liver qi stagnation. This herb should be added at the end of cooking, and cooked only briefly, as the active constituents evaporate or become deactivated by prolonged exposure to heat.

Niu Bang Zi (Fructus Arctii), acrid, bitter and cold, disperses wind-heat, clears the Lung, dispels phlegm, vents rashes, eliminates toxins, and reduces swelling. It is used when wind-heat has begun turning into Lung heat, with yellow sputum, incomplete eruption of rashes, sore throat, carbuncles and other toxic sores.

Chan Tui (Periostracum Cicadae) is sweet and cold. In addition to dispersing wind-heat to promote the eruption of measles and relieve itching, *Chan Tui* benefits the throat, restores normal voice, and benefits the eyes to remove superficial visual obstructions.

Chapter 1 summary

Sang Ye (Folium Mori) and ***Ju Hua*** (Flos Chrysanthemi) clear the head, dispel wind-heat, sedate the Liver and brighten the eyes. They treat wind-heat disorders involving dizziness, or Liver yang rising that causes red eyes, dizziness and vertigo.

Sang Ye is cooler, and functions more strongly to disperse exterior wind-heat. Thus, it is used more to relieve cough, moisten the Lung, cool blood and stop bleeding.

Ju Hua more strongly sedates rising Liver yang. It also eliminates toxins to treat sores and carbuncles.

Man Jing Zi (Fructus Viticis) disperses wind-heat in the head, relieving headache, clearing red eyes, and soothing painful, swollen gums. *Man Jing Zi* is also useful in treatment of *bi zheng* (painful obstruction syndrome).

Mu Zei (Herba Equiseti Hiemalis) clears wind-heat, brightens the eyes, removes superficial visual obstruction and treats wind and heat in the Liver channel that cause red eyes, excessive tearing and visual disturbances. *Mu Zei* stops rectal or hemorrhoidal bleeding.

Yi Zhi Xiang (Herba Vernoniae Cinereae) disperses wind-heat, clears Lung heat, and purges Liver fire. Thus, it treats sore throat, bronchitis, conjunctivitis and dysentery.

Ge Gen (Radix Puerariae), light and ascending in nature, relieves muscle tightness and pain in the upper body. It also relieves fever, facilitates the eruption of rashes, generates body fluids and relieves thirst.

Chai Hu (Radix Bupleuri) raises yang qi, relieves exterior conditions, treats *shaoyang* disorders and spreads Liver qi. It treats pathogenic factors trapped between the *taiyang* and *yangming* stages, manifesting in alternating chills and fever. Other indications for use of *Chai Hu* are: organ prolapse (such as the rectum and uterus), Liver qi stagnation with chest and hypochondriac distention, fullness and pain, irregular menstruation and pre-menstrual syndrome.

Sheng Ma (Rhizoma Cimicifugae) lifts yang qi and relieves exterior conditions. It clears heat, eliminates toxins, and promotes the eruption of rashes. Clinical indications include incomplete expression of rashes, sore throat, canker sores, and toxic sores and carbuncles. Compared to *Chai Hu*, *Sheng Ma* has similar but stronger properties to raise yang qi and is mostly used for rectal and uterine prolapse, as seen in *Bu Zhong Yi Qi Tang* (Tonify the Middle and Augment the Qi Decoction).

Dan Dou Chi (Semen Sojae Praeparatum) releases the exterior, induces perspiration and counters both wind-heat and wind-cold invasions. It also disperses heat in the body created by stagnation, to relieve irritability, insomnia or chest discomfort.

Wu Tian (Radix et Folium Viticis Quinatae) clears Lung heat, cools the blood and stops cough.

Fu Ping (Herba Spirodelae), acrid and cold in property, induces perspiration, relieves exterior conditions, and promotes water circulation. Clinical applications include edema, dysuria, incomplete eruption of rashes, itching of the skin, and wind-heat accompanied by fever and the absence of sweating.

Shuang Liu Huang (Herba Vernoniae Patulae) releases wind-heat from the exterior to treat common colds and influenza, and dispels heat from the Large Intestine to treat diarrhea.

Mao Zi Dun Tou (Herba Abutilon Indicum) dispels wind-heat from the exterior. It also opens sensory orifices by reducing swelling and abscesses. It treats common cold, deafness and tinnitus.

Chapter 1 summary

HERBS FROM OTHER FUNCTIONAL CATEGORIES WITH EXTERIOR-RELEASING FUNCTIONS

Name	Functional Category
Du Huo (Radix Angelicae Pubescentis)	Wind-Damp Dispelling Herbs (Chapter 4)
Jin Yin Hua (Flos Lonicerae)	Heat-Clearing Herbs (Chapter 2)
Ren Dong Teng (Caulis Lonicerae)	Heat-Clearing Herbs (Chapter 2)
Xi Xin (Herba Asari)	Interior-Warming Herbs (Chapter 7)

Chapter 2 — Heat-Clearing Herbs

清热药

Chapter 2 — Heat-Clearing Herbs

Chapter 2 清热药 — Heat-Clearing Herbs

Definition: Heat-clearing herbs address imbalances caused by excessive heat, whether mild or extreme, at various levels of pathological penetration of the body, by clearing heat, purging fire, or cooling organs or substances injured by heat.

Heat is a pathogenic factor in many disease patterns. Warmth, heat and fire refer to degrees of severity of the same pathological entity, with *warmth* being the mild expression, *heat* the moderate condition, and *fire* the extreme. Heat-clearing herbs address a range of heat disorders:

- invasion of heat from the exterior to the interior
- excess heat and fire affecting internal organs
- excess heat at *ying* (nutritive) and *xue* (blood) levels
- accumulation of damp-heat in various areas of the body
- febrile disorders
- formation of pus and abscesses in or outside of the body
- conditions characterized as deficiency heat

In general, cool herbs clear heat while cold herbs purge fire from the body.

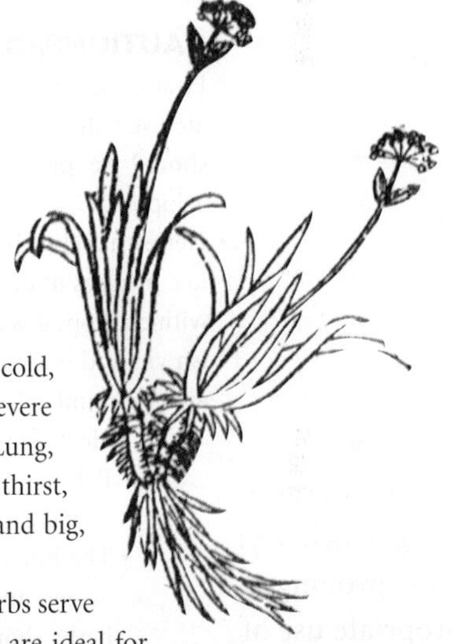

Zhi Mu (Radix Anemarrhenae)
Ben Cao Gang Mu (Materia Medica),
by Li Shi-Zhen, 1578 A.D.

SUBCATEGORIES OF ACTION

1. ***Heat-Clearing and Fire-Purging Herbs***: Usually sweet and cold, or bitter and cold, these herbs have strong therapeutic functions for treatment of moderate to severe cases of pathological conditions characterized by heat and fire affecting the Lung, Stomach, Heart, and Liver. Signs and symptoms: high fever, aversion to heat, thirst, restlessness, irritability, delirium, mania, red eyes, a yellow, dry tongue coat, and big, forceful pulse.
2. ***Heat-Clearing and Dampness-Drying Herbs***: Bitter, cold and drying, these herbs serve to clear heat, dry dampness, purge fire and eliminate toxins. Therefore, they are ideal for treating accumulations of damp-heat. Damp-heat in the intestines is characterized by symptoms such as burning diarrhea, dysentery, and hemorrhoids. Damp-heat in the Liver and Gallbladder creates jaundice, hypochondriac fullness and pain, and a bitter taste in the mouth. Damp-heat in the lower *jiao* gives rise to sensations of burning and pain during urination, genital itching, and yellow, turbid vaginal discharge in women. Other manifestations of damp-heat include eczema, abscess, swelling, ear infection, and suppurative diseases.
3. ***Heat-Clearing and Blood-Cooling Herbs***: The herbs that accomplish this are often cold with bitter, sweet, or salty tastes, and usually enter the Heart and Liver channels. These herbs clear heat and cool blood at the *ying* (nutritive) and *xue* (blood) levels, conditions characterized by restlessness, irritability, delirium, semiconsciousness, purpura and bleeding from various bodily orifices. Many herbs that clear heat and cool blood also nourish yin and promote the generation of body fluids.
4. ***Heat-Clearing and Toxin-Eliminating Herbs***: Heat and toxins imply infection and the presence of pus, abscesses, sores, and ulcerations, either internally or externally. With a wide range of therapeutic effects, these herbs commonly treat febrile diseases, diarrhea, dysentery, abscesses of internal organs, surface pus, burns, wounds, soreness and swelling of the throat, and similar imbalances.
5. ***Deficiency-Heat Clearing Herbs***: Deficiency heat is characterized by an underlying deficiency of yin with superficial manifestations of heat. Herbs that address deficiency heat are usually sweet and cold, and enter the Kidney and Liver channels. Deficiency heat signs and symptoms may indicate

Chapter 2 — Heat-Clearing Herbs

the presence of heat, but the actual cause of illness is deficiency of yin. Clinical manifestations include steaming bones sensations, warmth in the palms and soles, night sweats, dry throat and mouth, irritability, insomnia, red tongue with thin or no tongue coat, and thin, thready pulse. Herbs that clear deficiency heat also treat late stages of febrile disorders in which heat is lingering in the body, causing low-grade fever, tidal fevers, and/or sweating.

DIFFERENTIAL DIAGNOSIS AND TREATMENT

Optimal use of heat-clearing herbs requires careful differential diagnosis. Prior to prescribing heat-clearing herbs, one must determine the severity, location and characteristics of the heat.

- ***Severity*** of the pathogen may be classified as warmth, heat or fire. Warmth represents a mild condition, heat describes a moderate situation, and fire indicates a severe illness.
- ***Location*** must be accurate: heat may attack the exterior or the interior, individual organs, and *wei* (defensive), *qi* (energy), *ying* (nutritive), and *xue* (blood) levels.
- ***Characteristics*** of heat may be discerned in terms not just of temperature such as fire, but whether heat combines with other pathogens: damp-heat, toxic heat, or deficiency heat.

These diagnostic criteria are important in determining the selection of herbs of appropriate properties and potency to address the imbalance.

CAUTIONS/CONTRAINDICATIONS

- Heat-clearing herbs should be used only when needed. Overdose, prolonged use, or inappropriate use will damage the Spleen and Stomach, and consume yin and body fluids. Therefore, they should be prescribed carefully, and discontinued when the desired therapeutic results are achieved.
- Herbs that clear heat and dry dampness are drying in nature and will consume yin and body fluids. In cases of deficiency of the Spleen, Stomach, yin and body fluids, these herbs must be used with caution: it is advisable to add to the formula herbs that harmonize the middle *jiao*, or nourish yin and body fluids. In cases of cold and yang deficiency, bitter and cold heat-clearing herbs are contraindicated.
    - Heat-clearing herbs that are sweet and nourishing, such as *Sheng Di Huang* (Radix Rehmanniae), *Xuan Shen* (Radix Scrophulariae), and *Zhi Mu* (Radix Anemarrhenae), may create dampness and must be used with caution in cases of damp-heat.
    - The bitter, cold properties of herbs that clear heat and dry dampness may damage the Spleen and Stomach, while their drying properties may consume yin. Therefore, these herbs should be used with caution in cases of deficiency of Spleen, Stomach, and body fluids: for protection, herbs that harmonize the middle *jiao* or nourish yin must be combined in the formula.
    - Excess heat and deficiency heat are opposite conditions and require completely different treatment. Using bitter and cold herbs in cases of deficiency heat will deplete yin and cause further deterioration of the condition. Using sweet and cold herbs in cases of excess heat will create more dampness and heat, complicating the condition.
- Correct identification of the location of the heat imbalance is also extremely important. Use of herbs that clear heat from the *xue* (blood) level to treat heat in the *qi* (energy) level directs the heat further inward and worsens the condition. On the other hand, using herbs that clear heat from the *qi* level to treat heat in the *xue* level will not be effective and will further delay recovery from a severe illness.

Use caution in cases involving deficiency: overdose, prolonged or inappropriate use of heat-clearing herbs damage the Spleen and Stomach, and consume yin and body fluids.

PROCESSING

Heat-clearing herbs are generally used with little special processing or preparation.

PHARMACOLOGICAL EFFECTS

- **Antibiotic**: This includes antibacterial, antiviral and antifungal effects. More than 150 commonly-prescribed herbs have been tested for their antibiotic properties. The sensitivity of micro-

Chapter 2 — Heat-Clearing Herbs

organisms to the herbs is well established. Overall, researchers have concluded that herbs that clear heat and eliminate toxins have the most potent antibiotic effects. The benefits of using herbs to treat infections include a broad range of therapeutic actions and low risk of resistance, both of which may be attributed to the large number of bioactive components present within each herb, and the number of herbs present in each herbal formula.

- **Antibacterial**: Herbs with antibacterial action include *Jin Yin Hua* (Flos Lonicerae), *Lian Qiao* (Fructus Forsythiae), *Da Qing Ye* (Folium Isatidis), *Ban Lan Gen* (Radix Isatidis), *Pu Gong Ying* (Herba Taraxaci), *Zhi Mu* (Radix Anemarrhenae), *Zhi Zi* (Fructus Gardeniae), *Xia Ku Cao* (Spica Prunellae), *Huang Qin* (Radix Scutellariae), *Huang Lian* (Rhizoma Coptidis), *Huang Bai* (Cortex Phellodendri), *Mu Dan Pi* (Cortex Moutan), *Chi Shao* (Radix Paeoniae Rubrae), and *Qing Hao* (Herba Artemisiae Annuae).
- **Antiviral**: Herbs with antiviral effects are *Jin Yin Hua* (Flos Lonicerae), *Lian Qiao* (Fructus Forsythiae), *Da Qing Ye* (Folium Isatidis), *Ban Lan Gen* (Radix Isatidis), *Pu Gong Ying* (Herba Taraxaci), *She Gan* (Rhizoma Belamcandae), *Chuan Xin Lian* (Herba Andrographis), *Huang Qin* (Radix Scutellariae), and *Huang Bai* (Cortex Phellodendri).
- **Antifungal**: These include *Ren Dong Teng* (Caulis Lonicerae), *Bai Tou Weng* (Radix Pulsatillae), *Yu Xing Cao* (Herba Houttuyniae), *Huang Bai* (Cortex Phellodendri), *Xuan Shen* (Radix Scrophulariae), *Mu Dan Pi* (Cortex Moutan), *Zi Cao Gen* (Radix Lithospermi) and *Qing Hao* (Herba Artemisiae Annuae).

The sensitivity of micro-organisms to heating-clearing herbs is well established: many of these herbs have anti-bacterial, antiviral and antifungal effects.

- **Antineoplastic**: Many heat-clearing herbs have antineoplastic properties. While the exact mechanisms of this activity vary between herbs, the results include suppressed growth of cancer cells and enhanced immunity of host cells. Herbs with antineoplastic actions include *Qing Dai* (Indigo Naturalis), *Ya Dan Zi* (Fructus Bruceae), *Bai Hua She She Cao* (Herba Oldenlandia), *Ku Shen Gen* (Radix Sophorae Flavescentis), *Huang Lian* (Rhizoma Coptidis), *Xia Ku Cao* (Spica Prunellae), *Yu Xing Cao* (Herba Houttuyniae), *Ban Zhi Lian* (Herba Scutellariae Barbatae), and *Long Kui* (Herba Solanum Nigrum).
- **Antipyretic**: Fever is one of the main symptoms associated with infection. While elevation of body temperature is a defensive response, persistent high fever can cause a wide array of complications. The antipyretic effect of heat-clearing herbs is attributed to direct action on the central nervous system to reduce body temperature, or indirect action via treatment of infection. Herbs with distinct antipyretic action include *Shi Gao* (Gypsum Fibrosum), *Zhi Mu* (Radix Anemarrhenae), *Huang Qin* (Radix Scutellariae), *Huang Lian* (Rhizoma Coptidis), *Zhi Zi* (Fructus Gardeniae), *Da Qing Ye* (Folium Isatidis), *Jin Yin Hua* (Flos Lonicerae), *Lian Qiao* (Fructus Forsythiae), *Di Gu Pi* (Cortex Lycii), and others.
- **Anti-inflammatory**: Herbs that clear heat treat both acute and chronic inflammation. Generally speaking, these herbs are more effective for acute cases of inflammation characterized by swelling and increased capillary permeability. Examples include: *Jin Yin Hua* (Flos Lonicerae), *Lian Qiao* (Fructus Forsythiae), *She Gan* (Rhizoma Belamcandae), *Da Qing Ye* (Folium Isatidis), *Chuan Xin Lian* (Herba Andrographis), *Huang Lian* (Rhizoma Coptidis), *Huang Bai* (Cortex Phellodendri) and *Huang Qin* (Radix Scutellariae).

  Some herbs treat chronic cases of inflammation via stimulating the endocrine system to increase production of corticosteroids. When compared with oral steroids, herbs are gentler and less likely to cause side effects. Some examples are: *Chuan Xin Lian* (Herba Andrographis), *Shan Dou Gen* (Radix Sophorae Tonkinensis) and *Bai Hua She She Cao* (Herba Oldenlandia).

When treating chronic inflammation, herbs are gentler and less likely to cause side effects than oral steroids.

- **Immunologic**: Heat-clearing herbs have various effects on the immune system: some herbs potentiate both specific and non-specific immune response, other heat-clearing herbs suppress the immune system.
  - Herbs that stimulate the immune system by increasing the phagocytic activities of macrophages include *Huang Lian* (Rhizoma Coptidis), *Huang Qin* (Radix Scutellariae), *Zhi Zi* (Fructus Gardeniae), *Jin Yin Hua* (Flos Lonicerae), *Da Qing Ye* (Folium Isatidis), *Chuan Xin Lian* (Herba Andrographis), *Ye Ju Hua* (Flos Chrysanthemi Indici), and *Yu Xing Cao* (Herba Houttuyniae).

Chapter 2 — Heat-Clearing Herbs

- Herbs that enhance cellular immunity include *Bai Jiang Cao* (Herba cum Radice Patriniae), *Shan Dou Gen* (Radix Sophorae Tonkinensis), *Bai Hua She She Cao* (Herba Oldenlandia), *Huang Bai* (Cortex Phellodendri) and *Jin Yin Hua* (Flos Lonicerae).
- Herbs that suppress the immune system to treat allergy or auto-immune disorders include *Huang Qin* (Radix Scutellariae), *Huang Lian* (Rhizoma Coptidis), *Mu Dan Pi* (Cortex Moutan), and *Chuan Xin Lian* (Herba Andrographis).

- **Hematological:** Unchecked febrile disorders often progress to heat attacking the *ying* (nutritive) and *xue* (blood) levels, conditions associated with increased activities of platelets, and coagulation. Therefore, many herbs that clear heat inhibit the aggregation of platelets and slow the coagulation process.
  - Herbs with antiplatelet activity include *Chi Shao* (Radix Paeoniae Rubrae), *Ban Lan Gen* (Radix Isatidis), *Ye Ju Hua* (Flos Chrysanthemi Indici), *Niu Huang* (Calculus Bovis), and *Chuan Xin Lian* (Herba Andrographis).
  - An herb with anticoagulant activity is *Chi Shao* (Radix Paeoniae Rubrae).
  - One example of an herb with thrombolytic action is *Niu Huang* (Calculus Bovis).
- **Antihypertensive**: Many herbs that clear heat also act to lower blood pressure. The mechanism of action includes suppression of sympathetic stimulation, dilation of blood vessels, and diuresis. However, it is important to keep in mind that the antihypertensive actions of some of these herbs are only documented by *in vitro* studies via intravenous injection, and may not be replicated in clinical situations *in vivo*. Please refer to the monograph of each herb for additional details. Herbs with antihypertensive properties include *Huang Lian* (Rhizoma Coptidis), *Huang Qin* (Radix Scutellariae), *Zhi Zi* (Fructus Gardeniae), *Zhi Mu* (Radix Anemarrhenae), *Di Gu Pi* (Cortex Lycii), *Mu Dan Pi* (Cortex Moutan), *Niu Huang* (Calculus Bovis), *Xuan Shen* (Radix Scrophulariae), *Lian Qiao* (Fructus Forsythiae), *Shan Dou Gen* (Radix Sophorae Tonkinensis), *Xia Ku Cao* (Spica Prunellae), *Long Dan Cao* (Radix Gentianae), *Ye Ju Hua* (Flos Chrysanthemi Indici) and *Ban Bian Lian* (Herba Lobeliae Chinensis).
- **Hepatoprotective**: In addition to clearing heat, many herbs also act to lower liver enzyme levels to protect the liver. These herbs may treat elevated liver enzymes, hepatitis, and drug- or chemical-induced liver damage. Herbs with hepatoprotective activity include *Huang Qin* (Radix Scutellariae), *Lian Qiao* (Fructus Forsythiae), *Zhi Zi* (Fructus Gardeniae), *Bai Jiang Cao* (Herba cum Radice Patriniae), *Pu Gong Ying* (Herba Taraxaci), and *Long Dan Cao* (Radix Gentianae).
- **Cholagogic**: Herbs with cholagogic activity promote and regulate the normal production and release of bile acids, therefore minimizing liver- and gallbladder-related diseases. These herbs may be used to treat jaundice, cholecystitis, and cholelithiasis. Herbs with cholagogic actions include *Jin Yin Hua* (Flos Lonicerae), *Yin Chen Hao* (Herba Artemisiae Scopariae), and *Chuan Xin Lian* (Herba Andrographis).
- **Cardiotonic**: Herbs with cardiotonic influence stimulate the heart tissues to treat cardiovascular diseases. Cardiotonic herbs include *Lian Qiao* (Fructus Forsythiae), *Sheng Di Huang* (Radix Rehmanniae), *Xuan Shen* (Radix Scrophulariae), and *Zi Cao Gen* (Radix Lithospermi).

POTENTIAL HERB-DRUG INTERACTIONS

Antibiotic, antipyretic and anti-inflammatory properties are the primary pharmacological characteristics of heat-clearing herbs. Such herbs are commonly used to treat infection, fever and inflammation, all characterized by increase in body temperature. Generally speaking, heat-clearing herbs with these therapeutic effects are not known to interact adversely with drug therapies.

- **Antibiotics**: The concurrent use of herbs and drugs with antibiotic effects may enable these substances to exert a synergistic effect, or potentiate the effects of one another. The potentiating of antibiotic action offers a tremendous advantage, especially if the target micro-organism has high resistance or tolerance to standard pharmacological therapies. For example, the addition of *baicalin*, a component of *Huang Qin* (Radix Scutellariae), was effective in restoring the antibiotic potency of β-lactam antibiotics (such as ampicillin, amoxicillin, methicillin and cefotaxime) against β-lactam-resistant *Staphylococcus aureus* and methicillin-resistant *Staphylococcus aureus* (MRSA).[1]

Heat-clearing herbs in general are not known to interact adversely with drug therapies.

Chapter 2 — Heat-Clearing Herbs

- **Ciprofloxacin (Cipro)**: Some heat-clearing herbs and antibiotic drugs should not be combined. It has been shown that the absorption of ciprofloxacin (Cipro), a quinolone antibiotic, may be affected by concurrent use of *Pu Gong Ying* (Herba Taraxaci), due to the high mineral content of the latter. While the bioavailability of ciprofloxacin was not altered significantly, there were changes to other pharmacokinetic parameters.[2]
- **Antihypertensives**: Some heat-clearing herbs also reduce blood pressure. Thus, concurrent use of some herbs and drugs that affect blood pressure should be prescribed carefully and monitored closely to avoid potential fluctuations of blood pressure.

References

1. *J Pharm Pharmacol* 2000 Mar; 52(3):361-6
2. *Journal of Pharmaceutical Sciences*, 1999; June, 88(6):632-4

Section 1

— Heat-Clearing and Fire-Purging Herbs

Shi Gao (Gypsum Fibrosum)

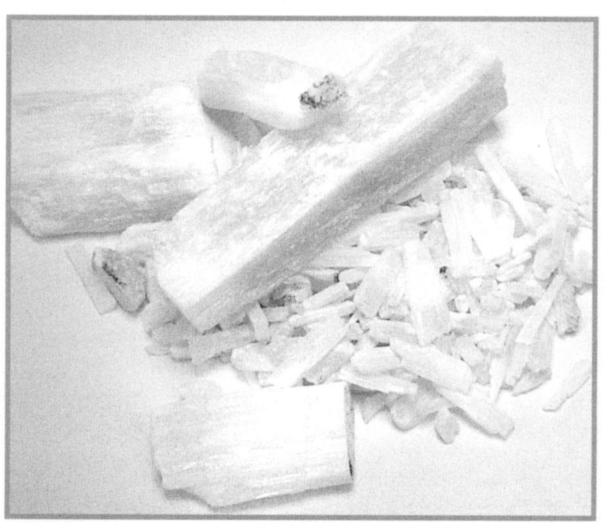

石膏

Pinyin Name: *Shi Gao*
Literal Name: "stone paste"
Alternate Chinese Names: *Ruan Shi Gao, Bai Hu*
Original Source: *Shen Nong Ben Cao Jing* (Divine Husbandman's Classic of the Materia Medica) in the second century
English Name: gypsum
Pharmaceutical Name: Gypsum Fibrosum
Properties: acrid, sweet, very cold
Channels Entered: Lung, Stomach

CHINESE THERAPEUTIC ACTIONS

1. Clears Heat, Sedates Fire, Relieves Irritability and Quenches Thirst

Excess heat in the *qi* (energy) level: Unlike other heat-clearing herbs that have a drying effect, *Shi Gao* (Gypsum Fibrosum) sedates fire, relieves irritability and quenches thirst without drying body fluids. It is most suitable for fire in the Lung and Stomach, characterized by high fever, extreme thirst with preference for cold drinks, profuse sweating, and forceful pulse. The condition is also referred to as 'heat in the *qi* (energy) level' according to the *Wei Qi Ying Xue Bian Zheng* (Defensive, Qi, Nutritive, Blood Differentiation).

- Fire in the Lung and Stomach, at the *qi* (energy) level: use *Shi Gao* with *Zhi Mu* (Radix Anemarrhenae) to clear heat, sedate fire, and moisten dryness. **Exemplar Formula:** *Bai Hu Tang* (White Tiger Decoction).
- Exterior wind-cold and interior heat: add *Ma Huang* (Herba Ephedrae) and *Gui Zhi* (Ramulus Cinnamomi). **Exemplar Formula:** *Da Qing Long Tang* (Major Bluegreen Dragon Decoction).
- Excessive heat in both *qi* (energy) and *xue* (blood) levels with continuous high fever and maculae: use this herb with *Mu Dan Pi* (Cortex Moutan), *Sheng Di Huang* (Radix Rehmanniae) and *Xuan Shen* (Radix Scrophulariae).
- Excessive heat with qi deficiency: combine it with *Ren Shen* (Radix Ginseng). **Exemplar Formula:** *Bai Hu Jia Ren Shen Tang* (White Tiger plus Ginseng Decoction).
- Excessive heat with qi and yin deficiencies: combine *Shi Gao* with *Ren Shen* (Radix Ginseng) and *Mai Men Dong* (Radix Ophiopogonis). **Exemplar Formula:** *Zhu Ye Shi Gao Tang* (Lophatherum and Gypsum Decoction).
- Toxic heat with infection: use it with *Huang Lian* (Rhizoma Coptidis), *Huang Qin* (Radix Scutellariae) and *Huang Bai* (Cortex Phellodendri). **Exemplar Formula:** *San Huang Shi Gao Tang* (Three-Yellow and Gypsum Decoction).
- Influenza, epidemic poliomyelitis, epidemic encephalitis B, with chills and high fever, headache, irritability, dry mouth, insomnia, and in severe cases, bleeding: add *Huang Lian* (Rhizoma Coptidis), *Zhi Zi* (Fructus Gardeniae), *Mu Dan Pi* (Cortex Moutan), *Chi Shao* (Radix Paeoniae Rubrae), and *Zhi Mu* (Radix

Shi Gao (Gypsum Fibrosum)

Anemarrhenae). **Exemplar Formula:** *Qing Wen Bai Du Yin* (Clear Epidemics and Overcome Toxin Decoction).

2. Clears Lung Heat

Excess heat in the Lung: Although *Shi Gao* does not relieve dyspnea or cough, it is essential in treating respiratory disorders caused by heat attacking the Lung. It sedates Lung heat and restores the ascending and descending functions of the Lung that have been impaired by heat. Clinical manifestations include: cough, dyspnea, wheezing, thirst, yellow sputum, red face, a rapid, forceful pulse and a red tongue. In western medicine, heat and toxins in the Lung closely resemble symptoms accompanying acute bronchitis, pneumonia, and pulmonary abscesses.

- Wheezing and dyspnea from Lung heat: add *Ma Huang* (Herba Ephedrae) and *Xing Ren* (Semen Armeniacae Amarum). **Exemplar Formula:** *Ma Xing Gan Shi Tang* (Ephedra, Apricot Kernel, Licorice, and Gypsum Decoction).
- Heat and toxins in the Lung: use *Shi Gao* with *Jin Yin Hua* (Flos Lonicerae), *Huang Qin* (Radix Scutellariae) and *Yu Xing Cao* (Herba Houttuyniae).

3. Clears Heat in the Stomach and Stomach Channel

Stomach Heat: When heat attacks the Stomach, Stomach qi rebels or reverses leading to nausea and vomiting. Heat may also attack the Stomach channel, leading to various problems along its pathway such as headache, orbital pain, toothache, oral ulcers, swelling and pain in the gums, stomatitis, canker sores, and similar heat conditions.

- Nausea and vomiting: add *Ban Xia* (Rhizoma Pinelliae) and *Zhu Ru* (Caulis Bambusae in Taenia).
- Heat attacking the Stomach channel: use this herb with *Sheng Di Huang* (Radix Rehmanniae), *Zhi Mu* (Radix Anemarrhenae) and *Niu Xi* (Radix Cyathulae seu Achyranthis). **Exemplar Formula:** *Yu Nu Jian* (Jade Woman Decoction).

4. Clears Heat and Promotes Healing of Sores, Burns and Eczema

The calcined form of *Shi Gao* has excellent properties to clear heat, treat necrosis and generate flesh. When applied topically, it promotes healing of sores by reducing swelling and bleeding. It can be administered topically or orally.

- Sores, burns and eczema: use calcined *Shi Gao* alone or with *Qing Dai* (Indigo Naturalis) and *Huang Bai* (Cortex Phellodendri).

DOSAGE

15 to 60 grams. The maximum dosage is 100 grams. For oral administration, use unprocessed *Shi Gao*. When it is used in decoction, it should be crushed into fine powder and pre-decocted for 20 to 30 minutes prior to adding other herbs. Since it is a mineral substance and has low solubility, its common dosage is larger than that for other herbs. For oral ingestion as powder, however, the dosage must be decreased, since solubility in decoction is no longer an issue. For topical administration, use calcined *Shi Gao* to promote healing.

CAUTIONS / CONTRAINDICATIONS

- Use of *Shi Gao* is contraindicated in patients who have qi deficiency, yin deficiency, Spleen yang deficiency, deficient cold of the Stomach, or fever due to yin deficiency.
- Because *Shi Gao* is very cold in thermal nature, it is not suitable for long-term use. Its use should be terminated as soon as the desired effect is achieved.

CHEMICAL COMPOSITION

($CaSO_4$+2 H_2O), CaO, SO_3, Al, Mg, Fe, Mn, Zn, Cu.[1]

PHARMACOLOGICAL EFFECTS

- **Antipyretic:** *Shi Gao* has antipyretic action but no diaphoretic effect. The antipyretic function of *Shi Gao* has a rapid onset, but only short duration of action. *Zhi Mu* (Radix Anemarrhenae), in comparison, has slower onset of action but much longer duration. Therefore, these two herbs are synergistic in action and are commonly combined.[2] **Exemplar Formula:** *Bai Hu Tang* (White Tiger Decoction).
- **Immunostimulant:** *Shi Gao* stimulates the immune system and increases phagocytic activity of macrophages. However, it does not have direct inhibitory effects on viruses or bacteria.[3]
- **Effect on healing:** Topical application of *Shi Gao* shortens the recovery time for rabbits with broken bones.[4]
- **Others:** *Shi Gao* has been shown to facilitate the passage of bile, shorten coagulation time, promote diuresis, and reduce spontaneous intake of water (thirst) in laboratory mice.[5]

CLINICAL STUDIES AND RESEARCH

- **Osteoarthrosis deformans endemica:** In Shanxi province, China, over 600 patients with osteoarthrosis deformans endemica were treated by oral ingestion of fine powder of *Shi Gao* at 1 to 3 grams per dose, twice daily. The study reported an overall rate of effectiveness of approximately 80%.[6]
- **Acute inflammation:** In one study, 126 patients with acute lymphadenitis, cellulitis or erysipelas were treated topically with an herbal formulation (3 parts of *Shi Gao* and 1 part China wood oil). The study excluded all

Shi Gao (Gypsum Fibrosum)

patients who had abscesses and ulcerations. The study reported satisfactory results.[7]

- **Burns:** In one study, 53 patients with burns were treated with fine powder of *Shi Gao* sprinkled on the affected area. The study reported a decrease in secretions, reduced incidence of infection, and shortened healing time.[8]
- **Acute sprain**: One report describes 15 patients with acute sprains who were treated with an herbal paste (fresh radish mixed with fine powder of *Shi Gao*) applied topically, with good results.[9]
- **Fever:** According to one report, 200 patients with high fever were treated with an herbal decoction (120 grams of *Shi Gao*, 3 grams of *Ma Huang* (Herba Ephedrae), and 3 grams of *Gui Zhi* (Ramulus Cinnamomi)). Of 200 patients, 181 showed a reduction in body temperature.[10]
- **Fever due to common colds or influenza:** Fifteen patients were treated with an herbal decoction (30 grams each of *Shi Gao* and *Ban Lan Gen* (Radix Isatidis)) with good results.[11]
- **Lobar pneumonia:** According to one report, 9 patients with lobar pneumonia were treated with *Bai Hu Tang* (White Tiger Decoction), with excellent results.[12]

TOXICOLOGY

Shi Gao has very little toxicity. No significant side effects were reported in doses up to 250 grams in humans.[13]

SUPPLEMENT

- 煆石膏 / 煅石膏 *Duan Shi Gao* (Gypsum Fibrosum Preparata), the calcined form of this substance, has excellent properties to clear heat, treat necrosis and generate flesh. It is generally used topically to reduce swelling and bleeding. *Duan Shi Gao* is generally not used internally because once calcined, it loses a major portion of its effectiveness in clearing heat and sedating fire. Furthermore, *Duan Shi Gao* has an astringent action and may cause stagnation and stasis in the middle *jiao*, and thus injure the Spleen and Stomach. In short, use unprocessed *Shi Gao* in decoction for oral ingestion, and calcined *Shi Gao* in powder for topical applications.

AUTHORS' COMMENTS

Shi Gao and *Han Shui Shi* (Mirabilite) both enter the Lung and Stomach to clear heat and sedate fire. *Shi Gao* is more effective to clear heat from *wei* (defense) and *qi* (energy) levels. *Han Shui Shi* is better to purge excess heat from the *xue* (blood) level.

Generally speaking, postpartum women experience deficiency and cold. However, *Shi Gao* can still be used if the diagnosis is heat in the *qi* (energy) level or in the Lung or Stomach. The same principle applies to patients recovering from febrile disorders. The key is to combine *Shi Gao* with tonic herbs such as *Ren Shen* (Radix Ginseng) or *Mai Men Dong* (Radix Ophiopogonis) so that heat can be cleared at the same time that the body is being tonified.

According to Dr. Zhang Xiao-Ping, the combination of *Shi Gao* and *Zhi Mu* (Radix Anemarrhenae) has excellent influence to lower plasma glucose levels to treat diabetes mellitus. These two herbs are especially effective in individuals with diabetes characterized by qi and yin deficiencies. However, it is important to note that high dosages are sometimes associated with hypoglycemia.

Dr. Zhang Xiao-Ping also states that the combination of *Shi Gao* and *Zhi Zi* (Fructus Gardeniae) is very effective to sedate Liver and Heart fire in hyperthyroid patients.

Dr. Shen Yen-Nan reports that fire in specific organs is effectively purged by key herbs, as listed here:

- Lung fire: *Huang Qin* (Radix Scutellariae) and *Sang Bai Pi* (Cortex Mori)
- Heart fire: *Huang Lian* (Rhizoma Coptidis)
- Stomach fire: *Shi Gao* (Gypsum Fibrosum)
- Liver fire: *Zhi Zi* (Fructus Gardeniae)
- Kidney fire: *Zhi Mu* (Radix Anemarrhenae)

References

1. *Xian Dai Zhong Yao Yao Li Xue* (Contemporary Pharmacology of Chinese Herbs), 1997; 284-285
2. *Zhong Yao Xue* (Chinese Herbology), 1998, 115:119
3. Ibid.
4. Ibid.
5. Ibid.
6. *Shan Xi Yi Yao* (Shanxi Medicine and Herbology), 1973; 4:17
7. *Zhong Hua Wai Ke Za Zhi* (Chinese Journal of External Medicine), 1960; 4:366
8. *Fu Jian Zhong Yi Yao* (Fujian Chinese Medicine and Herbology), 1960; 6:21
9. Ibid., 1981; 4:5
10. *Xin Zhong Yi* (New Chinese Medicine), 1980; 6:28
11. Ibid., 3:26
12. *Shang Hai Zhong Yi Yao Za Zhi* (Shanghai Journal of Chinese Medicine and Herbology), 1957; 4:23
13. *Chang Yong Zhong Yao Xian Dai Yan Jiu Yu Lin Chuan* (Recent Study & Clinical Application of Common Traditional Chinese Medicine), 1995; 57:601.

Zhi Mu (Radix Anemarrhenae)

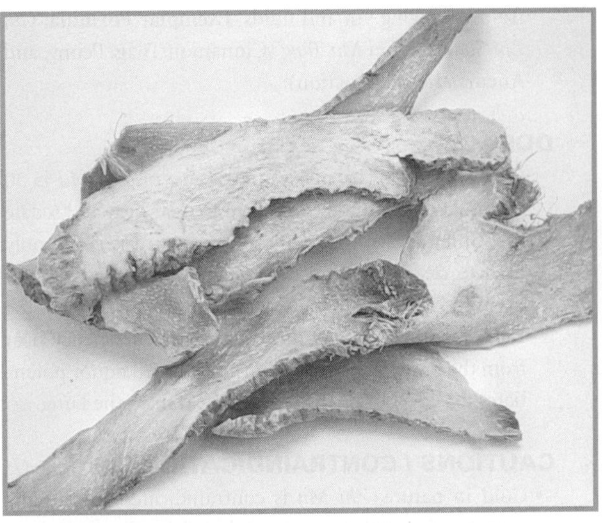

知母

Pinyin Name: *Zhi Mu*
Literal Name: "know about mother"
Alternate Chinese Names: *Mao Zhi Mu, Guang Zhi Mu, Zhi Mu Rou, Yan Zhi Mu*
Original Source: *Shen Nong Ben Cao Jing* (Divine Husbandman's Classic of the Materia Medica) in the second century
English Name: anemarrhena, common anemarrhena rhizome
Botanical Name: *Anemarrhena asphodeloides* Bge.
Pharmaceutical Name: Radix Anemarrhenae
Properties: bitter, sweet, cold
Channels Entered: Lung, Stomach, Kidney

CHINESE THERAPEUTIC ACTIONS

1. Clears Heat and Sedates Fire

Lung and Stomach fire: Excess heat in the *qi* (energy) level or the Lung and Stomach channels will manifest in symptoms of high fever, irritability, perspiration, thirst with desire for cold drinks, and forceful, rapid pulse. *Zhi Mu* (Radix Anemarrhenae), unlike most heat-clearing herbs such as *Huang Lian* (Rhizoma Coptidis) and *Huang Bai* (Cortex Phellodendri) that are drying in nature, can sedate fire and moisten dryness simultaneously. It is the herb of choice when body fluids have been injured by excess heat in the body, manifesting in symptoms such as thirst and excess perspiration.

- Heat in the *qi* (energy) level: combine *Zhi Mu* with *Shi Gao* (Gypsum Fibrosum) to clear heat. **Exemplar Formula:** *Bai Hu Tang* (White Tiger Decoction).

2. Nourishes Yin and Moistens Dryness

Cough due to Lung heat, yin deficiency, or Lung dryness: In addition to its heat-clearing function, *Zhi Mu* also nourishes yin, relieves irritability, and quenches thirst. It is most useful when excess heat is present internally in combination with heat damaging the body fluids.

- Cough with sticky yellow sputum due to Lung heat and yin deficiency: use *Zhi Mu* with *Chuan Bei Mu* (Bulbus Fritillariae Cirrhosae).
- Cough with excess Lung heat: combine it with *Huang Qin* (Radix Scutellariae) to clear heat.

3. Nourishes Yin and Clears Deficiency Fire

Liver and Kidney yin deficiencies: *Zhi Mu* is the ideal herb for patients experiencing yin-deficient fire because it has dual action to clear heat and nourish yin. Clinical applications include tidal fever, steaming bones sensations, irritability, *wu xin re* (five-center heat), and night sweats. It is an essential herb for the treatment of menopause.

- Yin-deficient fire: add *Huang Bai* (Cortex Phellodendri). **Exemplar Formulas:** *Zhi Bai Di Huang Wan* (Anemarrhena, Phellodendron, and Rehmannia Pill) and *Da Bu Yin Wan* (Great Tonify the Yin Pill).

4. Generates Fluids and Quenches Thirst

***Xiao ke* (wasting and thirsting) syndrome:** Deficiency fire damaging fluids can easily lead to thirst and dryness. *Zhi Mu* is commonly used for patients with *xiao ke* (wasting and thirsting) syndrome with thirst and increased water intake.

- Thirst due to heat in the Lung and Stomach damaging fluids: use *Zhi Mu* with *Shi Gao* (Gypsum Fibrosum), *Tian Hua Fen* (Radix Trichosanthis), *Wu Wei Zi* (Fructus Schisandrae Chinensis) and *Huang Qi* (Radix Astragali).

5. Neutralizes Unwanted Effects of Warm Herbs

Because warm or hot herbs are drying by nature, use of these herbs in large doses or over a long period of time may damage yin and body fluids. *Zhi Mu* is commonly used in combination with such warm or hot herbs to neutralize the unwanted side effects without compromising overall effectiveness.

- When *Huang Qi* (Radix Astragali) or other qi-tonic herbs must be used, yang rises, leading to dryness and heat. *Zhi Mu* can be used to neutralize this heat and moisten dryness.
- When *Fu Zi* (Radix Aconiti Lateralis Praeparata) and *Qiang Huo* (Rhizoma et Radix Notopterygii) are needed for treatment of *bi zheng* (painful obstruction syndrome), *Zhi Mu* can be used to prevent the two hot herbs

Zhi Mu (Radix Anemarrhenae)

from damaging yin and fluids. **Exemplar Formula:** *Gui Zhi Shao Yao Zhi Mu Tang* (Cinnamon Twig, Peony, and Anemarrhena Decoction).

DOSAGE

6 to 12 grams. The maximum dosage of *Zhi Mu* is 30 grams. Use the unprocessed form to clear heat and sedate fire. Bitter and cold, the unprocessed form is commonly used to clear heat from the Lung, Stomach and Kidney. Frying *Zhi Mu* with salt facilitates its entrance to the Kidney, and potentiates its effect to clear deficiency heat from the lower *jiao*. Frying with grain-based liquor potentiates the effect of *Zhi Mu* to clear heat from the Lung.

CAUTIONS / CONTRAINDICATIONS

- Cold in nature, *Zhi Mu* is contraindicated in patients with diarrhea, Spleen or Stomach deficiencies, or Kidney deficiency.

CHEMICAL COMPOSITION

Timosaponin, mangiferin, sarsasapogenin, markogenin, neogitogenin, anemarns A,B,C,D.[1]

PHARMACOLOGICAL EFFECTS

- **Antidiabetic:** In healthy rabbits, oral ingestion of *Zhi Mu* at 200 mg/kg decreased blood glucose levels between 18% and 30% for up to 6 hours. In rabbits with diabetes mellitus, oral ingestion of *Zhi Mu* at 500 mg/kg for 4 days reduced blood glucose levels and minimized atrophy of the pancreas. Anemarns A, B, C, and D all have antidiabetic effect, with B being the most potent.[2,3]
- **Antipyretic:** The antipyretic action of *Zhi Mu* has a slow onset but prolonged duration, while the same action of *Shi Gao* (Gypsum Fibrosum) has a rapid onset but short duration. Therefore, these two herbs have synergistic effects as they achieve immediate and prolonged antipyretic effects.[4] They are commonly combined, such as in *Bai Hu Tang* (White Tiger Decoction).
- **Antibiotic:** *Zhi Mu* has demonstrated inhibitory effects against *Staphylococcus aureus*, α- and β-hemolytic streptococcus, *Salmonella typhi, E. coli, Bacillus subtilis, Vibrio cholerae*, and *Pseudomonas* spp., *Mycobacterium* spp., and dermatophytes.[5,6]
- **Others:** *Zhi Mu* also displays antineoplastic and cholagogic activities.[7,8]

CLINICAL STUDIES AND RESEARCH

- **Prostatic hypertrophy:** In one study, 80 patients with prostatic hypertrophy were treated with an herbal formula with 86.3% reporting marked improvement. The formula contained *Zhi Mu* 20g, *Huang Bai* (Cortex Phellodendri) 20g, *Niu Xi* (Radix Cyathulae seu Achyranthis) 20g, *Dan Shen* (Radix Salviae Miltiorrhizae) 30 to 50g, *Da Huang* (Radix et Rhizoma Rhei) 10 to 15g, and *Yi Mu Cao* (Herba Leonuri) 50g.[9]
- **Acute rheumatism:** According to one report, 56 patients with acute-onset rheumatism were treated with an herbal formula with 71.4% effectiveness. The herbal formula contained *Zhi Mu* 30g, *Zhi Gan Cao* (Radix Glycyrrhizae Preparata) 15g, *Gui Zhi* (Ramulus Cinnamomi) 15g, *Shi Gao* (Gypsum Fibrosum) 50g, and *Geng Mi* (Semen Oryzae) 50g. Modifications to the formula were made if deemed necessary by the practitioner.[10]

HERB-DRUG INTERACTION

- **Antidiabetics:** It is prudent to use *Zhi Mu* with caution with insulin, sulfonylureas, and other antidiabetic medications. Though no interaction has been documented, the combination of antidiabetic herbs and drugs may have a synergistic effect, leading to hypoglycemia.[11] [Note: Examples of antidiabetic drugs include insulin, tolbutamide (Orinase), glipizide (Glucotrol), and glyburide (DiaBeta/Micronase).]

TOXICOLOGY

In rabbits, intravenous injection of a *Zhi Mu* preparation showed no toxicity at 0.5 ml, caused dyspnea and a small reduction in blood pressure at 1 to 3 ml, and led to respiratory depression and fatality at 7 ml.[12]

AUTHORS' COMMENTS

Depending on the other herbs with which it is combined, *Zhi Mu* has dual functions to clear excess or deficiency heat. It is used often because it nourishes fluids and clears heat simultaneously. Furthermore, *Zhi Mu* is often preferred over yin tonics, which are hard to digest and may cause dampness if not prescribed carefully.

Zhi Mu and *Shi Gao* (Gypsum Fibrosum) are often used synergistically to sedate fire and prevent the loss of yin. Sweet and cold, *Zhi Mu* clears heat, generates fluids and moistens dryness. It clears heat in all three *jiaos*, clearing Lung heat in the upper *jiao*, sedating Stomach fire in the middle *jiao*, and clearing deficiency fire of the Kidney in the lower *jiao*. Very cold in thermal nature, *Shi Gao* enters the *qi* (energy) level and is best in clearing excess heat in the Lung and Stomach. It is the herb of choice when clearing heat from the *qi* level manifesting in symptoms of high fever, extreme thirst with preference for cold drinks, profuse sweating and a forceful, rapid pulse. Together, *Zhi Mu* and *Shi Gao* sedate fire without drying yin.

Dr. Shen Yen-Nan reports that specific organs injured by fire can be treated with optimum results by key herbs, as follows:

Zhi Mu (Radix Anemarrhenae)

- Lung fire: *Huang Qin* (Radix Scutellariae) and *Sang Bai Pi* (Cortex Mori)
- Heart fire: *Huang Lian* (Rhizoma Coptidis)
- Stomach fire: *Shi Gao* (Gypsum Fibrosum)
- Liver fire: *Zhi Zi* (Fructus Gardeniae)
- Kidney fire: *Zhi Mu* (Radix Anemarrhenae)

References

1. *Xian Dai Zhong Yao Yao Li Xue* (Contemporary Pharmacology of Chinese Herbs), 1997; 286
2. *Ri Ben Yao Wu Xue Za Zhi* (Japan Journal of Pharmacology), 1971; 67(6):223p
3. *Planta med*, 1985; 51(2):100
4. *Zhong Yao Xue* (Chinese Herbology), 1998; 115:119
5. *Yao Xue Qing Bao Tong Xun* (Journal of Herbal Information), 1987; 5(4):62
6. *Zhong Hua Xin Yi Xue Bao* (Chinese Journal of New Medicine), 1950; 1(5):95
7. *Yao Xue Qing Bao Tong Xun* (Journal of Herbal Information), 1987; 5(4):62
8. *Chang Yong Zhong Yao Cheng Fen Yu Yao Li Shou Ce* (A Handbook of the Composition and Pharmacology of Common Chinese Drugs), 1994; 1240:1244
9. *Zhong Xi Yi Jie He Za Zhi* (Journal of Integrated Chinese and Western Medicine), 1988; 3:155
10. *Ji Lin Zhong Yi Yao* (Jilin Chinese Medicine and Herbology), 1992; (1):16
11. Chen, J. Recognition & prevention of herb-drug interactions, *Medical Acupuncture*, Fall/Winter 1998/1999; volume 10/number 2; 9-13
12. *Chang Yong Zhong Yao Xian Dai Yan Jiu Yu Lin Chuan* (Recent Study & Clinical Application of Common Traditional Chinese Medicine), 1995; 61:63

Qing Guo Gen (Radix Canarium Album)

青果根

Pinyin Name: *Qing Guo Gen*
Literal Name: "blue-green fruit root"
Alternate Chinese Names: *Gan Lan Gen, Jian Gan E Gen*
English Name: white olive root
Botanical Name: *Canarium album* (Lour.) Raeusch.
Pharmaceutical Name: Radix Canarium Album
Properties: sweet, sour, astringent, cool
Channels Entered: Lung, Stomach

CHINESE THERAPEUTIC ACTIONS

1. Clears the Lung, Benefits the Throat, Generates Body Fluids and Eliminates Toxins

Cough with profuse sputum, pharyngitis: *Qing Guo Gen* (Radix Canarium Album) reduces minor inflammation of the respiratory system involving sore throat, cough and profuse sputum.

- Cough with profuse sputum and pharyngitis: use *Qing Guo Gen* with *Fu Rong* (Radix Hibisci) and *Zao Xiu* (Rhizoma Paridis).
- Laryngitis: combine it with *Gu Zhi Hua* (Semen Oroxyli), *Pang Da Hai* (Semen Sterculiae Lychnophorae) and *Luo Han Guo* (Fructus Momordicae).

2. Strengthens the Spleen

Leukorrhea from Spleen deficiency: *Qing Guo Gen* treats leukorrhea from Spleen deficiency, indicated by clear or white vaginal discharge.

- Leukorrhea: use this herb with *Long Yan Hua* (Flos Longan) and *Bai Long Chuan Hua Tou* (Radix Clerodendron Paniculatum). It can also be used with *Wan Dai Tang* (End Discharge Decoction).

Stomach pain from Stomach qi deficiency: This type of pain caused by deficiency is typically dull, and can be temporarily reduced by applying pressure to the affected area.

- Stomach pain: use *Qing Guo Gen* with *Ren Shen* (Radix Ginseng), *Fu Ling* (Poria), *Bai Zhu* (Rhizoma Atractylodis Macrocephalae), and *Gan Cao* (Radix Glycyrrhizae).
- Dysentery from deficiency: combine it with *Feng Wei Cao* (Herba Pteris), *Huo Xiang* (Herba Agastache), *Hou Po* (Cortex Magnoliae Officinalis) and *Bai Zhu* (Rhizoma Atractylodis Macrocephalae).

DOSAGE

4.5 to 9 grams in decoction.

Han Shui Shi (Mirabilite)

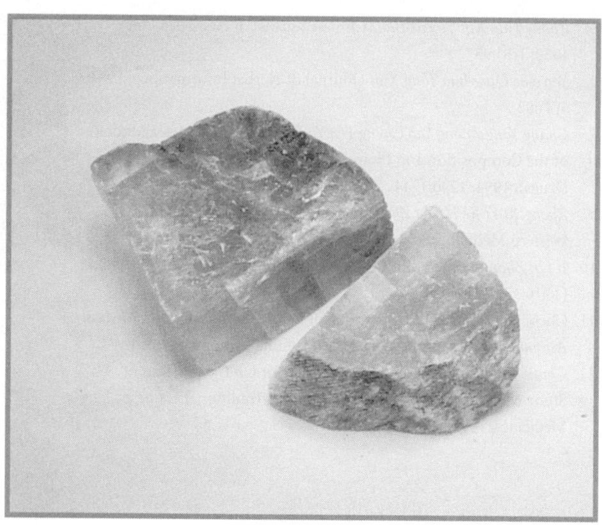

寒水石

Pinyin Name: *Han Shui Shi*
Literal Name: "cold water stone"
Alternate Chinese Names: *Ling Shui Shi, Yan Jing Shi*
Original Source: *Shen Nong Ben Cao Jing* (Divine Husbandman's Classic of the Materia Medica) in the second century
English Name: mirabilite crystal
Pharmaceutical Name: Mirabilite
Properties: salty, very cold
Channels Entered: Stomach, Kidney

CHINESE THERAPEUTIC ACTIONS

1. Clears Heat and Purges Fire

Han Shui Shi (Mirabilite) clears heat and purges fire from the *qi* (energy) level, a condition characterized by profuse perspiration, high fever, extreme thirst, and forceful pulse. It is also effective for treating heat attacking and covering the Pericardium, leading to delirium and semiconsciousness.

- Excess heat at the *qi* (energy) level: use *Han Shui Shi* with *Shi Gao* (Gypsum Fibrosum).
- Heat attacking and covering the Pericardium: combine it with herbs that function to open sensory orifices.

2. Topical Use to Sedate Fire and Toxins

Han Shui Shi is used topically to sedate fire and clear heat. Clinical applications include sore throat, stomatitis, burns, sores, infection and inflammation of the eyes, or other wounds with fire or heat components. *Han Shui Shi* is usually used individually in fine powder.

DOSAGE

10 to 15 grams. *Han Shui Shi* should be crushed into fine powder prior to oral or topical administration.

CAUTIONS / CONTRAINDICATIONS

- *Han Shui Shi* is contraindicated for patients with deficiency and cold of the Spleen and Stomach.

CHEMICAL COMPOSITION

Sodium sulfate.[1]

SUPPLEMENT

Two other substances are sometimes substituted for *Han Shui Shi*. It is important to be aware of their differences in clinical use.

- 寒水石 *Han Shui Shi* (Mirabilite), sodium sulfate, is the correct and standard substance. It is the most potent form, with maximum water solubility at 34° C. The saturated solution will yield crystalline precipitates when placed in cold water.
- 紅石膏 / 红石膏 *Hong Shi Gao* (Gypsum Rubrae), calcium sulfate, is sometimes used as a substitute. It has low water solubility and does not yield crystalline precipitates.
- 方解石 / 方解石 *Fang Jie Shi* (Calcitum), calcium carbonate, is the other substitute. It is insoluble in water and does not yield crystalline precipitates.

AUTHORS' COMMENTS

When *Mang Xiao* (Natrii Sulfas) in saturated solution is cooled below room temperature, *Han Shui Shi* (Mirabilite) is formed as the crystalline precipitate. *Han Shui Shi* (Mirabilite) and *Mang Xiao* (Natrii Sulfas) have similar functions but are not interchangeable. *Han Shui Shi* clears heat from the Stomach, while *Mang Xiao* has a much broader effect to clear heat from Lung, Stomach and Large Intestine.

References

1. *Zhong Yao Xue* (Chinese Herbology), 1998; 131:132

Tian Hua Fen (Radix Trichosanthis)

天花粉 天花粉

Pinyin Name: *Tian Hua Fen*
Literal Name: "sky pollen," "heavenly flower powder"
Alternate Chinese Names: *Hua Fen, Gua Lou Gen*
Original Source: *Shen Nong Ben Cao Jing* (Divine Husbandman's Classic of the Materia Medica) in the second century
English Name: trichosanthes root, snake gourd root
Botanical Name: *Trichosanthes kirilowii* Maxim. (*Gua Lou*); *Trichosanthes japonica* Regel (*Ri Ben Gua Lou*)
Pharmaceutical Name: Radix Trichosanthis
Properties: bitter, slightly sweet, cold
Channels Entered: Lung, Stomach

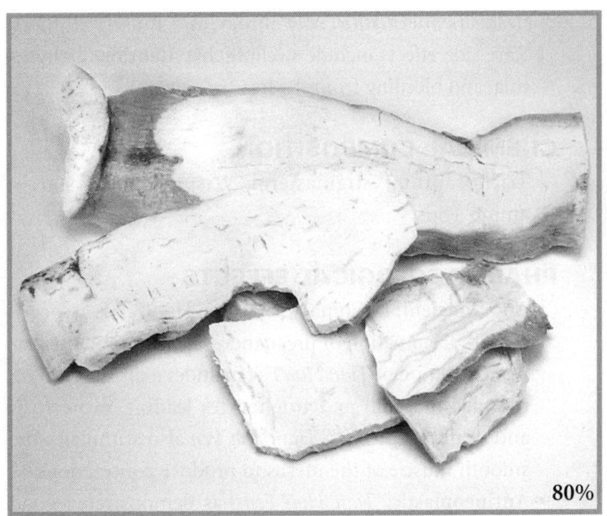
80%

CHINESE THERAPEUTIC ACTIONS

1. Clears Heat and Generates Body Fluids

Heat injuring the yin/body fluids: *Tian Hua Fen* (Radix Trichosanthis) is most effective for moistening the Lung and clearing Stomach fire. When internal heat remains untreated, it may create dryness or damage yin. Irritability, dry lips, mouth and tongue, and thirst with desire to drink cold beverages, are diagnostic keys for heat-damaged fluids. This herb is essential in treating patients suffering from *xiao ke* (wasting and thirsting) syndrome.

- Heat and dryness in the Lung and Stomach: use *Tian Hua Fen* with *Mai Men Dong* (Radix Ophiopogonis), *Zhi Mu* (Radix Anemarrhenae) and *Wu Wei Zi* (Fructus Schisandrae Chinensis). These herbs are commonly used to treat excessive thirst and excessive water intake due to upper *xiao ke* (wasting and thirsting) syndrome. **Exemplar Formula:** *Sha Shen Mai Dong Tang* (Glehnia and Ophiopogonis Decoction).
- Heat and dryness attacking the Lung with cough and thick, sticky sputum that is difficult to expectorate: use *Tian Hua Fen* with *Chuan Bei Mu* (Bulbus Fritillariae Cirrhosae), and *Sang Bai Pi* (Cortex Mori).
- Dryness with irritability: combine it with *Shi Hu* (Herba Dendrobii), *Yu Zhu* (Rhizoma Polygonati Odorati) and *Mai Men Dong* (Radix Ophiopogonis).
- *Xiao ke* (wasting and thirsting) syndrome, diabetes mellitus, diabetes insipidus, hyperthyroidism: use *Tian Hua Fen* with *Sheng Di Huang* (Radix Rehmanniae), *Shi Gao* (Gypsum Fibrosum) *Zhi Mu* (Radix Anemarrhenae), *Shan Yao* (Rhizoma Dioscoreae) and *Wu Wei Zi* (Fructus Schisandrae Chinensis).

2. Clears Heat, Dispels Pus

Carbuncles, abscesses and sores: Redness, swelling and pain with pus are signs of toxic heat accumulation. *Tian Hua Fen* is most effective in treating breast abscesses and is used both topically and internally for toxic heat problems.

- Skin abscesses and ulcerations: use *Tian Hua Fen* with *Jin Yin Hua* (Flos Lonicerae), *Chuan Bei Mu* (Bulbus Fritillariae Cirrhosae), and *Zao Jiao Ci* (Spina Gleditsiae). **Exemplar Formula:** *Zhen Ren Huo Ming Yin* (True Man Decoction to Revitalize Life).
- Abscess without ulceration or necrosis: combine this herb with *Chi Xiao Dou* (Semen Phaseoli) and vinegar, apply topically.
- Breast abscess: add *Ru Xiang* (Gummi Olibanum), *Gua Lou Shi* (Fructus Trichosanthis), *Bai Zhi* (Radix Angelicae Dahuricae), *Zhe Bei Mu* (Bulbus Fritillariae Thunbergii) and *Pu Gong Ying* (Herba Taraxaci).
- Swelling and pain of external injuries: use *Tian Hua Fen* with blood-activating herbs such as *Ru Xiang* (Gummi Olibanum). **Exemplar Formula:** *Fu Yuan Huo Xue Tang* (Revive Health by Invigorating the Blood Decoction).

DOSAGE

10 to 15 grams. The maximum dosage of *Tian Hua Fen* is 30 grams. This herb can be used in decoction or as topical powder.

CAUTIONS / CONTRAINDICATIONS

- Cold in nature, *Tian Hua Fen* should be used with caution in cases of deficiency and cold of the Spleen and Stomach.
- Use of *Tian Hua Fen* is contraindicated during pregnancy, as it may increase the risk of miscarriage.
- Concurrent use of *Tian Hua Fen* with *Wu Tou* (Radix Aconiti) or *Fu Zi* (Radix Aconiti Lateralis Praeparata) is contraindicated.
- Common side effects of *Tian Hua Fen* may include fever,

Tian Hua Fen (Radix Trichosanthis)

headache, dermatitis, sore throat, and muscle stiffness. Rare side effects include swelling, hypotension, arrhythmia, and bleeding from the liver or spleen.[1,2,3]

CHEMICAL COMPOSITION

Trichosanthin, stigmasterol, α-spinasterol, starch, amino acids.[4]

PHARMACOLOGICAL EFFECTS

- **Abortifacient:** In China, use of *Tian Hua Fen* is associated with termination of pregnancy. The proposed mechanism of action of *Tian Hua Fen* includes a direct effect on the placental villi and trophocytes leading to necrosis and death of the cells. *Tian Hua Fen* also stimulates the smooth muscle of the uterus to produce contractions.[5,6]
- **Antineoplastic:** *Tian Hua Fen* has demonstrated good results in treating cancer of the trophocyte. It is also effective in treating liver cancer with ascites in mice. It has not been shown to be effective for other types of cancer.[7]
- **Hyperglycemic:** Administration of *Tian Hua Fen* raises blood glucose levels in rabbits, especially in subjects that have been fasting.[8]
- **Antibiotic:** *Tian Hua Fen* has been shown to inhibit the activity of β-hemolytic streptococcus, *Diplococcus pneumoniae* and *Bacillus diphtheriae.* It also has an inhibiting influence on the replication of HIV virus *in vitro.*[9,10,11]

CLINICAL STUDIES AND RESEARCH

- **Abortion:** A preparation of *Tian Hua Fen* injected intramuscularly or into the amniotic sac has been used in over 10,000 patients seeking abortion in Shanghai, with 97% of the pregnancies terminated. In some cases, up to 150 hours passed before abortion occurred following *Tian Hua Fen* injection. Some patients experienced bleeding and allergic reactions. Injection of *Tian Hua Fen* into the amniotic sac was concluded to be more effective and cause fewer side effects than intramuscular injection. The women who received this treatment did not subsequently have trouble becoming pregnant, but did have a higher-than-average percentage of early delivery. Blood tests confirmed that traces of *Tian Hua Fen* may still be present in the patient up to six years following this procedure.[12]
- **Abortifacient:** Intramuscular injection of *Tian Hua Fen* has been effectively used in treatment of hydatid pregnancy, chorioepithelioma, and ectopic pregnancy.[13]

TOXICOLOGY

Moderate overdose of *Tian Hua Fen* in dogs (3 to 6 times the adult dose) is associated with lethargy, lack of energy, decreased food intake, and interference with heart, liver and kidney functions. Gross overdose (9 to 12 times the adult dose) for 1 to 2 weeks is associated with arrhythmia, necrosis of liver and kidney tissues, and death.[14]

AUTHORS' COMMENTS

Tian Hua Fen is commonly used in an herbal formula for treatment of diabetes mellitus. However, modern pharmacology confirms not only that *Tian Hua Fen* has no antidiabetic effect, but that it may in fact contribute to hyperglycemia. Two explanations have been offered to clarify this paradox.

- Diabetes is often diagnosed and treated as *xiao ke* (wasting and thirsting) syndrome, though it is not necessarily the same in all aspects. The diagnostic confirmation of diabetes mellitus is high blood glucose, while the diagnosis for *xiao ke* (wasting and thirsting) syndrome is the presence of polyuria, polydipsia, and polyphagia. These are two separate diagnoses. While *Tian Hua Fen* does not treat diabetes directly, it addresses yin deficiency that is present in both diabetes and *xiao ke* syndrome.
- The effect of an individual herb is different from that of an herbal formula. *Tian Hua Fen* may not lower blood glucose directly, but contributes to the overall treatment of diabetes mellitus by relieving the symptoms and complications.

Tian Hua Fen, Tian Men Dong (Radix Asparagi), and *Mai Men Dong* (Radix Ophiopogonis) have many similar functions to nourish yin and promote the generation of body fluids. *Tian Hua Fen* treats dryness caused by heat. *Tian Men Dong* treats Kidney yin-deficient fire with low-grade fever, night sweating and nocturnal emissions. *Mai Men Dong* treats Heart yin deficiency with fire due to heat in the *ying* (nutritive) level.

Dr. Hu Qing-Shan has successfully treated chronic granulocytic leukemia with this formula: *Tian Hua Fen* 40%, *Qing Dai* (Indigo Naturalis) 40%, *Niu Huang* (Calculus Bovis) 10%, and *Lu Hui* (Aloe) 10%. This is taken twice daily in 1.5 gram doses.

References

1. *Zhong Hua Yi Xue Za Zhi* (Chinese Journal of Medicine), 1976; (4):215
2. *Zhong Yao Yao Li Yu Ying Yong* (Pharmacology and Applications of Chinese Herbs), 1983: 149
3. *Zhong Xi Yi Jie He Za Zhi* (Journal of Integrated Chinese and Western Medicine), 1988; 8(8):461
4. *Xian Dai Zhong Yao Yao Li Xue* (Contemporary Pharmacology of Chinese Herbs), 1997; 289
5. *Wu Han Yi Xue Yuan Xue Bao* (Journal of Wuhan University School of Medicine), 1978; 19
6. Ibid., 1975(1):79
7. *Di Er Jun Yi Da Xue Xue Bao* (Journal of Second Military University of Medicine), 1980; (2):9
8. *Zhong Yao Xue* (Chinese Herbology), 1998; 123:125
9. *Zhong Yao Yao Li Yu Ying Yong* (Pharmacology and Applications of Chinese Herbs), 1983:149
10. *AIDS*, 1991; 5:865
11. *Proc Natl Acad Sci*, 1991; 88(15):6570

Tian Hua Fen (Radix Trichosanthis)

12. *Zhong Yao Yao Li Yu Ying Yong* (Pharmacology and Applications of Chinese Herbs), 1983
13. *Xin Yi Yao Xue Za Zhi* (New Journal of Medicine and Herbology), 1977; 10:45
14. *Chang Yong Zhong Yao Cheng Fen Yu Yao Li Shou Ce* (A Handbook of the Composition and Pharmacology of Common Chinese Drugs), 1994; 471:482

Lu Gen (Rhizoma Phragmitis)

蘆根　芦根

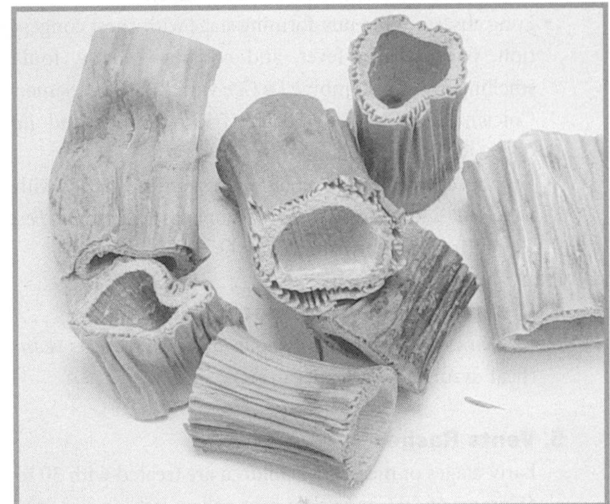

Pinyin Name: *Lu Gen*
Literal Name: "reed rhizome"
Alternate Chinese Names: *Wei Gen, Lu Zhu Gen*
Original Source: *Ming Yi Za Zhu* (Miscellaneous Records of Famous Physicians) by Tao Hong-Jing in 500 A.D.
English Name: phragmites root, reed rhizome
Botanical Name: *Phragmites communis* Trin.
Pharmaceutical Name: Rhizoma Phragmitis
Properties: sweet, cold
Channels Entered: Lung, Stomach

CHINESE THERAPEUTIC ACTIONS

1. Clears Heat and Promotes Generation of Body Fluids

Febrile disease injuring body fluids: Cold and sweet, *Lu Gen* (Rhizoma Phragmitis) clears heat and replenishes body fluids. It is most useful in treating patients with heat accompanied by fluid damage, characterized by fever, irritability, and thirst.

- Internal heat with thirst and dryness: use *Lu Gen* with *Tian Hua Fen* (Radix Trichosanthis) and *Mai Men Dong* (Radix Ophiopogonis).
- Internal heat with high fever: combine it with *Shi Gao* (Gypsum Fibrosum) and *Zhi Mu* (Radix Anemarrhenae).
- Wind-heat with thirst: add *Ju Hua* (Flos Chrysanthemi), *Jin Yin Hua* (Flos Lonicerae) and *Bo He* (Herba Menthae). **Exemplar Formulas:** *Sang Ju Yin* (Mulberry Leaf and Chrysanthemum Decoction) and *Yin Qiao San* (Honeysuckle and Forsythia Powder).
- Irritability: use *Lu Gen* with *Zhi Zi* (Fructus Gardeniae).

2. Clears Stomach Heat, Regulates Stomach Qi

Nausea and vomiting: When heat attacks the Stomach, it may damage yin and cause thirst. Furthermore, Stomach heat may also affect the normal circulation of Stomach qi, leading to qi reversal, manifesting in nausea and vomiting.

- Nausea, vomiting and thirst due to Stomach heat: use *Lu Gen* with *Zhu Ru* (Caulis Bambusae in Taenia) and *Pi Pa Ye* (Folium Eriobotryae).
- Thirst and perspiration: combine it with *Shi Gao* (Gypsum Fibrosum) and *Zhi Mu* (Radix Anemarrhenae).

3. Clears Lung Heat, Regulates Lung Qi

Lung heat with dryness: When heat attacks the Lung, it may damage yin and cause thirst and dry mouth, scanty, yellow, difficult-to-expectorate sputum, chest congestion, a tickling sensation in the throat, or, in severe cases, blood-streaked sputum. Furthermore, Lung heat may also affect the normal circulation of Lung qi, leading to qi reversal causing coughing.

- Cough and thirst caused by Lung heat: use *Lu Gen* with *Jie Geng* (Radix Platycodonis), *Xing Ren* (Semen Armeniacae Amarum) and *Sang Ye* (Folium Mori).
- Cough with thick and sticky sputum: use it with *Yi Yi Ren* (Semen Coicis), *Jin Yin Hua* (Flos Lonicerae), *Yu*

Lu Gen (Rhizoma Phragmitis)

Xing Cao (Herba Houttuyniae) and *Dong Gua Zi* (Semen Benincasae).

- Bronchitis with chest pain, congestion, the absence of perspiration, aversion to cold, fever: combine this herb with *Jing Jie* (Herba Schizonepetae), *Bo He* (Herba Menthae), and *Zi Su Ye* (Folium Perillae).
- Alternating chills and fever, chest congestion and pain: use it with *Chai Hu* (Radix Bupleuri) and *Qing Hao* (Herba Artemisiae Annuae).
- Blood-streaked sputum: use it with *Ou Jie* (Nodus Nelumbinis Rhizomatis), *Bai Mao Gen* (Rhizoma Imperatae) and *Bai Ji* (Rhizoma Bletillae).
- Lung abscess at the pus-forming stage with chest congestion, pain, cough, fever, and copious, bloody, foul-smelling sputum: combine *Lu Gen* with *Yi Yi Ren* (Semen Coicis), *Gua Lou Ren* (Semen Trichosanthis), and *Jie Geng* (Radix Platycodonis).
- Lung abscess during the suppuration stage: use *Lu Gen* with *Sha Shen* (Radix Glehniae seu Adenophorae), *Tian Hua Fen* (Radix Trichosanthis) and *Huang Qi* (Radix Astragali).

4. Clears Heat and Promotes Diuresis

Lu Gen clears heat and promotes diuresis. It treats *re lin* (heat dysuria) with scanty urine.

5. Vents Rashes

Early-stages of measles in children are treated with 30 to 60 grams of *Lu Gen* to clear heat, relieve itching and promote eruption of measles.

6. Relieves Food Poisoning

Lu Gen has a mild influence to treat food poisoning caused by ingestion of fish and crab. It also has mild action to relieve over-consumption of alcohol. Since its effect is rather mild, treatment in acute conditions requires combination with other herbs.

DOSAGE

10 to 30 grams of the dried herb. 15 to 60 grams of the fresh herb, with maximum (fresh) dosage of 100 grams. The fresh form of *Lu Gen* has a stronger function to clear heat and promote generation of body fluids.

CAUTIONS / CONTRAINDICATIONS

- Cold in nature, *Lu Gen* should be used with caution for patients who have deficiency and cold of the Spleen and Stomach.

CHEMICAL COMPOSITION

Amino acids, fatty acids, sterols, tocopherols, polyphenols, caffeic acid, gentisic acid, dioxane lignin, guaiacyl, syringyl, 4-hydroxyphenyl, 2,5-dimethoxy-p-benzoquinone, p-hydroxybenzaldehyde, syringaldehyde, coniferaldehyde, vanillic acid, ferulic acid, p-coumaric acid, coixol, asparagine, arabinose, xylose, glucose.[1]

PHARMACOLOGICAL EFFECTS

- **Gastrointestinal:** Preparations of *Lu Gen* have a mild inhibitory effect on the smooth muscle of the intestines by slowing down intestinal peristalsis.[2]
- **CNS suppressant:** It has a mild sedative effect on the central nervous system (CNS) in rats and mice. It also counters the excitation induced by caffeine.[3]

AUTHORS' COMMENTS

Lu Gen is a versatile herb that clears heat from the Lung in the upper *jiao*, from the Stomach in the middle *jiao*, and from the Urinary Bladder in the lower *jiao*.

References

1. *Chang Yong Zhong Yao Cheng Fen Yu Yao Li Shou Ce* (A Handbook of the Composition and Pharmacology of Common Chinese Drugs), 1994; 993-994
2. *Zhi Wu Yao You Xiao Cheng Fen Shou Ce* (Manual of Plant Medicinals and Their Active Constituents), 1986: 232, 1073
3. Ibid.

Zhu Ye (Herba Phyllostachys)

竹葉 竹叶

Pinyin Name: *Zhu Ye*
Literal Name: "bamboo leaves"
Alternate Chinese Names: *Xian Zhu Ye, Zhu Ye Juan Xin*
Original Source: *Ming Yi Za Zhu* (Miscellaneous Records of Famous Physicians) by Tao Hong-Jing in 500 A.D.
English Name: bamboo leaves
Botanical Name: *Phyllostachys nigra* (Lodd.) Munro var. *henonis* (Mitf.) Stapf. Ex Rendle
Pharmaceutical Name: Herba Phyllostachys
Properties: sweet, bland, cold
Channels Entered: Heart, Stomach, Lung

CHINESE THERAPEUTIC ACTIONS

1. Clears Heat, Relieves Irritability and Generates Body Fluids

Febrile disorders: *Zhu Ye* (Herba Phyllostachys) treats heat in the Heart and Stomach, manifesting in symptoms of irritability and thirst. The Heart opens to the tongue, thus excess heat accumulation in the Heart may lead to ulcers on the tongue, insomnia, and restless crying in children. Clinically, heat attacking the Heart is characterized by irritability, while heat attacking the Stomach is characterized by thirst.

- Heat attacking the Heart with irritability: use *Zhu Ye* with *Zhi Mu* (Radix Anemarrhenae) and *Mai Men Dong* (Radix Ophiopogonis).
- Heat attacking the Stomach with thirst and stomatitis: combine it with *Shi Gao* (Gypsum Fibrosum) and *Zhi Mu* (Radix Anemarrhenae).
- Heat attacking both Lung and Stomach: add *Mai Men Dong* (Radix Ophiopogonis), *Lu Gen* (Rhizoma Phragmitis) and *Tian Hua Fen* (Radix Trichosanthis).
- Wind-heat with thirst: add *Lian Qiao* (Fructus Forsythiae).
- Ulcers on the tongue: combine *Zhu Ye* with *Lian Zi Xin* (Plumula Nelumbinis).
- Restless crying in children: use this herb with *Gou Teng* (Ramulus Uncariae cum Uncis), and *Chan Tui* (Periostracum Cicadae).
- Delirium: add *Tian Zhu Huang* (Concretio Silicea Bambusae) and *Shi Chang Pu* (Rhizoma Acori).

2. Clears Heat and Promotes Diuresis

***Re lin* (heat dysuria):** *Zhu Ye* clears heat from both the Heart and Small Intestine. The Heart and Small Intestine are connected through their *zang fu* organ relationship. Disorder in one frequently affects the function of the other. Heat in the Heart is characterized by irritability, while heat in the Small Intestine is characterized by dysuria, burning sensations and pain accompanying urination.

- Dysuria arising from heat in the Small Intestine: add *Zhu Ye* to *Chuan Mu Tong* (Caulis Clematidis Armandii) and *Gan Cao* (Radix Glycyrrhizae). **Exemplar Formula:** *Dao Chi San* (Guide Out the Red Powder).

DOSAGE

6 to 15 grams. The maximum dosage of *Zhu Ye* is 30 grams. The fresh herb has a stronger heat-clearing function than the dried form.

CAUTIONS / CONTRAINDICATIONS

- Use *Zhu Ye* with caution during pregnancy.

AUTHORS' COMMENTS

Zhu Ye and *Dan Zhu Ye* (Herba Lophatheri) are two different herbs, though they have similar names and functions. *Zhu Ye* is stronger to clear heat from the Stomach and Heart. *Dan Zhu Ye* is stronger to clear heat and promote urination.

Dan Zhu Ye (Herba Lophatheri)

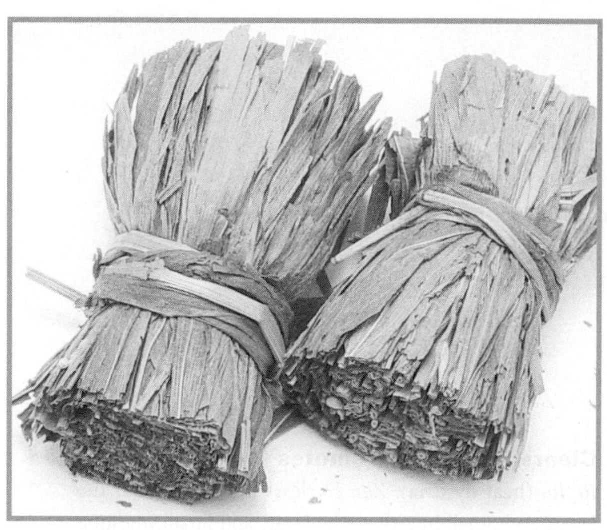

淡竹葉 淡竹叶

Pinyin Name: *Dan Zhu Ye*
Literal Name: "bland bamboo leaves"
Alternate Chinese Names: *Zhu Ye Mai Dong*
Original Source: *Ben Cao Gang Mu* (Materia Medica) by Li Shi-Zhen in 1578
English Name: lophatherum, common lophatherum
Botanical Name: *Lophatherum gracile* Brongn.
Pharmaceutical Name: Herba Lophatheri
Properties: sweet, bland, cold
Channels Entered: Heart, Stomach, Small Intestine

CHINESE THERAPEUTIC ACTIONS

1. Clears Heat and Relieves Irritability

Heat in the Heart and Stomach: Heat in these two organs manifests as irritability and thirst, respectively. *Dan Zhu Ye* (Herba Lophatheri) has an ascending and light nature that enters the *qi* (energy) level to treat febrile disorders.

- Heat attacking the Stomach with thirst and stomatitis: combine *Dan Zhu Ye* with *Shi Gao* (Gypsum Fibrosum) and *Zhi Mu* (Radix Anemarrhenae).
- Heat attacking both Lung and Stomach: combine it with *Mai Men Dong* (Radix Ophiopogonis), *Lu Gen* (Rhizoma Phragmitis) and *Tian Hua Fen* (Radix Trichosanthis).
- Ulcers on the tongue: combine *Dan Zhu Ye* with *Lian Zi Xin* (Plumula Nelumbinis).

2. Promotes Diuresis

***Lin zheng* (dysuria syndrome):** *Dan Zhu Ye* clears heat from both the Heart and Small Intestine. The Heart and Small Intestine are connected through their *zang fu* organ relationship. Disorder in one frequently affects the functioning of the other. Heat in the Heart may cause ulceration of the mouth and tongue, and heat in the Small Intestine may cause dysuria with burning sensations and pain accompanying urination.

- Dysuria because of heat in the Small Intestine: use *Dan Zhu Ye* with *Chuan Mu Tong* (Caulis Clematidis Armandii), *Che Qian Zi* (Semen Plantaginis) and *Sheng Di Huang* (Radix Rehmanniae).

DOSAGE

6 to 15 grams.

CAUTIONS / CONTRAINDICATIONS

- Use *Dan Zhu Ye* with caution during pregnancy.

CHEMICAL COMPOSITION

Arundoin, cylindrin, taraxerol, friedelin, β-sitosterol, organic acids, amino acids, and sugars.[1]

PHARMACOLOGICAL EFFECTS

- **Antipyretic:** In animal studies, *Dan Zhu Ye* has demonstrated antipyretic action similar to phenacetin. The active constituent that lowers temperature can be extracted with water, but not with alcohol.[2]
- **Diuretic:** In human studies, 10 grams of *Dan Zhu Ye* increased the elimination of water and chlorides. When compared to other diuretic herbs, such as *Fu Ling* (Poria), *Zhu Ling* (Polyporus) or *Chuan Mu Tong* (Caulis Clematidis Armandii), *Dan Zhu Ye* is weaker as a diuretic, but stronger in excretion of chlorides.[3,4]

HERB-DRUG INTERACTION

- **Diuretics:** *Dan Zhu Ye* has a diuretic effect. Though this potential interaction has not been documented, concurrent use with diuretic drugs may lead to increased elimination of water and/or electrolytes. [Note: Examples of diuretics include chlorothiazide, hydrochlorothiazide, furosemide (Lasix), bumetanide (Bumex), and torsemide (Demadex).][5]

TOXICOLOGY

The LD_{50} of *Dan Zhu Ye* in mice is 64.5 g/kg.[6]

References

1. *Chang Yong Zhong Yao Cheng Fen Yu Yao Li Shou Ce* (A Handbook of the Composition and Pharmacology of Common Chinese Drugs), 1994; 1639-1641

Dan Zhu Ye (Herba Lophatheri)

2. *Zhong Yao Yao Li Yu Ying Yong* (Pharmacology and Applications of Chinese Herbs), 1977:2253
3. Ibid.
4. *Zhong Yao Da Ci Dien* (Dictionary of Chinese Herbs), 1977:2253
5. Chen, J. Recognition & prevention of herb-drug interactions, *Medical Acupuncture*, Fall/Winter 1998/1999; volume 10/number 2; 9-13
6. *Zhong Yao Yao Li Yu Ying Yong* (Pharmacology and Applications of Chinese Herbs), 1977:2253

Zhi Zi (Fructus Gardeniae)

梔子 栀子

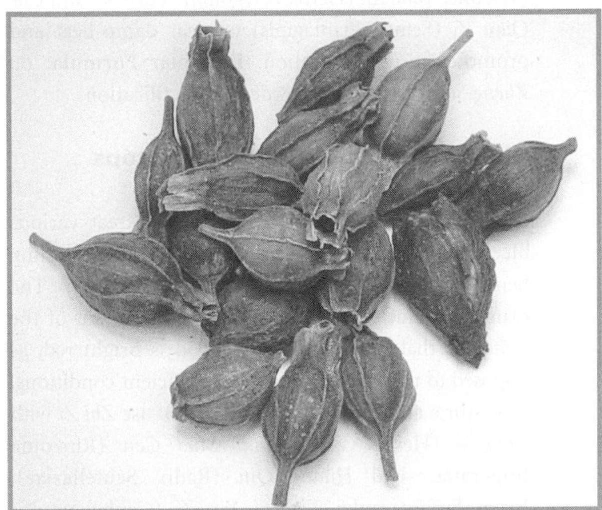

Pinyin Name: *Zhi Zi*
Alternate Chinese Names: *Shan Zhi Zi*
Original Source: *Shen Nong Ben Cao Jing* (Divine Husbandman's Classic of the Materia Medica) in the second century
English Name: gardenia, cape jasmine fruit
Botanical Name: *Gardenia jasminoides* Ellis.
Pharmaceutical Name: Fructus Gardeniae
Properties: bitter, cold
Channels Entered: Heart, Lung, Stomach, San Jiao

CHINESE THERAPEUTIC ACTIONS

1. Sedates Fire and Relieves Irritability

Febrile disorders: *Zhi Zi* (Fructus Gardeniae) is one of the most-commonly used herbs to clear heat and sedate fire from all three *jiaos*. It is most effective if heat and fire are prominent in the Heart, Lung and Stomach. Clinical applications include: heat affecting the Heart leading to irritability, frustration and restlessness; heat affecting the Stomach causing heartburn; heat affecting the Liver leading to irritability and Liver qi stagnation; severe heat and toxins attacking the interior creating high fever, irritability, short temper, delirium or semiconsciousness; and heat attacking the skin developing into carbuncles and furuncles with or without abscesses and ulceration. Other symptoms include: headache, red eyes, toothache, sore throat, ulcers on the tongue, constipation, and yellow urine.

- Irritability and heartburn: use *Zhi Zi* with *Dan Dou Chi* (Semen Sojae Praeparatum). **Exemplar Formula:** *Zhi Zi Chi Tang* (Gardenia and Soja Decoction).
- Irritability, short temper: combine it with *Chai Hu* (Radix Bupleuri), *Bai Shao* (Radix Paeoniae Alba) and *Mu Dan Pi* (Cortex Moutan). **Exemplar Formula:** *Jia Wei Xiao Yao San* (Augmented Rambling Powder).
- Depression with irritability: combine *Zhi Zi* with *Xiang Fu* (Rhizoma Cyperi), *Chuan Xiong* (Rhizoma Ligusticum Chuanxiong), and *Shen Qu* (Massa Fermentata). **Exemplar Formula:** *Yue Ju Wan* (Escape Restraint Pill).
- High fever, irritability, delirium or semiconsciousness: use this herb with *Huang Lian* (Rhizoma Coptidis), *Da Huang* (Radix et Rhizoma Rhei) and *Lian Qiao* (Fructus Forsythiae).
- Carbuncles and furuncles with or without abscesses and ulceration: use *Zhi Zi* topically or combine it with *Huang Lian* (Rhizoma Coptidis), *Da Huang* (Radix et Rhizoma Rhei) and *Lian Qiao* (Fructus Forsythiae). **Exemplar Formula:** *Qing Wen Bai Du Yin* (Clear Epidemics and Overcome Toxin Decoction).
- Constipation: add *Da Huang* (Radix et Rhizoma Rhei).

2. Drains Damp-Heat Downwards

Damp-heat in the Liver and Gallbladder: *Zhi Zi* enters the Liver and is commonly used to treat damp-heat in the middle *jiao*. Clinical manifestations include jaundice, infectious hepatitis, cholecystitis, and cholelithiasis.

- Jaundice, infectious hepatitis, cholecystitis, and cholelithiasis: use *Zhi Zi* with *Yin Chen Hao* (Herba Artemisiae Scopariae), and *Da Huang* (Radix et Rhizoma Rhei). **Exemplar Formula:** *Yin Chen Hao Tang* (Artemisia Scoparia Decoction).

***Re lin* (heat dysuria):** Symptoms of damp-heat in the lower *jiao* include urinary tract infection, and dysuria.

- Urinary tract infection: use *Zhi Zi* with *Hua Shi* (Talcum), *Bian Xu* (Herba Polygoni Avicularis), and *Che Qian Zi* (Semen Plantaginis) to clear damp-heat and promote normal urination. **Exemplar Formula:** *Ba Zheng San* (Eight-Herb Powder for Rectification).

3. Clears Heat, Cools Blood and Stops Bleeding

Bleeding: *Zhi Zi* is commonly used to treat various bleeding disorders characterized by heat, including hematuria, hemoptysis, hematemesis, and epistaxis. The primary characteristic of heat driving blood out of the vessels is that the color of the blood is bright red, as opposed to the light color found in deficient conditions.

- Hematuria and *xue lin* (bloody dysuria): use *Zhi Zi* with *Xiao Ji* (Herba Cirisii), *Bai Mao Gen* (Rhizoma Imperatae) and *Huang Qin* (Radix Scutellariae). **Exemplar Formula:** *Xiao Ji Yin Zi* (Cephalanoplos Decoction).
- Hematemesis and epistaxis: combine it with *Da Ji* (Herba seu Radix Cirsii Japonici), *Xiao Ji* (Herba Cirisii) and *Ce Bai Ye* (Cacumen Platycladi). **Exemplar Formula:** *Shi Hui San* (Ten Partially-charred Substance Powder).
- Hemoptysis: use it with *Ou Jie* (Nodus Nelumbinis Rhizomatis), *Bai Mao Gen* (Rhizoma Imperatae), *Bai Ji* (Rhizoma Bletillae), and *Ce Bai Ye* (Cacumen Platycladi).

4. Reduces Swelling and Relieves Pain

Traumatic injuries with swelling and bruises: *Zhi Zi* reduces swelling, disperses stagnation, and relieves pain. Clinical applications include sprains, strains, soft-tissue injuries, and other musculoskeletal injuries.

- Traumatic or sports injuries: mix *Zhi Zi* powder with water, rice-wine vinegar and egg white to apply topically on affected areas. This method is commonly used in rural areas of China to relieve bruises, swelling and pain.

DOSAGE

3 to 10 grams in decoction. The maximum dosage of *Zhi Zi* for internal use is 20 grams. The dosage for topical use varies depending on the size of the affected area and severity of the injury. For oral administration, fresh *Zhi Zi* functions more effectively to clear heat and sedate fire. When prepared with ginger, it more strongly relieves nausea and vomiting. Dry-fried *Zhi Zi* is warmer, and is less likely to damage the Spleen and Stomach. Charred *Zhi Zi* has stronger action to stop bleeding.

CAUTIONS / CONTRAINDICATIONS

- Bitter and cold in nature, *Zhi Zi* should be used with caution in patients who have deficiency and cold of the Spleen and Stomach, characterized by loose stools and decreased intake of food.
- Use of this herb may be associated with possible drowsiness and sedation. Therefore, individuals who take this herb should exercise caution if driving or operate heavy machinery.

CHEMICAL COMPOSITION

Gardenoside, geniposide, jeminoidin, genipin-1-β-D-gentiobioside, shanzhiside, genipin, geniposidic acid.[1,2]

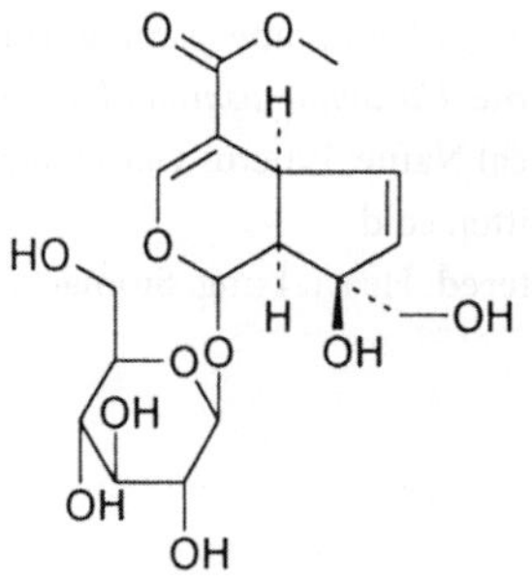

Gardenoside

PHARMACOLOGICAL EFFECTS

- **Analgesic and sedative:** Intravenous injection of geniposide has demonstrated mild analgesic effects in mice.[3]
- **Antihypertensive:** *Zhi Zi* has demonstrated marked antihypertensive action in numerous studies. It is effective via oral, intravenous or intraperitoneal injections; effective in cats, mice and rabbits; and in normal or anesthetized subjects. It has been proposed by some that the hypotensive effect of *Zhi Zi* is because of its stimulation of the parasympathetic nervous system. It has been stated by others that the hypotensive effect results from the decrease of cardiac contractility and cardiac output associated with *Zhi Zi*. Possibilities that have been ruled out include inhibition of adrenal cortical secretion and inhibition of the baroreceptor reflex. Lastly, its antihypertensive effect cannot be negated by intravenous injection of procaine.[4]
- **Hepatoprotective:** Administration of *Zhi Zi* is associated with a marked hepatoprotective function as it lowers serum bilirubin, liver enzymes, and prevents the death of hepatocytes. In one study, the use of *Zhi Zi* effectively reduced liver damage caused by carbon tetrachloride. It

Zhi Zi (Fructus Gardeniae)

also reduces the extent and severity of liver damage associated with acute jaundice in mice. In another study, the risk of acute onset of hepatitis associated with aminogalactose extract is significantly reduced if extract of *Zhi Zi* was given 24 to 48 hours earlier as prophylaxis.[5,6]

- **Cholagogic:** Geniposide has demonstrated marked effectiveness to stimulate the production of bile, enhance contraction of the gallbladder, and increase excretion of bile into the intestines in rats and rabbits. The effective dose for geniposide is 25 mg/kg, given orally or intravenously.[7]
- **Gastrointestinal:** One report states that 25 mg/kg of geniposide given orally decreases the secretion of gastric acid and increases the pH in the stomach in rats. Intravenous injection of 100 mg/kg of geniposide decreases peristalsis of the gastrointestinal system.[8]
- **CNS suppressant:** Intraperitoneal injection of an extract of *Zhi Zi* in rats has an inhibitory effect on the central nervous system (CNS). It decreased spontaneous activity, increased the sleeping time induced by barbiturates by up to 12 times, and decreased body temperature by 3°C for up to 7 hours.[9]
- **Antibiotic:** *Zhi Zi* has demonstrated inhibitory activity against *Staphylococcus aureus*, *Neisseria meningitidis*, and dermatophytes. The herbal decoction has demonstrated bactericidal action against leptospira and schistosoma.[10]

CLINICAL STUDIES AND RESEARCH

- **Musculoskeletal sprain and strain:** In one study, 407 patients with musculoskeletal injuries were treated topically with an herbal paste (*Zhi Zi* mixed with a small amount of water and rubbing alcohol). The herbal paste was placed on the affected area and changed every 2 to 5 days. Patients with bone fractures were disqualified from the study, and patients with dislocations had their joints adjusted prior to herbal treatment. Out of 407 patients, the average time required was 30 hours to relieve pain, 2.5 days to reduce swelling and inflammation, 7.8 days to relieve bruises, and 5.1 days to resume normal physical activities.[11]
- **Coronary artery disorders:** Patients with coronary artery disorders were treated with an herbal paste applied topically on the chest directly adjacent to the heart. The herbal paste was removed and re-applied every 3 days for the first week, then every 7 days thereafter. Out of 50 patients, 22 reported significant improvement and 22 reported moderate improvement. The herbal paste was made by mixing 12 grams each of *Zhi Zi* and *Tao Ren* (Semen Persicae) with 30 grams of honey.[12]
- **Analgesic:** In one report, 110 patients with various aches and pains were treated with an herbal paste topically, with good results. The herbal paste was made by mixing 10 grams each of *Zhi Zi* and *Da Huang* (Radix et Rhizoma Rhei) with paraffin oil and 75% rubbing alcohol.[13]

HERB-DRUG INTERACTION

- **Sedatives:** *Zhi Zi* has a sedative effect, and concurrent use with barbiturates may increase the drug-induced sleeping time.[14] [Note: Many categories of drugs induce sedation, such as antihistamines, narcotic analgesics, barbiturates, benzodiazepines and others.]

TOXICOLOGY

The LD_{50} for alcohol extract of *Zhi Zi* in mice is 107.4 g/kg via oral ingestion. For its isolated constituents, the LD_{50} for geniposide is 3 g/kg in mice via oral, intraperitoneal or intravenous administration. The LD_{50} for genipin is 237 mg/kg via oral ingestion, 190 mg/kg via intraperitoneal, and 153 mg/kg via intravenous injection.[15,16]

SUPPLEMENT

In addition to the fruit, other parts of *Zhi Zi* are also used for medicinal purposes, including

- 梔子仁 / 栀子仁 *Zhi Zi Ren* (Semen Gardeniae), the seeds, clears Heart fire and relieves irritability.
- 梔子皮 / 栀子皮 *Zhi Zi Pi* (Pericarpium Gardeniae), the skin, clears exterior heat.

AUTHORS' COMMENTS

Charred *Zhi Zi* is most effective in stopping bleeding as compared to unprocessed *Zhi Zi*. However, if the cause of bleeding is excessive heat driving blood out from the vessels, unprepared *Zhi Zi* should still be used, as charred *Zhi Zi* has lost most of its function to clear heat when it is turned into ashes.

Not only is *Zhi Zi* commonly used in clinical practice, its flower is also beautiful. According to ancient texts, the plant has the ability to clean the air and absorb toxins that may be harmful to the human body.

Dr. Shen Yen-Nan reports that specific organs injured by fire can be treated with optimum results by key herbs, as follows:

- Lung fire: *Huang Qin* (Radix Scutellariae) and *Sang Bai Pi* (Cortex Mori)
- Heart fire: *Huang Lian* (Rhizoma Coptidis)
- Stomach fire: *Shi Gao* (Gypsum Fibrosum)
- Liver fire: *Zhi Zi* (Fructus Gardeniae)
- Kidney fire: *Zhi Mu* (Radix Anemarrhenae)

References

1. *Xian Dai Zhong Yao Yao Li Xue* (Contemporary Pharmacology of Chinese Herbs), 1997; 292
2. Yan X, Zhou J, Xie G, *Traditional Chinese Medicines Molecular Structures, Natural Sources and Applications*; Ashgate, 1999; 2509
3. *Zhong Yao Zhi* (Chinese Herbology Journal), 1984; 578
4. *Zhong Yao Yao Li Yu Ying Yong* (Pharmacology and Applications of Chinese Herbs), 1983; 934
5. *Zhong Yao Xue* (Chinese Herbology), 1998; 126:128

Zhi Zi (Fructus Gardeniae)

6. *CA*, 1982; 97:16912n
7. *Zhong Yao Yao Li Yu Ying Yong* (Pharmacology and Applications of Chinese Herbs), 1983; 934
8. Ibid.
9. *Jiang Su Yi Yao* (Jiangsu Journal of Medicine and Herbology), 1976; (1):28
10. *Zhong Yao Zhi* (Chinese Herbology Journal), 1984; 578
11. *Zhong Yi Za Zhi* (Journal of Chinese Medicine), 1964; 12:450
12. *Zhong Ji Yi Kan* (Medium Medical Journal); 4:19
13. *Si Chuan Zhong Yi* (Sichuan Chinese Medicine), 1988; 9:11
14. *Jiang Su Yi Yao* (Jiangsu Journal of Medicine and Herbology), 1976; (1):28
15. *Zhong Cao Yao Xue* (Study of Chinese Herbal Medicine), 1980:1053
16. *Yao Xue Za Zhi* (Journal of Medicinals), 1974; 94(2):157

Xia Ku Cao (Spica Prunellae)

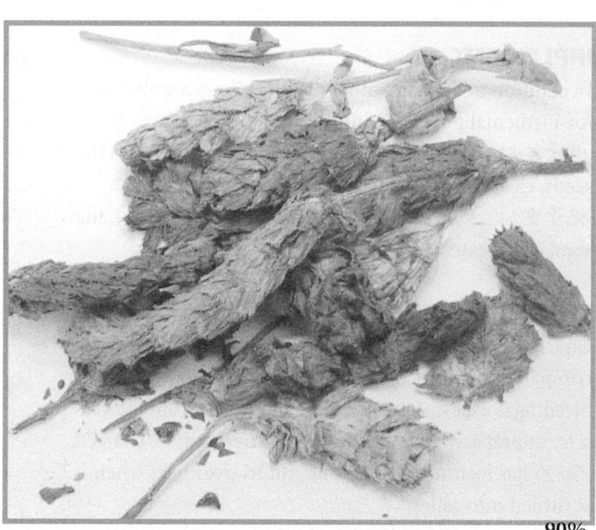

90%

夏枯草 夏枯草

Pinyin Name: *Xia Ku Cao*
Literal Name: "withered flower in summer," "summer withering grass"
Alternate Chinese Names: *Xia Ku Hua, Da Tou Hua*
Original Source: *Shen Nong Ben Cao Jing* (Divine Husbandman's Classic of the Materia Medica) in the second century
English Name: prunella, flower (fruit-spike) of common selfheal
Botanical Name: *Prunella vulgaris* L. (*Xia Ku Cao*)
Pharmaceutical Name: Spica Prunellae
Properties: bitter, acrid, cold
Channels Entered: Liver, Gallbladder

CHINESE THERAPEUTIC ACTIONS

1. Clears Liver Fire

Liver fire: Acrid and cold, *Xia Ku Cao* (Spica Prunellae) has dispersing and heat-clearing functions. It is commonly used to clear heat and sedate fire from the Liver and Gallbladder. Clinically, Liver fire flaring upwards is characterized by disorders of the eyes such as redness, swelling and pain in the eyes, photophobia, excessive tearing, headache and dizziness. Liver fire with blood deficiency is characterized by swelling and eye pain that worsens at night. Liver qi stagnation is characterized by hypochondriac fullness and pain, fidgeting, irritability, and emotional instability.

- Liver fire with eye disorders: use *Xia Ku Cao* with *Shi Jue Ming* (Concha Haliotidis), *Jue Ming Zi* (Semen Cassiae), and *Ju Hua* (Flos Chrysanthemi).
- Liver fire with blood deficiency: combine it with *Dang Gui* (Radicis Angelicae Sinensis), *Bai Shao* (Radix Paeoniae Alba), and *Xuan Shen* (Radix Scrophulariae).
- Liver qi stagnation: add *Xiang Fu* (Rhizoma Cyperi) and *Chai Hu* (Radix Bupleuri).

Xia Ku Cao can be used to treat severe liver disorders involving enlargement and inflammation of the liver, such as hepatitis and hepatomegaly, characterized by excessive heat and fire.

- Enlargement and inflammation of the liver: use this herb with *Yin Chen Hao* (Herba Artemisiae Scopariae), *Huang Bai* (Cortex Phellodendri) and *Dan Shen* (Radix Salviae Miltiorrhizae).

2. Clears Hot Phlegm, Disperses Stagnation, and Resolves Nodules

Scrofula, lipoma, swollen glands, goiter, lumps or nodules: In TCM, nodules are considered to be abnormal accumulations of heat, toxins and phlegm. When heat persists in the body over a long time, body fluids dry into phlegm masses or nodules. When accompanied by qi

Xia Ku Cao (Spica Prunellae)

stagnation, the masses harden and become immobile. *Xia Ku Cao* effectively resolves nodules by clearing heat and softening and dispersing qi and phlegm stagnation.

- Phlegm stagnation caused by heat and fire: use *Xia Ku Cao* with *Xuan Shen* (Radix Scrophulariae), *Mu Li* (Concha Ostreae) and *Kun Bu* (Thallus Laminariae seu Eckloniae).

3. Lowers Blood Pressure

Hypertension: *Xia Ku Cao* is commonly used to treat hypertension associated with Liver fire and Liver yang rising.

- Hypertension: use *Xia Ku Cao* with *Gou Teng* (Ramulus Uncariae cum Uncis), *Di Long* (Pheretima) and *Du Zhong* (Cortex Eucommiae).
- Redness, swelling and eye pain caused by hypertension: use it with *Ju Hua* (Flos Chrysanthemi), *Shi Jue Ming* (Concha Haliotidis) and *Chan Tui* (Periostracum Cicadae).

DOSAGE

10 to 15 grams. The maximum dosage of *Xia Ku Cao* is 100 grams. *Xia Ku Cao* may be used singly or in an herbal formula. The flower is commonly used as the medicinal part of the plant. The entire plant, however, does have stronger potency than the flower for lowering blood pressure.

CAUTIONS / CONTRAINDICATIONS

- Cold in thermal nature, *Xia Ku Cao* should be used with caution in patients with Spleen and Stomach deficiencies.

CHEMICAL COMPOSITION

Prunellin, oleanolic acid, ursolic acid, carotene, camphor, fenchone, rutin, hyperin, hyperside, delphinidin, cyanidin, caffeic acid, rosmarinic acid, deucosterol, β-amyrin.[1]

PHARMACOLOGICAL EFFECTS

- **Antihypertensive**: Both water and alcohol extracts of *Xia Ku Cao* have a rapid onset of effect in reducing blood pressure. This antihypertensive effect is generally attributed to vasodilation, though some reports indicate otherwise. In dogs with renal hypertension, daily administration of *Xia Ku Cao* was effective in reducing blood pressure. Unfortunately, blood pressure returned to previous levels upon discontinuation of herbal therapy. The stems, leaves, flowers and entire plant all have antihypertensive functions.[2,3]
- **Anti-inflammatory**: *Xia Ku Cao* has demonstrated marked anti-inflammatory action in rabbits. The exact mechanism of action is unclear, but is thought to be due in part to increased secretion of ACTH and/or glucocorticoids.[4]
- **Antibiotic:** *Xia Ku Cao* has demonstrated inhibitory effects against *Shigella* spp., *Salmonella typhi, E. coli, Pseudomonas aeruginosa, Mycobacterium tuberculosis, Streptococcus* spp., and dermatophytes.[5]
- **Effect on lipoma:** *Xia Ku Cao* has marked effectiveness in treating lipoma in animals. However, this therapeutic effect is only achieved with a large dosage of the herb, which is associated with toxic reactions.[6]
- **Smooth muscle stimulant:** *Xia Ku Cao* stimulates contractility of uterine and intestinal muscles.[7]

CLINICAL STUDIES AND RESEARCH

- **Hypertension:** Administration of *Xia Ku Cao* as a single herb in 42 patients showed good results for treatment of hypertension.[8]
- **Pulmonary tuberculosis:** In one study, 18 patients were treated with 60 grams of *Xia Ku Cao* taken as decoction. The effective rate was 78.5%.[9]

TOXICOLOGY

No abnormalities of internal organs or fatalities were observed following an oral bolus dose of a *Xia Ku Cao* preparation at 10 g/kg in mice.[10]

SUPPLEMENT

- 夏枯花 *Xia Ku Hua* (Flos Prunellae), first cited in the *Shen Nong Ben Cao Jing* (Divine Husbandman's Classic of the Materia Medica) in the second century, is acrid, cold and enters the Lung. Its main function is to dispel phlegm from the Lung to treat cases of lung abscess. Pharmacologically, it has both antibiotic and antihypertensive effects. *Xia Ku* Cao (Spica Prunellae) and *Xia Ku* Hua (Flos Prunellae) have essentially the same components and are often used interchangeably. *Xia Ku Cao*, however, is often considered more desirable and more potent than *Xia Ku Hua*. The dosage of *Xia Ku Hua* is 10 to 15 grams.

References

1. *Xian Dai Zhong Yao Yao Li Xue* (Contemporary Pharmacology of Chinese Herbs), 1997; 295
2. *Zhong Yao Yao Li Yu Ying Yong* (Pharmacology and Applications of Chinese Herbs), 1983:883
3. *Zhong Yao Xue* (Chinese Herbology), 1998; 128:130
4. Ibid.
5. *Zhong Cao Yao* (Chinese Herbal Medicine), 1989; 20(6):22
6. Ibid.
7. Ibid.
8. *Fu Jian Zhong Yi Yao* (Fujian Chinese Medicine and Herbology), 1959; 4:41
9. *Zhong Yi Za Zhi* (Journal of Chinese Medicine), 1961; 11:147
10. *Zhong Cao Yao* (Chinese Herbal Medicine), 1989; 20(6):22

Mi Meng Hua (Flos Buddlejae)

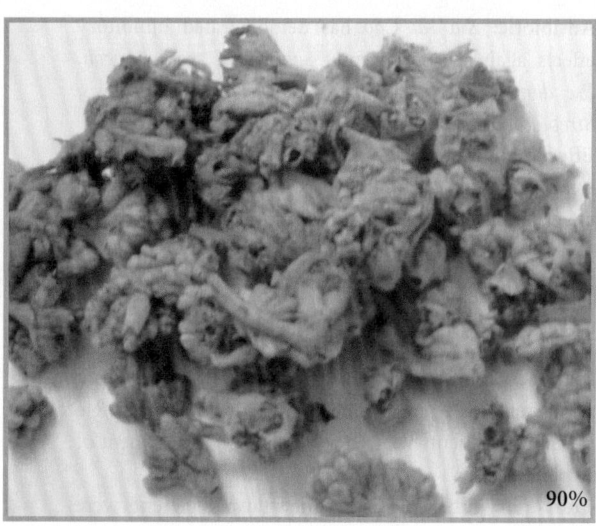

密蒙花 密蒙花

Pinyin Name: *Mi Meng Hua*
Literal Name: "dense-covered flower"
Alternate Chinese Names: *Meng Hua*
Original Source: *Kai Bao Ben Cao* (Materia Medica of the Kai Bao Era) by Ma Zhi in 973-974 A.D.
English Name: buddleja, pale butterfly bush flower
Botanical Name: *Buddleja officinalis* Maxim.
Pharmaceutical Name: Flos Buddlejae
Properties: sweet, cool
Channels Entered: Liver

CHINESE THERAPEUTIC ACTIONS

Clears Liver Heat, Brightens the Eyes and Removes Superficial Visual Obstruction

Eye Disorders: *Mi Meng Hua* (Flos Buddlejae) shows good results in treatment of eye disorders caused by either excess or deficiency syndromes. Eye disorders may be caused by Liver heat or wind-heat attacking the eyes, leading to redness, swelling and pain, photophobia, and excessive tearing. On the other hand, eye disorders may be caused by deficiency heat leading to dry eyes and dizziness. *Mi Meng Hua* is effective in treating both, when combined with other appropriate herbs.

- Eye disorders caused by wind-heat: use *Mi Meng Hua* with *Ju Hua* (Flos Chrysanthemi) and *Mu Zei* (Herba Equiseti Hiemalis).
- Eye disorders from Liver heat: use it with *Bai Ji Li* (Fructus Tribuli), *Shi Jue Ming* (Concha Haliotidis), *Jue Ming Zi* (Semen Cassiae) and *Gu Jing Cao* (Flos Eriocauli).
- Eye disorders caused by deficiency heat: combine it with *Gou Qi Zi* (Fructus Lycii), *Sha Yuan Zi* (Semen Astragali Complanati) and *Tu Si Zi* (Semen Cuscutae).
- Blurred vision from Liver deficiency: add *Shi Jue Ming* (Concha Haliotidis) and *Gou Qi Zi* (Fructus Lycii).
- Superficial visual obstruction: use *Mi Meng Hua* with *Mu Zei* (Herba Equiseti Hiemalis), *Ye Ming Sha* (Excrementum Vespertilionis Murini) and *Chan Tui* (Periostracum Cicadae).
- Itching eyes: use it with *Man Jing Zi* (Fructus Viticis), *Fang Feng* (Radix Saposhnikoviae), *Jing Jie* (Herba Schizonepetae) and *Ju Hua* (Flos Chrysanthemi).

DOSAGE

6 to 10 grams in decoction. The maximum dosage of *Mi Meng Hua* is 20 grams.

CHEMICAL COMPOSITION

Buddleoglucoside, linarin, acaciin, acacetin, p-methoxycinnamoylaucubin, p-methoxycinnamoylcatapol, catalposide, catalpol, aucubin, echinacoside, acteoside.[1,2]

Acacetin

PHARMACOLOGICAL EFFECTS

- **Antispasmodic:** Acacetin has a mild action to relieve muscle spasms in rats. When given as intravenous injection at 40 mg/kg, it relaxes the smooth muscle of the bile duct.[3]
- **Diuretic:** Intravenous injection of a *Mi Meng Hua* preparation increases urine output by up to 75% in rabbits within 25 to 30 minutes.[4]

CLINICAL STUDIES AND RESEARCH

- **Conjunctivitis:** According to one report, 10 patients with infectious hemorrhagic conjunctivitis were treated with an herbal formula, with complete recovery in 9 patients within 2 to 6 doses. The herbal formula contained *Mi Meng Hua* 9g, *Qing Xiang Zi* (Semen Celosiae) 9g, *Dang Gui* (Radicis Angelicae Sinensis) 9g, *Chi Shao* (Radix Paeoniae Rubrae) 9g, *Chai Hu* (Radix Bupleuri) 9g, *Niu Xi* (Radix Cyathulae seu Achyranthis) 9g, *Jie Geng* (Radix Platycodonis) 9g, *Jue Ming Zi* (Semen Cassiae) 9g, *Hong Hua* (Flos Carthami) 6g, *Chuan Xiong* (Rhizoma Ligustici Chuanxiong) 6g, *Tao Ren* (Semen Persicae) 12g, and *Sheng Di Huang* (Radix Rehmanniae)

Mi Meng Hua (Flos Buddlejae)

12g. Modifications included a larger dose of *Chai Hu* (Radix Bupleuri) for Liver qi stagnation, addition of *Mu Dan Pi* (Cortex Moutan) and *Di Gu Pi* (Cortex Lycii) for heat, and elimination of *Tao Ren* (Semen Persicae) during menses. The herbal formula was given as a decoction twice daily.[5]

- **Corneal ulcer:** In a clinical study, 121 patients with corneal ulcers were successfully treated using Chinese herbal medicine. Out of affected 129 eyes (several patients had ulcers in both eyes), the study reported complete recovery in 98 cases, moderate improvement in 22 cases, and no response in 9 cases. The herbal formula contained *Mi Meng Hua* 15g, *Huang Lian* (Rhizoma Coptidis) 15g, *Zi Cao Gen* (Radix Lithospermi) 15g, *Mu Zei* (Herba Equiseti Hiemalis) 20g, *Gu Jing Cao* (Flos Eriocauli) 20g, and *Qin Pi* (Cortex Fraxini) 20g. Modifications were made if deemed necessary. The herbs were cooked twice in 1500 ml of water for 20 minutes each time, and the two batches were mixed together and used as a topical application. The patients were instructed to soak a towel in the solution and apply the towel to the affected eye(s).[6]

HERB-DRUG INTERACTION

- **Diuretics:** *Mi Meng Hua* has a diuretic effect. Though this potential interaction has not been documented, concurrent use with diuretic drugs may lead to increased elimination of water and/or electrolytes. [Note: Examples of diuretics include chlorothiazide, hydrochlorothiazide, furosemide (Lasix), bumetanide (Bumex), and torsemide (Demadex).][7]

TOXICOLOGY

The LD_{50} for acacetin in mice is 933 mg/kg.[8]

References

1. *Chang Yong Zhong Yao Cheng Fen Yu Yao Li Shou Ce* (A Handbook of the Composition and Pharmacology of Common Chinese Drugs), 1994; 1646-1647
2. *The Merck Index* 12th edition, Chapman & Hall/CRCnetBASE/Merck, 2000
3. *Zhong Yao Da Ci Dien* (Dictionary of Chinese Herbs), 1977: 2264
4. Ibid.
5. *Hu Bei Yi Sheng* (Hubei Doctor), 1976; (5:42)
6. *Zhong Ji Yi Kan* (Medium Medical Journal), 1991; 26(11):63
7. Chen, J. Recognition & prevention of herb-drug interactions, *Medical Acupuncture*, Fall/Winter 1998/1999; volume 10/number 2; 9-13
8. *Zhong Yao Da Ci Dien* (Dictionary of Chinese Herbs), 1977: 2264

Qing Xiang Zi (Semen Celosiae)

青葙子 青葙子

Pinyin Name: *Qing Xiang Zi*
Alternate Chinese Names: *Ji Guan Qian*
Original Source: *Shen Nong Ben Cao Jing* (Divine Husbandman's Classic of the Materia Medica) in the second century
English Name: celosia argentea seed, feather cockscomb seed
Botanical Name: *Celosia argentea* L.
Pharmaceutical Name: Semen Celosiae
Properties: bitter, cool
Channels Entered: Liver

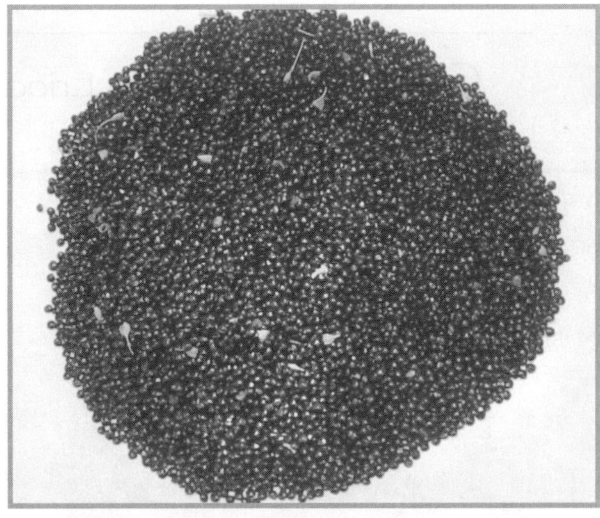

CHINESE THERAPEUTIC ACTIONS

1. Sedates Liver Fire and Benefits the Eyes

Eye disorders: *Qing Xiang Zi* (Semen Celosiae) treats eye disorders caused by Liver fire flaring upwards with symptoms such as redness, swelling and pain, photophobia, and excessive tearing.

Qing Xiang Zi (Semen Celosiae)

- Redness, swelling and eye pain due to Liver fire: use *Qing Xiang Zi* with *Jue Ming Zi* (Semen Cassiae) and *Xia Ku Cao* (Spica Prunellae).
- Redness, swelling and eye pain due to wind-heat: add *Mi Meng Hua* (Flos Buddlejae) and *Mu Zei* (Herba Equiseti Hiemalis).
- Night blindness: use *Qing Xiang Zi* with *Da Zao* (Fructus Jujubae).

2. Sedates Liver Fire and Lowers Blood Pressure

Hypertension: Clinical applications include Liver yang rising or Liver fire with headache, short temper and red eyes.

- Hypertension caused by Liver fire: use *Qing Xiang Zi* with *Xia Ku Cao* (Spica Prunellae), *Gou Teng* (Ramulus Uncariae cum Uncis) and *Shi Jue Ming* (Concha Haliotidis) to sedate Liver fire.
- Headache because of Liver fire: combine this herb with *Jue Ming Zi* (Semen Cassiae), *Huang Qin* (Radix Scutellariae) and *Xia Ku Cao* (Spica Prunellae).
- Epistaxis: apply decoction of *Qing Xiang Zi* topically into the nostrils.
- Eye disorders caused by wind-heat: use this herb with *Mi Meng Hua* (Flos Buddlejae) and *Mu Zei* (Herba Equiseti Hiemalis).

DOSAGE

6 to 15 grams in decoction. The maximum dosage of *Qing Xiang Zi* is 20 grams.

CAUTIONS / CONTRAINDICATIONS

- Cold in thermal nature, *Qing Xiang Zi* should be used with caution in patients with deficiency and cold of the Spleen and Stomach, qi and/or yang deficiency, and deficiency of the Liver or Kidney.
- *Qing Xiang Zi* dilates the pupils of the eyes. Therefore, it should be used with caution in individuals with eye disorders characterized by dilated pupils, such as in glaucoma.

CHEMICAL COMPOSITION

β-sitosterol, cholesteryl palmitate, 3,4-dihydroxyl benzaldehyde, p-hydroxyl benzoic acid, 3,4-dihydroxyl benzoic acid, nicotinic acid.[1]

PHARMACOLOGICAL EFFECTS

- **Antihypertensive:** *Qing Xiang Zi* has demonstrated moderate antihypertensive effects.[2]
- **Ophthalmic:** Decoction of *Qing Xiang Zi* given daily for 6 days lowered ocular pressure in rabbits.[3]
- **Antibiotic:** Decoction of *Qing Xiang Zi* has a strong inhibiting effect on *Pseudomonas aeruginosa*.[4]

References

1. *Chang Yong Zhong Yao Cheng Fen Yu Yao Li Shou Ce* (A Handbook of the Composition and Pharmacology of Common Chinese Drugs), 1994; 1166
2. *Zhong Yao Xue* (Chinese Herbology), 1998; 135:136
3. *Yun Nan Zhong Yi Za Zhi* (Yunan Journal of Chinese Medicine), 1990; 11(1):30
4. *Zhong Yao Zhi* (Chinese Herbology Journal), 1984; 443

Gu Jing Cao (Flos Eriocauli)

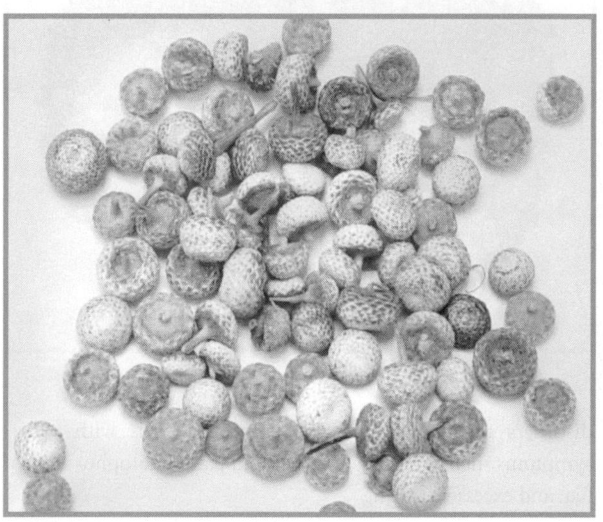

谷精草 谷精草

Pinyin Name: *Gu Jing Cao*
Literal Name: "grain essence herb"
Alternate Chinese Names: *Gu Jing Zhu, Dai Xing Cao*
Original Source: *Kai Bao Ben Cao* (Materia Medica of the Kai Bao Era) by Ma Zhi in 973-974 A.D.
English Name: eriocaulis, buerger pipewort flower
Botanical Name: *Eriocaulon buergerianum* Koern. (*Gu Jing Cao*); *Eriocaulon sieboldtianum* Seib. Et Zucc. (*Sai Gu Jing Cao*)
Pharmaceutical Name: Flos Eriocauli
Properties: sweet, neutral
Channels Entered: Liver, Stomach

Gu Jing Cao (Flos Eriocauli)

CHINESE THERAPEUTIC ACTIONS

Disperses Wind and Heat in the Liver Channel, Brightens the Eyes and Removes Superficial Visual Obstruction

Eye disorders caused by wind and heat in the Liver channel: Clinical manifestations include painful, swollen, red eyes, photophobia, excessive tearing, superficial visual obstructions, pterygium or spots in front of the eyes. These eye disorders can be attributed to both external wind-heat invasion and wind-heat attacking the Liver channel. *Gu Jing Cao* (Flos Eriocauli) can also be used for headache, toothache and sore throat caused by wind-heat invasion.

- Red eyes: use with *Ju Hua* (Flos Chrysanthemi), *Xia Ku Cao* (Spica Prunellae) and *Long Dan Cao* (Radix Gentianae).
- Itching of the eyes: add *Jing Jie* (Herba Schizonepetae) to *Gu Jing Cao*.
- Superficial visual obstruction: use it with *Chan Tui* (Periostracum Cicadae).

DOSAGE

6 to 10 grams in decoction.

CHEMICAL COMPOSITION

Phenolic compounds.[1]

PHARMACOLOGICAL EFFECTS

Antibiotic: Water decoction of *Gu Jing Cao* has an inhibiting effect *in vitro* against *Pseudomonas aeruginosa*, some dermatophytes, and pathogenic fungi.[2,3]

References

1. *CA*, 1991; 115:110604a
2. *Zhong Yao Xue* (Chinese Herbology), 1998; 133:134
3. *Xin Hua Ben Cao Gang Mu* (New Chinese Materia Medica), 1991; 579

Rui Ren (Semen Prinsepiae)

蕤仁 蕤仁

Pinyin Name: *Rui Ren*
Alternate Chinese Names: *Rui He, Rui Ren Rou, Rui Zi*
English Name: prinsepia seed, hedge prinsepia nut
Botanical Name: *Prinsepia uniflora* Batal
Pharmaceutical Name: Semen Prinsepiae
Properties: sweet, cool
Channels Entered: Liver

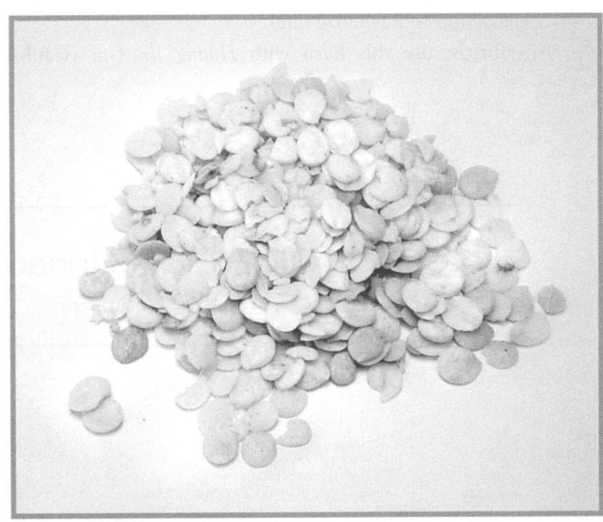

CHINESE THERAPEUTIC ACTIONS

Disperses Wind, Clears Heat, Clears the Liver and Brightens the Eyes

Acute conjunctivitis or acute keratitis: Acute disorders involving the eyes usually are caused by wind or heat in the Liver channel. *Rui Ren* (Semen Prinsepiae) treats both types of acute inflammation. However, it is not suitable for eye disorders caused by deficiencies of the Liver and Kidney, manifesting as diminished or blurred vision.

- Acute conjunctivitis or keratitis: use *Rui Ren* with *Qian Li Guang* (Herba Senecionis Scandens) and *Ma Bian Cao* (Herba Verbenae), and add to *Long Dan Xie Gan Tang* (Gentiana Decoction to Drain the Liver).

DOSAGE

4.5 to 9 grams in decoction.

CAUTIONS / CONTRAINDICATIONS

- Use of *Rui Ren* is contraindicated in patients with eye disorders caused by Liver and Kidney deficiencies.

Da Ding Huang (Caulis Euonymi)

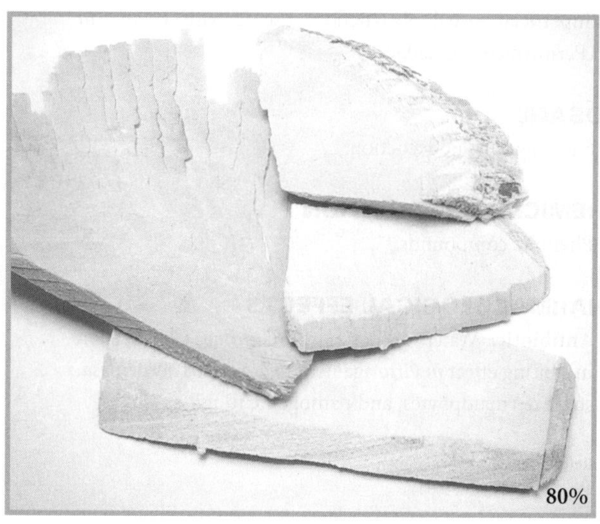

大疔黄

Pinyin Name: *Da Ding Huang*
Literal Name: "anti-inflammatory big furuncle"
English Name: euonymus
Botanical Name: *Euonymus echinata* Wall.
Pharmaceutical Name: Caulis Euonymi
Properties: bitter, cold
Channels Entered: Liver, Lung

CHINESE THERAPEUTIC ACTIONS

Reduces Inflammation and Eliminates Toxins

Da Ding Huang (Caulis Euonymi) is a cold herb that treats various conditions characterized by heat, inflammation and toxin.

- Toxic swellings, carbuncles and furuncles: combine *Da Ding Huang* with *Zhen Ren Huo Ming Yin* (True Man Decoction to Revitalize Life).
- Arthritis: use this herb with *Huang Jin Gui* (Caulis Vanieriae), *Mo Gu Xiao* (Caulis Hyptis Capitatae) and *Liu Zhi Huang* (Herba Solidaginis).

DOSAGE

6 to 15 grams in decoction.

CAUTIONS / CONTRAINDICATIONS

- Use *Da Ding Huang* with caution in patients with deficiency and cold of the Stomach and Spleen.

Ren Zhong Bai (Urinae Hominis Sedimen)

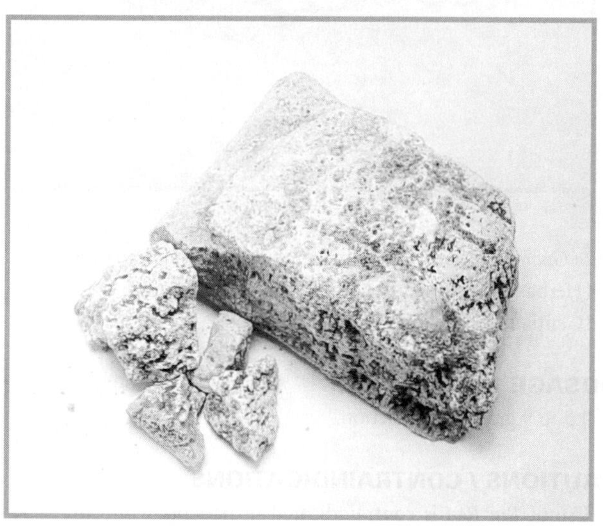

人中白

Pinyin Name: *Ren Zhong Bai*
Literal Name: "whiteness within man"
Original Source: *Shen Nong Ben Cao Jing* (Divine Husbandman's Classic of the Materia Medica) in the second century
English Name: human urine sediment
Zoological Name: *Homo sapiens* L. (*Ren Niao*)
Pharmaceutical Name: Urinae Hominis Sedimen
Properties: salty, neutral
Channels Entered: Liver, Kidney, San Jiao, Urinary Bladder

Ren Zhong Bai (Urinae Hominis Sedimen)

CHINESE THERAPEUTIC ACTIONS

Sedates Heat and Fire, Reduces Swelling, Stops Bleeding

Ren Zhong Bai (Urinae Hominis Sedimen) is used for a wide variety of conditions characterized by heat in the upper, middle and lower *jiaos*, including bleeding, soreness and swelling of the throat, ulceration of the mouth and gums, eczema, and headache.

- Edema: use *Ren Zhong Bai* as a sole remedy.
- Epistaxis: add it with *She Xiang* (Moschus).
- Frontal headache and migraine: use it with *Di Long* (Pheretima).

DOSAGE

3 to 6 grams.

CAUTIONS / CONTRAINDICATIONS

- Use of *Ren Zhong Bai* is contraindicated in cases of deficiency and cold of the Spleen and Stomach.

CHEMICAL COMPOSITION

Urea, sodium chloride, phosphoric acid, sulfuric acid, uric acid, hippuric acid, urobilin, and organic salts.[1]

References

1. *Dorland's Illustrated Medical Dictionary*, 1994; 1781

Shi Lian Zi (Herba Sinocrassulae Indicae)

石蓮子 石莲子

Pinyin Name: *Shi Lian Zi*
Literal Name: "stone lotus seed"
English Name: Indian sinocrassula
Botanical Name: *Sinocrassulae indicae*
Pharmaceutical Name: Herba Sinocrassulae Indicae
Properties: bitter, cold
Channels Entered: Large Intestine, Urinary Bladder, Stomach

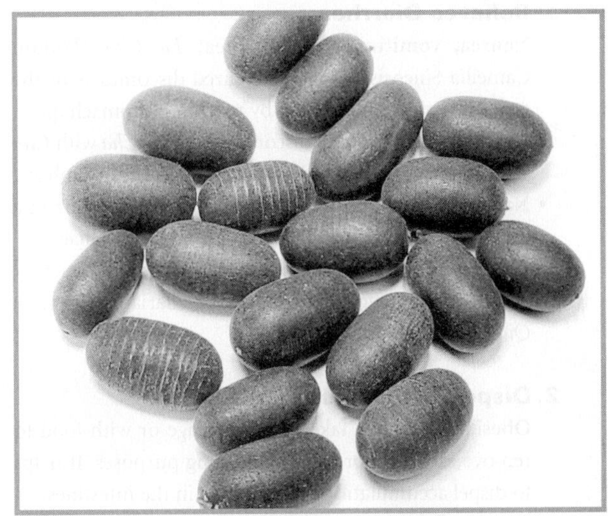

CHINESE THERAPEUTIC ACTIONS

Clears Heat

Shi Lian Zi (Herba Sinocrassulae Indicae) is a cold herb that clears heat from the Large Intestine, Urinary Bladder, and Stomach.

- Chronic dysentery: use *Shi Lian Zi* with *Feng Wei Cao* (Herba Pteris), *Huang Lian* (Rhizoma Coptidis), *Bai Tou Weng* (Radix Pulsatillae), *Huang Bai* (Cortex Phellodendri) and *Bai Shao* (Radix Paeoniae Alba).
- Chronic turbid urine: combine this herb with *Shui Ding Xiang* (Herba Ludwigiae Prostratae) and *Ya She Huang* (Herba Lippiae).
- Nausea, hiccups and vomiting due to qi reversal of the Stomach: use it with *Xuan Fu Hua* (Flos Inulae), *Ban Xia* (Rhizoma Pinelliae), *Sheng Jiang* (Rhizoma Zingiberis Recens) and *Dai Zhe Shi* (Haematitum).

DOSAGE

3 to 12 grams in decoction.

Lu Cha (Folium Camellia Sinensis)

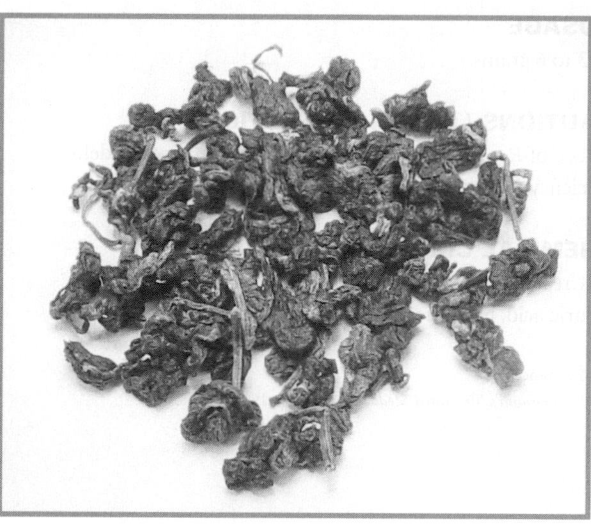

綠茶 绿茶

Pinyin Name: *Lu Cha*
Literal Name: "green tea"
English Name: green tea
Botanical Name: *Camellia sinensis* L. Kuntze (*Cha*)
Pharmaceutical Name: Folium Camellia Sinensis
Properties: bitter, cold
Channels Entered: Stomach

CHINESE THERAPEUTIC ACTIONS

1. Harmonizes the Stomach, Directs Rebellious Stomach Qi Downward and Relieves Diarrhea

Nausea, vomiting and diarrhea: *Lu Cha* (Folium Camellia Sinensis) treats generalized discomforts of the gastrointestinal tract caused by rebellious Stomach qi.

- General gastrointestinal discomfort: use *Lu Cha* with *Gan Cao* (Radix Glycyrrhizae) and *Da Zao* (Fructus Jujubae).
- Nausea and vomiting: add *Sheng Jiang* (Rhizoma Zingiberis Recens) and *Ban Xia* (Rhizoma Pinelliae).
- Diarrhea: combine this herb with *Ge Gen* (Radix Puerariae), *Huang Qin* (Radix Scutellariae) and *Lian Qiao* (Fructus Forsythiae).

2. Dispels Dampness

Obesity: *Lu Cha* is taken as a beverage or with food to remove excess fat or oil for slimming purposes. It helps to dispel accumulation of dampness in the intestines.

- Obesity: use *Lu Cha* with *Yi Yi Ren* (Semen Coicis) and *He Ye* (Folium Nelumbinis).

3. Clears the Head

Headache: *Lu Cha* clears the head and relieves headache. It is used as an adjuvant herb to prevent the drying, ascending and dispersing nature of diaphoretic herbs from harming the body.

- Headache: use this herb with *Bai Zhi* (Radix Angelicae Dahuricae), *Chuan Xiong* (Rhizoma Ligustici Chuanxiong), and *Qiang Huo* (Rhizoma et Radix Notopterygii). **Exemplar Formula:** *Chuan Xiong Cha Tiao San* (Ligusticum Chuanxiong Powder to be Taken with Green Tea).

DOSAGE

3 to 12 grams in decoction. *Lu Cha* can be consumed as tea up to 5 cups per day when used as a beverage.

CAUTIONS / CONTRAINDICATIONS

- Use with caution in cases with Stomach qi deficiency as *Lu Cha* may cause irritation when taken to the excess. Fermented or processed teas, such as black tea or oolong, are gentler on the stomach than unprocessed green tea.

CHEMICAL COMPOSITION

Caffeine, theobromine, theophylline, xanthine, theafolia, theaflavine, theaflavin acid, thearubigene, quercetin, kaempferol, myrecetin, chlorogenic acid, theogallin.[1,2]

(Structure: H_3C, CH_3, CH_3, O, O, N, N, N, N)

Caffeine

PHARMACOLOGICAL EFFECTS

- **CNS stimulant:** Administration of caffeine, one of the constituents of *Lu Cha*, is associated with stimulation of the central nervous system (CNS), leading to such effects as nervousness, insomnia, tachycardia, increased blood glucose and cholesterol levels, and high levels of stomach acid and heartburn.[3]
- **Antineoplastic:** Administration of *Lu Cha* is associated with beneficial results in subjects with cancer and undergoing chemotherapy. The polyphenol content of the herb may inhibit the formation of N-nitrosation by-products, which are known to be carcinogenic.[4]

Lu Cha (Folium Camellia Sinensis)

- **Effect on colon polyps:** In one study, consumption of *Lu Cha* was linked with decreased risk of developing adenomatous polyps of the sigmoid colon.[5]
- **Chemoprotective:** *Lu Cha* has chemoprotective effect, as pretreatment of animals with the herb suppressed the formation of experimentally-induced chromosome aberrations in bone marrow cells.[6]
- **Antimutagenic:** Various tea extracts (green tea, pauchong tea, oolong tea and black tea) and their components have demonstrated marked antimutagenic activity against N-methyl-N-nitro-N-nitrosoguanidine (MNNG), folpet, monocrotophos, and 2-acetylaminofluorene (AAF). Different teas have different effects against different chemical mutagens, and the differences in effect are attributed to the formation of different metabolites during various stages of tea fermentation.[7]
- **Cytoprotective:** *Lu Cha* extract and its phenolic compounds have been found to have marked cytoprotective effect. Specifically, the tea polyphenols protect liver cells against 1,4-naphthoquinone-induced liver toxicity in rats.[8]

CLINICAL STUDIES AND RESEARCH

- **Hypercholesterolemia:** In a clinical study, consumption of nine or more cups of *Lu Cha* per day was associated with a decrease in total cholesterol level but no decrease in triglycerides or HDL-cholesterol.[9]

HERB-DRUG INTERACTION

- **Oral contraceptives and cimetidine:** The effect of caffeine in *Lu Cha* may be potentiated when given in conjunction with oral contraceptives and cimetidine.[10]
- **Theophylline and ephedrine:** The combination of caffeine with theophylline and ephedrine may lead to increased thermogenesis, weight loss, agitation, tremors, and insomnia.[11]
- **Monoamine oxidase inhibitors (MAOI):** Combination of MAOI and excessive amounts of caffeine can cause hypertensive crisis.[12] [Note: Examples of MAOI include phenelzine (Nardil), tranylcypromine (Parnate), and isocarboxazid (Marplan).]
- **Antibiotics:** It has been reported that use of *Lu Cha* reversed MRSA and PRSA. Furthermore, it lowered minimum inhibitory concentration (MIC) of oxacillin and other β-lactams in MRSA.[13]

TOXICOLOGY

Increased consumption of caffeine in animals has been shown to be teratogenic. However, studies have been inconclusive about the effect of consumption of a moderate portion of the herb on the fetus.[14,15]

References

1. *Xian Dai Zhong Yao Yao Li Xue* (Contemporary Pharmacology of Chinese Herbs), 1997; 691
2. *The Merck Index* 12th edition, Chapman & Hall/CRCnetBASE/Merck, 2000
3. Tyler, V. *The New Honest Herbal. Philadelphia*, PA: G.F. Stickley Co., 1987
4. Wang, H et al., Inhibitory effect of Chinese tea on N-nitrosation *in vitro* and *in vivo*. *IARC Sci Publ*, 1991; 105:546
5. Kono, S. et al., Physical activity, dietary habits and adenomatous polyps of the sigmoid colon: a study of self-defense officials in Japan. *J Clin Epidemiol*, 1991; 44(11):1255
6. Imanishi, H. et al., Tea tannin components modify the induction of sister-chromatid exchanges and chromosome aberrations in mutagen-treated cultured mammalian cells and mice. *Mutat Res*, 1991; 259(1)79
7. *Food and Chemical Toxicology*. 37(6):569-79, 1999 Jun.
8. *Bioscience, Biotechnology and Biochemistry*. 61(11):1901-5, 1997 Nov.
9. Kono, S. et al., Green tea consumption and serum lipid profiles: a cross-sectional study in northern Kyushu, Japan. *Prev Med*, 1992; 21(4):526
10. Boyd, JR. *Facts and Comparison*. 1985
11. *Internat. J. Obesity*, 5:183-7, 1981
12. Brinker, Francis. *Herb Contraindications and Drug Interactions*, 1997; 84-85
13. Abascal K and Yarnell E, Herb and Drug Resistance – Clinical Implications of Research on Microbial Resistance to Antibiotics, *Alternative & Complementary Therapies*; vol 8, no 5, October 2002
14. Tyler, V. *The New Honest Herbal. Philadelphia*, PA: G.F. Stickley Co., 1987
15. Briggs G. et al., Drugs in Pregnancy and Lactation, ed. 3. Baltimore, MD: Williams and Wilkens, 1990

Wu Long Cha (Folium Camellia Sinensis Fermentata)

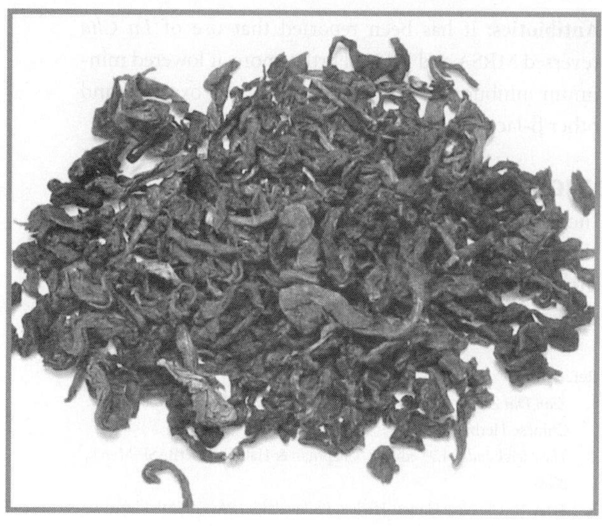

烏龍茶 乌龙茶

Pinyin Name: Wu Long Cha
English Name: oolong tea
Botanical Name: *Camellia sinensis* L. Kuntze (*Cha*)
Pharmaceutical Name: Folium Camellia Sinensis Fermentata
Properties: bitter, sweet, cool
Channels Entered: Heart, Lung, Stomach, Small Intestine

CHINESE THERAPEUTIC ACTIONS

1. Clears Heat and Detoxifies

Mild food poisoning: *Wu Long Cha* (Folium Camellia Sinensis Fermentata) contains tannic acid that can inhibit the spread of bacteria and therefore neutralizes the minor toxins present in many foods. Therefore, drinking tea can kill many of the bacteria and toxins that may cause various illnesses, mostly from food poisoning.

- Diarrhea with abdominal pain: use *Wu Long Cha* with *Huo Xiang* (Herba Agastache), *Huang Lian* (Rhizoma Coptidis), *Huang Qin* (Radix Scutellariae), *Ge Gen* (Radix Puerariae), *Pei Lan* (Herba Eupatorii) and *Da Suan* (Bulbus Alli Sativi).
- Vomiting: combine this herb with *Feng Wei Cao* (Herba Pteris), *Ban Xia* (Rhizoma Pinelliae), *Huang Qin* (Radix Scutellariae) and *Huang Lian* (Rhizoma Coptidis).

2. Promotes Diuresis

Edema: *Wu Long Cha* promotes diuresis to treat edema.

- Edema: use *Wu Long Cha* with *Fen Fang Ji* (Radix Stephaniae Tetandrae), *Huang Qi* (Radix Astragali), *Bai Zhu* (Rhizoma Atractylodis Macrocephalae) and *Fu Ling* (Poria).

3. Revives the *Shen* (Spirit), Clears the Head and Brightens the Eyes

Lassitude: *Wu Long Cha* functions to enhance alertness and relieve fatigue and weakness. It alleviates fatigue, weakness, withered *shen* (spirit), dizziness, hypersomnia, feelings of heaviness in the body, and inability to concentrate.

- Lassitude: combine it with *Xi Yang Shen* (Radix Panacis Quinquefolii), *Ci Wu Jia* (Radix et Caulis Acanthopanacis Senticosi), *Huang Qi* (Radix Astragali) and *Wu Wei Zi* (Fructus Schisandrae Chinensis).

Hangover: *Wu Long Cha* treats hangovers or alcohol poisoning.

- Hangover: use *Wu Long Cha* with *Ge Hua* (Flos Puerariae).

4. Dispels Grease

Intake of greasy food: *Wu Long Cha* promotes digestion and decreases absorption of grease and fats in the body. For this reason, it is customary in many cultures to drink a cup of tea after meals. All of the processed teas such as oolong, pu-er, and black tea are more effective in this than green tea, due to the fermentation process.

- Food stagnation: use it with *Shen Qu* (Massa Fermentata), *Shan Zha* (Fructus Crataegi), and *Mai Ya* (Fructus Hordei Germinatus).
- Excessive intake of greasy foods: combine it with *Chai Hu* (Radix Bupleuri), *Da Huang* (Radix et Rhizoma Rhei), *Zhi Shi* (Fructus Aurantii Immaturus), *Yin Chen Hao* (Herba Artemisiae Scopariae), *Bai Shao* (Radix Paeoniae Alba), *Ban Xia* (Rhizoma Pinelliae) and *Huang Qin* (Radix Scutellariae).

DOSAGE

3 to 12 grams in decoction.

CAUTIONS / CONTRAINDICATIONS

- *Wu Long Cha* should be used with caution in patients with deficiencies of the Spleen and Stomach. It should not be administered on an empty stomach.
- Patients with weak digestive systems should opt for fermented or processed teas such as oolong or black tea rather than the unprocessed green teas.

Wu Long Cha (Folium Camellia Sinensis Fermentata)

AUTHORS' COMMENTS

Lu Cha (Folium Camellia Sinensis) and *Wu Long Cha* (Folium Camellia Sinensis Fermentata) are derived from the same plant. *Lu Cha* is not fermented, while *Wu Long Cha* is. Refer to *Lu Cha* for additional details on chemical composition, pharmacological effects, clinical studies and research, and toxicology information for both herbs.

Xi Gua (Fructus Citrulli)

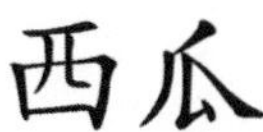

Pinyin Name: *Xi Gua*
Literal Name: "west fruit"
Alternate Chinese Names: *Han Gua*
Original Source: *Ri Yong Ben Cao* (Household Materia Medica) by Wu Rui in 1330
English Name: watermelon fruit
Botanical Name: *Citrullus vulgaris* Schrad.
Pharmaceutical Name: Fructus Citrulli
Properties: sweet, cold
Channels Entered: Heart, Stomach, Urinary Bladder

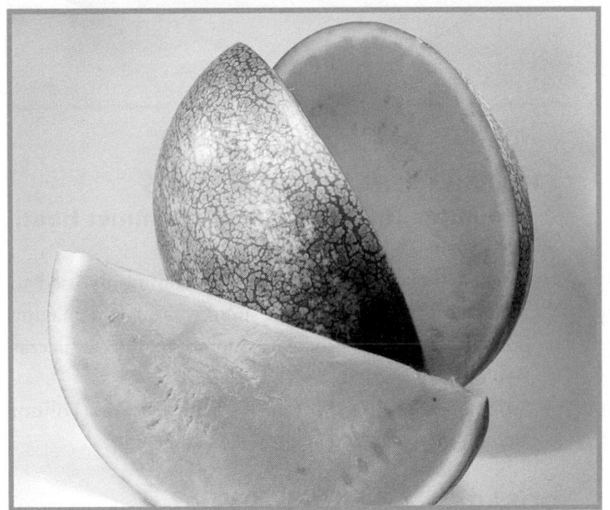

CHINESE THERAPEUTIC ACTIONS

Clears Summer-Heat, Relieves Thirst, Promotes Urination

Xi Gua (Fructus Citrulli) has an excellent ability to clear heat and dampness in summer. It is commonly used to treat summer-heat that has damaged body fluids, leading to irritability, thirst, and dysuria. It may be used individually or in combination with other herbs.

DOSAGE

15 to 30 grams.

CAUTIONS / CONTRAINDICATIONS

- Because of its sweet, cold nature, *Xi Gua* should be used with caution in cases of deficiency and cold of the Spleen and Stomach.

CHEMICAL COMPOSITION

Citrulline, arginine, betaine, lycopene, phytofluene, alanine, glutamic acid, carotene, sugars, vitamin C.[1]

PHARMACOLOGICAL EFFECTS

Diuretic: *Xi Gua* has a mild diuretic effect.[2]

AUTHORS' COMMENTS

Xi Gua is commonly known as "natural *Bai Hu Tang* (White Tiger Decoction)," as it has excellent influence to clear heat and promote the generation of body fluids.

References

1. *Zhong Yao Xue* (Chinese Herbology), 1998; 136
2. Ibid., 136:137

Xi Gua Pi (Pericarpium Citrulli)

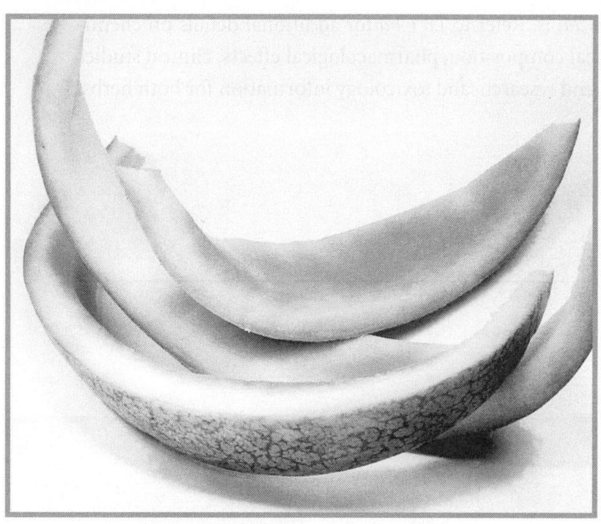

西瓜皮

Pinyin Name: *Xi Gua Pi*
Literal Name: "west fruit peel"
Original Source: *Dan Xi Xin Fa* (Teachings of [Zhu] Dan-Xi) by Zhu Zhen-Heng in 1481
English Name: watermelon peel, watermelon rind
Botanical Name: *Citrullus vulgaris* Schrad.
Pharmaceutical Name: Pericarpium Citrulli
Properties: sweet, cold
Channels Entered: Heart, Stomach, Urinary Bladder

CHINESE THERAPEUTIC ACTIONS

Promotes Urination, Clears Summer-Heat, Relieves Thirst

Xi Gua Pi (Pericarpium Citrulli) is commonly used to treat dysuria in cases which summer-heat is damaging body fluids. It may also be used topically to treat ulceration of the oral cavity.

- Summer-heat: use *Xi Gua Pi* with *He Ye* (Folium Nelumbinis) and *Jin Yin Hua* (Flos Lonicerae).

DOSAGE

15 to 30 grams.

CHEMICAL COMPOSITION

See *Xi Gua* (Fructus Citrulli).

SUPPLEMENT

- 西瓜翠皮 *Xi Gua Cui Pi* (Exocarpium Citrulli), the outermost layer of watermelon peel, is also used as a medicinal herb to clear heat and resolve summer dampness. It is used with *He Ye* (Folium Nelumbinis), *Jin Yin Hua* (Flos Lonicerae), and *Bian Dou Hua* (Flos Lablab Album) to treat exterior conditions in summer. The dosage is 5 to 10 grams.

AUTHORS' COMMENTS

Xi Gua (Fructus Citrulli) and *Xi Gua Pi* (Pericarpium Citrulli) clear summer-heat, relieve thirst, and promote urination, but to differing degrees:

- *Xi Gua* more effectively clears summer heat and dampness.
- *Xi Gua Pi* more strongly promotes urination.

Section 2

— Heat-Clearing and Dampness-Drying Herbs

Huang Qin (Radix Scutellariae)

黄芩 黃芩

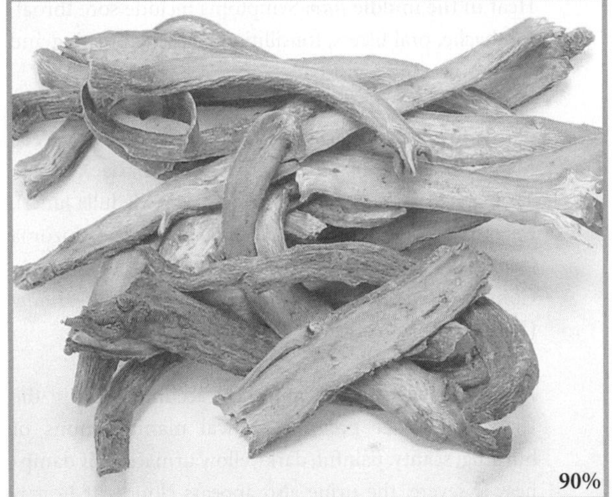
90%

Pinyin Name: *Huang Qin*
Alternate Chinese Names: *Lao Gen Zi Qin, Tiao Qin, Bei Qin, Pian Qin, Ku Qin*
Original Source: *Shen Nong Ben Cao Jing* (Divine Husbandman's Classic of the Materia Medica) in the second century
English Name: scute, scutellaria, baikal skullcap root
Botanical Name: *Scutellaria baicalensis* Georgi (*Huang Qin*); *Scutellaria amoena* C.H. Wright (*Xi Nan Huang Qin*); *Scutellaria rehderiana* Diels (*Gan Su Huang Qin*); *Scutellaria viscidula* Bge. (*Nian Mao Huang Qin*)
Pharmaceutical Name: Radix Scutellariae
Properties: bitter, cold
Channels Entered: Lung, Gallbladder, Stomach, Large Intestine

CHINESE THERAPEUTIC ACTIONS

1. Clears Heat and Dries Dampness

Damp-heat disorders: *Huang Qin* (Radix Scutellariae) treats a wide range of heat-related disorders characterized by fever, abdominal fullness, poor appetite, nausea, sensations of heaviness, thirst with no desire to drink, a red tongue with greasy, yellow coating, and rapid, slippery pulse.

- General damp-heat accumulation: use *Huang Qin* with *Hua Shi* (Talcum), *Tong Cao* (Medulla Tetrapanacis), and *Bai Dou Kou* (Fructus Amomi Rotundus).

Jaundice and hepatitis: Clinical applications for *Huang Qin* include jaundice with bright yellow skin, abdominal fullness, thirst, dysuria, a yellow, greasy tongue coating, and deep, slippery, rapid pulse.

- Jaundice: use *Huang Qin* with *Yin Chen Hao* (Herba Artemisiae Scopariae), *Zhi Zi* (Fructus Gardeniae) and *Da Huang* (Radix et Rhizoma Rhei).
- Infectious hepatitis with jaundice: use this herb with *Yin Chen Hao* (Herba Artemisiae Scopariae), *Huang Bai* (Cortex Phellodendri), *Zhi Zi* (Fructus Gardeniae), *Da Huang* (Radix et Rhizoma Rhei), *Che Qian Zi* (Semen Plantaginis), *Bing Lang* (Semen Arecae), charred *Shen Qu* (Massa Fermentata), charred *Shan Zha* (Fructus Crataegi), and charred *Mai Ya* (Fructus Hordei Germinatus).
- Infectious hepatitis without jaundice: combine *Huang Qin* with *Chuan Lian Zi* (Fructus Toosendan), *Cao Dou Kou* (Semen Alpiniae Katsumadai), *Lai Fu Zi* (Semen Raphani), *Hong Hua* (Flos Carthami), *Qian Cao* (Radix Rubiae), *Bai Ji Li* (Fructus Tribuli), *Zao Jiao Ci* (Spina Gleditsiae), *Bing Lang* (Semen Arecae), charred *Shen Qu* (Massa Fermentata), charred *Shan Zha* (Fructus Crataegi), and charred *Mai Ya* (Fructus Hordei Germinatus).

Huang Qin (Radix Scutellariae)

Dysentery caused by damp-heat in the Stomach and Intestines: Damp-heat accumulation in the gastrointestinal tract manifests in symptoms of dysentery, burning sensations in the anus after defecation, foul-smelling diarrhea, fever, heat sensations in the chest and abdomen, irritability, thirst with dry mouth, a yellow tongue coating and rapid pulse.

- Dysentery or diarrhea with burning sensations of the anus: use *Huang Qin* with *Huang Lian* (Rhizoma Coptidis) and *Bai Shao* (Radix Paeoniae Alba). **Exemplar Formula:** *Ge Gen Huang Qin Huang Lian Tang* (Kudzu, Coptis, and Scutellaria Decoction).

Heat in the middle *jiao*: Symptoms include sore throat, toothache, oral ulcers, tonsillitis, epigastric burning and discomfort, and constipation.

- Sore throat with lingering exterior symptoms: use *Huang Qin* with *Ban Lan Gen* (Radix Isatidis), *Bo He* (Herba Menthae), and *Xuan Shen* (Radix Scrophulariae).
- Toothache, oral ulcers: add *Deng Xin Cao* (Medulla Junci).
- Epigastric discomfort: add *Huang Lian* (Rhizoma Coptidis).
- Constipation: combine *Huang Qin* with *Da Huang* (Radix et Rhizoma Rhei).

***Re lin* (heat dysuria):** Damp-heat accumulation in the Urinary Bladder presents clinical manifestations of burning, scanty, painful, dark yellow urination. If dampness is severe, the urine also appears cloudy. If heat is severe, bleeding may occur.

- Burning dysuria: use *Huang Qin* with *Chuan Mu Tong* (Caulis Clematidis Armandii) and *Che Qian Zi* (Semen Plantaginis).
- *Shi-re lin* (damp-heat dysuria) with qi deficiency: combine this herb with *Shi Lian Zi* (Herba Sinocrassulae Indicae), *Che Qian Zi* (Semen Plantaginis) and *Huang Qi* (Radix Astragali) to tonify qi and clear damp-heat. **Exemplar Formula:** *Qing Xin Lian Zi Yin* (Lotus Seed Decoction to Clear the Heart).

2. Clears Heat and Sedates Fire

Lung heat: Bitter and cold, *Huang Qin* has excellent properties to clear heat and sedate fire in the Lung. Clinical manifestations include cough with yellow sputum, yellow nasal discharge, fever, dyspnea, dry mouth, sore throat, thirst, red tongue with yellow coating, and a rapid pulse.

- Cough with wheezing or dyspnea: use this herb with *Ma Huang* (Herba Ephedrae), *Xing Ren* (Semen Armeniacae Amarum) and *Shi Gao* (Gypsum Fibrosum). **Exemplar Formula:** *Ma Xing Gan Shi Tang* (Ephedra, Apricot Kernel, Licorice, and Gypsum Decoction).
- Chest congestion with profuse yellow sputum: combine it with *Gua Lou Shi* (Fructus Trichosanthis), *Sang Bai Pi* (Cortex Mori) and *Xing Ren* (Semen Armeniacae Amarum) to clear Lung heat and regulate qi circulation. **Exemplar Formula:** *Qing Qi Hua Tan Wan* (Clear the Qi and Transform Phlegm Pill).
- Cough due to heat: combine it with *Shi Gao* (Gypsum Fibrosum), *Zhi Zi* (Fructus Gardeniae), and *Sang Bai Pi* (Cortex Mori). **Exemplar Formula:** *Dun Sou San* (Long-Bout Cough Powder).
- Eye disorders with redness and pain: add *Dan Dou Chi* (Semen Sojae Praeparatum) and pork liver.

Excess heat in the *qi* (energy) level: Unremitting fever, or high fever in the *shaoyang* stage or entering the *yangming* stage. *Huang Qin* is excellent to clear heat in the upper *jiao* as well as clearing heat between different stages as it travels inward from the *taiyang* level.

- Excess heat with persistent high fever and irritability: use it with *Shi Gao* (Gypsum Fibrosum), *Zhi Mu* (Radix Anemarrhenae), and *Mu Dan Pi* (Cortex Moutan) .
- *Shaoyang* syndrome with alternation of fever and chills: combine it with *Chai Hu* (Radix Bupleuri) to clear heat from both the interior and exterior. **Exemplar Formula:** *Xiao Chai Hu Tang* (Minor Bupleurum Decoction).
- Cold and dampness at the exterior with heat in the interior: add *Qiang Huo* (Rhizoma et Radix Notopterygii) and other exterior-releasing herbs. **Exemplar Formula:** *Jiu Wei Qiang Huo Tang* (Nine-Herb Decoction with Notopterygium).

3. Clears Heat and Eliminates Toxins

Lesions, sores, ulcerations caused by toxic heat: *Huang Qin* is commonly used for disorders of the skin, eyes, throat, ears and nose.

- Lesions and sores with redness, swelling and pain: use *Huang Qin* with *Huang Lian* (Rhizoma Coptidis), *Huang Bai* (Cortex Phellodendri) and *Zhi Zi* (Fructus Gardeniae). **Exemplar Formula:** *Huang Lian Jie Du Tang* (Coptis Decoction to Relieve Toxicity).
- General heat and toxins: combine this herb with *Huang Lian* (Rhizoma Coptidis), *Lian Qiao* (Fructus Forsythiae) and *Pu Gong Ying* (Herba Taraxaci).

4. Cools Blood and Stops Bleeding

Bleeding: Clinical applications include hematemesis, cough with blood-streaked sputum, hematuria, gastrointestinal bleeding, and hypermenorrhea caused by heat driving blood out of the vessels. The charred form of *Huang Qin* has the strongest hemostatic effect.

- Hematemesis and epistaxis: use *Huang Qin* with *San Qi* (Radix Notoginseng), *Huai Hua* (Flos Sophorae) and *Bai Mao Gen* (Rhizoma Imperatae).

Huang Qin (Radix Scutellariae)

- Gastrointestinal bleeding: use it with *Huang Lian* (Rhizoma Coptidis) and *Fang Feng* (Radix Saposhnikoviae).

5. Calms and Stabilizes the Fetus

Restless fetus: *Huang Qin* stabilizes pregnancy by calming the fetus to relieve restlessness and constant kicking, a condition commonly described as heat in the womb.

- To calm the fetus: combine *Huang Qin* with *Bai Zhu* (Rhizoma Atractylodis Macrocephalae) and *Dang Gui* (Radicis Angelicae Sinensis).

DOSAGE

3 to 10 grams in decoction. The maximum dosage of *Huang Qin* is 30 grams. Use the fresh form to clear damp-heat in the Intestines; the dried, unprocessed form to clear heat and remove toxins; the dry-fried form to calm the fetus; the steamed with grain-based liquor form to clear Lung heat; and the charred form to stop bleeding.

CAUTIONS / CONTRAINDICATIONS

- Bitter and cold, *Huang Qin* should be used with caution as it may damage Stomach qi and injure Spleen yin.
- Patients with the following conditions should use *Huang Qin* with extreme caution: blood deficiency with abdominal pain, edema due to Spleen deficiency, loose stool because of Kidney deficiency, amenorrhea from blood deficiency, and unstable pregnancy caused by excess cold.

CHEMICAL COMPOSITION

Baicalin, baicalein, wogonin, wogonoside, chrysin, oroxylin A, oroxylin-A-glucuronide, skullcapflavone I, II; tenaxin II, koganebanacin, 7-melhoxy-baicalein, 2,5,8-trihydroxy-7-dimefhoxyflarone.[1,2]

Baicalein

PHARMACOLOGICAL EFFECTS

- **Antibiotic:** Baicalin has a wide-spectrum of inhibitory effect against *Staphylococcus aureus,* beta-hemolytic streptococcus, *Diplococcus pneumoniae, Pseudomonas aeruginosa, Bacillus dysenteriae, E. coli, Bordetella pertussis, Vibrio cholerae, Diplococcus meningitidis,* leptospira and various species of dermatophytes and influenza viruses. *Huang Qin* is most effective against *Staphylococcus aureus* and *Pseudomonas aeruginosa.* Furthermore, it was discovered that the effectiveness of standard antibiotics such as ampicillin, amoxicillin, methicillin and cefotaxime can be potentiated with addition of baicalin, a flavone isolated from the herb. With the addition of baicalin, the effectiveness of these beta-lactam antibiotics was restored against beta-lactam-resistant *Staphylococcus aureus* and methicillin-resistant *Staphylococcus aureus* (MRSA).[3,4]
- **Anti-inflammatory:** In laboratory studies, baicalin, baicalein, and extract of *Huang Qin* suppressed inflammation and swelling associated with allergic reactions in mice.[5]
- **Antipyretic:** Oral administration of *Huang Qin* decoction at the dosage of 2 g/kg has a marked effect to reduce temperature in rabbits with artificially-induced fever.[6]
- **Cholagogic and hepatoprotective:** In a laboratory study, both baicalin and baicalein have marked cholagogic influence to stimulate the production and excretion of bile acid in rabbits. In addition, baicalein has hepatoprotective effects.[7]
- **Antihypertensive:** *Huang Qin* lowers blood pressure through dilation of blood vessels and inhibition of the sympathetic nervous system.[8]
- **Others:** *Huang Qin* has mild sedative and diuretic effects.[9]

CLINICAL STUDIES AND RESEARCH

- **Hepatitis:** In one study, 268 patients with infectious or chronic hepatitis were treated with *Huang Qin* through oral administration and intramuscular injection. The duration of treatment was 1 month for both oral therapy (0.5 grams of baicalin three times daily) and injection therapy (60 to 120 mg of baicalin via intramuscular or intravenous injection). The effective rate was 63.6% for patients with infectious hepatitis and 73.3% for chronic hepatitis.[10]
- **Epidemic encephalitis:** One report states that 209 carriers of epidemic encephalitis were treated with 2 ml of 20% *Huang Qin* oral spray (equivalent to 0.4 grams of herb) with good effectiveness in all subjects.[11]
- **Scarlet fever:** Accordingly to one report, 9 grams of *Huang Qin* were given as herbal decoction two to three times daily for three days during the peak epidemic periods and showed good preventative influence in 1,577 healthy individuals.[12]
- **Hypertension:** Administration of 5 to 10 ml of a *Huang Qin* preparation three times daily showed good antihypertensive effect in 51 patients with hypertension.[13]
- **Trachoma:** In one study, 128 patients with trachoma were treated with 2% or 3% baicalin ophthalmic solution with a 97.1% rate of effectiveness.[14]

HERB-DRUG INTERACTION

- **Antibiotics:** Concurrent use of baicalin, a flavone isolated from *Huang Qin,* was found to have synergistic antibiotic

Huang Qin (Radix Scutellariae)

effect with beta-lactam antibiotics, such as ampicillin, amoxicillin, methicillin and cefotaxime. The addition of baicalin restored the effectiveness of these drugs against beta-lactam-resistant *Staphylococcus aureus* and methicillin-resistant *Staphylococcus aureus* (MRSA).[15]

TOXICOLOGY

While oral administration is associated with few unwanted side effects, intravenous injection of *Huang Qin* preparation has been linked with some toxic effects. The LD_{50} for baicalein via intraperitoneal injection is 3,081 mg/kg in mice. Oral administration of extract of *Huang Qin* at 15 g/kg did not cause nausea or vomiting in dogs. However, loose stools were observed following oral administration of *Huang Qin* at 5 g/kg for 8 weeks.[16,17]

AUTHORS' COMMENTS

Huang Qin, Huang Lian (Rhizoma Coptidis) and *Huang Bai* (Cortex Phellodendri) are commonly used to clear heat, sedate fire and dry dampness. Classic texts often describe *Huang Qin* to be most effective for Lung heat in the upper *jiao, Huang Lian* for Stomach fire in the middle *jiao* and *Huang Bai* for deficient Kidney fire in the lower *jiao*. This statement, however, is only a generalization, as all three herbs have many more functions.

According to Dr. Sam Liang, the combination of *Huang Qin, Huang Lian* (Rhizoma Coptidis), and *Da Huang* (Radix et Rhizoma Rhei), such as found in *San Huang Xie Xin Tang* (Three Yellows Decoction to Sedate the Epigastrium), used as a gargle is very effective to treat sore throat and stomatitis in HIV patients.

Dr. Shen Yen-Nan reports that specific organs injured by fire can be treated with optimum results by key herbs, as follows:

- Lung fire: *Huang Qin* (Radix Scutellariae) and *Sang Bai Pi* (Cortex Mori)
- Heart fire: *Huang Lian* (Rhizoma Coptidis)
- Stomach fire: *Shi Gao* (Gypsum Fibrosum)
- Liver fire: *Zhi Zi* (Fructus Gardeniae)
- Kidney fire: *Zhi Mu* (Radix Anemarrhenae)

There are four herbs commonly used to stabilize pregnancy:

- *Huang Qin* calms restless fetus caused by heat.
- *Sha Ren* (Fructus Amomi) regulates qi and calms restless fetus in the presence of qi stagnation and middle *jiao* deficiency.
- *Du Zhong* (Cortex Eucommiae) is most suitable to treat restless fetus caused by deficiency of the Kidney and Liver.
- *Bai Zhu* (Rhizoma Atractylodis Macrocephalae) treats restless fetus from Spleen qi deficiency.

References

1. *Xian Dai Zhong Yao Yao Li Xue* (Contemporary Pharmacology of Chinese Herbs), 1997; 299
2. *The Merck Index* 12th edition, Chapman & Hall/CRCnetBASE/Merck, 2000
3. *Zhong Yao Xue* (Chinese Herbology), 1988; 137:140
4. *J Pharm Pharmacol* 2000 Mar;52(3):361-6
5. *Chem Pharm Bull*, 1984; 32(7):2724
6. *Zhong Hua Yi Xue Za Zhi* (Chinese Journal of Medicine), 1956; 42(10):964
7. *Ri Ben Yao Wu Xue Za Zhi* (Japan Journal of Pharmacology), 1957; 53(6):215
8. *Zhong Yao Xue* (Chinese Herbology), 1988; 137:140
9. Ibid.
10. *Zhong Hua Nei Ke Za Zhi* (Chinese Journal of Internal Medicine), 1978; 2:127
11. *Zhong Yi Za Zhi* (Journal of Chinese Medicine), 1960; 6:20
12. *Zhong Cao Yao Tong Xun* (Journal of Chinese Herbal Medicine), 1972; 3:35
13. *Shang Hai Zhong Yi Yao Za Zhi* (Shanghai Journal of Chinese Medicine and Herbology), 1956; 1:24
14. *Zhong Cao Yao Tong Xun* (Journal of Chinese Herbal Medicine), 1978; 3:33
15. *J Pharm Pharmacol* 2000 Mar;52(3):361-6
16. *Xi An Yi Ke Da Xue Xue Bao* (Journal of Xian University School of Medicine), 1958; (5):30
17. *Sheng Li Xue Bao* (Physiology News), 1958; 22(3):249

Huang Lian (Rhizoma Coptidis)

黄連 黄连

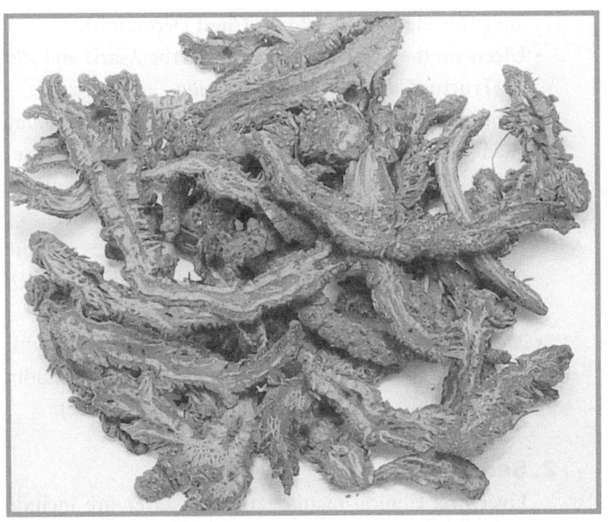

Pinyin Name: *Huang Lian*
Literal Name: "yellow connection," "yellow link"
Alternate Chinese Names: *Chuan Lian, Ya Lian, Wei Lian, Ji Zhua Lian*
Original Source: *Shen Nong Ben Cao Jing* (Divine Husbandman's Classic of the Materia Medica) in the second century
English Name: coptis, coptis root
Botanical Name: *Coptis chinensis* Franch. (*Huang Lian*); *Coptis deltoidea* C. Y. Cheng et Hsiao (*San Jiao Ye Huang Lian*); *Coptis teetoides* C. Y. Cheng. (*Yun Lian*); *Coptis omeiensis* (*Chen*) C. Y. Cheng (*E Mei Ye Lian*)
Pharmaceutical Name: Rhizoma Coptidis
Properties: bitter, cold
Channels Entered: Heart, Liver, Stomach, Large Intestine

CHINESE THERAPEUTIC ACTIONS

1. Clears Heat and Dries Dampness

Damp-heat in the Intestines: Very bitter, very cold, and extremely drying in nature, *Huang Lian* (Rhizoma Coptidis) is one of the strongest herbs to clear heat, dry dampness and eliminate toxins. It is commonly used to treat diarrhea or dysentery that may or may not contain pus and blood, burning sensations of the anus after defecation, foul-smelling stools, rectal tenesmus, feelings of incomplete evacuation, abdominal pain, epigastric distention and fullness, thirst with no desire to drink, vomiting or nausea, a slippery, rapid pulse, and a red tongue with greasy, yellow coating.

- Diarrhea or dysentery with burning sensations of the anus: combine *Huang Lian, Huang Bai* (Cortex Phellodendri), *Qin Pi* (Cortex Fraxini), and *Bai Tou Weng* (Radix Pulsatillae). **Exemplar Formula:** *Bai Tou Weng Tang* (Pulsatilla Decoction).
- Diarrhea with rectal tenesmus: use this herb with *Mu Xiang* (Radix Aucklandiae) and *Bing Lang* (Semen Arecae). **Exemplar Formula:** *Shao Yao Tang* (Peony Decoction).
- Diarrhea in exterior syndromes: combine with *Ge Gen* (Radix Puerariae). **Exemplar Formula:** *Ge Gen Huang Qin Huang Lian Tang* (Kudzu, Coptis, and Scutellaria Decoction).
- Diarrhea with bleeding: use *Huang Lian* with garlic.

Stomach heat: This condition is usually caused by frequent intake of spicy foods or a chronic state of Liver overacting on the Spleen and Stomach. Common symptoms and signs of Stomach heat include vomiting, nausea, gastric pain or burning sensations, acid regurgitation, foul breath, preference for cold drinks, constipation, hunger, swollen or painful gums, toothache, yellow and scanty urine with red tongue and yellow tongue coating. Heat in the Stomach reverses the normal downward flow of Stomach qi and causes nausea and vomiting. Heat enhances the digestive function of the Stomach and thus the patient feels constant hunger. Rising Stomach fire causes the burning epigastric pain, acid reflux, foul breath and swollen, painful gums.

- Nausea, vomiting and feelings of oppression in the chest: use *Huang Lian* with *Gan Jiang* (Rhizoma Zingiberis) and *Ban Xia* (Rhizoma Pinelliae). **Exemplar Formula:** *Ban Xia Xie Xin Tang* (Pinellia Decoction to Drain the Epigastrium).
- Nausea and vomiting from heat in the Stomach: use this herb with *Ban Xia* (Rhizoma Pinelliae) and *Zhu Ru* (Caulis Bambusae in Taenia).
- Gastric pain and ulcers due to Liver fire attacking the Stomach: combine it with *Wu Zhu Yu* (Fructus Evodiae), *Xiang Fu* (Rhizoma Cyperi) and *Yan Hu Suo* (Rhizoma Corydalis).
- Acid regurgitation: add *Hai Piao Xiao* (Endoconcha Sepiae) and *Zhe Bei Mu* (Bulbus Fritillariae Thunbergii).
- Bleeding peptic ulcer: use *Huang Lian* with *Bai Ji* (Rhizoma Bletillae) and *Wu Bei Zi* (Galla Chinensis).
- Feeling of fullness and oppression beneath the Heart with pain during palpation: use it with *Ban Xia* (Rhizoma Pinelliae) and *Gua Lou Shi* (Fructus Trichosanthis). **Exemplar Formula:** *Xiao Xian Xiong*

Huang Lian (Rhizoma Coptidis)

Tang (Minor Sinking Into the Chest Decoction).
- Ulcers on the tongue: add *Xi Xin* (Herba Asari) and *Zhi Zi* (Fructus Gardeniae) to *Huang Lian.*
- Toothache from Stomach fire: use it with *Sheng Di Huang* (Radix Rehmanniae), *Sheng Ma* (Rhizoma Cimicifugae) and *Bai Zhi* (Radix Angelicae Dahuricae). **Exemplar Formula:** *Qing Wei San* (Clear the Stomach Powder).
- Excessive hunger and thirst from Stomach fire: combine it with *Tian Hua Fen* (Radix Trichosanthis) and *Sheng Di Huang* (Radix Rehmanniae).
- *Xiao ke* (wasting and thirsting) syndrome: use it with *Shi Gao* (Gypsum Fibrosum), *Tian Hua Fen* (Radix Trichosanthis) and *Zhi Mu* (Radix Anemarrhenae).

2. Sedates Fire

Liver fire: Clinical manifestations of Liver fire include dizziness, headache, redness of the face and eyes, a bitter taste in the mouth, dry throat, short temper, irritability, insomnia or nightmares, burning hypochondriac pain, tinnitus, constipation, hematemesis or epistaxis, a red tongue with yellow coating, and a wiry, slippery and rapid pulse.
- Liver fire: use *Huang Lian* with *Wu Zhu Yu* (Fructus Evodiae), *Chai Hu* (Radix Bupleuri) and *Bai Shao* (Radix Paeoniae Alba).
- Red eyes due to Liver yang rising: use it with *Shi Jue Ming* (Concha Haliotidis), *Jue Ming Zi* (Semen Cassiae), *Long Dan Cao* (Radix Gentianae), *Mu Zei* (Herba Equiseti Hiemalis) and *Ye Ming Sha* (Excrementum Vespertilionis Murini).
- Photophobia, blurred vision, spots in front of the eyes, night blindness and acute conjunctivitis caused by Liver blood deficiency and Liver yang rising: use *Huang Lian* alone in decoction. It can also be used as an external wash for the eyes.

Heart fire: Insomnia, tongue ulcers, irritability, mania, incoherent speech, hematemesis, epistaxis, burning sensations in the chest, thirst, red face, dry stools, scanty yellow urine, red tongue tip, scarlet red tongue body, and rapid pulse are all symptoms and signs associated with Heart fire.
- Insomnia and irritability caused by Heart fire: use *Huang Lian* with *Zhu Sha* (Cinnabaris) and *Sheng Di Huang* (Radix Rehmanniae).
- Insomnia and irritability associated with Heart fire and deficiencies of yin and blood: combine it with *E Jiao* (Colla Corii Asini) and *Bai Shao* (Radix Paeoniae Alba).
- Hematemesis and rectal bleeding due to heat in the blood: use *Huang Lian* with *Huang Qin* (Radix Scutellariae) and *Da Huang* (Radix et Rhizoma Rhei).
- Aversion to heat and irritability due to excess heat and fire: add *Zhi Zi* (Fructus Gardeniae) and *Huang Qin* (Radix Scutellariae). **Exemplar Formula:** *Huang Lian Jie Du Tang* (Coptis Decoction to Relieve Toxicity).
- Delirium: use *Huang Lian* with *Shi Chang Pu* (Rhizoma Acori), *Tian Zhu Huang* (Concretio Silicea Bambusae), *Lian Qiao* (Fructus Forsythiae), and *Sheng Di Huang* (Radix Rehmanniae).

3. Clears Fire Toxin

Dermatological disorders arising from toxic fire: *Huang Lian* is commonly used to eliminate heat and toxins present at the skin level, characterized by abscesses and lesions. Apply the powder of this herb topically.
- Abscesses, lesions, carbuncles, furuncles, burns, swelling and inflammation due to heat toxins: use this herb with *Huang Qin* (Radix Scutellariae), *Da Huang* (Radix et Rhizoma Rhei) and *Lian Qiao* (Fructus Forsythiae) to clear heat and eliminate toxins. **Exemplar Formula:** *Huang Lian Jie Du Tang* (Coptis Decoction to Relieve Toxicity).

DOSAGE

2 to 10 grams in decoction. The maximum dosage of *Huang Lian* is 15 grams. *Huang Lian* has different functions depending on how it is processed:
- The unprocessed herb is stronger to clear heat, sedate fire and dry dampness.
- Frying with grain-based liquor gives *Huang Lian* an ascending function and diminishes its bitter and cold impact.
- Frying with *Sheng Jiang* (Rhizoma Zingiberis Recens) and *Wu Zhu Yu* (Fructus Evodiae) gives *Huang Lian* dispersing and ventilating functions, weakens its bitter and cold effects, and enhances its nausea-relieving function.
- Frying with pig bile enhances the effectiveness of *Huang Lian* to sedate fire of the Liver and Gallbladder.

CAUTIONS / CONTRAINDICATIONS

- *Huang Lian* is bitter, cold and drying. It must be used with caution in patients who have cold, yang deficiency, yin deficiency, or deficiency of the Spleen and Stomach.
- *Huang Lian* is relatively safe, but may be associated with the following side effects: allergic reaction, allergic rash, dizziness, headache, tinnitus, nausea, vomiting, palpitations, shortness of breath, abdominal fullness, diarrhea, and reduction of red blood cells.

CHEMICAL COMPOSITION

Berberine, coptisine, palmatine, jatrorrhizine, epiberberine, worenine, columbamine, magnoflorine.[1,2]

Huang Lian (Rhizoma Coptidis)

H_3CO OCH_3

Berberine

PHARMACOLOGICAL EFFECTS

- **Antibiotic:** *Huang Lian* has a broad spectrum of antibiotic effects against *Bacillus dysenteriae, Mycobacterium tuberculosis, Salmonella typhi, E. coli, Vibrio cholerae, Bacillus proteus, Pseudomonas aeruginosa, Diplococcus meningitidis, Staphylococcus aureus,* beta-hemolytic streptococcus, *Diplococcus pneumoniae, Corynebacterium diphtheriae, Bordetella pertussis, Bacillus anthracis,* and leptospira. The inhibitory effect is strongest against *E. coli, Mycobacterium tuberculosis,* and *Staphylococcus aureus.* Use of *Huang Lian* or its components individually is commonly associated with resistance. On the other hand, the use of *Huang Lian* within an herbal formula reportedly enhances its antibiotic effectiveness over tenfold with little incidence of resistance. Berberine, one of the components of *Huang Lian,* is most effective for gastrointestinal infection, but not for systemic infection, since it has poor absorption by the intestines and a short half-life. In addition to its antibacterial effect, *Huang Lian* also has antifungal and antiviral activities. According to one report, a 15% decoction of *Huang Lian* is effective against numerous pathogenic fungi and dermatophytes. Lastly, *Huang Lian* has an inhibitory effect against influenza and hepatitis viruses.[3,4,5]
- **Anti-inflammatory:** Oral administration of 50 mg/kg of berberine in rats has demonstrated a marked anti-inflammatory effect.[6]
- **Cardiovascular:** Intravenous injection of berberine at 0.1 to 6.0 mg/kg lowered blood pressure in anesthetized dogs, cats and rats. The mechanism of blood pressure reduction is dilation of the blood vessels and inhibition of secretion of the adrenal glands. Berberine also has antiarrhythmic actions.[7,8]
- **Antipyretic:** Intravenous injection of *Huang Lian* has demonstrated antipyretic effects in rabbits. Though the exact mechanism of action is unclear, it is related to cAMP in the central nervous system.[9]
- **Cholagogic:** *Huang Lian* and berberine act to increase production and decrease density of bile acid. Additionally, they reduce the plasma level of cholesterols.[10]
- **Antiulcer:** *Huang Lian* inhibits the secretion of gastric acid and is commonly used in conjunction with other herbs to treat peptic ulcers.[11]
- **Others:** *Huang Lian* has local anesthetic and antidiarrheal effects.[12]

CLINICAL STUDIES AND RESEARCH

- **Bacterial dysentery:** The use of *Huang Lian,* individually or in an herbal formula, was associated with excellent clinical results in treating over 1,000 patients with bacterial dysentery. The treatments showed marked effectiveness, a short treatment course, and low incidence of side effects.[13]
- **Acute gastroenteritis or enteritis:** An herbal formula (80% *Huang Lian* and 20% *Bai Dou Kou* (Fructus Amomi Rotundus)) was used to treat 100 patients with gastroenteritis at the dosage of 2 to 3 grams given four to six times daily. All patients reported marked improvement.[14]
- **Pulmonary tuberculosis:** In one study, 100 patients with pulmonary tuberculosis were treated with 0.3 grams of berberine three times daily for 3 months with good results.[15]
- **Suppurative otitis media:** An herbal solution (10% *Huang Lian* and 3% boric acid) was decocted twice and filtered. After cleaning the ears, the herbal solution was instilled in the affected ear three to four times daily. The effective rate was 50.8%.[16]
- **Arrhythmia:** One report describes 50 patients with hard-to-treat arrhythmia who were given 0.3 to 0.5 grams of berberine three to four times daily, with marked effectiveness in 40% of the patients.[17]
- **Hypertension:** Accordingly to one study, 88 hypertensive patients were treated with 0.6 to 1.8 grams of berberine three times daily with an effective rate of 70 to 93.3%.[18]
- **Osteomyelitis:** In one study, 87 patients with osteomyelitis were treated with *Huang Lian* decoction three times daily with a 100% success rate, with an average recovery period of 22.32 days. The decoction was prepared by cooking 65 grams of *Huang Lian* powder in 2,000 ml of boiling water for 15 minutes. The herb powder was not filtered out and no preservatives were added.[19]

HERB-DRUG INTERACTION

- **Cyclophosphamide**: It was reported in an *in vitro* study that the use of berberine in rats was effective in preventing cyclophosphamide-induced cystitis. According to the report, administration of berberine has a dose-dependent effect to block cyclophosphamide-induced bladder edema and hemorrhage, as well as nitric oxide metabolites increase in rat urine and plasma. The study suggested that berberine could be a potentially effective drug in the treatment of cyclophosphamide-induced cystitis, and provides bright hope for the prevention and treatment of cyclophosphamide urotoxicity.[20]

Huang Lian (Rhizoma Coptidis)

TOXICOLOGY

The LD_{50} for berberine in mice is 24.3 mg/kg via intraperitoneal injection, with respiratory depression as the main cause of death. In human, rare instances of fatality due to anaphylactic reaction have been reported after intravenous injection of berberine.[21] [Note: Anaphylactic shock is the most severe type of allergic reaction. Unfortunately, it is very difficult, if not impossible, to predict when patients will have such serious reactions. Though there is one case of anaphylactic reaction reported with injection of berberine, oral use of *Huang Lian* does not necessarily have a higher risk of allergy than other herbs.]

AUTHORS' COMMENTS

Huang Lian and *Suan Zao Ren* (Semen Zizyphi Spinosae) both treat insomnia. *Huang Lian* is used for excess fire in the Heart disturbing the *shen* (spirit) and *Suan Zao Ren* is used for Heart and Liver deficiencies with lack of nourishment to the Heart and *shen.*

Huang Lian (Rhizoma Coptidis) and *Hu Huang Lian* (Rhizoma Picrorhizae) have similar names and functions. *Huang Lian* clears excess heat with dampness and eliminates toxins to relieve sores and carbuncles. *Hu Huang Lian* is used for steaming bones sensations, *wu xin re* (five-center heat) and other deficiency heat symptoms.

Huang Lian, Chuan Mu Tong (Caulis Clematidis Armandii), *Mai Men Dong* (Radix Ophiopogonis), and *Tian Zhu Huang* (Concretio Silicea Bambusae) all clear the Heart and eliminate irritability.

- *Huang Lian* is used for febrile disease with excess fire in the Heart disturbing the *shen* (spirit), manifesting in irritability and insomnia.
- *Chuan Mu Tong* is a diuretic that clears damp-heat to relieve irritability with oral ulcers and yellow urine.
- *Mai Men Dong* is a tonic used for deficient Heart yin with heat that manifests as irritability and insomnia.
- *Tian Zhu Huang* dissolves hot phlegm and is best for irritability with spasms and convulsions.

Dr. Shen Yen-Nan reports that specific organs injured by fire can be treated with optimum results by key herbs, as follows:

- Lung fire: *Huang Qin* (Radix Scutellariae) and *Sang Bai Pi* (Cortex Mori)
- Heart fire: *Huang Lian* (Rhizoma Coptidis)
- Stomach fire: *Shi Gao* (Gypsum Fibrosum)
- Liver fire: *Zhi Zi* (Fructus Gardeniae)
- Kidney fire: *Zhi Mu* (Radix Anemarrhenae)

References

1. *Xian Dai Zhong Yao Yao Li Xue* (Contemporary Pharmacology of Chinese Herbs), 1997; 299
3. *The Merck Index* 12th edition, Chapman & Hall/CRCnetBASE/Merck, 2000
3. *Zhong Yao Xue* (Chinese Herbology), 1988, 140:144
4. *Zhong Hua Yi Xue Za Zhi* (Chinese Journal of Medicine), 1958; 44(9):888
5. *Zhong Xi Yi Jie He Za Zhi* (Journal of Integrated Chinese and Western Medicine), 1989; 9(8):494
6. *Yao Xue Za Zhi* (Journal of Medicinals), 1981, 101(10):883
7. *IRCS Med. Sci*, 1983; 11(7):570
8. *Zhong Yao Xue* (Chinese Herbology), 1988, 140:144
9. *Zhong Guo Bing Li Sheng Li Za Zhi* (Chinese Journal of Pathology and Biology), 1991; 7(3):264
10. *Zhong Yao Xue* (Chinese Herbology), 1988, 140:144
11. Ibid.
12. Ibid.
13. *Zhong Hua Nei Ke Za Zhi* (Chinese Journal of Internal Medicine), 1976; 4:219
14. *Si Chuan Yi Xue Yuan Xue Bao* (Journal of Sichuan School of Medicine), 1959; 1:102
15. *Zhe Jiang Zhong Yi Za Zhi* (Zhejiang Journal of Chinese Medicine), 1964; 10:51
16. *Zhong Hua Er Ke Za Zhi* (Chinese Journal of Pediatrics), 1954; 4:272
17. *Shi Yong Nei Ke Za Zhi* (Practical Journal of Internal Medicine), 1985; 11:587
18. *Zhong Hua Nei Ke Za Zhi* (Chinese Journal of Internal Medicine), 1960:2:117
19. *Zhong Xi Yi Jie He Za Zhi* (Journal of Integrated Chinese and Western Medicine), 1985; 10:604
20. Xu X, Malave A., Protective effect of berberine on cyclophosphamide-induced haemorrhagic cystitis in rats., Department of Pharmaceutical Sciences, College of Pharmacy, Nova Southeastern University, Fort Lauderdale, Florida 33328, USA.
21. *Zhong Yao Xue* (Chinese Herbology), 1988, 143

Huang Bai (Cortex Phellodendri)

黄柏

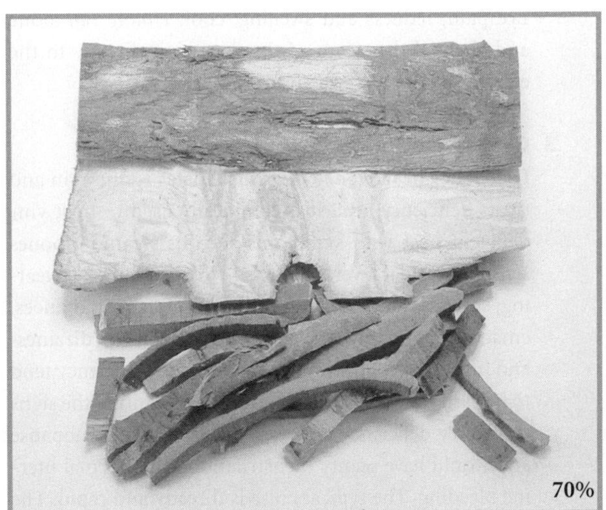

Pinyin Name: *Huang Bai*
Literal Name: "yellow fir"
Alternate Chinese Names: *Bai Pi, Huang Bo*
Original Source: *Shen Nong Ben Cao Jing* (Divine Husbandman's Classic of the Materia Medica) in the second century
English Name: phellodendron bark, Chinese cork tree bark, amur cork tree bark
Botanical Name: *Phellodendron amurense* Rupr. (*Guan Huang Bai*); *Phellodendron chinensis* Schneid. (*Chuan Huang Bai*)
Pharmaceutical Name: Cortex Phellodendri
Properties: bitter, cold
Channels Entered: Kidney, Urinary Bladder, Large Intestine

CHINESE THERAPEUTIC ACTIONS

1. Clears Heat and Dries Dampness

Damp-heat accumulation: Clinical manifestations of damp-heat include jaundice, dysentery, burning diarrhea, feelings of incomplete evacuation after defecation, bleeding hemorrhoids, yellow leukorrhea, dysuria, and *bi zheng* (painful obstruction syndrome) with swollen, burning joints. *Huang Bai* (Cortex Phellodendri) excels in clearing heat and drying dampness, especially from the lower *jiao*.

- Jaundice: combine *Huang Bai* with *Zhi Zi* (Fructus Gardeniae), *Da Huang* (Radix et Rhizoma Rhei) and *Yin Chen Hao* (Herba Artemisiae Scopariae). **Exemplar Formula:** *Yin Chen Hao Tang* (Artemisia Scoparia Decoction).
- Diarrhea: use it with *Huang Lian* (Rhizoma Coptidis), *Qin Pi* (Cortex Fraxini) and *Bai Tou Weng* (Radix Pulsatillae). **Exemplar Formula:** *Bai Tou Weng Tang* (Pulsatilla Decoction).
- Dysentery: use it with *Huang Lian* (Rhizoma Coptidis), *Mu Xiang* (Radix Aucklandiae), *Ma Chi Xian* (Herba Portulacae) and *Bai Shao* (Radix Paeoniae Alba).
- *Bi zheng* (painful obstruction syndrome) with swelling and burning pain: combine *Huang Bai* with *Cang Zhu* (Rhizoma Atractylodis), *Niu Xi* (Radix Cyathulae seu Achyranthis) and *Yi Yi Ren* (Semen Coicis).
- *Bi zheng* with sore and weak low back and knees: use it with *Du Zhong* (Cortex Eucommiae), *Dang Gui* (Radicis Angelicae Sinensis) and *Niu Xi* (Radix Cyathulae seu Achyranthis).
- *Lin zheng* (dysuria syndrome) or urinary tract infection: use it with *Bian Xu* (Herba Polygoni Avicularis) and *Chuan Mu Tong* (Caulis Clematidis Armandii).
- Hematuria: use charred *Huang Bai*, charred *Bai Mao Gen* (Rhizoma Imperatae), *Da Ji* (Herba seu Radix Cirsii Japonici), *Xiao Ji* (Herba Cirisii), and *Chuan Mu Tong* (Caulis Clematidis Armandii).
- Yellow leukorrhea: use it with *Zhi Zi* (Fructus Gardeniae), *Ze Xie* (Rhizoma Alismatis) and *Che Qian Zi* (Semen Plantaginis).
- Dysuria: combine it with *Bian Xu* (Herba Polygoni Avicularis), *Hua Shi* (Talcum) and *Chuan Mu Tong* (Caulis Clematidis Armandii).
- Bleeding hemorrhoid: use it with charred *Huai Hua* (Flos Sophorae), *Di Yu* (Radix Sanguisorbae) and *Fang Feng* (Radix Saposhnikoviae).

2. Sedates Fire and Eliminates Toxins

Accumulation of toxic heat: In addition to clearing heat and drying dampness, *Huang Bai* is used both internally and externally to sedate fire and eliminate toxins. Clinically, it is commonly used to treat abscesses, sores, carbuncles, ulcerations, eczema, lesions, burns, redness, and eye swelling and pain.

- Skin abscesses and lesions: use *Huang Bai* with *Huang Lian* (Rhizoma Coptidis) and *Lian Qiao* (Fructus Forsythiae). **Exemplar Formula:** *Huang Lian Jie Du Tang* (Coptis Decoction to Relieve Toxicity).
- Rash and eczema: use it with *Ku Shen Gen* (Radix Sophorae Flavescentis), *Chan Tui* (Periostracum Cicadae) and *Lian Qiao* (Fructus Forsythiae).
- Carbuncles or furuncles with abscesses and ulcerations: mix *Huang Bai* with *Zhu Dan* (Fel Porcus) and apply topically.
- Breast abscess: mix *Huang Bai* powder and egg whites, and apply topically.

Huang Bai (Cortex Phellodendri)

- Eye pain, redness and swelling: cook *Huang Bai* alone and channel the steam of the decoction directly to the eyes for maximum effectiveness.

3. Clears Deficiency Heat

Deficiency heat: *Huang Bai* consolidates Kidney yin and treats deficiency heat. It is commonly used to treat yin-deficient heat with symptoms such as steaming bones sensations, tidal fever, nocturnal emissions, night sweating, soreness and weakness of the lower back and knees, emaciation, dry throat, flushed cheeks, tinnitus, dizziness and insomnia. Men who have Kidney yin deficiency tend to be easily sexually aroused. Women exhibiting the signs of Kidney deficiency are often experiencing menopause and would have scanty menstruation or abnormal uterine bleeding. The typical pulse is thready and rapid. The tongue is usually dry, with a crack in the center.

- Kidney yin deficiency with deficiency heat: use *Huang Bai* with *Zhi Mu* (Radix Anemarrhenae) to clear deficiency heat without further damaging yin. **Exemplar Formula:** *Zhi Bai Di Huang Wan* (Anemarrhena, Phellodendron, and Rehmannia Pill).
- Severe signs of yin-deficient fire: add *Qing Hao* (Herba Artemisiae Annuae) and *Bie Jia* (Carapax Trionycis). **Exemplar Formula:** *Qing Hao Bie Jia Tang* (Artemisia Annua and Soft-shelled Turtle Shell Decoction).
- Kidney yin and yang deficiencies with yin-deficiency fire: use this herb with *Zhi Mu* (Radix Anemarrhenae), *Xian Mao* (Rhizoma Curculiginis), *Yin Yang Huo* (Herba Epimedii), and *Ba Ji Tian* (Radix Morindae Officinalis). **Exemplar Formula:** *Er Xian Tang* (Two-Immortal Decoction).
- Night sweating: combine *Huang Bai* with *Fu Xiao Mai* (Semen Tritici Aestivi Levis).
- Irritability: use it with *Long Gu* (Os Draconis) and *Mu Li* (Concha Ostreae).

DOSAGE

3 to 10 grams in decoction. The maximum dosage of *Huang Bai* is 30 grams. The unprocessed herb more effectively clears excess heat and eliminates toxins. The salt-fried herb more effectively clears deficiency heat from the Kidney. Frying with grain-based liquor enhances its function to clear Heart fire. The charred herb more strongly stops bleeding.

CAUTIONS / CONTRAINDICATIONS

- Bitter and cold, *Huang Bai* consumes yin and fluids and is not suitable for long-term use, especially in patients with deficiency and cold of the Spleen and Stomach.
- *Huang Bai* is contraindicated in patients with general yang deficiency, or Spleen or Kidney yang deficiency.

CHEMICAL COMPOSITION

Berberine, palmatine, jatrorrhizine, α-phellodendrine, β-phellodendrine menisperine, candicine, magnoflorine, limonin, obacunone.[1,2]

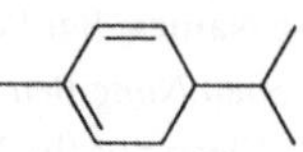

α-phellodendrine

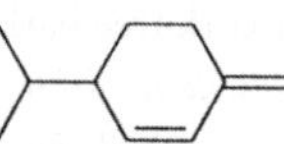

β-phellodendrine

PHARMACOLOGICAL EFFECTS

- **Antibiotic:** *Huang Bai* has demonstrated moderate antibiotic action against *Staphylococcus aureus, Diplococcus pneumoniae, Corynebacterium diphtheriae, Bacillus dysenteriae,* β-hemolytic streptococcus, *Diplococcus meningitidis, Vibrio cholerae, Bacillus anthracis,* dermatophytes and leptospira. The leaves, *Huang Bai Ye* (Folium Phellodendri), have demonstrated antiviral effect against herpes virus.[3,4,5]
- **Antihypertensive:** Xylopinin, derived from phellodendrine, has demonstrated marked effectiveness to lower blood pressure via its effect on the central nervous system.[6]
- **Antitussive and expectorant:** The essential oil of *Huang Bai* has demonstrated antitussive and expectorant effects.[7]

CLINICAL STUDIES AND RESEARCH

- **Chronic bacterial dysentery:** In one study, 40 patients with chronic bacterial dysentery were given 4 grams of *Huang Bai* pills (prepared from *Huang Bai* powder mixed with 10% ethanol) twice daily for 7 days, with marked response in all patients.[8]
- **Chronic bronchitis:** The combination of *Huang Bai* and *Ku Shen Gen* (Radix Sophorae Flavescentis) demonstrated satisfactory antitussive, expectorant, and antiasthmatic effects in 300 patients with chronic bronchitis.[9]

TOXICOLOGY

The LD_{50} for intraperitoneal injection of extract of *Huang Bai* is 2.7 g/kg in mice.[10]

AUTHORS' COMMENTS

Huang Bai does not have moistening or yin-tonifying functions. It is commonly used to clear deficiency heat of the Kidney and thus has been misconstrued by some to have yin-tonic functions. The reason Kidney yin can function properly after administrating *Huang Bai* is because of the ability of this herb to clear deficiency heat,

Huang Bai (Cortex Phellodendri)

thus the Kidney has a chance to restore water that would otherwise be 'burned up.' *Huang Bai* is drying in nature, and when improperly used or prescribed over a long period of time will damage yin. For that reason, it is often combined with other heat-clearing herbs such as *Zhi Mu* (Radix Anemarrhenae) that have moistening properties, so as to not damage the yin while clearing deficiency heat. If yin deficiency is severe, *Huang Bai* can be used with yin-tonic herbs to enhance their overall function.

References

1. *Xian Dai Zhong Yao Yao Li Xue* (Contemporary Pharmacology of Chinese Herbs), 1997; 310
2. Yan X, Zhou J, Xie G, *Traditional Chinese Medicines Molecular Structures, Natural Sources and Applications*; Ashgate, 1999; 5094
3. *Zhong Yao Da Ci Dien* (Dictionary of Chinese Herbs), 1977: 2032
4. *Zhong Cao Yao* (Chinese Herbal Medicine), 1985; 16(1):34
5. *Zhong Yao Xue* (Chinese Herbology), 1998; 144:146
6. *Zhong Guo Yao Li Xue Tong Bao* (Journal of Chinese Herbal Pharmacology), 1989; 10(5):385
7. *Zhong Cao Yao* (Chinese Herbal Medicine), 1981; 12(1):16
8. *Zhong Yi Za Zhi* (Journal of Chinese Medicine), 1959; 8:23
9. *Zhong Guo Zhong Xi Yi Jie He Za Zhi* (Chinese Journal of Integrative Chinese and Western Medicine), 1984; 4:222
10. *Yao Xue Xue Bao* (Journal of Herbology), 1962; 9(5):281

Ji Xue Cao (Herba Centellae)

積雪草 积雪草

Pinyin Name: *Ji Xue Cao*
Alternate Chinese Names: *Di Qian Cao, Ma Ti Cao, Han Ke Cao*
English Name: asiatic pennywort, gotu kola
Botanical Name: *Centella asiatica* (Linn.) Urban.
Pharmaceutical Name: Herba Centellae
Properties: acrid, bitter, cold
Channels Entered: Liver, Spleen, Kidney, Small Intestine, Large Intestine

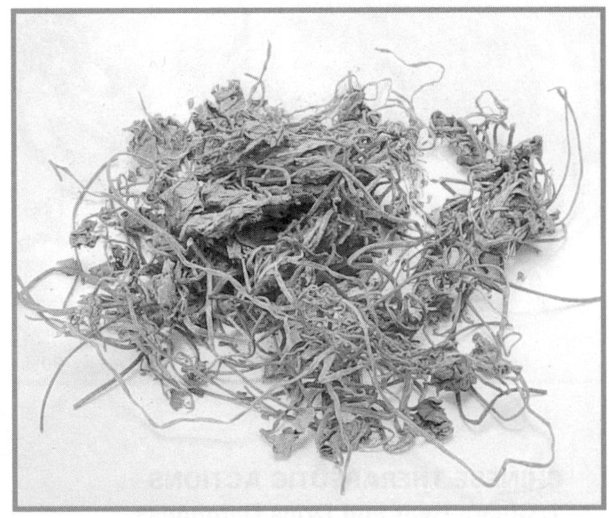

CHINESE THERAPEUTIC ACTIONS

1. Clears Damp-Heat

Enteritis, dysentery, abdominal pain: *Ji Xue Cao* (Herba Centellae) treats gastrointestinal disorders caused by accumulation of damp-heat.

- Enteritis, abdominal pain: use *Ji Xue Cao* with *Feng Wei Cao* (Herba Pteris), *Chuan Xin Lian* (Herba Andrographis), *Huang Lian* (Rhizoma Coptidis) and *Xian Feng Cao* (Herba Bidentis).
- Dysentery: use it with *Feng Wei Cao* (Herba Pteris), *Ge Gen* (Radix Puerariae), *Huang Qin* (Radix Scutellariae) and *Huang Lian* (Rhizoma Coptidis).
- Summer-heat stroke: combine it with *Feng Wei Cao* (Herba Pteris), *He Ye* (Folium Nelumbinis), *Shi Gao* (Gypsum Fibrosum) and *Zhi Mu* (Radix Anemarrhenae).

2. Cools Blood and Stops Bleeding

Bleeding due to heat in the *xue* (blood) level: *Ji Xue Cao* treats vomiting or uterine bleeding caused by heat in the blood.

3. Clears the Liver and Brightens the Eyes

Eye disorders: *Ji Xue Cao* treats eye disorders by clearing Liver heat. Clinical manifestations may include night blindness in children, inflammation, cataract, and glaucoma.

Ji Xue Cao (Herba Centellae)

DOSAGE

9 to 15 grams of dried *Ji Xue Cao*, 15 to 30 grams of the fresh herb, in decoction. It can also be crushed into herbal paste and applied topically.

CAUTIONS / CONTRAINDICATIONS

- Use *Ji Xue Cao* with caution during pregnancy due to its emmenagogic and abortifacient effects.[1]

CHEMICAL COMPOSITION

Asiatic acid, 3-glucosylquercetin, 3-glucosylkaempferol, asiaticoside, thankuniside, isothankuniside, madecassaside, brahmoside, brahminaside, brahmic acid, madasiatic acid, mesoinositol, centeilose.[2]

References

1. *Journal of Pharm. Sci.* 64:535-98, 1975
2. *Pharmazie* 1983;38(6):423) (*CA* 1969;71:1031d)

Long Dan Cao (Radix Gentianae)

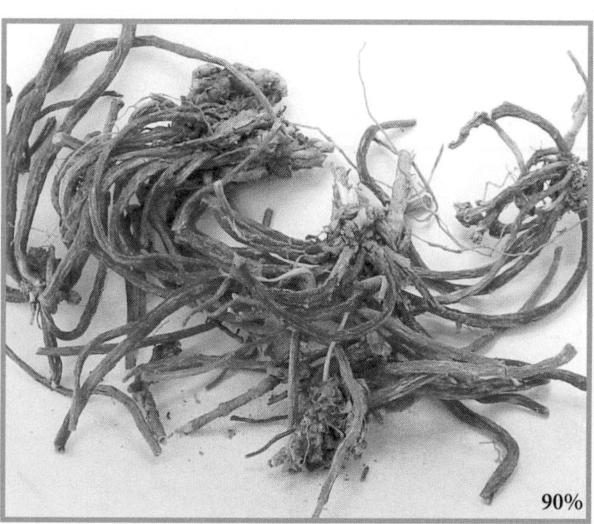

龍膽草 龙胆草

Pinyin Name: *Long Dan Cao*
Literal Name: "dragon gallbladder herb"
Alternate Chinese Names: *Long Dan, Dan Cao*
Original Source: *Shen Nong Ben Cao Jing* (Divine Husbandman's Classic of the Materia Medica) in the second century
English Name: gentiana
Botanical Name: *Gentiana scabra* Bunge. (*Long Dan Cao*); *Gentiana triflora* Pall. (*San Hua Long Dan*); *Gentiana manshurica* Kitag. (*Dong Bei Long Dan*); or *Gentiana rigescens* Franch. (*Jian Long Dan*)
Pharmaceutical Name: Radix Gentianae
Properties: bitter, cold
Channels Entered: Liver, Gallbladder, Stomach

CHINESE THERAPEUTIC ACTIONS

1. Clears Heat and Dries Dampness

Damp-heat in the Liver and Gallbladder: Damp-heat may affect not only the Liver and Gallbladder, but also the corresponding channels. Manifestations from affected Liver and Gallbladder organs include jaundice, eczema, thirst, no appetite, abdominal fullness, genital itching and swelling, foul-smelling yellow leukorrhea, and yellow, scanty urine. Damp-heat affecting the Liver and Gallbladder channels results in hypochondriac pain, headache, deafness, and red eyes. A bitter taste in the mouth is common to either level of involvement. *Long Dan Cao* (Radix Gentianae) effectively dispels damp-heat in the lower *jiao* and in the Liver channel (which travels through the genital region). It is excellent for treatment of sexually-transmitted diseases, infectious hepatitis, and jaundice with the above-mentioned symptoms.

- Damp-heat of the Liver and Gallbladder channels: use *Long Dan Cao* with *Chai Hu* (Radix Bupleuri), *Huang Qin* (Radix Scutellariae) and *Chuan Mu Tong* (Caulis Clematidis Armandii). **Exemplar Formula:** *Long Dan Xie Gan Tang* (Gentiana Decoction to Drain the Liver).
- Jaundice: combine this herb with *Yin Chen Hao* (Herba Artemisiae Scopariae), *Da Huang* (Radix et Rhizoma Rhei) and *Zhi Zi* (Fructus Gardeniae).

2. Sedates Liver Heat

Rising Liver fire: Clinical manifestations include high fever, burning hypochondriac pain, a bitter taste in the mouth, dry throat, redness of the eyes and face, deafness or severe tinnitus, ear pain or discharge, headache, irritability, short temper, insomnia or nightmares, and constipation

Long Dan Cao (Radix Gentianae)

with yellow urine. In severe cases, rising Liver yang may turn to Liver wind, manifesting in convulsions, seizures, and hematemesis or epistaxis.

- Seizures and convulsions: use *Long Dan Cao* with *Niu Huang* (Calculus Bovis), *Gou Teng* (Ramulus Uncariae cum Uncis) and *Huang Lian* (Rhizoma Coptidis).
- Redness, swelling and pain in the eyes: add *Ju Hua* (Flos Chrysanthemi) and *Jue Ming Zi* (Semen Cassiae).

DOSAGE

3 to 8 grams in decoction. The maximum dosage of *Long Dan Cao* is 15 grams. *Long Dan Cao* is commonly used internally (as decoction, pills or powder) or externally (as powder).

CAUTIONS / CONTRAINDICATIONS

- Use of *Long Dan Cao* is contraindicated in patients who have deficiency and cold of the Spleen and Stomach, qi deficiency, or blood deficiency.
- *Long Dan Cao* may be taken before meals. A small dose of *Long Dan Cao* taken before meals may stimulate the secretion of gastric acid and enhance digestion and absorption. In patients with a sensitive gastrointestinal system, however, *Long Dan Cao* may be taken with meals.
- *Long Dan Cao*, in large dosages, is sometimes associated with side effects such as headache, facial flushing, and dizziness.[1]
- Use of this herb may be associated with possible drowsiness and sedation. Therefore, individuals who take this herb should exercise caution if driving or operating heavy machinery.

CHEMICAL COMPOSITION

Gentiopicrin, gentiopicroside, sweroside, swertiamarin, amarogentin, amaroswerin, gentianine, gentianose, sucrose.[2,3]

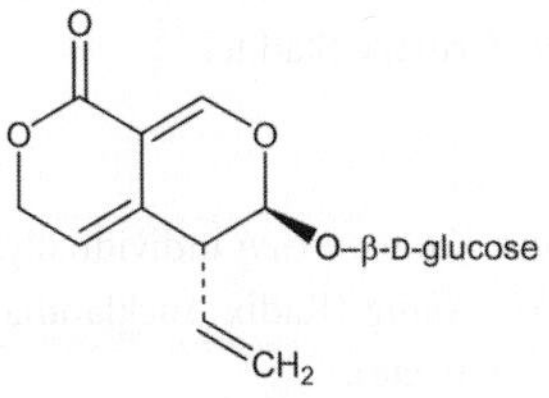

O–β-D-glucose
CH_2

Gentiopicroside

PHARMACOLOGICAL EFFECTS

- **Cholagogic:** Administration of *Long Dan Cao* via oral ingestion or intravenous injection has been shown to increase the production and excretion of bile in dogs.[4]
- **Hepatoprotective:** Gentiopicroside has shown hepatoprotective effects in mice, especially against carbon tetrachloride-induced liver damage.[5]
- **Diuretic:** Intravenous injection of *Long Dan Cao* at 10 g/kg increased the average urine output from 0.76 ml per 30 minutes to 2.64 ml per 30 minutes in rabbits.[6]
- **Effects on the CNS:** At small dosages, a preparation of *Long Dan Cao* has excitatory effects on the central nervous system (CNS); at large dosages, it has sedative and tranquilizing effects on the central nervous system. Furthermore, it was reported that a preparation of *Long Dan Cao* decreased spontaneous activity in mice and potentiated the sedative effect of barbiturates.[7]
- **Antibiotic:** *Long Dan Cao* has demonstrated inhibitory effects against *Pseudomonas aeruginosa, Bacillus proteus, Salmonella typhi, Diplococcus meningitidis, Staphylococcus aureus,* and some dermatophytes.[8]
- **Gastrointestinal:** Administration of gentiopicroside via gastric tube is associated with an increase in gastric acid secretion in dogs. It has no effect when given sublingually or via intravenous injection.[9]

CLINICAL STUDIES AND RESEARCH

- **Hepatitis:** In one report, 26 patients with chronic infectious hepatitis and persistent high liver enzymes levels were treated with an herbal formula with *Long Dan Cao* as the main herb, with good results.[10]
- **Encephalitis B:** According to one report, 23 patients with fever because of encephalitis B were treated with *Long Dan Cao* and standard western medicine. Patients who were conscious received 10 to 15 ml of 20% *Long Dan Cao* syrup three times daily. Patients who were unconscious or unable to take herbs orally received intramuscular injections three to four times daily. Out of 23 patients, 7 showed improvement, 15 returned to normal temperatures within 3 days, and 1 did not respond to the treatment.[11]

HERB-DRUG INTERACTION

- **Diuretics:** *Long Dan Cao* has a diuretic effect. Though this potential interaction has not been documented, concurrent use with diuretic drugs may lead to increased elimination of water and/or electrolytes.[12] [Note: Examples of diuretics include chlorothiazide, hydrochlorothiazide, furosemide (Lasix), bumetanide (Bumex), and torsemide (Demadex).]
- **Sedatives:** *Long Dan Cao* has a sedative effect and potentiates the effect of barbiturates.[13] [Note: Many categories of drugs induce sedation, such as antihistamines, narcotic analgesics, barbiturates, benzodiazepines and many others.]

TOXICOLOGY

The LD_{50} for genianine in mice is 460 mg/kg via oral ingestion, 500 mg/kg via subcutaneous injection, and 250 to 300 mg/kg via intravenous injection.[14]

Long Dan Cao (Radix Gentianae)

AUTHORS' COMMENTS

According to Dr. Jiao Shu-De, the dosage of *Long Dan Cao* has a significant implication on the potential effects and side effects. At a low dosage (less than 1 gram), it stimulates the stomach to increase the production of gastric acid and improves digestion. At a large dosage, it irritates the stomach and causes such side effects as nausea, vomiting, and lack of appetite.

References

1. *Zhong Yao Xue* (Chinese Herbology), 1998; 146:148
2. *Xian Dai Zhong Yao Yao Li Xue* (Contemporary Pharmacology of Chinese Herbs), 1997; 312
3. *The Merck Index* 12th edition, Chapman & Hall/CRCnetBASE/Merck, 2000
4. *Yun Nan Yi Yao* (Yunan Medicine and Herbology), 1991; 12(5):304
5. Ibid.
6. *Zhong Yao Yao Li Yu Ying Yong* (Pharmacology and Applications of Chinese Herbs), 1983; 295
7. Ibid.
8. Ibid.
9. *Zhong Yao Da Ci Dien* (Dictionary of Chinese Herbs), 1977: 624
10. *Shang Hai Zhong Yi Yao Za Zhi* (Shanghai Journal of Chinese Medicine and Herbology), 1965; 4:4
11. *Xin Yi Xue* (New Medicine), 1972; 8:11
12. Chen, J. Recognition & prevention of herb-drug interactions, *Medical Acupuncture*, Fall/Winter 1998/1999; volume 10/number 2; 9-13
13. *Zhong Yao Yao Li Yu Ying Yong* (Pharmacology and Applications of Chinese Herbs), 1983; 295
14. Ibid

Ku Shen Gen (Radix Sophorae Flavescentis)

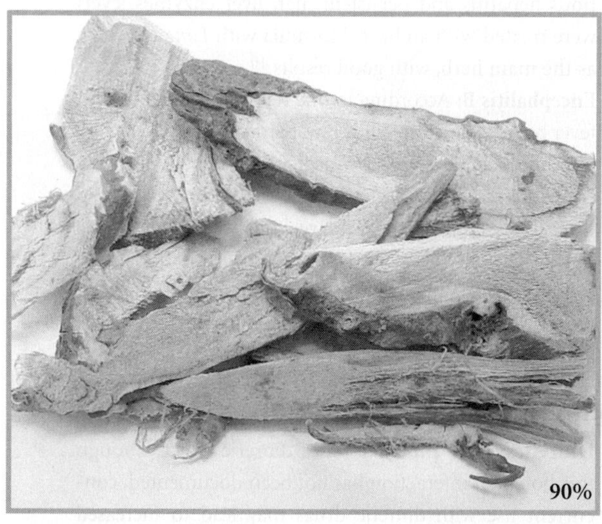

苦参根 苦參根

Pinyin Name: *Ku Shen Gen*
Literal Name: "bitter herb root," "bitter ginseng"
Alternate Chinese Names: *Ku Shen*
Original Source: *Shen Nong Ben Cao Jing* (Divine Husbandman's Classic of the Materia Medica) in the second century
English Name: sophora flavescens, light yellow sophora root
Botanical Name: *Sophora flavescens* Ait.
Pharmaceutical Name: Radix Sophorae Flavescentis
Properties: bitter, cold
Channels Entered: Heart, Liver, Stomach, Large Intestine, Urinary Bladder

CHINESE THERAPEUTIC ACTIONS

1. Clears Heat and Dries Dampness

Damp-heat in the lower *jiao*: *Ku Shen Gen* (Radix Sophorae Flavescentis) treats accumulation of damp-heat in the lower *jiao,* characterized by foul-smelling diarrhea, dysentery, foul-smelling yellow leukorrhea, genital itching, bleeding hemorrhoids, jaundice and various types of bleeding caused by heat driving blood out of the vessels.

- Jaundice: use *Ku Shen Gen* with *Zhi Zi* (Fructus Gardeniae), *Huang Bai* (Cortex Phellodendri) and *Long Dan Cao* (Radix Gentianae).
- Diarrhea: use *Ku Shen Gen* individually, or in combination with *Mu Xiang* (Radix Aucklandiae) and *Gan Cao* (Radix Glycyrrhizae).
- Yellow leukorrhea: combine it with *Huang Bai* (Cortex Phellodendri) and *She Chuang Zi* (Fructus Cnidii).
- Genital itching or vaginitis due to trichomonas infection: use this herb with *Huang Bai* (Cortex Phellodendri) and *She Chuang Zi* (Fructus Cnidii) as an herbal wash, and soak the affected area everyday for 10 minutes each time, at least 5 to 10 times total.
- Rectal bleeding caused by heat in the intestines, or hematemesis due to Stomach heat: use it with *Huai Hua*

Ku Shen Gen (Radix Sophorae Flavescentis)

(Flos Sophorae), and *Di Yu* (Radix Sanguisorbae).
- Hemorrhoid pain: add *Ku Lian Pi* (Cortex Meliae).

2. Dispels Wind, Kills Parasites, and Relieves Itching

Dermatological disorders: *Ku Shen Gen* is commonly used either internally or externally to treat dermatological disorders characterized by damp-heat. Clinical applications include itching, seepage, abscesses, urticaria, scabies, leprosy, genital itching, and similar skin problems.

- Skin itching with lesions and abscesses: use *Ku Shen Gen* with *Huang Bai* (Cortex Phellodendri), *She Chuang Zi* (Fructus Cnidii), and *Ming Fan* (Alumen), topically as herbal solution.
- Skin itching without lesions or abscesses: use it with *Chan Tui* (Periostracum Cicadae) and *Jing Jie* (Herba Schizonepetae).
- Genital itching: combine it with *She Chuang Zi* (Fructus Cnidii) as an herbal wash.
- Urticaria: use it with *Bai Xian Pi* (Cortex Dictamni), *Chi Shao* (Radix Paeoniae Rubrae), *Hong Hua* (Flos Carthami), *Sang Zhi* (Ramulus Mori), *Fang Feng* (Radix Saposhnikoviae), *Lian Qiao* (Fructus Forsythiae), *Chuan Shan Jia* (Squama Manis), *Zao Jiao Ci* (Spina Gleditsiae), *Chan Tui* (Periostracum Cicadae) and *She Tui* (Periostracum Serpentis).
- Genital sores: use *Ku Shen Gen* alone as an external wash.
- Leprosy: combine *Ku Shen Gen* with *Da Feng Zi* (Semen Hydnocarpi) and *Cang Er Zi* (Fructus Xanthii).

3. Promotes Urination

Damp-heat in the Urinary Bladder: *Ku Shen Gen* has heat-clearing and water-eliminating functions. It clears stagnation of damp-heat in the lower *jiao* to treat dysuria, with burning and pain sensations accompanying urination.

- Dysuria: use *Ku Shen Gen* individually, or use it with *Shi Wei* (Folium Pyrrosiae), *Che Qian Zi* (Semen Plantaginis) and *Pu Gong Ying* (Herba Taraxaci).
- Dysuria during pregnancy: use this herb with *Dang Gui* (Radicis Angelicae Sinensis) and *Bei Mu* (Bulbus Fritillaria).

DOSAGE

3 to 10 grams in decoction. The maximum dosage of *Ku Shen Gen* is 30 grams. Use a smaller dosage for decoction and large dosage (15 to 30 grams) for topical applications as an external wash. *Ku Shen Gen* is extremely bitter and is commonly associated with nausea and vomiting because of its taste. Therefore, capsules or tablets are preferred, to improve patient compliance.

CAUTIONS / CONTRAINDICATIONS

- *Ku Shen Gen* is contraindicated in patients who have deficiency and cold of the Spleen and Stomach.
- *Ku Shen Gen* is incompatible with *Li Lu* (Radix et Rhizoma Veratri) and should not be used concurrently.
- *Ku Shen Gen* antagonizes *Tu Si Zi* (Semen Cuscutae), *Lou Lu* (Radix Rhapontici) and *Bei Mu* (Bulbus Fritillaria), according to some traditional texts. The validity of this antagonism, however, has since been challenged.

OVERDOSAGE

Overdose of *Ku Shen Gen* is associated with adverse reactions such as irritability, muscle spasms and cramps, excitation, dyspnea, and in severe cases of gross overdose, respiratory failure.

TREATMENT OF OVERDOSAGE

Early-stage overdose (less than 4 hours) can be treated with emetic methods to eliminate the offending agent, or ingestion of activated charcoal to decrease absorption. Herbal decoction of 30 grams each of *Lu Dou* (Semen Phaseoli Radiati) and *Gan Cao* (Radix Glycyrrhizae) can also be administered for general detoxification purposes.[1]

CHEMICAL COMPOSITION

Alkaloids (matrine, oxymatrine, sophocarpine, sophoramine, sophoridine, sophoranol, anagyrine, N-methylcystisine, baptifoline), flavonoids (kushenols, kurarinol, formononetin), triterpenoids (soyasaponin).[2,3]

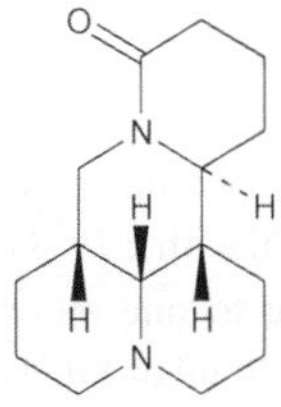

Matrine

PHARMACOLOGICAL EFFECTS

- **Antiarrhythmic:** *Ku Shen Gen* has demonstrated promise in the treatment of arrhythmia, especially if the condition is induced by excessive amounts of adrenaline or by aconite poisoning.[4]
- **Cardiovascular:** The alkaloids of *Ku Shen Gen* have been shown to dilate the blood vessels and increase blood perfusion to the cardiac muscles. In anesthetized rabbits, administration of *Ku Shen Gen* preparations lowered blood pressure, dilated peripheral blood vessels, and protected the heart from ischemia. In addition, it lowers blood cholesterol levels.[5,6]
- **Immunostimulant:** Intravenous or intramuscular injections of d-oxymatrine is associated with an increase in white blood cell count in mice.[7]
- **Respiratory:** *Ku Shen Gen* stimulates the beta receptors of

Ku Shen Gen (Radix Sophorae Flavescentis)

the sympathetic nervous system to relax the bronchioli and relieve asthma. Administration of alkaloids of *Ku Shen Gen* is over 90% effective in relieving asthma within one hour. *Ku Shen Gen* also has marked expectorant effect.[8,9]

- **Antibiotic:** *Ku Shen Gen* has demonstrated marked inhibitory action against *Bacillus dysenteriae, E. coli, Bacillus proteus,* β-hemolytic streptococcus, and *Staphylococcus aureus.*[10]
- **Antiparasitic:** *Ku Shen Gen* is effective against trichomonas infection, with effects comparable to *She Chuang Zi* (Fructus Cnidii).[11]
- **Antineoplastic:** Matrine, sophocarpine, and a decoction of *Ku Shen Gen* have demonstrated preliminary antineoplastic effects in laboratory mice.[12,13,14,15]

CLINICAL STUDIES AND RESEARCH

- **Bacterial dysentery:** In one study, 258 patients with bacterial dysentery were treated successfully with *Ku Shen Gen*, via tablets, decoction or injection.[16]
- **Chronic bronchitis or bronchial asthma:** A study of 517 patients with chronic bronchitis, wheezing and dyspnea were treated with *Ku Shen Gen* preparations with an 86.5% effective rate.[17]
- **Arrhythmia:** In one study, 100 patients with pre-ventricular contraction were treated with *Ku Shen Gen* injectable with good success. In another study, 167 patients with tachy-arrhythmia were treated with *Ku Shen Gen* with a 62% rate of effectiveness.[18]
- **Dermatological application:** Dermatological disorders in 148 patients, such as rashes, itching and eczema, were treated with *Ku Shen Gen* through intramuscular injection or oral decoction, with a 79% effective rate.[19]
- **Insomnia:** According to one report, 101 patients with insomnia were given 20 ml of *Ku Shen Gen* syrup (equivalent to 10 grams of herb) with good sedative/hypnotic effects. No significant side effects were reported.[20]

TOXICOLOGY

The LD_{50} for herbal extract of *Ku Shen Gen* in mice is 14.5 g/kg via oral ingestion and 14.4 g/kg via intramuscular injection.[21]

References

1. *Lin Chuan Shou Ce You Du Zhong Yao Shi Yong* (Clinical Handbook on Applications of Toxic Chinese Herbs), 1992; 45-46
2. *Xian Dai Zhong Yao Yao Li Xue* (Contemporary Pharmacology of Chinese Herbs), 1997; 312
3. *The Merck Index* 12th edition, Chapman & Hall/CRCnetBASE/Merck, 2000
4. *Shan Xi Xin Yi Yao* (New Medicine and Herbology of Shanxi), 1981; 10(4):58
5. *Zhong Guo Yao Li Xue Tong Bao* (Journal of Chinese Herbal Pharmacology), 1987; 8(6):501
6. *Zhong Yao Xue* (Chinese Herbology), 1998; 148:151
7. *Fang She Yi Xue* (Journal of Radiology), 1977; (1):8
8. *Zhong Yao Yao Li Yu Ying Yong* (Pharmacology and Applications of Chinese Herbs), 1983:101,639,642
9. *Zhong Guo Yao Li Tong Xun* (Journal of Chinese Herbal Studies), 1984; 1(3,4):304
10. *Zhong Yao Xue* (Chinese Herbology), 1998; 148:151
11. Ibid.
12. *Yao Xue Za Zhi* (Journal of Medicinals), 1961; 81:1635
13. *Bei Jing Yi Ke Da Xue Xue Bao* (Journal of Beijing University of Medicine), 1986; 18(2):127
14. *Zhong Hua Xue Yi Xue Za Zhi* (Chinese Journal on Study of Hematology), 1991; 12(2):89
15. *Zhong Guo Zhong Yao Za Zhi* (People's Republic of China Journal of Chinese Herbology), 1990; 15(10):49
16. *Zhong Cao Yao Tong Xun* (Journal of Chinese Herbal Medicine), 1972; 1:44
17. *Zhong Cheng Yao Yan Jiu* (Research of Chinese Patent Medicine), 1978; 4:46
18. *Xin Yi Yao Tong Xun* (Journal of New Medicine and Herbology), 1977; 7:24
19. *Zhong Cao Yao Tong Xun* (Journal of Chinese Herbal Medicine), 1976; 1:35
20. Ibid., 1979; 2:38
21. *Zhong Yao Yao Li Yu Ying Yong* (Pharmacology and Applications of Chinese Herbs), 1983; 101:639,642

Section 3

— Heat-Clearing and Blood-Cooling Herbs

Xi Jiao (Cornu Rhinoceri)

犀角 犀角

Pinyin Name: *Xi Jiao*
Alternate Chinese Names: *Xi Niu Jiao, Wu Xi Jiao*
Original Source: *Shen Nong Ben Cao Jing* (Divine Husbandman's Classic of the Materia Medica) in the second century
English Name: rhinoceros horn
Zoological Name: *Rhinoceros unicornis* L. (*Yin Du Xi*); *Rhinoceros sondaicus* Desmarest. (*Zhao Wa Xi*); *Rhinoceros sumatrensis* (Fischer) (*Su Men Da La Xi*); *Rhinoceros bicornis* L. (*Hei Xi*); *Rhinoceros simus* Burchell (*Bai Xi*)
Pharmaceutical Name: Cornu Rhinoceri
Properties: bitter, salty, cold
Channels Entered: Heart, Liver, Stomach
International Status: CITES I

CHINESE THERAPEUTIC ACTIONS

1. Cools the Blood and Stops Bleeding

Heat in the *xue* (blood) level: Excess heat can drive blood out of the vessels, causing bleeding, such as: epistaxis, hematemesis, hemoptysis, hematuria or hematochezia. *Xi Jiao* (Cornu Rhinoceri) enters the *xue* (blood) level and has historically been used to effectively treat the root cause of bleeding, by cooling the blood.

- Bleeding: use an appropriate substitute for *Xi Jiao* with *Sheng Di Huang* (Radix Rehmanniae), *Chi Shao* (Radix Paeoniae Rubrae) and *Mu Dan Pi* (Cortex Moutan).
- Severe bleeding: *Xi Jiao* would historically be combined with *Chi Shao* (Radix Paeoniae Rubrae), *Shi Gao* (Gypsum Fibrosum), *Bai Mao Gen* (Rhizoma Imperatae), *Da Ji* (Herba seu Radix Cirsii Japonici) and *Xiao Ji* (Herba Cirisii).

2. Eliminates Toxins and Clears Blotches on the Skin

Heat in the *ying* (nutritive) level: In addition to cooling blood, *Xi Jiao* sedates fire and eliminates toxins. It was commonly used to treat febrile disorders characterized by feverish sensations all over the body, dark-purplish macula and blotches on the skin, purpura and various kinds of bleeding. Heat and toxins attacking the throat is characterized by soreness, swelling and pain. Other signs may include fever that worsens at night, thirst with no desire to drink, irritability, insomnia, a scarlet red tongue and in severe cases, delirium.

- Febrile disorders: this substance would have been used with *Xuan Shen* (Radix Scrophulariae), *Shi Gao* (Gypsum Fibrosum) and *Da Qing Ye* (Folium Isatidis).
- Sore, swollen and painful throat: combine a similar substance with *Sheng Ma* (Rhizoma Cimicifugae), *Xuan Shen* (Radix Scrophulariae) and *Da Huang* (Radix et Rhizoma Rhei).

3. Calms the *Shen* (Spirit) and Extinguishes Liver Wind

Febrile disorders: In febrile disorders, heat travels inward as the disease progresses. As heat enters the *ying* (nutritive) and *xue* (blood) levels, it also affects the Heart and Liver. Clinical manifestations in this situation include unremitting high fever, irritability, insomnia, dark-purplish macula and blotches on the skin, hematemesis, epistaxis, muscle spasms and cramps, convulsions, delirium and mania. The Heart houses the *shen* (spirit): when it is invaded by heat, symptoms of insomnia,

Xi Jiao (Cornu Rhinoceri)

irritability and delirium may occur. The Liver controls the tendons: when Liver yang turns into Liver wind, convulsions occur.

- Delirium and mania in febrile disorders: *Xi Jiao* would be used with *Xuan Shen* (Radix Scrophulariae), *Dan Shen* (Radix Salviae Miltiorrhizae) and *Lian Qiao* (Fructus Forsythiae). **Exemplar Formula:** *Qing Ying Tang* (Clear the Nutrition Level Decoction).
- Convulsions in febrile disorders: combine a *Xi Jiao* substitute with *Ling Yang Jiao* (Cornu Saigae Tataricae), *Niu Huang* (Calculus Bovis) and *Bing Pian* (Borneolum Syntheticum).

HISTORICAL DOSAGE

0.5 to 1.5 grams in powder or pills, 2 to 6 grams in decoction. When used as powder, it was often taken with an herbal decoction.

CAUTIONS / CONTRAINDICATIONS

- *Xi Jiao* was used with caution during pregnancy as its cold nature could injure the fetus.
- *Xi Jiao* is counteracted by *Chuan Wu* (Radix Aconiti Preparata) and *Cao Wu* (Radix Aconiti Kusnezoffii).

CHEMICAL COMPOSITION

Keratin, cholesterol, calcium, guanidine derivatives.[1]

PHARMACOLOGICAL EFFECTS

- **Antiseizure and antiepileptic:** *Xi Jiao* is effective in preventing and treating seizures and epilepsy. In laboratory studies, it decreased fatalities from strychnine-induced seizures. It also prolonged sleeping time in mice induced by barbiturates. However, it does not counter the effects of pentylenetetrazol or caffeine.[2]
- **Cardiovascular:** A 10% water extract of *Xi Jiao* has demonstrated marked cardiotonic effect in frogs by direct stimulation of the cardiac muscle. It has positive inotropic and chronotropic effects, and it increases cardiac output. Overdose, however, may lead to paralysis of the cardiac muscle. In another study with anesthetized dogs and rabbits, intravenous injection of a decoction of *Xi Jiao* is associated with an initial rise of blood pressure, followed by a decline and then a gradual increase.[3]
- **Antipyretic:** *Xi Jiao* has a mixed effect in temperature regulation. It effectively reduces body temperature to normal in rabbits with fever artificially induced by *E. coli.* It is ineffective if the fever is artificially induced by injection of adrenaline.[4]
- **Immunologic:** Administration of *Xi Jiao* is associated with an initial decrease, followed by a substantial increase, of white blood cell counts.[5]
- **Smooth muscle stimulant:** It has a stimulating effect on the smooth muscles of the uterus and intestines.[6]

CLINICAL STUDIES AND RESEARCH

- **Hemorrhagic fever**: In one study, 450 patients with hemorrhagic fever were treated with satisfactory results using a modification of *Xi Jiao Di Huang Tang* (Rhinoceros Horn and Rehmannia Decoction). The exact formula contained *Xi Jiao* 9g, *Xian Di Huang* (Radix Rehmanniae Recens) 60 to 120g, *Chi Shao* (Radix Paeoniae Rubrae) 12g, *Mu Dan Pi* (Cortex Moutan) 12g, and *Da Huang* (Radix et Rhizoma Rhei) 15g. The formula was given as a decoction once daily. *Xi Jiao* was given as powder, to be mixed with the decoction immediately before ingestion.[7]

HERB-DRUG INTERACTION

- **Sedatives:** *Xi Jiao* has a sedative effect and potentiates the effect of barbiturates. However, it does not counter the effects of pentylenetetrazol or caffeine.[8]

SUPPLEMENT

- 水牛角 / 水牛角 *Shui Niu Jiao* (Cornu Bubali), the horn of water buffalo, was first cited in *Ming Yi Za Zhu* (Miscellaneous Records of Famous Physicians) by Tao Hong-Jing in 500 A.D. Today, *Shui Niu Jiao* is commonly used as a substitute for *Xi Jiao* since rhinoceros is an endangered species and commerce in *Xi Jiao* is illegal. *Shui Niu Jiao*, however, is much lower in potency and requires up to 8 to 10 times the normal dosage of *Xi Jiao* to achieve similar therapeutic effects. It is effective in treating patients with encephalitis B, high fever in infants and children, and thrombocytopenic purpura. This substance is usually used in decoctions. The appropriate dosage for *Shui Niu Jiao* is 20 to 40 grams.
- 黄牛角 / 黄牛角 *Huang Niu Jiao* (Cornu Bovis) is the horn from yellow cows, sometimes used as a substitute for *Xi Jiao.* In a clinical study of 414 cases, it effectively treated upper respiratory infection, pharyngitis, acute tonsillitis, acute hepatitis with jaundice and high fever.[9]
- 青牛角粉 / 青牛角粉 *Qing Niu Jiao Fen* (Cornu Bovis) is the powdered horn from black cows, also used as a substitute for *Xi Jiao*. In a clinical study, it effectively treated schizophrenia in up to 95.5% of the subjects. The treatment protocol started with 2 to 3 grams of powder with white sugar three times daily, and the dose was gradually increased each day. At the end of the 30-day treatment course, the dosage in some cases was up to 50 grams per day.[10]

AUTHORS' COMMENTS

Xi Jiao (Cornu Rhinoceri) is listed in Appendix I of the Convention on International Trade in Endangered

Xi Jiao (Cornu Rhinoceri)

Species of Wild Fauna and Flora (CITES). Trade in *Xi Jiao* is strictly prohibited. The discussion of *Xi Jiao* in this text is included only to offer 1) the accurate history of its critically important usage in traditional herbal medicine, and 2) models for appropriate usage of effective substitute substances (see Supplement). The information should not be interpreted as condoning illegal use of this endangered species. For more information, please refer to Appendix 10.

References

1. *Zhong Yao Xue* (Chinese Herbology), 1998; 154
2. Ibid., 154:156
3. *Chang Yong Zhong Yao Xian Dai Yan Jiu Yu Lin Chuan* (Recent Study & Clinical Application of Common Traditional Chinese Medicine), 1995; 100:102
4. Ibid.
5. *Zhong Yao Xue* (Chinese Herbology), 1998; 154:156
6. Ibid.
7. *Zhong Yi Za Zhi* (Journal of Chinese Medicine), 1985; 8:33
8. *Zhong Yao Xue* (Chinese Herbology), 1998; 154:156
9. *Shan Dong Zhong Yi Za Zhi* (Shandong Journal of Chinese Medicine), 1981; 39
10. *Tie Dao Yi Xue* (Tiedao Medicine), 1987; 5:264

Sheng Di Huang (Radix Rehmanniae)

生地黄

Pinyin Name: *Sheng Di Huang*
Literal Name: "fresh earth's yellowness"
Alternate Chinese Names: *Sheng Di, Huai Sheng Di, Huai Di Huang, Gan Di Huang*
Original Source: *Shen Nong Ben Cao Jing* (Divine Husbandman's Classic of the Materia Medica) in the second century
English Name: rehmannia, dried rehmannia rhizome, dried adhesive rehmannia rhizome
Botanical Name: *Rehmannia glutinosa* Libosch. F. *hueichingensis* (*Chao et Schih*) Hsiao. (*Huai Ching Di Huang*); *Rehmannia glutinosa* Libosch. (*Di Huang*)
Pharmaceutical Name: Radix Rehmanniae
Properties: sweet, bitter, cold
Channels Entered: Heart, Liver, Kidney

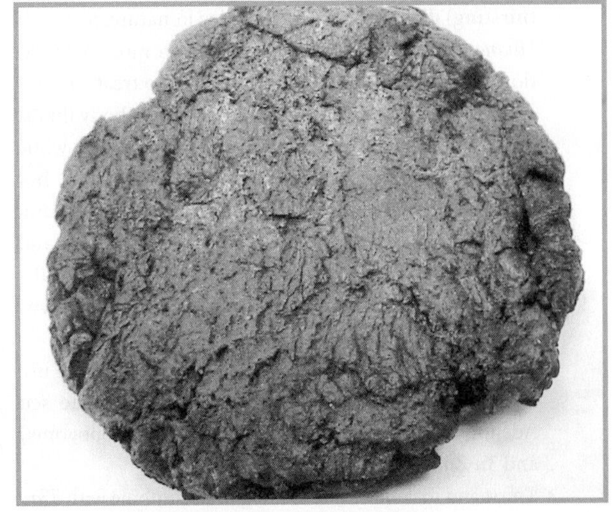

CHINESE THERAPEUTIC ACTIONS

1. Clears Heat and Cools the Blood

Sheng Di Huang (Radix Rehmanniae) treats heat invading the *ying* (nutritive) and *xue* (blood) levels, characterized by high fever, dry mouth and tongue, no thirst, restlessness and feverish sensations at night, delirium, and mania. The tongue is scarlet red.

- Heat in the *ying* (nutritive) and *xue* (blood) levels: use *Sheng Di Huang* with *Xuan Shen* (Radix Scrophulariae), and *Mai Men Dong* (Radix Ophiopogonis). **Exemplar Formula:** *Qing Ying Tang* (Clear the Nutrition Level Decoction).

Bleeding: Heat in the *xue* (blood) level forces blood out of the vessels, causing hematemesis, epistaxis, hematuria, gastrointestinal bleeding, purpura and excessive menstrual bleeding.

- Hematemesis and epistaxis: use *Sheng Di Huang* with *He Ye* (Folium Nelumbinis), *Ce Bai Ye* (Cacumen Platycladi) and *Ai Ye* (Folium Artemisiae Argyi). **Exemplar Formula:** *Si Sheng Wan* (Four-Fresh Pill).
- Gastrointestinal bleeding: use it with *Huang Qin* (Radix Scutellariae), *Huai Hua* (Flos Sophorae), *Di Yu* (Radix Sanguisorbae) and *Wu Mei* (Fructus Mume).

Sheng Di Huang (Radix Rehmanniae)

- Excessive menstrual bleeding: combine it with *Huang Qin* (Radix Scutellariae), *Dang Gui* (Radicis Angelicae Sinensis), *Ai Ye* (Folium Artemisiae Argyi) and *Ce Bai Ye* (Cacumen Platycladi).
- Purpura or bleeding with macula and blotches on the skin: add *Mu Dan Pi* (Cortex Moutan) and *Chi Shao* (Radix Paeoniae Rubrae).

Dermatological disorders: Heat in the *xue* (blood) level may also manifest as dermatological disorders, such as urticaria, rashes, and itching.

- Urticaria, rash and itching: use *Sheng Di Huang* with *Dang Gui* (Radicis Angelicae Sinensis), *Chan Tui* (Periostracum Cicadae), and *Fang Feng* (Radix Saposhnikoviae). **Exemplar Formula:** *Xiao Feng San* (Eliminate Wind Powder).

2. Nourishes Yin and Promotes Generation of Body Fluids

Febrile disorders injuring the yin, *xiao ke* (wasting and thirsting) disorders: Sweet and juicy in nature, *Sheng Di Huang* clears heat, nourishes yin and promotes generation of body fluids. It is commonly used to treat complications of excess heat in which heat is drying body fluids. Heat is often characterized by fever and irritability, while yin or fluid deficiency is characterized by thirst, hot flashes, a dry, cracked tongue with cracks, dry mouth, steaming bones sensations, dry cough, throat pain and soreness, and night sweating. This herb is especially effective in treating *xiao ke* (wasting and thirsting) syndrome with irritability and thirst.

- Thirst due to heat with Stomach yin deficiency: use *Sheng Di Huang* with *Sha Shen* (Radix Glehniae seu Adenophorae), *Mai Men Dong* (Radix Ophiopogonis) and *Yu Zhu* (Rhizoma Polygonati Odorati).
- Thirst and irritability due to Lung heat: combine with *Tian Hua Fen* (Radix Trichosanthis), *Huang Lian* (Rhizoma Coptidis), and *Ou Jie* (Nodus Nelumbinis Rhizomatis).
- *Xiao ke* (wasting and thirsting) syndrome: use it with *Huang Qi* (Radix Astragali), *Ge Gen* (Radix Puerariae) and *Tian Hua Fen* (Radix Trichosanthis).

Late-stages febrile disorders: These conditions are often characterized by the presence of heat with severe damage to yin and body fluids. Clinical manifestations include tidal fevers with feverish sensations at night but coldness in the morning. *Sheng Di Huang* is an excellent herb for treatment of chronic disorders with deficiency heat symptoms such as tidal fever, flushed cheeks, irritability, thirst, poor appetite, and *wu xin re* (five-center heat).

- Tidal fever with heat and yin deficiency: use *Sheng Di Huang* with *Zhi Mu* (Radix Anemarrhenae), *Qing Hao* (Herba Artemisiae Annuae) and *Bie Jia* (Carapax Trionycis) to clear yin-deficient heat. **Exemplar Formula:** *Qing Hao Bie Jia Tang* (Artemisia Annua and Soft-shelled Turtle Shell Decoction).

Constipation: *Sheng Di Huang* treats constipation caused by heat entering the Large Intestine and drying fluids.

- Constipation from heat drying fluids in the Large Intestine: combine this herb with *Xuan Shen* (Radix Scrophulariae) and *Mai Men Dong* (Radix Ophiopogonis).

***Lin zheng* (dysuria syndrome):** *Sheng Di Huang* is also used to address *lin zheng* arising from heat attacking the Small Intestine and Urinary Bladder.

- *Lin zheng* (dysuria syndrome) from heat attacking Small Intestine and Urinary Bladder: use it with *Zhu Ye* (Herba Phyllostachys), *Chuan Mu Tong* (Caulis Clematidis Armandii) and *Gan Cao* (Radix Glycyrrhizae).

DOSAGE

10 to 30 grams in decoction. The maximum dosage of *Sheng Di Huang* is 100 grams. Because it is rich and may cause stagnation, *Sheng Di Huang* is often processed with *Sheng Jiang* (Rhizoma Zingiberis Recens) juice or prescribed with a small portion of *Sha Ren* (Fructus Amomi) to avoid the buildup of dampness. Stir-frying *Sheng Di Huang* with grain-based liquor reduces the cold, greasy and stagnating nature of the herb. Charring *Sheng Di Huang* increases the hemostatic function. Once charred, however, the herb becomes less potent in heat-clearing and blood-cooling functions.

CAUTIONS / CONTRAINDICATIONS

Sweet and stagnating in nature, *Sheng Di Huang* may create dampness in the middle *jiao* and is contraindicated in patients with Spleen and Stomach qi or yang deficiencies or those with abdominal fullness or diarrhea.

CHEMICAL COMPOSITION

Catalpol, 6-o-acetylcatalpol, aucubin, melittoside, rehmanniosides A,B,C,D; rehmaglutins A,B,C,D; glutinoside, rehmannans A,B,C; stachyose, D-mannitol.[1]

PHARMACOLOGICAL EFFECTS

- **Anti-inflammatory:** In laboratory studies, water and alcohol extracts of *Sheng Di Huang* at 10 g/kg/day for 5 days showed marked effectiveness in reducing inflammation and swelling in mice.[2]
- **Endocrine:** Administration of *Sheng Di Huang* has a definite effect on the endocrine system. It has been shown that the ingestion of *Sheng Di Huang* increases the plasma levels of adrenocortical hormone, even in the presence of

Sheng Di Huang (Radix Rehmanniae)

dexamethasone. It has been proposed that *Sheng Di Huang* works by inhibiting the negative feedback from the dexamethasone to the pituitary gland. Other herbs that have shown similar influence include *Zhi Mu* (Radix Anemarrhenae) and *Gan Cao* (Radix Glycyrrhizae).[3]

- **Others:** *Sheng Di Huang* has demonstrated cardiotonic, antihypertensive, hemostatic, hepatoprotective, diuretic and antibiotic effects.[4]

CLINICAL STUDIES AND RESEARCH

- **Arthritis:** In one study, 23 patients with rheumatoid arthritis were treated with 90 grams of *Sheng Di Huang* per day given as herbal decoction, with good results.[5]
- **Urticaria:** Rashes and urticaria in 37 patients were treated with *Sheng Di Huang*, 90 grams per day given as herbal decoction, with good results.[6]
- **Vertebral hyperostosis:** In another study, 183 patients with hypertrophy of the spinal cord were treated with injections of *Sheng Di Huang* or *Wei Ling Xian* (Radix Clematidis). The study reported good results, with *Sheng Di Huang* showing more effectiveness than *Wei Ling Xian*.[7]

TOXICOLOGY

No fatalities were reported in mice following oral ingestion of water or alcohol extracts of *Sheng Di Huang* at 60 g/kg/day for 3 days. No fatalities were reported in rats following oral ingestion of water or alcohol extracts of *Sheng Di Huang* at 18 g/kg/day for 15 days. There was no evidence of damage to the internal organs.[8]

SUPPLEMENT

- 鮮地黄 / 鲜地黄 *Xian Di Huang* (Radix Rehmanniae Recens), first cited in *Shen Nong Ben Cao Jing* (Divine Husbandman's Classic of the Materia Medica) in the second century, is hydrated rehmannia freshly harvested from the ground. It can be preserved in moist sand for 2 to 4 months. The function of *Xian Di Huang* and *Sheng Di Huang* is similar except *Xian Di Huang* is colder and stronger in cooling the blood and generating body fluids to relieve thirst. Its tonic function is weaker. It is best used in cases involving high fever and bleeding. The normal dosage of *Xian Di Huang* is usually 20 to 60 grams. It can also be taken as juice.

AUTHORS' COMMENTS

Please refer to *Shu Di Huang* (Radix Rehmanniae Preparata) for comparisons of *Shu Di Huang* (Radix Rehmanniae Preparata), *Sheng Di Huang*, and *Xian Di Huang* (Radix Rehmanniae Recens).

References

1. *Chang Yong Zhong Yao Cheng Fen Yu Yao Li Shou Ce* (A Handbook of the Composition and Pharmacology of Common Chinese Drugs), 1994; 792-793
2. *Zhong Yao Yao Li Yu Ying Yong* (Pharmacology and Applications of Chinese Herbs), 1983: 400
3. *Zhong Yao Xue* (Chinese Herbology), 1998; 156:158
4. Ibid.
5. *Tian Jing Yi Xue Za Zhi* (Journal of Tianjing Medicine and Herbology), 1966; 3:209
6. Ibid.
7. *Xin Yi Yao Xue Za Zhi* (New Journal of Medicine and Herbology), 1975; 9:14
8. *Zhong Yao Yao Li Yu Ying Yong* (Pharmacology and Applications of Chinese Herbs), 1983; 400

Xuan Shen (Radix Scrophulariae)

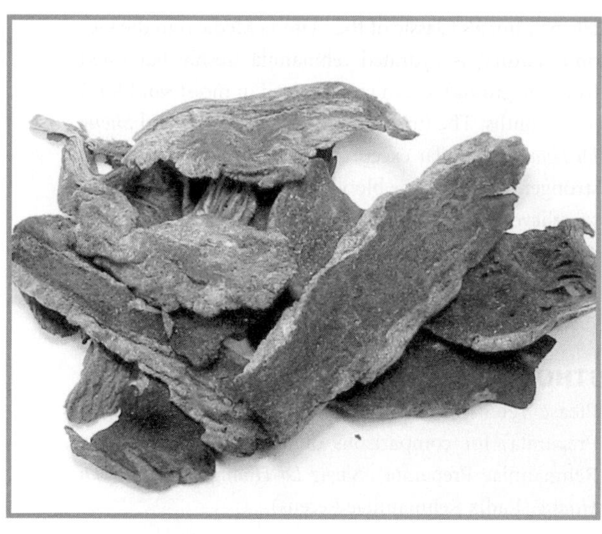

玄參 玄参

Pinyin Name: *Xuan Shen*
Literal Name: "dark root," "dark ginseng"
Alternate Chinese Names: *Yuan Shen, Hei Shen*
Original Source: *Shen Nong Ben Cao Jing* (Divine Husbandman's Classic of the Materia Medica) in the second century
English Name: scrophularia, figwort root
Botanical Name: *Scrophularia ningpoensis* Hemsl.
Pharmaceutical Name: Radix Scrophulariae
Properties: bitter, sweet, salty, cold
Channels Entered: Lung, Stomach, Kidney

CHINESE THERAPEUTIC ACTIONS

1. Clears Heat and Nourishes Yin

Heat in the *ying* (nutritive) level: Sweet, cold and moist in nature, *Xuan Shen* (Radix Scrophulariae) clears heat and nourishes yin. It is commonly used for situations where there is excess heat accompanied by consequent damage to yin or drying of body fluids. If heat enters the Lung and dries the fluids, symptoms will present as dry, non-productive cough, chest tightness, thirst, and dry mouth and throat. In febrile disorders where heat enters the *ying* (nutritive) level, attacks the Pericardium, and damages yin, symptoms will manifest as dry mouth, red tongue, delirium, and semiconsciousness.

- Lung heat with dryness: use *Xuan Shen* with *Bai He* (Bulbus Lilii), *Zhe Bei Mu* (Bulbus Fritillariae Thunbergii), and *Gan Cao* (Radix Glycyrrhizae). **Exemplar Formula:** *Bai He Gu Jin Tang* (Lily Bulb Decoction to Preserve the Metal).
- Heat entering the *ying* (nutritive) level and damaging yin: combine it with *Sheng Di Huang* (Radix Rehmanniae), and *Lian Qiao* (Fructus Forsythiae).

Heat in the *xue* (blood) level: This condition is characterized by purpura, dark-purplish blotches on the skin, caused by heat driving blood out of the vessels.

- Purpura or blotches: use *Xuan Shen* with *Sheng Ma* (Rhizoma Cimicifugae) and *Shui Niu Jiao* (Cornu Bubali).

2. Eliminates Toxins and Disperses Nodules

Toxic nodules and palpable masses: Toxic heat is characterized by swelling, pain, abscesses and ulceration. Clinically, *Xuan Shen* is often used to treat sore throat, scrofula, goiter, nodules due to phlegm stagnation, and skin lesions with abscesses or ulcerations. It is best for dry, swollen, painful throat caused by the rising of yin-deficient heat and toxicity, not sore throat from exterior wind-heat.

- Sore throat with dryness and pain: use this herb with *Jie Geng* (Radix Platycodonis) and *Gan Cao* (Radix Glycyrrhizae).
- Diphtheria: combine it with *Sheng Di Huang* (Radix Rehmanniae), *Mai Men Dong* (Radix Ophiopogonis), and *Mu Dan Pi* (Cortex Moutan). **Exemplar Formula:** *Yang Yin Qing Fei Tang* (Nourish the Yin and Clear the Lungs Decoction).
- Goiter, scrofula: add *Zhe Bei Mu* (Bulbus Fritillariae Thunbergii) and *Mu Li* (Concha Ostreae). **Exemplar Formula:** *Xiao Luo Wan* (Reduce Scrofula Pill).
- Suppurative inflammation: combine it with *Jin Yin Hua* (Flos Lonicerae), *Dang Gui* (Radicis Angelicae Sinensis) and *Gan Cao* (Radix Glycyrrhizae).
- Skin lesions with abscesses or ulcerations: use *Xuan Shen* with *Jin Yin Hua* (Flos Lonicerae), *Lian Qiao* (Fructus Forsythiae), and *Zi Hua Di Ding* (Herba Violae).

DOSAGE

10 to 15 grams in decoction. The maximum dosage of *Xuan Shen* is 50 grams. This herb is used internally or topically.

CAUTIONS / CONTRAINDICATIONS

- Cold in nature, *Xuan Shen* is contraindicated in patients who have dampness, deficiency and cold of the Spleen and Stomach.
- *Xuan Shen* is incompatible with *Li Lu* (Radix et Rhizoma Veratri).

CHEMICAL COMPOSITION

Scrophularin, iridioid, harpagoside, oleic acid, linoleic acid, and stearic acid.[1]

Xuan Shen (Radix Scrophulariae)

PHARMACOLOGICAL EFFECTS

- **Antihypertensive:** In dogs, cats, rabbits and other animals, water and alcohol extracts of *Xuan Shen* demonstrated antihypertensive action via vasodilation. Oral ingestion of a *Xuan Shen* decoction at 2 g/kg twice daily was effective in reducing blood pressure in dogs with renal hypertension. Intravenous injection of a *Xuan Shen* preparation dilated blood vessels, decreased heart rate, and increased urine output in mice. Alcohol extract of *Xuan Shen* increased blood flow to the coronary arteries and decreased oxygen requirement by the cardiac muscles.[2]
- **Antidiabetic:** Subcutaneous injection of *Xuan Shen* reduces blood glucose in rabbits.[3]
- **Antibiotic:** A 50% decoction of *Xuan Shen* has an inhibitory effect *in vitro* against *Staphylococcus aureus, Pseudomonas aeruginosa*, and some pathogenic fungi.[4]
- **Others:** *Xuan Shen* has sedative and antipyretic effects.[5]

CLINICAL STUDIES AND RESEARCH

- **Peeling of the skin**: According to one report, 50 patients with constant peeling of the skin were treated with an herbal tea once daily with good results. The herbal tea contained 30 grams each of *Xuan Shen* and *Sheng Di Huang* (Radix Rehmanniae).[6]

HERB-DRUG INTERACTION

- **Antidiabetics:** It is prudent to use *Xuan Shen* with caution with insulin, sulfonylureas, and other antidiabetic medications. Though the interaction has not been documented, the combination of antidiabetic herbs and drugs may have a synergistic effect, leading to hypoglycemia.[7] [Note: Examples of antidiabetic drugs include insulin, tolbutamide (Orinase), glipizide (Glucotrol), and glyburide (DiaBeta/Micronase).]

AUTHORS' COMMENTS

When combined appropriately with other herbs, *Xuan Shen* effectively treats sore throat from various causes. Because *Xuan Shen* eliminates toxins, it can be combined with *Bo He* (Herba Menthae) and *Niu Bang Zi* (Fructus Arctii) to treat initial stages of wind-heat where there are slight signs of toxicity. It can be used with *Mai Men Dong* (Radix Ophiopogonis) and *Lian Qiao* (Fructus Forsythiae) for sore and swollen throat from toxicity and heat. When combined with *Sheng Di Huang* (Radix Rehmanniae) and *Mai Men Dong* (Radix Ophiopogonis), *Xuan Shen* can treat sore and dry throat caused by rising of deficiency fire.

According to Dr. Zhang Xiao-Ping, the combination of *Xuan Shen* and *Cang Zhu* (Rhizoma Atractylodis) has an excellent effect to lower plasma glucose levels to treat diabetes mellitus patients. These two herbs are especially effective in individuals who have diabetes characterized by qi and yin deficiencies.

References

1. *Xian Dai Zhong Yao Yao Li Xue* (Contemporary Pharmacology of Chinese Herbs), 1997; 340
2. *Zhong Yao Yao Li Yu Ying Yong* (Pharmacology and Applications of Chinese Herbs), 1983: 370
3. *Zhong Yao Yao Li Du Li Yu Lin Chuan* (Pharmacology, Toxicology and Clinical Applications of Chinese Herbs), 1992; 50
4. *Zhong Yao Yao Li Yu Ying Yong* (Pharmacology and Applications of Chinese Herbs), 1983: 370
5. Ibid.
6. *Zhong Yuan Yi Kan* (Resource Journal of Chinese Medicine), 1984, 3:24
7. Chen, J. Recognition & prevention of herb-drug interactions, *Medical Acupuncture*, Fall/Winter 1998/1999; volume 10/number 2; 9-13

Mu Dan Pi (Cortex Moutan)

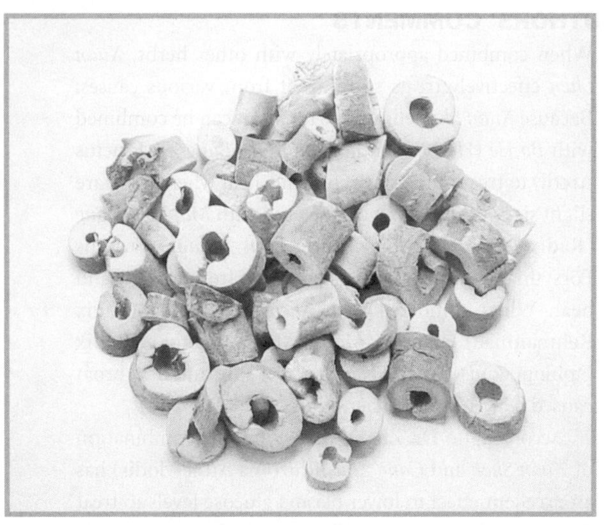

牡丹皮

Pinyin Name: *Mu Dan Pi*
Alternate Chinese Names: *Dan Pi, Fen Dan Pi, Mu Dan Gen Pi*
Original Source: *Shen Nong Ben Cao Jing* (Divine Husbandman's Classic of the Materia Medica) in the second century
English Name: moutan, tree peony bark
Botanical Name: *Paeonia suffruticosa* Andr.
Pharmaceutical Name: Cortex Moutan
Properties: bitter, acrid, cool
Channels Entered: Heart, Liver, Kidney

CHINESE THERAPEUTIC ACTIONS

1. Clears Heat and Cools Blood

Yin-deficient heat: *Mu Dan Pi* (Cortex Moutan) treats this imbalance to relieve steaming bones sensations, nighttime fevers, the absence of perspiration, and thirst. Typical patients with these symptoms are women experiencing menopause.

- Steaming bones sensations: use *Mu Dan Pi* with *Di Gu Pi* (Cortex Lycii), *Qing Hao* (Herba Artemisiae Annuae) and *Bie Jia* (Carapax Trionycis). **Exemplar Formula:** *Qing Hao Bie Jia Tang* (Artemisia Annua and Soft-shelled Turtle Shell Decoction).
- Menopause with yin deficiency and heat: use this herb with *Zhi Mu* (Radix Anemarrhenae) and *Sheng Di Huang* (Radix Rehmanniae).
- Spermatorrhea due to Kidney yin deficiency and heat: add *Ze Xie* (Rhizoma Alismatis), *Fu Ling* (Poria) and *Shan Zhu Yu* (Fructus Corni). **Exemplar Formula:** *Liu Wei Di Huang Wan* (Six-Ingredient Pill with Rehmannia).

Heat in the *xue* (blood) level: Maculae, bleeding-related blotches on the skin, purpura, hematemesis, hemoptysis, hematuria, and epistaxis are all commonly caused by heat driving the blood out of the vessels.

- Hematemesis and epistaxis because of heat in the *xue* (blood) level: use *Mu Dan Pi* with *Chi Shao* (Radix Paeoniae Rubrae) and *Sheng Di Huang* (Radix Rehmanniae).

Menstrual disorders: Clinical manifestations of heat affecting the *chong* (thoroughfare) and *ren* (conception) channels include hypermenorrhea, early menstruation, and epistaxis during menstruation. There are also forms of abnormal bleeding in which heat drives blood out of the vessels and thus creates shortened menstrual cycles, early menstruation or hypermenorrhea. Night fevers and morning or daytime chills are also common complaints. Often, premenstrual or postmenstrual feverish sensations may be present.

- Feverish sensations: use *Mu Dan Pi* with *Bai Shao* (Radix Paeoniae Alba), *Huang Qin* (Radix Scutellariae) and *Chai Hu* (Radix Bupleuri).

Liver yang rising or Liver fire: *Mu Dan Pi* treats hypertension, irritability, redness of the face and eyes, and short temper.

- Liver yang or Liver fire: use this herb with *Zhi Zi* (Fructus Gardeniae), *Chai Hu* (Radix Bupleuri) and *Bai Shao* (Radix Paeoniae Alba). **Exemplar Formula:** *Jia Wei Xiao Yao San* (Augmented Rambling Powder).

2. Invigorates Blood Circulation and Disperses Blood Stasis

Amenorrhea or abdominal masses: Because of blood stagnation, patients may experience amenorrhea and abdominal masses such as fibroids, tumors or other similar masses. *Mu Dan Pi*, cool in thermal property, can invigorate blood circulation and disperse blood stasis without drying the body, which is not characteristic of most blood-invigorating herbs.

- Amenorrhea or dysmenorrhea with severe pain, stagnation and heat: use *Mu Dan Pi* with *Tao Ren* (Semen Persicae), *Chi Shao* (Radix Paeoniae Rubrae) and *Fu Ling* (Poria) to activate blood circulation, remove blood stagnation and relieve pain. **Exemplar Formula:** *Gui Zhi Fu Ling Wan* (Cinnamon Twig and Poria Pill).

Bruises resulting from traumatic injuries: *Mu Dan Pi* can be used for the bruises, broken bones, inflammation, swelling and pain associated with traumatic injuries.

Mu Dan Pi (Cortex Moutan)

- Musculoskeletal injuries with inflammation, swelling, bruises and pain: use it with *Ru Xiang* (Gummi Olibanum), *Mo Yao* (Myrrha) and *Su Mu* (Lignum Sappan).

Abscess: *Mu Dan Pi* is a key herb in treating abscess, especially intestinal abscess or appendicitis.

- Suppurative inflammation: combine this herb with *Jin Yin Hua* (Flos Lonicerae), *Lian Qiao* (Fructus Forsythiae) and *Bai Zhi* (Radix Angelicae Dahuricae).
- Intestinal abscess with abdominal pain and mucus in the stool: use it with *Da Huang* (Radix et Rhizoma Rhei), *Tao Ren* (Semen Persicae) and *Dong Gua Zi* (Semen Benincasae). **Exemplar Formula:** *Da Huang Mu Dan Tang* (Rhubarb and Moutan Decoction).
- Acute appendicitis that has not suppurated, with fever, vomiting, and lower-right-quadrant pain: add *Da Huang* (Radix et Rhizoma Rhei), *Mang Xiao* (Natrii Sulfas), *Tao Ren* (Semen Persicae), *Dong Gua Zi* (Semen Benincasae) and *Chi Shao* (Radix Paeoniae Rubrae).

DOSAGE

6 to 12 grams in decoction. The maximum dosage of *Mu Dan Pi* is 30 grams. The unprocessed herb is stronger to clear heat and cool blood; the liquor-fried herb (with grain-based liquor) more strongly activates blood circulation and disperses blood stagnation; and the charred herb more effectively stops bleeding.

CAUTIONS / CONTRAINDICATIONS

- Cold in nature, *Mu Dan Pi* should be used with caution in patients who are experiencing deficiency and cold.
- Since *Mu Dan Pi* has blood-activating and stasis-removing functions, it is contraindicated in patients who are pregnant or have excessive bleeding during menstruation.

CHEMICAL COMPOSITION

Paeonol, paeonoside, paeonolide, paeoniflorin, benzoylpaeoniflorin, oxypaeoniflorin, benzoyloxypaeoniflorin, apiopaeonoside.[1,2]

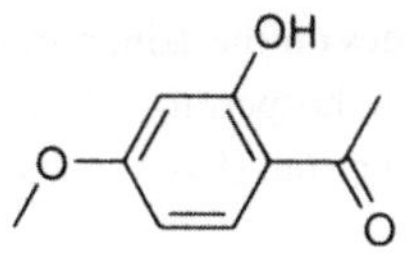

OH O

Paeonol

PHARMACOLOGICAL EFFECTS

- **Anti-inflammatory:** *Mu Dan Pi* has demonstrated strong anti-inflammatory actions, according to laboratory studies. The mechanism of the anti-inflammatory effect is attributed to inhibition of prostaglandin synthesis and decreased permeability of the blood vessels.[3,4]
- **Cardiovascular:** In anesthetized dogs, administration of *Mu Dan Pi* is associated with increased blood perfusion to the coronary arteries, decreased cardiac output and decreased load on the left ventricle. The herb has also been shown to have a protective effect against ischemia of the heart.[5,6]
- **Antihypertensive:** Decoction of *Mu Dan Pi* has prolonged antihypertensive effect in anesthetized dogs and rats. In dogs with essential and renal hypertension, oral ingestion of decoction of *Mu Dan Pi* at 5 to 10 g/kg/day for 7 days was effective in reducing blood pressure.[7]
- **Antibiotic:** *Mu Dan Pi* has demonstrated inhibitory influence against *Staphylococcus aureus,* β-hemolytic streptococcus, *Bacillus subtilis, E. coli, Shigella dysenteriae, Pseudomonas aeruginosa, Bacillus proteus, Diplococcus pneumoniae,* and *Vibrio cholerae.*[8]
- **Others:** *Mu Dan Pi* has analgesic, sedative, antiseizure, antipyretic and immune-enhancing effects.[9]

CLINICAL STUDIES AND RESEARCH

- **Allergic rhinitis:** In one study, 31 patients were treated with 50 ml of 10% *Mu Dan Pi* solution every night for 10 days with marked results. In another study, a preparation of *Mu Dan Pi* was used as topical solution three times daily in treating 140 patients with allergic rhinitis with an 87.1% effective rate.[10,11]
- **Purpura:** Anemic purpura in 32 patients was treated with an herbal formula with *Mu Dan Pi* with good results.[12]
- **Hypertension:** According to one report, 30 to 45 grams of *Mu Dan Pi* were cooked and the decoction was given in three equally-divided doses to 20 patients with hypertension, with marked effectiveness to lower blood pressure after approximately 5 days.[13]

TOXICOLOGY

No abnormalities were observed in liver, kidney, heart and blood exams following treatment of hypertension using *Mu Dan Pi* in dogs. The LD_{50} in mice for paeonol is 3,430 mg/kg for oral ingestion, 781 mg/kg for intraperitoneal injection, and 196 mg/kg for intravenous injection.[14]

SUPPLEMENT

- 牡丹葉 / 牡丹叶 *Mu Dan Ye* (Folium Moutan), the leaf of the same plant as *Mu Dan Pi,* can also be used to clear damp-heat from the intestines for indications such as bacterial dysentery. It was reported in one study that 29 patients with bacterial dysentery were treated with *Mu Dan Ye* with an effective rate of 96%. *Mu Dan Ye* was found to have inhibitory activities against *Shigella dysenteriae, Staphylococcus aureus,* and *Pseudomonas aeruginosa.*[15]

Mu Dan Pi (Cortex Moutan)

AUTHORS' COMMENTS

According to Dr. Xu Fu-He, *Mu Dan Pi* and *Zhi Zi* (Fructus Gardeniae) treat itching or heat sensations of the nipples when used internally and topically.

References

1. *Xian Dai Zhong Yao Yao Li Xue* (Contemporary Pharmacology of Chinese Herbs), 1997; 342
2. Yan X, Zhou J, Xie G, *Traditional Chinese Medicines Molecular Structures, Natural Sources and Applications*; Ashgate, 1999; 4941
3. *Sheng Yao Xue Za Zhi* (Journal of Raw Herbology), 1979; 33(3):178
4. *Zhong Guo Yao Ke Da Xue Xue Bao* (Journal of University of Chinese Herbology), 1990; 21(4):222
5. *Guo Wai Yi Xue Zhong Yi Zhong Yao Fen Ce* (Monograph of Chinese Herbology from Foreign Medicine), 1983; (3):5,1984;(5):54
6. *Shan Xi Yi Yao Za Zhi* (Shanxi Journal of Medicine and Herbology), 1984, 13(4):359
7. *Yao Xue Xue Bao* (Journal of Herbology), 8(6):250
8. *Zhong Yao Cai* (Study of Chinese Herbal Material), 1991; 14(2):41
9. *Zhong Yao Xue* (Chinese Herbology), 1998; 160:162
10. *Zhong Hua Er Bi Hou Ke Za Zhi* (Chinese Journal of ENT), 1957, 2:99
11. *Hu Nan Yi Yao Za Zhi* (Hunan Journal of Medicine and Herbology), 1983; (4):24
12. *Zhong Xi Yi Jie He Za Zhi* (Journal of Integrated Chinese and Western Medicine), 1985; 4:245
13. *Liao Ning Yi Xue Za Zhi* (Liaoning Journal of Medicine), 1960; (7):48
14. *He Han Yi Yao Xue Hui Zhi* (Hehan Journal of Medicine and Herbology), 1988; 5:214
15. *Zhong Cao Yao Tong Xun* (Journal of Chinese Herbal Medicine), 1976, 4:8

Chi Shao (Radix Paeoniae Rubrae)

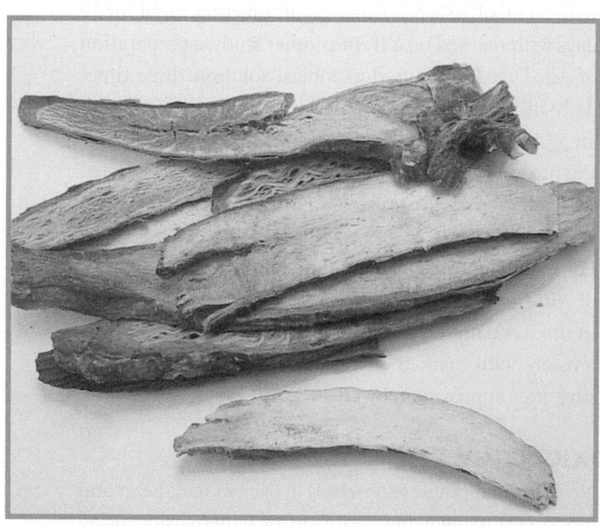

赤芍 赤芍

Pinyin Name: *Chi Shao*
Literal Name: "bright red peony"
Alternate Chinese Names: *Chi Shao Yao*
Original Source: *Shen Nong Ben Cao Jing* (Divine Husbandman's Classic of the Materia Medica) in the second century
English Name: red peony, red peony root
Botanical Name: *Paeonia veitchii* Lynch. (*Chuan Chi Shao*); *Paeonia abovata* Maxim. (*Cao Shao Yao*); *Paeonia lactiflora* Pall. (*Shao Yao*)
Pharmaceutical Name: Radix Paeoniae Rubrae
Properties: bitter, cool
Channels Entered: Liver

CHINESE THERAPEUTIC ACTIONS

1. Clears Heat, Cools Blood

Chi Shao (Radix Paeoniae Rubrae) treats various bleeding disorders caused by febrile disorders or heat attacking the *xue* (blood) level. Clinical manifestations include fever, macules or blotches on the skin, purpura, hematemesis, epistaxis and hematuria.

- Hematemesis or epistaxis: use *Chi Shao* with *Mu Dan Pi* (Cortex Moutan) and *Sheng Di Huang* (Radix Rehmanniae).
- Hematuria: combine it with *Xiao Ji* (Herba Cirisii), *Bai Mao Gen* (Rhizoma Imperatae), and *Qian Cao* (Radix Rubiae).
- Macules or blotches on the skin, purpura: use it with *Zi Cao Gen* (Radix Lithospermi), *Chan Tui* (Periostracum Cicadae), and *Hong Hua* (Flos Carthami).

2. Dispels Blood Stasis, Relieves Pain

Amenorrhea and dysmenorrhea: Blood stagnation in the uterus leads to amenorrhea or dysmenorrhea with blood clots. The blood is often dark in color, and pain is alleviated after clots have been dispelled.

- Amenorrhea or dysmenorrhea: use *Chi Shao* with *Dang Gui* (Radicis Angelicae Sinensis) and *Chuan Xiong* (Rhizoma Ligustici Chuanxiong).

Chi Shao (Radix Paeoniae Rubrae)

Bruises from traumatic injuries: Internal injuries in the chest and abdomen are associated with blood stagnation. Blood stagnation may also present as palpable masses in the abdomen. *Chi Shao* has excellent action to disperse blood stagnation, relieve pain, and reduce swelling.

- Blood stagnation in the chest: use *Chi Shao* with *Tao Ren* (Semen Persicae), *Hong Hua* (Flos Carthami) and *Chuan Xiong* (Rhizoma Ligustici Chuanxiong). **Exemplar Formula:** *Xue Fu Zhu Yu Tang* (Drive Out Stasis in the Mansion of Blood Decoction).
- Blood stagnation in the hypochondrium: add *Yan Hu Suo* (Rhizoma Corydalis), *Hong Hua* (Flos Carthami), *Wu Ling Zhi* (Excrementum Trogopteri seu Pteromi) and *Xiang Fu* (Rhizoma Cyperi). **Exemplar Formula:** *Ge Xia Zhu Yu Tang* (Drive Out Blood Stasis Below the Diaphragm Decoction).
- Blood stagnation in the lower abdomen: combine this herb with *Dang Gui* (Radicis Angelicae Sinensis), *Chuan Xiong* (Rhizoma Ligustici Chuanxiong), and *Pu Huang* (Pollen Typhae). **Exemplar Formula:** *Shao Fu Zhu Yu Tang* (Drive Out Blood Stasis in the Lower Abdomen Decoction).
- Palpable masses in the abdomen: use it with *Ru Xiang* (Gummi Olibanum), *Mo Yao* (Myrrha), *San Leng* (Rhizoma Sparganii) and *E Zhu* (Rhizoma Curcumae).

Post-stroke hemiplegia: This condition is caused by severe qi and blood stagnation in the channels and collaterals.

- Hemiplegia with deficiency: use *Chi Shao* with *Huang Qi* (Radix Astragali) and *Di Long* (Pheretima).

3. Reduces Swelling from Sores and Abscesses

In sores, swellings and abscesses due to heat and toxicity, the lesions are red and painful to the touch.

- Sores and abscesses: add *Jin Yin Hua* (Flos Lonicerae), *Ru Xiang* (Gummi Olibanum) and *Zao Jiao Ci* (Spina Gleditsiae). **Exemplar Formula:** *Zhen Ren Huo Ming Yin* (True Man Decoction to Revitalize Life).

4. Clears Heat and Relieves Eye Pain

Rising Liver yang: Clinical manifestations include redness, swelling and pain in the eyes.

- Redness, swelling and pain in the eyes: use *Chi Shao* with *Ju Hua* (Flos Chrysanthemi), *Mu Zei* (Herba Equiseti Hiemalis) and *Xia Ku Cao* (Spica Prunellae).

Heat in the Urinary Bladder: *Chi Shao* treats burning dysuria and hematuria.

- Burning dysuria: use this herb with *Che Qian Zi* (Semen Plantaginis) and *Hua Shi* (Talcum).
- Hematuria: combine it with *Bai Mao Gen* (Rhizoma Imperatae), and *Ou Jie* (Nodus Nelumbinis Rhizomatis).

DOSAGE

6 to 15 grams in decoction.

CAUTIONS / CONTRAINDICATIONS

- *Chi Shao* is contraindicated in patients with deficiency and cold.
- *Chi Shao* is incompatible with *Li Lu* (Radix et Rhizoma Veratri).

CHEMICAL COMPOSITION

Paeoniflorin, benzoylpaeoniflorin, oxypaeoniflorin, lactiflorin, daucosterol, d-catechin.[1,2]

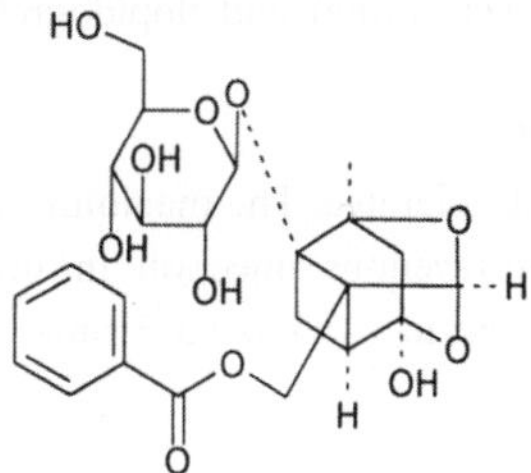

Paeoniflorin

PHARMACOLOGICAL EFFECTS

- **Antiplatelet:** Administration of *Chi Shao* has demonstrated effectiveness to inhibit platelet aggregation in rabbits.[3]
- **Hematological:** Administration of *Chi Shao* has been shown to inhibit thrombus formation in rats.[4]
- **Cardiovascular:** Administration of *Chi Shao* reduces blood pressure and dilates the coronary artery. It does not, however, influence the heart rate. Increased resistance to hypoxia is also observed in animals that receive *Chi Shao*.[5]
- **Antispasmodic:** *Chi Shao* has an inhibitory effect on the smooth muscles of the intestines and uterus as demonstrated in rats and guinea pigs.[6]
- **Effects on the central nervous system:** Paeoniflorin has mild sedative, antiseizure and antipyretic effects as demonstrated in animal models.[7]
- **Antibiotic:** *Chi Shao* has an inhibitory effect against *Salmonella typhi*, *Pseudomonas aeruginosa*, *E. coli*, *Staphylococcus aureus*, β-hemolytic streptococcus, *Diplococcus pneumoniae*, *Vibrio cholerae*, and some dermatophytes and viruses.[8]

CLINICAL STUDIES AND RESEARCH

- **Coronary artery disease:** In one study, 125 patients with coronary artery disease were treated with 40 grams of *Chi Shao* decoction three times daily, with satisfactory results.[9]
- **Cerebral thrombosis:** Intravenous infusion of *Chi Shao* injectables with D5W or D10W once daily was 92.01% effective for prevention of thrombus formation in 263 patients.[10]

Chi Shao (Radix Paeoniae Rubrae)

- **Cor pulmonale:** According to one report, 10 grams of *Chi Shao* given three times daily was effective in treating 30 patients with cor pulmonale.[11]

HERB-DRUG INTERACTION

- **Anticoagulant or antiplatelet drugs:** *Chi Shao* has antiplatelet action, and should be used with caution in patients who take anticoagulant or antiplatelet medications. Though this potential interaction has not been documented, this herb may potentiate the effect of drugs such as warfarin.[12] [Note: Examples of anticoagulants include heparin, warfarin (Coumadin) and enoxaparin (Lovenox); and examples of antiplatelets include aspirin, dipyridamole (Persantine), and clopidogrel (Plavix).]

TOXICOLOGY

Chi Shao is well-tolerated. The maximum safe dosage is 50 g/kg via intravenous injection in mice, which is roughly equivalent to 1,163 to 2,325 times the oral therapeutic dosage.[13]

AUTHORS' COMMENTS

Chi Shao (Radix Paeoniae Rubrae) and *Bai Shao* (Radix Paeoniae Alba) have similar names but different functions. Despite their differences, they are sometime used together in cases where there are concurrent excess and deficient conditions.

- *Chi Shao* invigorates blood and relieves stagnation. It sedates Liver fire and is dispersing in nature.
- *Bai Shao* nourishes blood and yin, softens the Liver, and is tonifying and consolidating in nature.

References

1. *Xian Dai Zhong Yao Yao Li Xue* (Contemporary Pharmacology of Chinese Herbs), 1997; 345
2. Yan X, Zhou J, Xie G, *Traditional Chinese Medicines Molecular Structures, Natural Sources and Applications*; Ashgate, 1999; 4939
3. *Zhong Xi Yi Jie He Za Zhi* (Journal of Integrated Chinese and Western Medicine), 1984; 4(12):745
4. Ibid., 1983; 2:109
5. *Zhong Cheng Yao Yan Jiu* (Research of Chinese Patent Medicine), 1980; 1:32
6. Ibid.
7. *Zhong Yao Xue* (Chinese Herbology), 1998; 162:164
8. Ibid.
9. *Zhong Ji Yi Kan* (Medium Medical Journal), 1984; 9:49
10. *Zhong Xi Yi Jie He Za Zhi* (Journal of Integrated Chinese and Western Medicine), 1986; 9:561
11. *He Nan Yi Ke Da Xue Xue Bao* (Journal of Henan University School of Medicine), 1987; 2:127
12. Chen, J. Recognition & prevention of herb-drug interactions, *Medical Acupuncture*, Fall/Winter 1998/1999; volume 10/number 2; 9-13
13. *Chang Yong Zhong Yao Cheng Fen Yu Yao Li Shou Ce* (A Handbook of the Composition and Pharmacology of Common Chinese Drugs), 1994; 1002-1015

Zi Cao Gen (Radix Lithospermi)

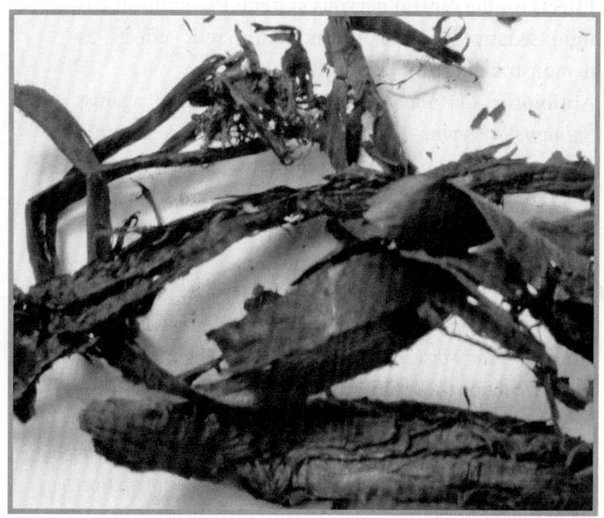

紫草根 紫草根

Pinyin Name: *Zi Cao Gen*
Literal Name: "purple herb root"
Alternate Chinese Names: *Zi Cao*
Original Source: *Shen Nong Ben Cao Jing* (Divine Husbandman's Classic of the Materia Medica) in the second century
English Name: lithospermum root
Botanical Name: *Lithospermum erythrorhizon* Sieb et Zucc. (*Zi Cao*); *Arnebiae euchroma* (*Xin Jiang Zi Cao*); *Arnebiae guttata* (*Nei Meng Zi Cao*)
Pharmaceutical Name: Radix Lithospermi
Properties: sweet, cold
Channels Entered: Heart, Liver

Zi Cao Gen (Radix Lithospermi)

CHINESE THERAPEUTIC ACTIONS

1. Cools Blood, Invigorates Blood Circulation, and Relieves Toxins

Incomplete eruption of measles: When there is lingering heat and toxicity in the *xue* (blood) level, measles cannot completely erupt, or the color of lesions may be dark red and purple. Cold in nature, *Zi Cao Gen* (Radix Lithospermi) cools the blood and eliminates heat and toxins from the blood. Clinically, it treats heat and toxins that are in the blood but are manifested in the skin, with such signs and symptoms as rashes, macula or blotches, and dark, purplish discoloration of the skin. Heat and toxicity may also affect the throat, leading to swelling and pain. Accompanying symptoms may include dry stools, fever and thirst.

- Macula or dark-purplish blotches with incomplete expression: use *Zi Cao Gen* with *Chan Tui* (Periostracum Cicadae), *Chi Shao* (Radix Paeoniae Rubrae) and *Lian Qiao* (Fructus Forsythiae).
- To prevent measles or to minimize the severity of symptoms: combine 3 to 6 grams of *Zi Cao Gen* with 1.3 to 3 grams of *Gan Cao* (Radix Glycyrrhizae) and serve as a decoction once a day for 3 to 7 days. It is recommended to begin this treatment within 5 days after contact with patients who have measles.
- Sore throat with swelling and pain: use it with *Lian Qiao* (Fructus Forsythiae) and *Shan Dou Gen* (Radix Sophorae Tonkinensis).

Bleeding: Heat in the blood may cause various types of bleeding, such as epistaxis and hematuria.

- Hematemesis or epistaxis: use *Zi Cao Gen* with *Sheng Di Huang* (Radix Rehmanniae), *Bai Guo* (Semen Ginkgo), *Fu Ling* (Poria) and *Mai Men Dong* (Radix Ophiopogonis).
- Hematuria: combine it with *Che Qian Zi* (Semen Plantaginis) and *Lian Qiao* (Fructus Forsythiae).
- General bleeding: add *Sheng Di Huang* (Radix Rehmanniae), *Xiao Ji* (Herba Cirisii), and *Bai Mao Gen* (Rhizoma Imperatae).

2. Eliminates Heat and Toxins from the Skin

Zi Cao Gen may be used topically or orally to eliminate heat and toxins from the skin. Clinical applications include carbuncles, furuncles, abscesses, lesions, eczema, cervical erosion, vaginal itching, and burns.

- Abscesses, lesions, ulceration: use this herb with *Dang Gui* (Radicis Angelicae Sinensis), *Xue Jie* (Sanguis Draconis), and *Bai Zhi* (Radix Angelicae Dahuricae), topically or internally.
- Burns with redness, swelling and pain: mix *Zi Cao Gen* with *Dang Gui* (Radicis Angelicae Sinensis), vinegar and sesame oil, and apply topically.
- Itching and irritation from insect bites: mix *Zi Cao Gen* with *Bai Zhi* (Radix Angelicae Dahuricae), *Dang Gui* (Radicis Angelicae Sinensis), *Gan Cao* (Radix Glycyrrhizae) and sesame oil, and apply topically.

3. Moistens the Intestines and Unblocks the Bowels

Constipation: *Zi Cao Gen* can be used for constipation or dry stools caused by heat in the blood.

- Constipation: use it with *Da Huang* (Radix et Rhizoma Rhei).

DOSAGE

3 to 10 grams in decoctions. The maximum dosage of *Zi Cao Gen* is 20 grams. *Zi Cao Gen* may be used internally as herbal decoction, or topically as cream or ointment. *Zi Cao Gen* cooked in boiling water has less antibiotic activity.

CAUTIONS / CONTRAINDICATIONS

Cold in nature, *Zi Cao Gen* is contraindicated in patients with diarrhea, or deficiency and cold of the Spleen and Stomach.

CHEMICAL COMPOSITION

Lithospermidin A, B; deoxyshikonin, dimethylacrylalkannin, acetylshikonin, dl-acetylalkannin, β-acetoxyisovalerylalkannin, dl-shikonin, β-hydroxyisovalerylalkannin, l-methoxy-acetylshikonin.[1]

PHARMACOLOGICAL EFFECTS

- **Antibiotic:** *Zi Cao Gen* has been shown to inhibit *Staphylococcus aureus, E. coli, Bacillus dysenteriae,* and some dermatophytes and influenza viruses. It also has an inhibitory effect against herpes virus. Lastly, it has shown effectiveness in HBsAg in patients with hepatitis B.[2]
- **Anti-inflammatory:** *Zi Cao Gen* has marked anti-inflammatory effects, and promotes healing in animals.[3]
- **Contraceptive:** *Zi Cao Gen* has demonstrated effectiveness as a contraceptive. Administration of extract of *Zi Cao Gen* inhibited the estrual cycle in rats. The effect was completely reversible upon discontinuation of treatment. In follow-up studies, it was determined that oral administration of *Zi Cao Gen* is associated with an inhibition of gonad-stimulating hormone and chorionic gonadotropin. The net result of such endocrine influence is decrease in weight of the ovaries and uterus.[4]
- **Cardiotonic:** In anesthetized rabbits and toads, administration of *Zi Cao Gen* from Xinjiang province (*Arnebiae Euchroma*) has a stimulating effect on the heart at low doses, and an inhibitory effect at high doses. Administration of *Zi Cao Gen* is associated with a sharp decline of blood pressure in anesthetized animals, but has no significant effect on awake subjects.[5]

Zi Cao Gen (Radix Lithospermi)

- **Gastrointestinal:** Oral administration of *Zi Cao Gen* decoction has a stimulating effect on the smooth muscle of the intestines, leading to contraction.[6]
- **Antineoplastic:** Preparations of *Zi Cao Gen* have shown antineoplastic effects by interfering with DNA synthesis of cancer cells at G2 phase. Preliminary tests showed that it is effective against chorioepithelioma, chorioadenoma and acute lymphocytic leukemia. It also decreases the incidence of breast cancer in mice.[7,8,9]

CLINICAL STUDIES AND RESEARCH

- **Measles:** *Zi Cao Gen* is used as preventative therapy against measles. However, results from most clinical studies showed mixed effectiveness.[10]
- **Birth Control:** One report describes that 1.8 grams of a *Zi Cao Gen* preparation were given to 102 women three times daily for 9 days, beginning after the last day of menstruation. Out of 102 patients, the rate of effectiveness was 82.4%.[11]
- **Hepatitis:** Good results were shown when 270 patients with non-icteric hepatitis or chronic hepatitis were injected intramuscularly with 2 ml of a 0.1% *Zi Cao Gen* preparation.[12]
- **Purpura:** In one study, 28 patients with purpura were treated with *Zi Cao Gen* with good results.[13]
- **Phlebitis:** There was close to a 100% rate of effectiveness when 25 patients with phlebitis were treated three times daily with a *Zi Cao Gen* preparation (each dose contains approximately 1.5 grams of the dried herb).[14]
- **Burns:** According to one report, 285 patients with burns were treated with *Zi Cao Gen* oil, with improvement in all patients. In another study 1,153 patients were treated with *Zi Cao Gen* oil. All but one patient showed significant improvement.[15,16]
- **Cervical erosion:** Topical application of *Zi Cao Gen* oil once every other day for 10 days per course of treatment was 96% effective in treating 100 cases of cervical erosion.[17]
- **Psoriasis:** Intramuscular injection of *Zi Cao Gen* demonstrated marked effectiveness in treating psoriasis in 50 patients.[18]

TOXICOLOGY

Oral administration of a *Zi Cao Gen* syrup at 5 to 15 mg/kg for 2 months resulted in no abnormalities of the internal organs. However, overdose of *Zi Cao Gen* in laboratory animals has been associated with such adverse reactions as pyuria, hematuria, proteinuria, and diarrhea. Such reactions are reversed 2 days following discontinuation of the herbs.[19]

References

1. *Xian Dai Zhong Yao Yao Li Xue* (Contemporary Pharmacology of Chinese Herbs), 1997; 349
2. *Zhong Cao Yao* (Chinese Herbal Medicine), 1986; 17(6):28
3. *Zhong Yao Xue* (Chinese Herbology), 1998; 164:167
4. *Chang Yong Zhong Yao Cheng Fen Yu Yao Li Shou Ce* (A Handbook of the Composition and Pharmacology of Common Chinese Drugs), 1994; 1673:1678
5. Ibid.
6. Ibid.
7. *Zhong Xi Yi Jie He Za Zhi* (Journal of Integrated Chinese and Western Medicine), 1990; 10(7):422
8. *Zhong Guo Mian Yi Xue Za Zhi* (Chinese Journal of Immunology), 1990; 6(3):154
9. *Zhong Liu Yu Fang Yan Jiu* (Tumor Prevention and Research), 1991; 18(2):71
10. *Zhong Yao Xue* (Chinese Herbology), 1998; 164:167
11. *Ha Er Bing Zhong Yi* (Haerbing Chinese Medicine), 1964; 2:30
12. *Zhong Cao Yao Tong Xun* (Journal of Chinese Herbal Medicine), 1972, 5:42
13. *Zhong Hua Nei Ke Za Zhi* (Chinese Journal of Internal Medicine), 1976; 6:339
14. *Bei Jing Yi Xue Yuan Xue Bao* (Journal of Beijing School of Medicine), 1978; 1:23
15. *Zhong Xi Yi Jie He Za Zhi* (Journal of Integrated Chinese and Western Medicine), 1986; 11:695
16. *Zhong Yi Za Zhi* (Journal of Chinese Medicine), 1988; 4:41
17. *Zhong Xi Yi Jie He Za Zhi* (Journal of Integrated Chinese and Western Medicine), 1986; 4:237
18. *Zhong Hua Pi Fu Ke Xue Za Zhi* (Chinese Journal of Dermatology), 1981; 1:40
19. *Chang Yong Zhong Yao Cheng Fen Yu Yao Li Shou Ce* (A Handbook of the Composition and Pharmacology of Common Chinese Drugs), 1994; 1673:1678

Fu Rong (Radix Hibisci)

芙蓉 芙蓉

Pinyin Name: *Fu Rong*
Alternate Chinese Names: *Shan Fu Rong, Gou Tou Fu Rong*
English Name: hibiscus root
Botanical Name: *Hibiscus taiwanensis*
Pharmaceutical Name: Radix Hibisci
Properties: acrid, cool
Channels Entered: Lung

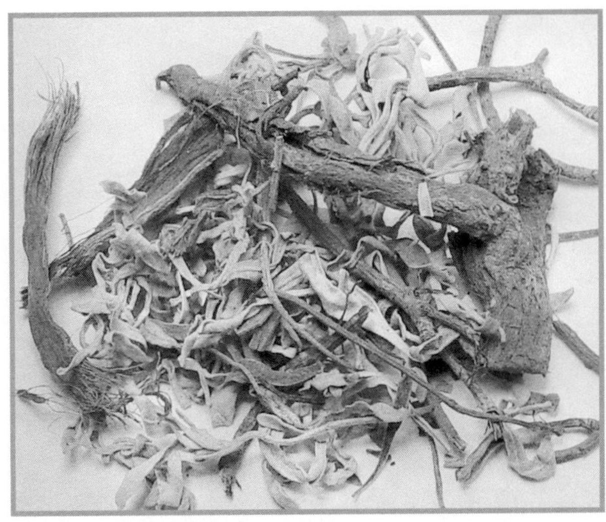

CHINESE THERAPEUTIC ACTIONS

1. Clears the Lung

Lung heat: Acrid and cool, *Fu Rong* (Radix Hibisci) clears Lung heat to relieve cough, dyspnea and yellow nasal discharge.

- Cough and dyspnea: use *Fu Rong* with *Da Qing Ye* (Folium Isatidis), *Pu Gong Ying* (Herba Taraxaci), *Huang Qin* (Radix Scutellariae), *Shi Gao* (Gypsum Fibrosum) and *Kuan Dong Hua* (Flos Farfarae).
- Sinusitis: use it with *Xin Yi Hua* (Flos Magnoliae) and *E Bu Shi Cao* (Herba Centipedae).

2. Reduces Inflammation and Relieves Pain

- Arthritis: combine *Fu Rong* with *Chuan Shan Long* (Rhizoma Dioscoreae Nipponicae) and *Yi Tiao Gen* (Radix Moghaniae).
- Hypermenorrhea and leukorrhea: use it with *Bai Long Chuan Hua Tou* (Radix Clerodendron Paniculatum) and *Ji Guan Hua* (Flos Celosiae Cristatae).
- Toxic swelling: apply *Fu Rong* topically.

DOSAGE

3 to 12 grams in decoction.

SUPPLEMENT

- 芙蓉葉 / 芙蓉叶 *Fu Rong Ye* (Folium Hibisci) treats dermatological disorders characterized by dampness, heat and toxins, such as carbuncles, furuncles and sores.

AUTHORS' COMMENTS

Most of the herbs that enter the Lung channel to treat respiratory disorders do not enter the nasal cavity. *Fu Rong* has the special characteristic of being able to treat nasal disorders such as allergies, rhinitis and sinusitis as well as clearing Lung heat.

Huang Teng (Caulis Fibraurea)

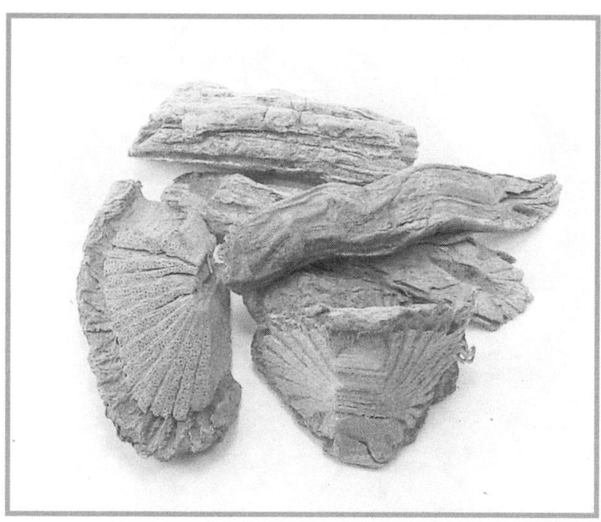

黄藤 黄藤

Pinyin Name: *Huang Teng*
Literal Name: "yellow vine"
Alternate Chinese Names: *Huang Teng Gen, Teng Gen*
English Name: fibraurea, common fibraurea stem
Botanical Name: *Fibraurea recisa* Pierre
Pharmaceutical Name: Caulis Fibraurea
Properties: bitter, cold
Channels Entered: Liver

CHINESE THERAPEUTIC ACTIONS

Clears Heat

Huang Teng (Caulis Fibraurea) treats Liver heat rising upwards, which may lead to elevated blood pressure. It also dispels wind from the exterior to relieve itching of the skin.

- Hypertension from Liver heat: use *Huang Teng* with *Sheng Di Huang* (Radix Rehmanniae), *Tu Fu Ling* (Rhizoma Smilacis Glabrae), and *Gou Ji* (Rhizoma Cibotii).
- Itching of the skin: combine it with *Ban Zhi Lian* (Herba Scutellariae Barbatae) and *Bai Hua She She Cao* (Herba Oldenlandia).

DOSAGE

3 to 15 grams in decoction.

CHEMICAL COMPOSITION

Palmatine, jatrorrhizine, pseudocolumbamine, fibrauin, fibralactone, fibranine, fibramine, columbamine, fiblecin, fibleucinoside, tinophylloloside.[1]

References

1. *Phytochemistry*, 1986; 25(4):905

Ji Guan Hua (Flos Celosiae Cristatae)

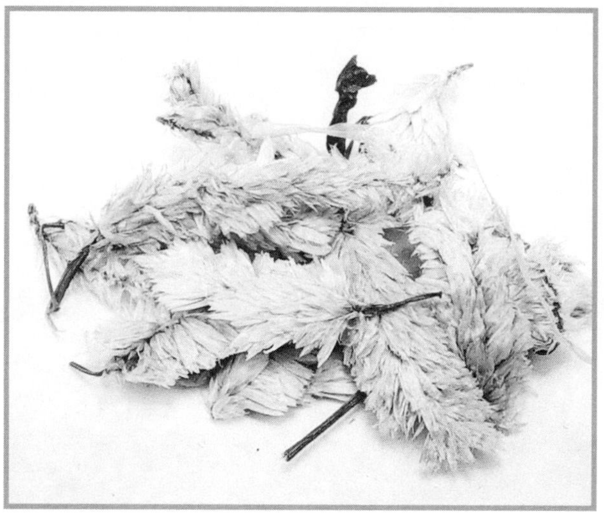

雞冠花 鸡冠花

Pinyin Name: *Ji Guan Hua*
Literal Name: "chicken crown flower"
Alternate Chinese Names: *Bai Ji Guan Hua, Ji Guan*
Original Source: *Ben Cao Gang Mu* (Materia Medica) by Li Shi-Zhen in 1578
English Name: celosia flower, cockscomb flower
Botanical Name: *Celosia cristata* L. (*Ji Guan*)
Pharmaceutical Name: Flos Celosiae Cristatae
Properties: sweet, cool
Channels Entered: Large Intestine, Liver

Ji Guan Hua (Flos Celosiae Cristatae)

CHINESE THERAPEUTIC ACTIONS

1. Clears Heat, Cools Blood and Stops Bleeding

Ji Guan Hua (Flos Celosiae Cristatae) clears heat and stops bleeding from various parts of the body.

- Hematemesis or epistaxis: use *Ji Guan Hua* with *Hua Rui Shi* (Ophicalcitum), *Ce Bai Ye* (Cacumen Platycladi) and charred *Pu Huang* (Pollen Typhae).
- Intestinal bleeding, hemorrhoidal bleeding due to heat: combine it with *Huai Hua* (Flos Sophorae), charred *Di Yu* (Radix Sanguisorbae), *Huang Lian* (Rhizoma Coptidis), *Mu Xiang* (Radix Aucklandiae), *Bai Shao* (Radix Paeoniae Alba) and *Da Huang* (Radix et Rhizoma Rhei).
- Uterine bleeding: add *Hua Rui Shi* (Ophicalcitum), *Bai Ji* (Rhizoma Bletillae) and *Wu Bei Zi* (Galla Chinensis).

2. Consolidates *Jing* (Essence) and Stops Diarrhea

Ji Guan Hua consolidates and retains body fluids, and stops diarrhea, dysentery, and vaginal discharge.

- Diarrhea or dysentery: use this herb with *Ge Gen* (Radix Puerariae), *Huang Lian* (Rhizoma Coptidis) and *Huang Qin* (Radix Scutellariae).
- White vaginal discharge: add *Long Yan Hua* (Flos Longan).

DOSAGE

6 to 12 grams. The charred form increases the warmth and binding effects of the herb, and is commonly used to stop bleeding, diarrhea, and leukorrhea.

CAUTIONS / CONTRAINDICATIONS

- Since *Ji Guan Hua* consolidates essence, it is not suitable for patients with dampness and heat accumulation, as it may retain these pathogens in the body.

Dong Qing Ye (Folium Ilexis)

冬青葉 冬青叶

Pinyin Name: *Dong Qing Ye*
Literal Name: "blue-green leaves in winter"
Alternate Chinese Names: *Gong Lau Ye, Si Ji Qing*
English Name: ilex
Botanical Name: *Ilex chinensis* Sims
Pharmaceutical Name: Folium Ilexis
Properties: bitter, astringent, cold
Channels Entered: Lung, Heart

CHINESE THERAPEUTIC ACTIONS

1. Dispels Heat and Toxins

Bitter and cold, *Dong Qing Ye* (Folium Ilexis) dispels heat and toxins from the Lung to treat bronchitis, pneumonia, and other respiratory tract infections. It also eliminates heat and toxins from the skin to address chronic, non-healing sores, lesions, and ulcerations.

2. Cools Blood, Stops Bleeding

Dong Qing Ye is used topically to stop bleeding.

DOSAGE

10 to 30 grams.

CHEMICAL COMPOSITION

Protocatechuic acid[1]

PHARMACOLOGICAL EFFECTS

- **Antibiotic:** *Dong Qing Ye* has an inhibitory action *in vitro* against *Pseudomonas aeruginosa, E. coli, Salmonella typhi, Bacillus subtilis,* and *Staphylococcus aureus.* The minimum inhibitory concentration for the herbs was 12.5 mg/ml.[2]

Dong Qing Ye (Folium Ilexis)

CLINICAL STUDIES AND RESEARCH

- **Burns:** Topical application of *Dong Qing Ye* has shown good results in facilitating healing, reducing discharge of pus from abscesses, and controlling infection.[3]

TOXICOLOGY

No abnormalities were observed following oral ingestion of *Dong Qing Ye* at 10 g/kg for 14 days. In an acute toxicology study, the LD_{50} was 233 g/kg via oral ingestion in mice.[4]

References

1. *Zhong Yao Da Ci Dien* (Dictionary of Chinese Herbs); 492-493
2. Ibid.
3. Ibid.
4. Ibid.

Section 4

— Heat-Clearing and Toxin-Eliminating Herbs

Jin Yin Hua (Flos Lonicerae)

金銀花 金银花

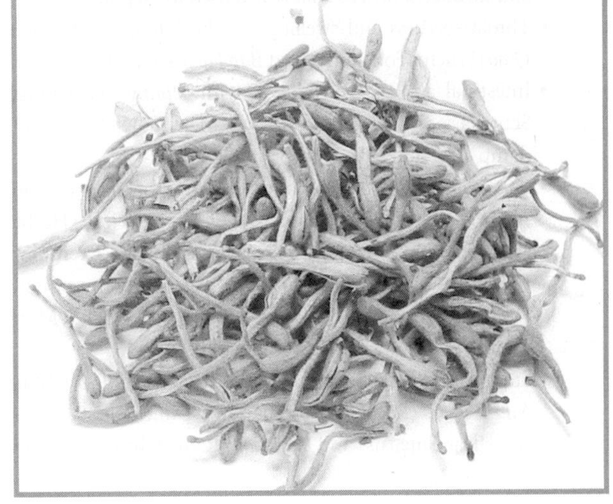

Pinyin Name: *Jin Yin Hua*

Literal Name: "golden silver flower"

Alternate Chinese Names: *Ren Dong Hua, Jin Hua, Er Hua, Shuang Hua*

Original Source: *Ming Yi Za Zhu* (Miscellaneous Records of Famous Physicians) by Tao Hong-Jing in 500 A.D.

English Name: lonicera flower, honeysuckle flower

Botanical Name: *Lonicera japonica* Thunb. (*Ren Dong*); *Lonicera hypoglauca* Miq. (*Hong Xian Ren Dong*); *Lonicera confusa* DC. (*Shan Yin Hua*); *Lonicera dasystyla* Rehd. (*Mao Hua Zhu Ren Dong*)

Pharmaceutical Name: Flos Lonicerae

Properties: sweet, cold

Channels Entered: Lung, Stomach, Large Intestine

CHINESE THERAPEUTIC ACTIONS

1. Clears Heat

Heat in various stages of febrile disorders: Combined with other appropriate herbs, *Jin Yin Hua* (Flos Lonicerae) can be used for treatment of many heat conditions. Clinical manifestations of heat include wind-heat and early-stage febrile disorders with sore throat, fever, perspiration and thirst; heat in the *qi* (energy) level showing as high fever, thirst, perspiration and forceful pulse; summer-heat with fever, heaviness sensations and heat stroke; and heat in the *ying* (nutritive) and *xue* (blood) levels with irritability, insomnia, bleeding, purpura or macules on the skin, with a scarlet red tongue. Though *Jin Yin Hua* is useful against all types of heat, it is most commonly used and most effective against the initial stages of febrile disorders, in which heat is in the upper *jiao*, at the *wei* (defense) and *qi* (energy) levels.

- Wind-heat and early-stage febrile disorders: use *Jin Yin Hua* with *Jing Jie* (Herba Schizonepetae), *Bo He* (Herba Menthae), and *Lian Qiao* (Fructus Forsythiae). **Exemplar Formula:** *Yin Qiao San* (Honeysuckle and Forsythia Powder).
- Pneumonia with heat signs: use it with *Xing Ren* (Semen Armeniacae Amarum), *Lian Qiao* (Fructus Forsythiae), and *Niu Bang Zi* (Fructus Arctii).
- Bronchitis with heat signs: combine it with *Shi Gao* (Gypsum Fibrosum), *Ma Huang* (Herba Ephedrae), *Xing Ren* (Semen Armeniacae Amarum) and *Gan Cao* (Radix Glycyrrhizae). **Exemplar Formula:** *Ma Xing Gan Shi Tang* (Ephedra, Apricot Kernel, Licorice, and Gypsum Decoction).
- Summer-heat: add *He Ye* (Folium Nelumbinis) and *Ju Hua* (Flos Chrysanthemi).
- Heat in the *qi* (energy) level with fever, irritability, thirst and forceful pulse: use *Jin Yin Hua* with *Shi Gao* (Gypsum Fibrosum) and *Zhi Mu* (Radix Anemarrhenae).
- Heat in the *ying* (nutritive) level with insomnia, irritability, blotches on the skin, dry mouth with dark-purplish

Jín Yín Hua (Flos Lonicerae)

tongue: use this herb with *Sheng Di Huang* (Radix Rehmanniae), *Xuan Shen* (Radix Scrophulariae) and *Dan Shen* (Radix Salviae Miltiorrhizae). **Exemplar Formula:** *Qing Ying Tang* (Clear the Nutrition Level Decoction).

2. Clears Heat and Eliminates Toxins

Sores and abscesses due to heat toxins: *Jin Yin Hua* is commonly used to clear heat and eliminate toxins from the interior and the exterior. The combination of heat and toxins in the interior is characterized by sore throat, swelling, intestinal abscesses and lung abscesses at various stages of development. Toxic heat in the exterior is characterized by all kinds of dermatological sores, lesions, ulcerations, warts and furuncles. *Jin Yin Hua* is also used for syphilis.

- Throat soreness and swelling: use *Jin Yin Hua* with *Lian Qiao* (Fructus Forsythiae) and *Ban Lan Gen* (Radix Isatidis).
- Intestinal abscess: combine it with *Huang Qin* (Radix Scutellariae) and *Yi Yi Ren* (Semen Coicis) to clear damp-heat and toxins in the intestines.
- Sores, lesions, carbuncles and ulceration of the skin: add *Ju Hua* (Flos Chrysanthemi), *Pu Gong Ying* (Herba Taraxaci), and *Zi Hua Di Ding* (Herba Violae). **Exemplar Formulas:** *Wu Wei Xiao Du Yin* (Five-Ingredient Decoction to Eliminate Toxins) and *Zhen Ren Huo Ming Yin* (True Man Decoction to Revitalize Life).
- Suppurative inflammation of the legs: use *Jin Yin Hua, Xuan Shen* (Radix Scrophulariae), *Dang Gui* (Radicis Angelicae Sinensis) and *Gan Cao* (Radix Glycyrrhizae) in large dosages.

3. Treats Diarrhea or Dysentery Caused by Toxic Heat

Diarrhea or dysentery: Heat and toxins attacking the intestines often leads to diarrhea or dysentery, and rectal tenesmus with or without the presence of mucus and blood.

- Diarrhea with mucus but no blood: use *Jin Yin Hua* with sugar.
- Diarrhea with blood: use *Jin Yin Hua* with brown sugar.
- Diarrhea or dysentery with mucus due to damp-heat and toxins: combine it with *Huang Lian* (Rhizoma Coptidis), *Huang Qin* (Radix Scutellariae), *Ge Gen* (Radix Puerariae), *Mu Xiang* (Radix Aucklandiae), *Ma Chi Xian* (Herba Portulacae) and *Bai Tou Weng* (Radix Pulsatillae).

DOSAGE

10 to 20 grams in decoction. In severe cases, the dosage of *Jin Yin Hua* can be increased up to 60 grams. Treatment of exterior conditions with *Jin Yin Hua* requires smaller dosages, while treatment of heat and toxins requires larger dosages. The charred form of this herb enhances hemostatic action for treating bloody diarrhea or bloody dysentery. Fresh *Jin Yin Hua* is more effective than the dried ones.

CHEMICAL COMPOSITION

Lonicein, loniceraflavone, loganin, tannin, chlorogenic acid, isochlorogenic acid, aromadendrene, linalool, geraniol, octanal, α-pinene, β-pinene, myrcene, 1,8-cineole, β-terpinene, hexenol, α-terpineol, neral, linalyl acetate, geranial, citronellol, terpinyl acetate, eugenol, β-eudesmol, geranyl acetate, α-copene, patchoulene, α-caryophyllene, β-caryophyllene, iso-bornyl acetate, farnesol, nerolidol.[1,2]

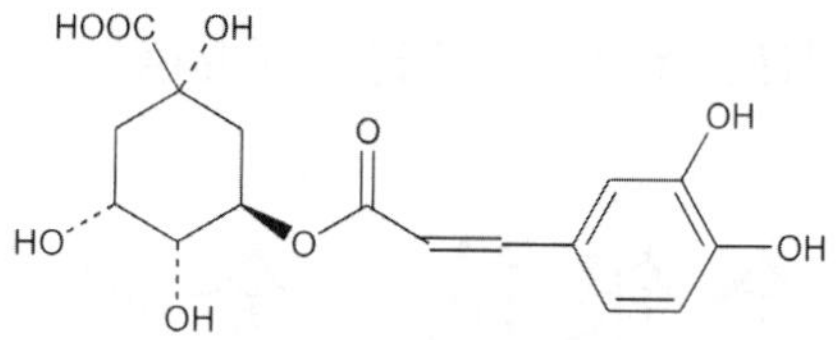

HOOC OH O OH HO O OH OH

Chlorogenic Acid

PHARMACOLOGICAL EFFECTS

- **Antibiotic:** *Jin Yin Hua* has demonstrated a broad spectrum of inhibitory actions against *Staphylococcus aureus,* β-hemolytic streptococcus, *E. coli, Bacillus dysenteriae, Vibrio cholerae, Salmonella typhi, Diplococcus pneumoniae, Diplococcus meningitidis, Pseudomonas aeruginosa,* and *Mycobacterium tuberculosis.* Chlorogenic acid and isochlorogenic acid have the strongest antibiotic effects. The fresh herb (just soaked in water) has a stronger antibiotic action than herbal decoction. The leaves have stronger antibiotic properties than the flowers.[3,4]
- **Anti-inflammatory and antipyretic:** *Jin Yin Hua* has demonstrated marked anti-inflammatory and antipyretic effects in mice and rabbits.[5]
- **CNS stimulant:** *Jin Yin Hua* has a mild stimulating influence on the central nervous system with one-sixth the potency of caffeine. The combination of *Jin Yin Hua* and caffeine showed no synergistic effect.[6]
- **Antihyperlipidemic:** Administration of 2.5 g/kg of *Jin Yin Hua* decreased absorption of cholesterol in the gastrointestinal tract in rats.[7]
- **Gastrointestinal:** Administration of a large dosage of *Jin Yin Hua* decoction is associated with increased motility of the stomach and the intestines. It also increases the excretion of bile acid and gastric acid.[8]

CLINICAL STUDIES AND RESEARCH

- **Appendicitis:** Administration of *Jin Yin Hua* via ionic penetration over 30 minutes daily for 10 to 20 treatments showed satisfactory results in 159 patients with appendicitis.[9]
- **Mastitis:** Administration of an herbal formula provided effective treatment for 10 patients with mastitis. The formula contained 45 grams of *Jin Yin Hua,* 15 grams of *Lu Jiao Shuang* (Cornu Cervi Degelatinatum), 12 grams of

Jin Yin Hua (Flos Lonicerae)

Wang Bu Liu Xing (Semen Vaccariae) and 1 cup of grain-based liquor.[10]

- **Common colds and influenza:** In one study, 1,150 patients with common colds or influenza were treated with *Yin Qiao San* (Honeysuckle and Forsythia Powder) with excellent results.[11]
- **Prevention of upper respiratory tract infections:** During the influenza season, administration of 1.2 ml of an herbal formula via inhalation of herbal vapor or instillation of herbal drops on the throat showed marked preventative effects in 393 children. The formula contained 60 grams of *Jin Yin Hua*, 60 grams of *Guan Zhong* (Rhizoma Dryopteridis), and 20 grams of *Gan Cao* (Radix Glycyrrhizae) cooked and concentrated to yield 120 ml of liquid extract.[12]

TOXICOLOGY

Oral ingestion of decoction of *Jin Yin Hua* is rarely associated with adverse reactions in rabbits, dogs, and other animals. The LD_{50} for extract of *Jin Yin Hua* in mice is 53 g/kg.[13]

References

1. *Chang Yong Zhong Yao Cheng Fen Yu Yao Li Shou Ce* (A Handbook of the Composition and Pharmacology of Common Chinese Drugs), 1994; 1264-1266
2. *The Merck Index* 12th edition, Chapman & Hall/CRCnetBASE/Merck, 2000
3. *Xin Yi Xue* (New Medicine), 1975; 6(3):155
4. *Jiang Xi Xin Yi Yao* (Jiangxi New Medicine and Herbology); 1960; (1):34
5. *Shan Xi Yi Kan* (Shanxi Journal of Medicine), 1960;(10):22
6. *CA*, 1961; 55:20218
7. *Ke Xue Chu Ban She* (Scientific Press), 1963:387
8. *Jiang Xi Xin Yi Yao* (Jiangxi New Medicine and Herbology); 1960;(1):34
9. *He Bei Yi Yao* (Hebei Medicine and Herbology), 1984; 3:168
10. *Zhong Yi Za Zhi* (Journal of Chinese Medicine), 1965; 10:47
11. *Guang Dong Zhong Yi* (Guangdong Chinese Medicine), 1962; 5:25
12. *Shang Hai Zhong Yi Yao Za Zhi* (Shanghai Journal of Chinese Medicine and Herbology), 1983; 9:27
13. *CA*, 1965; 63:18775e

Ren Dong Teng (Caulis Lonicerae)

忍冬藤 忍冬藤

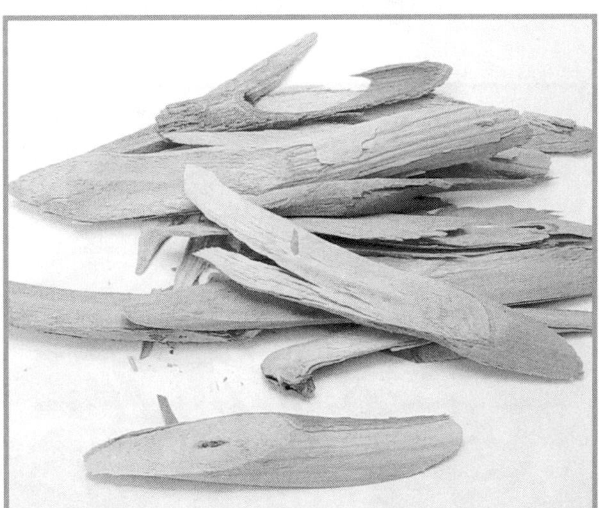

Pinyin Name: *Ren Dong Teng*
Literal Name: "tolerate winter vine," "winter-tolerating vine"
Alternate Chinese Names: *Yin Hua Teng*
Original Source: *Ming Yi Za Zhu* (Miscellaneous Records of Famous Physicians) by Tao Hong-Jing in 500 A.D.
English Name: lonicera vine, honeysuckle stem
Botanical Name: *Lonicera japonica* Thunb. (*Ren Dong*); *Lonicera hypoglauca* Miq. (*Hong Xian Ren Dong*); *Lonicera confusa* DC. (*Shan Yin Hua*); or *Lonicera dasystyla* Rehd. (*Mao Hua Zhu Ren Dong*)
Pharmaceutical Name: Caulis Lonicerae
Properties: sweet, cold
Channels Entered: Lung, Stomach

CHINESE THERAPEUTIC ACTIONS

1. Clears Heat and Releases the Exterior

Ren Dong Teng (Caulis Lonicerae) has mild ability to clear heat and release the exterior.

2. Clears Heat and Eliminates Toxins

Ren Dong Teng has milder action to clear heat and eliminate toxins.

Ren Dong Teng (Caulis Lonicerae)

3. Dispels Wind and Dampness from the Exterior

Ren Dong Teng dispels wind and dampness attacking the skin and muscles. Clinically, it treats itching caused by wind, or *bi zheng* (painful obstruction syndrome) from wind, dampness or heat.

- *Bi zheng* (painful obstruction syndrome) with swelling, redness and burning pain: use *Ren Dong Teng* with *Wei Ling Xian* (Radix Clematidis), *Qin Jiao* (Radix Gentianae Macrophyllae), *Qiang Huo* (Rhizoma et Radix Notopterygii), *Du Huo* (Radix Angelicae Pubescentis) and *Tou Gu Cao* (Caulis Impatientis).

DOSAGE

10 to 30 grams in decoction.

CHEMICAL COMPOSITION

Lonicein, luteolin-7-rhamnoglucoside, luteolin, lonicer-aflavone, loganin, tannins, chlorogenic acid, isochlorogenic acid.[1]

PHARMACOLOGICAL EFFECTS

- **Antibiotic:** *Ren Dong Teng* has demonstrated an inhibitory influence against *Staphylococcus aureus, Bacillus subtilis, Candida albicans, Salmonella typhi, Bacillus proteus, Bacillus dysenteriae,* and *H. suis.*[2]
- **Cardiovascular:** Luteolin increases systolic blood pressure, decreases diastolic pressure, and increases blood flow to the coronary artery in dogs.[3]
- **Antispasmodic:** Luteolin relieves spasms and cramps of the intestines and the respiratory tract.[4]

AUTHORS' COMMENTS

Both *Ren Dong Teng* (Caulis Lonicerae) and *Jin Yin Hua* (Flos Lonicerae) clear heat and release the exterior. *Ren Dong Teng* is milder in these actions.

References

1. *Xian Dai Zhong Yao Yao Li Xue* (Contemporary Pharmacology of Chinese Herbs), 1997; 210
2. *Ren Min Wei Sheng Chu Ban She* (Journal of People's Public Health), 1986:681
3. Ibid.
4. Ibid.

Lian Qiao (Fructus Forsythiae)

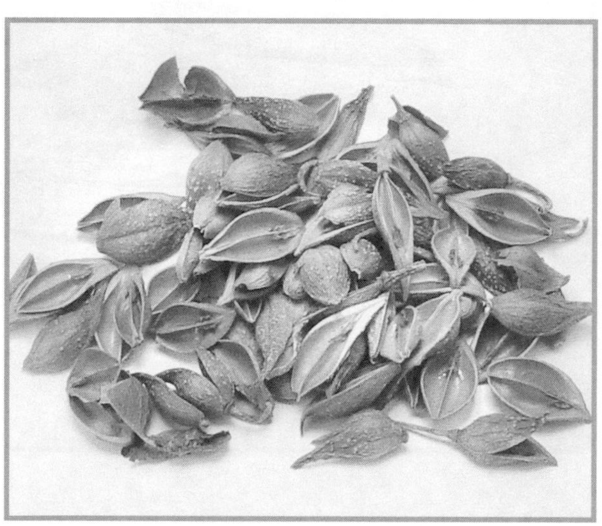

連翹 连翘

Pinyin Name: *Lian Qiao*
Alternate Chinese Names: *Lian Ke, Huang Hua Ban*
Original Source: *Shen Nong Ben Cao Jing* (Divine Husbandman's Classic of the Materia Medica) in the second century
English Name: forsythia, weeping forsythia capsule
Botanical Name: *Forsythia suspensa* (Thunb.) Vahl.
Pharmaceutical Name: Fructus Forsythiae
Properties: bitter, cool
Channels Entered: Lung, Heart, Gallbladder

CHINESE THERAPEUTIC ACTIONS

1. Clears Heat

Exterior wind-heat or early febrile disorders: Bitter and cold, *Lian Qiao* (Fructus Forsythiae) has ascending, floating and dispersing functions to clear heat and eliminate toxins. It is commonly used to treat exterior wind-heat or early-stage febrile disorders.

- Exterior wind-heat with sore throat: combine *Lian Qiao*

Lian Qiao (Fructus Forsythiae)

with *Jin Yin Hua* (Flos Lonicerae). **Exemplar Formula:** *Yin Qiao San* (Honeysuckle and Forsythia Powder).

- Early-stage febrile disorder with cough: add *Ju Hua* (Flos Chrysanthemi) and *Bo He* (Herba Menthae). **Exemplar Formula:** *Sang Ju Yin* (Mulberry Leaf and Chrysanthemum Decoction).

Interior heat affecting the Heart and Pericardium: *Lian Qiao* also treats heat attacking the Heart and Pericardium that is causing high fever, irritability, and delirium. In severe cases, rising Heart fire manifests in red, swollen eyes, sore throat, and ulcers on the tongue.

- Heat attacking the Heart and Pericardium: use *Lian Qiao* with *Lian Zi Xin* (Plumula Nelumbinis).
- Rising Heart fire: combine it with *Sheng Di Huang* (Radix Rehmanniae), *Shi Gao* (Gypsum Fibrosum) and *Xuan Shen* (Radix Scrophulariae).

Heat in the *ying* (nutritive) level: Heat forces blood out of the vessels, leading to subcutaneous bleeding, macula and purpura.

- Macula caused by heat in the *ying* (nutritive) level: use *Lian Qiao* with *Chi Shao* (Radix Paeoniae Rubrae), *Zi Cao Gen* (Radix Lithospermi) and *Da Zao* (Fructus Jujubae).

2. Clears Heat and Eliminates Toxins

Abscess: *Lian Qiao* is one of the most effective and commonly-used herbs for clearing heat and eliminating toxins from both the interior and the exterior. Heat and toxins in the interior are characterized by sore throat, swelling, and intestinal and lung abscesses in various stages of development. Heat and toxins in the exterior are characterized by sores, lesions, ulcerations, lumps, nodules and furuncles.

- Intestinal or lung abscesses: use this herb with *Jin Yin Hua* (Flos Lonicerae), *Ye Ju Hua* (Flos Chrysanthemi Indici) and *Pu Gong Ying* (Herba Taraxaci).
- Throat soreness and pain: combine it with *Shan Dou Gen* (Radix Sophorae Tonkinensis), *Jie Geng* (Radix Platycodonis) and *Gan Cao* (Radix Glycyrrhizae).
- Lumps and nodules: add *Xia Ku Cao* (Spica Prunellae). **Exemplar Formula:** *Xiao Luo Wan* (Reduce Scrofula Pill).

3. Promotes Urination

***Lin zheng* (dysuria syndrome):** *Lian Qiao* treats *lin zheng*, in which heat has invaded the Urinary Bladder and is causing burning dysuria or hematuria.

- Dysuria: use it with *Dan Zhu Ye* (Herba Lophatheri), *Chuan Mu Tong* (Caulis Clematidis Armandii) and *Che Qian Zi* (Semen Plantaginis).

DOSAGE

6 to 15 grams in decoction.

CAUTIONS / CONTRAINDICATIONS

- Use *Lian Qiao* with caution for patients experiencing diarrhea, or sores that are neither red nor painful.

CHEMICAL COMPOSITION

Lignoids: (phillyrin, phillygenin, (+)-pinorseinol, (+)-pinoresinol-β-D-glucoside), oleanolic acid, betulic acid, ursolic acid, rutin, forsythoside A, C, D; essential oils (α-pinene, β-pinene; terpinen-40ol; β-cymene).[1]

Phillyrin

PHARMACOLOGICAL EFFECTS

- **Antibiotic:** The essential oil of *Lian Qiao* has demonstrated a broad spectrum of inhibitory effects against *Staphylococcus aureus, Diplococcus pneumoniae, Bacillus dysenteriae,* α-hemolytic streptococcus, β-hemolytic streptococcus, *Neisseria catarrhalis, Salmonella typhi, E. coli, Mycobacterium tuberculosis, Bacillus proteus, Bordetella pertussis, Corynebacterium diphtheriae,* leptospira, and some dermatophytes and influenza viruses.[2]
- **Anti-inflammatory:** In guinea pigs, injection of *Lian Qiao* decreases the permeability of the blood vessels to reduce inflammation.[3]
- **Cardiovascular:** *Lian Qiao* has a mixed effect on blood pressure. In anesthetized cats in shock, intravenous injection of *Lian Qiao* (dosage equivalent to 8 g/kg of dried herb) is associated with increases of blood pressure and cardiac contraction. In another study with healthy subjects, injection of a water extract of *Lian Qiao* is associated with reduction in blood pressure.[4,5]
- **Others:** *Lian Qiao* also has hepatoprotective, antipyretic, antiemetic and diuretic effects.[6]

CLINICAL STUDIES AND RESEARCH

- **Nephropathy:** In one study, 8 patients with acute nephritis and 1 patient with tuberculosis of the kidney were treated with Chinese herbal formulas with good results. The treatment protocol was to cook 30 grams of *Lian Qiao* in water to yield 150 ml of final decoction, taken in equally-divided doses, three times daily, before meals. The dosage for children was adjusted accordingly. The duration of treatment was between 5 and 10 days. Patients were advised to avoid spicy and salty foods.[7]
- **Purpura:** According to one report, 1 patient with thrombocytopenic purpura and 2 patients with allergic purpura

Lian Qiao (Fructus Forsythiae)

were treated with Chinese herbs with satisfactory results. The treatment protocol was to cook 30 grams of *Lian Qiao* in water to yield 150 ml of final decoction, taken in equally-divided doses, three times daily, before meals.[8]

TOXICOLOGY

The LD_{50} of *Lian Qiao* in mice is 172.21 g/kg via oral ingestion, and 20.96 g/kg via intraperitoneal injection.[9]

References

1. *Xian Dai Zhong Yao Yao Li Xue* (Contemporary Pharmacology of Chinese Herbs), 1997; 214
2. *Shan Xi Xin Yi Yao* (New Medicine and Herbology of Shanxi), 1980; 9(11):51
3. *Ke Yan Tong Xun* (Journal of Science and Research), 1982; (3):35
4. Ibid.
5. *Zhong Yao Xue* (Chinese Herbology), 1998; 169:171
6. Ibid.
7. *Jiang Xi Yi Yao* (Jiangxi Medicine and Herbology), 1961; 7:18
8. *Guang Dong Zhong Yi* (Guangdong Chinese Medicine), 1960; 10:469
9. *Chang Yong Zhong Yao Cheng Fen Yu Yao Li Shou Ce* (A Handbook of the Composition and Pharmacology of Common Chinese Drugs), 1994; 1021:1027

Guan Ye Lian Qiao (Herba Hypericum)

貫葉連翹 贯叶连翘

Pinyin Name: *Guan Ye Lian Qiao*
Alternate Chinese Names: *Tu Lian Qiao, Guan Ye Jin Si Tao, Jin Si Tao*
Original Source: *Ben Cao Gang Mu Shi Yi* (Omissions from the Grand Materia Medica) by Zhao Xue-Min in 1765
English Name: St. John's Wort
Botanical Name: *Hypericum perforatum* L. (*Guan Ye Lian Qiao*)
Pharmaceutical Name: Herba Hypericum
Properties: bitter, acrid, astringent, neutral
Channels Entered: Liver

CHINESE THERAPEUTIC ACTIONS

1. Clears Heat, Eliminates Toxins

Toxic heat: *Guan Ye Lian Qiao* (Herba Hypericum) reduces swelling and inflammation to treat carbuncles, sores, snake and insect bites, and other disorders characterized by toxic heat.

- *Chang feng* (intestinal wind) with blood in the stools: combine *Guan Ye Lian Qiao* with dry-fried *Huai Hua* (Flos Sophorae) and *Zong Lu Pi* (Fibra Stipulae Trachycarpi).
- Urinary tract infection: use *Guan Ye Lian Qiao* as a single-herb remedy.
- Redness and swelling of the eyes: drink *Guan Ye Lian Qiao* as tea throughout the day.
- Snake and insect bites: ground the herb into paste and apply it topically.
- Tonsillitis: use the decoction as a gargle.

2. Stops Bleeding

Bleeding: *Guan Ye Lian Qiao* has an astringent effect to treat hemoptysis, hematemesis, and bleeding due to trauma.

- Hematemesis: add it to *Xian He Cao* (Herba Agrimoniae).
- Profuse uterine bleeding: use this herb with *Xian He Cao* (Herba Agrimoniae), *Han Lian Cao* (Herba Ecliptae), and charred *Pu Gong Ying* (Herba Taraxaci).

3. Dispels Wind-Damp

***Bi zheng* (painful obstruction syndrome):** *Guan Ye Lian Qiao* dispels wind-damp from the exterior to relieve muscle aches and pain.

- *Bi zheng*: use it with *Xun Gu Feng* (Herba Aristolochiae Mollissimae), *Shen Jin Cao* (Herba Lycopodii), *Mu Gua* (Fructus Chaenomelis), and *Ji Xue Teng* (Caulis Spatholobi).

4. Relieves Depression

Depression: *Guan Ye Lian Qiao* regulates Liver qi to treat depression. It may be used individually, or combined with *Yue Ju Wan* (Escape Restraint Pill).

Guan Ye Lian Qiao (Herba Hypericum)

DOSAGE

6 to 9 grams in decoction. *Guan Ye Lian Qiao* is used both internally and topically.

CAUTIONS / CONTRAINDICATIONS

- Use of *Guan Ye Lian Qiao* may be associated with increased photosensitivity.

CHEMICAL COMPOSITION

Hypericin, hyperforin, hyperin, pseudohypericin, protohypericin, cyclopseudohypericin, desmethylcyclopseudohypericin, emodinanthranol.[1,2]

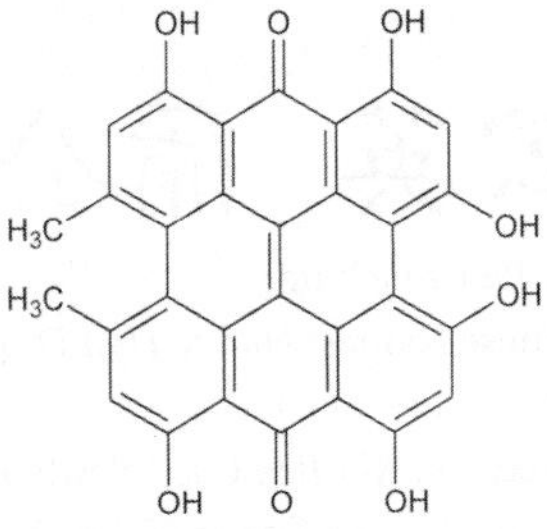

Hypericin

PHARMACOLOGICAL EFFECTS

- **Antitussive**: Intraperitoneal injection of hyperin in cats at 100 mg/kg had an antitussive effect.[3]
- **Analgesic**: Administration of hyperin is associated with an analgesic effect in mice.[4]
- **Antibiotic**: This herb has antibacterial action against *Staphylococcus aureus*, *Streptococcus pyogenes*, and *Streptococcus agalactiae*. In addition, hyperforin has an inhibitory effect against penicillin-resistant *Staphylococcus aureus* (PRSA) and methicillin-resistant *Staphylococcus aureus* (MRSA). Furthermore, hyperforin has antiviral action against herpes simplex virus, parainfluenza virus, vesicular stomatitis virus, and human cytomegalovirus.[5]
- **Antidepressant**: *Guan Ye Lian Qiao* extract has been shown to relieve depression by inhibiting the reuptake of serotonin and other neurotransmitters, such as norepinephrine and dopamine. Hyperforin is believed to be the main constituent responsible for the antidepressant activity.[6]

CLINICAL STUDIES AND RESEARCH

- **Depression**: *Guan Ye Lian Qiao* and fluoxetine demonstrated equivalent therapeutic effect for treatment of depression, according to a randomized, double-blind, comparative trial involving 149 outpatients with mild or moderate depression. The duration of treatment was 6 weeks. Patients in the herb group received 800 mg of *Guan Ye Lian Qiao* extract per day (5-7:1 extract, ethanol 60% solvent). Patients in the drug group received 20mg of fluoxetine.[7]

HERB-DRUG INTERACTION

- **SSRI's**: Since St. John's Wort and SSRI both inhibit the reuptake of serotonin, concurrent use of both the herb and the drug may lead to "serotonin syndrome" with symptoms such as sweating, tremor, flushing, confusion and agitation.[8] [Note: Examples of SSRI's include fluoxetine (Prozac), paroxetine (Paxil), sertraline (Zoloft), citalopram (Celexa), and fluvoxamine (Luvox).]
- **Antivirals**: It has been found that concurrent use of St. John's Wort and indinavir contributed to a 57% reduction in the area under the curve and an 81% decrease of the extrapolated 8-hour trough value for indinavir. The dose of St. John's Wort was 300 mg (standardized to 0.3% hypericin) three times daily, and the dose of indinavir was 800 mg every 8 hours.[9]
- **Digoxin (Lanoxin)**: St. John's Wort taken concomitantly with digoxin resulted in a significant decrease in digoxin C_{max}, C_{trough}, and AUC (area under the curve).[10]
- **Metabolic effect**: St. John's Wort may lower the plasma levels of many drugs, such as cyclosporine (Sandimmune/Neoral), ethinyloestradiol and desogestrel (combined oral contraceptive), theophylline (Theo-Dur), digoxin (Lanoxin), and indinavir (Crixivan). The proposed mechanism of this interaction is the induction of the cytochrome P-450 system of the liver by St. John's Wort, leading to increased metabolism and reduced plasma concentration of the drugs.[11]

TOXICOLOGY

The LD^{50} of hyperin in mice via intraperitoneal injection is 0.5 g/kg.[12]

AUTHORS' COMMENTS

Guan Ye Lian Qiao (Herba Hypericum) is commonly known as St. John's Wort. Historically in China, this herb was used as a heat-clearing agent, to treat various types of infectious and inflammatory conditions. In Europe, it was used more as a nerve tonic, to address anxiety, depression, and restlessness.

References

1. *Xian Dai Ben Cao Gang Mu* (Contemporary Materia Medica), 2000; 1759-1760
2. *The Merck Index* 12th edition, Chapman & Hall/CRCnetBASE/Merck, 2000
3. *Xian Dai Ben Cao Gang Mu* (Contemporary Materia Medica), 2000; 1759-1760
4. *Zhong Guo Yao Li Xue Tong Bao* (Journal of Chinese Herbal Pharmacology), 1986; 2(2):14
5. *CA*, 1972; 76:30830g) (*Planta Med*, 1990;56(6):651
6. Muller, WE et al., Hyperforin represents the neurotransmitter reuptake inhibiting constituent of Hypericum extract. *Pharmacopsychiatry* 1998 Jun;31 Suppl 1:16-21
7. Harrer, G et al., Comparison of equivalence between the St. John's

Wort extract LoHyp-57 and fluoxetine. *Arzneimittelforschung* 1999 Apr;(4):289-96

8. Muller WE, Schafer C er al., In-vitro-Studie uber Hypericum-Extrakt, Hyericin und Kampferol. *DAZ* 136(13):1015-1022.1996
9. Piscitelli, S et al., Indinavir concentration and St. John's Wort. *Lancet* 2000; 355:547-548
10. Andreas, J et al., Pharmacokinetic interaction of digoxin with an herbal extract from St. John's Wort. *Clinical Pharmacology & Therapeutics.* 1999;66:3380345
11. *PDR for Nutritional Supplements 1st Edition*, Medical Economics, 2001
12. *Xian Dai Ben Cao Gang Mu* (Contemporary Materia Medica), 2000; 1759-1760

Pu Gong Ying (Herba Taraxaci)

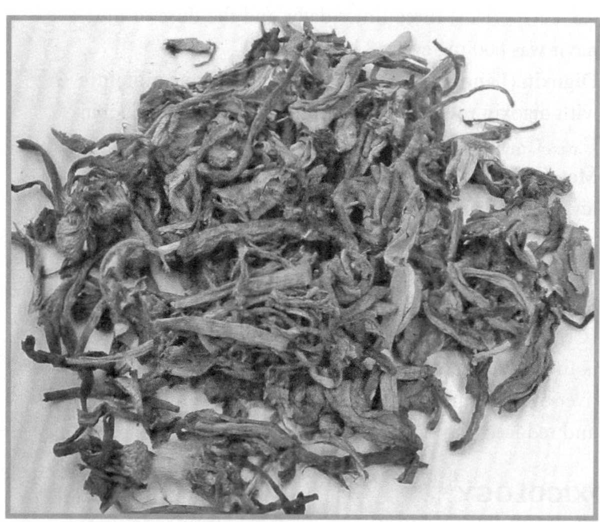

蒲公英 蒲公英

Pinyin Name: *Pu Gong Ying*

Alternate Chinese Names: *Huang Hua Di Ding, Pu Gong Ding, Puo Puo Ding*

Original Source: *Xin Xiu Ben Cao* (Newly Revised Materia Medica) by Su Jing in 657-659 A.D.

English Name: dandelion, Asian dandelion

Botanical Name: *Taraxacum mongolicum* Hand. –Mazz. (*Pu Gong Ying*)

Pharmaceutical Name: Herba Taraxaci

Properties: bitter, sweet, cold

Channels Entered: Liver, Stomach

CHINESE THERAPEUTIC ACTIONS

1. Clears Heat and Eliminates Toxins

Toxic heat accumulation: *Pu Gong Ying* (Herba Taraxaci) is commonly used to clear heat and toxins from both the exterior and the interior. External heat and toxins are characterized by sores, lesions, and ulcerations. Internal heat and toxins are characterized by abscesses, nodules, intestinal abscesses, breast lumps, parotitis and tonsillitis. Entering the Liver channel, *Pu Gong Ying* is excellent in treating the beginning stages of breast abscess or lumps involving redness and pain.

- Sores, lesions and ulceration of the skin: use *Pu Gong Ying* with *Zi Hua Di Ding* (Herba Violae), *Jin Yin Hua* (Flos Lonicerae) and *Ye Ju Hua* (Flos Chrysanthemi Indici). **Exemplar Formula:** *Wu Wei Xiao Du Yin* (Five-Ingredient Decoction to Eliminate Toxins).
- Breast lumps and abscesses: combine this herb with *Gua Lou Shi* (Fructus Trichosanthis), *Qing Pi* (Pericarpium Citri Reticulatae Viride), and *Lu Feng Fang* (Nidus Vespae).
- Intestinal abscesses: combine it with *Da Huang* (Radix et Rhizoma Rhei), *Bai Jiang Cao* (Herba cum Radice Patriniae) and *Mu Dan Pi* (Cortex Moutan).
- Lung abscesses: use it with *Yu Xing Cao* (Herba Houttuyniae) and *Jie Geng* (Radix Platycodonis).
- Nodules on the neck, goiter: add *Xia Ku Cao* (Spica Prunellae) and *Zhe Bei Mu* (Bulbus Fritillariae Thunbergii).
- Soreness and swelling of the throat: use *Pu Gong Ying* with *Xuan Shen* (Radix Scrophulariae) and *Ban Lan Gen* (Radix Isatidis).
- Eye redness, swelling and pain due to Liver heat: combine this herb with *Ju Hua* (Flos Chrysanthemi), *Xia Ku Cao* (Spica Prunellae) and *Huang Qin* (Radix Scutellariae).

2. Eliminates Damp-Heat

- Damp-heat jaundice: use *Pu Gong Ying* with *Yin Chen Hao* (Herba Artemisiae Scopariae), *Zhi Zi* (Fructus Gardeniae) and *Da Huang* (Radix et Rhizoma Rhei). **Exemplar Formula:** *Yin Chen Hao Tang* (Artemisia Scoparia Decoction).

Pu Gong Ying (Herba Taraxaci)

3. Promotes Urination

***Re lin* (heat dysuria):** Heat invading the Urinary Bladder manifests in burning pain on urination. In this case, the urine is usually scanty and yellow.

- *Re lin* (heat dysuria): use *Pu Gong Ying* with *Jin Qian Cao* (Herba Lysimachiae) and *Bai Mao Gen* (Rhizoma Imperatae).

DOSAGE

10 to 30 grams in decoction. A large dose of fresh *Pu Gong Ying* is usually crushed into paste for topical application.

CAUTIONS / CONTRAINDICATIONS

- Large dosages are sometimes associated with diarrhea.
- Use of *Pu Gong Ying* is contraindicated for yin sores or carbuncles where there is no redness and pain.

CHEMICAL COMPOSITION

Taraxacerin, taraxasterol, taraxicin, xanthoph.[1]

PHARMACOLOGICAL EFFECTS

- **Antibiotic:** *Pu Gong Ying* has bactericidal effects *in vitro* against *Staphylococcus aureus*, β-hemolytic streptococcus, *Diplococcus pneumoniae, Diplococcus meningitidis, Corynebacterium diphtheriae, Pseudomonas aeruginosa, Bacillus dysenteriae* and *Salmonella typhi*.[2]
- **Others:** *Pu Gong Ying* was noted to have immune-enhancing, hepatoprotective, diuretic and cholagogic effects.[3]

CLINICAL STUDIES AND RESEARCH

- **Acute tonsillitis:** In one report, 120 to 180 grams of *Pu Gong Ying* in decoction was successful in treating acute tonsillitis in 82 of 88 patients.[4]
- **Sore throat:** An herbal formula containing *Pu Gong Ying* and *Ban Lan Gen* (Radix Isatidis) was 98% effective in treating 45 patients with acute sore throat. The formula was cooked as decoction, with the steam channeled to the mouth for topical treatment of sore throat.[5]
- **Jaundice:** Oral and intramuscular injections of *Pu Gong Ying* were effective in lowering liver enzymes in 77 patients with icteric jaundice.[6]
- **Blurred vision:** *Pu Gong Ying* administered as oral decoction and ophthalmic solution three times daily was effective for treating patients with blurred vision. Out of 32 affected eyes, 8 showed significant improvement, 18 showed moderate improvement, and 6 showed no response.[7]
- **Burns:** An herbal paste made by mixing *Pu Gong Ying* with 75% rubbing alcohol was effective in treating 51 patients with infected burns.[8]
- **Parotitis:** Topical application of *Pu Gong Ying* every other day was found to be extremely effective in treating 40 patients with parotitis. The herbal paste was prepared by grinding 30 grams of the fresh herb (or 20 grams of dried herb) with one egg white. The resultant paste was applied to the affected area and covered with gauze.[9]

HERB-DRUG INTERACTION

- **Quinolone antibiotics:** It has been proposed that concurrent use of *Pu Gong Ying* and quinolone antibiotics may influence the bioavailability and disposition of the quinolone antibiotics. In one study, rats were divided into two groups with one receiving a single dose of ciprofloxacin and the other receiving both *Pu Gong Ying* and ciprofloxacin. Ciprofloxacin in plasma and urine was collected over 6 and 24 hours and evaluated by high performance liquid chromatography (HPLC). The results indicated that while the concurrent use of ciprofloxacin and *Pu Gong Ying* did not significantly alter the bioavailability of ciprofloxacin, it did lower the maximum plasma concentration (Cmax) by 73%, increase apparent volume of distribution by threefold, and increase terminal half-life from 1.96 to 5.71 hours. The decrease of maximum plasma concentration of ciprofloxacin has been attributed to the high mineral content of *Pu Gong Ying*.[10]

TOXICOLOGY

The LD_{50} for intravenous injection of *Pu Gong Ying* is 58.8 g/kg in mice.[11]

References

1. *Xian Dai Shi Yong Yao Xue* (Practical Applications of Modern Herbal Medicine), 1997; 223
2. *Zhong Yi Yao Xue Bao* (Report of Chinese Medicine and Herbology), 1991; (1):41
3. *Zhong Yao Xue* (Chinese Herbology), 1988; 171:172
4. *Xin Yi Yao Xue Za Zhi* (New Journal of Medicine and Herbology), 1977; 8:8
5. *Liao Ning Zhong Yi Za Zhi* (Liaoning Journal of Chinese Medicine), 1988; 9:27
6. *Zhong Yi Za Zhi* (Journal of Chinese Medicine), 1979; 12:55
7. *Tian Jing Yi Yao* (Tianjing Medicine and Herbology), 1974; 7:362
8. *Zhong Xi Yi Jie He Za Zhi* (Journal of Integrated Chinese and Western Medicine), 1987; 5:301
9. *New Medicine*, 1972; 10:49
10. *Journal of Pharmaceutical Sciences*, 1999; June, 88(6):632-4
11. *Zhong Yao Zhi* (Chinese Herbology Journal), 1988; 697

Zi Hua Di Ding (Herba Violae)

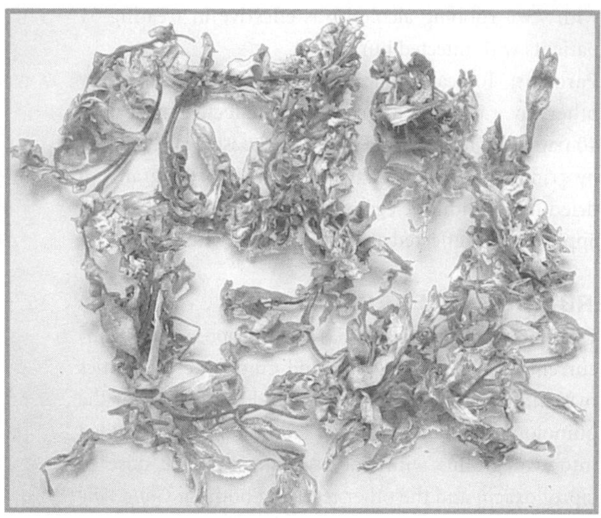

紫花地丁

紫花地丁

Pinyin Name: *Zi Hua Di Ding*

Literal Name: "purple flower earth herb," "purple flower earth spike"

Alternate Chinese Names: *Di Ding Cao, Di Ding*

Original Source: *Ben Cao Gang Mu* (Materia Medica) by Li Shi-Zhen in 1578

English Name: viola, tokyo violet herb

Botanical Name: *Viola yedoensis* Makino. (*Zi Hua Di Ding*)

Pharmaceutical Name: Herba Violae

Properties: bitter, acrid, cold

Channels Entered: Heart, Liver

CHINESE THERAPEUTIC ACTIONS

Clears Heat and Eliminates Toxins

Toxic heat: Bitter and cold, *Zi Hua Di Ding* (Herba Violae) has excellent properties to clear heat, eliminate toxins, reduce abscesses and cool blood. It can be used either internally or topically to reduce inflammation. It is also good for high fever and irritability accompanying bacterial infection.

- Furuncles, lesions, intestinal abscesses and erysipelas: combine *Zi Hua Di Ding* with *Pu Gong Ying* (Herba Taraxaci), *Jin Yin Hua* (Flos Lonicerae) and *Ye Ju Hua* (Flos Chrysanthemi Indici), internally or topically. **Exemplar Formula:** *Wu Wei Xiao Du Yin* (Five-Ingredient Decoction to Eliminate Toxins).
- Furuncles, lesions, intestinal abscesses and erysipelas with deficiencies of qi and blood: use this herb with *Pu Gong Ying* (Herba Taraxaci), *Jin Yin Hua* (Flos Lonicerae), *Ye Ju Hua* (Flos Chrysanthemi Indici), *Huang Qi* (Radix Astragali) and *Dang Gui* (Radicis Angelicae Sinensis).
- Snake or insect bites: *Zi Hua Di Ding* treats snake or insect bites by reducing swelling and toxicity. Apply fresh juice of *Zi Hua Di Ding* topically to the affected area.
- Redness, swelling and eye pain caused by Liver heat: add *Ju Hua* (Flos Chrysanthemi) and *Xia Ku Cao* (Spica Prunellae).

DOSAGE

10 to 20 grams in decoction. Fresh *Zi Hua Di Ding* is usually crushed into paste for topical application.

CAUTIONS / CONTRAINDICATIONS

- Use *Zi Hua Di Ding* with caution on yin sores, furuncles, abscesses and lesions where there is no redness or pain.

CHEMICAL COMPOSITION

Palmitic acid, p-hydroxybenzoic acid, trans-p-hydroxycinnamic acid, butanedioic acid, tetracosanoyl-p-hydroxyl phenthylamine, kaempferol-3-o-rhamnopyranoside.[1]

PHARMACOLOGICAL EFFECTS

- **Antibiotic:** Decoction of *Zi Hua Di Ding* has an inhibitory effect against *Pseudomonas aeruginosa, E. coli, Bacillus dysenteriae, Salmonella typhi, Staphylococcus aureus, Corynebacterium diphtheriae, Streptococcus* spp., *Diplococcus pneumoniae, Staphylococcus albus, Candida albicans, Bacillus proteus, Bacillus dysenteriae,* and leptospira.[2,3]
- **Others:** *Zi Hua Di Ding* has antipyretic and anti-inflammatory effects.[4]

References

1. *Chang Yong Zhong Yao Cheng Fen Yu Yao Li Shou Ce* (A Handbook of the Composition and Pharmacology of Common Chinese Drugs), 1994; 1667-1669
2. *Zhong Yao Zhi* (Chinese Herbology Journal), 1988:31
3. *Zhong Yi Yao Xue Bao* (Report of Chinese Medicine and Herbology), 1991; (2):47
4. *Zhong Yao Xue* (Chinese Herbology), 1998; 172:174

Ye Ju Hua (Flos Chrysanthemi Indici)

野菊花 野菊花

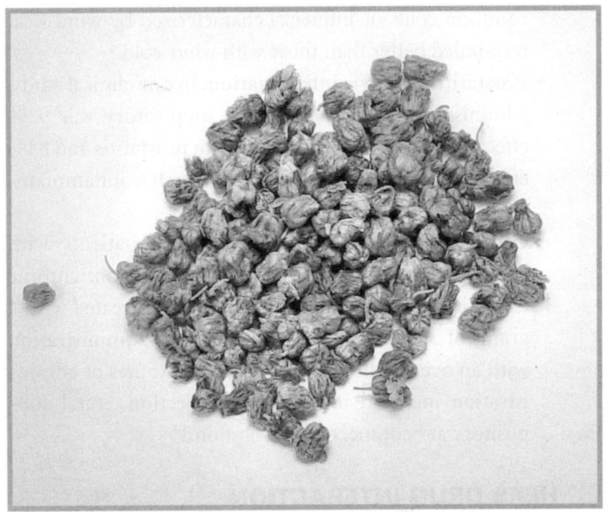

Pinyin Name: *Ye Ju Hua*
Literal Name: "wild chrysanthemum flower"
Original Source: *Shen Nong Ben Cao Jing* (Divine Husbandman's Classic of the Materia Medica) in the second century
English Name: wild chrysanthemum flower, flower of indian dendranthema
Botanical Name: *Chrysanthemum indicum* L.
Pharmaceutical Name: Flos Chrysanthemi Indici
Properties: bitter, acrid, cool
Channels Entered: Lung, Liver

CHINESE THERAPEUTIC ACTIONS

Clears Heat and Eliminates Toxins

Ye Ju Hua (Flos Chrysanthemi Indici) clears heat, eliminates toxins, and is commonly used to treat furuncles, carbuncles, sores, sore throat and red eyes.

- Carbuncles and furuncles: use *Ye Ju Hua* with *Pu Gong Ying* (Herba Taraxaci), *Zi Hua Di Ding* (Herba Violae) and *Jin Yin Hua* (Flos Lonicerae) internally or topically.
- Eye redness, swelling and pain: combine this herb with *Xia Ku Cao* (Spica Prunellae) and *Sang Ye* (Folium Mori) for use internally as an herbal decoction, or topically as an eyewash.
- Itching: use *Ye Ju Hua* alone internally as an herbal decoction or topically as an herbal wash.

DOSAGE

10 to 15 grams. *Ye Ju Hua* may be used both internally and externally.

CHEMICAL COMPOSITION

Essential oils 0.60-1.29% (camphor, α-pinene, carvone, eucalyptol, borneol), flavonoids (acaciin, linarin), chrysanthemin 0.42-0.45%, luteolin, acacetin.[1,2]

HO, OH, OH, OH, O, O

Luteolin

PHARMACOLOGICAL EFFECTS

- **Cardiovascular**: *Ye Ju Hua* has a marked influence on the cardiovascular system. In anesthetized cats, intravenous injection of alcohol extract of *Ye Ju Hua* increased blood perfusion to the coronary artery by up to 95% and lasted for approximately 40 minutes. In addition, it lowered the heart rate (by about 12%), decreased oxygen consumption by the cardiac muscle, and increased blood perfusion to other parts of the body, including the ears and kidneys. It has shown positive effectiveness in treatment of cardiac ischemia or angina in dogs.[3,4]
- **Antiplatelet**: Administration of *Ye Ju Hua* is associated with inhibition of platelet aggregation. The inhibition was concluded by the study to be 2.3 times stronger than the inhibition exerted by *Dan Shen* (Radix Salviae Miltiorrhizae).[5]
- **Antihypertensive**: Both water and alcohol extracts of *Ye Ju Hua* have demonstrated marked effectiveness to lower blood pressure. This was achieved with oral or intraperitoneal injections, in awake or anesthetized animals, such as rats, cats, and dogs. The duration of action was approximately 2 hours. There was no inhibition of the respiratory system. The proposed mechanisms of the antihypertensive effect include inhibition of adrenalin or dilation of the blood vessels.[6,7]
- **Antibiotic**: *Ye Ju Hua* has both antibacterial and antiviral functions against micro-organisms such as *Bacillus dysenteriae*, leptospira, influenza virus, herpes virus, and dermatophytes. The water decoction was found to have stronger antibiotic effect than alcohol decoction of the herb.[8,9,10,11]

CLINICAL STUDIES AND RESEARCH

- **Common colds and influenza:** In one report, 501 patients with common colds or influenza were treated by oral administration of *Ye Ju Hua* with good results. The treatment was more effective for those with chief complaints of fever, aversion to cold and headache, and less effective for those with cough. In addition, those with

Ye Ju Hua (Flos Chrysanthemi Indici)

common colds or influenza characterized by wind-heat responded better than those with wind-cold.[12]

- **Prostatitis or pelvic inflammation:** In one clinical study, administration of *Ye Ju Hua* as suppository was 93% effective in treating 175 patients with prostatitis and 84% effective in treating 131 patients with pelvic inflammatory disease.[13]
- **Others**: According to one report, 454 patients with chronic pelvic inflammation, cervical erosion, chronic enteritis, or acute bacterial dysentery were treated with 4 grams of *Ye Ju Hua* via various routes of administration with an overall effectiveness of 88.5%. Routes of administration included intramuscular injection, rectal suppository at bedtime, or oral solution.[14]

HERB-DRUG INTERACTION

- **Anticoagulant or antiplatelet drugs:** *Ye Ju Hua* has antiplatelet influence, and should be used with caution in patients who take anticoagulant or antiplatelet medications. Though this potential interaction has not been documented, this herb may potentiate the effect of drugs such as warfarin.[15] [Note: Examples of anticoagulants include heparin, warfarin (Coumadin) and enoxaparin (Lovenox); and examples of antiplatelets include aspirin, dipyridamole (Persantine), and clopidogrel (Plavix).]

AUTHORS' COMMENTS

Please refer to *Ju Hua* (Flos Chrysanthemi) for comparison and contrast of different types of chrysanthemum flowers.

References

1. *Xian Dai Zhong Yao Yao Li Xue* (Contemporary Pharmacology of Chinese Herbs), 1997; 260-261
2. *The Merck Index* 12th edition, Chapman & Hall/CRCnetBASE/Merck, 2000
3. *Zhong Cao Yao* (Chinese Herbal Medicine), 1984; 15(4):14
4. *Zhe Jiang Zhong Yi Yao* (Zhejiang Chinese Medicine and Herbology), 1979; (10):377
5. *Chang Yong Zhong Yao Cheng Fen Yu Yao Li Shou Ce* (A Handbook of the Composition and Pharmacology of Common Chinese Drugs), 1994; 1600:1603
6. *Sheng Li Xue Bao* (Physiology News), 1959; 23(3):254
7. *Chang Yong Zhong Yao Cheng Fen Yu Yao Li Shou Ce* (A Handbook of the Composition and Pharmacology of Common Chinese Drugs), 1994; 1600:1603
8. *Zhong Hua Yi Xue Za Zhi* (Chinese Journal of Medicine), 1962; 48(3):188
9. *Yi Yao Wei Sheng* (Medicine, Medicinals, and Sanitation), 1973; (2):63
10. *Xin Yi Yao Xue Za Zhi* (New Journal of Medicine and Herbology), 1973; (1):26
11. *Chang Yong Zhong Yao Cheng Fen Yu Yao Li Shou Ce* (A Handbook of the Composition and Pharmacology of Common Chinese Drugs), 1994; 1600:1603
12. *Shan Dong Zhong Yi Xue Yuan Xue Bao* (Journal of Shandong University School of Chinese Medicine), 1987; 3:58
13. *Zhong Yao Tong Bao* (Journal of Chinese Herbology), 1985; 7:45
14. Ibid., 1983; 4:39
15. Chen, J. Recognition & prevention of herb-drug interactions, *Medical Acupuncture*, Fall/Winter 1998/1999; volume 10/number 2; 9-13

Lou Lu (Radix Rhapontici)

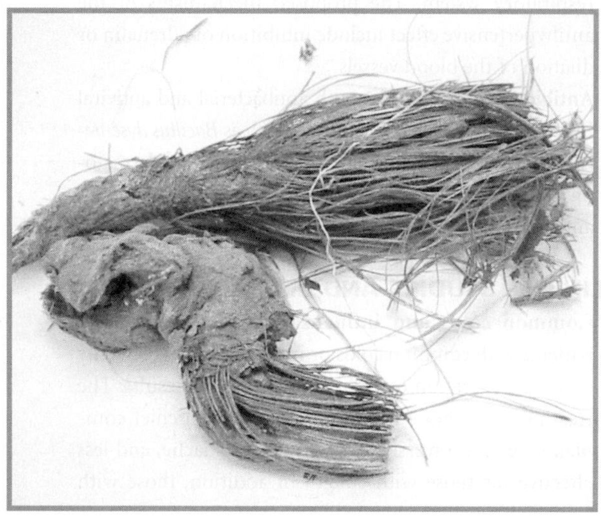

漏蘆 漏芦

Pinyin Name: *Lou Lu*
Literal Name: "leaking reed"
Original Source: *Shen Nong Ben Cao Jing* (Divine Husbandman's Classic of the Materia Medica) in the second century
English Name: rhaponticum, broadleaf globe thistle root
Botanical Name: *Rhaponticum uniflorum* (L.) DC. (*Chi Zhou Lou Lu*); *Echinops latifolius* Tausch (*Yu Zhou Lou Lu*)
Pharmaceutical Name: Radix Rhapontici
Properties: bitter, cold
Channels Entered: Stomach

Lou Lu (Radix Rhapontici)

CHINESE THERAPEUTIC ACTIONS

Clears Heat, Eliminates Toxins, Drains Abscesses, Promotes Lactation

Breast abscesses: *Lou Lu* (Radix Rhapontici) enters the *yangming* Stomach channel to treat breast abscesses formed by the accumulation of toxicity and heat.

- Swelling, pain and abscess of the breast: use *Lou Lu* with *Pu Gong Ying* (Herba Taraxaci), *Lian Qiao* (Fructus Forsythiae) and *Da Huang* (Radix et Rhizoma Rhei).
- Breast abscess with pus, that has ruptured: combine this herb with *Tian Hua Fen* (Radix Trichosanthis) and *Dang Gui* (Radicis Angelicae Sinensis).
- Breast abscess without pus, that has not ruptured: use *Lou Lu* with *Gua Lou Shi* (Fructus Trichosanthis), *Bai Zhi* (Radix Angelicae Dahuricae), *Pu Gong Ying* (Herba Taraxaci), and *Zao Jiao Ci* (Spina Gleditsiae).

Obstruction of lactation: *Lou Lu* promotes lactation in women who experience heat and toxicity blocking the channels. The affected breast is usually red and swollen. *Lou Lu* clears heat, eliminates toxins, disperses stagnation and reduces abscesses and swelling. This herb, however, should not be used for women whose lactation difficulties are caused by deficiency and cold.

- Insufficient milk production, or obstruction of milk flow, due to heat: use *Lou Lu* with *Wang Bu Liu Xing* (Semen Vaccariae) and *Chuan Shan Jia* (Squama Manis).

Dermatological disorders: *Lou Lu* treats sores, carbuncles, erysipelas, sore throat, and red, swollen and painful lesions caused by toxic heat.

- Dermatological disorders: use *Lou Lu* alone, or with appropriate heat-clearing and toxin-eliminating herbs.
- Sore throat: combine it with *Xuan Shen* (Radix Scrophulariae) and *Ban Lan Gen* (Radix Isatidis).

DOSAGE

5 to 12 grams in decoction.

CAUTIONS / CONTRAINDICATIONS

- Use of *Lou Lu* is not recommended in patients with insufficient milk, or lack of milk secretion because of qi and blood deficiencies.

CHEMICAL COMPOSITION

Echinopsine, hentriacontane, cardopatine, taxarerol acetate, essential oil.[1]

PHARMACOLOGICAL EFFECTS

- **Antioxidant:** *Lou Lu* has a strong antioxidant effect to maintain and protect the integrity of the cells. Antioxidant effect was observed in both water and alcohol extracts of the herb.[2]
- **Effect on the central nervous system:** In laboratory studies in mice, alcohol extract of *Lou Lu* inhibited the MAO-B activities in the brain.[3]

AUTHORS' COMMENTS

There are up to ten different herbs with the name "*Lou Lu*" given as an alternate name. For example, *Bai Tou Weng* (Radix Pulsatillae) is incorrectly used as *Lou Lu* (Radix Rhapontici) in certain regions in China. Therefore, when *Lou Lu* is prescribed, the desired substance should be properly specified.

References

1. *Chang Yong Zhong Yao Cheng Fen Yu Yao Li Shou Ce* (A Handbook of the Composition and Pharmacology of Common Chinese Drugs), 1994; 1780
2. *Zhong Xi Yi Jie He Za Zhi* (Journal of Integrated Chinese and Western Medicine), 1984; 4(11):686
3. *Zhong Yao Yao Li Yu Lin Chuan* (Pharmacology and Clinical Applications of Chinese Herbs), 1991; 7(6):24

Níu Huang (Calculus Bovis)

牛黄

Pinyin Name: *Niu Huang*
Literal Name: "cattle yellow"
Alternate Chinese Names: *Dan Huang, Ren Gong Niu Huang*
Original Source: *Shen Nong Ben Cao Jing* (Divine Husbandman's Classic of the Materia Medica) in the second century
English Name: cattle gallstone, bezoar
Zoological Name: *Bos taurus* domesticus Gmelin (*Niu Huang*)
Pharmaceutical Name: Calculus Bovis
Properties: bitter, cool
Channels Entered: Liver, Heart

CHINESE THERAPEUTIC ACTIONS

1. Clears Heat and Eliminates Toxins

Accumulation of heat toxins: *Niu Huang* (Calculus Bovis) treats accumulation of heat and toxins, a condition that refers to severe infection or inflammation.

- Sore, swollen throat, and ulcers on the throat or tongue: use *Niu Huang* with *Bing Pian* (Borneolum Syntheticum) and *Zhen Zhu* (Margarita) as powder. Apply topically.
- Boils, carbuncles, fibrocystic breast disorders and a wide variety of hot, painful swellings: combine it with *She Xiang* (Moschus), *Ru Xiang* (Gummi Olibanum) and *Mo Yao* (Myrrha).

2. Transforms Phlegm and Opens Orifices

Febrile disease with fire and phlegm in the Pericardium: Manic patients with this condition usually experience extreme psychological stimulation or anger. In this case, fire has turned the body fluids into phlegm; as phlegm is combined with fire it blocks the sensory orifices, causing *shen* (spirit) to be unable to reside peacefully in the Heart. Clinical manifestations include unconsciousness, delirious speech and high fever.

- Unconsciousness, delirious speech, high fever and convulsions: use *Niu Huang* with *She Xiang* (Moschus) and *Bing Pian* (Borneolum Syntheticum).

3. Arrests Tremors and Extinguishes Wind

Liver wind rising: Symptoms include convulsions, stroke, tremors, spasms, high fever, epilepsy, lockjaw, or fainting due to emotional distress.

- Liver wind rising: use *Niu Huang* with *She Xiang* (Moschus), *Gou Teng* (Ramulus Uncariae cum Uncis), *Quan Xie* (Scorpio) or *Tian Zhu Huang* (Concretio Silicea Bambusae).

DOSAGE

0.2 to 0.5 grams. *Niu Huang* is used mainly as pills or powder, as this substance is very expensive, and sometimes difficult to obtain.

CAUTIONS / CONTRAINDICATIONS

- *Niu Huang* should be used with caution during pregnancy, and in patients not presenting with excess heat.
- Though *Niu Huang* has very low toxicity, side effects and allergic reactions have been reported. Adverse reactions include eczema, mental disturbances, upper gastrointestinal bleeding, hematochezia, hematemesis, diarrhea, and wheezing.[1]
- Use of *Niu Huang* may be associated with possible drowsiness and sedation. Therefore, individuals who take this substance should exercise caution if driving or operating heavy machinery.

CHEMICAL COMPOSITION

Bile acid, bilirubin, cholesterol, amino acid.

PHARMACOLOGICAL EFFECTS

- **Effects on the central nervous system:** Administration of *Niu Huang* is associated with sedative, anticonvulsive and antipyretic effects. In one study, both *Niu Huang* and *Ren Gong Niu Huang* (Calculus Bovis Syntheticum) decreased spontaneous movement in mice. *Niu Huang* is also reported to counter the stimulation induced by caffeine and enhance the sedation caused by morphine and barbiturates. Though the exact mechanism of action is unclear, *Niu Huang* does have anticonvulsant effects, especially against convulsions induced by camphor or caffeine. Lastly, both *Niu Huang* and *Ren Gong Niu Huang* showed marked effectiveness against artificially-induced fever in rats and rabbits.[3,4,5,6]
- **Cardiovascular:** Administration of *Niu Huang* is associated with an inhibitory influence on the cardiovascular system characterized by a decrease of blood pressure and heart rate. Oral administration of 0.1 g/kg of *Niu Huang* significantly lowered blood pressure in mice with essential or renal hypertension. The hypotensive effect was reversed by atropine.[7,8]
- **Smooth muscle relaxant:** *Niu Huang* and *Ren Gong Niu*

Níu Huang (Calculus Bovis)

Huang (Calculus Bovis Syntheticum) have little effect on the normal contraction of the intestines. They do, however, relieve intestinal spasms and cramps by inhibiting the stimulation of smooth muscle by substances including (but not limited to) acetylcholine and barium chloride.[9]

- **Cholagogic:** According to studies in rabbits, administration of *Niu Huang* has a mild stimulating effect on the production and secretion of bile. The mild action is attributed to the mixed function of *Niu Huang* to simultaneously relax and contract the muscles and sphincter of the bile duct.[10]
- **Hematological:** Administration of *Niu Huang* is associated with an increase in red blood cell count in rabbits, with or without removal of the spleen. In another study, *Niu Huang* demonstrated a positive dose-effect relationship in treatment of anemia in rabbits.[11,12]
- **Anti-inflammatory:** Administration of *Niu Huang* via intraperitoneal injection once daily for 3 days was beneficial in treating ear inflammation in mice.[13]
- **Antibiotic:** *Niu Huang* inhibits *Mycobacterium tuberculosis* and *Staphylococcus aureus.*[14]

CLINICAL STUDIES AND RESEARCH

- **Infection:** In one clinical study, 476 patients with infections, such as upper respiratory infection, influenza, bronchitis, and pneumonia, were treated with a 75.2% success rate, using a preparation containing *Ren Gong Niu Huang* (Calculus Bovis Syntheticum).[15]

HERB-DRUG INTERACTION

- **Sedatives:** *Niu Huang* has a mild sedative effect. It reduces the stimulation induced by caffeine, and enhances the sedation caused by morphine and barbiturates.[16] [Note: Many categories of drugs induce sedation, such as antihistamines, narcotic analgesics, barbiturates, benzodiazepines and others.]

TOXICOLOGY

No fatalities were reported in mice following a bolus intraperitoneal injection of *Niu Huang* at 2 g/kg. No abnormalities were reported following intraperitoneal injection of *Niu Huang* at 0.6 g/kg daily for 6 days in mice. Nor were any abnormalities reported in rats following intraperitoneal injection of *Niu Huang* at 0.1 g/kg daily for 15 weeks.[17]

SUPPLEMENT

- 人工牛黄 *Ren Gong Niu Huang* (Calculus Bovis Syntheticum) is often used as a substitute for *Niu Huang* due to lack of supply of the natural substance. *Ren Gong Niu Huang* is produced by artificially inducing the production of stones in cattle or pigs. Clinical researches show that the pharmacological and therapeutic effects appear to be comparable to those of the original substance.

References

1. *Chang Yong Zhong Yao Cheng Fen Yu Yao Li Shou Ce* (A Handbook of the Composition and Pharmacology of Common Chinese Drugs), 1994; 557:566
2. *Xian Dai Zhong Yao Yao Li Xue* (Contemporary Pharmacology of Chinese Herbs), 1997; 277-278
3. *Zhong Cao Yao* (Chinese Herbal Medicine), 1988; 19(5):21
4. *Yao Xue Za Zhi* (Journal of Medicinals), 1967; 87:550
5. *Zhong Cheng Yao Yan Jiu* (Research of Chinese Patent Medicine), 1985; (10):26
6. *Zhong Guo Zhong Yao Za Zhi* (People's Republic of China Journal of Chinese Herbology), 199116(2):105
7. *Yao Xue Za Zhi* (Journal of Medicinals), 1965; 85(10):879
8. Ibid., 1966; 86(10):877
9. *Zhong Yao Cai Ke Ji* (Science and Technology of Chinese Herbal Material), 1984; (4):14
10. *Chang Yong Zhong Yao Cheng Fen Yu Yao Li Shou Ce* (A Handbook of the Composition and Pharmacology of Common Chinese Drugs), 1994; 13(3):676
11. *Dong Jing Yi Shi Xin Zhi* (Tokyo Journal of Medicine), 1931; (2749):2414
12. *Ri Ben Yao Wu Xue Za Zhi (Japanese Journal of Herbs)*, 1935; 21(1):23
13. *Zhong Yao Cai Ke Ji (Science and Technology of Chinese Herbal Material)*; 1984; (4):14
14. *Zhong Cheng Yao Yan Jiu (Research of Chinese Patent Medicine)*, 1985; (10):26
15. *Zhong Cao Yao Tong Xun (Journal of Chinese Herbal Medicine)*, 1972; 4:49
16. *Yao Xue Za Zhi (Journal of Medicinals)*, 1967; 87:550
17. *Zhong Guo Zhong Yao Za Zhi (People's Republic of China Journal of Chinese Herbology)*, 1991; 16(2):105

Zao Xiu (Rhizoma Paridis)

蚤休

Pinyin Name: *Zao Xiu*
Alternate Chinese Names: *Qi Ye Yi Zhi Hua, Chong Lou, Cao He Che*
English Name: paris rhizome
Botanical Name: *Paris polyphylla* Smith var. *yunnanensis* (Franch.) Hand. – Mazz.; *Paris polyphylla* Smith var. *chinensis* (Franch.) Hara.
Pharmaceutical Name: Rhizoma Paridis
Properties: bitter, cool
Channels Entered: Liver
Safety Index: slightly toxic

CHINESE THERAPEUTIC ACTIONS

1. Clears Heat and Eliminates Toxins

Toxic heat: Clinical manifestations include swollen and painful sores, scrofula, abscesses and carbuncles. *Zao Xiu* (Rhizoma Paridis) is extremely effective in eliminating various toxins. It is also effective in treating tonsillitis.

- Sores, abscesses and carbuncles: use *Zao Xiu* with *Jin Yin Hua* (Flos Lonicerae), *Ye Ju Hua* (Flos Chrysanthemi Indici) and *Huang Lian* (Rhizoma Coptidis).
- Scrofula: add *Xia Ku Cao* (Spica Prunellae).
- Tonsillitis: combine this herb with *Huang Qin* (Radix Scutellariae), *Chi Shao* (Radix Paeoniae Rubrae), *She Gan* (Rhizoma Belamcandae) and *Xuan Shen* (Radix Scrophulariae).

Snake bites: *Zao Xiu* is used topically to relieve the redness, swelling and pain associated with snake bites.

- Snake bites: mix *Zao Xiu* powder with vinegar and apply topically. It can also be taken orally with *Bai Hua She She Cao* (Herba Oldenlandia) in a decoction.

2. Reduces Swelling and Stops Pain

Traumatic injuries: Post-traumatic inflammation, swelling, redness, pain and bleeding are all treated by this herb.

- Traumatic injuries: use *Zao Xiu* alone topically. It can also be taken orally with *Ru Xiang* (Gummi Olibanum), *Mo Yao* (Myrrha) and *Yan Hu Suo* (Rhizoma Corydalis).

3. Extinguishes Liver Wind

Liver wind: Clinical manifestations include convulsions, dizziness, epilepsy, spasms and cramps.

- Liver wind: use *Zao Xiu* with *Chan Tui* (Periostracum Cicadae) and *Gou Teng* (Ramulus Uncariae cum Uncis).

DOSAGE

5 to 10 grams in decoction. Reduce the dosage if *Zao Xiu* is prescribed as powder or pills.

CAUTIONS / CONTRAINDICATIONS

Zao Xiu should be used with caution during pregnancy, and in patients with underlying deficiencies.

Xiong Dan (Fel Ursi)

熊膽 熊胆

Pinyin Name: *Xiong Dan*
Literal Name: "bear gallbladder"
Original Source: *Xin Xiu Ben Cao* (Newly Revised Materia Medica) by Su Jing in 657-659 A.D.
English Name: bear gallbladder
Zoological Name: *Ursus arctos* L. (*Zhong Xiong*); *Selenarctos thibetanus* G. Cuvier (*Hei Xiong*)
Pharmaceutical Name: Fel Ursi
Properties: bitter, cold
Channels Entered: Gallbladder, Heart, Liver
International Status: CITES I

Xiong Dan (Fel Ursi)

CHINESE THERAPEUTIC ACTIONS

1. Clears Heat and Eliminates Toxins

The bitter, cold nature of *Xiong Dan* (Fel Ursi) and its affinity for the Liver, Gallbladder and Heart channels made it one of the best substances historically for addressing excess pathogens attacking these regions. *Xiong Dan* would have been used either internally or topically to clear heat and eliminate toxins. Clinical applications include skin lesions, abscesses and ulcerations, sore throat, hemorrhoids, and jaundice.

- Sore throat due to toxic heat: *Xiong Dan* was combined with *Ban Lan Gen* (Radix Isatidis) and *Niu Bang Zi* (Fructus Arctii).
- Hemorrhoids due to accumulation of toxic heat and dampness: it was used with *Bing Pian* (Borneolum Syntheticum) topically to reduce swelling, pain and inflammation.
- Jaundice arising from damp-heat and toxins: it was combined with *Yin Chen Hao* (Herba Artemisiae Scopariae), *Zhi Zi* (Fructus Gardeniae) and *Da Huang* (Radix et Rhizoma Rhei).
- Topical use: this substance was used with *Bing Pian* (Borneolum Syntheticum) for swelling, pain and inflammation.

2. Extinguishes Liver Wind, Relieves Spasms

Liver wind: Clinical manifestations of Liver wind include muscle spasms and cramps, high fever, delirium, epilepsy, and childhood convulsions.

- Liver wind: *Xiong Dan* was used with *Zhu Sha* (Cinnabaris), *Yu Jin* (Radix Curcumae), and *Ming Fan* (Alumen).
- Childhood convulsions: add *Zhu Li* (Succus Bambusae).

3. Clears Liver Heat and Brightens the Eyes

Eye disorders: When Liver fire is present, clinical manifestations are redness, swelling and pain in the eyes, photophobia, excessive tearing, and visual obstruction.

- Eye disorders: *Xiong Dan* was used alone internally or topically.

DOSAGE

1.5 to 2.5 grams in powdered or pill form. *Xiong Dan* was used internally as pills or powder, and externally as drops. It was not generally used in decoctions.

CHEMICAL COMPOSITION

Tauroursodeoxycholic acid, taurocheuodeoxycholic acid, taurocholic acid, ursodeoxycholic acid, chenodeoxycholic acid, cholic acid, deoxycholic acid.[1]

PHARMACOLOGICAL EFFECTS

- **Cholagogic**: *Xiong Dan* stimulates the production and excretion of bile. It also dissolves gallstones.[2]
- **Others**: *Xiong Dan* has antibiotic, anti-inflammatory, antitussive, antiasthmatic, and antihypertensive effects.[3]

CLINICAL STUDIES AND RESEARCH

- **Renal hypertension:** Five patients with renal hypertension were treated with 0.5 grams of *Xiong Dan* powder, twice daily, with good results.[4]
- **Cholelithiasis:** In one study, 234 patients with cholesterol-predominant gallstones were treated with *Xiong Dan*. The dosages ranged from 0.75 to 1 gram, taken in 3 or 4 divided doses, for 3 to 18 months. At the conclusion of the study, 93 patients (39.7%) showed reduction or dissolution of gallstones.[5]

SUPPLEMENT

- 牛膽 / 牛胆 *Niu Dan* (Fel Bovis) - gallbladders from cattle, and 豬膽 / 猪胆 *Zhu Dan* (Fel Porcus) - gallbladders from pigs, have similar functions as *Xiong Dan* and are commonly used as its substitutes. *Niu Dan* and *Zhu Dan*, however, are weaker and require higher dosages to achieve the same therapeutic effect.

AUTHORS' COMMENTS

Xiong Dan (Fel Ursi) belongs in Appendix I of the Convention on International Trade in Endangered Species of Wild Fauna and Flora (CITES). Trade in *Xiong Dan* is strictly prohibited. The discussion of *Xiong Dan* in this text is included only to offer 1) the accurate history of its critically important usage in traditional herbal medicine, and 2) models for appropriate usage of effective substitute substances (see Supplement). The information should not be interpreted as condoning illegal use of this endangered species. For more information, please refer to Appendix 10.

References

1. *Xian Dai Zhong Yao Yao Li Xue* (Contemporary Pharmacology of Chinese Herbs), 1997; 271-272
2. *Zhong Yao Xue* (Chinese Herbology), 1998; 205:207
3. Ibid.
4. *Ha Er Bing Zhong Yi* (Haerbing Chinese Medicine), 1959; 6:4
5. *Lin Chuan Gan Dan Bing Za Zhi* (Clinical Journal of Hepatic and Gallbladder Diseases), 1988; 1:41

Bai Lian (Radix Ampelopsis)

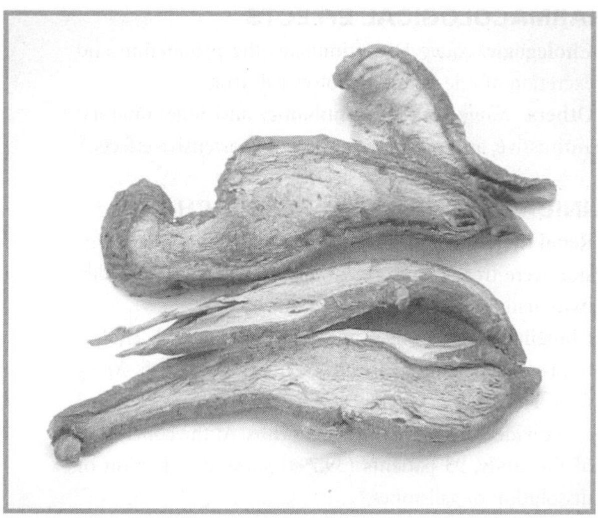

白蔹

Pinyin Name: *Bai Lian*
Original Source: *Shen Nong Ben Cao Jing* (Divine Husbandman's Classic of the Materia Medica) in the second century
English Name: ampelopsis, Japanese ampelopsis root
Botanical Name: *Ampelopsis japonica* (Thunb.) Makino (*Bai Lian*)
Pharmaceutical Name: Radix Ampelopsis
Properties: bitter, acrid, cool
Channels Entered: Heart, Stomach, Liver

CHINESE THERAPEUTIC ACTIONS

Clears Heat and Eliminates Toxins, Generates Flesh and Heals Wounds

Skin lesions: The bitter, cool attributes of *Bai Lian* (Radix Ampelopsis) help to reduce swelling, while the acrid quality of this herb helps to disperse stagnation. When used topically, it helps to heal ulcers by promoting the generation of flesh. Other clinical applications include carbuncles, sores, redness and swelling caused by damp-heat and toxicity.

- Sores, carbuncles, and other skin lesions: use *Bai Lian* with *Chi Xiao Dou* (Semen Phaseoli) and egg whites, and apply topically. Take with *Lian Qiao* (Fructus Forsythiae) internally.
- Burns: powdered *Bai Lian* can be applied topically as a single remedy.

DOSAGE

5 to 10 grams in decoctions.

CAUTIONS / CONTRAINDICATIONS

Bai Lian is incompatible with *Wu Tou* (Radix Aconiti).

Bai Xian Pi (Cortex Dictamni)

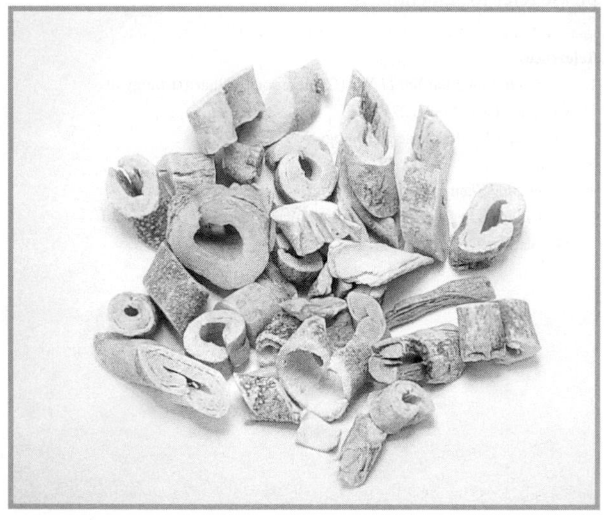

白鲜皮 白鮮皮

Pinyin Name: *Bai Xian Pi*
Literal Name: "white fresh bark"
Alternate Chinese Names: *Bai Tan*
Original Source: *Shen Nong Ben Cao Jing* (Divine Husbandman's Classic of the Materia Medica) in the second century
English Name: dictamnus, dense fruit pittany root bark
Botanical Name: *Dictamnus dasycarpus* Turcz. (*Bai Xian*)
Pharmaceutical Name: Cortex Dictamni
Properties: bitter, cold
Channels Entered: Spleen, Stomach

Bai Xian Pi (Cortex Dictamni)

CHINESE THERAPEUTIC ACTIONS

1. Clears Heat, Eliminates Toxins, and Alleviates Itching

Dermatological disorders caused by damp-heat: Clinically, *Bai Xian Pi* (Cortex Dictamni) is used most often to treat sores, carbuncles, rashes, eczema, ulceration, swelling and pain in the genital region, and similar conditions. In these cases, there is usually profuse oozing of fluids and ulceration of lesions.

- Dermatological disorders characterized by damp, heat and toxins: use *Bai Xian Pi* with *Ku Shen Gen* (Radix Sophorae Flavescentis), *Cang Zhu* (Rhizoma Atractylodis), and *Di Fu Zi* (Fructus Kochiae) internally as an herbal decoction, or topically as an herbal wash.

2. Clears Damp-Heat

Damp-heat jaundice: *Bai Xian Pi* clears damp-heat to treat jaundice.

- Damp-heat jaundice: use this herb with *Yin Chen Hao* (Herba Artemisiae Scopariae), *Da Huang* (Radix et Rhizoma Rhei), and *Zhi Zi* (Fructus Gardeniae). **Exemplar Formula:** *Yin Chen Hao Tang* (Artemisia Scoparia Decoction).

***Bi zheng* (painful obstruction syndrome):** *Bai Xian Pi* treats *bi zheng* caused by accumulation of heat and dampness manifesting in symptoms such as heaviness, redness and burning pain.

- *Bi zheng*: use it with *Ren Dong Teng* (Caulis Lonicerae) and *Wei Ling Xian* (Radix Clematidis).

DOSAGE

5 to 10 grams in decoction. *Bai Xian Pi* is used internally or topically.

CHEMICAL COMPOSITION

Alkaloid (dictamnine, skimmianine), triterpenoids (dictamnolactone, obacunone), dictamnolide, campesterol, sitosterol, limonoids, fraxinellore, limonin, rutaevin.[1,2]

N O OCH$_3$

Dictamnine

PHARMACOLOGICAL EFFECTS

- **Antifungal:** The water decoction of *Bai Xian Pi* has an inhibitory effect against various pathogenic fungi.[3]
- **Cardiovascular:** A small dose of dictamnine stimulates frog heart specimens, increasing cardiac contractility and cardiac output. It also causes constriction of blood vessels in rabbits.[4]

CLINICAL STUDIES AND RESEARCH

- **Suppurative dermatological disorders:** Topical application of *Bai Xian Pi* in fine powder form was 100% effective in treating 33 cases of suppurative dermatological disorders.[5]

HERB-DRUG INTERACTION

- **Antineoplastic drugs:** It has been proposed that obacunone, a component of *Bai Xian Pi*, may potentiate the effect of microtubule inhibitors. It was found that with the presence of obacunone, the cytotoxicity of vincristine, vinblastine and paclitaxel are all potentiated. However, there were no potentiating cytotoxic effects between obacunone and other antineoplastic drugs such as adriamycin, cisplatin or 5-florouracil.[6]

TOXICOLOGY

The LD_{50} for intraperitoneal injection of dictamnine is 150 to 250 mg/kg in mice.[7]

References

1. *Xian Dai Zhong Yao Yao Li Xue* (Contemporary Pharmacology of Chinese Herbs), 1997; 270
2. *The Merck Index* 12th edition, Chapman & Hall/CRCnetBASE/Merck, 2000
3. *Zhong Cao Yao Xue* (Study of Chinese Herbal Medicine), 1976: 527
4. Ibid.
5. *Chi Jiao Yi Shi Za Zhi* (Journal of Barefoot Doctors), 1975; 6:21
6. *Planta Med*, 2000 Feb; 66(1):74-6
7. *CA*, 1986; 104:62034p

2 HEAT-CLEARING HERBS

Qian Li Guang (Herba Senecionis Scandens)

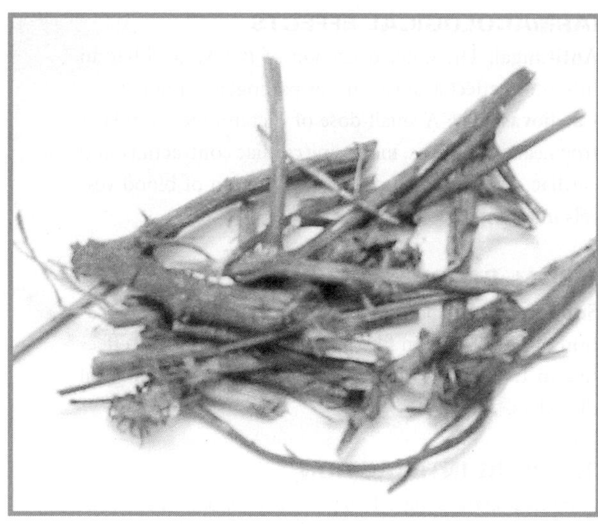

千里光

Pinyin Name: *Qian Li Guang*
Literal Name: "thousand mile brightness"
Alternate Chinese Names: *Qian Li Ji, Jiu Li Ming, Jiu Li Guang, Wu Teng Yi, Hu Die Yi, Ban Tian Lei, Tei Shao Chou*
Original Source: *Ben Cao Gang Mu Shi Yi* (Omissions from the Grand Materia Medica) by Zhao Xue-Min in 1765
English Name: senecio, climbing groundsel herb, ragwort herb
Botanical Name: *Senecio scandens* Buch.-Ham. (*Qian Li Guang*)
Pharmaceutical Name: Herba Senecionis Scandens
Properties: bitter, cold
Channels Entered: Lung, Liver, Large Intestine

CHINESE THERAPEUTIC ACTIONS

1. Clears Heat and Eliminates Toxins

Dermatological disorders: *Qian Li Guang* (Herba Senecionis Scandens) is used internally or externally to treat heat, toxicity and dampness in carbuncles, eczema, diarrhea, dysentery and intestinal abscesses.

- Dermatological disorders: use *Qian Li Guang* with *Ye Ju Hua* (Flos Chrysanthemi Indici), *Jin Yin Hua* (Flos Lonicerae) and *Pu Gong Ying* (Herba Taraxaci).
- Diarrhea, dysentery, or intestinal abscesses: combine it with *Huang Lian* (Rhizoma Coptidis) and *Huang Qin* (Radix Scutellariae).

2. Clears Liver Yang and Brightens the Eyes

Redness and swelling of the eyes: Liver yang rising can cause eye redness, pain and swelling. *Qian Li Guang* is often made into eyedrops to treat acute or chronic conjunctivitis, trachoma, keratitis, and corneal ulcers.

- Eye disorders: use *Qian Li Guang* alone as a wash.

DOSAGE

10 to 30 grams in decoction.

CHEMICAL COMPOSITION

Flavoxanthin, chrysanthemaxanthin, alkaloids, essential oils, flavonoids.[1]

PHARMACOLOGICAL EFFECTS

- **Antibiotic:** It has a broad spectrum of inhibitory activity against *Bacillus dysenteriae, Staphylococcus aureus, Salmonella typhi, Bacillus paratyphosus, Pseudomonas aeruginosa*, and *Diplococcus meningitidis*. The leaves and flowers have the strongest antibiotic effect, while the stems and roots have less.[2]

CLINICAL STUDIES AND RESEARCH

- **Inflammatory disorders:** In a clinical study, 1,338 patients suffering from inflammatory conditions were treated with three pills of *Qian Li Guang* (0.35 grams each) four times daily. Complete recovery was reported in 62% of the patients, improvement in 25%, and no response in 13%. Patients with acute tonsillitis, acute dysentery, acute enteritis, and acute appendicitis were most responsive to the treatment.[3]
- **Topical antibiotic:** Distillation of *Qian Li Guang* solution was used in place of rubbing alcohol to clean the skin. No infection was reported in over 1,600 patients with external injuries, and 24,000 patients who had intramuscular or subcutaneous injections.[4]

References

1. *Zhong Yao Xue* (Chinese Herbology), 1998; 217
2. Ibid.
3. *Zhong Cao Yao Tong Xun* (Journal of Chinese Herbal Medicine), 1971; 3:19
4. *Yi Yao Wei Sheng* (Medicine, Medicinals, and Sanitation), 1973; 2:19

Ji Gu Cao (Herba Abri)

雞骨草 鸡骨草

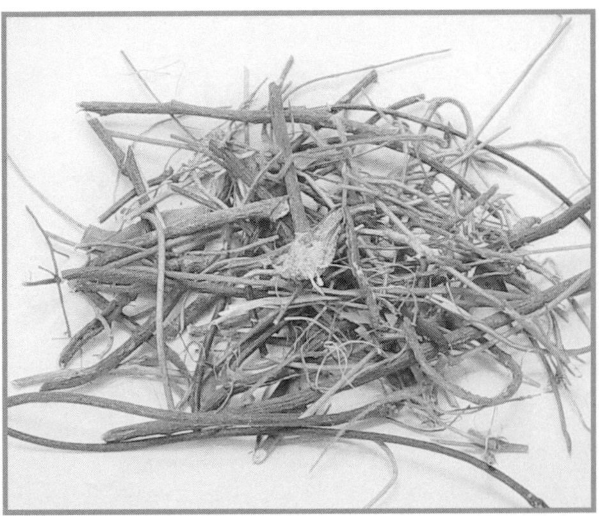

Pinyin Name: *Ji Gu Cao*
Literal Name: "chicken bone herb"
Original Source: *Ling Nan Cai Yao Lu* (Records of Picking Herbs in Guangdong)
English Name: Abrus
Botanical Name: *Arbus fruticulosus* Wall. Ex Wight et Arn. (*Guan Dong Xiang Si Zi*)
Pharmaceutical Name: Herba Abri
Properties: sweet, cool
Channels Entered: Liver, Gallbladder

CHINESE THERAPEUTIC ACTIONS

1. Clears Heat and Eliminates Toxins

Jaundice and infectious hepatitis caused by damp-heat: The sweet, cool nature of *Ji Gu Cao* (Herba Abri) and its affinity for the Liver and Gallbladder make it most useful to treat damp-heat jaundice and hepatitis.

- Jaundice and hepatitis: use *Ji Gu Cao* with *Yin Chen Hao* (Herba Artemisiae Scopariae), *Da Huang* (Radix et Rhizoma Rhei) and *Bai Hua She She Cao* (Herba Oldenlandia).

2. Drains Dampness and Disperses Stagnation

Traumatic injuries: *Ji Gu Cao* reduces the inflammation and pain associated with post-traumatic injuries with blood stagnation.

DOSAGE

6 to 15 grams.

CHEMICAL COMPOSITION

Abrine, choline, saponins, tannins, anthraquinone glycosides, β-sitosterol, stigmasterol, chrysophanol, physcion.[1]

PHARMACOLOGICAL EFFECTS

- **Hepatoprotective:** The saponins of *Ji Gu Cao* have been shown to protect the liver from carbon tetrachloride-induced damage in animals.[2]

CLINICAL STUDIES AND RESEARCH

- **Hepatitis:** In one study, 70 patients with various types of hepatitis were treated with a decoction of *Ji Gu Cao* (120 grams of fresh herb or 60 grams of dried herb) and sugar (60 grams) taken in two equally-divided doses daily. The dosage was reduced by half in children. Patients were instructed to continue the herbal treatment until the symptoms resolved. The study reported satisfactory results, with good responses observed in early stages of the disorder and in children. The herbal treatment was most effective if started early, and not effective for chronic cases of hepatitis.[3]

References

1. *Chang Yong Zhong Yao Cheng Fen Yu Yao Li Shou Ce* (A Handbook of the Composition and Pharmacology of Common Chinese Drugs), 1994; 1151
2. *Chem Pharm Bull*, 1990; 38(3)824
3. *Zhe Jiang Zhong Yi Za Zhi* (Zhejiang Journal of Chinese Medicine), 1960; 4:166

Ban Bian Lian (Herba Lobeliae Chinensis)

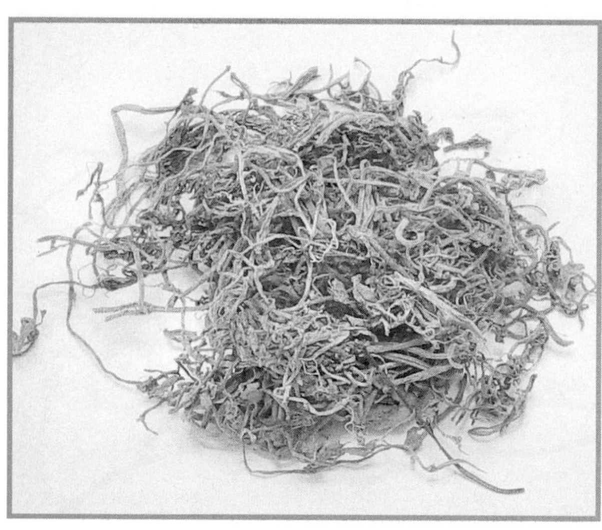

半邊蓮 半边莲

Pinyin Name: *Ban Bian Lian*
Literal Name: "half-sided lotus," "half-edged lily"
Alternate Chinese Names: *Ji Jie Suo, Ban Bian Ju*
Original Source: *Ben Cao Gang Mu* (Materia Medica) by Li Shi-Zhen in 1578
English Name: lobelia, Chinese lobelia herb
Botanical Name: *Lobelia chinensis* Lour. (*Ban Bian Lian*)
Pharmaceutical Name: Herba Lobeliae Chinensis
Properties: acrid, cold
Channels Entered: Heart, Lung, Small Intestine

CHINESE THERAPEUTIC ACTIONS

1. Clears Heat and Eliminates Toxins

Toxic heat: *Ban Bian Lian* (Herba Lobeliae Chinensis) treats various dermatological conditions characterized by heat and toxins. Clinical applications include stings and bites from bees, snakes, scorpions and centipedes. It is also effective for sores, swellings, lesions and ulcerations.

- Insect or snake bites: use *Ban Bian Lian* both internally and topically simultaneously. Also, combine it with *Huang Qin* (Radix Scutellariae), *Huang Lian* (Rhizoma Coptidis), *Jin Yin Hua* (Flos Lonicerae) and *Ye Ju Hua* (Flos Chrysanthemi Indici).
- Sores and lesions: use *Ban Bian Lian* with other herbs, internally or topically.

2. Regulates Water Circulation and Eliminates Water Retention

Edema: *Ban Bian Lian* regulates water circulation and reduces edema.

- Edema: use this herb with *Fu Ling* (Poria), *Zhu Ling* (Polyporus) and *Ze Xie* (Rhizoma Alismatis).

Ascites: *Ban Bian Lian* treats ascites whether caused by parasites or found in late stages of liver cirrhosis involving dysuria.

- Ascites: use *Ban Bian Lian* with *Hu Lu Ba* (Semen Trigonellae).

DOSAGE

10 to 20 grams of dried *Ban Bian Lian*, 30 to 60 grams of the fresh herb, in decoction.

CAUTIONS / CONTRAINDICATIONS

- *Ban Bian Lian* is contraindicated in patients who have edema caused by deficiency.

CHEMICAL COMPOSITION

Lobeline, lobelanine, lobelanidine, isolobelanine, lobelinin.[1]

PHARMACOLOGICAL EFFECTS

- **Respiratory:** *Ban Bian Lian* has a stimulating effect on the respiratory system. It has been shown to effectively reverse respiratory depression associated with the use of morphine in dogs. It is also effective in reversing respiratory depression induced by insect or snake venom.[2]
- **Diuretic:** Intravenous injection of *Ban Bian Lian* in anesthetized dogs is associated with a marked and prolonged diuretic effect.[3]
- **Antihypertensive:** Intravenous injection of a *Ban Bian Lian* preparation is associated with a marked and prolonged influence to lower blood pressure in anesthetized dogs. Similar effects may be observed following oral administration, but 10 to 20 times the normal dosage is required.[4]
- **Others:** *Ban Bian Lian* has diuretic, cholagogic, hemostatic, and antibiotic effects.

CLINICAL STUDIES AND RESEARCH

- **Schistosomal ascites:** In a clinical study, 120 patients with late-stage schistosomal ascites were treated with an herbal decoction with an overall effective rate of 83.3%. The treatment protocol was to administer the decoction once daily, for a total of 30 days. The herbal formula contained *Ban Bian Lian* 30g, *Dan Shen* (Radix Salviae Miltiorrhizae) 9g, *Dang Gui* (Radicis Angelicae Sinensis) 6g, *Fu Ling* (Poria) 12g, and *Bing Lang* (Semen Arecae) 6g.[5]
- **Snake bites:** According to one report, 14 snake bite patients recovered completely with herbal treatment.

Ban Bian Lian (Herba Lobeliae Chinensis)

The treatment protocol included both oral and topical administration of *Ban Bian Lian*. For oral ingestion, 30 to 120 grams of the herb was used to prepare the decoction, which was taken in equally-divided portions three times daily. For topical application, the fresh herb was crushed into paste and applied onto the affected area.[6]

HERB-DRUG INTERACTION

- **Diuretics:** *Ban Bian Lian* has a diuretic effect. Though no potential interaction has been documented, concurrent use with diuretic drugs may lead to increased elimination of water and/or electrolytes.[7] [Note: Examples of diuretics include chlorothiazide, hydrochlorothiazide, furosemide (Lasix), bumetanide (Bumex), and torsemide (Demadex).]

TOXICOLOGY

The LD_{50} for intravenous injection of a *Ban Bian Lian* preparation is 6.10 g/kg in mice. Symptoms of overdose included excitation, mania, and muscle contractions.[8]

References

1. *Xian Dai Zhong Yao Yao Li Xue* (Contemporary Pharmacology of Chinese Herbs), 1997; 775-776
2. *Zhong Yao Yao Li Yu Ying Yong* (Pharmacology and Applications of Chinese Herbs), 1983; 389
3. Ibid.
4. Ibid.
5. *Zhong Hua Nei Ke Za Zhi* (Chinese Journal of Internal Medicine), 1959; 5:406
6. *Zhong Hua Wai Ke Za Zhi* (Chinese Journal of External Medicine), 1960; 4:369
7. Chen, J. Recognition & prevention of herb-drug interactions, *Medical Acupuncture*, Fall/Winter 1998/1999; volume 10/number 2; 9-13
8. *Chang Yong Zhong Yao Cheng Fen Yu Yao Li Shou Ce* (A Handbook of the Composition and Pharmacology of Common Chinese Drugs), 1994;

Cha Chi Huang (Herba Stellariae Aquaticae)

茶匙癀

Pinyin Name: *Cha Chi Huang*
Alternate Chinese Names: *Ji Chang Cao, E Chang Cai, Chou Jin Cao, Ji Ran Cai, Ya Chang Cao, Niu Fan Lu, Ya Ran Cai*
English Name: stellaria
Botanical Name: *Stellaria aquatica* Scop.
Pharmaceutical Name: Herba Stellariae Aquaticae
Properties: acrid, slightly bitter, neutral
Channels Entered: Liver, Large Intestine, San Jiao

CHINESE THERAPEUTIC ACTIONS

1. Clears Heat and Eliminates Toxins

Cha Chi Huang (Herba Stellariae Aquaticae) has a potent and broad spectrum of heat-clearing and toxin-eliminating effects. It is commonly used to treat infection, inflammation, swelling, and other presentations of heat and toxins.

- Dysentery: use *Cha Chi Huang* with *Feng Wei Cao* (Herba Pteris), *Huang Lian* (Rhizoma Coptidis), *Bai Tou Weng* (Radix Pulsatillae), *Ge Gen* (Radix Puerariae) and *Huang Qin* (Radix Scutellariae).
- Chronic appendicitis: use it with *Zao Jiao Ci* (Spina Gleditsiae), *Chuan Shan Jia* (Squama Manis), *Dong Gua Zi* (Semen Benincasae), *Mu Dan Pi* (Cortex Moutan), and *Da Huang* (Radix et Rhizoma Rhei). The formulas *Zhen Ren Huo Ming Yin* (True Man Decoction to Revitalize Life) or *Da Huang Mu Dan Tang* (Rhubarb and Moutan Decoction) can also be used.
- Hypertension from Liver fire: combine this herb with *Gou Teng* (Ramulus Uncariae cum Uncis), *Ge Gen* (Radix Puerariae), *Che Qian Zi* (Semen Plantaginis) and *Xia Ku Cao* (Spica Prunellae).
- Sores, carbuncles and toxic swelling: use it with *Jin Yin Hua* (Flos Lonicerae), *Zi Cao Gen* (Radix Lithospermi), *Huang Qin* (Radix Scutellariae) and *Huang Lian* (Rhizoma Coptidis).

Cha Chi Huang (Herba Stellariae Aquaticae)

- Headache and eye disorders caused by Liver yang rising: use *Cha Chi Huang* with *Gou Teng* (Ramulus Uncariae cum Uncis), *Ge Gen* (Radix Puerariae), *Qing Xiang Zi* (Semen Celosiae) and *Xia Ku Cao* (Spica Prunellae).
- Palpable abdominal masses in postpartum women: combine it with *Dang Gui* (Radicis Angelicae Sinensis), *Chuan Xiong* (Rhizoma Ligustici Chuanxiong), *Tao Ren* (Semen Persicae), *Pao Jiang* (Rhizoma Zingiberis Preparatum) and *Zhi Gan Cao* (Radix Glycyrrhizae Preparata).
- Irregular menstruation: add it to *Tao Hong Si Wu Tang* (Four-Substance Decoction with Safflower and Peach Pit) or *Jia Wei Xiao Yao San* (Augmented Rambling Powder).
- General inflammation: incorporate it with *Hu Yao Huang* (Herba Leucas Mollissimae), *Hu Zhang* (Rhizoma Polygoni Cuspidati) and *Liu Zhi Huang* (Herba Solidaginis).

2. Invigorates Blood, Breaks Blood Stasis and Reduces Swelling

Cha Chi Huang treats disorders characterized by blood stagnation and swelling in the local area.

- Endometriosis or cervicitis: combine *Cha Chi Huang* with *Tao Ren* (Semen Persicae), *San Leng* (Rhizoma Sparganii), *E Zhu* (Rhizoma Curcumae), *Xiang Fu* (Rhizoma Cyperi), *Ya She Huang* (Herba Lippiae), *Pao Zai Cao* (Herba Physalis Angulatae), *Chuan Shan Jia* (Squama Manis), *Zao Jiao Ci* (Spina Gleditsiae) and *Mu Dan Pi* (Cortex Moutan).
- Hemorrhoids: use *Cha Chi Huang* alone as an external wash. It may also be combined with *Zao Jiao Ci* (Spina Gleditsiae). For best results, combine it with *Zhen Ren Huo Ming Yin* (True Man Decoction to Revitalize Life) and *Shao Yao Tang* (Peony Decoction).
- Swellings and abscesses: use it with *Jin Yin Hua* (Flos Lonicerae), *Zi Cao Gen* (Radix Lithospermi), *Da Huang* (Radix et Rhizoma Rhei), *Huang Lian* (Rhizoma Coptidis), *Huang Qin* (Radix Scutellariae) and *Gan Cao* (Radix Glycyrrhizae).

3. Promotes Urination

- Dysuria: use *Cha Chi Huang* with *Bian Xu* (Herba Polygoni Avicularis), *Qu Mai* (Herba Dianthi), *Che Qian Zi* (Semen Plantaginis), and *Shui Ding Xiang* (Herba Ludwigiae Prostratae) to promote the free flow of urine.

4. Promotes Lactation

- Blockage of lactation caused by inflammation and obstruction: combine *Cha Chi Huang* with *Chuan Shan Jia* (Squama Manis), *Wang Bu Liu Xing* (Semen Vaccariae), *Pu Gong Ying* (Herba Taraxaci) and *Chuan Mu Tong* (Caulis Clematidis Armandii).

DOSAGE

6 to 15 grams in decoction.

CAUTIONS / CONTRAINDICATIONS

- Use *Cha Chi Huang* with caution during pregnancy.
- *Cha Chi Huang* is contraindicated in patients who have weak constitutions.

Dao Di Wu Gong (Rhizoma Heliminthostachytis)

倒地蜈蚣　倒地蜈蚣

Pinyin Name: *Dao Di Wu Gong*
Literal Name: "upside-down centipede"
Alternate Chinese Names: *Di Wu Gong, Ru Di Wu Gong, Guo Lu Wu Gong, Di Ding Wu Gong*
English Name: Ceylan helminthostachys rhizome
Botanical Name: *Helminthostachys zeylanica* (L.) Hook
Pharmaceutical Name: Rhizoma Heliminthostachytis
Properties: bitter, cold
Channels Entered: Lung

Dao Di Wu Gong (Rhizoma Heliminthostachytis)

CHINESE THERAPEUTIC ACTIONS

Reduces Inflammation, Clears Heat, Eliminates Toxins, Reduces Swelling

Dao Di Wu Gong (Rhizoma Heliminthostachytis) clears heat, eliminates toxins, and reduces swelling and inflammation. It is generally combined with other herbs to enhance the heat-clearing effect.

- Stomatitis: crush and apply *Dao Di Wu Gong* topically. Internally, use this herb with *Huang Lian* (Rhizoma Coptidis), *Huang Qin* (Radix Scutellariae), *Zhi Zi* (Fructus Gardeniae), *Bo He* (Herba Menthae), *Lian Qiao* (Fructus Forsythiae), *Xuan Shen* (Radix Scrophulariae) and *Niu Bang Zi* (Fructus Arctii).
- Herpes zoster: crush the fresh herb to a paste consistency and apply topically to the affected area. For best results, internally, combine with *Zhen Ren Huo Ming Yin* (True Man Decoction to Revitalize Life) and *Zheng Gu Zi Jin Dan* (Purple and Gold Pill for Righteous Bones).
- Dysentery: crush and mix this herb with honey for topical application. For internal use, use with *Chuan Xin Lian* (Herba Andrographis), *Ji Xue Cao* (Herba Centellae), *Feng Wei Cao* (Herba Pteris) and *Bai Tou Weng* (Radix Pulsatillae).
- Joint pain throughout the body, caused by wind-heat invasion: add *Dao Di Wu Gong* to *Hong Gu She* (Radix Kadsura Japonicae).
- Fever with inflammation: use it with *Da Ding Huang* (Caulis Euonymi).

DOSAGE

6 to 15 grams in decoction.

CAUTIONS / CONTRAINDICATIONS

Dao Di Wu Gong should be used with caution for patients experiencing deficiency and coldness, because of its bitter, cold nature.

CHEMICAL COMPOSITION

Phosphorus, iron, calcium.

Jin Guo Lan (Radix Tinosporae)

金果欖 金果榄

Pinyin Name: *Jin Guo Lan*
Literal Name: "golden fruit"
Alternate Chinese Names: *Di Ku Dan, Jiu Niu Dan, Jin Niu Dan*
English Name: tinospora, arrow-shaped tinospora root, hairy stalk tinospora root
Botanical Name: *Tinospora capillipes* Gagn. (*Jin Guo Lan*); *Tinospora sagittata* Gagn. (*Qin Niu Dan*)
Pharmaceutical Name: Radix Tinosporae
Properties: bitter, cold
Channels Entered: Lung, Large Intestine

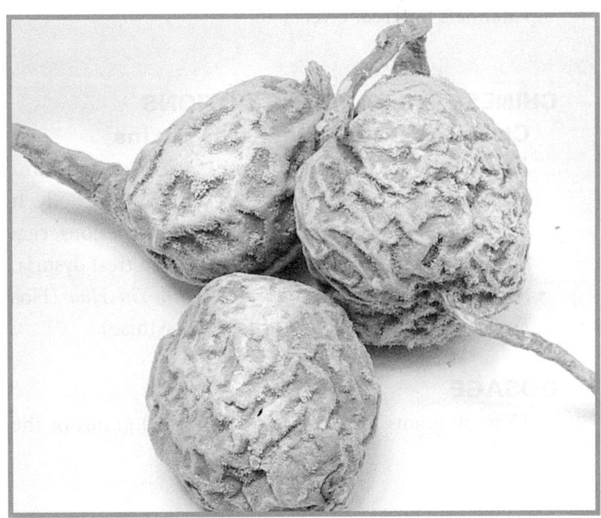

CHINESE THERAPEUTIC ACTIONS

Clears Heat, Eliminates Toxins

Bitter and cold, *Jin Guo Lan* (Radix Tinosporae) clears heat from the Lung and toxins from the throat. Clinically, it is used mainly for disorders of the throat, such as soreness, swelling, and abscesses. It is also effective for treating gastrointestinal disorders arising from Stomach heat, such as abdominal pain and diarrhea. When used topically, it is effective in treating various dermatological disorders, such as carbuncles, furuncles, sores, and ulcers.

- Sore throat: use *Jin Guo Lan* individually, or with *Ban*

Jin Guo Lan (Radix Tinosporae)

Lan Gen (Radix Isatidis) and *Da Qing Ye* (Folium Isatidis).

- Carbuncles and furuncles: mix it with vinegar and apply topically.

DOSAGE

3 to 9 grams.

CHEMICAL COMPOSITION

Flavonoids.[1]

CLINICAL STUDIES AND RESEARCH

Phlebitis: In one study, 7 out of 8 patients with phlebitis had good results when they were treated by topical application of herbs. The topical preparation was made by mixing *Jin Guo Lan* with 75% rubbing alcohol.[2]

References

1. *Zhong Yao Xue* (Chinese Herbology), 1998; 237
2. *Xin Yi Xue* (New Medicine), 1973; 1:25

Liu Ye (Folium Salicis Babylonicae)

柳葉 柳叶

Pinyin Name: *Liu Ye*
Literal Name: "willow leaves"
Alternate Chinese Names: *Liu Shu Ye*
English Name: weeping willow, Babylon weeping willow leaves
Botanical Name: *Salix babylonica*
Pharmaceutical Name: Folium Salicis Babylonicae
Properties: bitter, cold
Channels Entered: Liver

CHINESE THERAPEUTIC ACTIONS

Clears Heat and Eliminates Toxins

Liu Ye (Folium Salicis Babylonicae) clears heat and eliminates toxins, especially from the exterior of the body. It is used internally or topically to treat sores, lesions, carbuncles, and measles. It can also be used to treat dysuria.

- Sores and lesions: use *Liu Ye* with *Jin Yin Hua* (Flos Lonicerae) and *Lian Qiao* (Fructus Forsythiae).

DOSAGE

15 to 30 grams for dried *Liu Ye*, 30 to 60 grams of the fresh herb.

AUTHORS' COMMENTS

Willow bark, the bark from the Salix species, has been used in many cultures for treatment of fever and pain. Willow bark contains salicylic acid (1.5-12%) and salicin (0.1-2%). In fact, willow bark is the phytotherapeutic precursor to acetylsalicylic acid (aspirin), one of the most commonly used drugs in the world.

Bai Hua She She Cao (Herba Oldenlandia)

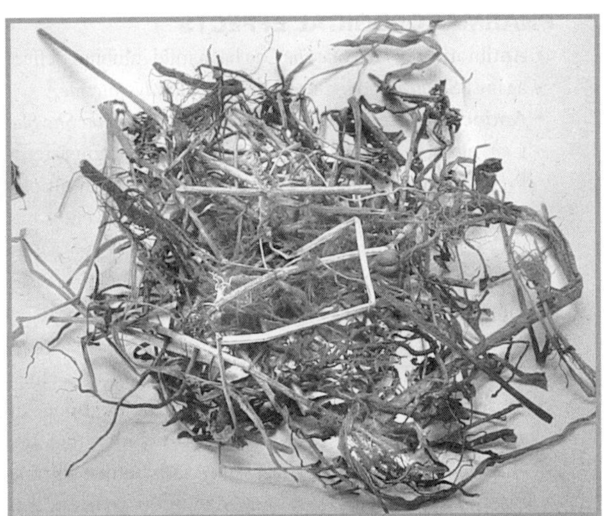

白花蛇舌草
白花蛇舌草

Pinyin Name: *Bai Hua She She Cao*
Literal Name: "white-flower snake tongue herb," "white-patterned snake's tongue herb"
Alternate Chinese Names: *She She Cao, Er Ye Lu*
Original Source: *Guangxi Zhong Yao Zhi* (Guangxi Journal of Chinese Herbal Medicines)
English Name: oldenlandia, spreading hedyotis herb
Botanical Name: *Oldenlandia diffusa* (Willd.) Roxb., [also known as *Hedyotis diffusa* (Willd.) Roxb.]
Pharmaceutical Name: Herba Oldenlandia
Properties: slightly bitter, sweet, cold
Channels Entered: Stomach, Large Intestine, Small Intestine

CHINESE THERAPEUTIC ACTIONS

1. Clears Heat, Eliminates Toxins, Reduces Abscesses

Toxic heat: *Bai Hua She She Cao* (Herba Oldenlandia) clears heat and eliminates toxins, and is commonly used both internally and topically. Clinical applications include intestinal abscesses, skin sores and carbuncles, sore throat, snake bite, tumors, cancer and hepatitis.

- Intestinal abscess: use *Bai Hua She She Cao* with *Hong Teng* (Caulis Sargentodoxae) and *Bai Jiang Cao* (Herba cum Radice Patriniae).
- Skin sores and carbuncles: use it with *Jin Yin Hua* (Flos Lonicerae), *Lian Qiao* (Fructus Forsythiae) and *Ye Ju Hua* (Flos Chrysanthemi Indici).
- Sore throat: combine it with *Xuan Shen* (Radix Scrophulariae), *Jie Geng* (Radix Platycodonis) and *Gan Cao* (Radix Glycyrrhizae).
- Snake bite: add it to *Ban Bian Lian* (Herba Lobeliae Chinensis) and *Zi Hua Di Ding* (Herba Violae), and apply topically.

Cancer: *Bai Hua She She Cao* has been used in recent years to treat various types of cancers. It is generally combined with other heat-clearing and toxins-eliminating herbs for optimal results.

- Cancer: use this herb with *Ban Zhi Lian* (Herba Scutellariae Barbatae), *Shan Ci Gu* (Pseudobulbus Cremastrae), *E Zhu* (Rhizoma Curcumae), *Shan Dou Gen* (Radix Sophorae Tonkinensis) and other antineoplastic herbs.
- Lung cancer: use *Bai Hua She She Cao* 60g, *Zi Cao Gen* (Radix Lithospermi) 60g, *Qian Hu* (Radix Peucedani) 30g, and *Niu Huang* (Calculus Bovis) 10g. The first three ingredients should be used in powdered extract form and mixed with powdered *Niu Huang* (Calculus Bovis). The dosage is 1.5 grams per dose, three times daily.
- Cancer of the esophagus, stomach and colon: use *Bai Hua She She Cao* 60g, *Huang Yao Zi* (Herba Dioscoreae Bulbiferae) 60g, *Shan Dou Gen* (Radix Sophorae Tonkinensis) 120g, *Bai Jiang Cao* (Herba cum Radice Patriniae) 120g, *Bai Xian Pi* (Cortex Dictamni) 120g, and *Xia Ku Cao* (Spica Prunellae) 120g. Powder and mix with honey to make pills. Administer 4 to 6 pills daily.

2. Drains Dampness

Lin zheng **(dysuria syndrome):** *Bai Hua She She Cao* drains dampness to relieve pain and burning sensations on urination. It also treats damp-heat jaundice.

- *Shi-re lin* (damp-heat dysuria): use *Bai Hua She She Cao* with *Bai Mao Gen* (Rhizoma Imperatae), *Che Qian Cao* (Herba Plantaginis) and *Shi Wei* (Folium Pyrrosiae).
- Damp-heat jaundice: combine it with *Yin Chen Hao* (Herba Artemisiae Scopariae), *Huang Bai* (Cortex Phellodendri) and *Zhi Zi* (Fructus Gardeniae).

DOSAGE

15 to 60 grams in decoction.

CHEMICAL COMPOSITION

Hentriacontane, stigmasterol, ursolic acid, oleanolic acid, β-sitosterol, β-sitosterol-D-glucoside, flavonoids.[1]

Bai Hua She She Cao (Herba Oldenlandia)

PHARMACOLOGICAL EFFECTS

- **Antibiotic:** *Bai Hua She She Cao* has a mild inhibitory effect against *Staphylococcus aureus* and *Bacillus dysenteriae*.[2]
- **Antineoplastic:** Reports on the effect of *Bai Hua She She Cao* against cancer cells have not been consistent. Preliminary reports indicate that it inhibits the multiplication of cancer cells, though its clinical effectiveness has yet to be confirmed.[3]
- **Antivenom:** Injection of *Bai Hua She She Cao* decreases mortality in mice bitten by poisonous snakes.[4]

CLINICAL STUDIES AND RESEARCH

- **Appendicitis:** A journal that evaluated the treatment of appendicitis in over 1,000 patients concluded that the effectiveness of Chinese herbs was satisfactory. Simple cases of appendicitis were treated with 60 grams of *Bai Hua She She Cao* in decoction, given through two to three equally-divided doses. In severe cases, the herbal treatments were modified to include *Hai Jin Sha* (Herba Lygodii), *Ye Ju Hua* (Flos Chrysanthemi Indici), or combined with *Da Huang Mu Dan Tang* (Rhubarb and Moutan Decoction), *Long Dan Xie Gan Tang* (Gentiana Decoction to Drain the Liver), or *Xian Fang Huo Ming Yin* (Sublime Formula for Sustaining Life).[5]
- **Snake bite:** According to one report, 19 snake bite patients were treated internally and topically with *Bai Hua She She Cao*, with complete recovery in all patients. The treatment protocol was to cook 15 grams of the herb in grain-based liquor, with 2/3 of the final solution given orally over 2 to 3 equally-divided doses, and 1/3 of the solution applied topically.[6]
- **Hepatitis:** In one study, 72 patients with acute icteric jaundice were treated with an herbal formula with 100% effectiveness. The average duration of hospitalization was 25.3 days. The herbal formula was given in syrup form. It contained 31.25 grams of *Bai Hua She She Cao*, 31.25 grams of *Xia Ku Cao* (Spica Prunellae), and 15.625 grams of *Gan Cao* (Radix Glycyrrhizae).[7]
- **Reduction of sperm production:** In a clinical study, 102 patients were treated with *Bai Hua She She Cao* for 3 weeks for evaluation of its effect on sperm production. The study reported that in 77% of patients, there was a 10-33% reduction of total sperm count.[8]
- **Cancer**: In one report, oral ingestion of *Bai Hua She She Cao* was found to have a dose-dependent effect to enhance macrophage function *in vitro* and inhibit tumor growth *in vivo*.[9]

AUTHORS' COMMENTS

Bai Hua She She Cao and *Tian Men Dong* (Radix Asparagi) have been used in combination to treat fibrocystic breast disorders, and cancers of the breast and the lymphatic system.

Diminished libido has been noted when *Bai Hua She She Cao* is prescribed at dosages in excess of 45 grams.

References

1. *Zhong Yao Xue* (Chinese Herbology), 1998; 204
2. Ibid., 204:205
3. Ibid.
4. Ibid.
5. *Zhong Yao Yao Li Yu Ying Yong* (Pharmacology and Applications of Chinese Herbs), 1983
6. *Guang Dong Yi Xue* (Guangdong Medicine); 1965; 2:11
7. *Zhong Cao Yao Tong Xun* (Journal of Chinese Herbal Medicine), 1978; 7:28
8. *Zhong Yao Xue* (Chinese Herbology), 1998; 204:205
9. Wong BY, Lau BH, Jia TY, Wan CP. Oldenlandia diffusa and Scutellaria barbata augment macrophage oxidative burst and inhibit tumor growth. *Cancer Biother Radiopharm* 1996 Feb;11(1):51-6

Tian Kui Zi (Radix Semiaquilegiae)

天葵子 天葵子

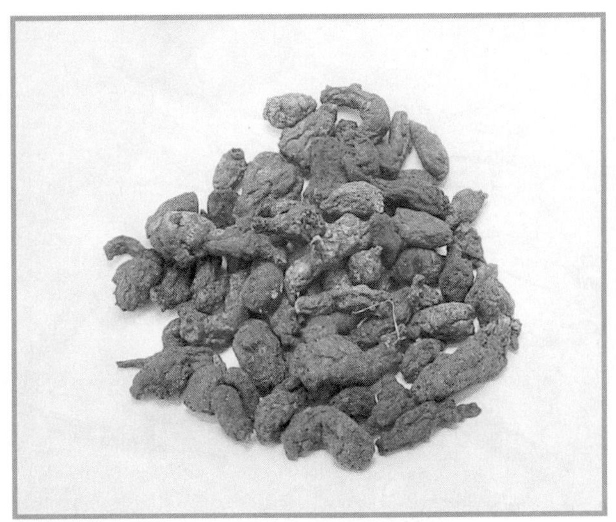

Pinyin Name: *Tian Kui Zi*

Alternate Chinese Names: *Tian Kui Gen, Zi Bei Tian Kui Zi, Qian Nian Lao Shu Shi*

Original Source: *Lei Gong Pao Zhi Lun* (Grandfather Lei's Discussions of Herb Preparation) by Lei Xiao in 470 A.D.

English Name: semiaquilegia, muskroot-like semiaquilegia root

Botanical Name: *Semiaquilegia adoxoides* (DC.) Mak. (*Tian Kui*)

Pharmaceutical Name: Radix Semiaquilegiae

Properties: sweet, bitter, cold

Channels Entered: Liver, Spleen, Urinary Bladder

CHINESE THERAPEUTIC ACTIONS

Clears Heat and Eliminates Toxins, Disperses Stagnation and Reduces Swelling

Tian Kui Zi (Radix Semiaquilegiae) resolves and reduces masses characterized by the presence of heat and toxins.

- Abscesses, sores and nodules: use *Tian Kui Zi* with *Jin Yin Hua* (Flos Lonicerae), *Ye Ju Hua* (Flos Chrysanthemi Indici), and *Zi Hua Di Ding* (Herba Violae). **Exemplar Formula:** *Wu Wei Xiao Du Yin* (Five-Ingredient Decoction to Eliminate Toxins).
- Breast abscesses, fibrocystic breast disorder with red, painful, palpable masses: use it with *Pu Gong Ying* (Herba Taraxaci) and *Lou Lu* (Radix Rhapontici).
- Scrofula: combine it with *Xia Ku Cao* (Spica Prunellae), *Xuan Shen* (Radix Scrophulariae) and *Mu Li* (Concha Ostreae).
- Cancer of the liver, breast, or lymph nodes: use this herb with *Ban Zhi Lian* (Herba Scutellariae Barbatae), *Bai Hua She She Cao* (Herba Oldenlandia) and *Zao Xiu* (Rhizoma Paridis).

DOSAGE

3 to 10 grams.

CAUTIONS / CONTRAINDICATIONS

Use *Tian Kui Zi* with caution in cases of deficiency and cold of the Spleen and Stomach.

CHEMICAL COMPOSITION

Alkaloids, amino acids, coumarin.[1]

SUPPLEMENT

- 紫背天葵 / 紫背天葵 *Zi Bei Tian Kui* (<u>Herba</u> Semiaquilegiae), first cited in *Lei Gong Pao Zhi Lun* (Grandfather Lei's Discussions of Herb Preparation) by Lei Xiao in 470 A.D., is the aerial part of the same plant as *Tian Kui Zi* (<u>Radix</u> Semiaquilegiae). *Zi Bei Tian Kui* has mild functions to dispel masses and treat nodules, carbuncles, and abscesses. The dosage of *Zi Bei Tian Kui* is 3 to 10 grams.

References

1. *Chang Yong Zhong Yao Cheng Fen Yu Yao Li Shou Ce* (A Handbook of the Composition and Pharmacology of Common Chinese Drugs), 1994; 503-504

Long Kui (Herba Solanum Nigrum)

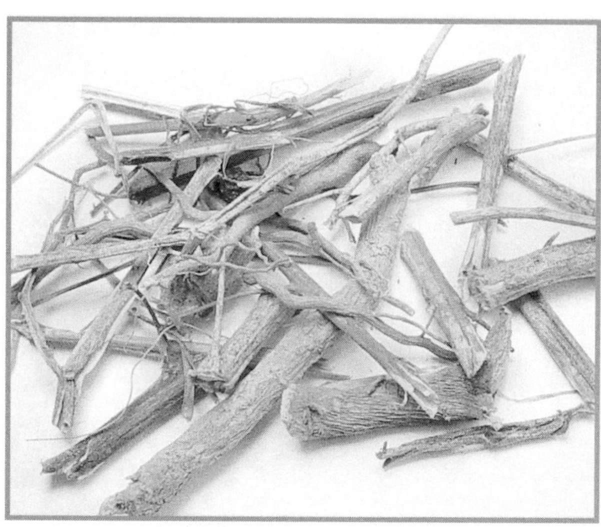

龍葵 龙葵

Pinyin Name: *Long Kui*
English Name: solanum
Botanical Name: *Solanum nigrum*
Pharmaceutical Name: Herba Solanum Nigrum
Properties: slightly bitter, cold
Channels Entered: Lung, Urinary Bladder
Safety Index: slightly toxic

CHINESE THERAPEUTIC ACTIONS

1. Clears Heat, Eliminates Toxins, Invigorates Blood Circulation and Reduces Swelling

Long Kui (Herba Solanum Nigrum) is a cold and potent herb that treats cases of severe heat and toxins. Clinical applications include cancer, sore and swollen throat, toxic swellings, carbuncles, and itching of eczema and sores.

- Cancer: use *Long Kui* with *Ban Zhi Lian* (Herba Scutellariae Barbatae).
- Sore and swollen throat: use it with *Da Qing Ye* (Folium Isatidis), *Ma Bo* (Lasiosphaera seu Calvatia) and *She Gan* (Rhizoma Belamcandae).
- Sores, carbuncles and toxic swellings: combine it with *Pu Gong Ying* (Herba Taraxaci), *Ye Ju Hua* (Flos Chrysanthemi Indici) and *Zi Hua Di Ding* (Herba Violae) both internally and externally.
- Itching of eczema or sores: add *Chan Tui* (Periostracum Cicadae) and *Jing Jie* (Herba Schizonepetae).

2. Promotes Urination

***Lin zheng* (dysuria syndrome):** *Long Kui* clears heat and treats dysuria.

- *Re lin* (heat dysuria), edema or dysuria: use *Long Kui* with *Ze Xie* (Rhizoma Alismatis), *Shi Wei* (Folium Pyrrosiae) and *Che Qian Cao* (Herba Plantaginis).

DOSAGE

15 to 30 grams.

CHEMICAL COMPOSITION

Solanigrine, solasnine, chaconine, solanine, solamargine, solasodamine, solavilline.[1]

TOXICOLOGY

Decoction of *Long Kui* is slightly toxic. The LD_{50} in rats is 144 g/kg via oral ingestion, 56.8 g/kg via intraperitoneal injection.

References

1. *Xian Dai Ben Cao Gang Mu* (Contemporary Materia Medica), 2000; 738

Ban Zhi Lian (Herba Scutellariae Barbatae)

半枝蓮 半枝莲

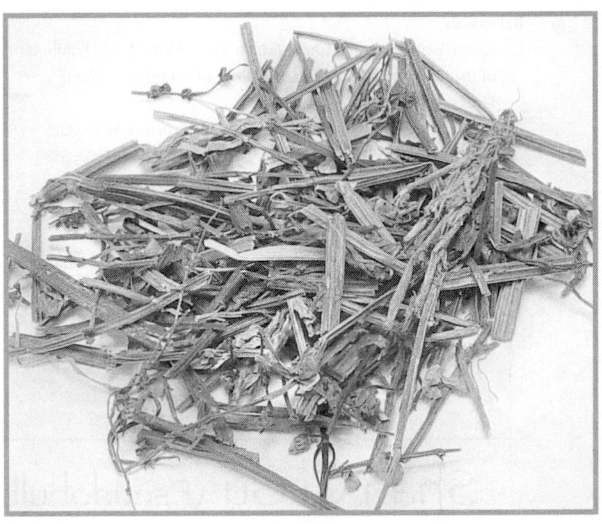

Pinyin Name: *Ban Zhi Lian*
Literal Name: "half-branch lotus"
Alternate Chinese Names: *Bing Tou Cao, Han Xin Cao, Ya Shua Cao*
Original Source: *Jiang Su Zhi Wu Zhi* (Jiangsu Journal of Botany)
English Name: scute barbata, barbed skullcap herb
Botanical Name: *Scutellaria barbata* D. Don. (*Ban Zhi Lian*)
Pharmaceutical Name: Herba Scutellariae Barbatae
Properties: acrid, slightly bitter, cool
Channels Entered: Liver, Lung, Stomach

CHINESE THERAPEUTIC ACTIONS

1. Clears Heat and Eliminates Toxins

Tumors characterized by heat and toxins: *Ban Zhi Lian* (Herba Scutellariae Barbatae) is most effective for cancers of the lung and gastrointestinal system.

- Cancer: use *Ban Zhi Lian* with other herbs with antineoplastic properties such as *Bai Hua She She Cao* (Herba Oldenlandia).

Lung abscess: Toxic heat accumulation with phlegm in the Lung results in lung abscesses.

- Lung abscess: use *Ban Zhi Lian* with *Yu Xing Cao* (Herba Houttuyniae).

2. Promotes Urination and Reduces Swelling

Water retention: *Ban Zhi Lian* treats *re lin* (heat dysuria) manifesting as painful urination with scanty yellow urine. In addition, this herb treats edema and ascites associated with liver cirrhosis. It promotes normal urination and reduces water accumulation.

- Liver cirrhosis with edema and ascites: use *Ban Zhi Lian* with *Ze Xie* (Rhizoma Alismatis), *Ban Bian Lian* (Herba Lobeliae Chinensis), and *Yu Mi Xu* (Stigma Maydis).
- Liver cancer: combine it with *Bie Jia* (Carapax Trionycis), *Dan Shen* (Radix Salviae Miltiorrhizae), and *Bai Shao* (Radix Paeoniae Alba).

3. Stops Bleeding

Bleeding: *Ban Zhi Lian* has a mild function to treat traumatic injuries, hematemesis, epistaxis and hematuria associated with blood stagnation.

DOSAGE

10 to 30 grams in decoction. The dosage for fresh *Ban Zhi Lian* should be doubled.

CHEMICAL COMPOSITION

Carthamidin, isocarthamidin, scutellarein, apigenin, luteolin, β-sitosterol, organic alkaloids.[1,2]

HO, OH, OH, O, OH, O

Carthamidin

PHARMACOLOGICAL EFFECTS

- **Antibiotic:** *Ban Zhi Lian* has inhibitory action against *Staphylococcus aureus, Salmonella typhi, Pseudomonas aeruginosa*, and *E. coli*.[3] Furthermore, apigenin and luteolin isolated from are selectively toxic to *S. aureus*, including the MRSA and methicillin-sensitive *S. aureus* strains.[4]
- **Antispasmodic:** Carthamidin inhibits contraction of smooth muscle.[5]
- **Antineoplastic**: *Ban Zhi Lian* has shown mild to moderate effectiveness in the treatment of acute leukemia.[6]

CLINICAL STUDIES AND RESEARCH

- **Cancer**: According to one report, oral ingestion of *Ban Zhi Lian* was found to have a dose-dependent effect to enhance macrophage function *in vitro* and inhibit tumor growth *in vivo*.[7]

TOXICOLOGY

The LD_{50} for intravenous injection of decoction of *Ban Zhi Lian* in mice is 6.10 g/kg (dosage of dried herb). The LD_{50} for oral administration of *Ban Zhi Lian* extract in rats is 75.1 g/kg (dosage of dried herb). No abnormalities were noted following intraperitoneal injection of 1 g/kg/day (dosage of dried herb) for three months.[8]

Ban Zhi Lian (Herba Scutellariae Barbatae)

References

1. *Chang Yong Zhong Yao Cheng Fen Yu Yao Li Shou Ce* (A Handbook of the Composition and Pharmacology of Common Chinese Drugs), 1994; 777-778
2. Yan X, Zhou J, Xie G, *Traditional Chinese Medicines Molecular Structures, Natural Sources and Applications*; Ashgate, 1999; 5983
3. *Ren Min Wei Sheng Chu Ban She* (Journal of People's Public Health), 1988:302
4. Sato Y, Suzaki S, et al. Phytochemical flavones isolated from Scutellaria barbata and antibacterial activity against methicillin-resistant Staphylococcus aureus. *J Ethnopharmacol* 2000 Oct;72(3):483-8
5. *Zhong Cao Yao* (Chinese Herbal Medicine), 1981; 12(2):19
6. *Ren Min Wei Sheng Chu Ban She* (Journal of People's Public Health), 1988:302
7. Wong BY, Lau BH, Jia TY, Wan CP. Oldenlandia diffusa and Scutellaria barbata augment macrophage oxidative burst and inhibit tumor growth. *Cancer Biother Radiopharm* 1996 Feb;11(1):51-6
8. *Zhong Yao Yao Li Yu Ying Yong* (Pharmacology and Applications of Chinese Herbs), 1983: 392

Shan Ci Gu (Pseudobulbus Cremastrae)

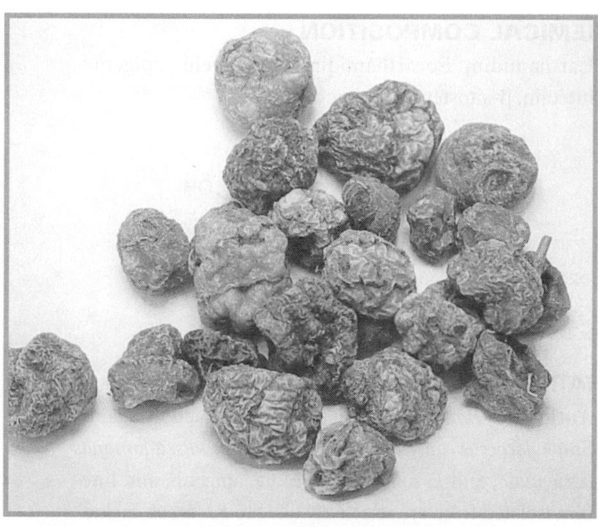

山慈姑

Pinyin Name: *Shan Ci Gu*
Literal Name: "benevolent aunt of the mountains"
Alternate Chinese Names: *Mao Ci Gu, Guang Ci Gu*
Original Source: *Jia You Ben Cao* (Materia Medica of the Jia You Era) by Zhang Yu-Xi and Su Song in 1057-1060
English Name: cremastra
Botanical Name: *Cremastra variabilis* (BL.) Nakai (*Du Juan Lan*); *Pleione bulbocodioides* (Franch.) Rolfe (*Du Suan Lan*)
Pharmaceutical Name: Pseudobulbus Cremastrae
Properties: acrid, cold
Channels Entered: Liver, Stomach
Safety Index: slightly toxic

CHINESE THERAPEUTIC ACTIONS

Clears Heat, Eliminates Toxins, Drains Abscesses, Dissipates Nodules

Toxic sores: *Shan Ci Gu* (Pseudobulbus Cremastrae) is applied topically or administered internally to treat ulcers, carbuncles, nodules, and toxic swellings and scrofula. It is also used to treat various types of cancer and tumors, such as carcinoma of the breast, cervix, esophagus, lung, stomach, and skin.

- Toxic sores: use *Shan Ci Gu* with *She Xiang* (Moschus) and *Da Ji* (Radix Euphorbiae seu Knoxiae).

DOSAGE

3 to 6 grams in decoction.

CAUTIONS / CONTRAINDICATIONS

- Use *Shan Ci Gu* with caution for patients having weak constitutions.

OVERDOSAGE

When used properly, *Shan Ci Gu* is only slightly toxic. However, overdose may result in nausea, vomiting, diarrhea, dehydration, abdominal pain, weakness, lethargy, hair loss, soreness and pain throughout the body, and mild suppression of the bone marrow and central nervous system. In serious cases, there may be severe muscle spasms and cramps throughout the entire body, leading to respiratory depression. Adverse reactions generally occur between 2 and 4 hours following ingestion of excessive amounts. In some cases, there may be a delay of

Shan Ci Gu (Pseudobulbus Cremastrae)

6 to 12 hours before the onset of symptoms. The toxic dose of *Shan Ci Gu* is between 15 and 45 grams.[1]

TREATMENT OF OVERDOSAGE

Vomiting and diarrhea associated with overdose of *Shan Ci Gu* are defensive reactions as they facilitate the elimination of the offending agent. However, excessive vomiting and diarrhea may deplete qi and body fluids. Excessive vomiting or diarrhea should be stopped once all the toxins are eliminated from the gastrointestinal tract.

Excessive vomiting may be relieved by taking 10 ml of fresh ginger juice mixed with 250 ml of vinegar. Excessive diarrhea may be treated with an herbal decoction of *Fang Feng* (Radix Saposhnikoviae) 15g, *Sheng Jiang* (Rhizoma Zingiberis Recens) 30g, *Rou Gui* (Cortex Cinnamomi) 6g, and small amounts of vinegar, sugar and salt.[2]

Administration of egg whites, milk or powdered *Ou Jie* (Nodus Nelumbinis Rhizomatis) is beneficial, as they provide protection for the digestive tract and decrease the absorption of *Shan Ci Gu*.

Purgative methods are sometimes used to facilitate elimination of the herb, such as 9 grams of *Dang Gui* (Radicis Angelicae Sinensis), 30 grams of *Da Huang* (Radix et Rhizoma Rhei), and 30 grams of *Yuan Ming Fen* (Matrii Sulfas Exsiccatus).[3]

CHEMICAL COMPOSITION

Glycomannan, colchicine, tulipin, alkaloids, starch.[4]

PHARMACOLOGICAL EFFECTS

- **Antineoplastic:** Subcutaneous injection of a *Shan Ci Gu* preparation in mice at 2 mg/kg has shown an inhibitory effect on the replication of cells.[5]

References

1. *Zhong Yao Bu Liang Fan Ying Yu Zhi Liao* (Adverse Reactions and Treatment of Chinese Herbal Medicine), 1996; 137:140
2. *Zhong Yao Du Li Xue* (Toxicology of Chinese Herbs); 1989, 41-43
3. *Lin Chuan Shou Ce You Du Zhong Yao Shi Yong* (Clinical Handbook on Applications of Toxic Chinese Herbs), 1992; 37-38
4. *Zhong Yao Xue* (Chinese Herbology), 1998; 210
5. *Chang Yong Zhong Yao Xian Dai Yan Jiu Yu Lin Chuan* (Recent Study & Clinical Application of Common Traditional Chinese Medicine), 1995; 165:166

Feng Wei Cao (Herba Pteris)

鳳尾草 风尾草

Pinyin Name: *Feng Wei Cao*
Literal Name: "phoenix tail herb"
Alternate Chinese Names: *Feng Huang Cao, Feng Wei Jue*
Original Source: *Zhi Wu Ming Shi Tu Kao* (Illustrated Guide for Nomenclature and Identification of Botanical Products)
English Name: pteris, Chinese brake, huguenot fern, serrulate brake, spider brake
Botanical Name: *Pteris multifida* Poir. (*Feng Wei Cao*)
Pharmaceutical Name: Herba Pteris
Properties: bitter, cold
Channels Entered: Large Intestine, Urinary Bladder

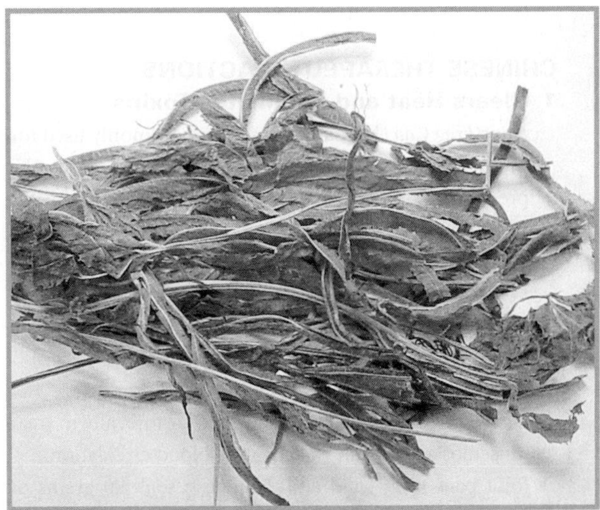

CHINESE THERAPEUTIC ACTIONS

1. Clears Heat, Drains Dampness and Reduces Inflammation

Feng Wei Cao (Herba Pteris) treats the accumulation of damp-heat in the Large Intestine and Urinary Bladder.

- Sore and swollen throat: use *Feng Wei Cao* with *Da Qing Ye* (Folium Isatidis) and *Ban Lan Gen* (Radix Isatidis).
- Dysentery, diarrhea: add *Ma Chi Xian* (Herba Portulacae).

Feng Wei Cao (Herba Pteris)

- Chronic appendicitis: combine *Feng Wei Cao* with *Bai Jiang Cao* (Herba cum Radice Patriniae) and *Yi Yi Ren* (Semen Coicis).
- *Lin zheng* (dysuria syndrome) and jaundice: use it with *Che Qian Cao* (Herba Plantaginis), *Hai Jin Sha* (Herba Lygodii) and *Huang Bai* (Cortex Phellodendri).

2. Cools the Blood and Eliminates Toxins

Feng Wei Cao treats heat and toxins in the blood, that are causing bleeding and cancer.

- Hematuria, blood in the stool, epistaxis: use *Feng Wei Cao* with *Xiao Ji* (Herba Cirisii), *Pu Huang* (Pollen Typhae) and *Di Yu* (Radix Sanguisorbae).
- Cancer: combine this herb with *Bai Hua She She Cao* (Herba Oldenlandia), *Ban Zhi Lian* (Herba Scutellariae Barbatae) and other herbs with antineoplastic properties.

DOSAGE

10 to 20 grams in decoctions.

Dong Ling Cao (Herba Rabdosiae)

冬凌草 冬凌草

Pinyin Name: *Dong Ling Cao*
Alternate Chinese Names: *Shan Xiang Cao, Bing Ling Cao*
Original Source: *Zhong Guo Yao Dian* (Dictionary of Chinese Medicine) in 1977
English Name: rabdosia, blush red rabdosia herb
Botanical Name: *Rabdosia rubescens* (Hemsl.) Hara; *Rabdosia japonica* (Burm. f) Hara var. *glaucocalyx* (Maxim) Hara; *Rabdosia japonica* Maxim
Pharmaceutical Name: Herba Rabdosiae
Properties: bitter, sweet, cool
Channels Entered: Liver, Spleen, Stomach

CHINESE THERAPEUTIC ACTIONS

1. Clears Heat and Eliminates Toxins

Dong Ling Cao (Herba Rabdosiae) is commonly used for the treatment of various disorders characterized by the presence of heat and toxins, such as sore throat, tonsillitis, and insect and snake bites.

- Headaches due to common cold: use 30 grams of *Dong Ling Cao* individually in decoction.

2. Activates Blood Circulation and Relieves Pain

Dong Ling Cao is used internally and/or topically to treat musculoskeletal pain by activating blood circulation.

- Joint pain from wind and dampness: soak 90 grams of *Dong Ling Cao* in 500 ml of grain-based liquor. Take 30 ml of the tincture twice daily, in the morning and at night.
- Joint pain: soak the affected area in the solution made by cooking 250 grams of the herb in water.

DOSAGE

30 to 60 grams in decoction.

CAUTIONS / CONTRAINDICATIONS

- *Dong Ling Cao* may cause gastrointestinal side effects, such as nausea, vomiting, diarrhea and abdominal distention.

CHEMICAL COMPOSITION

Rubescensine A, B, C, D; ludongnin, lushanrubescensin, quidongnin, xindongnin A, B; α-amyrin, circiliol.[1,2]

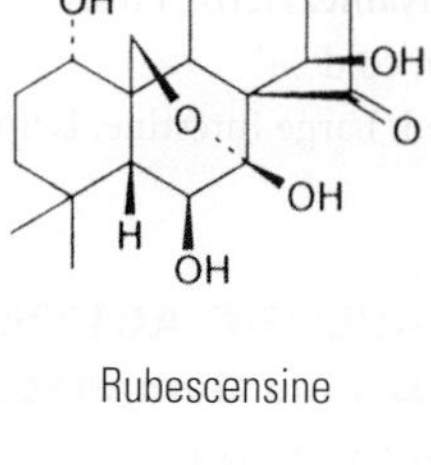

OH OH O O OH H OH

Rubescensine

Dong Ling Cao (Herba Rabdosiae)

PHARMACOLOGICAL EFFECTS

- **Antineoplastic**: The use of rubescensine A has been shown to have antineoplastic effects against esophageal cancer and liver cancer in rats. The herb was administered via injection. No significant suppression of the bone marrow was observed. In another report, the use of rubescensine A was associated with a dose-dependent inhibitory effect on stomach cancer cells (MGc80-3).[3,4]
- **Antibiotic effect**: *Dong Ling Cao* has moderate inhibitory action against 19 different micro-organisms, and is especially effective against gram-positive species. The minimum inhibitory concentration was 31 ug/ml, against *Staphylococcus aureus*.[5]

CLINICAL STUDIES AND RESEARCH

- **Esophageal and cardiac cancer**: In one study, 95 patients with middle-to-late stage esophageal and cardiac cancers were treated with preparations of *Dong Ling Cao*. Preparation I was made by mixing the herb with syrup (1:1 ratio); the treatment protocol was to give 20 to 30 ml three times daily for 2 to 3 months per course of treatment. Preparation II was made by incorporating 4.5 to 5 grams of the herb into one pill; the treatment protocol was to give 5 to 8 pills three times daily for 2 to 3 months per course of treatment. Preparation III was made by mixing 75 to 100 mg of rubescensine A in 500 ml of D5W; the treatment protocol was to infuse the preparation intravenously every other day until a total of 3,000 to 3,500 mg of the compound had been given. The study concluded that the rate of effectiveness was 26.7% for Preparation I, 27.6% for Preparation II, and 31.8% for Preparation III.[6]
- **Liver cancer**: According to one report, 31 patients with primary liver cancer were treated successfully with preparations of *Dong Ling Cao*. Improved appetite and reduced pain were reported in 80% of the subjects. The survival rate after treatment was 29.6% after 6 months, 12% after 1 year, and 10% after 2 years.[7]

TOXICOLOGY

In an acute toxicology study, the LD_{50} for rubescensine A was 55.8 mg/kg in mice via intraperitoneal injection. Daily administration of 5 to 10 mg/kg of rubescensine A for 10 days in rats via intraperitoneal injection did not cause any significant changes to body weight, red blood cells, white blood cells, platelets, kidney and liver functions.[8]

AUTHORS' COMMENTS

Dong Ling Cao is also used in a formulation for treatment of prostate cancer. The formula includes *Dong Ling Cao*, *Huang Qin* (Radix Scutellariae), *Da Qing Ye* (Folium Isatidis), *San Qi* (Radix Notoginseng), *Ju Hua* (Flos Chrysanthemi), *Ling Zhi* (Ganoderma), *Gan Cao* (Radix Glycyrrhizae) and saw palmetto berries (Semen Serenoa Repens).

References

1. *Xian Dai Ben Cao Gang Mu* (Contemporary Materia Medica); 885, 2000
2. Yan X, Zhou J, Xie G, *Traditional Chinese Medicines Molecular Structures, Natural Sources and Applications*; Ashgate, 1999; 4870
3. *Xian Dai Ben Cao Gang Mu* (Contemporary Materia Medica); 885, 2000
4. *Zhong Guo Yao Li Xue Bao* (Chinese Herbal Pharmacology Journal), 1986; (4):361
5. *Xian Dai Ben Cao Gang Mu* (Contemporary Materia Medica); 885, 2000
6. *Xian Dai Zhong Yao Yao Li Xue* (Contemporary Pharmacology of Chinese Herbs), 1997; 1468-1469
7. *He Nan Yi Xue Yuan Xue Bao* (Journal of Henan University of Medicine), 1976; (5):22
8. *Zhong Cao Yao Tong Xun* (Journal of Chinese Herbal Medicine), 1977; (10):5

Chui Pen Cao (Herba Sedi)

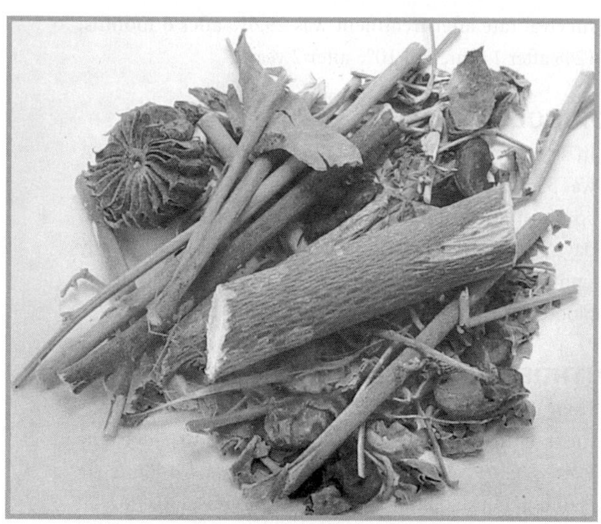

垂盆草 垂盆草

Pinyin Name: *Chui Pen Cao*
Alternate Chinese Names: *Fo Jia Cao, Gou Ya Cao, Shi Zi Jia*
English Name: sedum
Botanical Name: *Sedum sarmentosum* Bunge.
Pharmaceutical Name: Herba Sedi
Properties: sweet, bland, slightly sour, cool
Channels Entered: Liver, Gallbladder, Small Intestine

CHINESE THERAPEUTIC ACTIONS

1. Clears Heat and Eliminates Toxins

Carbuncles, cellulitis, toxic snake bites, burns, swollen throat: *Chui Pen Cao* (Herba Sedi) clears heat and toxins to treat these disorders. It is used alone internally or applied topically.

- Carbuncles, cellulitis, snake bites, burns: use *Chui Pen Cao* with *Ye Ju Hua* (Flos Chrysanthemi Indici), *Zi Hua Di Ding* (Herba Violae) and *Ban Bian Lian* (Herba Lobeliae Chinensis), applied to the affected area.

2. Dispels Dampness and Relieves Jaundice

Damp-heat jaundice: *Chui Pen Cao* clears damp-heat to relieve jaundice. It has recently been used to treat acute or chronic jaundice with or without infectious hepatitis. It also is effective in lowering liver enzymes.

- Damp-heat jaundice: use this herb with *Yin Chen Hao* (Herba Artemisiae Scopariae), *Zhi Zi* (Fructus Gardeniae) and *Da Huang* (Radix et Rhizoma Rhei).

DOSAGE

10 to 30 grams of dried *Chui Pen Cao*, 50 to 100 grams of the fresh herb.

CHEMICAL COMPOSITION

Sarmentosine, l-aspargine, l-aspartic acid, l-α-alanine, l-leucine, l-tyrosine, l-valine.[1]

PHARMACOLOGICAL EFFECTS

Chui Pen Cao has hepatoprotective and antibiotic effects.

TOXICOLOGY

No abnormalities of the blood, liver, kidney or other internal organs were reported following oral administration of *Chui Pen Cao* in dogs at 30 g/kg for 8 weeks. The LD_{50} of the herb via intraperitoneal injection in mice is 54.2 g/kg.[2]

References

1. *Xian Dai Zhong Yao Yao Li Xue* (Contemporary Pharmacology of Chinese Herbs), 1997; 282-283
2. Ibid.

Tu Fu Ling (Rhizoma Smilacis Glabrae)

土茯苓 土茯苓

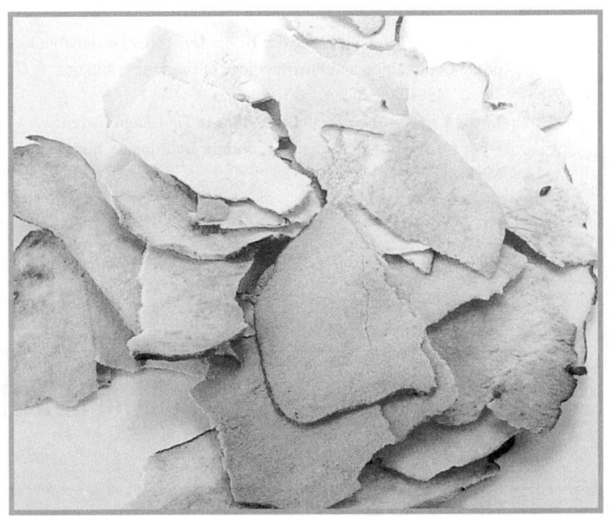

Pinyin Name: *Tu Fu Ling*
Original Source: *Ben Cao Gang Mu* (Materia Medica) by Li Shi-Zhen in 1578
English Name: smilax, glabrous greenbrier rhizome
Botanical Name: *Smilax glabra* Roxb. (*Tu Fu Ling*)
Pharmaceutical Name: Rhizoma Smilacis Glabrae
Properties: sweet, bland, neutral
Channels Entered: Liver, Stomach

CHINESE THERAPEUTIC ACTIONS

1. Eliminates Toxic Heat

Syphilis: *Tu Fu Ling* (Rhizoma Smilacis Glabrae) treats syphilis caused by toxic heat and dampness.

- Syphilis: use *Tu Fu Ling* alone in a large dose (70 grams or more), or use it with *Jin Yin Hua* (Flos Lonicerae), *Bai Xian Pi* (Cortex Dictamni) and *Gan Cao* (Radix Glycyrrhizae).

2. Dispels Toxic Heat from the Skin

Dermatological disorders: *Tu Fu Ling* treats rashes, carbuncles, psoriasis, ulcers and hot skin lesions characterized by heat and toxins attacking the skin.

- Rash, carbuncles or psoriasis: use *Tu Fu Ling* with *Di Fu Zi* (Fructus Kochiae), *Ku Shen Gen* (Radix Sophorae Flavescentis) and *Cang Zhu* (Rhizoma Atractylodis).

3. Promotes Normal Urination

***Lin zheng* (dysuria syndrome):** *Tu Fu Ling* dispels heat from the lower *jiao* to treat *re lin* (heat dysuria) with burning sensations and painful urination.

- *Re lin* (heat dysuria): combine this herb with *Bai Mao Gen* (Rhizoma Imperatae), *Pu Gong Ying* (Herba Taraxaci) and *Chuan Mu Tong* (Caulis Clematidis Armandii).

DOSAGE

15 to 60 grams in decoction.

CAUTIONS / CONTRAINDICATIONS

- It has been reported that concurrent use of *Tu Fu Ling* and tea may be associated with hair loss. [Note: The report did not specify the exact type of tea consumed.]

CHEMICAL COMPOSITION

Saponin, rutin, resin, octacosanal, 16-hentriacontanone.[1,2]

PHARMACOLOGICAL EFFECTS

- **Antineoplastic**: Administration of *Tu Fu Ling* has shown promising effects in the treatment of cancer. In animal studies, it is especially effective against cancers of the urinary bladder and liver.[3,4]

CLINICAL STUDIES AND RESEARCH

- **Syphilis:** In one clinical study, 400 patients with syphilis were treated with an herbal formula with satisfactory results. The treatment protocol was to cook *Tu Fu Ling* 60 to 120g, *Cang Er Zi* (Fructus Xanthii) 15g, *Bai Xian Pi* (Cortex Dictamni) 15g, and *Gan Cao* (Radix Glycyrrhizae) 3 to 9g, in water and have the patients take the decoction in three equally-divided doses daily, for 30 days.[5]
- **Leptospirosis:** According to one report, 80 patients with leptospirosis were treated with an herbal formula with good results. The formula contained *Tu Fu Ling* 60g and *Gan Cao* (Radix Glycyrrhizae) 9g. The dosage of *Tu Fu Ling* was increased to 150g in those who were otherwise healthy but had severe cases of leptospirosis. Other herbs, such as *Huang Qin* (Radix Scutellariae), *Yin Chen Hao* (Herba Artemisiae Scopariae), *Fen Fang Ji* (Radix Stephaniae Tetandrae), and *Ze Xie* (Rhizoma Alismatis), were added if deemed necessary.[6]

TOXICOLOGY

There was one reported case of severe dermatological allergic reaction associated with the use of *Tu Fu Ling*.[7]

AUTHORS' COMMENTS

According to Dr. Zhang Liang-Lin, *Tu Fu Ling* and *Bi Xie* (Rhizoma Dioscoreae Hypoglaucae) treat feelings of urinary bladder prolapse or burning sensations in the genitals.

Tu Fu Ling (Rhizoma Smilacis Glabrae)

References

1. *Chang Yong Zhong Yao Cheng Fen Yu Yao Li Shou Ce* (A Handbook of the Composition and Pharmacology of Common Chinese Drugs), 1994; 206-207
2. *Chang Yong Zhong Yao Xian Dai Yan Jiu Yu Lin Chuan* (Recent Study & Clinical Application of Common Traditional Chinese Medicine), 1995; 142
3. *Zhong Hua Yi Xue Za Zhi* (Chinese Journal of Medicine), 1987; 67(11):622
4. *Cancer*, 1986; 5(2):141
5. *Fu Jian Yi Za Zhi* (Fujian Journal of Chinese Medicine), 1960; 3:19
6. *Shan Xi Xin Yi Yao* (New Medicine and Herbology of Shanxi), 1972; 4:53
7. *Zhong Guo Yi Yao Xue Bao* (Chinese Journal of Medicine and Herbology), 1989; (4):29

Da Qing Ye (Folium Isatidis)

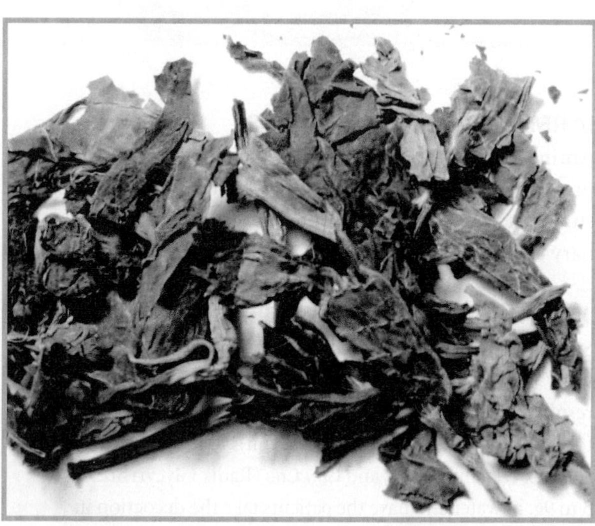

大青葉 大青叶

Pinyin Name: *Da Qing Ye*

Literal Name: "big green-blue leaves," "big green leaves"

Alternate Chinese Names: *Lan Ye*

Original Source: *Ming Yi Za Zhu* (Miscellaneous Records of Famous Physicians) by Tao Hong-Jing in 500 A.D.

English Name: isatis leaves, indigo woad leaves

Botanical Name: *Isatis tinctoria* L. (*Song Lan*); *Isatis indigotica* Fort. (*Cao Da Qing*); *Baphicacanthus cusia* Bremek. (*Ma Lan*); *Polygonum tinctorium* Ait. (*Liao Lan*); *Clerodendron cyrtophyllum* Turcz. (*Lu Bian Qing*).

Pharmaceutical Name: Folium Isatidis

Properties: bitter, very cold

Channels Entered: Heart, Lung, Stomach

CHINESE THERAPEUTIC ACTIONS

1. Clears Heat and Eliminates Toxins

Da Qing Ye (Folium Isatidis) is commonly used to clear heat and toxins from both the exterior or the interior, from the *qi* (energy) to the *xue* (blood) levels. Further, it is used for contagious epidemic febrile outbreaks. Bitter, cold, but not drying, *Da Qing Ye* has an excellent ability to clear heat and eliminate toxins without consuming yin.

Exterior wind-heat or early-stage febrile disorders: Clinical manifestations include high fever, sore throat and perspiration.

- Exterior wind-heat or early-stage febrile disorders: use *Da Qing Ye* with *Jin Yin Hua* (Flos Lonicerae), *Jing Jie* (Herba Schizonepetae), and *Niu Bang Zi* (Fructus Arctii).
- Throat soreness and pain: combine it with *Sheng Ma* (Rhizoma Cimicifugae), *Xuan Shen* (Radix Scrophulariae) and *Jin Yin Hua* (Flos Lonicerae).

Toxic heat: Clinical manifestations of toxic heat include measles, jaundice, encephalitis B, mumps, parotitis, scarlet fever, erysipelas, meningitis and any epidemic febrile disease that is contagious and manifests in high fever, purpura and, in severe cases, unconsciousness.

- Febrile disorders with excess heat and toxins, whether in the *qi* (energy), *ying* (nutritive), or the *xue* (blood) level: use *Da Qing Ye* with *Shi Gao* (Gypsum Fibrosum), *Xuan Shen* (Radix Scrophulariae) and *Sheng Di Huang* (Radix Rehmanniae).
- Jaundice: use this herb with *Yin Chen Hao* (Herba Artemisiae Scopariae) and *Da Huang* (Radix et Rhizoma Rhei).
- Parotitis: add it to *Huang Qin* (Radix Scutellariae) and *Ban Lan Gen* (Radix Isatidis).

2. Cools Blood and Eliminates Maculae

Bleeding: Heat in the *xue* (blood) level forcing blood out

Da Qing Ye (Folium Isatidis)

of its vessels can manifest in maculae, blotches on the skin, purpura, hematemesis and epistaxis.

- Heat in the blood: use *Da Qing Ye* with *Zhi Mu* (Radix Anemarrhenae), *Shi Gao* (Gypsum Fibrosum), *Xuan Shen* (Radix Scrophulariae) and *Zhi Zi* (Fructus Gardeniae).

DOSAGE

10 to 20 grams in decoction. *Da Qing Ye* is used internally or externally.

CAUTIONS / CONTRAINDICATIONS

- *Da Qing Ye* is contraindicated for patients who have deficiency and cold of the Spleen and Stomach.

CHEMICAL COMPOSITION

Indigo, indican, indirubin, fryptanthrin, glucobrassicin, neoglucobrassicin, glycobrassicin-1-sulzonate.[1,2]

H N O–β-D-glucose

Indican

PHARMACOLOGICAL EFFECTS

- **Antibiotic:** *Da Qing Ye* has broad-spectrum antibacterial, antiviral and antifungal effects. Decoction of *Da Qing Ye* is effective against *Staphylococcus aureus,* α-hemolytic streptococcus, *Diplococcus meningitidis, Salmonella typhi, E. coli, Corynebacterium diphtheriae, Bacillus dysenteriae,* leptospira, encephalitis B virus, and HBsAg. In addition, fryptanthrin has a strong effect against various pathogenic fungi, especially ones on the skin and feet.[3,4]
- **Antineoplastic:** Indirubin has been shown to have a positive inhibiting effect against cancer cells in treating leukemia, sarcoma, and lung cancer in mice.[5]
- **Anti-inflammatory:** *Da Qing Ye* has mild anti-inflammatory and antipyretic effects.[6]

CLINICAL STUDIES AND RESEARCH

- **Upper respiratory infection:** In one study, 168 children with upper respiratory infections were treated with *Da Qing Ye* with good results. Among these cases, 95 had common colds or influenza, 29 had acute laryngitis, 25 had bronchitis, and 19 had tonsillitis. The dosage of *Da Qing Ye* solution was 6 ml per dose (each 2 ml contains 3.125 grams of dried herb) for children over 3 years of age, given three to six times daily.[7]
- **Measles and pneumonia:** In one study, 150 patients with measles and pneumonia were treated with satisfactory results using an herbal syrup containing equal portions of *Da Qing Ye* and *Pu Gong Ying* (Herba Taraxaci). The patients were advised to take the syrup three times daily.[8]
- **Encephalitis B:** Decoction of *Da Qing Ye* was found to be effective in treating 51 cases of encephalitis B. The decoction was prepared by cooking 30 grams of *Da Qing Ye* in water to yield 100 ml of decoction. The decoction was given every 4 hours; dosage was 10 to 20 ml for children under 1 year of age, 30 ml for children between 1 and 5, 50 ml for children between 6 and 10, and 80 ml for children between 11 and 13. The patients were advised to continue taking the herbs for 2 to 3 days after the fever subsided.[9]

HERB-DRUG INTERACTION

- **Sulfonylurea antidiabetics and sulfonamide antibiotics:** Patients who are allergic to sulfonylureas and sulfonamides may also be allergic to *Qing Dai* (Indigo Naturalis), *Da Qing Ye* (Folium Isatidis) and *Ban Lan Gen* (Radix Isatidis), according to Dr. Zhang Xiao-Ping. [Note: Examples of sulfonylureas include tolbutamide (Orinase), glipizide (Glucotrol), and glyburide (DiaBeta/Micronase); and examples of sulfonamides include sulfadiazine, sulfisoxazole, sulfamethoxazole, trimethoprim/sulfamethoxazole (Bactrim/Septra), and erythromycin/sulfisoxazole (Pediazole).]

TOXICOLOGY

Oral ingestion of indirubin at 5 g/kg/day in mice showed no adverse reaction and resulted in no fatalities.[10]

References

1. *Xian Dai Zhong Yao Yao Li Xue* (Contemporary Pharmacology of Chinese Herbs), 1997; 217
2. *The Merck Index* 12th edition, Chapman & Hall/CRCnetBASE/Merck, 2000
3. *Zhong Yao Xue* (Chinese Herbology), 1998; 174:175
4. *Zhi Wu Yao You Xiao Cheng Fen Shou Ce* (Manual of Plant Medicinals and Their Active Constituents), 1986: 608,1084
5. Ibid.
6. *Zhong Yao Xue* (Chinese Herbology), 1998; 174:175
7. *Fu Jian Zhong Yi Yao* (Fujian Chinese Medicine and Herbology), 1965; 4:14
8. *Shang Hai Zhong Yi Yao Za Zhi* (Shanghai Journal of Chinese Medicine and Herbology), 1963; 2:23
9. *Fu Jian Zhong Yi Yao* (Fujian Chinese Medicine and Herbology), 1965; 4:11
10. *Xian Dai Zhong Yao Yao Li Xue* (Contemporary Pharmacology of Chinese Herbs), 1997; 217

Ban Lan Gen (Radix Isatidis)

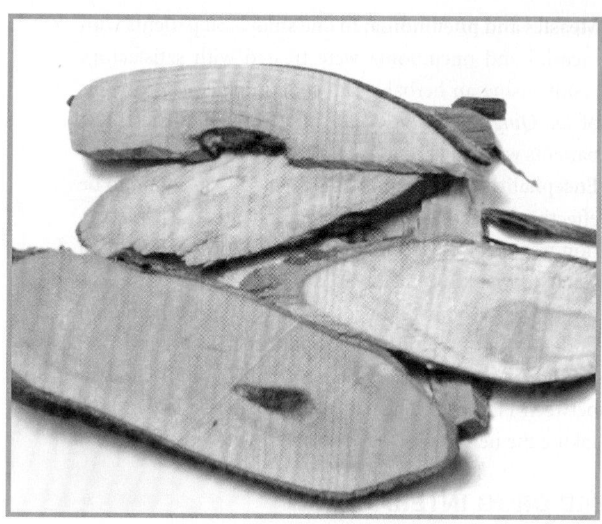

板藍根 板蓝根

Pinyin Name: *Ban Lan Gen*

Original Source: *Ben Cao Gang Mu* (Materia Medica) by Li Shi-Zhen in 1578

English Name: isatis root, indigo woad root

Botanical Name: *Isatis tinctoria* L. (*Song Lan*); *Isatis indigotica* Fort. (*Cao Da Qing*); *Baphicacanthus cusia* Bremek. (*Ma Lan*)

Pharmaceutical Name: Radix Isatidis

Properties: bitter, cold

Channels Entered: Heart, Stomach

CHINESE THERAPEUTIC ACTIONS

Clears Heat, Eliminates Toxins, Cools Blood and Benefits the Throat

Toxic heat: Bitter and cold, *Ban Lan Gen* (Radix Isatidis) has excellent properties to clear heat and eliminate toxins. It is commonly used to clear heat and toxins from both the exterior and the interior, and from the *qi* (energy) and *xue* (blood) levels. Commonly seen symptoms include fever, sore throat, tonsillitis, blotches on the skin, and flushed and swollen face, with feverish sensations. This herb can be used to treat encephalitis B, hepatitis, chickenpox, epidemic parotitis, and viral dermatitis including herpes simplex, herpes zoster, pityriasis rosea and flat warts. It is most commonly used to treat sore throat in febrile disorders.

- Febrile disorders: use *Ban Lan Gen* with *Lian Qiao* (Fructus Forsythiae), *Xuan Shen* (Radix Scrophulariae) and *Niu Bang Zi* (Fructus Arctii). **Exemplar Formula:** *Pu Ji Xiao Du Yin* (Universal Benefit Decoction to Eliminate Toxin).
- Exterior wind-heat or early-stage febrile disorders: use it with *Jin Yin Hua* (Flos Lonicerae), *Lian Qiao* (Fructus Forsythiae) and *Jing Jie* (Herba Schizonepetae).
- Sore throat: combine it with *Niu Bang Zi* (Fructus Arctii), *Xuan Shen* (Radix Scrophulariae), *Shan Dou Gen* (Radix Sophorae Tonkinensis) and *Ma Bo* (Lasiosphaera seu Calvatia).

DOSAGE

10 to 15 grams in decoction.

CAUTIONS / CONTRAINDICATIONS

- Oral use of *Ban Lan Gen* is relatively safe, with only occasional reports of gastrointestinal disturbances.
- Allergic reactions have been reported with both oral and intravenous administrations of this herb.

CHEMICAL COMPOSITION

Indican, indigo, indirubin, isatan B, uridine, hypoxanthine, uracil, salicylic acid, qingdainone, daucosterol, adenosine, kinetin.[1]

PHARMACOLOGICAL EFFECTS

- **Antibiotic**: *Ban Lan Gen* has demonstrated marked antibacterial effects *in vitro* against *Staphylococcus aureus, Diplococcus pneumoniae, E. coli, Salmonella typhi*, and leptospira. It is also effective against certain influenza viruses.[2]
- **Immunostimulant**: Intraperitoneal injection of a *Ban Lan Gen* preparation has been associated with an increased activity of natural killer (NK) cells in mice. However, there was no increased production of said cells observed.[3]
- **Antiplatelet**: Administration of a *Ban Lan Gen* preparation is associated with marked inhibition of platelet aggregation in rabbits.[4]

CLINICAL STUDIES AND RESEARCH

- **Upper respiratory tract infection**: *Ban Lan Gen* is commonly incorporated into herbal formulas for treatment of upper respiratory tract infection. In one clinical study, 46 patients with acute tonsillitis were treated with an herbal formula, with complete recovery in 40 patients, and moderate improvement in 6 patients. The herbal formula contained such herbs as *Ban Lan Gen, Ge Gen* (Radix Puerariae), *Bai Hua She She Cao* (Herba Oldenlandia), *Chai Hu* (Radix Bupleuri), *Lian Qiao* (Fructus Forsythiae), *Zhe Bei Mu* (Bulbus Fritillariae Thunbergii), *She Gan* (Rhizoma Belamcandae), and *Jing Jie* (Herba Schizonepetae).[5]
- **Encephalitis B**: Oral administration of *Ban Lan Gen* was found to be approximately 82% effective in treating patients with encephalitis B. There was an immediate reduction in body temperature.[6]

Ban Lan Gen (Radix Isatidis)

- **Hepatitis:** *Ban Lan Gen* has been used in various formulations for treatment of hepatitis. In one clinical trial with 53 patients, the combination of *Ban Lan Gen* and *Zhi Zi* (Fructus Gardeniae) was shown to be effective for treatment of icteric jaundice.[7]
- **Viral infection of the skin:** In a clinical study of 30 patients, administration of a *Ban Lan Gen* preparation was associated with marked effectiveness for treatment of herpes infection of the skin. The herbal preparation was applied topically to the affected area.[8]

HERB-DRUG INTERACTION

- **Sulfonylurea antidiabetics and sulfonamide antibiotics:** Patients who are allergic to sulfonylureas and sulfonamides may also be allergic to *Qing Dai* (Indigo Naturalis), *Da Qing Ye* (Folium Isatidis) and *Ban Lan Gen* (Radix Isatidis), according to Dr. Zhang Xiao-Ping. [Note: Examples of sulfonylureas include tolbutamide (Orinase), glipizide (Glucotrol), and glyburide (DiaBeta/Micronase); and examples of sulfonamides include sulfadiazine, sulfisoxazole, sulfamethoxazole, trimethoprim/sulfamethoxazole (Bactrim/Septra), and erythromycin/sulfisoxazole (Pediazole).]
- **Anticoagulant or antiplatelet drugs:** *Ban Lan Gen* has antiplatelet action, and should be used with caution in patients who take anticoagulant or antiplatelet medications. Though this potential interaction has not been documented, this herb may potentiate the effect of drugs such as warfarin.[9] [Note: Examples of anticoagulants include heparin, warfarin (Coumadin) and enoxaparin (Lovenox); examples of antiplatelets include aspirin, dipyridamole (Persantine), and clopidogrel (Plavix).]

AUTHORS' COMMENTS

Ban Lan Gen (Radix Isatidis) and *Da Qing Ye* (Folium Isatidis) are derived from the same plant and have many similar functions. *Ban Lan Gen* is stronger in eliminating heat and toxins to relieve sore throat. *Da Qing Ye* more strongly clears heat and cools the blood.

References

1. *Xian Dai Shi Yong Yao Xue* (Practical Applications of Modern Herbal Medicine), 1997; 219-220
2. *Zhong Cheng Yao Yan Jiu* (Research of Chinese Patent Medicine), 1987; 12:9
3. *Zhong Yao Yao Li Yu Ying Yong* (Pharmacology and Applications of Chinese Herbs), 1991; 7(2):22
4. *Zhong Yao Tong Bao* (Journal of Chinese Herbology), 1988; 13(2):31
5. *Zhong Yi Za Zhi* (Journal of Chinese Medicine), 1983; 24(11):19
6. *Xian Dai Shi Yong Yao Xue* (Practical Applications of Modern Herbal Medicine), 221
7. *Guang Xi Zhong Yi Yao* (Guangxi Chinese Medicine and Herbology), 1980; (3):13
8. *Jiang Xi Yi Yao* (Jiangxi Medicine and Herbology), 1989; 24(5):315
9. Chen, J. Recognition & prevention of herb-drug interactions, *Medical Acupuncture*, Fall/Winter 1998/1999; volume 10/number 2; 9-13

2 HEAT-CLEARING HERBS

Qing Dai (Indigo Naturalis)

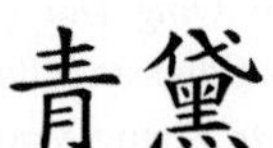

Pinyin Name: *Qing Dai*
Original Source: *Yao Xing Ben Cao* (Materia Medica of Medicinal Properties) by Zhen Quan in 600 A.D.
English Name: indigo, natural indigo
Botanical Name: *Isatis tinctoria* L. (*Song Lan*); *Isatis indigotica* Fort. (*Cao Da Qing*); *Baphicacanthus cusia* Bremek. (*Ma Lan*); *Polygonum tinctorium* Ait. (*Liao Lan*); *Clerodendron cyrtophyllum* Turcz. (*Lu Bian Qing*).
Pharmaceutical Name: Indigo Naturalis
Properties: salty, cold
Channels Entered: Liver, Lung, Stomach

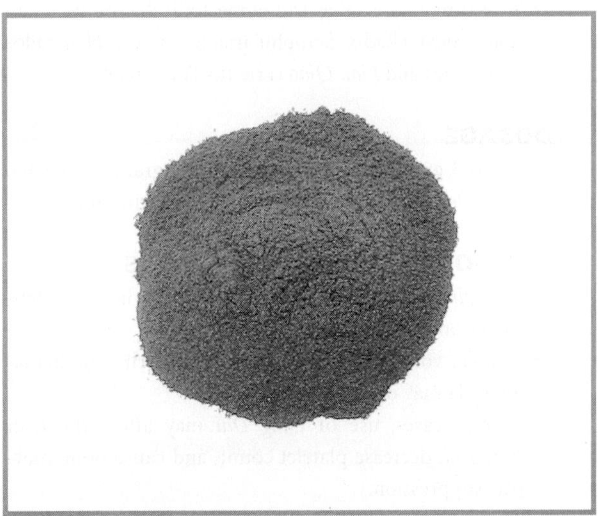

Qing Dai (Indigo Naturalis)

CHINESE THERAPEUTIC ACTIONS

1. Clears Heat and Eliminates Toxins

Convulsions arising from Liver wind: *Qing Dai* (Indigo Naturalis) is often used to treat childhood convulsions, and convulsions in adults accompanied by constipation, dizziness, delirium, incoherent speech, scanty yellow urine, and dysuria.

- Convulsions: use *Qing Dai* with *Niu Huang* (Calculus Bovis) and *Gou Teng* (Ramulus Uncariae cum Uncis).

Exemplar Formula: *Dang Gui Long Hui Wan* (Tangkuei, Gentiana, and Aloe Pill).

Lung heat: Clinical manifestations include cough, dyspnea, and profuse, thick, yellow sputum.

- Lung heat: use *Qing Dai* with *Gua Lou Ren* (Semen Trichosanthis), *Zhe Bei Mu* (Bulbus Fritillariae Thunbergii) and *Fu Hai Shi* (Pumice).

Eczema and oral ulcers

- Eczema and oral ulcers: use powdered *Qing Dai* with *Bing Pian* (Borneolum Syntheticum) and *Huang Bai* (Cortex Phellodendri), topically.

2. Cools Blood and Disperses Stagnation

Bleeding: Heat forcing blood out of the vessels may result in hematemesis, hemoptysis, epistaxis, and subcutaneous bleeding that manifests in blotches on the skin or purpura.

- Bleeding: use *Qing Dai* with *Ce Bai Ye* (Cacumen Platycladi) and *Bai Mao Gen* (Rhizoma Imperatae).
- Blotches on the skin: use it with *Shi Gao* (Gypsum Fibrosum), *Sheng Di Huang* (Radix Rehmanniae) and *Sheng Ma* (Rhizoma Cimicifugae).

Mumps, sore throat: Toxic heat accumulation in the throat results in mumps, sore throat and other painful sores.

- Sore throat: use *Qing Dai* alone topically, or use with *Xuan Shen* (Radix Scrophulariae), *Jin Yin Hua* (Flos Lonicerae) and *Lian Qiao* (Fructus Forsythiae).

DOSAGE

1.5 to 3 grams in decoctions, 0.6 to 1 gram in powder. *Qing Dai* can be used topically alone or with oil.

CAUTIONS / CONTRAINDICATIONS

- Use *Qing Dai* with caution in patients who have deficiency and cold of the Stomach.
- Nausea, vomiting, abdominal pain, diarrhea or hematochezia may occur with overdose.
- In rare cases, use of *Qing Dai* may affect the liver function, decrease platelet count, and cause bone marrow suppression.

CHEMICAL COMPOSITION

Indigotin, indirubin, qingdainone, isatin, tryptanthrin, qingdaiin, laccerol, isoindigo.[1]

PHARMACOLOGICAL EFFECTS

- **Antineoplastic**: The use of indirubin has been associated with moderate inhibitory influence against tumor cells in animals. Subcutaneous and intraperitoneal injections of indirubin at 200 mg/kg for 6 to 7 days were found to inhibit the growth of tumor cells in mice with lung and breast cancers.[2]
- **Antibiotic**: Decoction of *Qing Dai* has inhibitory influence against *Staphylococcus aureus*, *Bacillus anthracis* and *Vibrio cholerae*.[3]

CLINICAL STUDIES AND RESEARCH

- **Chronic granulocytic leukemia**: In a clinical study, 314 patients with chronic granulocytic leukemia were treated with indirubin. The treatment protocol was to administer 150 to 200 mg per day (maximum of 300 to 400 mg) of indirubin in three equally-divided doses for 30 to 180 days. The study reported an overall effective rate of 87.26%, with marked improvement in 59.87% of patients.[4]
- **Psoriasis**: According to one report, 35 patients with psoriasis were treated with 25 to 50 mg of indirubin daily for 8 weeks with good improvement. The study reported that indirubin exerted definite inhibition on psoriasis.[5]
- **Stomatitis**: In one study, 297 of 319 patients (92.92%) reported positive benefits after using topical application of an herbal formula for treatment of stomatitis. The treatment protocol was to apply the powder of *Qing Dai* and *Zhen Zhu* (Margarita) topically three times daily.[6]

HERB-DRUG INTERACTION

- **Sulfonylurea antidiabetics and sulfonamide antibiotics**: Patients who are allergic to sulfonylureas and sulfonamides may also be allergic to *Qing Dai* (Indigo Naturalis), *Da Qing Ye* (Folium Isatidis) and *Ban Lan Gen* (Radix Isatidis), according to Dr. Zhang Xiao-Ping. [Note: Examples of sulfonylureas include tolbutamide (Orinase), glipizide (Glucotrol), and glyburide (DiaBeta/Micronase); and examples of sulfonamides include sulfadiazine, sulfisoxazole, sulfamethoxazole, trimethoprim/sulfamethoxazole (Bactrim/Septra), and erythromycin/sulfisoxazole (Pediazole).]

TOXICOLOGY

No toxicity was reported following oral ingestion of indirubin by mice at 5 g/kg for 5 consecutive days. The LD_{50} for intraperitoneal injection of indirubin in mice is 1.1 to 2.0 g/kg. In a long-term toxicology study, indirubin was given to dogs orally at doses of 20, 100, and 200 mg/kg

Qing Dai (Indigo Naturalis)

for 6 months. The study reported poor appetite, diarrhea, hematochezia, and elevation of SGPT. At all three dose levels, however, there was no evidence of abnormalities of blood, bone marrow, kidney or heart functions.[7]

AUTHORS' COMMENTS

Qing Dai is the processed powder of *Da Qing Ye* (Folium Isatidis). *Qing Dai* has essentially the same functions as *Da Qing Ye*. However, its ability to cool blood is stronger, and it also dispels Lung heat.

The following formula by Dr. Hu Qing-Shan has been used to treat chronic granulocytic leukemia: *Qing Dai* 40%, *Tian Hua Fen* (Radix Trichosanthis) 40%, *Niu Huang* (Calculus Bovis) 10%, and *Lu Hui* (Aloe) 10%. Administer 1.5 grams in powder twice daily.

References

1. *Chang Yong Zhong Yao Cheng Fen Yu Yao Li Shou Ce* (A Handbook of the Composition and Pharmacology of Common Chinese Drugs), 1994; 1174-1175
2. Ibid., 1174-1177
3. *Zhong Yao Xue* (Chinese Herbology), 1998; 176-177
4. *Zhong Hua Xue Yi Xue Za Zhi* (Chinese Journal on Study of Hematology), 1980; 3:132
5. *Zhong Hua Yi Xue Za Zhi* (Chinese Journal of Medicine), 1987; 1:7
6. *Guang Zhou Yi Yao* (Guangzhou Medicine and Medicinals), 1987; 4:48
7. *Yao Xue Tong Bao* (Report of Herbology), 1983; 18(12):27

Zhu Zi Cao (Herba Euphorbiae Thymifoliae)

珠仔草 珠仔草

Pinyin Name: *Zhu Zi Cao*
Alternate Chinese Names: *Xiao Fei Yang Cao*
English Name: thymifolia
Botanical Name: *Euphorbia thymifolia* L.
Pharmaceutical Name: Herba Euphorbiae Thymifoliae
Properties: sweet, cool
Channels Entered: Liver, Lung

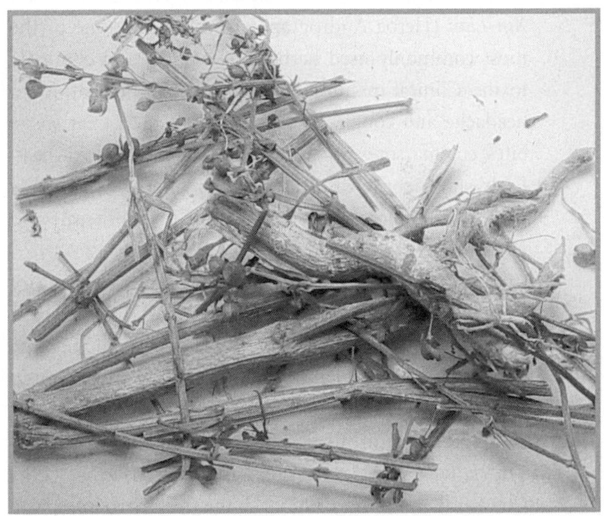

CHINESE THERAPEUTIC ACTIONS

1. Clears Heat, Eliminates Toxins, Cools Blood

Toxic heat: *Zhu Zi Cao* (Herba Euphorbiae Thymifoliae) treats toxic heat in the body that may manifest in various symptoms such as bronchitis, sore throat, hepatitis, pneumonia, dysentery or hematemesis.

- Bronchitis, sore throat, fever: use *Zhu Zi Cao* with *Xian Feng Cao* (Herba Bidentis), *Yi Zhi Xiang* (Herba Vernoniae Cinereae), and *Pao Zai Cao* (Herba Physalis Angulatae).
- Hematemesis with bright red blood: use this herb with *Ce Bai Ye* (Cacumen Platycladi).
- Hepatitis: combine it with *Huang Shui Qie* (Herba Solani) and *Hu Zhang* (Rhizoma Polygoni Cuspidati).
- Pneumonia: use it with *Da Qing Ye* (Folium Isatidis) and *Pao Zai Cao* (Herba Physalis Angulatae).
- Dysentery: add *Yu Xing Cao* (Herba Houttuyniae).

2. Promotes Urination

***Lin zheng* (dysuria syndrome):** *Zhu Zi Cao* is often used with *Bi Zi Cao* (Herba Pogonantheri Criniti) and *Shui Ding Xiang* (Herba Ludwigiae Prostratae) to promote urination and treat dysuria.

DOSAGE

3 to 15 grams.

Chuan Xin Lian (Herba Andrographis)

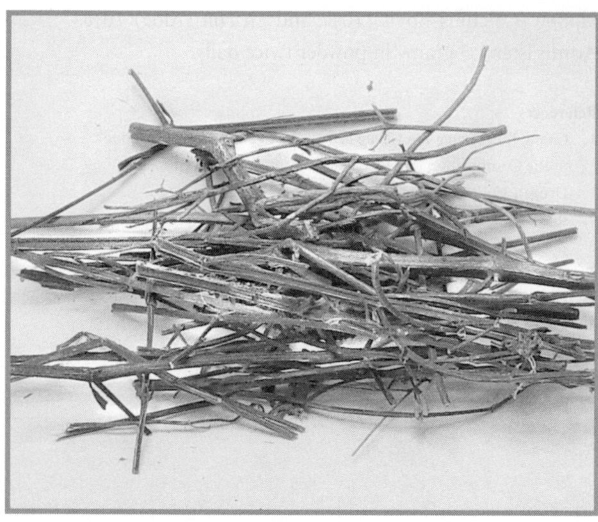

穿心蓮 穿心莲

Pinyin Name: *Chuan Xin Lian*

Literal Name: "penetrate the heart lotus," "thread-the-heart lotus"

Alternate Chinese Names: *Yi Jian Xi, Lan He Lian, Ku Dan Cao*

Original Source: *Ling Nan Cai Yao Lu* (Records of Picking Herbs in Guangdong)

English Name: andrographis, common andrographis herb

Botanical Name: *Andrographis paniculata* (Burm.f.) Nees. (*Chuan Xin Lian*)

Pharmaceutical Name: Herba Andrographis

Properties: bitter, cold

Channels Entered: Lung, Stomach, Large Intestine, Small Intestine

CHINESE THERAPEUTIC ACTIONS

1. Clears Heat and Eliminates Toxins

Accumulation of heat and toxins: In recent years, *Chuan Xin Lian* (Herba Andrographis) has become one of the most commonly-used herbs to clear heat and eliminate toxins. Clinical manifestations include sore throat, fever, headache and cough. It can also be used to treat snake bites, eczema, sores, and carbuncles that involve toxic heat.

- Early-stage febrile disorders: use this herb with *Jin Yin Hua* (Flos Lonicerae), *Ju Hua* (Flos Chrysanthemi) and *Niu Bang Zi* (Fructus Arctii).
- Cough due to Lung heat (including upper respiratory tract infection, bronchitis, or pneumonia), lung abscess, or sore throat: combine *Chuan Xin Lian* with *Yu Xing Cao* (Herba Houttuyniae) and *Jie Geng* (Radix Platycodonis).
- Eczema: apply powdered *Chuan Xin Lian* topically.
- Skin sores and carbuncles, or snake bite: use it with *Jin Yin Hua* (Flos Lonicerae) and *Ye Ju Hua* (Flos Chrysanthemi Indici). Or, mash the fresh herb into paste and apply topically.

2. Dries Dampness and Stops Diarrhea

Diarrhea or dysentery due to damp-heat: Symptoms may include rectal tenesmus, feelings of incomplete defecation, a burning sensation in the anus after defecation, diarrhea with mucus, and poor appetite.

- Diarrhea or dysentery due to damp-heat: use *Chuan Xin Lian* with *Ma Chi Xian* (Herba Portulacae) and *Jin Yin Hua* (Flos Lonicerae).

***Lin zheng* (dysuria syndrome)**: Clinical manifestations of *lin zheng* include frequent urinary urges, painful urination, and scanty yellow urine.

- *Re lin* (heat dysuria) with burning and pain: use *Chuan Xin Lian* with *Hu Zhang* (Rhizoma Polygoni Cuspidati), *Che Qian Zi* (Semen Plantaginis) and *Bai Mao Gen* (Rhizoma Imperatae).

DOSAGE

6 to 15 grams in decoction. *Chuan Xin Lian* is now commonly used in powder or capsule form at lower dosages.

CAUTIONS / CONTRAINDICATIONS

- *Chuan Xin Lian* is bitter and cold. Large dosages or long-term consumption may injure Stomach qi.
- *Chuan Xin Lian* must be used with caution during pregnancy, because of its abortifacient effect.[1]

CHEMICAL COMPOSITION

Andrographolide, neoandrographolide, deoxyandrographolide, ninandrographolide, deoxyandrographiside, andrographiside, andrographoside, homoandrographolide.[2,3]

Andrographolide

PHARMACOLOGICAL EFFECTS

- **Antibiotic**: *Chuan Xin Lian* has only a mild inhibitory

Chuan Xín Lían (Herba Andrographis)

effect *in vitro* against *Diplococcus pneumoniae* and β-hemolytic streptococcus. However, it is quite effective in treating infections *in vivo*. It has been proposed by many that its effectiveness in treating infections is due in part to its immune-enhancing effect.[4]

- **Antipyretic**: Andrographolide and neoandrographolide have antibiotic effects and are effective in reducing fever associated with infection.[5]
- **Anti-inflammatory**: In laboratory studies, administration of a preparation of *Chuan Xin Lian* is associated with stimulation of the adrenal cortex and secretion of corticosteroids, thereby exerting anti-inflammatory effects.[6]
- **Immunostimulant**: Decoction of *Chuan Xin Lian* enhances the immune system and increases the phagocytic activity of white blood cells.[7]
- **Antivenin**: Extract of *Chuan Xin Lian* may be used as an anti-snake venom, as it markedly delayed death of mice following snake bites. The exact mechanism of action is unclear.[8]
- **Abortifacient**: Intraperitoneal injection of *Chuan Xin Lian* terminated pregnancy in mice in the first, second or third trimester.[9]
- **Hepatoprotective and cholagogic**: *Chuan Xin Lian* increases the weight of the liver and the production and excretion of bile acid. In laboratory studies, andrographolide was effective in protecting the liver against foreign substances, such as carbon tetrachloride, and effectively lowered SGPT and SGOT.[10]
- **Cardiovascular**: Water extract of *Chuan Xin Lian* was found to have a marked effect on the cardiovascular system by decreasing the mean arterial blood pressure in a dose-dependent manner, without significant decrease in heart rate. Though the exact mechanism of action is unclear, it has been suggested that the hypotensive effect is related to α-adrenoceptors, not β-adrenoceptors.[11]

CLINICAL STUDIES AND RESEARCH

- **Nasosinusitis and rhinitis**: In one study, 242 patients with nasosinusitis and rhinitis were treated with 81% effectiveness using 1.8 grams of *Chuan Xin Lian* extract (6 pills per dose, 0.3 gram of herb per dose) internally, three times daily.[12]
- **Upper respiratory tract infection**: Injection of a *Chuan Xin Lian* preparation was used to treat 454 children with upper respiratory tract infection, with an 89.4% rate of effectiveness.[13]
- **Leptospirosis**: Andrographolide and deoxyandrographolide were used to treat 46 patients with leptospirosis, with an 87% rate of effectiveness.[14]

TOXICOLOGY

Intramuscular injection of *Chuan Xin Lian* was associated with one case of anaphylactic reaction.[15] [Note: Anaphylactic shock is the most severe type of allergic reaction. Unfortunately, it is very difficult, if not impossible, to predict when patients will have such serious reactions. Though there is one case of anaphylactic reaction reported in response to injection, oral use of *Chuan Xin Lian* does not necessarily have a higher risk of allergy than other herbs.]

References

1. *Bei Jing Yi Xue Yuan Xue Bao* (Journal of Beijing School of Medicine), 1979; (2):79
2. *Xian Dai Zhong Yao Yao Li Xue* (Contemporary Pharmacology of Chinese Herbs), 1997; 240-241
3. *The Merck Index* 12th edition, Chapman & Hall/CRCnetBASE/Merck, 2000
4. *Zhong Yao Xue* (Chinese Herbology), 1998, 178:179
5. *Zhong Yao Zhi* (Chinese Herbology Journal), 1988; 560
6. *Yao Xue Tong Bao* (Report of Herbology), 1982; 17(4):3
7. *Zhong Yao Yao Li Yu Ying Yong* (Pharmacology and Applications of Chinese Herbs), 1983:824
8. *Indian J Pharm Sci*, 1978; 40(4):132
9. *Bei Jing Yi Xue Yuan Xue Bao* (Journal of Beijing School of Medicine), 1979; (2):79
10. *Res Der Indigenous Drugs*, 1989:147
11. *Journal of Ethnopharmacology*. 56(2):97-101, 1997 Apr.
12. *Xin Yi Xue* (New Medicine), 1984; 9:481
13. *Zhong Cao Yao Tong Xun* (Journal of Chinese Herbal Medicine), 1978; 10:27
14. *Xin Yi Yao Xue Za Zhi* (New Journal of Medicine and Herbology), 1973; 7:7
15. *Xin Yi Xue* (New Medicine), 1972; 11:53

Yu Xing Cao (Herba Houttuyniae)

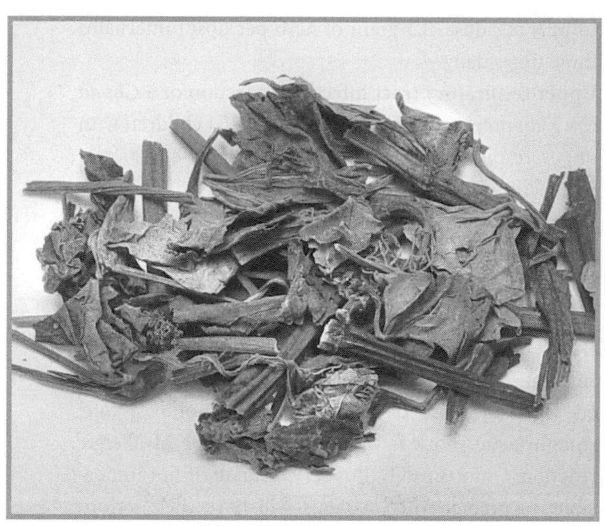

魚腥草 鱼腥草

Pinyin Name: *Yu Xing Cao*
Literal Name: "fishy-smelling herb"
Original Source: *Ming Yi Za Zhu* (Miscellaneous Records of Famous Physicians) by Tao Hong-Jing in 500 A.D.
English Name: houttuynia, heart-leaf houttuynia
Botanical Name: *Houttuynia cordata* Thunb. (*Ji Cai*)
Pharmaceutical Name: Herba Houttuyniae
Properties: acrid, cool
Channels Entered: Lung

CHINESE THERAPEUTIC ACTIONS

1. Clears Heat, Eliminates Toxins and Drains Pus

Lung abscess: Acrid and cool, *Yu Xing Cao* (Herba Houttuyniae) dispels heat and toxins, and drains abscesses and pus. It is commonly used to treat various lung infections, lung abscesses with coughing, or vomiting with mucus and blood.

- Lung abscess: use *Yu Xing Cao* with *Jie Geng* (Radix Platycodonis), *Huang Qin* (Radix Scutellariae), and *Lu Gen* (Rhizoma Phragmitis).
- Cough caused by Lung heat: use it with *Zhi Mu* (Radix Anemarrhenae), *Zhe Bei Mu* (Bulbus Fritillariae Thunbergii), and *Sang Bai Pi* (Cortex Mori).

Sores and skin lesions from heat and toxins: *Yu Xing Cao* is used both internally and topically to treat skin infections.

- Sores and skin lesions: combine it with *Ye Ju Hua* (Flos Chrysanthemi Indici), *Lian Qiao* (Fructus Forsythiae) and *Pu Gong Ying* (Herba Taraxaci), for use internally or topically.

Various infections: *Yu Xing Cao* effectively treats infection of the internal organs. Clinical applications include pneumonia, acute or chronic bronchitis and enteritis.

- Pneumonia, acute or chronic bronchitis: use this herb with *Xing Ren* (Semen Armeniacae Amarum), *Shi Gao* (Gypsum Fibrosum) and *Huang Qin* (Radix Scutellariae).
- Enteritis: add *Bai Jiang Cao* (Herba cum Radice Patriniae).

2. Promotes Normal Urination

***Lin zheng* (dysuria syndrome)**: *Yu Xing Cao* drains heat and dampness from the lower *jiao* to promote normal urination and relieve *lin zheng*, urinary tract infection with frequent urinary urges, and scanty yellow urine.

- *Shi lin* (stone dysuria): use this herb with *Hai Jin Sha* (Herba Lygodii), *Shi Wei* (Folium Pyrrosiae) and *Jin Qian Cao* (Herba Lysimachiae).
- *Re lin* (heat dysuria): combine it with *Che Qian Zi* (Semen Plantaginis) and *Chuan Mu Tong* (Caulis Clematidis Armandii).

DOSAGE

15 to 30 grams in decoction. *Yu Xing Cao* should be decocted for only a short period of time. Double the dosage if the fresh form is used. *Yu Xing Cao* may be used topically, as a fresh herb crushed into paste, or as an herbal solution to be used as a rinse.

CHEMICAL COMPOSITION

Essential oil 0.022 to 0.025% (decanoylacetaldehyde, methyl nonyl ketone, laurinaldehyde, α-pinene, myrcene, limonene, linalool, citronellol, citral, 1,8-cineol, ocimene, carvacrol, thymol), flavonoids (quercetin, isoquercitrin, quercitrin, reynoutrin, hyperin, rutin, cordarine). Houttuynium is the synthetic sodium derivative of decanoylacetaldehyde.[1]

PHARMACOLOGICAL EFFECTS

- **Antibiotic**: *Yu Xing Cao* has a broad spectrum of action to inhibit *Staphylococcus aureus*, β-hemolytic streptococcus, *Diplococcus pneumoniae*, *Neisseria catarrhalis*, *Corynebacterium diphtheriae*, *Bacillus proteus*, *Bacillus dysenteriae*, leptospira, dermatophytes and some influenza viruses.[2,3]
- **Immunostimulant**: Administration of *Yu Xing Cao* in rabbits is associated with an increase in phagocytic activities by the white blood cells, and an increase of serum properdin.[4]

Yu Xing Cao (Herba Houttuyniae)

- **Others**: *Yu Xing Cao* has anti-inflammatory, diuretic, analgesic, antitussive, and hemostatic effects.[5,6]

CLINICAL STUDIES AND RESEARCH

- **Pneumonia**: In one study, 25 of 28 patients with pneumonia showed complete recovery following an herbal treatment containing 30 grams of *Yu Xing Cao* and 15 grams of *Jie Geng* (Radix Platycodonis). The herbs were cooked in water to yield 200 ml of decoction. Patients were given 30 ml per dose, three to four times daily. Those with a profuse amount of thick sputum were also treated with inhalation of a 5% *Yu Xing Cao* solution.[7]
- **Chronic bronchitis**: In a clinical study, 190 patients with chronic bronchitis were divided into two groups and treated with houttuynium. In the first group, the study reported a 78% rate of effectiveness with intramuscular injection. In the second group, the study reported a 76.7% from oral ingestion of houttuynium.[8]
- **Inflammation**: Good results were reported when 183 patients with various inflammatory disorders were treated with houttuynium. The various disorders treated included cervicitis, pelvic inflammatory disease, pneumonia, pulmonary abscesses, and others.[9]
- **Nephrotic syndrome**: Five patients with nephrotic syndrome were treated with 100 grams of *Yu Xing Cao* in tea or decoction form, with good results.[10]
- **Leptospirosis**: A study reported that 15 to 30 grams of *Yu Xing Cao* per day was effective in prevention of leptospirosis in 1,603 patients. *In vitro* studies also showed that *Yu Xing Cao* inhibits leptospira.[11]
- **Cervical erosion**: Treatment of 679 patients with cervical erosion resulted in 86.2 to 99.3% effectiveness, using topical application of an herbal formula. The formula was prepared by mixing houttuynium, *Bing Pian* (Borneolum Syntheticum) and coconut oil.[12]
- **Atrophic sinusitis**: Nasal distillation of a *Yu Xing Cao* solution was used to treat 33 patients with atrophic sinusitis with satisfactory results.[13]
- **Angioma**: A preparation of *Yu Xing Cao* was reported to be 90.8% effective in treating 55 patients with angioma.[14]

TOXICOLOGY

Yu Xing Cao has very little toxicity. Injection in animals of doses up to 200 times the normal human dose for one week did not result in any abnormalities or fatalities.[15]

There was one instance of anaphylactic reaction associated with intramuscular injection of *Yu Xing Cao*.[16] [Note: Anaphylactic shock is the most severe type of allergic reaction. Unfortunately, it is very difficult, if not impossible, to predict when patients will have such serious reactions. Though there is one case of anaphylactic reaction reported with injection, oral use of *Yu Xing Cao* does not necessarily have a higher risk of allergy than other herbs.]

AUTHORS' COMMENTS

Yu Xing Cao, literally known as 'fishy-smelling herb,' has a distinct smell when freshly harvested from the ground. Therefore, the usual assumption is that the decoction must be difficult to swallow. However, decoction of this herb is dark red, and rather fragrant, without any unpleasant odor.

References

1. *Xian Dai Zhong Yao Yao Li Xue* (Contemporary Pharmacology of Chinese Herbs), 1997; 252-253
2. *Chang Yong Zhong Yao Cheng Fen Yu Yao Li Shou Ce* (A Handbook of the Composition and Pharmacology of Common Chinese Drugs), 1994; 1286:1289
3. *Zhong Yao Xue* (Chinese Herbology), 1998; 187:189
4. *Xin Yi Yao Xue Za Zhi* (New Journal of Medicine and Herbology), 1973; (7):25
5. *Chang Yong Zhong Yao Cheng Fen Yu Yao Li Shou Ce (A Handbook of the Composition and Pharmacology of Common Chinese Drugs)*, 1994; 1286:1289
6. *Zhong Yao Xue (Chinese Herbology)*, 1998; 187:189
7. *Zhong Hua Nei Ke Za Zhi (Chinese Journal of Internal Medicine)*, 1963; 3:250
8. *Xin Yi Yao Xue Za Zhi (New Journal of Medicine and Herbology)*, 1973; 7:25
9. *Xin Yi Xue (New Medicine)*, 1979; 12:601
10. *Shan Xi Zhong Yi (Shanxi Chinese Medicine)*, 1988; 2:20
11. *Xin Yi Yao Xue Za Zhi (New Journal of Medicine and Herbology)*, 1975; 6:49
12. *Shang Hai Zhong Yi Yao Za Zhi (Shanghai Journal of Chinese Medicine and Herbology)*, 1983; 3:24
13. *Xin Yi Yao Xue Za Zhi (New Journal of Medicine and Herbology)*, 1977; 7:34
14. *Jiang Xi Yi Xue Yuan Xue Bao (Medical Journal of Jiangxi University of Medicine)*, 1987; 1:50
15. *He Nan Zhong Yi (Henan Chinese Medicine)*, 1986; (6):39
16. *Guang Xi Chi Jiao Yi Shen (Guangxi Barefoot Doctor)*, 1978; 3:25

She Gan (Rhizoma Belamcandae)

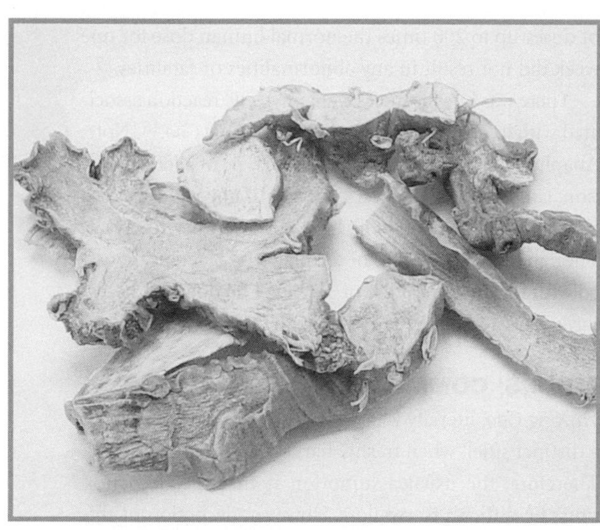

射干

Pinyin Name: *She Gan*
Literal Name: "arrow shaft," "shooting dryness"
Alternate Chinese Names: *Wu San, Bian Zhu*
Original Source: *Shen Nong Ben Cao Jing* (Divine Husbandman's Classic of the Materia Medica) in the second century
English Name: belamcanda, blackberry lily rhizome
Botanical Name: *Belamcanda chinensis* (L.) DC. (*She Gan*)
Pharmaceutical Name: Rhizoma Belamcandae
Properties: bitter, cold
Channels Entered: Lung

CHINESE THERAPEUTIC ACTIONS

1. Clears Heat and Eliminates Toxins

Sore throat: *She Gan* (Rhizoma Belamcandae) treats sore throat by eliminating heat, toxins and phlegm. Severe cases of sore throat caused by heat and toxins are characterized by sharp pain, redness of the affected area, swollen throat and excruciating pain when swallowing. Profuse phlegm and labored breathing with throttling sound are also common presentations of heat and toxins affecting the Lung.

- Sore throat with profuse phlegm: use *She Gan* with *Huang Qin* (Radix Scutellariae), *Jie Geng* (Radix Platycodonis) and *Gan Cao* (Radix Glycyrrhizae).
- Sore throat due to heat and toxins: combine it with *Sheng Ma* (Rhizoma Cimicifugae), *Ma Bo* (Lasiosphaera seu Calvatia), and *Xuan Shen* (Radix Scrophulariae).

2. Eliminates Phlegm and Relieves Wheezing

Dyspnea, cough with profuse sputum: Bitter, cold and dispersing in nature, *She Gan* dissolves sputum and relieves wheezing caused by accumulation of heat and phlegm in the Lung.

- Dyspnea, cough with profuse yellow sputum: use *She Gan* with *Sang Bai Pi* (Cortex Mori) and *Jie Geng* (Radix Platycodonis).
- Dyspnea, cough with profuse white or clear sputum: combine this herb with *Xi Xin* (Herba Asari), *Ban Xia* (Rhizoma Pinelliae) and *Sheng Jiang* (Rhizoma Zingiberis Recens).

DOSAGE

6 to 10 grams in decoction.

CAUTIONS / CONTRAINDICATIONS

- *She Gan* is contraindicated during pregnancy.
- Use *She Gan* with caution for patients who have deficiency and cold of the Spleen and Stomach.

CHEMICAL COMPOSITION

Tectoridin, tectorigenin, irigenin, belamcadin, iridin, mangiferin, iristectorin A, B; tectoruside, embinin.[1]

PHARMACOLOGICAL EFFECTS

- **Antiviral**: According to one report, 100% extract of *She Gan* has an inhibitory effect on dermatophytes and influenza viruses.[2]

CLINICAL STUDIES AND RESEARCH

- **Galacturia**: In a clinical study, 87 patients with galacturia were treated with decoction of *She Gan* three times daily with an 85.1% rate of effectiveness. Depending on the individual, the dosage was between 12 and 25 grams. In another study, 104 patients with galacturia were treated with a *She Gan* preparation with 90.4% effectiveness. Those with uncomplicated galacturia received *She Gan* 15g; those with a chronic condition received *She Gan* 15g, *Chuan Xiong* (Rhizoma Ligustici Chuanxiong) 9g, and *Chi Shao* (Radix Paeoniae Rubrae) 12g; and those with galacturia and hematuria received *She Gan* 15g, *Sheng Di Huang* (Radix Rehmanniae) 15g, and *Xian He Cao* (Herba Agrimoniae) 15g.[3,4]

TOXICOLOGY

The LD_{50} for alcohol extract of *She Gan* (1:1) in mice via oral ingestion is 66.78 g/kg.[5]

She Gan (Rhizoma Belamcandae)

AUTHORS' COMMENTS

She Gan and *Shan Dou Gen* (Radix Sophorae Tonkinensis) have similar actions to clear heat. *She Gan* has a stronger function to dispel phlegm and disperse stagnation. *Shan Dou Gen* has a stronger function to sedate fire.

She Gan and *Ma Bo* (Lasiosphaera seu Calvatia) have similar functions to clear Lung heat. *She Gan* sedates Lung heat and disperses phlegm. It is best for heat-type cough with profuse phlegm. *Ma Bo* clears Lung heat and benefits the throat. It is used for sore throat, loss of voice and cough caused by heat and toxicity affecting the descending functions of the Lung.

References

1. *Xian Dai Zhong Yao Yao Li Xue* (Contemporary Pharmacology of Chinese Herbs), 1997; 239
2. *Zhong Yao Yao Li Yu Ying Yong* (Pharmacology and Applications of Chinese Herbs), 1990; 6(6):28
3. *Zhong Yi Za Zhi* (Journal of Chinese Medicine), 1986; 11:66
4. Ibid.
5. *Zhong Yao Yao Li Yu Lin Chuan* (Pharmacology and Clinical Applications of Chinese Herbs), 1990; 6(6):28

Shan Dou Gen (Radix Sophorae Tonkinensis)

山豆根

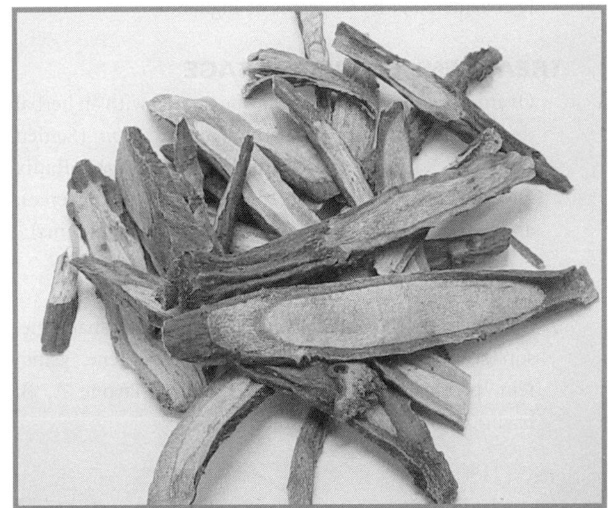

Pinyin Name: *Shan Dou Gen*
Literal Name: "mountain bean root"
Alternate Chinese Names: *Guan Dou Gen, Nan Dou Gen*
Original Source: *Kai Bao Ben Cao* (Materia Medica of the Kai Bao Era) by Ma Zhi in 973-974 A.D.
English Name: sophora root, tonkin sophora root
Botanical Name: *Sophora tonkinensis* Gagnep. (*Yue Nan Hui*); *Sophora subprostrata* Chun et. T. Chen (*Guan Dou Gen*)
Pharmaceutical Name: Radix Sophorae Tonkinensis
Properties: bitter, cold
Channels Entered: Lung
Safety Index: slightly toxic

CHINESE THERAPEUTIC ACTIONS

1. Clears Heat and Eliminates Toxins

Sore throat: *Shan Dou Gen* (Radix Sophorae Tonkinensis) treats sore throat and reduces pain, as it has marked effectiveness to clear heat and eliminate toxins.

- Mild sore throat: use *Shan Dou Gen* individually as an herbal decoction or herbal gargle.
- Severe sore throat: use it with *Xuan Shen* (Radix Scrophulariae), *She Gan* (Rhizoma Belamcandae) and *Ban Lan Gen* (Radix Isatidis).

2. Treats Cancer, Abscesses, and Carbuncles

Shan Dou Gen treats throat or lung cancer, sores, and abscesses and carbuncles characterized by heat and toxins.

- Sore throat: use this herb with *Jin Yin Hua* (Flos Lonicerae), *Lian Qiao* (Fructus Forsythiae), and *Huang Lian* (Rhizoma Coptidis).
- Throat or lung cancers: combine it with *Ban Zhi Lian* (Herba Scutellariae Barbatae) and *Bai Hua She She Cao* (Herba Oldenlandia).

3. Relieves Jaundice

In the past, *Shan Dou Gen* was used for damp-heat jaundice. However, it is no longer used for this function today as there are other herbs that are more effective.

DOSAGE

6 to 10 grams in decoction. *Shan Dou Gen* is used as a gargle or as powder on affected areas.

Shan Dou Gen (Radix Sophorae Tonkinensis)

CAUTIONS / CONTRAINDICATIONS

- *Shan Dou Gen* is contraindicated in patients with deficiency and cold of the Spleen and Stomach characterized by decreased appetite and loose stools.

OVERDOSAGE

Overdose of *Shan Dou Gen* is characterized by varying degrees of abdominal pain, dizziness, nausea, vomiting, pale face, increased or decreased heart rate, headache, weakness of the extremities, tremor, profuse perspiration, increased blood pressure, and loss of balance. Gross overdose is characterized by difficulty in breathing, spasms and cramps of the extremities, purple lips and face, and delirium. In severe cases, there may be respiratory depression and death. Such adverse reactions occur because *Shan Dou Gen* is a strong stimulant and may interfere with normal functions of the nervous and respiratory systems. Side effects have been observed in dosages as low as 12 grams. The lethal dosage is generally considered to be 60 grams or higher.

TREATMENT OF OVERDOSAGE

Overdose of *Shan Dou Gen* may be treated with an herbal decoction containing 60 grams of *Lu Dou* (Semen Phaseoli Radiati), 30 grams of *Gan Cao* (Radix Glycyrrhizae), 24 grams of *Jin Yin Hua* (Flos Lonicerae), and 9 grams of *Chuan Xin Lian* (Herba Andrographis).[1]

CHEMICAL COMPOSITION

Alkaloids (matrine, oxymatrine, methylcytisine, anagyrine, sophocarpine), flavonoids (sophoradochromene, genistein, pterocarpine, trifolirhizin, sophoraflavone A, B, bayin), sophoradin, sophoranone.[2,3]

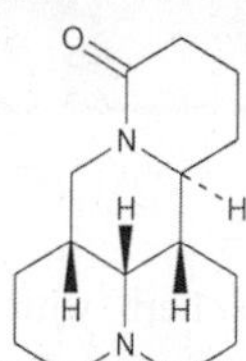

Matrine

PHARMACOLOGICAL EFFECTS

- **Antiarrhythmic**: Administration of *Shan Dou Gen* via intramuscular or intraperitoneal injections has been found to be effective in treating animals with drug-induced arrhythmias. *Shan Dou Gen* has a negative chronotropic and positive inotropic effect on the right ventricle of the heart in guinea pigs.[4]
- **Immunostimulant**: Administration of *Shan Dou Gen* orally in mice is associated with an increase of IgM and IgG.[5]
- **CNS suppressant:** The alkaloids of *Shan Dou Gen* have a marked inhibitory effect on the central nervous system (CNS), leading to sedation, analgesia, and lowered body temperature in mice. It is also effective in preventing and treating drug-induced seizures.[6]
- **Antiasthmatic**: Alkaloids of *Shan Dou Gen*, such as matrine, oxymatrine, methylcytisine, anagyrine, and sophocarpine have shown marked antiasthmatic effects. By comparison to aminophylline, oxymatrine has similar but prolonged antiasthmatic effects.[7,8]
- **Antipyretic**: Matrine, oxymatrine, and sophocarpine have all demonstrated marked ability to reduce body temperature in mice. The exact mechanism of action is unclear.[9]
- **Hepatoprotective**: Reports have indicated that administration of *Shan Dou Gen* is associated with a hepatoprotective function by lowering the liver enzymes and minimizing liver damage caused by carbon tetrahydrochloride.[10]
- **Antiulcer**: The alcohol extract of *Shan Dou Gen* inhibits the secretion of gastric acid in rats. Components with this action included sophoradin and sophoranone.[11]
- **Antineoplastic**: Administration of *Shan Dou Gen* via oral or intraperitoneal routes has been associated with antineoplastic effects in mice, especially against uterine, abdominal and liver cancers. The antineoplastic components of the herb have been identified as the alkaloids of the herb, such as matrine, oxymatrine, and sophocarpine.[12,13]
- **Antibiotic**: *Shan Dou Gen* has an inhibitory effect against *Bacillus dysenteriae, Bacillus proteus, E. coli, Staphylococcus aureus*, and *Pseudomonas aeruginosa*.[14]

CLINICAL STUDIES AND RESEARCH

- **Sore throat**: An herbal formula containing *Shan Dou Gen, Lian Qiao* (Fructus Forsythiae), *She Gan* (Rhizoma Belamcandae) and *Tian Hua Fen* (Radix Trichosanthis) was evaluated for its effectiveness in treatment of sore throat. Out of 120 patients who took 15 doses of the formula, 84 reported complete recovery, 30 showed marked improvement, and 6 had no response. The overall rate of effectiveness was 95%.[15]
- **Hepatitis**: Injection of a *Shan Dou Gen* preparation containing primarily alkaloids was 91.8% effective in 402 patients with hepatitis. The study reported that most patients showed a significant reduction of liver enzymes within 2 to 4 weeks.[16]
- **Arrhythmia**: Eleven patients with arrhythmia were treated with 40 grams of *Shan Dou Gen* with marked improvement in 7 patients, improvement in 3 patients, and no results in 1 patient.[17]

TOXICOLOGY

Shan Dou Gen is slightly toxic. In a toxicology study in mice, the LD_{50} of decoction of *Shan Dou Gen* via intraperitoneal injection is 15.6 g/kg.[18]

Shan Dou Gen (Radix Sophorae Tonkinensis)

SUPPLEMENT

- 北豆根 *Bei Dou Gen* (Rhizoma Menispermi), *Menispermum dahuricum* DC., is sometimes used as a substitute for *Shan Dou Gen* in northern China. Bitter and cold, *Bei Dou Gen* clears heat and toxins. It is commonly used to treat throat soreness and pain. The recommended dosage of *Bei Dou Gen* is 3 to 10 grams.

References

1. *Zhong Yao Bu Liang Fan Ying Yu Zhi Liao* (Adverse Reactions and Treatment of Chinese Herbal Medicine), 1996; 123:125
2. *Xian Dai Shi Yong Yao Xue* (Practical Applications of Modern Herbal Medicine), 1997; 226
3. Yan X, Zhou J, Xie G, *Traditional Chinese Medicines Molecular Structures, Natural Sources and Applications*; Ashgate, 1999; 4904
4. *Zhong Guo Yao Li Xue Bao* (Chinese Herbal Pharmacology Journal), 1990; 11(3):253
5. *Guo Wai Yi Xue Zhong Yi Zhong Yao Fen Ce* (Monograph of Chinese Herbology from Foreign Medicine), 1989; 11(2):59
6. *Zhong Yao Yao Li Yu Lin Chuan* (Pharmacology and Clinical Applications of Chinese Herbs), 1987; (9):645
7. *Xi Bei Yi Yao Za Zhi* (Northwest Journal of Herbal Medicine), 1989; 4(4):12
8. *Zhong Yao Yao Li Yu Ying Yong* (Pharmacology and Applications of Chinese Herbs), 1985; 195
9. *Zhong Xi Yi Jie He Za Zhi* (Journal of Integrated Chinese and Western Medicine), 1982; 5(2):108
10. *Xian Dai Shi Yong Yao Xue* (Practical Applications of Modern Herbal Medicine), 1988; 5(1):7
11. *Guo Wai Yi Yao Zhi Wu Yao Fen Ce* (Monograph of Foreign Botanical Medicine), 1980; (1):43
12. *Zhong Guo Yi Xue Ke Xue Xue Bao* (Journal of Chinese Medical Science University), 1988; 10(1):39
13. *Zhong Xi Yi Jie He Za Zhi* (Journal of Integrated Chinese and Western Medicine), 1982; 2(1):42
14. *Xian Dai Shi Yong Yao Xue* (Practical Applications of Modern Herbal Medicine), 1988; 5(1):7
15. *Zhong Yi Yao Yan Jiu* (Research of Chinese Medicine and Herbology), 1991; (4):54
16. *Yao Xue Tong Bao* (Report of Herbology), 1983; (10):37
17. *Hu Bei Zhong Yi Za Zhi* (Hubei Journal of Chinese Medicine), 1989; (4):16
18. *Guang Zhou Zhong Yi Xue Yuan Xue Bao* (Journal of Guangzhou University of Chinese Medicine), 1982; (4):27

Ma Bo (Lasiosphaera seu Calvatia)

馬勃 马勃

Pinyin Name: *Ma Bo*
Original Source: *Ming Yi Za Zhu* (Miscellaneous Records of Famous Physicians) by Tao Hong-Jing in 500 A.D.
English Name: lasiosphaera (puffball)
Botanical Name: *Lasiosphaera fenzlii* Reich. (*Tuo Pi Ma Bo*); *Calvatia gigantea* (Batsch ex Pers.) Lloyd. (*Da Ma Bo*); *Calvatia lilacina* (Mont. et Ber.) Lloyd (*Zi She Ma Bo*)
Pharmaceutical Name: Lasiosphaera seu Calvatia
Properties: acrid, neutral to cool
Channels Entered: Lung

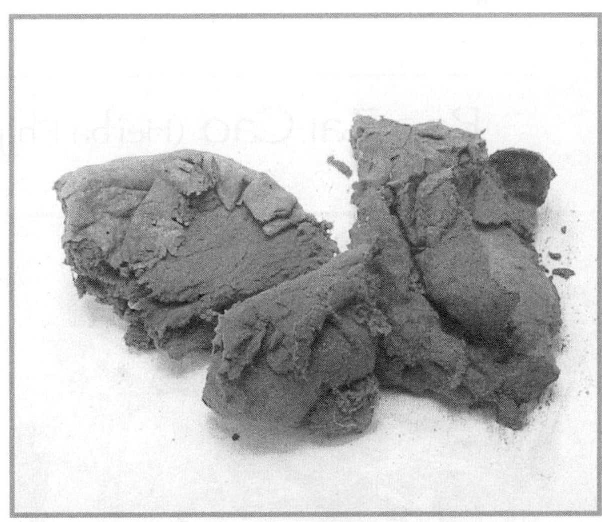

CHINESE THERAPEUTIC ACTIONS

1. Clears the Lung, Benefits the Throat, and Eliminates Toxins

Sore throat: *Ma Bo* (Lasiosphaera seu Calvatia) enters the Lung and is commonly used to clear heat and eliminate toxins from the upper body. It treats Lung heat with cough, a sore, swollen, red throat, and loss of voice. *Ma Bo* cools the blood and is best for the type of sore throat involving bleeding or ulceration. Other symptoms may include redness and swelling of the face, and fever.

Ma Bo (Lasiosphaera seu Calvatia)

Disorders exhibiting such symptoms may include infectious parotitis and tonsillitis.

- Throat swelling and pain: use *Ma Bo* with *Xuan Shen* (Radix Scrophulariae), *She Gan* (Rhizoma Belamcandae) and *Ban Lan Gen* (Radix Isatidis).
- Sore throat: sprinkle *Ma Bo* onto the affected area.
- Loss of voice: use it with *Gu Zhi Hua* (Semen Oroxyli) and *Chan Tui* (Periostracum Cicadae).

2. Stops Bleeding

Bleeding: *Ma Bo*, used internally or topically, stops bleeding caused by heat driving blood out of the vessels. Clinical applications include epistaxis and hematemesis. This herb is also used topically for frostbite or bleeding resulting from sports injuries.

- Epistaxis and hematemesis: combine it with *Bai Mao Gen* (Rhizoma Imperatae), *Ou Jie* (Nodus Nelumbinis Rhizomatis) and *Ce Bai Ye* (Cacumen Platycladi).

DOSAGE

3 to 6 grams in decoction. *Ma Bo* should be wrapped in cheesecloth prior to cooking. *Ma Bo* can be placed directly on the throat in powder form to reduce swelling and pain.

CHEMICAL COMPOSITION

Gemmatein, urea.[1]

PHARMACOLOGICAL EFFECTS

- **Hemostatic**: Constituents of *Ma Bo* have a mild influence to stop bleeding.[2]
- **Antibiotic**: This substance has an inhibitory effect against *Staphylococcus aureus*, *Pseudomonas aeruginosa*, *Bacillus proteus*, and *Diplococcus pneumoniae*.[3]

CLINICAL STUDIES AND RESEARCH

- **Bleeding**: *Ma Bo* has shown good results in stopping bleeding in patients with bleeding from the oral cavity.[4]
- **Post-surgical bleeding**: Topical application of 1 to 4 grams of *Ma Bo* powder has shown marked hemostatic effect both during and after surgery.[5]
- **External use**: Topical application of powdered *Ma Bo* was effective in treatment of external injury and frostbite.[6]

References

1. *Zhong Yao Xue* (Chinese Herbology), 1998; 192-193
2. Ibid.
3. Ibid.
4. *Zhong Hua Kou Qiang Ke Za Zhi* (Chinese Journal of Stomatology), 1960; 3:143
5. *Zhong Xi Yi Jie He Za Zhi* (Journal of Integrated Chinese and Western Medicine), 1985; 10:601
6. *Jiang Su Zhong Yi* (Jiangsu Chinese Medicine), 1963; 2:19

Pao Zai Cao (Herba Physalis Angulatae)

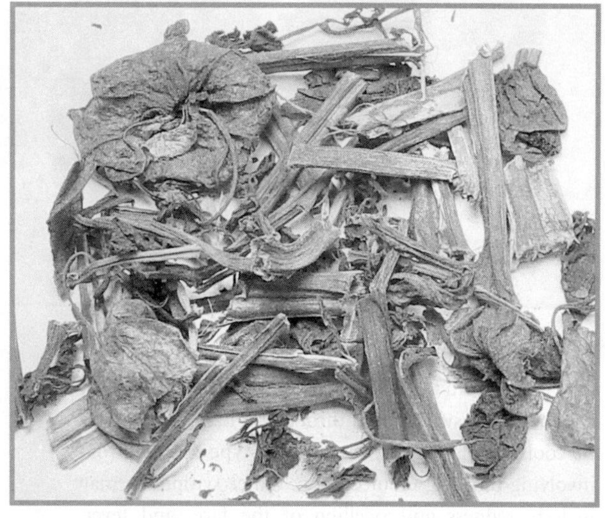

炮仔草 炮仔草

Pinyin Name: *Pao Zai Cao*
Alternate Chinese Names: *Deng Long Cao, Ding Ren Zai Cao, Gua Jin Deng, Gui Deng Long*
English Name: physalis angulata
Botanical Name: *Physalis angulata* L.
Pharmaceutical Name: Herba Physalis Angulatae
Properties: bitter, cool
Channels Entered: Lung, Urinary Bladder, Liver, Kidney

Pao Zai Cao (Herba Physalis Angulatae)

CHINESE THERAPEUTIC ACTIONS

1. Clears Heat, Arrests Cough

Pao Zai Cao (Herba Physalis Angulatae) clears heat from the Lung to treat coughing and sore throat.

- Wind-heat with cough and sore throat: use *Pao Zai Cao* with *Yi Zhi Xiang* (Herba Vernoniae Cinereae), *Da Qing Ye* (Folium Isatidis) and *Ya She Huang* (Herba Lippiae).

2. Reduces Inflammation and Eliminates Toxins

- Gynecological disorders from inflammation, such as dysmenorrhea or inflammation of the uterus, fallopian tubes and ovaries: use *Pao Zai Cao* with *Hu Yao Huang* (Herba Leucas Mollissimae), *Ma Bian Cao* (Herba Verbenae), *Yi Mu Cao* (Herba Leonuri) and *Ya She Huang* (Herba Lippiae).
- *Chang feng* (intestinal wind) with bright bleeding from the rectum before passage of stools, and abdominal pain: use this herb with *Qing Mu Xiang* (Radix Aristolochiae) and *Ma Ti Jin* (Herba Dichondrae Repentis).
- Oral sores, stomatitis because of Stomach heat: use it with *Xian Feng Cao* (Herba Bidentis), *Huang Lian* (Rhizoma Coptidis) and *Lu Gen* (Rhizoma Phragmitis).
- Snake bite or toxic swelling and pain: apply *Pao Zai Cao* topically.

DOSAGE

3 to 15 grams in decoction.

CAUTIONS / CONTRAINDICATIONS

- *Pao Zai Cao* is contraindicated during pregnancy.

Dao Diao Jin Zhong (Melothria Maderospatana)

倒吊金鐘
倒吊金钟

Pinyin Name: *Dao Diao Jin Zhong*
Alternate Chinese Names: *Feng Fang Ran*
English Name: melothria
Botanical Name: *Melothria maderaspatana* M.J. Roem.
Pharmaceutical Name: Melothria Maderospatana
Properties: sweet, bitter, cool
Channels Entered: Lung, Liver, Urinary Bladder

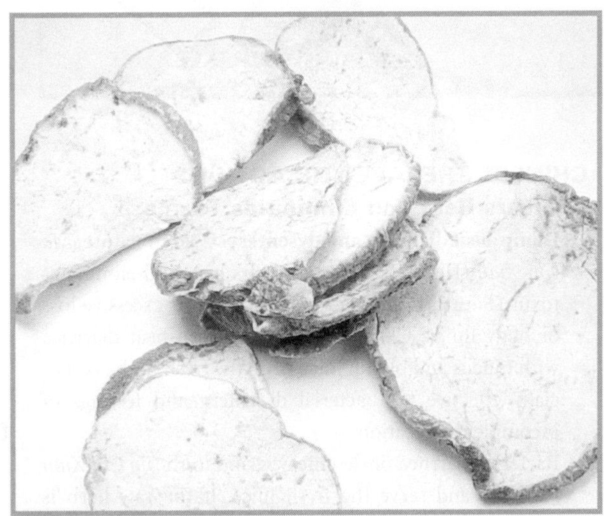

CHINESE THERAPEUTIC ACTIONS

Clears Heat, Eliminates Toxins and Relieves Pain

Febrile disorders, jaundice, dysuria, fetal toxicosis, various toxic swellings, lung abscesses: *Dao Diao Jin Zhong* (Melothria Maderospatana) treats a wide range of disorders caused by heat and toxicity.

- Lung abscess: use *Dao Diao Jin Zhong* with *Pu Gong Ying* (Herba Taraxaci), *Bai Jiang Cao* (Herba cum Radice Patriniae) and *Da Qing Ye* (Folium Isatidis).
- Febrile disorders with irritability and stifling sensations in the chest: use it with *Xian Feng Cao* (Herba Bidentis) and *Ji Xue Cao* (Herba Centellae).
- Jaundice: add it to *Yin Chen Hao* (Herba Artemisiae Scopariae).
- Dysuria or frequent urinary urges: combine this herb with *Shui Ding Xiang* (Herba Ludwigiae Prostratae) and *Shan Pu Tao* (Radix Vitis Amurensis).
- Toxic swelling: use it with *Hu Yao Huang* (Herba Leucas Mollissimae), *Shu Wei Huang* (Herba Rostellulariae), and *Cha Chi Huang* (Herba Stellariae Aquaticae).

Dao Diao Jin Zhong (Melothria Maderospatana)

DOSAGE

3 to 12 grams in decoction.

CAUTIONS / CONTRAINDICATIONS

- Use with caution for patients with Spleen deficiency.

Ma Chi Xian (Herba Portulacae)

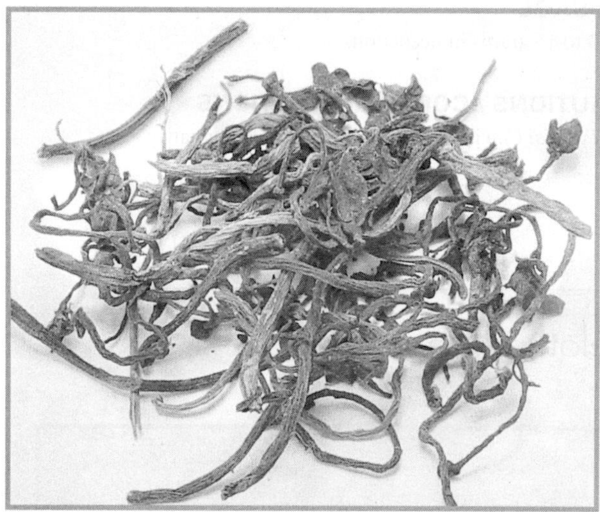

馬齒莧 马齿苋

Pinyin Name: *Ma Chi Xian*
Literal Name: "horse's teeth amaranth"
Alternate Chinese Names: *Ma Chi Cai*
Original Source: *Xin Xiu Ben Cao* (Newly Revised Materia Medica) by Su Jing in 657-659 A.D.
English Name: portulaca
Botanical Name: *Portulaca oleracea* L. (*Ma Chi Xian*)
Pharmaceutical Name: Herba Portulacae
Properties: sour, cold
Channels Entered: Large Intestine, Liver

CHINESE THERAPEUTIC ACTIONS

1. Clears Heat and Eliminates Toxins

Damp-heat diarrhea and dysentery: Cold in nature, *Ma Chi Xian* (Herba Portulacae) clears heat and eliminates toxins. Sour-tasting, *Ma Chi Xian* prevents excessive loss of body fluids. Clinically, it treats damp-heat diarrhea with mucus and blood. Juice from the fresh herb is especially effective for bacterial dysentery and feelings of incomplete defecation.

- Bacterial diarrhea or dysentery: grind fresh *Ma Chi Xian* for juice and serve the fresh juice. If the raw herb is unavailable, post-decoct *Ma Chi Xian* and serve it with garlic, or use it as decoction with *Huang Lian* (Rhizoma Coptidis) and *Huang Qin* (Radix Scutellariae).
- White leukorrhea with or without the presence of blood: use it with *Hai Piao Xiao* (Endoconcha Sepiae).
- Intestinal abscess: combine this herb with *Pu Gong Ying* (Herba Taraxaci).
- Heat and toxins in the skin: use *Ma Chi Xian* topically.
- Sores, hemorrhoids, lesions, ulcerations, or eczema due to toxic heat: use the crushed paste of fresh *Ma Chi Xian*, apply topically.

2. Cools Blood, Stops Bleeding, Treats *Lin Zheng* (Dysuria Syndrome)

Bleeding: *Ma Chi Xian* cools the blood and treats various kinds of bleeding from the lower body, such as profuse menstrual bleeding, *xue lin* (bloody dysuria) and *re lin* (heat dysuria). *Ma Chi Xian* is used as a single-herb treatment, or is combined with other hemostatic herbs.

DOSAGE

9 to 15 grams for the dried herb, 30 to 60 grams for the fresh herb, in decoction. *Ma Chi Xian* is commonly used both internally and topically.

CHEMICAL COMPOSITION

Nor-adrenaline 0.25%, l-noradrenaline, dopamine, malic acid, citric acid, glutamic acid, aspartic acid, alanine, galacturonic acid, arabinose, galactose, rhamnose, betacyanin, oleracin I, II; ferulic acid, β-amyrin, lupeol, nicotinic acid, tocopherol, β-carotene.[1]

PHARMACOLOGICAL EFFECTS

- **Antibiotic**: The water extract of *Ma Chi Xian* has an inhibitory effect *in vitro* against *Bacillus dysenteriae*;

Ma Chi Xian (Herba Portulacae)

while an alcohol extract of the herb is effective against *E. coli*, *Salmonella typhi*, *Staphylococcus aureus* and some dermatophytes.[2]

- **Uterine stimulant**: Extract of *Ma Chi Xian* has a stimulating effect on the smooth muscles of the intestines and uterus in rats, rabbits, and guinea pigs. It leads to increased peristalsis of the intestines and contraction of the uterus. It was noted in another study that *Ma Chi Xian* has mixed effects on the uterus. While the stem may stimulate the uterus and lead to contraction, the leaves may inhibit the uterus and lead to relaxation.[3,4,5]

CLINICAL STUDIES AND RESEARCH

- **Bacterial dysentery**: Patients with acute and chronic dysentery were treated with a 50% decoction of *Ma Chi Xian* with marked effectiveness. The study reported 89.12% effectiveness in 331 patients with acute bacterial dysentery, and 83.62% effectiveness in 403 patients with chronic bacterial dysentery. The treatment protocol was to give 40 ml of the decoction three times daily, for 7 to 14 days per course of treatment. The dosage and duration of treatment were increased for those who did not initially respond.[6]
- **Whooping cough**: In one study, 54 patients with whooping cough showed satisfactory responses following an herbal treatment. The treatment protocol was to give 100 ml of 50% *Ma Chi Xian* syrup in equally-divided portions four times daily over three days.[7]
- **Parasitic infection**: Hookworm infestations in 41 patients were treated with an herbal decoction with a 87.8% rate of complete recovery. The treatment protocol was to cook 90 grams of fresh *Ma Chi Xian* in two bowls of water. After simmering to evaporate 20% of the water, the decoction was filtered out and 15 grams each of clear vinegar and white sugar were added. The patients were given the decoction once daily, before bedtime.[8]
- **Vitiligo**: After topical application of herbs in 125 patients with vitiligo, 91.2% of patients reported some improvement and 45.6% showed complete recovery. The treatment protocol was to mix the juice of *Ma Chi Xian* with sugar and vinegar. Patients were asked to apply the herbal formulation topically and stay in the sun. The duration of sunbath was not specified.[9]
- **Suppurative dermatological diseases**: Concurrent administration of *Ma Chi Xian* orally and topically was reported to be very effective in treating various suppurative dermatological disorders.[10]
- **Cervical erosion**: In a clinical study, 212 patients with cervical erosion were treated with an herbal formula for 20 days, with an overall success rate of 97.2%. The herbal formula was prepared by cooking 3,500 grams of *Ma Chi Xian* and 500 grams of *Gan Cao* (Radix Glycyrrhizae) in water to yield 300 ml of final decoction. The pills were made by adding 2,000 grams of starch to 300 ml of decoction. Patients were instructed to take 2 grams of herbs in pills twice daily, for two courses (20 days) of treatment.[11]
- **Uterine bleeding**: Intramuscular injection of *Ma Chi Xian* was effective in treating over 500 patients with various causes of uterine bleeding, including but not limited to postpartum bleeding, cesarean section, miscarriage, and abortion.[12]
- **Others**: According to one report, 60 grams of *Ma Chi Xian* and 30 grams of brown sugar cooked in decoction were found to be effective in treating 4 cases of hematuria, 98 cases of urinary tract infection, 32 cases of bacterial infection, 39 cases of enteritis, and 112 cases of suppurative dermatological disorders.[13]

References

1. *Chang Yong Zhong Yao Cheng Fen Yu Yao Li Shou Ce* (A Handbook of the Composition and Pharmacology of Common Chinese Drugs), 1994; 446-447
2. *Ji Lin Zhong Yi Yao* (Jilin Chinese Medicine and Herbology), 1985; 3:28
3. Ibid.
4. *Zhong Cao Yao Tong Xun* (Journal of Chinese Herbal Medicine), 1972; 1:32
5. *Zhong Yao Xue* (Chinese Herbology), 1998; 194:196
6. *Fu Jian Zhong Yi Yao* (Fujian Chinese Medicine and Herbology), 1959; 6:1
7. *Shang Hai Zhong Yi Yao Za Zhi* (Shanghai Journal of Chinese Medicine and Herbology), 1959; 3:40
8. *Xin Yi Yao Xue Za Zhi* (New Journal of Medicine and Herbology); 1973; 8:30
9. *Guang Xi Zhong Yi Yao* (Guangxi Chinese Medicine and Herbology), 1978; 4:38
10. *Zhong Hua Wai Ke Za Zhi* (Chinese Journal of External Medicine), 1959; 7:645
11. *Tian Jing Yi Yao* (Tianjing Medicine and Herbology), 1973; 2:5
12. *Zhong Cao Yao Tong Xun* (Journal of Chinese Herbal Medicine), 1972; 1:32
13. *Si Chuan Yi Xue* (Sichuan Medicine), 1982; 2:97

Qin Pi (Cortex Fraxini)

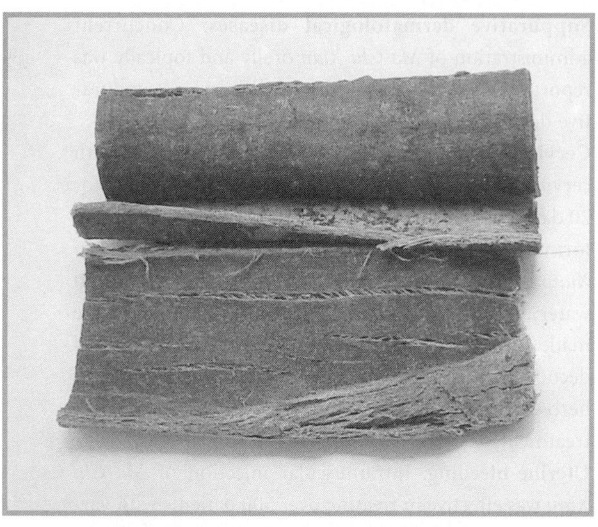

秦皮

Pinyin Name: *Qin Pi*
Alternate Chinese Names: *La Shu Pi*
Original Source: *Shen Nong Ben Cao Jing* (Divine Husbandman's Classic of the Materia Medica) in the second century
English Name: fraxinus, ash bark
Botanical Name: *Fraxinus rhynchophylla* Hance. (*Ku Li Bai La Shu*); *Fraxinus chinensis* Roxb. (*Bai La Shu*); *Fraxinus bungeana* DC. (*Bai La Shu*); *Fraxinus chinensis* Roxb. var. *acuminata*. (*Jien Ye Bai La Shu*)
Pharmaceutical Name: Cortex Fraxini
Properties: bitter, cold
Channels Entered: Gallbladder, Liver, Large Intestine

CHINESE THERAPEUTIC ACTIONS

1. Clears Heat, Eliminates Toxins, and Dries Dampness

Diarrhea and dysentery due to damp-heat: *Qin Pi* (Cortex Fraxini) has a unique ability to concurrently purge damp-heat and retain body fluids. It is commonly used to treat diarrhea or dysentery involving rectal tenesmus, abdominal pain, hematochezia, a yellow, greasy tongue coating, and thirst with no desire to drink.

- Diarrhea or dysentery with rectal tenesmus due to damp-heat: use *Qin Pi* with *Bai Tou Weng* (Radix Pulsatillae) and *Huang Lian* (Rhizoma Coptidis). **Exemplar Formula**: *Bai Tou Weng Tang* (Pulsatilla Decoction).

Damp-heat leukorrhea: *Qin Pi* treats foul-smelling yellow, turbid leukorrhea.

- Damp-heat leukorrhea: use this herb with *Mu Dan Pi* (Cortex Moutan).

2. Clears Liver Fire and Brightens the Eyes

Eye disorders caused by Liver yang rising: Clinical manifestations include eye redness, swelling, and pain, photophobia, tearing upon exposure to wind, and superficial visual obstruction.

- Eye redness and swelling due to Liver fire: use *Qin Pi* alone as a wash, or combine it with *Jue Ming Zi* (Semen Cassiae), *Mu Zei* (Herba Equiseti Hiemalis) and *Ju Hua* (Flos Chrysanthemi).

3. Redirects Lung Qi to Relieve Cough and Wheezing

Cough or dyspnea: *Qin Pi* clears Lung heat and causes Lung qi to descend to treat cough, wheezing and dyspnea. It can be used individually or in combination with other herbs.

DOSAGE

6 to 12 grams in decoction.

CAUTIONS / CONTRAINDICATIONS

- *Qin Pi* should be used with caution in patients with deficiency and cold of the Spleen and Stomach.

CHEMICAL COMPOSITION

Coumarin (aesculin, aesculetin, fraxin, fraxetin, fraximol, fraxidin, isofraxidin, cichorin), tannin.[1,2]

Fraxin

Fraxetin

PHARMACOLOGICAL EFFECTS

- **Antibiotic:** *Qin Pi* has demonstrated inhibitory action against *Staphylococcus aureus, Bacillus dysenteriae, E. coli, Neisseria catarrhalis*, and α-hemolytic streptococcus.[3,4]

Qin Pi (Cortex Fraxini)

- **Respiratory**: Aesculetin and fraxin from *Qin Pi* have demonstrated marked antitussive, expectorant, and antiasthmatic effects in animals.[5]
- **Anti-inflammatory**: Aesculin has demonstrated definite anti-inflammatory influence, possibly through an increased secretion of corticosteroids from the adrenal glands.[6]
- **Others**: *Qin Pi* has sedative, analgesic, antiseizure, and diuretic effects.

CLINICAL STUDIES AND RESEARCH

- **Bacterial dysentery**: Fifty patients with bacterial dysentery were treated with an 80% success rate using an herbal formulation containing *Qin Pi*.[7]
- **Chronic bronchitis**: In one study, 530 patients with chronic bronchitis were treated through inhalation of steam from *Qin Pi* decoction. The treatment demonstrated marked antitussive, antiasthmatic and expectorant results in 92.9% of the patients.[8]

TOXICOLOGY

No fatalities were reported following intraperitoneal injection of aesculetin in mice at 3 g/kg.[9]

SUPPLEMENT

- 核桃楸皮 *He Tao Qiu Pi* (Cortex Juglans), *Juglans mandshurica* Maxim., is bitter and cold. It clears heat, eliminates toxins, stops diarrhea and dysentery, and treats eye infections. The dosage of *He Tao Qiu Pi* is 4.5 to 9 grams in decoction. *Qin Pi* (Cortex Fraxini) is sometimes substituted incorrectly with *He Tao Qiu Pi* (Cortex Juglans). Though these two herbs have some overlapping characteristics, they should not be used interchangeably as there are also significant differences.

References

1. *Xian Dai Zhong Yao Yao Li Xue* (Contemporary Pharmacology of Chinese Herbs), 1997; 258
2. *The Merck Index* 12th edition, Chapman & Hall/CRCnetBASE/Merck, 2000
3. *Zhi Wu Yao You Xiao Cheng Fen Shou Ce* (Manual of Plant Medicinals and Their Active Constituents), 1986; 419,467,942
4. *Zhong Yao Xue* (Chinese Herbology), 1998; 197:199
5. *Zhi Wu Yao You Xiao Cheng Fen Shou Ce* (Manual of Plant Medicinals and Their Active Constituents), 1986; 419,467,942
6. *Zhong Yao Xue* (Chinese Herbology), 1998; 197:199
7. Ibid.
8. *Zhong Cao Yao Tong Xun* (Journal of Chinese Herbal Medicine), 1973; 1:21
9. *Zhi Wu Yao You Xiao Cheng Fen Shou Ce* (Manual of Plant Medicinals and Their Active Constituents), 1986; 419,467,942

Bai Tou Weng (Radix Pulsatillae)

白頭翁 白头翁

Pinyin Name: *Bai Tou Weng*
Literal Name: "white-headed gentleman"
Original Source: *Shen Nong Ben Cao Jing* (Divine Husbandman's Classic of the Materia Medica) in the second century
English Name: pulsatilla, Chinese pulsatilla root
Botanical Name: *Pulsatilla chinensis* (Bge.) Regel (*Bai Tou Weng*)
Pharmaceutical Name: Radix Pulsatillae
Properties: bitter, cold
Channels Entered: Large Intestine

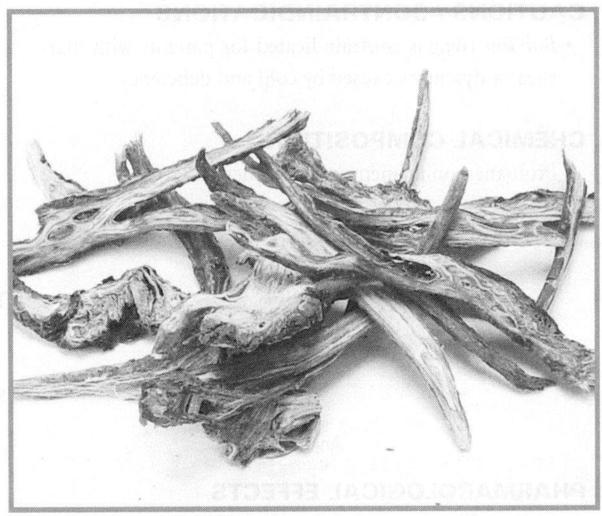

Bai Tou Weng (Radix Pulsatillae)

CHINESE THERAPEUTIC ACTIONS

Clears Heat, Eliminates Toxins, and Cools Blood

Diarrhea, dysentery: These conditions are characterized by damp-heat in the Large Intestine causing bloody diarrhea or dysentery. *Bai Tou Weng* (Radix Pulsatillae) is an essential herb in treating amoebic dysentery. Other symptoms may include rectal tenesmus, abdominal pain and frequent urges to defecate.

- Diarrhea or dysentery with mucus and blood caused by damp-heat: use *Bai Tou Weng* with *Huang Lian* (Rhizoma Coptidis), *Huang Bai* (Cortex Phellodendri) and *Qin Pi* (Cortex Fraxini). **Exemplar Formula:** *Bai Tou Weng Tang* (Pulsatilla Decoction).

Hemorrhoids from damp-heat and toxicity:

- Hemorrhoids: use *Bai Tou Weng* internally or topically.
- Bleeding hemorrhoids: combine it with *Di Yu* (Radix Sanguisorbae), charred *Huai Hua* (Flos Sophorae) and charred *Huang Qin* (Radix Scutellariae).

Scrofula:

- Scrofula: use *Bai Tou Weng* internally or topically, as a single-herb remedy or in a formula.

Febrile malarial disorders:

- Febrile malarial disorders: use *Bai Tou Weng* with *Chai Hu* (Radix Bupleuri), *Huang Qin* (Radix Scutellariae) and *Bing Lang* (Semen Arecae).

DOSAGE

6 to 15 grams in decoction.

CAUTIONS / CONTRAINDICATIONS

- *Bai Tou Weng* is contraindicated for patients with diarrhea or dysentery caused by cold and deficiency.

CHEMICAL COMPOSITION

Protoanemonin, anemonin, ranunculin.[1,2]

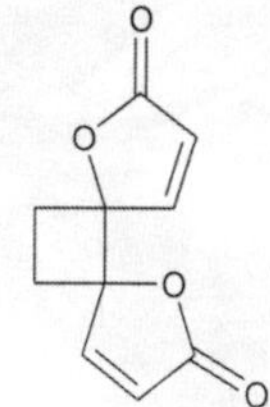

Anemonin

PHARMACOLOGICAL EFFECTS

- **Antiamebic**: *Bai Tou Weng* has an inhibitory effect against amoeba *in vitro* and *in vivo*, but only at large doses. In one study, decoction of *Bai Tou Weng* at 1 g/kg for 6 days effectively treated amoebic dysentery in mice. However, the treatment was ineffective when the dosage was reduced to 0.3 g/kg.[3]
- **Antibiotic**: The fresh juice, decoction and alcohol extract of *Bai Tou Weng* have all shown an inhibitory effect against *Staphylococcus aureus, Pseudomonas aeruginosa, Bacillus dysenteriae, Salmonella typhi, Bacillus subtilis, Corynebacterium diphtheriae, Mycobacterium tuberculosis, Candida albicans*, and others.[4]
- **Others**: *Bai Tou Weng* has cardiotonic, sedative, and analgesic effects.[5]

CLINICAL STUDIES AND RESEARCH

- **Amoebic dysentery**: In one report, 26 patients with amoebic dysentery were treated with a 100% success rate using a 50% decoction of *Bai Tou Weng*. The dosage was 5 to 10 ml, three times daily, for a total of 60 to 300 ml.[6]
- **Scrofula**: Thirty patients with scrofula were treated with good results, using a decoction of *Bai Tou Weng*. The treatment protocol was to cook 30 grams of *Bai Tou Weng* in water, and take the final decoction in four equally-divided doses.[7]
- **Uterine bleeding**: In one study, 106 patients with uterine bleeding were treated with a 93.4% rate of effectiveness using an herbal decoction. The herbal formula contained 90 grams of *Bai Tou Weng*, and 60 grams each of *Di Yu* (Radix Sanguisorbae) and white sugar, with other herbs as deemed necessary.[8]
- **Toothache**: According to one report, 25 patients with toothache were treated with good results using a decoction of *Bai Tou Weng*, one to three times daily.[9]
- **Dermatitis**: In one study, 107 patients with dermatitis were treated with topical application of *Bai Tou Weng*, with complete recovery in 66 cases, significant improvement in 23 cases, moderate improvement in 12 cases, and no response in 6 cases. The treatment protocol was to soak fresh *Bai Tou Weng* leaves in water, gently rub the soaked leaves on the skin, then cover the affected area with gauze. Apply gentle had pressure to the skin for 20 minutes. Patients generally report a warm, burning sensation, which lasts approximately 20 minutes.[10]

TOXICOLOGY

Decoction of *Bai Tou Weng* has very low toxicity.[11]

SUPPLEMENT

- 白頭翁莖/白头翁茎 *Bai Tou Weng Jing* (Caulis Pulsatillae) and 白頭翁葉/白头翁叶 *Bai Tou Weng Ye* (Folium Pulsatillae) have antirheumatic functions, cardiotonic effects, and are slightly toxic. The root, *Bai Tou Weng* (Radix Pulsatillae), on the other hand, has antibiotic effects and is commonly used to treat bacterial or

Bai Tou Weng (Radix Pulsatillae)

amoebic dysentery. The stems and leaves of this plant are not interchangeable with the root, as their functions and properties are significantly different.

AUTHORS' COMMENTS

Bai Tou Weng, *Huang Lian* (Rhizoma Coptidis), and *Qin Pi* (Cortex Fraxini) are commonly used to treat diarrhea and dysentery.

- *Bai Tou Weng* clears heat and toxins from the blood. It has antibiotic effects against amoebae.
- *Huang Lian* clears heat and dries up dampness. It has antibiotic effects against bacteria.
- *Qin Pi* dispels damp-heat and preserves body fluids in the intestines. It has antibiotic effects against bacteria.

References

1. *Xian Dai Zhong Yao Yao Li Xue* (Contemporary Pharmacology of Chinese Herbs), 1997; 752
2. *The Merck Index* 12th edition, Chapman & Hall/CRCnetBASE/Merck, 2000
3. *Wu Han Yi Xue Yuan Xue Bao* (Journal of Wuhan University School of Medicine), 1958; (1):1
4. *CA*, 1948; 42:4228a
5. *Zhong Yao Xue* (Chinese Herbology), 1998; 195:197
6. *Xin Zhong Yao Xue* (New Chinese Herbal Medicine), 1956; 10:11
7. *Si Chuan Zhong Yi* (Sichuan Chinese Medicine), 1987; 5:33
8. *Hu Bei Zhong Yi Za Zhi* (Hubei Journal of Chinese Medicine), 1987; 4:22
9. *Zhong Guo Yi Yuan Yao Xue Za Zhi* (Chinese Hospital Journal of Herbology), 1987; 9:391
10. *Xin Yi Xue* (New Medicine), 1975; 12:57
11. *Wu Han Yi Xue Yuan Xue Bao* (Journal of Wuhan University School of Medicine), 1958; (1):1

Ya Dan Zi (Fructus Bruceae)

鴉膽子 鸦胆子

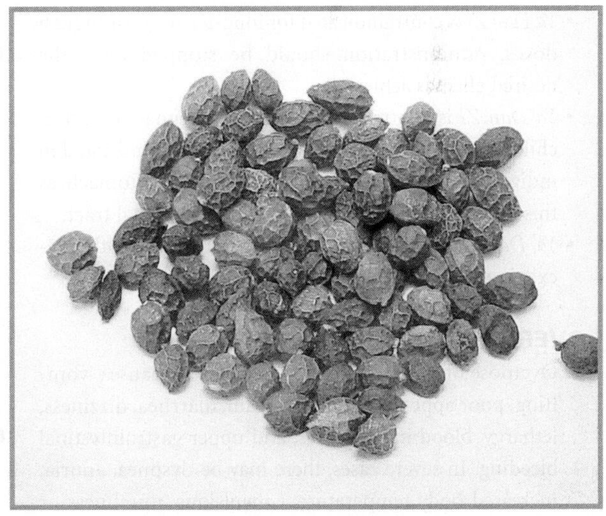

Pinyin Name: *Ya Dan Zi*
Literal Name: "duck's gallbladder seed"
Alternate Chinese Names: *Ku Shen Zi*
Original Source: *Ben Cao Gang Mu Shi Yi* (Omissions from the Grand Materia Medica) by Zhao Xue-Min in 1765
English Name: brucea seed, java brucea fruit
Botanical Name: *Brucea javanica* (L.) Merr. (*Ya Dan Zi*)
Pharmaceutical Name: Fructus Bruceae
Properties: bitter, cold
Channels Entered: Large Intestine, Liver
Safety Index: slightly toxic

CHINESE THERAPEUTIC ACTIONS

1. Clears Heat and Eliminates Toxins

Dysentery: *Ya Dan Zi* (Fructus Bruceae) is especially effective for treatment of chronic intermittent dysentery, in which there seem to be periods of rest and recurrence over a period of one to two years. This herb is taken on an empty stomach during attacks, and Spleen tonic herbs are taken during remission periods. *Ya Dan Zi* is also good for rectal tenesmus with dysentery containing blood and mucus, and dysentery caused by protozoans and amoebas.

- Bloody dysentery: wrap *Ya Dan Zi* inside *Long Yan Rou* (Arillus Longan) for oral consumption.

Ya Dan Zi (Fructus Bruceae)

2. Treats Malaria

Ya Dan Zi treats malaria characterized by alternating fever and chills, in which each episode may last 2 to 3 days.

- Malaria: use *Ya Dan Zi* in capsules for 3 to 5 days.

3. Treats Cancer

Ya Dan Zi is used in treatment of cancers of the colon, breast, esophagus, stomach, cervix and rectum that are caused by toxic heat.

4. Softens Hardness

Ya Dan Zi is used topically to soften nodules and hardnesses. Indications include warts and corns. For treatment of warts and corns, crush the herb and mix with grain-based liquor, make it into a paste, and apply topically.

DOSAGE

The dosage of *Ya Dan Zi* is 10 to 15 seeds for malaria, and 10 to 30 seeds for dysentery. Remove the shells and use only the seeds. This extremely bitter herb is not suitable for decoction. Instead, it is often given in capsule or tablet form; or wrapped inside *Long Yan Rou* (Arillus Longan) to mask the bitter taste. *Ya Dan Zi* is also used in powder form at the dosage of 1.5 to 2 grams.

CAUTIONS / CONTRAINDICATIONS

- *Ya Dan Zi* is contraindicated for long-term use or in high doses. Administration should be stopped once the desired effect is achieved.
- *Ya Dan Zi* is contraindicated during pregnancy, and in children and elderly patients. It is also contraindicated in individuals with deficiency of the Spleen and Stomach, as this herb is very irritating to the gastrointestinal tract.
- *Ya Dan Zi* is contraindicated in individuals with pre-existing liver and kidney disorders.

OVERDOSAGE

Overdose of *Ya Dan Zi* is characterized by nausea, vomiting, poor appetite, abdominal pain, diarrhea, dizziness, lethargy, blood in the stools, and upper gastrointestinal bleeding. In severe cases, there may be dyspnea, anuria, increased body temperature, convulsions, numbness or paralysis of the extremities, kidney and liver damage, and unconsciousness. Adverse reactions usually occur within 20 to 60 minutes after ingestion of the herbs. Overdose in adults may occur following ingestion of 50 seeds of *Ya Dan Zi*.

TREATMENT OF OVERDOSAGE

Overdose may be treated with general or specific methods using herbal decoction:

- Overdose in general can be treated with an herbal decoction given three times daily, with the following ingredients: *Gan Cao* (Radix Glycyrrhizae) 12g, *Lu Dou* (Semen Phaseoli Radiati) 15 to 30g, and *Lu Gen* (Rhizoma Phragmitis) 50 to 80g.
- Overdose with upper gastrointestinal bleeding should be treated with an herbal decoction of *Gan Cao* (Radix Glycyrrhizae) 50g, *Yuan Zhi* (Radix Polygalae) 9g, *Sha Shen* (Radix Glehniae seu Adenophorae) 15g, charred *Di Yu* (Radix Sanguisorbae) 9g, *Xue Yu Tan* (Crinis Carbonisatus) 9g, and *San Qi* (Radix Notoginseng) 2g.[1]

CHEMICAL COMPOSITION

Glyceroltrioleate, oleic acid, linoleic acid, bruceantin, bruceanlinol, bruceine A, B, C; dehydro brucein A, brusatol, bruceine C, D; yadanzioside A, F, and I; bruceoside A and B.[2,3,4]

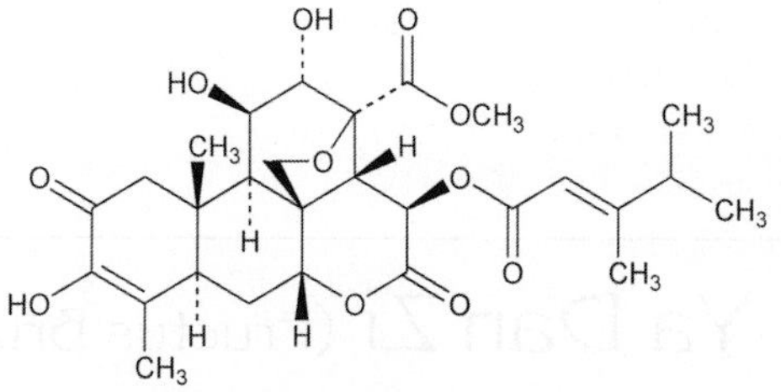

Bruceantin

PHARMACOLOGICAL EFFECTS

- **Antiamebic**: Bruceantin and bruceine C have both demonstrated marked effectiveness against *Entamoeba histolitica*.[5]
- **Antimalarial**: Many constituents of *Ya Dan Zi* have demonstrated marked antimalarial action, including but not limited to bruceantin, bruceanlinol, bruceine A, B, and C; dehydro brucein A, brusatol, bruceine D, yadanzioside A, F, and I.[6]
- **Antineoplastic**: Many components of *Ya Dan Zi* have demonstrated antineoplastic effects, such as bruceoside A and B.[7]

CLINICAL STUDIES AND RESEARCH

- **Amoebic dysentery**: Sixty-five patients with amoebic dysentery were treated with *Ya Dan Zi* with approximately 94% effectiveness. The patients were given the herbs in both capsule (three times daily) and liquid (once daily) forms for 10 days per course of treatment.[8]
- **Malaria**: Good results were reported when 27 patients with malaria were treated with *Ya Dan Zi*. The treatment protocol was to grind 12 seeds into fine powder and place it in capsules. Patients were instructed to take the capsules three times daily on an empty stomach. This treatment was effective against many types of malaria, especially those in which the outbreaks take place during daytime.[9]

Ya Dan Zi (Fructus Bruceae)

- **Warts**: In one study, 3 to 5 grams of *Ya Dan Zi* crushed into powder and soaked in 75% alcohol overnight was effective as a topical agent for treating warts. The solution was applied to the affected area two to three times daily.[10]
- **Cancer**: In a multi-center study, 388 patients with esophageal, stomach, rectal, and cervical cancers were treated with intravenous injection of *Ya Dan Zi*. The study reported an overall effectiveness of 71.6% in terms of prolonging life.[11]

TOXICOLOGY

One instance of anaphylactic reaction was reported following the use of *Ya Dan Zi*. The clinical presentation included numbness of the extremities, perspiration, cyanotic face, urinary and bowel incontinence, dyspnea, and unconsciousness.[12] [Note: Anaphylactic shock is the most severe type of allergic reaction. Unfortunately, it is very difficult, if not impossible, to predict when patients will have such serious reactions. Though there has been one case of anaphylactic reaction reported, use of *Ya Dan Zi* does not necessarily have a higher risk of allergy than other herbs.]

References

1. *Zhong Yao Bu Liang Fan Ying Yu Zhi Liao* (Adverse Reactions and Treatment of Chinese Herbal Medicine), 1996; 220:222
2. *Xian Dai Zhong Yao Yao Li Xue* (Contemporary Pharmacology of Chinese Herbs), 1997; 767
3. *Chang Yong Zhong Yao Cheng Fen Yu Yao Li Shou Ce* (A Handbook of the Composition and Pharmacology of Common Chinese Drugs), 1994; 1409
4. *The Merck Index* 12th edition, Chapman & Hall/CRCnetBASE/Merck, 2000
5. *Planata Med*, 1986; (2):108
6. *J Nat Prod*, 1987; 50 (1):41
7. *Zhong Yao Xue* (Chinese Herbology), 1998; 199:201
8. *Zhong Yi Za Zhi* (Journal of Chinese Medicine), 1956; 1:16
9. *Yi Yao Xue* (Study of Medicine and Medicinals), 1952; 1:28
10. *Zhong Yao Tong Bao* (Journal of Chinese Herbology), 1986; 9:59
11. *Zhong Guo Yi Yao Bao* (Chinese Journal of Medicine and Medicinals), 1985
12. *Zhong Yao Bu Liang Fan Ying Yu Zhi Liao* (Adverse Reactions and Treatment of Chinese Herbal Medicine), 1996; 220:222

Hong Teng (Caulis Sargentodoxae)

紅藤 红藤

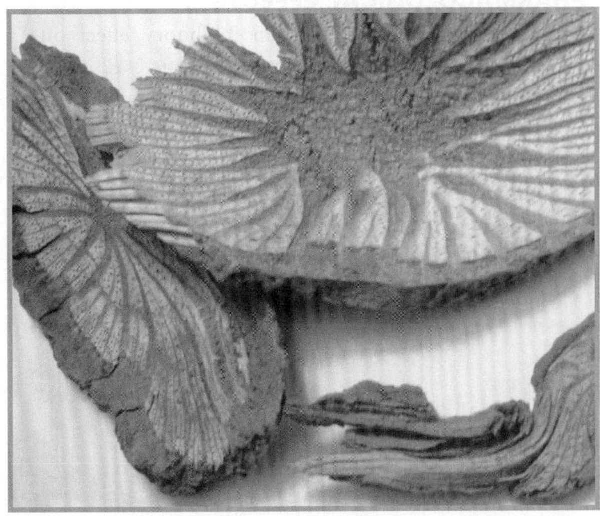

Pinyin Name: *Hong Teng*
Literal Name: "red vine"
Alternate Chinese Names: *Da Xue Teng, Xue Teng, Huo Xue Teng*
Original Source: *Tu Jing Ben Cao* (Illustrated Classic of the Materia Medica) by Su Song in 1061
English Name: sargentodoxa vine
Botanical Name: *Sargentodoxa cuneata* Rehd. et Wils. (*Da Xue Teng*)
Pharmaceutical Name: Caulis Sargentodoxae
Properties: bitter, neutral
Channels Entered: Large Intestine

CHINESE THERAPEUTIC ACTIONS

1. Clears Heat and Eliminates Toxins

Intestinal abscess: *Hong Teng* (Caulis Sargentodoxae) clears heat, eliminates toxins, activates blood circulation and relieves pain. It is one of the most commonly used herbs to treat intestinal abscesses characterized by accumulation of

Hong Teng (Caulis Sargentodoxae)

heat and toxins, and stagnation of qi and blood. *Hong Teng* is also effective for treatment of appendicitis.

- Intestinal abscess: use *Hong Teng* with *Da Huang* (Radix et Rhizoma Rhei), *Lian Qiao* (Fructus Forsythiae), *Pu Gong Ying* (Herba Taraxaci) and *Mu Dan Pi* (Cortex Moutan). **Exemplar formula**: *Da Huang Mu Dan Tang* (Rhubarb and Moutan Decoction).
- Appendicitis: use this herb with *Jin Yin Hua* (Flos Lonicerae), *Zi Hua Di Ding* (Herba Violae), and *Pu Gong Ying* (Herba Taraxaci).

2. Dispels Stasis and Relieves Pain

Blood stagnation: *Hong Teng* treats sharp pain caused by blood stasis. Clinical applications include *bi zheng* (painful obstruction syndrome), traumatic or sports injuries, and menstrual pain.

- Pain: combine it with *Dang Gui* (Radicis Angelicae Sinensis), *Chi Shao* (Radix Paeoniae Rubrae), *Wu Ling Zhi* (Excrementum Trogopteri seu Pteromi), and *Pu Huang* (Pollen Typhae).

DOSAGE

10 to 15 grams in decoction. The maximum dosage of *Hong Teng* is 30 grams. It is commonly used as an herbal decoction or herbal wine.

CHEMICAL COMPOSITION

Tannin, emodin, physcion, daucosteral, β-sitosterol, salidroside, liriodendrin.[1,2]

PHARMACOLOGICAL EFFECTS

- **Antibiotic**: *Hong Teng* has an inhibitory effect on *Staphylococcus aureus*, β-streptococcus, *E. coli*, *Pseudomonas aeruginosa*, and *Neisseria catarrhalis*.[3]
- **Cardiovascular**: According to numerous *in vitro* and *in vivo* studies, administration of *Hong Teng* is associated with inhibition of platelet aggregation, increased blood perfusion to the coronary artery, inhibited formation of thrombin, and elevated plasma levels of cAMP.[4]

CLINICAL STUDIES AND RESEARCH

- **Appendicitis**: In one study, acute non-complicated appendicitis in 1,213 patients was treated with an herbal preparation, with over 90% effectiveness. The herbal preparation contained extracts of *Hong Teng*, *Pu Gong Ying* (Herba Taraxaci), *Da Huang* (Radix et Rhizoma Rhei), and *Hou Po* (Cortex Magnoliae Officinalis). Excipients included starch and magnesium stearate.[5]
- **Acute mastitis**: In a clinical study, decoction of 60 to 90 grams of *Hong Teng* taken in two equally-divided doses was effective in treating patients with acute mastitis. Out of 24 cases, 21 showed complete recovery, 2 showed moderate improvement, and 1 had no response.[6]

AUTHORS' COMMENTS

Hong Teng (Caulis Sargentodoxae) and *Ji Xue Teng* (Caulis Spatholobi) are sometimes used interchangeably in certain parts of China. Both herbs invigorate blood circulation, open channels and collaterals, and relieve pain. The difference, however, is that *Hong Teng* treats intestinal abscess while *Ji Xue Teng* invigorates and tonifies blood. These two herbs have some similarities yet significantly distinct functions, and should not be confused or substituted casually for each other.

According to Dr. Zhang Liang-Lin, *Hong Teng*, *Bai Jiang Cao* (Herba cum Radice Patriniae), *Yi Yi Ren* (Semen Coicis) and *Gan Cao* (Radix Glycyrrhizae) work synergistically to drain dampness and dispel excessive vaginal discharge.

References

1. *Chang Yong Zhong Yao Cheng Fen Yu Yao Li Shou Ce* (A Handbook of the Composition and Pharmacology of Common Chinese Drugs), 1994; 213-214
2. *Zhong Yao Xue* (Chinese Herbology), 1998; 201-202
3. Ibid.
4. Ibid.
5. *Zhong Hua Yi Xue Za Zhi* (Chinese Journal of Medicine), 1972; 1:34
6. *Zhong Yi Za Zhi* (Journal of Chinese Medicine), 1984; 8:27

Bai Jiang Cao (Herba cum Radice Patriniae)

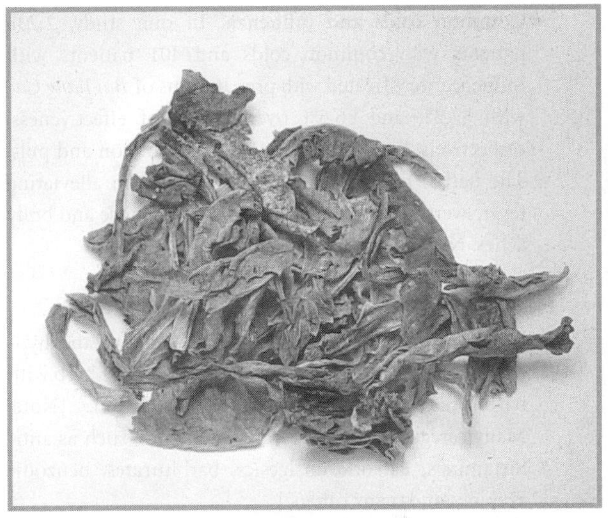

敗醬草 败酱草

Pinyin Name: *Bai Jiang Cao*
Literal Name: "spoiled paste herb"
Alternate Chinese Names: *Bai Jiang, Ku Cai*
Original Source: *Shen Nong Ben Cao Jing* (Divine Husbandman's Classic of the Materia Medica) in the second century
English Name: thlaspi, dahurian patrinia herb, white flower patrinia
Botanical Name: *Patrinia scabiosaefolia* Fisch. Ex Link. (*Huang Hua Bai Jiang*); *Patrinia villosa* Juss. (*Bai Hua Bai Jiang*)
Pharmaceutical Name: Herba cum Radice Patriniae
Properties: acrid, bitter, cool
Channels Entered: Stomach, Large Intestine, Liver

CHINESE THERAPEUTIC ACTIONS

1. Clears Heat, Eliminates Toxins, Drains Pus and Abscesses

Abscess: Acrid, bitter and cold, *Bai Jiang Cao* (Herba cum Radice Patriniae) is commonly used to eliminate heat and toxins with or without the accompanying formation of abscesses. Clinical applications include intestinal or lung abscesses and various swellings, sores, lesions and pain. This herb is especially effective in the treatment of intestinal abscess.

- Intestinal abscesses with pus: use *Bai Jiang Cao* with *Fu Zi* (Radix Aconiti Lateralis Praeparata) and *Yi Yi Ren* (Semen Coicis).
- Intestinal abscesses with no pus: use this herb with *Jin Yin Hua* (Flos Lonicerae), *Da Huang* (Radix et Rhizoma Rhei) and *Mu Dan Pi* (Cortex Moutan).
- Lung abscess with fever, and cough with mucus and blood: combine *Bai Jiang Cao* with *Yu Xing Cao* (Herba Houttuyniae), *Huang Qin* (Radix Scutellariae) and *Jie Geng* (Radix Platycodonis).

2. Resolves Bruises and Relieves Pain

Chest and abdominal pain: *Bai Jiang Cao* enters the blood to eliminate blood stasis and relieve pain. It is commonly used to treat chest and abdominal pain, abdominal fullness and masses due to blood stasis, or postpartum abdominal pain caused by blood stasis.

- Blood stasis: combine it with *Wu Ling Zhi* (Excrementum Trogopteri seu Pteromi) and *Xiang Fu* (Rhizoma Cyperi).

DOSAGE

6 to 15 grams in decoction.

CAUTIONS / CONTRAINDICATIONS

- *Bai Jiang Cao* is contraindicated in patients experiencing abdominal pain from cold and deficiency.
- Use of *Bai Jiang Cao* may be associated with possible drowsiness and sedation. Therefore, individuals who take this herb should exercise caution if driving or operating heavy machinery.

CHEMICAL COMPOSITION

Villoside, loganin, morroniside, patrinoside, scabioside, oleanolic acid, hederagenin, daucosterol.[1]

PHARMACOLOGICAL EFFECTS

- **Sedative and hypnotic**: Both alcohol extract and essential oil of *Bai Jiang Cao* have demonstrated marked sedative and hypnotic effects. They also potentiate the effect of barbiturates. The sedative and hypnotic effect of *Bai Jiang Cao* is approximately double that of *Xie Cao* (Radix et Rhizoma Valerianae).[2]
- **Hepatoprotective**: *Bai Jiang Cao* promotes the generation of hepatocytes and prevents mutation.[3]
- **Antibiotic**: *Bai Jiang Cao* has an inhibitory effect against *Staphylococcus aureus, Staphylococcus albus, Corynebacterium diphtheriae*, and influenza viruses.[4]

CLINICAL STUDIES AND RESEARCH

- **Insomnia**: In a clinical study, 406 patients with insomnia characterized by neurasthenia were treated with alcohol tincture, alcohol extract, and essential oil of *Bai Jiang Cao*. The study reported that the essential oil was most effective, with a success rate of over 50%. The results with alcohol tincture and alcohol extract were less satisfactory.[5]

Bai Jiang Cao (Herba cum Radice Patriniae)

- **Common colds and influenza**: In one study, 2,233 patients with common colds and 401 patients with influenza were treated with preparations of *Bai Jiang Cao* with 82.2% and 86.5% overall rates of effectiveness, respectively. Dosage forms included decoction and pills. The herbal treatment was most effective in alleviating fever, aversion to cold, stuffy nose, runny nose and body aches. No significant side effects were reported.[6]

HERB-DRUG INTERACTION

- **Sedatives:** *Bai Jiang Cao* has marked sedative and hypnotic effects. Concurrent administration of the herb with barbiturates will lead to prolonged sedation.[7] [Note: Many categories of drugs induce sedation, such as antihistamines, narcotic analgesics, barbiturates, benzodiazepines and many others.]

References

1. *Chang Yong Zhong Yao Xian Dai Yan Jiu Yu Lin Chuan* (Recent Study & Clinical Application of Common Traditional Chinese Medicine), 1995; 159
2. *Zhong Yao Xue* (Chinese Herbology), 1998; 202:203
3. Ibid.
4. Ibid.
5. *Bei Jing Zhong Yi* (Beijing Chinese Medicine), 1982; 3:30
6. *Zhong Cao Yao* (Chinese Herbal Medicine); 1981; 3:143
7. *Zhong Yao Xue* (Chinese Herbology), 1998; 202:203

Hu Yao Huang (Herba Leucas Mollissimae)

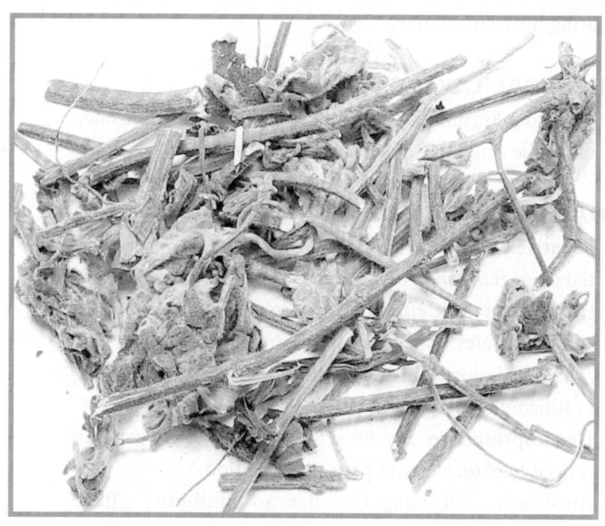

虎咬癀

Pinyin Name: *Hu Yao Huang*
Alternate Chinese Names: *Bai Hua Cao*
English Name: leucas
Botanical Name: *Leucas mollissima* Wall. var. *chinensis* Benth
Pharmaceutical Name: Herba Leucas Mollissimae
Properties: bitter, cool
Channels Entered: Large Intestine, Small Intestine, Lung

CHINESE THERAPEUTIC ACTIONS

1. Clears Heat and Eliminates Toxins

Hu Yao Huang (Herba Leucas Mollissimae) has general and broad-ranging heat-clearing effects. It treats infection and inflammation in many parts of the body.

- Enteritis: use *Hu Yao Huang* with *Ma Bian Cao* (Herba Verbenae), *Pao Zai Cao* (Herba Physalis Angulatae), and *Xian Feng Cao* (Herba Bidentis). It can be combined with *Ge Gen Huang Qin Huang Lian Tang* (Kudzu, Coptis, and Scutellaria Decoction) for best results.
- Appendicitis: use this herb with *Ma Bian Cao* (Herba Verbenae), *Da Huang* (Radix et Rhizoma Rhei), *Mu Dan Pi* (Cortex Moutan), and *Dong Gua Zi* (Semen Benincasae).
- Dysentery: combine it with *Feng Wei Cao* (Herba Pteris) and *Chuan Xin Lian* (Herba Andrographis), or with *Ge Gen Huang Qin Huang Lian Tang* (Kudzu, Coptis, and Scutellaria Decoction).
- Lung heat with cough: add *Fu Rong* (Radix Hibisci) and *Da Qing Ye* (Folium Isatidis).

Hu Yao Huang (Herba Leucas Mollissimae)

- Leukorrhea: use *Hu Yao Huang* with *Yi Mu Cao* (Herba Leonuri), *Long Yan Hua* (Flos Longan) and *Bai Guo* (Semen Ginkgo).
- Summer-heat stroke: combine it with *Feng Wei Cao* (Herba Pteris), *He Ye* (Folium Nelumbinis), *Ji Xue Cao* (Herba Centellae), *Shi Gao* (Gypsum Fibrosum) and *Zhi Mu* (Radix Anemarrhenae).
- Jaundice: use it with *Yin Chen Hao* (Herba Artemisiae Scopariae), *Da Huang* (Radix et Rhizoma Rhei) and *Zhi Zi* (Fructus Gardeniae).

2. Invigorates Blood Circulation, Promotes Diuresis

- Uterine infection: use *Hu Yao Huang* with *Ma Bian Cao* (Herba Verbenae), *Feng Wei Cao* (Herba Pteris), and *Xian Feng Cao* (Herba Bidentis).
- Nephritis, dysuria: use it with *Hai Jin Sha* (Herba Lygodii), *Jin Qian Cao* (Herba Lysimachiae) and *Bai Mao Gen* (Rhizoma Imperatae).

DOSAGE

6 to 15 grams in decoction.

CAUTIONS / CONTRAINDICATIONS

- *Hu Yao Huang* is contraindicated during pregnancy.

Huang Shui Qie (Herba Solani)

黄水茄 黄水茄

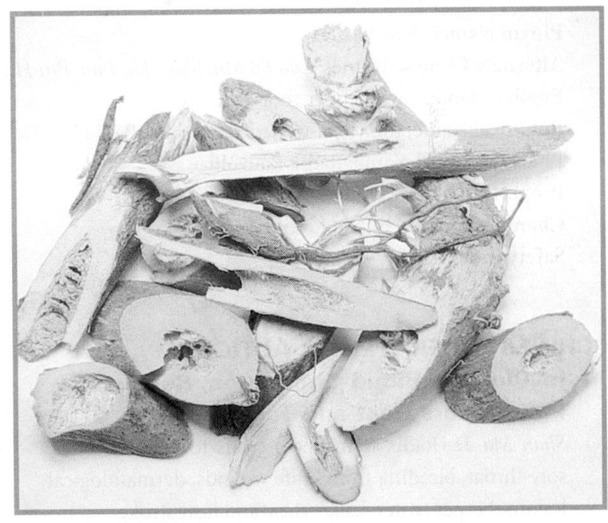

Pinyin Name: *Huang Shui Qie*
Alternate Chinese Names: *Huang Guo Qie*
English Name: solanum
Botanical Name: *Solanum xanthocarpum* Schrad. et Wendl. (*Huang Guo Qie*)
Pharmaceutical Name: Herba Solani
Properties: acrid, bitter, cold
Channels Entered: Liver

CHINESE THERAPEUTIC ACTIONS

Anchors Liver Yang, Eliminates Toxins, Reduces Inflammation and Relieves Pain

Liver fire: *Huang Shui Qie* (Herba Solani) treats various disorders caused by Liver fire. It is a strong toxin-eliminating herb that has been recently used for hepatitis A, B and C.

- Hepatitis: use *Huang Shui Qie* with *Hua Shi Cao* (Herba Orthosiphon Aristatus), *Bai Jiang Cao* (Herba cum Radice Patriniae), *Hu Zhang* (Rhizoma Polygoni Cuspidati) and *Hu Yao Huang* (Herba Leucas Mollissimae).
- Liver cirrhosis: use it with *Zhi Zi* (Fructus Gardeniae), *Wu Tian* (Radix et Folium Viticis Quinatae), and *Hu Zhang* (Rhizoma Polygoni Cuspidati). For best result, use it with *Xue Fu Zhu Yu Tang* (Drive Out Stasis in the Mansion of Blood Decoction).
- Eye disorders caused by excess conditions: combine this

Huang Shui Qie (Herba Solani)

herb with *Qian Li Guang* (Herba Senecionis Scandens), *Xia Ku Cao* (Spica Prunellae) and *Jue Ming Zi* (Semen Cassiae).

- Sinusitis: use it with *Fu Rong* (Radix Hibisci) and *Wu Tian* (Radix et Folium Viticis Quinatae).
- Itchy skin and various dermatological disorders: use it with *Fang Feng* (Radix Saposhnikoviae), *Jing Jie* (Herba Schizonepetae), *Ku Shen Gen* (Radix Sophorae Flavescentis), *Bai Hua She She Cao* (Herba Oldenlandia) and *Ban Zhi Lian* (Herba Scutellariae Barbatae).
- Pleuritis and edema: combine it with *Ding Shu Xiu* (Herba Elephantopus Scaber) and *Shan Pu Tao* (Radix Vitis Amurensis).

DOSAGE

3 to 9 grams in decoction.

CHEMICAL COMPOSITION

Solasonine, solamargine, solasurine, solasodine, methyl caffeate, caffeic acid.[1]

References

1. *J Chem Soc Pak* 1983; 5(2):99

Shan Ma Ti (Radix Rauvolfiae)

山馬蹄 山马蹄

Pinyin Name: *Shan Ma Ti*
Alternate Chinese Names: *Luo Fu Mu, Shan Hu Jiao, Bai Hua Lian, Du Gou Yao*
English Name: devil pepper root
Botanical Name: *Rauvolfia verticillata* (Lour.) Baill (*Luo Fu Mu*)
Pharmaceutical Name: Radix Rauvolfiae
Properties: bitter, cold
Channels Entered: Lung, Liver, Heart
Safety Index: slightly toxic

CHINESE THERAPEUTIC ACTIONS

1. Invigorates Blood Circulation, Relieves Pain, Clears Heat and Toxins

Shan Ma Ti (Radix Rauvolfiae) treats toxic snake bites, sore throat, bleeding from knife wounds, dermatological lesions, herpes zoster, leukorrhea, and heat stroke.

- Toxic snake bites or bleeding from knife wounds: crush the leaves of *Shan Ma Ti* and apply topically.
- Sore throat: use it with *Da Qing Ye* (Folium Isatidis), *She Gan* (Rhizoma Belamcandae) and *Zao Xiu* (Rhizoma Paridis).
- Dermatological lesions: combine it with *Ku Shen Gen* (Radix Sophorae Flavescentis), *Ren Dong Teng* (Caulis Lonicerae), *Wan Dian Jin* (Radix Ilicis Asprellae), and *Dao Di Wu Gong* (Rhizoma Heliminthostachytis). It can also be used alone as an external wash.
- Herpes zoster: add *Ma Bian Cao* (Herba Verbenae) and *Qi Li San* (Seven-Thousandths of a Tael Powder).
- Leukorrhea: use *Shan Ma Ti* with *Ji Guan Hua* (Flos Celosiae Cristatae) and *Bai Long Chuan Hua Tou* (Radix Clerodendron Paniculatum).
- Heat stroke: combine it with *Hu Yao Huang* (Herba Leucas Mollissimae) and *Feng Wei Cao* (Herba Pteris).

2. Anchors Rising Liver Yang and Lowers Blood Pressure

- Hypertension: use *Shan Ma Ti* with *Cha Chi Huang* (Herba Stellariae Aquaticae), *Tian Ma* (Rhizoma Gastrodiae), *Gou Teng* (Ramulus Uncariae cum Uncis), *Xia Ku Cao* (Spica Prunellae), and *Xi Xian Cao* (Herba Siegesbeckiae).

DOSAGE

3 to 15 grams in decoction.

Shan Ma Ti (Radix Rauvolfiae)

CAUTIONS / CONTRAINDICATIONS

Shan Ma Ti is contraindicated in patients with weak digestive systems, or in cases of qi and blood deficiencies.

CHEMICAL COMPOSITION

Serpine, raujemidine, aricine, isoreserpiline, yohimbine isomer, reserpiline, reserpine.[1,2]

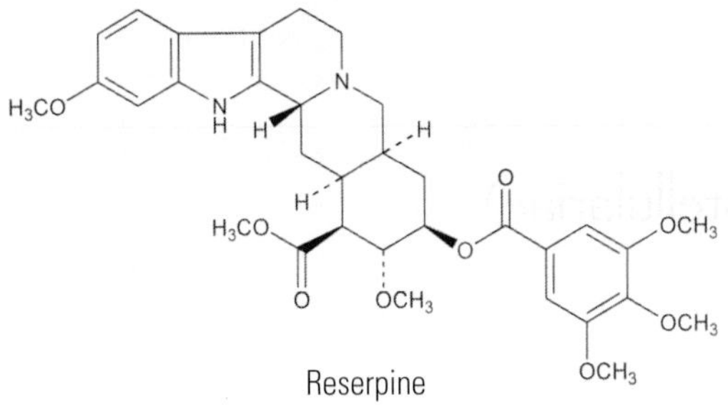

Reserpine

References

1. *J Org Chem* 1958; 21:923
2. *Rev Cubana Farm* 1982; 16(3):251:316

Pu Yin (Radix Wikstroemia Indica)

埔銀 埔银

Pinyin Name: *Pu Yin*
Alternate Chinese Names: *Jiu Xin Yao, Liao Ge Wang, Jin Yao Dai, Shan Pu Run*
English Name: Indian stringbush
Botanical Name: *Wikstroemia indica* C.A. Mey.
Pharmaceutical Name: Radix Wikstroemia Indica
Properties: bitter, cold
Channels Entered: Lung, Liver
Safety Index: toxic

CHINESE THERAPEUTIC ACTIONS

Clears Heat, Eliminates Toxins, Breaks Masses and Dispels Water

Pu Yin (Radix Wikstroemia Indica) has a general effect to clear heat and eliminate toxins.

- Pneumonia, tonsillitis, scrofula: use *Pu Yin* with *Da Qing Ye* (Folium Isatidis), *Ban Lan Gen* (Radix Isatidis) and *Zao Jiao* (Fructus Gleditsiae).
- Liver cirrhosis with ascites: add it with *Bai Jiang Cao* (Herba cum Radice Patriniae) to *Xue Fu Zhu Yu Tang* (Drive Out Stasis in the Mansion of Blood Decoction).
- Gout, arthritis: use it with *Yi Tiao Gen* (Radix Moghaniae).
- Carbuncles and toxic lesions: Apply *Pu Yin* topically.

DOSAGE

3 to 9 grams.

CAUTIONS / CONTRAINDICATIONS

- *Pu Yin* is contraindicated during pregnancy and for those experiencing deficiency and cold.

OVERDOSAGE

Vomiting, abdominal pain, diarrhea, swelling of the throat, difficult respiration, and unconsciousness has been associated with overdose of *Pu Yin*.

TREATMENT OF OVERDOSAGE

Overdose of *Pu Yin* is treated with administration of

Pu Yin (Radix Wikstroemia Indica)

milk or egg whites with decoction of 30 grams of *Jie Geng* (Radix Platycodonis). Another formula that is also beneficial contains *Shi Chang Pu* (Rhizoma Acori) 30g, *Hei Dou* (Semen Glycine Max) 15g, *Lu Gen* (Rhizoma Phragmitis) 120g, *Bai Mao Gen* (Rhizoma Imperatae) 30g and *Jin Yin Hua* (Flos Lonicerae) 15g.

AUTHORS' COMMENTS

According to Dr. Cheng Jian-Hua, *Pu Yin* treats lung and liver cancer when taken internally, and skin cancer when applied topically.

Shu Wei Huang (Herba Rostellulariae)

鼠尾癀

Pinyin Name: *Shu Wei Huang*
Alternate Chinese Names: *Jue Chuang, Ci Wei Huang, Su Wei Hong*
English Name: rostellularia, justicia
Botanical Name: *Rostellularia procumbens* (L.); *Justicia procumbens* (L.)
Pharmaceutical Name: Herba Rostellulariae
Properties: bitter, cold
Channels Entered: Liver, Lung

CHINESE THERAPEUTIC ACTIONS

Regulates Qi, Invigorates Blood and Reduces Inflammation

Shu Wei Huang (Herba Rostellulariae) moves qi and blood circulation to clear heat and reduce inflammation.

- Wind-heat invasion causing sore throat: use *Shu Wei Huang* with *Da Qing Ye* (Folium Isatidis) and *Ban Lan Gen* (Radix Isatidis).
- Scrofula: combine *Shu Wei Huang* with *Xia Ku Cao* (Spica Prunellae).
- Summer-heat stroke: use it with *Feng Wei Cao* (Herba Pteris), *Hu Yao Huang* (Herba Leucas Mollissimae), *Shi Gao* (Gypsum Fibrosum) and *Zhi Mu* (Radix Anemarrhenae).
- Sores, carbuncles, cellulitis, toxic swellings: combine this herb with *Pao Zai Cao* (Herba Physalis Angulatae), *Xian Feng Cao* (Herba Bidentis), *Zao Jiao Ci* (Spina Gleditsiae), *Chuan Shan Jia* (Squama Manis), *Fang Feng* (Radix Saposhnikoviae), *Bai Zhi* (Radix Angelicae Dahuricae), *Tian Hua Fen* (Radix Trichosanthis), *Jin Yin Hua* (Flos Lonicerae) and *Lian Qiao* (Fructus Forsythiae) for internal use. Externally, use it with *Pao Zai Cao* (Herba Physalis Angulatae) and *Xian Feng Cao* (Herba Bidentis).
- Gonorrhea or sexually-transmitted diseases caused by damp-heat with yellow discharge: combine *Shu Wei Huang* with *Long Dan Cao* (Radix Gentianae), *Huang Qin* (Radix Scutellariae), *Che Qian Zi* (Semen Plantaginis), *Chuan Mu Tong* (Caulis Clematidis Armandii), *Niu Xi* (Radix Cyathulae seu Achyranthis), *Bian Xu* (Herba Polygoni Avicularis), and *Qu Mai* (Herba Dianthi).

DOSAGE

5 to 15 grams

CAUTIONS / CONTRAINDICATIONS

- Use *Shu Wei Huang* with caution in patients with deficiency and cold of the Spleen and Stomach.
- *Shu Wei Huang* is contraindicated during pregnancy.

Xiang Si Cao (Herba Eupatorii Formosani)

相思草 相思草

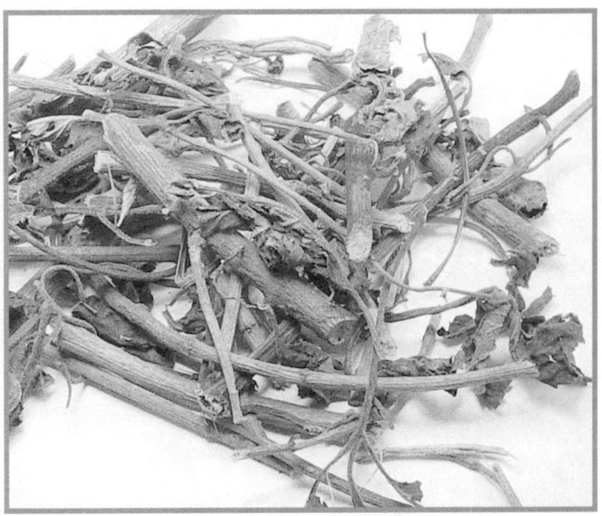

Pinyin Name: *Xiang Si Cao*
Alternate Chinese Names: *Liu Yue Xue, Shan Ze Lan, Da Ben Bai Hua Zai Cao, Jian Wei Feng*
English Name: eupatorium
Botanical Name: *Eupatorium formosanu*
Pharmaceutical Name: Herba Eupatorii Formosani
Properties: neutral, cool
Channels Entered: Lung, Large Intestine, Urinary Bladder

CHINESE THERAPEUTIC ACTIONS

Clears Heat, Eliminates Toxins, Reduces Swelling, Opens Channels and Promotes Urination

Xiang Si Cao (Herba Eupatorii Formosani) has a general effect to clear heat, eliminate toxins, and reduce accumulation of water.

- Acute appendicitis, abdominal pain: use *Xiang Si Cao* with *Xian Feng Cao* (Herba Bidentis), *Dong Gua Zi* (Semen Benincasae), *Da Huang* (Radix et Rhizoma Rhei) and *Mu Dan Pi* (Cortex Moutan).
- Pleurisy: use it with *Wang Bu Liu Xing* (Semen Vaccariae), *Hong Hua* (Flos Carthami), *Tao Ren* (Semen Persicae), *Chi Shao* (Radix Paeoniae Rubrae), *Chuan Xiong* (Rhizoma Ligustici Chuanxiong), *Da Qing Ye* (Folium Isatidis), *Pu Gong Ying* (Herba Taraxaci), and *Ban Lan Gen* (Radix Isatidis).
- Pneumonia: combine it with *Wan Dian Jin* (Radix Ilicis Asprellae), *Da Qing Ye* (Folium Isatidis), *Yu Xing Cao* (Herba Houttuyniae), *Yi Zhi Xiang* (Herba Vernoniae Cinereae), *Pu Gong Ying* (Herba Taraxaci), and *Huang Qin* (Radix Scutellariae).
- Leukemia: add *Bai Hua She She Cao* (Herba Oldenlandia) and *Ban Zhi Lian* (Herba Scutellariae Barbatae).
- High uric acid: combine this herb with *Shan Pu Tao* (Radix Vitis Amurensis), *Shui Ding Xiang* (Herba Ludwigiae Prostratae), and *Ding Shu Xiu* (Herba Elephantopus Scaber).
- Diabetes: add *Huang Shui Qie* (Herba Solani), *Yu Mi Xu* (Stigma Maydis), *Shi Gao* (Gypsum Fibrosum) and *Zhi Mu* (Radix Anemarrhenae).
- Hypertension: use it with *Xia Ku Cao* (Spica Prunellae), *Tian Ma* (Rhizoma Gastrodiae) and *Jue Ming Zi* (Semen Cassiae).

DOSAGE

6 to 30 grams in decoction.

Ya She Huang (Herba Lippiae)

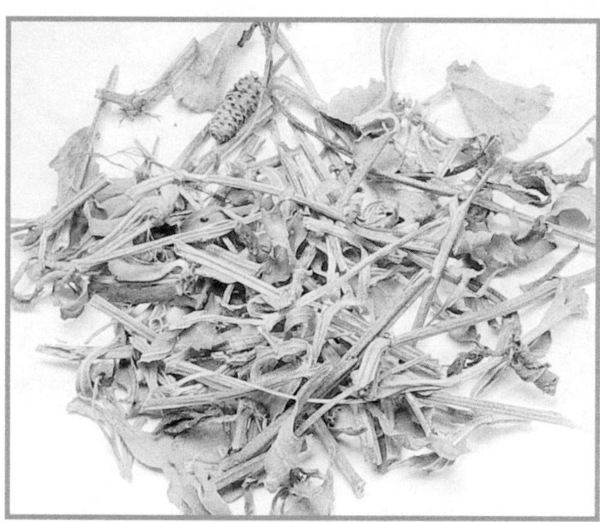

鴨舌癀 鸭舌癀

Pinyin Name: *Ya She Huang*
Literal Name: "duck tongue yellow"
Alternate Chinese Names: *Ya Zuai Huang, Shi Chi*
English Name: lippia
Botanical Name: *Lippia nodiflora* (Linn.) L.C. Richard.
Pharmaceutical Name: Herba Lippiae
Properties: acrid, bitter, cool
Channels Entered: Liver, Kidney
Safety Index: slightly toxic

CHINESE THERAPEUTIC ACTIONS

Regulates Menstruation and Reduces Inflammation

Ya She Huang (Herba Lippiae) effectively clears heat and reduces inflammation. It is commonly used for treating gynecological disorders.

- Irregular menstruation, amenorrhea or menstrual pain because of blood stagnation and heat in the lower *jiao*: use *Ya She Huang* with *Shao Fu Zhu Yu Tang* (Drive Out Blood Stasis in the Lower Abdomen Decoction).
- White discharge: combine it with *Ji Guan Hua* (Flos Celosiae Cristatae) and *Ma Chi Xian* (Herba Portulacae).
- Infertility due to chronic inflammation of the pelvic cavity: use this herb with *Feng Wei Cao* (Herba Pteris), *Ya She Huang* (Herba Lippiae), *Ma Bian Cao* (Herba Verbenae), *Hong Hua* (Flos Carthami), *Mu Dan Pi* (Cortex Moutan), *Tao Ren* (Semen Persicae), and *Chi Shao* (Radix Paeoniae Rubrae). *Long Dan Xie Gan Tang* (Gentiana Decoction to Drain the Liver) can also be added to enhance the overall effect.
- Gonorrhea: use it with *Feng Wei Cao* (Herba Pteris) and *Yi Mu Cao* (Herba Leonuri). Combine it with *Ba Zheng San* (Eight-Herb Powder for Rectification) to enhance the overall effect.
- Herpes zoster: apply *Ya She Huang* powder externally.
- Tonsillitis, parotitis, upper respiratory infection or toxic swelling: use it with *Da Qing Ye* (Folium Isatidis), *Ma Bo* (Lasiosphaera seu Calvatia) and *Shu Wei Huang* (Herba Rostellulariae).

DOSAGE

6 to 15 grams in decoction.

CHEMICAL COMPOSITION

Flavonoids.

Lu Dou (Semen Phaseoli Radiati)

綠豆 绿豆

Pinyin Name: *Lu Dou*
Literal Name: "green beans"
Original Source: *Kai Bao Ben Cao* (Materia Medica of the Kai Bao Era) by Ma Zhi in 973-974 A.D.
English Name: mung beans, phaseolus
Botanical Name: *Phaseolus radiatus* L. (*Lu Dou*)
Pharmaceutical Name: Semen Phaseoli Radiati
Properties: sweet, cold
Channels Entered: Heart, Stomach

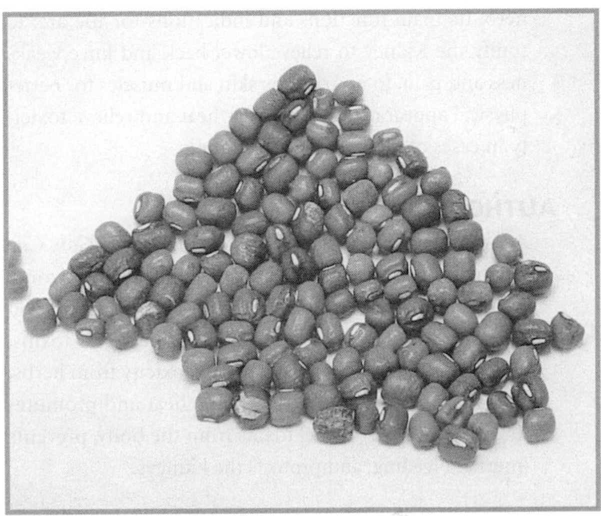

CHINESE THERAPEUTIC ACTIONS

1. Clears Heat, Relieves Toxicity

Lu Dou (Semen Phaseoli Radiati) is commonly used to dispel heat and toxins from the exterior of the body, treating disorders such as carbuncles, furuncles, sores, and ulcers. It is also an effective antidote for the overdose of many toxic substances.

- Heat and toxins on the exterior: use *Lu Dou* as a single-herb remedy for internal consumption. This herb can also be applied topically in combination with *Da Huang* (Radix et Rhizoma Rhei), *Bo He* (Herba Menthae) and honey.
- Overdose of *Ba Dou* (Fructus Crotonis) and *Fu Zi* (Radix Aconiti Lateralis Praeparata) causing irritation and thirst: use *Lu Dou* individually. It can also be combined with *Huang Lian* (Rhizoma Coptidis) and *Gan Cao* (Radix Glycyrrhizae) for a stronger effect.

2. Dispels Summer-Heat and Relieves Thirst

Lu Dou is commonly used as food or dessert in the summertime to clear heat, relieve thirst, alleviate restlessness, and lower body temperature. It is also effective to prevent heat stroke due to summer-heat.

DOSAGE

15 to 30 grams. *Lu Dou* may safely be used up to 120 grams in decoction in decoction.

CAUTIONS / CONTRAINDICATIONS

- *Lu Dou* should be used with caution in patients with deficiency and cold of the Spleen and Stomach characterized by loose stools.

CHEMICAL COMPOSITION

Phosphatidyl choline, phosphatidylethanolamine, phosphatidylinositol, phosphatidylglycerol, phosphatidylserine, phosphatidic acid, protein, carbohydrates, calcium, phosphorus, iron, vitamin A, B, C.[1]

CLINICAL STUDIES AND RESEARCH

- **Pesticide poisoning**: Three farmers experiencing pesticide poisoning were treated with an herbal solution with complete recovery after 3 doses. The herbal solution was prepared by soaking 500 grams of finely-powdered *Lu Dou* with 60 grams of salt in 2,000 ml of water for several minutes. The residue of the herbs was filtered out prior to ingestion of the herbal solution.[2]
- **Heat stroke**: According to one report, heat stroke in summer can be prevented by ingestion of an herbal formula that contains 500 grams of *Lu Dou*, and 30 grams of *Gan Cao* (Radix Glycyrrhizae), cooked in 5,000 ml of water to yield the final decoction. The herbal decoction may be taken warm or cold.[3]

SUPPLEMENT

- 綠豆衣 / 绿豆衣 *Lu Dou Yi* (Pericarpium Phaseoli Radiati), first cited in *Kai Bao Ben Cao* (Materia Medica of the Kai Bao Era) by Ma Zhi in 973-974 A.D., is the outer skin of the seed. *Lu Dou Yi* is sweet and cold, and enters the Heart and Stomach. In comparison with *Lu Dou*, *Lu Dou Yi* has similar but weaker functions to clear summer-heat and dampness and eliminate toxins. The dosage is 6 to 12 grams.
- 黑豆 *Hei Dou* (Semen Glycine Max), also referred to as black bean or black soybean, is another commonly used

Lu Dou (Semen Phaseoli Radiati)

herb. Its main functions and indications for use are: to tonify the Kidney to relieve lower back and knee weakness and pain, to nourish the skin and muscles for better physical appearance, and to clear heat and relieve toxicity in cases of overdose and poisoning.

AUTHORS' COMMENTS

According to Dr. Zhang Xue-Wen, *Lu Dou*, *Gan Cao* (Radix Glycyrrhizae), and *Bai Mao Gen* (Rhizoma Imperatae) are an effective combination to treat food poisoning. *Lu Dou* and *Gan Cao* clear heat and toxins, and are commonly used to eliminate toxicity from herbs, drugs and food. *Bai Mao Gen* clears heat and promotes diuresis to quickly dispel toxins from the body, prevents internal bleeding, and protects the kidneys.

References

1. *Chang Yong Zhong Yao Xian Dai Yan Jiu Yu Lin Chuan* (Recent Study & Clinical Application of Common Traditional Chinese Medicine), 1995; 168-169
2. *Zhe Jiang Zhong Yi Za Zhi* (Zhejiang Journal of Chinese Medicine), 1965; 7:7
3. *Zhong Yao Tong Bao* (Journal of Chinese Herbology), 1985; 5:9

He Ye (Folium Nelumbinis)

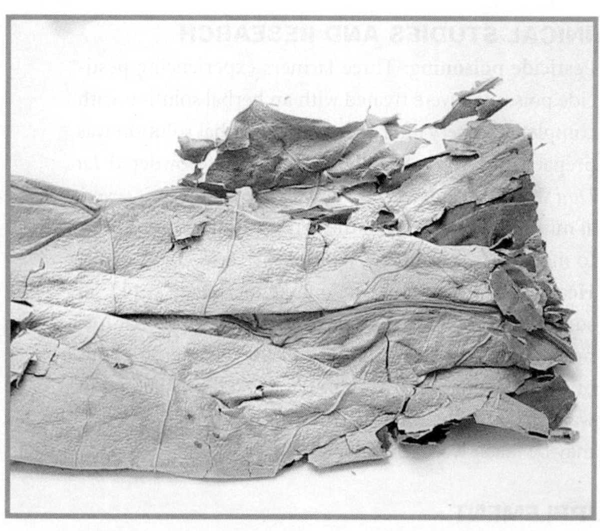

荷葉 荷叶

Pinyin Name: *He Ye*
Literal Name: "lotus leaves"
Alternate Chinese Names: *Ou Ye*
Original Source: *Shi Liao Ben Cao* (Materia Medica of Diet Therapy) by Meng Shan in the seventh Century
English Name: lotus leaf
Botanical Name: *Nelumbo nucifera* Gaertn. (*Lian*)
Pharmaceutical Name: Folium Nelumbinis
Properties: bitter, astringent, neutral
Channels Entered: Heart, Liver, and Spleen

CHINESE THERAPEUTIC ACTIONS

1. Clears Summer-Heat and Dissolves Dampness

Summer-heat: *He Ye* (Folium Nelumbinis) clears summer-heat and dampness, a condition characterized by fever, irritability, sweating, and scanty urine.

- Summer-heat and dampness: use *He Ye* with *Jin Yin Hua* (Flos Lonicerae), *Bian Dou Hua* (Flos Lablab Album), *Xi Gua* (Fructus Citrulli) and *Hou Po* (Cortex Magnoliae Officinalis).
- Obesity: cook *He Ye* and *Yi Yi Ren* (Semen Coicis) together and drink daily as tea.

2. Stops Bleeding

Bleeding: *He Ye* treats bleeding disorders. It is commonly used with other herbs that have hemostatic functions.

He Ye (Folium Nelumbinis)

DOSAGE

3 to 10 grams. Unprocessed *He Ye* functions more effectively to clear heat. The charred herb more strongly stops bleeding.

CAUTIONS / CONTRAINDICATIONS

- *He Ye* should be used with caution if the cause of bleeding is cold.

AUTHORS' COMMENTS

There are eight parts of the lotus plant that are used as medicines. Please refer to *Lian Zi* (Semen Nelumbinis) for complete description.

Section 5

— Deficiency-Heat Clearing Herbs

Qing Hao (Herba Artemisiae Annuae)

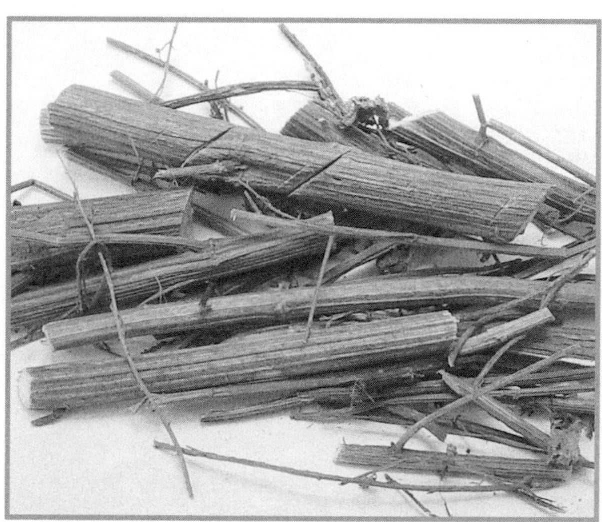

青蒿 青蒿

Pinyin Name: *Qing Hao*
Literal Name: "bluegreen artemisia"
Original Source: *Shen Nong Ben Cao Jing* (Divine Husbandman's Classic of the Materia Medica) in the second century
English Name: artemisia, sweet wormwood herb
Botanical Name: *Artemisia annua* L. (*Huang Hua Hao*); *Artemisia apiacea* Hance (*Qing Hao*)
Pharmaceutical Name: Herba Artemisiae Annuae
Properties: bitter, acrid, cold
Channels Entered: Liver, Gallbladder, Stomach

CHINESE THERAPEUTIC ACTIONS

1. Clears Heat and Treats Malaria

Malaria with alternating chills and fever: *Qing Hao* (Herba Artemisiae Annuae) is traditionally used to clear heat, summer-heat or damp-heat. However, its most distinct function is in the treatment of malaria, where its effectiveness is confirmed by both historical data and modern pharmacology. *Qing Hao* can be used individually or in combination with other herbs to treat malaria and relieve alternation of fever and chills. Fresh *Qing Hao* given as juice is most effective for this application.

- Malaria: use a large dose of fresh *Qing Hao* by itself.
- Malaria with nausea, vomiting and feelings of oppression in the chest due to damp-heat: use this herb with *Huang Qin* (Radix Scutellariae) and *Ban Xia* (Rhizoma Pinelliae). **Exemplar Formula**: *Hao Qin Qing Dan Tang* (Artemisia Annua and Scutellaria Decoction to Clear the Gallbladder).
- Malaria with alternating chills and fever: add *Qing Hao* to *Xiao Chai Hu Tang* (Minor Bupleurum Decoction).

2. Clears Yin-Deficient Heat

Yin-deficient heat: Clinical manifestations of yin-deficient heat include steaming-bones sensations with no perspiration, tidal fever, unremitting low-grade fever, *wu xin re* (five-center heat), thirst, soreness and weakness of the lower back and knees, and irritability. *Qing Hao* has distinct ventilating and dispersing functions without consuming yin or body fluids. Therefore, it is commonly used to clear heat in patients who have an underlying yin deficiency.

- Yin-deficient heat: use *Qing Hao* with *Bie Jia* (Carapax Trionycis), *Zhi Mu* (Radix Anemarrhenae), and *Qin Jiao* (Radix Gentianae Macrophyllae).

3. Cools Blood

Late-stage febrile disorders: Clinically, the patient will experience feelings of warmth at night and chills in the morning, constant feelings of warmth or low-grade fever, thirst, flushed face, irritability, and an absence of perspiration. *Qing Hao* is commonly used to treat chronic febrile disorders where the heat factor has entered the *ying* (nutritive) level.

Qing Hao (Herba Artemisiae Annuae)

- Heat in the *ying* (nutritive) level with constant feverish sensations: use *Qing Hao* with *Bie Jia* (Carapax Trionycis), *Mu Dan Pi* (Cortex Moutan) and *Sheng Di Huang* (Radix Rehmanniae). **Exemplar Formula:** *Qing Hao Bie Jia Tang* (Artemisia Annua and Soft-shelled Turtle Shell Decoction).

4. Clears Summer-Heat or Damp-Heat

Qing Hao treats summer-heat or damp-heat characterized by fever, with or without perspiration, heavy limbs, and a stifling sensation in the chest. Fresh *Qing Hao* is most effective for this application.

- Summer-heat or damp-heat: use this herb with *He Ye* (Folium Nelumbinis).
- Summer-heat or damp-heat in infants or children with fever and dysuria: add *Che Qian Cao* (Herba Plantaginis).

5. Clears Liver Heat and Brightens the Eyes

Eye disorders: *Qing Hao* treats Liver Yang rising that is causing red eyes, dizziness, and photophobia.

- Disorders of the eyes: use *Qing Hao* with *Ju Hua* (Flos Chrysanthemi), *Shi Jue Ming* (Concha Haliotidis), *Jue Ming Zi* (Semen Cassiae) and *Huang Qin* (Radix Scutellariae).

Damp-heat jaundice: Accompanying symptoms may include dysuria and scanty, yellow urine.

- Jaundice: use *Qing Hao* with *Yin Chen Hao* (Herba Artemisiae Scopariae), *Huang Bai* (Cortex Phellodendri), *Che Qian Zi* (Semen Plantaginis) and *Zhi Zi* (Fructus Gardeniae).

DOSAGE

3 to 10 grams in decoction. *Qing Hao* should only be cooked for a short period of time as a decoction. *Qing Hao* may be used in decoctions or as juice squeezed from the fresh herb. The fresh herb squeezed into juice is often more effective than decoction, as the active constituents have not been destroyed by heat.

CAUTIONS / CONTRAINDICATIONS

- *Qing Hao* should be used with caution in patients who have deficiency and cold of the Spleen and Stomach.
- *Qing Hao* should be cooked only for a short period of time, as heat may make the herb less effective.

CHEMICAL COMPOSITION

Artemisinin, arteannuin, essential oils 0.20-0.25% (artemisia ketone, isoartemisia ketone, camphene, β-pinene, β-caryophyllene, l-camphor).[1,2]

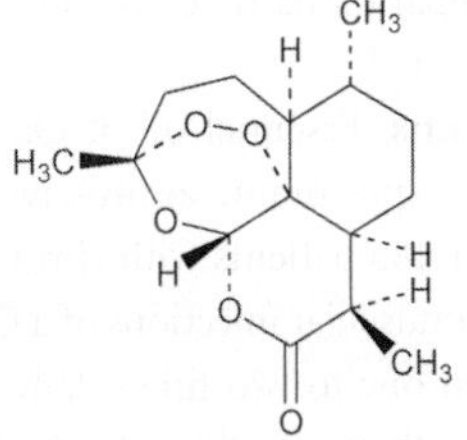

Artemisinin

PHARMACOLOGICAL EFFECTS

- **Antimalarial:** Artemisinin has demonstrated excellent effectiveness against malarial parasites. It is one of the most powerful schizonticidal agents to treat falciparum malaria. The mechanism of this antimalarial effect is believed to be associated with the blocked utilization of host erythrocyte protein by the plasmodium, causing starvation and death. However, this compound is not effective as a prophylactic agent because it affects neither the sexual nor the exoerythrocytic forms of the plasmodium.[3,4,5]
- **Antibiotic:** Decoction of *Qing Hao* has been shown to inhibit *Staphylococcus aureus, Neisseria catarrhalis, Bacillus anthracis, Corynebacterium diphtheriae, Pseudomonas aeruginosa, Bacillus dysenteriae,* and *Mycobacterium tuberculosis.* The essential oil of *Qing Hao* is effective against some dermatophytes.[6,7]
- **Antihypertensive:** Intravenous injection of arteannuin in rabbits lowered blood pressure, decreased heart rate, inhibited contraction of the cardiac muscle, and decreased blood perfusion to the coronary artery. In another study, intravenous injection of *Qing Hao* at 20 mg/kg was effective in treating aconitine-induced arrhythmias in rabbits.[8,9]
- **Antipyretic:** Injection of *Qing Hao* was effective in reducing body temperature in rabbits with artificially-induced fevers.[10]
- **Cholagogic:** *Qing Hao* has been shown to increase the production and excretion of bile in rats.[11]

CLINICAL STUDIES AND RESEARCH

- **Malaria:** The use of *Qing Hao* in treatment of malaria is well-established. In one study, 488 patients with malaria were treated with preparations of *Qing Hao* with close to 100% effectiveness. In another study, 125 patients with malaria were treated with preparations of *Qing Hao* three hours prior to the onset of illness. *Qing Hao* was administered as decoction (the herbs were cooked for no more than 15 minutes), tea (the herbs were soaked in 60° C water for 24 hours), and juice (the fresh herbs were put through a juicer). The dosage was 120 grams of fresh *Qing Hao*. The success rate was approximately 80%. Lastly, a study including 2,009 patients with malaria demonstrated that the participants were effectively

Qing Hao (Herba Artemisiae Annuae)

treated with preparations of *Qing Hao* through intramuscular injection.[14]

- **Chronic bronchitis**: Essential oil of *Qing Hao* demonstrated marked expectorant, antitussive and antiasthmatic effects in 1,485 patients with chronic bronchitis.[15]
- **High fever**: Intramuscular injections of a *Qing Hao* preparation were given one to two times daily to 126 patients with high fever, with an effective rate of 68.25%.[16]

HERB-DRUG INTERACTION

- **Azole antifungals and calcium channel blockers:** Artelinic acid (AL), a water-soluble artemisinin analogue for treatment of multi-drug resistant malaria, is metabolized to the active metabolite dihydroqinghaosu (DQHS) solely by liver enzyme CYP3A4/5. In human liver microsomes, ketoconazole and miconazole were potent competitive inhibitors of DQHS formation. Verapamil is a non-competitive inhibitor of DQHS formation in human liver microsomes. Therefore, it has been suggested that azole antifungals and calcium channel blockers may present clinically significant herb-drug interactions with *Qing Hao*.[17] [Note: Examples of azole antifungals include griseofulvin (Gris-PEG), nystatin (Mycostatin), ketoconazole (Nizoral), fluconazole (Diflucan), and itraconazole (Sporanox); and examples of calcium channel blockers include nifedipine (Procardia/Adalat), amlodipine (Norvasc), diltiazem (Cardizem), and verapamil (Calan/Isoptin/Verelan).]

TOXICOLOGY

Qing Hao has shown few adverse reactions in toxicology studies. In acute toxicology studies, the LD_{50} was not determined as no fatalities were observed in the subjects. In chronic toxicology studies, no abnormalities were reported in heart, liver, kidney, and other vital organs following long-term administration.[18]

AUTHORS' COMMENTS

According to the World Health Organization (WHO), over 1.5 million malaria patients in southeast Asia and Latin America were treated with artemisinin, a constituent of *Qing Hao*. In China, *falciparum plasmodium* resistance to chloroquine is 84.6%, but only 2.2-2.4% to artemisinin. Thus, artemisinin has completely replaced chloroquine and quinine as drugs of choice for treatment of malaria. However, it is important to keep in mind that while artemisinin is effective as a drug for treatment, it is not effective as a casual prophylactic agent.[19]

According to Dr. Cheng Chun-Fu, the decoction of *Qing Hao* and *Mang Xiao* (Natrii Sulfas) used to wash the scalp, relieves itching and dandruff and treats hair loss. This topical combination also clears redness, itching and rashes in the axillary and genital areas.

References

1. *Xian Dai Zhong Yao Yao Li Xue* (Contemporary Pharmacology of Chinese Herbs), 1997; 353
2. *The Merck Index* 12th edition, Chapman & Hall/CRCnetBASE/Merck, 2000
3. *Ann Froo Med Parasito*, 1985; 79(4):367
4. *Trans Roy Soc Trop Med Hyg*, 1983; 77(4):522
5. Huang, K. *The Pharmacology of Chinese Herbs 2nd Edition*, CRC Press, 1999; 450-452
6. *Chang Yong Zhong Yao Cheng Fen Yu Yao Li Shou Ce* (A Handbook of the Composition and Pharmacology of Common Chinese Drugs), 1994; 1167:1173
7. *Zhong Hua Pi Fu Ke Xue Za Zhi* (Chinese Journal of Dermatology), 1988; 21(2):75
8. *Xin Zhong Yi* (New Chinese Medicine), 1979; (6):51
9. Ibid., 1980; (1):37
10. *Zhong Yao Yao Li Yu Ying Yong* (Pharmacology and Applications of Chinese Herbs), 1983:59
11. *Zhong Yao Xue* (Chinese Herbology), 1998; 240:242
12. *Guang Xi Yi Xue* (Guangxi Medicine), 1984; 3:117
13. *Shan Xi Xin Yi Yao* (New Medicine and Herbology of Shanxi), 1975; 3:19
14. *Yao Xue Tong Bao* (Report of Herbology), 1979; 2:49
15. *Zhong Cao Yao* (Chinese Herbal Medicine), 1980; 12:576
16. *Hu Bei Zhong Yi Za Zhi* (Hubei Journal of Chinese Medicine), 1983; 2:17
17. *Xenobiotica*. 29(7):703-17, 1999 Jul
18. *Xian Dai Zhong Yao Yao Li Xue* (Contemporary Pharmacology of Chinese Herbs), 1997; 359
19. Huang, K. *The Pharmacology of Chinese Herbs 2nd Edition*, CRC Press, 1999; 450-452

Bai Wei (Radix Cynanchi Atrati)

白薇 白薇

Pinyin Name: *Bai Wei*
Literal Name: "white rose"
Alternate Chinese Names: *Shen Nong Ben Cao Jing* (Divine Husbandman's Classic of the Materia Medica) in the second century
English Name: cynanchum, blackened swallowwort root, versicolorous swallowwort root
Botanical Name: *Cynanchum atratum* Bge. (*Bai Wei*); *Cynanchum versicolor* Bge. (*Man Sheng Bai Wei*)
Pharmaceutical Name: Radix Cynanchi Atrati
Properties: bitter, salty, cold
Channels Entered: Stomach, Liver

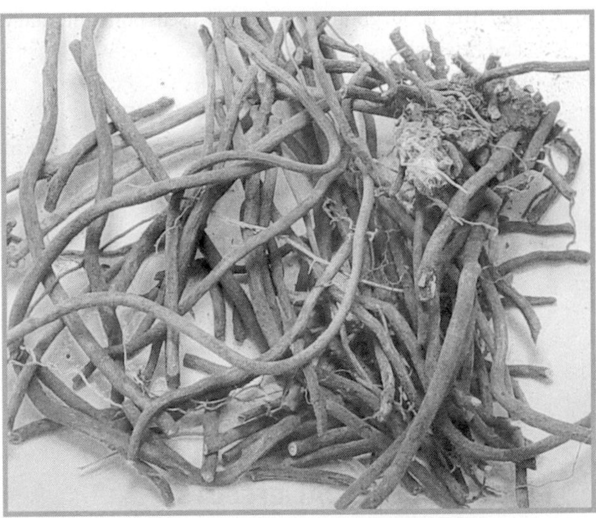

CHINESE THERAPEUTIC ACTIONS

1. Clears Heat and Cools Blood

Heat in the *ying* (nutritive) level: Bitter and cold in nature, *Bai Wei* (Radix Cynanchi Atrati) clears heat and cools blood. It treats both deficiency heat and excess heat. Deficiency heat is often characterized by yin or blood deficiency caused by chronic illness. *Bai Wei* is most helpful in the recovery stage of febrile disorders: in these cases, the high fever has subsided, but injured yin causes difficulties for the body in restoring normal qi, and yin-deficient heat signs persist. The most common signs and symptoms include unremitting low-grade fever, *wu xin re* (five-center heat), flushed face, irritability and steaming bones sensations, poor appetite, and in severe cases, heat sensations at night and cold sensations in the morning.

- Late-stage febrile disorders characterized by lingering fever due to yin deficiency and heat: use *Bai Wei* with *Di Gu Pi* (Cortex Lycii), *Mai Men Dong* (Radix Ophiopogonis) and *Sheng Di Huang* (Radix Rehmanniae).
- Fever, steaming bones sensations and night sweats because of yin-deficient heat: use it with *Di Gu Pi* (Cortex Lycii) to dispel yin-deficient heat.

Heat in postpartum women: Other clinical manifestations of heat include nausea, irritability, feverish sensations, enuresis or burning urination. *Bai Wei* enters the *chong* (thoroughfare) and *ren* (conception) channels to clear heat in the *xue* (blood) level. Deficiency heat symptoms in postpartum women are often the result of sudden loss of blood.

- Postpartum fever due to blood deficiency and heat: use this herb with *Dang Gui* (Radicis Angelicae Sinensis) and *Ren Shen* (Radix Ginseng) to clear heat and nourish qi and blood.

Exterior wind-heat or Lung heat: *Bai Wei* can be used to treat wind-heat in the exterior or Lung heat with or without an underlying yin deficiency. The chief manifestations are cough with fever and yellow phlegm.

- Exterior wind-heat syndrome with underlying yin deficiency: combine *Bai Wei* with *Bo He* (Herba Menthae), *Dan Dou Chi* (Semen Sojae Praeparatum) and *Yu Zhu* (Rhizoma Polygonati Odorati).
- Cough due to Lung heat: use this herb with *Zhe Bei Mu* (Bulbus Fritillariae Thunbergii), *Qian Hu* (Radix Peucedani) and *Pi Pa Ye* (Folium Eriobotryae).

2. Cools the Blood and Promotes Urination

***Lin zheng* (dysuria syndrome)**: *Bai Wei* cools the blood and promotes normal urination. It is commonly used to treat burning and painful urination caused by *xue lin* (bloody dysuria) with heat.

- Postpartum dysuria: combine *Bai Wei* and *Bai Shao* (Radix Paeoniae Alba).
- *Xue lin* (bloody dysuria) with heat: use it with *Hua Shi* (Talcum), *Chuan Mu Tong* (Caulis Clematidis Armandii) and *Sheng Di Huang* (Radix Rehmanniae).
- Prostate inflammation caused by heat in the lower *jiao*: combine it with *Che Qian Zi* (Semen Plantaginis) and *Hua Shi* (Talcum).

3. Eliminates Heat and Toxins

Presentations of heat and toxins include sore throat, skin lesions and abscesses, snake bites and similar ailments. *Bai Wei* may be used internally or topically to eliminate heat and toxins.

DOSAGE

3 to 12 grams in decoction. The maximum dosage of

Bai Wei (Radix Cynanchi Atrati)

Bai Wei is 30 grams. *Bai Wei* is used both internally and externally.

CAUTIONS / CONTRAINDICATIONS

- Cold in nature, *Bai Wei* should be used with caution in patients with deficiency and cold of the Spleen and Stomach, characterized by loose stools or decreased intake of food.
- *Bai Wei* should be used with caution in patients who do not have heat in the blood.

CHEMICAL COMPOSITION

Cynatratoside A, B, C, D, E, F; atratoside A, B, C, D; cynarersicoside C, D; neocynanversicoside, glaucogenin D.[1]

PHARMACOLOGICAL EFFECTS

- **Cardiovascular:** Preparations of *Bai Wei* have shown positive inotropic and negative chronotropic effects. It is effective in treating congestive heart failure.[2]
- **Antibiotic:** It has an inhibitory effect *in vitro* against *Diplococcus pneumoniae.*[3]

CLINICAL STUDIES AND RESEARCH

- **Hemiplegia:** In one study, 3 patients with hemiplegia were treated with great success using an herbal decoction given once or twice daily. The herbal formula contained 15 grams of *Bai Wei*, 9 grams of *Ze Lan* (Herba Lycopi), and 6 grams of *Chuan Shan Jia* (Squama Manis).[4]

AUTHORS' COMMENTS

Historically, *Bai Wei* has been used as a key herb in treatment of malaria. However, while *Bai Wei* addresses the symptoms of deficiency heat, it does not have antimalarial action to treat the cause of this illness. Thus, *Bai Wei* is no longer used for treatment of malaria, but only for management of deficiency heat in post-febrile conditions.

References

1. *Chang Yong Zhong Yao Cheng Fen Yu Yao Li Shou Ce* (A Handbook of the Composition and Pharmacology of Common Chinese Drugs), 1994; 764-765
2. *Zhong Yao Yao Li Du Li Yu Lin Chuan* (Pharmacology, Toxicology and Clinical Applications of Chinese Herbs), 1992; 57
3. Ibid.
4. *Guang Dong Zhong Yi* (Guangdong Chinese Medicine), 1962; 9:31

Di Gu Pi (Cortex Lycii)

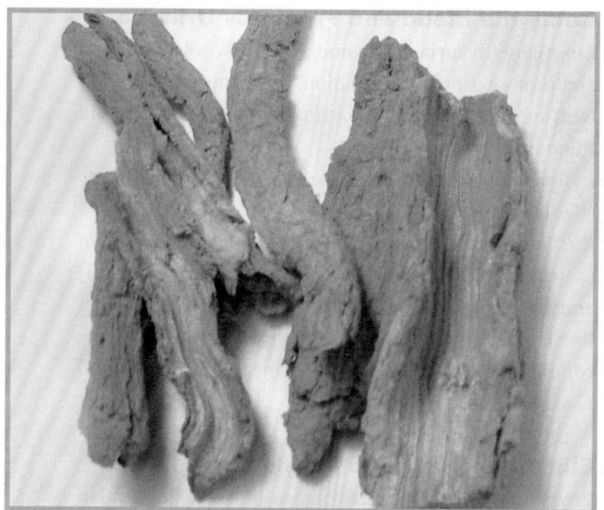

地骨皮 地骨皮

Pinyin Name: *Di Gu Pi*
Literal Name: "ground bone skin," "earth bone bark"
Alternate Chinese Names: *Gou Qi Gen Pi*
Original Source: *Shen Nong Ben Cao Jing* (Divine Husbandman's Classic of the Materia Medica) in the second century
English Name: lycium root bark, barbary wolfberry root bark, Chinese wolfberry root bark
Botanical Name: *Lycium barbarum* (*Ning Xia Gou Ji*); *Lycium chinense* Mill (*Mu Gou Ji*)
Pharmaceutical Name: Cortex Lycii
Properties: sweet, bland, cold
Channels Entered: Lung, Kidney

CHINESE THERAPEUTIC ACTIONS

1. Cools Blood and Relieves Steaming Bones Sensation

Yin deficiency with heat in the blood: *Di Gu Pi* (Cortex Lycii) enters the bones, clears heat from within, and relieves steaming bones sensations and night sweats.

- Steaming bones sensation with tidal fever and night sweats caused by yin deficiency and heat: use *Di Gu Pi*

Di Gu Pi (Cortex Lycii)

with *Zhi Mu* (Radix Anemarrhenae), *Bie Jia* (Carapax Trionycis) and *Qin Jiao* (Radix Gentianae Macrophyllae).

- *Gan ji* (infantile malnutrition) with heat sensations: use this herb with *Zhi Mu* (Radix Anemarrhenae) and *Bie Jia* (Carapax Trionycis).
- Fever, irritability and steaming bones sensation due to heat in the muscles and the bones: combine it with *Fang Feng* (Radix Saposhnikoviae) and *Gan Cao* (Radix Glycyrrhizae).

***Xiao ke* (wasting and thirsting) syndrome**: When heat damages body fluids over a long period of time, patients with *xiao ke* syndromes experience thirst, dry mouth, irritability and polyuria. *Di Gu Pi* is especially good for the type of thirst that cannot be relieved by water intake.

- *Xiao ke* syndrome: use *Di Gu Pi* with *Tian Hua Fen* (Radix Trichosanthis), *Sheng Di Huang* (Radix Rehmanniae), *Zhi Mu* (Radix Anemarrhenae) and *Shi Gao* (Gypsum Fibrosum).
- *Xiao ke* syndrome with constant thirst and water ingestion: combine this herb with *Lu Gen* (Rhizoma Phragmitis), *Mai Men Dong* (Radix Ophiopogonis), *Tian Hua Fen* (Radix Trichosanthis) and *Da Zao* (Fructus Jujubae).

Toothache from rising deficient Kidney fire: For patients with Kidney yin deficiency, fire may attack the Kidney channel, as heat travels upwards and causes toothache. Sweet, cold and moistening, *Di Gu Pi* clears various yin-deficient heat conditions.

- Toothache: add *Di Gu Pi* to *Zhi Bai Di Huang Wan* (Anemarrhena, Phellodendron, and Rehmannia Pill).

2. Clears Lung Heat

Cough due to Lung heat: *Di Gu Pi* is effective in treating cough, wheezing and dyspnea due to Lung heat. It is also effective for treatment of Lung heat with fluid damage. When heat travels down to the paired organ of Lung, the Large Intestine, constipation or dry stools occur.

- Cough, wheezing and dyspnea: use this herb with *Sang Bai Pi* (Cortex Mori) and *Gan Cao* (Radix Glycyrrhizae). **Exemplar Formula**: *Xie Bai San* (Drain the White Powder).
- Constipation: combine it with *Da Huang* (Radix et Rhizoma Rhei), *Gua Lou Shi* (Fructus Trichosanthis) and *Xing Ren* (Semen Armeniacae Amarum).

3. Clears Heat, Cools Blood, and Stops Bleeding

Bleeding: *Di Gu Pi* commonly treats various bleeding disorders characterized by heat in the blood forcing blood out of the vessels. It clears heat, cools the blood, and stops bleeding.

- Hematemesis and epistaxis due to heat in the blood: use this herb with *Bai Mao Gen* (Rhizoma Imperatae), *Ou Jie* (Nodus Nelumbinis Rhizomatis) and *Ce Bai Ye* (Cacumen Platycladi) to cool blood and stop bleeding.
- Hematuria: use it with *Gou Qi Zi* (Fructus Lycii) in powder form.
- Cough with blood-streaked sputum: use it with *Mai Men Dong* (Radix Ophiopogonis) and *Ce Bai Ye* (Cacumen Platycladi).

DOSAGE

6 to 15 grams in decoction. The maximum dosage of *Di Gu Pi* is 60 grams.

CAUTIONS / CONTRAINDICATIONS

- Cold in nature, *Di Gu Pi* should be used with caution in patients who have deficiency and cold of the Spleen and Stomach, characterized by loose stools.
- *Di Gu Pi* is contraindicated for patients with exterior wind-cold or wind-heat conditions.
- Use *Di Gu Pi* with caution in patients who have true cold but false heat.

CHEMICAL COMPOSITION

Betaine, lyciumins A, B; kukoamine A, lyciumamide, cinnamic acid.[1]

PHARMACOLOGICAL EFFECTS

- **Antibiotic**: *Di Gu Pi* has been shown to inhibit the activity of typhoid, paratyphoid and shigella.[2]
- **Antihypertensive**: Intravenous injection of a *Di Gu Pi* preparation in anesthetized dogs, cats and rats lowered blood pressure by 53%, 67%, and 27%, respectively. Alcohol extracts of *Di Gu Pi* and kukoamine A also have antihypertensive effects. Lyciumins A and B are angiotensin converting enzyme (ACE) inhibitors, and have marked effects to lower blood pressure.[3]
- **Antipyretic**: Both oral and intravenous administrations of water and alcohol extracts of *Di Gu Pi* have marked effectiveness in reducing body temperature in rabbits.[4]
- **Antidiabetic**: Oral ingestion of decoction of *Di Gu Pi* at 8 g/kg lowered blood glucose in healthy rabbits by 14% for up to 7 or 8 hours.[5]

CLINICAL STUDIES AND RESEARCH

- **Hypertension:** In one study, primary hypertension patients were treated with *Di Gu Pi* (decoction of 60 grams of the herb with a small quantity of sugar) once every other day for 5 doses per course of treatment, for a total of 2 to 3 courses. Out of 50 patients, 40% showed marked improvement and 94% showed some improvement.[6]
- **Diabetes mellitus:** According to one report, 16 patients with diabetes mellitus were treated with a twice-daily regimen that consisted of *Di Gu Pi* (50 grams of herb in

Di Gu Pi (Cortex Lycii)

decoction), 100 mg of vitamin C and 100 mg of vitamin B1 injected intramuscularly. The study reported satisfactory results.[7]

- **Corns:** In one study, 25 patients with corns were successfully treated with a topical herbal preparation made with 6 grams of *Di Gu Pi* and 3 grams of *Hong Hua* (Flos Carthami) crushed into a fine powder and mixed with sesame oil and flour. After the outer layer of the corn was removed, the herbs were applied topically and covered with gauze. The herbs were removed and re-applied every two days.[8]

HERB-DRUG INTERACTION

- **Antidiabetics:** It is prudent to use *Di Gu Pi* with caution with insulin, sulfonylureas, and other antidiabetic medications, as the combination may have synergistic effects, leading to hypoglycemia. [Note: Examples of antidiabetic drugs include insulin, tolbutamide (Orinase), glipizide (Glucotrol), and glyburide (DiaBeta/Micronase).][9]

TOXICOLOGY

The LD_{50} for intraperitoneal injection of a *Di Gu Pi* preparation in mice is 12.8 g/kg.[10]

AUTHORS' COMMENTS

Di Gu Pi and *Sang Bai Pi* (Cortex Mori) both clear heat, but from different parts of the body. *Di Gu Pi* sedates Lung fire and clears heat in the *xue* (blood) level. *Sang Bai Pi* clears Lung heat and sedates fire from the *qi* (energy) level. Their differences make them useful together to eliminate heat in both *xue* (blood) and *qi* (energy) levels.

References

1. *Xian Dai Zhong Yao Yao Li Xue* (Contemporary Pharmacology of Chinese Herbs), 1997; 363
2. *Zhong Yao Xue* (Chinese Herbology), 1998; 244:245
3. *CA*, 1990; 112:14538g
4. *Yi Xue Zhong Yang Za Zhi* (Central Journal of Medicine), 1967; 223:664
5. *Zhong Cao Yao Xue* (Study of Chinese Herbal Medicine), 1980; 978
6. *Guang Xi Yi Xue* (Guangxi Medicine), 1983; 3:46
7. *Shang Hai Zhong Yi Yao Za Zhi* (Shanghai Journal of Chinese Medicine and Herbology), 1984; 9:11
8. *Xin Zhong Yi* (New Chinese Medicine), 1974; 4:39
9. Chen, J. Recognition & prevention of herb-drug interactions, *Medical Acupuncture*, Fall/Winter 1998/1999; volume 10/number 2; 9-13
10. *Zhong Cao Yao Xue* (Study of Chinese Herbal Medicine), 1980; 978

Yin Chai Hu (Radix Stellariae)

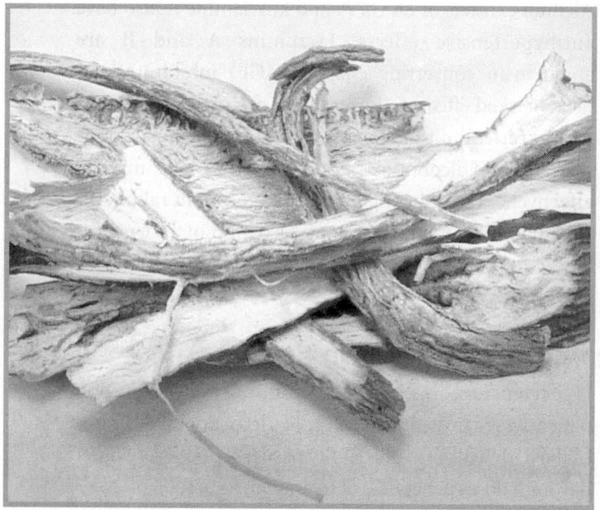

銀柴胡 银柴胡

Pinyin Name: *Yin Chai Hu*
Literal Name: "silver barbarian kindling"
Alternate Chinese Names: *Yin Hu*
Original Source: *Ben Cao Gang Mu* (Materia Medica) by Li Shi-Zhen in 1578
English Name: stellaria root, starwort root
Botanical Name: *Stellaria dichotoma* L. var. *lanceolata* Bge. (*Yin Chai Hu*)
Pharmaceutical Name: Radix Stellariae
Properties: sweet, cool
Channels Entered: Liver, Stomach

CHINESE THERAPEUTIC ACTIONS

1. Clears Deficiency Heat

Yin-deficient heat: Because it is not bitter and only cool (not cold) in nature, *Yin Chai Hu* (Radix Stellariae) is an excellent herb to clear deficiency heat without damaging yin. It is commonly used to treat yin-deficient heat char-

Yin Chai Hu (Radix Stellariae)

acterized by night sweats, steaming bones sensations, irritability, *wu xin re* (five-center heat), flushed cheeks and tidal fever.

- Yin-deficient heat with night sweats and steaming-bones sensation: use *Yin Chai Hu* with *Di Gu Pi* (Cortex Lycii), *Qing Hao* (Herba Artemisiae Annuae) and *Bie Jia* (Carapax Trionycis).
- Febrile disorders with tidal fever, thin body frame, dry skin and nails: add *Bie Jia* (Carapax Trionycis).

2. Clears Heat

***Gan ji* (infantile malnutrition):** *Yin Chai Hu* is commonly used to treat malnutrition in infants due to accumulation of heat. Clinical applications of *Yin Chai Hu* include malnutrition, fever, enlarged abdomen, and weight loss.

- *Gan ji* with fever: use it with *Dang Shen* (Radix Codonopsis), *Zhi Zi* (Fructus Gardeniae), *Hu Huang Lian* (Rhizoma Picrorhizae), and *Huang Qin* (Radix Scutellariae).

DOSAGE

3 to 10 grams in decoction. The maximum dosage of *Yin Chai Hu* is 20 grams.

CAUTIONS / CONTRAINDICATIONS

- *Yin Chai Hu* is contraindicated in patients who have exterior wind-cold conditions, or in patients who have blood deficiency without heat signs.

CHEMICAL COMPOSITION

Saponins.[1]

AUTHORS' COMMENTS

Yin Chai Hu (Radix Stellariae) and *Chai Hu* (Radix Bupleuri) have similar names and functions. Both clear heat and reduce fever. *Yin Chai Hu* is most effective for treating deficiency heat and fever, such as tidal fever, steaming-bones sensations, night sweats due to yin-deficient heat, and *gan ji* (infantile malnutrition) with fever. *Chai Hu*, on the other hand, is more effective for treating *shaoyang* syndrome with alternating chills and fever. Furthermore, *Chai Hu* functions to raise yang qi and regulate Liver qi stagnation.

References

1. *Zhong Yao Xue* (Chinese Herbology), 1998; 246

Hu Huang Lian (Rhizoma Picrorhizae)

胡黄連 胡黄连

Pinyin Name: *Hu Huang Lian*
Literal Name: "barbarian yellow connection," "barbarian yellow link"
Original Source: *Xin Xiu Ben Cao* (Newly Revised Materia Medica) by Su Jing in 657-659 A.D.
English Name: picrorhiza, figwort flower rhizome
Botanical Name: *Picrorrhiza kurrooa* Royle ex Benth. (*Hu Huang Lian*); *Picrorrhiza scrophulariaeflora* Pennell. (*Xi Zhang Hu Huang Lian*)
Pharmaceutical Name: Rhizoma Picrorhizae
Properties: bitter, cold
Channels Entered: Heart, Liver, Stomach, Large Intestine

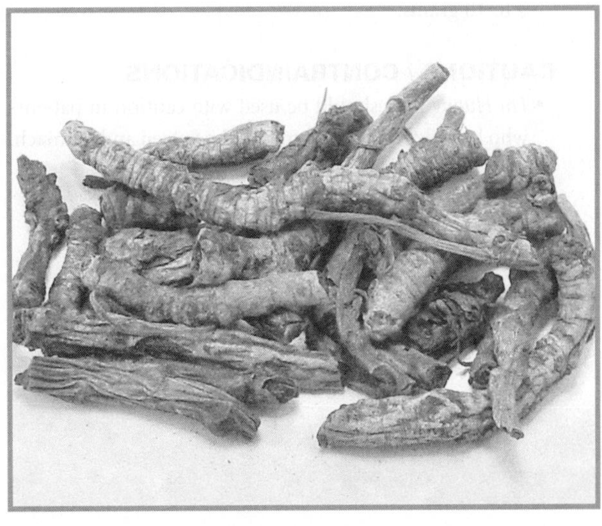

Hu Huang Lian (Rhizoma Picrorhizae)

CHINESE THERAPEUTIC ACTIONS

1. Clears Deficiency Heat

Yin-deficient heat: *Hu Huang Lian* (Rhizoma Picrorhizae) is commonly used to dispel yin-deficient heat, characterized by steaming bones sensations, tidal fever, and night sweating.

- Yin-deficient heat: use *Hu Huang Lian* with *Yin Chai Hu* (Radix Stellariae), *Di Gu Pi* (Cortex Lycii) and *Zhi Mu* (Radix Anemarrhenae).

***Gan ji* (infantile malnutrition)**: *Hu Huang Lian* treats malnutrition in infants due to accumulation of heat, characterized by malnutrition, fever, enlarged abdomen, and weight loss.

- *Gan ji* with fever: use this herb with *Bai Zhu* (Rhizoma Atractylodis Macrocephalae), *Shan Zha* (Fructus Crataegi), and *Shi Jun Zi* (Fructus Quisqualis) to strengthen the Spleen and clear heat. **Exemplar Formula**: *Jin Jian Fei Er Wan* (Golden Pills to Construct a Fat Child).

2. Clears Heat and Dries Dampness

Bitter and cold, *Hu Huang Lian* treats disorders characterized by damp-heat, such as diarrhea, dysentery, abscesses and lesions.

- Bloody dysentery: use this herb with *Wu Mei* (Fructus Mume) and *Fu Long Gan* (Terra Flava Usta).
- Chronic diarrhea: combine it with *Gan Jiang* (Rhizoma Zingiberis).
- Hemorrhoids: take *Hu Huang Lian* with goose gallbladder.

DOSAGE

3 to 10 grams.

CAUTIONS / CONTRAINDICATIONS

- *Hu Huang Lian* should be used with caution in patients who have deficiency and cold of the Spleen and Stomach.

CHEMICAL COMPOSITION

Kutkin, picroside I, picroside II, kutkoside, D-mannitol, vanillic acid, kutkiol, kutkisterol, apocynin, picroside, putkoside, kurroside.[1]

PHARMACOLOGICAL EFFECTS

- **Cholagogic**: Vanilloylcatalpol, a derivative of picroside II, markedly increases production and excretion of bile in mice. It also has hepatoprotective effects, especially against carbon tetrachloride.[2]
- **Antibiotic**: *Hu Huang Lian* has been shown to inhibit the growth of some dermatophytes and pathogenic fungi.[3]

CLINICAL STUDIES AND RESEARCH

- **Bacterial dysentery**: In one study, 45 patients with bacterial dysentery were treated with 2 to 6 grams of powdered *Hu Huang Lian* in three equally-divided doses daily, with excellent success.[4]

AUTHORS' COMMENTS

Hu Huang Lian (Rhizoma Picrorhizae) and *Huang Lian* (Rhizoma Coptidis) have similar names, but different functions. *Hu Huang Lian* primarily clears deficiency heat. *Huang Lian* mainly clears excess, such as damp-heat.

Hu Huang Lian has similar effects to those of *Yin Chai Hu* (Radix Stellariae) to clear deficiency heat, but is stronger than *Yin Chai Hu*.

References

1. *Xian Dai Zhong Yao Yao Li Xue* (Contemporary Pharmacology of Chinese Herbs), 1997; 364
2. *Guo Wai Yi Xue Zhong Yi Zhong Yao Fen Ce* (Monograph of Chinese Herbology from Foreign Medicine), 1989; 11(1):56
3. *Zhong Hua Pi Fu Ke Xue Za Zhi* (Chinese Journal of Dermatology), 1957; (4):286
4. *Guang Dong Zhong Yi* (Guangdong Chinese Medicine), 1960; 4:187

Chapter 2 summary — Heat-Clearing Herbs

SECTION 1: HEAT-CLEARING AND FIRE-PURGING HERBS

Name	Similarities	Differences
Shi Gao (Gypsum Fibrosum)	Sedate excess fire in the Stomach and Lung	Strongly clears excess heat
Zhi Mu (Radix Anemarrhenae)		Nourishes yin, moistens dryness
Qing Guo Gen (Radix Canarium Album)		Generates body fluids, strengthens Spleen
Han Shui Shi (Mirabilite)		Treats burns when used externally
Tian Hua Fen (Radix Trichosanthis)	Clear heat, generate body fluids	Dispels pus
Lu Gen (Rhizoma Phragmitis)		Clears Stomach and Lung heat
Zhu Ye (Herba Phyllostachys)		Relieves dysuria
Dan Zhu Ye (Herba Lophatheri)		Relieves dysuria
Zhi Zi (Fructus Gardeniae)	Clear fire in the Liver and Gallbladder	Cools blood, eliminates toxins, dries dampness; for heat in all three *jiaos*
Xia Ku Cao (Spica Prunellae)		Disperses nodules and scrofulae due to Liver qi stagnation
Mi Meng Hua (Flos Buddlejae)	Sedate Liver, treat eye disorders	Sedates Liver fire
Qing Xiang Zi (Semen Celosiae)		Sedates Liver fire
Gu Jing Cao (Flos Eriocauli)		Disperses wind-heat in the Liver channel
Rui Ren (Semen Prinsepiae)		Clears the Liver, brightens the eyes
Da Ding Huang (Caulis Euonymi)	Clear heat, purge fire	Eliminates toxins, reduces inflammation
Ren Zhong Bai (Urinae Hominis Sedimen)		Stops bleeding
Shi Lian Zi (Herba Sinocrassulae Indicae)		Relieves irritability, stops dysentery
Lu Cha (Folium Camellia Sinensis)	Clear heat, promote diuresis	Clears Stomach heat, dispels dampness, relieves headache
Wu Long Cha (Folium Camellia Sinensis Fermentata)		Clears heat, relieves headache
Xi Gua (Fructus Citrulli)		Relieves thirst
Xi Gua Pi (Pericarpium Citrulli)		Promotes urination, clears heat

General Characteristics of Heat-Clearing and Fire-Purging Herbs:

Taste: sweet, bitter
Thermal property: cool, cold
Channels entered: Lung, Stomach, Heart, Liver
Therapeutic actions: clear heat and purge fire

These herbs are mainly used to sedate excess heat in the *qi* (energy) level or excess heat in the Lung or Stomach. Excess conditions include excess heat, excess fire, or Lung or Stomach heat.

Shi Gao (Gypsum Fibrosum) and ***Zhi Mu*** (Radix Anemarrhenae) are the most commonly used herbs to clear heat, sedate fire, dispel irritability and relieve thirst, and are often used together for synergistic effect, such as in *Bai Hu Tang* (White Tiger Decoction). They are used for excess heat in the *qi* (energy) level with symptoms of high fever, irritability and thirst. They also clear Lung heat to relieve cough and dyspnea.

Shi Gao is stronger in clearing heat and descending fire. It should only be used in cases of excess heat.

Chapter 2 summary

Zhi Mu clears heat and moistens the Lung simultaneously, and clears heat and purges fire in both excess and deficiency conditions.

Qing Guo Gen (Radix Canarium Album) eliminates heat and toxins from the throat, and promotes generation of fluids.

Han Shui Shi (Mirabilite), like *Shi Gao* (Gypsum Fibrosum), clears heat and purges fire. However, it is not used as often as *Shi Gao*, since it does not clear the Lung or relieve dyspnea and cough.

Tian Hua Fen (Radix Trichosanthis) and ***Zhi Mu*** (Radix Anemarrhenae) are commonly used to clear heat in individuals with underlying deficiencies.

Tian Hua Fen clears heat, generates body fluids, relieves thirst and alleviates consumption of body fluids by febrile disorders.

Zhi Mu is stronger to clear heat and purge fire.

Lu Gen (Rhizoma Phragmitis) and ***Zhu Ye*** (Herba Phyllostachys) clear interior and exterior heat and reduce irritability.

Lu Gen generates body fluids, relieves thirst, clears Stomach heat to stop vomiting, and dispels Lung heat to eliminate phlegm and abscess.

Zhu Ye clears Heart heat and promotes diuresis.

Zhu Ye (Herba Phyllostachys) and ***Dan Zhu Ye*** (Herba Lophatheri) clear heat and promote diuresis.

Zhu Ye more directly clears Heart and Stomach fire.

Dan Zhu Ye more effectively clears heat and promotes diuresis.

Zhi Zi (Fructus Gardeniae) effectively clears excess heat or damp-heat at *qi* (energy) or *xue* (blood) levels, from all three *jiaos*. Externally, it disperses stagnation, reduces swelling and treats sprains and strains.

Zhi Zi (Fructus Gardeniae) and ***Xia Ku Cao*** (Spica Prunellae) effectively clear heat from the Liver and Gallbladder.

Zhi Zi exerts a broader effect as it clears heat from all three *jiaos*.

Xia Ku Cao is more focused on clearing heat from the Liver and Gallbladder.

Xia Ku Cao (Spica Prunellae), ***Mi Meng Hua*** (Flos Buddlejae), ***Qing Xiang Zi*** (Semen Celosiae), ***Gu Jing Cao*** (Flos Eriocauli), and ***Rui Ren*** (Semen Prinsepiae) all sedate Liver fire and treat various disorders of the eyes, such as redness, swelling and pain.

Xia Ku Cao is best for pain in the eyeball, especially during the night, caused by Liver fire and qi stagnation.

Mi Meng Hua nourishes the Liver, moistens dryness and treats eye disorders caused by excess or deficiency conditions.

Qing Xiang Zi and *Gu Jing Cao* treat eye disorders caused by excess heat and Liver fire.

Rui Ren helps eye disorders characterized by excess, but not by deficiency.

Da Ding Huang (Caulis Euonymi), ***Ren Zhong Bai*** (Urinae Hominis Sedimen) and ***Shi Lian Zi*** (Herba Sinocrassulae Indicae) clear heat and purge fire.

Da Ding Huang is most effective to reduce inflammation and eliminate toxins.

Ren Zhong Bai clears heat from the upper, middle and lower *jiaos* to stop bleeding.

Shi Lian Zi clears heat from the Heart to relieve irritability, and heat from the Large Intestine to treat dysentery.

Chapter 2 summary

Lu Cha (Folium Camellia Sinensis), ***Wu Long Cha*** (Folium Camellia Sinensis Fermentata), ***Xi Gua*** (Fructus Citrulli) and ***Xi Gua Pi*** (Pericarpium Citrulli) clear heat and promote diuresis.

Lu Cha and *Wu Long Cha* are derived from the same plant, and have essentially the same functions to treat Stomach disorders (nausea, vomiting and diarrhea), clear the head, and brighten the eyes. *Lu Cha* is the unprocessed tea leaf while *Wu Long Cha* is the fermented leaf.

Xi Gua and *Xi Gua Pi* are derived from the same plant, and function to clear heat and promote urination. *Xi Gua* more effectively clears heat and relieves thirst. *Xi Gua Pi* more strongly promotes urination.

SECTION 2: HEAT-CLEARING AND DAMPNESS-DRYING HERBS

Name	Similarities	Differences
Huang Qin (Radix Scutellariae)	Clear heat, sedate fire, eliminate toxins, dry dampness	Clears heat from upper *jiao*, sedates Lung heat, stabilizes fetus
Huang Lian (Rhizoma Coptidis)		Clears heat from middle *jiao*, clears fire in the Heart, Liver, Stomach and Large Intestine
Huang Bai (Cortex Phellodendri)		Clears deficiency Kidney fire and lower *jiao* heat
Ji Xue Cao (Herba Centellae)		Cools blood and stops bleeding, clears the Liver, brightens eyes
Long Dan Cao (Radix Gentianae)	Clear heat, dry dampness	Sedates damp-heat in the Liver and Gallbladder channels, dispels damp-heat from lower *jiao*
Ku Shen Gen (Radix Sophorae Flavescentis)		Dispels damp-heat from lower *jiao*, used externally to relieve itching

General Characteristics of Heat-Clearing and Dampness-Drying Herbs:

Taste: bitter
Thermal property: cold
Channels entered: Liver, Gallbladder, Large Intestine, Small Intestine
Therapeutic actions: clear heat, sedate fire, dry dampness

Theses herbs treat disorders characterized by heat, fire and dampness, such as hepatitis, jaundice, dysentery, hemorrhoids, infections, sores, abscesses, and others.

Huang Qin (Radix Scutellariae), ***Huang Lian*** (Rhizoma Coptidis) and ***Huang Bai*** (Cortex Phellodendri) are known as the "*san huang*," literally 'three yellows.' Bitter, cold and drying in nature, all three herbs clear heat, dry dampness, sedate fire and eliminate toxins. They treat various damp-heat and toxic heat syndromes.

Huang Qin more effectively clears heat from the upper *jiao*. It clears Lung heat, stops bleeding, promotes diuresis, and stabilizes the fetus.

Huang Lian more effectively clears heat from the middle *jiao*. It sedates fire in the Stomach, Large Intestine, Heart and Liver. *Huang Lian* is the strongest of the "three yellows."

Huang Bai more effectively clears heat from the lower *jiao*. It treats lower *jiao* damp-heat with leukorrhea, edema, heat in the lower body and jaundice. It clears both excess and deficiency heat.

Huang Bai (Cortex Phellodendri) and ***Zhi Mu*** (Radix Anemarrhenae) are commonly combined because of their excellent synergistic effect to consolidate yin and clear deficiency heat.

Huang Bai dries dampness, eliminates toxins, and dispels damp-heat in the lower *jiao*.

Zhi Mu is nourishing and clears deficiency fire of the Kidney.

Ji Xue Cao (Herba Centellae) eliminates damp-heat, cools blood to stop bleeding, and clears Liver heat to brighten the eyes. However, it is not as potent as the "three yellows" and is rarely used.

Chapter 2 summary

Long Dan Cao (Radix Gentianae) and ***Xia Ku Cao*** (Spica Prunellae) clear the Liver, brighten the eyes, and sedate Liver fire involving red, painful and swollen eyes.

Long Dan Cao is very cold and very drying. It is one of the strongest herbs to sedate Liver fire and dry dampness. It also is excellent for symptoms associated with Liver fire flaring upwards or damp-heat in the Liver channel in the lower *jiao*. This herb is reserved for use only in excess conditions.

Xia Ku Cao, milder in action, clears heat and disperses stagnation simultaneously. It treats goiter, nodules and masses, and relieves eye pain caused by Liver heat or Liver qi stagnation.

Ku Shen Gen (Radix Sophorae Flavescentis) dries dampness and kills parasites, treating damp-heat in the lower *jiao* as found in dysentery, jaundice, yellow leukorrhea, *re lin* (heat dysuria), or itching skin and eczema. Today, *Ku Shen Gen* is also being used to treat dyspnea, arrhythmia and elevated white blood cell counts.

SECTION 3: HEAT-CLEARING AND BLOOD-COOLING HERBS

Name	Similarities	Differences
Xi Jiao (Cornu Rhinoceri)	Clear heat,	Eliminates toxins, clears the Heart, extinguishes Liver wind
Sheng Di Huang (Radix Rehmanniae)	cool blood	Nourishes yin, promotes generation of body fluids
Xuan Shen (Radix Scrophulariae)		Nourishes yin, purges fire, eliminates toxins
Mu Dan Pi (Cortex Moutan)		Invigorates blood circulation, purges Liver fire, clears Heart fire
Chi Shao (Radix Paeoniae Rubrae)		Invigorates blood circulation, purges Liver fire, relieves pain
Zi Cao Gen (Radix Lithospermi)		Eliminates toxins, promotes eruption of measles
Fu Rong (Radix Hibisci)		Clears Lung heat, reduces inflammation and pain
Huang Teng (Caulis Fibraurea)		Dispels wind from the exterior
Ji Guan Hua (Flos Celosiae Cristatae)		Stops bleeding
Dong Qing Ye (Folium Ilexis)		Clears heat, eliminates toxins

General Characteristics of Heat-Clearing and Blood-Cooling Herbs:

Taste: bitter, sweet, salty
Thermal property: cold
Channels entered: Heart, Liver
Therapeutic actions: clear heat, cool blood

These herbs clear heat and cool blood at the *ying* (nutritive) and *xue* (blood) levels, conditions characterized by restlessness, irritability, delirium, high fever, altered consciousness, purpura, and bleeding.

Xi Jiao (Cornu Rhinoceri) cools blood, stops bleeding, eliminates toxins, clears the Heart and extinguishes Liver wind. It has historically been excellent for treatment of heat in the blood characterized by high fever with delirium and incoherent speech, purpura, and reckless movement of blood (with bleeding from the nose and the mouth). *Shui Niu Jiao* (Cornu Bubali) is now used as a substitute, because *Xi Jiao* is an endangered animal and its use is prohibited.

Sheng Di Huang (Radix Rehmanniae) and ***Xuan Shen*** (Radix Scrophulariae) both nourish the yin and cool the blood simultaneously. They are used for heat in the *ying* (nutritive) and *xue* (blood) levels characterized by purple blotches on the skin, bleeding, yin-deficient heat, thirst and body fluid deficiency.

Sheng Di Huang has a stronger tonic function to nourish yin and generate body fluids.

Xuan Shen is more effective to eliminate toxins, dispel heat, and treat sore throat, scrofula and goiter.

Chapter 2 summary

Mu Dan Pi (Cortex Moutan) and ***Chi Shao*** (Radix Paeoniae Rubrae) cool and invigorate blood circulation, clear heat in the *ying* (nutritive) and *xue* (blood) levels with purpura, hematemesis, bleeding and amenorrhea.

Mu Dan Pi more strongly clears Heart fire and cools blood to treat yin-deficient heat.

Chi Shao more effectively clears Liver fire, regulates blood circulation, and relieves pain caused by heat and blood stagnation.

Mu Dan Pi (Cortex Moutan) and ***Di Gu Pi*** (Cortex Lycii) clear deficiency heat and treat steaming bones sensations.

Mu Dan Pi is better for treating steaming bones sensations without perspiration

Di Gu Pi is more effective for alleviating steaming bones sensations with perspiration.

Zi Cao Gen (Radix Lithospermi) cools the blood, promotes eruption of measles and treats purple blotches on the skin caused by heat in the vessels. Used externally, it treats burns, ulcerations and eczema.

Fu Rong (Radix Hibisci) cools the blood, clears heat from the Lung, and reduces inflammation and pain.

Huang Teng (Caulis Fibraurea) cools the blood, clears heat from the Liver, and lowers blood pressure.

Ji Guan Hua (Flos Celosiae Cristatae) clears heat, cools blood, stops bleeding, and stops the loss of fluids from the lower *jiao*, such as found in diarrhea, dysentery, and vaginal discharge.

Dong Qing Ye (Folium Ilexis) clears heat and eliminates toxins, cools blood and stops bleeding.

SECTION 4: HEAT-CLEARING AND TOXIN-ELIMINATING HERBS

Name	Similarities	Differences
Jin Yin Hua (Flos Lonicerae)	Clear heat, eliminate toxins, reduce abscesses, sores, and swellings	Treats wind-heat, summer-heat, dysentery, and intestinal abscesses
Ren Dong Teng (Caulis Lonicerae)		Dispels wind, dampness and heat from the exterior
Lian Qiao (Fructus Forsythiae)		Sedates heart fire, treats nodules/abscesses
Guan Ye Lian *Qiao* (Herba Hypericum)		Stops bleeding, dispels wind-damp
Pu Gong Ying (Herba Taraxaci)		Treats breast abscesses
Zi Hua Di Ding (Herba Violae)		Treats skin lesions, snake bites
Ye Ju Hua (Flos Chrysanthemi Indici)		Treats skin and eye disorders
Lou Lu (Radix Rhapontici)		Treats breast disorders
Niu Huang (Calculus Bovis)		Disperses wind, dispels phlegm
Zao Xiu (Rhizoma Paridis)		Extinguishes Liver wind, disperses blood stagnation
Xiong Dan (Fel Ursi)		Extinguishes Liver wind and Liver yang rising
Bai Lian (Radix Ampelopsis)		Treats burns
Bai Xian Pi (Cortex Dictamni)		Relieves damp-heat itching and jaundice
Qian Li Guang (Herba Senecionis Scandens)		Brightens the eyes and treats eye disorders
Ji Gu Cao (Herba Abri)		Treats jaundice, *bi zheng* (painful obstruction syndrome)
Ban Bian Lian (Herba Lobeliae Chinensis)		Treats snake bites, bee stings, ascites
Cha Chi Huang (Herba Stellariae Aquaticae)		Invigorates blood circulation and eliminates blood stagnation
Dao Di Wu Gong (Rhizoma Heliminthostachytis)		Reduces swelling and inflammation
Jin Guo Lan (Radix Tinosporae)		Clears damp-heat from the skin
Liu Ye (Folium Salicis Babylonicae)		Clears heat and toxins from the skin

Chapter 2 summary

Name	Similarities	Differences
Bai Hua She She Cao (Herba Oldenlandia)	Clear heat, eliminate toxins, treat cancer	Promotes urination to treat dysuria
Tian Kui Zi (Radix Semiaquilegiae)		Promotes urination, reduces abscesses
Long Kui (Herba Solanum Nigrum)		Promotes urination to alleviate edema
Ban Zhi Lian (Herba Scutellariae Barbatae)		Promotes urination
Shan Ci Gu (Pseudobulbus Cremastrae)		Reduces masses
Feng Wei Cao (Herba Pteris)		Dispels damp-heat
Dong Ling Cao (Herba Rabdosiae Rubescentis)		Invigorates blood circulation to relieve pain
Chui Pen Cao (Herba Sedi)	Clear heat, eliminate toxins, dispel dampness	Treats jaundice and hepatitis
Tu Fu Ling (Rhizoma Smilacis Glabrae)		Treats syphilis
Da Qing Ye (Folium Isatidis)	Clear heat, eliminate toxins, cool blood, disperse spots on the skin	Treats infectious respiratory disorders and purpura, cools blood
Ban Lan Gen (Radix Isatidis)		Relieves sore throat
Qing Dai (Indigo Naturalis)		Sedates Liver fire and Lung heat
Zhu Zi Cao (Herba Enphorbiae Thymifoliae)		Treats toxic heat
Chuan Xin Lian (Herba Andrographis)	Clear heat, eliminate toxins from the Lung	Strongly eliminates toxins, clears damp-heat in the lower *jiao*
Yu Xing Cao (Herba Houttuyniae)		Dispels Lung abscesses
She Gan (Rhizoma Belamcandae)		Treats sore throat, phlegm and cough
Shan Dou Gen (Radix Sophorae Tonkinensis)		Treats sore throat, reduces swellings, treats cancer
Ma Bo (Lasiosphaera seu Calvatia)		Stops bleeding
Pao Zai Cao (Herba Physalis Angulatae)		Relieves cough, promotes diuresis
Dao Diao Jin Zhong (Melothria Maderospatana)		Relieves pain
Ma Chi Xian (Herba Portulacae)	Clear heat, eliminate toxins, treat dysentery and diarrhea	Treats sores, carbuncles, eczema, bacterial dysentery; alleviates feeling of incomplete evacuation
Qin Pi (Cortex Fraxini)		Sedates Liver yang rising, treats bacterial dysentery
Bai Tou Weng (Radix Pulsatillae)		Treats amoebic and bacterial dysentery with toxic heat, mucus and blood
Ya Dan Zi (Fructus Bruceae)		Treats malaria, cancer, and amoebic dysentery
Hong Teng (Caulis Sargentodoxae)	Clear heat, eliminate toxins, treat intestinal abscess	Invigorates blood circulation, relieves pain
Bai Jiang Cao (Herba cum Radice Patriniae)		Dispels pus
Hu Yao Huang (Herba Leucas Mollissimae)		Promotes diuresis, invigorates blood circulation
Huang Shui Qie (Herba Solani)	Clear heat, eliminate toxins	Clears Liver fire, reduces inflammation and relieves pain
Shan Ma Ti (Radix Rauvolfiae)		Anchors Liver yang
Pu Yin (Radix Wikstroemia Indica)		Breaks masses, eliminates water accumulation
Shu Wei Huang (Herba Rostellulariae)		Regulates qi, invigorates blood
Xiang Si Cao (Herba Eupatorii Formosani)		Opens channels and collaterals, promotes urination
Ya She Huang (Herba Lippiae)		Regulates menstruation, reduces inflammation
Lu Dou (Semen Phaseoli Radiati)	Clear summer-heat	Detoxifies other herbs, relieves thirst
He Ye (Folium Nelumbinis)		Stops bleeding

General Characteristics of Heat-Clearing and Toxin-Eliminating Herbs:

Taste: bitter
Thermal property: cold
Channels entered: varies
Therapeutic actions: clear heat, eliminate toxins, treat sores and abscesses

Chapter 2 summary

Herbs in this category have a wide range of therapeutic effect in treating disorders characterized by heat and toxins, such as febrile disorders, infection, inflammation, diarrhea, dysentery, sores, abscesses, ulcers, burns, cancer, and many others.

Jin Yin Hua (Flos Lonicerae) and ***Lian Qiao*** (Fructus Forsythiae) are the most commonly used herbs for clearing heat and eliminating toxins. They disperse wind-heat and clear heat in the *qi* (energy) and *xue* (blood) levels, treat febrile disorders or symptoms related to toxic heat accumulation.

Jin Yin Hua disperses wind-heat, clears summer-heat and treats dysentery and intestinal abscesses. It is better for toxic heat attacking the entire body.

Lian Qiao clears heat, dispels stagnant heat in the chest and diaphragm, and cools blood to relieve blotches on the skin. It is better for toxic heat isolated to a local area. *Lian Qiao* is one of the most important herbs for treatment of abscesses.

Jin Yin Hua (Flos Lonicerae) and ***Ren Dong Teng*** (Caulis Lonicerae) are derived from the same plant.

Jin Yin Hua has stronger effects to clear heat, eliminate toxins and release the exterior.

Ren Dong Teng, weaker overall, is used much less than *Jin Yin Hua*.

Lian Qiao (Fructus Forsythiae) and ***Guan Ye Lian Qiao*** (Herba Hypericum) both clear heat, eliminate toxins, and treat sores and abscesses.

Lian Qiao is more potent, and is effective for toxic heat affecting the interior and exterior.

Guan Ye Lian Qiao is less effective, and is generally reserved for topical use.

Pu Gong Ying (Herba Taraxaci), ***Zi Hua Di Ding*** (Herba Violae), ***Ye Ju Hua*** (Flos Chrysanthemi Indici), and ***Lou Lu*** (Radix Rhapontici) clear heat, eliminate toxins, and treat sores. All three herbs have a wide range of applications to treat internal and external disorders.

Pu Gong Ying is effective for sores and abscesses of the skin, breast, lung, intestines, throat, and other parts of the body.

Zi Hua Di Ding treats abscesses, sores and snake bites.

Ye Ju Hua is most effective for skin, eye and cardiovascular disorders.

Lou Lu is more effective for breast fibroids and abscesses than for other uses.

Niu Huang (Calculus Bovis) has numerous functions that make it useful for many disorders. It clears heat and eliminates toxins to treat carbuncles and cellulitis, extinguishes wind to relieve spasms and tremors, and disperses phlegm and opens orifices to treat high fevers with delirium. As one of the more potent and expensive herbs, it is used in small quantities and only in pill form for maximum therapeutic benefit and cost effectiveness.

Zao Xiu (Rhizoma Paridis) clears heat, eliminates toxins, extinguishes Liver wind, and treats seizures, epilepsy, carbuncles, swellings and sores, snake bites, the pain of blood stagnation, and bleeding from external injuries.

Xiong Dan (Fel Ursi) has long been revered for its potency to clear heat, eliminate toxins, relieve spasms, and brighten the eyes. Historical clinical applications included sores, carbuncles, swellings, convulsions, tremors, redness, and eye swelling and pain. *Xiong Dan* was used internally or externally. *Xiong Dan*, bear gallbladder, is not only very expensive, it is difficult to find and unwise to pursue: most bears are protected or endangered species. *Zhu Dan* (Fel Porcus), pig gallbladder, is often used as an alternative.

Bai Lian (Radix Ampelopsis) and ***Bai Xian Pi*** (Cortex Dictamni) clear heat and are used both internally and externally to treat sores, furuncles and carbuncles.

Bai Lian treats burns.

Bai Xian Pi dispels dampness and relieves itching and jaundice.

Chapter 2 summary

Qian Li Guang (Herba Senecionis Scandens) clears heat, eliminates toxins, treats sores, carbuncles and eczema, and brightens the eyes to treat redness, swelling and pain.

Ji Gu Cao (Herba Abri) clears heat, eliminates toxins, drains dampness, disperses stagnation, and treats jaundice and *bi zheng* (painful obstruction syndrome).

Ban Bian Lian (Herba Lobeliae Chinensis) and ***Ban Zhi Lian*** (Herba Scutellariae Barbatae) clear heat, eliminate toxins, promote diuresis to reduce swelling, and treat carbuncles, swellings, toxic snake bites and edema.

Ban Bian Lian relieves snake bites and promotes diuresis to relieve edema.

Ban Zhi Lian has strong antibiotic action and is commonly used for cancer.

Cha Chi Huang (Herba Stellariae Aquaticae) clears heat, eliminates toxins, invigorates blood circulation and eliminates blood stagnation. Clinical applications include dysentery, sores, carbuncles, toxic swellings, endometriosis, cervicitis, hemorrhoids and other conditions characterized by general inflammation.

Dao Di Wu Gong (Rhizoma Heliminthostachytis) clears heat, eliminates toxins, and reduces swelling and inflammation.

Jin Guo Lan (Radix Tinosporae) clears heat and toxins from the Lung and the skin.

Liu Ye (Folium Salicis Babylonicae) clears heat and toxins from the exterior of the body.

Bai Hua She She Cao (Herba Oldenlandia), ***Tian Kui Zi*** (Radix Semiaquilegiae), ***Long Kui*** (Herba Solanum Nigrum), ***Ban Zhi Lian*** (Herba Scutellariae Barbatae), ***Shan Ci Gu*** (Pseudobulbus Cremastrae), ***Feng Wei Cao*** (Herba Pteris) and ***Dong Ling Cao*** (Herba Rabdosiae Rubescentis) clear heat, eliminate toxin, and have promising antineoplastic activities for treatment of cancer. In addition, many of these herbs promote normal urination and treat dysuria.

Bai Hua She She Cao clears heat, eliminates toxins, and treats toxic sores, intestinal abscesses, sore throat, toxic snake bites, dysentery, and cancers of the breast and the lymphatic system.

Tian Kui Zi and *Long Kui* have similar functions to clear heat, disperse stagnation, and reduce swelling.

Ban Zhi Lian has a strong effect to clear heat toxins to treat cancers of the lung and the gastrointestinal tract.

Shan Ci Gu eliminates toxins and treats carbuncles, cellulitis, and cancers of the breast, cervix, esophagus, lungs, stomach, and skin.

Feng Wei Cao eliminates toxicity and dries dampness to treat diarrhea, sore throat, and jaundice.

Dong Ling Cao clears heat and toxins to treat esophageal, stomach, liver, and prostate cancers.

Chui Pen Cao (Herba Sedi) and ***Tu Fu Ling*** (Rhizoma Smilacis Glabrae) eliminate toxins, dispel dampness, and treat swelling and carbuncles.

Chui Pen Cao treats damp-heat jaundice and hepatitis.

Tu Fu Ling treats syphilis with damp-heat in the lower *jiao*.

Da Qing Ye (Folium Isatidis) and ***Ban Lan Gen*** (Radix Isatidis) are derived from different parts of the same plant. Both cool the blood, eliminate toxins and treat febrile disorders and purple blotches on the skin. They have shown excellent antibiotic effects and are used frequently for infectious diseases, especially infections of the upper respiratory tract.

Da Qing Ye is cooler and more dispersing in nature. It clears both exterior and interior heat, and disperses heat in the *qi* (energy) and *xue* (blood) levels to cool blood.

Ban Lan Gen is more clearing and descending in nature. It eliminates toxins and relieves sore throat.

Chapter 2 summary

Qing Dai (Indigo Naturalis), a processed derivative of ***Da Qing Ye*** (Folium Isatidis), cools the blood, eliminates toxins, clears the Liver, and eliminates wind. It is also used externally to treat eczema and mumps.

Zhu Zi Cao (Herba Enphorbiae Thymifoliae) clears heat, eliminates toxins, and cools blood. Its clinical applications include bronchitis, sore throat, hepatitis, pneumonia, dysentery and hematemesis.

Chuan Xin Lian (Herba Andrographis) clears heat, eliminates toxins and dries dampness. It treats dysentery, coughing caused by heat, sore throat and other febrile disorders.

Yu Xing Cao (Herba Houttuyniae) clears heat and eliminates toxins, and is one of the best herbs for treatment of lung abscesses. It has a wide range of applications, including but not limited to cough caused by heat, *re lin* (heat dysuria), dysentery, diarrhea, carbuncles and swelling.

She Gan (Rhizoma Belamcandae), ***Shan Dou Gen*** (Radix Sophorae Tonkinensis), and ***Ma Bo*** (Lasiosphaera seu Calvatia) clear heat, eliminate toxins, and treat severe soreness, swelling and pain of the throat.

She Gan dispels phlegm, relieves sore throat, and arrests dyspnea.

Shan Dou Gen more strongly eliminates toxins and reduces swelling.

Ma Bo relieves severe sore throat, stops bleeding, and helps with wound healing.

Pao Zai Cao (Herba Physalis Angulatae) and ***Dao Diao Jin Zhong*** (Melothria Maderospatana) clear heat and eliminate toxins from the Lung to treat disorders of the Lung with coughing, phlegm, and abscesses. They are also effective for cases of heat and toxins attacking the Urinary Bladder and Kidney, such as in dysuria, toxic swellings and gynecological disorders caused by inflammation.

Ma Chi Xian (Herba Portulacae), ***Qin Pi*** (Cortex Fraxini), ***Bai Tou Weng*** (Radix Pulsatillae) and ***Ya Dan Zi*** (Fructus Bruceae) all clear heat, eliminate toxins and treat dysentery.

Ma Chi Xian treats bacterial dysentery with feelings of incomplete evacuation. It also treats uterine bleeding and carbuncles with swelling.

Qin Pi treats bacterial dysentery with its astringent effect. It also treats coughing accompanied by redness and pain of the eyes.

Bai Tou Weng treats both amoebic and bacterial dysentery.

Ya Dan Zi is effective for amoebic dysentery only. However, it also treats malaria, cancer and warts when used externally.

Hong Teng (Caulis Sargentodoxae), ***Bai Jiang Cao*** (Herba cum Radice Patriniae) and ***Hu Yao Huang*** (Herba Leucas Mollissimae) clear heat, eliminate toxins, invigorate blood circulation, and have excellent functions to treat abscesses of the intestines, such as enteritis, appendicitis, and dysentery.

Hong Teng disperses stagnation, relieves pain, and treats traumatic pain, dysmenorrhea and the pain associated with *bi zheng* (painful obstruction syndrome).

Bai Jiang Cao functions more effectively to dispel pus.

Hu Yao Huang promotes urination to treat dysuria and nephritis.

Huang Shui Qie (Herba Solani), ***Shan Ma Ti*** (Radix Rauvolfiae), ***Pu Yin*** (Radix Wikstroemia Indica), ***Shu Wei Huang*** (Herba Rostellulariae), ***Xiang Si Cao*** (Herba Eupatorii Formosani) and ***Ya She Huang*** (Herba Lippiae) have general effectiveness in clearing heat and eliminating toxins. Many of these herbs are only found in southeast China. Therefore, despite having excellent functions, they are not cited in most texts, and are so far underused in clinical practice.

Chapter 2 summary

Huang Shui Qie and *Shan Ma Ti* clear Liver fire and sedate Liver yang.

Pu Yin has a special effect to break masses and eliminate water accumulation, as is found in liver cirrhosis with ascites.

Shu Wei Huang regulates qi and blood circulation.

Xiang Si Cao and *Ya She Huang* treat a variety of inflammatory conditions.

Lu Dou (Semen Phaseoli Radiati) and ***He Ye*** (Folium Nelumbinis) clear summer-damp-heat.

Lu Dou eliminates toxins and treats sores and carbuncles. Used during the summertime, it relieves summer-heat, irritability and thirst. It is also used as an antidote to treat the toxicity associated with *Ba Dou* (Fructus Crotonis) and *Fu Zi* (Radix Aconiti Lateralis Praeparata).

He Ye stops bleeding in cases of yang deficiency.

SECTION 5: DEFICIENCY-HEAT CLEARING HERBS

Name	Similarities	Differences
Qing Hao (Herba Artemisiae Annuae)	Clear deficiency heat	Treats malaria
Bai Wei (Radix Cynanchi Atrati)		Cools blood
Di Gu Pi (Cortex Lycii)		Clears Lung heat
Yin Chai Hu (Radix Stellariae)		Treats deficiency heat
Hu Huang Lian (Rhizoma Picrorhizae)		Dries dampness, eliminates toxins

General Characteristics of Deficiency-Heat Clearing Herbs:

Taste: sweet
Thermal property: cold
Channels entered: Kidney, Liver
Therapeutic actions: clear deficient heat

These herbs treat deficiency heat with symptoms and signs such as steaming bones sensations, warmth in the palms and soles, night sweats, hot flashes, afternoon fever, dry throat and mouth, irritability, insomnia, a red tongue with thin or no tongue coat, and thin, thready pulse.

Qing Hao (Herba Artemisiae Annuae) clears deficiency heat, and is the best herb for treatment of malaria. It relieves summer-heat and exterior conditions common during the summer.

Bai Wei (Radix Cynanchi Atrati) clears deficiency heat in febrile disorders caused by exterior pathogenic invasion, and treats *lin zheng* (dysuria syndrome) and sores.

Di Gu Pi (Cortex Lycii) clears deficiency heat and Lung heat, cools blood, stops bleeding and relieves thirst and irritability.

Yin Chai Hu (Radix Stellariae) and ***Hu Huang Lian*** (Rhizoma Picrorhizae) clear deficiency heat, steaming bones sensations, and tidal fever.

Yin Chai Hu clears deficiency heat.

Hu Huang Lian dries dampness, eliminates toxins and treats dysentery and diarrhea.

Hu Huang Lian (Rhizoma Picrorhizae) and ***Huang Lian*** (Rhizoma Coptidis) are from different geographic regions but both clear heat, dry dampness and eliminate toxins.

Hu Huang Lian clears deficiency heat.

Huang Lian sedates excess fire, damp-heat and toxic heat.

Chapter 2 summary

HERBS FROM OTHER FUNCTIONAL CATEGORIES WITH HEAT-CLEARING FUNCTIONS

Name	Functional Category
Bai Mao Gen (Rhizoma Imperatae)	Stop-Bleeding Herbs (Chapter 11)
Bing Pian (Borneolum Syntheticum)	Orifice-Opening Herbs (Chapter 16)
Da Huang (Radix et Rhizoma Rhei)	Downward Draining Herbs (Chapter 3)
Deng Xin Cao (Medulla Junci)	Water-Regulating and Damp-Resolving Herbs (Chapter 6)
Fan Xie Ye (Folium Sennae)	Downward Draining Herbs (Chapter 3)
Gou Teng (Ramulus Uncariae cum Uncis)	Liver-Calming and Wind-Extinguishing Herbs (Chapter 15)
Guan Zhong (Rhizoma Dryopteridis)	Antiparasitic Herbs (Chapter 10)
Hu Zhang (Rhizoma Polygoni Cuspidati)	Blood-Invigorating and Stasis-Removing Herbs (Chapter 12)
Hua Shi (Talcum)	Water-Regulating and Damp-Resolving Herbs (Chapter 6)
Huang Yao Zi (Herba Dioscoreae Bulbiferae)	Phlegm-Resolving and Coughing- and Wheezing-Relieving Herbs (Chapter 13)
Jiao Gu Lan (Rhizoma seu Herba Gynostemmatis)	Tonic Herbs (Chapter 17)
Ju Hua (Flos Chrysanthemi)	Exterior-Releasing Herbs (Chapter 1)
Jue Ming Zi (Semen Cassiae)	Liver-Calming and Wind-Extinguishing Herbs (Chapter 15)
Lian Zi (Semen Nelumbinis)	Astringent Herbs (Chapter 18)
Lian Zi Xin (Plumula Nelumbinis)	Astringent Herbs (Chapter 18)
Lu Hui (Aloe)	Downward Draining Herbs (Chapter 3)
Ma Bian Cao (Herba Verbenae)	Blood-Invigorating and Stasis-Removing Herbs (Chapter 12)
Mang Xiao (Natrii Sulfas)	Downward Draining Herbs (Chapter 3)
Niu Bang Zi (Fructus Arctii)	Exterior-Releasing Herbs (Chapter 1)
Nu Zhen Zi (Fructus Ligustri Lucidi)	Tonic Herbs (Chapter 17)
Shi Hu (Herba Dendrobii)	Tonic Herbs (Chapter 17)
Yi Mu Cao (Herba Leonuri)	Blood-Invigorating and Stasis-Removing Herbs (Chapter 12)
Yu Jin (Radix Curcumae)	Blood-Invigorating and Stasis-Removing Herbs (Chapter 12)
Zhu Li (Succus Bambusae)	Phlegm-Resolving and Coughing- and Wheezing-Relieving Herbs (Chapter 13)
Zhu Ru (Caulis Bambusae in Taenia)	Phlegm-Resolving and Coughing- and Wheezing-Relieving Herbs (Chapter 13)

Chapter 3

— Downward Draining Herbs

泻下药

Chapter 3 — Downward Draining Herbs

Chapter 3 泻下药 — Downward Draining Herbs

Definition: "Downward draining" describes the action of substances that eliminate pathogenic factors and conditions via purgative, laxative or cathartic means.

Herbs that drain downward are commonly used to treat internal accumulations of pathogenic factors, or excess conditions. The terms 'pathogenic factors' or 'excess conditions' in this context refer to internal heat, cold, or dampness, and to manifestations of constipation, food stagnation, intestinal obstruction, and water accumulation. These conditions interfere with normal physiological functioning of the body and cause illness. Herbs that drain downward remove the pathogens or blockages and thus assist the body in resuming its normal functions. These substances are categorized as purgatives, moist laxatives, or harsh expellants (cathartics), all of which eliminate pathogenic factors via defecation and/or urination.

Draining downward treats internal accumulations of pathogens, including constipation, ascites, and water accumulation.

SUBCATEGORIES OF ACTION

1. ***Purgatives***: These herbs function to strongly induce defecation and eliminate constipation and accumulations of excess in the body. Cold purgatives are bitter and cold, and treat accumulations of heat and fire in the body. Warm purgatives are acrid and warm, and treat acute conditions of cold accumulation in the body. Purgative herbs are commonly prescribed with qi-regulating herbs, as the accumulation of excess is usually accompanied by stagnation of qi. Purgative herbs are sometimes combined with qi or blood tonics for chronic and habitual constipation in elderly patients who have weak constitutions.
2. ***Moist laxatives***: Most herbs in this subcategory are sweet and nourishing seeds that contain significant amounts of lipids to moisten the bowels and relieve constipation. They are most suitable in treatment of mild to moderate cases of constipation that do not require strong purgatives or harsh cathartics. Moist laxatives are most beneficial for treatment of constipation in elderly patients, or patients with weak constitutions, or deficiency of blood or body fluids. Herbs that regulate qi, tonify blood and nourish yin are commonly combined with moist laxatives to enhance their overall effectiveness.
3. ***Harsh expellants (cathartics)***: Mostly bitter, cold and toxic, these herbs eliminate pathogenic factors from the body by strongly promoting bowel movement and urination. Because these herbs are extremely harsh and have toxic aspects, they must be reserved for treatment of individuals who are otherwise strong enough to tolerate such approaches. Clinical applications include severe constipation, ascites, and water accumulation. It is also recommended that a small quantity of tonic herbs be combined in the formula to prevent damage to the body from loss of essential components along with removal of pathogenic factors.

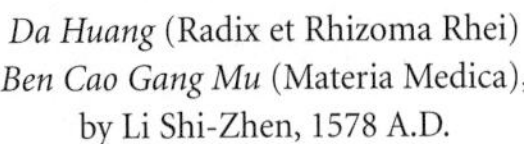

Da Huang (Radix et Rhizoma Rhei)
Ben Cao Gang Mu (Materia Medica), by Li Shi-Zhen, 1578 A.D.

DIFFERENTIAL DIAGNOSIS AND TREATMENT

Diagnosis of constipation is simple and straightforward, based on information obtained during patient intake. The absence of bowel movement, or difficulty in voiding the bowels, possibly accompanied by fullness, bloating, pain, fever or local inflammation, are some of the factors to consider. Once this diagnosis is made, optimal treatment requires determination of both the severity of constipation and the underlying condition of the patient. While moist laxatives are sufficient for mild to moderate cases, strong purgatives and harsh cathartics may be required for severe constipation. Determining the underlying condition of the patient is also important: weak,

Chapter 3 — Downward Draining Herbs

deficient or elderly patients, or menstruating or postpartum women may not be able to safely tolerate purgatives and cathartics. Other conditions combined with constipation may require careful differential diagnosis and treatment. While most cases can be categorized as the effects of excess heat or excess cold in the interior, other complications may also be present. Therefore, it is often necessary to combine herbs that drain downward with substances to address complicating factors.

Purgatives and harsh expellants (cathartics) should be used with extreme caution in elderly patients, and menstruating, pregnant or postpartum women.

CAUTIONS/CONTRAINDICATIONS

Purgatives and harsh expellants (cathartics) should be used with extreme caution in elderly patients, in menstruating, pregnant or postpartum women, and patients with qi, blood, yin, or yang deficiencies.

PROCESSING

Purgative and harsh cathartic substances may require special processing and preparation to both preserve their functions and minimize unwanted side effects. Specific details are listed in each herb monograph.

PHARMACOLOGICAL EFFECTS

- **Laxative:** Many herbs in this category promote bowel movement. Mechanisms of action include osmotic effect to increase the content of water in the intestines; stimulating action to increase the speed of intestinal peristalsis; and moistening influence to promote bowel movement.
- **Diuretic**: Many herbs in this category regulate water circulation and eliminate water accumulation. Herbs with diuretic action include *Gan Sui* (Radix Euphorbiae Kansui), *Da Ji* (Radix Euphorbiae seu Knoxiae), *Shang Lu* (Radix Phytolaccae), and *Qian Niu Zi* (Semen Pharbitidis).
- **Antibiotic**: Some downward-draining herbs have broad-spectrum antibiotic activities to kill bacteria, viruses, and dermatophytes, such as *Da Huang* (Radix et Rhizoma Rhei), *Lu Hui* (Aloe) and *Fan Xie Ye* (Folium Sennae).
- **Cholagogic**: Some herbs increase the production of bile by the liver and excretion of bile acids by the gallbladder, including substances such as *Mang Xiao* (Natrii Sulfas) and *Da Huang* (Radix et Rhizoma Rhei).
- **Hemostatic**: Some herbs may be used to stop bleeding, such as *Da Huang* (Radix et Rhizoma Rhei) and *Fan Xie Ye* (Folium Sennae).

POTENTIAL HERB-DRUG INTERACTIONS

- Downward-draining herbs are well recognized for their purgative and laxative effects. While proper use of these herbs effectively treats constipation, inappropriate use may lead to diarrhea, dehydration and electrolyte imbalance. Therefore, individuals ingesting such herbs should receive adequate amounts of water and electrolytes, and should be monitored for warning signs such as spasms and cramps.
- Downward draining herbs should be used with caution in patients taking pharmaceutical laxatives and diuretics, as these drugs also contribute to the elimination of water and electrolytes. The inappropriate or excessive combination of herbs and pharmaceuticals in this case might cause or exaggerate diarrhea, dehydration, and electrolyte imbalance.

Section 1

— Purgatives

Da Huang (Radix et Rhizoma Rhei)

大黄

Pinyin Name: *Da Huang*
Literal Name: "big yellow," "greater yellow root"
Alternate Chinese Names: *Jiang Jun, Chuan Jun, Jin Wen*
Original Source: *Shen Nong Ben Cao Jing* (Divine Husbandman's Classic of the Materia Medica) in the second century
English Name: rhubarb root
Botanical Name: *Rheum palmatum* L. (*Zhang Ye Da Huang*); *Rheum tanguticum* Maxim ex Balf. (*Tang Gu Te Da Huang*); or *Rheum officinale* Baill. (*Da Huang*)
Pharmaceutical Name: Radix et Rhizoma Rhei
Properties: bitter, cold
Channels Entered: Spleen, Stomach, Large Intestine, Liver, Heart

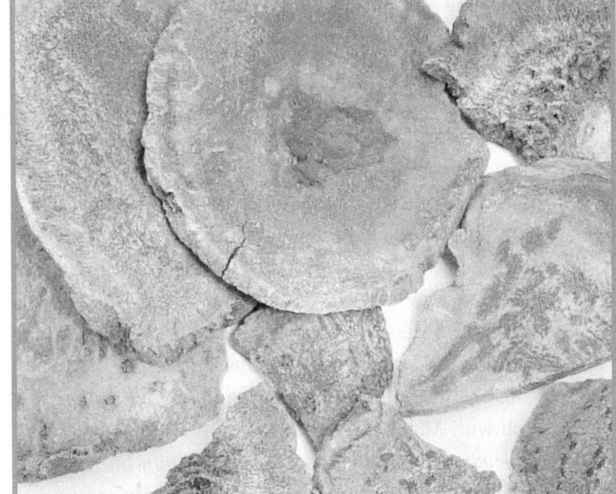

CHINESE THERAPEUTIC ACTIONS

1. Attacks Accumulations by Purging Downwards

Constipation: *Da Huang* (Radix et Rhizoma Rhei) has excellent purgative properties to treat a wide variety of accumulations, including constipation, epigastric distention, fullness and abdominal pain that worsens with pressure and palpation. Bitter, cold and descending in nature, *Da Huang* is best used to treat constipation caused by excess heat. It also treats excess heat in the *fu* (hollow) organs during the *yangming* stage of illness, a condition characterized by high fever, delirium, semi-consciousness, and convulsions. *Da Huang* purges the accumulation and eliminates heat, thereby relieving the condition and preserving yin.

Da Huang is often combined with *Mang Xiao* (Natrii Sulfas) to treat excess-type constipation caused by heat. *Mang Xiao* is salty and softens the stool while *Da Huang* has a strong purgative effect to drive out stagnation. Both *Da Huang* and *Mang Xiao* clear heat in the *xue* (blood) level. These two herbs are the chief ingredients in the primary formula for treatment of constipation, *Da Cheng Qi Tang* (Major Order the Qi Decoction).

Heat and qi stagnation often accompany constipation. The purgative effect of *Da Huang* is greatly enhanced by adding qi-regulating herbs such as *Hou Po* (Cortex Magnoliae Officinalis) and *Zhi Shi* (Fructus Aurantii Immaturus). Typical symptoms that require addition of these herbs include abdominal bloating, distention and pain. A larger dose of *Da Huang* should be used if heat and constipation are more severe than the bloating, distention and pain.

- Severe constipation due to accumulation of excess heat: use *Da Huang* with *Mang Xiao* (Natrii Sulfas), *Hou Po* (Cortex Magnoliae Officinalis) and *Zhi Shi* (Fructus Aurantii Immaturus) to soften the hardness, relieve constipation and purge excess heat. **Exemplar Formula:** *Da Cheng Qi Tang* (Major Order the Qi Decoction).
- Moderate constipation from accumulation of heat: use it with *Huo Ma Ren* (Fructus Cannabis), *Xing Ren* (Semen

Da Huang (Radix et Rhizoma Rhei)

Armeniacae Amarum) and honey. **Exemplar Formula:** *Ma Zi Ren Wan* (Hemp Seed Pill).

Severe constipation sometimes presents as extremely dry, hard, fecal matter obstructing the large intestine. Attempts to defecate result only in the passage of clear, foul-smelling liquid, without expelling solid stools. Abdominal pain persists despite passage of liquids.

- Severe constipation with passage of liquid but no solid stool: use *Da Huang* with *Mang Xiao* (Natrii Sulfas) to soften the stool, moisten the intestines, and relieve constipation.

In addition to excess heat, constipation is often accompanied by complications, such as qi deficiency, blood deficiency, fluid deficiency, or Spleen yang deficiency. Optimal therapy requires concurrent focus on treatment of the disease without damaging the body, by using purgatives and tonics together. Such concurrent treatment ensures that purgative herbs will not damage the body, and tonic herbs will not cause further stagnation.

- Excess heat in the *fu* (hollow) organs during the *yangming* stage of illness with qi and blood deficiencies: use *Da Huang* with *Ren Shen* (Radix Ginseng) and *Dang Gui* (Radicis Angelicae Sinensis) to tonify qi and blood. **Exemplar Formula:** *Huang Long Tang* (Yellow Dragon Decoction).
- Constipation with heat consuming body fluids: use this herb with *Mai Men Dong* (Radix Ophiopogonis), *Sheng Di Huang* (Radix Rehmanniae) and *Xuan Shen* (Radix Scrophulariae) to nourish yin and promote generation of body fluids.
- Constipation with Spleen yang deficiency and accumulation of cold: combine it with *Ren Shen* (Radix Ginseng) and *Gan Cao* (Radix Glycyrrhizae) to tonify the Spleen, and *Fu Zi* (Radix Aconiti Lateralis Praeparata) and *Gan Jiang* (Rhizoma Zingiberis) to dispel cold.
- Habitual constipation with deficiency: combine it with honey and seeds such as *Huo Ma Ren* (Fructus Cannabis) and *Xing Ren* (Semen Armeniacae Amarum) to lubricate the intestines and thus facilitate passage of stools.

Dysentery: *Da Huang* is also used in treatment of late-stage dysentery, when there is accumulation of damp-heat after numerous episodes of diarrhea characterized by rectal tenesmus and feelings of incomplete evacuation after defecation. To complete the treatment, *Da Huang* clears and purges the remaining accumulation of damp-heat in the intestines, preventing chronic complications.

- Dysentery: cook *Da Huang* with grain-based liquor.
- Dysentery with excess damp-heat: use it with *Huang Lian* (Rhizoma Coptidis), *Huang Qin* (Radix Scutellariae) and *Bai Shao* (Radix Paeoniae Alba).
- Chronic dysentery with accumulation of damp-heat and Spleen yang deficiency: combine this herb with *Fu Zi* (Radix Aconiti Lateralis Praeparata) and *Gan Jiang* (Rhizoma Zingiberis).

Parasites: *Da Huang* is commonly used with antiparasitic herbs or formulas to enhance the expulsion of parasites.

2. Purges Fire

Da Huang has an excellent ability to purge excess fire whether constipation is present or not. Clinical indications include excessive fire flaring upward, attacking the head, and leading to headache, red eyes, sore throat, swelling and pain of the gums, and oral ulcers.

- Excess upward flaring of heat attacking the head: use *Da Huang* with *Mang Xiao* (Natrii Sulfas), *Zhi Zi* (Fructus Gardeniae), *Huang Qin* (Radix Scutellariae), and *Lian Qiao* (Fructus Forsythiae) to clear heat from the head and the upper *jiao*. **Exemplar Formula:** *Liang Ge San* (Cool the Diaphragm Powder).
- Liver fire with headaches, irritability, convulsions and constipation: combine this herb with *Long Dan Cao* (Radix Gentianae), *Zhi Zi* (Fructus Gardeniae) and *Xia Ku Cao* (Spica Prunellae).

Da Huang cools the blood, stops bleeding, and treats various bleeding disorders caused by heat and fire attacking the *xue* (blood) level. The blood is usually bright red and generally profuse in these cases. Since *Da Huang* has a strong purgative function, it is unique in that it purges heat and stops bleeding without leaving blood stasis behind. It may be used individually or in combination with other herbs that tonify yin or clear heat.

- Epistaxis and hematemesis because of Heart fire: use this herb with *Huang Lian* (Rhizoma Coptidis) and *Huang Qin* (Radix Scutellariae).
- Hematemesis due to chronic weakness and deficiency: use *Da Huang* powder with juice from *Sheng Di Huang* (Radix Rehmanniae).
- Upper gastrointestinal tract bleeding: ingest powdered *Da Huang* alone.

3. Clears Heat and Eliminates Toxins

Da Huang is commonly used internally or topically to clear heat and eliminate toxins. Indications for internal use include intestinal abscesses, and for topical use include cellulitis, swelling, abscesses, carbuncles and burns.

- Intestinal abscess: use *Da Huang* with *Mu Dan Pi* (Cortex Moutan), *Tao Ren* (Semen Persicae), *Mang Xiao* (Natrii Sulfas) and *Hong Teng* (Caulis Sargentodoxae). **Exemplar Formula:** *Da Huang Mu Dan Tang* (Rhubarb and Moutan Decoction).

Da Huang (Radix et Rhizoma Rhei)

- Cellulitis on the back with constipation and a forceful pulse: ingest this herb with *Bai Zhi* (Radix Angelicae Dahuricae) as powder, decoction or in combination with scallion and grain-based liquor.
- Burns: mix powdered *Da Huang* with sesame oil and apply topically.

4. Activates Blood Circulation and Removes Blood Stasis

Da Huang has two unique functions in activating blood circulation and removing blood stasis. First, it eliminates blood stasis and bruises through its purgative function; then it clears heat related to the stasis. Clinical applications include amenorrhea due to blood stasis, postpartum blood stasis, palpable abdominal masses and blood stasis due to external or traumatic injuries. It is often used for amenorrhea accompanied by dry skin, emaciation, poor appetite, lower abdominal fullness, night sweating and withered *shen* (spirit).

- Blood stasis: use *Da Huang* individually or in herbal combinations.
- Moderate blood stasis: combine it with *Tao Ren* (Semen Persicae), *Hong Hua* (Flos Carthami), *Dang Gui* (Radicis Angelicae Sinensis) and *Chuan Xiong* (Rhizoma Ligustici Chuanxiong).
- Severe blood stasis: add *Shui Zhi* (Hirudo) and *Meng Chong* (Tabanus).
- Chronic blood stasis with qi and blood deficiencies: use *Da Huang* with *Ren Shen* (Radix Ginseng) and *E Jiao* (Colla Corii Asini).
- Amenorrhea: add *Meng Chong* (Tabanus) and *Di Bie Chong* (Eupolyphaga).

5. Clears Damp-Heat and Promotes Diuresis

Da Huang treats water accumulation in patients who have no deficiencies. It is commonly combined with diuretic or cathartic herbs to dispel water, clear damp-heat and promote normal urination. Additionally, *Da Huang* drains damp-heat and is an important herb in treating jaundice.

- Water accumulation characterized by edema and abdominal fullness: use it with *Fen Fang Ji* (Radix Stephaniae Tetandrae) and *Ting Li Zi* (Semen Descurainiae seu Lepidii).
- Accumulation of water and heat in the chest: combine it with *Gan Sui* (Radix Euphorbiae Kansui) and *Mang Xiao* (Natrii Sulfas).
- *Re lin* (heat dysuria): add *Chuan Mu Tong* (Caulis Clematidis Armandii), *Che Qian Zi* (Semen Plantaginis) and *Zhi Zi* (Fructus Gardeniae). **Exemplar Formula:** *Ba Zheng San* (Eight-Herb Powder for Rectification).
- Damp-heat jaundice: use *Da Huang* with *Yin Chen Hao* (Herba Artemisiae Scopariae) and *Zhi Zi* (Fructus Gardeniae). **Exemplar Formula:** *Yin Chen Hao Tang* (Artemisia Scoparia Decoction).
- Damp-heat throughout the body: combine it with *Huang Lian* (Rhizoma Coptidis) and *Huang Qin* (Radix Scutellariae). **Exemplar Formula:** *San Huang Xie Xin Tang* (Three Yellows Decoction to Sedate the Epigastrium).

Da Huang also treats chronic accumulation of phlegm heat characterized by cough, dyspnea, mania, disorientation and other symptoms associated with hot phlegm misting the Heart.

DOSAGE

5 to 10 grams; up to 15 to 20 grams in severe cases. Reduce the dosage of *Da Huang* by half when using as powder internally. *Da Huang* should be cooked for only a short period of time (thus, added at the end of decoction and cooked for only 5 to 10 minutes) to preserve its purgative function. Frying with grain-based liquor enhances its function to clear heat from the upper body, activate blood circulation and remove blood stasis, but weakens its effect to treat constipation. Charred *Da Huang* has a stronger hemostatic function.

Ingestion of *Da Huang* is often associated with nausea and vomiting, since this herb is bitter and irritating to the stomach. If the patient vomits after drinking a decoction containing *Da Huang*, let the decoction cool to room temperature. Before giving the patient the cooled decoction, serve a cup of a decoction composed of 1 gram of *Da Huang* and 1 gram of *Gan Cao* (Radix Glycyrrhizae), wait 15 minutes, and then administer the original decoction.

Because the components of *Da Huang* responsible for purgative actions are extremely sensitive to heat, its potency is heavily dependant on the processing methods. In one study, the purgative effect of *Da Huang* was evaluated using different preparations. The ED_{50} (effective dose) was 0.18 g/kg for fresh *Da Huang*, 0.25 g/kg for the vinegar-processed herb, 0.26 g/kg for herb processed with grain-based liquor, 3.42 g/kg for herb decocted with grain-based liquor, 7.26 g/kg for herb decocted with vinegar, and >12.00 g/kg for charred *Da Huang*.[1]

CAUTIONS / CONTRAINDICATIONS

- Extremely bitter and cold, *Da Huang* may damage the Spleen and Stomach and should be used with caution. Possible side effects may include nausea, vomiting and poor appetite.
- Use of *Da Huang* is contraindicated in patients who do not have constipation or blood stagnation.
- Use *Da Huang* with caution in patients who are menstruating, or in postpartum women without stasis.

Da Huang (Radix et Rhizoma Rhei)

- *Da Huang* is contraindicated in patients with qi and blood deficiencies, and in pregnancy.
- Nursing mothers should take *Da Huang* with great caution as it may enter breast milk, causing diarrhea in the infant.

OVERDOSAGE

In humans, the use of *Da Huang* is relatively safe. However, with overdose, adverse reactions such as diarrhea, nausea, vomiting, dizziness, and abdominal pain may occur. In one study with 30 subjects, oral administration of 3 grams of *Da Huang* three times daily for 5 days caused adverse reactions such as diarrhea, abdominal pain, vomiting, nausea, and borborygmus.[2]

TREATMENT OF OVERDOSAGE

Overdosage associated with *Da Huang* can be treated symptomatically using acupuncture, moxa and herbs. Adequate intake of fluids during treatment with *Da Huang* is important to avoid dehydration.

CHEMICAL COMPOSITION

Sennoside A,B,C,D,E,F; emodin, aloe-emodin, chrysophanol, rhein, physcion, rhein-8-mono-β-D-glucoside, physcion monoglucoside, aloe-emodin-8-monoglucoside, emodin monoglucoside, chrysophanol monoglucoside.[3,4]

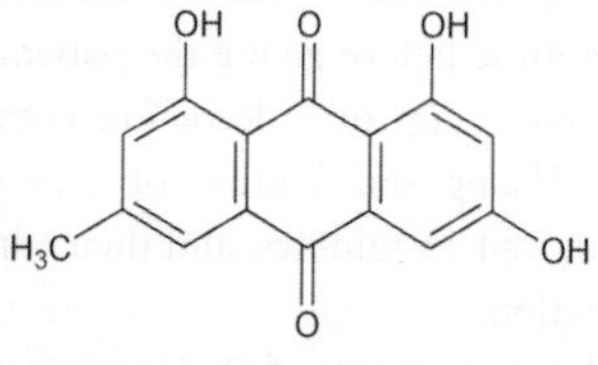

Emodin

PHARMACOLOGICAL EFFECTS

- **Laxative:** *Da Huang* has a remarkable purgative effect. Sennoside A, aloe-emodin, and rhein are components most responsible for this purgative action. *Da Huang* works directly on the large intestine to increase contraction and peristalsis. However, the purgative effect does not occur until 6 to 8 hours after oral ingestion, which indicates that the herb must be absorbed systemically before it exerts its effect on the large intestine. It has no effect on the small intestine and will not interfere with normal absorption of nutrients. Interestingly, *Da Huang* contains a small amount of tannin that may cause constipation if used repeatedly for a prolonged period of time.[5]
- **Hepatoprotective:** *Da Huang* has a hepatoprotective effect, especially against carbon tetrachloride-induced liver damage. In mice with acute icteric jaundice, administration of *Da Huang* was effective in reducing the extent of liver damage (necrosis of hepatocytes), while the placebo group made no comparable progress.[6]
- **Cholagogic:** Intravenous injection of alcohol extract of *Da Huang* was effective in increasing the excretion of bile in dogs and cats within 5 to 15 minutes. The peak effect was observed after 8 to 10 minutes, and the duration of action was approximately 30 minutes.[7]
- **Hemostatic:** Intraperitoneal injection of *Da Huang* was effective in stopping bleeding in mice. The hemostatic effect is attributed to the herb's ability to increase viscosity of the blood and to facilitate aggregation of platelets.[8,9]
- **Antibiotic:** *Da Huang* has a broad spectrum antibiotic effect. It is most effective against the streptococcus and staphylococcus species of bacteria. It also inhibits the activity of *Corynebacterium diphtheriae, Bacillus subtilis, Salmonella typhi,* and *Bacillus dysenteriae.* Constituents responsible for the antibiotic effect include emodin, rhein, and aloe-emodin.[10]
- **Cardiovascular:** Administration of *Da Huang* has various impacts on the cardiovascular system. In one study, intravenous injection reduced blood pressure by 20% and heart rate by 12% in mice. In another study, administration of a *Da Huang* preparation to anesthetized dogs is associated with a decrease in oxygen consumption of the cardiac muscle, and with reduction of heart rate and peripheral resistance.[11,12]
- **Nephroprotective:** Decoction of *Da Huang* effectively reduces blood urea nitrogen (BUN) and creatinine as demonstrated in both *in vitro* and *in vivo* studies.[13]
- **Others:** Administration of *Da Huang* is associated with antipyretic, analgesic, and anti-inflammatory effects.[14]

CLINICAL STUDIES AND RESEARCH

- **Nephropathy:** Twenty patients with various degrees of renal impairment were treated with an herbal formula with marked reduction of blood urea nitrogen (BUN) and creatinine levels. Treatment was most effective in mild-to-moderate cases of renal impairment. The herbal formula contained *Da Huang* 30 to 60g (10g if post-decocted), calcined *Mu Li* (Concha Ostreae) 30g, and *Pu Gong Ying* (Herba Taraxaci) 20g. The treatment protocol was to instill 600 to 800 ml of herbal decoction as a rectal enema one to two times daily. Most patients had between 4 and 6 bowel movements per day.[15]
- **Upper gastrointestinal bleeding:** In one clinical study, 890 patients with upper gastrointestinal bleeding were treated with 3 grams of powdered *Da Huang* (in pills or syrup) three times daily, with a 97% rate of effectiveness. The average time required to stop bleeding was 2 days, as determined by hemoccult testing. All other herbs and drugs were discontinued for the duration of the study. In severe cases of bleeding, supportive treatments such as intravenous fluids

Da Huang (Radix et Rhizoma Rhei)

and blood transfusion were administered.[16]

- **Acute pancreatitis:** According to one report, 100 patients with pancreatitis were treated with *Da Huang* with great success. Initial treatment included decoction of 30 to 60 grams of *Da Huang* every 1 to 2 hours until symptoms returned to normal. After the patients stabilized, they were switched to tablets of *Da Huang,* 3 grams twice daily. The total dosage of *Da Huang* per patient was 450 grams. The study reported close to 100% effectiveness. The time required was 2 days for normalization of amylase in urine and 3 days for relief of pain.[17]
- **Enteritis:** Patients with hemorrhagic necrotic enteritis were treated with good results using 24 to 30 grams of fresh unprocessed *Da Huang* two to three times daily. The study reported improvement in 12 of 14 patients after 2 to 6 doses, with relief of pain and diminished amount of hematochezia.[18]
- **Constipation:** One report cites 72 patients with cerebral vascular accident (11 due to hemorrhage and 61 due to embolism) that were admitted to the hospital and treated for related constipation with an herbal decoction, with good results. Records indicated that all patients had greasy or dry yellow tongue coats, and had passed no bowel movements within the previous four days. The herbal prescription contained *Da Huang* 12g, *Mang Xiao* (Natrii Sulfas) 10g, *Zhi Shi* (Fructus Aurantii Immaturus) 9g, and *Gan Cao* (Radix Glycyrrhizae) 6g, cooked to yield a final decoction of 200 ml. The decoction was divided into 2 doses, taken 2 hours apart. Most people responded within 1 to 2 doses.[19]
- **Hyperlipidemia:** A preparation of *Da Huang* given three times daily for 3 weeks was 76% effective in reducing plasma triglycerides and β-lipoprotein levels in 47 patients.[20]
- **Acute icteric hepatitis:** According to one report, 80 cases of acute icteric hepatitis were treated with a large dosage of *Da Huang* with a 95% rate of effectiveness based on symptomatic evaluation and improvement of liver function. The treatment protocol was 50 grams of *Da Huang* for adults, and 25 to 30 grams for children, given as decoction one time daily.[21]
- **Tonsillitis:** In a clinical study, 22 patients with acute tonsillitis experienced complete recovery within 2 to 4 days, using *Da Huang*. The treatment protocol was to soak fresh *Da Huang* in 250 ml of hot water and drink the solution every 2 hours as needed. Each set of herbs could be used up to four times before replacement. The dosage of *Da Huang* was 15 grams for adults, and 8 to 10 grams for children.[22] In another study, 40 children with acute tonsillitis were treated with an 85% success rate using 6 to 9 grams of *Da Huang* soaked in hot water, every 2 hours.[23]

HERB-DRUG INTERACTION

- **Cardiac glycosides:** Prolonged use of *Da Huang* may cause loss of potassium, leading to increased toxicity of cardiac glycosides, such as digoxin (Lanoxin).[24]

TOXICOLOGY

In acute toxicology studies in mice, the LD_{50} for decoction of *Da Huang* via oral ingestion is 153 g/kg. In chronic toxicology studies in mice, administration of *Da Huang* on a long-term basis may cause severe diarrhea, inhibition of the immune system, and decrease in weight of the reproductive organs.[25,26]

AUTHORS' COMMENTS

Da Huang is the key herb in treating excess-type constipation involving heat. Constipation may cause various toxins to be absorbed by the intestines, thus causing symptoms of fever, delirium, headache, and in severe cases, unconsciousness. *Da Huang* restores normal bodily metabolism by purging the excess accumulation and thus preventing further absorption of toxins and accumulation of heat.

Da Huang has the unique characteristic of being able to simultaneously treat both constipation and dysentery. For treatment of constipation, its main function is to dispel stagnation and induce bowel movement by purging heat accumulation in the intestines. The initial stage of dysentery includes diarrhea with a feeling of incomplete evacuation and rectal tenesmus caused by damp-heat. *Da Huang* is used in this case to treat the root of the problem, namely damp-heat. Use of *Da Huang* is necessary to purge damp-heat to ensure successful and complete recovery. If antidiarrheal herbs are used, the condition may improve slightly but may turn from acute to chronic dysentery as the pathogenic factors are trapped in the intestines. Though constipation and dysentery may manifest in completely different symptoms, the cause of stagnation and heat is the same. For that reason, *Da Huang* can be used for both cases.

It may seem paradoxical that, although *Da Huang* has descending properties, it is used in treatment of disorders of the head such as red eyes, sore throat, swollen and painful gums, hematemesis, and epistaxis. It may be helpful to consider that these symptoms are caused by a flaring up of heat, not by heat accumulation in the local region. In these cases, instead of choosing herbs that go to the head, it is better to choose an herb such as *Da Huang* that has descending properties to bring the flaring up of fire back down.

According to Dr. Zhang Xiao-Ping, a small amount of the downward-directing *Da Huang,* used for patients with hypertension, sedates rising Liver fire.

Da Huang (Radix et Rhizoma Rhei)

References

1. *Zhong Yao Tong Bao* (Journal of Chinese Herbology), 1983; 8:20
2. *Zhong Yi Yao Xue Bao* (Report of Chinese Medicine and Herbology), 1990; (5):48
3. *Xian Dai Zhong Yao Yao Li Xue* (Contemporary Pharmacology of Chinese Herbs), 1997; 368-369
4. *The Merck Index* 12th edition, Chapman & Hall/CRCnetBASE/Merck, 2000
5. *Zhong Yao Xue* (Chinese Herbology), 1998; 251:256
6. *Zhong Guo Zhong Yao Za Zhi* (People's Republic of China Journal of Chinese Herbology), 1989; 14(10):46
7. *Xin Yi Yao Xue Za Zhi* (New Journal of Medicine and Herbology), 1974; (5):34
8. *Zhong Cao Yao* (Chinese Herbal Medicine), 1981; 12(10):31
9. Ibid., 1986; 17(11):27
10. *Zhong Yao Xue* (Chinese Herbology), 1998; 251:256
11. *Chang Yong Zhong Yao Cheng Fen Yu Yao Li Shou Ce* (A Handbook of the Composition and Pharmacology of Common Chinese Drugs), 1994; 226:323
12. *Zhong Guo Zhong Yao Za Zhi* (People's Republic of China Journal of Chinese Herbology), 1989; 14(10):46
13. *Chang Yong Zhong Yao Xian Dai Yan Jiu Yu Lin Chuan* (Recent Study & Clinical Application of Common Traditional Chinese Medicine), 1995; 181:190
14. *Chang Yong Zhong Yao Cheng Fen Yu Yao Li Shou Ce* (A Handbook of the Composition and Pharmacology of Common Chinese Drugs), 1994; 226:323
15. *Zhong Yi Za Zhi* (Journal of Chinese Medicine), 1981; 9:21
16. *Zhong Xi Yi Jie He Za Zhi* (Journal of Integrated Chinese and Western Medicine), 1982; 2:85
17. Ibid.
18. *Fu Jian Zhong Yi Yao* (Fujian Chinese Medicine and Herbology), 1985; 1:36
19. *Zhong Xi Yi Jie He Za Zhi* (Journal of Integrated Chinese and Western Medicine), 1983; 1:19
20. *Shang Hai Zhong Yi Yao Za Zhi* (Shanghai Journal of Chinese Medicine and Herbology), 1988; 8:2
21. *Zhong Xi Yi Jie He Za Zhi* (Journal of Integrated Chinese and Western Medicine), 1983; 1:19
22. *Fu Jian Zhong Yi Yao* (Fujian Chinese Medicine and Herbology), 1987; 2:43
23. *Zhong Xi Yi Jie He Za Zhi* (Journal of Integrated Chinese and Western Medicine), 1987; 11:695
24. Brinker, Francis. *The Toxicology of Botanical Medicines,* rev. 2nd ed., 1996
25. *Zhong Xi Yi Jie He Za Zhi* (Journal of Integrated Chinese and Western Medicine), 1985; 5(11):691
26. *Zhong Yi Yao Xue Bao* (Report of Chinese Medicine and Herbology), 1990; (5):48

Mang Xiao (Natrii Sulfas)

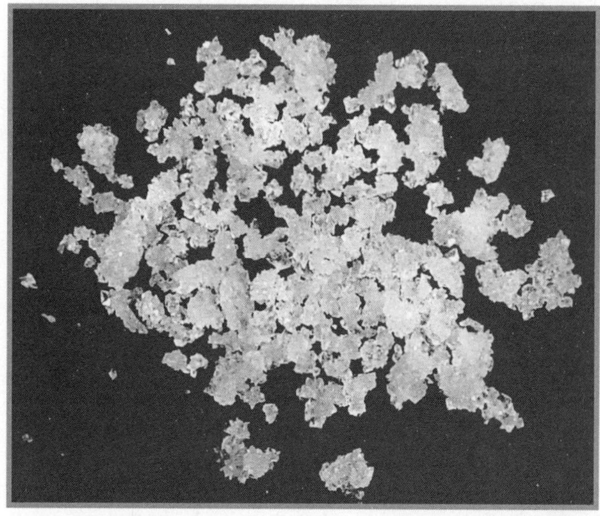

芒硝 芒硝

Pinyin Name: *Mang Xiao*
Alternate Chinese Names: *Pi Xiao, Ma Ya Xiao*
Original Source: *Ming Yi Za Zhu* (Miscellaneous Records of Famous Physicians) by Tao Hong-Jing in 500 A.D.
English Name: sodium sulfate, mirabilite, mirabilitum
Pharmaceutical Name: Natrii Sulfas
Properties: salty, bitter, cold
Channels Entered: Lung, Stomach, Large Intestine

CHINESE THERAPEUTIC ACTIONS

1. Purges Excess, Softens Hardness

Constipation due to excess heat accumulation in the Large Intestine: Bitter, salty and cold, *Mang Xiao* (Natrii Sulfas) treats constipation by softening hardness, eliminating stagnation and purging heat. *Mang Xiao* moistens the intestines, softens the stool and is best for constipation characterized by dry, hard stools.

- Severe constipation due to accumulation of excess heat: use *Mang Xiao* with *Da Huang* (Radix et Rhizoma Rhei),

Mang Xiao (Natrii Sulfas)

Hou Po (Cortex Magnoliae Officinalis) and *Zhi Shi* (Fructus Aurantii Immaturus) to soften hardness, relieve constipation and purge excess heat. **Exemplar Formula:** *Da Cheng Qi Tang* (Major Order the Qi Decoction).

- Moderate constipation due to accumulation of excess heat: combine this herb with *Da Huang* (Radix et Rhizoma Rhei) and *Gan Cao* (Radix Glycyrrhizae). **Exemplar Formula:** *Tiao Wei Cheng Qi Tang* (Regulate the Stomach and Order the Qi Decoction).

2. Clears Heat and Sedates Fire

Externally contracted febrile diseases: *Mang Xiao* clears heat from the Lung and Stomach, that is often characterized by high fever, irritability, thirst, delirium and constipation.

- Heat in the Lung and Stomach: use *Mang Xiao* with *Da Huang* (Radix et Rhizoma Rhei), *Huang Qin* (Radix Scutellariae), and *Zhi Zi* (Fructus Gardeniae).

Cough, mania and upper back pain caused by hot phlegm: Stagnation of phlegm in the body creates secondary heat and fire. Phlegm and heat attacking the Lung lead to cough, dyspnea and yellow sticky sputum; phlegm and heat obstructing the channels and collaterals cause swelling and pain in the upper body and the extremities; and phlegm and heat misting the Heart leads to delirium and mania.

- Phlegm and heat in the Lung: use *Mang Xiao* with *Huang Qin* (Radix Scutellariae), *Qing Dai* (Indigo Naturalis) and *Gua Lou Ren* (Semen Trichosanthis).
- Phlegm and heat obstructing the channels and collaterals: combine this herb with *Ban Xia* (Rhizoma Pinelliae), *Fu Ling* (Poria) and *Zhi Ke* (Fructus Aurantii).
- Phlegm and heat misting the Heart: also add *Dai Zhe Shi* (Haematitum), *Da Huang* (Radix et Rhizoma Rhei), *Ban Xia* (Rhizoma Pinelliae) and *Yu Jin* (Radix Curcumae). Or, use *Mang Xiao* instead of salt when cooking vegetables.

Nodules, lumps, abscesses and swellings characterized by heat and toxins: When applied topically, *Mang Xiao* clears heat, softens hardness, and reduces abscesses and swelling. It treats breast lumps with redness and swelling that have no pus discharge. It is used topically to stop lactation, and treat oral ulcers and sore throat.

- Breast lumps without pus: apply *Mang Xiao* topically to soften nodules and reduce swellings.
- For cessation of lactation: apply *Mang Xiao* topically.
- Oral ulcers and sore throat: combine it with *Peng Sha* (Borax), *Bing Pian* (Borneolum Syntheticum) and *Zhu Sha* (Cinnabaris), and apply topically.

DOSAGE

10 to 15 grams. Dissolve in hot water or herbal decoction immediately before administration.

CAUTIONS / CONTRAINDICATIONS

- *Mang Xiao* is contraindicated in patients who have deficiency and cold of the Spleen and Stomach.
- Use of *Mang Xiao* is contraindicated during pregnancy.
- Use of *Mang Xiao* topically for breast abscess in a nursing mother may lead to decreased (or termination of) lactation. Therefore, it should be used only if necessary, and discontinued immediately when the desired effect is achieved.

CHEMICAL COMPOSITION

Hydrated sodium sulfate ($Na_2SO_4+10H_2O$) 96-98%, sodium chloride, magnesium chloride, magnesium sulfate, calcium sulfate.[1]

PHARMACOLOGICAL EFFECTS

- **Laxative:** *Mang Xiao* is an osmotic agent and has a marked purgative effect. Following oral administration, it remains in the gastrointestinal system and is not absorbed systemically. As an osmotic agent, it increases water content and pressure in the intestines, thus inducing peristalsis and bowel movement. *Mang Xiao* is most effective when taken with a large amount of water. The laxative effect is usually achieved within 4 to 6 hours following oral ingestion.[2]

CLINICAL STUDIES AND RESEARCH

- **Cessation of lactation:** Lactation was successfully terminated in 33 women following topical application of *Mang Xiao*. The treatment protocol was to use 200 grams of powdered *Mang Xiao* covered with gauze, applied equally to both breasts for 24 hours. The same protocol may be repeated one or two times more if necessary.[3]
- **Rectal disorders:** In one study, 4,834 patients with various rectal disorders, including but not limited to hemorrhoids and colitis, were treated with a 3% *Mang Xiao* soaking solution, with good results.[4]

SUPPLEMENT

There are three types of this medicinal substance: *Po Xiao* (Sal Glauberis), *Mang Xiao* (Natrii Sulfas), and *Yuan Ming Fen* (Matrii Sulfas Exsiccatus).

- 樸硝 / 朴硝 *Po Xiao* (Sal Glauberis) is the crude form of sodium sulfate. Because of impurities, it is often used only topically for swellings and nodules.
- 芒硝 / 芒硝 *Mang Xiao* (Natrii Sulfas), sodium sulfate, is used both internally and topically. *Mang Xiao* is derived by dissolving *Po Xiao* in warm water, and filtering out the impurities.
- 元明粉 *Yuan Ming Fen* (Matrii Sulfas Exsiccatus) is the

Mang Xiao (Natrii Sulfas)

purest form and is best used as powder for oral ingestion, or used topically for sore throat, oral ulcers and eye disorders. *Yuan Ming Fen* is less effective as a laxative, compared to *Mang Xiao*, and weaker in clearing heat.

AUTHORS' COMMENTS

Da Huang (Radix et Rhizoma Rhei) and *Mang Xiao* are commonly prescribed together to treat excess-type constipation caused by heat. From the traditional Chinese medicine perspective, they work synergistically because *Da Huang* has a strong purgative effect to drive out stagnation and *Mang Xiao* softens the stool and facilitates the passage of stools. From a pharmacological perspective, they work synergistically because *Da Huang* increases intestinal peristalsis, and *Mang Xiao* increases bowel fluid content, to achieve bowel movements. In short, these two substances are the strongest pair of herbs to treat constipation.

Mang Xiao is an osmotic agent that has a marked purgative effect. Since it does not require systemic absorption for its action, it has an immediate onset of purgative effect. For this reason, *Mang Xiao* is sometimes used as the substance of choice to induce evacuation of intestinal contents in cases of ingestion of poisonous or toxic substances.

References

1. *Xian Dai Zhong Yao Yao Li Xue* (Contemporary Pharmacology of Chinese Herbs), 1997; 379
2. *Chang Yong Zhong Yao Xian Dai Yan Jiu Yu Lin Chuan* (Recent Study & Clinical Application of Common Traditional Chinese Medicine), 1995; 190:192
3. *Zhong Hua Fu Chan Ke Za Zhi* (Chinese Journal of OB/GYN), 1957; 5:401
4. *Hu Bei Zhong Yi Xue Yuan Xue Bao* (Journal of Hubei University of Medicine), 1983; 1:21

Fan Xie Ye (Folium Sennae)

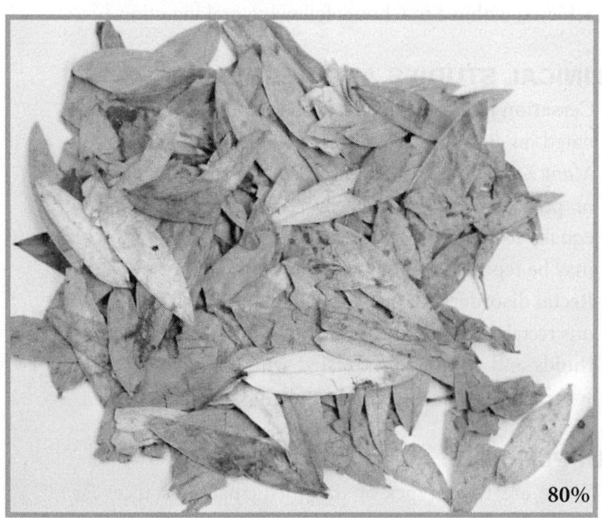
80%

番瀉葉 番泻叶

Pinyin Name: *Fan Xie Ye*
Literal Name: "barbarian purgative leaves," "purgative leaves of the foreigners"
Original Source: *Zhong Guo Yao Xue Da Ci Dian* (Grand Dictionary of Chinese Herbal Medicine) in 1935
English Name: senna leaves
Botanical Name: *Cassia angustifolia* Vahl. (*Xia Ye Fan Xie*); *Cassia acutifolia* Del. (*Jian Ye Fan Xie*)
Pharmaceutical Name: Folium Sennae
Properties: sweet, bitter, cold
Channels Entered: Large Intestine

CHINESE THERAPEUTIC ACTIONS

Purges Downward, Clears Heat

Fan Xie Ye (Folium Sennae) purges accumulation and clears heat. It is commonly used to relieve constipation caused by heat and stagnation. Clinical applications include relieving acute or chronic constipation, and cleansing the intestines prior to x-ray or abdominal surgery.

- Mild constipation: soak *Fan Xie Ye* in hot water and serve as tea.
- Moderate constipation: use it with *Hou Po* (Cortex Magnoliae Officinalis) and *Zhi Shi* (Fructus Aurantii Immaturus).

DOSAGE

1.5 to 3.0 grams when used as a mild laxative. The

maximum dosage of *Fan Xie Ye* is 5 to 10 grams. This herb is usually steeped in hot water for no more than 15 minutes, and consumed as tea.

CAUTIONS / CONTRAINDICATIONS

- *Fan Xie Ye* must be used with extreme caution for patients who are weak, pregnant or nursing.
- This herb promotes blood circulation to the lower body and thus should be used with caution in patients who are menstruating or have hemorrhoids.

OVERDOSAGE

Overdose of *Fan Xie Ye* is associated with nausea, vomiting, abdominal pain, numbness of the lips, mouth and extremities, swelling of the hands and fingers, dizziness and loss of balance. In severe cases, there may be labored breathing, tonic-clonic contraction of the extremities, locked jaws, clenched fists, foaming at the mouth, and unconsciousness.[1]

TREATMENT OF OVERDOSAGE

Overdose or adverse reactions associated with *Fan Xie Ye* are treated symptomatically using acupuncture, moxa and herbs. Adequate intake of fluids is important to avoid dehydration.

CHEMICAL COMPOSITION

Sennoside A,B,C,D; rhein, aloe-emodin, chrysophanol.[2,3]

Sennoside A

PHARMACOLOGICAL EFFECTS

- **Laxative:** Sennoside A and B both have marked laxative effects. Following oral administration, these substances are absorbed systemically, and converted to active components. They then exert their laxative effect on the large intestine.[4]
- **Antibiotic:** It has an inhibitory effect on *E. coli*, *Bacillus dysenteriae*, *Bacillus proteus*, *Candida albicans*, and some pathogenic fungi.[5]
- **Hemostatic:** Oral administration of *Fan Xie Ye* powder helps to stop bleeding. The hemostatic effect is attributed to increased platelet activities.[6]

CLINICAL STUDIES AND RESEARCH

- **Intestinal obstruction:** In one study, 106 patients with acute intestinal obstruction were treated with gastric lavage of stomach contents, followed by a decoction of 15 to 30 grams of *Fan Xie Ye*. The study reported an overall effective rate of 69.8%. Of those who responded to the treatment, over 90% showed laxative action within 24 hours. Surgery was performed on those who did not respond.[7]
- **Pancreatitis:** Patients with pancreatitis were treated with a standard therapy of 10 grams of *Fan Xie Ye* in capsules three times daily. The same treatment was repeated for those who did not have a bowel movement within 24 hours. Complete recovery was reported in most of 100 patients with acute pancreatitis within 2 to 4 days.[8]
- **Cholecystitis and cholelithiasis:** In one study, 49 patients with cholecystitis and/or cholelithiasis were treated with 10 grams of *Fan Xie Ye* in capsules three times daily with great success. In another study, 20 patients with cholecystitis and/or cholelithiasis were treated with 10 gram of *Fan Xie Ye* in capsules, three times daily with good results.[9,10]
- **Gastrointestinal bleeding:** One study describes 346 patients with gastric or duodenal bleeding characterized by hematemesis or hematochezia who were treated with *Fan Xie Ye* with a 94.2% success rate. Bleeding stopped after approximately 2 to 3 days. All patients were treated with a standard therapy of 10 grams of *Fan Xie Ye* in capsules, three times daily.[11]
- **Constipation:** According to another study, 137 patients with constipation were treated with a 95.1% rate of effectiveness using *Fan Xie Ye* soaked in hot water to make tea. The dosage was 3 to 6 grams for moderate constipation, and 10 grams for severe constipation. The study also noted that the treatment was effective for constipation in elderly, hypertensive, postpartum, or post-surgical patients.[12]
- **Post-surgical constipation:** Administration of 4 grams of *Fan Xie Ye* soaked in hot water effectively induced bowel movement and restored intestinal functioning within 24 hours. The overall rate of effectiveness was 95.6% for 276 post-surgical patients.[13]

HERB-DRUG INTERACTION

- **Diuretics:** Overuse of *Fan Xie Ye* aggravates loss of potassium associated with the use of diuretic drugs.[14] [Note: Examples of diuretics include chlorothiazide, hydrochlorothiazide, furosemide (Lasix), bumetanide (Bumex), and torsemide (Demadex).]
- **Cardiac glycosides:** Excessive loss of potassium increases toxicity of cardiac glycosides, such as digoxin (Lanoxin).[15]

TOXICOLOGY

The LD_{50} for sennoside in mice is 1.4 g/kg, which is

Fan Xie Ye (Folium Sennae)

equivalent to 36.3 g/kg of *Fan Xie Ye*, or approximately 300 times the normal adult dose.[16,17]

AUTHORS' COMMENTS

Besides treating constipation, *Fan Xie Ye* has been used effectively in the treatment of acute pancreatitis, cholecystitis and gastrointestinal bleeding.

Fan Xie Ye and *Da Huang* (Radix et Rhizoma Rhei) both purge downward and treat constipation due to heat. Similarly, both are to be used with caution or are contraindicated in pregnant, lactating and menstruating women. However, the primary and only function of *Fan Xie Ye* is to purge heat and relieve constipation. *Da Huang*, besides its purgative function, also purges fire, eliminates toxins, and disperses blood stagnation.

References

1. *Zhong Yao Bu Liang Fan Ying Yu Zhi Liao* (Adverse Reactions and Treatment of Chinese Herbal Medicine), 1996; 192:194
2. *Xian Dai Zhong Yao Yao Li Xue* (Contemporary Pharmacology of Chinese Herbs), 1997; 374
3. *The Merck Index* 12th edition, Chapman & Hall/CRCnetBASE/Merck, 2000
4. *Ri Ben Yao Wu Xue Za Zhi* (Japan Journal of Pharmacology), 1963; (4):91
5. *Zhong Hua Pi Fu Ke Xue Za Zhi* (Chinese Journal of Dermatology), 1959; (4):286
6. *Ke Ji Tong Bao* (Newspaper of Science and Technology), 1985; (3):48
7. *Zhong Xi Yi Jie He Za Zhi* (Journal of Integrated Chinese and Western Medicine), 1976; 2:38
8. *Ji Lin Zhong Yi Yao* (Jilin Chinese Medicine and Herbology), 1983; 4:29
9. *Zhong Yi Za Zhi* (Journal of Chinese Medicine), 1986; 11:56
10. Ibid.
11. Ibid.
12. *Zhong Yao Tong Bao* (Journal of Chinese Herbology), 1987; 7:51
13. *Zhong Guo Xiang Cun Xin Xi* (Suburb Doctors of China), 1988; 1:35
14. P.F.D'Arcy: *Adverse Reactions And Interactions With Herbal Medicine. Part 2 – Drug Interactions.* Adverse Drug React. Toxicol. Rev. 1993, 12(3) 147-162 © Oxford University Press 1993
15. Brinker, Francis. *The Toxicology of Botanical Medicines*, rev. 2nd ed., 1996
16. *Zhong Xi Yi Jie He Za Zhi* (Journal of Integrated Chinese and Western Medicine), 1986; (8):445
17. *Zhong Yi Za Zhi* (Journal of Chinese Medicine), 1980; 6:24

Lu Hui (Aloe)

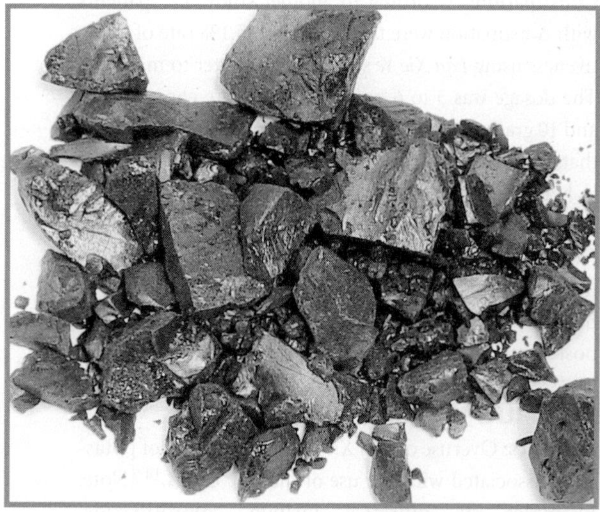

蘆薈 芦荟

Pinyin Name: *Lu Hui*

Alternate Chinese Names: *Xiang Dan*

Original Source: *Yao Xing Ben Cao* (Materia Medica of Medicinal Properties) by Zhen Quan in 600 A.D.

English Name: aloe

Botanical Name: *Aloe vera* L. (*Ku La Suo Lu Hui*); *Aloe ferox* Mill (*Hao Wang Jiao Lu Hui*)

Pharmaceutical Name: Aloe

Properties: bitter, cold

Channels Entered: Liver, Large Intestine

CHINESE THERAPEUTIC ACTIONS

1. Purges Downwards

Excess-type constipation: *Lu Hui* (Aloe) is most effective if constipation is accompanied by heat attacking the Heart and leading to irritability and insomnia. The purgative action removes the source of the heat so that the Heart energy can settle.

- Constipation with irritability and insomnia: use *Lu Hui* with *Zhu Sha* (Cinnabaris).

Lu Hui (Aloe)

2. Clears Liver Fire

Liver fire: Excess Liver fire is characterized by symptoms such as headache, hypochondriac pain, red eyes, dizziness, irritability, constipation and infantile convulsions.

- Liver fire: use *Lu Hui* with *Long Dan Cao* (Radix Gentianae), *Zhi Zi* (Fructus Gardeniae) and *Qing Dai* (Indigo Naturalis). **Exemplar Formula:** *Dang Gui Long Hui Wan* (Tangkuei, Gentiana, and Aloe Pill).
- Infantile convulsions with Liver heat and phlegm: use this herb with *Dan Nan Xing* (Arisaema cum Bile) and *Chuan Bei Mu* (Bulbus Fritillariae Cirrhosae).
- Hepatitis: use a small dose of *Lu Hui* as the guiding herb with others herbs that clear damp-heat from the Liver, such as *Chai Hu* (Radix Bupleuri) and *Huang Qin* (Radix Scutellariae).

3. Kills Parasites

Intestinal parasites: *Lu Hui* kills roundworm and ringworm to treat malnutrition caused by intestinal parasites in infants and children.

- Intestinal parasites: use powdered *Lu Hui* and *Shi Jun Zi* (Fructus Quisqualis) in equal portions and serve with rice water.
- *Gan ji* (infantile malnutrition) with intestinal parasites and Spleen deficiency: combine it with *Ren Shen* (Radix Ginseng) and *Bai Zhu* (Rhizoma Atractylodis Macrocephalae).

Lu Hui can also be used topically to treat itching due to parasites, or to chronic skin disorders that do not respond to other treatments.

- Itching due to parasites: apply powdered *Lu Hui* and *Gan Cao* (Radix Glycyrrhizae) topically.
- Hemorrhoids: apply *Lu Hui* and *Bing Pian* (Borneolum Syntheticum) topically.

DOSAGE

0.6 to 1.5 grams in powder, capsules or pills. Decoction is not recommended, as *Lu Hui* is extremely bitter and has an unpleasant smell.

CAUTIONS / CONTRAINDICATIONS

- *Lu Hui* is contraindicated during pregnancy, and in cases of deficiency and cold of the Spleen and Stomach.

CHEMICAL COMPOSITION

Alon, aloe-emodin.[1]

PHARMACOLOGICAL EFFECTS

- **Laxative:** Alon has a marked laxative effect.[2]
- **Antibiotic:** Water extract of *Lu Hui* has various degrees of inhibitory action against pathogenic fungi and dermatophytes.[3]
- **Antineoplastic:** Alcohol extract of *Lu Hui* has demonstrated preliminary ability to inhibit the growth of cancer cells.[4]

HERB-DRUG INTERACTION

- **Cardiac glycosides:** Overuse of *Lu Hui* may cause potassium depletion, leading to increased toxicity of cardiac glycosides, such as digoxin (Lanoxin).[5]

TOXICOLOGY

No fatalities or bodily abnormalities were reported following intramuscular injection of *Lu Hui* continuously for six months (daily dosage was equivalent to 10 mg/kg of bulk herb). There was, however, necrosis of tissue at the injection site.[6]

AUTHORS' COMMENTS

Classic text states that *Lu Hui* can be used to treat overdose of *Ba Dou* (Fructus Crotonis).

References

1. *Xian Dai Zhong Yao Yao Li Xue* (Contemporary Pharmacology of Chinese Herbs), 1997; 381
2. *Zhi Wu Yao You Xiao Cheng Fen Shou Ce* (Manual of Plant Medicinals and Their Active Constituents), 1986; 44
3. *Zhong Yao Xue* (Chinese Herbology), 1998; 260:261
4. *Chang Yong Zhong Yao Cheng Fen Yu Yao Li Shou Ce* (A Handbook of the Composition and Pharmacology of Common Chinese Drugs), 1994; 989:992
5. Brinker, Francis. *The Toxicology of Botanical Medicines*, rev. 2nd ed., 1996
6. *Zhong Guo Zhong Yao Za Zhi* (People's Republic of China Journal of Chinese Herbology), 1989; 14(2):42

Ba Dou (Fructus Crotonis)

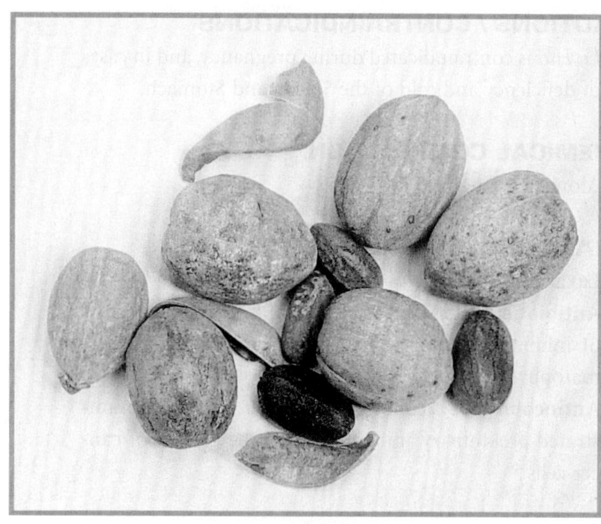

巴豆

Pinyin Name: *Ba Dou*
Literal Name: "clinging bean"
Alternate Chinese Names: *Ba Ji, Gang Zi, Jiang Zi*
Original Source: *Shen Nong Ben Cao Jing* (Divine Husbandman's Classic of the Materia Medica) in the second century
English Name: croton fruit, croton seed
Botanical Name: *Croton tiglium* L. (*Ba Dou*)
Pharmaceutical Name: Fructus Crotonis
Properties: acrid, hot
Channels Entered: Stomach, Large Intestine
Safety Index: toxic

CHINESE THERAPEUTIC ACTIONS

1. Purges Cold Accumulation

Food stagnation or constipation due to cold: *Ba Dou* (Fructus Crotonis) is one of the strongest cathartic herbs that purges abdominal stagnation caused by cold. It is best for patients who exhibit the following symptoms: sudden abdominal and epigastric fullness, distention, piercing pain and constipation. It is frequently used for acute intestinal obstruction.

- Acute intestinal obstruction: use *Ba Dou* with *Da Huang* (Radix et Rhizoma Rhei) and *Gan Jiang* (Rhizoma Zingiberis).

2. Eliminates Water Accumulation

Ascites: use it with *Xing Ren* (Semen Armeniacae Amarum) as a pill for late stage ascites due to schistosomal cirrhosis.

3. Eliminates Phlegm

Obstruction of the throat due to phlegm accumulation: *Ba Dou* induces vomiting and expels phlegm obstruction of the throat that is causing suffocation, dyspnea, and profuse sputum.

Lung abscess with profuse sputum: *Ba Dou* dispels sputum when used with *Jie Geng* (Radix Platycodonis) and *Bei Mu* (Bulbus Fritillaria).

4. Stops Diarrhea

Chronic diarrhea due to cold: The dry-fried form of *Ba Dou* treats diarrhea due to cold accumulation in the abdomen. It is imperative to ensure that the dry-fried form does not contain any essential oil, which may worsen the diarrhea.

5. Kills Parasites and Heals Ulceration

Ba Dou can be used topically to treat ulcerations, sores, scabies, abscesses, and swelling and other dermatological disorders. *Ba Dou* should not be applied to the head, face or the genital areas.

- Skin disorders: use it topically with *Xiong Huang* (Realgar) as a paste. If the sore has not ulcerated, use *Ba Dou* with *Ru Xiang* (Gummi Olibanum) and *Mo Yao* (Myrrha) to promote eruption and healing.

DOSAGE

0.1 to 0.3 grams in capsule, powder or pill forms. For treatment of food stagnation in infants between 6 to 12 months of age, the dosage should not exceed 0.09 gram. For treatment of diarrhea, use only the dry-fried form of *Ba Dou* that does not have any essential oils.

CAUTIONS / CONTRAINDICATIONS

- *Ba Dou* is toxic, and is one of the most potent cathartics. It must be used with extreme caution, and only when necessary.
- Do not serve *Ba Dou* decoction with hot beverages as it will enhance the purgative function of the herb.
- *Ba Dou* is contraindicated in pregnancy, as it may irritate the uterus and cause abortion.
- *Ba Dou* antagonizes *Qian Niu Zi* (Semen Pharbitidis).
- According to classic texts, it is incompatible with *Qian Niu Zi* (Semen Pharbitidis).
- Direct contact between *Ba Dou* and the skin or mucous membranes may lead to dermatitis, itching, burning sensations, swelling and other allergic reactions. Therefore, topical application to the face or genital areas is contraindicated.[1]

Ba Dou (Fructus Crotonis)

OVERDOSAGE

Overdose generally occurs within 1 to 3 hours after ingestion. Clinical manifestations include nausea, vomiting, burning sensations of the mouth and throat, poor appetite, severe abdominal pain, hematemesis, hematochezia, rectal tenesmus, and profuse diarrhea with the presence of mucus and blood. *Ba Dou* is also toxic to the kidneys and may cause such symptoms as hematuria, dysuria, anuria and proteinuria. Severe overdose is characterized by hypotension, cyanotic face, rapid heartbeat but weak pulse, dyspnea, decreased body temperature, respiratory depression, and in severe cases, shock.[2]

TREATMENT OF OVERDOSAGE

Many methods have been used successfully for treatment of overdose:

- An herbal decoction of *Ban Lan Gen* (Radix Isatidis) and sugar.
- Administration of 60 to 120 ml of peanut oil.
- An herbal decoction with 12 grams of *Xuan Shen* (Radix Scrophulariae) and 15 grams of *Shi Chang Pu* (Rhizoma Acori) administered every four hours for a total of 3 to 4 doses.
- An herbal decoction with 150 grams of *Lu Dou* (Semen Phaseoli Radiati), 9 grams of *Huang Bai* (Cortex Phellodendri), and 9 grams of *Gan Cao* (Radix Glycyrrhizae) given every three hours for a total of 2 to 4 doses.
- An herbal decoction with *Huang Lian* (Rhizoma Coptidis), *Huang Bai* (Cortex Phellodendri), *Bai Shao* (Radix Paeoniae Alba), *Che Qian Zi* (Semen Plantaginis) and *Shi Hu* (Herba Dendrobii) may be prescribed to counteract the side effects of *Ba Dou.*
- Diarrhea can be treated with administration of a cold decoction containing *Huang Lian* (Rhizoma Coptidis) and *Huang Bai* (Cortex Phellodendri), with cold congee.
- Dermatitis can be resolved by applying a solution of *Huang Lian* topically.[3]

CHEMICAL COMPOSITION

Croton resin, phorbol, crotonic acid, cocarcinogen, crotin, crotonoside, ricinine.[4]

PHARMACOLOGICAL EFFECTS

- **Cathartic:** *Ba Dou* has a stimulating effect on the mucous membranes of the intestines, leading to increased secretion, peristalsis, and bowel movements within 30 minutes to 3 hours.[5]
- **Antibiotic:** Decoction of *Ba Dou* has an inhibitory effect against *Pseudomonas aeruginosa*, *Staphylococcus aureus*, and *Corynebacterium diphtheriae*.[6]
- **Analgesic:** Essential oil of *Ba Dou* administered via oral, subcutaneous or intraperitoneal injection, has an analgesic effect in mice. The exact mechanism of action is unclear.[7]
- **Antineoplastic:** Extract of *Ba Dou* had an inhibiting effect on the growth of cancer cells in mice with sarcoma, cervical cancer, and skin cancer.[8,9,10]

CLINICAL STUDIES AND RESEARCH

- **Intestinal obstruction:** According to one report, 40 out of 50 patients with intestinal obstructions were treated with a preparation of *Ba Dou*, with complete recovery. The treatment protocol stated that *Ba Dou* must be prepared by extracting and discarding the essential oil prior to use. The dosage of the herb was 150 to 300 mg. Most patients showed relief within a short period of time. However, a second dose within 3 to 4 hours was repeated if necessary.[11]

TOXICOLOGY

Ingestion of 20 drops of *Ba Dou* oil is lethal in humans. In guinea pigs, injection of *Ba Dou* oil led to proteinuria and hematuria.[12]

References

1. *Zhong Yao Da Ci Dien* (Dictionary of Chinese Herbs), 1975; 502
2. *Zhong Yao Bu Liang Fan Ying Yu Zhi Liao* (Adverse Reactions and Treatment of Chinese Herbal Medicine), 1996; 176:179
3. Ibid.
4. *Xian Dai Zhong Yao Yao Li Xue* (Contemporary Pharmacology of Chinese Herbs), 1997; 358
5. *Zhong Yao Xue* (Chinese Herbology), 1998; 262:264
6. *Zhong Yao Yao Li Yu Ying Yong* (Pharmacology and Applications of Chinese Herbs), 1983; 236
7. Ibid.
8. *Zhong Yi Yao Yan Jiu Can Kao* (Research and Discussion of Chinese Medicine and Herbology), 1979; (2):48
9. *Science*, 1976:191(4227):571
10. *CA*, 1980; 92:140lt
11. *Tian Jing Yi Yao* (Tianjing Medicine and Herbology), 1974; 7:341
12. *Zhong Yao Yao Li Yu Ying Yong* (Pharmacology and Applications of Chinese Herbs), 1983; 236

Section 2

— Moist Laxatives

Huo Ma Ren (Fructus Cannabis)

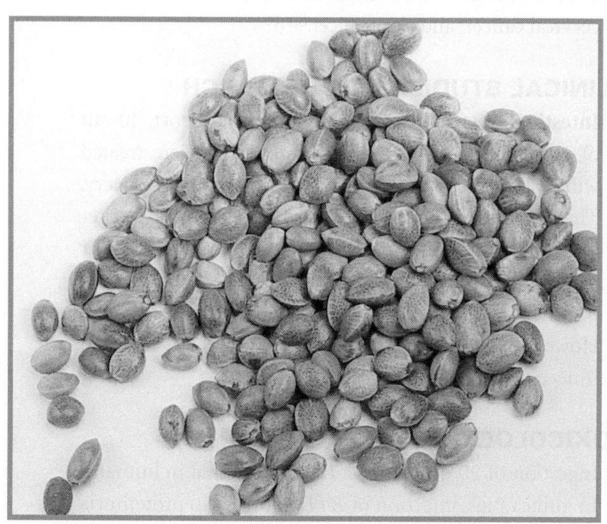

火麻仁

Pinyin Name: *Huo Ma Ren*
Literal Name: "fire hemp seeds"
Alternate Chinese Names: *Da Ma Ren, Da Ma Zi, Ma Zi Ren*
Original Source: *Shen Nong Ben Cao Jing* (Divine Husbandman's Classic of the Materia Medica) in the second century
English Name: linum, hemp seed, cannabis seed, marijuana seed
Botanical Name: *Cannabis sativa* L. (*Da Ma*)
Pharmaceutical Name: Fructus Cannabis
Properties: sweet, neutral
Channels Entered: Spleen, Stomach, Large Intestine

CHINESE THERAPEUTIC ACTIONS

1. Lubricates the Intestines

Constipation: *Huo Ma Ren* (Fructus Cannabis), rich in oil, lubricates the intestines and relieves constipation. It is most effective in treating constipation in postpartum women or geriatric patients, characterized by dry stools, generalized weakness and deficiency of body fluids.

- Constipation due to deficiency of body fluids: use *Huo Ma Ren* with *Yu Li Ren* (Semen Pruni), *Gua Lou Ren* (Semen Trichosanthis) and *Xing Ren* (Semen Armeniacae Amarum).
- Constipation with blood deficiency: use it with *Dang Gui* (Radicis Angelicae Sinensis) and *Shu Di Huang* (Radix Rehmanniae Preparata).
- Constipation with yin deficiency: add *Mai Men Dong* (Radix Ophiopogonis) and *Sheng Di Huang* (Radix Rehmanniae).
- Constipation with qi deficiency: combine *Huo Ma Ren* with *Huang Qi* (Radix Astragali) and *Dang Shen* (Radix Codonopsis).
- Habitual constipation: combine it with *Tao Ren* (Semen Persicae) and *Dang Gui* (Radicis Angelicae Sinensis). **Exemplar Formula:** *Run Chang Wan* (Moisten the Intestines Pill).
- Severe constipation due to general deficiency: use it with *Da Huang* (Radix et Rhizoma Rhei), *Hou Po* (Cortex Magnoliae Officinalis) and *Zhi Shi* (Fructus Aurantii Immaturus). **Exemplar Formula:** *Ma Zi Ren Wan* (Hemp Seed Pill).

2. Moistens Dryness, Benefits the Hair

Huo Ma Ren has a moistening effect that promotes hair growth and treats dry hair.

- Hair loss with blood deficiency: apply *Huo Ma Ren* essential oil topically on the scalp. Take *He Shou Wu* (Radix Polygoni Multiflori) orally.
- Hair loss or dry hair: use *Huo Ma Ren* as a rinse or shampoo.
- Scalp ulcers: mix *Huo Ma Ren* powder with water and honey, apply topically.

DOSAGE

10 to 15 grams. *Huo Ma Ren* seeds should be crushed

Huo Ma Ren (Fructus Cannabis)

prior to cooking. Dry-frying the herb minimizes toxicity and maximizes extraction of active components. *Huo Ma Ren* is also used topically as a powder or essential oil.

CAUTIONS / CONTRAINDICATIONS

- Avoid use of the unprocessed herb, as it is slightly toxic.

OVERDOSAGE

Overdose of *Huo Ma Ren* is characterized by symptoms and signs such as nausea, vomiting, diarrhea, numb extremities, muscle spasms, irritability, restlessness, convulsions, cramps, dilation of the pupils, increased heart rate, drowsiness, headache, dizziness, pale face, blurred vision, tremor, semiconsciousness and delirium. These reactions generally occur within 2 hours of the time of ingestion.

TREATMENT OF OVERDOSAGE

Overdose may be treated by ingestion of milk or egg whites to reduce absorption of the herb. If necessary, gastric lavage using 1:5000 potassium permanganate, or administration of activated charcoal, reduces absorption. Intravenous fluids, balancing electrolytes, and other symptomatic treatment may also be beneficial.[1]

CHEMICAL COMPOSITION

Cannabinol, trigonelline, isoleucin betaine, muscarin.[2,3]

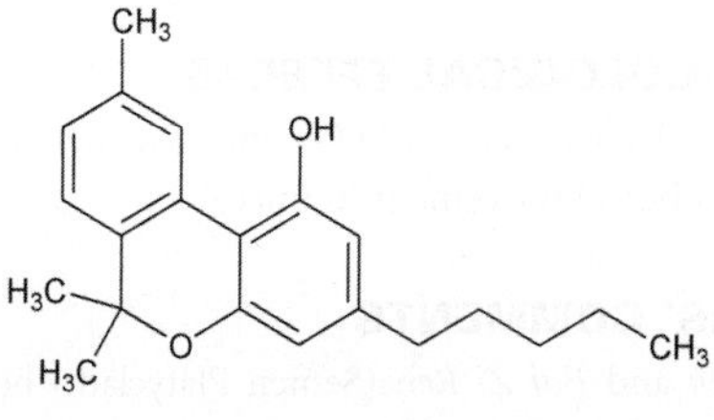

Cannabinol

PHARMACOLOGICAL EFFECTS

- **Laxative:** *Huo Ma Ren* stimulates the intestines, increases peristalsis, and promotes bowel movement.[4]
- **Antihypertensive:** Alcohol extract of *Huo Ma Ren* has a mild tendency to lower blood pressure in cats and rabbits.[5]
- **Antihyperlipidemic:** Continuous administration of *Huo Ma Ren* for 4 weeks significantly reduced plasma cholesterol levels in rats, compared to the placebo group.[6]

AUTHORS' COMMENTS

Cannabis is a highly regulated substance in many countries. Fresh seeds are generally designated a controlled substance, since they can be planted and propagated. But after processing, the seeds can no longer germinate and thus are not considered a controlled substance. Therefore, most countries require that the seeds be fully processed prior to importation.

Huo Ma Ren and *Yu Li Ren* (Semen Pruni) both treat constipation. *Huo Ma Ren* generates fluids, moistens the intestines and relieves constipation. *Yu Li Ren* regulates Large Intestine qi to relieve constipation.

Huo Ma Ren (Fructus Cannabis) and *Hu Ma Ren* (Semen Sesami Nigrum) have similar pinyin names, but completely different functions. *Huo Ma Ren* generates body fluids and treats constipation. *Hu Ma Ren* tonifies the Liver and Kidney, and nourishes blood and *jing* (essence) to moisten dryness. [Note: *Hu Ma Ren* is an alternate name of *Hei Zhi Ma*.]

References

1. *Zhong Yao Bu Liang Fan Ying Yu Zhi Liao* (Adverse Reactions and Treatment of Chinese Herbal Medicine), 1996; 125:126
2. *Xian Dai Zhong Yao Yao Li Xue* (Contemporary Pharmacology of Chinese Herbs), 1997; 383
3. *The Merck Index* 12th edition, Chapman & Hall/CRCnetBASE/Merck, 2000
4. *Zhong Yao Xue* (Chinese Herbology), 1998; 265:266
5. *Zhong Cao Yao Xue* (Study of Chinese Herbal Medicine), 1976; 110
6. *Guang Xi Yi Xue Yuan Xue Bao* (Journal of Guangxi University of Medicine), 1984; 1(4):20

Yu Li Ren (Semen Pruni)

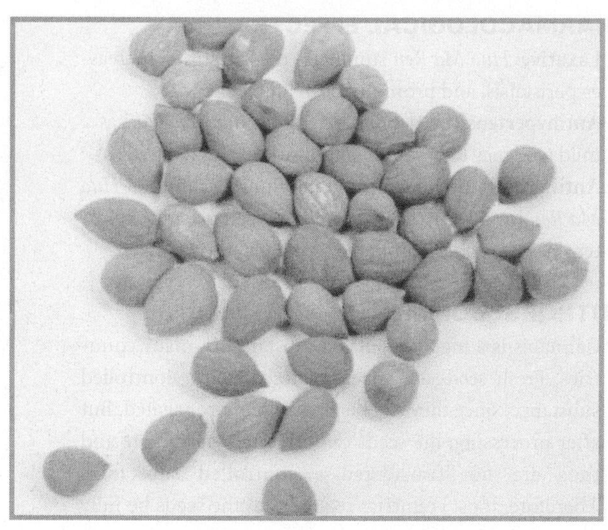

郁李仁

Pinyin Name: *Yu Li Ren*
Literal Name: "constrained plum pit"
Original Source: *Shen Nong Ben Cao Jing* (Divine Husbandman's Classic of the Materia Medica) in the second century
English Name: prunus seed, Chinese dwarf cherry seed, bunge cherry seed, dwarf flowering cherry seed, Chinese bushcherry seed, downy cherry seed
Botanical Name: *Prunus humilis* Bge. (*Ou Li*); *Prunus japonica* Thunb. (*Yu Li*); *Prunus tomentosa* Thunb. (*Mao Ying Tao*)
Pharmaceutical Name: Semen Pruni
Properties: acrid, bitter, sweet, neutral
Channels Entered: Spleen, Large Intestine, Small Intestine

CHINESE THERAPEUTIC ACTIONS

1. Moistens the Intestines and Relieves Constipation

Yu Li Ren (Semen Pruni), rich in oil, lubricates the intestines and relieves constipation. It is most effective in treating constipation characterized by dry stools, general dryness and weakness, or deficiency of body fluids or blood.

- Constipation: combine *Yu Li Ren, Huo Ma Ren* (Fructus Cannabis), *Bai Zi Ren* (Semen Platycladi) and *Xing Ren* (Semen Armeniacae Amarum).
- Constipation with blood deficiency: combine it with *Sheng Di Huang* (Radix Rehmanniae), *Dang Gui* (Radicis Angelicae Sinensis), and *He Shou Wu* (Radix Polygoni Multiflori).

2. Regulates Water and Reduces Swelling

Yu Li Ren regulates water circulation and treats edema-related abdominal fullness.

- Abdominal fullness with edema: add *Sang Bai Pi* (Cortex Mori), *Chi Xiao Dou* (Semen Phaseoli) and *Chen Pi* (Pericarpium Citri Reticulatae).

Yu Li Ren regulates qi and is used for cough and dyspnea.

DOSAGE

5 to 10 grams in decoction. *Yu Li Ren* seeds should be crushed prior to decoction.

CHEMICAL COMPOSITION

Amygadin, saponin (0.96%), lipids (58.3-74.2%), organic acid.[1]

PHARMACOLOGICAL EFFECTS

- **Laxative:** Decoction of *Yu Li Ren* increases peristalsis and promotes bowel movement in mice.[2]

AUTHORS' COMMENTS

Yu Li Ren and *Bai Zi Ren* (Semen Platycladi) both treat constipation. *Yu Li Ren* is better for dry stools caused by generalized dryness, whereas *Bai Zi Ren* is better for constipation caused by blood deficiency and intestinal dryness.

References

1. *Chang Yong Zhong Yao Cheng Fen Yu Yao Li Shou Ce* (A Handbook of the Composition and Pharmacology of Common Chinese Drugs), 1994; 1215
2. *Zhong Yao Tong Bao* (Journal of Chinese Herbology), 1988; 13(8):43

Section 3

— Harsh Expellants (Cathartics)

Gan Sui (Radix Euphorbiae Kansui)

甘遂

Pinyin Name: *Gan Sui*
Literal Name: "sweet process"
Original Source: *Shen Nong Ben Cao Jing* (Divine Husbandman's Classic of the Materia Medica) in the second century
English Name: euphorbia, gansui root, kansui root
Botanical Name: *Euphorbia kansui* T. N. Liou ex T. P. Wang. (*Gan Sui*)
Pharmaceutical Name: Radix Euphorbiae Kansui
Properties: bitter, sweet, cold
Channels Entered: Lung, Kidney, Large Intestine
Safety Index: toxic

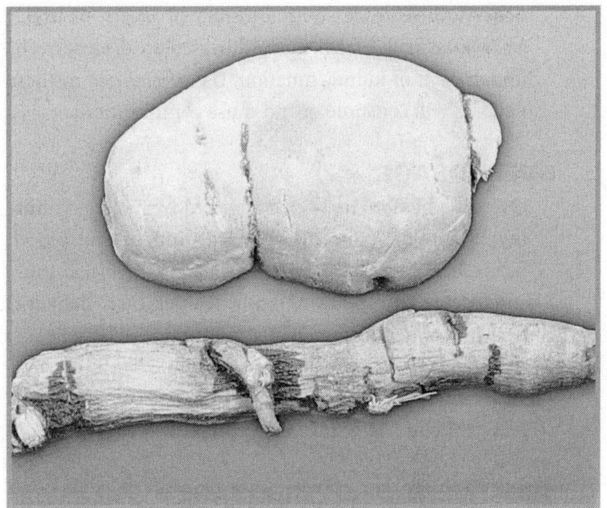

CHINESE THERAPEUTIC ACTIONS

1. Purges Downwards and Eliminates Water Accumulation

Gan Sui (Radix Euphorbiae Kansui) has an extremely strong purgative effect to drive out water accumulation. It treats ascites, characterized by water accumulation in the abdominal and chest regions with edema of the face and extremities.

- Ascites: use *Gan Sui* with *Qian Niu Zi* (Semen Pharbitidis).
- Water retention in the chest and hypochondrium: use it with *Da Ji* (Radix Euphorbiae seu Knoxiae) and *Bai Jie Zi* (Semen Sinapis).
- Water retention with heat in the chest: add *Da Huang* (Radix et Rhizoma Rhei) and *Mang Xiao* (Natrii Sulfas).
- Intestinal obstruction with fluid retention: combine *Gan Sui* with *Da Huang* (Radix et Rhizoma Rhei), *Hou Po* (Cortex Magnoliae Officinalis) and *Tao Ren* (Semen Persicae).

2. Eliminates Phlegm

Gan Sui treats seizures and epilepsy caused by phlegm and heat stagnation.

- Seizures and epilepsy due to phlegm stagnation: use it with *Da Huang* (Radix et Rhizoma Rhei), *Dai Zhe Shi* (Haematitum) and *Ban Xia* (Rhizoma Pinelliae).

DOSAGE

0.5 to 1.0 gram in powder or pill form. Unprocessed *Gan Sui* is more toxic; the vinegar-fried herb is less toxic. Since *Gan Sui* has low water solubility, it is less effective when cooked in an herbal decoction, compared to when delivered in powder or as pills. Therefore, the powder should be added to the strained decoction before ingestion.

CAUTIONS / CONTRAINDICATIONS

- *Gan Sui* is incompatible with *Gan Cao* (Radix Glycyrrhizae), according to classic texts.
- *Gan Sui* is extremely irritating to the gastrointestinal tract. Individuals with sensitive stomachs should take

Gan Sui (Radix Euphorbiae Kansui)

Gan Sui in capsules, or in conjunction with *Da Zao* (Fructus Jujubae) tea.

- *Gan Sui* is a potent cathartic. It must be used with extreme caution, and only when necessary. It should not be given for an extended period of time. The dosage should not exceed the recommended amount.
- *Gan Sui* is suitable only for symptomatic relief in acute cases of ascites and constipation.
- Treatment with *Gan Sui* should be alternated with use of herbs that tonify the Spleen, to prevent over-consumption of qi.
- *Gan Sui* is contraindicated for patients who are pregnant, weak, have qi, blood, yin or yang deficiencies, have a tendency to bleed excessively, a history of ulcers, or upper gastrointestinal bleeding, cardiovascular disorders, or impairment of kidney function. Use of *Gan Sui* in these patients will consume qi and cause complications.

OVERDOSAGE

Overdose of *Gan Sui* is characterized by nausea, vomiting, abdominal pain, diarrhea with mucus and blood, headache, dizziness, palpitations, decreased blood pressure, delirium, decreased body temperature, dehydration, unconsciousness, dilated pupils, and convulsions. Adverse reactions usually occur within 30 minutes to 2 hours after ingestion. Overdose may occur at doses between 9 and 15 grams.[1]

TREATMENT OF OVERDOSAGE

- General detoxification: administer an herbal decoction of 30 grams of *Lu Dou* (Semen Phaseoli Radiati), 9 grams of *Huang Bai* (Cortex Phellodendri), and 6 grams of *Huang Lian* (Rhizoma Coptidis).
- Nausea and vomiting: administer an herbal decoction of *Sheng Jiang* (Rhizoma Zingiberis Recens) or *Da Zao* (Fructus Jujubae).
- Continuous diarrhea: administer an herbal decoction of 9 grams of *Ren Shen* (Radix Ginseng) and 6 grams of *Huang Lian* (Rhizoma Coptidis).

CHEMICAL COMPOSITION

Euphorbone, euphorbol, kanzuiol, euphol, ingenol, 13-oxyingenol, kansuinine A, B.[2]

PHARMACOLOGICAL EFFECTS

- **Cathartic:** *Gan Sui* stimulates the intestines, promotes peristalsis, and relieves constipation. Fresh *Gan Sui* has potent cathartic and toxic effects. Processing with vinegar reduces both cathartic and toxic effects.[3]
- **Abortifacient:** Intramuscular injection of alcohol extract of *Gan Sui* induces abortion in mice.[4]

CLINICAL STUDIES AND RESEARCH

- **Intestinal obstruction:** In one clinical study, 50 patients with intestinal obstruction (due to roundworms in 24 cases) were treated with 0.3 gram of *Gan Sui* powder, repeated in 2 to 4 hours. Of 50 cases, 44 experienced complete recovery.[5]
- **Abortion:** In China, a large-scale study demonstrated the efficacy of using a low dose of *Gan Sui* to induce abortion, for women seeking to terminate pregnancy. Over 6,000 women received intra-amniotic injection of a 50% *Gan Sui* solution. The low dosage (0.4 to 1.0 ml) showed effectiveness within 26 to 28 hours in 99.31-100% of these cases.[6]

TOXICOLOGY

The LD_{50} for alcohol extract of *Gan Sui* via intraperitoneal injection is 346.1 mg/kg in mice.[7]

AUTHORS' COMMENTS

In comparison with *Da Ji* (Radix Euphorbiae seu Knoxiae), *Gan Sui* has similar but stronger purgative effects.

References

1. *Zhong Yao Bu Liang Fan Ying Yu Zhi Liao* (Adverse Reactions and Treatment of Chinese Herbal Medicine), 1996; 231:232
2. *Xian Dai Zhong Yao Yao Li Xue* (Contemporary Pharmacology of Chinese Herbs), 1997; 388
3. *Zhong Yao Xue* (Chinese Herbology), 1998; 1976; 3:40
4. Ibid.
5. *Xin Zhong Yi* (New Chinese Medicine), 1976; 3:40
6. *Yi Xue Yan Jiu Tong Xun* (Report of Medical Studies), 1985; 4:114
7. *Chang Yong Zhong Yao Xian Dai Yan Jiu Yu Lin Chuan* (Recent Study & Clinical Application of Common Traditional Chinese Medicine), 1995; 198:200

Da Ji (Radix Euphorbiae seu Knoxiae)

大戟

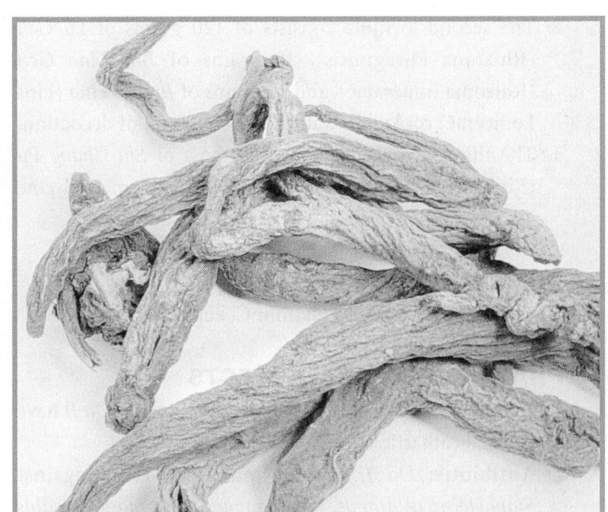

Pinyin Name: *Da Ji*
Literal Name: "big lance from the capital"
Alternate Chinese Names: *Xia Ma Xian, Long Hu Cao, Jiu Tou Shi Zi Cao, Gu Zhang Cao, Tian Ping Yi Zhi Xiang*
Original Source: *Shen Nong Ben Cao Jing* (Divine Husbandman's Classic of the Materia Medica) in the second century
English Name: euphorbia, knoxia
Botanical Name: *Euphorbia pekinensis* Rupr. (*Jing Da Ji*); *Knoxia valerianoides* Thorel et. Pitard. (*Hong Da Ji*)
Pharmaceutical Name: Radix Euphorbiae seu Knoxiae
Properties: bitter, acrid, cold
Channels Entered: Spleen, Kidney, Large Intestine
Safety Index: extremely toxic

CHINESE THERAPEUTIC ACTIONS

1. Purges Downwards and Eliminates Water Accumulation

Edema, ascites and water accumulation in the chest cavity: *Da Ji* (Radix Euphorbiae seu Knoxiae) has a strong purgative function to drive out water accumulation. It treats ascites, characterized by water accumulation in the abdominal and chest regions, involving edema of the face and extremities.

- Ascites: cook *Da Ji* with *Da Zao* (Fructus Jujubae), and eat the *Da Zao*.
- Liver cirrhosis with ascites: use *Da Ji* individually as decoction or powder.

2. Reduces Swelling and Disperses Nodules

Da Ji, used internally or topically, reduces swelling and disperses nodules. Clinical applications include sores, abscesses, lesions, and scrofula.

DOSAGE

1.5 to 3.0 grams in decoction, 0.5 to 1.0 gram in powder. *Da Ji* should be processed with vinegar to reduce toxicity.

CAUTIONS / CONTRAINDICATIONS

- *Da Ji* is incompatible with *Gan Cao* (Radix Glycyrrhizae), according to classic texts.
- *Da Ji* has potent purgative action and must be used with caution and only when necessary.
- *Da Ji* is contraindicated for patients who are pregnant, weak, have qi, blood, yin or yang deficiencies, have a tendency to bleed excessively, a history of ulcers, or upper gastrointestinal bleeding, cardiovascular disorders, or impairment of kidney function.
- Treatment of ascites with *Da Ji* should be alternated with use of herbs that tonify the Spleen to prevent over-consumption of qi.

OVERDOSAGE

Overdose of *Da Ji* may occur by direct contact or following systemic absorption. Dermatitis may occur with direct skin contact, and conjunctivitis with direct eye contact. Systemic reaction following oral ingestion includes redness and swelling of the mouth and throat, nausea, vomiting, headache, drowsiness, abdominal pain, diarrhea, decreased blood pressure, dehydration, and electrolyte imbalance. Overdose or prolonged use of *Da Ji* may cause bleeding and semiconsciousness. In severe cases, there may be hematemesis, hematochezia, dilation of the pupils, severe muscle spasms and cramps, and respiratory depression. Overall, gastrointestinal irritation is the most common side effect.

TREATMENT OF OVERDOSAGE

Administration of *Da Ji* is sometimes associated with nausea and vomiting, which can be alleviated by giving *Sheng Jiang* (Rhizoma Zingiberis Recens) or *Da Zao* (Fructus Jujubae) decoction.

Three herbal treatments have been used successfully to clear *Da Ji* overdose:

1. The first formula contains 30 grams of *Che Qian Zi* (Semen Plantaginis) and 30 grams of *Bai Mao Gen* (Rhizoma Imperatae) cooked in water to yield 300 ml of decoction.

Da Ji (Radix Euphorbiae seu Knoxiae)

2. The second formula consists of 120 grams of *Lu Gen* (Rhizoma Phragmitis), 30 grams of *Bai Mao Gen* (Rhizoma Imperatae), and 15 grams of *Jin Yin Hua* (Flos Lonicerae) cooked in water to yield 200 ml of decoction.
3. The third formula contains 30 grams of *Shi Chang Pu* (Rhizoma Acori) and 15 grams of *Hei Dou* (Semen Glycine Max) cooked in water to yield 200 ml of decoction.[1]

CHEMICAL COMPOSITION

Euphorbon, alkaloids, vitamin C, euphorbia A, B, C.[2]

PHARMACOLOGICAL EFFECTS

- **Cathartic:** Both water and alcohol extracts of *Da Ji* have marked cathartic effects.[3]
- **Antibiotic:** *Da Ji* has an inhibitory effect against *Staphylococcus aureus, Pseudomonas aeruginosa, Bacillus dysenteriae, Diplococcus pneumoniae*, and β-hemolytic streptococcus.[4]

SUPPLEMENT

There are two distinct herbs used as the purgative '*Da Ji*:'

- 紅大戟 / 红大戟 *Hong Da Ji* (Radix Knoxiae) is the one most commonly used, and more strongly reduces swelling and nodules.
- 京大戟 *Jing Da Ji* (Radix Euphorbiae Pekinensis) is stronger in dispelling water.

AUTHORS' COMMENTS

Da Ji (Radix Euphorbiae seu Knoxiae) and *Da Ji* (Herba seu Radix Cirsii Japonici) have identical pinyin names, but are two distinct herbs with completely different functions. *Da Ji* (Radix Euphorbiae seu Knoxiae) has cathartic properties and treats excess conditions. *Da Ji* (Herba seu Radix Cirsii Japonici) exerts hemostatic action and stops bleeding. To avoid errors and confusion, one must specify which "*Da Ji*" is to be used, whether in written or verbal communication.

Da Ji (Radix Euphorbiae seu Knoxiae) has similar effects to those of *Gan Sui* (Radix Euphorbiae Kansui), but is stronger than *Gan Sui*.

References

1. *Zhong Yao Bu Liang Fan Ying Yu Zhi Liao* (Adverse Reactions and Treatment of Chinese Herbal Medicine), 1996; 135:137
2. *Chang Yong Zhong Yao Xian Dai Yan Jiu Yu Lin Chuan* (Recent Study & Clinical Application of Common Traditional Chinese Medicine), 1995; 200-201
3. *Zhong Yao Xue* (Chinese Herbology), 1998; 269:271
4. Ibid.

Yuan Hua (Flos Genkwa)

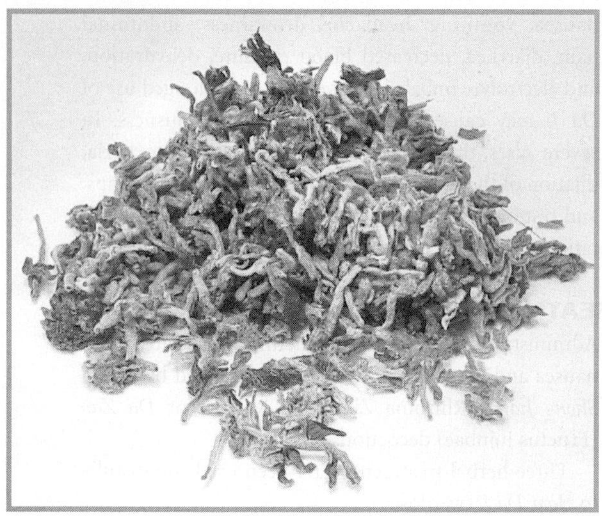

芫花 芫花

Pinyin Name: *Yuan Hua*

Alternate Chinese Names: *Lao Shu Hua, Tou Tong Hua, Du Yu*

Original Source: *Shen Nong Ben Cao Jing* (Divine Husbandman's Classic of the Materia Medica) in the second century

English Name: genkwa flower, lilac daphne flower bud

Botanical Name: *Daphne genkwa* Sieb. et Zucc. (*Yuan Hua*)

Pharmaceutical Name: Flos Genkwa

Properties: acrid, bitter, warm

Channels Entered: Lung, Kidney, Large Intestine

Safety Index: toxic

Yuan Hua (Flos Genkwa)

CHINESE THERAPEUTIC ACTIONS

1. Purges Stagnation and Eliminates Water Accumulation

Ascites, edema and water retention in the chest: *Yuan Hua* (Flos Genkwa) treats excess-type water accumulation in the chest and abdominal region involving edema of the face and extremities.

- Ascites and edema: use *Yuan Hua* with *Gan Sui* (Radix Euphorbiae Kansui), *Da Huang* (Radix et Rhizoma Rhei), *Ting Li Zi* (Semen Descurainiae seu Lepidii) and *Ba Dou* (Fructus Crotonis) in pill form.
- Bloating and abdominal distention caused by parasites: use this herb with *Zhi Ke* (Fructus Aurantii).

2. Eliminates Phlegm, Relieves Cough

Yuan Hua treats chronic bronchitis caused by cold phlegm obstruction. Use *Yuan Hua* alone and mix with sugar before serving.

3. Kills Parasites, Drains Abscesses

Dermatological disorders: *Yuan Hua* treats tinea capitis, carbuncles on the head, eczema, mastitis and various ulcerations and sores.

- Dermatological disorders: use *Yuan Hua* as powder and apply topically with *Xiong Huang* (Realgar) and lard.
- Mastitis: boil an egg in water with *Yuan Hua*, eat the egg, and drink the decoction.

4. Stops Pain

- Toothache: apply *Yuan Hua* topically as powder.
- Pain due to qi and blood stagnation: use it with *Yan Hu Suo* (Rhizoma Corydalis).

DOSAGE

1.5 to 3 grams in decoction. 0.5 to 1 gram in powdered form. Unprocessed *Yuan Hua* has drastic, toxic effects. Frying it with vinegar reduces this toxicity, and minimizes side effects such as diarrhea and abdominal pain.

CAUTIONS / CONTRAINDICATIONS

- *Yuan Hua*, a potent purgative, must be used with extreme caution, only when necessary. It is only suitable for symptomatic relief in acute cases of ascites and constipation.
- *Yuan Hua* is contraindicated if the patient shows poor appetite, fatigue or weakness. Prolonged use, or usage of this herb for patients with deficiency, or overdose, may consume qi and may cause bleeding and semiconsciousness.
- *Yuan Hua* is contraindicated in patients who are pregnant, weak, have deficiencies or a tendency toward excessive bleeding, a history of ulcers, upper gastrointestinal bleeding, cardiovascular disorders, or impaired kidney function.
- *Yuan Hua* is incompatible with *Gan Cao* (Radix Glycyrrhizae), according to classic texts.
- Treatment of ascites with *Yuan Hua* should be alternated with use of herbs that tonify the Spleen to prevent overconsumption of qi.
- Administration of *Yuan Hua* is sometimes associated with nausea and vomiting that can be alleviated by giving *Sheng Jiang* (Rhizoma Zingiberis Recens) or *Da Zao* (Fructus Jujubae).

CHEMICAL COMPOSITION

Genkwanin, apigenin, yuankanin, luteolin, genkwadaphnin, yuanhuacine, sitosterol, benzoic acid.[1]

PHARMACOLOGICAL EFFECTS

- **Cathartic:** Both water and alcohol extracts of *Yuan Hua* stimulate the intestines to increase peristalsis and promote bowel movement. At large doses, however, they may instead have an inhibiting effect.[2]
- **Antitussive and expectorant:** Inhalation therapy using *Yuan Hua* solution has marked antitussive and expectorant effects in mice. The mechanism of action has been attributed to its ability to reduce inflammation and decrease viscosity of the sputum.[3]
- **Analgesic:** Decoction of *Yuan Hua* has a mild-to-moderate analgesic action via its effect on the central nervous system.[4]
- **Antibiotic:** Vinegar- or alcohol-processed *Yuan Hua* inhibits *Diplococcus pneumoniae*, β-hemolytic streptococcus, and influenza virus.[5]
- **Diuretic:** In a placebo-controlled laboratory study, oral administration of decoction of *Yuan Hua* at 10 g/kg significantly increased the excretion of water and sodium. At 20 g/kg, there was an increased excretion of water, sodium, and potassium. No effect was observed at 5 to 10 g/kg.[6]

CLINICAL STUDIES AND RESEARCH

- **Frostbite:** Patients with early-stage frostbite characterized by swelling, pain and itching were treated with topical application of an herbal solution, with good results. The treatment protocol was to cook 15 grams each of *Yuan Hua* and *Gan Cao* (Radix Glycyrrhizae) in water to yield 2,000 ml of the final solution. Patients were instructed to soak the affected area in the warm solution for 30 minutes twice daily for 2 to 3 days. Patients were instructed not to drink the solution, as *Yuan Hua* and *Gan Cao* are incompatible for oral ingestion.[7]
- **Chronic bronchitis:** In one study, 231 patients with chronic bronchitis were treated with preparations of *Yuan Hua*, with an overall effective rate of 91.34%. The treatment protocol was to administer 0.5 to 1.0 gram the herbs two to three times daily for 10 days per course of treatment, with 3 to 5 days of rest between each course, for a total of 3 courses of treatment. The study also noted

Yuan Hua (Flos Genkwa)

that those with uncomplicated bronchitis (without wheezing and dyspnea) characterized by cold were most responsive to the treatment.[8]

- **Abortion:** According to one report, an intra-amniotic injection of an alcohol extract of *Yuan Hua* was used in 2,674 women seeking abortion in the second trimester of pregnancy, with 99.4% experiencing termination of pregnancy. Adverse reactions reported following this procedure included one case each of peritonitis, necrosis of the myometrium, stillbirth, and acute renal failure.[9]
- **Hepatitis:** Administration of water-extract of *Yuan Hua* was found effective in treating 20 patients with acute infectious hepatitis, 12 patients with chronic hepatitis, and 8 patients with drug-induced hepatitis.[10]

TOXICOLOGY

The LD_{50} of *Yuan Hua* in mice via oral ingestion is 17.78 g/kg for water extract, 14.05 g/kg for alcohol extract, and 8.48 g/kg for vinegar-processed extract. The LD_{50} of *Yuan Hua* in mice via intraperitoneal injection is 9.25 g/kg for water extract, 7.07 g/kg for alcohol extract, and 1.0 g/kg for vinegar-processed extract. Therefore, it can be inferred that processing with vinegar reduces the toxicity of *Yuan Hua*.[11,12,13]

AUTHORS' COMMENTS

Yuan Hua has similar actions to purge stagnation and eliminate water accumulation to that of *Gan Sui* (Radix Euphorbiae Kansui) and *Da Ji* (Radix Euphorbiae seu Knoxiae). *Gan Sui* is the strongest of the three.

References

1. *Chang Yong Zhong Yao Cheng Fen Yu Yao Li Shou Ce* (A Handbook of the Composition and Pharmacology of Common Chinese Drugs), 1994; 960-961
2. *Zhe Jiang Zhong Yi Yao* (Zhejiang Chinese Medicine and Herbology), 1978; (6):27
3. *Zhong Cao Yao Tong Xun* (Journal of Chinese Herbal Medicine), 1973; (5):7
4. *Zhong Yao Tong Bao* (Journal of Chinese Herbology), 1986; 11(4):49
5. *Zhong Cao Yao Tong Xun* (Journal of Chinese Herbal Medicine), 1973; (5):7
6. *Yao Xue Xue Bao* (Journal of Herbology), 1966; 13(6):454
7. *Zhong Cheng Yao Yan Jiu* (Research of Chinese Patent Medicine), 1981; 2:44
8. *Zhong Cao Yao Tong Xun* (Journal of Chinese Herbal Medicine), 1973; 5:7
9. *Xin Yi Xue* (New Medicine), 1985; 4:178
10. *Tian Jing Yi Yao Tong Xun* (Publication of Tianjing Medicine and Herbology), 1971; (8):7
11. *Hu Nan Yi Xue Yuan Xue Bao* (Medical Journal of Hunan University of Medicine), 1960; (7):30
12. *Zhong Cao Yao Tong Xun* (Journal of Chinese Herbal Medicine), 1973; (5):7
13. *Zhe Jiang Zhong Yi Yao* (Zhejiang Chinese Medicine and Herbology), 1978; (6):27

Qian Niu Zi (Semen Pharbitidis)

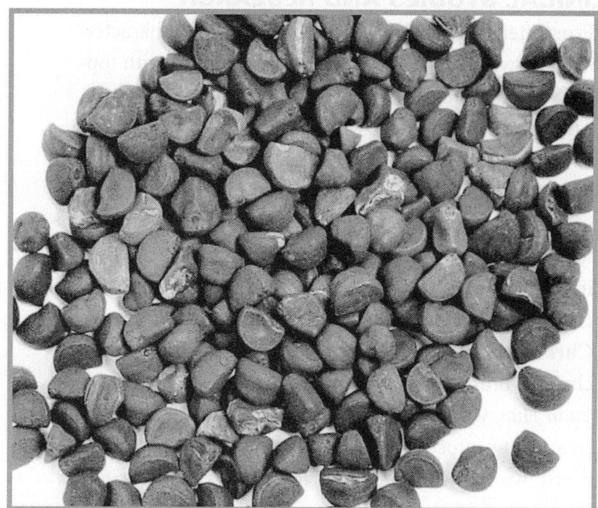

牽牛子 牵牛子

Pinyin Name: *Qian Niu Zi*
Literal Name: "cowherd seeds"
Alternate Chinese Names: *Hei Bai Niu, Er Niu, La Ba Hua Zi*
Original Source: *Ming Yi Za Zhu* (Miscellaneous Records of Famous Physicians) by Tao Hong-Jing in 500 A.D.
English Name: pharbitis, pharbitis seed, morning glory seed
Botanical Name: *Pharbitis nil* (L.) Choisy. (*Lie Ye Qian Niu*); *Pharbitis purpurea* (L.) Voigt (*Yuan Ye Qian Niu*)
Pharmaceutical Name: Semen Pharbitidis
Properties: bitter, acrid, cold
Channels Entered: Lung, Kidney, Large Intestine
Safety Index: toxic

Qian Niu Zi (Semen Pharbitidis)

CHINESE THERAPEUTIC ACTIONS

1. Purges Downward and Promotes Diuresis

Qian Niu Zi (Semen Pharbitidis) purges and eliminates accumulations through defecation and urination. Clinical applications include ascites and edema. This herb should be used only for excess conditions and in patients who are not deficient in qi, blood or yin.

- Mild edema: use powdered *Qian Niu Zi* as a single-herb remedy.
- Ascites and edema with qi stagnation: use it with *Mu Xiang* (Radix Aucklandiae) and *Hou Po* (Cortex Magnoliae Officinalis).
- Edema in children: combine it with *Qing Pi* (Pericarpium Citri Reticulatae Viride) or *Mu Xiang* (Radix Aucklandiae).
- Nephritis with edema, or liver cirrhosis with ascites: use this herb with *Sheng Jiang* (Rhizoma Zingiberis Recens), *Da Zao* (Fructus Jujubae) and brown sugar to make pills.

2. Redirects Lung Qi and Eliminates Phlegm

Qian Niu Zi treats acute coughing and wheezing caused by phlegm stagnation in the chest and abnormal rising of qi. Clinical manifestations of this syndrome include wheezing, dyspnea, fullness of the chest, labored breathing, flared nostrils and a throttling sound in the throat because of the presence of sputum.

- Cough and wheezing: use it with *Da Huang* (Radix et Rhizoma Rhei) and *Bing Lang* (Semen Arecae).

3. Reduces Stagnation and Purges Constipation

Qian Niu Zi treats constipation through its purgative action. A small dosage treats constipation or food stagnation, while a large dosage leads to watery diarrhea.

- Constipation: use it with *Tao Ren* (Semen Persicae).
- Severe constipation: add *Da Huang* (Radix et Rhizoma Rhei).

4. Kills Parasites

Qian Niu Zi kills intestinal parasites, and is especially effective against roundworm and tapeworm. Since this herb has both antiparasitic and purgative functions, it kills and expels intestinal parasites simultaneously. Addition of purgative herbs to expel parasites is not necessary.

- Intestinal parasitic infestation: use it with *Bing Lang* (Semen Arecae) and other antiparasitic herbs.

DOSAGE

3 to 10 grams in decoction, 1.5 to 3.0 grams as powder. Fresh *Qian Niu Zi* is more potent, but also has more side effects. The dry-fried herb is milder, and has fewer side effects. Dry-fried *Qian Niu Zi* is considered the preferred form, as it has fewer side effects, moderated purgative action, and when cooked in a decoction, a more complete extraction of active components.

CAUTIONS / CONTRAINDICATIONS

- Use of *Qian Niu Zi* is contraindicated during pregnancy, or in cases of Stomach qi deficiency.
- According to some classic texts, it is incompatible with *Ba Dou* (Fructus Crotonis).

OVERDOSAGE

Early reaction to overdose of *Qian Niu Zi* (Semen Pharbitidis) is characterized by dizziness, headache, severe vomiting, abdominal pain and diarrhea, green watery stools with mucous, increased heart rate (up to 120 beats per minute), impaired speech, fever, blood and cells in the urine, and deep thready pulse. Late or severe reaction is characterized by fever, unconsciousness, cold extremities, with purple lips, skin and nails, and shortness of breath.[1]

Overdose of *Qian Niu Zi* may damage the gastrointestinal and urinary tracts and the central nervous system. The herb may be irritating to the gastrointestinal tract and may increase intestinal peristalsis, leading to symptoms such as nausea, vomiting, abdominal pain, diarrhea, and blood and mucus in the stools. Irritation may also occur in the urinary tract, leading to increased urination and hematuria. In severe cases, overdose may disturb the central nervous system, leading to impaired speech and unconsciousness. Adverse reactions to *Qian Niu Zi* are usually associated with doses between 15 and 45 grams. One case of fatality was documented following gross overdose of 195 grams.[2]

TREATMENT OF OVERDOSAGE

Most patients will have severe vomiting with overdose of *Qian Niu Zi*, so the emetic method is often ineffective and unnecessary. Instead, treatment should be focused on minimizing absorption of the offending agent, which can be achieved with administration of 12 grams of *Wu Bei Zi* (Galla Chinensis) in powder, 6 egg whites, and 60 grams of honey all mixed with warm water. An herbal decoction with 120 grams of *Lu Dou* (Semen Phaseoli Radiati) can also be used in place of water, to rehydrate the body and eliminate the toxin.

One formula that has been successfully used for treatment of overdose include *Huang Qi* (Radix Astragali) 30g, *Xian He Cao* (Herba Agrimoniae) 30g, *Dang Shen* (Radix Codonopsis) 15g, *Bai Zhu* (Rhizoma Atractylodis Macrocephalae) 9g, *Fu Ling* (Poria) 9g, *Zhi Zi* (Fructus Gardeniae) 9g, and *Huang Lian* (Rhizoma Coptidis) 6g.

If the adverse reaction is characterized by continuous diarrhea leading to severe weakness and fatigue, an

Qian Niu Zi (Semen Pharbitidis)

herbal decoction of *Chi Shi Zhi* (Halloysitum Rubrum) 30g, *Gan Cao* (Radix Glycyrrhizae) 15g, and *Geng Mi* (Semen Oryzae) 30g should be given.

Patients with hematuria should be treated twice daily with a decoction of *San Qi* (Radix Notoginseng) 6g, *Gan Cao* (Radix Glycyrrhizae) 15g, *Sheng Di Huang* (Radix Rehmanniae) 30g, and *Xi Jiao* (Cornu Rhinoceri) 9g. [Note: *Shui Niu Jiao* (Cornu Bubali) should be used in place of *Xi Jiao*, a protected animal.] This is served at room temperature.

Adverse reactions characterized by altered consciousness and impaired speech should be treated with herbs that open the sensory orifices, such as *Fang Feng* (Radix Saposhnikoviae) 15g, *Bai Fu Zi* (Rhizoma Typhonii) 15g, *Dan Nan Xing* (Arisaema cum Bile) 15g, *Gan Cao* (Radix Glycyrrhizae) 10g, *Yuan Zhi* (Radix Polygalae) 6g, *Zhu Li* (Succus Bambusae) 3 spoonfuls, *Sheng Jiang* (Rhizoma Zingiberis Recens) 3 spoonfuls of juice, and *Niu Huang* (Calculus Bovis) 0.3g.[3]

CHEMICAL COMPOSITION

Pharbitin 2%, pharbitic acid C, D; lysergol, chanoclavine, penniclavine, isopenniclavine, elymoclavine, gibberellin, gibberellin glucoside.[4]

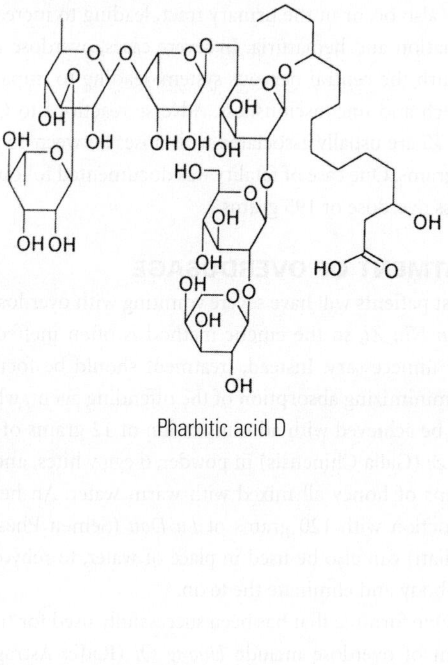

Pharbitic acid D

PHARMACOLOGICAL EFFECTS

- **Cathartic:** *Qian Niu Zi* stimulates intestinal peristalsis and promotes bowel movement. It must be processed at a low temperature or by soaking in alcohol. It is ineffective if cooked at a high temperature.[5]
- **Antiparasitic:** *Qian Niu Zi* has antiparasitic action against roundworms derived from pigs, according to *in vitro* studies.[6]

CLINICAL STUDIES AND RESEARCH

- **Epilepsy:** In one clinical study, 115 patients with epilepsy were treated with preparations of *Qian Niu Zi* for 3 months with 56.7% effectiveness.[7]

AUTHORS' COMMENTS

Traditionally, *Qian Niu Zi* has been separated into white and black seeds. The white seeds were supposed to be stronger in descending Lung qi and eliminating phlegm, and the black seeds were supposed to be stronger in dispelling water. However, contemporary research has shown that there is no effective difference between the two. Thus, they are no longer classified as separate herbs.

References

1. *Zhong Yao Du Li Xue* (Toxicology of Chinese Herbs), 123-124, 1989
2. *Zhong Yao Bu Liang Fan Ying Yu Zhi Liao* (Adverse Reactions and Treatment of Chinese Herbal Medicine), 1996; 163:164
3. *Zhong Yao Du Li Xue* (Toxicology of Chinese Herbs), 123-124, 1989
4. *Xian Dai Zhong Yao Yao Li Xue* (Contemporary Pharmacology of Chinese Herbs), 1997; 384
5. *Zhong Yao Zhi* (Chinese Herbology Journal), 1984; 523
6. Ibid.
7. *Zhong Hua Nei Ke Za Zhi* (Chinese Journal of Internal Medicine), 1977; 6:323

Shang Lu (Radix Phytolaccae)

商陸 商陆

Pinyin Name: *Shang Lu*
Literal Name: "commerce continent"
Alternate Chinese Names: *Bai Mu Ji, Shan Luo Bo, Ye Luo Bo*
Original Source: *Shen Nong Ben Cao Jing* (Divine Husbandman's Classic of the Materia Medica) in the second century
English Name: phytolacca, poke root, pokeberry root
Botanical Name: *Phytolacca acinosa* Roxb. (*Shang Lu*)
Pharmaceutical Name: Radix Phytolaccae
Properties: bitter, cold
Channels Entered: Lung, Kidney, Large Intestine
Safety Index: toxic

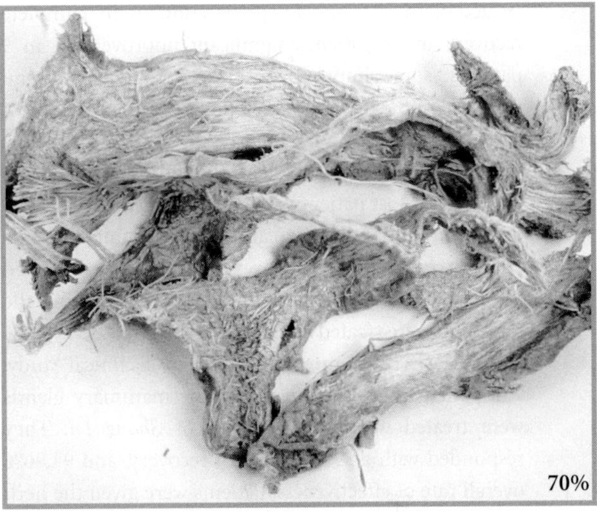
70%

CHINESE THERAPEUTIC ACTIONS

1. Eliminates Water Accumulation

Ascites, edema: *Shang Lu* (Radix Phytolaccae) has a potent ability to eliminate water accumulation to treat ascites and edema.

- Ascites and edema: use *Shang Lu* with *Ze Xie* (Rhizoma Alismatis), *Chi Xiao Dou* (Semen Phaseoli), *Da Fu Pi* (Pericarpium Arecae) and *Bing Lang* (Semen Arecae).

2. Reduces Swelling and Disperses Stagnation

Shang Lu may be crushed and applied topically to treat swelling and nodules.

DOSAGE

5 to 10 grams in decoction. Processing with vinegar decreases the toxicity of *Shang Lu*.

CAUTIONS / CONTRAINDICATIONS

- *Shang Lu* is contraindicated during pregnancy, due to its toxicity.
- *Gan Cao* (Radix Glycyrrhizae) and *Lu Dou* (Semen Phaseoli Radiati) are generally prescribed with *Shang Lu* to minimize its toxicity.

OVERDOSAGE

Overdose of *Shang Lu* is characterized by nausea, vomiting, diarrhea, headache, slurred speech, irritability or muscle twitching. In severe cases, there may be a sudden drop in blood pressure, unconsciousness, dilation of pupils, and heart failure.

TREATMENT OF OVERDOSAGE

Overdose of *Shang Lu* can be treated by emetic methods within the first 4 hours, followed by administration of egg whites or rice porridge. An herbal decoction that has been used successfully includes *Shi Chang Pu* (Rhizoma Acori) 9g, *Huang Bai* (Cortex Phellodendri) 9g, *Chuan Lian Zi* (Fructus Toosendan) 9g, and *Yan Hu Suo* (Rhizoma Corydalis) 12g.[1]

Adverse reactions characterized by abdominal pain, diarrhea, and fever can be treated with an herbal decoction containing *Fang Feng* (Radix Saposhnikoviae) 15g, *Gan Cao* (Radix Glycyrrhizae) 15g, *Rou Gui* (Cortex Cinnamomi) 3g, and *Lu Dou* (Semen Phaseoli Radiati) 60g.[2]

CHEMICAL COMPOSITION

Phytolaccagenin, phytolaccoside A,B,D,E,F,D_2; jaligonic acid.[3]

PHARMACOLOGICAL EFFECTS

- **Diuretic:** Administration of *Shang Lu* has different effects on different subjects. In anesthetized dogs, it has no effect on diuresis or blood pressure. In frogs and toads, it has significant diuretic and vasodilating effects.[4]
- **Antitussive and expectorant:** Both water and alcohol extracts of *Shang Lu* have antitussive and expectorant effects.[5]
- **Antibiotic:** Both water and alcohol extracts of *Shang Lu* inhibit *Bacillus dysenteriae, Diplococcus pneumoniae*, and some dermatophytes.[6]

CLINICAL STUDIES AND RESEARCH

- **Chronic bronchitis:** A study on treatment of chronic bronchitis reported that alcohol extract of *Shang Lu* has marked antitussive, expectorant, and antiasthmatic effects. It was noted that *Shang Lu* was especially effective in patients who have adrenal cortical insufficiency.[7]
- **Psoriasis:** In one report, 40 patients with psoriasis were

Shang Lu (Radix Phytolaccae)

treated with a *Shang Lu* preparation, with complete recovery in 12 patients, significant improvement in 9 patients, some improvement in 11 patients, and no response in 8 patients. *Shang Lu* was steamed in a pressure cooker for 2 hours, then baked until dry. Patients were given 3 grams of the herb three times daily, for 10 to 60 days. Most patients showed improvement 20 to 30 days after initiation of treatment. No significant side effects were reported. However, 2 patients reported atropine-like side effects within 2 hours of taking the herb, and were treated accordingly.[8]

- **Hyperplasia of mammary glands:** In a clinical study, 253 patients with hyperplasia of the mammary glands were treated with a preparation of *Shang Lu.* They responded with a 37.15% rate of recovery, and 94.86% overall rate of effectiveness. Patients were given the herb in pills three times daily, starting with 3 grams per dose and gradually increasing to 10 grams per dose.[9]

TOXICOLOGY

The LD_{50} for *Shang Lu* in mice via oral administration is 26 g/kg for water solution, 28 g/kg for water decoction, and 46.5 g/kg for alcohol tincture. Cooking the herb in boiling water for 2 hours decreased the toxicity.[10]

AUTHORS' COMMENTS

There are two types of *Shang Lu*: white and red. The white type is the standard herb used by pharmacies. The red type is toxic and may cause diarrhea and bleeding, leading to death. The red type is twice as toxic as the white type.

Shang Lu and *Ren Shen* (Radix Ginseng) are similar in physical appearance, but exert completely different effects. Proper care must be taken to ensure that they are appropriately identified and not used incorrectly.

Shang Lu is a mild cathartic in comparison with others within this category.

References

1. *Lin Chuan Shou Ce You Du Zhong Yao Shi Yong* (Clinical Handbook on Applications of Toxic Chinese Herbs), 1992; 154-155
2. *Zhong Yao Du Li Xue* (Toxicology of Chinese Herbs), 1989; 146-147
3. *Xian Dai Zhong Yao Yao Li Xue* (Contemporary Pharmacology of Chinese Herbs), 1997; 390
4. *Zhong Yao Cai* (Study of Chinese Herbal Material), 1991; 14(3):46
5. *Zhong Cao Yao* (Chinese Herbal Medicine), 1984; 15(12):22
6. *Zhong Yao Yao Li Yu Du Li Za Zhi* (Journal of Pharmacology and Toxicology of Chinese Herbs), 1992; 6(3):221
7. *Yao Wu Fen Xi Za Zhi* (Journal of Herbal Analysis), 1983; 3(1):31
8. *Zhong Yi Za Zhi* (Journal of Chinese Medicine), 1984; 12:38
9. *Zhong Cao Yao* (Chinese Herbal Medicine), 1985; 3:22
10. *Zhong Yao Cai* (Study of Chinese Herbal Material), 1991; 14(3):46

Chapter 3 summary

— Downward Draining Herbs

SECTION 1: PURGATIVES

Name	Similarities	Differences
Da Huang (Radix et Rhizoma Rhei)	Purgative, downward draining	Sedates fire, eliminates toxins, and invigorates the blood to relieve stagnation
Mang Xiao (Natrii Sulfas)		Softens hardness, sedates fire
Fan Xie Ye (Folium Sennae)		Milder, used for habitual constipation
Lu Hui (Aloe)		Sedates Liver fire, kills parasites
Ba Dou (Fructus Crotonis)		For cold type constipation, dispels water and phlegm, and is used externally to kill parasites

General Characteristics of Purgatives:

Taste: bitter
Thermal property: cold
Channels entered: Large Intestine
Therapeutic actions: clear heat, sedate fire, purge stagnation and relieve constipation

Purgative herbs primarily treat constipation and stagnation in the Large Intestine, caused by or accompanied by heat, fire, toxins, or hardness. These strong herbs should be reserved for severe constipation in patients who are strong and otherwise healthy. They should be used only with extreme caution for weak individuals or those experiencing generalized deficiencies.

Da Huang (Radix et Rhizoma Rhei) is the most widely-used purgative. It sedates fire, clears toxins, invigorates blood circulation, eliminates blood stasis, and purges accumulation. Extremely bitter and cold, *Da Huang* should be reserved for heat and excess conditions. It can be used for constipation due to excess cold, provided that appropriate warming herbs are added. Processing methods and time influence the purgative intensity of *Da Huang*: use of the unprocessed form and/or post-decoction maintains a strong purgative effect, while using the processed form or exposing it to prolonged cooking weakens its purgative effect.

Mang Xiao (Natrii Sulfas) purges downward, clears heat and is used primarily to soften hardness, that is, to soften dry stools to facilitate passage. Used externally, *Mang Xiao* softens hard nodules or masses, especially in the breasts. Dissolved in water and applied topically, it treats various oral disorders such as sores or lesions caused by heat. The decocted form is not recommended for topical application.

Da Huang (Radix et Rhizoma Rhei) and ***Mang Xiao*** (Natrii Sulfas) are frequently paired together for their synergistic effect to treat constipation.

Fan Xie Ye (Folium Sennae), quite similar to *Da Huang* (Radix et Rhizoma Rhei), addresses constipation caused by heat and treats acute gastrointestinal bleeding. It has been used to cleanse the colon prior to x-ray examination or surgery. *Fan Xie Ye* may be taken as tea simply by soaking the herb in hot water.

Lu Hui (Aloe) treats constipation resulting from Liver fire. It also kills parasites in children to treat concurrent malnutrition, and, when applied externally, kills parasites, relieves itching and treats

Chapter 3 summary

stubborn dermatological disorders. Because it is extremely bitter, this herb is often made into pills or administered in capsules. Decocting this herb is not recommended.

Ba Dou (Fructus Crotonis), the only purgative listed here that is acrid, hot and toxic, addresses constipation arising from cold accumulation. It strongly purges downward, removing intestinal obstruction ('opening' the intestines), and purging water to reduce ascites or edema. *Ba Dou* induces vomiting, stops drooling of saliva, treats lung abscesses and throat obstruction caused by phlegm. Additionally, the action of this herb can rise or descend, depending on how it is combined and administered.

SECTION 2: MOIST LAXATIVES

Name	Similarities	Differences
Huo Ma Ren (Fructus Cannabis)	Lubricate the bowels, promote defecation	Moistens dryness, nourishes hair and kills parasites
Yu Li Ren (Semen Pruni)		Promotes diuresis, reduces swelling

General Characteristics of Moist Laxatives:

Taste: sweet
Thermal property: neutral
Channels entered: Spleen, Stomach, Large Intestine, Small Intestine
Therapeutic actions: lubricate the bowels to relieve constipation

Moist laxatives lubricate the Large Intestine, facilitating the passage of stools. Milder and gentler than purgatives, these more suitably treat constipation caused by deficiency: weak constitution, body fluid deficiency or blood deficiency.

Huo Ma Ren (Fructus Cannabis) and ***Yu Li Ren*** (Semen Pruni) are the most commonly used substances with these attributes.

Huo Ma Ren moistens dryness.

Yu Li Ren promotes diuresis, reduces swelling and treats edema while contributing to lubrication of the bowels.

SECTION 3: HARSH EXPELLANTS (CATHARTICS)

Name	Similarities	Differences
Gan Sui (Radix Euphorbiae Kansui)	Strongly purge stool and water from the body	Toxic, strongest in purging water
Da Ji (Radix Euphorbiae seu Knoxiae)		Toxic, weaker in purging water
Yuan Hua (Flos Genkwa)		Dispels water accumulation in the thoracic area, used externally to kill parasites
Qian Niu Zi (Semen Pharbitidis)		Promotes diuresis, reduces stagnation and kills roundworms and pinworms
Shang Lu (Radix Phytolaccae)		Reduces swelling and disperses stagnation when used externally

General Characteristics of Harsh Expellants (Cathartics):

Taste: bitter
Thermal property: cold
Channels entered: varies
Therapeutic actions: promote bowel movement and urination
Safety index: many are toxic

Chapter 3 summary

Harsh expellants (cathartics) have potent effects to purge downwards, for treatment of severe constipation, ascites, and water accumulation. They must be used with great caution, especially in elderly patients, menstruating, pregnant, or postpartum women, or patients deficient in qi, blood or yin. Clinically, these herbs are rarely used.

Gan Sui (Radix Euphorbiae Kansui), ***Da Ji*** (Radix Euphorbiae seu Knoxiae), and ***Yuan Hua*** (Flos Genkwa) have strong cathartic effects to treat edema, ascites and pleurisy. They are used mainly to remove water from the abdominal cavity. Processing these herbs with vinegar decreases their toxicity.

Gan Sui, strongest in driving out water accumulation, has significant toxicity and side effects. It treats mania and epilepsy caused by phlegm accumulation. Because the active constituents of this herb do not dissolve in water, it is most suitable for dispensing in pill or powdered form. Decocting *Gan Sui* dramatically decreases its potency.

Da Ji purges water accumulation, dissolves stagnation, reduces swelling, and treats toxic carbuncles and swellings.

Yuan Hua purges water and dispels phlegm to relieve cough. Used externally, it kills parasites and reduces swellings and abscesses.

Qian Niu Zi (Semen Pharbitidis) and ***Shang Lu*** (Radix Phytolaccae) have diuretic functions.

Qian Niu Zi purges water and treats edema when used in large doses. Small doses relieve stagnation and promote bowel movement. It also sedates Lung qi, dispels phlegm accumulation and treats cough and dyspnea due to phlegm accumulation. It kills parasites when used externally. Unprocessed *Qian Niu Zi* is stronger than the processed form.

Shang Lu (Radix Phytolaccae), used internally, treats edema; and externally, reduces swelling and disperses stagnation. *Shang Lu* is stronger than *Gan Sui* in dispelling water.

HERBS FROM OTHER FUNCTIONAL CATEGORIES WITH DOWNWARD DRAINING FUNCTIONS

Name	Functional Category
Bai Zi Ren (Semen Platycladi)	*Shen*-Calming Herbs (Chapter 14)
Dang Gui (Radicis Angelicae Sinensis)	Tonic Herbs (Chapter 17)
Dong Kui Zi (Semen Malvae)	Water-Regulating and Damp-Resolving Herbs (Chapter 6)
Feng Mi (Mel)	Tonic Herbs (Chapter 17)
Gua Lou Ren (Semen Trichosanthis)	Phlegm-Dissolving and Coughing/Relieve Relieving Herbs (Chapter 13)
He Shou Wu (Radix Polygoni Multiflori)	Tonic Herbs (Chapter 17)
Jue Ming Zi (Semen Cassiae)	Liver-Calming and Wind-Extinguishing Herbs (Chapter 15)
Rou Cong Rong (Herba Cistanches)	Tonic Herbs (Chapter 17)
Tao Ren (Semen Persicae)	Blood-Invigorating and Stasis-Removing Herbs (Chapter 12)
Xing Ren (Semen Armeniacae Amarum)	Phlegm-Resolving and Coughing- and Wheezing-Relieving Herbs (Chapter 13)

Chapter 4

— Wind-Damp Dispelling Herbs

祛风湿药

Chapter 4 — Wind-Damp Dispelling Herbs

Chapter 4

— Wind-Damp Dispelling Herbs

Definition: Herbs that dispel wind and dampness eliminate these pathogenic factors from muscles and joints to relieve obstruction and pain associated with *bi zheng* (painful obstruction syndrome).

Wind, cold and dampness are environmental factors responsible for causing *bi zheng* (painful obstruction syndrome), characterized by stagnation and pain attacking muscles, joints, tendons and bones. In addition to dispelling wind, cold and dampness, these herbs relieve pain, relax muscles and tendons, open the channels and collaterals, and strengthen tendons and bones. Signs and symptoms of wind-damp affecting the muscles and joints include muscle aches and pain, muscle spasms and cramps, weakness and pain of the lower back and knees, numbness and atrophy of the muscles, and paralysis. Clinical applications of herbs that dispel wind and dampness include treatment of arthritis, arthralgia, sciatica, bone spurs, and post-stroke complications such as hemiplegia and paralysis.

Wind-damp dispelling herbs are generally acrid and bitter, qualities that disperse wind and dry dampness, respectively. These substances are either warm or cold, to treat cold or hot *bi zheng* (painful obstruction syndrome). Most of these herbs enter the Liver and Kidney, as these are the organs that control tendons and bones.

Wind-damp dispelling herbs eliminate pathogens from muscles and joints in disorders such as arthritis, arthralgia, sciatica, bone spurs, and post-stroke complications.

SUBCATEGORIES OF ACTION

Herbs that dispel wind and dampness are generally acrid and bitter, to disperse and drain pathogenic factors. Most enter the Liver and Kidney channels to strengthen soft tissue and promote healing. They are commonly considered in three subcategories:

1. ***Dispel wind and damp to relieve pain***: These herbs strongly dispel exterior pathogenic factors of wind, cold and damp in patients who have no interior deficiency. The same herbs relieve pain.
2. ***Open peripheral channels and collaterals***: These herbs eliminate stagnation to address chronic and stubborn *bi zheng* (painful obstruction syndrome), characterized by decreased range of movement of the joints, decreased mobility of the extremities, bodily numbness, hemiplegia and paralysis.
3. ***Dispel wind and damp by strengthening the tendons and bones***: In addition to dispelling wind, cold and damp, these herbs enter the Liver and Kidney channels to tonify the tendons and bones. They are most effective for treating chronic cases of *bi zheng* (painful obstruction syndrome) characterized by weakness, deficiency and atrophy of the soft tissues.

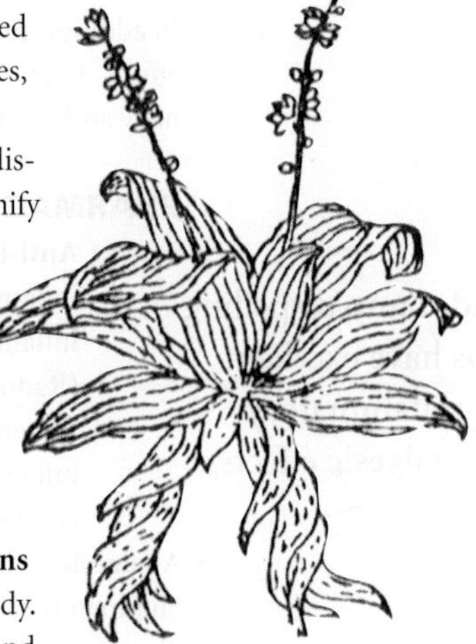

Qin Jiao (Radix Gentianae Macrophyllae)
Ben Cao Gang Mu (Materia Medica),
by Li Shi-Zhen, 1578 A.D.

DIFFERENTIAL DIAGNOSIS AND TREATMENT

Bi zheng (painful obstruction syndrome) is usually caused by exterior factors, interior conditions, or the combination of both. **Exterior factors** refers to environmental pathogenic factors, namely wind, cold and dampness. **Interior conditions** refers to imbalances affecting the constitution and internal health of the body. Individuals with constitutional deficiencies, such as deficiency of *wei* (defensive) and *zheng* (upright) *qi*, are more susceptible to the invasion of wind, cold and dampness than those who are hearty and robust. There are several different types of *bi zheng* (painful obstruction syndrome):

Chapter 4 — Wind-Damp Dispelling Herbs

- *Xing bi* (mobile painful obstruction) is caused by wind attacking the body. Similar to wind that is light and mobile, *xing bi* is characterized by pain in the upper body, specifically pain that travels from one area to another.
- *Tong bi* (extremely painful obstruction) is characterized by cold. Similar to cold that is stationary and constricting, *tong bi* is distinguished by severe pain at a fixed location. This type of pain intensifies with exposure to cold, and is relieved by exposure to warmth.
- *Zhuo bi* (fixed painful obstruction) often occurs when damp affects specific, fixed area(s). Similar to dampness that is heavy and sinking, *zhuo bi* is characterized by pain and swelling in the lower extremities.
- *Re bi* (heat painful obstruction) is characterized by local redness, swelling, burning sensations and pain. The development of heat is often caused by prolonged obstruction of the channels and collaterals by wind, cold or damp.
- *Wan bi* (stubborn painful obstruction) generally occurs after chronic or repetitive injuries to the same areas, causing stiffness, numbness, and lack of mobility.
- *Wei bi* (atrophic painful obstruction) is caused by deficiency of the Liver and Kidney, with such presentations as atrophy, weakness and pain of the muscles and bones.
- *Xue bi* (blood painful obstruction) describes *bi zheng* (painful obstruction syndrome) related to blood. Dull pain may be caused by blood deficiency and its inability to nourish the tendons and bones. Sharp pain is often related to blood stagnation blocking the channels and collaterals.
- *Zhou bi* (generalized painful obstruction) is characterized by generalized pain that also affects the bones and joints.

CAUTIONS/CONTRAINDICATIONS

- Bitter, warm, aromatic and drying herbs may consume yin and blood and should be used with caution in patients experiencing deficiency of yin and/or blood.
- Herbs that dispel wind and dampness are contraindicated in cases of endogenous Liver wind. External wind and internal wind have very different clinical presentations, and require distinctly different treatments.

PROCESSING

Because of the chronic nature of *bi zheng* (painful obstruction syndrome) ailments, dosage forms are often changed from decoction to herbal wines, pills, or tablets to improve patient compliance. In addition to the actions of the herbs, the alcohol of the wines provides dispersing and analgesic effects. Grain-based liquor is the solvent of choice. Alcohol-based tinctures are used both internally and externally.

PHARMACOLOGICAL EFFECTS

Wind-damp dispelling herbs have excellent anti-inflammatory and analgesic effects.

- **Anti-inflammatory**: Wind-damp dispelling herbs are excellent substances to reduce inflammation. The mechanisms of this action vary depending on the herb. Some reduce inflammation and swelling by decreasing permeability of the capillaries, such as *Du Huo* (Radix Angelicae Pubescentis) and *Wu Jia Pi* (Cortex Acanthopanacis); others stimulate the endocrine system to increase the secretion of corticosteroids that, in turn, reduce inflammation, such as *Qin Jiao* (Radix Gentianae Macrophyllae) and *Lei Gong Teng* (Radix Tripterygii Wilfordii).
- **Analgesic**: These herbs have varying degrees of analgesic activity. *Qing Feng Teng* (Caulis Sinomenii) relieves pain via its effect on the central nervous system. Prolonged use of *Qing Feng Teng* is associated with tolerance, but not dependence. *Fen Fang Ji* (Radix Stephaniae Tetandrae) also has a marked analgesic effect. On a weight-to-weight comparison, the analgesic effect of the pure alkaloids of *Fen Fang Ji* is approximately 1/8th the strength of morphine.
- **Immunosuppressive**: Some herbs exert inhibitory influences on the immune system, leading to suppressed phagocytic activity of macrophages, and decreased production of T-lymphocytes, IgM, and IgG. Herbs with such actions include *Lei Gong Teng* (Radix Tripterygii Wilfordii), *Du*

Huo (Radix Angelicae Pubescentis), *Qing Feng Teng* (Caulis Sinomenii), and *Xi Xian Cao* (Herba Siegesbeckiae).

- **Antipyretic**: Herbs with antipyretic properties include *Qin Jiao* (Radix Gentianae Macrophyllae) and *Fen Fang Ji* (Radix Stephaniae Tetandrae).
- **Sedative**: Sedative herbs include *Qin Jiao* (Radix Gentianae Macrophyllae), *Ci Wu Jia* (Radix et Caulis Acanthopanacis Senticosi), *Qing Feng Teng* (Caulis Sinomenii), and *Xu Chang Qing* (Radix Cynanchi Paniculati).

POTENTIAL HERB-DRUG INTERACTIONS

- **Analgesics and anti-inflammatories**: Herbs that dispel wind and dampness are usually characterized by pronounced analgesic and anti-inflammatory activity. While their mechanisms of action vary, there is little or no documentation of any incidents of adverse interaction between analgesic and anti-inflammatory herbs and drug therapy.
- **Antiplatelets and anticoagulants**: Some herbs in this category, such as *Du Huo* (Radix Angelicae Pubescentis), mildly inhibit platelet aggregation, and should be taken with caution by patients who are using anticoagulant or antiplatelet drugs.[1]
- **Sedatives**: Some herbs have sedative and hypnotic effects, and should be used with caution with drugs exerting similar actions, to avoid causing excessive drowsiness and sedation. Furthermore, individuals who take such herbs should exercise caution if driving or operating heavy machinery.

References

1. *108th Convention of Japanese Herbology Convention*, 1988

Section 1

– Wind-Damp Dispelling and Pain-Relieving Herbs

Du Huo (Radix Angelicae Pubescentis)

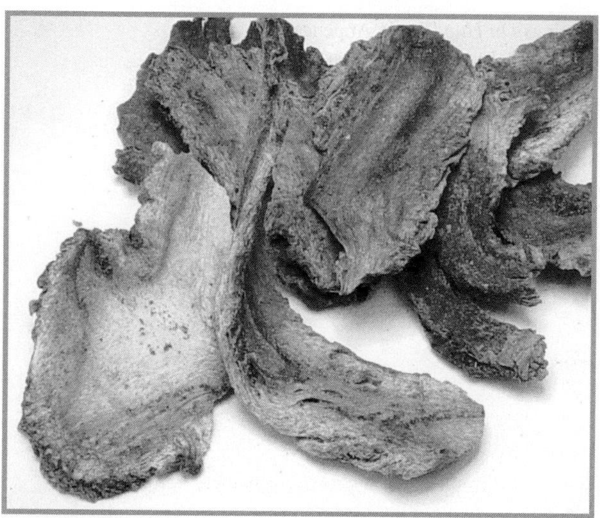

獨活 独活

Pinyin Name: *Du Huo*
Literal Name: "self-reliant existence"
Alternate Chinese Names: *Xiang Du Huo*
Original Source: *Shen Nong Ben Cao Jing* (Divine Husbandman's Classic of the Materia Medica) in the second century
English Name: pubescent angelica root, double teeth pubescent angelica root
Botanical Name: *Angelica pubescens* Maxim. F. biserrata Shan et Yuan. (*Mao Dang Gui*)
Pharmaceutical Name: Radix Angelicae Pubescentis
Properties: acrid, bitter, warm
Channels Entered: Liver, Kidney, Urinary Bladder

CHINESE THERAPEUTIC ACTIONS

1. Dispels Wind and Dampness to Relieve Pain

***Bi zheng* (painful obstruction syndrome):** Wind, cold and dampness are responsible for the majority of *bi zheng* afflictions. These pathogens block the channels and collaterals and lead to stagnation of qi and blood. Acrid, bitter and warm, *Du Huo* (Radix Angelicae Pubescentis) enters the peripheral channels and collaterals to dispel wind, cold and dampness. It relieves various acute and chronic aches and pains of the muscles and joints. Furthermore, *Du Huo* enters the Liver and Kidney channels and benefits the tendons and bones. Clinically, *Du Huo* treats such disorders as muscle and joint aches and pains, low back pain, weak knees, and muscle atrophy. This herb is best for pain in the lower body (back and knees).

- Low back pain and weak knees: use *Du Huo* with *Sang Ji Sheng* (Herba Taxilli), *Du Zhong* (Cortex Eucommiae) and *Dang Gui* (Radicis Angelicae Sinensis) to tonify the Liver and Kidney. **Exemplar Formula:** *Du Huo Ji Sheng Tang* (Angelica Pubescens and Taxillus Decoction).

***Shaoyin* stage headache and toothache:**

- Headache: combine *Du Huo* with *Xi Xin* (Herba Asari) and *Chuan Xiong* (Rhizoma Ligustici Chuanxiong).
- Toothache: prepare *Du Huo* individually in an herbal decoction, to be used for gargling while warm.
- Toothache and swollen gums due to wind-heat or Stomach heat: use it with *Shi Gao* (Gypsum Fibrosum), *Sheng Di Huang* (Radix Rehmanniae) and *Sheng Ma* (Rhizoma Cimicifugae).

Dermatological disorders:

- Rash and itching: use *Du Huo* with *Fang Feng* (Radix Saposhnikoviae) and *Di Fu Zi* (Fructus Kochiae).

2. Releases the Exterior

Wind-cold disorder with dampness: Acrid, dispersing and warm, *Du Huo* dispels the pathogenic factors wind, cold or dampness from the exterior. Clinically, it treats exterior wind-cold with dampness characterized by symptoms such as aversion to cold, fever, headache, sensations of heaviness, and muscle aches and pain.

Du Huo (Radix Angelicae Pubescentis)

- Muscle aches and pain due to exterior wind, cold and dampness: use *Du Huo* with *Qiang Huo* (Rhizoma et Radix Notopterygii), *Fang Feng* (Radix Saposhnikoviae), and *Gao Ben* (Rhizoma Ligustici). **Exemplar Formula:** *Qiang Huo Sheng Shi Tang* (Notopterygium Decoction to Overcome Dampness).

DOSAGE

3 to 10 grams.

CAUTIONS / CONTRAINDICATIONS

- Drying in nature, *Du Huo* should be used with caution in patients who have yin and/or blood deficiencies.
- *Du Huo* is contraindicated for patients who have internal Liver wind.
- Overdose of *Du Huo* is sometimes associated with increased photosensitivity.

CHEMICAL COMPOSITION

Osthole, columbianetin, columbianctin acetate, bergapten, columbianadin, xanthotoxin, isoimperatorin, angelol B, anpubesol, umbelliferone, columbianctin-β-D-glucopyranoside, and isoangelol.[1,2]

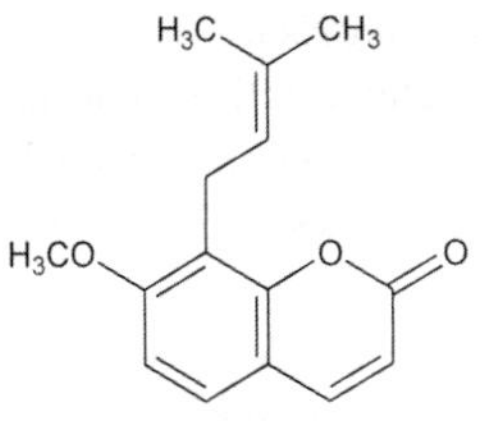

Osthole

PHARMACOLOGICAL EFFECTS

- **Analgesic and anti-inflammatory:** Intraperitoneal injection of *Du Huo* at 2 g/kg has demonstrated marked analgesic and anti-inflammatory effects in mice. It also has a mild sedative effect in mice and rats.[3]
- **Antihypertensive:** *Du Huo* herbal decoction has been shown to have marked antihypertensive action in anesthetized dogs and cats. However, the duration of action is rather short, lasting only 1 to 2 hours.[4]
- **Antiplatelet:** Some constituents isolated from *Du Huo* have demonstrated a mild inhibitory effect on platelet aggregation in mice.[5]
- **Gastrointestinal:** *Du Huo* has demonstrated efficacy in treating peptic ulcers and relieving intestinal spasms in rabbits.[6]
- **Antibiotic:** *Du Huo* has been shown to have an inhibitory effect on *Mycobacterium tuberculosis, E. coli, Bacillus dysenteriae, Salmonella typhi, Pseudomonas aeruginosa,* and *Vibrio cholerae.*[7]
- **Respiratory:** Osthole, an constituent isolated from *Du Huo*, has a non-specific relaxant effect on the trachea by inhibiting the cAMP and cGMP phosphodiesterases, as concluded by an *in vitro* study with guinea-pig trachea. The proposed mechanism of action of osthole is suppression of the contraction response curves of tracheal smooth muscle caused by carbachol, prostaglandin F2 alpha (PGF2 alpha), U46619 (thromboxane A2 analogue) and leukotriene C4 (LTC4), in a concentration-dependent manner. The relaxant actions of osthole were not affected by propranolol, glibenclamide, or removal of the tracheal epithelium.[8]

CLINICAL STUDIES AND RESEARCH

- **Chronic tracheitis:** According to one report, 450 patients with chronic tracheitis were treated with an herbal decoction (9 grams of *Du Huo* and 15 grams of brown sugar) divided equally and taken three to four times daily. The rate of effectiveness was 73.7%.[9]
- **Vitiligo:** In one study, 307 patients with vitiligo were treated with topical application of a *Du Huo* preparation in conjunction with UV ray therapy. The treatment was 54.4% effective.[10]
- **Psoriasis:** According to one report, 92 patients with psoriasis were treated with a *Du Huo* preparation and UV ray therapy. The herb was given after meals, and the UV ray therapy was administered 1.5 to 2 hours after herbal therapy. The rate of effectiveness was 66.3%.[11]

HERB-DRUG INTERACTION

- **Anticoagulant or antiplatelet drugs:** Since components of *Du Huo* have an inhibitory effect on platelet aggregation, *Du Huo* should be given with caution to patients who are taking anticoagulant or antiplatelet drugs.[12] [Note: Examples of anticoagulants include heparin, warfarin (Coumadin) and enoxaparin (Lovenox); and examples of antiplatelets include aspirin, dipyridamole (Persantine), and clopidogrel (Plavix).]

TOXICOLOGY

The LD_{50} in rats via intramuscular injection is 160 mg/kg for xanthotoxin and 945 mg/kg for bergapten. Toxic effects due to gross overdose in mice are liver and kidney damage.[13]

AUTHORS' COMMENTS

Du Huo (Radix Angelicae Pubescentis) and *Qiang Huo* (Rhizoma et Radix Notopterygii) share functions to dispel wind, dry dampness, relieve pain, and treat *bi zheng* (painful obstruction syndrome). They were used interchangeably in the early history of traditional Chinese medicine; in fact, they were not separated as two distinct

Du Huo (Radix Angelicae Pubescentis)

herbs until the *Tang* dynasty. By contrast, *Du Huo* is more commonly used to dispel wind, cold and dampness from the lower body to relieve pain; while *Qiang Huo* is more commonly used to release the exterior and treat aches and pains in the upper body.

References

1. *Xian Dai Zhong Yao Yao Li Xue* (Contemporary Pharmacology of Chinese Herbs), 1997; 400
2. *The Merck Index* 12th edition, Chapman & Hall/CRCnetBASE/Merck, 2000
3. *Zhong Yao Yao Li Yu Ying Yong* (Pharmacology and Applications of Chinese Herbs), 1983; 796
4. *Shan Dong Yi Xue Yuan Xue Bao* (Journal of Shandong University School of Medicine), 1959; (1):43
5. *108th Convention of Japanese Herbology Convention*, 1988
6. *Zhong Yao Xue* (Chinese Herbology), 1998; 281:283
7. *Zhong Yao Yao Li Yu Ying Yong* (Pharmacology and Applications of Chinese Herbs), 1983; 796
8. *Naunyn-Schmiedebergs Archives of Pharmacology*. 349(2):202-8, 1994 Feb.
9. *Wu Han Xin Zhong Yi* (Wuhan New Chinese Medicine), 1971; 3:24
10. *Lin Chuan Pi Fu Ke Za Zhi* (Journal of Clinical Dermatology), 1982; 3:122
11. *Zhong Hua Yi Liao Za Zhi* (Journal of Chinese Therapies), 1983; 3:144
12. Chen, J. Recognition & prevention of herb-drug interactions, *Medical Acupuncture*, Fall/Winter 1998/1999; volume 10/number 2; 9-13
13. *Thromb Haemostasis*, 1989; 62(3):996

Wei Ling Xian (Radix Clematidis)

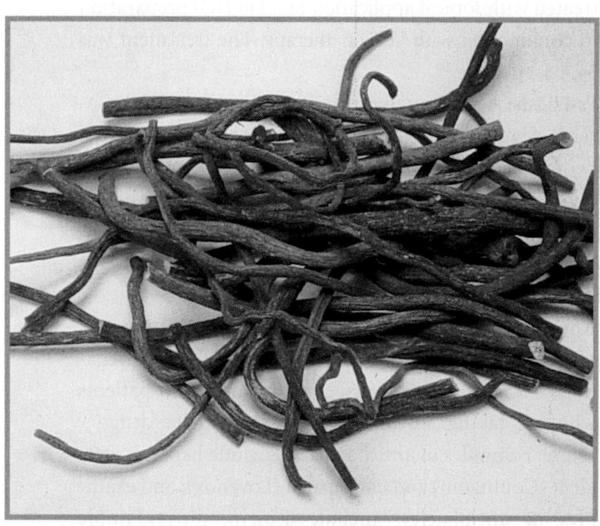

威靈仙 威灵仙

Pinyin Name: *Wei Ling Xian*

Literal Name: "mighty curative immortal," "powerful soul root," "awesome spiritual immortal"

Alternate Chinese Names: *Ling Xian, Tie Jiao Wei Ling Xian*

Original Source: *Xin Xiu Ben Cao* (Newly Revised Materia Medica) by Su Jing in 657-659 A.D.

English Name: clematis, Chinese clematis root, six-petal clematis root

Botanical Name: *Clematis chinensis* Osbeck (*Wei Ling Xian*); *Clematis hexapetala* Pall. (*Mian Tuan Tie Xian Lian*); *Clematis manshurica* Rupr. (*Dong Bei Tie Xian Lian*)

Pharmaceutical Name: Radix Clematidis

Properties: acrid, salty, warm

Channels Entered: Urinary Bladder

CHINESE THERAPEUTIC ACTIONS

1. Dispels Wind and Dampness, Opens Channels and Collaterals, Relieves Pain

***Bi zheng* (painful obstruction syndrome):** Acrid and warm, *Wei Ling Xian* (Radix Clematidis) has excellent dispersing and penetrating functions. It disperses and dispels wind and dampness from the muscles, penetrates and opens peripheral channels and collaterals, and relieves *bi zheng*. Clinically, it is best for musculoskeletal pain, spasms and cramps of the muscles, numbness and pain in the extremities, and difficulty with extension and flexion.

- Low back pain or leg pain: combine *Wei Ling Xian* with *Du Huo* (Radix Angelicae Pubescentis) and warm rice wine.
- Musculoskeletal pain caused by accumulation of wind and dampness or external injuries: use this herb with *Rou Gui* (Cortex Cinnamomi) and *Dang Gui* (Radicis Angelicae Sinensis).

2. Treats Fish Bones Blocking the Throat

Fish bones blocking the throat: *Wei Ling Xian* treats

Wei Ling Xian (Radix Clematidis)

obstruction caused by fish bones lodged in the throat that cannot be swallowed or cleared by vomiting. Combine *Wei Ling Xian*, *Sha Ren* (Fructus Amomi) and sugar. A small amount of vinegar can also be added to the decoction. Swallow the decoction slowly.

Lastly, *Wei Ling Xian* disperses stagnation and accumulations to treat hiccups, phlegm obstruction, and distention, when combined with appropriate herbs.

DOSAGE

5 to 10 grams. Use up to 30 grams of *Wei Ling Xian* to treat obstruction of fish bones in the throat.

CAUTIONS / CONTRAINDICATIONS

- The penetrating action of *Wei Ling Xian* is so strong that it should be used with caution in women who are pregnant, or in patients with generalized weakness, or who have deficiency of qi and/or blood.
- Topical application of *Wei Ling Xian* has been associated with adverse dermatological reactions such as rash, swelling, itching, and pain.[1]

OVERDOSAGE

Though uncommon, incidences of gastrointestinal bleeding caused by overdose of *Wei Ling Xian* have been reported.[2]

CHEMICAL COMPOSITION

Protoanemonin, anemonin, anemonol.[3]

PHARMACOLOGICAL EFFECTS

- **Gastrointestinal:** Administration of *Wei Ling Xian* is associated with increased peristalsis of smooth muscle in the gastrointestinal tract in anesthetized dogs.[4]
- **Cardiovascular:** Water extract of *Wei Ling Xian* has a protective effect against lack of oxygen and blood perfusion to the cardiac muscles in rats.[5]
- **Abortifacient:** Alcohol extract of *Wei Ling Xian* may induce abortion in mice in the second trimester.[6]

CLINICAL STUDIES AND RESEARCH

- **Obstruction by fish bones:** Obstruction caused by fish bones in the throat is commonly treated by administering a decoction of *Wei Ling Xian*, due in part to its effect of relaxing the pharynx to facilitate passage of the bone. In one study, 104 patients with such obstructions were treated with decoction of *Wei Ling Xian* with or without vinegar, with an overall 87.6% rate of effectiveness.[7]
- **Hypertrophic spondylitis:** According to one report, 65 patients with hypertrophic spondylitis were treated with intramuscular injection or trigger point injection of a *Wei Ling Xian* preparation, with marked success.[8]
- **Nausea:** Over 60 patients with nausea were treated with greater than 90% effectiveness, using an herbal decoction containing 30 grams each of *Wei Ling Xian* and honey.[9]
- **Cholelithiasis:** Oral administration of a decoction of 30 to 60 grams of *Wei Ling Xian* was reportedly 87% effective in treating 120 patients with cholelithiasis.[10]

AUTHORS' COMMENTS

According to Dr. He Zi-Jun, herbs such as *Wei Ling Xian* and *Shi Chang Pu* (Rhizoma Acori) are effective for male patients with ejaculation difficulties, as the herbs have penetrating effects to open closed orifices.

Dr. Guan You-Bo states that *Wei Ling Xian*, *Bai Shao* (Radix Paeoniae Alba), *Gan Cao* (Radix Glycyrrhizae), and *Mu Gua* (Fructus Chaenomelis) alleviate the pain and numbness associated with bone spurs of the neck, spine and heels.

Classic texts state that *Wei Ling Xian* "dissolves" fish bones that are obstructing the throat. This statement, however, is not strictly correct, since this herb does not literally "dissolve" fish bones. Instead, *Wei Ling Xian* relaxes the throat muscles, thereby helping to dislodge the obstruction.

References

1. *Zhong Yi Yao Xue Bao* (Report of Chinese Medicine and Herbology), 1978; 2:43
2. *Zhe Jiang Zhong Yi Za Zhi* (Zhejiang Journal of Chinese Medicine), 1991; 26(10):464
3. *Xian Dai Zhong Yao Yao Li Xue* (Contemporary Pharmacology of Chinese Herbs), 1997; 403
4. *Zhong Yao Xue* (Chinese Herbology), 1998; 283:285
5. *Ha Er Bing Yi Ke Da Xue Xue Bao* (Journal of Haerbing University of Medicine), 1980; (2):7
6. *Zhong Yao Xue* (Chinese Herbology), 1998; 283:285
7. *Xin Yi Xue* (New Medicine), 1973; 3:144
8. *Zhong Cao Yao Tong Xun* (Journal of Chinese Herbal Medicine), 1979; 7:13
9. *Zhong Cheng Yao Yan Jiu* (Research of Chinese Patent Medicine), 1982; 2:46
10. *He Nan Zhong Yi* (Henan Chinese Medicine), 1987; 6:22

Fen Fang Ji (Radix Stephaniae Tetandrae)

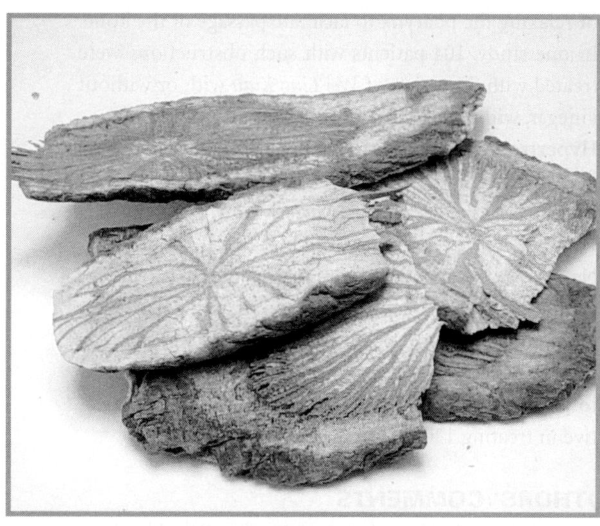

粉防己

Pinyin Name: *Fen Fang Ji*
Alternate Chinese Names: *Han Fang Ji, Fang Ji*
Original Source: *Shen Nong Ben Cao Jing* (Divine Husbandman's Classic of the Materia Medica) in the second century
English Name: stephania, four-stamen stephania root
Botanical Name: *Stephania tetrandra* S. Moore (*Fen Fang Ji*)
Pharmaceutical Name: Radix Stephaniae Tetandrae
Properties: acrid, bitter, cold
Channels Entered: Urinary Bladder, Lung, Kidney
Safety Index: Safe

CHINESE THERAPEUTIC ACTIONS

1. Dispels Wind and Dampness to Relieve Pain

***Bi zheng* (painful obstruction syndrome):** Acrid and bitter, *Fen Fang Ji* (Radix Stephaniae Tetandrae) is an excellent herb to dispel wind and dampness, eliminate stagnation from the channels and collaterals, and relieve pain. Because it is cold and has diuretic effects, it is best for the type of pain caused by heat and dampness.

- *Bi zheng* caused by dampness and heat: use *Fen Fang Ji* with *Yi Yi Ren* (Semen Coicis) and *Can Sha* (Excrementum Bombycis Mori).
- *Bi zheng* from cold and dampness: use it with *Wu Tou* (Radix Aconiti), *Gui Zhi* (Ramulus Cinnamomi), and *Bai Zhu* (Rhizoma Atractylodis Macrocephalae).

2. Promotes Diuresis

Edema: *Fen Fang Ji* regulates water circulation and promotes normal urination. It clears damp-heat in the lower *jiao* and is commonly used to treat edema, ascites, leg *qi* and other disorders associated with water accumulation.

- Edema accompanying deficiency: use *Fen Fang Ji* with *Huang Qi* (Radix Astragali), *Bai Zhu* (Rhizoma Atractylodis Macrocephalae) and *Fu Ling* (Poria).
- Dysuria and constipation due to water accumulation: combine it with *Jiao Mu* (Semen Zanthoxyli Bungeani), *Ting Li Zi* (Semen Descurainiae seu Lepidii) and *Da Huang* (Radix et Rhizoma Rhei).
- Leg *qi*: use this herb with *Fu Ling* (Poria), *Huang Qi* (Radix Astragali), *Gui Zhi* (Ramulus Cinnamomi) and *Gan Cao* (Radix Glycyrrhizae).

DOSAGE

4.5 to 9 grams.

CAUTIONS / CONTRAINDICATIONS

- Bitter and cold, *Fen Fang Ji* is damaging to the middle *jiao* and should be used with caution in patients with yin deficiency, in patients having no signs of damp-heat, or in patients with deficiency and cold of the Spleen and Stomach.

CHEMICAL COMPOSITION

1.2 to 2.3% tetrandrine ($C_{38}H_{42}N_2O_6$), fenfangjine, cyclanoline, menisine, menisidine, oxofangchirine, stephenanthrine, stepholidine, bisbenzylisoquinoline.[1,2]

Tetrandrine

PHARMACOLOGICAL EFFECTS

- **Cardiovascular:** *Fen Fang Ji* has been shown to lower blood pressure, dilate coronary blood vessels, increase blood perfusion to cardiac muscles, and decrease oxygen consumption of cardiac muscles. Tetrandrine has an antiarrhythmic effect.[3]
- **Analgesic and anti-inflammatory:** *Fen Fang Ji* has demonstrated marked analgesic, anti-inflammatory, and antipyretic effects. Some studies have shown *Fen Fang Ji* to be more potent in its analgesic effect than *Yan Hu Suo* (Rhizoma Corydalis), but less potent than morphine.[4]
- **Antispasmodic:** *Fen Fang Ji* has been shown to have a relaxant effect on smooth muscle.[5]

Fen Fang Ji (Radix Stephaniae Tetandrae)

CLINICAL STUDIES AND RESEARCH

- **Hypertension:** Intravenous infusion of fenfangjine lowered blood pressure in 84.07% of patients. Of 270 patients, 256 received the herbs via intravenous injection and 14 via oral ingestion. The study also indicated that this treatment was effective for patients in hypertensive crisis.[6]
- **Coronary artery disorders:** Intravenous injections of an herbal preparation (2 to 3 mg/kg of fenfangjine A with 20 ml of normal saline) were administered twice daily for 2 weeks. The study concluded this therapy to be effective for patients with coronary artery disorder with hypertension.[7]
- **Silicosis:** In one study, 33 patients were treated with 200 to 300 mg of tetrandrine, three times daily after meals, for a total of 3 years, with marked improvement. The first and second courses of treatment were each 6 months, separated by 3-to-6 month intervals of rest. The third and fourth courses of treatment were 3 months each, with 2 months of rest.[8]
- **Lung cancer:** Intravenous injections of an herbal preparation (180 to 300 mg of fenfangjine A mixed with normal saline or D5W) were given to 97 patients with lung cancer, with promising results. Fenfangjine A appeared to have an inhibitory effect on the DNA and RNA of the cancer cells.[9]

HERB-DRUG INTERACTION

- **Diuretics:** *Fen Fang Ji* has a diuretic effect. Though this potential interaction has not been documented as an actual occurrence, concurrent use with diuretic drugs may lead to increased elimination of water and/or electrolytes.[10] [Note: Examples of diuretics include chlorothiazide, hydrochlorothiazide, furosemide (Lasix), bumetanide (Bumex), and torsemide (Demadex).]

SUPPLEMENT

- 木防己 *Mu Fang Ji* (Radix Cocculi Trilobi), *Cocculus trilobus* (Thunb) DC, promotes the circulation of water and eliminates water accumulation. Though *Mu Fang Ji* is similar in name to *Fen Fang Ji* or *Han Fang Ji*, it must not be confused with or used interchangeably with either of these herbs. Proper identification must be made prior to prescribing and dispensing this herb. [Note: Historically, '*Mu Fang Ji*' was used as an alternate name for *Fen Fang Ji* or *Han Fang Ji*, contributing to confusion.]

  Fen Fang Ji and *Han Fang Ji* both refer to the plant *Stephania tetrandra*. *Fen Fang Ji* is the standard pinyin name according to *Zhong Hua Ren Min Gong He Guo Yao Dian* (Chinese Herbal Pharmacopoeia by People's Republic of China) published in 2000. *Han Fang Ji* is the pinyin name used by most contemporary doctors and herbalists.

AUTHORS' COMMENTS

Fen Fang Ji (Radix Stephaniae Tetandrae) and *Guang Fang Ji* (Radix Aristolochiae Fangchi), despite similar names and functions, have completely different toxicological profiles and should never be used interchangeably. Please refer to *Guang Fang Ji* for additional details on toxicology.

References

1. *Xian Dai Zhong Yao Yao Li Xue* (Contemporary Pharmacology of Chinese Herbs), 1997; 282-283, 1997; 405-410
2. *The Merck Index* 12th edition, Chapman & Hall/CRCnetBASE/Merck, 2000
3. *Zhong Yao Xue* (Chinese Herbology), 1998; 285-287
4. Ibid.
5. Ibid.
6. *Wu Han Yi Xue Za Zhi* (Wuhan Journal of Medicine), 1964; 5:358
7. *Zhong Hua Nei Ke Za Zhi* (Chinese Journal of Internal Medicine), 1985; 11:682
8. *Chinese Journal of Tuberculosis and Respiratory Tract Disorders*, 1981; 6:321
9. *Zhong Yi Za Zhi* (Journal of Chinese Medicine), 1980; 3:597
10. Chen, J. Recognition & prevention of herb-drug interactions, *Medical Acupuncture*, Fall/Winter 1998/1999; volume 10/number 2; 9-13

Guang Fang Ji (Radix Aristolochiae Fangchi)

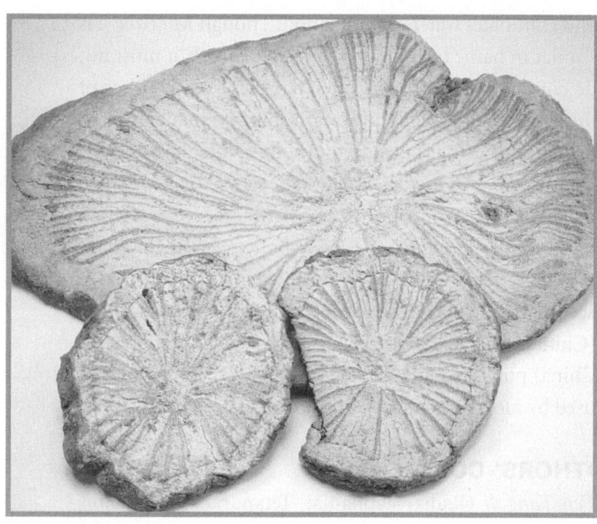

廣防己 广防己

Pinyin Name: *Guang Fang Ji*
Original Source: *Shen Nong Ben Cao Jing* (Divine Husbandman's Classic of the Materia Medica) in the second century
English Name: aristolochia root, fangchi root, southern fangchi root
Botanical Name: *Aristolochia fangchi* Y.C. Wu ex L.D.
Pharmaceutical Name: Radix Aristolochiae Fangchi
Properties: acrid, bitter, cold
Channels Entered: Urinary Bladder, Lung
Safety Index: toxic

CHINESE THERAPEUTIC ACTIONS

1. Dispels Wind and Dampness to Relieve Pain

***Bi zheng* (painful obstruction syndrome):** Acrid, bitter, and cold, *Guang Fang Ji* (Radix Aristolochiae Fangchi) treats *bi zheng* characterized by damp-heat or wind-damp.

2. Promotes Diuresis

Edema: *Guang Fang Ji* regulates water circulation and promotes normal urination. It treats edema in the legs, and dysuria.

DOSAGE

4.5 to 9 grams.

CAUTIONS / CONTRAINDICATIONS

- Use with caution in patients having deficiency and cold of the Spleen and Stomach.

CHEMICAL COMPOSITION

Aristolochic acid I, II.[1,2]

COOH
NO_2
OCH_3

Aristolochic Acid

PHARMACOLOGICAL EFFECTS

- **Anti-inflammatory**: Aristolochic acid has an anti-inflammatory action via its regulatory effect in prostaglandin synthesis.[3]
- **Immunostimulant**: In a human study, administration of aristolochic acid at a dosage of 0.9 mg/kg for 3 days was associated with increased phagocytic activities.[4]

TOXICOLOGY

Guang Fang Ji is toxic and its use should be avoided. The toxic component of *Guang Fang Ji* is generally believed to be aristolochic acid. *Guang Fang Ji* has been shown to have a toxic effect on the liver, kidneys and adrenal glands. Therefore, it is particularly contraindicated in patients who have impairment of these organs. It should be used with extreme caution in patients who are taking hepatotoxic or nephrotoxic medications.

According to one report in the early 1990s, a weight loss clinic in Belgium treated a group of women with a slimming preparation that contained a blend of pharmaceuticals and herbs: fenfluramine, diethylpropion, cascara powder, belladonna extract, acetazolamide, "*Fang Ji*" and *Hou Po* (Cortex Magnoliae Officinalis). In those who ingested this preparation, 33 cases of nephropathy were reported initially. To date, more than 100 cases of nephropathy have been reported. Many hypotheses have been published on why there was an "outbreak" of nephropathy in Belgium. Some suggest that the primary reason for nephropathy was the substitution of *Guang Fang Ji* (Radix Aristolochiae Fangchi) for *Fen Fang Ji* (Radix Stephaniae Tetandrae). Some believe the culprit to be the concurrent use of *Guang Fang Ji* (containing aristolochic acid) with another potential nephrotoxin, acetazolamide. Others propose that the main reason for the outbreak was the use of *Guang Fang Ji* in powder (uncooked) instead of decoction (cooked). Decoction is believed to be a much safer mode of administration because the concentration of aristolochic acid is much lower in decoction, since it has low water solubility.[5,6]

Guang Fang Ji (Radix Aristolochiae Fangchi)

AUTHORS' COMMENTS

Guang Fang Ji (Radix Aristolochiae Fangchi) and *Fen Fang Ji* (Radix Stephaniae Tetandrae) have similar names and functions. *Guang Fang Ji* more effectively dispels wind and dampness to treat *bi zheng* (painful obstruction syndrome). *Fen Fang Ji* more strongly promotes diuresis to treat edema. Despite their similarities, these two herbs, have completely different toxicological profiles and should never be used interchangeably.

References

1. *Chang Yong Zhong Yao Cheng Fen Yu Yao Li Shou Ce* (A Handbook of the Composition and Pharmacology of Common Chinese Drugs), 1994; 898-899
2. *The Merck Index* 12th edition, Chapman & Hall/CRCnetBASE/Merck, 2000
3. McGuffin M, Hobbs C, et al. *Botanical Safety Handbook*, CRC Press, 1997; 131-132
4. Ibid.
5. Depierreux M, et al. Pathological aspects of a newly-described nephropathy related to the prolonged use of Chinese herbs. *American Journal of Kidney Diseases*, Aug 1994; vol. 24(2):172-80
6. Vanherweghem JL et al. Rapidly progressive interstitial fibrosis in young women: association with slimming regimen including Chinese herbs. *Lancet* 1993; 341:387-91

Xu Chang Qing (Radix Cynanchi Paniculati)

徐長卿 徐长卿

Pinyin Name: *Xu Chang Qing*
Original Source: *Shen Nong Ben Cao Jing* (Divine Husbandman's Classic of the Materia Medica) in the second century
English Name: paniculate swallowwort root
Botanical Name: *Cynanchum paniculatum* (Bge.) Kitag. (*Xu Chang Qing*)
Pharmaceutical Name: Radix Cynanchi Paniculati
Properties: acrid, warm
Channels Entered: Liver, Stomach

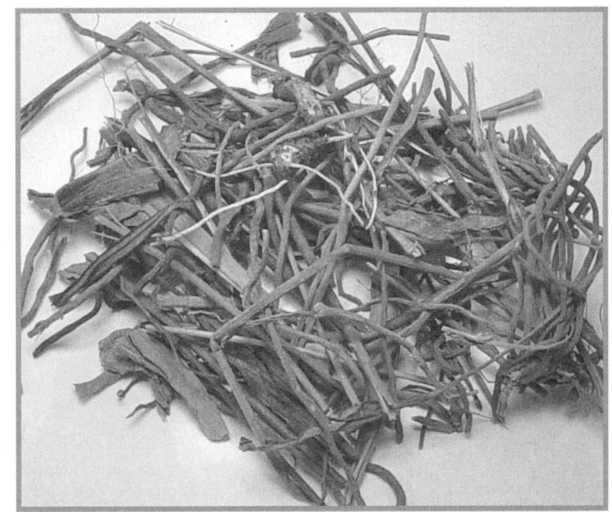

CHINESE THERAPEUTIC ACTIONS

1. Dispels Wind and Relieves Pain

***Bi zheng* (painful obstruction syndrome):** *Xu Chang Qing* (Radix Cynanchi Paniculati) is widely used with other herbs to treat pain caused by wind-damp, qi stagnation, cold accumulation and blood stagnation. It has also been used recently to treat trauma-related, cancer-related and post-surgical pain.

- *Bi zheng* due to wind and dampness: use *Xu Chang Qing* with *Wei Ling Xian* (Radix Clematidis) and *Wu Jia Pi* (Cortex Acanthopanacis).
- Back pain and soreness: use it with *Du Zhong* (Cortex Eucommiae), *Xu Duan* (Radix Dipsaci) and *Du Huo* (Radix Angelicae Pubescentis).
- Epigastric and abdominal pain: combine it with *Gao Liang Jiang* (Rhizoma Alpiniae Officinarum) and *Xiang Fu* (Rhizoma Cyperi).
- Trauma-related pain and menstrual cramps: use it with *Wu Ling Zhi* (Excrementum Trogopteri seu Pteromi) and *Tao Ren* (Semen Persicae).

2. Relieves Itching and Eliminates Toxins

Itching of the skin: *Xu Chang Qing* has a strong effect to dispel wind and relieve itching. It is commonly used for eczema, wind rashes and other dermatological disorders where itching is the predominant sign.

Xu Chang Qing (Radix Cynanchi Paniculati)

- Itching: use *Xu Chang Qing* with *Ku Shen Gen* (Radix Sophorae Flavescentis), *Di Fu Zi* (Fructus Kochiae) and *Bai Xian Pi* (Cortex Dictamni), both internally and topically.

Sores, carbuncles, and snake bites: *Xu Chang Qing* eliminates toxins and can be used for swelling and pain caused by toxins.

- Snake bite, sores and carbuncles: use this herb with *Ban Bian Lian* (Herba Lobeliae Chinensis) and *Ye Ju Hua* (Flos Chrysanthemi Indici).

DOSAGE

3 to 10 grams in decoction, 1.5 to 3 grams in powdered form. *Xu Chang Qing* may be prescribed up to 10 to 20 grams when the entire plant is used. Because this herb is aromatic or acrid in nature, it should not be cooked for a prolonged period of time.

CHEMICAL COMPOSITION

Paeonol, isopaeonol, cynapanoside A,B,C; cynatratoside B.[1]

PHARMACOLOGICAL EFFECTS

- **Analgesic:** Intraperitoneal injection of *Xu Chang Qing* at 10 g/kg in mice showed marked analgesic action that started 10 minutes after injection, and lasted for up to 60 minutes.[2]
- **Sedative:** Intraperitoneal injection of *Xu Chang Qing* at 5 to 10 g/kg in mice showed marked sedative effects by decreasing spontaneous movement and reaction to external stimuli, for up to 60 minutes.[3]
- **Effect on temperature regulation:** Intraperitoneal injection of a *Xu Chang Qing* preparation at 3 g/kg lowered body temperature by approximately 0.9° C for up to 30 minutes.[4]

TOXICOLOGY

The LD_{50} for intraperitoneal injection of *Xu Chang Qing* is 32.93 g/kg in mice.[5]

References

1. *Xian Dai Zhong Yao Yao Li Xue* (Contemporary Pharmacology of Chinese Herbs), 1997; 459
2. *Xin Yi Yao Xue Za Zhi* (New Journal of Medicine and Herbology), 1973; (10):30
3. Ibid.
4. *Zhong Cao Yao* (Chinese Herbal Medicine), 1983; 14(10):26
5. *Xin Yi Yao Xue Za Zhi* (New Journal of Medicine and Herbology), 1973; (10):30

Can Sha (Excrementum Bombycis Mori)

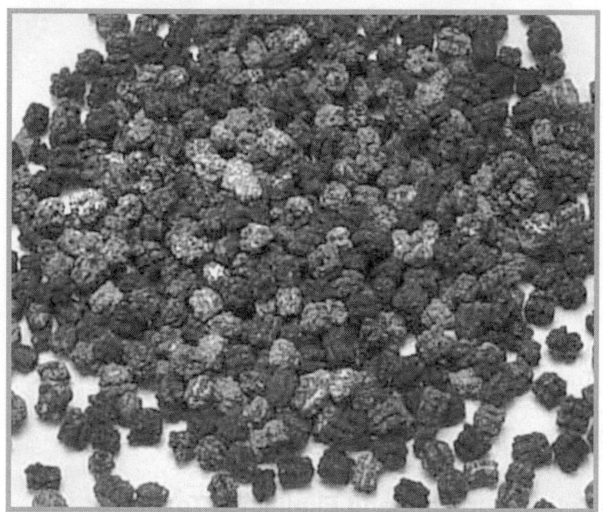

蠶砂 蚕砂

Pinyin Name: *Can Sha*
Literal Name: "silkworm sand"
Alternate Chinese Names: *Can Shi, Yuan Can Sha, Wan Can Sha*
Original Source: *Ming Yi Za Zhu* (Miscellaneous Records of Famous Physicians) by Tao Hong-Jing in 500 A.D.
English Name: silkworm droppings, silkworm feces
Zoological Name: *Bombyx mori* L. (*Jia Can*)
Pharmaceutical Name: Excrementum Bombycis Mori
Properties: sweet, acrid, warm
Channels Entered: Liver, Spleen, Stomach

CHINESE THERAPEUTIC ACTIONS

1. Dispels Wind and Dampness

***Bi zheng* (painful obstruction syndrome) and itching skin:** Acrid and warm, *Can Sha* (Excrementum Bombycis Mori) dispels wind, dries dampness, and opens peripheral channels and collaterals. Clinically, it

Can Sha (Excrementum Bombycis Mori)

treats disorders characterized by accumulation of wind and dampness in the extremities, such as *bi zheng*, muscle aches and pain, itching and eczema.

- *Bi zheng* due to wind-damp: use *Can Sha* with *Fen Fang Ji* (Radix Stephaniae Tetandrae), *Yi Yi Ren* (Semen Coicis) and *Lian Qiao* (Fructus Forsythiae).
- Hemiplegia: place *Can Sha* in a cotton bag, heat it thoroughly with steam, then place the bag directly on the affected area.
- Headache from accumulation of dampness: use this herb with *Bai Zhi* (Radix Angelicae Dahuricae) and *Chuan Xiong* (Rhizoma Ligustici Chuanxiong).
- Itching, eczema and other dermatological disorders: use *Can Sha* internally or topically.

2. Dissolves Turbidity and Dampness, Harmonizes the Stomach

Vomiting, diarrhea, headache and abdominal cramps: *Can Sha* dissolves dampness from the middle *jiao* and harmonizes the Spleen and Stomach. It relieves nausea, vomiting, spasms, cramps and pain.

- Nausea, vomiting and abdominal cramps: use *Can Sha* with *Mu Gua* (Fructus Chaenomelis), *Wu Zhu Yu* (Fructus Evodiae) and *Huang Qin* (Radix Scutellariae).
- Headache due to turbidity and accumulated dampness: use this herb with *Bai Zhi* (Radix Angelicae Dahuricae) and *Chuan Xiong* (Rhizoma Ligustici Chuanxiong).

DOSAGE

5 to 10 grams.

CHEMICAL COMPOSITION

Phytol, β-sitosterol, ergosterol, bombiprenone, protocatechuric acid, caffeic acid.[1]

CLINICAL STUDIES AND RESEARCH

- **Urticaria:** In one study, 19 patients with urticaria were treated with satisfactory results using both oral and topical applications of *Can Sha*. The oral treatment protocol was to cook 60 grams of this substance in water and take the decoction twice daily. The topical solution was prepared by cooking 120 grams of *Can Sha* in water and applying the decoction topically as an herbal wash, twice daily, for 20 minutes per treatment.[2]
- **Profuse menstrual bleeding:** Profuse menstrual bleeding may be effectively treated by ingesting 6 grams of charred *Can Sha* with grain-based liquor.[3]
- **Leukopenia:** In one report, 265 patients with leukopenia were treated with a preparation of *Can Sha* three times daily, for 30 days per course of treatment, with an 88.7% overall rate of effectiveness.[4]

References

1. *Xian Dai Zhong Yao Yao Li Xue* (Contemporary Pharmacology of Chinese Herbs), 1997; 463
2. *Zhe Jiang Zhong Yi Yao* (Zhejiang Chinese Medicine and Herbology), 1976; 2:47
3. *Zhong Yi Za Zhi* (Journal of Chinese Medicine), 1964; 3:24
4. *Yi Xue Yan Jiu Tong Xun* (Report of Medical Studies), 1988; 4:23

Song Jie (Lignum Pini Nodi)

松節 松节

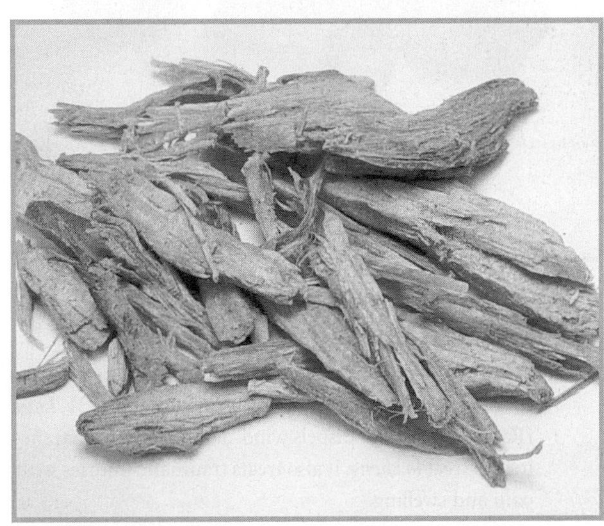

Pinyin Name: *Song Jie*
Literal Name: "pine joint"
Alternate Chinese Names: *Ma Wei Song, You Song Jie*
Original Source: *Ming Yi Za Zhu* (Miscellaneous Records of Famous Physicians) by Tao Hong-Jing in 500 A.D.
English Name: knotty pine
Botanical Name: *Pinus tabulaeformis* Carr. (*Mu You Song*); *Pinus massoniana* Lamb. (*Ma Wei Song*)
Pharmaceutical Name: Lignum Pini Nodi
Properties: bitter, warm
Channels Entered: Liver

Song Jie (Lignum Pini Nodi)

CHINESE THERAPEUTIC ACTIONS

Dispels Wind, Dries Dampness and Relieves Pain

Bi zheng **(painful obstruction syndrome), traumatic injuries:** Typical manifestations include fixed, deep pain in the joints with difficulty flexing or moving. *Song Jie* (Lignum Pini Nodi) has a warm, drying nature that makes it useful for dispelling pain caused by cold and dampness. *Song Jie* is often soaked in grain-based liquor and used with pepper to potentiate its effect to eliminate stagnation and relieve pain.

- *Bi zheng*: use *Song Jie* with *Hai Feng Teng* (Caulis Piperis Kadsurae), *Du Huo* (Radix Angelicae Pubescentis) and *Dang Gui* (Radicis Angelicae Sinensis).
- Trauma-related pain: use it with *Ru Xiang* (Gummi Olibanum), *Mo Yao* (Myrrha) and *Su Mu* (Lignum Sappan).

DOSAGE

10 to 15 grams.

CHEMICAL COMPOSITION

α-pinene, β-pinene, resin.[1]

SUPPLEMENT

- 松葉 / 松叶 *Song Ye* (Folium Pini), first cited in *Ming Yi Za Zhu* (Miscellaneous Records of Famous Physicians) by Tao Hong-Jing in 500 A.D., is the leaf of the same plant as *Song Jie*. *Song Ye* is bitter and warm, and dispels wind and dries dampness. It also kills parasites and stops itching. The recommended dose for *Song Ye* is 6 to 15 grams.
- 松果 *Song Guo* (Fructus Pini), first cited in *Ming Yi Za Zhu* (Miscellaneous Records of Famous Physicians) by Tao Hong-Jing in 500 A.D., is the fruit or pine cone of the same plant as *Song Jie*. *Song Guo* is bitter and warm. It dispels wind, dries dampness, moistens the intestines and relieves pain. The recommended dosage of *Song Guo* is 6 to 10 grams.

References

1. *Zhong Yao Xue* (Chinese Herbology), 1998; 307-308

Qi Ye Lian (Radix Schefflerae)

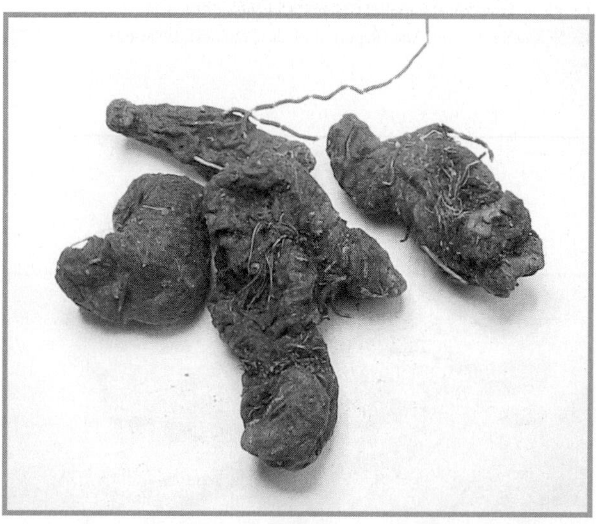

七葉蓮 七叶莲

Pinyin Name: *Qi Ye Lian*
Literal Name: "seven-leaf lotus"
Alternate Chinese Names: *Qi Ye Teng, Qi Jia Pi*
English Name: schefflera, scandent schefflera root, Taiwan schefflera root
Botanical Name: *Schefflera arboricola* Hayata; *Schefflera kwangsiensis* Merr. Ex Li.
Pharmaceutical Name: Radix Schefflerae
Properties: bitter, acrid, warm
Channels Entered: Liver

CHINESE THERAPEUTIC ACTIONS

Dispels Wind-Damp, Relieves Pain

Bi zheng **(painful obstruction syndrome):** *Qi Ye Lian* (Radix Schefflerae) dispels wind-damp from the extremities to treat *bi zheng*. It also treats traumatic injuries with pain and swelling.

- *Bi zheng*: fry *Qi Ye Lian* with grain-based liquor, and apply it topically.
- Traumatic injuries: grind the herb into paste and apply topically.

Qi Ye Lian (Radix Schefflerae)

DOSAGE

10 to 15 grams. *Qi Ye Lian* is used both internally and externally.

CAUTIONS / CONTRAINDICATIONS

- *Qi Ye Lian* should be used with caution during pregnancy.

CHEMICAL COMPOSITION

Organic acid, mucic acid, fumaric acid, butanedioic acid.[1]

PHARMACOLOGICAL EFFECTS

- **Analgesic**: *Qi Ye Lian* has a marked analgesic effect, which is achieved with oral ingestion, intramuscular injection, and trigger point injection of the herb.[2]

CLINICAL STUDIES AND RESEARCH

- **Pain:** *Qi Ye Lian* has been used *in vivo* to treat various disorders involving pain, including kidney stones, gallstones, fractured bones, pancreatitis, and arthritis.[3]
- **Anesthesia:** Injection of *Qi Ye Lian* into ear points was effective in patients requiring extensive dental work, such as tooth extraction. The rate of effectiveness was 89.4% among 112 patients.[4]

References

1. *Xian Dai Zhong Yao Yao Li Xue* (Contemporary Pharmacology of Chinese Herbs, 1997; 482)
2. *Zhong Yao Da Ci Dien* (Dictionary of Chinese Herbs), 1975; 17-18
3. Ibid.
4. Ibid.

Lei Gong Teng (Radix Tripterygii Wilfordii)

雷公藤 雷公藤

Pinyin Name: *Lei Gong Teng*
Literal Name: "thunder vine"
Original Source: *Zhong Guo Yao Ci Dian* (Journal of Chinese Medicinal Plants)
English Name: tripterygium, common broad lily root
Botanical Name: *Tripterygium wilfordii* Hook. f. (*Lei Gong Teng*)
Pharmaceutical Name: Radix Tripterygii Wilfordii
Properties: bitter, acrid, cool
Channels Entered: Liver
Safety Index: toxic

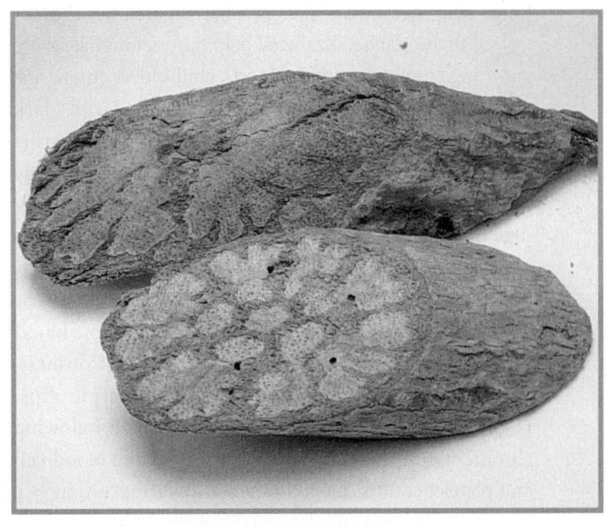

CHINESE THERAPEUTIC ACTIONS

1. Dispels Wind and Dampness

***Bi zheng* (painful obstruction syndrome):** *Lei Gong Teng* (Radix Tripterygii Wilfordii) relieves pain and reduces swelling, in patients who have swollen joints and difficulty moving. It can be used alone or with other antirheumatic herbs.

- *Bi zheng*: use *Lei Gong Teng* with *Fen Fang Ji* (Radix Stephaniae Tetandrae).

2. Kills Parasites and Eliminates Toxins

Maggots, rats and snake venom: *Lei Gong Teng* is used topically as an antitoxin for wounds infested by maggots, or caused by rat or snake bites.

DOSAGE

5 to 12 grams. Peel and discard the root bark of *Lei Gong Teng* before decocting. Prolonged decoction (between one and two hours) is recommended to decrease its toxicity. *Lei Gong Teng* should be taken after meals.

Lei Gong Teng (Radix Tripterygii Wilfordii)

CAUTIONS / CONTRAINDICATIONS

- *Lei Gong Teng* is contraindicated in pregnancy.
- It should be used with caution in geriatric and pediatric patients.
- It should also be used with caution for patients with heart, stomach and spleen disorders.
- *Lei Gong Teng* is toxic, and should not be used for patients who have compromised hepatic functions.[1]

OVERDOSAGE

The entire tripterygium plant is toxic. The toxicity of the root and bark is greater than that of other parts of the plant. The fresh form is more toxic than the dried form that has been stored for at least a year. Toxic signs include local irritation of the gastrointestinal tract, damage to the central nervous system, internal bleeding and necrosis of the organs. In severe cases, gross overdose of *Lei Gong Teng* may cause bleeding in the stomach, intestines, liver and lungs. Other symptoms include dizziness, dry mouth, palpitations, necrosis of mucous membranes and irregular menstruation.

Any adverse reactions generally occur within 2 to 3 hours after ingestion of the herb. Early reaction is characterized by headache, dizziness, palpitation, fatigue, severe vomiting (sometimes with blood), chills, fever (up to 40° C), continuous abdominal pain, diarrhea (with dark watery stools), generalized aches and pain, tachycardia and irregular heart rhythms. In some cases, patients may present with frequent urination with urgency, and feelings of stabbing pain during urination. Other patients may exhibit delayed symptoms after 2 to 3 days, such as low back pain, hair loss, facial edema, decreased or increased urinary output, and in severe cases, low blood pressure, low body temperature, altered consciousness, convulsions, difficult respiration and purple lips. Hematological disorders have also been noted following chronic use of the herb, with decreased white blood cell and platelet counts due to bone marrow suppression.[2]

TREATMENT OF OVERDOSAGE

Early-stage overdose (within 4 hours of ingestion) should be treated with emetic methods or gastric lavage to eliminate the offending agent from the body. Successful cases of detoxification have been reported using gastric lavage, even with gross overdose.[3]

Systemic reaction to the herb is generally treated with *Feng Wei Cao* (Herba Pteris) or *San Qi* (Radix Notoginseng) given as decoction.[4]

While this herb is toxic to humans, it has no toxicity for goats and rabbits. It was found that goats or rabbits that consume *Lei Gong Teng* regularly have developed resistance and antibodies to the toxicity of the herb. The consumption of fresh blood (200 to 300 ml) from goats and rabbits has been used successfully to treat overdose of the herb, using the rationale that the blood of these two animals contains substances that antidote the herb.[5]

CHEMICAL COMPOSITION

Alkaloids (wilfordine, wilforine, wilforidine, wilforgine, wilfortrine, wilforzine, wilformine, wilfornine, euonine, celacinnine, celafurine, celabenzine, neowilforine, regilidine), terpenoids (triptolide T13, tripdiolide, tripterolide, triptonide, triptolidenol T9, hypolide, triptonoterpenol, triptophenolide methylether, neotriptophenolide, isotriptophenolide, isoneotriptophenolide, triptonoterpene, triptonoterpene methylether, tripdioltonide, tripdiolide T8, triptriolide T11, triptolide T10, wilforlide A T1, triptotriterpenoidal lactone A, wilforlide B, triptotriterpenic acid A T3, triptotriterpenic acid B T2, triptoterpenic acid C T28, selaspermic acid, wilfornide, triptofordin A,B,C-1,C-2, D).[6]

PHARMACOLOGICAL EFFECTS

- **Antiviral:** Sesquiterpenes isolated from *Lei Gong Teng* were found to have moderate virucidal activity against several enveloped viruses including HSV-1, HCMV, measles virus and influenza A virus. The mechanism of action has been attributed to the suppressed viral protein synthesis of infected cells at early steps of viral replication and exerted inhibition of translation of the transcripts of the immediate early genes.[7]
- **Antiarthritic:** According to *in vitro* studies, administration of an extract of *Lei Gong Teng* once daily for 14 days exhibited a marked effect to suppress the development of arthritis, antibody production and delayed-type hypersensitivity to Type II collagen. On the other hand, therapeutic administration of the herbal extract did not affect the clinical course of the disease.[8]

CLINICAL STUDIES AND RESEARCH

- **Rheumatoid arthritis**: In one study, the combination of *Lei Gong Teng* and *Fen Fang Ji* (Radix Stephaniae Tetandrae) was found to have a powerful suppressive effect on human immune responses for treatment of rheumatoid arthritis. The mechanisms of action included inhibition of prostaglandin E2 secretion from monocytes, and inhibited IL-1, IL-6, IL-8, and tumor necrosis factor-alpha.[9]
- **Glomerulonephritis**: According to one study, administration of *Lei Gong Teng* was shown to reduce proteinuria in 102 patients with glomerulonephritis. The treatment protocol was to administer 15 to 18 grams of the herb per day, for a total of one to nine months of treatment. The rate of effectiveness was 72.5%.[10]

Lei Gong Teng (Radix Tripterygii Wilfordii)

TOXICOLOGY

While the side effects of *Lei Gong Teng* are related mostly to gastrointestinal upset, infertility and suppression of lymphocyte proliferation, one fatality has been reported. After ingesting the herb, the patient developed hypovolemic shock and cardiac damage, and died three days later. There was no information available on the prior physical condition of the deceased nor what dosage of the herb was consumed.[11]

AUTHORS' COMMENTS

According to Dr. Zhu Fang-Shou, *Lei Gong Teng* is excellent for rheumatoid arthritis, various *bi zheng* (painful obstruction syndrome) imbalances, and the pain associated with bone spurs. However, because *Lei Gong Teng* is toxic, the daily dose should be kept between 5 and 12 grams, with a maximum of 15 grams. In addition, *Lei Gong Teng* should be cooked for at least 60 minutes, before the addition of other herbs, and then cooked for another 15 minutes. Side effects are minimal when this herb is prescribed following the proper dosage and preparation. *Lei Gong Teng* is contraindicated in patients with pre-existing cardiovascular or hepatic disorders.

References

1. *Int J Cardiol*, 1995 April; 49(2):173-7
2. *Zhong Yao Du Li Xue* (Toxicology of Chinese Herbs), 1989; 154-155
3. *Wu Han Yi Xue Yuan Xue Bao* (Journal of Wuhan University School of Medicine), 1981; 4-67
4. *Hu Nan Yi Yao Za Zhi* (Hunan Journal of Medicine and Herbology), 1977; 5:3
5. *Zhong Yao Du Li Xue* (Toxicology of Chinese Herbs), 1989; 156-157
6. *Xian Dai Zhong Yao Yao Li Xue* (Contemporary Pharmacology of Chinese Herbs), 1997; 413
7. *Journal of Antimicrobial Chemotherapy*. 37(4):759-68, 1996 Apr.
8. *Immunopharmacology*. 39(2):117-26, 1998 May
9. Chang, W-Y, et al. *The Effects of Traditional Antirheumatic Herbal Medicines on Immune Response Cells. The Journal of Rheumatology* 1997; 24:3
10. *Zhong Hua Nei Ke Za Zhi* (Chinese Journal of Internal Medicine), 1981; 20(4):216
11. *Int J Cardiol*, 1995 April; 49(2):173-7

Qin Jiao (Radix Gentianae Macrophyllae)

秦艽 秦艽

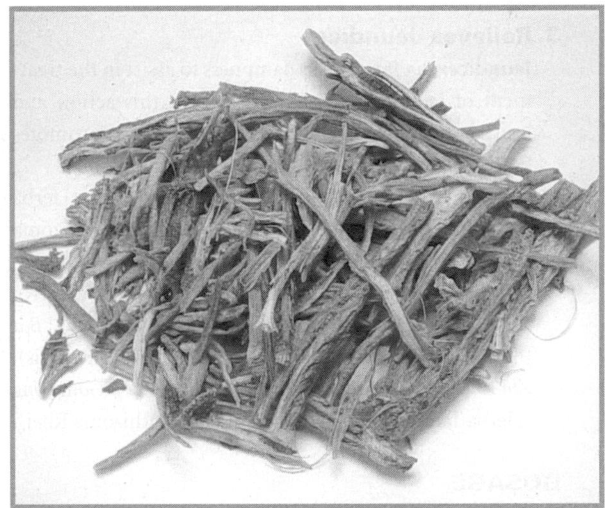

Pinyin Name: *Qin Jiao*
Alternate Chinese Names: *Zuo Qin Jiao*
Original Source: *Shen Nong Ben Cao Jing* (Divine Husbandman's Classic of the Materia Medica) in the second century
English Name: gentiana macrophylla root
Botanical Name: *Gentiana macrophylla* Pall. (*Qin Jiao*); *Gentiana straminea* Maxim. (*Ma Hua Qin Jiao*); *Gentiana crassicaulis* Duthie ex Burk. (*Cu Jin Qin Jiao*); *Gentiana dahurica* Fisch. (*Xiao Qin Jiao*)
Pharmaceutical Name: Radix Gentianae Macrophyllae
Properties: bitter, acrid, cool
Channels Entered: Stomach, Liver, Gallbladder

CHINESE THERAPEUTIC ACTIONS

1. Dispels Wind and Dampness, Opens Channels and Collaterals, Relaxes the Sinews

***Bi zheng* (painful obstruction syndrome):** Acrid and bitter, *Qin Jiao* (Radix Gentianae Macrophyllae) has a dispersing nature that dispels dampness and opens peripheral channels and collaterals. It treats musculoskeletal and joint disorders, whether acute or chronic, hot or cold in nature. Since *Qin Jiao* is cool, it is most effective for *bi zheng* caused by heat, with redness, swelling and inflammation. It also relieves stiffness and

Qín Jiāo (Radix Gentianae Macrophyllae)

tightness of the joints.

- Hot *bi zheng* with redness, swelling and pain: use *Qin Jiao* with *Fen Fang Ji* (Radix Stephaniae Tetandrae), *Zhi Mu* (Radix Anemarrhenae) and *Ren Dong Teng* (Caulis Lonicerae).
- Cold *bi zheng* with pain and difficulty moving: use *Qin Jiao* with *Du Huo* (Radix Angelicae Pubescentis), *Gui Zhi* (Ramulus Cinnamomi) and *Fu Zi* (Radix Aconiti Lateralis Praeparata).
- Paralysis and post-stroke complications: use it with *Tian Ma* (Rhizoma Gastrodiae), *Dang Gui* (Radicis Angelicae Sinensis) and *Chuan Xiong* (Rhizoma Ligustici Chuanxiong).

2. Clears Deficiency Heat

Steaming bones sensations, tidal fever: Unlike other herbs that dispel wind-damp, *Qin Jiao* is not drying in nature. This makes it an excellent herb to clear deficiency heat without consuming yin or body fluids. Other typical signs of yin deficiency include afternoon fever, flushed cheeks, emaciation, night sweats, a dry and red tongue with a crack in the center, and a thready, rapid pulse.

- Deficiency heat characterized by steaming bones sensations and tidal fever: use *Qin Jiao* with *Qing Hao* (Herba Artemisiae Annuae), *Zhi Mu* (Radix Anemarrhenae), and *Bie Jia* (Carapax Trionycis). **Exemplar Formula:** *Qin Jiao Bie Jia San* (Gentiana Macrophylla and Soft-shelled Turtle Shell Powder).

3. Relieves Jaundice

Jaundice: *Qin Jiao* dispels dampness to assist in the treatment of jaundice. It is rather mild in this action and must be combined with other herbs. It also promotes bowel movement and dispels water accumulation.

- Jaundice: use this herb with *Yin Chen Hao* (Herba Artemisiae Scopariae), *Da Huang* (Radix et Rhizoma Rhei) and *Zhi Zi* (Fructus Gardeniae).
- Infectious hepatitis with jaundice: combine it with *Yin Chen Hao* (Herba Artemisiae Scopariae), *Huang Bai* (Cortex Phellodendri), *Che Qian Zi* (Semen Plantaginis), *Zhi Zi* (Fructus Gardeniae), *Fu Ling* (Poria), *Pu Gong Ying* (Herba Taraxaci) and *Da Huang* (Radix et Rhizoma Rhei).

DOSAGE

5 to 10 grams in decoction.

CAUTIONS / CONTRAINDICATIONS

- Use *Qin Jiao* with caution in patients with deficiency and cold of the Spleen and Stomach, or those with loose stools.
- Use of this herb may be associated with drowsiness and sedation. Therefore, individuals who take this herb should exercise caution if driving or operating heavy machinery.

CHEMICAL COMPOSITION

Gentianine, gentianidine, gentiopieroside, gentianel, homoorientin, sapoknaretin.[1]

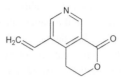

Gentianine

PHARMACOLOGICAL EFFECTS

- **Anti-inflammatory:** Gentianine has shown marked anti-inflammatory action via stimulation of the endocrine system to increase the secretion of hormones by the adrenal glands.[2]
- **Sedative:** Administration of *Qin Jiao* has demonstrated sedative effects via inhibition of the central nervous system in mice and rats. It also prolonged sleeping time when combined with barbiturates. However, a high dose of *Qin Jiao* is sometimes associated with excitation of the central nervous system.[3]
- **Cardiovascular:** Gentianine has been shown to lower blood pressure and decrease heart rate in guinea pigs, dogs and rabbits. The antihypertensive effect has a short duration, but is not affected by injection of atropine.[4]
- **Hyperglycemic:** Administration of gentianine is associated with an increase in blood glucose levels in mice. The mechanism of the hyperglycemic effect is attributed to stimulation of the endocrine system. When the adrenal glands of subjects were removed, gentianine could no longer raise blood glucose levels.[5]

CLINICAL STUDIES AND RESEARCH

- **Acute infantile jaundice or infectious hepatitis:** Twenty patients with jaundice or hepatitis characterized by heat were given *Qin Jiao*, *Huang Qin* (Radix Scutellariae) and *Lian Qiao* (Fructus Forsythiae); and patients with jaundice or hepatitis characterized by dampness were given *Qin Jiao*, *Cang Zhu* (Rhizoma Atractylodis), *Bai Zhu* (Rhizoma Atractylodis Macrocephalae) and *Hou Po* (Cortex Magnoliae Officinalis). Each course of treatment was 14 days. Positive results were reported in both groups.[6]
- **Tooth extraction:** *Qin Jiao* and *Fen Fang Ji* (Radix Stephaniae Tetandrae) showed marked analgesic and anti-inflammatory effectiveness in 26 patients who had tooth extractions. The herbs were given as 300 mg capsules, with equal amounts of each herb. All patients received 2 capsules 30 minutes prior to the procedure, and every 6 hours after the procedure for 3 days.[7]

HERB-DRUG INTERACTION

- **Sedatives:** *Qin Jiao* has an inhibitory effect on the central

Qin Jiao (Radix Gentianae Macrophyllae)

nervous system to induce sedation. It potentiates the sedative effect of barbiturates.[8] [Note: Many categories of drugs induce sedation, such as antihistamines, narcotic analgesics, barbiturates, benzodiazepines and many others.]

TOXICOLOGY

The LD_{50} for gentianine in mice is 480 mg/kg via oral administration, 350 mg/kg via intraperitoneal, and 250 to 300 mg/kg via intravenous injections.[9]

AUTHORS' COMMENTS

Dr. Wei Jia states that *Qin Jiao* is one of the best herbs to relieve joint pain associated with weather changes.

References

1. *Xian Dai Zhong Yao Yao Li Xue* (Contemporary Pharmacology of Chinese Herbs), 1997; 398
2. *Chang Yong Zhong Yao Cheng Fen Yu Yao Li Shou Ce* (A Handbook of the Composition and Pharmacology of Common Chinese Drugs), 1994; 1479:1482
3. *Zhong Yao Yao Li Yu Ying Yong* (Pharmacology and Applications of Chinese Herbs), 1983; 854:297
4. Ibid.
5. *Yao Xue Xue Bao* (Journal of Herbology), 1965; 12(6):357
6. *Shang Hai Zhong Yi Yao Za Zhi* (Shanghai Journal of Chinese Medicine and Herbology), 1965; 7:10
7. *Zhijin Medicine*, 1987; 1:73
8. *Zhong Yao Yao Li Yu Ying Yong* (Pharmacology and Applications of Chinese Herbs), 1983; 854:297
9. *Sheng Li Xue Bao* (Physiology News), 1959; 23(4):311

Hong Gu She (Radix Kadsura Japonicae)

紅骨蛇 红骨蛇

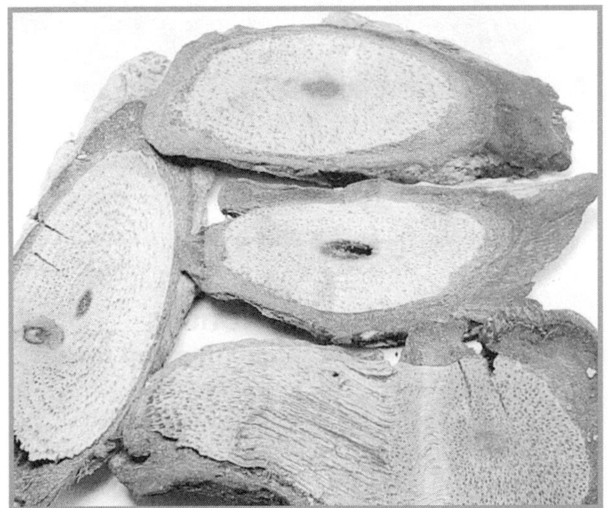

Pinyin Name: *Hong Gu She*
Literal Name: "red bone snake"
Alternate Chinese Names: *Hong Gu She Tou*
English Name: kadsura
Botanical Name: *Kadsura japonica* Dun
Pharmaceutical Name: Radix Kadsura Japonicae
Properties: acrid, bitter, cool
Channels Entered: Lung, Liver, Stomach

CHINESE THERAPEUTIC ACTIONS

1. Relieves Pain

Hong Gu She (Radix Kadsura Japonicae) opens the peripheral channels and collaterals to alleviate pain, relax the tendons, and relieve spasms and cramps.

- Wind-heat with headache and body aches: use *Hong Gu She* with *Dao Di Wu Gong* (Rhizoma Heliminthostachytis).
- Postpartum exterior invasion: use it with *Ji Xiang Teng* (Caulis Paederiae).

2. Reduces Swelling and Inflammation

Diarrhea with abdominal pain and vomiting: use *Hong Gu She* with *Ji Xue Cao* (Herba Centellae) and *Xian Feng Cao* (Herba Bidentis).

- Dizziness with an imbalance in the inner ear due to deficiency: combine this herb with *Suan Zao Ren* (Semen Zizyphi Spinosae), *Shan Yao* (Rhizoma Dioscoreae), *Dang Gui* (Radicis Angelicae Sinensis), and *Long Yan Rou* (Arillus Longan).
- Dizziness with an imbalance in the inner ear due to excess: use *Hong Gu She* with *Ban Xia* (Rhizoma Pinelliae), *Bai Zhu* (Rhizoma Atractylodis Macrocephalae), *Tian Ma* (Rhizoma Gastrodiae), *Gou Teng* (Ramulus Uncariae cum Uncis), *Long Dan Cao*

Hong Gu She (Radix Kadsura Japonicae)

(Radix Gentianae) and *Huang Qin* (Radix Scutellariae).
- Diabetes: add *Gou Qi Gen* (Radix Lycii).

DOSAGE

3 to 9 grams.

CHEMICAL COMPOSITION

Xyloglucoronit $(C_{11}H_{16}O_{10})_5$.

Tou Gu Cao (Caulis Impatientis)

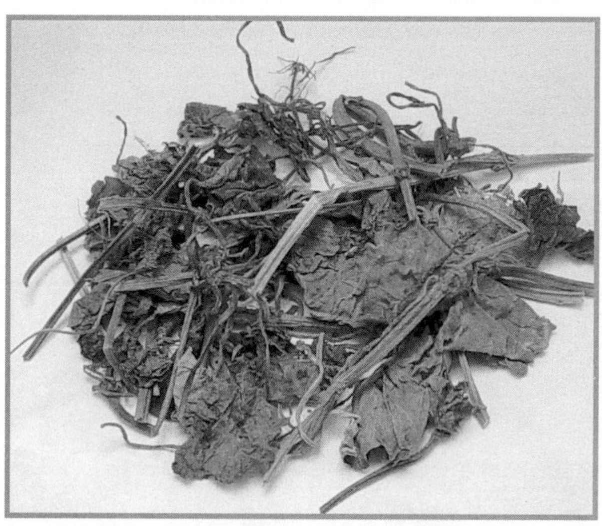

透骨草 透骨草

Pinyin Name: *Tou Gu Cao*
Literal Name: "penetrate the bone herb"
English Name: garden balsam
Botanical Name: *Impatiens balsamina* Line
Pharmaceutical Name: Caulis Impatientis
Properties: bitter, slightly sweet and acrid, cool
Channels Entered: Liver, Spleen, Kidney

CHINESE THERAPEUTIC ACTIONS

1. Invigorates Blood Circulation and Breaks Blood Stasis

Tou Gu Cao (Caulis Impatientis) treats external and traumatic injuries characterized by bruises, swelling, inflammation, blood stasis and pain. In addition to moving blood stagnation, it reduces swelling and promotes generation of tissues.

- Trauma-related pain and bleeding: use *Tou Gu Cao* with *Ru Xiang* (Gummi Olibanum), *Mo Yao* (Myrrha) and *Chi Shao* (Radix Paeoniae Rubrae).

2. Clears Heat, Eliminates Toxins, Cools Blood and Relieves Pain

- Toxic sores, carbuncles and swellings: apply *Tou Gu Cao* topically.
- Burns: apply it topically.
- Hematemesis, abnormal uterine bleeding, epistaxis and hematuria due to heat: use this herb with *Zhi Zi* (Fructus Gardeniae), *Pu Huang* (Pollen Typhae), *Huang Qin* (Radix Scutellariae), and *Huai Hua* (Flos Sophorae).

3. Drains Damp-Heat

- Acute jaundice with hepatitis, fever, poor appetite and hepatomegaly: use *Tou Gu Cao* with *Cang Zhu* (Rhizoma Atractylodis), *Hou Po* (Cortex Magnoliae Officinalis), *Huang Bai* (Cortex Phellodendri), *Long Dan Cao* (Radix Gentianae) and *Xia Ku Cao* (Spica Prunellae). Formulas to combine with this herb included *Long Dan Xie Gan Tang* (Gentiana Decoction to Drain the Liver) and *Jia Wei Xiao Yao San* (Augmented Rambling Powder).

DOSAGE

10 to 20 grams in decoction.

AUTHORS' COMMENTS

There are three different herbs with the pinyin names "*Tou Gu Cao*:" Caulis Impatientis, Caulis Leptostachya and Caulis Speranskla Tuberculata. Detailed information on the properties and uses of Caulis Leptostachya and Caulis Speranskla Tuberculata was unavailable at the time of publication.

Yi Wu Gen (Radix Elaeagni)

宜梧根

Pinyin Name: *Yi Wu Gen*
English Name: elaeagnus
Botanical Name: *Elaeagnus oldhamii* Maxim
Pharmaceutical Name: Radix Elaeagni
Properties: bland, cool
Channels Entered: Liver

CHINESE THERAPEUTIC ACTIONS

1. Dispels Wind and Dampness

***Bi zheng* (painful obstruction syndrome):** *Yi Wu Gen* (Radix Elaeagni) dispels wind and dampness to relieve *bi zheng*, muscle aches, and pain.

- *Bi zheng*: use *Yi Wu Gen* with *Huang Jin Gui* (Caulis Vanieriae) and *Wan Dian Jin* (Radix Ilicis Asprellae).
- Weakness of extremities: use it with *Yi Tiao Gen* (Radix Moghaniae), *Wang Bu Liu Xing* (Semen Vaccariae), *Ji Xue Teng* (Caulis Spatholobi) and *Gu Sui Bu* (Rhizoma Drynariae).
- Chronic arthritis: combine it with *Ding Shu Xiu* (Herba Elephantopus Scaber), *Xiao Jin Ying* (Fructus Rosae Cymosae) and *Bai Long Chuan Hua Tou* (Radix Clerodendron Paniculatum).
- Postpartum exterior wind invasion: add *Da Feng Teng* (Caulis Sinomenii).

2. Reduces Swelling and Dispels Stagnation

- Traumatic injury: use *Yi Wu Gen* with *San Qi* (Radix Notoginseng), *Ru Xiang* (Gummi Olibanum), *Mo Yao* (Myrrha), *Chuan Shan Long* (Rhizoma Dioscoreae Nipponicae) and *Yi Tiao Gen* (Radix Moghaniae).

DOSAGE

3 to 9 grams.

Hai Fu Rong (Herba Limonium Wrightii)

海芙蓉 海芙蓉

Pinyin Name: *Hai Fu Rong*
Alternate Chinese Names: *Huang Hua Shi Cong Rong, Hai Huang Jin*
English Name: limonium
Botanical Name: *Limonium wrightii* (Hance) O. Ktze var. *luteum* (Hara)
Pharmaceutical Name: Herba Limonium Wrightii
Properties: acrid, bitter, cold
Channels Entered: Liver, Kidney

CHINESE THERAPEUTIC ACTIONS

1. Dispels Wind and Dampness

***Bi zheng* (painful obstruction syndrome):** *Hai Fu Rong* (Herba Limonium Wrightii) treats *bi zheng* caused by heat. The chief characteristics of this imbalance include redness, burning and swelling of the joints. This herb is also used to treat arthritis and neuralgia.

- Arthritis, neuralgia: use *Hai Fu Rong* with *Ji Xiang Teng* (Caulis Paederiae), *Da Feng Teng* (Caulis Sinomenii) and *Qin Jiao* (Radix Gentianae Macrophyllae).

Traumatic Injuries: *Hai Fu Rong* relieves pain associated with traumatic injuries, with redness, local inflammation and bruises.

- Pain of traumatic injuries: use it with *Huang Jin Gui* (Caulis Vanieriae) and *E Bu Shi Cao* (Herba Centipedae).

2. Lowers Blood Pressure

- **Hypertension:** use *Hai Fu Rong* with *Cha Chi Huang* (Herba Stellariae Aquaticae) and *Xia Ku Cao* (Spica Prunellae).

DOSAGE

3 to 12 grams.

Qing Feng Teng (Caulis Sinomenii)

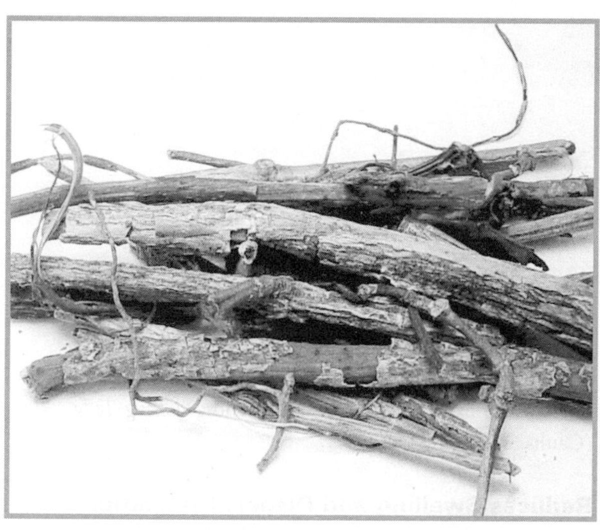

青風藤 青风藤

Pinyin Name: *Qing Feng Teng*
Literal Name: "blue-green wind vine"
Alternate Chinese Names: *Da Feng Teng, Feng Teng, Lao Teng, Hai Feng Teng*
Original Source: *Tu Jing Ben Cao* (Illustrated Classic of the Materia Medica) by Su Song in 1061
English Name: sinomenium, Orient vine stem, Japanese sabia stem
Botanical Name: *Sinomenium acutum* (Thunb.) Rehd. et Wils. (*Qing Teng*), *Sinomenium acutum* (Thunb.) Rehd. et Wils. var. *cinoreum* Rehd. et Wils. (*Mao Qing Teng*)
Pharmaceutical Name: Caulis Sinomenii
Properties: bitter, neutral
Channels Entered: Liver

CHINESE THERAPEUTIC ACTIONS

Dispels Wind and Relieves Pain

***Bi zheng* (painful obstruction syndrome):** *Qing Feng Teng* (Caulis Sinomenii) dispels wind and dampness, opens the channels and relieves pain. It is often used for patients experiencing joint tightness and pain with swelling. This herb also treats leg *qi*. It is used alone or with other antirheumatic herbs in grain-based liquor or in decoction.

- Arthroncus of the knee, rheumatoid arthritis: use *Qing Feng Teng* with *Huang Jin Gui* (Caulis Vanieriae), *Rou Cong Rong* (Herba Cistanches), *Chuan Niu Xi* (Radix Cyathulae), *Xu Duan* (Radix Dipsaci), *Gu Sui Bu* (Rhizoma Drynariae) and *Yi Wu Gen* (Radix Elaeagni).
- Back pain, soreness of tendons and muscles, infantile paralysis or hemiplegia: use *Qing Feng Teng* both as a tea and as a bath for soaking.

DOSAGE

6 to 12 grams.

CHEMICAL COMPOSITION

Sinomenine, sinoacutine, disinomenine, magnoflorine, N-acetylsinomenine.[1,2]

Sinomenine

PHARMACOLOGICAL EFFECTS

- **Analgesic and anti-inflammatory:** *Qing Feng Teng* has demonstrated marked analgesic and anti-inflammatory effectiveness. Although the exact mechanism is unclear, it has been proposed that it works via stimulation of the endocrine system, which consequently increases production of adrenal hormones. In laboratory studies, the analgesic effect was estimated to be 1/10th – 2/5th that of morphine. However, in comparison with morphine, there is no evidence of dependence associated with use of *Qing Feng Teng*, and tolerance develops much more slowly.[3]
- **Antihypertensive:** Administration of *Qing Feng Teng* is associated with a rapid decline of blood pressure. Repeated dosing, however, is associated with tolerance. The exact mechanism of this action is unclear.[4]
- **Antitussive:** Marked antitussive effect was demonstrated in rats and cats.[5]

CLINICAL STUDIES AND RESEARCH

- **Arthritis:** Administration of *Qing Feng Teng* was reported to be effective for treating pain in 93.4% of 311 patients. The herb was given in various dosage forms, including injection, decoction, and pills. Full details of the study were unavailable.[6]
- **Arrhythmia:** In a clinical study, 60 patients with various arrhythmia problems were treated with a preparation of *Qing Feng Teng* for 2 weeks, with satisfactory results.[7]

TOXICOLOGY

Rare cases of eczema and neutropenia have been reported following the use of *Qing Feng Teng*.[8]

Qing Feng Teng (Caulis Sinomenii)

References

1. *Xian Dai Zhong Yao Yao Li Xue* (Contemporary Pharmacology of Chinese Herbs), 1997; 445
2. *The Merck Index* 12th edition, Chapman & Hall/CRCnetBASE/Merck, 2000.
3. *Zhong Yao Xue* (Chinese Herbology), 1998; 303
4. Ibid.
5. Ibid.
6. *Zhong Cao Yao Tong Xun* (Journal of Chinese Herbal Medicine), 1979; 11:40
7. *Xi An Yi Ke Da Xue Xue Bao* (Journal of Xian University School of Medicine), 1988; 2:133
8. *Shan Xi Zhong Yi* (Shanxi Chinese Medicine), 1987; 2:54

Ma An Teng (Herba Ipomoea Pes-caprae)

馬鞍藤 马鞍藤

Pinyin Name: *Ma An Teng*
Alternate Chinese Names: *Er Ye Hong Su*
English Name: beach morning glory
Botanical Name: *Ipomoea pres-caprae* (L.) Sweet.
Pharmaceutical Name: Herba Ipomoea Pes-caprae
Properties: acrid, bitter, neutral
Channels Entered: Liver, Kidney, Large Intestine

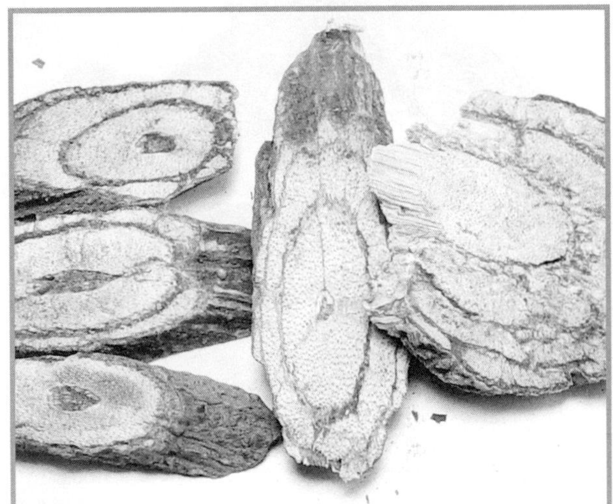

CHINESE THERAPEUTIC ACTIONS

1. Dispels Wind and Dampness

***Bi zheng* (painful obstruction syndrome):** *Ma An Teng* (Herba Ipomoea Pes-caprae) dispels wind and dampness to treat arthritis, rheumatoid arthritis, and soreness and pain in the back, tendons and bones.

- Arthritis, rheumatoid arthritis: use *Ma An Teng* with *Po Bu Zi Ye* (Folium Cordia Dichotoma), *Gou Teng* (Ramulus Uncariae cum Uncis), *Ji Xue Teng* (Caulis Spatholobi) and *Dang Gui* (Radicis Angelicae Sinensis).
- Soreness and pain in the back, tendons and bones: combine it with *Wan Dian Jin* (Radix Ilicis Asprellae) and *Huang Jin Gui* (Caulis Vanieriae).

2. Reduces Carbuncles and Disperses Nodules

- Nodules, carbuncles, furuncles and swelling: apply *Ma An Teng* externally.
- Bleeding hemorrhoids: use it with *Zhen Ren Huo Ming Yin* (True Man Decoction to Revitalize Life) and *Huai Hua* (Flos Sophorae).

DOSAGE

3 to 12 grams.

Section 2 — Wind-Damp Dispelling and Channel- and Collateral-Opening Herbs

Mu Gua (Fructus Chaenomelis)

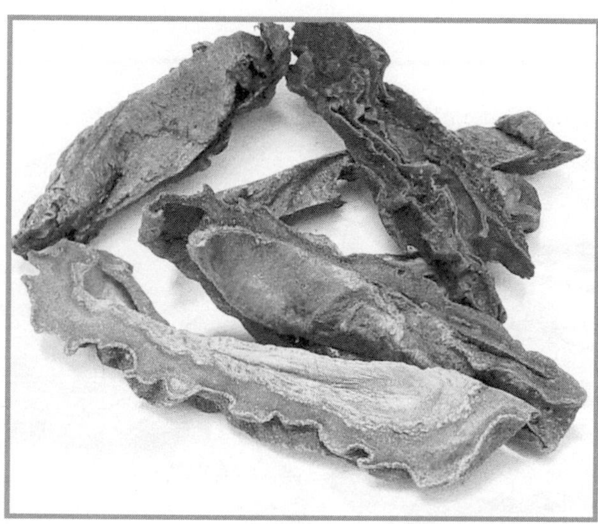

木瓜

Pinyin Name: *Mu Gua*
Literal Name: "wood fruit," "wood melon"
Alternate Chinese Names: *Zuo Pi Mu Gua, Guan Pi Mu Gua, Xuan Mu Gua*
Original Source: *Ming Yi Za Zhu* (Miscellaneous Records of Famous Physicians) by Tao Hong-Jing in 500 A.D.
English Name: chaenomeles, papaya
Botanical Name: *Chaenomeles lagenaria* (Loisel.) Koidz. (*Zhou Pi Mu Gua*); *Chaenomeles sinensis* (Thouin) Koehne (*Guang Pi Mu Gua*).
Pharmaceutical Name: Fructus Chaenomelis
Properties: sour, warm
Channels Entered: Liver, Spleen

CHINESE THERAPEUTIC ACTIONS

1. Relaxes Sinews, Opens Channels and Collaterals

***Bi zheng* (painful obstruction syndrome), stiffness and spasms of the sinews:** Warm yet not drying, sour yet not astringent, *Mu Gua* (Fructus Chaenomelis) enters the Liver to nourish the muscles and tendons. It is one of the most commonly used herbs to treat musculoskeletal disorders characterized by muscle cramps, spasms, and stiffness. *Mu Gua* is useful in treatment of both acute and chronic conditions, and is most effective for treating the lower body.

- Muscle stiffness and spasms with difficult movement: use *Mu Gua* with *Ru Xiang* (Gummi Olibanum), *Mo Yao* (Myrrha) and *Sheng Di Huang* (Radix Rehmanniae).
- Muscle spasms due to blood deficiency: combine it with *Dang Gui* (Radicis Angelicae Sinensis) and *Bai Shao* (Radix Paeoniae Alba).
- Weakness and atrophy of muscles in the lower extremities: use it with *Du Huo* (Radix Angelicae Pubescentis).

Leg *qi* with edema, swelling and pain:

- Leg *qi* with swelling and pain in the lower extremities: add *Mu Gua* to *Wu Zhu Yu* (Fructus Evodiae), *Zi Su Ye* (Folium Perillae) and *Bing Lang* (Semen Arecae).

2. Dissolves Dampness and Harmonizes the Stomach

Vomiting, diarrhea and cramps: *Mu Gua* dissolves dampness from the middle *jiao* and harmonizes the Spleen and Stomach to relieve nausea, vomiting and abdominal pain. Its sour taste helps to generate body fluids, so *Mu Gua* is also useful for treating severe abdominal cramps, or calf muscle and lower leg cramps following excessive loss of fluids from vomiting.

- Nausea, vomiting and cramps: use *Mu Gua* with *Xiao Hui Xiang* (Fructus Foeniculi) and *Wu Zhu Yu* (Fructus Evodiae).

Mu Gua (Fructus Chaenomelis)

3. Promotes Digestion

Indigestion or food stagnation: *Mu Gua* has mild action to promote digestion and relieve food stagnation.

Degenerative gastritis: Because of its sour taste, *Mu Gua* has been used to promote gastric secretion in patients with degenerative gastritis where there is atrophy of the gastric glands.

DOSAGE

6 to 12 grams.

CHEMICAL COMPOSITION

Oleanolic acid, malic acid, saponins, tannins.[1]

PHARMACOLOGICAL EFFECTS

- **Hepatoprotective:** Administration of *Mu Gua* in mice had a marked protective effect on the liver by lowering elevated liver enzyme levels and preventing the death of hepatocytes.[2]
- **Antineoplastic:** *Mu Gua* was found to have an inhibiting effect on the growth of cancer cells in mice.[3]

CLINICAL STUDIES AND RESEARCH

- **Icteric jaundice:** According to one report, 70 patients with acute icteric jaundice were treated with 5 to 10 grams of *Mu Gua* three times daily, with marked improvement. Therapeutic benefits included symptomatic improvement, relief of jaundice, and improvement of liver function.[4]
- **Acute bacterial dysentery:** Administration of 5 pills of a preparation of *Mu Gua* (equivalent to approximately 5-6 grams of dried herb) to patients with acute bacterial dysentery three times daily for 5 to 7 days, was 96.28% effective. The study also reported complete recovery in 85.98% of these cases.[5]

SUPPLEMENT

The following are other species of herbs from various regions of China that have been used for the same function as *Mu Gua: Xi Nan Mu Gua* (Fructus Chaenomeles Lagenaria Cathayensis), *Wei Shi Mu Gua* (Fructus Chaenomeles Lagenaria Wilsonii), *Chiu Mu Gua* (Fructus Chaenomeles Speciosa), *Mao Ye Mu Gua* (Fructus Chaenomeles Cathayensis), and *Xi Zhang Mu Gua* (Fructus Chaenomeles Thibetica).

AUTHORS' COMMENTS

Dr. Chang Jie-An states that *Mu Gua* helps patients who suffer from diarrhea or loose stools containing undigested food. These patients exhibit weak digestive functions, in which diarrhea occurs immediately following intake of greasy, cold or raw food. *Mu Gua* contains digestive enzymes and is sour, which binds the intestines to control diarrhea.

References

1. *Xian Dai Zhong Yao Yao Li Xue* (Contemporary Pharmacology of Chinese Herbs), 1997; 434-435
2. *Fu Jian Zhong Yi Yao* (Fujian Chinese Medicine and Herbology), 1985; 16(6):35
3. *Zhong Cao Yao Tong Xun* (Journal of Chinese Herbal Medicine), 1975; (6)18
4. *Fu Jian Zhong Yi Yao* (Fujian Chinese Medicine and Herbology), 1987; 2:24
5. *Zhong Hua Yi Xue Za Zhi* (Chinese Journal of Medicine), 1984; 11:689

Luo Shi Teng (Caulis Trachelospermi)

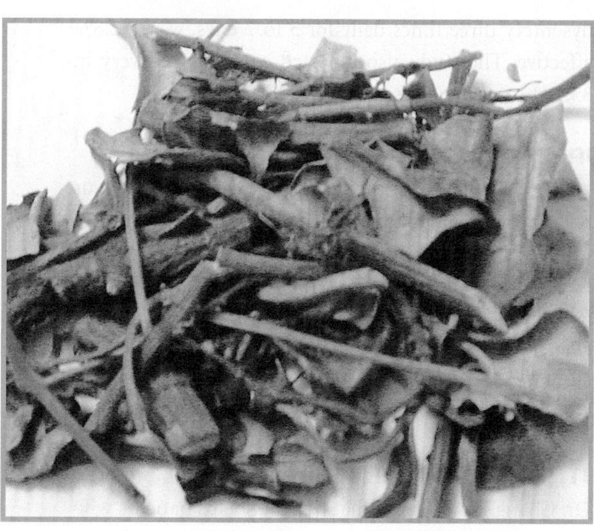

絡石藤 络石藤

Pinyin Name: *Luo Shi Teng*
Literal Name: "collateral stone vine"
Alternate Chinese Names: *Luo Shi*
Original Source: *Shen Nong Ben Cao Jing* (Divine Husbandman's Classic of the Materia Medica) in the second century
English Name: star jasmine vine, Chinese star jasmine stem, confederate jasmine stem
Botanical Name: *Trachelospermum jasminoides* (Lindl.) Lem. (*Luo Shi*)
Pharmaceutical Name: Caulis Trachelospermi
Properties: bitter, cool
Channels Entered: Heart, Liver

CHINESE THERAPEUTIC ACTIONS

1. Dispels Wind, Opens Channels and Collaterals

***Bi zheng* (painful obstruction syndrome):** *Luo Shi Teng* (Caulis Trachelospermi) treats musculoskeletal pain, and muscle spasms and cramps caused by wind obstructing the channels and collaterals. Since *Luo Shi Teng* is cool in thermal property, it is most effective for *bi zheng* caused by heat.

- *Bi zheng*: use *Luo Shi Teng* with *Wu Jia Pi* (Cortex Acanthopanacis) and *Niu Xi* (Radix Cyathulae seu Achyranthis) with other herbs to strengthen the sinews in herbal decoction.
- Pain and spasms of the extremities: add *Ren Dong Teng* (Caulis Lonicerae).

2. Cools Blood, Reduces Swelling

Sore throat: *Luo Shi Teng* cools blood and reduces swelling and inflammation. It treats soreness and swelling of the throat, and abscesses and sores on the skin.

- Sore and swollen throat: cook *Luo Shi Teng* alone and slowly sip the herbal decoction.

Abscesses and sores:

- Skin abscesses and sores: use *Luo Shi Teng* with *Zao Jiao Ci* (Spina Gleditsiae), *Gua Lou Shi* (Fructus Trichosanthis), and *Ru Xiang* (Gummi Olibanum).

DOSAGE

6 to 15 grams. *Luo Shi Teng* is commonly used as decoction or herbal wine.

CHEMICAL COMPOSITION

Coronaridine, voacangine, 19-epi-voacangavine, ibogaine, tabernaemontanine, vobasine, apigenin, campesterol, arctiin, tracheloside, nortracheloside, matairesinoside, dambonitol, cymarose.[1,2]

Arctiin

PHARMACOLOGICAL EFFECTS

- **Antibiotic:** Decoction of *Luo Shi Teng* has an inhibitory effect on *Salmonella typhi*, *Staphylococcus aureus*, and *Bacillus dysenteriae*.[3]
- **Cardiovascular:** At low doses, arctiin stimulates the central nervous system to increase the rate of respiration. At high doses, it inhibits the central nervous system to decrease respiration rate, dilate blood vessels and decrease blood pressure.[4]

References

1. *Chang Yong Zhong Yao Cheng Fen Yu Yao Li Shou Ce* (A Handbook of the Composition and Pharmacology of Common Chinese Drugs), 1994; 1473-1474
2. Yan X, Zhou J, Xie G, *Traditional Chinese Medicines Molecular Structures, Natural Sources and Applications*; Ashgate, 1999; 432
3. *Zhong Cao Yao Xue* (Study of Chinese Herbal Medicine), 1976: 867
4. *Chang Yong Zhong Yao Cheng Fen Yu Yao Li Shou Ce* (A Handbook of the Composition and Pharmacology of Common Chinese Drugs), 1994; 1473:1474

Sang Zhi (Ramulus Mori)

桑枝

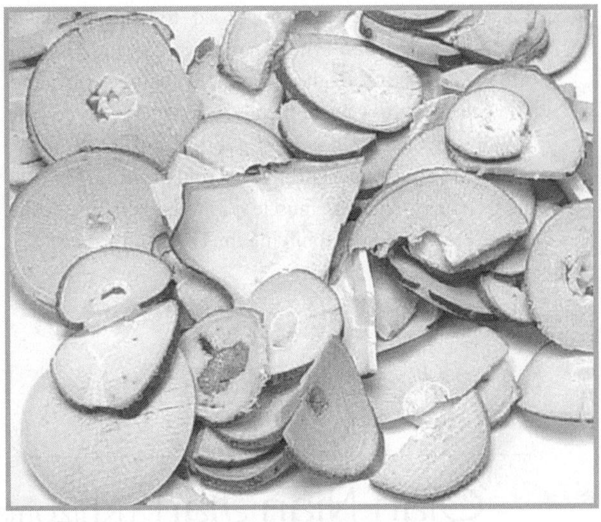

Pinyin Name: *Sang Zhi*
Literal Name: "mulberry twigs"
Original Source: *Tu Jing Ben Cao* (Illustrated Classic of the Materia Medica) by Su Song in 1061
English Name: mulberry twig
Botanical Name: *Morus alba* L. (*Sang Shu*)
Pharmaceutical Name: Ramulus Mori
Properties: bitter, neutral
Channels Entered: Liver

CHINESE THERAPEUTIC ACTIONS

1. Dispels Wind, Opens Channels and Collaterals

***Bi zheng* (painful obstruction syndrome), tightness and spasms of the limbs:** *Sang Zhi* (Ramulus Mori) dispels wind and dampness, opens peripheral channels and collaterals, and benefits the joints. Clinically, it treats *bi zheng*, muscle aches and pain, and muscle spasms and cramps. It is most effective for *bi zheng* caused by heat, with pain in the upper extremities.

- Wind-heat *bi zheng* of the shoulder and arms: use *Sang Zhi* as a single herb.
- Generalized *bi zheng*: use it with *Fen Fang Ji* (Radix Stephaniae Tetandrae), *Wei Ling Xian* (Radix Clematidis), and *Du Huo* (Radix Angelicae Pubescentis).
- Hemiplegia or post-stroke paralysis: use a large dosage of this herb.

2. Promotes Diuresis and Reduces Swelling

Edema: *Sang Zhi* regulates water circulation to treat edema and dysuria involving painful limbs.

DOSAGE

10 to 30 grams. Unprocessed *Sang Zhi* has a slow and moderate overall action. Frying it with grain-based liquor will enhance its effect to dispel wind and dampness, open channels and collaterals, and relieve pain.

CHEMICAL COMPOSITION

Mulberrin, mulberrochromene, cyclomulberrin, cyclomulberrochromene, morin, dihydromorin, dihydrokaempferol, maclurin.[1]

PHARMACOLOGICAL EFFECTS

- **Antibiotic:** *Sang Zhi* has an inhibiting influence against *Staphylococcus aureus*, *Bacillus dysenteriae*, *Salmonella typhi*, and numerous pathogenic fungi.[2,3]
- **Others:** It has antihypertensive, antineoplastic and spasmolytic effects.[4,5]

CLINICAL STUDIES AND RESEARCH

- **Tendonitis:** In one study, patients with tendonitis of the elbow were treated with herbal formulas. Of 15 patients, there was complete recovery in 10 cases, marked improvement in 4 cases, and no response in 1 case. The patients were instructed to take one dose daily of an herbal formula that contained *Sang Zhi* 20g, *Ji Xue Teng* (Caulis Spatholobi) 30g, *Wei Ling Xian* (Radix Clematidis) 30g, *Dang Gui* (Radicis Angelicae Sinensis) 20g, *Qiang Huo* (Rhizoma et Radix Notopterygii) 15g, *Gui Zhi* (Ramulus Cinnamomi) 15g, *Bai Shao* (Radix Paeoniae Alba) 15g, *Jiang Huang* (Rhizoma Curcumae Longae) 15g, *Fang Feng* (Radix Saposhnikoviae) 15g, and *Xi Xin* (Herba Asari) 5g (post-decocted). Modifications were made if deemed necessary by adding *Huang Qi* (Radix Astragali) 20g for right shoulder pain; *He Shou Wu* (Radix Polygoni Multiflori) 20g for left shoulder pain; *Ru Xiang* (Gummi Olibanum) 15g and *Mo Yao* (Myrrha) 15g for severe pain; *Quan Xie* (Scorpio) 5g and *Jiang Can* (Bombyx Batryticatus) 10g for numbness; *Xu Duan* (Radix Dipsaci) 20g and *Sang Ji Sheng* (Herba Taxilli) 15g for low back pain; and *Chuan Shan Jia* (Squama Manis) 10g and *Wu Shao She* (Zaocys) 15g for a chronic non-healing condition.[6]

AUTHORS' COMMENTS

Sang Zhi, *Gui Zhi* (Ramulus Cinnamomi), *Niu Xi* (Radix Cyathulae seu Achyranthis) and *Mu Gua* (Fructus

Sang Zhi (Ramulus Mori)

Chaenomelis) are commonly used to treat *bi zheng* (painful obstruction syndrome). *Sang Zhi* and *Gui Zhi* are most effective for the upper body; while *Niu Xi* and *Mu Gua* (Fructus Chaenomelis) are most effective for the lower body. *Sang Zhi* is most effective for hot *bi zheng*; while *Gui Zhi* is most effective for cold *bi zheng*. *Mu Gua* treats pain by relieving muscle spasms and cramps; while *Niu Xi* treats pain by tonifying the Liver and Kidney.

References

1. *Xian Dai Zhong Yao Yao Li Xue* (Contemporary Pharmacology of Chinese Herbs), 1997; 502
2. *Tetrahedron Lett*, 1979; (48):4675
3. *Zhi Wu Yao You Xiao Cheng Fen Shou Ce* (Manual of Plant Medicinals and Their Active Constituents), 1986; 734:735
4. *Chang Yong Zhong Yao Cheng Fen Yu Yao Li Shou Ce* (A Handbook of the Composition and Pharmacology of Common Chinese Drugs), 1994; 1554:1555
5. *Zhong Yao Xue* (Chinese Herbology), 1998; 295:296
6. *Hei Long Jiang Zhong Yi Yao* (Heilongjiang Chinese Medicine and Herbology), 1991; (1):27

Qian Nian Jian (Rhizoma Homalomenae)

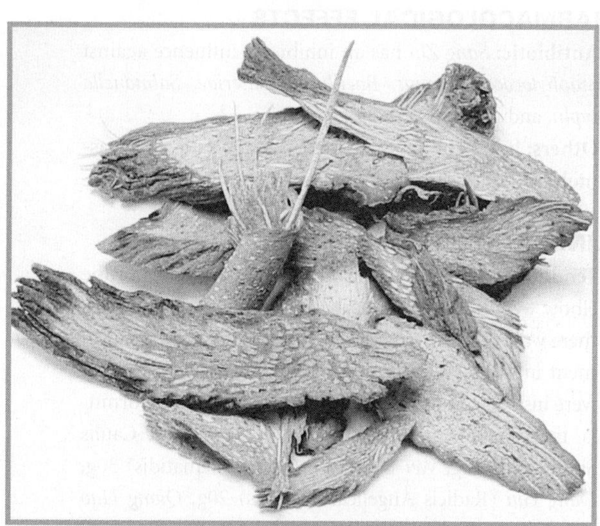

千年健

Pinyin Name: *Qian Nian Jian*

Literal Name: "thousand year vitality," "thousand years of health"

Original Source: *Ben Cao Gang Mu Shi Yi* (Omissions from the Grand Materia Medica) by Zhao Xue-Min in 1765

English Name: homalomena, obscured homalomena rhizome

Botanical Name: *Homalomena occulta* (Lour.) Schott (*Qian Nian Jian*)

Pharmaceutical Name: Rhizoma Homalomenae

Properties: bitter, acrid, warm

Channels Entered: Kidney, Liver

CHINESE THERAPEUTIC ACTIONS

Dispels Wind and Dampness, Strengthens Tendons and Bones

***Bi zheng* (painful obstruction syndrome), numbness and tightness of tendons:** Acrid, bitter and warm, *Qian Nian Jian* (Rhizoma Homalomenae) dispels wind and dampness and opens peripheral channels and collaterals. Furthermore, it strengthens tendons and bones to relieve pain deep inside the extremities. It treats both acute and chronic pain, such as coldness and pain of the low back and knee, and numbness and spasms in the lower extremities. *Qian Nian Jian* is most suitable for elderly patients with weakness in the tendons and bones, and numbness and tightness in limbs and joints.

- Muscle and joint pain: use *Qian Nian Jian* with *Luo Shi Teng* (Caulis Trachelospermi), *Hai Feng Teng* (Caulis Piperis Kadsurae), and *Niu Xi* (Radix Cyathulae seu Achyranthis).
- *Bi zheng* in the elderly: use this herb with *Du Huo* (Radix Angelicae Pubescentis), *Wu Jia Pi* (Cortex Acanthopanacis), *Shu Di Huang* (Radix Rehmanniae Preparata), *Xu Duan* (Radix Dipsaci) and other tonic herbs, to remedy deficiencies.

DOSAGE

5 to 10 grams. *Qian Nian Jian* is commonly used as herbal wine, as pills, or in decoction.

OVERDOSAGE

There have been two reported cases of overdose of *Qian Nian Jian*. The adverse reactions reported following ingestion included nausea, vomiting, dizziness, convulsions, unconsciousness, and urinary and bowel incontinence.

Qian Nian Jian (Rhizoma Homalomenae)

Both patients were treated with gastric lavage, followed by ingestion of a *Gan Cao* (Radix Glycyrrhizae) decoction, and recovered shortly thereafter.[1]

CHEMICAL COMPOSITION

α-pinene, β-pinene, limonene, geranial, geraniol, nerol, linalool, β-terpineol, patchouli alcohol, isoborneol, cedrol, 4-cadinene.[2]

PHARMACOLOGICAL EFFECTS

Antibiotic: Essential oil of *Qian Nian Jian* has a mild antibiotic effect *in vitro*.[3]

References

1. *Fu Jian Zhong Yi Yao* (Fujian Chinese Medicine and Herbology), 1963; 5:28
2. *Chang Yong Zhong Yao Cheng Fen Yu Yao Li Shou Ce* (A Handbook of the Composition and Pharmacology of Common Chinese Drugs), 1994, 398-399
3. *Yao Xue Tong Bao* (Report of Herbology), 1984, 19(12):22

Hai Feng Teng (Caulis Piperis Kadsurae)

海風藤 海风藤

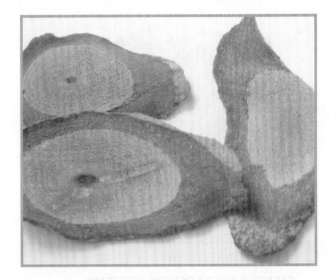

Pinyin Name: *Hai Feng Teng*
Literal Name: "sea wind vine"
Original Source: *Ben Cao Zai Xin* (Renewed Materia Medica)
English Name: kadsura stem, futokadsura stem, kadsura pepper stem
Botanical Name: *Piper futokadsura* Sieb. et Zucc. (*Feng Teng*); *Piper wallichii* (Miq); *Piper kadsura* (choisy) Ohwi
Pharmaceutical Name: Caulis Piperis Kadsurae
Properties: acrid, bitter, slightly warm
Channels Entered: Liver

CHINESE THERAPEUTIC ACTIONS

Dispels Wind-Dampness, Opens Channels and Collaterals

***Bi zheng* (painful obstruction syndrome), traumatic injuries:** Acrid, warm and dispersing in nature, *Hai Feng Teng* (Caulis Piperis Kadsurae) treats painful joints, spasms and pain of the lower back and knees. It also alleviates pain from traumatic injury.

- *Bi zheng*: use *Hai Feng Teng* with *Gui Zhi* (Ramulus Cinnamomi), *Qin Jiao* (Radix Gentianae Macrophyllae), *Dang Gui* (Radicis Angelicae Sinensis) and other blood-invigorating herbs.

DOSAGE

5 to 10 grams.

CHEMICAL COMPOSITION

Futoenone, futoamide, futoguinol, α-pinene, β-pinene, limonene.[1]

PHARMACOLOGICAL EFFECTS

- **Cardiovascular:** Administration of *Hai Feng Teng* is associated with decreased vascular resistance, increased blood perfusion to the coronary artery and peripheral parts of the body, and decreased blood pressure. It shows promise for treatment of coronary artery disease and cerebral thrombosis.[2]

CLINICAL STUDIES AND RESEARCH

- **Coronary artery disease and angina:** Intravenous infusion of a *Hai Feng Teng* preparation in 250 ml of D10W once daily for 14 days produced good results in treating

Hai Feng Teng (Caulis Piperis Kadsurae)

56 patients with coronary artery disease and angina.[3]

- **Cerebral thrombosis:** Intravenous infusion of a *Hai Feng Teng* preparation in 500 ml of D10W once daily showed an overall 83.9% rate of effectiveness in 87 patients with cerebral thrombosis.[4] In another study, 50 patients with cerebral thrombosis or embolism were treated with *Hai Feng Teng* with an 86.1% rate of effectiveness.[5]

References

1. *Xian Dai Zhong Yao Yao Li Xue* (Contemporary Pharmacology of Chinese Herbs), 1997; 440-441
2. *Zhong Guo Zhong Yao Za Zhi* (People's Republic of China Journal of Chinese Herbology), 1989; 14(11):43
3. *Zhong Xi Yi Jie He Za Zhi* (Journal of Integrated Chinese and Western Medicine), 1983; 5:271
4. *Zhong Yao Xue* (Chinese Herbology), 1998; 3:180
5. *Zhong Hua Shen Jing Jing Shen Ke Za Zhi* (Chinese Journal of Neurology and Psychiatry), 1979; 3:160

Hai Tong Pi (Cortex Erythrinae)

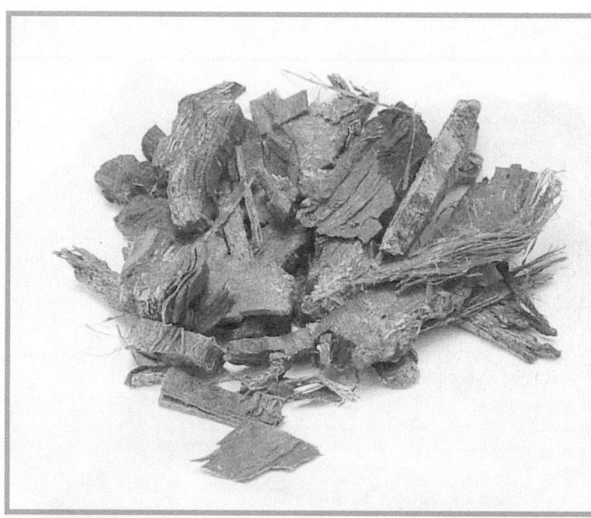

海桐皮

Pinyin Name: *Hai Tong Pi*

Original Source: *Hai Yao Ben Cao* (Materia Medica of Herbs from [Across the] Seas) by Li Xun in 907-960 A.D.

English Name: erythrina, Oriental variegated coral bean bark, Himalayan coral bean bark

Botanical Name: *Erythrina variegata* L. var. *orientalis* (L.) Merr. (*Ci Tong*)

Pharmaceutical Name: Cortex Erythrinae

Properties: bitter, acrid, neutral

Channels Entered: Liver

CHINESE THERAPEUTIC ACTIONS

1. Dispels Wind and Dampness, Opens Channels and Collaterals

***Bi zheng* (painful obstruction syndrome):** Acrid, bitter, drying and dispersing in nature, *Hai Tong Pi* (Cortex Erythrinae) dispels wind and dampness and opens peripheral channels and collaterals. It treats various musculoskeletal disorders, such as muscle aches and pain, spasms and cramps, and pain in the low back. It has a moderate pain-relieving action, and must be combined with other herbs for full effectiveness.

- Lower body aches and pains with dampness and heat: use *Hai Tong Pi* with *Bi Xie* (Rhizoma Dioscoreae Hypoglaucae) and *Chuan Mu Tong* (Caulis Clematidis Armandii).
- Chronic joint pain due to wind, cold and dampness: use this herb with *Niu Xi* (Radix Cyathulae seu Achyranthis) and *Qiang Huo* (Rhizoma et Radix Notopterygii).
- Pain and swelling of the joints: add *Gui Zhi* (Ramulus Cinnamomi).

2. Kills Parasites and Relieves Itching

Used topically, *Hai Tong Pi* kills parasites and relieves itching. It treats itchy skin lesions and infections.

- Itchy skin lesions and infections: use *Hai Tong Pi* with *She Chuang Zi* (Fructus Cnidii) and *Da Huang* (Radix et Rhizoma Rhei). Cook as decoction for use as a topical herbal wash. Or, place the herbs in alcohol and apply the tincture to the affected area.

DOSAGE

6 to 12 grams. *Hai Tong Pi* is commonly used internally as a decoction. It is also used topically by mixing the powdered herb with water and applying the resultant paste to the affected areas.

Hai Tong Pi (Cortex Erythrinae)

CAUTIONS / CONTRAINDICATIONS

- *Hai Tong Pi* should be used with caution in cases of blood deficiency.

CHEMICAL COMPOSITION

Erythraline, amino acids, organic acids.[1]

PHARMACOLOGICAL EFFECTS

- **Antibiotic:** *Hai Tong Pi* inhibits *Staphylococcus aureus*, some pathogenic fungi and dermatophytes.[2]

References

1. *Chang Yong Zhong Yao Xian Dai Yan Jiu Yu Lin Chuan* (Recent Study & Clinical Application of Common Traditional Chinese Medicine), 1995; 238
2. Ibid.

Xun Gu Feng (Herba Aristolochiae Mollissimae)

尋骨風 寻骨风

Pinyin Name: *Xun Gu Feng*
Literal Name: "wind that searches the bone"
English Name: aristolochia
Botanical Name: *Aristolochia mollissima* Hance
Pharmaceutical Name: Herba Aristolochiae Mollissimae
Properties: acrid, bitter, neutral
Channels Entered: Liver

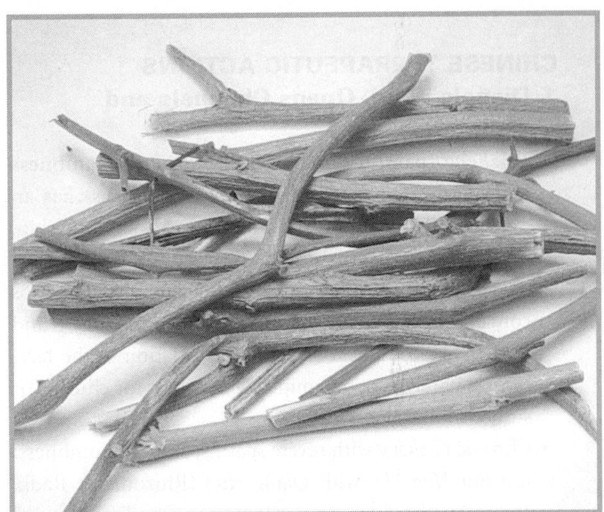

CHINESE THERAPEUTIC ACTIONS

Dispels Wind-Dampness, Opens Channels and Collaterals and Relieves Pain

***Bi zheng* (painful obstruction syndrome), traumatic injuries:** Acrid and dispersing in nature, *Xun Gu Feng* (Herba Aristolochiae Mollissimae) treats joint pain, numbness of the limbs, spasms, cramps, and pain associated with traumatic injuries. It is often used with other antirheumatic herbs to enhance the overall function of the formula. It is also used alone in decoction or herbal wine.

Xun Gu Feng is also effective to treat stomach pain and toothache.

DOSAGE

10 to 15 grams.

CHEMICAL COMPOSITION

Aristolochic acid A,D; aristolactone, mollislactone, allantoin, β-sitosterol, 9-ethoxy-aristolactam, 9-ethoxy-aristolactone, neo-aristolactone.[1]

TOXICOLOGY

The LD_{50} for oral administration of *Xun Gu Feng* via decoction in mice is 64.11 g/kg.[2]

Xun Gu Feng contains a trace amount of aristolochic acid. For more information on the toxicology of this compound, please refer to *Guang Fang Ji* (Radix Aristolochiae Fangchi) or *Guan Mu Tong* (Caulis Aristolochiae Manshuriensis).

References

1. *Xian Dai Zhong Yao Yao Li Xue* (Contemporary Pharmacology of Chinese Herbs), 1997; 165
2. *Yi Xue Xue Bao* (Report of Medicine), 1984; 19(6):405

Bai Hua She (Bungarus Parvus)

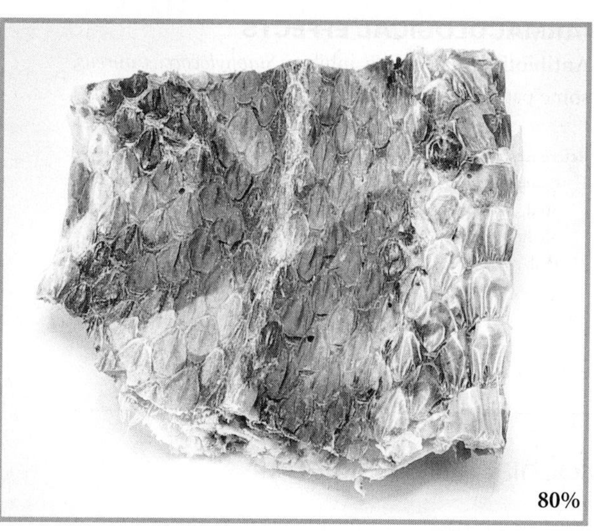
80%

白花蛇 白花蛇

Pinyin Name: *Bai Hua She*

Literal Name: "white flower snake," "white-patterned snake"

Original Source: *Lei Gong Pao Zhi Lun* (Grandfather Lei's Discussions of Herb Preparation) by Lei Xiao in 470 A.D.

English Name: bungarus

Zoological Name: *Bungarus multicinctus* Blyth (*Yin Huan She*)

Pharmaceutical Name: Bungarus Parvus

Properties: sweet, salty, warm

Channels Entered: Liver

Safety Index: toxic

CHINESE THERAPEUTIC ACTIONS

1. Dispels Wind, Opens Channels and Collaterals

***Bi zheng* (painful obstruction syndrome), numbness and paralysis:** *Bai Hua She* (Bungarus Parvus) has an excellent dispersing function that travels along the skin, enters the internal organs and penetrates to the bone. It dispels wind, opens channels and collaterals, and stops convulsions. Clinical applications include *bi zheng* and post-stroke complications such as deviation of the face, muscle paralysis and hemiplegia. It is best for chronic or stubborn numbness and pain.

- Chronic *bi zheng* with severe spasms, pain, or numbness: use *Bai Hua She* with *Qiang Huo* (Rhizoma et Radix Notopterygii), *Fang Feng* (Radix Saposhnikoviae), and *Qin Jiao* (Radix Gentianae Macrophyllae).
- *Bi zheng* due to wind and dampness: use it with *Tian Ma* (Rhizoma Gastrodiae), *Jing Jie* (Herba Schizonepetae) and *Bo He* (Herba Menthae).
- Post-stroke complications such as muscle paralysis and hemiplegia: combine it with *Quan Xie* (Scorpio), *Tian Ma* (Rhizoma Gastrodiae) and *Dang Gui* (Radicis Angelicae Sinensis).

2. Dispels Wind from the Skin

Bai Hua She dispels wind from the skin to treat dermatological disorders, such as itching, rash, tinea, chronic non-healing ulcers and other skin disorders.

- Itching and rashes: use it with *Dang Gui* (Radicis Angelicae Sinensis), *He Shou Wu* (Radix Polygoni Multiflori) and *Bai Shao* (Radix Paeoniae Alba).

3. Stops Convulsions

Bai Hua She dispels wind from the muscles to relieve muscle cramps and spasms. It also treats seizures, convulsions, acute and chronic childhood convulsions, tetanus, and wind-stroke.

- Tetanus: use *Bai Hua She* with *Wu Shao She* (Zaocys) and *Wu Gong* (Scolopendra).

DOSAGE

3 to 10 grams in decoction, 1.0 to 1.5 grams in powder form. *Bai Hua She* is also used as a medicinal wine. Frying with grain-based liquor will reduce its odor, prevent spoilage, and potentiate its effect to treat *bi zheng* (painful obstruction syndrome).

CAUTIONS / CONTRAINDICATIONS

- Use *Bai Hua She* with caution in patients with yin deficiency or blood dryness, or individuals at risk for endogenous wind rising because of blood deficiency.

CHEMICAL COMPOSITION

Guanoside, α-bungarotoxin, β-bungarotoxin, protein, lipids.[1]

PHARMACOLOGICAL EFFECTS

- **Hematological:** Administration of *Bai Hua She* is associated with antiplatelet and anticoagulant effects.[2]
- **Analgesic:** Administration of *Bai Hua She* is associated with marked analgesic effects in rats. The snake venom at 0.188 mg/kg is approximately three to four times more potent than morphine at 1 mg/kg. In addition, the use of snake venom is not associated with tolerance or dependence, and is effective for pain from many causes, including nerve pain and cancer.[3]

Bai Hua She (Bungarus Parvus)

CLINICAL STUDIES AND RESEARCH

- **Clotting disorders:** *Bai Hua She* has a marked anticoagulant effect and is commonly used to treat patients with various clotting disorders, such as angiitis, arteritis, phlebitis, and Raynaud's disease.[4,5]
- **Coronary artery disorders:** Intravenous infusion of a *Bai Hua She* preparation once daily was beneficial in treating 50 patients with coronary artery disorders.[6]
- **Pain:** Oral administration of a *Bai Hua She* preparation was effective in treating 484 pain patients, with good results and few side effects. Tolerance and dependence were not observed.[7] In another study, intramuscular injection or trigger point injection of a *Bai Hua She* preparation was effective in treating 467 patients with various sources of pain, such as headache, neuropathic pain, or rheumatism. The overall rate of effectiveness was 81.8%.[8]

HERB-DRUG INTERACTION

- **Anticoagulant or antiplatelet drugs:** *Bai Hua She* has antiplatelet and anticoagulant effects, and should be used with caution in patients who take anticoagulant or antiplatelet medications. Though no examples of this potential interaction have not been documented, this herb may potentiate the effect of drugs such as warfarin. [Note: Examples of anticoagulants include heparin, warfarin (Coumadin) and enoxaparin (Lovenox); and examples of antiplatelets include aspirin, dipyridamole (Persantine), and clopidogrel (Plavix).][9]

SUPPLEMENT

- 蘄蛇 / 蕲蛇 *Qi She* (Agkistrodon), *Agkistrodon acutus* (Gunther), is sometimes used as a substitute for *Bai Hua She* (Bungarus Parvus). Both substances have very similar therapeutic effects.

AUTHORS' COMMENTS

Bai Hua She and *Wu Shao She* (Zaocys) are very similar in function and indications. *Bai Hua She* is stronger, but slightly toxic; *Wu Shao She* is weaker, but not toxic.

References

1. *Xian Dai Zhong Yao Yao Li Xue* (Contemporary Pharmacology of Chinese Herbs), 1997; 439
2. *Zhong Yao Xue* (Chinese Herbology), 1998; 301:302
3. Ibid.
4. *Yao Xue Tong Bao* (Report of Herbology), 1985; 5:33
5. Ibid., 1988; 1:45
6. *He Bei Yi Yao* (Hebei Medicine and Herbology), 1988; 2:45
7. *Zhong Cao Yao* (Chinese Herbal Medicine), 1981; 12:41
8. Ibid., 1986; 1:7
9. Chen, J. Recognition & prevention of herb-drug interactions, *Medical Acupuncture*, Fall/Winter 1998/1999; volume 10/number 2; 9-13

Wu Shao She (Zaocys)

烏蛸蛇 乌蛸蛇

Pinyin Name: *Wu Shao She*
Literal Name: "black-striped snake"
English Name: zaocys, black snake
Zoological Name: *Zaocys dhumnades* (Cantor) (*Wu Shao She*)
Pharmaceutical Name: Zaocys
Properties: sweet, salty, neutral
Channels Entered: Spleen, Liver

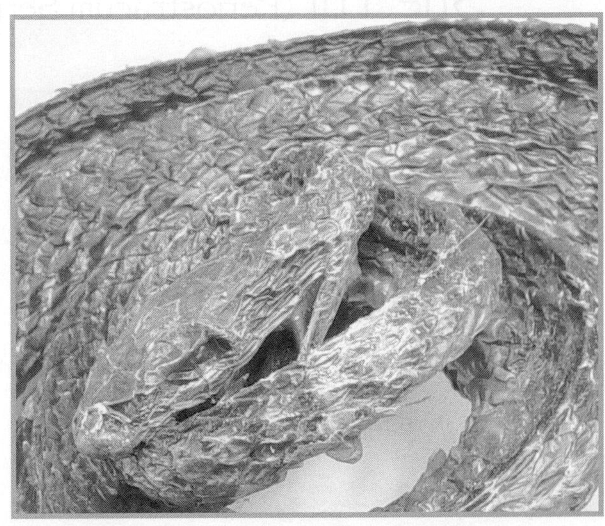

Wu Shao She (Zaocys)

CHINESE THERAPEUTIC ACTIONS

1. Dispels Wind, Opens Channels and Collaterals

***Bi zheng* (painful obstruction syndrome):** *Wu Shao She* (Zaocys) has an excellent dispersing action that enters the internal organs and penetrates to the skin. It dispels wind, opens channels and collaterals, and stops convulsions. Clinical applications include *bi zheng*, and post-stroke complications such as deviation of the face, muscle paralysis and hemiplegia.

- *Bi zheng*: use *Wu Shao She* with *Di Long* (Pheretima).

2. Stops Convulsions

Wu Shao She dispels wind from the muscles to relieve cramps and spasms. It treats seizures, convulsions, tetanus, and wind-stroke.

- Convulsions: use it with *Wu Gong* (Scolopendra) and *Quan Xie* (Scorpio).

DOSAGE

5 to 10 grams in decoction, 2 to 3 grams as powder. Frying with grain-based liquor reduces the odor, prevents spoilage, and potentiates its effect to treat *bi zheng* (painful obstruction syndrome).

CHEMICAL COMPOSITION

Lipids, 17 various amino acids.[1]

PHARMACOLOGICAL EFFECTS

- **Anti-inflammatory:** Injection of water and alcohol extracts of *Wu Shao She* reduced swelling and inflammation in rats.[2]
- **Analgesic:** Alcohol extract of *Wu Shao She* at 40 mg/kg showed marked analgesic effects in rats.[3]
- **Sedative:** Intraperitoneal injection of *Wu Shao She* was associated with a marked sedative effect in mice. The potency is similar to phenobarbital.[4]
- **Antiseizure:** Intraperitoneal injection of *Wu Shao She* in mice has a similar antiseizure influence to that of phenobarbital.[5]

TOXICOLOGY

The LD_{50} for *Wu Shao She* in mice is 166.2 g/kg for water extract and 20.41 g/kg for alcohol extract. Adverse reactions caused by overdose included muscle stiffness, diminished or absent physical activity, and respiratory depression.[6]

References

1. *Chang Yong Zhong Yao Cheng Fen Yu Yao Li Shou Ce* (A Handbook of the Composition and Pharmacology of Common Chinese Drugs), 1994; 581
2. *Zhe Jiang Yao Xue* (Zhejiang Journal of Chinese Herbology), 1986; 3(4):4
3. Ibid.
4. Ibid.
5. Ibid.
6. Ibid

She Tui (Periostracum Serpentis)

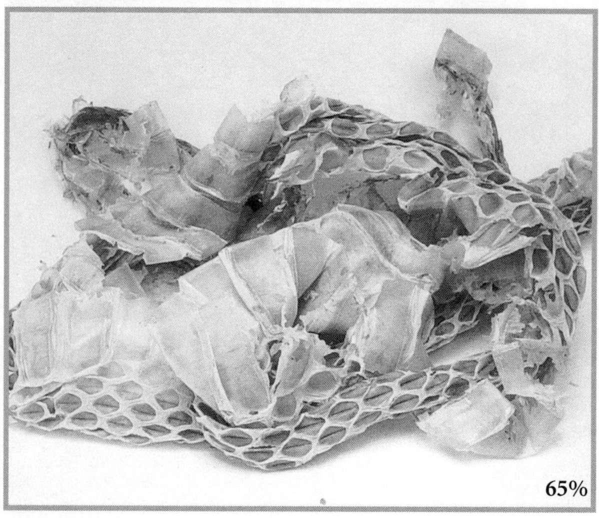
65%

蛇蜕

Pinyin Name: *She Tui*
Literal Name: "snake skin slough"
Alternate Chinese Names: *Long Yi*
English Name: sloughed snake skin
Zoological Name: *Elaphe taeniurus* Cope. (*Hei Mei Jin She*); *Elaphe carinata* (Guenther) (*Jin She*)
Pharmaceutical Name: Periostracum Serpentis
Properties: sweet, salty, neutral
Channels Entered: Liver

She Tui (Periostracum Serpentis)

CHINESE THERAPEUTIC ACTIONS

1. Dispels Wind and Stops Spasms

She Tui (Periostracum Serpentis) dispels wind to stop seizures and convulsions in children.

2. Dispels Wind from the Skin

She Tui dispels wind from the skin to relieve itching.

- Itching and rash: use it with *Chan Tui* (Periostracum Cicadae), *Sheng Di Huang* (Radix Rehmanniae) and *Dang Gui* (Radicis Angelicae Sinensis).

3. Benefits the Eyes

She Tui improves vision and treats pterygium or disorders of the cornea.

- Pterygium or disorders of the cornea: combine it with *Chan Tui* (Periostracum Cicadae) and *Bai Ji Li* (Fructus Tribuli).

DOSAGE

2 to 3 grams in decoction, 0.3 to 0.6 gram as powder. Frying *She Tui* with grain-based liquor reduces its odor, prevents spoilage, and potentiates its effect to treat *bi zheng* (painful obstruction syndrome).

CHEMICAL COMPOSITION

Ossein, fatty acids, amino acids.[1]

PHARMACOLOGICAL EFFECTS

- **Anti-inflammatory:** Intravenous injection of a *She Tui* preparation is associated with marked reduction of inflammation and swelling. The peak effect is reached approximately 2 hours after the injection. The anti-inflammatory effect of *She Tui* is similar to that of indomethacin. Oral ingestion showed no tendency to reduce inflammation in rats.[2]

References

1. *Xian Dai Zhong Yao Yao Li Xue* (Contemporary Pharmacology of Chinese Herbs), 1997; 455
2. *Guo Wai Yi Xue Zhong Yi Zhong Yao Fen Ce* (Monograph of Chinese Herbology from Foreign Medicine), 1981

Xia Tian Wu (Rhizoma Corydalis Decumbentis)

夏天無 夏天无

Pinyin Name: *Xia Tian Wu*
Literal Name: "not in summer"
English Name: decumbent corydalis rhizome
Botanical Name: *Corydalis decumbens* (Thunb.) Pers.
Pharmaceutical Name: Rhizoma Corydalis Decumbentis
Properties: acrid, bitter, warm
Channels Entered: Liver

CHINESE THERAPEUTIC ACTIONS

1. Dispels Wind and Dampness

***Bi zheng* (painful obstruction syndrome):** *Xia Tian Wu* (Rhizoma Corydalis Decumbentis) treats joint pain and/or paralysis and numbness. It is used alone or with other herbs that dispel wind-dampness.

2. Invigorates Blood Circulation and Stops Pain

Trauma-related pain, epigastric and abdominal pain: *Xia Tian Wu* strongly relieves pain and invigorates blood. It is used alone or with other herbs that dispel wind-dampness.

DOSAGE

5 to 15 grams. Decrease the dosage when using *Xia Tian Wu* as a powder or in pills.

CAUTIONS / CONTRAINDICATIONS

- Use of *Xia Tian Wu* is sometimes associated with nausea, vomiting and gastrointestinal disturbance.

CHEMICAL COMPOSITION

Tetrahydropalmatine, protopine, bulbocapnine, adlumidine, bicuculline, palmatine, decumbenine, corlumidine, berberine, jatrorrhizine, hydrastinine, corydaline, decumbenine, hydroxyhydrastine.[1,2]

Xia Tian Wu (Rhizoma Corydalis Decumbentis)

Tetrahydropalmatine

PHARMACOLOGICAL EFFECTS

- **Cardiovascular:** Injection of *Xia Tian Wu* in anesthetized dogs is associated with dilation of blood vessels, decreased vascular resistance, and increased blood perfusion to peripheral parts of the body. The vasodilating effect is not countered by injection of atropine.[3,4]
- **Antiplatelet:** Injection of *Xia Tian Wu* is associated with an inhibitory effect on aggregation of platelets in rats.[5]
- **Analgesic:** Tetrahydropalmatine is present in both *Xia Tian Wu* and *Yan Hu Suo* (Rhizoma Corydalis). For a complete explanation of western therapeutic properties, please refer to the *Yan Hu Suo* monograph.

CLINICAL STUDIES AND RESEARCH

- **Pain management:** Administration of *Xia Tian Wu* is associated with a marked reduction of pain. Greater than 90% effectiveness was reported in 88 patients with wind-damp *bi zheng* (painful obstruction syndrome), 46 patients with acute back injury, and 60 patients with chronic lower back and leg injuries. Routes of administration varied, but included trigger point injection, and administration of suspension or pills.[6,7,8]

HERB-DRUG INTERACTION

- **Anticoagulant or antiplatelet drugs:** *Xia Tian Wu* exerts antiplatelet action, and should be used with caution in patients who take anticoagulant or antiplatelet medications. Though no examples of this potential interaction have been documented, this herb may potentiate the effect of drugs such as warfarin. [Note: Examples of anticoagulants include heparin, warfarin (Coumadin) and enoxaparin (Lovenox); and examples of antiplatelets include aspirin, dipyridamole (Persantine), and clopidogrel (Plavix).][9]

TOXICOLOGY

The LD_{50} for *Xia Tian Wu* in mice is 24.04 g/kg via subcutaneous injection, and 7.63 g/kg via intravenous injection.[10]

AUTHORS' COMMENTS

Xia Tian Wu (Rhizoma Corydalis Decumbentis) has long been used as a replacement for *Yan Hu Suo* (Rhizoma Corydalis), since both herbs belong in the same genus and have similar analgesic effects.

References

1. *Xian Dai Zhong Yao Yao Li Xue* (Contemporary Pharmacology of Chinese Herbs), 1997; 1514
2. *The Merck Index* 12th edition, Chapman & Hall/CRCnetBASE/Merck, 2000
3. *Zhong Yao Zhi* (Chinese Herbology Journal), 1979: 72
4. *Zhong Cao Yao Tong Xun* (Journal of Chinese Herbal Medicine), 1976; 56(1):62
5. *Zhong Guo Yao Li Xue Tong Bao* (Journal of Chinese Herbal Pharmacology), 1988; 4(5):301
6. *Zhong Cao Yao Tong Xun* (Journal of Chinese Herbal Medicine), 1970; (4):43
7. *Zhong Yuan Yi Kan* (Resource Journal of Chinese Medicine), 1989; (6):19
8. *Jiang Xi Yi Yao* (Jiangxi Medicine and Herbology), 1982; (4):60
9. Chen, J. Recognition & prevention of herb-drug interactions, *Medical Acupuncture*, Fall/Winter 1998/1999; volume 10/number 2; 9-13
10. *Zhong Cao Yao Tong Xun* (Journal of Chinese Herbal Medicine), 1976; 56(1):62

Chuan Shan Long (Rhizoma Dioscoreae Nipponicae)

穿山龍 穿山龙

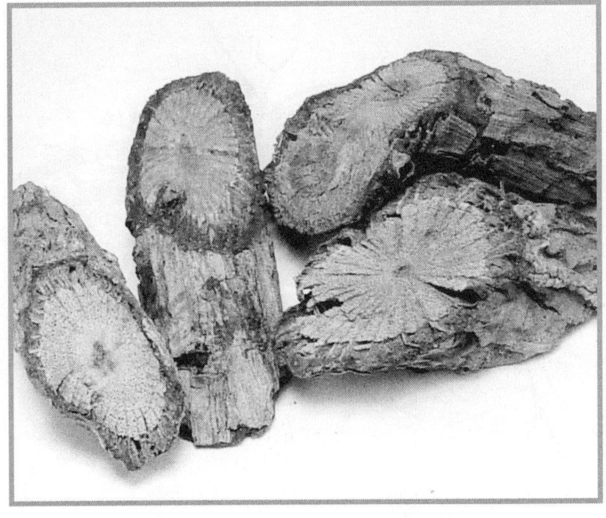

Pinyin Name: *Chuan Shan Long*
Literal Name: "penetrate mountain dragon"
Original Source: *Dong Bei Zhi Wu Zhi* (Northeast Journal of Herbal Medicine)
English Name: dioscorea nipponica
Botanical Name: *Dioscorea nipponica* Makino. (*Chuan Long Shu*)
Pharmaceutical Name: Rhizoma Dioscoreae Nipponicae
Properties: bitter, cool
Channels Entered: Liver, Lung

CHINESE THERAPEUTIC ACTIONS

1. Dispels Wind and Dampness, Invigorates Blood and Opens Channels and Collaterals

***Bi zheng* (painful obstruction syndrome):** *Chuan Shan Long* (Rhizoma Dioscoreae Nipponicae) relieves painful joints with numbness and difficulty of movement. It also alleviates the pain of traumatic injuries. It is often used alone or with other herbs that dispel wind-dampness, in grain-based liquor or in decoction.

***Xiong bi* (painful obstruction of the chest):** *Chuan Shan Long* invigorates blood circulation, opens channels and collaterals, and treats *xiong bi* caused by blood stagnation. Clinical applications include coronary artery disease and angina.

2. Relieves Cough and Dissolves Phlegm

Cough and wheezing due to Lung heat: Being cool in thermal property, *Chuan Shan Long* is good for treatment of respiratory disorders manifesting in cough, dyspnea and wheezing caused by heat.

- Cough and wheezing: use it with *Gua Lou Shi* (Fructus Trichosanthis) and *Huang Qin* (Radix Scutellariae).

DOSAGE

10 to 15 grams.

CHEMICAL COMPOSITION

Dioscin, diosgenin.[1]

TOXICOLOGY

No abnormalities in mice were observed following oral administration of *Chuan Shan Long* at 60 to 180 mg/kg for 7 weeks. The maximum dose for oral administration of *Chuan Shan Long* in mice is 15.6 g/kg. The LD_{50} for intravenous injection of a *Chuan Shan Long* preparation is 750 mg/kg in mice.[2]

References

1. *Xian Dai Zhong Yao Yao Li Xue* (Contemporary Pharmacology of Chinese Herbs), 1997; 472
2. *Zhong Yao Yao Li Yu Ying Yong* (Pharmacology and Applications of Chinese Herbs), 1983; 817

Lao Guan Cao (Herba Erodii seu Geranii)

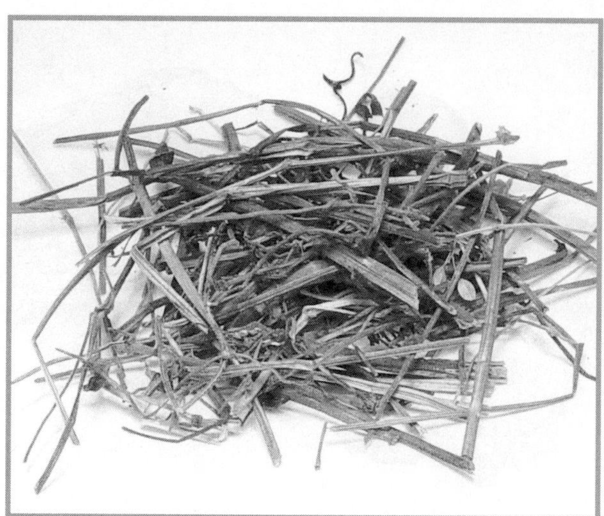

老鸛草 老鸛草

Pinyin Name: *Lao Guan Cao*
Literal Name: "old crane herb"
English Name: erodium, geranium, common heron's bill herb, wilford crane's bill herb
Botanical Name: *Erodium stephanianum* Willd.; *Geranium wilfordii* Maxim.
Pharmaceutical Name: Herba Erodii seu Geranii
Properties: acrid, bitter, neutral
Channels Entered: Liver, Large Intestine

CHINESE THERAPEUTIC ACTIONS

1. Dispels Wind and Dampness

***Bi zheng* (painful obstruction syndrome):** *Lao Guan Cao* (Herba Erodii seu Geranii) relaxes the tendons and invigorates circulation in the channels and collaterals. It relieves joint pain, numbness of the limbs, soreness and pain of the sinews, difficulty of movement, and trauma-related pain.

- *Bi zheng*: use *Lao Guan Cao* with *Sang Zhi* (Ramulus Mori), *Ji Xue Teng* (Caulis Spatholobi) and *Dang Gui* (Radicis Angelicae Sinensis).

2. Stops Diarrhea

Diarrhea or dysentery caused by damp-heat: *Lao Guan Cao* treats acute or chronic diarrhea or dysentery.

- Diarrhea or dysentery: add *Di Jin Cao* (Herba Euphorbiae Humifusae).

DOSAGE

10 to 30 grams.

CHEMICAL COMPOSITION

Geraniol, geraniin.[1]

TOXICOLOGY

The LD_{50} for oral injection of *Lao Guan Cao* is 99 g/kg in mice.[2]

References

1. *Xian Dai Zhong Yao Yao Li Xue* (Contemporary Pharmacology of Chinese Herbs), 1997; 443
2. *Shan Xi Xin Yi Yao* (New Medicine and Herbology of Shanxi), 1978; (6):44

Shen Jin Cao (Herba Lycopodii)

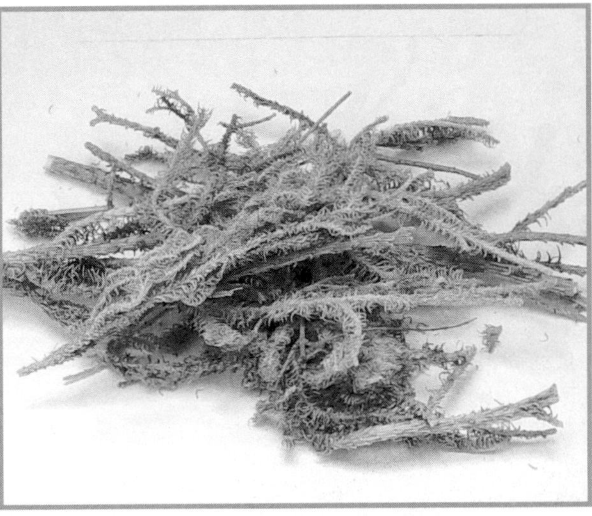

伸筋草 伸筋草

Pinyin Name: *Shen Jin Cao*
Literal Name: "stretch the tendon herb"
Alternate Chinese Names: *Da Shen Jin, Da Shen Jin Teng*
Original Source: *Ben Cao Shi Yi* (Omissions from the [Classic of the] Materia Medica) by Chen Cang-Qi in 741 A.D.
English Name: lycopodium, common club moss, wolf's claw club moss
Botanical Name: *Lycopodium clavatum* L. (*Shi Song*); *Lycopodium cernnum* L. (*Sheng Jin Cao*); *Smilax nipponica* Miq. (*Da Shen Jin*)
Pharmaceutical Name: Herba Lycopodii
Properties: bitter, acrid, warm
Channels Entered: Liver

CHINESE THERAPEUTIC ACTIONS

Dispels Wind and Dampness, Relaxes the Tendons and Sinews, Opens the Channels and Collaterals

***Bi zheng* (painful obstruction syndrome):** *Shen Jin Cao* (Herba Lycopodii) is acrid, warm and dispersing in nature. It treats tightness of the tendons involving difficulty of movement and painful joints. It also treats trauma-related pain.

- *Bi zheng*: use *Shen Jin Cao* with *Tou Gu Cao* (Caulis Impatientis), *Sang Zhi* (Ramulus Mori) and *Wu Jia Pi* (Cortex Acanthopanacis).
- Trauma-related pain: add *Lian Qian Cao* (Herba Glechomae).

DOSAGE

6 to 15 grams.

CAUTIONS / CONTRAINDICATIONS

- *Shen Jin Cao* is contraindicated in pregnant women.

CHEMICAL COMPOSITION

Lycopodine, clavatine, clavolonine, fawcettiine, fawcettimine, deacetylfawcettiine, dihydrolycopodine, clavalonine, clavatoxine, nicotine, dehydrolycopodine, vanillic acid, ferulic acid, azelaic acid, oleic acid, and lycopodic acid.[1]

PHARMACOLOGICAL EFFECTS

- **Antipyretic:** Administration of both water and alcohol extracts of *Shen Jin Cao* is associated with a reduction of body temperature in rabbits.[2]

References

1. *Chang Yong Zhong Yao Cheng Fen Yu Yao Li Shou Ce* (A Handbook of the Composition and Pharmacology of Common Chinese Drugs), 1994; 1071-1072
2. *Zhong Yao Zhi* (Chinese Herbology Journal), 1988: 423

Xi Xian Cao (Herba Siegesbeckiae)

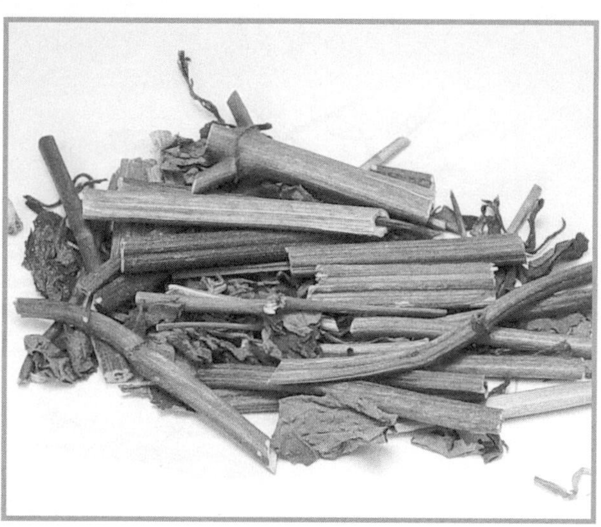

豨薟草 豨莶草

Pinyin Name: *Xi Xian Cao*
Alternate Chinese Names: *Xi Xian*
Original Source: *Xin Xiu Ben Cao* (Newly Revised Materia Medica) by Su Jing in 657-659 A.D.
English Name: siegesbeckia
Botanical Name: *Siegesbeckia orientalis* L. (*Xi Xian*); *Siegesbeckia pubescens* Mak. (*Xian Geng Xi Xian*); *Siegesbeckia glabrescens* Mak. (*Mao Geng Xi Xian*)
Pharmaceutical Name: Herba Siegesbeckiae
Properties: bitter, cold
Channels Entered: Kidney, Liver

CHINESE THERAPEUTIC ACTIONS

1. Dispels Wind and Dampness, Opens Channels and Collaterals

***Bi zheng* (painful obstruction syndrome), numbness, spasms and paralysis:** *Xi Xian Cao* (Herba Siegesbeckiae) benefits the sinews, and dispels wind and dampness, treating *bi zheng* and musculoskeletal disorders. Furthermore, it opens peripheral channels and collaterals, and treats muscle spasms and cramps, muscle weakness and paralysis. This herb is often processed with grain-based liquor or made into honey pills to reduce side effects that may occur due to its cold and bitter nature.

- *Bi zheng*: use *Xi Xian Cao* with *Wei Ling Xian* (Radix Clematidis).

2. Clears Heat and Eliminates Toxins

Xi Xian Cao clears heat and toxins from the skin to treat various dermatological disorders caused by wind, damp and heat, such as sores, itching and rashes. Historically, *Xi Xian* Cao is also used to treat jaundice and malaria.

- Dermatological disorders: use *Xi Xian Cao* internally or topically.

3. Lowers Blood Pressure

Hypertension: *Xi Xian Cao* is now being used to treat hypertension due to heat.

- Hypertension: combine with *Chou Wu Tong* (Folium Clerodendri Trichotomi).

DOSAGE

10 to 15 grams. *Xi Xian Cao* processed with grain-based liquor is stronger for treatment of *bi zheng* (painful obstruction syndrome). The fresh herb more effectively clears heat and eliminates toxins.

CAUTIONS / CONTRAINDICATIONS

- *Xi Xian Cao* should be used with extreme caution in pregnant women and in children, as it may suppress normal development.[1]

CHEMICAL COMPOSITION

Darutoside, darutigenol, neodarutoside.[2]

PHARMACOLOGICAL EFFECTS

- **Anti-inflammatory:** Oral administration of a preparation of *Xi Xian Cao* for 10 days effectively reduced swelling in the legs of rats.[3]
- **Antihypertensive:** Water and alcohol extracts of *Xi Xian Cao* dilated the blood vessels and reduced blood pressure in cats and rabbits. The duration of action is approximately 1.5 hours.[4]
- **Immunosuppressive:** Administration of *Xi Xian Cao* is associated with an inhibitory effect on the immune system in mice. Daily administration of the decoction reduced both cellular and humoral immunities.[5]
- **Antibiotic:** It has an inhibitory effect against *Staphylococcus aureus, E. coli, Pseudomonas aeruginosa, Bacillus dysenteriae, Salmonella typhi*, and *Staphylococcus albus*.[6]

CLINICAL STUDIES AND RESEARCH

- ***Bi zheng* (painful obstruction syndrome):** Good results were reported when 100 grams of *Xi Xian Cao* and 30 grams of *Dang Gui* (Radicis Angelicae Sinensis) were used to treat *bi zheng* and other musculoskeletal disorders caused by wind-damp.[7]

TOXICOLOGY

The LD_{50} for intravenous injection of *Xi Xian Cao* in mice is equivalent to 45.54 g/kg of dried herb. Via

Xi Xian Cao (Herba Siegesbeckiae)

intraperitoneal injection, mice can tolerate up to 400 times the normal adult dose.[8]

References
1. *Zhong Guo Zhong Yao Za Zhi* (People's Republic of China Journal of Chinese Herbology), 1989; 14(3):44
2. *Xian Dai Zhong Yao Yao Li Xue* (Contemporary Pharmacology of Chinese Herbs), 1997; 411
3. *Zhong Yao Yao Li Yu Ying Yong* (Pharmacology and Applications of Chinese Herbs), 1983; 1221
4. Ibid.
5. *Zhong Guo Zhong Yao Za Zhi* (People's Republic of China Journal of Chinese Herbology), 1989; 14(3):44
6. *Phytochemistry*, 1979; 18(5):894
7. *Shang Hai Zhong Yi Yao Za Zhi* (Shanghai Journal of Chinese Medicine and Herbology), 1982; 9:33
8. *Guang Xi Zhong Yi Yao* (Guangxi Chinese Medicine and Herbology), 1990; 13(4):44

Chou Wu Tong (Folium Clerodendri Trichotomi)

臭梧桐

Pinyin Name: *Chou Wu Tong*
Literal Name: "stinky Chinese parasol tree"
Alternate Chinese Names: *Ba Jiao Wu Tong, Ai Tong Zi*
Original Source: *Tu Jing Ben Cao* (Illustrated Classic of the Materia Medica) by Su Song in 1061
English Name: glory bower leaves, harlequin glorybower leaves, hairy clerodendron
Botanical Name: *Clerodendron trichotomum* Thunb.
Pharmaceutical Name: Folium Clerodendri Trichotomi
Properties: acrid, bitter, sweet, cool
Channels Entered: Liver

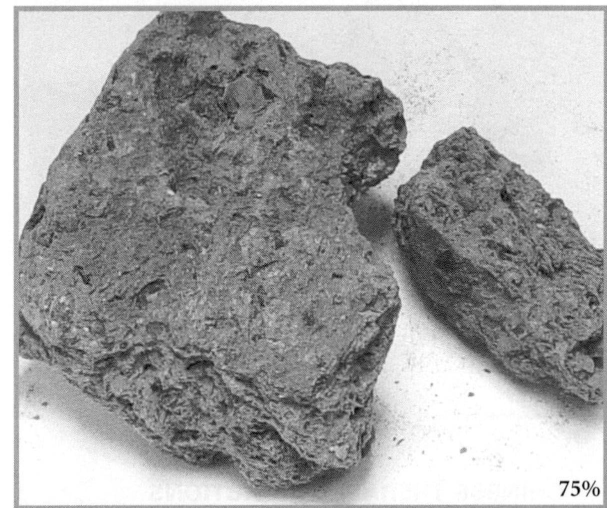
75%

CHINESE THERAPEUTIC ACTIONS

1. Dispels Wind-Damp

***Bi zheng* (painful obstruction syndrome):** *Chou Wu Tong* (Folium Clerodendri Trichotomi) treats musculoskeletal pain, numbness of the extremities, paralysis and hemiplegia. *Chou Wu Tong*, when used topically as a wash or soak, effectively treats eczema and itching of the skin.

- *Bi zheng*: use *Chou Wu Tong* with *Xi Xian Cao* (Herba Siegesbeckiae).

2. Lowers Blood Pressure

Hypertension: *Chou Wu Tong* lowers blood pressure to treat hypertension. This herb is most effective if the leaves are harvested before the flowers bloom. *Chou Wu Tong* should not be cooked at a high temperature or for a prolonged period of time, as processing with heat makes the herb less effective.

- Hypertension: combine with *Xi Xian Cao* (Herba Siegesbeckiae).

DOSAGE

5 to 15 grams. Fresh *Chou Wu Tong* harvested before the flowers bloom is most effective for treatment of hypertension.

CHEMICAL COMPOSITION

Clerodendtin, meso-inositol, clerodendronin A, B.[1]

PHARMACOLOGICAL EFFECTS

- *Chou Wu Tong* has been shown to have antihypertensive, sedative and analgesic effects.[2]

CLINICAL STUDIES AND RESEARCH

- **Malaria:** In one study, 226 patients were treated with a

Chou Wu Tong (Folium Clerodendri Trichotomi)

preparation of *Chou Wu Tong*, with good results.[3]

- **Hypertension:** A preparation of *Chou Wu Tong* given three to four times daily had an 81.87% rate of effectiveness in treating 171 patients with hypertension.[4]

References

1. *Xian Dai Zhong Yao Yao Li Xue* (Contemporary Pharmacology of Chinese Herbs), 1997; 457
2. *Zhong Yao Xue* (Chinese Herbology), 1998; 290:291
3. *Zhong Yi Za Zhi* (Journal of Chinese Medicine), 1961; 5:31
4. *Shang Hai Zhong Yi Yao Za Zhi* (Shanghai Journal of Chinese Medicine and Herbology), 1957; 3:6

Huang Jin Gui (Caulis Vanieriae)

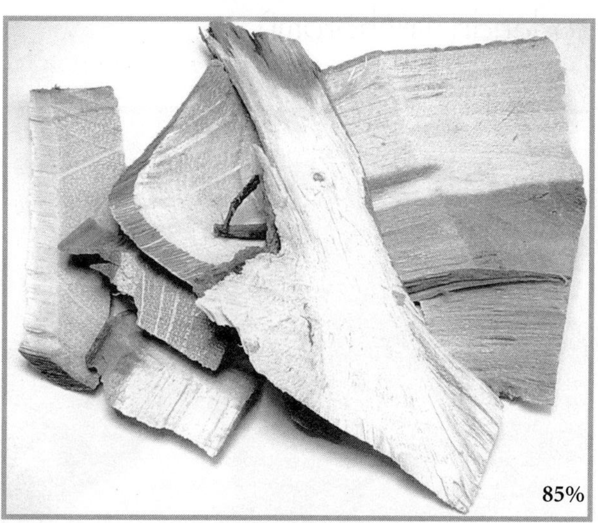
85%

黄金桂

Pinyin Name: *Huang Jin Gui*
Alternate Chinese Names: *Ci Ge Zi, Xiang Gang Zhe Shu*
English Name: vanieria
Botanical Name: *Vanieria gerontogea* Sieb. et Zucc.
Pharmaceutical Name: Caulis Vanieriae
Properties: bland, cool
Channels Entered: Liver, Kidney

CHINESE THERAPEUTIC ACTIONS

Relieves Pain

Huang Jin Gui (Caulis Vanieriae) dispels wind, invigorates blood circulation, opens channels and collaterals, clears heat, eliminates toxins, reduces swelling and relieves pain.

- Trauma-related pain: use *Huang Jin Gui* with *Wan Dian Jin* (Radix Ilicis Asprellae), *Zou Ma Tai* (Rhizoma Ardisiae), *Du Zhong* (Cortex Eucommiae), *Chuan Niu Xi* (Radix Cyathulae) and *Wang Bu Liu Xing* (Semen Vaccariae).
- *Bi zheng* (painful obstruction syndrome), rheumatoid arthritis: use this herb with *Rou Cong Rong* (Herba Cistanches), *Chuan Niu Xi* (Radix Cyathulae), and *Xu Duan* (Radix Dipsaci).
- Neuralgia: combine it with *Chuan Shan Long* (Rhizoma Dioscoreae Nipponicae) and *Jin Bu Huan* (Herba Lycopodii Serrati).

DOSAGE

5 to 30 grams in decoction.

Liu Zhi Huang (Herba Solidaginis)

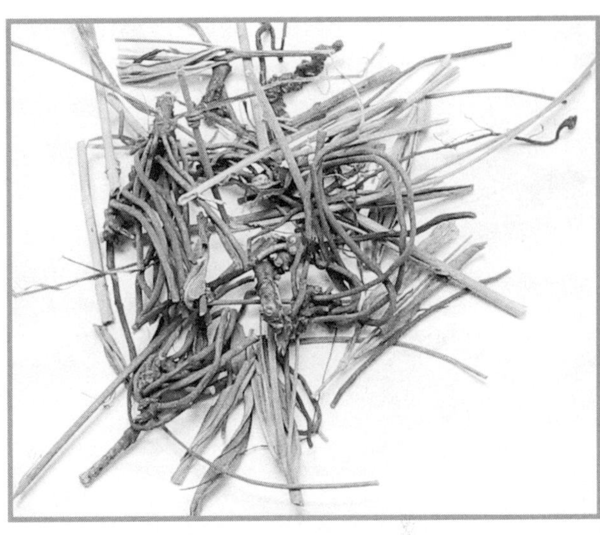

柳枝癀

Pinyin Name: *Liu Zhi Huang*
Alternate Chinese Names: *Yi Zhi Huang Hua, Ye Huang Ju*
English Name: solidago
Botanical Name: *Solidago virga-aurea* L. var. *leiocapa* (Benth.) A. Gray.
Pharmaceutical Name: Herba Solidaginis
Properties: bitter, sweet, cold
Channels Entered: Lung, Liver, Kidney

CHINESE THERAPEUTIC ACTIONS

1. Relieves Pain, Reduces Inflammation, and Opens Channels and Collaterals

Liu Zhi Huang (Herba Solidaginis) effectively opens channels and collaterals to relieve pain and reduce inflammation.

- Trauma-related pain or tightness of tendons: use *Liu Zhi Huang* with *Mo Gu Xiao* (Caulis Hyptis Capitatae), *Huang Jin Gui* (Caulis Vanieriae), *Yi Tiao Gen* (Radix Moghaniae), *Ru Xiang* (Gummi Olibanum), *Mo Yao* (Myrrha), *Mu Gua* (Fructus Chaenomelis) and *Bai Shao* (Radix Paeoniae Alba).

2. Reduces Swelling and Eliminates Toxins

- Jaundice: use *Liu Zhi Huang* with *Shui Ding Xiang* (Herba Ludwigiae Prostratae), *Zhi Zi* (Fructus Gardeniae), *Da Huang* (Radix et Rhizoma Rhei) and *Yin Chen Hao* (Herba Artemisiae Scopariae).
- Influenza, sore throat, tonsillitis: use this herb with *Yi Zhi Xiang* (Herba Vernoniae Cinereae) and *Ban Lan Gen* (Radix Isatidis).
- Tinea unguium, athlete's foot: apply *Liu Zhi Huang* topically.

DOSAGE

3 to 12 grams.

CHEMICAL COMPOSITION

Essential oil, saponins, flavones, rutin.

AUTHORS' COMMENTS

According to Dr. Chang Wei-Yen, *Liu Zhi Huang*, *Huang Jin Gui* (Caulis Vanieriae) and *Mo Gu Xiao* (Caulis Hyptis Capitatae) should always be used together for synergistic action to reduce inflammation and relieve pain of the spine.

Yi Tiao Gen (Radix Moghaniae)

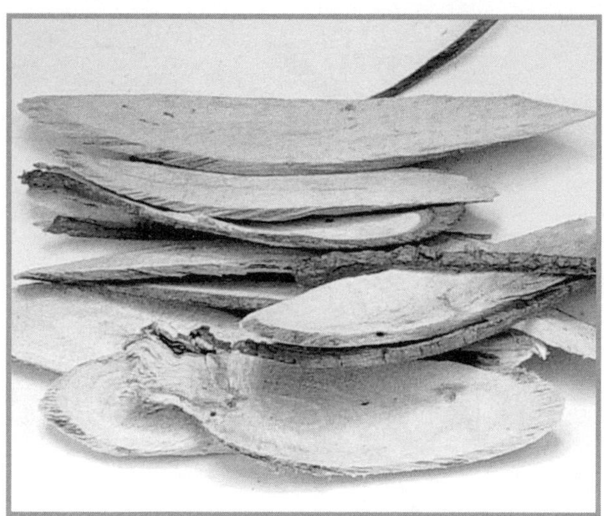

一條根 一条根

Pinyin Name: *Yi Tiao Gen*
Alternate Chinese Names: *Qian Jin Ba, Chou Kong Zai*
English Name: moghania
Botanical Name: *Moghania lineate* (L.) O. Kuntze
Pharmaceutical Name: Radix Moghaniae
Properties: acrid, warm
Channels Entered: Liver, Kidney

CHINESE THERAPEUTIC ACTIONS

Dispels Wind and Dampness, Opens Channels and Collaterals

***Bi zheng* (painful obstruction syndrome):** *Yi Tiao Gen* (Radix Moghaniae) enters the channels and collaterals to treat musculoskeletal pain, stiffness and soreness.

- *Bi zheng*, tendon and bone pain: use *Yi Tiao Gen* with *Chuan Shan Long* (Rhizoma Dioscoreae Nipponicae), *Huang Jin Gui* (Caulis Vanieriae) and *Niu Xi* (Radix Cyathulae seu Achyranthis).
- Sore legs from Liver and Kidney yin deficiencies: use this herb with *Chun Gen Pi* (Cortex Ailanthi), *Xu Duan* (Radix Dipsaci), *Gui Zhi* (Ramulus Cinnamomi), *Mu Gua* (Fructus Chaenomelis), *Du Huo* (Radix Angelicae Pubescentis), *Sang Ji Sheng* (Herba Taxilli) and *Du Zhong* (Cortex Eucommiae).
- Fractured bones: combine *Yi Tiao Gen* with *Xu Duan* (Radix Dipsaci), *Du Zhong* (Cortex Eucommiae) and *Zi Ran Tong* (Pyritum) to help with healing of bones.
- Sciatica: use it with *Xi Xian Cao* (Herba Siegesbeckiae), *Po Bu Zi Ye* (Folium Cordia Dichotoma), *Ru Xiang* (Gummi Olibanum) and *Mo Yao* (Myrrha).

DOSAGE

3 to 12 grams.

CAUTIONS / CONTRAINDICATIONS

- Use with caution in patients who have weak digestive systems.

Section 3 — Wind-Damp Dispelling and Tendon- and Bone-Strengthening Herbs

Sang Ji Sheng (Herba Taxilli)

桑寄生

Pinyin Name: *Sang Ji Sheng*
Literal Name: "mulberry parasite," "mulberry parasitic herb"
Alternate Chinese Names: *Guang Ji Sheng, Bei Ji Sheng, Liu Ji Sheng*
Original Source: *Shen Nong Ben Cao Jing* (Divine Husbandman's Classic of the Materia Medica) in the second century
English Name: taxillus, Chinese taxillus
Botanical Name: *Taxillus chinensis* (DC.) Danser
Pharmaceutical Name: Herba Taxilli
Properties: bitter, neutral
Channels Entered: Liver, Kidney

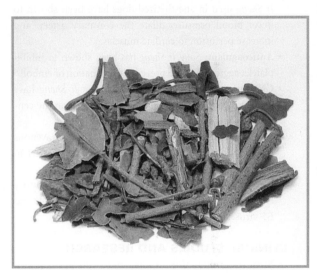

CHINESE THERAPEUTIC ACTIONS

1. Tonifies the Liver and Kidney, Strengthens Sinews and Bones, Dispels Wind-Dampness

***Bi zheng* (painful obstruction syndrome), soreness and weakness of the lower back and knees:** The Liver governs the tendons, and the Kidney governs the bones. Yin deficiency in these two organs will lead to chronic *bi zheng* with accumulation of wind-damp. *Sang Ji Sheng* (Herba Taxilli) is essential in treating elderly patients or yin-deficient patients with chronic lower back and knee weakness, soreness and pain. Other symptoms include tightness and weakness of sinews and tendons, joint pain, and in severe cases, atrophy of bones and tendons.

- Lower back and knee soreness and weakness: combine *Sang Ji Sheng* with *Du Zhong* (Cortex Eucommiae), *Du Huo* (Radix Angelicae Pubescentis) and *Chuan Niu Xi* (Radix Cyathulae). **Exemplar Formula:** *Du Huo Ji Sheng Tang* (Angelica Pubescens and Taxillus Decoction).

2. Calms the Fetus

Restless fetus: *Sang Ji Sheng*, with its tonic nature, is used for restless fetus associated with yin and blood deficiencies. Other symptoms may include bleeding and back pain.

- Restless fetus, back pain due to yin and blood deficiencies: combine *Sang Ji Sheng* with *Xu Duan* (Radix Dipsaci), *Dang Gui* (Radicis Angelicae Sinensis) and *Du Zhong* (Cortex Eucommiae).
- Bleeding after miscarriage: use this herb with *E Jiao* (Colla Corii Asini) and charred *Ai Ye* (Folium Artemisiae Argyi) to stop bleeding.

DOSAGE

10 to 20 grams.

CHEMICAL COMPOSITION

Quercetin, avicullarin, coriamyrtin, tutin, coratin, d-catechin, quercitrin, hyperin, hyperoside.[1,2]

Sang Ji Sheng (Herba Taxilli)

Avicullarin

PHARMACOLOGICAL EFFECTS

- **Cardiovascular:** Both water and alcohol extracts of *Sang Ji Sheng* used in anesthetized dogs have been shown to lower blood pressure, dilate the coronary artery, and increase perfusion to cardiac muscles.[3]
- **Anticoagulant:** *Sang Ji Sheng* has been shown to inhibit platelet aggregation and prevent the formation of emboli.[4]
- **CNS suppressant:** Preparations of *Sang Ji Sheng* have been shown to exert an inhibitory influence on the central nervous system (CNS).[5]
- **Diuretic:** Avicullarin, given orally or via intravenous injection, has demonstrated a marked diuretic effect in anesthetized dogs.[6]
- **Antiviral:** *Sang Ji Sheng* has demonstrated an inhibitory effect against many ECHO 6.9, coxsackie A9, B4, and B5 viruses.[7]

CLINICAL STUDIES AND RESEARCH

- **Myocardial infarction:** In one study, 180 patients with myocardial infarction were treated with intravenous injection of a *Sang Ji Sheng* preparation. One ml of *Sang Ji Sheng* injectable was equivalent to 2 grams of fresh herb. The intravenous solution was prepared by mixing 12 ml of *Sang Ji Sheng* in injectable form with 20 ml of 25% glucose solution; or by mixing 18 ml of injectable *Sang Ji Sheng* with 250 ml of a 5% glucose solution. The intravenous solution was administered once daily for 14 days with improvement noted in 82.8% of the subjects.[8]
- **Myocardial infarction:** According to one report, 54 patients with past histories of myocardial infarction were treated with *Sang Ji Sheng* tea (using 40 grams of herb per dose) twice daily for 6 weeks. Improvement was noted in 76% of subjects.[9]
- **Chronic tracheitis:** In one study, 200 patients with chronic tracheitis were treated with an herbal decoction, with 42 patients reporting marked improvement and 69 experiencing moderate improvement. The herbal formula was prepared by cooking 9 grams of *Sang Ji Sheng*, and 4.5 grams of *Chen Pi* (Pericarpium Citri Reticulatae) in 200 ml of water.[10]
- **Poliomyelitis:** Intramuscular injections of an herbal preparation (equal parts of *Sang Ji Sheng* and *Yin Yang Huo* (Herba Epimedii)) were given to poliomyelitis patients with promising results.[11]

HERB-DRUG INTERACTION

- **Anticoagulant or antiplatelet drugs:** Since *Sang Ji Sheng* has been shown to inhibit aggregation of platelets, it should be used with caution in patients who take anticoagulant or antiplatelet medications.[12] [Note: Examples of anticoagulants include heparin, warfarin (Coumadin) and enoxaparin (Lovenox); and examples of antiplatelets include aspirin, dipyridamole (Persantine), and clopidogrel (Plavix).]
- **Diuretics:** *Sang Ji Sheng* has a diuretic effect. Though no examples of adverse interaction have been documented, concurrent use with diuretic drugs may lead to increased elimination of water and/or electrolytes.[13] [Note: Examples of diuretics include chlorothiazide, hydrochlorothiazide, furosemide (Lasix), bumetanide (Bumex), and torsemide (Demadex).]

TOXICOLOGY

The LD_{50} for intraperitoneal injection of avicullarin in mice is 1.17 g/kg. The cause of fatality included seizures and respiratory depression.[14]

AUTHORS' COMMENTS

Taxillus chinensis is the standard name and official source for *Sang Ji Sheng.*[15] The previous names, such as *Loranthus parasiticus, Loranthus yadorik*, and *Viscum coloratum*, are no longer used.

Other traditional texts have reported *Sang Ji Sheng* to be able to treat disorders such as hair loss, looseness of teeth and insufficient breast milk.

Sang Ji Sheng and *Wu Jia Pi* (Cortex Acanthopanacis) both tonify the Liver and the Kidney to treat *bi zheng* (painful obstruction syndrome). They differ in that *Sang Ji Sheng* also calms a restless fetus, while *Wu Jia Pi* is a diuretic that treats edema.

Sang Ji Sheng and *Du Zhong* (Cortex Eucommiae) both treat low back pain. However, *Sang Ji Sheng* dispels wind-damp and tonifies blood to treat pain. *Du Zhong* tonifies qi and strengthens soft tissues to relieve pain. Their differences are complimentary, thus, they are often used as a pair.

References

1. *Xian Dai Zhong Yao Yao Li Xue* (Contemporary Pharmacology of Chinese Herbs), 1997; 433
2. Yan X, Zhou J, Xie G, *Traditional Chinese Medicines Molecular Structures, Natural Sources and Applications*; Ashgate, 1999; 533
3. *Zhong Yao Yao Li Yu Ying Yong* (Pharmacology and Applications of Chinese Herbs), 1983; 950
4. *Zhong Yao Xue* (Chinese Herbology), 1998; 296:297

Sang Ji Sheng (Herba Taxilli)

5. Ibid.
6. *Zhong Yao Yao Li Yu Ying Yong* (Pharmacology and Applications of Chinese Herbs), 1983; 950
7. Ibid.
8. *Yi Yao Gong Ye* (Pharmaceutical Industry), 1977; 3:39
9. *Xin Yi Yao Xue Za Zhi* (New Journal of Medicine and Herbology), 1974; 3:16
10. *Xin Yi Xue* (New Medicine), 1973; 10:498
11. *Zhong Cao Yao Tong Xun* (Journal of Chinese Herbal Medicine), 1972; 2:28
12. Chen, J. Recognition & prevention of herb-drug interactions, *Medical Acupuncture*, Fall/Winter 1998/1999; volume 10/number 2; 9-13
13. Ibid.
14. *Zhong Guo Yi Yuan Yao Xue Za Zhi* (Chinese Hospital Journal of Herbology), 1988; 8(3):1
15. *Zhong Hua Ren Min Gong He Guo Yao Dian* (Chinese Herbal Pharmacopoeia by People's Republic of China), 2000

Wu Jia Pi (Cortex Acanthopanacis)

五加皮

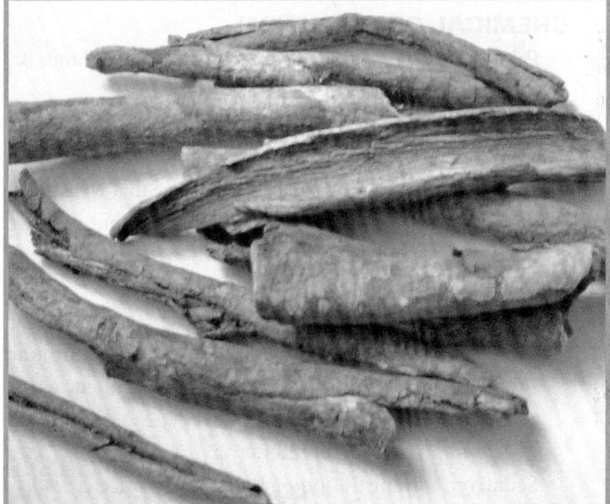

Pinyin Name: *Wu Jia Pi*

Literal Name: "five plus bark," "bark of five additions"

Alternate Chinese Names: *Nan Wu Jia Pi*

Original Source: *Shen Nong Ben Cao Jing* (Divine Husbandman's Classic of the Materia Medica) in the second century

English Name: acanthopanax, acanthopanax root bark, slender style acanthopanax root bark

Botanical Name: *Acanthopanax gracilistylus* W.W. Smith (*Xi Zhu Wu Jia*); substitutes include *Acanthopanax sessiliforus* (*Duan Geng Wu Jia; Wu Geng Wu Jia*); *Acanthopanax henryi* (*Zao Ye Wu Jia*); *Acanthopanax giraldii* (*Hong Mao Wu Jia*); *Acanthopanax leucorrhizus* (*Teng Wu Jia*); and *Acanthopanax setchuenensis* (*Shu Wu Jia*). Acanthopanax is also referred to as Eleutherococcus in literature.

Pharmaceutical Name: Cortex Acanthopanacis

Properties: acrid, bitter, warm

Channels Entered: Kidney, Liver

CHINESE THERAPEUTIC ACTIONS

1. Dispels Wind and Dampness, Strengthens Bones and Tendons

***Bi zheng* (painful obstruction syndrome), weakness and soreness of the back and knees:** *Wu Jia Pi* (Cortex Acanthopanacis) dispels wind and dampness to relieve muscle aches and pain. It also tonifies the Kidney and Liver to strengthen bones and tendons. Clinical applications include *bi zheng* due to wind, cold or dampness, muscle spasms and cramps due to excess or deficient conditions, and weakness of the low back and knees due to Liver and Kidney deficiencies. It is especially useful for elderly patients who have muscular atrophy, or for children who have delayed development of motor functions. For daily intake, this herb is commonly used alone, as an herbal wine.

- *Bi zheng* due to wind, cold or dampness: use *Wu Jia Pi* with *Mu Gua* (Fructus Chaenomelis) and *Chuan Niu Xi* (Radix Cyathulae).
- Traumatic injuries with bruises or broken bones: use it with *Zi Ran Tong* (Pyritum), *Di Bie Chong* (Eupolyphaga) and *Ru Xiang* (Gummi Olibanum).
- Delayed motor development in children: combine this herb with *Mu Gua* (Fructus Chaenomelis), *Chuan Niu Xi* (Radix Cyathulae), *Sang Ji Sheng* (Herba Taxilli), and *Xu Duan* (Radix Dipsaci).

Wu Jia Pi (Cortex Acanthopanacis)

2. Dispels Water Retention

Edema: *Wu Jia Pi* regulates water circulation to treat edema and dysuria.

- Edema: add *Fu Ling Pi* (Cortex Poria), *Da Fu Pi* (Pericarpium Arecae), and *Sheng Jiang Pi* (Pericarpium Zingiberis Recens) to this herb. **Exemplar Formula:** *Wu Pi Yin* (Five-Peel Decoction).

DOSAGE

5 to 10 grams.

CAUTIONS / CONTRAINDICATIONS

- Use of *Wu Jia Pi* may be associated with drowsiness and sedation. Therefore, individuals who take this herb should exercise caution if driving or operating heavy machinery.

CHEMICAL COMPOSITION

Palmitic acid, linolenic acid, tannin, vitamin A, vitamin B.[1]

PHARMACOLOGICAL EFFECTS

- **Adaptogenic:** Administration of *Wu Jia Pi* is associated with a marked adaptogenic effect. In mice that were given the herb daily for 9 days, there was a significant increase in swimming endurance compared to the performance of the placebo group that did not receive any herbs.[2]
- **Immunostimulant:** Administration of *Wu Jia Pi* has shown marked effectiveness in enhancing the immune system. Therapeutic benefits include elevated white blood cell count, increased phagocytic activity, and increased production of interferon.[3]
- **Sedative:** Administration of *Wu Jia Pi* to mice is associated with only mild sedative effects. However, it potentiates the sedative effect of barbiturates and leads to prolonged sleeping time.[4]
- **Anti-inflammatory and analgesic:** Intraperitoneal injection of *Wu Jia Pi* has marked anti-inflammatory and analgesic effects in rats. In another study, oral administration of alcohol extract of *Wu Jia Pi* reduced pain and swelling for up to five hours, with peak effect at hours two and three.[5,6]
- **Vasodilative:** *Wu Jia Pi* dilates blood vessels to increase blood perfusion to the coronary artery and thus decrease blood pressure.[7]
- **Others:** *Wu Jia Pi* also has antitussive, expectorant, antiasthmatic and antineoplastic properties.[8]

CLINICAL STUDIES AND RESEARCH

- **Leukopenia:** Two separate clinical trials have shown administration of *Wu Jia Pi* to be effective in treating patients with leukopenia.[9,10]
- **Cerebral thrombosis:** The combination of oral decoction and intravenous infusion of *Wu Jia Pi* once daily was beneficial in treating 20 patients with cerebral thrombosis.[11]
- **Hypotension:** A preparation of *Wu Jia Pi* given three times daily for 20 days was beneficial in treatment of hypotension.[12]

HERB-DRUG INTERACTION

- **Sedatives:** *Wu Jia Pi* has a mild sedative effect, and potentiates the sedative effect of barbiturates.[13] [Note: Many categories of drugs induce sedation, such as antihistamines, narcotic analgesics, barbiturates, benzodiazepines and many others.]

TOXICOLOGY

No fatalities were reported following oral administration of *Wu Jia Pi* at 480 g/kg/day for 3 days in mice.[14]

SUPPLEMENT

- 北五加皮 *Bei Wu Jia Pi* (Cortex Periploca Sepium Radicis), *Periploca sepium* Bge., is sometimes incorrectly used as a substitute for *Wu Jia Pi* (Cortex Acanthopanacis), as both have a similar appearance and smell. These two herbs are completely different in function and should not be used interchangeably. *Bei Wu Jia Pi*, literally meaning '*Wu Jia Pi* from the north,' grows in the northern regions of China. *Bei Wu Jia Pi* has cardiotonic and diuretic functions; it is also toxic, and its use requires only a small dosage. *Wu Jia Pi*, also known as *Nan Wu Jia Pi*, literally meaning '*Wu Jia Pi* from the south,' grows in southern parts of China.

AUTHORS' COMMENTS

Wu Jia Pi and *Sang Ji Sheng* (Herba Taxilli) both tonify the Liver and Kidney to treat *bi zheng* (painful obstruction syndrome). They differ in that *Wu Jia Pi* is also a diuretic that treats edema, whereas *Sang Ji Sheng* can calm a restless fetus.

References

1. *Zhong Guo Yi Yuan Yao Xue Za Zhi* (Chinese Hospital Journal of Herbology), 1988; 8(3):1
2. *Zhong Cao Yao* (Chinese Herbal Medicine), 1987; 18(3):28
3. *Zhong Yao Xue* (Chinese Herbology), 1998; 297:300
4. *Zhong Cao Yao* (Chinese Herbal Medicine), 1987; 18(3):28
5. *Zhong Guo Yao Li Xue Tong Bao* (Journal of Chinese Herbal Pharmacology), 1986; 2(2):21
6. *Zhong Cheng Yao Yan Jiu* (Research of Chinese Patent Medicine), 1984; 10:22
7. *Zhong Cao Yao* (Chinese Herbal Medicine), 1987; 18(3):28
8. Ibid.
9. *Guang Xi Yi Xue Yuan Xue Bao* (Journal of Guangxi University of Medicine), 1978; 3:1
10. *Hu Bei Zhong Yi Za Zhi* (Hubei Journal of Chinese Medicine), 1982; 6:52
11. *Gan Su Zhong Yi Xue Yuan Xue Bao* (*Journal of Gansu University of Chinese Medicine*), 1988; 1:27
12. *Zhong Cheng Yao Yan Jiu* (*Research of Chinese Patent Medicine*), 1985; 12:43
13. *Zhong Cao Yao* (*Chinese Herbal Medicine*), 1987; 18(3):28
14. *Zhong Cheng Yao Yan Jiu* (*Research of Chinese Patent Medicine*), 1985; (4):41

Hu Gu (Os Tigris)

虎骨 虎骨

Pinyin Name: *Hu Gu*
Literal Name: "tiger bone"
Original Source: *Ming Yi Za Zhu* (Miscellaneous Records of Famous Physicians) by Tao Hong-Jing in 500 A.D.
English Name: tiger bone
Zoological Name: *Pathera tigris* L. (*Hu*)
Pharmaceutical Name: Os Tigris
Properties: acrid, warm
Channels Entered: Liver, Kidney
International Status: CITES I

CHINESE THERAPEUTIC ACTIONS

Dispels Wind, Relieves Pain, Strengthens Sinews and Bones

***Bi zheng* (painful obstruction syndrome), weakness and soreness of the back and knees:** Dispersing, warming and tonifying in nature, *Hu Gu* (Os Tigris) was historically used to open channels and collaterals, tonify the Liver and Kidney, strengthen the sinews and bones, and stop pain. It best treated migratory pain, spasms and cramps caused by deficiencies of the Liver and Kidney. *Hu Gu* was the substance of choice when treating weakness and soreness of the lower back and knees, and for cold pain in the bones.

- *Bi zheng*, weakness and soreness of the back and knees: *Hu Gu* was used alone as a medicinal wine, or with *Mu Gua* (Fructus Chaenomelis), *Niu Xi* (Radix Cyathulae seu Achyranthis) and *Wu Jia Pi* (Cortex Acanthopanacis).

DOSAGE

3 to 6 grams. *Hu Gu* was used as powder, pills or herbal tincture. Unprocessed *Hu Gu* is hard, and has a distinct odor. It was necessary to dry-fry *Hu Gu* or fry it with sesame oil to eliminate the odor and facilitate extraction of the active constituents. Preparation of the substance was done at a moderate temperature: processing at high temperatures or under high pressure reduces the effectiveness of the resultant substance.

CHEMICAL COMPOSITION

Calcium, protein, amino acids.[1]

PHARMACOLOGICAL EFFECTS

- **Anti-inflammatory:** Administrating *Hu Gu* or *Gou Gu* (Os Canitis) in powdered form showed marked effectiveness to stop inflammation and reduce permeability of the capillaries. The mechanism of its anti-inflammatory effect is attributed to stimulation of the endocrine system and increased production of hormones by the adrenal glands.[2]
- **Sedative and analgesic:** Both *Hu Gu* and *Gou Gu* (Os Canitis) have shown sedative and analgesic effects in rats.[3]

SUPPLEMENT

- 豬骨 / 猪骨 *Zhu Gu* (Os Porcus) – bones from pigs, and 狗骨 / 狗骨 *Gou Gu* (Os Canitis) – bones from dogs, are generally used today as a replacement for *Hu Gu*. They have similar functions to *Hu Gu*, but are not as strong.

AUTHORS' COMMENTS

Hu Gu is listed in Appendix I of the Convention on International Trade in Endangered Species of Wild Fauna and Flora (CITES). Trade in *Hu Gu* is strictly prohibited. The discussion of *Hu Gu* in this text is included only to offer 1) the accurate history of its critically important usage in traditional herbal medicine, and 2) models for appropriate usage of effective substitute substances (see Supplement). The information should not be interpreted as condoning illegal use of this endangered species. For more information, please refer to Appendix 10.

References

1. *Zhong Yao Xue* (Chinese Herbology), 1998; 300-301
2. Ibid.
3. Ibid.

Lu Han Cao (Herba Pyrolae)

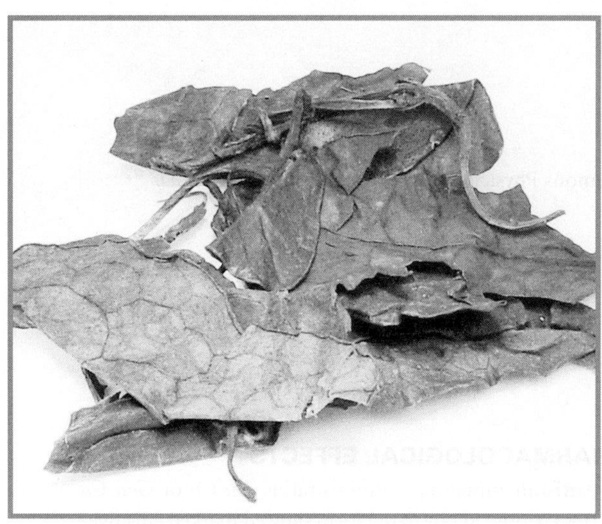

鹿含草 鹿含草

Pinyin Name: *Lu Han Cao*
Alternate Chinese Names: *Lu Xian Cao, Lu Shou Cha*
Original Source: *Ben Cao Gang Mu* (Materia Medica) by Li Shi-Zhen in 1578
English Name: pyrola
Botanical Name: *Pyrola rotundifolia L.* (*Lu Ti Cao*); *Pyrola calliantha* (*Lu Ti Cao*); *Pyrola decorata* (*Pu Tong Lu Ti Cao*)
Pharmaceutical Name: Herba Pyrolae
Properties: sweet, bitter, warm
Channels Entered: Liver, Kidney

CHINESE THERAPEUTIC ACTIONS

1. Dispels Wind-Dampness, Strengthens Tendons and Bones

***Bi zheng* (painful obstruction syndrome):** *Lu Han Cao* (Herba Pyrolae) dispels wind-dampness and tonifies the Liver and Kidney. It treats *bi zheng* with low back pain and degeneration of the tendons and bones, caused by Kidney and Liver deficiencies. It alleviates weakness and soreness of the joints accompanied by cold sensations. It is also used for bone spurs.

- Soreness, weakness and coldness of the lower back and knees: use *Lu Han Cao* with *Du Zhong* (Cortex Eucommiae), *Niu Xi* (Radix Cyathulae seu Achyranthis) and *Tu Si Zi* (Semen Cuscutae).
- Bone spurs: combine it with *Po Bu Zi Ye* (Folium Cordia Dichotoma), *Yin Yang Huo* (Herba Epimedii), *Gu Sui Bu* (Rhizoma Drynariae) and *Ji Xue Teng* (Caulis Spatholobi).

2. Tonifies Lung and Kidney

Chronic cough, asthma due to Kidney deficiency: *Lu Han Cao* has a mild effect to moisten the Lung. It is best for chronic respiratory disorders such as dry, feeble cough, or asthma from Kidney deficiency.

3. Stops Bleeding

Bleeding: When combined with other hemostatic herbs, *Lu Han Cao* treats epistaxis, hematemesis, hypermenorrhea and abnormal uterine bleeding. Crush the fresh form of this herb into a paste to be applied topically, to stop local bleeding due to traumatic injuries.

4. Nourishes the Heart and Stops Perspiration

Lu Han Cao stops palpitations and night sweating associated with yin deficiency.

DOSAGE

10 to 30 grams in decoction, pills or powder.

CHEMICAL COMPOSITION

Arbutin, chimaphillin, einulsin.[1]

HERB-DRUG INTERACTION

- **Aminoglycosides**: In one study, compound injection of *Lu Han Cao* and *Huang Qi* (Radix Astragali) in guinea pigs was found to be effective in preventing the ototoxicity and nephrotoxicity associated with use of aminoglycosides.[2] [Note: Examples of aminoglycosides include gentamicin, tobramycin, amikacin.]

TOXICOLOGY

The LD_{50} for intravenous injection of *Lu Han Cao* is 9.73/kg in mice. No abnormalities were observed in mice following oral administration of *Lu Han Cao* at 60 g/kg for one week.[3]

References

1. *Xian Dai Zhong Yao Yao Li Xue* (Contemporary Pharmacology of Chinese Herbs), 1997; 448
2. Xuan, W., Dong, M., and Dong, M. *Annals of Otology, Rhinology and Laryngology*, May 1995, vol. 104(5): 374-80
3. *Zhong Cao Yao Tong Xun* (Journal of Chinese Herbal Medicine), 1976; (7):12

Shi Nan Teng (Ramulus Piper)

石南藤 石南藤

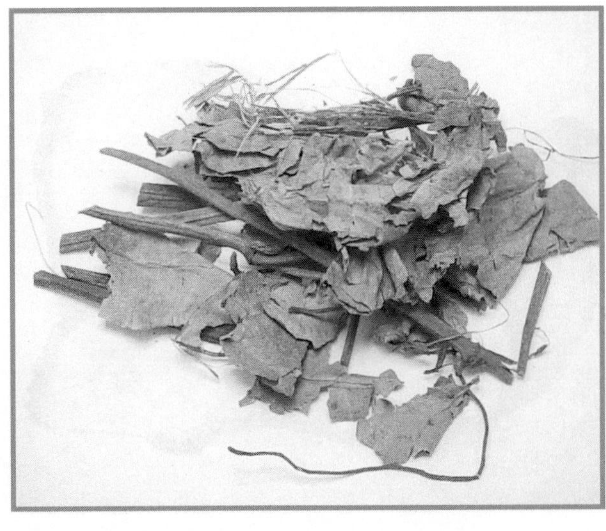

Pinyin Name: *Shi Nan Teng*
Alternate Chinese Names: *Nan Teng, Ding Gong Teng*
English Name: piper vine
Botanical Name: *Piper wallichii* Hand.-Mazz. var. *hupehense* Hang.-Mazz.; *Piper aurantiacum* Wall.ex C.DC.; *Piper puberulum* (Benth.) Maxim.
Pharmaceutical Name: Ramulus Piper
Properties: acrid, warm
Channels Entered: Liver, Lung, Kidney

CHINESE THERAPEUTIC ACTIONS

1. Dispels Wind-Cold Invasion, Strengthens the Back and Legs

- *Bi zheng* (painful obstruction syndrome) due to wind-cold, weak legs: use *Shi Nan Teng* (Ramulus Piper) with *Chuan Shan Long* (Rhizoma Dioscoreae Nipponicae), *Du Zhong* (Cortex Eucommiae), *Xu Duan* (Radix Dipsaci) and *Du Huo* (Radix Angelicae Pubescentis).

2. Arrests Cough

- Cough with dyspnea due to wind-cold: combine *Shi Nan Teng* with *Xiao Qing Long Tang* (Minor Bluegreen Dragon Decoction).

DOSAGE

6 to 20 grams.

CAUTIONS / CONTRAINDICATIONS

- Use *Shi Nan Teng* with caution in patients with deficiency and cold of the Spleen and Stomach.

Zou Ma Tai (Rhizoma Ardisiae)

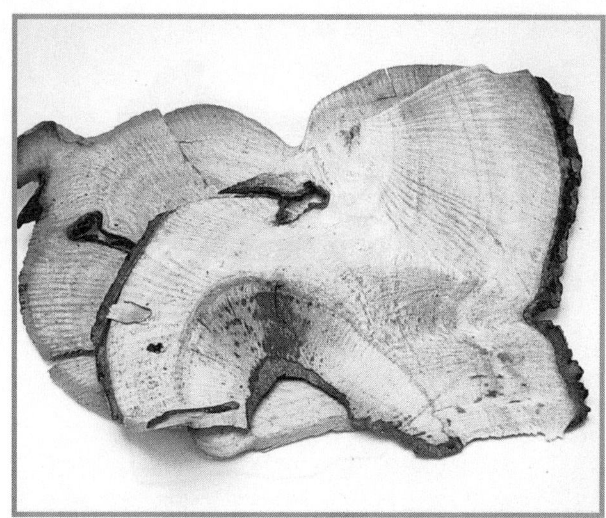

走馬胎 走马胎

Pinyin Name: *Zou Ma Tai*
Alternate Chinese Names: *Ma Tai, Shuang Ma Tai*
English Name: ardisia root, giant leaf ardisia rhizome
Botanical Name: *Ardisia gigantifolia* Stapf.
Pharmaceutical Name: Rhizoma Ardisiae
Properties: acrid, neutral
Channels Entered: Lung, Stomach, Spleen, Large Intestine

CHINESE THERAPEUTIC ACTIONS

1. Dispels Wind

Exterior condition: *Zou Ma Tai* (Rhizoma Ardisiae) treats wind-heat or wind-cold invasions. It is also commonly used for exterior invasion in postpartum patients.

- Wind-heat: use *Zou Ma Tai* with *Da Qing Ye* (Folium Isatidis).
- Wind-cold: use this herb with *Gui Zhi* (Ramulus Cinnamomi).

2. Generates Flesh, Strengthens Bones and Tendons

- Arthritis or numbness and pain in the extremities in the elderly: use this herb with *Qian Nian Jian* (Rhizoma Homalomenae), and *Ji Xiang Teng* (Caulis Paederiae).

3. Strengthens the Stomach and Regulates the Digestive Track

- Dysentery: add *Feng Wei Cao* (Herba Pteris).

DOSAGE

3 to 12 grams.

AUTHORS' COMMENTS

Zou Ma Tai, used externally, treats toxic swellings.

Chapter 4 summary

— Wind-Damp Dispelling Herbs

SECTION 1: WIND-DAMP DISPELLING AND PAIN-RELIEVING HERBS

Name	Similarities	Differences
Du Huo (Radix Angelicae Pubescentis)	Dispel wind-dampness, alleviate pain	Mostly addresses lower body pain
Wei Ling Xian (Radix Clematidis)		Treats fish bones obstructing the throat
Fen Fang Ji (Radix Stephaniae Tetandrae)		Promotes diuresis and reduces swelling
Xu Chang Qing (Radix Cynanchi Paniculati)		Treats traumatic injuries, relieves itching and toxic snake bites
Can Sha (Excrementum Bombycis Mori)		Harmonizes Stomach, disperses turbidity to treat vomiting, relieves itching and eczema when used externally
Song Jie (Lignum Pini Nodi)		Relieves pain associated with *bi zheng* (painful obstruction syndrome) and trauma
Qi Ye Lian (Radix Schefflerae)		Relieves pain associated with *bi zheng* (painful obstruction syndrome) and trauma
Lei Gong Teng (Radix Tripterygii Wilfordii)		Toxic, kills parasites and treats snake bites
Qin Jiao (Radix Gentianae Macrophyllae)		Clears deficiency heat and relieves jaundice
Hong Gu She (Radix Kadsura Japonicae)		Cools blood, reduces inflammation and pain, relieves spasms and cramps
Tou Gu Cao (Caulis Impatientis)		Invigorates blood circulation, dispels blood stagnation
Yi Wu Gen (Radix Elaeagni)		Reduces swelling and eliminates stagnation
Hai Fu Rong (Herba Limonium Wrightii)		Lowers blood pressure
Qing Feng Teng (Caulis Sinomenii)		Reduces swelling and pain
Ma An Teng (Herba Ipomoea Pes-caprae)		Reduces carbuncles and disperses nodules

General Characteristics of Wind-Damp Dispelling and Pain-Relieving Herbs:

Taste: acrid, bitter
Thermal property: varies
Channels entered: Kidney, Liver
Therapeutic actions: disperse wind, cold, and damp; and relieve pain

These herbs dispel wind, cold and damp to treat muscle aches and pains, spasms and cramps, and weakness and pain of the lower back and knees.

Du Huo (Radix Angelicae Pubescentis) is most suitable for back pain due to excess-type wind-damp invasion with coldness. In addition, it has a strong effect to relieve pain and release the exterior. *Du Huo*, however, does not have a tonic effect, and is therefore not suitable by itself for patients who are weak or deficient. *Du Huo* is combined with *Sang Ji Sheng* (Herba Taxilli) to treat chronic back pain due to deficiency.

Wei Ling Xian (Radix Clematidis), extremely penetrating in nature, opens channels and collaterals, and treats fish bones lodged in the throat.

Fen Fang Ji (Radix Stephaniae Tetandrae), in addition to having an antirheumatic effect, promotes diuresis and reduces swelling. Cold in thermal property, it relieves pain, regulates water circulation, and relieves edema.

Chapter 4 summary

Xu Chang Qing (Radix Cynanchi Paniculati) dispels wind and relieves pain. In addition to alleviating arthritis pain, it treats trauma-related pain, epigastric and abdominal pain and toothache. It relieves the itching of various dermatological disorders and detoxifies snake bites.

Can Sha (Excrementum Bombycis Mori) treats vomiting, diarrhea and cramps, dispels dampness and relieves itching.

Song Jie (Lignum Pini Nodi) and ***Qi Ye Lian*** (Radix Schefflerae) dispel wind-damp, relieves pain, and most suitable for *bi zheng* (painful obstruction syndrome) and traumatic injuries.

Lei Gong Teng (Radix Tripterygii Wilfordii) strongly dispels wind-dampness, relieves pain, and treats arthritis. However, it is toxic and should be used with caution.

Qin Jiao (Radix Gentianae Macrophyllae) dispels wind-dampness and clears deficiency heat to relieve jaundice, lowers blood pressure and soothes itching.

Hong Gu She (Radix Kadsura Japonicae) relieves spasms and cramps to reduce inflammation and pain.

Tou Gu Cao (Caulis Impatientis) invigorates blood circulation, dispels blood stagnation, and is especially effective for pain associated with blood stagnation.

Yi Wu Gen (Radix Elaeagni) relieves pain accompanied by swelling and inflammation.

Hai Fu Rong (Herba Limonium Wrightii) and ***Qing Feng Teng*** (Caulis Sinomenii) have a generalized effect to dispel wind-dampness and relieve pain.

Ma An Teng (Herba Ipomoea Pes-caprae) dispels wind-dampness, relieves pain, and dispels heat and toxins from the exterior to reduce carbuncles and nodules.

SECTION 2: WIND-DAMP DISPELLING AND CHANNELS- AND COLLATERALS-OPENING HERBS

Name	Similarities	Differences
Mu Gua (Fructus Chaenomelis)	Dispel wind-dampness and open channels and collaterals	Relaxes tendons, dissolves dampness, harmonizes Stomach
Luo Shi Teng (Caulis Trachelospermi)		Cools blood, reduces swelling for swollen throat
Sang Zhi (Ramulus Mori)		Relieves pain and stiffness of extremities
Qian Nian Jian (Rhizoma Homalomenae)		Relieves stiff and numb extremities
Hai Feng Teng (Caulis Piperis Kadsurae)		Relieves pain associated with *bi zheng* (painful obstruction syndrome) and trauma
Hai Tong Pi (Cortex Erythrinae)		Treats dermatological disorders when used externally
Xun Gu Feng (Herba Aristolochiae Mollissimae)		Relieves pain associated with *bi zheng* (painful obstruction syndrome) and trauma
Bai Hua She (Bungarus Parvus)		Strongly opens channels, and extinguishes wind to relieve convulsions
Wu Shao She (Zaocys)		Opens channels, and extinguishes wind to relieve convulsions
She Tui (Periostracum Serpentis)		Extinguishes wind to relieve itching, convulsions and superficial visual obstruction
Xia Tian Wu (Rhizoma Corydalis Decumbentis)		Invigorates blood circulation, treats trauma-related injuries; also relieves abdominal and epigastric pain
Chuan Shan Long (Rhizoma Dioscoreae Nipponicae)		Invigorates blood circulation to treat *xiong bi* (painful obstruction of the chest); relieves cough, dispels hot phlegm

Chapter 4 summary

Name	Similarities	Differences
Lao Guan Cao (Herba Erodii seu Geranii)		Stops damp-heat diarrhea
Shen Jin Cao (Herba Lycopodii)		Eases tendons that are tight from chronic *bi zheng* (painful obstruction syndrome)
Xi Xian Cao (Herba Siegesbeckiae)		Clears heat, eliminates toxins, relieves carbuncles, swellings and eczema
Chou Wu Tong (Folium Clerodendri Trichotomi)		Relieves skin itching and eczema
Huang Jin Gui (Caulis Vanieriae)		Opens channels and collaterals, reduces swelling and pain
Liu Zhi Huang (Herba Solidaginis)		Opens channels and collaterals, reduces swelling and pain
Yi Tiao Gen (Radix Moghaniae)		Opens channels and collaterals

General Characteristics of Wind-Damp Dispelling and Channels- and Collaterals-Opening Herbs:

Taste: acrid, bitter
Thermal property: varies
Channels entered: Kidney, Liver
Therapeutic actions: relieve pain; reduce stiffness, soreness, and swelling; and restore mobility

These herbs open peripheral channels and collaterals to treat chronic, stubborn *bi zheng* (painful obstruction syndrome) accompanied by decreased range of joint motion, decreased mobility of extremities, numbness, hemiplegia and paralysis.

Mu Gua (Fructus Chaenomelis) and ***Can Sha*** (Excrementum Bombycis Mori) treat vomiting, diarrhea and cramps.

Mu Gua more effectively relaxes tendons and opens the collaterals, and treats swelling and pain in the legs.

Can Sha dispels dampness and relieves itching.

Luo Shi Teng (Caulis Trachelospermi), ***Sang Zhi*** (Ramulus Mori), and ***Qian Nian Jian*** (Rhizoma Homalomenae) dispel wind and open the collaterals, and are most suitable to treat *bi zheng* (painful obstruction syndrome) caused by wind-dampness, with tightness and cramping of the tendons.

Luo Shi Teng is slightly cold, cools the blood, reduces swelling and treats swollen throat, swellings or carbuncles.

Sang Zhi is neutral, and treats pain in the upper limbs.

Qian Nian Jian is warm, and relieves muscle stiffness and numbness.

Hai Feng Teng (Caulis Piperis Kadsurae), ***Hai Tong Pi*** (Cortex Erythrinae) and ***Xun Gu Feng*** (Herba Aristolochiae Mollissimae) dispel wind, open the collaterals and relieve pain, and are mostly used to treat pain, spasms and tightness from wind-dampness.

Hai Feng Teng relieves pain associated with trauma and *bi zheng* (painful obstruction syndrome).

Hai Tong Pi treats pain in the lower back.

Xun Gu Feng also treats stomach pain and toothache.

Bai Hua She (Bungarus Parvus) and ***Wu Shao She*** (Zaocys) treat chronic stubborn pain, numbness, spasms or itching. They also extinguish wind and treat convulsions and tetany.

Bai Hua She is stronger but also more toxic.

Wu Shao She is not toxic but is less potent in action.

Chapter 4 summary

She Tui (Periostracum Serpentis) extinguishes wind, stops convulsions, relieves itching, and treats superficial visual obstruction. It is weaker than *Bai Hua She* (Bungarus Parvus) and *Wu Shao She* (Zaocys).

Xia Tian Wu (Rhizoma Corydalis Decumbentis) and ***Chuan Shan Long*** (Rhizoma Dioscoreae Nipponicae) dispel wind, open collaterals, and relieve pain and spasms.

Xia Tian Wu treats hemiplegia and paralysis and has a strong pain-relieving effect.

Chuan Shan Long treats *xiong bi* (painful obstruction of the chest).

Lao Guan Cao (Herba Erodii seu Geranii) dispels wind-dampness and opens collaterals to treat pain and spasms, and stops damp-heat diarrhea.

Shen Jin Cao (Herba Lycopodii) opens channels and collaterals, treating pain in the extremities, such as is found in trauma or *bi zheng* (painful obstruction syndrome).

Xi Xian Cao (Herba Siegesbeckiae) treats numbness and tightness of the extremities, and eliminates toxins to heal carbuncles and sores.

Chou Wu Tong (Folium Clerodendri Trichotomi) dispels wind-dampness, lowers blood pressure, and relieves itching.

Huang Jin Gui (Caulis Vanieriae) and ***Liu Zhi Huang*** (Herba Solidaginis) are both excellent to dispel wind-dampness, open channels and collaterals, and reduce swelling and inflammation. They are commonly used together for synergistic benefit.

Yi Tiao Gen (Radix Moghaniae) dispels wind-dampness and opens channels and collaterals.

SECTION 3: WIND-DAMP DISPELLING AND TENDON- AND BONE-STRENGTHENING HERBS

Name	Similarities	Differences
Sang Ji Sheng (Herba Taxilli)	Dispel wind-damp, strengthen tendons and bones	Stabilizes fetus
Wu Jia Pi (Cortex Acanthopanacis)		Promotes diuresis and reduces swelling
Hu Gu (Os Tigris)		Strongly relieves pain and dispels wind
Lu Han Cao (Herba Pyrolae)		Tonifies Lung and Kidney for chronic cough or asthma, stops bleeding
Shi Nan Teng (Ramulus Piper)		Strengthens back and legs
Zou Ma Tai (Rhizoma Ardisiae)		Strengthens tendons and bones

General Characteristics of Wind-Damp Dispelling and Tendon- and Bone-Strengthening Herbs:

Taste: acrid, bitter

Thermal property: warm

Channels entered: Kidney, Liver

Therapeutic actions: dispel wind, damp, cold; and tonify tendons and bones

These herbs tonify the Liver and Kidney to treat chronic *bi zheng* (painful obstruction syndrome) characterized by pain, weakness, deficiency and atrophy of soft tissues.

Sang Ji Sheng (Herba Taxilli) is often used with ***Du Huo*** (Radix Angelicae Pubescentis) to treat back pain. Together, they have excellent synergistic action as both address deficiency and excess conditions, in chronic or acute situations.

Sang Ji Sheng tonifies the Liver and Kidney to strengthen the sinews and bones.

Du Huo dispels wind-damp-cold from the exterior to relieve pain.

Chapter 4 summary

Wu Jia Pi (Cortex Acanthopanacis), besides having an antirheumatic effect, promotes diuresis and reduces swelling. It tonifies the Kidney and Liver to strengthen tendons and bones.

Hu Gu (Os Tigris), no longer a legal substance, has shown historically that it strongly dispels wind-damp, relieves pain, and strengthens tendons and bones. Use of *Hu Gu* is prohibited since tiger is an endangered animal. Bones from pigs or cattle are generally used as substitutes.

Lu Han Cao (Herba Pyrolae) dispels wind-dampness and tonifies the Liver and Kidney. It also tonifies the Lung to relieve deficiency cough and dyspnea. It stops epistaxis and uterine bleeding.

Shi Nan Teng (Ramulus Piper) and ***Zou Ma Tai*** (Rhizoma Ardisiae) dispel wind-dampness and strengthen soft tissues.

Shi Nan Teng is more specific for the back and legs.

Zou Ma Tai strengthens tendons and bones throughout the body.

HERBS FROM OTHER FUNCTIONAL CATEGORIES WITH WIND-DAMP DISPELLING FUNCTIONS

Name	Functional Category
Ba Ji Tian (Radix Morindae Officinalis)	Tonic Herbs (Chapter 17)
Bai Long Chuan Hua Tou (Radix Clerodendron Paniculatum)	Water-Regulating and Damp-Resolving Herbs (Chapter 6)
Bai Zhi (Radix Angelicae Dahuricae)	Exterior-Releasing Herbs (Chapter 1)
Bi Xie (Rhizoma Dioscoreae Hypoglaucae)	Water-Regulating and Damp-Resolving Herbs (Chapter 6)
Cang Er Zi (Fructus Xanthii)	Exterior-Releasing Herbs (Chapter 1)
Cang Zhu (Rhizoma Atractylodis)	Aromatic Damp-Dissolving Herbs (Chapter 5)
Cao Wu (Radix Aconiti Kusnezoffii)	Interior-Warming Herbs (Chapter 7)
Chuan Mu Tong (Caulis Clematidis Armandii)	Water-Regulating and Damp-Resolving Herbs (Chapter 6)
Chuan Wu (Radix Aconiti Preparata)	Interior-Warming Herbs (Chapter 7)
Chuan Xiong (Rhizoma Ligusticum Chuanxiong)	Blood-Invigorating and Stasis-Removing Herbs (Chapter 12)
Dang Gui (Radicis Angelicae Sinensis)	Tonic Herbs (Chapter 17)
Di Long (Pheretima)	Liver-Calming and Wind-Extinguishing Herbs (Chapter 15)
Du Zhong (Cortex Eucommiae)	Tonic Herbs (Chapter 17)
Fang Feng (Radix Saposhnikoviae)	Exterior-Releasing Herbs (Chapter 1)
Fu Zi (Radix Aconiti Lateralis Praeparata)	Interior-Warming Herbs (Chapter 7)
Gou Ji (Rhizoma Cibotii)	Tonic Herbs (Chapter 17)
Gu Sui Bu (Rhizoma Drynariae)	Tonic Herbs (Chapter 17)
Gui Zhi (Ramulus Cinnamomi)	Exterior-Releasing Herbs (Chapter 1)
Ji Xue Teng (Caulis Spatholobi)	Blood-Invigorating and Stasis-Removing Herbs (Chapter 12)
Jiang Huang (Rhizoma Curcumae Longae)	Blood-Invigorating and Stasis-Removing Herbs (Chapter 12)
Mo Yao (Myrrha)	Blood-Invigorating and Stasis-Removing Herbs (Chapter 12)
Niu Xi (Radix Cyathulae seu Achyranthis)	Blood-Invigorating and Stasis-Removing Herbs (Chapter 12)
Qiang Huo (Rhizoma et Radix Notopterygii)	Exterior-Releasing Herbs (Chapter 1)
Rou Gui (Cortex Cinnamomi)	Interior-Warming Herbs (Chapter 7)
Ru Xiang (Gummi Olibanum)	Blood-Invigorating and Stasis-Removing Herbs (Chapter 12)
Wu Tou (Radix Aconiti)	Interior-Warming Herbs (Chapter 7)
Xi Xin (Herba Asari)	Interior-Warming Herbs (Chapter 7)
Xian Mao (Rhizoma Curculiginis)	Tonic Herbs (Chapter 17)
Xu Duan (Radix Dipsaci)	Tonic Herbs (Chapter 17)
Yi Yi Ren (Semen Coicis)	Water-Regulating and Damp-Resolving Herbs (Chapter 6)
Yin Yang Huo (Herba Epimedii)	Tonic Herbs (Chapter 17)

Chapter 5

— Aromatic Damp-Dissolving Herbs

芳香化湿药

Chapter 5 — Aromatic Damp-Dissolving Herbs

Chapter 5

芳香化湿药

— Aromatic Damp-Dissolving Herbs

Definition: Aromatic and fragrant, these herbs enhance the function of the Spleen to dissolve, dry or disperse dampness, transforming and transporting substances that would otherwise accumulate to cause damp imbalance or obstruction.

"Dampness" refers to the environmental pathogenic factor that tends to accumulate in the middle *jiao* and obstruct the normal transforming and transporting functions of the Spleen and Stomach. Symptoms of the presence of dampness include fullness and distention of the epigastrium and abdomen, nausea, vomiting, poor appetite, heaviness of the extremities, loose stools, and a thick, greasy tongue coat. Acrid, bitter, warm and drying, many of these herbs enter and strengthen the Spleen and Stomach, to activate qi circulation, dissolve dampness, and improve the Spleen's transformation and transportation activities.

Aromatic damp-dissolving herbs work for restoration of Spleen and Stomach transformation and transportation activities.

DIFFERENTIAL DIAGNOSIS AND TREATMENT

Dampness may be divided into damp-cold or damp-heat: each condition must be treated accordingly. Because accumulation of dampness is often accompanied by stagnation, it is beneficial to use herbs that simultaneously activate the qi. Accumulation of dampness may also lead to edema; therefore, herbs that regulate water circulation may be added.

CAUTIONS/CONTRAINDICATIONS

Long-term use of warming and drying herbs may consume yin and body fluids. Thus, they should not be used for very long in patients with such deficiencies. This applies in particular to *Cang Zhu* (Rhizoma Atractylodis), *Hou Po* (Cortex Magnoliae Officinalis) and *Cao Guo* (Fructus Tsaoko), herbs with the strongest drying abilities.

PROCESSING

Most of these herbs are aromatic and contain large percentages of essential oils that evaporate easily. Therefore, they should be added towards the end or at the close of cooking to avoid loss of active components and potency from over-cooking, a process known as post-decoction.

These herbs are post-decocted to avoid loss of active components and potency.

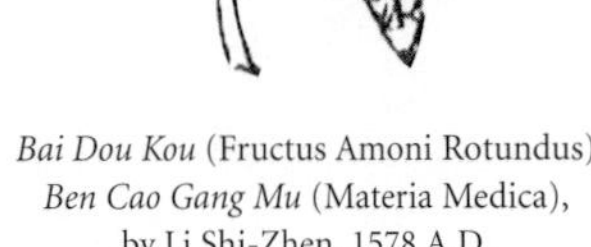

Bai Dou Kou (Fructus Amoni Rotundus)
Ben Cao Gang Mu (Materia Medica),
by Li Shi-Zhen, 1578 A.D.

PHARMACOLOGICAL EFFECTS

- **Gastrointestinal:** Many aromatic damp-dissolving substances stimulate the gastrointestinal system to increase peristalsis of the intestines and production of gastric acid, to treat indigestion, fullness and distention of the abdomen, and abdominal spasms and cramps.
- **Antibiotic**: Some of these herbs have antibiotic actions, such as *Cang Zhu* (Rhizoma Atractylodis), *Hou Po* (Cortex Magnoliae Officinalis), *Huo Xiang* (Herba Agastache), *Bai Bu* (Radix Stemonae) and *Sha Ren* (Fructus Amomi).

Chapter 5 — Aromatic Damp-Dissolving Herbs

POTENTIAL HERB-DRUG INTERACTIONS

- **Antiulcer:** Aromatic and damp-resolving herbs may stimulate the digestive system to produce more stomach acid and increase peristalsis. Therefore, they should be used with caution in patients who are taking histamine-2 receptor antagonists (such as ranitidine or famotidine) or proton-pump inhibitors (such as omeprazole or lansoprazole).
- **Antiplatelets and anticoagulants:** Some herbs, such as *Hou Po* (Cortex Magnoliae Officinalis) and *Sha Ren* (Fructus Amomi), have anticoagulant properties and should be used with caution for patients using anticoagulant or antiplatelet drugs.[1,2]

References

1. *CA*, 1988; 109:86013k
2. *Zhong Yao Yao Li Yu Lin Chuan* (Pharmacology and Clinical Applications of Chinese Herbs), 1990; 6(5):32

Cang Zhu (Rhizoma Atractylodis)

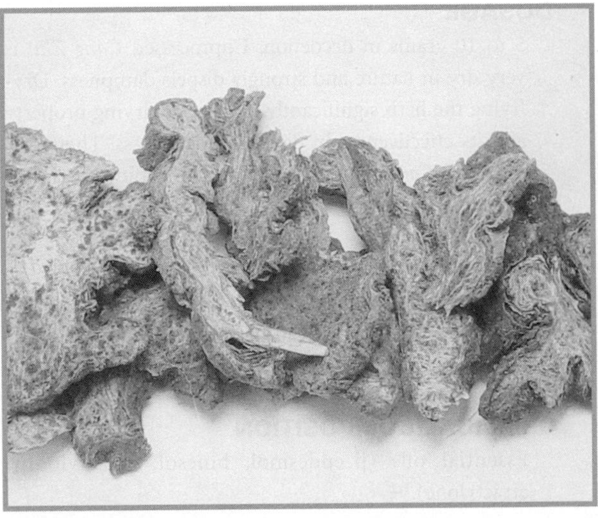

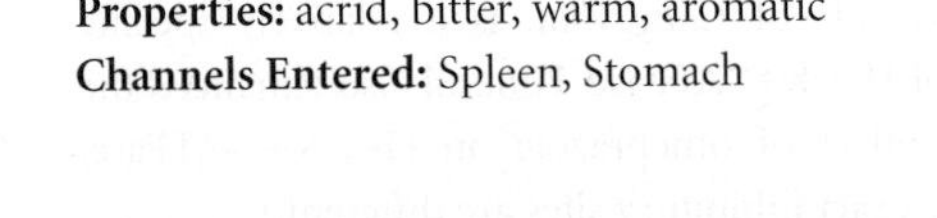

Pinyin Name: *Cang Zhu*
Literal Name: "gray rhizome," "gray essence"
Original Source: *Jing Shi Zheng Lei Bei Ji Ben Cao* (Differentiation and Application of Materia Medica) by Tang Shen-Wei in 1082
English Name: atractylodes, sword-like atractylodes rhizome, Chinese atractylodes rhizome
Botanical Name: *Atractylodes lancea* (Thunb.) DC. (*Nan Cang Zhu*); *Atractylodes chinensis* (DC.) Koidz. (*Bei Cang Zhu*)
Pharmaceutical Name: Rhizoma Atractylodis
Properties: acrid, bitter, warm, aromatic
Channels Entered: Spleen, Stomach

CHINESE THERAPEUTIC ACTIONS

1. Dries Dampness, Strengthens the Spleen

Aromatic and drying in nature, *Cang Zhu* (Rhizoma Atractylodis) dries dampness and strengthens the Spleen. It is commonly used when the accumulation of dampness impairs the Spleen's transformation and transportation functioning, leading to epigastric and abdominal fullness and distention, nausea, vomiting, loose stools, diarrhea, feeling of heaviness of the body and extremities, and a greasy tongue coat.

- Accumulation of dampness in the Spleen: use *Cang Zhu* with *Hou Po* (Cortex Magnoliae Officinalis) and *Chen Pi* (Pericarpium Citri Reticulatae). **Exemplar Formula:** *Ping Wei San* (Calm the Stomach Powder).
- Diarrhea due to accumulation of dampness: use *Cang Zhu* (Rhizoma Atractylodis) individually, or in combination with *Shen Qu* (Massa Fermentata) and *Hua Jiao* (Pericarpium Zanthoxyli).
- Infantile diarrhea with food stagnation: add *Shan Zha* (Fructus Crataegi).
- Infantile diarrhea from damp-heat: add *Hua Shi* (Talcum).
- Infantile diarrhea from deficiency and cold: use it with *Gan Jiang* (Rhizoma Zingiberis).
- Chronic accumulation of dampness in the Spleen with hypochondriac pain, acid reflux, and poor appetite: add *Da Zao* (Fructus Jujubae).

2. Induces Perspiration, Dispels Wind-Dampness

Cang Zhu dispels wind-cold with dampness, characterized by fever, chills, headache, body aches, the absence of perspiration, and nasal obstruction.

- Wind-cold with dampness: use this herb with *Chuan Xiong* (Rhizoma Ligustici Chuanxiong), *Bai Zhi* (Radix Angelicae Dahuricae), *Qiang Huo* (Rhizoma et Radix Notopterygii) and *Xi Xin* (Herba Asari).

Cang Zhu treats febrile disorders with dampness, characterized by persistent fever, heavy sensations of the body, feelings of chest oppression, and thirst with no desire to drink.

- Febrile disorders with dampness: add it to *Bai Hu Tang* (White Tiger Decoction).

***Bi zheng* (painful obstruction syndrome):** This condition is often caused by obstruction of wind, cold or dampness. *Cang Zhu* dispels wind and dampness to relieve pain.

- *Bi zheng* with swelling and pain caused by dampness: use *Cang Zhu* with *Fen Fang Ji* (Radix Stephaniae Tetandrae) and *Yi Yi Ren* (Semen Coicis).
- *Bi zheng* with knee pain and swelling, muscle weakness or atrophy, and difficulty walking because of damp-heat in the lower half of the body: use this herb with *Huang Bai* (Cortex Phellodendri). **Exemplar Formula:** *Er Miao San* (Two-Marvel Powder).
- Musculoskeletal disorders of the arms and shoulders caused by phlegm stagnation: combine *Cang Zhu* with *Bai Zhu* (Rhizoma Atractylodis Macrocephalae). **Exemplar Formula:** *Er Zhu Tang* (Two Atractylodes Decoction).

3. Benefits the Eyes

Night blindness or diminished vision: Traditionally, *Cang Zhu* is used with food to treat eye disorders.

- Cataracts, glaucoma and night blindness: use it with *Hei Zhi Ma* (Semen Sesami Nigrum).
- Night blindness: cook *Cang Zhu* with pig or goat liver and take daily as food.

Cang Zhu (Rhizoma Atractylodis)

DOSAGE

5 to 10 grams in decoction. Unprocessed *Cang Zhu* is very dry in nature and strongly dispels dampness. Dry-frying the herb significantly reduces its drying property and its effectiveness in dispelling dampness. Therefore, dry-fried *Cang Zhu* is generally used to bind the intestines and stop diarrhea.

CAUTIONS / CONTRAINDICATIONS

- Use *Cang Zhu* with caution for patients with yin-deficient heat, or patients who have spontaneous perspiration due to *wei* (defensive) *qi* deficiency.

CHEMICAL COMPOSITION

Essential oils (β-eudesmol, hinesol, atractylodin, atractylone).[1,2]

OH

Hinesol

PHARMACOLOGICAL EFFECTS

- **Hepatoprotective:** Decoction of *Cang Zhu* has marked hepatoprotective functions, especially against carbon tetrachloride, in mice.[3]
- **Antidiabetic:** Both water and alcohol extracts of *Cang Zhu* administered for 10 days demonstrated consistent antidiabetic effects. Seven to fourteen days after cessation of administration of the herb, the blood glucose levels started to increase again, but were still lower than previous levels.[4]
- **Antibiotic:** *Cang Zhu* has been shown to kill *Staphylococcus aureus*, some dermatophytes, and some viruses.[5]
- **Genitourinary:** Decoction of *Cang Zhu* did not have a diuretic effect in rats. It did, however, increase the excretion of sodium and chloride in the urine.[6]
- **Gastrointestinal:** Administration of *Cang Zhu* relieved spasms and cramps in mice intestines by blocking stimulation of the parasympathetic nervous system.[7]
- **Cardiovascular:** Intravenous injection of *Cang Zhu* is associated with increased blood pressure at low doses, but decreased blood pressure at high doses.[8]

CLINICAL STUDIES AND RESEARCH

- **Infantile rickets:** One report describes 120 infants between 2 and 3 years of age who were treated orally with 0.066 ml of essential oil of *Cang Zhu*, three times daily for 1 to 2 weeks, with an 85.4% rate of effectiveness.[9] In another study, 1,006 infants were treated with *Cang Zhu* syrup (contains 4.5 grams of *Cang Zhu*) twice daily for 15 days. According to the study, 541 patients (53.8%) showed marked improvement, 340 patients (33.7%) showed moderate improvement, and 125 patients (12.4%) had no response.[10]
- **Prevention of respiratory tract infections:** Incense made of *Cang Zhu* and *Ai Ye* (Folium Artemisiae Argyi) was burned in schools where there were widespread respiratory tract infections, with good preventative results.[11]
- **Gastric prolapse:** Daily ingestion of 20 grams of *Cang Zhu* as tea was found to be effective in treating prolapse of the stomach.[12]

HERB-DRUG INTERACTION

- **Omeprazole:** It has been suggested that hinesol, one of the components of *Cang Zhu,* is a relatively specific inhibitor of H+, K+ -ATPase. Hinesol also enhanced the inhibitory effect of omeprazole on H+, K+ -ATPase, though the exact inhibitory sites are different.[13]
- **Antidiabetics:** It is prudent to use *Cang Zhu* with caution with insulin, sulfonylureas, and other antidiabetic medications. Though the potential interaction has not been documented, the combination of antidiabetic herbs and drugs may have a synergistic effect, leading to hypoglycemia.[14] [Note: Examples of antidiabetic drugs include insulin, tolbutamide (Orinase), glipizide (Glucotrol), and glyburide (DiaBeta/Micronase).]
- **Diuretics:** *Cang Zhu* has a diuretic effect. Though this potential interaction has not been documented, concurrent use of this herb with diuretic drugs may lead to increased elimination of water and/or electrolytes.[15] [Note: Examples of diuretics include chlorothiazide, hydrochlorothiazide, furosemide (Lasix), bumetanide (Bumex), and torsemide (Demadex).]

AUTHORS' COMMENTS

Optimal treatment of headaches requires use of channel-guiding herbs to deliver the therapeutic effect of the herbs to the affected area. The following is a list of the commonly used channel-guiding herbs:

- *Taiyang* channels: *Qiang Huo* (Rhizoma et Radix Notopterygii)
- *Shaoyang* channels: *Chai Hu* (Radix Bupleuri)
- *Yangming* channels: *Bai Zhi* (Radix Angelicae Dahuricae)
- *Taiyin* channels: *Cang Zhu* (Rhizoma Atractylodis)
- *Shaoyin* channels: *Xi Xin* (Herba Asari)
- *Jueyin* channels: *Wu Zhu Yu* (Fructus Evodiae)

References

1. *Xian Dai Zhong Yao Yao Li Xue* (Contemporary Pharmacology of Chinese Herbs), 1997; 517-518
2. Yan X, Zhou J, Xie G, *Traditional Chinese Medicines Molecular Structures, Natural Sources and Applications*; Ashgate, 1999; 5404
3. *Guo Wai Yi Yao Zhi Wu Yao Fen Ce* (Monograph of Foreign

Cang Zhu (Rhizoma Atractylodis)

Botanical Medicine), 1985; (2):54
4. *Zhong Hua Yi Xue Za Zhi* (Chinese Journal of Medicine), 19858; 44(2):150
5. *Zhong Yao Xue* (Chinese Herbology), 1998; 318:320
6. *Yao Xue Xue Bao* (Journal of Herbology), 1966; 15(6):454
7. *Zhong Cheng Yao Yan Jiu* (Research of Chinese Patent Medicine), 1983; (7):25
8. *Chang Yong Zhong Yao Cheng Fen Yu Yao Li Shou Ce* (A Handbook of the Composition and Pharmacology of Common Chinese Drugs), 1994; 979:985
9. *Zhong Yao Tong Bao* (Journal of Chinese Herbology), 1986; 11:58
10. *Chi Jiao Yi Shi Za Zhi* (Journal of Barefoot Doctors), 1979; 10:14
11. *Yi Xue Qing Kuang Jiao Liu* (Medical Information Exchange), 1974; 2:end
12. *Zhong Cheng Yao Yan Jiu* (Research of Chinese Patent Medicine), 1992; 2:60
13. *Biochem Pharmacol* 2000, April 1:59(7):881-6
14. Chen, J. Recognition & prevention of herb-drug interactions, *Medical Acupuncture*, Fall/Winter 1998/1999; volume 10/number 2; 9-13
15. Ibid.

Hou Po (Cortex Magnoliae Officinalis)

厚朴

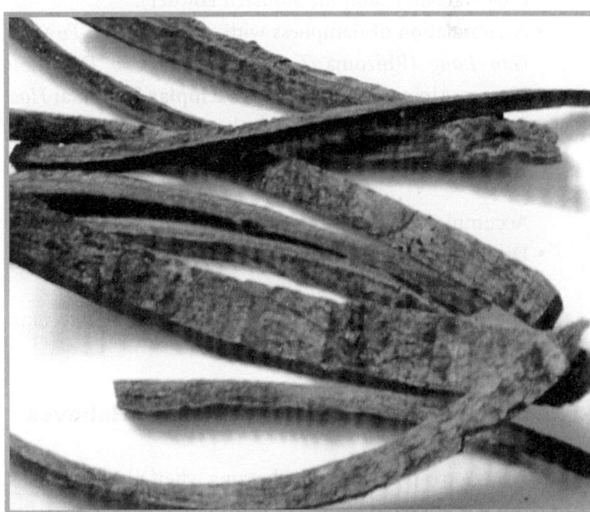

Pinyin Name: *Hou Po*
Alternate Chinese Names: *Chuan Po, Lie Po, Chi Po*
Original Source: *Shen Nong Ben Cao Jing* (Divine Husbandman's Classic of the Materia Medica) in the second century
English Name: magnolia bark
Botanical Name: *Magnolia officinalis* Rehd. et. Eils. (*Hou Po*); *Magnolia officinalis* Rehd. et. Wils. var *blioba* Rehd. et Wils. (*Ao Ye Hou Po*)
Pharmaceutical Name: Cortex Magnoliae Officinalis
Properties: bitter, acrid, warm, aromatic
Channels Entered: Large Intestine, Lung, Spleen, Stomach

CHINESE THERAPEUTIC ACTIONS

1. Regulates Qi and Reduces Stagnation

Stagnation of the middle *jiao*: Acrid, warm and dispersing in nature, *Hou Po* (Cortex Magnoliae Officinalis) is an excellent herb to promote movement of qi and reduce stagnation. It is the key herb for treatment of qi stagnation of the Spleen and Stomach that is causing epigastric and abdominal fullness and distention, loss of appetite, and poor digestion. It is an indispensable herb when treating bloating, distention and other related signs of qi stagnation.

- Qi stagnation of the Spleen and Stomach: use *Hou Po* with *Bai Zhu* (Rhizoma Atractylodis Macrocephalae), *Zhi Ke* (Fructus Aurantii) and *Sheng Jiang* (Rhizoma Zingiberis Recens). Serve with grain-based liquor.
- Stagnation of qi with cold in the Spleen and Stomach: combine this herb with *Gui Zhi* (Ramulus Cinnamomi), *Fu Zi* (Radix Aconiti Lateralis Praeparata) and *Gan Jiang* (Rhizoma Zingiberis) to warm the middle *jiao*.
- Hypochondriac pain due to Liver qi stagnation: use it with *Qing Pi* (Pericarpium Citri Reticulatae Viride) and *Chuan Lian Zi* (Fructus Toosendan).

Food stagnation: Food stagnation leads to qi stagnation that impairs the normal transformation and transportation functions of the Spleen and Stomach. This causes poor digestion, and in severe cases, abdominal pain and constipation.

- Food stagnation: use *Hou Po* with *Shan Zha* (Fructus Crataegi), *Mai Ya* (Fructus Hordei Germinatus), and *Shen Qu* (Massa Fermentata) to promote digestion.
- Food stagnation with abdominal pain and constipation: add *Da Huang* (Radix et Rhizoma Rhei) and *Zhi Shi* (Fructus Aurantii Immaturus). **Exemplar Formulas:** *Da Cheng Qi Tang* (Major Order the Qi Decoction) and *Xiao*

Hou Po (Cortex Magnoliae Officinalis)

Cheng Qi Tang (Minor Order the Qi Decoction).

- Paralytic ileus: use a larger dosage of *Hou Po* with *Da Huang* (Radix et Rhizoma Rhei) and *Zhi Shi* (Fructus Aurantii Immaturus).

2. Regulates Qi Circulation and Dries Dampness

In addition to regulating qi circulation of the Spleen and Stomach, *Hou Po* dries dampness. Clinically, qi stagnation with accumulation of dampness in the middle *jiao* is characterized by epigastric and abdominal fullness, nausea, vomiting, decreased intake of food, and a greasy tongue coat.

- Accumulation of dampness with qi stagnation: use *Hou Po* with *Cang Zhu* (Rhizoma Atractylodis) and *Chen Pi* (Pericarpium Citri Reticulatae). **Exemplar Formula:** *Ping Wei San* (Calm the Stomach Powder).
- Accumulation of dampness with cold: use *Hou Po* with *Gan Jiang* (Rhizoma Zingiberis) and *Cao Dou Kou* (Semen Alpiniae Katsumadai). **Exemplar Formula:** *Hou Po Wen Zhong Tang* (Magnolia Bark Decoction for Warming the Middle).

Accumulation of dampness may also cause diarrhea.

- Diarrhea due to cold and dampness: use *Hou Po* with *Gan Jiang* (Rhizoma Zingiberis).
- Diarrhea due to heat and dampness: add *Huang Lian* (Rhizoma Coptidis).

3. Descends Qi, Dissolves Phlegm, Relieves Wheezing

Hou Po treats cough and wheezing when phlegm blocks the normal circulation of qi in the Lung. It is best for tightness in the chest, dyspnea, and cough and wheezing accompanied by profuse phlegm.

- Cough and wheezing due to excess in the upper *jiao* (phlegm obstruction in the Lung), with deficiency in the lower *jiao* (Kidney deficiency): use it with *Su Zi* (Fructus Perillae), *Rou Gui* (Cortex Cinnamomi) and *Dang Gui* (Radicis Angelicae Sinensis). **Exemplar Formula:** *Su Zi Jiang Qi Tang* (Perilla Fruit Decoction for Directing Qi Downward).
- Cough and wheezing due to wind-cold: combine *Hou Po* with *Xing Ren* (Semen Armeniacae Amarum), *Gui Zhi* (Ramulus Cinnamomi), and *Sheng Jiang* (Rhizoma Zingiberis Recens).

DOSAGE

3 to 10 grams in decoction. Bitter, acrid and warm, unprocessed *Hou Po* is sometimes irritating to the throat and may cause nausea. After it has been processed with *Sheng Jiang* (Rhizoma Zingiberis Recens), this herb has reduced bitterness and stimulatory effect, and is less likely to cause nausea and stomach discomfort.

CAUTIONS / CONTRAINDICATIONS

- Use *Hou Po* with caution during pregnancy, or in cases of qi deficiency.

CHEMICAL COMPOSITION

Essential oils (machilol), magnolol, magnocurarine, magnoloside.[1,2]

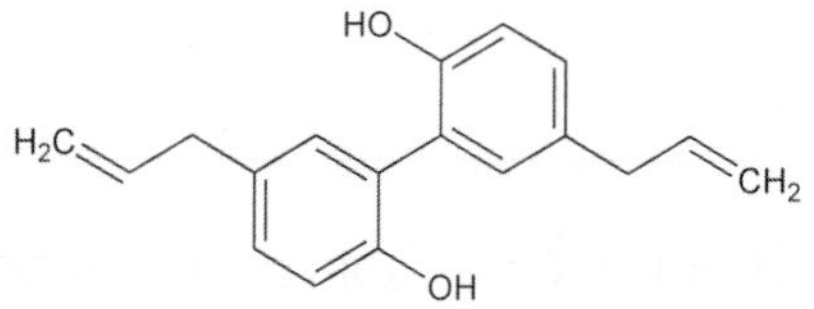

HO, H_2C, CH_2, OH

Magnolol

PHARMACOLOGICAL EFFECTS

- **Gastrointestinal:** Administration of *Hou Po* in various forms has shown an inhibitory influence on the gastrointestinal system, leading to decreased secretion of gastric acid and reduced contractions in the duodenum.[3,4]
- **Anticoagulant:** Magnolol has a mild anticoagulant effect.[5]
- **CNS suppressant:** Extract of *Hou Po* given via intraperitoneal and oral administration has demonstrated an inhibiting effect on the central nervous system (CNS). The exact mechanism of action is unclear, but may be related to GABA receptors.[6]
- **Antihypertensive:** Intravenous injection of magnocurarine at 3 mg/kg in cats lowered blood pressure by 20 mmHg for 10 minutes.[7]
- **Respiratory:** Decoction of *Hou Po* has a stimulating effect on the respiratory system at small doses, but an inhibiting effect at large doses.[8]
- **Antibiotic:** Extract of *Hou Po* has an inhibitory effect against *Streptococcus matuans, Staphylococcus aureus, Bacillus subtilis, Diplococcus pneumoniae*, and *Bacillus dysenteriae*.[9,10,11]

CLINICAL STUDIES AND RESEARCH

- **Post-surgical bloating:** Prior to hysterectomy, 5 to 10 grams of *Hou Po* were given to 36 women. The study reported that the patients were much less likely to experience abdominal bloating following surgery.[12]

HERB-DRUG INTERACTION

- **Anticoagulant or antiplatelet drugs:** *Hou Po* has a mild anticoagulant effect, and should be used with caution in patients who take anticoagulant or antiplatelet medications.[13] [Note: Examples of anticoagulants include heparin, warfarin (Coumadin) and enoxaparin (Lovenox); and examples of antiplatelets include aspirin,

Hou Po (Cortex Magnoliae Officinalis)

dipyridamole (Persantine), and clopidogrel (Plavix).]

TOXICOLOGY

The LD_{50} for decoction of *Hou Po* is 6.12 g/kg in mice via intraperitoneal injection, and 4.25 g/kg in cats via intravenous injection. No fatalities were recorded following a bolus dose of decoction of *Hou Po* at 60 g/kg in mice.[14,15]

SUPPLEMENT

- 厚朴花 / 厚朴花 *Hou Po Hua* (Flos Magnoliae Officinalis), first cited in *Yin Pian Xin Can* (New References of Prepared Medicines), is derived from the flower of the same plant as *Hou Po*. *Hou Po Hua* regulates Liver qi and treats Liver and Stomach qi stagnation manifesting in poor appetite, dull epigastric fullness and pain. *Hou Po Hua* is slightly milder in its overall function than *Hou Po*, but is less drying in nature. *Hou Po Hua* is better for qi stagnation of the upper and middle *jiaos* while *Hou Po* is better for qi stagnation of the middle and lower *jiaos*. The dosage for *Hou Po Hua* is 3 to 6 grams.

AUTHORS' COMMENTS

Hou Po regulates qi, warms the middle *jiao* and dries dampness. It is one of the most important herbs used to treat fullness and distention. It treats food stagnation, accumulated dampness, and cold and qi stagnation causing abdominal discomfort. It has been used recently for post-surgical abdominal bloating, and prior to administering anesthesia for hysterectomy, to prevent abdominal bloating.

Hou Po is quite strong in its qi-regulating function. Some describe its potent effect as "breaking open the qi." Therefore, when this herb is used improperly, *yuan* (source) *qi* can be injured. It should be used with caution for deficient patients with bloating so it does not injure the qi. This caution does not prohibit the use of *Hou Po* for deficient patients altogether, it simply indicates that the dosage should be decreased and/or it should be combined with qi tonics such as *Ren Shen* (Radix Ginseng) and *Gan Cao* (Radix Glycyrrhizae).

Some records have shown that this herb helps to unblock the yang when used in a small dosage. When used in large dosages, it breaks open qi.

References

1. *Xian Dai Zhong Yao Yao Li Xue* (Contemporary Pharmacology of Chinese Herbs), 1997; 521
2. *The Merck Index* 12th edition, Chapman & Hall/CRCnetBASE/Merck, 2000
3. *Guo Wai Yi Yao Zhi Wu Yao Fen Ce* (Monograph of Foreign Botanical Medicine), 1988; 10(1):43
4. *J of Nat Prod*, 1991; 54(3):816
5. *CA*, 1988; 109:86013k
6. *Yao Xue Tong Bao* (Report of Herbology), 1985; 20(9):522
7. *Yao Jian Gong Zuo Tong Xun* (Journal of Herbal Preparations), 1980; 10(4):154
8. *Zhong Yao Xue* (Chinese Herbology), 1998; 320:323
9. *Planta med*, 1982; 44(2):100
10. *Yao Jian Gong Zuo Tong Xun* (Journal of Herbal Preparations), 1980; 10(4):209
11. *Xin Hua Ben Cao Gang Mu* (New Chinese Materia Medica), 1988; 58
12. *Xin Yi Yao Xue Za Zhi* (New Journal of Medicine and Herbology), 1973; 4:25
13. Chen, J. Recognition & prevention of herb-drug interactions, *Medical Acupuncture*, Fall/Winter 1998/1999; volume 10/number 2; 9-13
14. *Chang Yong Zhong Yao Cheng Fen Yu Yao Li Shou Ce* (A Handbook of the Composition and Pharmacology of Common Chinese Drugs), 1994; 1961; 2:42
15. *Xin Yi Yao Xue Za Zhi* (New Journal of Medicine and Herbology), 1975; (3):42

Huo Xiang (Herba Agastache)

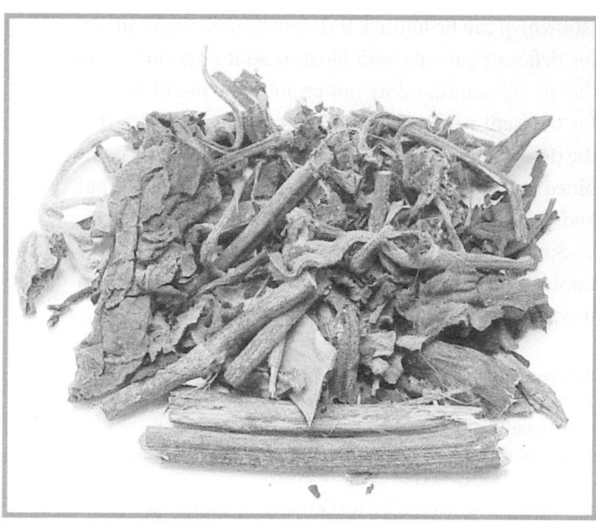

藿香 藿香

Pinyin Name: *Huo Xiang*
Literal Name: "aromatic bean leaf"
Original Source: *Ming Yi Za Zhu* (Miscellaneous Records of Famous Physicians) by Tao Hong-Jing in 500 A.D.
English Name: agastache, wrinkled giant hyssop
Botanical Name: *Agastache rugosus* (Fisch. et. Mey.) O. Ktze. (*Huo Xiang*)
Pharmaceutical Name: Herba Agastache
Properties: acrid, slightly warm, aromatic
Channels Entered: Spleen, Stomach, Lung

CHINESE THERAPEUTIC ACTIONS

1. Dispels Damp, Releases the Exterior and Relieves Summer-Damp

Accumulation of dampness: Aromatic and acrid, *Huo Xiang* (Herba Agastache) is very strong and quite drying in nature. It harmonizes the middle *jiao* and is an excellent herb to dispel summer-dampness from both the interior and exterior. When summer-dampness is stagnant in the middle *jiao*, the normal transformation and transportation functions of the Spleen and Stomach are affected, leading to symptoms such as abdominal and epigastric fullness and distention, poor appetite, nausea, vomiting, diarrhea, and greasy tongue coat.

- Summer-heat and damp stagnation in the middle *jiao*: use *Huo Xiang* with *Cang Zhu* (Rhizoma Atractylodis), *Hou Po* (Cortex Magnoliae Officinalis), and *Ban Xia* (Rhizoma Pinelliae). **Exemplar Formula:** *Bu Huan Jin Zheng Qi San* (Rectify the Qi Powder Worth More than Gold).
- Initial stage of dampness attacking the *qi* (energy) level with fever, feelings of heaviness, chest oppression, nausea, a dense feeling in the mouth (profuse accumulation of thick, sticky saliva and phlegm) and absence of thirst: combine *Huo Xiang* with *Hua Shi* (Talcum), *Yin Chen Hao* (Herba Artemisiae Scopariae) and *Huang Qin* (Radix Scutellariae).

Summer-damp: *Huo Xiang* dispels summer-dampness from the exterior. When summer-damp is accompanied by wind-cold, patients may have fever, chills, headache, feelings of chest oppression, abdominal fullness, nausea, vomiting, diarrhea and fatigue.

- Summer-dampness with wind-cold: use this herb with *Zi Su Ye* (Folium Perillae) and *Bai Zhi* (Radix Angelicae Dahuricae).

Summer-heat and dampness: This condition is characterized by fever, heavy sensations in the extremities, a feeling of oppression in the chest, abdominal fullness, dysuria, and constipation.

- Summer-heat and dampness: use *Huo Xiang* with *Hua Shi* (Talcum), *Yin Chen Hao* (Herba Artemisiae Scopariae) and *Huang Qin* (Radix Scutellariae).

2. Relieves Nausea and Vomiting

Huo Xiang does an excellent job of harmonizing the Stomach and relieving nausea and vomiting. It is most suitable for patients experiencing dampness and turbidity in the middle *jiao*.

- Nausea and vomiting: use *Huo Xiang* individually, or in combination with *Ban Xia* (Rhizoma Pinelliae).
- Nausea and vomiting from damp-heat: use it with *Huang Lian* (Rhizoma Coptidis) and *Zhu Ru* (Caulis Bambusae in Taenia).
- Nausea and vomiting with Spleen and Stomach deficiencies: add *Dang Shen* (Radix Codonopsis) and *Gan Cao* (Radix Glycyrrhizae).
- Nausea and vomiting during pregnancy: combine this herb with *Ban Xia* (Rhizoma Pinelliae) and *Sha Ren* (Fructus Amomi).

3. Treats Fungal Infection

Topical use of *Huo Xiang* has demonstrated effectiveness in treatment of fungal infections of the hands and feet.

- Fungal infection: combine *Huo Xiang* with *Da Huang* (Radix et Rhizoma Rhei), *Zao Fan* (Melanterite), and *Huang Jing* (Rhizoma Polygonati). Soak the herbs in vinegar for 1 week and filter out the solution. Soak the affected area in the herbal solution once daily for 30 minutes.

Huo Xiang (Herba Agastache)

DOSAGE

5 to 10 grams. Double the dosage if the fresh form is used. *Huo Xiang* is commonly used internally as decoction or tea, or topically. Due to its aromatic nature, *Huo Xiang* is generally added to the decoction at the end of the cooking process, to preserve its effectiveness.

CHEMICAL COMPOSITION

Essential oil 1.5%, patchoulialcohol, cinnamic aldehyde, benzaldehyde, eugenol, patchoulipyridine, epiguaipyridine, β-elemene, caryophyllene, alloaromadendrene, γ-patchoulene, α-guaiene, γ-guaiene, α-patchoulene.[1]

PHARMACOLOGICAL EFFECTS

- **Antibiotic:** It has a broad spectrum antibiotic effect against *Candida albicans, Staphylococcus aureus, Pseudomonas aeruginosa, E. coli, Bacillus dysenteriae*, α-hemolytic streptococcus, *Bacillus dysenteriae, Diplococcus pneumoniae*, and some dermatophytes.[2]
- **Gastrointestinal:** *Huo Xiang* increases the secretion of gastric acid and promotes digestion.[3]

CLINICAL STUDIES AND RESEARCH

- **Infantile diarrhea:** In one study, 112 infants with diarrhea were treated with herbal decoctions, with complete recovery in all cases. The primary herbal formula contained *Huo Xiang* 6g, *Cang Zhu* (Rhizoma Atractylodis) 6g, *Che Qian Zi* (Semen Plantaginis) 9g, *Hou Po* (Cortex Magnoliae Officinalis) 4g, *Chen Pi* (Pericarpium Citri Reticulatae) 4g, *Gan Cao* (Radix Glycyrrhizae) 3g, *Sheng Jiang* (Rhizoma Zingiberis Recens) 3 pieces, *Da Zao* (Fructus Jujubae) 5 to 7 pieces, and others as deemed necessary.[4]

SUPPLEMENT

- 廣藿香 / 广藿香 *Guang Huo Xiang* (Herba Pogostemonis) is derived from the plant *Pogostemon cablin* (Blanco) Benth. It is commonly used as a substitute for *Huo Xiang*, because it has similar functions and applications. The dosage for *Guang Huo Xiang* is 3 to 9 grams.

References

1. *Xian Dai Zhong Yao Yao Li Xue* (Contemporary Pharmacology of Chinese Herbs), 1997; 523-524
2. *Zhong Yao Xue* (Chinese Herbology), 1998; 323:324
3. Ibid.
4. *Fu Jian Zhong Yi Yao* (Fujian Chinese Medicine and Herbology), 1984; (1):13

Pei Lan (Herba Eupatorii)

佩蘭 佩兰

Pinyin Name: *Pei Lan*
Literal Name: "wearing orchid," "ornamental orchid"
Original Source: *Shen Nong Ben Cao Jing* (Divine Husbandman's Classic of the Materia Medica) in the second century
English Name: eupatorium, fortune eupatorium
Botanical Name: *Eupatorium fortunei* Turcz. (*Lan Cao*)
Pharmaceutical Name: Herba Eupatorii
Properties: acrid, neutral, aromatic
Channels Entered: Spleen, Stomach, Lung

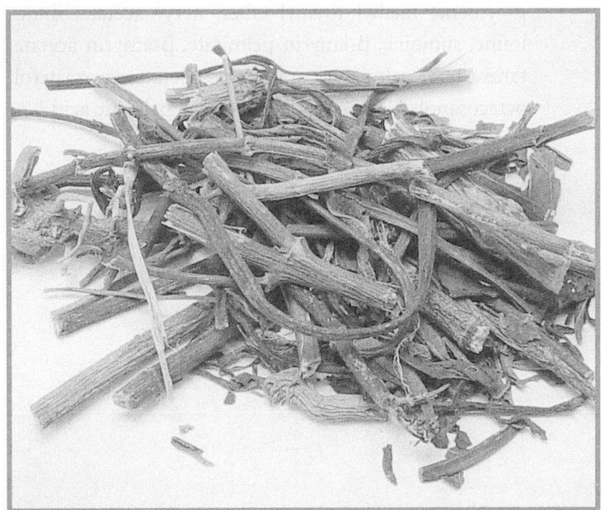

Pei Lan (Herba Eupatorii)

CHINESE THERAPEUTIC ACTIONS

1. Dissolves Dampness and Dispels Summer-Damp

Aromatic and acrid, *Pei Lan* (Herba Eupatorii) dispels summer-damp with or without heat from the middle *jiao.*

- Summer-dampness: use *Pei Lan* with *Huo Xiang* (Herba Agastache), *Cang Zhu* (Rhizoma Atractylodis), *Hou Po* (Cortex Magnoliae Officinalis), and *Bai Dou Kou* (Fructus Amomi Rotundus).
- Summer-heat and dampness: use it with *Hua Shi* (Talcum), *Huang Qin* (Radix Scutellariae), and *Yi Yi Ren* (Semen Coicis).

2. Eliminates Damp-Heat from the Spleen

Damp-heat accumulation in the Spleen: This disorder is caused by excessive intake of fatty food, that leads to accumulation of heat and dampness in the Spleen, causing symptoms such as a sweet and greasy taste in the mouth, epigastric and abdominal fullness and distention, thick sticky saliva or sputum with bubbles, and foul breath.

- Early stage damp-heat accumulation: use *Pei Lan* alone.
- Chronic accumulation of damp-heat: combine it with *Tian Hua Fen* (Radix Trichosanthis), *Mai Men Dong* (Radix Ophiopogonis) and *Huang Lian* (Rhizoma Coptidis) to nourish yin, promote the generation of body fluids, and clear heat.

DOSAGE

5 to 10 grams in decoctions. Double the dosage when using fresh *Pei Lan.*

CHEMICAL COMPOSITION

p-cymene, methyl thymyl ether, neryl acetate, lindelofine, supinine, β-amyrin palmitate, β-amyrin acetate, taraxasteryl palmitate, taraxasteryl acetate, taraxasterol, octacosanol, stigmasterol, β-sitosterol, palmitic acid.[1]

PHARMACOLOGICAL EFFECTS

- **Antibiotic:** Decoction of *Pei Lan* exerts antibacterial activities against *Corynebacterium diphtheriae, Staphylococcus aureus,* sarcinae, *Bacillus proteus,* and *Salmonella typhi*; and the essential oil has an antiviral effect against influenza viruses.[2]

CLINICAL STUDIES AND RESEARCH

- **Snake bite:** In one report, 30 patients with snake bite were treated with a topical application of *Pei Lan,* with marked improvement of 8 cases within 2 days, 12 cases within 3 days, and 10 cases within 4 days. The treatment protocol was to first remove the snake venom, clean the affected area, and apply fresh herbal paste of *Pei Lan* topically. The herbal paste was removed and re-applied every 2 to 3 days.[3]

AUTHORS' COMMENTS

Pei Lan and *Huo Xiang* (Herba Agastache) are both acrid and aromatic, and dispel dampness and summer-dampness, and awaken the Spleen. These herbs are frequently used together to treat dampness accumulation in the middle *jiao* that manifests in nausea, vomiting, heavy sensations of the limbs, fatigue and possibly some exterior symptoms. *Pei Lan* has a mild exterior-relieving function. It is best for retention of dampness and turbidity manifesting in chest oppression and a sweet taste in the mouth with profuse thick and sticky saliva. By contrast, *Huo Xiang* more effectively disperses dampness in the middle *jiao* manifesting as nausea, vomiting and a thick, greasy tongue coating.

References

1. *Chang Yong Zhong Yao Cheng Fen Yu Yao Li Shou Ce* (A Handbook of the Composition and Pharmacology of Common Chinese Drugs), 1994; 1256-1257
2. *Zhong Yao Tong Bao* (Journal of Chinese Herbology), 1983; 8(6):30
3. *Guang Xi Zhong Yi Yao* (Guangxi Chinese Medicine and Herbology), 1985; 4:43

Sha Ren (Fructus Amomi)

砂仁

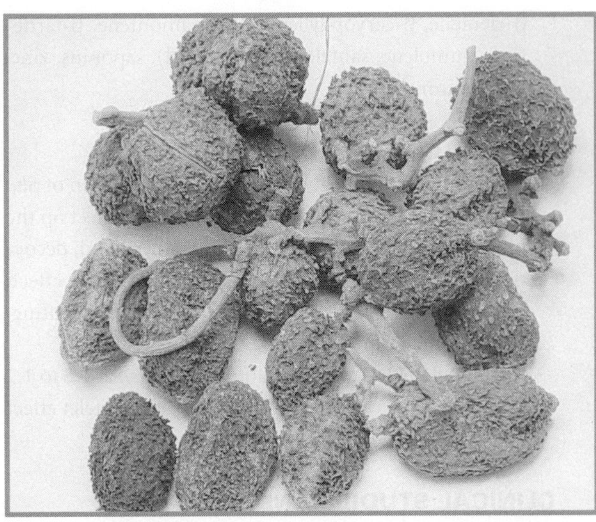

Pinyin Name: *Sha Ren*
Literal Name: "sand seeds"
Alternate Chinese Names: *Suo Sha Mi, Chun Sha Ren*
Original Source: *Yao Xing Ben Cao* (Materia Medica of Medicinal Properties) by Zhen Quan in 600 A.D.
English Name: amomum, villous amomum fruit
Botanical Name: *Amomum villosum* Lour. (*Yang Chun Sha*); *Amomum xanthioides* Wall. (*Suo Sha*)
Pharmaceutical Name: Fructus Amomi
Properties: acrid, warm, aromatic
Channels Entered: Spleen, Stomach

CHINESE THERAPEUTIC ACTIONS

1. Regulates Qi, Dissolves Dampness, Strengthens the Spleen

Accumulation of dampness: Acrid, warm and aromatic, *Sha Ren* (Fructus Amomi) treats disorders characterized by Spleen and Stomach qi stagnation accompanied by an accumulation of dampness. *Sha Ren* not only dispels dampness in these organs, it also restores their normal transportation and transformation functions. Damp accumulation in the middle *jiao* is characterized by epigastric and abdominal distention and pain, lack of appetite, nausea, and vomiting. *Sha Ren* is often used with tonic herbs to offset their possible side effect of indigestion.

- Spleen and Stomach qi stagnation: use *Sha Ren* with *Mu Xiang* (Radix Aucklandiae).
- Spleen and Stomach qi stagnation with indigestion: use this herb with *Zhi Shi* (Fructus Aurantii Immaturus) and *Bai Zhu* (Rhizoma Atractylodis Macrocephalae).
- Food stagnation with indigestion (acid regurgitation with rotten food smell): combine it with *Lai Fu Zi* (Semen Raphani), *Shan Zha* (Fructus Crataegi) and *Zhi Shi* (Fructus Aurantii Immaturus).
- Accumulation of dampness in the middle *jiao*: use *Sha Ren* with *Cang Zhu* (Rhizoma Atractylodis), *Hou Po* (Cortex Magnoliae Officinalis) and *Bai Dou Kou* (Fructus Amomi Rotundus).
- Spleen and Stomach deficiency: use it with *Ren Shen* (Radix Ginseng) and *Bai Zhu* (Rhizoma Atractylodis Macrocephalae).

2. Warms the Middle, Stops Diarrhea

Diarrhea: *Sha Ren* is warm and is thus most suitable for addressing cold and damp accumulation in the middle *jiao* manifesting as diarrhea.

- Cold, damp diarrhea: use *Sha Ren* with *Gan Jiang* (Rhizoma Zingiberis) and *Fu Zi* (Radix Aconiti Lateralis Praeparata).

3. Stabilizes Pregnancy

Sha Ren calms the fetus and stabilizes pregnancy. It is commonly used to treat bleeding, abdominal pain, severe nausea and vomiting, and restless fetus associated with an unstable pregnancy.

- Bleeding and abdominal pain during pregnancy: use *Sha Ren* (Fructus Amomi) individually.
- Severe nausea and vomiting during pregnancy: add *Ban Xia* (Rhizoma Pinelliae).
- Restless fetus: use this herb with *Bai Zhu* (Rhizoma Atractylodis Macrocephalae) and *Su Geng* (Caulis Perillae).
- Unstable pregnancy due to Kidney deficiency: combine it with *Sang Ji Sheng* (Herba Taxilli), *Du Zhong* (Cortex Eucommiae) and *Xu Duan* (Radix Dipsaci).

DOSAGE

3 to 6 grams. *Sha Ren* should be added last to the decoction, as prolonged cooking destroys its effectiveness. The fresh herb has a stronger function than the dried herb to regulate qi, reduce distention, and relieve pain. Salt-fried *Sha Ren* functions more effectively to descend qi, calm the fetus, and stop frequent urination or diarrhea.

CAUTIONS / CONTRAINDICATIONS

- *Sha Ren* is contraindicated in patients with yin-deficient heat.
- Oral ingestion of *Sha Ren* is sometimes associated with allergic reactions.[1]

CHEMICAL COMPOSITION

Essential oils (α-thujene, alloocimene, ocimene,

Sha Ren (Fructus Amomi)

β-elemene, β-caryophyllene, β-bergamontene, β-farnesene, humulene, santalol, palmitic acid), saponins, zinc, copper, iron.[2]

PHARMACOLOGICAL EFFECTS

- **Gastrointestinal:** In laboratory studies, decoction of *Sha Ren* at a low concentration has a stimulating effect on the intestines of rats and rabbits. On the other hand, decoction at a high concentration has an inhibiting effect. Clinically, *Sha Ren* is commonly used to relieve bloating, spasms, and pain.[3]
- **Antiplatelet:** Oral administration of *Sha Ren* at 0.6 to 1.2 g/kg in rabbits is associated with a mild antiplatelet effect 15, 30, 60 and 90 minutes after ingestion.[4]

CLINICAL STUDIES AND RESEARCH

- **Nausea:** Eleven patients with nausea were treated orally with 2 grams of powdered *Sha Ren* three times daily, with good results.[5]
- **Peptic ulcer disease:** In one study, 43 patients with gastric or duodenal ulcers were treated effectively using *Sha Ren* in powdered form. The treatment protocol was to give 1.5 grams twice daily for 1 week, and 1.5 grams once daily for another week. The patients were given one day of rest between the two courses of treatment. The study reported significant improvement in symptoms such as epigastric pain, abdominal distention, and acid reflux.[6]

HERB-DRUG INTERACTION

- **Anticoagulant or antiplatelet drugs:** *Sha Ren* has antiplatelet action, and should be used with caution in patients who take anticoagulant or antiplatelet medications. Though this potential interaction has not been documented, this herb may potentiate the effect of drugs such as warfarin. [Note: Examples of anticoagulants include heparin, warfarin (Coumadin) and enoxaparin (Lovenox); and examples of antiplatelets include aspirin, dipyridamole (Persantine), and clopidogrel (Plavix).][7]

TOXICOLOGY

In one study, oral administration of decoction of *Sha Ren* at 25 g/kg in 10 mice for 3 days showed no signs of toxicity and caused no fatalities. In another study, no abnormalities were observed in liver and kidney functions following oral administration of *Sha Ren* decoction in 10 rats at 1.62 g/kg for 30 days.[8]

SUPPLEMENT

- 砂仁殼 / 砂仁壳 *Sha Ren Ke* (Pericarpium Amomi), first cited in *Ben Cao Gang Mu* (Materia Medica) by Li Shi-Zhen in 1578 A.D., is derived from the shell of the same fruit as *Sha Ren*. The taste, properties and functions of *Sha Ren Ke* are similar to but weaker than those of *Sha Ren*. *Sha Ren Ke* is more suitable for less severe cases of qi stagnation in the middle *jiao* manifesting in epigastric and abdominal fullness, distention and poor appetite. The recommended dosage of *Sha Ren Ke* is 3 to 5 grams.

AUTHORS' COMMENTS

There are four herbs that are commonly used to stabilize pregnancy, each having a particular influence:

- *Sha Ren* (Fructus Amomi) regulates qi and calms restless fetus in the presence of qi stagnation and middle *jiao* deficiency.
- *Du Zhong* (Cortex Eucommiae) is most suitable to treat restless fetus caused by deficiency of the Kidney and Liver.
- *Huang Qin* (Radix Scutellariae) calms restless fetus caused by heat.
- *Bai Zhu* (Rhizoma Atractylodis Macrocephalae) treats restless fetus from Spleen qi deficiency.

References

1. *Jiang Su Zhong Yi Za Zhi* (Jiangsu Journal of Chinese Medicine), 1983; (10):442
2. *Chang Yong Zhong Yao Cheng Fen Yu Yao Li Shou Ce* (A Handbook of the Composition and Pharmacology of Common Chinese Drugs), 1994; 1393-1398
3. *Zhong Yao Xue* (Chinese Herbology), 1998; 326:327
4. *Zhong Yao Yao Li Yu Lin Chuan* (Pharmacology and Clinical Applications of Chinese Herbs), 1990; 6(5):32
5. *Zhong Yao Xue* (Chinese Herbology), 1998; 326:327
6. *Fu Jian Zhong Yi Yao* (Fujian Chinese Medicine and Herbology), 1983; (6):36
7. Chen, J. Recognition & prevention of herb-drug interactions, *Medical Acupuncture*, Fall/Winter 1998/1999; volume 10/number 2; 9-13
8. *Fu Jian Zhong Yi Yao* (Fujian Chinese Medicine and Herbology), 1985; (1):44

Bai Dou Kou (Fructus Amomi Rotundus)

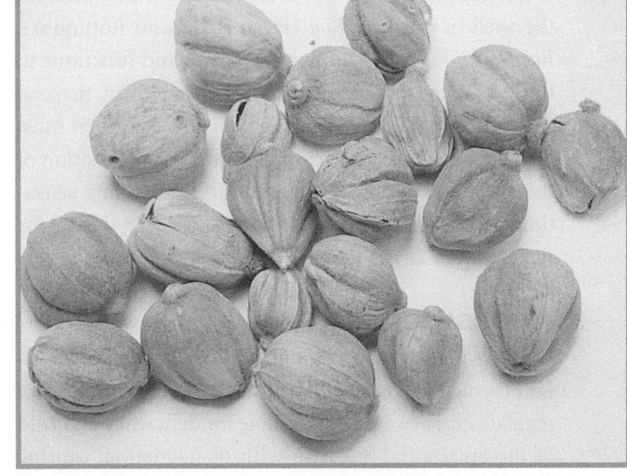

白豆蔻 白豆蔻

Pinyin Name: *Bai Dou Kou*
Alternate Chinese Names: *Dou Kou*
Literal Name: "white cardamon"
Original Source: *Ben Cao Shi Yi* (Omissions from the [Classic of the] Materia Medica) by Chen Cang-Qi in 741 A.D.
English Name: amomum, cardamon
Botanical Name: *Amomum kravanh* Pirre ex Gagnep. (*Bai Dou Kou*); *Amomum compactum* Soland ex Maton (*Zhao Wa Bai Dou Kou*)
Pharmaceutical Name: Fructus Amomi Rotundus
Properties: acrid, warm, aromatic
Channels Entered: Lung, Spleen, Stomach

CHINESE THERAPEUTIC ACTIONS

1. Regulates Qi, Dissolves Dampness, Strengthens the Stomach

Acrid, aromatic and warm, *Bai Dou Kou* (Fructus Amomi Rotundus) moves the qi and dissolves dampness from the interior and exterior. Accumulation of dampness in the interior, or the middle *jiao*, prevents the Spleen and Stomach from performing their normal transportation and transformation functions, leading to epigastric and abdominal fullness, distention and poor appetite.

- Accumulation of dampness in the middle *jiao*: use *Bai Dou Kou* with *Cang Zhu* (Rhizoma Atractylodis), *Hou Po* (Cortex Magnoliae Officinalis) and *Chen Pi* (Pericarpium Citri Reticulatae).

Some exterior syndromes, namely damp-heat febrile disorders, are sometimes complicated by an accumulation of dampness. If there is more dampness than heat, patients will experience chest congestion, lack of appetite, and a feeling of heaviness in the body and extremities. If there is more heat than dampness, patients may experience persistent fever, thick, yellow tongue coating and dysuria.

- Exterior syndrome with more dampness than heat: use *Bai Dou Kou* with *Xing Ren* (Semen Armeniacae Amarum), *Yi Yi Ren* (Semen Coicis) and *Hou Po* (Cortex Magnoliae Officinalis).
- Exterior syndrome with more heat than dampness: combine this herb with *Huang Qin* (Radix Scutellariae), *Hua Shi* (Talcum), and *Zhu Ling* (Polyporus).

2. Warms the Stomach, Relieves Nausea

Bai Dou Kou warms the Stomach, dispels cold, and relieves nausea. It treats abdominal pain, nausea, vomiting, and other conditions characterized by cold in the Stomach. It is safe for pregnant women and for infants with such conditions.

- Nausea and vomiting: use it with *Ban Xia* (Rhizoma Pinelliae) and *Huo Xiang* (Herba Agastache).
- Vomiting in infants: treat by using the powder of *Bai Dou Kou, Sha Ren* (Fructus Amomi) and *Gan Cao* (Radix Glycyrrhizae).

DOSAGE

3 to 6 grams. *Bai Dou Kou* should be ground into powder and added towards the end of decocting, as prolonged cooking destroys its effectiveness. The decoction should be served immediately, while warm, for maximum effect. Since essential oils of *Bai Dou Kou* are quite volatile, dry-frying the herb significantly decreases its potency.

CAUTIONS / CONTRAINDICATIONS

- Use of *Bai Dou Kou* is contraindicated in patients with yin or blood deficiency.

CHEMICAL COMPOSITION

Essential oils (1,8-cineol, α-terpineol, α-pinene, β-pinene, humalene, caryophyllene, mycene, p-cymene, humalene epoxide, sabinene, limonene, terpinene-4-ol, myrtenol); saponin, starch.[1,2]

PHARMACOLOGICAL EFFECTS

- **Gastrointestinal:** Administration of *Bai Dou Kou* is associated with increased secretion of gastric acid, increased intestinal peristalsis, and decreased vomiting.[3]

SUPPLEMENT

- 白豆蔻殼/白豆蔻壳 *Bai Dou Kou Ke* (Pericarpium

Bai Dou Kou (Fructus Amomi Rotundus)

Amomi Rotundus), first cited in *Ben Cao Gang Mu* (Materia Medica) by Li Shi-Zhen in 1578, is derived from the shell of *Bai Dou Kou* (Fructus Amomi Rotundus). *Bai Dou Kou Ke* has similar properties and functions to those of *Bai Dou Kou*, but is not as warm in thermal property and milder in potency. *Bai Dou Kou Ke* is most suitable for dampness accumulation and qi stagnation of the chest and abdomen manifesting in a stifling sensation of the chest and poor appetite. Common dosage for *Bai Dou Kou Ke* is 3 to 5 grams.

AUTHORS' COMMENTS

Bai Dou Kou (Fructus Amomi Rotundus) and *Rou Dou Kou* (Semen Myristicae) both warm the middle *jiao* and regulate qi. They are both suitable for deficiency and cold of the Spleen and Stomach with qi stagnation, causing symptoms such as epigastric and abdominal fullness and pain, diarrhea, and vomiting.

- *Bai Dou Kou* regulates qi and relieves nausea and vomiting. It is used more commonly to dry middle *jiao* dampness and relieve abdominal fullness and poor appetite.
- *Rou Dou Kou* is also an astringent and stops chronic diarrhea (especially early morning diarrhea caused by Spleen and Kidney yang deficiencies).

Bai Dou Kou (Fructus Amomi Rotundus), *Rou Dou Kou* (Semen Myristicae), and *Cao Dou Kou* (Semen Alpiniae Katsumadai) have similar pinyin names, but different functions. To avoid confusion, they should not be abbreviated as "*Dou Kou*."

- *Bai Dou Kou* regulates qi, dissolves dampness, and strengthens the Stomach
- *Rou Dou Kou* binds the intestines and stops diarrhea.
- *Cao Dou Kou* warms the middle *jiao* and dries dampness.

References

1. *Chang Yong Zhong Yao Xian Dai Yan Jiu Yu Lin Chuan* (Recent Study & Clinical Application of Common Traditional Chinese Medicine), 1995; 248-249
2. *Xian Dai Ben Cao Gang Mu* (Contemporary Materia Medica), 2000; 823
3. *Zhong Yao Xue* (Chinese Herbology), 1998; 248:249

Cao Guo (Fructus Tsaoko)

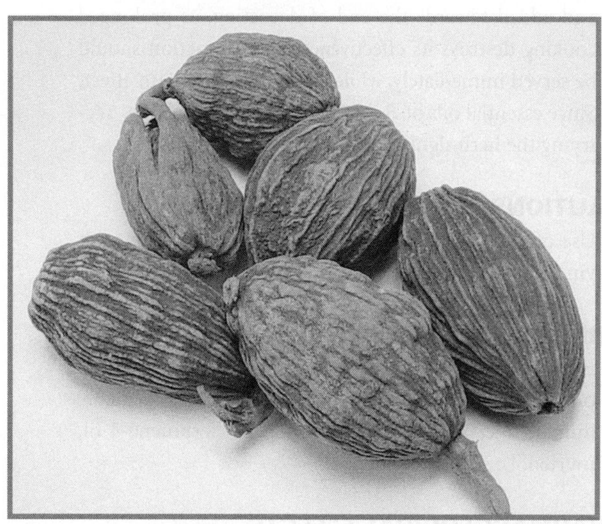

草果 草果

Pinyin Name: *Cao Guo*
Literal Name: "grass fruit"
Original Source: *Yin Shan Zheng Yao* (Correct Guide to Eating and Drinking)
English Name: tsaoko fruit
Botanical Name: *Amomum tsao-ko* Crevost et Lemaire (*Cao Guo*)
Pharmaceutical Name: Fructus Tsaoko
Properties: acrid, warm, aromatic
Channels Entered: Spleen, Stomach

CHINESE THERAPEUTIC ACTIONS

1. Warms the Middle *Jiao*, Dries Dampness

Accumulation of cold and damp in the middle *jiao*: *Cao Guo* (Fructus Tsaoko) treats abdominal coldness and pain, abdominal fullness, nausea, vomiting, diarrhea, and greasy tongue coating.

- Accumulation of damp and cold (more damp) in the middle *jiao*: use *Cao Guo* with *Cang Zhu* (Rhizoma

Cao Guo (Fructus Tsaoko)

Atractylodis), *Hou Po* (Cortex Magnoliae Officinalis) and *Huo Xiang* (Herba Agastache).

- Accumulation of cold and damp (more cold) in the middle *jiao*: add *Wu Zhu Yu* (Fructus Evodiae) and *Gan Jiang* (Rhizoma Zingiberis).

2. Treats Malaria

Warm and drying, *Cao Guo* treats malaria characterized by cold and dampness.

- Malaria: use it with *Chang Shan* (Radix Dichroae), *Bing Lang* (Semen Arecae), and *Zhi Mu* (Radix Anemarrhenae).

DOSAGE

3 to 6 grams. Frying *Cao Guo* with *Sheng Jiang* (Rhizoma Zingiberis Recens) increases its effectiveness to warm the interior, dispel cold, and relieve pain.

CAUTIONS / CONTRAINDICATIONS

- Warm and drying, *Cao Guo* consumes body fluids and thus is contraindicated in patients with yin deficiency or blood deficiency.

CHEMICAL COMPOSITION

Geraniol.[1,2]

CH3 CH3
H3C OH

Geraniol

PHARMACOLOGICAL EFFECTS

- **Respiratory:** Components isolated from *Cao Guo* have demonstrated antitussive, expectorant, and antiasthmatic effects.[3]
- **Antibiotic:** Preparations of *Cao Guo* inhibit the growth of some bacteria and pathogenic fungi.[4]

TOXICOLOGY

The LD_{50} for geraniol is 4.8 g/kg in rats via oral administration, and 50 mg/kg in rabbits via intravenous injection.[5]

AUTHORS' COMMENTS

Cao Guo has effects similar to but slightly weaker than *Cao Dou Kou* (Semen Alpiniae Katsumadai).

References

1. *Zhi Wu Yao You Xiao Cheng Fen Shou Ce* (Manual of Plant Medicinals and Their Active Constituents), 1986: 427,498,833,834
2. *The Merck Index* 12th edition, Chapman & Hall/CRCnetBASE/Merck, 2000
3. *Zhi Wu Yao You Xiao Cheng Fen Shou Ce* (Manual of Plant Medicinals and Their Active Constituents), 1986: 427,498,833,834
4. *Chang Yong Zhong Yao Cheng Fen Yu Yao Li Shou Ce* (A Handbook of the Composition and Pharmacology of Common Chinese Drugs), 1994; 1376:1377
5. *Zhi Wu Yao You Xiao Cheng Fen Shou Ce* (Manual of Plant Medicinals and Their Active Constituents), 1986: 427,498,833,834

Cao Dou Kou (Semen Alpiniae Katsumadai)

草豆蔻 草豆蔻

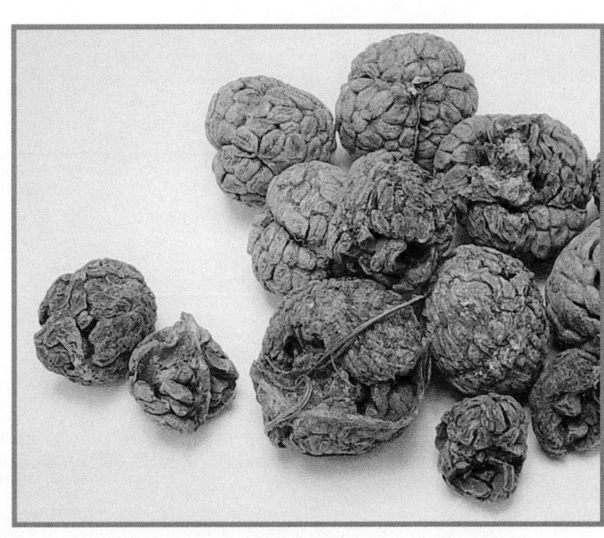

Pinyin Name: *Cao Dou Kou*
Literal Name: "grass cardamom"
Original Source: *Ming Yi Za Zhu* (Miscellaneous Records of Famous Physicians) by Tao Hong-Jing in 500 A.D.
English Name: katsumadai, katsumada galangal seed
Botanical Name: *Alpinia katsumadai* Hayata (*Cao Dou Kou*)
Pharmaceutical Name: Semen Alpiniae Katsumadai
Properties: acrid, warm, aromatic
Channels Entered: Spleen, Stomach

Cao Dou Kou (Semen Alpiniae Katsumadai)

CHINESE THERAPEUTIC ACTIONS

Warms the Middle *Jiao,* Dries Dampness

Cao Dou Kou (Semen Alpiniae Katsumadai) treats accumulation of cold and dampness in the middle *jiao* characterized by abdominal coldness and pain, vomitus of clear liquids, lack of appetite, loose stools and a white, greasy tongue coat.

- Accumulation of cold and damp in the middle *jiao*: use *Cao Dou Kou* with *Wu Zhu Yu* (Fructus Evodiae) and *Gao Liang Jiang* (Rhizoma Alpiniae Officinarum).
- Accumulation of damp in the middle *jiao*: use it with *Cang Zhu* (Rhizoma Atractylodis) and *Hou Po* (Cortex Magnoliae Officinalis).
- Chronic diarrhea due to deficiency and cold: add *Rou Gui* (Cortex Cinnamomi), *Gan Jiang* (Rhizoma Zingiberis), and *Rou Dou Kou* (Semen Myristicae).
- Nausea and vomiting due to accumulation of cold phlegm: combine this herb with *Ban Xia* (Rhizoma Pinelliae), *Chen Pi* (Pericarpium Citri Reticulatae) and *Sheng Jiang* (Rhizoma Zingiberis Recens).

DOSAGE

3 to 6 grams in decoction. *Cao Dou Kou* should be added at the close of cooking, as prolonged cooking destroys its effectiveness.

CAUTIONS / CONTRAINDICATIONS

- *Cao Dou Kou* is contraindicated in patients who have yin or blood deficiencies.

CHEMICAL COMPOSITION

Essential oil, alpinetin, 7-hydroxy-5-methoxyflavanone, cardamonin, 2,4-dihydroxy-6-methoxychalcone.[1]

PHARMACOLOGICAL EFFECTS

- **Antibiotic:** Decoction of *Cao Dou Kou* has an inhibitory effect *in vitro* against *Staphylococcus aureus, Bacillus dysenteriae,* and *E. coli.*[2]
- **Gastrointestinal:** A low dose of a *Cao Dou Kou* decoction has a stimulating effect on the intestines, while a large dose of the decoction has an inhibiting effect.[3]

AUTHORS' COMMENTS

Cao Dou Kou (Semen Alpiniae Katsumadai), *Bai Dou Kou* (Fructus Amomi Rotundus), and *Rou Dou Kou* (Semen Myristicae) have similar pinyin names, but different functions. To avoid confusion, they should not be abbreviated as "*Dou Kou*."

- *Cao Dou Kou* warms the middle *jiao* and dries dampness.
- *Bai Dou Kou* regulates qi, dissolves dampness, and strengthens the Stomach
- *Rou Dou Kou* binds the intestines and stops diarrhea.

References

1. *Chang Yong Zhong Yao Xian Dai Yan Jiu Yu Lin Chuan* (Recent Study & Clinical Application of Common Traditional Chinese Medicine), 1995; 249
2. *Zhong Yao Xue* (Chinese Herbology), 1998; 328:329
3. Ibid.

Chapter 5 summary — Aromatic Damp-Dissolving Herbs

Name	Similarities	Differences
Cang Zhu (Rhizoma Atractylodis)	Strong aromatic properties to dry	Strongly dries dampness, strengthens the Spleen, dispels wind-dampness
Hou Po (Cortex Magnoliae Officinalis)	dampness	Regulates qi, breaks stagnation, relieves bloating and distention, descends Lung qi to relieve dyspnea
Huo Xiang (Herba Agastache)	Dissolve dampness, relieve summer-heat	Dissolves dampness from middle *jiao*, stops vomiting, releases exterior
Pei Lan (Herba Eupatorii)		Mildly releases the exterior
Sha Ren (Fructus Amomi)	Invigorate qi circulation,	Warms the middle *jiao* to treat diarrhea due to coldness, stabilizes the fetus
Bai Dou Kou (Fructus Amomi Rotundus)	dissolve dampness	Dissolves dampness in the middle and upper *jiaos*, most suitable for initial stages of vomiting
Cao Guo (Fructus Tsaoko)	Dry dampness,	Dries dampness, treats malaria
Cao Dou Kou (Semen Alpiniae Katsumadai)	warm middle *jiao*	Strengthens the Spleen and Stomach

General Characteristics of Aromatic Damp-Dissolving Herbs:

Taste: acrid, bitter
Thermal property: warm and drying
Channels entered: Spleen and Stomach
Therapeutic actions: dissolve dampness, eliminate damp-heat, harmonize the Spleen and Stomach

These aromatic herbs regulate qi, dissolve dampness, and strengthen the Spleen. They are mainly used to treat dampness obstructing the middle *jiao*, summer-dampness, damp-heat and other symptoms related to disharmony of the Spleen and Stomach.

Cang Zhu (Rhizoma Atractylodis) and ***Hou Po*** (Cortex Magnoliae Officinalis), strongest in drying dampness, are the chief herbs used for dry dampness obstructing the middle *jiao*. They are often used together for synergistic effects.

Cang Zhu is one of the most important herbs to dry dampness as it is useful in treatment of both external and internal disorders. It induces perspiration and treats external conditions characterized by accumulation of wind-damp in the muscle and skin level, such as *bi zheng* (painful obstruction syndrome). Internally, it dries dampness, strengthens the Spleen and dispels dampness obstructing the middle *jiao*. It can be combined with bitter and cold herbs like *Huang Bai* (Cortex Phellodendri) to treat damp-heat in the lower *jiao*. Also, this herb brightens the vision and treats cataracts, glaucoma and night blindness.

Hou Po disperses stagnation and relieves epigastric and abdominal fullness and distention. It treats cold accumulation, obstruction by dampness, food stagnation and qi stagnation that are individually or jointly causing bloating, fullness and distention. It regulates qi, warms the middle *jiao*. and disperses fullness caused by cold accumulation with qi stagnation. It redirects Lung qi to relieve dyspnea, cough and phlegm.

Huo Xiang (Herba Agastache) and ***Pei Lan*** (Herba Eupatorii) dissolve dampness and relieve summer-heat.

Chapter 5 summary

Huo Xiang is warm, and more strongly dries dampness. It also harmonizes the Stomach to relieve vomiting. When used topically, *Huo Xiang* treats dermatological disorders, such as fungal infection.

Pei Lan is neutral and mostly used to treat damp-heat accumulation in the middle *jiao* that impairs Spleen function. It also has a mild function to release the exterior.

Sha Ren (Fructus Amomi) and ***Bai Dou Kou*** (Fructus Amomi Rotundus) regulate qi, dissolve dampness and treat dampness obstructing the middle *jiao* accompanied by Spleen and Stomach qi stagnation.

Sha Ren more strongly relieves diarrhea due to cold in the Spleen, and stabilizes the fetus.

Bai Dou Kou more effectively stops vomiting caused by cold and dampness accumulation in the middle *jiao*.

Cao Guo (Fructus Tsaoko) and ***Cao Dou Kou*** (Semen Alpiniae Katsumadai) warm the middle *jiao* and dry dampness, and treat cold and dampness in the Spleen and Stomach.

Cao Guo more strongly dries dampness, and treats malaria.

Cao Dou Kou, acrid and aromatic, strengthens the Spleen.

HERBS FROM OTHER FUNCTIONAL CATEGORIES WITH DAMP-DISSOLVING FUNCTIONS

Name	Functional Category
Bai Zhu (Rhizoma Atractylodis Macrocephalae)	Tonic Herbs (Chapter 17)
Bian Dou (Semen Lablab Album)	Tonic Herbs (Chapter 17)
Chen Pi (Pericarpium Citri Reticulatae)	Qi-Regulating Herbs (Chapter 8)
Shi Chang Pu (Rhizoma Acori)	Orifice-Opening Herbs (Chapter 16)
Xiang Ru (Herba Elsholtziae seu Moslae)	Exterior-Releasing Herbs (Chapter 1)
Zhang Nao (Camphora)	Substances for Topical Application (Chapter 20)

Chapter 6

— Water-Regulating and Damp-Resolving Herbs

利水渗湿药

Chapter 6 – Water-Regulating and Damp-Resolving Herbs

Chapter 6

— Water-Regulating and Damp-Resolving Herbs

Definition: Substances that regulate water and resolve dampness act to normalize water circulation, eliminate water accumulation and drain dampness.

These herbs function to promote normal urination, increase urinary output, and eliminate bodily accumulation of water and dampness. They are primarily used to treat *lin zheng* (dysuria syndrome), dysuria, anuria, edema, and phlegm accumulation. Other applications include jaundice, sores, febrile disorders, *bi zheng* (painful obstruction syndrome), and leukorrhea.

SUBCATEGORIES OF ACTION

1. ***Promote diuresis***: These sweet and/or bland herbs, neutral or cool, promote diuresis and are commonly used to treat accumulations of water, dampness and phlegm.
2. ***Drain damp-heat***: These herbs are either bitter or sweet, and cold. In addition to promoting diuresis, they drain damp-heat, and are commonly used to treat dysuria, infection in the genito-urinary tract, or stones in the urinary tract.

Differential Diagnosis and Treatment:
Treatment of Water Element disorders requires careful *zang-fu* differential diagnosis. The ***Lung***, ***Spleen*** and ***Kidney*** control the circulation of water:

the ***Spleen*** absorbs water,
the ***Lung*** distributes water, and
the ***Kidney*** eliminates water.

When these organs fail to carry out their normal functions, disease occurs. **Spleen yang deficiency** results in unabsorbed water accumulating in the body as dampness, rather than being efficiently absorbed or processed. **Lung qi deficiency** permits water to accumulate in the Lung and skin, instead of being appropriately distributed. **Kidney yang deficiency** manifests in dysuria and water accumulating in the lower extremities, rather than being promptly eliminated. **Urinary Bladder qi deficiency**, failing to maintain proper volume of urinary output, compromises proper water circulation and contributes to fluid build-up.

Complicating factors include increasing levels of combined damp and heat (aptly renamed 'damp-heat') in the lower *jiao*, hematuria, and the formation of urinary calculi [with the resultant inflammation and pain known as '*shi lin*' (stone dysuria)]. Therefore, in addition to selecting herbs that regulate water and drain dampness to address the primary syndrome, successful treatment requires correct diagnosis of any complications, and corresponding modification of herbal choices.

Yin Chen Hao (Herba Artemisiae Scopariae)
Ben Cao Gang Mu (Materia Medica),
by Li Shi-Zhen, 1578 A.D.

Appropriate treatment to remove (that is, 'drain') accumulations, or to transform damp or phlegm into valuable circulating fluids, may alleviate blockages of qi flow or restore generation of yang energy and thus allow the key organs to regain correct functioning. However, a superior practitioner will be alert to assess whether qi- and/or yang-tonifying herbs are necessary with (or following) treatment of the damp, phlegm, damp-heat or combined accumulations.

Chapter 6 –Water-Regulating and Damp-Resolving Herbs

CAUTIONS/CONTRAINDICATIONS

Decreased urinary output may be the result of *either* accumulation of water in the body *or* deficiency of yin and body fluids. Herbs that regulate water and drain dampness may further deplete yin and body fluids, thus causing further injury to individuals already experiencing these deficiencies.

PROCESSING

Timing of harvest and methods of preparation have a significant impact on the clinical effectiveness of these herbs; so it is wise to observe any processing advice available. Some examples: to achieve maximum therapeutic effectiveness, *Ze Xie* (Rhizoma Alismatis) should be harvested in the fall and winter, but not in the summer. *Ban Bian Lian* (Herba Lobeliae Chinensis) should be harvested prior to flowering. Preparations of fresh or alcohol-processed *Ze Xie* have a much stronger diuretic action than salt-processed *Ze Xie*.

PHARMACOLOGICAL EFFECTS

- **Diuretic**: Many herbs are quite potent in increasing urinary output. While the diuretic influence of these herbs may not strongly affect healthy individuals, it has a significant impact on individuals experiencing edema or chronic nephritis. Herbs with diuretic action include *Fu Ling* (Poria), *Zhu Ling* (Polyporus), *Ze Xie* (Rhizoma Alismatis), *Ban Bian Lian* (Herba Lobeliae Chinensis), *Yu Mi Xu* (Stigma Maydis), *Chuan Mu Tong* (Caulis Clematidis Armandii), *Bian Xu* (Herba Polygoni Avicularis), *Qu Mai* (Herba Dianthi), *Jin Qian Cao* (Herba Lysimachiae) and *Yin Chen Hao* (Herba Artemisiae Scopariae).
- **Antibiotic**: Many herbs inhibit the growth or activity of bacteria, fungi and parasites.
  - Herbs with antibacterial properties include *Fu Ling* (Poria), *Ze Xie* (Rhizoma Alismatis), *Ban Bian Lian* (Herba Lobeliae Chinensis), *Zhu Ling* (Polyporus), *Che Qian Zi* (Semen Plantaginis), *Bian Xu* (Herba Polygoni Avicularis), *Jin Qian Cao* (Herba Lysimachiae), *Yin Chen Hao* (Herba Artemisiae Scopariae), *Qu Mai* (Herba Dianthi), and *Chi Xiao Dou* (Semen Phaseoli).
  - Herbs with antifungal effects include *Che Qian Zi* (Semen Plantaginis), *Chuan Mu Tong* (Caulis Clematidis Armandii), *Bian Xu* (Herba Polygoni Avicularis), *Di Fu Zi* (Fructus Kochiae) and *Yin Chen Hao* (Herba Artemisiae Scopariae).
  - Among antiparasitic herbs are *Che Qian Zi* (Semen Plantaginis) and *Yin Chen Hao* (Herba Artemisiae Scopariae).
- **Cholagogic**: Some herbs promote bile secretion, among them: *Yin Chen Hao* (Herba Artemisiae Scopariae), *Ban Bian Lian* (Herba Lobeliae Chinensis), *Yu Mi Xu* (Stigma Maydis), *Bian Xu* (Herba Polygoni Avicularis), and *Jin Qian Cao* (Herba Lysimachiae).
- **Metabolic influence**: *Ze Xie* (Rhizoma Alismatis), *Yin Chen Hao* (Herba Artemisiae Scopariae) and others may lower blood cholesterol and triglyceride levels.

Many water-regulating and damp-resolving herbs have potent influence to increase the elimination of water and electrolytes.

POTENTIAL HERB-DRUG INTERACTIONS

- **Diuretics**: Herbs that regulate water and transform dampness often have diuretic characteristics to eliminate the accumulation of excess water in the body. Therefore, it is prudent to avoid combining these herbs with drugs that exert diuretic effects, as there may be additive or synergistic results. Combination therapy may lead to excessive loss of fluids and electrolytes.[1]

References

1. Chen, J. Recognition & prevention of herb-drug interactions, *Medical Acupuncture*, Fall/Winter 1998/1999; volume 10/number 2; 9-13

Fu Ling (Poria)

茯苓 茯苓

Pinyin Name: *Fu Ling*
Alternate Chinese Names: *Yun Ling*
Original Source: *Shen Nong Ben Cao Jing* (Divine Husbandman's Classic of the Materia Medica) in the second century
English Name: poria, indian bread, tuckahoe
Botanical Name: *Poria cocos* (Schw.) Wolf (*Fu Ling*)
Pharmaceutical Name: Poria
Properties: sweet, bland, neutral
Channels Entered: Heart, Spleen, Kidney

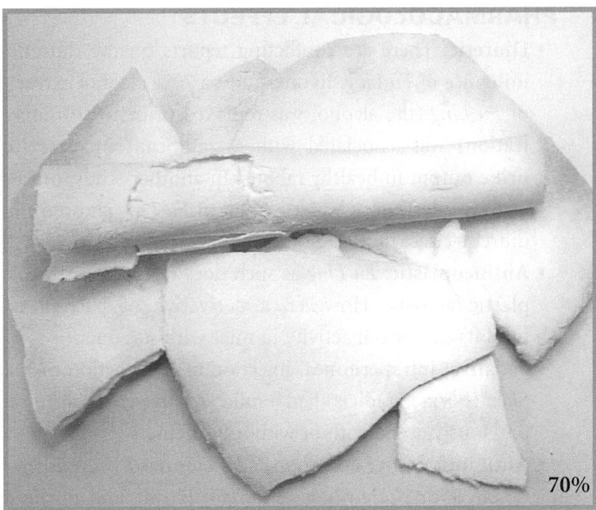
70%

CHINESE THERAPEUTIC ACTIONS

1. Promotes Urination and Resolves Dampness

Accumulation of water and dampness: Because of its neutral thermal property, *Fu Ling* (Poria) is frequently used to promote urination and eliminate dampness without damaging qi. It is commonly used to treat edema, fullness and distention, dysuria, and internal accumulations of water or phlegm. Because it is neutral, *Fu Ling* is useful for conditions that are excess or deficient, hot or cold.

- Dysuria: combine *Fu Ling* with *Zhu Ling* (Polyporus) and *Ze Xie* (Rhizoma Alismatis). **Exemplar Formula:** *Wu Lin San* (Five-Ingredient Powder for Painful Urinary Dysfunction).
- Edema caused by Spleen and Kidney yang deficiencies: use this herb with *Fu Zi* (Radix Aconiti Lateralis Praeparata) and *Sheng Jiang* (Rhizoma Zingiberis Recens).
- Edema with dysuria: combine it with *Bai Zhu* (Rhizoma Atractylodis Macrocephalae) and *Gui Zhi* (Ramulus Cinnamomi).
- Phlegm accumulation: add *Zhu Ling* (Polyporus) and *Ze Xie* (Rhizoma Alismatis).
- Phlegm accumulation with Spleen deficiency: increase dosage of *Fu Ling*, or add *Bai Zhu* (Rhizoma Atractylodis Macrocephalae).
- Phlegm accumulation with vertigo: combine it with *Bai Zhu* (Rhizoma Atractylodis Macrocephalae) and *Tian Ma* (Rhizoma Gastrodiae).

2. Strengthens the Spleen

Spleen qi deficiency: Spleen qi deficiency is the leading cause of accumulation of dampness in the body. *Fu Ling* strengthens and tonifies the Spleen to treat edema, loose stools, fatigue, poor appetite and lack of energy.

- Loose stools because of Spleen qi deficiency: combine this herb with *Ren Shen* (Radix Ginseng) and *Bai Zhu* (Rhizoma Atractylodis Macrocephalae). **Exemplar Formula:** *Shen Ling Bai Zhu San* (Ginseng, Poria and Atractylodes Macrocephala Powder).
- Irritable bowel syndrome from Spleen qi deficiency: add *Gui Zhi* (Ramulus Cinnamomi), *Bai Shao* (Radix Paeoniae Alba), *Gan Cao* (Radix Glycyrrhizae), *Bai Zhu* (Rhizoma Atractylodis Macrocephalae), *Mu Xiang* (Radix Aucklandiae), *Rou Dou Kou* (Semen Myristicae) and *Wu Zhu Yu* (Fructus Evodiae).

3. Calms the *Shen* (Spirit)

***Shen* disturbance:** *Fu Ling* calms the *shen* to treat insomnia and palpitations caused either by deficiency of the Heart and Spleen, or by phlegm obstructing the Heart.

- Insomnia and palpitations caused by deficiency of the Heart and Spleen: combine *Fu Ling* with *Dang Shen* (Radix Codonopsis), *Long Yan Rou* (Arillus Longan), and *Suan Zao Ren* (Semen Zizyphi Spinosae).
- Insomnia and palpitations because of phlegm obstructing the Heart: use it with *Shi Chang Pu* (Rhizoma Acori) and *Yuan Zhi* (Radix Polygalae Tenufoliae).

DOSAGE

10 to 15 grams in decoction.

CAUTIONS / CONTRAINDICATIONS

- Use *Fu Ling* with caution in patients with yin deficiency and/or spermatorrhea.

CHEMICAL COMPOSITION

Pachymose, pachyman, pachymaran, tumulosic acid, poriaic acid A, B, C.[1]

Fu Ling (Poria)

PHARMACOLOGICAL EFFECTS

- **Diuretic**: There are conflicting reports on the diuretic influence of *Fu Ling*. In one study, a 70% alcohol extract of *Fu Ling* (the alcohol was removed prior to administration) was associated with a significant increase in urine output in healthy rabbits. In another study, intravenous injection of water extract of *Fu Ling* showed no diuretic effect in dogs or mice.[2]
- **Antineoplastic**: *Fu Ling* as such does not have antineoplastic activity. However, a derivative of pachyman inhibits cancer cell activity in mice with sarcoma.[3]
- **Sedative**: Intraperitoneal injection of a decoction of *Fu Shen* (Poria Paradicis) had a mild sedative effect in mice previously dosed with or without caffeine.[4]
- **Antibiotic**: Water decoction of *Fu Ling* has a bacteriostatic effect on *Staphylococcus aureus*, *E. coli*, and *Bacillus proteus*, and the alcohol-extracted form has a bactericidal effect against leptospira.[5,6]

CLINICAL STUDIES AND RESEARCH

- **Edema**: Thirty patients with edema were treated with a preparation of *Fu Ling*, with marked effectiveness in 23 cases and moderate effectiveness in 7 cases. The herbs were given in the form of cookies, each containing at least 30% (3.5 grams) *Fu Ling*. The treatment protocol was to ingest 8 cookies, three times daily for 7 days, for each course of treatment. The dosage was adjusted for children. All other diuretics were discontinued prior to herbal treatment.[7]
- **Tumor**: A preparation of *Fu Ling* was evaluated for its antineoplastic effect in 70 patients in an oncology hospital in Fuzhou, China. Some patients received herbal treatment only, while others used it in conjunction with chemotherapy, radiation, and/or surgery. It was observed that *Fu Ling* strengthens the body, enhances the immune system, improves liver and kidney functions, improves appetite, supports increased body weight, and minimizes the adverse reactions associated with chemotherapy.[8]
- **Schizophrenia**: In one study, 53 patients with chronic schizophrenia were treated with 60 grams of *Fu Ling* in decoction once daily for 1 to 3 months. The study reported complete recovery in 3 cases, moderate improvement in 11 cases, slight improvement in 16 cases, and no response in 23 cases.[9]

HERB-DRUG INTERACTION

- **Ethanol:** In an *in vitro* study, a traditional Chinese medicinal preparation including *Fu Ling*, *Ren Shen* (Radix Ginseng), *Yuan Zhi* (Radix Polygalae Tenufoliae), and *Shi Chang Pu* (Rhizoma Acori) was found to reduce the ethanol-induced impairment of memory registration. It also ameliorated the scopolamine-induced memory registration deficit. These results suggest that this herbal preparation ameliorates the impairment effect of ethanol on learning and memory processes.[10]
- **Diuretics:** Although no documented cases of this interaction have been reported, it is prudent to avoid combination of herbs and drugs that exert diuretic effects, as there may be additive or synergistic effects. Combination therapy may lead to excessive loss of fluid and electrolytes.[11] [Note: Examples of diuretics include chlorothiazide, hydrochlorothiazide, furosemide (Lasix), bumetanide (Bumex), and torsemide (Demadex).]

TOXICOLOGY

No significant adverse reactions or side effects were reported following toxicology studies in dogs. When *Fu Ling* was given to mice for 2 weeks at a dosage 500 times the normal adult dose, a slight decrease in body weight and increase in white blood cell counts was noted.[12,13]

SUPPLEMENT

Various segments of this fungal herb have differing functions and names.

- 茯苓皮 / 茯苓皮 *Fu Ling Pi* (Cortex Poria), the outer layer, is the better choice to eliminate dampness. It has the same properties and taste as *Fu Ling*. The strongest functions of *Fu ling Pi* are to dispel edema and promote urination. It is commonly combined with *Sheng Jiang Pi* (Pericarpium Zingiberis Recens), *Sang Bai Pi* (Cortex Mori) and *Da Fu Pi* (Pericarpium Arecae). Recommended dose in decoctions for *Fu Ling Pi* is 10 to 15 grams.
- 白茯苓 / 白茯苓 *Bai Fu Ling* (Poria Alba), the inner part, functions best to strengthen the Spleen. *Bai Fu Ling* and *Fu Ling* are generally considered to be interchangeable names for the same herb.
- 赤茯苓 / 赤茯苓 *Chi Fu Ling* (Poria Rubrae), the outer, light red layer, treats damp-heat. It treats *re lin* (heat dysuria).
- 茯神 / 茯神 *Fu Shen* (Poria Paradicis), the innermost part surrounding the root, has stronger *shen* (spirit)-calming influence to treat insomnia, forgetfulness and palpitations.

AUTHORS' COMMENTS

Fu Ling is a fungus that may be thinly sliced, in typical white 'curls,' or cut into blocks approximately 2 cm thick. For decoctions, select the thin cut: the greater exposed surface area of the curls permits maximum extraction of active constituents. The dense nature of the block cut prevents full penetration by the water during cooking. Even after cooking, a block of *Fu Ling* may be completely dry in the center.

Fu Ling and *Zhu Ling* (Polyporus) both are commonly

Fu Ling (Poria)

used to regulate water. *Fu Ling* dispels dampness and benefits the Heart and Spleen; therefore it is often added to tonic herbs to promote restored organ function. *Zhu Ling* has a stronger diuretic function than *Fu Ling* but does not serve as a tonic. It is used mostly to dispel dampness but does not restore the body's ability to regulate water.

In the past, *Fu Ling* was coated with *Zhu Sha* (Cinnabaris) at times for the purpose of calming the *shen* (spirit). However, this is rarely done now.

References

1. *Xian Dai Zhong Yao Yao Li Xue* (Contemporary Pharmacology of Chinese Herbs), 1997; 529
2. *Chang Yong Zhong Yao Cheng Fen Yu Yao Li Shou Ce* (A Handbook of the Composition and Pharmacology of Common Chinese Drugs), 1994; 1383:1391
3. *Zhong Cao Yao Xue* (Study of Chinese Herbal Medicine), 1976:15
4. *Zhong Yao Da Ci Dien* (Dictionary of Chinese Herbs), 1977:1596
5. Ibid.
6. *Zhong Yao Cai* (Study of Chinese Herbal Material), 1985; (2):36
7. *Shang Hai Zhong Yi Yao Za Zhi* (Shanghai Journal of Chinese Medicine and Herbology), 1986; 8:25
8. *Zhong Xi Yi Jie He Za Zhi* (Journal of Integrated Chinese and Western Medicine), 1985; 2:115
9. *Zhong Xi Yi Yao Za Zhi* (Journal of Chinese and Western Medicine), 1982; 5:14
10. *Biological and Pharmaceutical Bulletin.* 17(11):1472-6, 1994 Nov
11. Chen, J. Recognition & prevention of herb-drug interactions, *Medical Acupuncture*, Fall/Winter 1998/1999; volume 10/number 2; 9-13
12. *Fu Jian Yi Yao Za Zhi* (Fujian Journal of Medicine and Herbology), 1988; 10(1):29
13. *Bei Jing Yi Xue Yuan Xue Bao* (Journal of Beijing School of Medicine), 1984; 16(1):48

Zhu Ling (Polyporus)

豬苓 猪苓

Pinyin Name: *Zhu Ling*
Literal Name: "pig's fungus"
Alternate Chinese Names: *Zhu Shi Ling*
Original Source: *Shen Nong Ben Cao Jing* (Divine Husbandman's Classic of the Materia Medica) in the second century
English Name: polyporus
Botanical Name: *Polyporus umbellatus* (Pers.) Fries (*Zhu Ling*)
Pharmaceutical Name: Polyporus
Properties: sweet, bland, neutral
Channels Entered: Kidney, Urinary Bladder

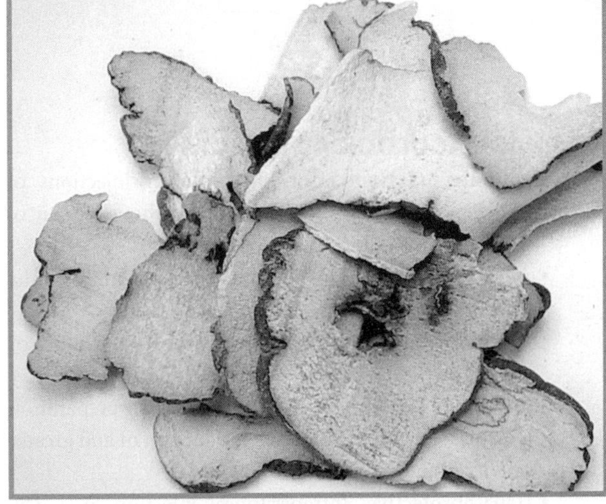

CHINESE THERAPEUTIC ACTIONS

Promotes Urination and Resolves Dampness

Accumulation of water and dampness: Bland and neutral, *Zhu Ling* (Polyporus) promotes urination, eliminates dampness and water accumulation, and treats edema, scanty urine, jaundice, diarrhea, and *lin zheng* (dysuria syndrome).

- Generalized edema: use *Zhu Ling* individually
- Edema arising from Spleen deficiency: use it with *Fu Ling* (Poria), *Ze Xie* (Rhizoma Alismatis) and *Bai Zhu* (Rhizoma Atractylodis Macrocephalae).
- Fever, dysuria, thirst, and irritability caused by accumulation of water and heat with yin deficiency: use *Zhu Ling* with *Hua Shi* (Talcum) and *E Jiao* (Colla Corii Asini). **Exemplar Formula:** *Zhu Ling Tang* (Polyporus Decoction).
- *Lin zheng* (dysuria syndrome) resulting from dampness and heat: use it with *Chuan Mu Tong* (Caulis Clematidis Armandii), *Che Qian Zi* (Semen Plantaginis) and *Hua Shi* (Talcum).
- Diarrhea caused by cold-damp accumulation in the intestines: combine it with *Rou Dou Kou* (Semen Myristicae) and *Huang Bai* (Cortex Phellodendri).

Zhu Ling (Polyporus)

- Epigastric distention and fullness: use it with *Bian Xu* (Herba Polygoni Avicularis), *Qu Mai* (Herba Dianthi), *Chuan Mu Tong* (Caulis Clematidis Armandii) and *Hua Shi* (Talcum).
- Jaundice: combine *Zhu Ling* with *Yin Chen Hao* (Herba Artemisiae Scopariae), *Zhi Zi* (Fructus Gardeniae), *Huang Bai* (Cortex Phellodendri), *Ze Xie* (Rhizoma Alismatis) and *Da Huang* (Radix et Rhizoma Rhei).

DOSAGE

5 to 10 grams.

CAUTIONS / CONTRAINDICATIONS

- *Zhu Ling* is not recommended for patients with dizziness caused by yin deficiency, or those experiencing thirst and dampness.

CHEMICAL COMPOSITION

Ergosterol, biotin, polyporenic acid A, C; polyporusterone.[1,2]

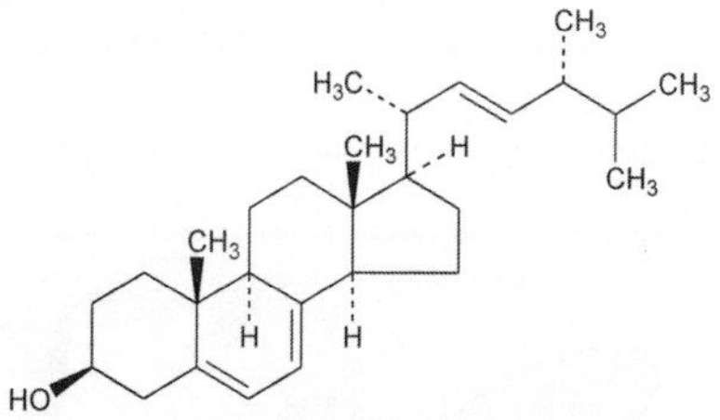

Ergosterol

PHARMACOLOGICAL EFFECTS

- **Diuretic**: Intravenous or intramuscular injections of *Zhu Ling* decoction in dogs increases the excretion of water, sodium, chloride, and potassium.[3]
- **Antineoplastic**: A preparation of *Zhu Ling* inhibited the growth of cancer cells in mice with liver cancer.[4]
- **Antibiotic**: Alcohol extract of *Zhu Ling* has an inhibitory influence on *Staphylococcus aureus* and *E. coli.*[5]
- **Immunologic**: Administration of a *Zhu Ling* preparation is associated with an increased production of and greater activity in the T-cells.[6]
- **Hepatoprotective**: Intraperitoneal injection of a *Zhu Ling* preparation has a protective effect against carbon tetrachloride-induced hepatitis in rats.[7,8]

CLINICAL STUDIES AND RESEARCH

- **Tumor**: Administration of a *Zhu Ling* preparation was associated with a positive effect in enhancing the immune system and suppressing the growth of cancer cells in 200 patients with lung cancer, 40 patients with leukemia, and 68 patients with liver, nose or throat cancers. No significant side effects were reported.[9]
- **Psoriasis:** Intramuscular injections of *Zhu Ling* twice daily for 2 weeks or more was effective in treating psoriasis patients. Out of 265 cases, 83 showed complete remission, 67 showed moderate improvement, 79 showed slight improvement, and 36 had no response. Out of 83 cases who were in complete remission, 13 later had a recurrence. The overall rate of effectiveness was 86.4%.[10]
- **Chronic viral hepatitis**: Intramuscular injection of a *Zhu Ling* preparation was effective in treating 359 patients with chronic viral hepatitis. The treatment protocol was 20 days of therapy followed by 10 days of rest, for a total of 3 months per course of treatment. Therapeutic effects included symptomatic improvement and a decrease in liver enzyme levels. No significant side effects or adverse reactions were reported.[11]

HERB-DRUG INTERACTION

- **Diuretics:** Although no documented cases of this interaction have been reported, it is prudent to avoid combination of herbs and drugs that exert diuretic effects, as there may be additive or synergistic effects, possibly leading to excessive loss of fluids and electrolytes.[12] [Note: Examples of diuretics include chlorothiazide, hydrochlorothiazide, furosemide (Lasix), bumetanide (Bumex), and torsemide (Demadex).]

TOXICOLOGY

No fatalities or organ abnormalities were reported in mice following a bolus dose of *Zhu Ling* at 2,000 times the normal adult dose, or after continuous administration for 28 days at 100 times the normal adult dose.[13]

AUTHORS' COMMENTS

Zhu Ling has similar diuretic functions to those of *Fu Ling* (Poria), but is stronger. See Authors' Comment, *Fu Ling*.

References

1. *Xian Dai Zhong Yao Yao Li Xue* (Contemporary Pharmacology of Chinese Herbs), 1997; 533
2. *The Merck Index* 12th edition, Chapman & Hall/CRCnetBASE/Merck, 2000
3. *Yao Xue Xue Bao* (Journal of Herbology), 1964; 11(12):815
4. *Yao Xue Tong Bao* (Report of Herbology), 1985; (2):74
5. *Zhong Yao Xue* (Chinese Herbology), 1998, 334:336
6. *Zhong Guo Mian Yi Xue Za Zhi* (Chinese Journal of Immunology), 1991; 7(3):185
7. *Zhong Guo Yao Li Xue Tong Bao* (Journal of Chinese Herbal Pharmacology), 1988; 9(4):345
8. *Zhong Yao Yao Li Yu Lin Chuan* (Pharmacology and Clinical Applications of Chinese Herbs), 1989; 5(3):37
9. *Zhong Xi Yi Jie He Za Zhi* (Journal of Integrated Chinese and Western Medicine), 1984; 5:285
10. Ibid.
11. *Zhong Xi Yi Jie He Za Zhi* (Journal of Integrated Chinese and Western Medicine), 1988; 3:141
12. Chen, J. Recognition & prevention of herb-drug interactions, *Medical Acupuncture*, Fall/Winter 1998/1999; volume 10/number 2; 9-13
13. *Yao Xue Tong Bao* (Report of Herbology), 1985; 20(2):74

Ze Xie (Rhizoma Alismatis)

澤瀉 泽泻

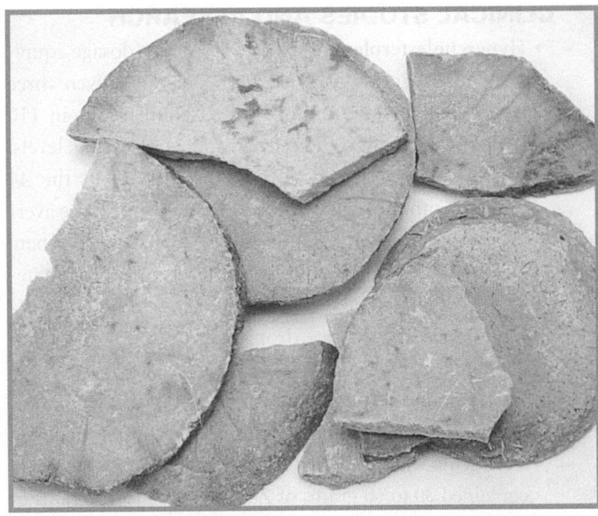

Pinyin Name: *Ze Xie*
Literal Name: "marsh drain"
Original Source: *Shen Nong Ben Cao Jing* (Divine Husbandman's Classic of the Materia Medica) in the second century
English Name: alisma, Oriental water plantain rhizome
Botanical Name: *Alisma orientalis* (Sam.) Juzep. (*Ze Xie*)
Pharmaceutical Name: Rhizoma Alismatis
Properties: sweet, bland, cold
Channels Entered: Kidney, Urinary Bladder

CHINESE THERAPEUTIC ACTIONS

1. Regulates Water Circulation and Resolves Dampness

Water and dampness accumulation: *Ze Xie* (Rhizoma Alismatis) has a potent function to regulate water circulation and resolve dampness. It treats edema, *lin zheng* (dysuria syndrome), urinary disorders, vertigo, and other disorders characterized by accumulation of water and dampness.

- Generalized edema: use *Ze Xie* with *Fu Ling* (Poria) and *Zhu Ling* (Polyporus).
- Edema in pregnancy: use it with *Sang Bai Pi* (Cortex Mori), *Zhi Ke* (Fructus Aurantii), *Sang Ji Sheng* (Herba Taxilli), *Fu Ling* (Poria) and *Da Fu Pi* (Pericarpium Arecae).
- *Shi lin* (stone dysuria): combine it with *Hai Jin Sha* (Herba Lygodii), *Jin Qian Cao* (Herba Lysimachiae), *Niu Xi* (Radix Cyathulae seu Achyranthis), *Ze Lan* (Herba Lycopi), *Dong Kui Zi* (Semen Malvae) and *Zhu Ling* (Polyporus).
- *Shi-re lin* (damp-heat dysuria): combine this herb with *Hua Shi* (Talcum) and *Che Qian Zi* (Semen Plantaginis).
- *Gao lin* (cloudy dysuria): use it with *Fu Ling* (Poria), *Hai Jin Sha* (Herba Lygodii), *Hua Shi* (Talcum) and *Bi Xie* (Rhizoma Dioscoreae Hypoglaucae).
- Vertigo, dizziness, and tinnitus due to phlegm accumulation: use it with *Bai Zhu* (Rhizoma Atractylodis Macrocephalae).
- Damp-heat in the Liver and Gallbladder, manifesting in jaundice, red eyes, hypochondriac pain, nausea, poor appetite, and scanty dark urine: combine *Ze Xie* with *Chai Hu* (Radix Bupleuri), *Long Dan Cao* (Radix Gentianae), *Huang Qin* (Radix Scutellariae), *Yin Chen Hao* (Herba Artemisiae Scopariae), *Qing Dai* (Indigo Naturalis) and *Che Qian Zi* (Semen Plantaginis).

2. Clears Deficiency Fire from the Kidney

Ze Xie treats spermatorrhea, nocturnal emissions, and premature ejaculation, which are symptoms commonly associated with the rising fire from Kidney yin deficiency.

- Deficiency fire from the Kidney: use *Ze Xie* with *Sheng Di Huang* (Radix Rehmanniae), *Zhi Mu* (Radix Anemarrhenae) and *Huang Bai* (Cortex Phellodendri).

DOSAGE

5 to 10 grams. Use up to 15, 18 or even 30 grams of *Ze Xie* in severe cases. The unprocessed herb greatly strengthens the Spleen and regulates water, and is commonly used for treating edema, dysuria, and jaundice. Frying *Ze Xie* with salt enhances its effect of nourishing yin, purging heat and regulating water circulation. Salt-fried *Ze Xie* is commonly used to treat knee and lower back weakness and pain. Dry-frying the herb enhances its strengthening influence on the Spleen, commonly helping to resolve diarrhea and vertigo.

CHEMICAL COMPOSITION

Alisol A, alisol B, alisol A monoacetate, alisol B monoacetate, alisol C monoacetate, epialisol A, alismol, alismoxide, alismin, starch, protein, essential oil.[1]

PHARMACOLOGICAL EFFECTS

- **Diuretic:** Administration of *Ze Xie* is associated with marked diuretic effects. However, it is not clear whether there is also an increase in excretion of sodium and potassium.[2]
- **Antihyperlipidemic:** In one study, *Ze Xie* was effective in treating hyperlipidemia, arteriosclerosis and fatty liver.[3]
- **Antihypertensive:** Intravenous injection of an extract of *Ze Xie* had a mild antihypertensive effect that lasted approximately 30 minutes.[4]

Ze Xie (Rhizoma Alismatis)

CLINICAL STUDIES AND RESEARCH

- **Hypercholesterolemia:** Extract of *Ze Xie* (dosage equivalent to 27 grams of dried herb per day) given three times daily for one month showed good results in 110 patients with high cholesterol and triglyceride levels. There was a 9% reduction of these levels in the 44 patients with the highest cholesterol levels, with the average dropping from 258.4 mg/dL to 235.2 mg/dL. There was a 10% or higher reduction of levels in approximately 50% of all patients. Of 103 patients with high triglyceride levels, the average dropped from 337.1 mg/dL to 258.0 mg/dL.[5]
- **Dizziness and vertigo:** In one study, 55 patients with dizziness and vertigo reported complete recovery following treatments with an herbal decoction. The herbal formula contained 30 to 60 grams of *Ze Xie* and 10 to 15 grams of *Bai Zhu* (Rhizoma Atractylodis Macrocephalae). The patients were instructed to take the decoction twice daily. The duration of treatment was between 1 and 9 days.[6]

HERB-DRUG INTERACTION

- **Diuretics:** Although no documented cases of this interaction have been reported, it is prudent to avoid combination of herbs and drugs that exert diuretic effects, as there may be additive or synergistic effects. Combination therapy may lead to excessive loss of fluids and electrolytes. [Note: Examples of diuretics include chlorothiazide, hydrochlorothiazide, furosemide (Lasix), bumetanide (Bumex), and torsemide (Demadex).][7]

TOXICOLOGY

Oral administration of an extract of *Ze Xie* at 1 g/kg and 2 g/kg in rats (20 and 40 times the normal adult dose, respectively) for 3 months showed no tendency to cause abnormalities of the internal organs. The LD_{50} for an alcohol extract of *Ze Xie* in rats is 0.98 g/kg via intravenous injection and 1.27 g/kg via intraperitoneal injection.[8]

AUTHORS' COMMENTS

Tonic herbs may create unnecessary heat in the body, causing the formation and rising of Kidney fire. *Ze Xie* is frequently combined with tonic herbs to prevent this side effect, such as in *Liu Wei Di Huang Wan* (Six-Ingredient Pill with Rehmannia).

Ze Xie, *Zi Su Ye* (Folium Perillae), *Shi Chang Pu* (Rhizoma Acori), and *Shan Zha* (Fructus Crataegi) taken as tea on a daily basis, are effective to reduce body weight and lower cholesterol levels.

References

1. *Xian Dai Zhong Yao Yao Li Xue* (Contemporary Pharmacology of Chinese Herbs), 1997; 537
2. *Sheng Yao Xue Za Zhi* (Journal of Raw Herbology), 1982; 36(2):150
3. He, XY. Effects of alisma plantago l. on hyperlipidemia, arteriosclerosis and fatty liver. *Chinese Journal of Modern Developments in Traditional Medicine.* 1(2):114-7, Oct. 1981
4. *Zhong Yao Yao Li Yu Ying Yong* (Pharmacology and Applications of Chinese Herbs), 1983: 718
5. *Zhong Hua Yi Xue Za Zhi* (Chinese Journal of Medicine), 1976; 11:693
6. *He Bei Zhong Yi Za Zhi* (Hebei Journal of Chinese Medicine), 1988; 6:14
7. Chen, J. Recognition & prevention of herb-drug interactions, *Medical Acupuncture*, Fall/Winter 1998/1999; volume 10/number 2; 9-13
8. *Zhong Yao Yao Li Yu Ying Yong* (Pharmacology and Applications of Chinese Herbs), 1983: 718

Yi Yi Ren (Semen Coicis)

薏苡仁 薏苡仁

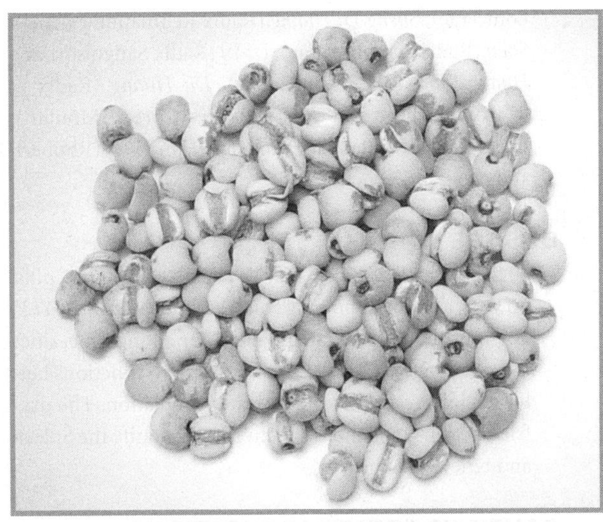

Pinyin Name: *Yi Yi Ren*
Alternate Chinese Names: *Mi Ren, Yi Ren, Yi Mi*
Original Source: *Shen Nong Ben Cao Jing* (Divine Husbandman's Classic of the Materia Medica) in the second century
English Name: coix seeds, Job's tears
Botanical Name: *Coix lacryma-jobi* L. var. *ma-yuen* (Roman) Stapf (*Yi Yi*)
Pharmaceutical Name: Semen Coicis
Properties: sweet, bland, cool
Channels Entered: Spleen, Stomach, Lung

CHINESE THERAPEUTIC ACTIONS

1. Strengthens the Spleen and Resolves Dampness

Dampness accumulation due to Spleen deficiency: Clinical presentations of this imbalance include leg *qi*, damp febrile disorders, edema, and *lin zheng* (dysuria syndrome). The sweet, bland, cool properties of *Yi Yi Ren* (Semen Coicis) make it particularly useful to strengthen the Spleen and address imbalances including dampness and other water element difficulties.

- Accumulation of dampness and Spleen deficiency: combine *Yi Yi Ren* with *Bai Zhu* (Rhizoma Atractylodis Macrocephalae), *Fu Ling* (Poria), *Bian Dou* (Semen Lablab Album) and *Chi Xiao Dou* (Semen Phaseoli).
- Shortness of breath due to water accumulation: use this herb in combination with *Yu Li Ren* (Semen Pruni).
- *Re lin* (heat dysuria): use it with *Che Qian Zi* (Semen Plantaginis) and *Hua Shi* (Talcum).
- *Shi lin* (stone dysuria): add *Hai Jin Sha* (Herba Lygodii) and *Jin Qian Cao* (Herba Lysimachiae).
- Deficiency of the Spleen and Stomach, with loose stools and decreased food intake: combine this herb with *Ren Shen* (Radix Ginseng), *Bai Zhu* (Rhizoma Atractylodis Macrocephalae) and *Shan Yao* (Rhizoma Dioscoreae).
- Damp febrile disorders with feelings of oppression in the chest, lack of appetite, and a thick, greasy tongue coat: use it with *Xing Ren* (Semen Armeniacae Amarum), *Bai Dou Kou* (Fructus Amomi Rotundus) and *Hou Po* (Cortex Magnoliae Officinalis).

2. Resolves Dampness and Relieves Pain

***Bi zheng* (painful obstruction syndrome):** *Yi Yi Ren* eliminates dampness from the muscles to relieve pain. It is best for tightness and spasms of the tendons restricting flexibility. It also effectively treats muscle, joint and tendon pain caused by accumulated dampness.

- *Bi zheng* due to dampness: cook *Yi Yi Ren* and rice as porridge on a daily basis.
- *Bi zheng* due to the accumulation of wind and dampness at the exterior: use it with *Ma Huang* (Herba Ephedrae), *Xing Ren* (Semen Armeniacae Amarum) and *Gan Cao* (Radix Glycyrrhizae).
- *Bi zheng* due to wind and dampness: combine it with *Ma Huang* (Herba Ephedrae), *Gui Zhi* (Ramulus Cinnamomi), and *Cang Zhu* (Rhizoma Atractylodis). **Exemplar Formula:** *Yi Yi Ren Tang* (Coicis Decoction).
- *Wei* (atrophy) syndrome and muscle weakness due to damp-heat: add it to *Cang Zhu* (Rhizoma Atractylodis), *Huang Bai* (Cortex Phellodendri) and *Niu Xi* (Radix Cyathulae seu Achyranthis). **Exemplar Formula:** *Si Miao San* (Four-Marvel Powder).

3. Clears Heat and Dispels Pus

By entering the Lung channel with its cooling influence, *Yi Yi Ren* treats lung abscesses characterized by purulent, thick sputum containing pus and blood, and cough with nasal discharge. It also treats intestinal abscesses, by virtue of the organ partnership between the Lung and Large Intestine.

- Lung abscess: use *Yi Yi Ren* with *Dong Gua Zi* (Semen Benincasae) and *Tao Ren* (Semen Persicae).
- Suppurated lung abscesses with profuse, thick, bloody sputum: add *Jie Geng* (Radix Platycodonis) and *Bai Ji* (Rhizoma Bletillae).
- Intestinal abscess: combine this herb with *Mu Dan Pi* (Cortex Moutan), *Tao Ren* (Semen Persicae) and *Bai Jiang Cao* (Herba cum Radice Patriniae).
- Acute appendicitis: use it with *Jin Yin Hua* (Flos

Yi Yi Ren (Semen Coicis)

Lonicerae), *Sheng Di Huang* (Radix Rehmanniae), *Xuan Shen* (Radix Scrophulariae), *Di Yu* (Radix Sanguisorbae), *Huang Qin* (Radix Scutellariae), *Da Huang* (Radix et Rhizoma Rhei) and *Mu Dan Pi* (Cortex Moutan). **Exemplar Formula:** *Da Huang Mu Dan Tang* (Rhubarb and Moutan Decoction).

DOSAGE

10 to 30 grams. *Yi Yi Ren* may be taken as decoction, pills, powder, and food (porridge or other preparations). *Yi Yi Ren* must be taken at large dosages for a long time, since it is relatively mild. The unprocessed herb functions better to clear heat and regulate water circulation. The dry-fried herb has enhanced effectiveness to tonify the Spleen and relieve diarrhea.

CAUTIONS / CONTRAINDICATIONS

- Use *Yi Yi Ren* with caution in patients with spermatorrhea and polyuria.
- *Yi Yi Ren* is contraindicated during pregnancy.

CHEMICAL COMPOSITION

Coixol, coixenolide, coixan A, B, C; protein, lipids.[1]

PHARMACOLOGICAL EFFECTS

- **Antineoplastic**: Alcohol extract of *Yi Yi Ren* is associated with mild antineoplastic action according to some *in vitro* studies.[2]
- **Effects on muscles**: Administration of essential oil of *Yi Yi Ren* is associated with an inhibitory effect on the skeletal muscle, a stimulating effect on the smooth muscle of the uterus, and varied effects on the smooth muscle of the intestines.[3]
- **Sedative, analgesic and antipyretic** properties have been observed, in relatively mild degrees.[4]

CLINICAL STUDIES AND RESEARCH

- **Flat Warts**: In one study, patients with flat warts were treated with 60 grams of *Yi Yi Ren* taken daily as food, for 7 to 16 days. Out of 23 patients, 11 showed complete recovery, 6 showed mild improvement, and 6 showed no response.[5]

SUPPLEMENT

- 薏苡根 / 薏苡根 *Yi Yi Gen* (Radix Coicis), first cited in the *Shen Nong Ben Cao Jing* (Divine Husbandman's Classic of the Materia Medica) in the second century, is derived from the same plant as *Yi Yi Ren* (Semen Coicis). Bitter, sweet and cold, *Yi Yi Gen* clears heat and dispels dampness. Clinical applications include *re lin* (heat dysuria), *xue lin* (bloody dysuria), edema and lung abscesses. It also dispels roundworms. Suggested dosage for *Yi Yi Gen* is 10 to 15 grams. When using this herb in the fresh form, the dosage is 30 to 60 grams. *Yi Yi Gen* is contraindicated during pregnancy.

AUTHORS' COMMENTS

Yi Yi Ren is one of the most helpful herbs for treatment of acne. It is combined with *Qing Shang Fang Feng Tang* (Clear the Upper and Guard the Wind Decoction) to treat acne with whiteheads. It is used with *Huang Lian Shang Qing Wan* (Coptis Pills to Clear the Upper) to treat acne pustules that are red and inflamed.

According to Dr. Yin Hui-He, when treating patients with Large Intestine disorders that manifest in pus or blood in the stools, accompanied by feelings of incomplete evacuation after defecation, herbs such as *Yi Yi Ren* (Semen Coicis), *Tao Ren* (Semen Persicae), *Dong Gua Zi* (Semen Benincasae) and *Huang Qin* (Radix Scutellariae) are useful. They enter the Lung, the paired organ of the Large Intestine, and drain dampness. This principle can also be applied when treating inflammatory bowel disorders.

References

1. *Xian Dai Zhong Yao Yao Li Xue* (Contemporary Pharmacology of Chinese Herbs), 1997; 542
2. *Zhong Yao Xue* (Chinese Herbology), 1998; 337-339
3. Ibid.
4. Ibid.
5. *Zhong Hua Pi Fu Ke Xue Za Zhi* (Chinese Journal of Dermatology), 1959; 1:34

Che Qian Zi (Semen Plantaginis)

車前子 车前子

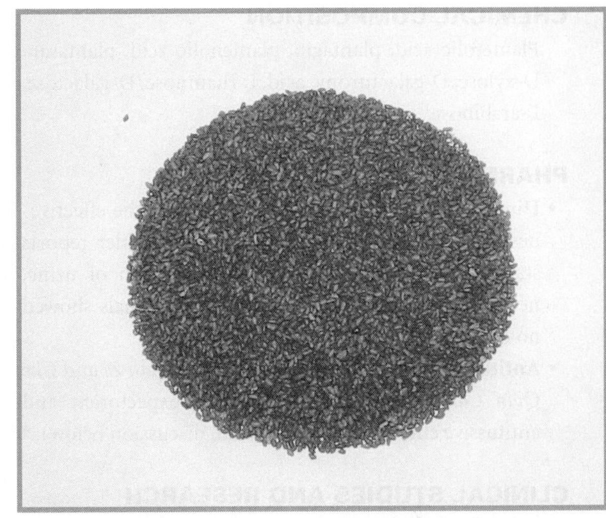

Pinyin Name: *Che Qian Zi*
Literal Name: "seed in front of cart," "seed-before-cart," "before the cart seeds"
Original Source: *Shen Nong Ben Cao Jing* (Divine Husbandman's Classic of the Materia Medica) in the second century
English Name: plantago seed, asiatic plantain seed, plantain seed
Botanical Name: *Plantago asiatica* L. (*Che Qian*); *Plantago depressa* Willd (*Ping Che Qian*)
Pharmaceutical Name: Semen Plantaginis
Properties: sweet, cold
Channels Entered: Kidney, Urinary Bladder, Liver, Lung

CHINESE THERAPEUTIC ACTIONS

1. Clears Damp-Heat and Resolves Dampness

***Lin zheng* (dysuria syndrome) and edema:** Sweet and cold, *Che Qian Zi* (Semen Plantaginis) dispels damp-heat from the lower *jiao*. It treats edema and *re lin* (heat dysuria). Clinical manifestations include: burning dysuria, urgency with inability to urinate, painful urination, and dribbling urination with pain and swelling.

- *Shi-re lin* (damp-heat dysuria): use *Che Qian Zi* with *Chuan Mu Tong* (Caulis Clematidis Armandii), *Hua Shi* (Talcum) and *Zhi Zi* (Fructus Gardeniae). **Exemplar Formula:** *Ba Zheng San* (Eight-Herb Powder for Rectification).
- Edema: use this herb with *Bai Zhu* (Rhizoma Atractylodis Macrocephalae), *Fu Ling* (Poria) and *Ze Xie* (Rhizoma Alismatis).

2. Resolves Dampness and Stops Diarrhea

Dampness accumulation in the intestines causing diarrhea: *Che Qian Zi* consolidates and hardens the stool by promoting urination. It is usually used alone in powder form for this purpose.

- Diarrhea due to summer-damp: use *Che Qian Zi* with *Xiang Ru* (Herba Elsholtziae seu Moslae) and *Huo Xiang* (Herba Agastache).
- Diarrhea with dysuria: use it with *Bai Zhu* (Rhizoma Atractylodis Macrocephalae) and *Fu Ling* (Poria).
- Summer diarrhea in children: combine it with *Dang Shen* (Radix Codonopsis), *Bai Zhu* (Rhizoma Atractylodis Macrocephalae), *Gan Cao* (Radix Glycyrrhizae), *Fu Ling* (Poria) and *Chen Pi* (Pericarpium Citri Reticulatae).

3. Clears Liver Heat and Benefits the Eyes

Eye disorders: *Che Qian Zi* treats eye problems caused by Liver fire, and headaches provoked by Liver yang rising.

- Eye redness, swelling and pain from Liver fire: use this herb with *Huang Lian* (Rhizoma Coptidis), *Jue Ming Zi* (Semen Cassiae), *Man Jing Zi* (Fructus Viticis), *Sang Ye* (Folium Mori), *Mi Meng Hua* (Flos Buddlejae) and *Ju Hua* (Flos Chrysanthemi).
- Headache due to Liver yang rising: combine it with herbs that anchor Liver yang, such as *Shi Jue Ming* (Concha Haliotidis).

Dizziness and blurred vision due to Liver and Kidney deficiencies: *Che Qian Zi* supports healing of deficiency-induced eye disorders.

- Dizziness and blurred vision: add *Shu Di Huang* (Radix Rehmanniae Preparata), *Shi Hu* (Herba Dendrobii), *Gou Qi Zi* (Fructus Lycii) and *Tu Si Zi* (Semen Cuscutae).

4. Clears the Lung and Dissolves Phlegm

Cough due to Lung heat: *Che Qian Zi* treats cough with thick yellow sputum caused by Lung heat.

- Cough from Lung heat: use it with *Huang Qin* (Radix Scutellariae), *Yu Xing Cao* (Herba Houttuyniae), and *Bei Mu* (Bulbus Fritillaria).
- Lung yin deficiency cough: add *Mai Men Dong* (Radix Ophiopogonis) and *Nan Sha Shen* (Radix Adenophorae).

DOSAGE

5 to 10 grams. Place *Che Qian Zi* in cheesecloth when decocting to maximize cooking efficiency (this prevents the seeds from floating to the top and sides of the cooking pot). Frying the herb with salt directs the effects to the lower parts of the body, thus enhancing its tonic influence on the Liver and Kidney. In addition, frying with salt facilitates and increases extraction of active components.

Che Qian Zi (Semen Plantaginis)

CHEMICAL COMPOSITION

Planterolic acid, plantagin, plantenolic acid, plantasan, D-xylose, D-galacturonic acid, L-rhamnose, D-galactose, L-arabinose.[1]

PHARMACOLOGICAL EFFECTS

- **Diuretic:** There are conflicting reports on the effectiveness of *Che Qian Zi* as a diuretic. While older reports stated that the herb may increase excretion of urine, newer reports on healthy humans and animals showed no diuretic effect.[2,3]
- **Antitussive and expectorant:** Both *Che Qian Zi* and *Che Qian Cao* (Herba Plantaginis) have expectorant and antitussive effects (see supplemental discussion below).[4]

CLINICAL STUDIES AND RESEARCH

- **Infantile diarrhea**: In one study, 63 of 69 infants with diarrhea showed complete recovery within 1 to 2 days following treatment using an herbal decoction containing 30 grams of *Che Qian Zi* and a small amount of sugar.[5]

HERB-DRUG INTERACTION

- **Absorption:** *Che Qian Zi* may reduce the absorption of oral medications, such as lithium.[6] It may also inhibit the absorption of carbohydrates, thus requiring the adjustment of insulin dosage in diabetic patients.[7]
- **Diuretics:** Although no documented cases of this interaction have been reported, it is prudent to avoid combination of herbs and drugs that exert diuretic effects, as there may be additive or synergistic effects. Combination therapy may lead to excessive loss of fluids and electrolytes. [Note: Examples of diuretics include chlorothiazide, hydrochlorothiazide, furosemide (Lasix), bumetanide (Bumex), and torsemide (Demadex).][8]

TOXICOLOGY

No abnormalities were noted following oral administration of *Che Qian Zi* in rats at 2 to 3 g/kg for 28 days and in dogs at 3 to 5 g/kg for 3 weeks.[9]

SUPPLEMENT

- 車前草 / 车前草 *Che Qian Cao* (Herba Plantaginis), first cited in *Shen Nong Ben Cao Jing* (Divine Husbandman's Classic of the Materia Medica) in the second century, is the entire plant that produces the seeds called *Che Qian Zi*. *Che Qian Cao* is sweet, cold and enters the Liver, Kidney, Lung, and Small Intestine channels. It has functions similar to those of *Che Qian Zi* to dispel water, clear heat, brighten the eyes, dispel phlegm and stop coughing. Clinical applications of *Che Qian Cao* include edema, *lin zheng* (dysuria syndrome), redness and swelling of the eyes, and Lung heat with cough. It is most effective for ulcers or acute diarrhea or dysentery caused by toxic heat. Recommended dosage for *Che Qian Cao* is 10 to 15 grams. When using the fresh form, double the dosage. *Che Qian Cao* is also used as a topical substance to treat ulcers and sores.

  Che Qian Cao has been used to effectively treat bacterial dysentery. According to one report, 88 patients with acute or chronic bacterial dysentery were treated with an herbal decoction, with 71.6% showing complete recovery and a total of 84% showing marked improvement. The herbal decoction contained 100% fresh *Che Qian Cao*. Patients were instructed to take 60 to 120 ml per dose, three times daily (or every 4 hours), for 7 to 10 days. Some patients received up to 200 ml per dose and some were treated for up to one month.[10]

AUTHORS' COMMENTS

There are many species of plantago within the family of Plantaginaceae. In traditional Chinese medicine, *Plantago depressa* and *Plantago asiatica* are the two commonly-used species, for they are widely available on the Asian continent. Beyond the Asian continent, *Plantago psyllium* and *Plantago arenaria* can be found in Spain, and *Plantago ovata* is found in southern Europe and northern Africa. According to the literature, all species of plantago have similar functions and indications and can be used interchangeably. Therapeutic effects include diuresis, promotion of regular bowel movement, and antibacterial and antifungal effects.

References

1. *Xian Dai Zhong Yao Yao Li Xue* (Contemporary Pharmacology of Chinese Herbs), 1997; 546
2. *Zhong Yao Da Ci Dien* (Dictionary of Chinese Herbs), 1975: 403
3. *Zhong Yao Xue* (Chinese Herbology), 1998; 340:341
4. Ibid.
5. *Zhong Xi Yi Jie He Za Zhi* (Journal of Integrated Chinese and Western Medicine), 1987; 11:697
6. Brinker, Francis. *Herb Contraindications and Drug Interactions*, 1997; 74-75
7. Wichtl, M. *Herbal Drugs and Phytopharmaceuticals*, 1994
8. Chen, J. Recognition & prevention of herb-drug interactions, *Medical Acupuncture*, Fall/Winter 1998/1999; volume 10/number 2; 9-13
9. *Zhong Yao Da Ci Dien* (Dictionary of Chinese Herbs), 1975: 401
10. *Zhong Hua Nei Ke Za Zhi* (Chinese Journal of Internal Medicine), 1960; 4:351

Hua Shi (Talcum)

滑石 滑石

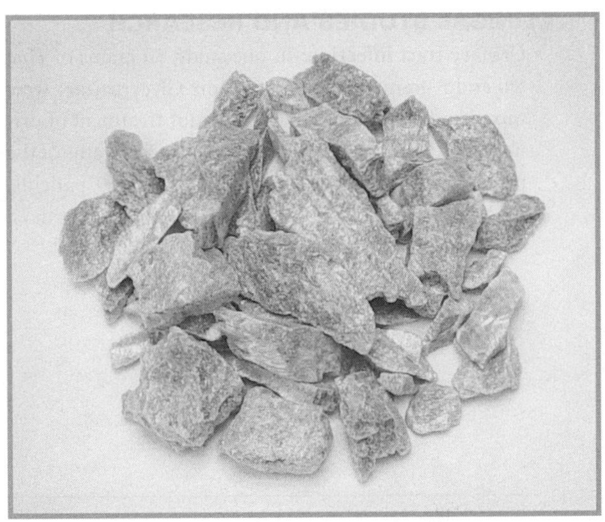

Pinyin Name: *Hua Shi*
Literal Name: "slippery rock"
Alternate Chinese Names: *Fei Hua Shi*
Original Source: *Shen Nong Ben Cao Jing* (Divine Husbandman's Classic of the Materia Medica) in the second century
English Name: talc
Pharmaceutical Name: Talcum
Properties: sweet, bland, cold
Channels Entered: Stomach, Urinary Bladder

CHINESE THERAPEUTIC ACTIONS

1. Clears Heat and Resolves Dampness

***Lin zheng* (dysuria syndrome):** Cold in nature, *Hua Shi* (Talcum) enters the Urinary Bladder channel to clear heat and promote normal diuresis. It is one of the most commonly used herbs in treatment of various *lin zheng*.

- *Re lin* (heat dysuria) with burning and pain during urination: combine *Hua Shi* with *Chuan Mu Tong* (Caulis Clematidis Armandii). **Exemplar Formula:** *Ba Zheng San* (Eight-Herb Powder for Rectification).
- *Shi-re lin* (damp-heat dysuria) with pain and cloudy urine: add *Che Qian Zi* (Semen Plantaginis), *Zhi Zi* (Fructus Gardeniae) and *Chuan Mu Tong* (Caulis Clematidis Armandii).
- *Shi lin* (stone dysuria): use it with *Jin Qian Cao* (Herba Lysimachiae), *Hai Jin Sha* (Herba Lygodii) and *Shi Wei* (Folium Pyrrosiae).
- *Xue lin* (bloody dysuria): combine it with *Da Ji* (Herba seu Radix Cirsii Japonici), *Ce Bai Ye* (Cacumen Platycladi), and *Bai Mao Gen* (Rhizoma Imperatae).

2. Clears Summer-Heat

Hua Shi clears summer-heat to treat irritability, thirst, dysuria and watery diarrhea.

- Summer-heat: combine *Hua Shi* with *Gan Cao* (Radix Glycyrrhizae) at a six-to-one ratio. **Exemplar Formula:** *Liu Yi San* (Six-to-One Powder).
- Heatstroke with vomiting and diarrhea: use *Hua Shi* with *Huo Xiang* (Herba Agastache), *Pei Lan* (Herba Eupatorii), *Zhu Ru* (Caulis Bambusae in Taenia) and *Ban Xia* (Rhizoma Pinelliae).
- Damp febrile disorder obstructing the *qi* (energy) level with unremitting fever, heavy sensations of the body and limbs, poor appetite, listlessness with thick, greasy coating and slippery pulse: add *Huang Qin* (Radix Scutellariae) and *Tong Cao* (Medulla Tetrapanacis).

3. Topical Use to Clear Heat and Dry Dampness

Dermatological disorders: Clinical applications include eczema, rash, athlete's foot, sudamen, and other damp skin disorders.

- Dermatological disorders: use *Hua Shi* with *Duan Shi Gao* (Gypsum Fibrosum Preparata). Apply as powder, topically.

DOSAGE

10 to 15 grams. *Hua Shi* should be wrapped in cheesecloth for decoction.

CAUTIONS / CONTRAINDICATIONS

- Use care when giving *Hua Shi* to patients who have Spleen deficiency, spermatorrhea, polyuria and/or febrile disorders with consequent consumption of body fluids.

CHEMICAL COMPOSITION

$Mg_3(Si_4O_{10})(OH)_2$ [1]

PHARMACOLOGICAL EFFECTS

- **Effects on skin and mucous membranes:** *Hua Shi* has small particles and a large surface area. Applied externally, *Hua Shi* absorbs large amounts of chemicals and toxins to protect the skin from irritation. Taken internally, *Hua Shi* protects the stomach lining from gastritis, suppresses nausea and vomiting, and reduces the absorption of toxins through the intestinal tract.[2]

Hua Shi (Talcum)

CLINICAL STUDIES AND RESEARCH

- **Urinary tract infection:** In one study, 30 grams of *Hua Shi* and 5 grams of *Gan Cao* (Radix Glycyrrhizae) were mixed and ground into fine powder for treatment of urinary tract infections. Patients were given 5.8 grams of the powder with warm water twice daily. Of 10 patients, most experienced complete recovery within 3 to 4 days, although some required up to 6 days of treatment.[3]

TOXICOLOGY

Hua Shi increases the incidence of granulomas in the abdomen, rectum and vagina. When used topically in the vagina as a contraceptive, *Hua Shi* increases the risk of uterine fibroids by three-fold.[4]

References

1. *Xian Dai Zhong Yao Yao Li Xue* (Contemporary Pharmacology of Chinese Herbs), 1997; 596
2. *Zhong Yao Xue* (Chinese Herbology), 1998; 341:343
3. *Liao Ning Yi Yao* (Liaoning Medicine and Herbology), 1976; (2):69
4. *Zhong Yao Xue* (Chinese Herbology), 1998; 341:343

Chuan Mu Tong (Caulis Clematidis Armandii)

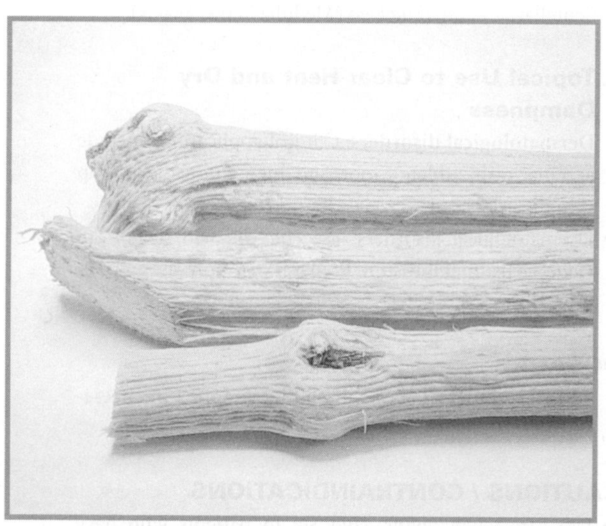

川木通

Pinyin Name: *Chuan Mu Tong*
Literal Name: "open-ended wood from Sichuan"
Alternate Chinese Names: *Mu Tong*
Original Source: *Shen Nong Ben Cao Jing* (Divine Husbandman's Classic of the Materia Medica) in the second century
English Name: clematis, armand clematis stem, anemone clematis stem
Botanical Name: *Clematis armandii* Franch. (*Xiao Mu Tong*); *Clematis montana* Buch.-Ham. (*Xiu Chiu Teng*)
Pharmaceutical Name: Caulis Clematidis Armandii
Properties: bitter, cold
Channels Entered: Urinary Bladder, Heart, Small Intestine
Safety Index: Safe

CHINESE THERAPEUTIC ACTIONS

1. Promotes Urination

***Lin zheng* (dysuria syndrome):** *Chuan Mu Tong* (Caulis Clematidis Armandii) is commonly used to treat dysuria characterized by burning sensations and pain during urination, indicating an accumulation of damp-heat in the Urinary Bladder.

- *Shi-re lin* (damp-heat dysuria): combine *Chuan Mu Tong* with *Che Qian Zi* (Semen Plantaginis), *Zhi Zi* (Fructus Gardeniae), *Hua Shi* (Talcum), and *Da Huang* (Radix et Rhizoma Rhei).
- *Xue lin* (bloody dysuria): add *Pu Huang* (Pollen Typhae) and *Ou Jie* (Nodus Nelumbinis Rhizomatis) to *Chuan Mu Tong.*
- *Shi lin* (stone dysuria): use it with *Jin Qian Cao* (Herba Lysimachiae) and *Hai Jin Sha* (Herba Lygodii).

2. Sedates Heart and Small Intestine Fire

Heart fire: *Chuan Mu Tong* treats ulcerations of the tongue and mouth, irritability, and burning urination caused by heat in the Heart and Small Intestine channels (paired organs in *zang fu* relationship).

- Heat or fire in the Heart and Small Intestine: add *Sheng Di Huang* (Radix Rehmanniae), *Zhu Ye* (Herba Phyllostachys), *Gan Cao* (Radix Glycyrrhizae), *Deng Xin Cao* (Medulla Junci) and *Zhi Zi* (Fructus Gardeniae).

Chuan Mu Tong (Caulis Clematidis Armandii)

3. Opens Channels to Relieve Pain

Chuan Mu Tong is used as a single-herb remedy to relieve pain or *bi zheng* (painful obstruction syndrome) with blood stagnation in the channels.

4. Promotes Lactation

Insufficient lactation: *Chuan Mu Tong* is often cooked with pig's feet and soy sauce and served as a food to promote lactation in nursing mothers.

- To promote secretion of breast milk: use this herb with *Chuan Shan Jia* (Squama Manis) and *Wang Bu Liu Xing* (Semen Vaccariae).

DOSAGE

3 to 6 grams in decoction.

CHEMICAL COMPOSITION

Climontanoside B.[1]

PHARMACOLOGICAL EFFECTS

- **Diuretic:** Oral ingestion or intravenous injection of a decoction of *Chuan Mu Tong* creates marked diuretic results in rabbits.[2]

CLINICAL STUDIES AND RESEARCH

- ***Bi zheng* (painful obstruction syndrome):** Four patients with chronic numbness and pain were treated with a decoction of *Chuan Mu Tong* and experienced relief from pain within four doses. The decoction was prepared by cooking 50 to 75 grams of *Chuan Mu Tong* in water to yield 50 to 100 ml of tea. The patients were given 25 to 30 ml of decoction per dose, two to three times daily.[3]
- ***Lin zheng* (dysuria syndrome):** According to one report, 58 patients with *lin zheng* were treated with great success using an herbal formula containing *Chuan Mu Tong* 20g, *Huang Qin* (Radix Scutellariae) 20g, *Che Qian Zi* (Semen Plantaginis) 20g, *Long Dan Cao* (Radix Gentianae) 15g, *Dang Gui* (Radicis Angelicae Sinensis) 15g, *Chai Hu* (Radix Bupleuri) 15g, *Ze Xie* (Rhizoma Alismatis) 15g, *Zhi Zi* (Fructus Gardeniae) 15g, *Sheng Di Huang* (Radix Rehmanniae) 25g, and *Gan Cao* (Radix Glycyrrhizae) 5g.[4]

SUPPLEMENT

"*Mu Tong*" may be derived from the following plants: clematis and akebia.

- 川木通 *Chuan Mu Tong* (Caulis Clematidis Armandii): *Clematis armandii* and *Clematis montana* are known as "*Chuan Mu Tong*," and are the most common botanical sources of "*Mu Tong*." They originate from the Sichuan and Guizhou areas. *Chuan Mu Tong* is now used as the preferred source of "*Mu Tong*."
- 五葉木通 / 五叶木通 *Wu Ye Mu Tong* (Caulis Akebia Quinata) is not used frequently. The botanical name is *Akebia quinata* (Thunb.) Decue.
- 三葉木通 / 三叶木通 *San Ye Mu Tong* (Caulis Akebia Trifoliata) is also not used frequently. The botanical name is *Akebia trifoliata* (Thunb.) Koidz.
- 白木通 *Bai Mu Tong* (Caulis Akebia Trifoliata Australis) is also not used frequently. The botanical name is *Akebia trifoliata* (Thunb.) Koidz. var. *australis* (Diels) Rehd.

AUTHORS' COMMENTS

Chuan Mu Tong and *Ze Xie* (Rhizoma Alismatis) both have diuretic action. *Chuan Mu Tong* more effectively dispels heat in the Heart and Small Intestine, whereas *Ze Xie* (Rhizoma Alismatis) more strongly clears damp-heat from the Liver and Kidney channels.

According to Dr. Wang Shi-Xiang, when treating *bi zheng* (painful obstruction syndrome), the use of *Chuan Mu Tong* (Caulis Clematidis Armandii) may cause nausea and vomiting. *Gan Cao* (Radix Glycyrrhizae) and *Chen Pi* (Pericarpium Citri Reticulatae) are added to counter these side effects.

Chuan Mu Tong (Caulis Clematidis Armandii), *Mai Men Dong* (Radix Ophiopogonis), *Huang Lian* (Rhizoma Coptidis), and *Tian Zhu Huang* (Concretio Silicea Bambusae) all clear the Heart and eliminate irritability.

- *Chuan Mu Tong* is a diuretic that clears damp-heat to relieve irritability with oral ulcers and yellow urine.
- *Mai Men Dong* is a tonic used for deficient Heart yin with heat that manifests as irritability and insomnia.
- *Huang Lian* is used for febrile disease with excess fire in the Heart disturbing *shen* (spirit), thus manifesting in irritability and insomnia.
- *Tian Zhu Huang* dissolves hot phlegm and is best for irritability with spasms and convulsions.

References

1. *Int. J. Crude Drugs Res*, 1990; 28(1):39
2. *Chang Yong Zhong Yao Xian Dai Yan Jiu Yu Lin Chuan* (Recent Study & Clinical Application of Common Traditional Chinese Medicine), 1995; 267:269
3. *Liao Ning Zhong Yi Za Zhi* (Liaoning Journal of Chinese Medicine), 1977; (1); 18
4. *Ji Lin Zhong Yi Yao* (Jilin Chinese Medicine and Herbology), 1991; (2):12

Guan Mu Tong (Caulis Aristolochiae Manshuriensis)

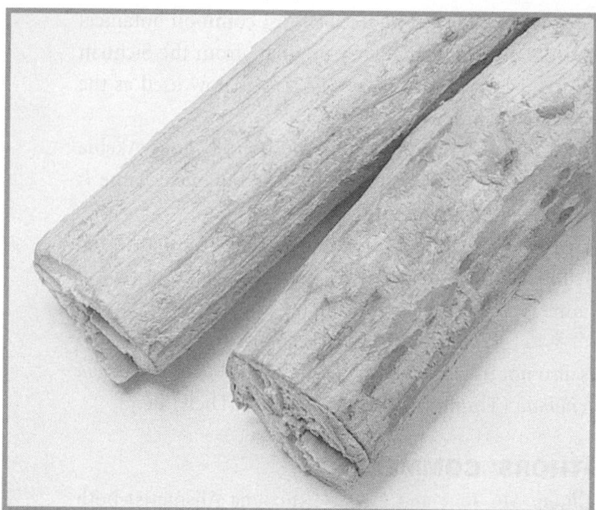

關木通 关木通

Pinyin Name: *Guan Mu Tong*
Literal Name: "open-ended wood from Guan"
Alternate Chinese Names: *Dong Bei Ma Dou Ling*
Original Source: *Shen Nong Ben Cao Jing* (Divine Husbandman's Classic of the Materia Medica) in the second century
English Name: aristolochia stem, Manchurian dutchman's pipe stem
Botanical Name: *Aristolochia manshuriensis* Kom. (*Dong Bei Ma Dou Ling; Guan Mu Tong*)
Pharmaceutical Name: Caulis Aristolochiae Manshuriensis
Properties: bitter, cold
Channels Entered: Urinary Bladder, Heart, Small Intestine
Safety Index: toxic

CHINESE THERAPEUTIC ACTIONS

1. Promotes Urination

***Lin zheng* (dysuria syndrome):** *Guan Mu Tong* (Caulis Aristolochiae Manshuriensis) has historically been used to treat dysuria, particularly the accumulation of damp-heat in the Urinary Bladder, characterized by a burning sensation and pain during urination.

- *Lin zheng* due to damp-heat: this herb was combined with *Che Qian Zi* (Semen Plantaginis), *Zhi Zi* (Fructus Gardeniae), *Hua Shi* (Talcum), and *Da Huang* (Radix et Rhizoma Rhei).
- *Xue lin* (bloody dysuria): used with *Pu Huang* (Pollen Typhae) and *Ou Jie* (Nodus Nelumbinis Rhizomatis).
- *Shi lin* (stone dysuria): combined with *Jin Qian Cao* (Herba Lysimachiae) and *Hai Jin Sha* (Herba Lygodii).

2. Sedates Heart and Small Intestine Fire

Heart fire: *Guan Mu Tong* has been used to treat ulcerations of the mouth and tongue, irritability and burning urination caused by heat in the Heart and Small Intestine, *zang fu* partners.

- Heat in the Heart and Small Intestine: used with *Sheng Di Huang* (Radix Rehmanniae), *Zhu Ye* (Herba Phyllostachys), *Gan Cao* (Radix Glycyrrhizae), *Deng Xin Cao* (Medulla Junci) and *Zhi Zi* (Fructus Gardeniae).

DOSAGE

3 to 6 grams in decoction.

CAUTIONS / CONTRAINDICATIONS

- *Guan Mu Tong* is contraindicated during pregnancy, and in cases of compromised kidney function.
- Do not use *Guan Mu Tong* in large doses, or for prolonged periods of time.

OVERDOSAGE

Overdose of *Guan Mu Tong* may cause upper abdominal discomfort, nausea, vomiting, diarrhea, abdominal distention, poor appetite, headache, chest congestion, facial edema, palpitations, frequent urination, low back pain, edema of the entire body, dysuria, anuria, increased blood pressure, hematuria, delirium, proteinuria, cylindruria, increased protein nitrogen in blood and urine, and hyperkalemia. In severe cases, overdose of *Guan Mu Tong* (over 60 grams) has been associated with nephropathy.[1,2]

CHEMICAL COMPOSITION

Aristolochic acid A, D; aristoloside, magnoflorine, β-sitosterol, oleanolic acid, hederagenin, sodium, potassium, chloride, iron, zinc, copper.[3,4]

COOH, NO_2, OCH_3

Aristolochic Acid

PHARMACOLOGICAL EFFECTS

- **Diuretic:** Oral ingestion of *Guan Mu Tong* in rats demonstrates marked diuretic influence, increasing

Guan Mu Tong (Caulis Aristolochiae Manshuriensis)

elimination of water, sodium, potassium and chloride.[5]

- **Cardiovascular:** Intravenous injection stimulates the cardiac muscle of frog specimens, increasing the contractile force of the heart.[6]
- **Antibiotic**: Aristolochic acid tablets (0.15 mg per tablet) are commercially available for treatment of infection. The recommended dose for treatment of infection is 1 to 2 tablets three times daily.[7]

CLINICAL STUDIES AND RESEARCH

- **Urinary stones**: In one study, 132 patients with urinary tract stones were treated with an herbal formula, with a 76.3% success rate in passing the stones. Time required to pass the stones varied from 6 to 73 days. The herbal formula contained *Guan Mu Tong*, *Qu Mai* (Herba Dianthi), *Bian Xu* (Herba Polygoni Avicularis), *Che Qian Zi* (Semen Plantaginis), *Hua Shi* (Talcum), *Zhi Zi* (Fructus Gardeniae), *Jin Qian Cao* (Herba Lysimachiae), *Hai Jin Sha* (Herba Lygodii), and *Ji Nei Jin* (Endothelium Corneum Gigeriae Galli).[8]
- **Urinary stones**: In another study, 215 patients with urinary stones were treated with an herbal decoction on a daily basis, with 127 patients successfully (58.9%) passing the stones. The herbal formula included *Guan Mu Tong*, *Qu Mai* (Herba Dianthi), *Zhi Zi* (Fructus Gardeniae), *Jin Qian Cao* (Herba Lysimachiae), *Ji Nei Jin* (Endothelium Corneum Gigeriae Galli), *Hu Po* (Succinum), *Sheng Di Huang* (Radix Rehmanniae), *Huai Niu Xi* (Radix Achyranthis Bidentatae), *Huang Bai* (Cortex Phellodendri), *Hai Jin Sha* (Herba Lygodii) and *Gan Cao* (Radix Glycyrrhizae).[9]

SUPPLEMENT

- 關木通 / 关木通 *Guan Mu Tong* (Caulis Aristolochiae Manshuriensis), 大葉馬兜鈴 / 大叶马兜铃 *Da Ye Ma Dou Ling* (Caulis Aristolochia Kaempferi), and 淮通馬兜鈴 / 淮通马兜铃 *Huai Tong Ma Dou Ling* (Caulis Aristolochia Moupinensis) are sometimes used.

The use of aristolochia types of "*Mu Tong*" is strongly discouraged because of toxicity associated with aristolochic acid.[10,11]

AUTHORS' COMMENTS

It is wise to be able to discern various types of "*Mu Tong*." Visual inspection shows that *Guan Mu Tong* (Caulis Aristolochiae Manshuriensis), the undesirable species, is long and round, approximately 1 – 2 meters in length by 1 – 6 centimeters in diameter. The outer layer is grayish-yellow or light brown in color. It has enlarged joints in-between parts of the plant and a distinct camphor-like odor. By contrast, *Chuan Mu Tong* (Caulis Clematidis Armandii) or *Chuan Mu Tong* (Caulis Clematidis Montana) is long and round, 50 to 100 cm in length, and 2 to 3.5 cm in diameter. The outer layer is light to dark yellow/brown in color. It has no joints and no odor.[12]

References

1. *Zhe Jiang Zhong Yi Za Zhi* (Zhejiang Journal of Chinese Medicine), 1965; 12:32
2. Lord GM, Tagore R, Cook T, Gower P, Pusey CD. Nephropathy caused by Chinese herbs in the UK. *The Lancet* August 7, 1999; 354:481-482,494
3. *Zhong Cao Yao* (Chinese Herbal Medicine), 1986; 17(8):11
4. *The Merck Index* 12th edition, Chapman & Hall/CRCnetBASE/Merck, 2000
5. *Zhong Hua Yi Xue Za Zhi* (Chinese Journal of Medicine), 1961; 47(1):7
6. *Yao Xue Xue Bao* (Journal of Herbology), 1956; 4(3):175
7. Huang, Kee Chang, *The Pharmacology of Chinese Herbs, 2nd edition*, CRC Press, 1999, 80-81
8. *Hei Long Jiang Zhong Yi Yao* (Heilongjiang Chinese Medicine and Herbology), 1991; 5:30
9. *Hu Nan Zhong Yi Za Zhi* (Hunan Journal of Chinese Medicine), 1987; 3(2):8
10. Goshi T, ed. *Pharmacopoeia of the People's Republic of China* 1992; 16-17 and 304-05
11. Zheng HZ, Dong ZH et al. *Modern Study of Chinese Medicine.* October 1997.vol 1. 936:954
12. Ibid.

Tong Cao (Medulla Tetrapanacis)

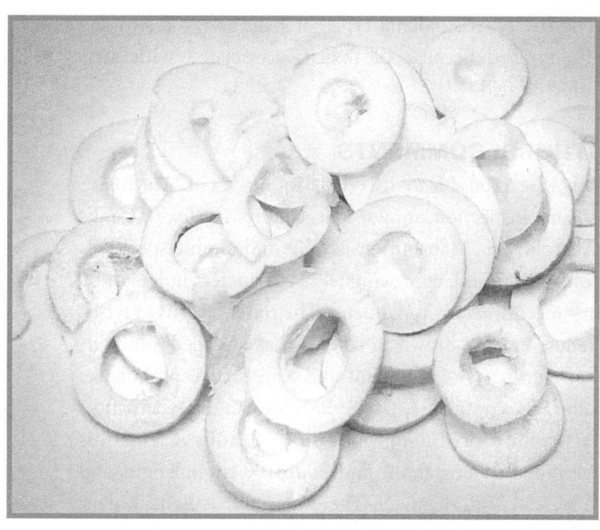

通草 通草

Pinyin Name: *Tong Cao*
Literal Name: "unblocking herb"
Original Source: *Ben Cao Shi Yi* (Omissions from the [Classic of the] Materia Medica) by Chen Cang-Qi in 741 A.D.
English Name: tetrapanax, rice paper plant pith
Botanical Name: *Tetrapanax papyriferus* (Hook.) K. Koch (*Tong Tuo Mu*)
Pharmaceutical Name: Medulla Tetrapanacis
Properties: sweet, bland, cool
Channels Entered: Lung, Stomach

CHINESE THERAPEUTIC ACTIONS

1. Promotes Urination and Resolves Dampness

Tong Cao (Medulla Tetrapanacis) treats *lin zheng* (dysuria syndrome) by promoting urination and resolving dampness. Clinical manifestations include painful and/or dribbling urination with heat sensations.

- Dysuria and pain caused by damp-heat in the Urinary Bladder: add *Tong Cao* to *Shi Wei* (Folium Pyrrosiae) and *Qu Mai* (Herba Dianthi).
- Painful urination, turbid cloudy urine, and heaviness of the body due to damp-heat: use *Tong Cao* with *Bai Dou Kou* (Fructus Amomi Rotundus), *Hua Shi* (Talcum) and *Yi Yi Ren* (Semen Coicis).
- Edema with dysuria: combine it with *Fen Fang Ji* (Radix Stephaniae Tetandrae), *Fu Ling* (Poria), *Zhu Ling* (Polyporus), and *Da Fu Pi* (Pericarpium Arecae).
- Damp febrile disorders with sensations of heaviness of the body, the absence of thirst, oppression in the chest, afternoon fever and dysuria: add *Yi Yi Ren* (Semen Coicis), *Hua Shi* (Talcum), *Ban Xia* (Rhizoma Pinelliae), *Hou Po* (Cortex Magnoliae Officinalis) and *Bai Dou Kou* (Fructus Amomi Rotundus).

2. Promotes Lactation

Tong Cao promotes secretion of breast milk in nursing mothers.

- To promote lactation, combine *Tong Cao* in decoction with *Chuan Shan Jia* (Squama Manis) and *Wang Bu Liu Xing* (Semen Vaccariae).

DOSAGE

2 to 5 grams. Use 15 to 18 grams of *Tong Cao* when the intent is to promote lactation.

CAUTIONS / CONTRAINDICATIONS

- Use of *Tong Cao* is not recommended for pregnant women.

CHEMICAL COMPOSITION

Uronic acid, galactose, galacturonic acid, glucose, xylose, lipid 1.70%, protein 1.10%, fiber 48.73%, total ash content 5.95%.[1]

PHARMACOLOGICAL EFFECTS

- **Diuretic:** Administration of *Tong Cao* is associated with an increase in excretion of water, sodium, chloride and potassium in rats.[2]

HERB-DRUG INTERACTION

- **Diuretics:** *Tong Cao* has a diuretic effect. Though this potential interaction has not been documented, concurrent use with diuretic drugs may lead to increased elimination of water and/or electrolytes.[3] [Note: Examples of diuretics include chlorothiazide, hydrochlorothiazide, furosemide (Lasix), bumetanide (Bumex), and torsemide (Demadex).]

SUPPLEMENT

- 梗通草 / 梗通草 *Geng Tong Cao* (Ramulus Aeschynomene Indica), first cited in *Ben Cao Zheng Yi* (Truth and False Information of Materia Medica) by Zhang Shan-Lei in 1920, has functions, and properties similar to those of *Tong Cao*. *Geng Tong Cao* promotes diuresis, treats *lin zheng* (dysuria syndrome) and promotes lactation. Recommended dosage of *Geng Tong Cao* is 3 to 6 grams.

AUTHORS' COMMENTS

Tong Cao and *Chuan Mu Tong* (Caulis Clematidis Armandii) both promote lactation. However, *Tong Cao* is

Tong Cao (Medulla Tetrapanacis)

sweet and is often preferred over *Chuan Mu Tong*, which is bitter. Other foods commonly used with or without *Tong Cao* and/or *Chuan Mu Tong* to promote lactation include pig's feet, fish, peanuts and papaya.

References

1. *Chang Yong Zhong Yao Cheng Fen Yu Yao Li Shou Ce* (A Handbook of the Composition and Pharmacology of Common Chinese Drugs), 1994; 1560-1561
2. *Zhong Yao Cai* (Study of Chinese Herbal Material), 1991; 14(9):40
3. Chen, J. Recognition & prevention of herb-drug interactions, *Medical Acupuncture*, Fall/Winter 1998/1999; volume 10/number 2; 9-13

Deng Xin Cao (Medulla Junci)

燈心草 灯心草

Pinyin Name: *Deng Xin Cao*
Literal Name: "lamp wick herb"
Alternate Chinese Names: *Deng Xin, Deng Cao*
Original Source: *Kai Bao Ben Cao* (Materia Medica of the Kai Bao Era) by Ma Zhi in 973-974 A.D.
English Name: juncus, rush
Botanical Name: *Juncus offusus* L. var. *decipiens* Buchen. (*Deng Xin Cao*)
Pharmaceutical Name: Medulla Junci
Properties: sweet, bland, cool
Channels Entered: Heart, Lung, Small Intestine

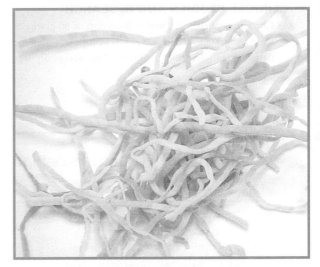

CHINESE THERAPEUTIC ACTIONS

1. Promotes Urination to Treat *Lin Zheng* (Dysuria Syndrome)

***Re lin* (heat dysuria)**: Because it is cool, *Deng Xin Cao* (Medulla Junci) effectively treats urinary disorders arising from accumulated damp and heat in the lower *jiao*. Its diuretic effect, however, is relatively mild and must be supplemented with other herbs for maximum effect. *Deng Xin Cao* also promotes urination and treats generalized edema or edema from nephritis.

- Dysuria: add this herb to *Dan Zhu Ye* (Herba Lophatheri) and *Che Qian Cao* (Herba Plantaginis).
- Generalized edema: use a large dose of *Deng Xin Cao*.
- Edema due to nephritis: combine it with *Che Qian Cao* (Herba Plantaginis) and *Bai Mao Gen* (Rhizoma Imperatae).

2. Clears Heart Heat and Sedates Fire

***Shen* (spirit) disturbance:** *Deng Xin Cao* clears Heart fire and treats related symptoms. Clinical applications include insomnia, irritability, and infantile crying at night.

- Insomnia and irritability: combine this herb with *Zhu Sha* (Cinnabaris), *Suan Zao Ren* (Semen Zizyphi Spinosae) and *Fu Shen* (Poria Paradicis).
- Infantile crying at night: add *Suan Zao Ren* (Semen Zizyphi Spinosae), *Xiao Mai* (Fructus Tritici) and *Fu Shen* (Poria Paradicis).

3. Clears Lung Heat

Throat inflammation: *Deng Xin Cao* treats sore throat caused by heat in the Lung. Use charred *Deng Xin Cao* either internally or topically to relieve pain.

- Apply the powdered herb topically: administer by conveying the powder through the mouth (such as by pouring or blowing through a straw) to apply directly to the mucous membranes of the throat.

4. Cools Blood, Stops Bleeding

Charred *Deng Xin Cao* cools blood and stops bleeding.

Deng Xin Cao (Medulla Junci)

DOSAGE

1.5 to 2.5 grams in decoction or pills. Unprocessed *Deng Xin Cao* clears heat and regulates water circulation. The charred herb cools blood and stops bleeding.

CAUTIONS / CONTRAINDICATIONS

- Use of *Deng Xin Cao* is contraindicated for patients with deficiency and cold in the middle *jiao*, or in cases of urinary incontinence.

CHEMICAL COMPOSITION

Araban, xylan, methyl pentosan, luteolin, luteolin-7-glucoside, tripeptide, effusol.[1]

CLINICAL STUDIES AND RESEARCH

- **Chronic nephritis:** An herbal decoction of 60 grams of fresh *Deng Xin Cao* and 300 grams of tofu was used for patients with chronic nephritis. The decoction was administered once daily for 30 days per course of treatment. A one-week rest was given before continuing, if more than one course was necessary. Out of 30 patients, the study reported complete recovery in 16 cases, significant improvement in 8 cases, slight improvement in 2 cases, and no response in 4 cases.[2]

AUTHORS' COMMENTS

Deng Xin Cao and *Zhu Ye* (Herba Phyllostachys) both clear Heart fire and promote diuresis. *Deng Xin Cao* is better for *lin zheng* (dysuria syndrome) with burning and painful urination. *Zhu Ye* more effectively sedates Heart fire to treat irritability and insomnia.

References

1. *Xian Dai Zhong Yao Yao Li Xue* (Contemporary Pharmacology of Chinese Herbs), 1997; 581
2. *Fu Zhou Yi Yao* (Fuzhou Medicine and Medicinals), 1983; (3):30

Di Fu Zi (Fructus Kochiae)

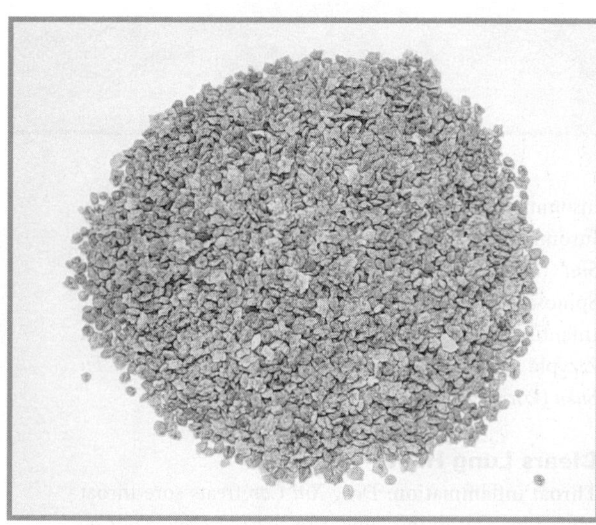

地膚子 地肤子

Pinyin Name: *Di Fu Zi*
Literal Name: "earth skin seed"
Alternate Chinese Names: *Luo Sao Zi, Di Kui, Di Mai*
Original Source: *Shen Nong Ben Cao Jing* (Divine Husbandman's Classic of the Materia Medica) in the second century
English Name: kochia, belvedere fruit, broom cypress fruit
Botanical Name: *Kochia scoparia* (L.) schrad. (*Di Fu*)
Pharmaceutical Name: Fructus Kochiae
Properties: sweet, bitter, cold
Channels Entered: Urinary Bladder, Kidney

CHINESE THERAPEUTIC ACTIONS

1. Clears Damp-Heat and Promotes Urination

***Lin zheng* (dysuria syndrome)**: *Di Fu Zi* (Fructus Kochiae) clears damp-heat and promotes urination. It is commonly used to treat *shi-re lin* (damp-heat dysuria) with burning, scanty, dark urine.

- *Shi-re lin* (damp-heat dysuria): use *Di Fu Zi* with *Che Qian Zi* (Semen Plantaginis), *Hua Shi* (Talcum) and *Chuan Mu Tong* (Caulis Clematidis Armandii).
- Urinary tract infection during pregnancy: use *Di Fu Zi* alone.
- Urinary tract infection or bladder infection: combine it with *Zhu Ling* (Polyporus), *Che Qian Zi* (Semen Plantaginis), *Tong Cao* (Medulla Tetrapanacis) and *Gan Cao* (Radix Glycyrrhizae).

Di Fu Zi (Fructus Kochiae)

2. Dispels Dampness to Relieve Itching

Di Fu Zi dispels dampness from the skin to relieve the itching and inflammation of eczema, scabies, urticaria, and other dermatological disorders. It also effectively treats genital itching. It is commonly used internally or topically as a powder or wash.

- Itching: use this herb with *Bai Xian Pi* (Cortex Dictamni), *Ku Shen Gen* (Radix Sophorae Flavescentis) and *She Chuang Zi* (Fructus Cnidii). Apply topically in powdered form.
- Eczema: combine it with *Mu Dan Pi* (Cortex Moutan), *Bai Xian Pi* (Cortex Dictamni), *Huang Bai* (Cortex Phellodendri) and *Jin Yin Hua* (Flos Lonicerae), in decoction.
- Urticaria with redness and itching: combine it with *Jin Yin Hua* (Flos Lonicerae), *Fang Feng* (Radix Saposhnikoviae), *Bo He* (Herba Menthae), *Ju Hua* (Flos Chrysanthemi) and *Huang Bai* (Cortex Phellodendri) for internal use.
- Eye redness and pain: use *Di Fu Zi* as a tea with *Jue Ming Zi* (Semen Cassiae), *Qing Xiang Zi* (Semen Celosiae) and *Gu Jing Cao* (Flos Eriocauli).

DOSAGE

10 to 15 grams.

CHEMICAL COMPOSITION

Oleanolic acid, ecdysteroid, triterpenoid saponins, alkaloids.[1]

PHARMACOLOGICAL EFFECTS

- **Antibiotic:** Water extract of *Di Fu Zi* has an inhibitory effect *in vitro* on some dermatophytes and pathogenic fungi.[2]

References

1. *Xian Dai Zhong Yao Yao Li Xue* (Contemporary Pharmacology of Chinese Herbs), 1997; 577
2. *Yun Nan Zhong Yao Zhi* (Yunan Journal of Chinese Herbal Medicine), 1990; 244

Bian Xu (Herba Polygoni Avicularis)

萹蓄

Pinyin Name: *Bian Xu*
Alternate Chinese Names: *Bian Zhu, Dao Sheng Cao, Niu Bian Cao*
Original Source: *Shen Nong Ben Cao Jing* (Divine Husbandman's Classic of the Materia Medica) in the second century
English Name: common knotgrass herb
Botanical Name: *Polygonum aviculare* L. (*Bian Xu*)
Pharmaceutical Name: Herba Polygoni Avicularis
Properties: bitter, cool
Channels Entered: Urinary Bladder

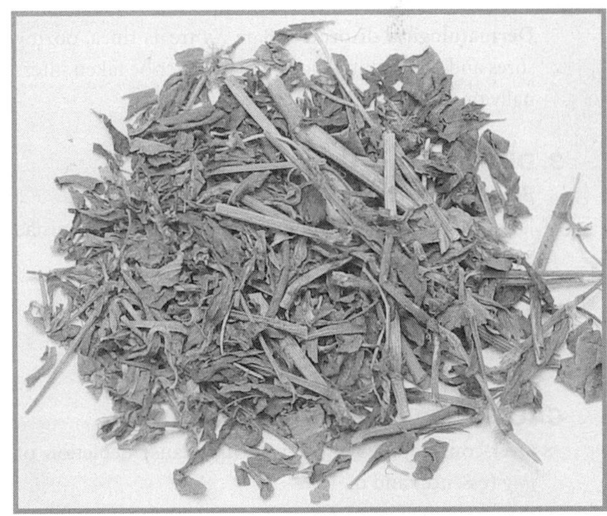

CHINESE THERAPEUTIC ACTIONS

1. Promotes Diuresis

***Lin zheng* (dysuria syndrome)**: *Bian Xu* (Herba Polygoni Avicularis) dispels damp-heat and promotes urination. It is commonly used to treat *re lin* (heat dysuria) with burning and pain. It also is effective in treating urethral calculi.

- *Shi-re lin* (damp-heat dysuria) with burning sensations and pain during urination: use *Bian Xu* with *Chuan Mu Tong* (Caulis Clematidis Armandii), *Che Qian Zi* (Semen Plantaginis), *Zhi Zi* (Fructus Gardeniae) and *Hua Shi* (Talcum). **Exemplar Formula:** *Ba Zheng San* (Eight-Herb Powder for Rectification).
- *Xue lin* (bloody dysuria) with hematuria: use this herb

Bian Xu (Herba Polygoni Avicularis)

with *Xiao Ji* (Herba Cirisii), *Pu Huang* (Pollen Typhae) and *Bai Mao Gen* (Rhizoma Imperatae).
- *Shi lin* (stone dysuria) with kidney stones: use it with *Jin Qian Cao* (Herba Lysimachiae) and *Hai Jin Sha* (Herba Lygodii).

Jaundice: *Bian Xu* treats jaundice caused by the accumulation of damp-heat in the Liver and Gallbladder.
- Jaundice: use this herb with *Da Huang* (Radix et Rhizoma Rhei), *Yin Chen Hao* (Herba Artemisiae Scopariae) and *Zhi Zi* (Fructus Gardeniae).

2. Kills Parasites

Parasites: *Bian Xu* kills parasites, especially roundworm and hookworm.
- Parasites: use the vinegar-fried form of *Bian Xu* with *Shi Jun Zi* (Fructus Quisqualis), *Wu Mei* (Fructus Mume) and *Hua Jiao* (Pericarpium Zanthoxyli).
- Anal itching caused by parasites: use *Bian Xu* decoction as a topical wash.
- Genital itching: use it with *Di Fu Zi* (Fructus Kochiae) and *Ku Shen Gen* (Radix Sophorae Flavescentis) topically as a powder or wash.
- Eczema: combine it with *Cang Zhu* (Rhizoma Atractylodis), *Huang Bai* (Cortex Phellodendri), *Bai Xian Pi* (Cortex Dictamni) and *Ku Shen Gen* (Radix Sophorae Flavescentis).

Dermatological disorders: *Bian Xu* treats tinea, oozing sores and damp skin lesions. It can either be taken internally or applied topically.

3. Dispels Damp-Heat

Bian Xu treats jaundice caused by damp-heat.
- Jaundice: use it with *Yin Chen Hao* (Herba Artemisiae Scopariae) and *Zhi Zi* (Fructus Gardeniae).

DOSAGE

10 to 15 grams.

CAUTIONS / CONTRAINDICATIONS

- Over-consumption of *Bian Xu* may cause depletion of *jing* (essence) and qi.

CHEMICAL COMPOSITION

Avicularin, quercitrin, d-catechol, gallic acid, caffeic acid, oxalic acid, silicic acid, cholorogenic acid, p-coumaric acid.[1]

PHARMACOLOGICAL EFFECTS

- **Diuretic:** Decoction of *Bian Xu* at 20 g/kg increased the excretion of water, sodium and potassium in rats.[2]
- **Antibiotic:** Decoction of *Bian Xu* has an inhibitory influence on *Bacillus dysenteriae*, *Staphylococcus aureus*, and *Pseudomonas aeruginosa*.[3]
- **Antihypertensive:** Intravenous injection of water or alcohol extracts of *Bian Xu* lowered blood pressure in dogs, rabbits, and cats. The antihypertensive effect is attributed to increased urine output.[4]

CLINICAL STUDIES AND RESEARCH

- **Acute bacterial dysentery:** An herbal syrup of *Bian Xu* containing 1 g/ml of the herb was used to treat patients with acute bacterial dysentery; 50 ml of the syrup was administered two to three times daily. Out of 108 patients, there was complete recovery in 104 cases and moderate improvement in 4 cases. The average was one day for reduction of body temperature, four days for relief of abdominal pain, and five days for return of normal bowel movement. No adverse reaction was reported during the treatment period. In a follow-up evaluation of 36 patients between 1 and 12 months after treatment, there were only 2 cases of recurrence.[5]
- **Toothache:** A decoction of 50 to 100 grams of *Bian Xu* given in two equally-divided doses effectively treated toothache. Of 81 patients, 80 reported relief of pain within 2 to 3 days after the treatment.[6]

HERB-DRUG INTERACTION

- **Diuretics:** *Bian Xu* has a diuretic effect. Though this potential interaction has not been documented, concurrent use with diuretic drugs may lead to increased elimination of water and/or electrolytes.[7] [Note: Examples of diuretics include chlorothiazide, hydrochlorothiazide, furosemide (Lasix), bumetanide (Bumex), and torsemide (Demadex).]

TOXICOLOGY

Bian Xu may cause dermatitis or gastrointestinal disturbance when used as food for horses and sheep.[8]

References

1. *Xian Dai Zhong Yao Yao Li Xue* (Contemporary Pharmacology of Chinese Herbs), 1997; 556
2. *Chang Yong Zhong Yao Cheng Fen Yu Yao Li Shou Ce* (A Handbook of the Composition and Pharmacology of Common Chinese Drugs), 1994; 1665:1667
3. *Yi Xue Xue Bao* (Report of Medicine), 1983; 18(9):700
4. *Chang Yong Zhong Yao Cheng Fen Yu Yao Li Shou Ce* (A Handbook of the Composition and Pharmacology of Common Chinese Drugs), 1994; 1665:1667
5. *Zhong Cao Yao Tong Xun* (Journal of Chinese Herbal Medicine), 1972; 2:24
6. *Shan Xi Zhong Yi* (Shanxi Chinese Medicine), 1986; 1:28
7. Chen, J. Recognition & prevention of herb-drug interactions, *Medical Acupuncture*, Fall/Winter 1998/1999; volume 10/number 2; 9-13
8. *Zhong Yao Yao Li Xue* (Study of Chinese Herbology), 1986; 127

Qu Mai (Herba Dianthi)

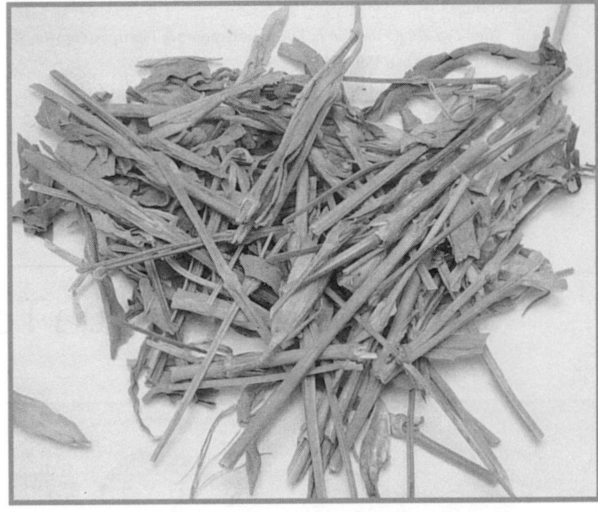

瞿麥 瞿麦

Pinyin Name: *Qu Mai*
Alternate Chinese Names: *Ju Mai*
Original Source: *Shen Nong Ben Cao Jing* (Divine Husbandman's Classic of the Materia Medica) in the second century
English Name: dianthus, lilac pink, Chinese pink, rainbow pink
Botanical Name: *Dianthus superbus* L. (*Qu Mai*); *Dianthus chinensis* L. (*Shi Zhu*)
Pharmaceutical Name: Herba Dianthi
Properties: bitter, cold
Channels Entered: Urinary Bladder, Heart, Small Intestine

CHINESE THERAPEUTIC ACTIONS

1. Promotes Diuresis

***Lin zheng* (dysuria syndrome):** *Qu Mai* (Herba Dianthi) regulates water circulation and is one of the most commonly used herbs to treat *shi-re lin* (damp-heat dysuria). The tip of *Qu Mai* has the strongest diuretic action compared to the stem and body.

- *Re lin* (heat dysuria) with burning and pain during urination: use *Qu Mai* with *Che Qian Zi* (Semen Plantaginis) and *Hua Shi* (Talcum). **Exemplar Formula:** *Ba Zheng San* (Eight-Herb Powder for Rectification).
- *Xue lin* (bloody dysuria) with hematuria: combine this herb with *Xiao Ji* (Herba Cirisii), *Pu Huang* (Pollen Typhae) and *Bai Mao Gen* (Rhizoma Imperatae).
- *Shi lin* (stone dysuria): add *Jin Qian Cao* (Herba Lysimachiae), *Ji Nei Jin* (Endothelium Corneum Gigeriae Galli) and *Hai Jin Sha* (Herba Lygodii).

2. Invigorates Blood Circulation and Regulates Menstruation

Amenorrhea: *Qu Mai* enters the *xue* (blood) level to clear heat. It helps amenorrhea, or menstrual cramps due to blood clots.

- Amenorrhea: use it with *Dan Shen* (Radix Salviae Miltiorrhizae), *Chi Shao* (Radix Paeoniae Rubrae) and *Yi Mu Cao* (Herba Leonuri).
- Blood clots: combine it with *Tao Ren* (Semen Persicae), *Chuan Xiong* (Rhizoma Ligustici Chuanxiong), *Hong Hua* (Flos Carthami) and *Niu Xi* (Radix Cyathulae seu Achyranthis).

Difficult Labor: *Qu Mai* invigorates blood circulation and is used to induce or further the progress of labor.

DOSAGE

5 to 10 grams.

CAUTIONS / CONTRAINDICATIONS

- Use of *Qu Mai* is contraindicated in pregnant women, as it stimulates contraction of the uterus.

CHEMICAL COMPOSITION

Eugenol, phenyethylalcohol, methylsalicylate, homorientin, dianthus saponin, gyposgenin.[1]

PHARMACOLOGICAL EFFECTS

- **Diuretic:** Water decoction of *Qu Mai* at 2 g/kg increased the excretion of water and chloride in rabbits.[2]
- **Uterine stimulant:** Alcohol extract of *Qu Mai* has a stimulating effect on the uterus in anesthetized rabbits, leading to uterine contraction.[3]
- **Others:** It also has a stimulating effect on the gastrointestinal system and an inhibitory effect on the cardiovascular system.[4]

CLINICAL STUDIES AND RESEARCH

- **Edema:** An herbal tea prepared by soaking 100 grams of *Qu Mai* in a sealed bottle of hot water for 60 minutes was used to treat patients with edema. The study reported satisfactory results in over 100 cases.[5]

HERB-DRUG INTERACTION

- **Diuretics:** *Qu Mai* has a diuretic effect. Though this potential interaction has not been documented, concurrent use with diuretic drugs may lead to increased elimination of water and/or electrolytes.[6] [Note: Examples of diuretics include chlorothiazide, hydrochlorothiazide, furosemide (Lasix), bumetanide (Bumex), and torsemide (Demadex).]

Qu Mai (Herba Dianthi)

References
1. *Xian Dai Zhong Yao Yao Li Xue* (Contemporary Pharmacology of Chinese Herbs), 1997; 558
2. *Zhong Yao Xue* (Chinese Herbology), 1998; 353:354
3. *Tian Jing Yi Yao* (Tianjing Medicine and Herbology), 1983; (5):268
4. *Zhong Yao Xue* (Chinese Herbology), 1998; 353:354
5. *Xiang Cun Yi Xue* (Suburban Medicine), 1996; 11:34
6. Chen, J. Recognition & prevention of herb-drug interactions, *Medical Acupuncture*, Fall/Winter 1998/1999; volume 10/number 2; 9-13

Bai Long Chuan Hua Tou (Radix Clerodendron Paniculatum)

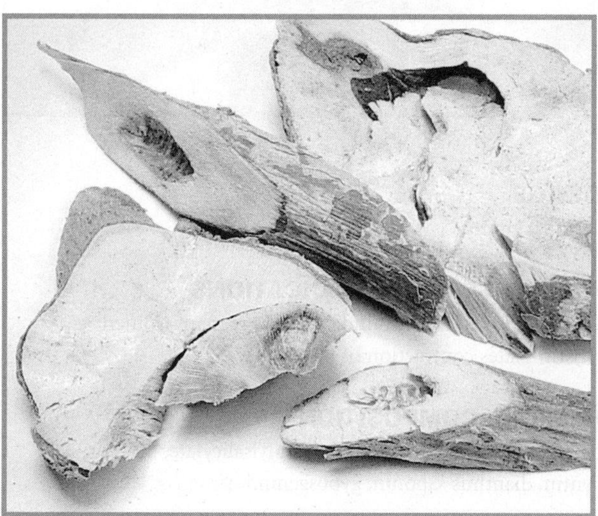

白龍船花頭
白龙船花头

Pinyin Name: *Bai Long Chuan Hua Tou*
Alternate Chinese Names: *Long Chuan Hua, Bai Long Chuan Tou, Bai Long Chuan Gen*
Original Source: *Tai Wan Min Jian Yao* (Folk Medicine of Taiwan) by Gao Mu-Chun in 1985
English Name: clerodendron, scarlet glory bower
Botanical Name: *Clerodendron paniculatum* L. (*Bai Long Chuan*)
Pharmaceutical Name: Radix Clerodendron Paniculatum
Properties: slightly bitter, warm
Channels Entered: Lung, Liver, Kidney

CHINESE THERAPEUTIC ACTIONS

1. Regulates Menstruation and Resolves Vaginal Discharge

Bai Long Chuan Hua Tou (Radix Clerodendron Paniculatum) treats gynecological disorders by regulating menstruation.

- White vaginal discharge: use this herb with *Ma Chi Xian* (Herba Portulacae), *Ji Guan Hua* (Flos Celosiae Cristatae) and *Long Yan Hua* (Flos Longan).
- Yellow vaginal discharge, with or without blood: combine it with *Huang Bai* (Cortex Phellodendri) and *Long Dan Cao* (Radix Gentianae).
- Irregular menstruation caused by blood stagnation and water retention: add *Rou Dou Gen* (Radix Myristicae) and *Yi Mu Cao* (Herba Leonuri) to *Bai Long Chuan Hua Tou*.

2. Dispels Wind and Dampness

- *Bi zheng* (painful obstruction syndrome) caused by wind-dampness: use *Bai Long Chuan Hua Tou* with *Gui Zhi* (Ramulus Cinnamomi), *Huang Qin* (Radix Scutellariae), *Huang Bai* (Cortex Phellodendri), *Chi Fu Ling* (Poria Rubrae) and *Cang Zhu* (Rhizoma Atractylodis).

3. Regulates Qi and Promotes Urination

Bai Long Chuan Hua Tou controls frequent urination in patients with diabetes mellitus.

- Diabetes with polyuria caused by Kidney yin deficiency: add this herb to the formula *Liu Wei Di Huang Wan* (Six-Ingredient Pill with Rehmannia).
- Diabetes with polyuria from Kidney yang deficiency: combine it with the classic formula *Ba Wei Di Huang Wan* (Eight-Ingredient Pill with Rehmannia).

DOSAGE

3 to 12 grams in decoction.

Ding Shu Xiu (Herba Elephantopus Scaber)

丁豎杇 丁竖杇

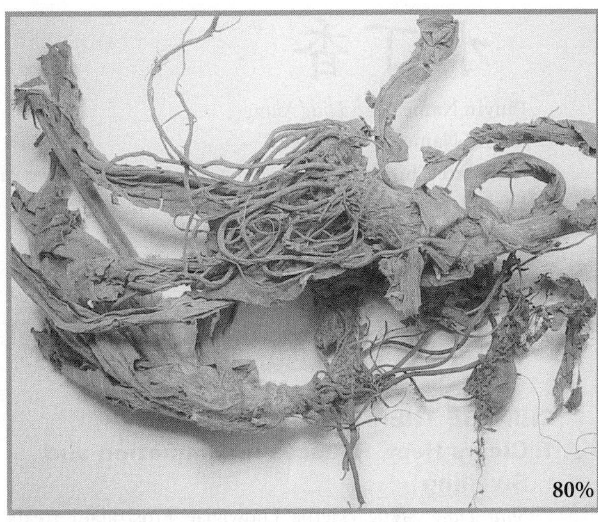
80%

Pinyin Name: *Ding Shu Xiu*
Alternate Chinese Names: *Xi Ben Deng Shu Xiu, Hong Shu Xiu, Tian Jie Cai, Ku Di Dan*
English Name: elephantopi
Botanical Name: *Elephantopus scaber* L.
Pharmaceutical Name: Herba Elephantopus Scaber
Properties: sweet, bitter, cold
Channels Entered: Liver, Kidney, Large Intestine

CHINESE THERAPEUTIC ACTIONS

1. Promotes Urination and Reduces Swelling

Water accumulation: *Ding Shu Xiu* (Herba Elephantopus Scaber) is often used for generalized edema, edema of the face and limbs, leg *qi*, and swelling as seen in patients with nephritis and hydronephrosis.

- Nephritis: use *Ding Shu Xiu* with *Shui Ding Xiang* (Herba Ludwigiae Prostratae), *Bian Xu* (Herba Polygoni Avicularis), *Qu Mai* (Herba Dianthi), *Hua Shi* (Talcum), *Gan Cao* (Radix Glycyrrhizae), *Chuan Mu Tong* (Caulis Clematidis Armandii) and *Yu Mi Xu* (Stigma Maydis).
- Edema: combine it with *Mo Gu Xiao* (Caulis Hyptis Capitatae), *Bian Xu* (Herba Polygoni Avicularis), *Qu Mai* (Herba Dianthi), *Yi Yi Ren* (Semen Coicis), *Huang Qi* (Radix Astragali), *Fen Fang Ji* (Radix Stephaniae Tetandrae) and *Yu Mi Xu* (Stigma Maydis).
- Gout: use it with *Wan Dian Jin* (Radix Ilicis Asprellae), *Shui Ding Xiang* (Herba Ludwigiae Prostratae) and *Shan Pu Tao* (Radix Vitis Amurensis).

2. Clears Heat and Eliminates Toxins

Ding Shu Xiu addresses various kinds of painful swelling, *chang feng* (intestinal wind) with bleeding from the rectum during or before a bowel movement, and hemorrhoidal bleeding.

- Bleeding hemorrhoids: use this herb with *Feng Wei Cao* (Herba Pteris).

3. Relieves Pain

- Headache or migraine headache: use *Ding Shu Xiu* with *Ma Bian Cao* (Herba Verbenae), *Hu Zhang* (Rhizoma Polygoni Cuspidati), *Chuan Xiong* (Rhizoma Ligustici Chuanxiong), *Bai Zhi* (Radix Angelicae Dahuricae), *Chai Hu* (Radix Bupleuri) and *Gan Cao* (Radix Glycyrrhizae).

DOSAGE

6 to 15 grams in decoction.

Shui Ding Xiang (Herba Ludwigiae Prostratae)

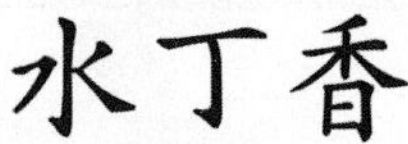

Pinyin Name: *Shui Ding Xiang*
Literal Name: "water clove"
Alternate Chinese Names: *Shui Xiang Liao, Shui Deng Xiang*
English Name: ludwigia, climbing seed box
Botanical Name: *Ludwigia prostrata* Roxb.
Pharmaceutical Name: Herba Ludwigiae Prostratae
Properties: sweet, bland, very cold
Channels Entered: Kidney, Urinary Bladder

CHINESE THERAPEUTIC ACTIONS

1. Clears Heat, Reduces Inflammation and Swelling

Shui Ding Xiang (Herba Ludwigiae Prostratae) treats sore throat, dysentery and toothache by clearing heat and reducing inflammation.

- Sore throat: use *Shui Ding Xiang* with *Yi Zhi Xiang* (Herba Vernoniae Cinereae), *Shu Wei Huang* (Herba Rostellulariae), *Ban Lan Gen* (Radix Isatidis), *Jin Yin Hua* (Flos Lonicerae), and *Da Qing Ye* (Folium Isatidis).
- Dysentery: combine it with *Feng Wei Cao* (Herba Pteris), *Ge Gen* (Radix Puerariae), *Huang Qin* (Radix Scutellariae), *Huang Lian* (Rhizoma Coptidis), *Mu Xiang* (Radix Aucklandiae), *Bing Lang* (Semen Arecae) and *Bai Shao* (Radix Paeoniae Alba).
- Toothache: use *Shui Ding Xiang* with *Shi Gao* (Gypsum Fibrosum), *Zhi Mu* (Radix Anemarrhenae) and *Xi Xin* (Herba Asari). The herbs may be taken orally as a decoction, or applied as a topical paste to the affected area.

2. Promotes Urination

Shui Ding Xiang treats disorders characterized by accumulation of water and heat. Clinical applications include infection of the genitourinary system, and hypertension.

- Chronic nephritis, cystitis and urinary tract infection: use it with *Ze Xie* (Rhizoma Alismatis), *Pao Zai Cao* (Herba Physalis Angulatae) and *Ya She Huang* (Herba Lippiae).
- *Lin zheng* (dysuria syndrome), hematuria, or hematochezia: combine it with *Tong Cao* (Medulla Tetrapanacis), *Bian Xu* (Herba Polygoni Avicularis) and *Da Ji* (Herba seu Radix Cirsii Japonici).
- Itching of the skin with redness and swelling: use *Shui Ding Xiang* topically or internally with *Hu Yao Huang* (Herba Leucas Mollissimae), *Shu Wei Huang* (Herba Rostellulariae) and *Xian Feng Cao* (Herba Bidentis).
- Hypertension: combine this herb with *Hu Zhang* (Rhizoma Polygoni Cuspidati), *Cha Chi Huang* (Herba Stellariae Aquaticae) and *Shan Pu Tao* (Radix Vitis Amurensis).

DOSAGE

6 to 18 grams in decoction

CAUTIONS / CONTRAINDICATIONS

- Use *Shui Ding Xiang* with caution in patients who have deficiency and cold of Spleen and Stomach.
- Use *Shui Ding Xiang* with caution in patients experiencing yin deficiency.

Mo Gu Xiao (Caulis Hyptis Capitatae)

有骨消 有骨消

Pinyin Name: *Mo Gu Xiao*
Alternate Chinese Names: *Mo Gu Xiao Gen, Qi Ye Gen, Mo Gu Gen, Mo Gu Shao*
English Name: hyptis
Botanical Name: *Hyptis capitata; Sambucus formosana* Nakai
Pharmaceutical Name: Caulis Hyptis Capitatae
Properties: bland, cold
Channels Entered: Liver, Kidney

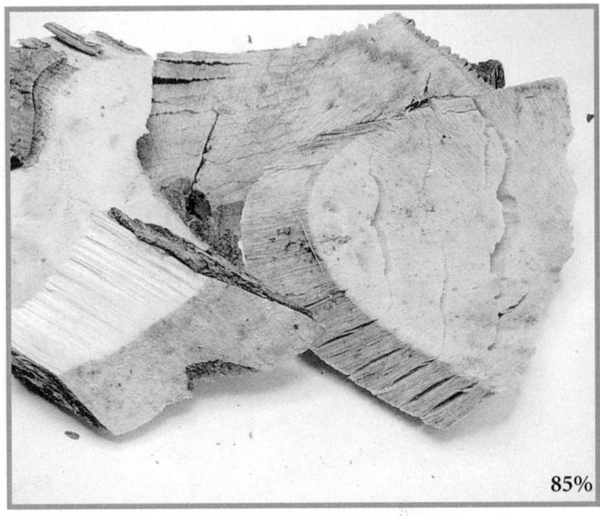
85%

CHINESE THERAPEUTIC ACTIONS

1. Promotes Diuresis, Clears Heat, Reduces Swelling and Inflammation

- Edema resulting from nephritis: use *Mo Gu Xiao* (Caulis Hyptis Capitatae) with *Shui Ding Xiang* (Herba Ludwigiae Prostratae), and *Ding Shu Xiu* (Herba Elephantopus Scaber). If the patient is deficient and cold, use this herb with the formula *Ba Wei Di Huang Wan* (Eight-Ingredient Pill with Rehmannia).
- Renal hypertension: combine it with *Cha Chi Huang* (Herba Stellariae Aquaticae), *Hu Zhang* (Rhizoma Polygoni Cuspidati), *Du Zhong* (Cortex Eucommiae) and *Sang Ji Sheng* (Herba Taxilli).

2. Unblocks Stagnation and Relieves Pain

- *Bi zheng* (painful obstruction syndrome), arthritis, neuralgia, sciatica: add *Huang Jin Gui* (Caulis Vanieriae), *Chuan Shan Long* (Rhizoma Dioscoreae Nipponicae) and *Yi Tiao Gen* (Radix Moghaniae).

3. Drains Abscesses and Promotes Healing and Generation of New Flesh

- Skin lesions and ulceration: apply *Mo Gu Xiao* topically.
- Swelling and abscesses from unknown causes: combine it with *Da Qing Ye* (Folium Isatidis), *Ren Dong Teng* (Caulis Lonicerae), *Xian Feng Cao* (Herba Bidentis) and *Zao Jiao Ci* (Spina Gleditsiae).
- Foot odor: use *Mo Gu Xiao* topically.

DOSAGE

5 to 15 grams in decoction.

CAUTIONS / CONTRAINDICATIONS

- Use *Mo Gu Xiao* carefully for patients with deficiency and cold of the Spleen and Stomach.

AUTHORS' COMMENTS

According to Dr. Chang Wei-Yen, *Mo Gu Xiao* should be used with *Huang Jin Gui* (Caulis Vanieriae) and *Liu Zhi Huang* (Herba Solidaginis) to treat arthritis, neuritis, sciatica and pain along the spine.

Xian Feng Cao (Herba Bidentis)

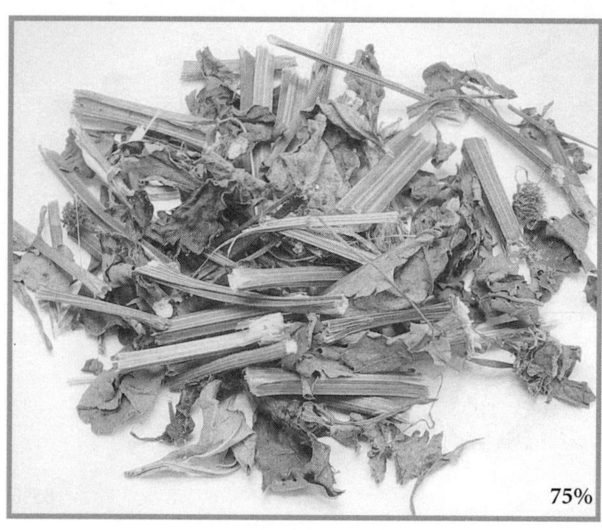
75%

咸豐草 咸丰草

Pinyin Name: *Xian Feng Cao*
Alternate Chinese Names: *Tong Zhi Cao, Bai Hua Puo Puo Zeng, Fu Yin Tou, Han Feng Cao, Nan Feng Cao, Chia Za Bo*
English Name: bidens
Botanical Name: *Bidens pilosa* L. var. *minor* (Bl.) Sherff.
Pharmaceutical Name: Herba Bidentis
Properties: bland, cold
Channels Entered: Kidney, Small Intestine, Urinary Bladder

CHINESE THERAPEUTIC ACTIONS

1. Reduces Inflammation, Clears Heat and Promotes Urination

- Appendicitis: combine *Xian Feng Cao* (Herba Bidentis) with *Da Huang Mu Dan Tang* (Rhubarb and Moutan Decoction).
- Nephritis: use it with *Ding Shu Xiu* (Herba Elephantopus Scaber), *Bian Xu* (Herba Polygoni Avicularis), *Qu Mai* (Herba Dianthi), *Bi Zi Cao* (Herba Pogonantheri Criniti) and *Shui Ding Xiang* (Herba Ludwigiae Prostratae).
- Dysentery: combine it with *Feng Wei Cao* (Herba Pteris), *Ji Xue Cao* (Herba Centellae), *Ge Gen* (Radix Puerariae), *Huang Qin* (Radix Scutellariae) and *Huang Lian* (Rhizoma Coptidis).
- Urinary tract infection or cystitis: use *Xian Feng Cao* with *Yu Xing Cao* (Herba Houttuyniae), *Pao Zai Cao* (Herba Physalis Angulatae), *Ya She Huang* (Herba Lippiae), *Huang Bai* (Cortex Phellodendri), *Che Qian Zi* (Semen Plantaginis) and *Bai Mao Gen* (Rhizoma Imperatae).
- Hepatitis: use this herb with *Bai Jiang Cao* (Herba cum Radice Patriniae), *Hu Zhang* (Rhizoma Polygoni Cuspidati), *Bai Hua She She Cao* (Herba Oldenlandia), *Huang Shui Qie* (Herba Solani), *Ban Lan Gen* (Radix Isatidis) and *Hua Shi Cao* (Herba Orthosiphon Aristatus).
- Diabetes: use *Xian Feng Cao* with *Yu Mi Xu* (Stigma Maydis).

2. Reduces Swelling, Drains Pus and Promotes Generation of Tissues

- Hemorrhoids: use *Xian Feng Cao* with *Zao Jiao Ci* (Spina Gleditsiae). It can also be added to formulas such as *Zhen Ren Huo Ming Yin* (True Man Decoction to Revitalize Life), *Shao Yao Tang* (Peony Decoction), or *Yi Zi Tang* (Yi Word Decoction).
- Toxic swellings: apply *Xian Feng Cao* externally.

DOSAGE

6 to 15 grams in decoction

CAUTIONS / CONTRAINDICATIONS

- Administer *Xian Feng Cao* carefully for patients with deficiency and cold of the Spleen and Stomach.

AUTHORS' COMMENTS

Xian Feng Cao can be used as an iced beverage or tea in summertime to relieve summer-heat.

Bi Zi Cao (Herba Pogonantheri Criniti)

筆仔草 笔仔草

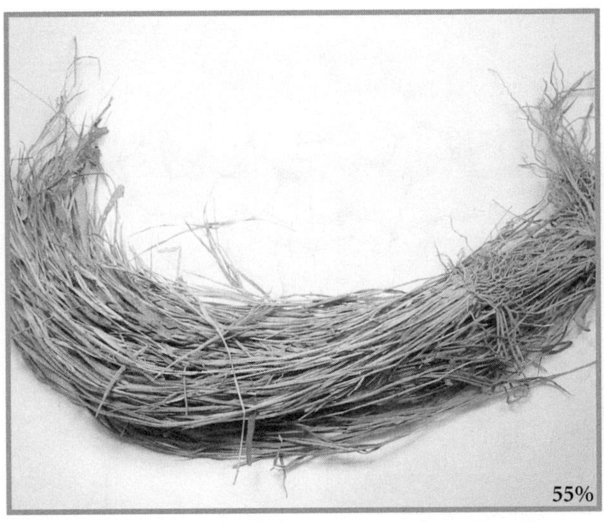
55%

Pinyin Name: *Bi Zi Cao*
Alternate Chinese Names: *Jin Si Cao, Wen Bi Cao, Hong Mao Cao*
English Name: crinite pogonatherum
Botanical Name: *Pogonantherum crinitum* (Thunb.) Kunth
Pharmaceutical Name: Herba Pogonantheri Criniti
Properties: sweet, cool
Channels Entered: Kidney, Urinary Bladder

CHINESE THERAPEUTIC ACTIONS

Clears Heat and Dispels Water

Because of its sweet and cool nature, and entrance to the Kidney and Urinary Bladder channels, *Bi Zi Cao* (Herba Pogonantheri Criniti) treats a wide variety of disorders caused by heat and water retention, such as diabetes, leukorrhea, spermatorrhea, urinary tract infection, cystitis, and nephritis.

- Diabetes with polyuria: use *Bi Zi Cao* with *Bai Guo* (Semen Ginkgo) and *Yu Mi Xu* (Stigma Maydis).
- White leukorrhea: combine it with *Bai Guo* (Semen Ginkgo) and *Ji Guan Hua* (Flos Celosiae Cristatae).
- Turbid urine due to dampness or Kidney yang deficiency: use it with *Hai Jin Sha* (Herba Lygodii), or add it to *Sang Piao Xiao San* (Mantis Egg-Case Powder).
- Urinary tract infection, cystitis, nephritis: use this herb with *Che Qian Cao* (Herba Plantaginis), *Bai Mao Gen* (Rhizoma Imperatae), *Bian Xu* (Herba Polygoni Avicularis) and *Shui Ding Xiang* (Herba Ludwigiae Prostratae).

DOSAGE

5 to 12 grams in decoction.

Dong Gua Zi (Semen Benincasae)

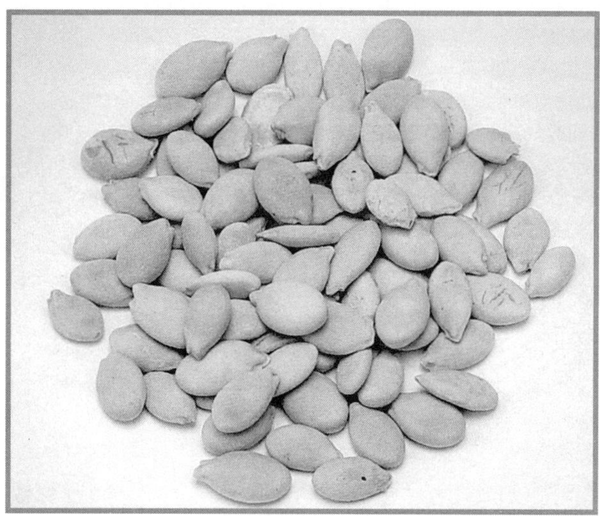

冬瓜子

Pinyin Name: *Dong Gua Zi*
Literal Name: "winter melon seed"
Alternate Chinese Names: *Bai Gua Zi, Dong Gua Ren, Gua Ban, Bai Dong Gua Zi, Gua Zi*
Original Source: *Shen Nong Ben Cao Jing* (Divine Husbandman's Classic of the Materia Medica) in the second century
English Name: benincasa, Chinese wax gourd seed
Botanical Name: *Benincasa hispida* (Thunb.) Cogn. (*Dong Gua*)
Pharmaceutical Name: Semen Benincasae
Properties: sweet, cool
Channels Entered: Lung, Stomach, Small Intestine, Large Intestine

CHINESE THERAPEUTIC ACTIONS

1. Clears Heat, Dissolves Phlegm, and Eliminates Pus

Dong Gua Zi (Semen Benincasae), by virtue of its sweet, cold nature, and access to the Lung, Stomach and Large and Small Intestines, is useful in treating lung and intestinal abscesses. Other applications include cough, edema, phlegm, and bronchitis.

- Lung abscess with foul-smelling sputum: use *Dong Gua Zi* with *Jie Geng* (Radix Platycodonis), *Yu Xing Cao* (Herba Houttuyniae), *Lian Qiao* (Fructus Forsythiae), *Yi Yi Ren* (Semen Coicis), *Jin Yin Hua* (Flos Lonicerae) and *Da Qing Ye* (Folium Isatidis).
- Bronchitis with cough, yellow sputum and sore throat: use it with *Bo He* (Herba Menthae), *Xing Ren* (Semen Armeniacae Amarum), *Qian Hu* (Radix Peucedani), *Niu Bang Zi* (Fructus Arctii) and *She Gan* (Rhizoma Belamcandae).
- Bronchitis with dry cough and possibly scanty blood-streaked sputum: combine it with *Xing Ren* (Semen Armeniacae Amarum), *Ban Xia* (Rhizoma Pinelliae), *Sheng Di Huang* (Radix Rehmanniae), *Nan Sha Shen* (Radix Adenophorae), *Chuan Bei Mu* (Bulbus Fritillariae Cirrhosae), *Ce Bai Ye* (Cacumen Platycladi) and *Qian Cao* (Radix Rubiae).
- Intestinal abscess: use this herb with *Da Huang* (Radix et Rhizoma Rhei) and *Mu Dan Pi* (Cortex Moutan). **Exemplar Formula:** *Da Huang Mu Dan Tang* (Rhubarb and Moutan Decoction).

2. Promotes Diuresis

Edema: *Dong Gua Zi* is a relatively mild herb that treats edema caused by nephritis and dysuria. It should be combined with other herbs to enhance its effectiveness.

- Edema: use this herb with *Fu Ling* (Poria), *Ze Xie* (Rhizoma Alismatis) and *Zhu Ling* (Polyporus).
- Lower body edema with burning sensations and swelling: use it with *Niu Xi* (Radix Cyathulae seu Achyranthis), *Mu Gua* (Fructus Chaenomelis), *Fen Fang Ji* (Radix Stephaniae Tetandrae) and *Yi Yi Ren* (Semen Coicis).
- Summer damp-heat: combine *Dong Gua Zi* with *Pei Lan* (Herba Eupatorii), *Huo Xiang* (Herba Agastache) and *Hua Shi* (Talcum).
- Dysuria: use it with *Hua Shi* (Talcum), *Zhu Ling* (Polyporus) and *Che Qian Zi* (Semen Plantaginis).

DOSAGE

10 to 15 grams. Unprocessed *Dong Gua Zi* has a stronger effect to dissolve phlegm, dispel pus and abscesses, regulate water circulation, and treat edema. Dry-fried *Dong Gua Zi* functions better to warm the Spleen and Stomach, and eliminate dampness. In addition, dry-frying this herb facilitates the extraction of its active components.

CAUTIONS / CONTRAINDICATIONS

- Use *Dong Gua Zi* carefully for patients with diarrhea caused by deficiency and cold of the Spleen and Stomach.

AUTHORS' COMMENTS

According to Dr. Yin Hui-He, when treating patients with Large Intestine disorders that manifest in pus or blood in the stools, accompanied by feelings of incomplete evacuation after defecation, the practitioner can combine *Dong Gua Zi* (Semen Benincasae) with *Yi Yi Ren* (Semen Coicis), *Tao Ren* (Semen Persicae), and *Huang Qin* (Radix Scutellariae). This combination enters the Lung, the paired organ of the Large Intestine, and drains dampness. This principle, of treating the Lung to influence the Large Intestine, can also be applied when treating inflammatory bowel disorders.

Shan Pu Tao (Radix Vitis Amurensis)

山葡萄 山葡萄

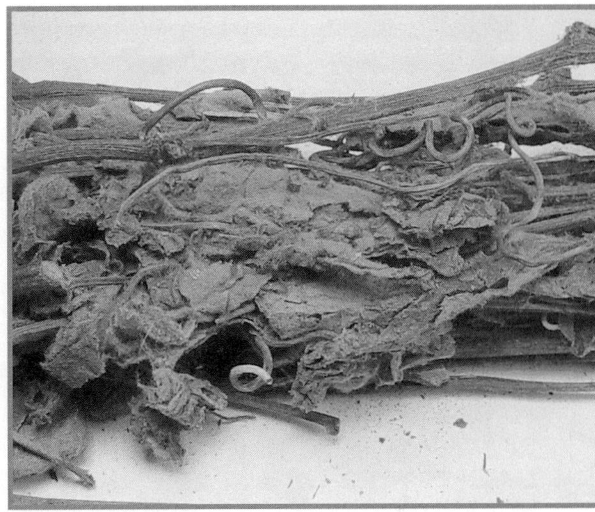

Pinyin Name: *Shan Pu Tao*
Literal Name: "mountain grape"
Alternate Chinese Names: *Xiao Pu Tao, Xiao Ben Shan Pu Tao, Shan Teng Teng Yang*
English Name: viticis
Botanical Name: *Vitis amurensis, Vitis adstricta*
Pharmaceutical Name: Radix Vitis Amurensis
Properties: sweet, cold
Channels Entered: Lung, Liver, Kidney

CHINESE THERAPEUTIC ACTIONS

1. Promotes Diuresis

Edema: *Shan Pu Tao* (Radix Vitis Amurensis) dispels accumulations of water to treat edema.

- Edema arising from deficiency: use *Shan Pu Tao* with *Fen Fang Ji* (Radix Stephaniae Tetandrae), *Huang Qi* (Radix Astragali), *Fu Ling* (Poria), *Gui Zhi* (Ramulus Cinnamomi), *Ze Xie* (Rhizoma Alismatis) and *Zhu Ling* (Polyporus).
- Edema due to excess: combine it with *Shui Ding Xiang* (Herba Ludwigiae Prostratae), *Ding Shu Xiu* (Herba Elephantopus Scaber), *Zhu Ling* (Polyporus), *Chuan Mu Tong* (Caulis Clematidis Armandii) and *Fu Ling* (Poria).

2. Tonifies the Kidney, Brightens the Eyes and Benefits the Liver

- Cataracts: use the fresh juice of *Shan Pu Tao* as eye drops.
- Eye disorders (conjunctivitis or others) caused by excess conditions: add *Gou Qi Gen* (Radix Lycii), *Qian Li Guang* (Herba Senecionis Scandens), *Qing Xiang Zi* (Semen Celosiae), *Shu Wei Huang* (Herba Rostellulariae) and *Niao Bu Su* (Ramus Kalopanax Pictus).
- Blood deficiency in children with malnutrition or delayed growth: use *Shan Pu Tao* with *Ren Shen* (Radix Ginseng), *Bai Zhu* (Rhizoma Atractylodis Macrocephalae), *Gan Cao* (Radix Glycyrrhizae), *Fu Ling* (Poria), *Dang Gui* (Radicis Angelicae Sinensis), *Shu Di Huang* (Radix Rehmanniae Preparata), *Chuan Xiong* (Rhizoma Ligustici Chuanxiong) and *Bai Shao* (Radix Paeoniae Alba).

3. Disperses Swelling, Eliminates Toxins

- Initial stages of fibrocystic breast disorders with swelling and pain, aversion to cold and fever: use *Shan Pu Tao* with *Wang Bu Liu Xing* (Semen Vaccariae), *Pu Gong Ying* (Herba Taraxaci), *Lu Feng Fang* (Nidus Vespae) and *Chuan Shan Jia* (Squama Manis).
- Red or white vaginal discharge: combine this herb with *Bai Long Chuan Hua Tou* (Radix Clerodendron Paniculatum) and *Ji Guan Hua* (Flos Celosiae Cristatae).

DOSAGE

6 to 18 grams in decoction.

Ma Ti Jin (Herba Dichondrae Repentis)

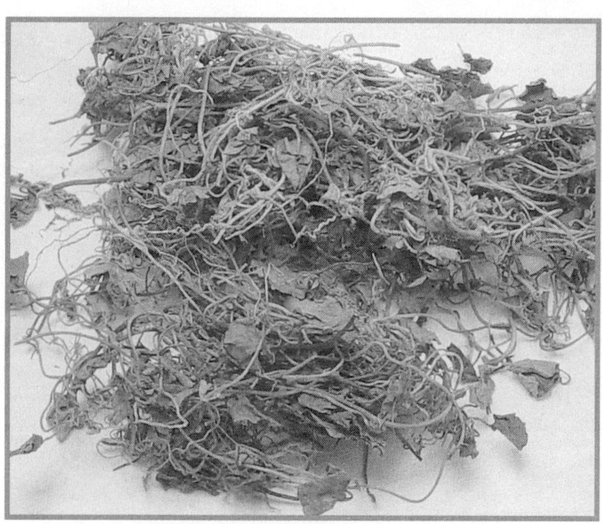

馬蹄金 马蹄金

Pinyin Name: *Ma Ti Jin*
Alternate Chinese Names: *He Bao Cao, Jin Suo Chi, Ma Cha Jin, Xiao Ying Feng Cao*
English Name: dichondra
Botanical Name: *Dichondra repens* Forst.
Pharmaceutical Name: Herba Dichondrae Repentis
Properties: bitter, acrid, cool
Channels Entered: Liver, Lung

CHINESE THERAPEUTIC ACTIONS

1. Clears Heat and Eliminates Toxins

Toxic heat: *Ma Ti Jin* (Herba Dichondrae Repentis) treats various disorders such as jaundice, dysentery, fetal toxicosis and infectious hepatitis.

- Jaundice: use *Ma Ti Jin* with *Zhi Zi* (Fructus Gardeniae), *Da Huang* (Radix et Rhizoma Rhei) and *Yin Chen Hao* (Herba Artemisiae Scopariae).
- Dysentery: combine it with *Feng Wei Cao* (Herba Pteris) and *Chuan Xin Lian* (Herba Andrographis).
- Infectious hepatitis: add *Huang Shui Qie* (Herba Solani), *Hua Shi Cao* (Herba Orthosiphon Aristatus) and *Hu Zhang* (Rhizoma Polygoni Cuspidati).

2. Invigorates Blood Circulation and Dispels Water

- Urinary stones: use *Ma Ti Jin* with *Wang Bu Liu Xing* (Semen Vaccariae), *Jin Qian Cao* (Herba Lysimachiae) and *Hai Jin Sha* (Herba Lygodii).
- Edema due to nephritis: use this herb with *Wan Dian Jin* (Radix Ilicis Asprellae), *Shan Pu Tao* (Radix Vitis Amurensis) and *Shui Ding Xiang* (Herba Ludwigiae Prostratae).

DOSAGE

3 to 12 grams

CAUTIONS / CONTRAINDICATIONS

- Use of *Ma Ti Jin* with salt is not recommended as the combination will cause water retention.

Jin Qian Cao (Herba Lysimachiae)

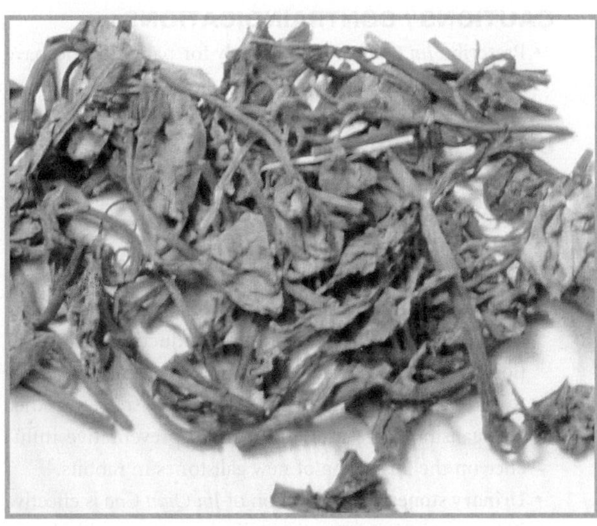

金錢草 金钱草

Pinyin Name: *Jin Qian Cao*

Literal Name: "gold money herb," "golden coin grass"

Alternate Chinese Names: *Da Jin Qian Cao, Si Chuan Da Jin Qian Cao, Jiang Su Jin Qian Cao, Lian Qian Cao, Pian Di Xiang, Ru Xiang Teng, Jiu Li Xiang, Ban Chi Lian, Pian Di Jin Lian*

Original Source: *Ben Cao Shi Yi* (Omissions from the [Classic of the] Materia Medica) by Chen Cang-Qi in 741 A.D.

English Name: lysimachia, loose strife herb

Botanical Name: *Lysimachia christinae* Hance (*Si Chuan Da Jin Qian Cao*); *Glechoma longituba* (*Nakai*) Kupr. (*Lian Qian Cao*); *Desmodium styracifolium* (Osb.) Merr. (*Guan Jin Qian Cao*); *Hydrocotyle sibthorpioides* Lam. var. *batrachium* (Hance) Hand. – Mazz. (*Jiang Xi Jin Qian Cao*); *Dichondra repens* Forst. (*Si Chuan Xiao Jin Qian Cao*); *Glechoma hederacea* (*Jiang Su Jin Qian Cao*).

Pharmaceutical Name: Herba Lysimachiae

Properties: sweet, salty, cool

Channels Entered: Urinary Bladder, Gallbladder, Kidney, Liver

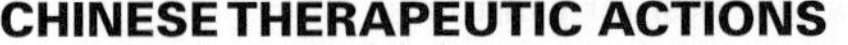

CHINESE THERAPEUTIC ACTIONS

1. Clears Damp-Heat and Treats Dysuria

***Shi lin* (stone dysuria):** *Jin Qian Cao* (Herba Lysimachiae) clears damp-heat and is commonly used to treat various *lin zheng* (dysuria syndromes). It is most effective for treating *shi lin* (stone dysuria) and *re lin* (heat dysuria). This is an indispensable herb for treatment of urinary stones.

- Kidney or urinary stones: use *Jin Qian Cao* with *Hai Jin Sha* (Herba Lygodii), *Shi Wei* (Folium Pyrrosiae), *Che Qian Zi* (Semen Plantaginis) and *Chuan Mu Tong* (Caulis Clematidis Armandii).
- Kidney or urinary stones formed because of Kidney deficiency, along with low back pain and soreness of the knees: use this herb with *Sang Ji Sheng* (Herba Taxilli), *Xu Duan* (Radix Dipsaci) and *Gou Qi Zi* (Fructus Lycii).

2. Clears Damp-Heat from the Liver and Gallbladder

Gallstones: *Jin Qian Cao* is an excellent herb to treat gallstones. In addition, it addresses various disorders characterized by damp-heat in the Liver and Gallbladder such as jaundice and hepatitis.

- Gallstones: use *Jin Qian Cao* with *Yin Chen Hao* (Herba Artemisiae Scopariae), *Huang Qin* (Radix Scutellariae), *Da Huang* (Radix et Rhizoma Rhei), *Chai Hu* (Radix Bupleuri), *Ji Nei Jin* (Endothelium Corneum Gigeriae Galli), *Chuan Lian Zi* (Fructus Toosendan) and *Yu Jin* (Radix Curcumae).
- Gallstones from Liver qi stagnation with hypochondriac pain, distention, chest fullness, emotional instability, and frequent sighing: use this herb with *Xiang Fu* (Rhizoma Cyperi), *Chuan Lian Zi* (Fructus Toosendan), *Mu Xiang* (Radix Aucklandiae) and *Yu Jin* (Radix Curcumae).
- Gallstones caused by blood stagnation, with fixed colicky pain and petechiae on the tongue: combine it with *Wu Ling Zhi* (Excrementum Trogopteri seu Pteromi), *Pu Huang* (Pollen Typhae), *Yan Hu Suo* (Rhizoma Corydalis), *Ru Xiang* (Gummi Olibanum) and *Mo Yao* (Myrrha).
- Jaundice: use it with *Yin Chen Hao* (Herba Artemisiae Scopariae), *Zhi Zi* (Fructus Gardeniae) and *Da Huang* (Radix et Rhizoma Rhei).

3. Clears Heat and Eliminates Toxins

Jin Qian Cao clears heat and toxins from the skin, as found in sores, lesions and snake bites. The fresh form of this herb can be mashed and applied topically, or juiced for internal use.

- Sores and lesions: use this herb with *Ye Ju Hua* (Flos Chrysanthemi Indici) and *Pu Gong Ying* (Herba Taraxaci), internally or topically.

DOSAGE

15 to 30 grams. The maximum dosage for *Jin Qian Cao* is 60 grams.

Jin Qian Cao (Herba Lysimachiae)

CAUTIONS / CONTRAINDICATIONS

- Prescribe *Jin Qian Cao* cautiously for patients who have diarrhea due to Spleen deficiency.

CHEMICAL COMPOSITION

Quercetin, quercetin-3-glucoside, kaempferol, kaempferol-3-O-galactoside.[1]

PHARMACOLOGICAL EFFECTS

- **Cholagogic:** Administration of *Jin Qian Cao* is associated with a marked increase in the production and excretion of bile acid in rats. It has also shown marked effectiveness in treating dogs for severe pain from jaundice and gallstones. In addition, it has a preventative influence on the formation of new gallstones in rabbits.[2]
- **Urinary stones:** The decoction of *Jin Qian Cao* is effective in preventing and treating urinary stones, with better action against kidney stones than bladder stones. Furthermore, different species of this herb serve to markedly increase the excretion of bladder and kidney stones. *Jiang Su Jin Qian Cao* (Herba Glechoma Hederacea) has a marked diuretic action in rabbits; and *Guang Jin Qian Cao* (Herba Desmodii Styracifolii) and *Si Chuan Xiao Jin Qian Cao* (Herba Dichondra Repens) increase the excretion of urine and sodium in rats.[3]
- **Cardiovascular:** An intravenous injection of water-extracted *Guang Jin Qian Cao* (Herba Desmodii Styracifolii) in anesthetized dogs increased blood perfusion to the heart and the kidneys by 197.4%.[4]
- **Antibiotic:** Both water and alcohol extracts of *Jiang Su Jin Qian Cao* (Herba Glechoma Hederacea) inhibit the growth of *Corynebacterium diphtheriae*, *Staphylococcus aureus*, *Bacillus subtilis*, and *E. coli*. Alcohol extract of *Guang Jin Qian Cao* (Herba Desmodii Styracifolii), but not the water extract, has an inhibitory effect against *Candida albicans*.[5]

CLINICAL STUDIES AND RESEARCH

- **Cholelithiasis:** Four cases of cholelithiasis were successfully treated with a preparation of *Jin Qian Cao*.[6]
- **Infection of the bile duct:** Decoction of *Jin Qian Cao* given once daily, for 30 days per course of treatment, for a total of 2 to 3 months, was 76.9% effective in treating 52 patients with non-bacterial infection of the bile duct. Those with low-grade fevers received 30 grams of herb per day, others received 10 to 20 grams per day.[7]
- **Hemorrhoids:** A decoction of *Jin Qian Cao* was used to effectively treat 30 patients with hemorrhoids. Most patients responded within 1 to 3 doses. The dosage used was 100 grams for the fresh herb, and 50 grams for the dried herb.[8]

HERB-DRUG INTERACTION

- **Diuretics:** *Jin Qian Cao* has a diuretic effect. Though there are no documented instances of this potential interaction, concurrent use with diuretic drugs may lead to increased elimination of water and/or electrolytes. [Note: Examples of diuretics include chlorothiazide, hydrochlorothiazide, furosemide (Lasix), bumetanide (Bumex), and torsemide (Demadex).][9]

TOXICOLOGY

No abnormalities were observed in dogs or mice following oral administration of decoction of *Jin Qian Cao* at 200 times the normal adult dose. No fatalities were reported following oral administration of *Jiang Su Jin Qian Cao* (Herba Glechoma Hederacea) at 20 g/kg/day for 6 days in rats. An oral bolus dose of *Jiang Su Jin Qian Cao* at 100 grams increased respiratory rates, but did not change blood pressure levels in dogs.[10]

SUPPLEMENT

Various species of this herb have been used as the medicinal herb in China. The following list includes the three most commonly used forms and their special applications:

- 四川大金錢草 / 四川大金钱草 *Si Chuan Da Jin Qian Cao* (Herba Lysimachia Christinae) clears heat and eliminates toxins, and is best for gallstones.
- 連錢草 / 连钱草 *Lian Qian Cao* (Herba Glechomae) clears heat and eliminates toxins, and is best for kidney stones.
- 廣金錢草 / 广金钱草 *Guang Jin Qian Cao* (Herba Desmodii Styracifolii) is best for kidney stones.

AUTHORS' COMMENTS

According to Dr. Liu Du-Zhou, the combination of *Jin Qian Cao* and *Chui Pen Cao* (Herba Sedi) serves to reduce elevated liver enzyme levels.

References

1. *Xian Dai Zhong Yao Yao Li Xue* (Contemporary Pharmacology of Chinese Herbs), 1997; 562
2. *Zhong Yao Yao Li Yu Ying Yong* (Pharmacology and Applications of Chinese Herbs), 1983: 696
3. *Guang Xi Zhong Yi Yao* (Guangxi Chinese Medicine and Herbology), 1990; 13(6):40
4. *Zhong Yao Yao Li Yu Ying Yong* (Pharmacology and Applications of Chinese Herbs), 1983: 696
5. Ibid.
6. *Zhong Yi Za Zhi* (Journal of Chinese Medicine), 1958; 11:749
7. *Bei Jing Zhong Yi* (Beijing Chinese Medicine), 1985; 1:26
8. *Zhong Guo Gang Chang Bing Za Zhi* (Chinese Journal of Proctology), 1986; 2:48
9. Chen, J. Recognition & prevention of herb-drug interactions, *Medical Acupuncture*, Fall/Winter 1998/1999; volume 10/number 2; 9-13
10. *Zhong Yao Yao Li Yu Ying Yong* (Pharmacology and Applications of Chinese Herbs), 1983: 696

Hai Jin Sha (Herba Lygodii)

海金砂

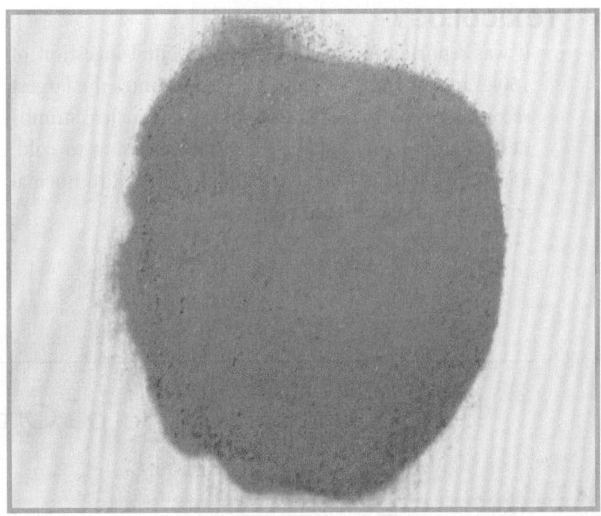

Pinyin Name: *Hai Jin Sha*
Literal Name: "golden sand of the sea"
Original Source: *Jia You Ben Cao* (Materia Medica of the Jia You Era) by Zhang Yu-Xi and Su Song in 1057-1060
English Name: lygodium spores
Botanical Name: *Lygodium japonicum* (Thunb.) Sw. (*Hai Jin Sha*)
Pharmaceutical Name: Herba Lygodii
Properties: sweet, bland, cold
Channels Entered: Urinary Bladder, Small Intestine

CHINESE THERAPEUTIC ACTIONS

1. Promotes Diuresis, Dispels Stones

Urinary stones and *lin zheng* (dysuria syndrome): *Hai Jin Sha* (Herba Lygodii) promotes urination and dispels urinary stones. It can be used for dysuria with burning sensations, hematuria, turbid, cloudy urine or urinary stones.

- Damp-heat in the Urinary Bladder: use *Hai Jin Sha* with *Huang Bai* (Cortex Phellodendri), *Zhi Zi* (Fructus Gardeniae) and *Che Qian Zi* (Semen Plantaginis).
- *Xue lin* (bloody dysuria): combine this herb with *Sheng Di Huang* (Radix Rehmanniae) and *Pu Huang* (Pollen Typhae).
- *Shi lin* (stone dysuria): use it with *Jin Qian Cao* (Herba Lysimachiae), *Ji Nei Jin* (Endothelium Corneum Gigeriae Galli) and *Shi Wei* (Folium Pyrrosiae).
- *Shi lin* (stone dysuria) with back pain from deficiency: combine *Hai Jin Sha* with *Sang Ji Sheng* (Herba Taxilli), *Xu Duan* (Radix Dipsaci), *Gou Ji* (Rhizoma Cibotii), *Du Zhong* (Cortex Eucommiae), *Ru Xiang* (Gummi Olibanum) and *Mo Yao* (Myrrha).
- *Gao lin* (cloudy dysuria): add this herb to *Hua Shi* (Talcum) and *Gan Cao* (Radix Glycyrrhizae).

Gallstones: With its ability to dispel stones, *Hai Jin Sha* is commonly used to treat gallstones.

- Gallstones: use it with *Yu Jin* (Radix Curcumae), *Jin Qian Cao* (Herba Lysimachiae), and *Ji Nei Jin* (Endothelium Corneum Gigeriae Galli).

2. Eliminates Water Accumulation and Reduces Swelling

Dampness accumulation: *Hai Jin Sha* can treat distention and fullness in the abdomen when it is caused by damp in the middle *jiao* blocking the Spleen's ability to dispel dampness. Clinical manifestations include severe abdominal fullness with bloating, dyspnea with inability to lie flat, generalized edema and swelling.

- Dampness accumulation: use *Hai Jin Sha* with *Qian Niu Zi* (Semen Pharbitidis) and *Gan Sui* (Radix Euphorbiae Kansui).

DOSAGE

6 to 15 grams. *Hai Jin Sha* should be wrapped in cheesecloth to maximize saturation when cooking in decoctions.

CAUTIONS / CONTRAINDICATIONS

- Do not prescribe *Hai Jin Sha* for patients experiencing deficiency but having no accumulation of damp-heat.

CHEMICAL COMPOSITION

Trans-p-coumaric acid, caffeic acid, lygodin.[1]

PHARMACOLOGICAL EFFECTS

- **Genitourinary:** In anesthetized dogs, injection of *Hai Jin Sha* is associated with increased pressure and motility of the urinary tract.[2]
- **Others:** *Hai Jin Sha* also has cholagogic and antibiotic effects.

CLINICAL STUDIES AND RESEARCH

- **Urinary stones:** Seven patients with stones in the urinary tract were treated with an herbal formula containing *Hai Jin Sha*, *Jin Qian Cao* (Herba Lysimachiae), *Qu Mai* (Herba Dianthi), *Hua Shi* (Talcum), *Che Qian Zi* (Semen Plantaginis), *Chuan Mu Tong* (Caulis Clematidis Armandii), *Chuan Niu Xi* (Radix Cyathulae), and *Zhi Gan Cao* (Radix Glycyrrhizae Praeparata). After 10 days of herbal treatment, stones were eliminated in all patients.[3]

Hai Jin Sha (Herba Lygodii)

TOXICOLOGY

It was reported in one case that accidental ingestion of 150 grams of *Hai Jin Sha* (which is ten times the largest recommended dosage) caused side effects such as numbness of the tongue, nausea, headache, aversion to cold, and frequent urination. The patient returned to normal after symptomatic treatment.[4]

References

1. *Xian Dai Zhong Yao Yao Li Xue* (Contemporary Pharmacology of Chinese Herbs), 1997; 568
2. *Xin Zhong Yi* (New Chinese Medicine), 1985; (6):51
3. *Zhe Jiang Zhong Yi Za Zhi* (Zhejiang Journal of Chinese Medicine), 1983; (11):493
4. *An Hui Yi Xue* (Anhui Medicine), 1987; 8(1):34

Hua Shi Cao (Herba Orthosiphon Aristatus)

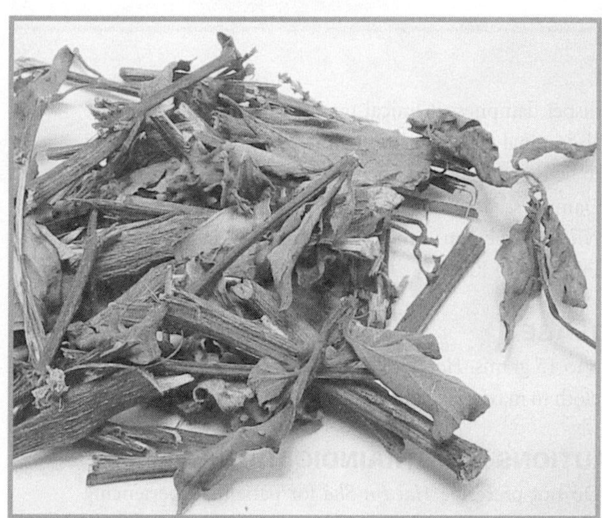

化石草 化石草

Pinyin Name: *Hua Shi Cao*
Literal Name: "dissolve stone herb"
Alternate Chinese Names: *Mao Xu Cao, Shen Cha, Yao Zi Cao, Nan Yang Cao*
English Name: orthosiphon, cat's whiskers
Botanical Name: *Orthosiphon aristatus; Orthosiphon grandiflorus*
Pharmaceutical Name: Herba Orthosiphon Aristatus
Properties: bitter, cold
Channels Entered: Liver, Kidney, Urinary Bladder

CHINESE THERAPEUTIC ACTIONS

1. Promotes Urination, Reduces Inflammation and Dissolves Stones

Nephritis, edema and urinary stones, gallstones, and hepatitis: *Hua Shi Cao* (Herba Orthosiphon Aristatus) enters the Kidney and Urinary Bladder to clear heat and promote diuresis. It also treats gallstones and hepatitis.

- Nephritis with edema: use this herb with *Wan Dian Jin* (Radix Ilicis Asprellae) and *Shan Pu Tao* (Radix Vitis Amurensis).
- Urinary stones: combine it with *Jin Qian Cao* (Herba Lysimachiae), *Hai Jin Sha* (Herba Lygodii), *Shi Wei* (Folium Pyrrosiae) or with the combination *Ba Zheng San* (Eight-Herb Powder for Rectification).
- Gallstones: use *Hua Shi Cao* with *Yu Jin* (Radix Curcumae), *Hai Jin Sha* (Herba Lygodii) and *Jin Qian Cao* (Herba Lysimachiae).
- Hepatitis: use it with *Bai Jiang Cao* (Herba cum Radice Patriniae), *Huang Shui Qie* (Herba Solani) and *Hu Zhang* (Rhizoma Polygoni Cuspidati).

2. Lowers Blood Pressure

- Hypertension: use *Hua Shi Cao* with *Shui Ding Xiang* (Herba Ludwigiae Prostratae) and *Ji Xue Cao* (Herba Centellae).

DOSAGE

6 to 18 grams in decoction

CAUTIONS / CONTRAINDICATIONS

- *Hua Shi Cao* should be used with caution for individuals who have Spleen and Stomach deficiencies.

CHEMICAL COMPOSITION

Potassium, sodium.

Shi Wei (Folium Pyrrosiae)

石韋 石韦

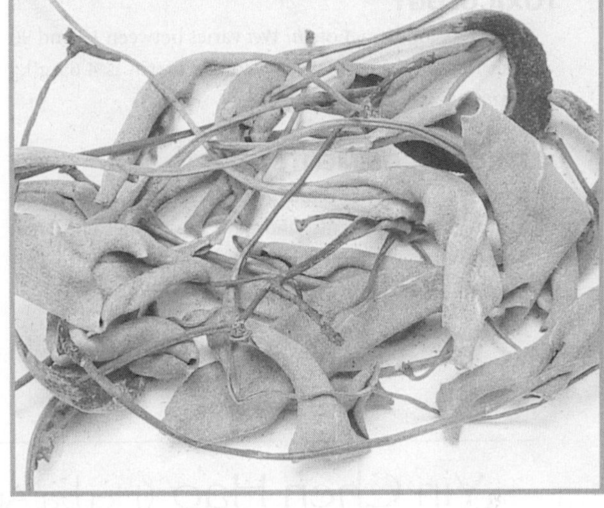

Pinyin Name: *Shi Wei*
Literal Name: "stone reed"
Alternate Chinese Names: *Shi Lan, Shi Pi*
Original Source: *Shen Nong Ben Cao Jing* (Divine Husbandman's Classic of the Materia Medica) in the second century
English Name: pyrrosia, shearer's pyrrosia leaf, Japanese felt fern
Botanical Name: *Pyrrosia sheareri* (Bak.) Ching (*Lu Shan Shi Wei*); *Pyrrosia petiolosa* (Christ) Ching (*Bing Shi Wei*); *Pyrrosia lingua* (Thunb.) Farw. (*Shi Wei*)
Pharmaceutical Name: Folium Pyrrosiae
Properties: bitter, sweet, cool
Channels Entered: Urinary Bladder, Lung

CHINESE THERAPEUTIC ACTIONS

1. Promotes Diuresis

***Lin zheng* (dysuria syndrome) and edema:** *Shi Wei* (Folium Pyrrosiae) dispels damp-heat and promotes urination. It is commonly used to treat various kinds of *lin zheng*. In addition, it regulates water circulation and treats edema.

- *Re lin* (heat dysuria): use *Shi Wei* with *Che Qian Zi* (Semen Plantaginis) and *Chuan Mu Tong* (Caulis Clematidis Armandii).
- *Shi lin* (stone dysuria): combine it with *Jin Qian Cao* (Herba Lysimachiae), *Hai Jin Sha* (Herba Lygodii) and *Hua Shi* (Talcum).
- *Xue lin* (bloody dysuria): use it with *Bai Mao Gen* (Rhizoma Imperatae), *Zhi Zi* (Fructus Gardeniae) and *Pu Huang* (Pollen Typhae).
- Edema: add *Che Qian Zi* (Semen Plantaginis), *Ze Xie* (Rhizoma Alismatis), and *Fu Ling* (Poria).

2. Dissolves Phlegm and Relieves Cough

Cough: *Shi Wei* treats cough with profuse sputum. It sedates heat in the *qi* (energy) level and also in the Lung channel. The decocted form of this herb is best for treatment of chronic bronchitis with cough and phlegm.

- Cough: use powdered *Shi Wei* and *Bing Lang* (Semen Arecae), served with *Sheng Jiang* (Rhizoma Zingiberis Recens) juice.
- Cough with yin deficiency: combine it with *Zhi Mu* (Radix Anemarrhenae).

3. Stops Bleeding

Bleeding: *Shi Wei* has a hemostatic effect and is commonly used to treat epistaxis, hematemesis, hypermenorrhea, and bleeding from trauma.

- Bleeding: use *Shi Wei* alone.

DOSAGE

5 to 10 grams, up to 15 to 30 grams of *Shi Wei* in severe cases.

CHEMICAL COMPOSITION

Isomangiferin, kaempferol, quercetin, isoquercitrin, trifolin, β-sitosterol, diploloptene, chlorogenic acid.[1]

PHARMACOLOGICAL EFFECTS

- **Expectorant:** The water decoction of *Shi Wei* decreased the secretion of mucus in the respiratory tract. However, it showed only minimal expectorant effect at 15 g/kg via intraperitoneal injection or 50 g/kg via oral ingestion.[2]
- **Antitussive:** Oral administration of isomangiferin has marked antitussive action in mice, but is not as potent when compared to codeine.[3]
- **Antiviral:** Preparations of *Shi Wei* have shown marked inhibitory effectiveness against herpes simplex virus I.[4]

CLINICAL STUDIES AND RESEARCH

- **Chronic tracheitis:** *Shi Wei* was used individually or in an herbal combination for treatment of 552 patients with chronic tracheitis. Of those who received only *Shi Wei* for 20 days, 22% of patients showed improvement. Of those who received *Shi Wei* in an herbal combination, 56.6% showed significant improvement. The study reported that most patients began to benefit from the treatment within 1 to 2 days, characterized by a decrease in the amount and viscosity of the sputum.[5]

Shi Wei (Folium Pyrrosiae)

TOXICOLOGY

The LD_{50} for extract of *Shi Wei* varies between 17 and 90 g/kg for mice. The LD_{50} for isomangiferin is 4.65 g/kg in mice.[6,7]

AUTHORS' COMMENTS

Recent research has shown *Shi Wei* to be effective in treating cancer patients who have low white blood cell counts after receiving chemotherapy or radiation. It helps to increase the white blood cell count.

References

1. *Xian Dai Zhong Yao Yao Li Xue* (Contemporary Pharmacology of Chinese Herbs), 1997; 569
2. *Yi Yao Yan Jiu Tong Xun* (Research Journal of Medicine and Medicinals), 1973; (10):32
3. *Yi Yao Gong Ye* (Pharmaceutical Industry), 1973; (6):1
4. *Zhong Guo Yao Li Xue Tong Bao* (Journal of Chinese Herbal Pharmacology), 1989; 10(1):85
5. *Shang Hai Ren Min Chu Ban She* (People's Press of Shanghai), 1973
6. *Zhong Yao Da Ci Dien* (Dictionary of Chinese Herbs), 1977; 579
7. *Zhong Cao Yao Xue* (Study of Chinese Herbal Medicine), 1976:59

Yin Chen Hao (Herba Artemisiae Scopariae)

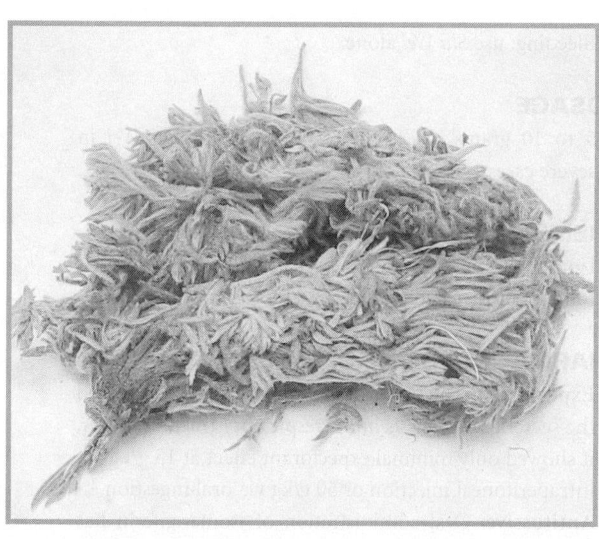

茵陳蒿 茵陈蒿

Pinyin Name: *Yin Chen Hao*
Literal Name: "mattress old wormwood"
Alternate Chinese Names: *Yin Chen, Mian Yin Chen*
Original Source: *Shen Nong Ben Cao Jing* (Divine Husbandman's Classic of the Materia Medica) in the second century
English Name: artemisia scoparia, virgate wormwood, capillary wormwood
Botanical Name: *Artemisia scoparia* Waldst. et Kit. (*Bin Hao*); *Artemisia capillaris* Thunb. (*Yin Chen Hao*)
Pharmaceutical Name: Herba Artemisiae Scopariae
Properties: bitter, cool
Channels Entered: Liver, Spleen, Gallbladder, Stomach

CHINESE THERAPEUTIC ACTIONS

1. Dispels Damp-Heat to Treat Jaundice

Jaundice: *Yin Chen Hao* (Herba Artemisiae Scopariae) is one of the most commonly used and most effective herbs for treating jaundice. It is most suitable for the yang-type jaundice in which the skin appears to be bright orange-yellow. *Yin Chen Hao*, when combined properly with other herbs, also addresses yin-type jaundice in which the skin appears dull, lusterless and yellow.

- Jaundice due to damp-heat with fever, bright yellow discoloration of the skin, dark, scanty urine: use *Yin Chen Hao* with *Zhi Zi* (Fructus Gardeniae) and *Da Huang* (Radix et Rhizoma Rhei). **Exemplar Formula:** *Yin Chen Hao Tang* (Artemisia Scoparia Decoction).
- Jaundice caused more by dampness with dysuria: use it with *Wu Ling San* (Five-Ingredient Powder with Poria). **Exemplar Formula:** *Yin Chen Wu Ling San* (Artemisia Scoparia and Five-Ingredient Powder with Poria).
- Jaundice from damp-cold with dark yellow discoloration of the skin, aversion to cold, and abdominal distention: use this herb with *Gan Jiang* (Rhizoma Zingiberis) and *Fu Zi* (Radix Aconiti Lateralis Praeparata).

Damp-heat in the Liver: Manifestations include cholecystitis, infectious hepatitis and liver cirrhosis. With its cooling thermal property, *Yin Chen Hao* dispels damp-heat from the Liver and Gallbladder with or without manifestations of jaundice. It helps in the secretion of bile and aids in the generation of liver cells.

- Cholecystitis or cholelithiasis: use *Yin Chen Hao* with *Chai Hu* (Radix Bupleuri), *Jin Qian Cao* (Herba Lysimachiae), *Yu Jin* (Radix Curcumae) and *Da Huang*

Yin Chen Hao (Herba Artemisiae Scopariae)

(Radix et Rhizoma Rhei).

- Hepatitis: combine it with *Huang Qin* (Radix Scutellariae), *Jin Qian Cao* (Herba Lysimachiae), *Bai Hua She She Cao* (Herba Oldenlandia) and *Chai Hu* (Radix Bupleuri).
- Liver cirrhosis: add *Bai Hua She She Cao* (Herba Oldenlandia) and *Hu Zhang* (Rhizoma Polygoni Cuspidati).

2. Treats Damp-Heat Febrile Disorders

Damp-heat febrile disorders: *Yin Chen Hao* dispels damp-heat in febrile disorders characterized by fever, muscle aches and pain, feelings of oppression in the chest, abdominal distention, yellow urine and constipation.

- Febrile disorders with damp-heat: use this herb with *Hua Shi* (Talcum), *Huang Qin* (Radix Scutellariae), and *Bai Dou Kou* (Fructus Amomi Rotundus). **Exemplar Formula**: *Gan Lu Xiao Du Dan* (Sweet Dew Special Pill to Eliminate Toxin).

3. Dispels Damp-Heat from the Exterior

Dermatological disorders: *Yin Chen Hao* dispels damp-heat from the exterior and treats various dermatological disorders, including urticaria, eczema, rashes, oozing sores, and more.

- Dermatological disorders due to damp-heat: use *Yin Chen Hao* with *Bai Xian Pi* (Cortex Dictamni), *Di Fu Zi* (Fructus Kochiae) and *Ku Shen Gen* (Radix Sophorae Flavescentis), either internally or topically.

DOSAGE

10 to 30 grams.

CAUTIONS / CONTRAINDICATIONS

- *Yin Chen Hao* is contraindicated if there is no damp-heat present.

CHEMICAL COMPOSITION

Capillanol, capillarin, capillarisin, capillartemisin A, B; capillene, chlorogenic acid, caffeic acid, phydroxya cetophenone, 6,7-dimethoxycoumarin.[1,2]

Capillarin

PHARMACOLOGICAL EFFECTS

- **Cholagogic:** A stimulating effect on gallbladder function was observed in dogs following administration of *Yin Chen Hao* in various preparation forms, including but not limited to water extract, alcohol extract, and essential oil.[3]
- **Hepatoprotective:** In one laboratory study, subcutaneous injection of a decoction of *Yin Chen Hao* showed a marked protective effect against carbon chloride-induced liver damage. In another study, oral administration of decoction of *Yin Chen Hao* stimulated the activity of cytochrome P-450 and increased the weight of the liver in mice. Lastly, *Yin Chen Hao Tang* (Artemisia Scoparia Decoction) was effective in reducing SGPT and SGOT levels.[4]
- **Antihypertensive:** Both water and alcohol extracts of *Yin Chen Hao* lowered blood pressure in anesthetized rats, cats and rabbits. While its effect was not negated by atropine, *Yin Chen Hao* did not lower blood pressure elevated by adrenalin. The duration of antihypertensive action following intravenous injection is approximately 120 to 160 minutes.[5]
- **Antihyperlipidemic:** Administration of a decoction of *Yin Chen Hao* at 3 g/kg/day for 2 to 3 weeks lowered both plasma cholesterols and β-lipoproteins in rabbits.[6]
- **Antibiotic:** Decoction of *Yin Chen Hao* has varying degrees of inhibitory effectiveness against such pathogens as *Mycobacterium tuberculosis, Corynebacterium diphtheriae, Bacillus anthracis, Salmonella typhi, Pseudomonas aeruginosa, E. coli, Bacillus dysenteriae, Bacillus subtilis, Staphylococcus aureus, Diplococcus meningitidis*, and influenza virus. The essential oil of the herb is effective against dermatophytes.[7,8]
- **Antipyretic:** Intraperitoneal injection of *Yin Chen Hao* effectively lowered body temperature for approximately 3 to 4 hours in rats with artificially-induced fever.[9,10]
- *Yin Chen Hao* also demonstrated mild diuretic and antiparasitic effects.[11]

CLINICAL STUDIES AND RESEARCH

- **Hepatitis:** Decoction of 30 to 45 grams of *Yin Chen Hao* given three times daily was prescribed for treatment of 32 cases of acute infectious hepatitis. The study reported excellent treatment results, with marked reduction of fever, jaundice, and of the size of the liver. The duration of treatment ranged from 3 to 15 days, with an average of 7 days.[12]
- **Parasitic infestation of the bile duct:** According to one study, 50 patients with parasitic infestation of the bile duct were treated with an herbal decoction with good success. The formula contained 30 to 60 grams of *Yin Chen Hao*. Also, *Jin Yin Hua* (Flos Lonicerae), *Lian Qiao* (Fructus Forsythiae), *Pu Gong Ying* (Herba Taraxaci) and others were added if infection was present.[13]
- **Hypercholesterolemia:** Daily consumption of 15 grams of *Yin Chen Hao* as a tea for one month per course of treatment was effective in reducing serum cholesterol levels. Of 82 patients, the study reported an average reduction of 42.4 mg/dL, or a 14.3% decrease, per person.[14]
- **Topical fungal infection:** Topical application of essential oil of *Yin Chen Hao* twice daily for four weeks was effec-

Yin Chen Hao (Herba Artemisiae Scopariae)

tive for skin and foot fungal infections.[15]

TOXICOLOGY

Overdose of capillarin is characterized by lethargy and salivation. The LD_{50} for capillarin in mice is 262.5 mg/kg via intraperitoneal injection.[16,17]

SUPPLEMENT

- 鈴茵陳 / 铃茵陈 *Ling Yin Chen* (Herba Siphonostegia Chinensis), an herb with a similar pinyin name as *Yin Chen Hao*, is sometimes used as a substitute. However, these are two completely different herbs and should not be used interchangeably.

References

1. *Xian Dai Zhong Yao Yao Li Xue* (Contemporary Pharmacology of Chinese Herbs), 1997; 571
2. Yan X, Zhou J, Xie G, *Traditional Chinese Medicines Molecular Structures, Natural Sources and Applications*; Ashgate, 1999; 855
3. *Sheng Yao Xue Za Zhi* (Journal of Raw Herbology), 1978; 32(2):177
4. *Guo Wai Yi Xue Zhong Yi Zhong Yao Fen Ce* (Monograph of Chinese Herbology from Foreign Medicine), 1986; 8(5):22
5. *Zhi Wu Yao You Xiao Cheng Fen Shou Ce* (Manual of Plant Medicinals and Their Active Constituents), 1986; 172; 173; 584; 940
6. *Zhong Yao Yao Li Yu Ying Yong* (Pharmacology and Applications of Chinese Herbs), 1990; 15(6):52
7. Ibid.
8. *Zhong Yao Xue* (Chinese Herbology), 1998; 355:357
9. *Planta Med*, 1984; 46(1):84
10. *Yao Xue Tong Bao* (Report of Herbology), 1987; 22(10):590
11. *Zhong Yao Xue* (Chinese Herbology), 1998; 355:357
12. *Fu Jian Zhong Yi Yao* (Fujian Chinese Medicine and Herbology), 1959; 7:42
13. *Shan Dong Yi Kan* (Shandong Medical Journal), 1965; 12:44
14. *Zhong Yi Za Zhi* (Journal of Chinese Medicine), 1980; 1:39
15. *Si Chuan Zhong Cao Yao Tong Xun* (Sichuan Journal of Chinese Herbology), 1976; 3:28
16. *Yao Xue Tong Bao* (Report of Herbology), 1987; 22(10):590
17. *Zhi Wu Yao You Xiao Cheng Fen Shou Ce* (Manual of Plant Medicinals and Their Active Constituents), 1986; 172, 173, 584, 940

Bi Xie (Rhizoma Dioscoreae Hypoglaucae)

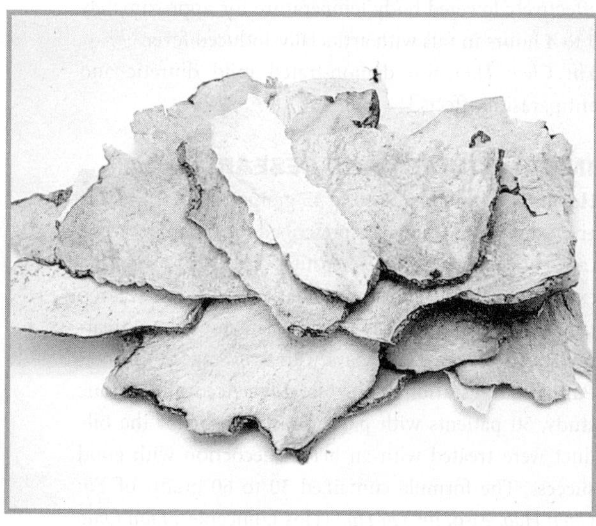

萆薢

Pinyin Name: *Bi Xie*
Alternate Chinese Names: *Zhu Mu, Chi Jie, Fen Bie Xie*
Original Source: *Shen Nong Ben Cao Jing* (Divine Husbandman's Classic of the Materia Medica) in the second century
English Name: tokoro
Botanical Name: *Dioscorea hypoglauca* palibin (*Fen Bi Xie*); *Dioscorea septemloba* Thunb. (*Mian Bi Xie*); *Dioscorea futschauensis* Uline (*Fu Zhou Shu Yu*)
Pharmaceutical Name: Rhizoma Dioscoreae Hypoglaucae
Properties: bitter, neutral
Channels Entered: Urinary Bladder, Liver, Stomach

CHINESE THERAPEUTIC ACTIONS

1. Separates Clear from Turbid

Gao lin **(cloudy dysuria)**: *Bi Xie* (Rhizoma Dioscoreae Hypoglaucae) dispels dampness and treats disorders characterized by cloudy, turbid, milky urine with white patches or bloody streaks. Burning sensations and pain during urination, and a red tongue with yellow tongue coating are all manifestations of damp-heat in the lower *jiao*. Other manifestations may include: frequent urge to urinate, urinary incontinence, cystitis, and acute inflammation of the urethra. Cloudy and turbid urine, urinary frequency and *lack* of burning sensation and pain are manifestations of yang deficiency.

- Cloudy urine from damp-heat: use *Bi Xie* with *Che Qian*

Bi Xie (Rhizoma Dioscoreae Hypoglaucae)

Zi (Semen Plantaginis), *Huang Bai* (Cortex Phellodendri) and *Hua Shi* (Talcum).

- Cloudy urine caused by yang deficiency: combine it with *Wu Yao* (Radix Linderae), *Yi Zhi Ren* (Fructus Alpiniae Oxyphyllae) and *Shi Chang Pu* (Rhizoma Acori). **Exemplar Formula:** *Bi Xie Fen Qing Yin* (Dioscorea Hypoglauca Decoction to Separate the Clear).

Leukorrhea: Accumulation of dampness in the lower *jiao* results in turbid, white vaginal discharge.

- Leukorrhea from dampness: use *Bi Xie* with *Fu Ling* (Poria) and *Bai Zhu* (Rhizoma Atractylodis Macrocephalae).

2. Dispels Wind and Dampness

***Bi zheng* (painful obstruction syndrome):** *Bi Xie* treats excess or deficient *bi zheng*, such as those characterized by cold and dampness (that worsen in cold and rainy weather), heat and dampness (worse in hot weather), or Kidney deficiency (weakness and soreness of the joints, especially the lower back and knees).

- *Bi zheng*: use *Bi Xie* with *Du Huo* (Radix Angelicae Pubescentis), *Chuan Xiong* (Rhizoma Ligustici Chuanxiong), and *Wei Ling Xian* (Radix Clematidis).
- *Bi zheng* due to cold and dampness: combine it with *Fu Zi* (Radix Aconiti Lateralis Praeparata) and *Gui Zhi* (Ramulus Cinnamomi).
- *Bi zheng* from heat and dampness: add *Qin Jiao* (Radix Gentianae Macrophyllae), *Yi Yi Ren* (Semen Coicis) and *Fen Fang Ji* (Radix Stephaniae Tetandrae).
- Low back pain and weak knees caused by Kidney deficiency: use this herb with *Du Zhong* (Cortex Eucommiae), *Xu Duan* (Radix Dipsaci) and *Niu Xi* (Radix Cyathulae seu Achyranthis).

DOSAGE

10 to 15 grams.

CAUTIONS / CONTRAINDICATIONS

- Use *Bi Xie* with caution in patients with Kidney yin deficiency.

CHEMICAL COMPOSITION

Dioscin, gracillin, dioscoreasapotoxin A, B; tokoronin, yononin, diosgenin, tokorogenin, yamoogenin, yonogenin, kogagenin, igagenin.[1]

CLINICAL STUDIES AND RESEARCH

- **Nephritis:** A study reported good results in 14 patients with nephritis who took 24 to 36 grams of an herbal formula with hot water, two to three times daily, before meals. No contraindications were listed for this formula. The herbal formula contained 500g each of *Bi Xie*, *Huang Bai* (Cortex Phellodendri), *Zhi Mu* (Rhizoma Anemarrhenae Asphodeloidis), *Ze Xie* (Rhizoma Alismatis), *Fu Ling* (Poria), *Yi Zhi Ren* (Fructus Alpiniae Oxyphyllae), and *Mu Dan Pi* (Cortex Moutan), ground into fine powder, mixed, and made into pills.[2]
- **Urinary tract infection:** In another study, 32 patients with urinary tract infections were treated with an herbal decoction containing *Bi Xie*, with complete recovery in 18 cases, marked improvement in 13 cases, and no response in 1 case. The overall effective rate was 97.6%. The treatment protocol was: one dose of the decoction daily for 3 days per course of treatment. The herbal decoction contained *Bi Xie* 20g, *Fu Ling* (Poria) 30g, *Hua Shi* (Talcum) 30g, *Cang Zhu* (Rhizoma Atractylodis) 15g, *Huang Bai* (Cortex Phellodendri) 15g, *Che Qian Zi* (Semen Plantaginis) 15g, *Qu Mai* (Herba Dianthi) 15g, *Chuan Mu Tong* (Caulis Clematidis Armandii) 10g, *Bian Xu* (Herba Polygoni Avicularis) 10g, *Zhi Zi* (Fructus Gardeniae) 10g, *Da Huang* (Radix et Rhizoma Rhei) 10g, *Gan Cao* (Radix Glycyrrhizae) 3g, and other herbs as deemed necessary.[3]

References

1. *Chang Yong Zhong Yao Xian Dai Yan Jiu Yu Lin Chuan* (Recent Study & Clinical Application of Common Traditional Chinese Medicine), 1995; 270
2. *Zhong Yi Za Zhi* (Journal of Chinese Medicine), 1959; (6):21
3. *Zhe Jiang Zhong Yi Za Zhi* (Zhejiang Journal of Chinese Medicine), 1992; 27(2):59

Dong Gua Pi (Exocarpium Benincasae)

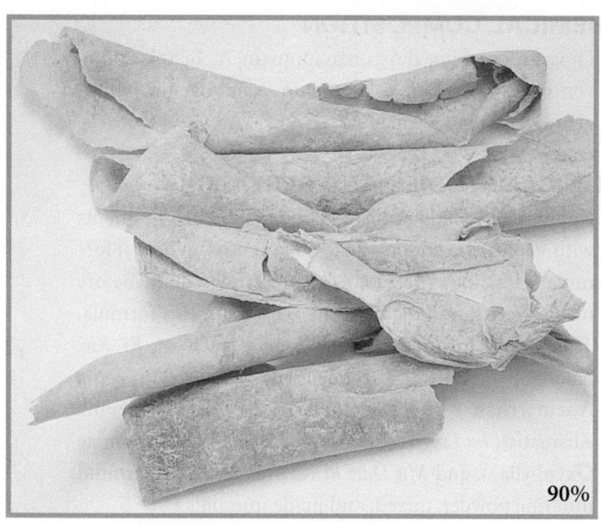
90%

冬瓜皮

Pinyin Name: *Dong Gua Pi*
Literal Name: "wintermelon peel"
Original Source: *Kai Bao Ben Cao* (Materia Medica of the Kai Bao Era) by Ma Zhi in 973-974 A.D.
English Name: benincasa peel
Botanical Name: *Benincasa hispida* (Thunb.) Cogn. (*Dong Gua*)
Pharmaceutical Name: Exocarpium Benincasae
Properties: sweet, bland, cool
Channels Entered: Lung, Small Intestine

CHINESE THERAPEUTIC ACTIONS

Promotes Diuresis and Reduces Edema

Edema: *Dong Gua Pi* (Exocarpium Benincasae) dispels the accumulation of water and clears heat simultaneously. It is mainly used for edema caused by damp-heat, and is relatively mild when used alone. Therefore, it is often used in combination with other diuretic herbs to enhance its effect.

- Edema: use *Dong Gua Pi* with *Fu Ling* (Poria), *Chi Xiao Dou* (Semen Phaseoli), and *Bai Mao Gen* (Rhizoma Imperatae).

DOSAGE

15 to 30 grams in decoction.

Chi Xiao Dou (Semen Phaseoli)

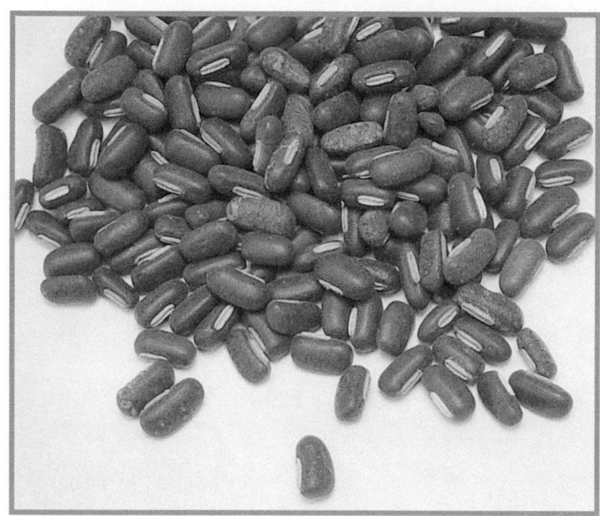

赤小豆

Pinyin Name: *Chi Xiao Dou*
Literal Name: "red little bean," "dark red little bean"
Alternate Chinese Names: *Hong Dou, Ci Dou, Zhu Xiao Dou*
Original Source: *Shen Nong Ben Cao Jing* (Divine Husbandman's Classic of the Materia Medica) in the second century
English Name: phaseolus, rice bean, adsuki bean
Botanical Name: *Phaseolus calcaratus* Roxb. (*Chi Xiao Dou*); *Phaseolus angularis* Wight (*Chi Dou*)
Pharmaceutical Name: Semen Phaseoli
Properties: sweet, sour, neutral
Channels Entered: Heart, Small Intestine

Chi Xiao Dou (Semen Phaseoli)

CHINESE THERAPEUTIC ACTIONS

1. Promotes Diuresis and Reduces Swelling

Chi Xiao Dou (Semen Phaseoli) regulates water circulation and treats disorders characterized by the accumulation of water, such as edema, ascites, and leg *qi*. *Chi Xiao Dou* can be used as a single-herb remedy, or combined with other diuretic herbs.

- Generalized edema with constipation: use *Chi Xiao Dou* with *Sang Bai Pi* (Cortex Mori) and *Zi Su Ye* (Folium Perillae), or take alone as food, instead of rice.
- Edema caused by nephritis or malnutrition, and ascites from liver cirrhosis: cook this herb with carp and take it as food on a daily basis.
- Leg *qi* with edema: use *Chi Xiao Dou* alone internally, and externally as a soak.

2. Clears Damp-Heat, Relieves Jaundice

Jaundice: *Chi Xiao Dou* has a mild action for treatment of jaundice caused by the accumulation of damp-heat.

3. Eliminates Toxins and Drains Pus

Erysipelas or toxic swellings and carbuncles: *Chi Xiao Dou* eliminates heat and toxins from the skin to treat dermatological disorders such as sores, erysipelas, lesions and carbuncles. This herb drains pus, reduces swelling, and enhances recovery.

- Swellings and abscesses that have not ulcerated: mix *Chi Xiao Dou* with egg whites, honey or vinegar, and apply topically. Re-apply as it dries.
- External injuries with bruises and sprains: apply the herb topically.

DOSAGE

10 to 30 grams. *Chi Xiao Dou* can be used in decoctions, pills, or as a powder. It can be taken internally or applied topically. It is also consumed as a food (congee or porridge).

CAUTIONS / CONTRAINDICATIONS

- *Chi Xiao Dou* is contraindicated for yin-deficient patients or those without dampness.

CHEMICAL COMPOSITION

α-globulin, β-globulin, carbohydrates, fatty acid, saponin, vitamin A, B_1, B_2.[1]

CLINICAL STUDIES AND RESEARCH

- **Mumps:** Seven patients with mumps were treated by topical application of *Chi Xiao Dou*, with positive results. The topical application was prepared by grinding 50 to 70 pieces of *Chi Xiao Dou* and mixing the powder with water, egg white, or honey.[2]
- **Sprain or strain with bruises:** Fifty-two patients with swelling and bruises due to sprain or strain were treated with a topical application of *Chi Xiao Dou*, with good results within 1 or 2 doses. The treatment protocol was to apply the herbal paste, leave it on, and remove it after 24 hours. The herbal paste was prepared by mixing the finely-powdered herb with cold water.[3]
- **Insufficient lactation:** Twenty patients experiencing insufficient production of breast milk were treated with a decoction of 240 grams of *Chi Xiao Dou* twice daily for 3 to 5 days, with good results.[4]

SUPPLEMENT

- 相思子 *Xiang Si Zi* (Semen Abrus Precatoris), *Abrus precatoris* L., is sometimes used in error as *Chi Xiao Dou* because of their similar appearances. *Chi Xiao Dou* is dark red in color, while *Xiang Si Zi* is half-red, half-black. These herbs should not be used interchangeably since *Xiang Si Zi* is toxic, and responsible for some reported instances of accidental poisoning.[5]

References

1. *Xian Dai Zhong Yao Yao Li Xue* (Contemporary Pharmacology of Chinese Herbs), 1997; 578-579
2. *Ha Er Bing Zhong Yi* (Haerbing Chinese Medicine), 1965; 9:32
3. *Zhong Xi Yi Jie He Za Zhi* (Journal of Integrated Chinese and Western Medicine), 1985; 10:630
4. *Chi Jiao Yi Shi Za Zhi* (Journal of Barefoot Doctors), 1975; 12:593
5. *Zhong Yao Xue* (Chinese Herbology), 1998; 359:360

Yu Mi Xu (Stigma Maydis)

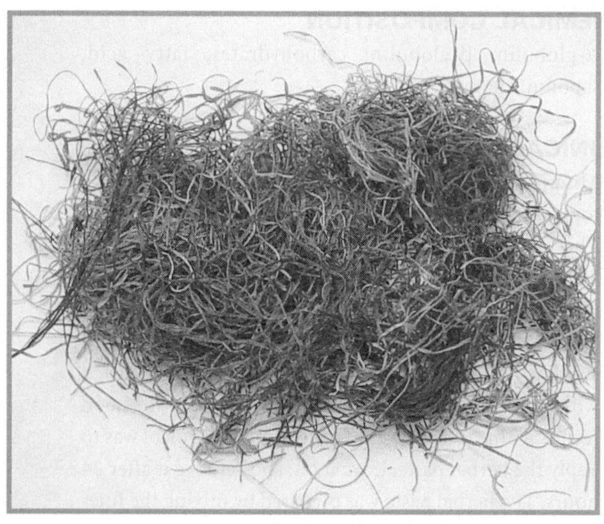

玉米鬚 玉米须

Pinyin Name: *Yu Mi Xu*
Literal Name: "corn silk," "jade rice whiskers"
Alternate Chinese Names: *Bao Mi Xu, Bang Zi Mao, Yu Mi Xin, Yu Mi Rui*
Original Source: *Zhen Nan Ben Cao* (Materia Medica of South Yunnan) by Lan Mao in Qing Dynasty
English Name: corn silk, corn stigma
Botanical Name: *Zea mays* L. (*Yu Shu Shu*)
Pharmaceutical Name: Stigma Maydis
Properties: sweet, bland, neutral
Channels Entered: Urinary Bladder, Kidney, Liver

CHINESE THERAPEUTIC ACTIONS

1. Promotes Diuresis, Treats Edema and Dysuria

Edema and dysuria: *Yu Mi Xu* (Stigma Maydis) regulates water circulation and reduces swelling. It is effective in addressing edema and dysuria arising from nephritis.

- Edema: use 6 grams of *Yu Mi Xu* alone.
- Nephritis with edema: use a large dosage of *Yu Mi Xu* alone, or in combination with *Ze Xie* (Rhizoma Alismatis) and *Bai Zhu* (Rhizoma Atractylodis Macrocephalae).
- Dysuria with stones: combine this herb with *Che Qian Zi* (Semen Plantaginis) and *Hai Jin Sha* (Herba Lygodii).
- Diabetes mellitus: use 30 grams of *Yu Mi Xu* in decoction.
- Hypertension: use it with *Xi Gua Pi* (Pericarpium Citrulli).

2. Clears Damp-Heat from the Liver and Gallbladder

Yu Mi Xu dispels damp-heat from the Liver and Gallbladder to treat infectious hepatitis, cholecystitis, cholelithiasis and hypertension.

- Hepatitis, cholecystitis, and cholelithiasis caused by damp-heat: use *Yu Mi Xu* with *Jin Qian Cao* (Herba Lysimachiae), *Yin Chen Hao* (Herba Artemisiae Scopariae), *Yu Jin* (Radix Curcumae) and *Ji Nei Jin* (Endothelium Corneum Gigeriae Galli).
- Hypertension: use *Yu Mi Xu* alone or with *Tian Ma* (Rhizoma Gastrodiae) and *Gou Teng* (Ramulus Uncariae cum Uncis).

DOSAGE

15 to 30 grams, up to 45 to 60 grams of *Yu Mi Xu* in severe cases.

CHEMICAL COMPOSITION

Crytoxanthin, resin, saponins, alkaloids, ascorbic acid, vitamin K, sitosterol, stigmasterol, malic acid, palmitic acid, tartaric acid, oxalic acid, pantothenic acid.[1]

PHARMACOLOGICAL EFFECTS

- **Diuretic:** Administration of *Yu Mi Xu* has been associated with an increase in excretion of urine and chloride in humans and rabbits.[2]
- **Antihypertensive:** Intravenous injection of a preparation of *Yu Mi Xu* in dogs has been associated with reduction of blood pressure. Continuous administration for 3 weeks, however, showed no permanent change of the animals' blood pressure.[3]
- **Cholagogic:** *Yu Mi Xu* stimulates production and excretion of bile acid. It also decreases the viscosity of bile.[4,5]
- **Others:** *Yu Mi Xu* has antidiabetic and hemostatic effects.[6]

CLINICAL STUDIES AND RESEARCH

- **Chronic nephritis:** In one clinical study, patients with chronic nephritis were treated with long-term therapy of *Yu Mi Xu*. The treatment protocol was to cook 50 grams of the herb in 600 ml of water for 20 to 30 minutes, to yield 300 to 400 ml of decoction. All 300 to 400 ml of the decoction were to be consumed at once, or as several doses daily. After 15 days to 6 months of continuous treatment in 9 patients with chronic nephritis, 3 showed complete recovery, 2 showed some improvement, 4 showed no change. Positive improvements were reduction of edema, improvement of kidney function and remission of proteinuria. No significant side effects were reported.[7]

HERB-DRUG INTERACTION

- **Warfarin (Coumadin):** *Yu Mi Xu* contains vitamin K,

Yu Mi Xu (Stigma Maydis)

which may reduce the anticoagulant effect of warfarin. Therefore, concurrent use of the herb and the drug should be monitored carefully to avoid the formation of blood clots.[8]

- **Diuretics:** *Yu Mi Xu* has a diuretic effect. Though this potential interaction has not been documented, concurrent use with diuretic drugs may lead to increased elimination of water and/or electrolytes. [Note: Examples of diuretics include chlorothiazide, hydrochlorothiazide, furosemide (Lasix), bumetanide (Bumex), and torsemide (Demadex).][9]

TOXICOLOGY

Yu Mi Xu is very well-tolerated. The lethal dose in rabbits is 250 mg/kg via intravenous injection. The effective dose for diuretic action, however, is only 1.5 mg/kg. No toxic injury to the heart, lungs, or other vital organs was observed at 1.5 mg/kg.[10]

References

1. *Xian Dai Zhong Yao Yao Li Xue* (Contemporary Pharmacology of Chinese Herbs), 1997; 560
2. *Zhong Yao Xue* (Chinese Herbology), 1998; 362:363
3. *Zhong Yao Da Ci Dien* (Dictionary of Chinese Herbs); 1037
4. *Zhong Yao Xue* (Chinese Herbology), 1998; 362:363
5. *Zhong Yao Da Ci Dien* (Dictionary of Chinese Herbs); 1037
6. *Zhong Yao Xue* (Chinese Herbology), 1998; 362:363
7. *Zhong Hua Yi Xue Za Zhi* (Chinese Journal of Medicine), 1956; 10:922
8. Chen, J. Recognition & prevention of herb-drug interactions, *Medical Acupuncture*, Fall/Winter 1998/1999; volume 10/number 2; 9-13
9. Ibid.
10. *Zhong Yao Da Ci Dien* (Dictionary of Chinese Herbs); 1037

Ze Qi (Herba Euphorbiae Helioscopiae)

澤漆 泽漆

Pinyin Name: *Ze Qi*
Literal Name: "marsh lacquer"
Original Source: *Shen Nong Ben Cao Jing* (Divine Husbandman's Classic of the Materia Medica) in the second century
English Name: euphorbia
Botanical Name: *Euphorbia helioscopia* L. (*Ze Qi*)
Pharmaceutical Name: Herba Euphorbiae Helioscopiae
Properties: sweet, bitter, acrid, cool
Channels Entered: Large Intestine, Small Intestine, Lung
Safety Index: toxic

CHINESE THERAPEUTIC ACTIONS

1. Promotes Circulation of Water, Reduces Edema

Edema or ascites: *Ze Qi* (Herba Euphorbiae Helioscopiae) strongly promotes water circulation and eliminates water stagnation.

- Water stagnation: use *Ze Qi* with *Ze Xie* (Rhizoma Alismatis), *Chi Fu Ling* (Poria Rubrae), and *Sang Bai Pi* (Cortex Mori).

2. Dissolves Phlegm, Stops Cough

Ze Qi treats cough and wheezing accompanied by profuse sputum. It is also beneficial in treatment of chronic tracheitis.

- Cough and wheezing with sputum: use it with *Ban Xia* (Rhizoma Pinelliae), *Bai Qian* (Rhizoma Cynanchi Stauntonii), *Huang Qin* (Radix Scutellariae), and *Gan Cao* (Radix Glycyrrhizae).

3. Dissolves Phlegm, Disperses Nodules

Ze Qi dissolves nodules and hardnesses characterized by accumulation and hardening of phlegm. It may be used individually or in an herbal combination; internally or topically.

DOSAGE

5 to 10 grams. For external use, cook *Ze Qi* until it turns into a thick paste, and apply topically.

Ze Qi (Herba Euphorbiae Helioscopiae)

CAUTIONS / CONTRAINDICATIONS

- Do not use *Ze Qi* in cases of qi and blood deficiencies.
- Direct contact of *Ze Qi* to skin or mucous membranes may cause irritation, redness, and discomfort.

CHEMICAL COMPOSITION

Quercetin, quercetin-5,3-di-D-galactoside, heliosin, quercetin-3-o-digalactoside, hyperoside, dihydrofucosterol, phasin, helioscopiol, euphorbin, calcium maltale.[1]

PHARMACOLOGICAL EFFECTS

- **Antibiotic:** A preparation of *Ze Qi* at high concentration (50:1) has an inhibitory effect against *Mycobacterium tuberculosis*.[2]
- **Others:** It has expectorant, antitussive, and antipyretic effects.[3]

CLINICAL STUDIES AND RESEARCH

- **Chronic tracheitis:** In one report, extract of *Ze Qi* was used to treat 232 patients with chronic tracheitis two to four times daily for 10 days. The study reported marked improvement in 36% of the cases, and moderate improvement in 52% of the cases. Therapeutic benefits included decreased amounts of both sputum and coughing. Side effects such as stomach discomfort and upper abdominal pain were reported in 16 cases. Seven patients dropped out of the study as a result of gastrointestinal disturbances.[4]

TOXICOLOGY

No fatalities were reported following oral ingestion of *Ze Qi* by mice at 125 g/kg.[5]

References

1. *Xian Dai Zhong Yao Yao Li Xue* (Contemporary Pharmacology of Chinese Herbs), 1997; 584
2. *Zhong Yao Xue* (Chinese Herbology), 1998; 360:362
3. Ibid.
4. *Zhong Cheng Yao Yan Jiu* (Research of Chinese Patent Medicine), 1981; 5:27
5. *Chang Yong Zhong Yao Xian Dai Yan Jiu Yu Lin Chuan* (Recent Study & Clinical Application of Common Traditional Chinese Medicine), 1995; 275:276

Dong Kui Zi (Semen Malvae)

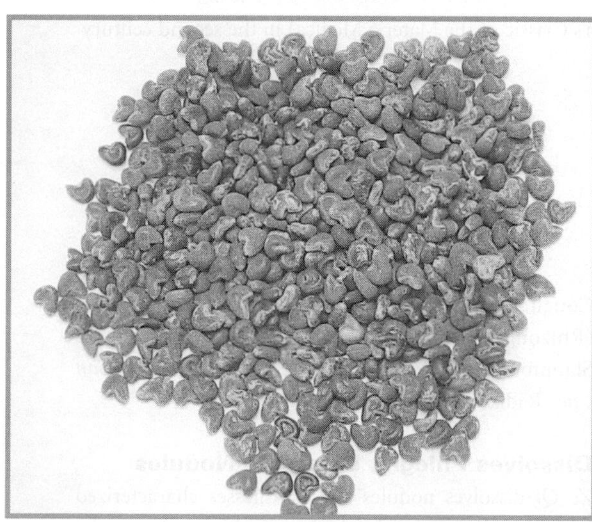

冬葵子 冬葵子

Pinyin Name: *Dong Kui Zi*
Alternate Chinese Names: *Dong Kui Guo, Kui Zi*
Original Source: *Shen Nong Ben Cao Jing* (Divine Husbandman's Classic of the Materia Medica) in the second century
English Name: malva
Botanical Name: *Malva verticillata* L. (*Dong Kui Zi*)
Pharmaceutical Name: Semen Malvae
Properties: sweet, cold
Channels Entered: Urinary Bladder, Large Intestine, Small Intestine

CHINESE THERAPEUTIC ACTIONS

1. Regulates Water Circulation

***Lin zheng* (dysuria syndrome) and edema:** *Dong Kui Zi* (Semen Malvae) regulates water circulation to promote normal urination.

- Generalized dysuria: use *Dong Kui Zi* as a single-herb remedy.
- Dysuria due to accumulation of heat in the Urinary Bladder: combine this herb with *Che Qian Zi* (Semen Plantaginis), *Chuan Mu Tong* (Caulis Clematidis

Dong Kui Zi (Semen Malvae)

Armandii) and *Huang Bai* (Cortex Phellodendri).

- Edema, sensations of heaviness, dysuria during pregnancy: use it with *Fu Ling* (Poria).
- Urinary stones: combine it with *Hai Jin Sha* (Herba Lygodii), *Jin Qian Cao* (Herba Lysimachiae), *Ze Xie* (Rhizoma Alismatis), *Ze Lan* (Herba Lycopi) and *Niu Xi* (Radix Cyathulae seu Achyranthis).

2. Promotes Lactation

Blocked lactation: *Dong Kui Zi* promotes lactation in postpartum women who have breast distention and pain due to stagnation in the channels and collaterals.

- Insufficient lactation with breast pain and swelling: use *Dong Kui Zi* with *Wang Bu Liu Xing* (Semen Vaccariae) and *Chuan Shan Jia* (Squama Manis); or, take *Dong Kui Zi* and *Sha Ren* (Fructus Amomi) as powder, chased by warm grain-based liquor.
- Fibrocystic breast disorder: use this herb with *Bai Zhi* (Radix Angelicae Dahuricae), *Gua Lou Shi* (Fructus Trichosanthis), *Lou Lu* (Radix Rhapontici), *Lu Feng Fang* (Nidus Vespae) and *Chi Shao* (Radix Paeoniae Rubrae).

3. Moistens the Intestines, Relieves Constipation

Constipation: *Dong Kui Zi* treats constipation due to insufficient fluids in the Large Intestine. It is best for patients experiencing both frequent urination and constipation. It is commonly combined with other herbs in the purgative or moist laxative categories to maximize its effectiveness.

DOSAGE

10 to 15 grams.

CAUTIONS / CONTRAINDICATIONS

- Use *Dong Kui Zi* carefully in pregnant women, or in patients who have deficiency and cold of the Spleen and Stomach.

CHEMICAL COMPOSITION

Lipids, protein, sugars, starch.[1]

TOXICOLOGY

There has been one case report of an adverse reaction associated with the use of *Dong Kui Zi*. After taking two doses of a decoction containing the herb, the patient reported diplopia, visual disturbance, excitation, and delirium. Administration of the herbs was immediately discontinued and the patient was treated symptomatically. All adverse reactions resolved within 24 hours.[2]

SUPPLEMENT

- 苘麻子 *Qing Ma Zi* (Semen Abutili): In the past, malva and albutilon were both used as the botanical source for "*Dong Kui Zi.*" Today, however, these plants are separately identified as having distinct and different functions that are not interchangeable in clinical usage. Efforts are being made to separate these two sources, to avoid confusion. The more updated and accurate terminologies are *Dong Kui Zi* (Semen Malvae) and *Qing Ma Zi* (Semen Abutili). *Dong Kui Zi* is derived from *Malva verticillata,* while *Qing Ma Zi* is derived from *Abutilon theophrastii* or *Abutilon avicennae*. Clinically, *Dong Kui Zi* (Semen Malvae) is commonly used to treat dysuria and constipation, and *Qing Ma Zi* (Semen Abutili) treats dysuria and dysentery.[3]

References

1. *Chang Yong Zhong Yao Cheng Fen Yu Yao Li Shou Ce* (A Handbook of the Composition and Pharmacology of Common Chinese Drugs), 1994; 735
2. *Si Chuan Zhong Yi* (Sichuan Chinese Medicine), 1984; (1):57
3. *Zhong Yao Xue* (Chinese Herbology), 1998; 363:364

Chapter 6 summary

— Water-Regulating and Damp-Resolving Herbs

Name	Similarities	Differences
Fu Ling (Poria)	Promote diuresis, treat edema and *lin zheng* (dysuria syndrome)	Strengthens the Spleen, calms the *shen* (spirit)
Zhu Ling (Polyporus)		Exerts a stronger diuretic function than the others
Ze Xie (Rhizoma Alismatis)		Strongly promotes diuresis, treats vertigo and dizziness caused by accumulation of dampness
Yi Yi Ren (Semen Coicis)		Strengthens the Spleen, treats *bi zheng* (painful obstruction syndrome) due to dampness, and clears heat to expel pus
Che Qian Zi (Semen Plantaginis)	Clear heat, promote diuresis, treat *shi-re lin* (damp-heat dysuria)	Clears heat from the Liver and Lung
Hua Shi (Talcum)		Clears summer-heat, clears heat and promotes healing of damp sores when used externally
Chuan Mu Tong (Caulis Clematidis Armandii)		Sedates Heart fire, promotes lactation
Tong Cao (Medulla Tetrapanacis)		Promotes lactation, weaker in clearing heat
Deng Xin Cao (Medulla Junci)		Clears Heart fire
Di Fu Zi (Fructus Kochiae)		Treats damp sores and relieves itching
Bian Xu (Herba Polygoni Avicularis)		Kills parasites and relieves itching
Qu Mai (Herba Dianthi)		Invigorates blood circulation, opens channels and collaterals, treats amenorrhea
Bai Long Chuan Hua Tou (Radix Clerodendron Paniculatum)		Regulates menstruation and treats abnormal vaginal discharge
Ding Shu Xiu (Herba Elephantopus Scaber)		Reduces swelling
Shui Ding Xiang (Herba Ludwigiae Prostratae)		Cools blood
Mo Gu Xiao (Caulis Hyptis Capitatae)		Unblocks stagnation to relieve pain
Xian Feng Cao (Herba Bidentis)		Reduces swelling and inflammation
Bi Zi Cao (Herba Pogonantheri Criniti)		Promotes normal urination
Dong Gua Zi (Semen Benincasae)		Clears heat, dissolves phlegm, and eliminates pus
Shan Pu Tao (Radix Vitis Amurensis)		Tonifies the Kidney and benefits the eyes
Ma Ti Jin (Herba Dichondrae Repentis)		Invigorates blood circulation
Jin Qian Cao (Herba Lysimachiae)	Dispel dampness, treat *re lin* (heat dysuria) and *shi lin* (stone dysuria)	Dispels gallstones and urinary stones, reduces jaundice
Hai Jin Sha (Herba Lygodii)		Treats *lin zheng* (dysuria syndrome)
Hua Shi Cao (Herba Orthosiphon Aristatus)		Lowers blood pressure
Shi Wei (Folium Pyrrosiae)		Dissolves phlegm and relieves cough
Yin Chen Hao (Herba Artemisiae Scopariae)	Regulate water, promote diuresis, reduce edema	Treats jaundice
Bi Xie (Rhizoma Dioscoreae Hypoglaucae)		Dispels dampness and treats cloudy urine, treats arthritis
Dong Gua Pi (Exocarpium Benincasae)		Reduces edema
Chi Xiao Dou (Semen Phaseoli)		Treats jaundice, clears toxins, treats abscesses and swellings
Yu Mi Xu (Stigma Maydis)		Treats dysuria and damp-heat in the Liver and Gallbladder
Ze Qi (Herba Euphorbiae Helioscopiae)		Dispels phlegm to relieve cough and disperse nodules
Dong Kui Zi (Semen Malvae)		Promotes lactation and treats constipation

Chapter 6 summary

General Characteristics of Water-Regulating and Damp-Resolving Herbs:

Taste: sweet, bland or bitter
Thermal property: neutral to cold
Channels entered: Kidney, Urinary Bladder
Therapeutic actions: promote diuresis, reduce swelling, treat *lin zheng* (dysuria syndrome)

These herbs regulate water and resolve dampness to treat dysuria, leukorrhea, edema, phlegm or damp accumulation, jaundice, damp sores, damp-heat disorders, and *bi zheng* (painful obstruction syndrome).

Fu Ling (Poria), *Zhu Ling* (Polyporus), ***Ze Xie*** (Rhizoma Alismatis) and ***Yi Yi Ren*** (Semen Coicis) promote diuresis to treat edema, dysuria, edema, and water accumulation.

Fu Ling strengthens the Spleen, addressing Spleen deficiency with accumulation of dampness by dispelling dampness and reducing swelling. Its ability to treat the symptoms and the cause of the disease makes it one of the most commonly prescribed herbs for these imbalances.

Zhu Ling and *Ze Xie* both have stronger diuretic action but do not strengthen the Spleen.

Ze Xie treats dizziness and vertigo caused by phlegm accumulation.

Yi Yi Ren strengthens the Spleen and is most suited for use in patients with Spleen deficiency and damp accumulation. It clears heat and dispels pus, thus is useful in treating lung and/or intestinal abscesses. It also treats *bi zheng* (painful obstruction syndrome).

Che Qian Zi (Semen Plantaginis) and ***Hua Shi*** (Talcum) commonly address *shi-re lin* (damp-heat dysuria) and *re lin* (heat dysuria). Both are sweet and cold, clear heat, dispel dampness, and consolidate loose stools by promoting urination of excess water.

Che Qian Zi, stronger in clearing heat, clears Liver fire and brightens the eyes, clears Lung heat and dissolves phlegm. The entire plant clears heat, promotes diuresis and is especially good at clearing heat to eliminate toxins.

Hua Shi clears summer-heat and dampness, and is used in the summer for febrile disorders resulting from heat and dampness. As a topical, *Hua Shi* clears heat to treat eczema, damp sores, rashes and other dermatological disorders.

Chuan Mu Tong (Caulis Clematidis Armandii), bitter and cold, strongly promotes diuresis, promotes lactation, and clears Heart fire. It also opens the channels and treats *bi zheng* (painful obstruction syndrome).

Tong Cao (Medulla Tetrapanacis) and ***Deng Xin Cao*** (Medulla Junci) are sweet, bland and cool.

Tong Cao has a milder heat-clearing effect to treat *shi-re lin* (damp-heat dysuria).

Deng Xin Cao dispels dampness and treats *shi-re lin* (damp-heat dysuria) and *shi lin* (stone dysuria).

Di Fu Zi (Fructus Kochiae) and ***Bian Xu*** (Herba Polygoni Avicularis) dispel dampness, relieve itching and treat sores, furuncles and other dermatological disorders.

Di Fu Zi relieves itching, eczema, and urticaria.

Bian Xu kills parasites, particularly roundworm and hookworm.

Qu Mai (Herba Dianthi) treats various types of *lin zheng* (dysuria syndrome). It also invigorates blood circulation to regulate menstruation.

Bai Long Chuan Hua Tou (Radix Clerodendron Paniculatum), ***Ding Shu Xiu*** (Herba Elephantopus Scaber) and ***Shui Ding Xiang*** (Herba Ludwigiae Prostratae) promote diuresis to treat water accumulation, and dispel wind and damp to relieve pain.

Bai Long Chuan Hua Tou dispels wind and damp to relieve pain.

Ding Shu Xiu relieves headache and migraine.

Shui Ding Xiang clears heat, reduces swelling and inflammation.

Chapter 6 summary

Mo Gu Xiao (Caulis Hyptis Capitatae) and ***Xian Feng Cao*** (Herba Bidentis) promote generation of new flesh.

Mo Gu Xiao unblocks stagnation to promote generation of flesh.

Xian Feng Cao reduces swelling and inflammation to promote generation of flesh.

Bi Zi Cao (Herba Pogonantheri Criniti) treats dysuria caused by a wide variety of disorders, as in urinary tract infection, cystitis, and nephritis.

Dong Gua Zi (Semen Benincasae) clears the Lung to dispel phlegm and abscesses, and treats cough or lung abscesses caused by Lung heat, or by intestinal abscesses.

Shan Pu Tao (Radix Vitis Amurensis) tonifies the Liver and the Kidney to brighten the eyes.

Ma Ti Jin (Herba Dichondrae Repentis) invigorates blood circulation to enhance its effectiveness in regulating water.

Jin Qian Cao (Herba Lysimachiae), ***Hai Jin Sha*** (Herba Lygodii), ***Hua Shi Cao*** (Herba Orthosiphon Aristatus) and ***Shi Wei*** (Folium Pyrrosiae) display excellent abilities to resolve dampness, promote urination, dispel damp-heat, and treat *shi lin* (stone dysuria). These herbs are often used together to dissolve and dispel stones.

Jin Qian Cao is the most effective herb for dissolving both gallstones and kidney stones.

Hai Jin Sha is effective to treat both kinds of stones, but also clears heat and eliminates toxins.

Hua Shi Cao addresses both gallstones and kidney stones, as well as hepatitis and nephritis.

Shi Wei reduces edema, and is used for kidney stones but not for gallstones. It also resolves phlegm.

Yin Chen Hao (Herba Artemisiae Scopariae) is essential in treatment of both yin- and yang-type jaundice. It treats gallstones and cholecystitis (with or without jaundice), clears heat, dispels dampness and treats various dermatological disorders caused by damp-heat.

Chi Xiao Dou (Semen Phaseoli) promotes diuresis, reduces swelling and treats jaundice. Externally, it eliminates toxins, expels pus and reduces swelling and carbuncles.

Yu Mi Xu (Stigma Maydis) clears damp-heat from the Liver and Gallbladder, treating hepatitis, cholecystitis and gallstones caused by damp-heat.

Bi Xie (Rhizoma Dioscoreae Hypoglaucae) is an essential herb to separate clear urine from turbid urine. Clinically, it treats nephritis and urinary tract infections, and dispels wind and dampness in *bi zheng* (painful obstruction syndrome).

Dong Gua Pi (Exocarpium Benincasae) is used strictly to regulate water and relieve edema.

Ze Qi (Herba Euphorbiae Helioscopiae) treats cough with phlegm and sputum, or nodules of phlegm stagnation.

Dong Kui Zi (Semen Malvae) promotes lactation and relieves constipation.

Chapter 6 summary

HERBS FROM OTHER FUNCTIONAL CATEGORIES WITH WATER-REGULATING AND DAMP-RESOLVING FUNCTIONS

Name	Functional Category
Bai Mao Gen (Rhizoma Imperatae)	Stop-Bleeding Herbs (Chapter 11)
Bai Zhu (Rhizoma Atractylodis Macrocephalae)	Tonic Herbs (Chapter 17)
Ban Bian Lian (Herba Lobeliae Chinensis)	Heat-Clearing Herbs (Chapter 2)
Fen Fang Ji (Radix Stephaniae Tetandrae)	Wind-Damp Dispelling Herbs (Chapter 4)
Fu Ping (Herba Spirodelae)	Exterior-Releasing Herbs (Chapter 1)
Huang Qi (Radix Astragali)	Tonic Herbs (Chapter 17)
Ma Huang (Herba Ephedrae)	Exterior-Releasing Herbs (Chapter 1)
Qian Niu Zi (Semen Pharbitidis)	Downward Draining Herbs (Chapter 3)
Shang Lu (Radix Phytolaccae)	Downward Draining Herbs (Chapter 3)
Ting Li Zi (Semen Descurainiae seu Lepidii)	Phlegm-Resolving and Coughing- and Wheezing-Relieving Herbs (Chapter 13)
Xiang Ru (Herba Elsholtziae seu Moslae)	Exterior-Releasing Herbs (Chapter 1)
Yi Mu Cao (Herba Leonuri)	Blood-Invigorating and Stasis-Removing Herbs (Chapter 12)
Ze Lan (Herba Lycopi)	Blood-Invigorating and Stasis-Removing Herbs (Chapter 12)

Chapter 7

— Interior-Warming Herbs

温里药

Chapter 7 — Interior-Warming Herbs

Chapter 7

温里药

— Interior-Warming Herbs

Definition: Herbs that warm the interior, as the name implies, warm the interior of the body and dispel cold.

Cold disorders may affect the exterior or interior of the body. When cold attacks the exterior, acrid and warm herbs dispel cold and release the exterior. When cold affects the interior, acrid and hot herbs dispel cold and restore internal warmth. Interior-warming herbs are acrid, bitter and warm. They dispel interior cold and fortify yang to treat excess cold attacking the interior, or yang deficiency leading to invasion of cold. Herbs that warm the interior may serve one or more of the following functions:

- dispel cold to relieve epigastric and abdominal pain
- warm the ***Spleen*** and ***Stomach*** to treat nausea, vomiting, diarrhea and dysentery
- strengthen yang to relieve aversion to cold, cold extremities, pale face, clear urine, pale tongue with white coat, and deep, thready pulse
- restore yang in individuals experiencing yang collapse, with extreme coldness of the extremities, polyuria with clear urine, profuse perspiration, and failing pulse.

Interior-warming herbs restore normal functioning of the internal organs.

SUBCATEGORIES OF ACTION

Herbs that warm the interior are not divided into subcategories, but they do individually enter different organs and treat different patterns of illness. It is important to keep in mind that each herb has distinct properties and indications for use. Some are extremely potent and restore collapsed yang, while others are mild to moderate in potency and gradually dispel cold and warm yang.

Though **interior-warming** herbs and **yang-tonifying** herbs are identified in separate categories, they share many similarities amid their differences. Interior-warming herbs primarily warm Heart and Spleen yang to drive out excess cold, while yang-tonifying herbs mainly replenish Kidney yang, blood, and *jing* (essence), and strengthen tendons and bones.

- Interior-warming herbs are usually acrid, warm or hot, and drying. Some interior-warming herbs are sweet, salty and moistening in nature to help tonify the yang and benefit the *jing* (essence), blood, bones and tendons. These herbs enter the Heart, Spleen and Kidney to warm the organs and dispel internal cold. This treats excess cold, Heart and Kidney yang deficiencies, invasion of cold, and yang qi trapped by excess invasion of cold.
- Yang-tonifying herbs are mostly sweet, salty, and warm, and they enter the Kidney channel to treat Kidney yang deficiency and related symptoms. The salty taste signifies that the herbs enter the Kidney channel and the sweet taste denotes the tonic nature of the herbs.

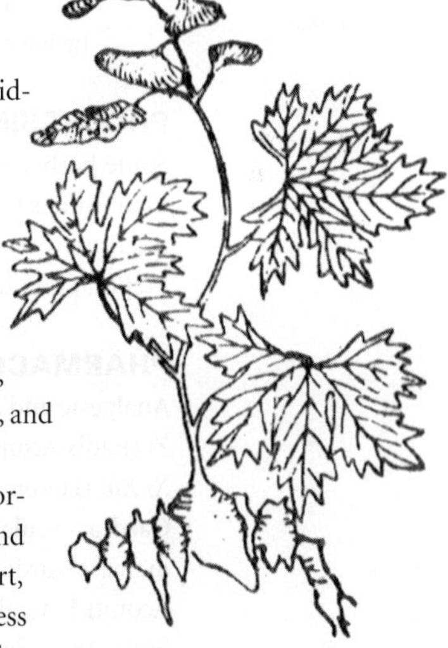

Fu Zi (Radix Aconiti Lateralis Praeparata) *Ben Cao Gang Mu* (Materia Medica), by Li Shi-Zhen, 1578 A.D.

DIFFERENTIAL DIAGNOSIS AND TREATMENT

Correct differential diagnosis requires assessment of the affected location, the severity of cold excess and yang deficiency, and awareness of whether the illness is acute, chronic, or an acute flare-up of a chronic condition.

Location: Assessment of the location of cold excess requires discerning whether the pathogen is at the exterior or has penetrated to the interior. External cold requires the use of exterior-releasing herbs, while internal cold requires the use of interior-warming herbs.

Chapter 7 — Interior-Warming Herbs

Severity: Assessment of the location and severity of yang deficiency refers to determining which organ is affected, and whether yang is merely deficient, or on the verge of collapse. The ***Spleen, Stomach*** and ***Kidney*** are the organs most vulnerable to yang deficiency. In addition to herbs that warm the interior, herbs that tonify yang should be added as well.

Acute or **chronic**: Acute conditions often involve the collapse of yang, characterized by symptoms such as extreme coldness of the extremities, profuse perspiration, and a failing pulse. Such conditions require immediate and aggressive treatment to revive the patient. Chronic conditions often involve simultaneous cold excess and yang deficiency. Symptoms that indicate internal cold and yang deficiency include epigastric and abdominal pain, vomiting, hiccups, poor appetite, diarrhea or loose stools, intolerance to cold, coldness of the extremities, pale complexion, clear polyuria, pale tongue with a thin, white coating, and a deep, thready pulse. Exact symptoms vary depending on the organs affected. Therefore, optimal treatment requires continuous and gentle therapy to dispel cold and to warm yang.

Interior-warming herbs primarily warm Heart and Spleen yang. *Yang-tonifying* herbs mainly replenish Kidney yang, blood, and *jing* (essence).

CAUTIONS/CONTRAINDICATIONS

- Acrid, warm and drying, interior-warming herbs are contraindicated in cases of excess heat and in yin deficiency. They must be used with caution for patients with deficiencies of body fluids or blood, patients who are bleeding, or who have true heat masked by false cold.
- Some of these herbs should be used with caution during pregnancy.
- Do not prescribe at larger than appropriate dosage or use these herbs for an extended period of time.

Note: Patients experiencing conditions of extreme cold may vomit after drinking the interior-warming decoction. To avoid this, either add some heat-clearing herbs to the formula or have the patient drink the decoction when it has cooled to room temperature.

PROCESSING

Some herbs that warm the interior are toxic and must be processed separately before decocting, to minimize the risk of side effects and adverse reactions. Examples of interior-warming herbs that require processing include *Fu Zi* (Radix Aconiti Lateralis Praeparata), *Chuan Wu* (Radix Aconiti Preparata) and *Cao Wu* (Radix Aconiti Kusnezoffii).

PHARMACOLOGICAL EFFECTS

- **Analgesic and anesthetic:** Varying degrees of analgesic strength are represented in herbs such as *Fu Zi* (Radix Aconiti Lateralis Praeparata), *Rou Gui* (Cortex Cinnamomi), *Wu Zhu Yu* (Fructus Evodiae), *Xi Xin* (Herba Asari), *Hua Jiao* (Pericarpium Zanthoxyli) and *Ding Xiang* (Flos Caryophylli).
- **Cardiovascular:** Interior-warming herbs have positive inotropic and chronotropic actions to increase cardiac contractility, dilate blood vessels, and increase cardiac output. *Fu Zi* (Radix Aconiti Lateralis Praeparata) is one of the strongest herbs to increase heart rate and contractile force. In addition, both *Fu Zi* and *Rou Gui* (Cortex Cinnamomi) dilate the coronary arteries, increase blood perfusion to cardiac muscle, and increase cardiac output. Other herbs with cardiotonic effects include *Gan Jiang* (Rhizoma Zingiberis), *Hu Jiao* (Fructus Piper), and *Wu Zhu Yu* (Fructus Evodiae).
- **Gastrointestinal:** Many interior-warming herbs stimulate the gastrointestinal system to increase the production and secretion of saliva and gastric acid, improve digestion and absorption, and increase peristalsis of the intestines.

  Substances that increase the release of saliva and gastric acid include *Gan Jiang* (Rhizoma Zingiberis), *Ding Xiang* (Flos Caryophylli), and *Gao Liang Jiang* (Rhizoma Alpiniae Officinarum).

  Herbs that increase peristalsis of the intestines include *Gan Jiang* (Rhizoma Zingiberis), *Ding Xiang* (Flos Caryophylli), *Wu Zhu Yu* (Fructus Evodiae), and *Hu Jiao* (Fructus Piper).

Chapter 7 — Interior-Warming Herbs

Interior-warming herbs that exert antiulcer actions include *Gan Jiang* (Rhizoma Zingiberis), *Rou Gui* (Cortex Cinnamomi), *Wu Zhu Yu* (Fructus Evodiae), *Fu Zi* (Radix Aconiti Lateralis Praeparata), *Hua Jiao* (Pericarpium Zanthoxyli), *Xiao Hui Xiang* (Fructus Foeniculi) and *Ding Xiang* (Flos Caryophylli).

- **Antibiotic:** Some inhibit the activity of dermatophytes, such as *Rou Gui* (Cortex Cinnamomi), *Gan Jiang* (Rhizoma Zingiberis), *Ding Xiang* (Flos Caryophylli), and *Xiao Hui Xiang* (Fructus Foeniculi).

POTENTIAL HERB-DRUG INTERACTIONS

- **Analgesics:** While the analgesic effect is not completely understood, it is clear that these herbs do not cause drowsiness, and therefore will not accentuate sedation when combined with drugs having sedative and/or hypnotic properties.
- **Cardiovascular agents:** Interior-warming herbs have marked positive inotropic and chronotropic effects, with one example being *Fu Zi* (Radix Aconiti Lateralis Praeparata).[1] Thus, they should be used with caution in patients having certain cardiovascular disorders (such as arrhythmia) or who are on certain medications (such as digoxin or thyroid supplements).
- **Antiulcers:** Lastly, many herbs in this category stimulate the gastrointestinal system to increase production of gastric acid, such as *Ding Xiang* (Flos Caryophylli). Therefore, some of these herbs may counter the effects of certain drugs such as histamine-2 receptor antagonists (such as ranitidine or famotidine) or proton-pump inhibitors (such as omeprazole or lansoprazole).

References

1. *Zhong Yao Tong Bao* (Journal of Chinese Herbology), 1988; 13(6):40

Fu Zi (Radix Aconiti Lateralis Praeparata)

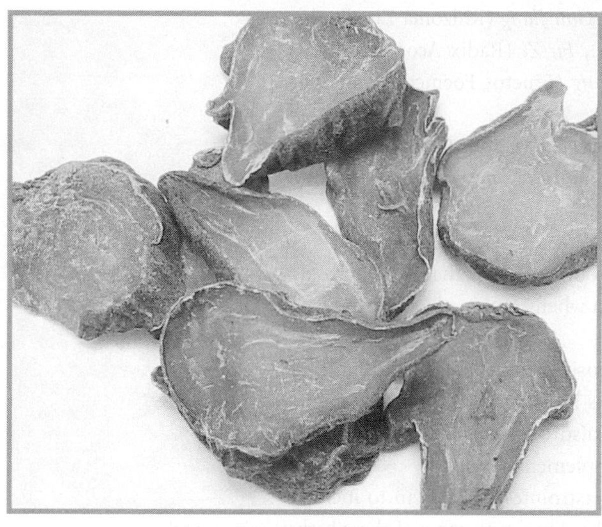

附子

Pinyin Name: *Fu Zi*
Literal Name: "appendage"
Original Source: *Shen Nong Ben Cao Jing* (Divine Husbandman's Classic of the Materia Medica) in the second century
English Name: aconite, prepared daughter root of common monks' hood
Botanical Name: *Aconitum carmichaeli* Debx. (*Wu Tou*)
Pharmaceutical Name: Radix Aconiti Lateralis Praeparata
Properties: acrid, hot
Channels Entered: Heart, Kidney, Spleen
Safety Index: toxic

CHINESE THERAPEUTIC ACTIONS

1. Restores Depleted Yang

Yang failure: Acrid and hot, *Fu Zi* (Radix Aconiti Lateralis Praeparata) is used in emergency situations in which there is a complete void of yang energy in the body. This critical condition is characterized by profuse perspiration with clear and cold sweats, intolerance of cold, faint respiration, icy extremities, diarrhea containing undigested food, and faint or imperceptible pulse. *Fu Zi* restores depleted yang by tonifying Heart yang, thus opening channels and collaterals, and by tonifying Kidney yang to augment fire.

- Intolerance of cold, icy extremities, and diarrhea with undigested food because of depleted yang: use *Fu Zi* with *Gan Jiang* (Rhizoma Zingiberis) and *Gan Cao* (Radix Glycyrrhizae). **Exemplar Formula:** *Si Ni Tang* (Frigid Extremities Decoction).
- Profuse perspiration with shortness of breath and increased respiration due to depletion of yang with qi escaping the body: add *Ren Shen* (Radix Ginseng).
- Shock or heart failure: *Fu Zi* is used as an injectable substance in China for this application.
- Lower body edema, dysuria: combine *Fu Zi* with *Fu Ling* (Poria).

2. Tonifies Yang, Augments Fire

Fu Zi treats any type of yang deficiency, as it warms all of the organs and opens all of the channels and collaterals. The organs that are most susceptible to yang deficiency are Kidney, Spleen and Heart.

Kidney yang deficiency: Kidney yang deficiency, the most severe of yang deficiencies, is characterized by cold extremities (especially the lower extremities), intolerance to cold, weakness, coldness and soreness of the low back and knees, impotence, frequent urination (especially during the night), clear polyuria, pale complexion, cough, and wheezing. Secondary symptoms may include impotence or spermatorrhea, profuse and clear leukorrhea, diarrhea (especially during the early morning), edema and infertility.

- Kidney yang deficiency: use *Fu Zi* with *Rou Gui* (Cortex Cinnamomi) and *Shu Di Huang* (Radix Rehmanniae Preparata). **Exemplar Formula:** *You Gui Wan* (Restore the Right [Kidney] Pill), or *Ba Wei Di Huang Wan* (Eight-Ingredient Pill with Rehmannia).
- Infertility: use this herb with *Lu Jiao* (Cornu Cervi), *Shu Di Huang* (Radix Rehmanniae Preparata), *Rou Gui* (Cortex Cinnamomi), *Tu Si Zi* (Semen Cuscutae), *Yang Qi Shi* (Actinolitum), *Ba Ji Tian* (Radix Morindae Officinalis), *Dang Gui* (Radicis Angelicae Sinensis) and *Gou Qi Zi* (Fructus Lycii).
- Impotence: combine it with *Tu Si Zi* (Semen Cuscutae), *Yin Yang Huo* (Herba Epimedii) and *Rou Gui* (Cortex Cinnamomi).

Spleen yang deficiency: Spleen yang deficiency is more severe than Spleen qi deficiency. Patients suffering from this disorder manifest all signs of Spleen qi deficiency, plus abdominal fullness, coldness and dull pain, decreased intake of food, loose stools or diarrhea, edema, profuse watery leukorrhea, cold limbs and a preference for pressure and warmth applied to the abdomen.

- Spleen yang deficiency: use *Fu Zi* with *Ren Shen* (Radix Ginseng), *Gan Jiang* (Rhizoma Zingiberis) and *Bai Zhu* (Rhizoma Atractylodis Macrocephalae). **Exemplar Formula:** *Fu Zi Li Zhong Tang* (Prepared Aconite Pill to Regulate the Middle).

Fu Zi (Radix Aconiti Lateralis Praeparata)

- Spleen and Kidney yang deficiency with edema: use it with *Bai Zhu* (Rhizoma Atractylodis Macrocephalae) and *Fu Ling* (Poria). **Exemplar Formula:** *Zhen Wu Tang* (True Warrior Decoction).

Heart yang deficiency: Clinical manifestations include palpitations, shortness of breath, chest pain, dull purplish complexion, cold extremities, a flabby, pale or dark purple tongue, and a deep, weak pulse. In the range of Heart conditions, Heart qi deficiency is least serious, followed by Heart yang deficiency, and then Heart yang collapse being most serious.

- Heart yang deficiency: use *Fu Zi* with *Ren Shen* (Radix Ginseng) and *Gui Zhi* (Ramulus Cinnamomi).
- Heart yang collapse with vomiting, fading pulse, icy extremities and profuse perspiration: combine this herb with *Gan Jiang* (Rhizoma Zingiberis), *Zhi Gan Cao* (Radix Glycyrrhizae Preparata) and *Ren Shen* (Radix Ginseng).
- Shock: use it with *Ren Shen* (Radix Ginseng), *Mai Men Dong* (Radix Ophiopogonis), and *Wu Wei Zi* (Fructus Schisandrae Chinensis) as a decoction, administered through the nose.
- Yang deficiency with exterior wind-cold: use this herb with *Ma Huang* (Herba Ephedrae) and *Xi Xin* (Herba Asari).

3. Warms Channels, Disperses Cold and Dampness, Relieves Pain

***Bi zheng* (painful obstruction syndrome) due to cold:** *Fu Zi* dispels cold and dampness from the peripheral channels and collaterals to treat *bi zheng*.

- *Bi zheng* caused by cold and dampness: use *Fu Zi* with *Gui Zhi* (Ramulus Cinnamomi), *Bai Zhu* (Rhizoma Atractylodis Macrocephalae), and *Gan Cao* (Radix Glycyrrhizae).
- Joint and muscle pain, numbness and difficulty of movement: use it with *Qiang Huo* (Rhizoma et Radix Notopterygii), *Du Huo* (Radix Angelicae Pubescentis), *Wei Ling Xian* (Radix Clematidis), and *Sang Ji Sheng* (Herba Taxilli).

Menstrual Pain: *Fu Zi* can be used with *Dang Gui* (Radicis Angelicae Sinensis), *Wu Ling Zhi* (Excrementum Trogopteri seu Pteromi), and *Yan Hu Suo* (Rhizoma Corydalis) for menstrual pain caused by cold.

Yin sores: *Fu Zi* disperses cold and opens collaterals to facilitate the healing of yin sores that do not ulcerate, or ulcerate but do not heal.

- Yin sores: use *Fu Zi* with *Ren Shen* (Radix Ginseng) and *Huang Qi* (Radix Astragali).

DOSAGE

The normal dosage is 3 to 15 grams. *Fu Zi* must be pre-decocted for 30 to 60 minutes.

There are two major schools of thought regarding appropriate dosages of *Fu Zi*. Some scholars have proposed dosages of up to 100 grams for severe cases. Others proposed small dosages only.

When prescribing this herb, the condition of the individual must be taken into consideration. An individual with a weak constitution will react to the toxicity of *Fu Zi* even when it is prescribed at a low dose. Another individual with a stronger constitution and thus higher tolerance may not experience adverse effects even at a large dose. This difference in response depends on the individual constitution as well as geographic, weather and lifestyle differences. In some areas of China, *Fu Zi* is commonly used with other vegetables to make stew. Naturally, these people will have higher tolerance for the toxicity of *Fu Zi*. In short, the dosage should be selected cautiously according to the condition of each patient.

Fu Zi is generally sold in the processed form only, as the unprocessed form is quite toxic. Though there are multiple ways to process this herb, the most common way is for the manufacturer to cook the herb at boiling temperature for 4 to 6 hours before drying and distribution. Prior to use, the patient should again pre-decocted *Fu Zi* for 30 to 60 minutes before the addition of other herbs.

Use of unprocessed *Fu Zi*, or overdose of the herb, are responsible for the majority of possible adverse reactions. Proper processing reduces the toxicity of *Fu Zi* to between 1/2000 and 1/4000th of the toxicity of the unprocessed herb.[1]

CAUTIONS / CONTRAINDICATIONS

- *Fu Zi* is contraindicated during pregnancy.
- *Fu Zi* is contraindicated in patients with yang excess and yin deficiency (also referred to as false cold and true heat).
- Some classic texts have suggested that *Fu Zi* is incompatible with *Bei Mu* (Bulbus Fritillaria), *Ban Xia* (Rhizoma Pinelliae), *Gua Lou Shi* (Fructus Trichosanthis), *Bai Ji* (Rhizoma Bletillae), and *Bai Lian* (Radix Ampelopsis).
- Consumption of alcohol is contraindicated with *Fu Zi*, as absorption of the toxic elements will be greatly enhanced.
- Side effects and adverse reactions are usually due to overdose, to improper processing, or to inappropriate combination with other herbs, and/or inaccurate diagnosis.

OVERDOSAGE

Signs and symptoms of *Fu Zi* overdose include involuntary salivation, nausea, vomiting, diarrhea, dizziness,

Fu Zi (Radix Aconiti Lateralis Praeparata)

blurred vision, dry mouth, vertigo, numbness of the body and extremities, slowed pulse, difficulty breathing, twitching limbs, convulsions, disorientation, urinary and fecal incontinence, decreased blood pressure and body temperature, arrhythmia, tachyarrhythmia, bradycardia, and possible death.[2]

One text divided *Fu Zi* overdose into acute and chronic cases. Symptoms in acute cases are described as numbness, tremor, irregularity, and deterioration. Numbness is characterized by numbness starting at the lips, tongue, and mouth, and gradually spreading to the body and extremities. Tremor is characterized by involuntary movement and tremor of the tongue and extremities, which will impair normal speech and movement. Irregularity describes the heart rate and rhythm, which may be fast, slow, knotted, or unpredictable. Lastly, deterioration refers to compromise in all aspects of physical functioning, with altered consciousness, weak respiration, extremely weak pulse, hypotension, and extreme coldness of the extremities. Chronic cases of overdose are characterized by numbness of the legs, dysuria, painful urination, and blurred vision.[3]

A hospital-based study in Hong Kong reported that up to 61% of all serious poisonings attributed to herbal medicines were associated with the use of various types of aconite root. The study, however, did not clearly describe whether the toxic reactions were due to overdosage, incorrect use, accidental ingestion, or other causes.[4]

TREATMENT OF OVERDOSAGE

Rou Gui (Cortex Cinnamomi) is usually used to reverse early-stage overdose within 4 to 6 hours of the ingestion of *Fu Zi*. According to one report, acute *Fu Zi* poisoning in 14 patients was treated by oral ingestion of *Rou Gui* tea that was prepared by soaking 5 to 10 grams of the herb in hot water. The tea should induce vomiting of the toxin within 5 to 15 minutes, and relieve overall symptoms within 15 to 30 minutes. If toxic symptoms persist, repeat the process by using 3 to 5 grams of *Rou Gui* in tea. Resolution of poisoning is characterized by warmth at the extremities, increased contractility of the heart, and gradual sensory recovery from numbness of the mouth, lips, and extremities.[5]

Overdose of *Fu Zi* can also be treated with a decoction containing *Sheng Jiang* (Rhizoma Zingiberis Recens), *Gan Cao* (Radix Glycyrrhizae), *Gan Jiang* (Rhizoma Zingiberis), *Lu Dou* (Semen Phaseoli Radiati), *Hei Dou* (Semen Glycine Max), *Huang Lian* (Rhizoma Coptidis), *Ren Shen* (Radix Ginseng) and *Huang Qi* (Radix Astragali). The dosage of each of the herbs will vary depending on the specific condition of the patient.

Overdose characterized by irregular heartbeat can be treated with a decoction of 20 grams of *Ku Shen Gen* (Radix Sophorae Flavescentis) and 10 grams of *Gan Cao* (Radix Glycyrrhizae).

Overdose characterized by extreme coldness of the extremities, extremely weak pulse, and shortness of breath, can be treated with a decoction of *Ren Shen* (Radix Ginseng), *Gan Cao* (Radix Glycyrrhizae), and *Gan Jiang* (Rhizoma Zingiberis).

[Note: Gross overdose of *Fu Zi* is potentially life-threatening. Therefore, treatment of overdose should be performed carefully, and only by qualified health-care professionals.]

CHEMICAL COMPOSITION

Aconitine, mesaconitine, hypaconitine, isodelphinine, benzoylmesaconitine, coryneine, atisines, aminophenols, neoline, 15-α-hydroxyneoline, higenamine, dl-demethyl coclaurine, salsolinol.[6,7]

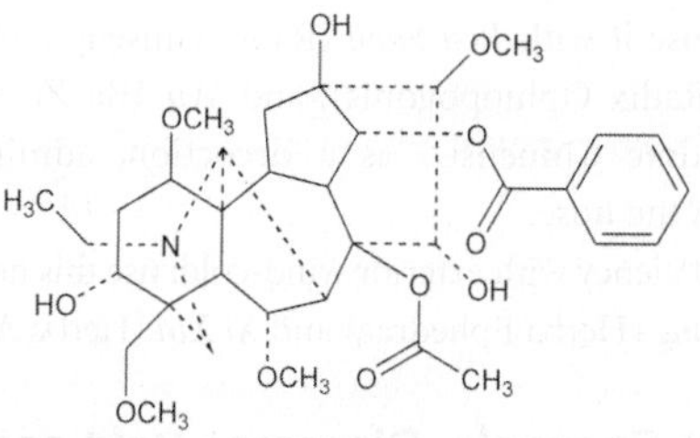

Aconitine

PHARMACOLOGICAL EFFECTS

- **Cardiovascular:** Administration of *Fu Zi* is associated with positive inotropic and chronotropic effects. In animal experiments, intravenous injection of *Fu Zi* increased cardiac contractility, dilated blood vessels, and increased cardiac output. It also increases heart rate and treats patients with bradycardia or bradyarrhythmia. Experiments in cats and rats have also shown *Fu Zi* to be beneficial in the treatment of shock, as it increases blood pressure and cardiac contraction.[8]
- **Anti-inflammatory:** Oral administration of a 20% *Fu Zi* decoction at the dosage of 2.5 ml/100g in rats has demonstrated marked effectiveness to reduce inflammation and swelling in the joints. The exact mechanism of action is unclear. Some studies show that it stimulates secretions by the adrenal cortex, leading to anti-inflammatory activity. Other studies, however, show that *Fu Zi* has anti-inflammatory influence even in animals whose adrenal glands have been removed.[9]
- **Analgesic:** Intraperitoneal injection of *Fu Zi* significantly increased pain tolerance in mice and rats.[10]

CLINICAL STUDIES AND RESEARCH

- **Abdominal coldness and pain during pregnancy:** A

Fu Zi (Radix Aconiti Lateralis Praeparata)

classic text reported that *Fu Zi* was used to treat 4 women who were 4 months pregnant with coldness in the lower abdominal region, abdominal distention and pain, and aversion to cold. All 4 women had previous history of early deliveries. The diagnosis according to traditional Chinese medicine was coldness in the internal organs requiring the use of warm herbs. After herbal treatment, the symptoms improved and all delivered after full-term pregnancies.[11] [Note: The use of *Fu Zi* is generally considered contraindicated during pregnancy. This is a rare report that discussed the use of *Fu Zi* during pregnancy. This should not be attempted unless the benefit clearly outweighs the risks.]

- **Deficiency syndrome:** According to one report, 13 patients with generalized deficiency were treated with injections of *Fu Zi* one time daily at night for 2 weeks per course of treatment, with a total of 1 to 2 courses. The study reported an overall improvement of symptoms, and was especially effective in patients characterized by yang deficiency.[12]

HERB-DRUG INTERACTION

- **Antiarrhythmics:** Patients who have a past history of cardiovascular disorders or are taking antiarrhythmic medications should take *Fu Zi* with extreme caution.[13] [Note: Examples of antiarrhythmics include quinidine, procainamide (Pronestyl), disopyramide (Norpace), flecainide (Tambocor), propafenone (Rythmol), and amiodarone (Cordarone).]

TOXICOLOGY

The LD_{50} for unprocessed *Fu Zi* in mice is 5.49 g/kg via oral administration and 0.49 g/kg via intravenous injection. The LD_{50} for processed *Fu Zi* is 161 g/kg via oral administration and 3.516 g/kg via intravenous injection. The LD_{50} for water extract of *Fu Zi* in mice is 26.30 g/kg.[14,15]

AUTHORS' COMMENTS

Fu Zi is an extremely important herb to tonify yang, and there is no other herb in the entire pharmacopoeia with equivalent functions that can be used as a substitute. However, it should also be used with great caution, as it has a relatively narrow range of safety.

There is a saying: "*Fu Zi* is not hot without *Gan Jiang* (Rhizoma Zingiberis)." When used together, the two herbs have a synergistic interaction that enhances the warming influence of the formula, compared to when either is used alone. *Gan Jiang* also decreases the toxicity of *Fu Zi*.

Fu Zi is generally used in combination with other herbs that increase the therapeutic effect and minimize potential side effects. For example, the use of *Fu Zi* as a single herb treatment for its cardiotonic effect is not appropriate, as it only has moderate potency, short duration and numerous side effects. However, when combined with *Gan Cao* (Radix Glycyrrhizae) or *Gan Jiang* (Rhizoma Zingiberis), the combination has more potent cardiotonic effect and prolonged duration of action. Furthermore, the addition of these two herbs will decrease the potential for side effects of *Fu Zi* by just over fourfold.

Fu Zi, extremely acrid and hot, is highly effective in restoring yang and warming the body. It is an important herb for treating yang deficiency with excess accumulation of cold. In cases of yang collapse, this herb is indispensable in restoring life, or the vital yang, to the body. However, because of the powerful effect this herb exerts, accurate diagnosis is essential. Essential indications for the use of *Fu Zi* include: a flabby, pale tongue with a white or greasy coating, a thready, weak pulse or deep and slow pulse, a bland taste in the mouth with no desire to drink, cold limbs, intolerance to cold, soreness, coldness and weakness of the lower back and knees; and clear polyuria.

Fu Zi can be used in patients with mixed yin and yang symptoms. *Fu Zi* is often combined with warm herbs such as *Rou Gui* (Cortex Cinnamomi), *Gan Jiang* (Rhizoma Zingiberis), *Gan Cao* (Radix Glycyrrhizae), *Bai Zhu* (Rhizoma Atractylodis Macrocephalae), *Ren Shen* (Radix Ginseng), *Huang Qi* (Radix Astragali) and other qi-tonic or interior-warming herbs. However, it is also used with cold herbs such as *Da Huang* (Radix et Rhizoma Rhei) to treat cold-type constipation. It is combined with *Huang Lian* (Rhizoma Coptidis) to treat epigastric fullness due to yang deficiency. The combination of *Fu Zi* and *Yin Chen Hao* (Herba Artemisiae Scopariae) treats yin-type jaundice caused by cold and dampness. With *Long Dan Cao* (Radix Gentianae), it treats damp-heat in the Liver and Gallbladder affecting a yang-deficient Spleen. To nourish blood or stop bleeding due to yang deficiency, *Fu Zi* can be combined with *Sheng Di Huang* (Radix Rehmanniae). Also, interestingly, it can also be used in Heart yang deficiency patients who have febrile disorders.

References

1. *Zhong Yao Xue* (Chinese Herbology), 1998; 367-371
3. *Yao Xue Xue Bao* (Journal of Herbology), 1983; 18(5):394
3. *Zhong Yao Du Li Xue* (Toxicology of Chinese Herbs), 94-98, 1989
4. *Vet Human Toxicol*, 1995 April 37(2)
5. *Xin Zhong Yi* (New Chinese Medicine), 1987; 5:53
6. *Xian Dai Zhong Yao Yao Li Xue* (Contemporary Pharmacology of Chinese Herbs), 1997; 600
7. *The Merck Index* 12th edition, Chapman & Hall/CRCnetBASE/Merck, 2000
8. *Yao Xue Xue Bao* (Journal of Herbology), 1983; 18(5):394)
9. *Zhong Yao Tong Bao* (Journal of Chinese Herbology), 1988; 13(6):40
10. *Zhong Guo Zhong Yao Za Zhi* (People's Republic of China Journal of Chinese Herbology), 1992; 17(2):104

7 INTERIOR-WARMING HERBS

Fu Zi (Radix Aconiti Lateralis Praeparata)

11. *Zhong Yi Za Zhi* (Journal of Chinese Medicine), 1964; 5:10
12. *Zhong Xi Yi Jie He Za Zhi* (Journal of Integrated Chinese and Western Medicine), 1985; 4:219
13. Chen, J. Recognition & prevention of herb-drug interactions, *Medical Acupuncture*, Fall/Winter 1998/1999; volume 10/number 2; 9-13
14. *Zhong Yao Xue* (Chinese Herbology), 1993; 137
15. *Zhong Yao Yao Li Yu Ying Yong* (Pharmacology and Applications of Chinese Herbs), 1983; 575

Chuan Wu (Radix Aconiti Preparata)

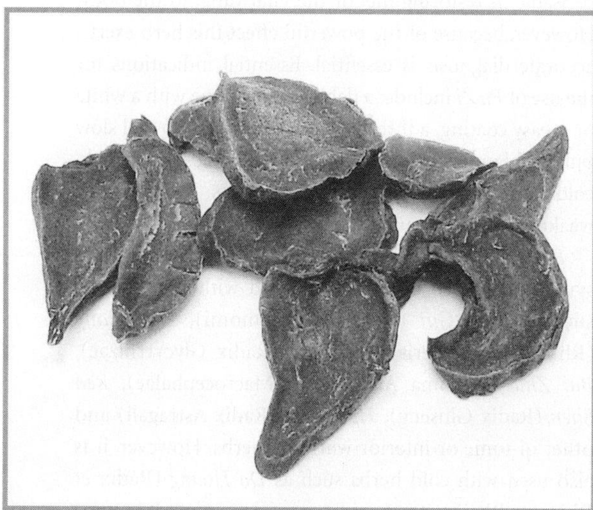

川烏 川乌

Pinyin Name: *Chuan Wu*
Literal Name: "crow's head from Sichuan"
Original Source: *Shen Nong Ben Cao Jing* (Divine Husbandman's Classic of the Materia Medica) in the second century
English Name: aconite wutou, Sichuan aconite, mother root of common monks' hood
Botanical Name: *Aconitum carmichaeli* Debx. (*Chuan Wu*)
Pharmaceutical Name: Radix Aconiti Preparata
Properties: acrid, bitter, hot
Channels Entered: Heart, Liver, Spleen
Safety Index: extremely toxic

CHINESE THERAPEUTIC ACTIONS

1. Dispels Wind, Disperses Cold, and Relieves Pain

***Bi zheng* (painful obstruction syndrome):** *Chuan Wu* (Radix Aconiti Preparata) is acrid and hot and has excellent properties to dispel wind, disperse cold, and relieve pain. It treats pain characterized by wind and dampness, such as headache, abdominal and musculoskeletal pain. *Chuan Wu* is often combined with blood-activating herbs to enable it to treat various kinds of pain.

- Aching and pain in the joints and muscles: apply *Chuan Wu* topically as a plaster or analgesic ointment with *Cao Wu* (Radix Aconiti Kusnezoffii) and *Ma Qian Zi* (Semen Strychni).
- Joint pain with difficulty in extension and flexion: use it with *Ma Huang* (Herba Ephedrae), *Bai Shao* (Radix Paeoniae Alba) and *Huang Qi* (Radix Astragali).
- Muscle spasms and pain with difficulty in movement, because of damp-cold or blood stagnation: use it with *Cao Wu* (Radix Aconiti Kusnezoffii), *Di Long* (Pheretima), *Ru Xiang* (Gummi Olibanum) and *Mo Yao* (Myrrha).
- Coldness and pain in the low back and legs: mix powdered *Chuan Wu* with vinegar and ingest internally or apply topically.
- Headache: use this herb with *Dan Nan Xing* (Arisaema cum Bile), *Sheng Jiang* (Rhizoma Zingiberis Recens) and plums, as a decoction.
- Headache: mix and crush *Chuan Wu*, *Dan Nan Xing* (Arisaema cum Bile) and *Cong Bai* (Bulbus Allii Fistulosi), and apply topically on the acupuncture point *Taiyang*.
- Angina, severe pain in the chest radiating to the back: use this herb with *Fu Zi* (Radix Aconiti Lateralis Praeparata), *Hua Jiao* (Pericarpium Zanthoxyli), *Gan Jiang* (Rhizoma Zingiberis) and *Chi Shi Zhi* (Halloysitum Rubrum).
- Hernia due to cold: use *Chuan Wu* with *Xiao Hui Xiang* (Fructus Foeniculi) and *Feng Mi* (Mel).

2. Reduces Swellings and Treats Abscesses and Lesions

Yin sores: Acrid, dispersing and warm in nature, *Chuan Wu* is commonly used topically for chronic cases of abscesses and lesions. It helps to reduce swellings, and promotes healing of ulcerated sores. It is most suitable for stubborn sores that do not ulcerate or those that have ulcerated but do not heal.

Chuan Wu (Radix Aconiti Preparata)

- Abscess and ulceration: use *Chuan Wu* with *Tian Nan Xing* (Rhizoma Arisaematis), *Chuan Bei Mu* (Bulbus Fritillariae Cirrhosae), *Tian Hua Fen* (Radix Trichosanthis), and *Fu Rong* (Radix Hibisci). Mix with vinegar and apply topically.

3. Treats Unconsciousness Caused by Phlegm Stagnation

According to *Tai Ping Hui Min He Ji Ju Fang* (Imperial Grace Formulary of the Tai Ping Era), unprocessed *Chuan Wu*, unprocessed *Fu Zi* (Radix Aconiti Lateralis), unprocessed *Tian Nan Xing* (Rhizoma Arisaematis), and *Mu Xiang* (Radix Aucklandiae) can be used to treat cases of unconsciousness, deviation of the eyes and mouth, and a roaring sound of phlegm in the throat. [Note: This is an extremely **rare** exception for which one would use the unprocessed forms of *Chuan Wu*, *Fu Zi* and *Tian Nan Xing*. The unprocessed forms of these three herbs are all very toxic.]

DOSAGE

1.5 to 4.5 grams. To reduce toxicity prior to oral administration, *Chuan Wu* is cooked by the manufacturer at boiling temperature for 4 to 6 hours, before drying and distribution. It must again be pre-decocted by the patient for 30 to 60 minutes before the addition of other herbs. Properly prepared, this herb should not have a bitter taste or numbing effect when placed in the mouth.

CAUTIONS / CONTRAINDICATIONS

- *Chuan Wu* is contraindicated in pregnancy.
- *Chuan Wu* is incompatible with *Bei Mu* (Bulbus Fritillaria), *Gua Lou Shi* (Fructus Trichosanthis), *Ban Xia* (Rhizoma Pinelliae), *Bai Ji* (Rhizoma Bletillae) and *Bai Lian* (Radix Ampelopsis).
- Use of the fresh or unprocessed form of aconite should be strictly prohibited because of toxicity. Herbs of the aconite family must be processed to reduce toxicity, which can be lowered to 1/2000 to 1/4000th of that of the unprocessed herb. Concurrent use of alcohol must also be prohibited to avoid increased absorption of toxic components.[1]
- Even with appropriate indications and dosage, *Chuan Wu* should be used with other herbs, such as *Gan Cao* (Radix Glycyrrhizae), *Sheng Jiang* (Rhizoma Zingiberis Recens) or honey, to minimize toxicity,.

OVERDOSAGE

Overdose of *Chuan Wu* is associated with cardiovascular side effects, such as arrhythmia, ventricular tachycardia, ventricular fibrillation and cardiac arrest.[2] Adverse reactions associated with *Chuan Wu* are usually divided into three types: mild, moderate and severe.

- **Mild** reactions are characterized by feelings of numbness, warmth and swelling of the mouth, lips, and fingers, nausea, salivation, abdominal pain, vomiting, hurried respiration, and feelings of oppression in the chest. Reactions often occur within 15 to 30 minutes after ingestion of the herbs, with the patient remaining conscious the entire time.
- **Moderate** reactions are characterized by irritability, perspiration, spasms and cramps of the extremities, speech impairment, dyspnea, hypotension, low body temperature, pale face, cold skin and extremities, and slow and irregular pulse.
- **Severe** reactions are characterized by altered consciousness, purple discoloration of the lips and mouth, extremely weak pulse, urinary and bowel incontinence, and irregular heartbeat.

The toxicity of *Chuan Wu* is usually attributed to aconitine, which has a marked stimulating action followed by an inhibiting effect on the central nervous system and cardiovascular system. Aconitine is absorbed through the gastrointestinal tract and eliminated by the kidneys.[3]

A hospital-based study in Hong Kong reported that up to 61% of all serious poisonings due to herbal medicines were associated with the use of various types of aconite root. The study, however, did not clearly describe whether the toxic reactions were due to overdosage, incorrect use, accidental ingestion, or other causes.[4]

TREATMENT OF OVERDOSAGE

Mild cases of adverse reaction can be relieved by ingestion of 120 grams of honey dissolved in water. Other herbs that have been documented to relieve the toxicity of *Chuan Wu* include *Huang Lian* (Rhizoma Coptidis), *Jin Yin Hua* (Flos Lonicerae), *Hei Dou* (Semen Glycine Max), *Lu Dou* (Semen Phaseoli Radiati), *Gan Cao* (Radix Glycyrrhizae), and *Sheng Jiang* (Rhizoma Zingiberis Recens). Irregular heartbeat caused by *Chuan Wu* can be treated with 30 grams of *Ku Shen* (Radix Sophorae Flavescentis) in decoction.

Please refer to *Fu Zi* (Radix Aconiti Lateralis Praeparata) for additional information on treatment of aconite overdose.

[Note: Gross overdose of *Chuan Wu* is potentially a life-threatening situation. Therefore, treatment of overdose should be performed carefully, and only by qualified healthcare professionals.]

CHEMICAL COMPOSITION

Aconitine, hypaconitine, mesaconitine, talatigamine, carmichaeline, 14-acetyltateizamine, isotalatizidine, karakoline, neoline, lipoaconitine, lipohpaconitine, lipomesaconitine, lipodeoxyaconitine.[5]

Chuan Wu (Radix Aconiti Preparata)

PHARMACOLOGICAL EFFECTS

- **Cardiovascular**: Administration of *Chuan Wu* has a profound and direct effect on the contractile force and rhythm of the heart. Use of unprocessed *Chuan Wu* is often associated with increased heart rate, irregular heart rate, and in severe cases, cardiac arrest. Use of the processed herb (prolonged cooking at high temperature) is associated with increased contractile force of the heart.[6]
- **Analgesic and anti-inflammatory**: *Chuan Wu* has demonstrated marked analgesic and anti-inflammatory effects. In laboratory experiments in mice, the use of aconitine was associated with significant reduction of pain and inflammation. The analgesic effect of aconitine is related to its effect on the central nervous system. The anti-inflammatory effect of aconitine is stronger than aspirin, and its mechanism of action is unrelated to the production of steroids from the adrenal glands.[7]

CLINICAL STUDIES AND RESEARCH

- **Arthritis:** In one study, 150 patients with arthritis caused by wind and dampness were treated with an herbal preparation with a 92.4% overall rate of effectiveness. The formula was given three times daily, and contained *Chuan Wu*, *Cao Wu* (Radix Aconiti Kusnezoffii), *Qiang Huo* (Rhizoma et Radix Notopterygii), *Du Huo* (Radix Angelicae Pubescentis), *Fu Zi* (Radix Aconiti Lateralis Praeparata), *Ru Xiang* (Gummi Olibanum), *Mo Yao* (Myrrha), *Dang Gui* (Radicis Angelicae Sinensis), *Chuan Niu Xi* (Radix Cyathulae), *Ma Huang* (Herba Ephedrae), *Gui Zhi* (Ramulus Cinnamomi), *Wu Gong* (Scolopendra), *Chuan Xiong* (Rhizoma Ligustici Chuanxiong), and *Ma Qian Zi* (Semen Strychni).[8]
- **Inflammation of the shoulder:** According to one report, 10 out of 11 patients with shoulder inflammation experienced complete recovery using an herbal formula that contained 10 grams of *Chuan Wu* (Radix Aconiti Preparata). The formula was given in decoction, twice daily, in the morning and at night, for 6 to 15 days.[9]

HERB-DRUG INTERACTION

- **Antiarrhythmics:** Patients who have a past history of cardiovascular disorders or are taking antiarrhythmic medications should take *Chuan Wu* with extreme caution.[10] [Note: Examples of antiarrhythmics include quinidine, procainamide (Pronestyl), disopyramide (Norpace), flecainide (Tambocor), propafenone (Rythmol), and amiodarone (Cordarone).]

TOXICOLOGY

See *Fu Zi* (Radix Aconiti Lateralis Praeparata).

SUPPLEMENT

- 烏頭 / 乌头 *Wu Tou* (Radix Aconiti) is the inclusive name for *Chuan Wu* (Radix Aconiti Preparata) and *Cao Wu* (Radix Aconiti Kusnezoffii). In the original documentation of this herb in *Shen Nong Ben Cao Jing* (Divine Husbandman's Classic of the Materia Medica) in the second century, no distinction was made between *Chuan Wu* and *Cao Wu*. Later in history, the aconites from the Sichuan province were given the name *Chuan Wu*, and the rest, grown in other regions or wild became known as *Cao Wu*. Interestingly, in the original text, it was stated that *Wu Tou* can be used in hunting. The juice of *Wu Tou* applied to the tip of an arrow will induce paralysis when the arrow penetrates the prey.

AUTHORS' COMMENTS

Chuan Wu is an extremely valuable herb to dispel cold and relieve pain. However, it should also be used with great caution, as it has a relatively narrow range of safety.

References

1. *Zhong Yao Xue* (Chinese Herbology)
2. *Forensic Science International*, 1994 June 28; 55-8
3. *Zhong Yao Du Li Xue* (Toxicology of Chinese Herbs); 35-38, 1989
4. *Vet Human Toxicol*, 1995 April 37(2)
5. *Xian Dai Zhong Yao Yao Li Xue* (Contemporary Pharmacology of Chinese Herbs), 1997; 425
6. Ibid.
7. Ibid.
8. *Nei Meng Gu Zhong Yi Yao* (Traditional Chinese Medicine and Medicinals of Inner Magnolia), 1986; (3):7
9. Ibid.
10. Chen, J. Recognition & prevention of herb-drug interactions, *Medical Acupuncture*, Fall/Winter 1998/1999; volume 10/number 2; 9-13

Cao Wu (Radix Aconiti Kusnezoffii)

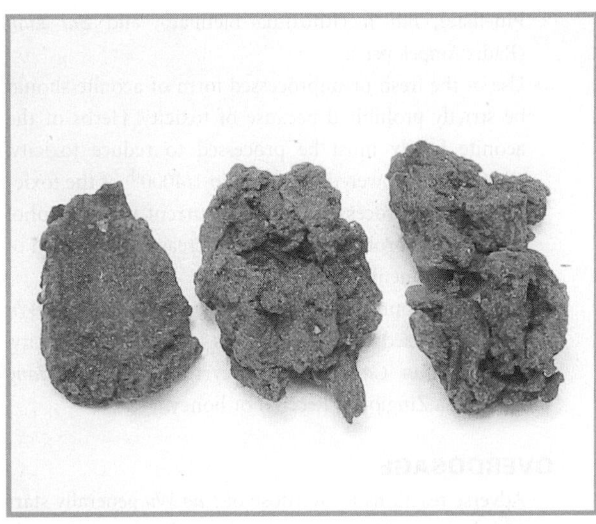

草烏 草乌

Pinyin Name: *Cao Wu*
Original Source: *Shen Nong Ben Cao Jing* (Divine Husbandman's Classic of the Materia Medica) in the second century
English Name: aconite tsaowu, Kusnezoff monks' hood root
Botanical Name: *Aconitum kusnezoffii* Reichb. (*Cao Wu*)
Pharmaceutical Name: Radix Aconiti Kusnezoffii
Properties: acrid, bitter, hot
Channels Entered: Heart, Liver, Spleen
Safety Index: extremely toxic

CHINESE THERAPEUTIC ACTIONS

1. Dispels Wind, Disperses Cold, and Relieves Pain

***Bi zheng* (painful obstruction syndrome):** Acrid and hot, *Cao Wu* (Radix Aconiti Kusnezoffii) is an excellent herb to dispel wind, disperse cold, and relieve pain. It treats pain characterized by wind and dampness, such as headache, abdominal pain, and musculoskeletal pain. Herbs in the blood-activating category are often combined with this herb to further enable it to treat various kinds of pain.

- Muscle spasms and pain with difficulty in movement because of cold-damp or blood stagnation: use *Cao Wu* with *Chuan Wu* (Radix Aconiti Preparata), *Di Long* (Pheretima), *Ru Xiang* (Gummi Olibanum) and *Mo Yao* (Myrrha).
- Atrophy due to wind and dampness: use this herb with *Wu Ling Zhi* (Excrementum Trogopteri seu Pteromi).
- Shortness of breath, coldness and pain in the chest and abdomen due to excess cold: use this herb with *Chi Shi Zhi* (Halloysitum Rubrum).
- Angina, severe pain in the chest radiating to the back: combine it with *Fu Zi* (Radix Aconiti Lateralis Praeparata), *Hua Jiao* (Pericarpium Zanthoxyli), *Gan Jiang* (Rhizoma Zingiberis) and *Chi Shi Zhi* (Halloysitum Rubrum).
- Hernia due to cold: use *Cao Wu* with honey.
- *Bi zheng* (painful obstruction syndrome): combine *Cao Wu* with *Chuan Wu* (Radix Aconiti Preparata) and *Ma Qian Zi* (Semen Strychni), and use topically in plasters or analgesic ointments.

2. Reduces Swellings and Treats Abscesses and Lesions

Yin sores: Acrid, dispersing and warm in nature, *Cao Wu* is commonly used topically for chronic cases of abscesses and lesions. It helps to reduce swelling and promote healing of ulcerated sores. It is most suitable for stubborn sores that do not ulcerate or ulcerated lesions with an inability to heal.

- Cellulitis with hard swelling: mix the powder of *Cao Wu* with *Dan Nan Xing* (Arisaema cum Bile), *Ban Xia* (Rhizoma Pinelliae) and *Lang Du* (Radix Euphorbiae Fischerianae). If mixed with the appropriate heat-clearing, toxin-eliminating herbs, this topical application can treat all types of toxic sores and swellings.
- Abscess and ulceration: use it with *Tian Nan Xing* (Rhizoma Arisaematis), *Chuan Bei Mu* (Bulbus Fritillariae Cirrhosae), *Tian Hua Fen* (Radix Trichosanthis), and *Fu Rong* (Radix Hibisci). Mix with vinegar and apply topically three times daily.

DOSAGE

1.5 to 3.0 grams. To reduce toxicity prior to oral administration, *Cao Wu* is cooked by the manufacturer at boiling temperature for 4 to 6 hours, before drying and distribution. It must again be pre-decocted by the patient for 30 to 60 minutes before the addition of other herbs. Properly prepared, this herb should not have a bitter taste or numbing effect when placed in the mouth.

CAUTIONS / CONTRAINDICATIONS

- *Cao Wu* is contraindicated in pregnancy.
- *Cao Wu* is incompatible with *Bei Mu* (Bulbus Fritillaria), *Gua Lou Shi* (Fructus Trichosanthis), *Ban Xia* (Rhizoma

Cao Wu (Radix Aconiti Kusnezoffii)

Pinelliae), *Bai Ji* (Rhizoma Bletillae), and *Bai Lian* (Radix Ampelopsis).

- Use of the fresh or unprocessed form of aconite should be strictly prohibited because of toxicity. Herbs of the aconite family must be processed to reduce toxicity, which can be lowered to 1/2000 to 1/4000th of the toxicity of the unprocessed herb. Concurrent use of alcohol must also be prohibited to avoid increased absorption of toxic components.[1]
- Even with appropriate indication and dosage, *Cao Wu* should be used with other herbs to minimize toxicity, such as *Gan Cao* (Radix Glycyrrhizae), *Sheng Jiang* (Rhizoma Zingiberis Recens) or honey.

OVERDOSAGE

Adverse reactions to overdose of *Cao Wu* generally start 10 minutes to 3 hours after ingestion. Symptoms include numbness and burning sensations of the tongue and oral cavity, dry mouth, nausea, vomiting, dizziness, blurred vision, numbness of the body and extremities, decreased heart rate, difficulty breathing, and muscle spasms of the arms and legs.

Overdose of *Cao Wu* and *Chuan Wu* (Radix Aconiti Carmichaeli Preparata) is associated with cardiovascular side effects, such as arrhythmia, ventricular tachycardia, ventricular fibrillation and cardiac arrest.[2]

A hospital-based study in Hong Kong reported that up to 61% of all serious poisonings attributed to herbal medicines were associated with the use of various types of aconite root. The study, however, did not clearly describe whether the toxic reactions were due to overdosage, incorrect use, accidental ingestion, or other causes.[3]

TREATMENT OF OVERDOSAGE

Please refer to *Fu Zi* (Radix Aconiti Lateralis Praeparata) and *Chuan Wu* (Radix Aconiti Preparata) for information on treatment of aconite overdose.

[Note: Gross overdose of *Cao Wu* is potentially a life-threatening situation. Therefore, treatment of overdose should be performed carefully, and only by qualified healthcare professionals.]

CHEMICAL COMPOSITION

Aconitine, hypaconitine, mesaconitine, talatigamine, beiwutine, 14-acetyltateizamine, isotalatizidine, karakoline, neoline, lipoaconitine, lipohpaconitine, lipomesaconitine, lipodeoxyaconitine.[4]

HERB-DRUG INTERACTION

- **Antiarrhythmics:** Patients who have a past history of cardiovascular disorders or are taking antiarrhythmic medications should take *Cao Wu* with extreme caution. [Note: Examples of antiarrhythmics include quinidine, procainamide (Pronestyl), disopyramide (Norpace), flecainide (Tambocor), propafenone (Rythmol), and amiodarone (Cordarone).][5]

TOXICOLOGY

The LD_{50} of unprocessed *Cao Wu* in mice is 0.19 g/kg for intraperitoneal injection, and 0.16 g/kg for intravenous injection. The LD_{50} of the processed herb (cooked for 6 hours) in mice is 41.59 g/kg via intraperitoneal injection.[6]

AUTHORS' COMMENTS

In their unprocessed form, the three aconites, *Cao Wu* (Radix Aconiti Kusnezoffii), *Chuan Wu* (Radix Aconiti Preparata) and *Fu Zi* (Radix Aconiti Lateralis Praeparata) are all toxic when ingested by humans. Properly processed, prepared, combined with other herbs and prescribed, these herbs are among the life-saving substances of Chinese medicine. Although unprocessed *Cao Wu* is the most toxic of the three, this does not mean it is less valuable clinically.

Cao Wu is an extremely valuable herb to dispel cold and relieve pain. However, it should also be used with great caution as it has a relatively narrow range of safety.

References

1. *Zhong Yao Xue* (Chinese Herbology), 1998; 367-371
2. *Forensic Science International*, 1994 June 28; 55-8
3. *Vet Human Toxicol*, 1995 April 37(2)
4. *Xian Dai Zhong Yao Yao Li Xue* (Contemporary Pharmacology of Chinese Herbs), 1997; 450
5. Chen, J. Recognition & prevention of herb-drug interactions, *Medical Acupuncture*, Fall/Winter 1998/1999; volume 10/number 2; 9-13
6. *Lin Chuan Shou Ce You Du Zhong Yao Shi Yong* (Clinical Handbook on Applications of Toxic Chinese Herbs), 1992; 22:23

Rou Gui (Cortex Cinnamomi)

肉桂

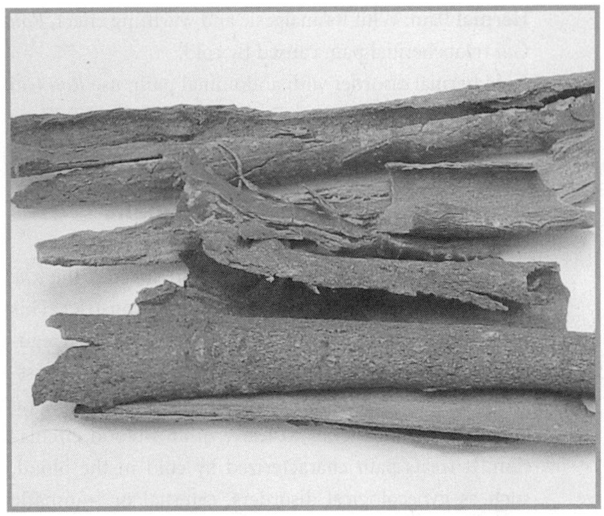

Pinyin Name: *Rou Gui*
Alternate Chinese Names: *Gui Pi, Guan Gui*
Original Source: *Shen Nong Ben Cao Jing* (Divine Husbandman's Classic of the Materia Medica) in the second century
English Name: cinnamon bark, cassia bark
Botanical Name: *Cinnamomum cassia* Presl. (*Rou Gui*)
Pharmaceutical Name: Cortex Cinnamomi
Properties: acrid, sweet, hot
Channels Entered: Heart, Kidney, Liver, Spleen

CHINESE THERAPEUTIC ACTIONS

1. Tonifies Kidney Yang, Augments *Ming Men* (Life Gate) Fire

Declining *ming men* (life gate) fire: *Rou Gui* (Cortex Cinnamomi) treats a wide variety of disorders characterized by Kidney yang deficiency and insufficient *ming men* fire. This condition is characterized by intolerance to cold, cold extremities, weakness, soreness and coldness of the low back and knees, impotence, lack of libido, polyuria and loose stools. In addition, Kidney deficiency affects the Lung. Kidney deficiency and its inability to grasp qi downwards causes symptoms such as wheezing, dyspnea, profuse phlegm and cold extremities. Cold in the lower *jiao* may manifest as false yang rising, with symptoms of dizziness, flushed face, sore throat and coldness of the lower extremities. Fortifying in nature, *Rou Gui* is not dispersing and is one of the best herbs to warm the yang of the lower *jiao*.

- Kidney yang deficiency: use *Rou Gui* with *Fu Zi* (Radix Aconiti Lateralis Praeparata), *Shu Di Huang* (Radix Rehmanniae Preparata) and *Shan Zhu Yu* (Fructus Corni). **Exemplar Formula:** *You Gui Wan* (Restore the Right [Kidney] Pill), or *Ba Wei Di Huang Wan* (Eight-Ingredient Pill with Rehmannia).
- Asthma or wheezing: use it with *Fu Zi* (Radix Aconiti Lateralis Praeparata) and *Liu Huang* (Sulfur).
- Impotence: combine it with *Lu Rong* (Cornu Cervi Pantotrichum), *Shu Di Huang* (Radix Rehmanniae Preparata), *Tu Si Zi* (Semen Cuscutae), *Shan Zhu Yu* (Fructus Corni), *Yin Yang Huo* (Herba Epimedii), *Rou Cong Rong* (Herba Cistanches) and *Ba Ji Tian* (Radix Morindae Officinalis).
- Lack of libido: use this herb with *Dang Gui* (Radicis Angelicae Sinensis), *Shu Di Huang* (Radix Rehmanniae Preparata), *Bai Shao* (Radix Paeoniae Alba), *Chuan Xiong* (Rhizoma Ligustici Chuanxiong), *Xiang Fu* (Rhizoma Cyperi), *Ai Ye* (Folium Artemisiae Argyi), *Fu Zi* (Radix Aconiti Lateralis Praeparata), *Zi Shi Ying* (Fluoritum), *Wu Zhu Yu* (Fructus Evodiae) and *Wu Yao* (Radix Linderae).
- Edema due to Kidney yang deficiency: use *Rou Gui* with *Shu Di Huang* (Radix Rehmanniae Preparata), *Shan Yao* (Rhizoma Dioscoreae), *Niu Xi* (Radix Cyathulae seu Achyranthis), *Fu Ling* (Poria), *Fu Zi* (Radix Aconiti Lateralis Praeparata), *Ze Xie* (Rhizoma Alismatis) and *Che Qian Zi* (Semen Plantaginis). **Exemplar Formula:** *Ji Sheng Shen Qi Wan* (Kidney Qi Pill from Formulas that Aid the Living).

2. Dispels Cold, Warms the Spleen and Relieves Pain

Epigastric and abdominal coldness and pain, vomiting or diarrhea: *Rou Gui* warms the middle *jiao* and treats digestive disorders that are cold in nature. The volatile oils in this herb have a mild stimulating effect to promote digestion, dispel gas and relieve spasmodic pain in the stomach and intestines.

- Epigastric and abdominal coldness and pain: use *Rou Gui* individually as powder or in pills.
- Deficiency and cold of the Spleen and Stomach with abdominal pain and diarrhea: use this herb with *Gao Liang Jiang* (Rhizoma Alpiniae Officinarum), *Bi Ba* (Fructus Piperis Longi) and *Pao Jiang* (Rhizoma Zingiberis Preparatum).
- Chronic diarrhea: add *Gan Jiang* (Rhizoma Zingiberis), *Bai Zhu* (Rhizoma Atractylodis Macrocephalae) and *Chen Pi* (Pericarpium Citri Reticulatae).
- Chronic dysentery or enteritis: use this herb with *Huang Lian* (Rhizoma Coptidis).

Rou Gui (Cortex Cinnamomi)

Hernial Pain: With its analgesic and warming effect, *Rou Gui* treats hernial pain caused by cold.

- Cold hernial disorder with abdominal pain: use *Rou Gui* with *Wu Zhu Yu* (Fructus Evodiae) and *Xiao Hui Xiang* (Fructus Foeniculi).

3. Dispels Cold, Relieves Pain, Opens Channels and Vessels

Coldness in the channels: When cold invades the *xue* (blood) level, the channels and collaterals constrict. This results in blood stagnation, causing symptoms of irregular menstruation, amenorrhea, dysmenorrhea and postpartum pain. *Rou Gui* infuses warmth to the peripheral channels and collaterals to move qi and blood circulation. It treats pain characterized by cold in the blood, such as gynecological disorders, external or traumatic injuries, or obstruction of cold and dampness in the channels and collaterals. This herb dilates the central and peripheral vessels and increases blood circulation.

- Irregular menstruation, amenorrhea, and postpartum abdominal pain: use *Rou Gui* with *Dang Gui* (Radicis Angelicae Sinensis) and *Chuan Xiong* (Rhizoma Ligustici Chuanxiong).
- Hypochondriac pain due to Liver qi stagnation: use it with *Yu Jin* (Radix Curcumae) and *Chuan Xiong* (Rhizoma Ligustici Chuanxiong).
- External or traumatic injury with blood stasis, feelings of oppression and pain in the abdomen: combine this herb with *Dang Gui* (Radicis Angelicae Sinensis), *Hong Hua* (Flos Carthami), *Ru Xiang* (Gummi Olibanum) and *Mo Yao* (Myrrha).
- *Bi zheng* (painful obstruction syndrome) due to cold and dampness in the channels and collaterals: use *Rou Gui* with *Qiang Huo* (Rhizoma et Radix Notopterygii), *Du Huo* (Radix Angelicae Pubescentis) and *Dang Gui* (Radicis Angelicae Sinensis).

Yin sores: *Rou Gui* warms the channels and collaterals to treat deep-rooted sores. It promotes the generation of flesh and enhances recovery.

- Yin sores: use *Rou Gui* with *Shu Di Huang* (Radix Rehmanniae Preparata), *Lu Jiao Jiao* (Gelatinum Cornu Cervi), *Ma Huang* (Herba Ephedrae) and *Bai Jie Zi* (Semen Sinapis).
- Sores with pus but no ulceration: use this herb with *Huang Qi* (Radix Astragali) and *Dang Gui* (Radicis Angelicae Sinensis).

4. Encourages Production of Qi and Blood

A small quantity of *Rou Gui* is often added to qi and blood tonics to enhance the movement of yang qi in the body and encourage the production of blood and qi. **Exemplar Formula:** *Ren Shen Yang Ying Tang* (Ginseng Decoction to Nourish the Nutritive Qi) and *Shi Quan Da Bu Tang* (All-Inclusive Great Tonifying Decoction).

DOSAGE

2 to 5 grams in herbal decoction, 1 to 2 grams in herbal powder. *Rou Gui* should be added in the last 5 to 10 minutes of the cooking process, to avoid loss of active constituents from over-exposure to heat.

CAUTIONS / CONTRAINDICATIONS

- Use of *Rou Gui* is contraindicated during pregnancy, or in cases of excess heat, yin-deficient fire, or bleeding caused by heat in the blood.
- *Rou Gui* is counteracted by *Chi Shi Zhi* (Halloysitum Rubrum).
- *Rou Gui* is hot, and generally considered to be an herb with pure yang energy. When used improperly for patients affected by pathogenic heat, or prescribed in excessive amounts, it can induce rising of fire, resulting in a flushed face, red eyes, dry mouth and tongue and, in severe cases, bleeding.

OVERDOSAGE

Overdose of *Rou Gui* is characterized by disturbances to the gastrointestinal and urinary tract systems. Clinical manifestations include nausea, vomiting, abdominal pain, dysuria, anuria, burning sensations on urination, proteinuria, flushed face, dizziness, blurred vision, and numbness of the tongue.[1]

CHEMICAL COMPOSITION

Cinnamic aldehyde, cinnamic acid, cinnamyl acetate, phenylpropyl acetate, cinncassiol-A, -B, -C1, -C2, -C3; cinnzeylanine, cinnzeylanol.[2]

PHARMACOLOGICAL EFFECTS

- **Cardiovascular:** Intravenous administration of *Rou Gui* is associated with a marked reduction in blood pressure, a decrease in heart rate, peripheral vasodilation, and decreased vessel resistance, within 3 to 5 minutes after injection. The cardiovascular system returned to normal after 15 minutes.[3]
- **Sedative and analgesic:** Essential oil of *Rou Gui* demonstrates marked analgesic and sedative actions in rats.[4]
- **Gastrointestinal:** Essential oil of *Rou Gui* has a mild stimulating effect on the gastrointestinal system. It increases the secretion of saliva and gastric acid, enhances digestive functioning, and relieves intestinal spasms and pain.[5]

Rou Gui (Cortex Cinnamomi)

- **Immunostimulant:** Subcutaneous injection of a *Rou Gui* preparation for 5 days increased the white blood cell count by 150 to 200% in dogs.[6]
- **Antibiotic:** *Rou Gui* has an inhibitory effect on dermatophytes, pathogenic fungi, and many gram-positive bacteria.[7]

CLINICAL STUDIES AND RESEARCH

- **Low back pain:** According to one report, 102 patients with low back pain characterized by Kidney yang deficiency were treated with 5 grams of *Rou Gui* powder twice daily for 3 weeks, with a 98% rate of effectiveness. Dry mouth and constipation were the most common side effects.[8]
- **Psoriasis:** Nineteen patients were treated with a *Rou Gui* preparation three times daily for 4 to 8 weeks, with significant improvement in 7 patients, marked improvement in 2 patients, slight improvement in 7 patients, and no response in 2 patients. Overall, the preparation had a 91.2% effective rate.[9]

TOXICOLOGY

The LD_{50} for intravenous injection of *Rou Gui* decoction in mice is 18.48 +/- 1.80 g/kg.[10]

SUPPLEMENT

- 桂心 *Gui Xin* (Cortex Rasus Cinnamomi) is the thin layer of tree cortex that remains after the outer layer of bark has been removed. *Gui Xin* is not drying in nature and is best used for Heart and Kidney yang deficiencies.
- 土肉桂 *Tu Rou Gui* (Cortex Cinnamomum Burmannii), derived from the plant *Cinnamomum burmannii* (Nees) Bl. (*Tian Zhu Gui*), is the type of cinnamon used for cooking to add flavor. It is acrid and warm and warms the Spleen and Stomach. However, it is mild in nature and cannot be used therapeutically to warm the body. *Rou Gui*, derived from the plant *Cinnamomum cassia* Presl., is much stronger and has the therapeutic potency to warm the body and dispel cold.

AUTHORS' COMMENTS

Rou Gui (Cortex Cinnamomi) and *Gui Zhi* (Ramulus Cinnamomi) are derived from different parts of the same plant. *Rou Gui* is the bark of the tree trunk. *Gui Zhi* is the tips of the branches. Both function to disperse coldness, warm the channels and assist the yang. However, *Rou Gui* is acrid, hot and descending in nature to warm the Kidney. *Gui Zhi* is acrid, warm and ascending in nature to disperse wind-cold and open the channels and collaterals in the four limbs.

Rou Gui and *Fu Zi* (Radix Aconiti Lateralis Praeparata) are two of the most important interior-warming herbs. *Rou Gui* has a slower onset than *Fu Zi* but has pure yang energy. It is more tonifying in nature and is suitable for long-term use with other tonic herbs to revitalize the body. *Fu Zi* is strong and fast-acting in nature, and is most suitable in cases where yang qi has collapsed and treatment needs to be initiated immediately to revive the patient.

Rou Gui and *Gan Jiang* (Rhizoma Zingiberis) are both interior-warming herbs, but have different functions and applications. *Rou Gui* enters the lower *jiao* to tonify Kidney yang. *Gan Jiang* warms the middle *jiao* and disperses cold from the Spleen and Stomach.

Rou Gui is often added to formulas to treat yin sores. Yin sores are often the results of yang deficiency that has caused stagnation of phlegm, and coldness. Over a long period of time, this stagnation becomes toxic and obstructs the channels, tendons and joints. *Rou Gui* is acrid, dispersing and warming in nature, and can open the channels by dispersing coldness. It enters both the *qi* (energy) and *xue* (blood) levels to strengthen the body's yang qi and thus break open stagnation.

References

1. *Zhong Yao Bu Liang Fan Ying Yu Zhi Liao* (Adverse Reactions and Treatment of Chinese Herbal Medicine), 1996; 172:173
2. *Xian Dai Zhong Yao Yao Li Xue* (Contemporary Pharmacology of Chinese Herbs), 1997; 606
3. *Zhong Yao Tong Bao* (Journal of Chinese Herbology), 1981; 6(5):32
4. *Zhi Wu Yao You Xiao Cheng Fen Shou Ce* (Manual of Plant Medicinals and Their Active Constituents), 1986; 218
5. *Zhong Yao Xue* (Chinese Herbology), 1998; 373:376
6. *Zhong Yao Yao Li Yu Ying Yong* (Pharmacology and Applications of Chinese Herbs), 1983;443
7. Ibid.
8. *Zhong Xi Yi Jie He Za Zhi* (Journal of Integrated Chinese and Western Medicine), 1984; 2:115
9. *He Nan Yi Xue Yuan Xue Bao* (Journal of Henan University of Medicine), 1981; 2:385
10. *Zhong Yao Yao Li Yu Ying Yong* (Pharmacology and Applications of Chinese Herbs), 1983:443

Gan Jiang (Rhizoma Zingiberis)

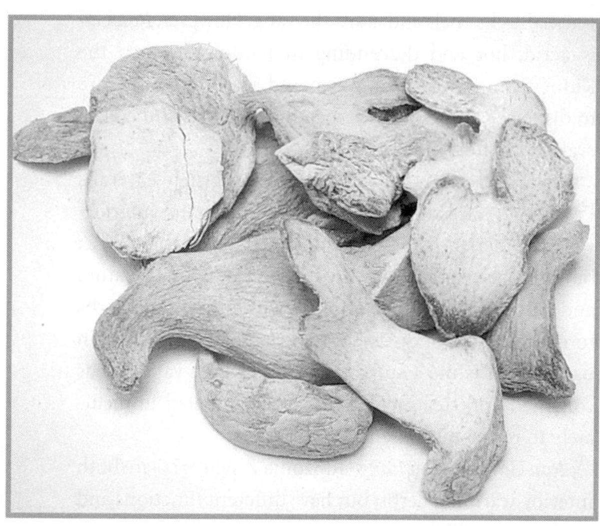

乾薑 干姜

Pinyin Name: *Gan Jiang*
Literal Name: "dry ginger"
Original Source: *Shen Nong Ben Cao Jing* (Divine Husbandman's Classic of the Materia Medica) in the second century
English Name: dried ginger
Botanical Name: *Zingiber officinale* Rosc. (*Jiang*)
Pharmaceutical Name: Rhizoma Zingiberis
Properties: acrid, hot
Channels Entered: Heart, Lung, Spleen, Stomach

CHINESE THERAPEUTIC ACTIONS

1. Warms the Middle *Jiao*

Spleen and Stomach cold syndrome: *Gan Jiang* (Rhizoma Zingiberis) warms the Spleen and Stomach to dispel cold from the middle *jiao*. The cause of this cold may be an invasion of cold from the exterior, or yang deficiency of the Spleen. Common manifestations include epigastric and abdominal coldness and pain, nausea, vomiting, and diarrhea.

- Spleen and Stomach cold syndromes: use *Gan Jiang* with *Ren Shen* (Radix Ginseng) and *Bai Zhu* (Rhizoma Atractylodis Macrocephalae). **Exemplar Formula:** *Li Zhong Tang* (Regulate the Middle Decoction).
- Continuous diarrhea due to Spleen and Kidney yang deficiencies: use it with *Fu Zi* (Radix Aconiti Lateralis Praeparata) and *Bu Gu Zhi* (Fructus Psoraleae).
- Chronic diarrhea damaging yin, with pus and blood in the stools, and other mixed hot and cold signs: use this herb with *Huang Lian* (Rhizoma Coptidis) and *E Jiao* (Colla Corii Asini).
- Dry heaves or vomiting of saliva because of accumulation of cold in the Stomach: combine it with *Ban Xia* (Rhizoma Pinelliae).

2. Restores Depleted Yang

Yang collapse: *Gan Jiang* tonifies yang and expels cold. When combined with *Fu Zi* (Radix Aconiti Lateralis Praeparata), *Gan Jiang* enhances the overall effect of *Fu Zi* to restore depleted yang, and minimizes its toxicity. These two herbs are often paired together for their synergistic action. Classic texts stated that "*Fu Zi* is not warm without *Gan Jiang*."

3. Warms the Lung, Dissolves Phlegm

Cough and dyspnea due to cold accumulation: *Gan Jiang* warms the Spleen to stop the production of damp, and warms the Lung to eliminate the accumulation of phlegm. It is commonly used to treat accumulation of cold and fluids in the Lung characterized by cough and wheezing, aversion to cold, and profuse watery sputum.

- Accumulation of cold and fluids in the Lung: use *Gan Jiang* with *Ma Huang* (Herba Ephedrae), *Xi Xin* (Herba Asari) and *Wu Wei Zi* (Fructus Schisandrae Chinensis). **Exemplar Formula:** *Xiao Qing Long Tang* (Minor Bluegreen Dragon Decoction).
- Coughing due to rebellious qi rising upwards: combine this herb with *Zao Jiao* (Fructus Gleditsiae) and *Gui Zhi* (Ramulus Cinnamomi).

4. Warms the Channels, Stops Bleeding

Bleeding due to deficiency and cold: *Gan Jiang* treats various kinds of bleeding caused by deficiency and cold: hematemesis, hematochezia, hypermenorrhea or abnormal menstrual bleeding. This type of bleeding is characterized by the presence of blood that is dark in color, and thin in consistency. These patients usually have cold extremities, a pale tongue, and a thready pulse.

- Bleeding due to deficiency and cold: use *Gan Jiang* with *Ren Shen* (Radix Ginseng), *Ai Ye* (Folium Artemisiae Argyi) and *Bai Zhu* (Rhizoma Atractylodis Macrocephalae).
- Hematemesis because of deficiency and cold: use charred *Gan Jiang* as a single-herb treatment. Some records have shown good results when this herb is mixed with children's urine to stop hematemesis.
- Hematochezia and profuse menstrual bleeding: use this herb with *Bai Zhu* (Rhizoma Atractylodis Macrocephalae).

Gan Jiang (Rhizoma Zingiberis)

5. Dispels Cold and Dampness

Gan Jiang treats the sensation of heaviness, coldness and pain in the back and lower body, characterized by cold and dampness.

- Accumulation of cold and damp in the lower body: use *Gan Jiang* with *Fu Ling* (Poria), *Bai Zhu* (Rhizoma Atractylodis Macrocephalae) and *Gan Cao* (Radix Glycyrrhizae).

DOSAGE

3 to 10 grams in herbal decoction.

CAUTIONS / CONTRAINDICATIONS

- *Gan Jiang* is contraindicated in cases of interior heat with yin deficiency, or heat in the blood.
- Use *Gan Jiang* with caution during pregnancy as large quantities may have an abortifacient effect.[1]

CHEMICAL COMPOSITION

Essential oils 1.2-2.8% (zingberol, zingiberene, bisabolene, α-curcumene, α-farnesene, β-farnesene, linalool, cineole, β-sesouiphellandrene), gingerol, shogaol, zingerone, dihydroginerol, hexyhydrocurcumin, L-pipecolic acid.[2]

PHARMACOLOGICAL EFFECTS

- **Gastrointestinal:** *Gan Jiang* has a mild stimulating effect on the gastrointestinal system to increase peristalsis.[3] Furthermore, oral administration of a 10% decoction of *Gan Jiang* in mice has demonstrated a protective effect on the gastrointestinal system, by stimulating the production of stomach mucous membranes. It also increased stomach acid secretion and intestinal activity.[4]
- **Antiemetic:** According to one report, 30 ml of 10 to 50% *Gan Jiang* solution has a marked effect to relieve artificially-induced nausea and vomiting in dogs.[5]
- **Stimulant:** Alcohol extract of *Gan Jiang* has a stimulating effect on the central nervous system, cardiovascular system, and respiratory system in dogs.[6]
- **Effect on temperature regulation:** Administration of *Gan Jiang* was ineffective in prolonging the survival time in mice kept in an environment of under 18° to 20° C.[7]

CLINICAL STUDIES AND RESEARCH

- **Cold syndrome:** In one report, 34 patients with a complex syndrome (characterized by coldness, according to traditional Chinese medicine) were treated by an herbal decoction. The clinical presentation of symptoms included epigastric pain, acid regurgitation, epigastric and abdominal fullness, borborygmus, diarrhea, chest pain, dizziness, cough, wheezing, abdominal coldness and pain with menstruation, slow pulse, pale tongue, white tongue coat, aversion to cold, no thirst, and no fever. The herbal formula contained 9 to 15 grams each of *Gan Jiang* and *Gan Cao* (Radix Glycyrrhizae). Patients with mild to moderate conditions responded within 1 to 2 doses, while those with more severe conditions required 3 to 5 doses.[8]

TOXICOLOGY

The LD_{50} for oral ingestion of *Gan Jiang* decoction in mice is 250 g/kg.[9]

SUPPLEMENT

- 炮薑 / 炮姜 *Pao Jiang* (Rhizoma Zingiberis Preparatum), processed ginger, is bitter and astringent. It is the herb of choice to warm channels and stop bleeding. It is often used in patients experiencing bleeding from deficiency and cold.

AUTHORS' COMMENTS

Gan Jiang (Rhizoma Zingiberis), *Pao Jiang* (Rhizoma Zingiberis Preparatum), and *Sheng Jiang* (Rhizoma Zingiberis Recens) have similar yet different functions.

- *Gan Jiang* is acrid and hot, and it warms the middle *jiao* to restore normal digestive functions. It treats interior cold.
- *Pao Jiang* is bitter and astringent, and it warms channels and stops bleeding. It treats deficiency and cold.
- *Sheng Jiang* is acrid and warm, and it warms the middle *jiao* to relieve nausea and vomiting. It treats exterior wind-cold.

References

1. Brinker, Francis. *Herb Contraindications and Drug Interactions*, 1997; 51
2. *Xian Dai Zhong Yao Yao Li Xue* (Contemporary Pharmacology of Chinese Herbs), 1997; 610-611
3. *Zhong Yao Xue* (Chinese Herbology), 1998; 376:378
4. *Zhong Cao Yao* (Chinese Herbal Medicine), 1988; 13(11):17
5. *Zhong Yao Xue* (Chinese Herbology), 1998; 378-380
6. Ibid., 1998; 376:378
7. *Zhong Guo Zhong Yao Za Zhi* (People's Republic of China Journal of Chinese Herbology), 1991; 16(3):32
8. *Zhong Yi Za Zhi* (Journal of Chinese Medicine), 1965; 11:6
9. *Sheng Yao Xue Za Zhi* (Journal of Raw Herbology), 1983; 37(1):73

Wu Zhu Yu (Fructus Evodiae)

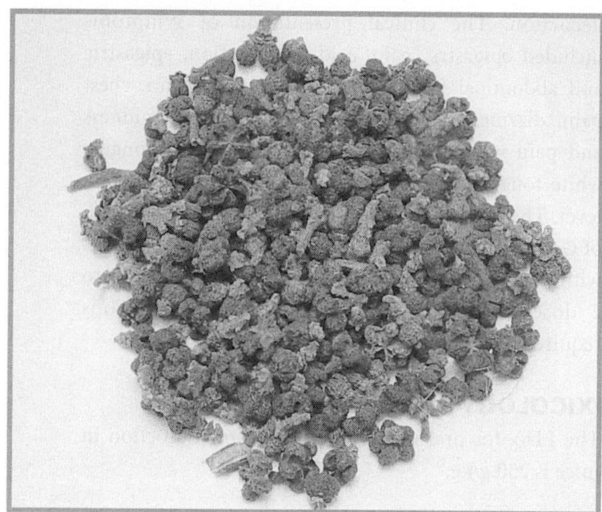

吴茱萸 吳茱萸

Pinyin Name: *Wu Zhu Yu*

Literal Name: "Wu-Zhu's fruit," "evodia of Wu"

Original Source: *Shen Nong Ben Cao Jing* (Divine Husbandman's Classic of the Materia Medica) in the second century

English Name: evodia, medicinal evodia fruit

Botanical Name: *Evodia rutaecarpa* (Juss.) Benth. (*Wu Zhu Yu*); *Evodia rutaecarpa* (Juss.) Benth. var. *officinalis* (Dode) Huang (*Shi Hu*); *Evodia rutaecarpa* (Juss.) Benth. var. *bodinieri* (Dode) Huang (*Shu Mao Wu Zhu Yu*)

Pharmaceutical Name: Fructus Evodiae

Properties: acrid, bitter, hot

Channels Entered: Liver, Spleen, Stomach

Safety Index: slightly toxic

CHINESE THERAPEUTIC ACTIONS

1. Dispels Cold, Dries Dampness, Activates Qi Circulation, Relieves Pain

Epigastric and abdominal pain, and *jueyin* headache: *Wu Zhu Yu* (Fructus Evodiae) treats pain characterized by stagnation of cold, damp and qi. It dispels cold to relieve epigastric and abdominal pain. It warms and dispels cold in the *jueyin* Liver channel and relieves hernial pain, dysmenorrhea, leg *qi* and vertex headache. This is the best herb for migraine or vertex headaches with nausea and vomiting, as it warms the deficient middle *jiao* and dispels cold in the Liver and Stomach channels.

- Epigastric and abdominal pain due to cold and dampness: use *Wu Zhu Yu* with *Gan Jiang* (Rhizoma Zingiberis) and *Gui Zhi* (Ramulus Cinnamomi).
- Cold hernial pain or abdominal pain: use it with *Xiao Hui Xiang* (Fructus Foeniculi) and *Wu Yao* (Radix Linderae).
- Menstrual pain due to cold in the womb: combine it with *Ai Ye* (Folium Artemisiae Argyi), *Gui Zhi* (Ramulus Cinnamomi), *Dang Gui* (Radicis Angelicae Sinensis), *Xiang Fu* (Rhizoma Cyperi), *Wu Ling Zhi* (Excrementum Trogopteri seu Pteromi) and *Yan Hu Suo* (Rhizoma Corydalis).
- Leg *qi* caused by accumulation of cold and dampness: use this herb with *Mu Gua* (Fructus Chaenomelis) and *Bing Lang* (Semen Arecae).
- Vertex or migraine headaches: combine it with *Ren Shen* (Radix Ginseng) and *Sheng Jiang* (Rhizoma Zingiberis Recens). **Exemplar Formula:** *Wu Zhu Yu Tang* (Evodia Decoction).
- Hernial pain: use *Wu Zhu Yu* with *Wu Yao* (Radix Linderae), *Qing Pi* (Pericarpium Citri Reticulatae Viride), *Ju He* (Semen Citri Rubrum), *Xiao Hui Xiang* (Fructus Foeniculi), and *Li Zhi He* (Semen Litchi).

2. Spreads the Liver, Descends Qi

Acid reflux, vomiting: *Wu Zhu Yu* is one of the most effective herbs to treat vomiting and acid reflux caused by Liver overacting on the Stomach. Other symptoms may include hypochondriac pain, stomach pain and nausea.

- Acid reflux after meals due to deficiency and cold of the Stomach: use *Wu Zhu Yu* individually, or with *Gan Jiang* (Rhizoma Zingiberis).
- Nausea, vomiting, stomach pain with acid regurgitation due to deficiency and cold of the Stomach: use this herb with *Sheng Jiang* (Rhizoma Zingiberis Recens), *Ban Xia* (Rhizoma Pinelliae), *Gao Liang Jiang* (Rhizoma Alpiniae Officinarum), *Huo Xiang* (Herba Agastache) and *Sha Ren* (Fructus Amomi).
- Acid reflux, stomach pain, hypochondriac pain with foul breath due to Liver heat overacting on the Stomach: use *Wu Zhu Yu* with *Huang Lian* (Rhizoma Coptidis). The dose of *Huang Lian* should be five times greater than that of *Wu Zhu Yu*. **Exemplar Formula:** *Zuo Jin Wan* (Left Metal Pill).

3. Warms Middle *Jiao*, Relieves Diarrhea

Diarrhea or dysentery due to cold and dampness: *Wu Zhu Yu* treats chronic diarrhea from accumulation of cold and dampness, or from deficiency and cold of the Spleen and Kidney. Patients with accumulation of cold and dampness have diarrhea throughout the day, while patients with deficiency and cold of the Spleen and Kidney experience diarrhea in the early morning hours.

Wu Zhu Yu (Fructus Evodiae)

- Chronic diarrhea from deficiency and cold of the Spleen and Kidney: combine *Wu Zhu Yu* with *Rou Dou Kou* (Semen Myristicae), *Bu Gu Zhi* (Fructus Psoraleae) and *Wu Wei Zi* (Fructus Schisandrae Chinensis). **Exemplar Formula:** *Si Shen Wan* (Four-Miracle Pill).
- Chronic dysentery because of the accumulation of cold and dampness affecting the Spleen: use this herb with *Huang Lian* (Rhizoma Coptidis) and *Bai Shao* (Radix Paeoniae Alba).

4. Directs Fire Downwards

Hypertension, oral ulcers: *Wu Zhu Yu* treats heat conditions, such as ulceration of the tongue and mouth, and hypertension, by directing heat downwards.

- Oral ulcers and hypertension: mix powdered *Wu Zhu Yu* with vinegar and place it on the center of the soles of the feet.
- Eczema or sores on the scalp: apply *Wu Zhu Yu* in liquid form topically, or mix the powder of the herb with water and apply topically.

DOSAGE

1.5 to 5 grams. Unprocessed *Wu Zhu Yu* is often used topically, while the processed herb is often used internally. Processing is done by cooking the herb with *Gan Cao* (Radix Glycyrrhizae) to eliminate its drying effect and toxicity.

CAUTIONS / CONTRAINDICATIONS

- *Wu Zhu Yu* is contraindicated in cases of yin deficiency with heat.
- *Wu Zhu Yu* is not recommended for long-term use, or for use in large doses, due to toxicity.

OVERDOSAGE

Overdose of *Wu Zhu Yu* is characterized by severe abdominal pain, diarrhea, visual disturbance, hair loss, chest oppression, headache, dizziness and rashes.

TREATMENT OF OVERDOSAGE

General overdose of *Wu Zhu Yu* can be treated with 15 grams of *Huang Lian* (Rhizoma Coptidis) in decoction. For visual disturbance or hair loss, use a decoction taken twice daily, consisting of *Shi Hu* (Herba Dendrobii) 15g, *Huang Qin* (Radix Scutellariae) 9g, *Gu Jing Cao* (Flos Eriocauli) 15g, *Ju Hua* (Flos Chrysanthemi) 12g, *Gou Qi Zi* (Fructus Lycii) 15g, *Sheng Di Huang* (Radix Rehmanniae) 9g and *Gan Cao* (Radix Glycyrrhizae) 6g.[1]

CHEMICAL COMPOSITION

Evodiamine, rutaecarpine, evocarpine, hydroxyevodiomine, wuchuyine, dihydrorutaecarpine, 14-formyldihydrorutaecarpine, quinolone, N,N-dimethyl-5-methoxytryptamine, N-methylanthranylamide, dl-synephrine, evodene, ocimene, evodin, evodol, goshuynic acid, evodinone, evogin, evodine, jangomolide.[2,3]

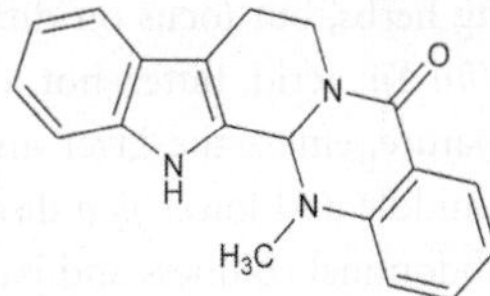

Evodiamine

PHARMACOLOGICAL EFFECTS

- **Antiulcer:** According to various animal studies, administration of *Wu Zhu Yu* is associated with marked effectiveness in preventing and treating stomach ulcers by reducing gastric acid secretion.[4]
- **Antiemetic:** Decoction of *Wu Zhu Yu* has an antiemetic effect on pigeons, although the effect was not statistically significant.[5]
- **Antidiarrheal:** Decoction of *Wu Zhu Yu* at dosages of 10 to 20 g/kg has a slow onset but a prolonged duration of action for treatment of diarrhea in mice.[6]
- **Analgesic:** Several components of *Wu Zhu Yu* have demonstrated analgesic effects.[7]
- **Cardiovascular:** According to various animal studies, injection of a *Wu Zhu Yu* preparation is associated with a positive inotropic effect, a negative chronotropic effect and a marked decrease in blood pressure. The herb has a rapid onset and a prolonged duration of action on the cardiovascular system. The preparation contained *Wu Zhu Yu*, *Ren Shen* (Radix Ginseng) and *Da Zao* (Fructus Jujubae).[8]
- **Effects on the uterus:** *Wu Zhu Yu* has a mixed effect on the uterus. Some constituents induce contraction while others induce relaxation.[9]
- **Antibiotic:** Decoction of *Wu Zhu Yu* has an inhibitory effect on *Pseudomonas aeruginosa*, *Staphylococcus aureus*, and some dermatophytes.[10]

CLINICAL STUDIES AND RESEARCH

- **Ulceration of the mouth:** In one study, 256 patients with oral ulcerations were treated by topical application of *Wu Zhu Yu* with 96.48% effectiveness. The herbal preparation was made by mixing the powdered herb with vinegar to form a paste. The treatment protocol was to place the herbal paste on *Yongquan* (KI 1) bilaterally for 24 hours.[11]
- **Eczema:** Over 1,100 eczema patients were treated by topical application of an herbal powder containing 30 grams of *Wu Zhu Yu*, 21 grams of *Hai Piao Xiao* (Endoconcha Sepiae), and 6 grams of *Liu Huang* (Sulfur). The treatment protocol was to sprinkle the herbal powder on the

Wu Zhu Yu (Fructus Evodiae)

affected area and cover it with gauze, every other day. The study reported over 95% success in treatment.[12]

AUTHORS' COMMENTS

Wu Zhu Yu and *Gan Jiang* (Rhizoma Zingiberis) are both interior-warming herbs, but focus on different parts of the body. *Wu Zhu Yu*, acrid, bitter, hot, dispersing and descending in nature, enters the Liver and Stomach to primarily treat middle and lower *jiao* disorders such as epigastric and abdominal coldness and pain, hernia and dysmenorrhea. *Gan Jiang*, acrid, hot and dry, enters the Spleen, Stomach, Heart and Lung. Its main effects are focused on the upper and middle *jiaos* to disperse coldness, warm the interior and dispel phlegm to treat dyspnea, phlegm, wheezing and yang collapse symptoms.

Wu Zhu Yu and *Gao Ben* (Rhizoma Ligustici) are both acrid and hot, and treat vertex headaches. *Wu Zhu Yu* enters the *jueyin* Liver channel and is best at dispelling cold, relieving pain and regulating Liver qi circulation. It is best for vertex headache with vomiting or nausea because of coldness and phlegm accumulation. *Gao Ben* enters the *taiyang* Urinary Bladder channel and is best at dispelling wind, cold, and damp and relieving pain. It is for vertex headaches associated with wind-cold invasion.

Optimal treatment of headache requires the use of channel-guiding herbs to deliver the therapeutic effect of the herbs to the affected area. The following is a list of commonly used channel-guiding herbs:

- *Taiyang* channels: *Qiang Huo* (Rhizoma et Radix Notopterygii)
- *Shaoyang* channels: *Chai Hu* (Radix Bupleuri)
- *Yangming* channels: *Bai Zhi* (Radix Angelicae Dahuricae)
- *Taiyin* channels: *Cang Zhu* (Rhizoma Atractylodis)
- *Shaoyin* channels: *Xi Xin* (Herba Asari)
- *Jueyin* channels: *Wu Zhu Yu* (Fructus Evodiae)

References

1. *Zhong Yao Bu Liang Fan Ying Yu Zhi Liao* (Adverse Reactions and Treatment of Chinese Herbal Medicine), 1996; 218:220
2. *Xian Dai Zhong Yao Yao Li Xue* (Contemporary Pharmacology of Chinese Herbs), 1997; 608
3. *The Merck Index* 12th edition, Chapman & Hall/CRCnetBASE/Merck, 2000
4. *Zhong Yao Yao Li Du Li Yu Lin Chuan* (Pharmacology, Toxicology and Clinical Applications of Chinese Herbs), 1988; 4(3):9
5. Ibid.
6. *Zhong Yao Cai* (Study of Chinese Herbal Material), 1991; 14(3):39
7. *Zhong Yao Xue* (Chinese Herbology), 1998; 378:380
8. *Zhong Yao Yao Li Du Li Yu Lin Chuan* (Pharmacology, Toxicology and Clinical Applications of Chinese Herbs), 1991; 7(2):1
9. *Zhong Yao Xue* (Chinese Herbology), 1998; 378:380
10. Ibid.
11. *Shan Dong Yi Kan* (Shandong Medical Journal), 1965; 3:23
12. *Zhong Cao Yao Tong Xun* (Journal of Chinese Herbal Medicine), 1971; 3:46

Xi Xin (Herba Asari)

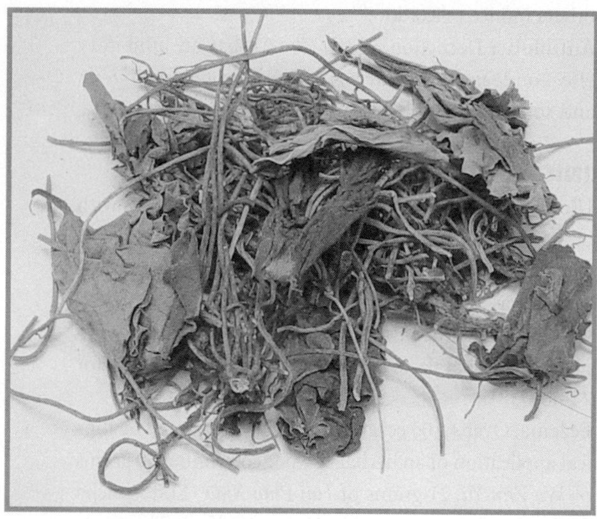

細辛 细辛

Pinyin Name: *Xi Xin*

Literal Name: "thin-acrid," "fine-pungent"

Alternate Chinese Names: *Xiao Xin, Shao Xin, Bei Xi Xin, Liao Xi Xin*

Original Source: *Shen Nong Ben Cao Jing* (Divine Husbandman's Classic of the Materia Medica) in the second century

English Name: asarum, Chinese wild ginger, Manchurian wild ginger, Seoul wild ginger, Siebold wild ginger

Botanical Name: *Asarum heteropoides* Fr. var. *mandshuricum* (Maxim.) Kitag. (*Bei Xi Xin*); *Asarum sieboldii* Miq. (*Hua Xi Xin*)

Pharmaceutical Name: Herba Asari

Properties: acrid, warm

Channels Entered: Lung, Heart, Kidney

Safety Index: slightly toxic

Xi Xin (Herba Asari)

CHINESE THERAPEUTIC ACTIONS

1. Dispels Wind, Disperses Cold and Relieves Pain

Pain (headache, arthritis or abdominal pain): Extremely acrid and warm, *Xi Xin* (Herba Asari) dispels wind and cold from the exterior. It is commonly used to treat headache, *bi zheng* (painful obstruction syndrome), abdominal pain, and various aches and pains caused by wind, cold, and/or dampness. *Xi Xin* enters the Kidney channel and dispels cold from the *shaoyin* channel to relieve lower-abdominal pain and coldness of the lower extremities, a bland taste in the mouth, and no desire to drink.

- Headache due to wind: use *Xi Xin* with *Chuan Xiong* (Rhizoma Ligustici Chuanxiong), *Jing Jie* (Herba Schizonepetae), *Fang Feng* (Radix Saposhnikoviae), and *Qiang Huo* (Rhizoma et Radix Notopterygii). **Exemplar Formula:** *Chuan Xiong Cha Tiao San* (Ligusticum Chuanxiong Powder to be Taken with Green Tea).
- *Bi zheng* (painful obstruction syndrome) with wind, cold and/or dampness obstructing the channels and collaterals: use this herb with *Chuan Xiong* (Rhizoma Ligustici Chuanxiong) and *Fang Feng* (Radix Saposhnikoviae).
- Chronic low back and knee pain with Kidney and Liver deficiencies: use *Xi Xin* with *Du Zhong* (Cortex Eucommiae) and *Sang Ji Sheng* (Herba Taxilli). **Exemplar Formula:** *Du Huo Ji Sheng Tang* (Angelica Pubescens and Taxillus Decoction).
- Abdominal pain, coldness of the lower extremities, pale tongue, no thirst: combine this herb with *Fu Zi* (Radix Aconiti Lateralis Praeparata) and *Rou Gui* (Cortex Cinnamomi).
- Chest pain due to cold and qi stagnation: use it with *Xie Bai* (Bulbus Allii Macrostemonis), *Gui Zhi* (Ramulus Cinnamomi) and *Dan Shen* (Radix Salviae Miltiorrhizae).

2. Dispels Wind-Cold from the Exterior

Exterior wind-cold syndrome: *Xi Xin* releases the exterior and dispels wind and cold. It is most effective for exterior cold syndromes with headache, severe muscle aches and pain.

- Exterior wind-cold conditions with headache and body aches: use *Xi Xin* with *Fang Feng* (Radix Saposhnikoviae), *Qiang Huo* (Rhizoma et Radix Notopterygii) and *Chuan Xiong* (Rhizoma Ligustici Chuanxiong) to dispel wind-cold. **Exemplar Formula:** *Jiu Wei Qiang Huo Tang* (Nine-Herb Decoction with Notopterygium).
- Exterior wind-cold syndrome with underlying yang deficiency: use this herb with *Ma Huang* (Herba Ephedrae) and *Fu Zi* (Radix Aconiti Lateralis Praeparata) to dispel wind-cold and tonify yang. Common signs and symptoms associated with this condition include aversion to cold, fever, desire to assume the fetal position, and deep pulse. **Exemplar Formula:** *Ma Huang Fu Zi Xi Xin Tang* (Ephedra, Asarum, and Prepared Aconite Decoction).

3. Warms the Lung and Resolves Phlegm

Coldness and phlegm accumulation in the Lung: Clinical presentation includes cough, dyspnea, wheezing, stifling sensations in the chest, and profuse white or clear sputum. Patients who show this pattern usually have chronic water metabolism problems with congested phlegm in the Lung, and a weak Spleen. When exposed to wind-cold, the Lung's ability to facilitate water passage is impaired. This results in congested fluids in the Lung, which manifest in symptoms of dyspnea, wheezing, cough, stifling sensations in the chest and profuse white or clear sputum. *Xi Xin*, with its strong acrid and warm properties, is one of the most commonly-used herbs to dispel dampness and cold in the Lung to restore normal functioning of respiration and transportation of fluids.

- Exterior wind-cold or Lung cold: use *Xi Xin* with *Ma Huang* (Herba Ephedrae), *Gan Jiang* (Rhizoma Zingiberis), and *Wu Wei Zi* (Fructus Schisandrae Chinensis) to dispel wind-cold and disperse Lung cold. **Exemplar Formula:** *Xiao Qing Long Tang* (Minor Bluegreen Dragon Decoction).

4. Opens Sensory Orifices

Nasal obstruction or unconsciousness due to stroke: This condition involves blockage of two sensory pathways, the nose and the *shen* (spirit). *Xi Xin* has a strong dispersing function to penetrate blockages to relieve nasal congestion or restore consciousness.

- Nasal obstruction: apply *Xi Xin* topically to the nostrils.
- Nasal obstruction with a clear nasal discharge: use this herb with *Xin Yi Hua* (Flos Magnoliae) and *Bai Zhi* (Radix Angelicae Dahuricae).
- Unconsciousness: blow *Xi Xin* powder into the nostrils to restore consciousness.

5. Promotes Healing of Oral Ulceration

- Oral lesions or ulcerations: use *Xi Xin* alone, or in combination with *Huang Lian* (Rhizoma Coptidis).

6. Relieves Toothache

- Toothache due to cold: use *Xi Xin* with *Bai Zhi* (Radix Angelicae Dahuricae) to make a gargle, or apply the powder of these two herbs topically.
- Toothache due to heat, with swollen and red gums associated with rising Stomach fire: use this herb with *Shi Gao* (Gypsum Fibrosum) and *Huang Qin* (Radix Scutellariae).

DOSAGE

1 to 3 grams in decoction, 0.5 to 2.0 grams in powder. *Xi*

Xi Xin (Herba Asari)

Xin should never be prescribed in excess of the recommended dosage. Classic texts specifically state that the dose of *Xi Xin* in decoction should never exceed one *qian* (3.125 grams). *Xi Xin* should be applied sparingly when used topically.

Xi Xin is extremely dangerous when used in larger quantities than suggested, or if used in powder form. The safrole in the essential oil of *Xi Xin* is responsible for the toxicity of this herb, which can be reduced or removed by cooking.[1]

CAUTIONS / CONTRAINDICATIONS

- *Xi Xin* is incompatible with *Li Lu* (Radix et Rhizoma Veratri).
- *Xi Xin* is contraindicated in patients with febrile disorders, yin deficiency, yang excess, cough or wheezing due to yin deficiency, headache due to blood deficiency or wind-heat, and perspiration from qi deficiency.

OVERDOSAGE

Adverse reaction associated with overdose of *Xi Xin* is generally observed 1 to 2 hours after ingestion, but may occur within 30 minutes. Early symptoms include headache, increased pressure sensations in the head, nausea, vomiting, perspiration, thirst, red face, restlessness, anxiety, stiff neck, dilated pupils, hurried respiration rate (up to 53 times per minute), elevated body temperature (up to 45° C), elevated blood pressure (up to 150-170/110-130 mmHg), tachycardia (up to 123 beats per minute), and forceful rapid pulse. As the reaction progresses, patients may also exhibit general tremors, muscle stiffness, clenched jaw, mania, jaundice, and in severe cases, anuria, unconsciousness, and respiratory depression.[2]

TREATMENT OF OVERDOSAGE

Early-stage overdose can be treated with emetic methods, followed by ingestion of milk, egg whites or activated charcoal.

Overdose of *Xi Xin* can be differentiated into different types and treated accordingly. Overdose characterized by headache with increased pressure, perspiration, red face, dilated pupils, increased heart rate, and a forceful, rapid pulse should be treated with herbs that clear heat and eliminate toxins, such as 250 grams of *Lu Dou* (Semen Phaseoli Radiati), with a small amount of salt.

Overdose characterized by yellow discoloration of the skin, yellow urine, and a red tongue with a yellow tongue coating should be treated with herbs that clear heat and relieve jaundice, such as an herbal decoction with *Jin Yin Hua* (Flos Lonicerae) 15g, *Sheng Ma* (Rhizoma Cimicifugae) 15g, *San Qi* (Radix Notoginseng) 3g, *Mu Dan Pi* (Cortex Moutan) 12g, *Yin Chen Hao* (Herba Artemisiae Scopariae) 15g, *Che Qian Zi* (Semen Plantaginis) 15g, and *Hu Zhang* (Rhizoma Polygoni Cuspidati) 15g.

Overdose characterized by delirium, muscle stiffness and convulsions, rapid respiration, and a red tongue with a yellow tongue coating should be treated by clearing heat and toxins from the *ying* (nutritive) and *xue* (blood) levels, such as with an herbal decoction that contains *Xi Yang Shen* (Radix Panacis Quinquefolii) 3g, *Wu Wei Zi* (Fructus Schisandrae Chinensis) 3g, *Mai Men Dong* (Radix Ophiopogonis) 9g, *Shi Gao* (Gypsum Fibrosum) 24g, *Gan Cao* (Radix Glycyrrhizae) 30g, and *Ling Yang Jiao* (Cornu Saigae Tataricae) 3g.

CHEMICAL COMPOSITION

Essential oils 2.39-3.80% (methyl eugenol, safrole, asaricin, eucarvone), higenamine, aristolochic acid.[3,4]

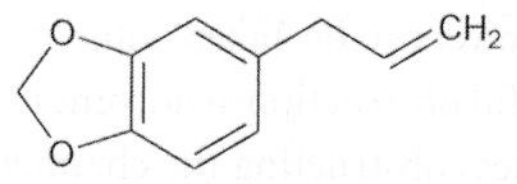

Safrole

PHARMACOLOGICAL EFFECTS

- **Respiratory:** Many constituents of *Xi Xin* stimulate the respiratory system. Intravenous injection of alcohol extract of *Xi Xin* effectively reversed morphine-induced respiratory depression in rabbits. *Xi Xin* may also increase lung capacity for 15 to 30 minutes. Methyleugenol has a bronchodilating effect in mice.[5]
- **Cardiovascular:** Administration of an alcohol extract of *Xi Xin* is associated with increased heart rate and increased cardiac output in laboratory experiments.[6]
- **Antibiotic:** *Xi Xin* has an inhibitory effect against *Streptococcus* spp., *Shigella* spp., and *Salmonella typhi*.[7]
- **Anti-inflammatory:** Essential oil of *Xi Xin* has a marked effect to reduce inflammation associated with increased vascular permeability caused by PGE2. In laboratory experiments, intraperitoneal injection of essential oil of *Xi Xin* at 0.24 ml/kg effectively reduced swelling in the legs of rats.[8]
- **Anesthetic:** Essential oil of *Xi Xin* produces a local anesthetic effect in rabbits when injected locally. The anesthetic effect of *Xi Xin* is comparable to that of 1% novacaine.[9]

CLINICAL STUDIES AND RESEARCH

- **Aphthous ulcers:** *Xi Xin* in the form of topical paste was used in one study to treat 106 patients with aphthous ulcers. The herbal paste was made from 9 to 15 grams of powder mixed with water and glycerin, and placed on the navel for at least three days. The rate of effectiveness was 93.4%.[10]
- **Angina:** In one study, 281 patients with coronary artery disease and angina were treated with an herbal sublingual

Xi Xin (Herba Asari)

spray with pain relief achieved within 5 minutes in 64.8% of the cases. The therapeutic effect was concluded to be similar to that of nitroglycerin. The herbal spray contained 50 ml of essential oil of *Xi Xin,* and 16 grams of *Bing Pian* (Borneolum Syntheticum), dissolved in 600 ml of 95% alcohol.[11]

TOXICOLOGY

In animal experiments, the LD_{50} for essential oil of *Xi Xin* in mice is 1.2 ml/kg via intraperitoneal injection. Respiratory paralysis was associated with overdose.[12]

Xi Xin belongs in the Aristolochiaceae family, and has been found to contain trace amounts of aristolochic acid. For more information on the toxicology of this compound, please refer to the monographs on *Guang Fang Ji* (Radix Aristolochiae Fangchi) or *Guan Mu Tong* (Caulis Aristolochiae Manshuriensis).

SUPPLEMENT

- 土細辛 / 土细辛 *Tu Xi Xin* (Herba Asarum Forbgesii), derived from the same genus as *Xi Xin,* has actions that are similar to this herb but weaker.

AUTHORS' COMMENTS

Xi Xin has potent effect to dispel wind-cold from the exterior and warm the interior. Depending on the reference, it has been classified as either an exterior-releasing herb or an interior-warming herb.

Xi Xin and *Ma Huang* (Herba Ephedrae) both function to warm the body and dispel wind-cold.

- *Xi Xin* is penetrating in nature and more strongly warms the body while mainly relieving pain of headaches, body-wide muscle aches, and pain caused by wind-cold.
- *Ma Huang* is dispersing in nature and more effectively disperses wind and releases exterior conditions. It is the strongest herb for treating wheezing and dyspnea in wind-cold invasions where there is no perspiration.

Optimal treatment of headache requires use of channel-guiding herbs to deliver the therapeutic effect of the herbs to the affected area. The following is a list of commonly used channel-guiding herbs:

- *Taiyang* channels: *Qiang Huo* (Rhizoma et Radix Notopterygii)
- *Shaoyang* channels: *Chai Hu* (Radix Bupleuri)
- *Yangming* channels: *Bai Zhi* (Radix Angelicae Dahuricae)
- *Taiyin* channels: *Cang Zhu* (Rhizoma Atractylodis)
- *Shaoyin* channels: *Xi Xin* (Herba Asari)
- *Jueyin* channels: *Wu Zhu Yu* (Fructus Evodiae)

References

1. *Shang Hai Zhong Yi Yao Za Zhi* (Shanghai Journal of Chinese Medicine and Herbology), 1987; 9:2
2. *Zhong Yao Du Li Xue* (Toxicology of Chinese Herbs), 1989;110-111
3. *Xian Dai Zhong Yao Yao Li Xue* (Contemporary Pharmacology of Chinese Herbs), 1997; 49
4. *The Merck Index* 12th edition, Chapman & Hall/CRCnetBASE/Merck, 2000
5. *Zhong Yao Yao Li Yu Ying Yong* (Pharmacology and Applications of Chinese Herbs), 1983; 724
6. *Yao Xue Xue Bao* (Journal of Herbology), 1981; 16(10):24
7. *Zhong Yao Zhi* (Chinese Herbology Journal), 1988: 117
8. *Yao Xue Xue Bao* (Journal of Herbology), 1982; 17(1):12
9. *Zhong Yao Xue* (Chinese Herbology), 1998, 380:382
10. *Zhong Hua Kou Qiang Ke Za Zhi* (Chinese Journal of Stomatology), 1960; 2:75
11. *Xin Yi Yao Xue Za Zhi* (New Journal of Medicine and Herbology), 1977; 1:13
12. *Yao Xue Xue Bao* (Journal of Herbology), 1982; 17(1):12

Hua Jiao (Pericarpium Zanthoxyli)

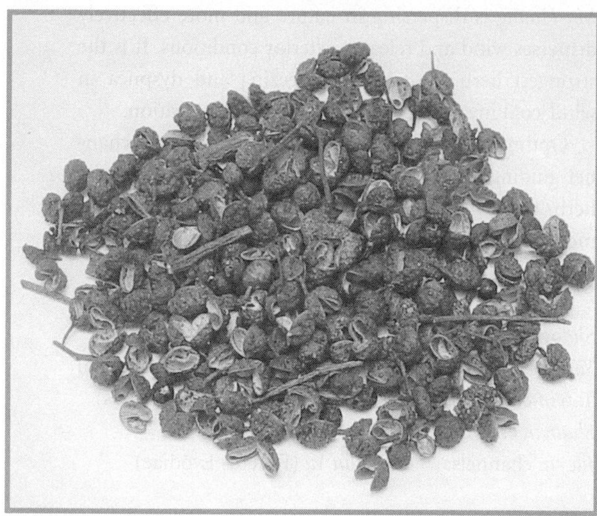

花椒 花椒

Pinyin Name: *Hua Jiao*
Literal Name: "flower pepper"
Alternate Chinese Names: *Qin Jiao, Shu Jiao, Chuan Jiao, Ba Jiao, Hong Jiao, Da Hong Pao*
Original Source: *Shen Nong Ben Cao Jing* (Divine Husbandman's Classic of the Materia Medica) in the second century
English Name: zanthoxylum, prickly ash pepper tree peel, bunge prickly ash peel
Botanical Name: *Zanthoxylum bungeanum* Maxim. (*Hua Jiao*); *Zanthoxylum schinifolium* Sieb. et Zucc. (*Qing Jiao*); Various other species that are used interchangeably include *Zanthoxylum simulans* Hance. (*Ye Hua Jiao*), *Zanthoxylum planispinum* Sieb. et Zucc. (*Zhu Ye Jiao*); *Zanthoxylum avicennae* (Lam.) DC. (*Lei Dang*); and *Zanthoxylum simulans* Hance var. *podocarpum* (Hemsl.) Huang (*Bing Guo Hua Jiao*).
Pharmaceutical Name: Pericarpium Zanthoxyli
Properties: acrid, hot
Channels Entered: Kidney, Spleen, Stomach
Safety Index: slightly toxic

CHINESE THERAPEUTIC ACTIONS

1. Warms the Middle *Jiao,* Stops Pain and Relieves Diarrhea

Epigastric and abdominal coldness and pain, toothache, diarrhea: *Hua Jiao* (Pericarpium Zanthoxyli) warms the Spleen and Stomach to treat excess accumulation of cold in the middle *jiao.*

- Coldness and pain in the chest with vomiting and inability to eat: use *Hua Jiao* with *Gan Jiang* (Rhizoma Zingiberis), *Ren Shen* (Radix Ginseng) and *Yi Tang* (Saccharum Granorum). **Exemplar Formula:** *Da Jian Zhong Tang* (Major Construct the Middle Decoction).
- Coldness and pain in the epigastric and abdominal regions: dry fry *Hua Jiao* and apply it to the affected area to disperse cold.
- Diarrhea due more to cold than to dampness: use this herb with *Fu Zi* (Radix Aconiti Lateralis Praeparata) and *Gan Jiang* (Rhizoma Zingiberis).
- Diarrhea due more to dampness than to cold: combine it with *Cang Zhu* (Rhizoma Atractylodis) and *Hou Po* (Cortex Magnoliae Officinalis).
- Toothache: apply *Hua Jiao* topically to the affected tooth and gums.

2. Kills Parasites

Parasites and itching of the skin: *Hua Jiao* treats parasitic infestations in the intestines that are causing vomiting and abdominal pain. It also treats parasitic infection of the skin manifesting in pruritus and eczema.

- Vomiting and abdominal pain due to roundworms: use *Hua Jiao* individually, or combine it with *Wu Mei* (Fructus Mume) and *Huang Lian* (Rhizoma Coptidis).
- Intestinal obstruction by parasites: fry *Hua Jiao* with cooking oil and use it daily with meals.
- Pruritis, genital itching and eczema: use it with *Ku Shen Gen* (Radix Sophorae Flavescentis) and *Di Fu Zi* (Fructus Kochiae).

DOSAGE

2 to 5 grams in herbal decoction. *Hua Jiao* may be used both internally and topically.

CAUTIONS / CONTRAINDICATIONS

- *Hua Jiao* is contraindicated in the presence of excess fire, or of yin deficiency.
- Use *Hua Jiao* with caution during pregnancy.

CHEMICAL COMPOSITION

Essential oils (limonene, 1,8-cineol, myrcene), skimmianine, kokusaginine, haplopine, herniarin, xanthoxylin.[1]

Hua Jiao (Pericarpium Zanthoxyli)

PHARMACOLOGICAL EFFECTS

- **Anesthetic and analgesic:** Water extract of *Hua Jiao* has local anesthetic and analgesic effects as demonstrated in mice. Prolonged use is associated with tolerance.[2]
- **Antiulcer:** Water extract of *Hua Jiao* at 5 to 10 g/kg acts to prevent and treat stomach ulcers in mice. However, it only achieved 22% effectiveness.[3]
- **Antidiarrheal:** Water extract of *Hua Jiao* at 5 to 10 g/kg has an antidiarrheal effect. In mice, *Hua Jiao* effectively delays the onset and shortens the duration of diarrhea, when diarrhea is induced by ingestion of *Fan Xie Ye* (Folium Sennae).[4]
- **Antibiotic:** It has an inhibitory effect against β-hemolytic streptococcus, *Staphylococcus aureus*, *Diplococcus pneumoniae*, *Bacillus dysenteriae*, *Salmonella typhi*, and some dermatophytes.[5]

CLINICAL STUDIES AND RESEARCH

- **Intestinal obstruction:** Eight children with intestinal obstructions caused by roundworms were treated with *Hua Jiao*, with satisfactory results. Pain relief was achieved within 15 to 30 minutes, followed by defecation of stool with roundworms.[6]
- **Inhibition of lactation:** According to one report, 163 women who wanted to stop lactation immediately after labor were treated with one 400 mg capsule of *Hua Jiao* three times daily for 3 to 4 days, with a 93.9% rate of effectiveness. The herbal capsule was prepared by grinding the herb into powder and placing it in capsules.[7]

TOXICOLOGY

The LD_{50} for skimmianine is 150 to 250 mg/kg in mice.[8]

SUPPLEMENT

- 椒目 *Jiao Mu* (Semen Zanthoxyli Bungeani), first cited in the *Ben Cao Jing Ji Zhu* (Collection of Commentaries on the Classic of the Materia Medica) by Tao Hong-Jing in 480-498 A.D., is bitter, cold, toxic, and enters the Spleen and Urinary Bladder. It regulates water circulation to relieve edema, and eliminates water accumulation in the Lung to facilitate breathing. Clinically, it treats dysuria and edema with its mild diuretic effect. It is also used to treat accumulation of water in the Lung with symptoms such as wheezing, dyspnea, edema, drum-like distention of the abdomen, and phlegm invading the Lung causing dyspnea and wheezing with an inability to lie down. It was demonstrated in one clinical study of 958 patients with wheezing and dyspnea that a preparation of *Jiao Mu* given three times daily for 7 to 10 days per course of treatment was effective in 78.5% of patients. The herbal preparation was described as having a rapid onset of action, good therapeutic effect, few side effects, and a wide range of clinical applications. The regular dose for *Jiao Mu* is 2 to 5 grams.[9]

AUTHORS' COMMENTS

Hua Jiao (Pericarpium Zanthoxyli) and *Hu Jiao* (Fructus Piper) have similar pinyin names. However, they should not be confused, as they are two different herbs with differing characteristics and actions.

References

1. *Xian Dai Zhong Yao Yao Li Xue* (Contemporary Pharmacology of Chinese Herbs), 1997; 613-614
2. *Zhong Guo Zhong Yao Za Zhi* (People's Republic of China Journal of Chinese Herbology), 1991; 16(8):493
3. Ibid.
4. Ibid.
5. *Zhong Yao Xue* (Chinese Herbology), 1998; 382:384
6. *Zhong Yi Za Zhi* (Journal of Chinese Medicine), 4:21
7. *Di Er Jun Yi Da Xue Xue Bao* (Journal of Second Military University of Medicine), 1987; 3:232
8. *Zhi Wu Yao You Xiao Cheng Fen Shou Ce* (Manual of Plant Medicinals and Their Active Constituents), 1986; 123:969
9. *Zhong Yi Za Zhi* (Journal of Chinese Medicine), 1987; 12:19

Gao Liang Jiang (Rhizoma Alpiniae Officinarum)

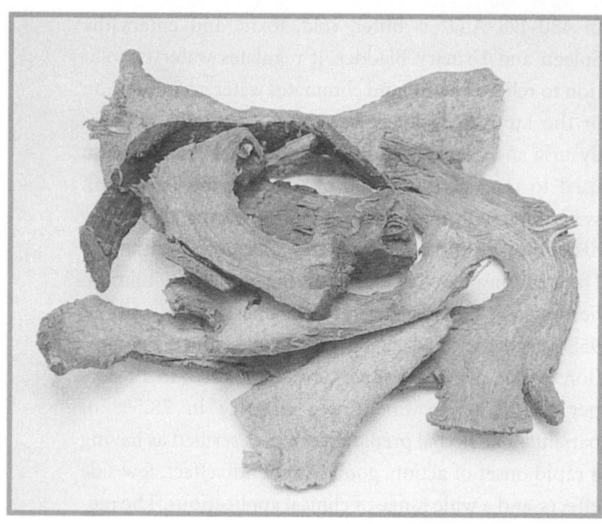

高良薑 高良姜

Pinyin Name: *Gao Liang Jiang*
Original Source: *Ming Yi Za Zhu* (Miscellaneous Records of Famous Physicians) by Tao Hong-Jing in 500 A.D.
English Name: alpinia, galanga, lesser galangal rhizome
Botanical Name: *Alpinia officinarum* Hance. (*Gao Liang Jiang*)
Pharmaceutical Name: Rhizoma Alpiniae Officinarum
Properties: acrid, hot
Channels Entered: Spleen, Stomach

CHINESE THERAPEUTIC ACTIONS

Warms the Spleen and Stomach

The major strength of *Gao Liang Jiang* (Rhizoma Alpiniae Officinarum) is in dispelling cold from the middle *jiao* to treat epigastric and abdominal pain, nausea, vomiting, food stagnation, intestinal cramps and diarrhea. It can be used alone, or with other interior-warming herbs to enhance the overall effect.

- Coldness and pain in the epigastric and abdominal region: use *Gao Liang Jiang* with *Pao Jiang* (Rhizoma Zingiberis Preparatum) and *Wu Zhu Yu* (Fructus Evodiae).
- Sharp, stabbing pain in the chest and abdomen: use it with *Rou Gui* (Cortex Cinnamomi) and *Dang Gui* (Radicis Angelicae Sinensis).
- Intestinal cramps: combine it with *Hou Po* (Cortex Magnoliae Officinalis), *Dang Gui* (Radicis Angelicae Sinensis), *Rou Gui* (Cortex Cinnamomi) and *Sheng Jiang* (Rhizoma Zingiberis Recens). **Exemplar Formula:** ***Liang Fu Wan*** (Galangal and Cyperus Pill).
- Accumulation of cold with Liver qi stagnation: use this herb with *Xiang Fu* (Rhizoma Cyperi).
- Nausea and vomiting due to cold: use it with *Gan Jiang* (Rhizoma Zingiberis), *Ban Xia* (Rhizoma Pinelliae), *Su Zi* (Fructus Perillae), *Ding Xiang* (Flos Caryophylli), *Rou Gui* (Cortex Cinnamomi) and *Wu Zhu Yu* (Fructus Evodiae).
- Abdominal hernial pain: add *Xiao Hui Xiang* (Fructus Foeniculi).
- Acute diarrhea from Spleen and Kidney yang deficiencies: use *Gao Liang Jiang* with *Fu Zi* (Radix Aconiti Lateralis Praeparata) and *Rou Gui* (Cortex Cinnamomi).
- Chronic diarrhea from deficiency and cold: combine it with *Bu Gu Zhi* (Fructus Psoraleae) and *Li Zhong Tang* (Regulate the Middle Decoction).

DOSAGE

3 to 10 grams.

CAUTIONS / CONTRAINDICATIONS

- *Gao Liang Jiang* is contraindicated in cases of interior heat with yin deficiency.

CHEMICAL COMPOSITION

Essential oils 0.5 to 1.5% (cineol, methy cinnamate, eugenol, pinene, cadinene, galangol), flavonoids (galangin, kampferide, kaempferol, quercetin, isorhamnetin).[1]

PHARMACOLOGICAL EFFECTS

- **Gastrointestinal:** *Gao Liang Jiang* has various effects on the gastrointestinal system. Both water and alcohol extracts of the herb have demonstrated marked analgesic and cholagogic effects. In addition, both have shown marked preventative and treatment effects on peptic ulcers and diarrhea. The water extract of the herb also has an inhibitory effect on the gastrointestinal system, as it decreases intestinal peristalsis.[2]
- **Analgesic:** *Gao Liang Jiang* may be used to treat angina, as it has a rapid onset of analgesic effect.[3]
- **Antibiotic:** It has an inhibitory effect on *Bacillus anthracis*, *Corynebacterium diphtheriae*, *Diplococcus pneumoniae*, *Salmonella typhi*, *Staphylococcus aureus*, β-hemolytic streptococcus, and *Mycobacterium tuberculosis hominis.*[4]

TOXICOLOGY

Water extract of *Gao Liang Jiang* administered orally at the dosage of 120 g/kg for 7 days did not contribute to any fatalities in mice. The LD_{50} for alcohol extract of the herb via the oral route was 4.2 +/- 0.4 ml/kg in mice.[5]

Gao Liang Jiang (Rhizoma Alpiniae Officinarum)

SUPPLEMENT

- 紅豆蔻 / 红豆蔻 *Hong Dou Kou* (Fructus Alphiniae Galangae), first cited in the *Yao Xing Ben Cao* (Materia Medica of Medicinal Properties) by Zhen Quan in 600 A.D., is derived from the fruit of the same plant as *Gao Liang Jiang*. *Hong Dou Kou* is acrid and warm, enters the Spleen and Stomach and warms the Lung, dispels coldness, awakens the Spleen, dries dampness, aids digestion, stops pain and eliminates alcohol toxins. Common applications include epigastric and abdominal coldness and pain, vomiting, diarrhea, and no desire to drink or eat. *Hong Dou Kou* can also be used topically to treat toothache caused by wind and cold. The recommended dosage of *Hong Dou Kou* is 3 to 6 grams. It is contraindicated in patients with yin-deficient heat.

AUTHORS' COMMENTS

Gao Liang Jiang and *Gan Jiang* (Rhizoma Zingiberis) both warm the middle *jiao* and dispel cold. *Gao Liang Jiang* is stronger in warming the Stomach, dispersing cold and relieving pain. It is most suitable for cold directly attacking the middle, injuring the Stomach, and resulting in epigastric and abdominal fullness and pain. *Gan Jiang* is stronger in warming the Spleen to stop diarrhea. It is suitable for deficiency and cold of the middle *jiao* with epigastric and abdominal coldness and pain, loose stools and decreased food intake.

References

1. *Xian Dai Zhong Yao Yao Li Xue* (Contemporary Pharmacology of Chinese Herbs), 1997; 624
2. *Zhong Yao Cai* (Study of Chinese Herbal Material), 1991; 14(10):37
3. *Zhong Yao Tong Bao* (Journal of Chinese Herbology), 1986; 11(7):54
4. *Zhong Yao Xue* (Chinese Herbology), 1998; 384:385
5. *CA*, 1987; 88:46079C

Ding Xiang (Flos Caryophylli)

丁香

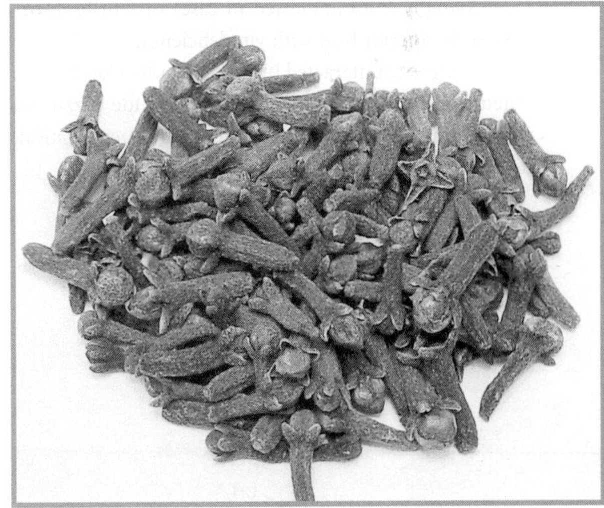

Pinyin Name: *Ding Xiang*
Literal Name: "t-shaped aroma," "spike fragrance"
Alternate Chinese Names: *Gong Ding Xiang, Xiong Ding Xiang*
Original Source: *Yao Xing Ben Cao* (Materia Medica of Medicinal Properties) by Zhen Quan in 600 A.D.
English Name: clove
Botanical Name: *Eugenia caryophyllata* Thunb. (*Ding Xiang*)
Pharmaceutical Name: Flos Caryophylli
Properties: acrid, warm
Channels Entered: Kidney, Spleen, Stomach

CHINESE THERAPEUTIC ACTIONS

1. Warms the Middle *Jiao,* Relieves Pain and Reverses Rising Stomach Qi

Epigastric and abdominal coldness and pain, vomiting, hiccups: *Ding Xiang* (Flos Caryophylli) is the key herb for treating abnormal rising of Stomach qi caused by coldness that is manifesting in vomiting, nausea and hiccups. Other clinical applications include epigastric and abdominal coldness and pain, abdominal fullness and distention that occurs when the individual is exposed to cold.

- Coldness and pain in the epigastric and abdominal regions: use *Ding Xiang* with *Rou Gui* (Cortex Cinnamomi) and *Gan Jiang* (Rhizoma Zingiberis).
- Nausea and vomiting due to Stomach cold: use it with *Ban Xia* (Rhizoma Pinelliae) and *Sheng Jiang* (Rhizoma Zingiberis Recens).

Ding Xiang (Flos Caryophylli)

- Hiccups due to Stomach cold: add *Shi Di* (Calyx Kaki).
- Hiccups due to deficiency and cold: use *Ding Xiang* with *Ren Shen* (Radix Ginseng) or *Dang Shen* (Radix Codonopsis).
- Morning sickness in pregnant women: combine it with *Ren Shen* (Radix Ginseng) and *Huo Xiang* (Herba Agastache).
- Diarrhea due to deficiency or cold: use this herb with *Gan Jiang* (Rhizoma Zingiberis), *Ren Shen* (Radix Ginseng), *Bai Zhu* (Rhizoma Atractylodis Macrocephalae) and *Rou Dou Kou* (Semen Myristicae).

2. Tonifies Kidney Yang

Ding Xiang treats impotence, cold body and extremities, and weakness and soreness of the back and knees caused by Kidney yang deficiency.

- Kidney yang deficiency: use *Ding Xiang* with *Fu Zi* (Radix Aconiti Lateralis Praeparata), *Rou Gui* (Cortex Cinnamomi) and *Ba Ji Tian* (Radix Morindae Officinalis).

Ding Xiang, soaked in rubbing alcohol and applied topically, has been used to treat various fungal infections.

DOSAGE

2 to 5 grams.

CAUTIONS / CONTRAINDICATIONS

- *Ding Xiang* is contraindicated in cases of febrile disorders, or in interior heat with yin deficiency.
- *Ding Xiang* is counteracted by *Yu Jin* (Radix Curcumae).
- Potential side effects of *Ding Xiang* include dizziness, palpitations, chest oppression, headache, perspiration, decreased blood pressure, and skin rash.[1]

CHEMICAL COMPOSITION

Essential oils 16–19% (eugenol, caryophyllene, acetyleugenol), α-caryophyllene, chavicol.[2,3]

OH, OCH_3, CH_2

Eugenol

PHARMACOLOGICAL EFFECTS

- **Gastrointestinal:** *Ding Xiang* promotes digestion by increasing bile and gastric acid secretions.[4]
- **Antibiotic:** *Ding Xiang* has an inhibiting effect against *Vibrio cholerae, Bacillus anthracis, Salmonella typhi, Corynebacterium diphtheriae, Bacillus dysenteriae, E. coli, Bacillus subtilis*, and *Staphylococcus aureus*.[5]
- **Analgesic:** Essential oil of *Ding Xiang* applied topically has an analgesic effect to relieve toothache.[6]
- **Antitoxin:** Potassium cyanide and sodium nitrate poisoning can be treated by administration of *Ding Xiang*. According to animal studies, intraperitoneal injection of *Ding Xiang* was beneficial in prolonging the survival time in mice that were given 4 mg/kg of potassium cyanide via intravenous injection. Similar beneficial effects were observed in mice poisoned with 800 mg/kg of sodium nitrate.[7]
- **Antiasthmatic:** Essential oil of *Ding Xiang* has a marked antiasthmatic effect, with a duration of action of approximately 6 hours.[8]

CLINICAL STUDIES AND RESEARCH

- **Fungal infection:** According to one report, 31 patients who had fungal infection for two years or more were treated topically with an herbal tincture applied to the affected area three times daily for 2 to 5 days, with excellent results. Most patients began to notice improvement after 2 to 3 days, with complete recovery achieved within 3 to 5 days. The incidence of recurrence was approximately 20%. The herbal tincture was prepared by soaking 15 grams of *Ding Xiang* in 100 ml of 70% alcohol for 48 hours.[9]

SUPPLEMENT

- 母丁香 *Mu Ding Xiang* (Fructus Caryophylli), first cited in *Ming Yi Za Zhu* (Miscellaneous Records of Famous Physicians) by Tao Hong-Jing in 500 A.D., is derived from the fruit of the same plant as *Ding Xiang*. Both herbs have the same taste, functions and indications. *Mu Ding Xiang* has a weaker but longer-lasting therapeutic effect. The recommended dosage of *Mu Ding Xiang* is 2 to 5 grams.
- 丁香皮 *Ding Xiang Pi* (Cortex Caryophylli), the bark from the same plant as *Ding Xiang*, is used to dispel cold and relieve pain.

References

1. *Hua Xi Kou Qiang Yi Xue Za Zhi* (Huaxi Journal of Stomatology), 1990; 4:275
2. *Xian Dai Zhong Yao Yao Li Xue* (Contemporary Pharmacology of Chinese Herbs), 1997; 622
3. *The Merck Index* 12th edition, Chapman & Hall/CRCnetBASE/Merck, 2000
4. *Chang Yong Zhong Yao Cheng Fen Yu Yao Li Shou Ce* (A Handbook of the Composition and Pharmacology of Common Chinese Drugs), 1994; 1:10
5. *Zhong Cao Yao Xue* (Study of Chinese Herbal Medicine), 1976; 707
6. *Zhong Yao Xue* (Chinese Herbology), 1998; 386:387
7. *Chang Yong Zhong Yao Cheng Fen Yu Yao Li Shou Ce* (A Handbook of the Composition and Pharmacology of Common Chinese Drugs), 1994; 1:10
8. *Yao Xue Xue Bao* (Journal of Herbology), 1987; 22(3):179
9. *Zhong Hua Pi Fu Ke Xue Za Zhi* (Chinese Journal of Dermatology), 1963; 1:17

Hu Jiao (Fructus Piper)

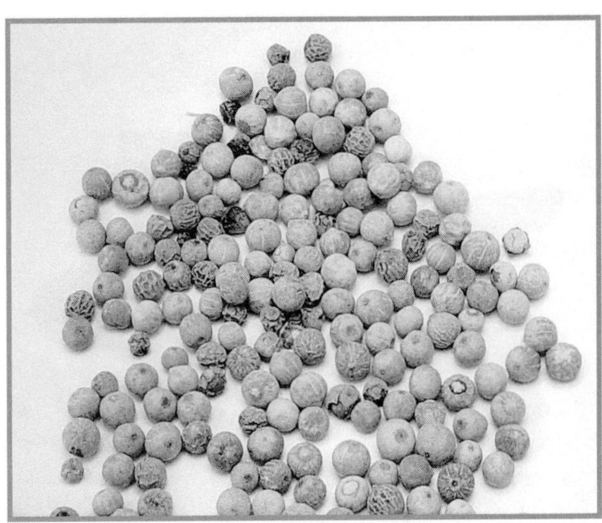

胡椒

Pinyin Name: *Hu Jiao*
Literal Name: "barbarian pepper"
Alternate Chinese Names: *Bai Chuan, Hei Chuan*
Original Source: *Xin Xiu Ben Cao* (Newly Revised Materia Medica) by Su Jing in 657-659 A.D.
English Name: pepper, black pepper
Botanical Name: *Piper nigrum* L. (*Hu Jiao*)
Pharmaceutical Name: Fructus Piper
Properties: acrid, hot
Channels Entered: Stomach, Large Intestine

CHINESE THERAPEUTIC ACTIONS

Warms the Middle and Relieves Pain

Hu Jiao (Fructus Piper) disperses cold in the gastrointestinal system and relieves vomiting, nausea, epigastric and abdominal cold and pain, poor appetite and diarrhea.

- Gastrointestinal symptoms due to cold: use *Hu Jiao* with *Sheng Jiang* (Rhizoma Zingiberis Recens), and *Gao Liang Jiang* (Rhizoma Alpiniae Officinarum).
- Vomiting and nausea: use it with *Ban Xia* (Rhizoma Pinelliae) and *Sheng Jiang* (Rhizoma Zingiberis Recens).

The powder of *Hu Jiao* can be applied to the umbilicus to warm the middle *jiao*, or applied topically for toothache.

DOSAGE

2 to 3 grams in decoction, 0.5 to 1 gram in powder.

CAUTIONS / CONTRAINDICATIONS

- *Hu Jiao* is contraindicated in patients with yin deficiency or heat.
- *Hu Jiao* should be used with caution during pregnancy, due to its abortifacient effect.[1]

CHEMICAL COMPOSITION

Piperonal, dihydrocarveol, caryo-phyllene oxide, cryptone, transpinocarrol, piperine, piperyline, piperoleine A, B, C; piperanine.[2]

CLINICAL STUDIES AND RESEARCH

- **Diarrhea:** In a clinical study, 209 infants with diarrhea were treated with topical application of *Hu Jiao,* with a 81.3% rate of effectiveness. The treatment protocol was to grind 1 to 2 pieces of *Hu Jiao* and apply the powder to the umbilicus, cover with gauze, and change the application every 24 hours. The treatment may be repeated two to three times if necessary.[3]

AUTHORS' COMMENTS

Hu Jiao (Fructus Piper) and *Hua Jiao* (Pericarpium Zanthoxyli) have similar pinyin names. However, they should not be confused, as they are two different herbs, with differing characteristics and actions.

References

1. Brinker, Francis. *The Toxicology of Botanical Medicines,* rev. 2nd ed., 1996
2. *Xian Dai Zhong Yao Yao Li Xue* (Contemporary Pharmacology of Chinese Herbs), 1997; 630
3. *He Bei Zhong Yi* (Hebei Chinese Medicine), 1985; 4:23

Bi Ba (Fructus Piperis Longi)

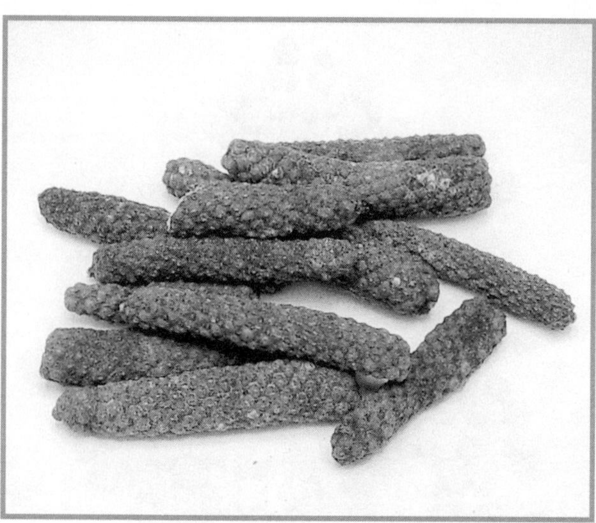

蓽茇 荜茇

Pinyin Name: *Bi Ba*
Original Source: *Xin Xiu Ben Cao* (Newly Revised Materia Medica) by Su Jing in 657-659 A.D.
English Name: long pepper
Botanical Name: *Piper longum* L. (*Bi Ba*)
Pharmaceutical Name: Fructus Piperis Longi
Properties: acrid, hot
Channels Entered: Stomach, Large Intestine

CHINESE THERAPEUTIC ACTIONS

Warms Middle *Jiao*, Relieves Pain

Bi Ba (Fructus Piperis Longi), hot and acrid, dispels cold in the middle *jiao*. It is often cooked with porridge to dispel cold from the Spleen and Stomach to relieve epigastric and abdominal pain, nausea, vomiting, poor appetite, diarrhea and dysentery.

- Cold in the Spleen and Stomach: use *Bi Ba* with *Rou Gui* (Cortex Cinnamomi), *Pao Jiang* (Rhizoma Zingiberis Preparatum) and *Gao Liang Jiang* (Rhizoma Alpiniae Officinarum).
- Deficiency of the Spleen and Stomach: use this herb with *Ren Shen* (Radix Ginseng) and *Bai Zhu* (Rhizoma Atractylodis Macrocephalae).
- Nausea and vomiting arising from cold phlegm in the Stomach: use it with *Ban Xia* (Rhizoma Pinelliae) and *Sheng Jiang* (Rhizoma Zingiberis Recens).
- Epigastric and abdominal fullness and distention: use this herb with *Mu Xiang* (Radix Aucklandiae) and *Hou Po* (Cortex Magnoliae Officinalis).
- Toothache: use it with *Hu Jiao* (Fructus Piper) and apply topically as powder.

DOSAGE

2 to 5 grams. *Bi Ba* is used both internally and topically.

CAUTIONS / CONTRAINDICATIONS

- *Bi Ba* is contraindicated in cases of yin-deficient heat or excess heat.

CHEMICAL COMPOSITION

Piperine, piperlongumine, piplartin, sesamine.[1]

PHARMACOLOGICAL EFFECTS

- **Antibiotic:** *Bi Ba* has an inhibitory influence on *Staphylococcus aureus, Bacillus subtilis, Mycobacterium tuberculosis, Bacillus dysenteriae, Salmonella typhi,* and *Bacillus cereus.*[2]
- **Anticonvulsant:** Intraperitoneal injection of *Bi Ba* has marked effectiveness to prevent seizures and convulsions in rats, with potency similar to phenytoin and trimethadione.[3]
- **Cardiovascular:** *Bi Ba* dilates blood vessels and causes feelings of warmth in the body and the extremities. Essential oil of the herb is associated with increased resistance of the cardiac muscle to hypoxia.[4] Lastly, piperlongumine and piplartin at 0.1 mg/kg have a marked effect to lower blood pressure in rabbits and rats.[5]

TOXICOLOGY

Long-term administration of *Bi Ba* at therapeutic dosage for 9 months showed no abnormality in the liver, kidneys, lungs, or other internal organs. The LD_{50} for piperine via intraperitoneal injection in rats is 348.6 mg/kg.[6]

References

1. *Xian Dai Zhong Yao Yao Li Xue* (Contemporary Pharmacology of Chinese Herbs), 1997; 616
2. *Zhong Yao Zhi* (Chinese Herbology Journal), 1984; 508
3. *Zhi Wu Yao You Xiao Cheng Fen Shou Ce* (Manual of Plant Medicinals and Their Active Constituents), 1986; 954:836:838
4. *Zhong Yao Xue* (Chinese Herbology), 1998; 389:390
5. *Zhong Cao Yao* (Chinese Herbal Medicine), 1992; 23(4):197
6. *Zhong Yi Za Zhi* (Journal of Chinese Medicine), 1981; (12):65

Bi Cheng Qie (Fructus Litseae)

蓽澄茄 荜澄茄

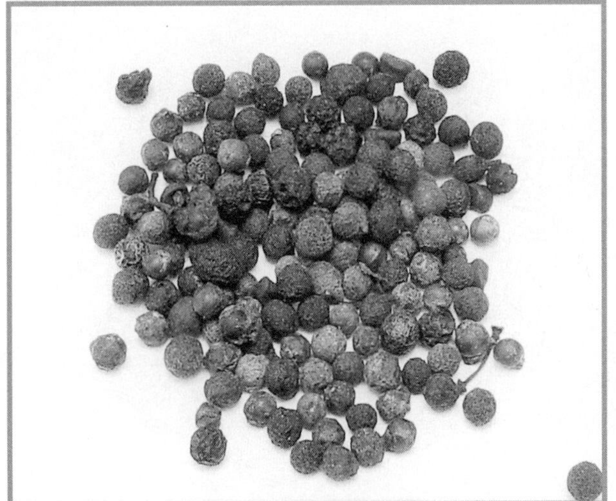

Pinyin Name: *Bi Cheng Qie*
Alternate Chinese Names: *Cheng Qie*
Original Source: *Hai Yao Ben Cao* (Materia Medica of Herbs from [Across the] Seas) by Li Xun in 907-960 A.D.
English Name: litsea
Botanical Name: *Litsea cubeba* (Lour.) Pers. (*Shan Ji Jiao*); *Piper cubeba* L. (*Bi Cheng Qie*)
Pharmaceutical Name: Fructus Litseae
Properties: acrid, warm
Channels Entered: Spleen, Stomach, Kidney, Urinary Bladder

CHINESE THERAPEUTIC ACTIONS

1. Warms the Middle *Jiao* and Relieves Pain

Epigastric and abdominal pain and coldness, vomiting, diarrhea: *Bi Cheng Qie* (Fructus Litseae) warms the middle *jiao*, stops pain, promotes digestion and treats cold-related gastrointestinal disorders.

- Hiccups, poor appetite: use *Bi Cheng Qie* with *Sheng Jiang* (Rhizoma Zingiberis Recens) and *Shen Qu* (Massa Fermentata).
- Vomiting and nausea: use it with *Gao Liang Jiang* (Rhizoma Alpiniae Officinarum) and *Bai Dou Kou* (Fructus Amomi Rotundus).
- Hernial pain: combine it with *Wu Zhu Yu* (Fructus Evodiae) and *Xiang Fu* (Rhizoma Cyperi).

2. Dispels Cold in the Urinary Bladder

Dysuria or turbid urine: *Bi Cheng Qie* dispels cold in the Kidney and Urinary Bladder. It is excellent for deficiency and cold of the lower *jiao* that manifest in symptoms of dysuria and turbid urine.

Bi Cheng Qie is used to relieve toothache, when applied topically as powder.

DOSAGE

2 to 5 grams.

CAUTIONS / CONTRAINDICATIONS

- *Bi Cheng Qie* is contraindicated in cases of yin deficiency and heat.

CHEMICAL COMPOSITION

Essential oils 2-6% (citral, limonene, citronellal, camphene, methylheptenone, α-pinene, methylheptylketone), cubebaol.[1]

References

1. *Xian Dai Zhong Yao Yao Li Xue* (Contemporary Pharmacology of Chinese Herbs), 1997; 617-618

Xiao Hui Xiang (Fructus Foeniculi)

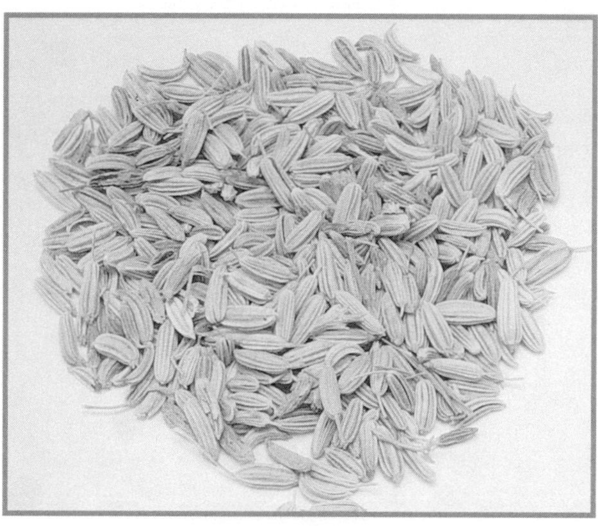

小茴香 小茴香

Pinyin Name: *Xiao Hui Xiang*
Alternate Chinese Names: *Gu Hui Xiang*
Original Source: *Yao Xing Ben Cao* (Materia Medica of Medicinal Properties) by Zhen Quan in 600 A.D.
English Name: fennel seed, fennel fruit
Botanical Name: *Foeniculum vulgare* Mill. (*Hui Xiang*)
Pharmaceutical Name: Fructus Foeniculi
Properties: acrid, warm
Channels Entered: Liver, Kidney, Spleen, Stomach

CHINESE THERAPEUTIC ACTIONS

1. Disperses Cold, Warms the Liver and Kidney, Relieves Pain

Abdominal pain, hernial pain: *Xiao Hui Xiang* (Fructus Foeniculi) treats hernial disorders by dispelling cold from the Liver and Kidney channels. Clinical applications include abdominal pain, prolapse sensations in the abdomen, and testicular swelling and pain.

- Hernia: use *Xiao Hui Xiang* with *Li Zhi He* (Semen Litchi), *Chuan Lian Zi* (Fructus Toosendan), and *Wu Yao* (Radix Linderae).
- Cold hernial disorders: use it with *Wu Zhu Yu* (Fructus Evodiae), *Rou Gui* (Cortex Cinnamomi) and *Chen Xiang* (Lignum Aquilariae Resinatum). *Xiao Hui Xiang* can also be heated and applied topically to the scrotum and abdomen.
- Heat-related hernial disorders with heat symptoms and burning pain: use this herb with *Chuan Lian Zi* (Fructus Toosendan), *Zhi Zi* (Fructus Gardeniae) and *Huang Qin* (Radix Scutellariae).
- Swelling and hardness of the scrotum: combine it with *Li Zhi He* (Semen Litchi) and *Chen Pi* (Pericarpium Citri Reticulatae).

2. Warms the Kidney, Relieves Pain

Low back pain caused by Kidney deficiency: The lower back houses the Kidney; when Kidney energy is deficient, patients will feel soreness, weakness and pain. *Xiao Hui Xiang* warms the Kidney and relieves pain.

- Low back pain: use this herb with *Du Zhong* (Cortex Eucommiae), *Hu Lu Ba* (Semen Trigonellae), and *Bu Gu Zhi* (Fructus Psoraleae).

3. Regulates Qi, Improves Appetite

Epigastric, hypochondriac, abdominal and intercostal pain, vomiting and decreased intake of food: *Xiao Hui Xiang* treats qi stagnation in the middle *jiao*, characterized by bloating pain in different parts of the abdomen, lack of appetite, nausea, abdominal fullness after meals, indigestion and vomiting.

- Qi stagnation in the middle *jiao*: use *Xiao Hui Xiang* with *Gan Jiang* (Rhizoma Zingiberis) and *Mu Xiang* (Radix Aucklandiae).
- Indigestion and fullness after meals: combine it with *Shen Qu* (Massa Fermentata), *Sha Ren* (Fructus Amomi) and *Mai Ya* (Fructus Hordei Germinatus).

DOSAGE

3 to 8 grams. Unprocessed *Xiao Hui Xiang* has the strongest function to regulate qi. Salt-fried *Xiao Hui Xiang* has moderate acrid and dispersing effects. Frying with salt also increases its effect to warm the Kidney and Liver, to treat disorders of the lower *jiao*, such as hernial pain.

CAUTIONS / CONTRAINDICATIONS

- Use *Xiao Hui Xiang* with caution in cases of yin deficiency with fire.
- Use *Xiao Hui Xiang* with caution during pregnancy because of its emmenagogic effect.[1]

CHEMICAL COMPOSITION

Essential oil 3-6% (trans-anethole, limonene, fenchone, estragole, γ-terpinene, α-pinene, mycene, β-pinene, camphor, camphene, methoxyphenyl acetone, sabinene, α-phellandrene, p-cymene, cineole, 4-terpineol, transfenchol acetate, anethole, anisaldenyde), petroselinic acid.[2]

PHARMACOLOGICAL EFFECTS

- **Gastrointestinal:** *Xiao Hui Xiang* has various effects on

Xiao Hui Xiang (Fructus Foeniculi)

the gastrointestinal system. It stimulates smooth muscle to increase peristalsis. It also exerts an inhibitory effect on the secretion of gastric acid.[3]

- **Effect on the liver:** It was found in one study that continuous administration of essential oil of *Xiao Hui Xiang* for 10 days increases the weight of the liver. It has been proposed that the herb may promote the regeneration of liver cells.[4]

CLINICAL STUDIES AND RESEARCH

- **Incarcerated hernia:** In one study, 7 children and 8 adult patients diagnosed with incarcerated hernia were treated with *Xiao Hui Xiang* with marked effectiveness. The treatment protocol was to soak the herb in hot water prior to ingestion. The dosage was 15 grams for adults, and 7.5 grams for children. Relief was achieved within 1 to 2 doses in 13 out of 15 patients. Those who did not report relief 15 minutes after the first dose were given the second dose. Those who did not report relief 30 minutes after the second dose were treated with surgical intervention.[5]
- **Hydrocele of tunica vaginalis:** Patients with hydrocele of tunica vaginalis were treated with an herbal remedy with good results. The herbal treatment was to dry fry 15 grams of *Xiao Hui Xiang*, 4.5 grams of salt, and 2 duck eggs into a pancake and take daily at bedtime with warm rice wine for 4 days per course of treatment, followed by 2 days of rest in between each course. Multiple courses of treatment may be necessary depending on the condition of each patient. Most patients reported a mild sore sensation and a gradual decrease in the size of the scrotum. Of 64 patients, 59 had complete recovery, 1 showed improvement, and 4 had no response.[6]

HERB-DRUG INTERACTION

- **Ciprofloxacin:** It has been suggested that the absorption and disposition of ciprofloxacin in rats may be affected when given concurrently with *Xiao Hui Xiang*. In one study, rats were divided into two groups with one receiving ciprofloxacin only and the other receiving both ciprofloxacin and *Xiao Hui Xiang*. Blood and urine samples were collected after 6 and 24 hours and analyzed by HPLC. Compared with the control group, the study found that there was a decrease of maximum plasma concentration by 83%, of area under the curve by 48%, and of urinary recovery by 43% in the treatment group. Furthermore, the apparent volume of distribution and terminal half-life were both increased. The mechanism of the herb-drug interaction was attributed to the high content of metal cations present in the herb. The researchers concluded that if the two agents are to be used concurrently, an adequate dosing interval is required to ensure efficacy of ciprofloxacin.[7]

SUPPLEMENT

- 蒔蘿 / 莳萝 *Shi Luo* (Fructus Anethum Graveolens), first cited in the *Shen Nong Ben Cao Jing* (Divine Husbandman's Classic of the Materia Medica) in the second century, is aromatic, has a similar physical appearance, and is sometimes substituted for *Xiao Hui Xiang*. Despite similar appearance and past history of interchangeable use, they are not identical herbs and should not be confused as such. *Shi Luo* is smaller and rounder, while *Xiao Hui Xiang* is longer, with a stronger fragrance.

References

1. Brinker, Francis. *Herb Contraindications and Drug Interactions*, 1997; 47
2. *Xian Dai Zhong Yao Yao Li Xue* (Contemporary Pharmacology of Chinese Herbs), 1997; 628
3. *Zhong Cao Yao* (Chinese Herbal Medicine), 1989; 20(7):41
4. Ibid.
5. *Zhong Hua Wai Ke Za Zhi* (Chinese Journal of External Medicine), 1959; 7:657
6. *Zhong Ji Yi Kan* (Medium Medical Journal), 1960; 5:11
7. Zhu, M et al. Effect of oral administration of fennel (*Foeniculum vulgare*) on ciprofloxacin absorption and disposition in the rat. *Journal of Pharmacy and Pharmacology*, v.51, n.12, Dec., 1999: 1391-1396

Da Hui Xiang (Fructus Anisi Stellati)

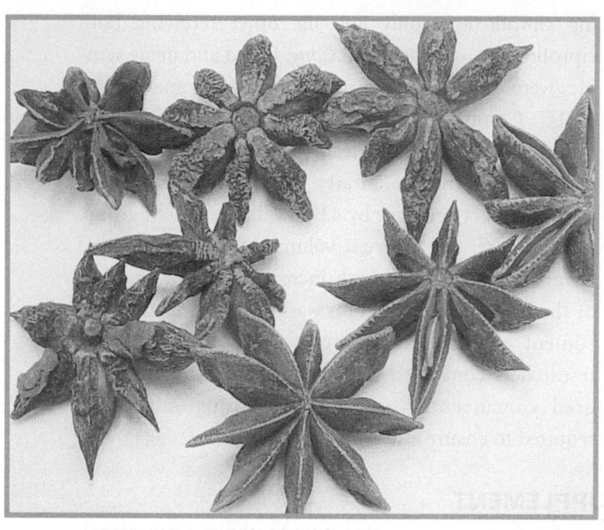

大茴香 大茴香

Pinyin Name: *Da Hui Xiang*
Alternate Chinese Names: *Ba Jiao Hui Xiang, Ba Jiao, Da Ba Jiao*
Original Source: *Ben Cao Pin Hui Jing Yao* (Essentials of Materia Medica) by Liu Wen-Tai in 1505
English Name: star anise
Botanical Name: *Illicium verum* Hook. F. (*Ba Jiao Hui Xiang*)
Pharmaceutical Name: Fructus Anisi Stellati
Properties: acrid, sweet, warm
Channels Entered: Liver, Kidney, Spleen

THERAPEUTIC ACTIONS

1. Disperses Cold, Warms the Liver and Kidney, Relieves Pain

Da Hui Xiang (Fructus Anisi Stellati) treats abdominal pain, hernial pain, prolapse, swelling and pain in the scrotum.

- Hernia: use *Da Hui Xiang* with *Ru Xiang* (Gummi Olibanum), *Li Zhi He* (Semen Litchi), *Chuan Lian Zi* (Fructus Toosendan), *Wu Yao* (Radix Linderae), *Wu Zhu Yu* (Fructus Evodiae) and *Rou Gui* (Cortex Cinnamomi).

2. Warms the Kidney, Relieves Pain

Da Hui Xiang is especially good for prickly pain in the low back from Kidney deficiency. To ensure maximum effectiveness, *Da Hui Xiang* is usually fried with salt to facilitate entry to the Kidney.

- Low back pain: use salt-fried *Da Hui Xiang* with *Du Zhong* (Cortex Eucommiae) and *Mu Xiang* (Radix Aucklandiae) and serve with grain-based liquor.

3. Regulates Qi, Improves Appetite

Da Hui Xiang treats qi stagnation in the middle *jiao* characterized by bloating pain, lack of appetite, vomiting and nausea.

- Gastrointestinal disorders: use it with *Mu Xiang* (Radix Aucklandiae), *Sha Ren* (Fructus Amomi) and *Gan Jiang* (Rhizoma Zingiberis).

DOSAGE

3 to 8 grams.

CAUTIONS / CONTRAINDICATIONS

- Use *Da Hui Xiang* cautiously in the presence of yin deficiency with fire.

CHEMICAL COMPOSITION

Trans-anethole, anisaldehyde, cineole, eslragole, aniske-tone, carene, feniculine, α-pinene, p-cymene.[1]

SUPPLEMENT

- 莽草 / 莽草 *Mang Cao* (Fructus Illicium Lanceolatum), having a similar appearance to *Da Hui Xiang*, is sometimes incorrectly used as a substitute. *Mang Cao* is toxic, and its use has been linked with adverse reactions such as dizziness, nausea, vomiting, twitching and convulsions. These two herbs can be identified by careful examination. *Mang Cao* has ten to thirteen parts with sharp curving tips, is thin, lusterless, bland in taste, and numbs the tongue after being in the mouth for a period of time. *Da Hui Xiang* has only eight parts with dull tips, is thick, lustrous and sweet. When placed side-by-side, *Mang Cao* appears to be smaller than *Da Hui Xiang*.

AUTHORS' COMMENTS

Da Hui Xiang (Fructus Anisi Stellati) has similar functions to those of *Xiao Hui Xiang* (Fructus Foeniculi). In fact, these two herbs are commonly used together for treatment of hernial disorders.

Da Hui Xiang is often used as a cooking spice. The essential oil of this herb is also used in toothpaste, soaps and cosmetics.

References

1. *Xian Dai Zhong Yao Yao Li Xue* (Contemporary Pharmacology of Chinese Herbs), 1997; 616

Chapter 7 summary

— Interior-Warming Herbs

Herb	Similarities	Differences
Fu Zi (Radix Aconiti Lateralis Praeparata)	Disperse cold, relieve pain	Warms body yang, restores *ming men* (life gate) fire, treats yang collapse
Chuan Wu (Radix Aconiti Preparata)		Strongly relieves pain
Cao Wu (Radix Aconiti Kusnezoffii)		Strongly relieves pain
Rou Gui (Cortex Cinnamomi)		Warms Kidney yang, disperses cold in the *xue* (blood) level
Gan Jiang (Rhizoma Zingiberis)		Warms Spleen and Lung yang, stops bleeding.
Wu Zhu Yu (Fructus Evodiae)	Disperse cold and relieve pain, warm the middle *jiao*	Relieves acid regurgitation, *jueyin* headache
Xi Xin (Herba Asari)		Dispels wind-cold, dissolves phlegm and opens orifices
Hua Jiao (Pericarpium Zanthoxyli)		Stops vomiting and hiccups, relieves toothache
Gao Liang Jiang (Rhizoma Alpiniae Officinarum)		Stops diarrhea
Ding Xiang (Flos Caryophylli)		Relieves hiccups
Hu Jiao (Fructus Piper)		Stops diarrhea, kills parasites
Bi Ba (Fructus Piperis Longi)		Stops diarrhea
Bi Cheng Qie (Fructus Litseae)		Dispels cold from the Urinary Bladder
Xiao Hui Xiang (Fructus Foeniculi)		Treats hernia
Da Hui Xiang (Fructus Anisi Stellati)		Treats hernia

General Characteristics of Interior-Warming Herbs:

Taste: acrid
Thermal property: warm to hot
Channels entered: Heart, Spleen, Stomach, Kidney
Therapeutic actions: warm the interior and the organs

Interior-warming herbs warm the interior and relieve pain, warm the Spleen and Stomach to relieve gastrointestinal disorders, warm the middle *jiao* to relieve abdominal discomfort, warm the Liver and the Kidney to relieve hernia and back pain, reverse qi rebellion and assist in restoring the yang. Clinical presentations of cold in the interior include aversion to cold, cold extremities, pale face, clear urine, pale tongue with white coat, and deep, thready pulse.

Fu Zi (Radix Aconiti Lateralis Praeparata), ***Chuan Wu*** (Radix Aconiti Preparata), ***Cao Wu*** (Radix Aconiti Kusnezoffii), ***Rou Gui*** (Cortex Cinnamomi), and ***Gan Jiang*** (Rhizoma Zingiberis) all have strong interior-warming, pain-relieving and cold-dispersing functions. Except for *Chuan Wu* and *Cao Wu*, all of them assist in restoring yang in the body.

Fu Zi (Radix Aconiti Lateralis Praeparata), ***Chuan Wu*** (Radix Aconiti Preparata) and ***Cao Wu*** (Radix Aconiti Kusnezoffii) are three aconite herbs with potent interior-warming properties.

Fu Zi restores yang in severe cases such as collapse of yang with icy extremities, fading pulse, profuse sweating and pale or cyanotic complexion. It treats coldness caused by yang deficiency or invasion of excess cold. It is especially effective for Kidney, Spleen and Heart yang deficiencies. It also dispels cold and dampness from the limbs to treat *bi zheng* (painful obstruction syndrome).

Chapter 7 summary

Chuan Wu and *Cao Wu* are stronger than *Fu Zi* in dispelling wind and cold and relieving pain. They are most suitable for *bi zheng* (painful obstruction syndrome), headache and abdominal pain. They can also be used topically to treat yin sores.

All three herbs are toxic, with *Cao Wu* being the most toxic, followed by *Chuan Wu* and *Fu Zi.* All should be pre-decocted for at least an hour to reduce toxicity. They should never be prescribed or administered in unprocessed form.

Rou Gui (Cortex Cinnamomi) is important in warming the *ming men* (life gate) fire. It is often used with *Fu Zi* (Radix Aconiti Lateralis Praeparata) to supplement Kidney yang and fading *ming men* fire. Clinical applications of this herb include abdominal coldness and pain, amenorrhea, dysmenorrhea or postpartum abdominal pain. *Rou Gui* is often added to tonic formulas to enhance production of qi and blood. Used topically, *Rou Gui* treats yin sores. While *Fu Zi* needs prolonged decoction to remove toxicity, prolonged decoction for *Rou Gui* is not advised, as this will reduce the effectiveness of the herb as volatile oils evaporate.

Gan Jiang (Rhizoma Zingiberis), the main herb for dispelling cold in the middle *jiao*, treats vomiting, nausea, diarrhea, abdominal coldness and pain caused by cold and deficiency in the Spleen and Stomach. *Gan Jiang* is often used with *Fu Zi* (Radix Aconiti Lateralis Praeparata) for synergistic effect. Furthermore, *Gan Jiang* helps to decrease the toxicity of *Fu Zi,* making the combination an ideal pair, maximizing the therapeutic effect while minimizing side effects. *Gan Jiang* warms the Lung to treat cough and dyspnea from cold and phlegm accumulation.

In summary, *Fu Zi* (Radix Aconiti Lateralis Praeparata), *Rou Gui* (Cortex Cinnamomi) and *Gan Jiang* (Rhizoma Zingiberis) all assist yang in the body.

Fu Zi warms the whole body.

Rou Gui more strongly warms Kidney yang.

Gan Jiang more effectively warms the Spleen and Stomach.

Wu Zhu Yu (Fructus Evodiae) and ***Xi Xin*** (Herba Asari) disperse cold and relieve pain.

Wu Zhu Yu is hot, dry and enters the Liver channel, and is used mainly for *jueyin* headache, hernial pain, dysmenorrhea and pain from leg *qi* caused by cold invasion of the Liver channel. *Wu Zhu Yu* directs rebellious qi downwards to treat acid regurgitation and vomiting. It treats diarrhea when mixed with vinegar and applied to the soles of the feet. *Wu Zhu Yu* also treats hypertension and oral sores. By comparison to *Xi Xin*, *Wu Zhu Yu* more strongly sends qi downwards.

Xi Xin has strong analgesic properties and dispels wind, treating *bi zheng* (painful obstruction syndrome), wind-cold headache and toothache. *Xi Xin* also warms the Lung to treat dyspnea and wheezing involving phlegm caused by cold in the Lung. By comparison to *Wu Zhu Yu*, *Xi Xin* more effectively disperses stagnation.

Hua Jiao (Pericarpium Zanthoxyli), ***Gao Liang Jiang*** (Rhizoma Alpiniae Officinarum) and ***Ding Xiang*** (Flos Caryophylli) warm the middle *jiao* and relieve pain, treating epigastric and abdominal coldness and pain, vomiting and diarrhea.

Hua Jiao warms the Spleen and Stomach to stop vomiting and hiccups.

Gao Liang Jiang warms the Spleen and Stomach to treat coldness of the abdomen accompanied by vomiting and diarrhea.

Ding Xiang warms the Stomach to treat hiccups, vomiting and nausea, and it warms Kidney yang.

Hu Jiao (Fructus Piper), ***Bi Ba*** (Fructus Piperis Longi) and ***Bi Cheng Qie*** (Fructus Litseae) have similar functions to warm the middle *jiao*, dispel cold and relieve pain in the abdomen, and treat vomiting, diarrhea and toothache.

Chapter 7 summary

Xiao Hui Xiang (Fructus Foeniculi) and ***Da Hui Xiang*** (Fructus Anisi Stellati) disperse coldness in the lower *jiao* via the Liver and Kidney channels. They are essential herbs to treat hernia and scrotal prolapse, warm the low back, dispel cold, and relieve soreness and pain.

HERBS FROM OTHER FUNCTIONAL CATEGORIES WITH INTERIOR-WARMING FUNCTIONS

Name	Functional Category
Ai Ye (Folium Artemisiae Argyi)	Stop-Bleeding Herbs (Chapter 11)
Gui Zhi (Ramulus Cinnamomi)	Exterior-Releasing Herbs (Chapter 1)
Sheng Jiang (Rhizoma Zingiberis Recens)	Exterior-Releasing Herbs (Chapter 1)

Chapter 8

— Qi-Regulating Herbs

理气药

Chapter 8 — Qi-Regulating Herbs

Chapter 8 理气药 — Qi-Regulating Herbs

Definition: Herbs that regulate qi function to promote normal circulation of qi, correct reversed flow of qi, and eliminate qi stagnation.

The proper, natural circulation of qi is essential to health. Qi brings energy to all parts of the body, and leads the circulation of blood. Without proper flow of qi, appropriate blood circulation is not possible. When normal qi circulation is disrupted, the flow of qi becomes impaired or reversed, and the resultant qi stagnation may cause illness. Without appropriate qi flow, the body's organs are not able to carry out their normal ascending, descending or dispersing functions. In addition, disruption of normal qi flow interferes with delivery of energy and nutrients to various parts of the body.

SUBCATEGORIES OF ACTION

Acrid, bitter and warm, herbs that regulate qi tend to disperse and move. Most herbs enter the Lung, Liver, and Spleen/Stomach to treat related disorders. The major functions of herbs that regulate qi are to promote the normal circulation of qi, correct reversed flow of qi, expand the chest, arrest wheezing, and relieve pain.

1. ***Herbs that regulate Lung qi***: The Lung is responsible for acquiring qi from nature via breathing. The main manifestations of Lung qi stagnation include stifling sensations in the chest, coughing, dyspnea and wheezing.
2. ***Herbs that regulate Liver qi***: The responsibility of the Liver is to promote smooth flow of qi. The chief negative emotion associated with the Liver is anger. The primary clinical manifestations of Liver qi stagnation include emotional disturbances, stress, irritability, anger, hypochondriac distention or pain, hernial pain, breast distention and tenderness (with or without palpable masses), irregular menstruation and loss of appetite.
3. ***Herbs that regulate Spleen and Stomach qi***: The Spleen is responsible for transformation of food into qi, while the Stomach is responsible for receiving and digesting this food. When qi is impaired in these organs, the following symptoms may occur: nausea, vomiting, hiccups, epigastric and abdominal bloating, fullness and pain, acid regurgitation, belching, poor appetite and irregular bowel movements.

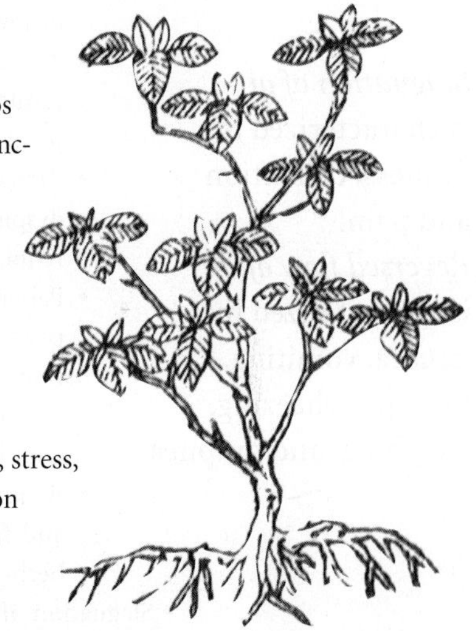

Mu Xiang (Radix Aucklandiae)
Ben Cao Gang Mu (Materia Medica), by Li Shi-Zhen, 1578 A.D.

Clinical Presentations of Abnormal Flow of Qi:

Organ Affected:	Clinical Presentation
Lung	cough, wheezing, dyspnea, shortness of breath
Liver	hypochondriac distention and pain, feelings of oppression in the chest, hernial pain, breast distention and pain, formation of nodules and cysts, irregular menstruation, and painful menstruation
Spleen and *Stomach*	fullness and distention of the epigastrium and abdomen, acid reflux, nausea, vomiting, reduced food intake, and irregular bowel movements

Qi-regulating herbs enter the Lung, Liver, and Spleen/Stomach to disperse and move qi.

Chapter 8 — Qi-Regulating Herbs

DIFFERENTIAL DIAGNOSIS AND TREATMENT

Disorders of qi may be assessed based on the location of the imbalance and the characteristics of the qi. Qi disorders are found in the organs most susceptible to qi stagnation and qi reversal, namely the Lung, Liver and Spleen/Stomach. Assessment of its characteristics determines whether the disorder is stagnation of qi or reversed flow of qi. The location of the imbalance is revealed by differing clinical presentations. It is also important to be aware of other complications that may occur as a result of qi stagnation.

The main characteristics of qi disorders include qi stagnation and reversed flow of qi.

- ***Qi stagnation*** may be caused by constrained emotions, disharmony of cold and heat, accumulated dampness and phlegm, blood stagnation and improper dietary intake. Most qi-stagnation sufferers manifest symptoms of bloating, pain, distention and stifling sensations. The hallmark symptoms of qi stagnation are fullness, distention and pain. Qi stagnation interrupts the smooth flow of qi and can cause it to move in the opposite direction from its appropriate flow.
- ***Reversed flow of qi*** is characterized by nausea, vomiting, hiccups, wheezing, coughing, and dyspnea. Assessment of location determines which organ is affected.

Stagnation of qi is characterized by fullness, distention and pain. *Reversed flow of qi* is characterized by nausea, vomiting, hiccups, wheezing, coughing, and dyspnea.

There are many complications that occur as a result of, or in addition to, stagnation of qi or reversed flow of qi.

- *Attack of wind-cold,* in addition to affecting the exterior, may also constrict the Lung, resulting in dyspnea, cough or wheezing, and production of white phlegm. Optimal treatment requires use of herbs to dispel wind-cold and regulate qi.
- *Attack of wind-heat,* in addition to affecting the exterior, may invade the Lung, resulting in dyspnea, cough or wheezing and production of yellow phlegm. Optimal treatment requires use of herbs to dispel wind-heat, clear Lung heat, and regulate qi.
- Patients with chronic asthma often have a *deficiency of Kidney qi,* that leads to the inability of Kidney qi to grasp Lung qi and pull it downward. Classic symptoms of this condition include feeble respiration characterized by comparatively longer exhalations and shorter inhalations. Optimal treatment requires the use of herbs that tonify Kidney qi in addition to herbs to move and/or redirect qi downward.
- *Accumulation of dampness in the middle jiao* is characterized by poor appetite, indigestion, and fullness in the abdomen. Optimal treatment requires concurrent use of aromatic herbs to dry dampness, with herbs that regulate qi.
- Stagnation of qi often occurs simultaneously with *stagnation of blood,* as proper flow of the one cannot occur without the other. Therefore, herbs that regulate qi are commonly used with herbs that regulate blood.
- *Food stagnation and indigestion* lead to qi stagnation. Optimal treatment requires concurrent use of digestive herbs and qi-regulating herbs.
- *Qi deficiency* is generally treated with both qi-tonic and qi-regulating herbs to ensure the maximum tonic effect without accumulation of dampness.
- *Hernia due to stagnation of cold and qi* is treated with herbs that warm the channels, regulate qi, and relieve pain.

CAUTIONS/CONTRAINDICATIONS

- Qi-regulating herbs are drying in nature, and should be used with caution for patients who have qi and/or yin deficiencies, or those who suffer from yin deficiency caused by febrile disorders.

PHARMACOLOGICAL EFFECTS

- **Gastrointestinal***:* Herbs that regulate qi have various effects on the gastrointestinal system.

Inhibiting: Herbs that inhibit the gastrointestinal tract relax the smooth muscles and slow intestinal peristalsis. Clinical applications include treatment of nausea, vomiting, diarrhea, borborygmus, intestinal spasms and cramps, and other conditions characterized by hyperactivity of the gastrointestinal system. Herbs that inhibit the gastrointestinal system include *Chen Pi* (Pericarpium Citri Reticulatae), *Qing Pi* (Pericarpium Citri Reticulatae Viride), *Zhi Shi* (Fructus Aurantii Immaturus), *Zhi Ke* (Fructus Aurantii), *Wu Yao* (Radix Linderae), *Mu Xiang* (Radix Aucklandiae), *Xiang Fu* (Rhizoma Cyperi) and *Chen Xiang* (Lignum Aquilariae Resinatum).

Stimulating: Herbs that stimulate the gastrointestinal tract increase intestinal peristalsis and contractile force. Clinical applications include treatment of fullness and distention of the abdomen, and indigestion, constipation and other disorders characterized by lack of activity of the gastrointestinal system. These herbs include *Zhi Shi* (Fructus Aurantii Immaturus), *Zhi Ke* (Fructus Aurantii), and *Chuan Lian Zi* (Fructus Toosendan).

Regulating: Some herbs have both inhibiting and stimulating actions to regulate the gastrointestinal tract, such as *Zhi Shi* (Fructus Aurantii Immaturus) and *Zhi Ke* (Fructus Aurantii).

Generating gastric acid: Some herbs stimulate and increase the production of gastric acid, as do *Zhi Shi* (Fructus Aurantii Immaturus), *Xiang Fu* (Rhizoma Cyperi), *Fo Shou* (Fructus Citri Sarcodactylis), *Mu Xiang* (Radix Aucklandiae), *Wu Yao* (Radix Linderae) and *Chen Xiang* (Lignum Aquilariae Resinatum).

Generating bile acid: Among the herbs that increase the production and release of bile are *Chen Xiang* (Lignum Aquilariae Resinatum), *Chen Pi* (Pericarpium Citri Reticulatae), *Qing Pi* (Pericarpium Citri Reticulatae Viride), and *Xiang Fu* (Rhizoma Cyperi).

- **Respiratory**: Some herbs dilate the bronchi to relieve wheezing and dyspnea, including *Chen Pi* (Pericarpium Citri Reticulatae), *Qing Pi* (Pericarpium Citri Reticulatae Viride), *Fo Shou* (Fructus Citri Sarcodactylis), *Mu Xiang* (Radix Aucklandiae), *Wu Yao* (Radix Linderae) and *Chen Xiang* (Lignum Aquilariae Resinatum). Others, like *Xiang Fu* (Rhizoma Cyperi), stimulate the lungs to increase the rate of respiration.
- **Cardiovascular**: Herbs that regulate qi have various effects on the cardiovascular system.

  Some increase contractility of the heart and lower blood cholesterol levels, as do *Chen Pi* (Pericarpium Citri Reticulatae), *Qing Pi* (Pericarpium Citri Reticulatae Viride), and *Mu Xiang* (Radix Aucklandiae).

  Among those that restore normal rhythms of the heart to treat arrhythmia are *Tan Xiang* (Lignum Santali Albi) and *Gan Song* (Radix seu Rhizoma Nardostachys).

  Some increase blood perfusion to the coronary arteries, including *Qing Pi* (Pericarpium Citri Reticulatae Viride) and *Zhi Shi* (Fructus Aurantii Immaturus).

  Some dilate the peripheral blood vessels to decrease blood pressure, such as *Fo Shou* (Fructus Citri Sarcodactylis) and *Mu Xiang* (Radix Aucklandiae).
- **Central nervous system**: Some herbs exert sedative and analgesic effects, such as *Xiang Fu* (Rhizoma Cyperi) and *Gan Song* (Radix seu Rhizoma Nardostachys).
- **Effect on the uterus**: Herbs that regulate qi may stimulate or inhibit the smooth muscle of the uterus. *Zhi Shi* (Fructus Aurantii Immaturus) stimulates the uterus to increase contractions. *Xiang Fu* (Rhizoma Cyperi) inhibits it to relieve spasms and pain.
- **Antibiotic**: Many of these herbs inhibit the growth of bacteria, viruses and dermatophytes, including *Mu Xiang* (Radix Aucklandiae), *Chen Xiang* (Lignum Aquilariae Resinatum), *Wu Yao* (Radix Linderae), *Chuan Lian Zi* (Fructus Toosendan), and *Xiang Fu* (Rhizoma Cyperi).
- **Metabolic**: Some herbs, such as *Li Zhi He* (Semen Litchi), lower blood glucose levels.

POTENTIAL HERB-DRUG INTERACTIONS

- **Antiulcer drugs**: Some qi-regulating herbs that stimulate the gastrointestinal system, increasing the production of gastric acid, may counter the effects of certain drugs such as histamine-2 receptor antagonists (such as ranitidine or famotidine) or proton-pump inhibitors (such as omeprazole or lansoprazole).
- **Sympathomimetics**: Some herbs that move qi may exert stimulant influence. For example, *Chen Pi* (Pericarpium Citri Reticulatae), *Qing Pi* (Pericarpium Citri Reticulatae Viride), *Zhi Shi* (Fructus Aurantii Immaturus) and *Zhi Ke* (Fructus Aurantii) all contain components that stimulate the sympathetic nervous system. Therefore, such herbs should be used with caution in

Chapter 8 — Qi-Regulating Herbs

patients who take medications for pre-existing conditions such as hypertension, diabetes mellitus, hyperthyroidism, and seizures.[1,2]

- **Cardiovascular agents:** Some qi-regulating herbs stimulate the cardiovascular system and increase blood pressure, while others dilate the blood vessels to decrease blood pressure. Therefore, these herbs should be used with caution in patients taking cardiovascular medications.

References

1. *Zhong Yao Yao Li Yu Ying Yong* (Pharmacology and Applications of Chinese Herbs), 1983; 586
2. *Xian Dai Zhong Yao Yao Li Xue* (Contemporary Pharmacology of Chinese Herbs), 1997; 636

Chen Pi (Pericarpium Citri Reticulatae)

陳皮 陈皮

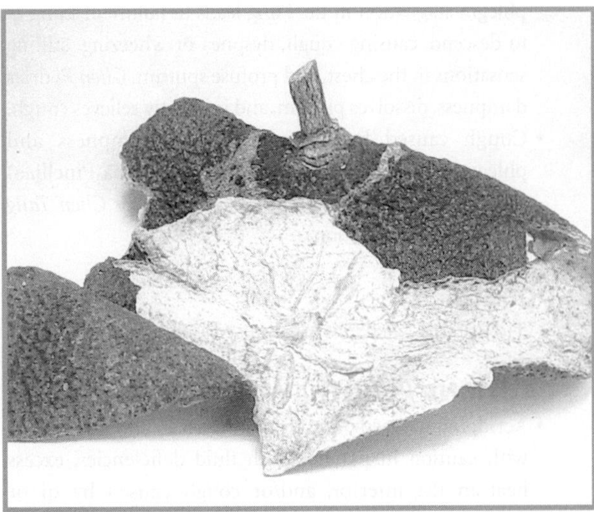

Pinyin Name: *Chen Pi*
Literal Name: "aged peel"
Alternate Chinese Names: *Ju Pi, Guang Chen Pi, Xin Hui Pi*
Original Source: *Shen Nong Ben Cao Jing* (Divine Husbandman's Classic of the Materia Medica) in the second century
English Name: citrus peel, orange peel, tangerine peel
Botanical Name: *Citrus reticulata* Blanco. (*Ju*)
Pharmaceutical Name: Pericarpium Citri Reticulatae
Properties: acrid, bitter, warm
Channels Entered: Lung, Spleen

CHINESE THERAPEUTIC ACTIONS

1. Regulates Qi, Adjusts the Middle *Jiao*

Qi stagnation of the Spleen and Stomach: Qi stagnation creates an upwards reversal of qi, leading to nausea and vomiting. *Chen Pi* (Pericarpium Citri Reticulatae) has moving and descending properties to treat disharmony of the middle *jiao* that manifests in abdominal fullness and distention, belching, nausea, and vomiting. One aspect of disharmony of the middle *jiao* is characterized by the Liver over-acting on the Spleen, resulting in abdominal pain and diarrhea.

- Qi stagnation of the Spleen and Stomach: use *Chen Pi* with *Zhi Shi* (Fructus Aurantii Immaturus) and *Mu Xiang* (Radix Aucklandiae).
- Nausea and vomiting due to rising Stomach qi: use it with *Sheng Jiang* (Rhizoma Zingiberis Recens), *Zhu Ru* (Caulis Bambusae in Taenia), and *Ban Xia* (Rhizoma Pinelliae).
- Abdominal pain with diarrhea caused by the Liver over-acting on the Spleen: combine it with *Bai Zhu* (Rhizoma Atractylodis Macrocephalae), *Bai Shao* (Radix Paeoniae Alba) and *Fang Feng* (Radix Saposhnikoviae). **Exemplar Formula:** *Tong Xie Yao Fang* (Important Formula for Painful Diarrhea).
- Nausea, vomiting, and epigastric fullness and distention arising from Stomach heat: use this herb with *Huang Lian* (Rhizoma Coptidis) and *Chuan Lian Zi* (Fructus Toosendan).
- Nausea, vomiting, and epigastric fullness and distention caused by Stomach cold: use it with *Wu Yao* (Radix Linderae) and *Gao Liang Jiang* (Rhizoma Alpiniae Officinarum).
- Thick, white tongue coating with no desire to drink: combine *Chen Pi* with *Cang Zhu* (Rhizoma Atractylodis) and *Fu Ling* (Poria).

2. Regulates Spleen and Stomach Qi

Indigestion from Spleen and Stomach deficiencies: *Chen Pi* regulates qi circulation of the Spleen and Stomach and treats indigestion with bloating, and distention or poor appetite.

- Indigestion: use *Chen Pi* with *Dang Shen* (Radix Codonopsis), *Bai Zhu* (Rhizoma Atractylodis Macrocephalae), *Shen Qu* (Massa Fermentata), *Shan Zha* (Fructus Crataegi), *Mai Ya* (Fructus Hordei Germinatus) and *Zhi Gan Cao* (Radix Glycyrrhizae Preparata).
- Diarrhea due to Spleen and Stomach deficiencies: use it with *Bai Zhu* (Rhizoma Atractylodis Macrocephalae), *Fu Ling* (Poria) and *Bai Shao* (Radix Paeoniae Alba) to relieve pain and stop diarrhea.

3. Dries Dampness, Dissolves Phlegm

Damp accumulation in the middle *jiao*: *Chen Pi* warms yang in the middle *jiao* to eliminate the accumulation of dampness and phlegm, a condition characterized by feelings of oppression in the chest, abdominal fullness, loss of appetite, fatigue, loose stools, and a thick, greasy tongue coat. *Chen Pi* is also added to various tonic formulas to aid in their digestion and prevent stagnation.

- Accumulation of dampness in the middle *jiao*: use *Chen Pi* with *Cang Zhu* (Rhizoma Atractylodis) and *Hou Po* (Cortex Magnoliae Officinalis). **Exemplar Formula:** *Ping Wei San* (Calm the Stomach Powder).
- Accumulation of phlegm in the middle *jiao*: combined this herb with *Ban Xia* (Rhizoma Pinelliae).

4. Relieves Cough

Cough with phlegm: Damp obstruction of the middle *jiao* arising from inadequate functioning of the Spleen leads to accumulation of phlegm in the Lung. The qi and

Chen Pi (Pericarpium Citri Reticulatae)

phlegm stagnation in the Lung leads to failure of Lung qi to descend, causing cough, dyspnea or wheezing, stifling sensations in the chest, and profuse sputum. *Chen Pi* dries dampness, dissolves phlegm, and indirectly relieves cough.

- Cough caused by accumulation of dampness and phlegm: use *Chen Pi* with *Ban Xia* (Rhizoma Pinelliae) and *Fu Ling* (Poria). **Exemplar Formula:** *Er Chen Tang* (Two-Cured Decoction).

DOSAGE

3 to 9 grams. *Chen Pi* is usually used as decoction or in pills.

CAUTIONS / CONTRAINDICATIONS

- Acrid, bitter, warm, and drying, *Chen Pi* should be used with caution in patients with fluid deficiencies, excess heat in the interior, and/or cough caused by qi or yin deficiencies.
- It should be used with extreme caution in hematemesis.
- Long-term use of *Chen Pi* may consume *yuan* (source) *qi*.

CHEMICAL COMPOSITION

Hesperidin, nobiletin, limonene, α-pinene, β-pinene, β-phellandrene, tangeretin.[1,2,3]

Hesperidin

PHARMACOLOGICAL EFFECTS

- **Gastrointestinal:** Injection of *Chen Pi* has been shown to stimulate contraction of smooth muscle and to increase intestinal peristalsis.[4]
- **Antiasthmatic:** Herbal decoction of *Chen Pi* has been shown to dilate the bronchi in rabbits.[5]
- **Anti-inflammatory:** Intraperitoneal administration of *Chen Pi* has shown ability to decrease permeability of the blood vessels and reduce inflammation in mice with inflammation or allergy.[6]
- **Cardiovascular:** Intravenous injection of *Chen Pi* increases the contractility and cardiac output of the heart without significant changes to the heart rate. It also dilates the coronary artery. At larger doses, however, there is a decrease in heart rate and contractility. In other studies, injection of *Chen Pi* demonstrated an increase in blood pressure in rats. However, the duration of effectiveness was rather short, as blood pressure returned to normal after 3 minutes. Repeated injection is associated with repeated increase in blood pressure.[7,8]

CLINICAL STUDIES AND RESEARCH

- **Acute mastitis:** An herbal decoction with 30 grams of *Chen Pi* and 6 grams of *Gan Cao* (Radix Glycyrrhizae) successfully treated 85 out of 88 patients with acute mastitis.[9]
- **Chronic bronchitis:** Patients with chronic bronchitis characterized by severe coughing at night were treated with an herbal decoction with good success. Out of 33 patients, 17 showed marked improvement, 14 experienced moderate improvement, and 2 showed no response. The herbal formula contained *Chen Pi* 6g, *Ban Xia* (Rhizoma Pinelliae) 6g, *Fu Ling* (Poria) 10g, *Dang Gui* (Radicis Angelicae Sinensis) 20g, *Gan Cao* (Radix Glycyrrhizae) 6g, and *Sheng Jiang* (Rhizoma Zingiberis Recens) 3 pieces.[10]
- **Cholelithiasis:** A preparation of *Chen Pi* has demonstrated effectiveness in dissolving gallstones in 134 patients with cholelithiasis.[11]
- **Burns:** Topical application of *Chen Pi* paste several times daily showed marked effectiveness in patients with first- and second-degree burns. The proposed mechanisms of action include analgesic, anti-inflammatory, and astringent functions.[12]

TOXICOLOGY

No significant adverse reaction was reported following administration of a 50% *Chen Pi* herbal decoction at the dosage of 3 ml/kg in dogs. The LD_{50} for mice is approximately 850 mg/kg following intravenous injection of hesperidin, and 780 mg/kg following intravenous injection of tangeretin.[13]

SUPPLEMENT

- 橘紅 / 橘红 *Ju Hong* (Exocarpium Citri Rubrum), also known as *Yun Pi* and *Yun Hong*, was first cited in *Yi Xue Qi Yuan* (Origins of the Medicine) by Zhang Yuan-Su in Yuan Dynasty. *Ju Hong* is derived from the outermost peel of oranges. It is bitter, acrid, warm, and enters the Lung and Stomach. It functions to regulate qi, open the middle *jiao*, and dry dampness. It treats cough with profuse sputum or food stagnation with no heat symptoms. In comparison to *Chen Pi*, *Ju Hong* has a stronger drying and aromatic effect. Recommended dosage of *Ju Hong* is 3 to 10 grams.
- 橘絡 / 橘络 *Ju Luo* (Fibra Citri Rubrum), also known as *Ju Si* and *Ju Jin*, was first cited in *Yi Xue Qi Yuan* (Origins of the Medicine) by Zhang Yuan-Su in Yuan Dynasty. *Ju Luo* is the inside of the orange peel and is white and vein-like in appearance. It is sweet, bitter and neutral. Its primary functions are to open the channels and collaterals, regulate qi and dissolve phlegm. It is most suitable to address phlegm obstruction in the channels and collaterals, or cough with chest and hypochondriac pain. The

Chen Pi (Pericarpium Citri Reticulatae)

recommended dosage of *Ju Luo* is 3 to 5 grams.

- 橘葉 / 橘叶 *Ju Ye* (Folium Citri Rubrum), first cited in *Zhen Nan Ben Cao* (Materia Medica of South Yunnan) by Lan Mao in Qing Dynasty, is orange tree leaves. It is acrid, bitter and neutral. It regulates Liver qi, reduces swelling, and disperses stagnation. Clinical applications include hypochondriac pain, breast abscesses and palpable masses and/or tumors. The recommended dosage of *Ju Ye* is 6 to 10 grams.
- 橘核 *Ju He* (Semen Citri Rubrum), also known as *Ju Zi He, Ju Zi Ren* and *Ju Ren*, was first cited in *Ri Hua Zi Ben Cao* (Materia Medica of Ri Hua-Zi) by Ri Hua-Zi in 713 A.D. *Ju He* is orange seed. It is bitter and neutral. It disperses nodules, activates qi circulation, and relieves pain. It is often used to treat Liver qi stagnation with phlegm obstruction, such as hernia, pain and swelling of the testes, mastitis, and nodules of the breast. *Ju He* may be used internally as decoction or powder, or topically as cream or ointment. Frying it with salt directs its functions to the Kidney, and enhances its effect to treat hernia, and testicular swelling and pain. The dosage of *Ju He* is 3 to 10 grams.
- 化橘紅 / 化橘红 *Hua Ju Hong* (Exocarpium Citri Grandis), also known as *Hua Zhou Ju Hong, Hua Pi*, and *You Pi Ju Hong*, was first cited in *Ben Cao Gang Mu Shi Yi* (Omissions from the Grand Materia Medica) by Zhao Xue-Min in 1765. *Hua Ju Hong*, derived from *Citri grandis* 'Tomentosa' or *Citri grandis* (L.) Osbeck, is the dried outermost rind of pummelo. It is bitter, warm, acrid, and enters the Lung, Spleen and Stomach. It regulates qi, opens the middle *jiao*, dries dampness, dissolves phlegm, and relieves food stagnation. It is used for cough with profuse sputum with no heat signs. The recommended dosage of *Hua Ju Hong* is 3 to 10 grams. *Hua Ju Hong* should be used with caution in patients with qi and yin deficiencies. *Hua Ju Hong* is also known as *Hua Ju Pi*.

AUTHORS' COMMENTS

Chen Pi, literally "aged peel," implies that the longer it is stored and aged, the stronger its functions. *Chen Pi* is also known as *Ju Pi*, literally "orange peel." *Guang Chen Pi*, the herb grown in Guangzhou province, is often considered to be the best type of *Chen Pi*.

Chen Pi primarily treats Lung and Spleen imbalances by regulating qi and drying dampness. However, it can be used to enhance the function of other herbs. According to *Ben Cao Gang Mu* (Materia Medica), *Chen Pi* "tonifies when combined with tonics, purges when combined with purgatives, moves upwards when added to herbs with ascending effects, and downwards if added to herbs with descending effects."

References

1. *Zhong Yao Yao Li Yu Ying Yong* (Pharmacology and Applications of Chinese Herbs), 1983; 567
2. *Xian Dai Zhong Yao Yao Li Xue* (Contemporary Pharmacology of Chinese Herbs), 1997; 640
3. *The Merck Index* 12th edition, Chapman & Hall/CRCnetBASE/Merck, 2000
4. *Jiang Su Zhong Yi Za Zhi* (Jiangsu Journal of Chinese Medicine), 1981; (3):61
5. *Shang Hai Yi Yao Za Zhi* (Shanghai Journal of Medicine and Herbology), 1957; (3):148
6. *Zhong Yao Yao Li Yu Ying Yong* (Pharmacology and Applications of Chinese Herbs), 1983; 567
7. *Journal of Pharmacol Exp Ther*, 1940; 69:309
8. *Jiang Su Zhong Yi Za Zhi* (Jiangsu Journal of Chinese Medicine), 1981; (3):61
9. *Zhong Hua Wai Ke Za Zhi* (Chinese Journal of External Medicine), 1959; 4:362
10. *Zhe Jiang Zhong Yi Za Zhi* (Zhejiang Journal of Chinese Medicine), 1985; 1:18
11. *Zhong Xi Yi Jie He Za Zhi* (Journal of Integrated Chinese and Western Medicine), 1985; 10:591
12. *Chi Jiao Yi Shi Za Zhi* (Journal of Barefoot Doctors), 1975; 4:11
13. *Zhong Yao Yao Li Yu Ying Yong* (Pharmacology and Applications of Chinese Herbs), 1983; 567

Qing Pi (Pericarpium Citri Reticulatae Viride)

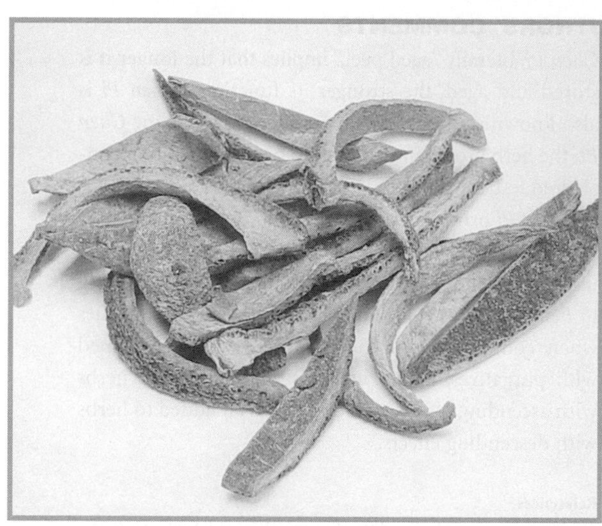

青皮

Pinyin Name: *Qing Pi*
Literal Name: "blue-green peel," "green peel"
Alternate Chinese Names: *Qing Ju Pi, Xiao Qing Pi*
Original Source: *Tu Jing Ben Cao* (Illustrated Classic of the Materia Medica) by Su Song in 1061
English Name: citrus viride, immature orange peel, green tangerine peel
Botanical Name: *Citrus reticulata* Blanco. (*Ju*)
Pharmaceutical Name: Pericarpium Citri Reticulatae Viride
Properties: bitter, acrid, warm
Channels Entered: Liver, Gallbladder, Stomach

CHINESE THERAPEUTIC ACTIONS

1. Spreads Liver Qi, Breaks Up Qi Stagnation

Liver qi stagnation: Clinical symptoms include hypochondriac distention and pain, breast distention and pain, breast nodules, and hernia. There may also be emotional distress, frequent sighing, irritability, irregular menstruation and pre-menstrual syndrome, abdominal bloating or pain, poor appetite, and reversal of Stomach qi causing hiccups, belching, nausea or vomiting. Patients with Liver qi stagnation often become agitated easily. *Qing Pi* (Pericarpium Citri Reticulatae Viride) enters the Liver and Gallbladder channels to spread Liver qi and break up qi stagnation. *Qing Pi* is relatively strong, suitable for patients with strong constitutions or acute conditions.

- Hypochondriac pain: use *Qing Pi* with *Chai Hu* (Radix Bupleuri) and *Yu Jin* (Radix Curcumae).
- Breast distention and pain, or breast nodules: use it with *Chai Hu* (Radix Bupleuri), *Xiang Fu* (Rhizoma Cyperi) and *Wang Bu Liu Xing* (Semen Vaccariae).
- Cold-type hernia and abdominal pain: combine it with *Wu Yao* (Radix Linderae), *Xiao Hui Xiang* (Fructus Foeniculi), and *Mu Xiang* (Radix Aucklandiae).
- Intestinal prolapse, feeling of genital prolapse or testicular swelling due to chronic orchitis: use this herb with *Wu Yao* (Radix Linderae), *Chuan Lian Zi* (Fructus Toosendan), *Xiao Hui Xiang* (Fructus Foeniculi), *Mu Xiang* (Radix Aucklandiae) and *Bing Lang* (Semen Arecae).

2. Disperses Nodules, Resolves Stagnation

Food stagnation: This manifests as indigestion, epigastric or abdominal fullness, distention and pain, belching marked by a sour or rotten smell, acid regurgitation, constipation or diarrhea with foul or rotten smell. *Qing Pi* effectively eliminates food stagnation.

- Food stagnation and indigestion: combine *Qing Pi* with *Shan Zha* (Fructus Crataegi), *Mai Ya* (Fructus Hordei Germinatus) and *Shen Qu* (Massa Fermentata).

Mass formation due to qi or blood stasis: *Qing Pi* is often used with qi- and blood-invigorating herbs to enhance the overall function of breaking stagnation that manifestes as masses, nodules or tumors.

- Nodules caused by qi or blood stasis: use this herb with *San Leng* (Rhizoma Sparganii), *E Zhu* (Rhizoma Curcumae), and *Yu Jin* (Radix Curcumae).

DOSAGE

3 to 10 grams in decoction. *Qing Pi* may also be used in pills or powder. The unprocessed herb has a strong, drastic action to move qi and break up qi stagnation. Vinegar-processing moderates the strong effect and minimizes possible side effects.

CAUTIONS / CONTRAINDICATIONS

- Use *Qing Pi* with caution for patients with qi deficiency, as the strong dispersing quality may consume qi.
- Long-term use or large doses of *Qing Pi* are not recommended.

CHEMICAL COMPOSITION

Hesperidin, nobiletin, limonene, α-pinene, β-pinene, β-phellandrene.[1]

PHARMACOLOGICAL EFFECTS

- **Gastrointestinal:** Injection of *Qing Pi* relieves spasms and cramps by inhibiting the contraction of smooth muscles of the stomach, intestines, and gallbladder.[2]
- **Respiratory:** *Qing Pi* has demonstrated marked antitussive,

Qing Pi (Pericarpium Citri Reticulatae Viride)

expectorant, and antiasthmatic properties in animals. Intravenous injection of *Qing Pi* dilates the bronchi and prevents bronchial constriction for up to one hour.[3]

- **Sympathomimetic:** *Qing Pi* stimulates both the central nervous system and the cardiovascular system. In one study, *Qing Pi* administered via intravenous injection increased both blood pressure and respiration rate, while oral administration showed little effect. Furthermore, repeated injection within a short period of time may contribute to tolerance. Clinically, *Qing Pi* injection (equivalent bulk herb dose of 1 g/kg) has an effect similar to but more prolonged than that of 10 mcg/kg of epinephrine.[4]

CLINICAL STUDIES AND RESEARCH

- **Shock:** Patients in shock due to infection, allergy or cardiovascular conditions were treated with intravenous infusion of *Qing Pi* in D5W. Out of 22 patients, 17 showed marked improvement and 5 showed moderate improvement. All patients responded with significant increases in blood pressure, without adverse reactions.[5]
- **Supraventricular tachycardia:** Patients with supraventricular tachycardia were treated with intravenous infusion of 4 ml of *Qing Pi* injectable (equivalent to 4 grams of bulk herb) in 40 ml of D5W. Out of 49 patients, 42 regained normal sinus rhythm within a short period of time. No adverse reactions were reported.[6]

AUTHORS' COMMENTS

Qing Pi (Pericarpium Citri Reticulatae Viride) and *Chen Pi* (Pericarpium Citri Reticulatae) both are warm, regulate qi and resolve stagnation of food, qi and phlegm. Both can be used for epigastric and abdominal fullness, distention, pain, vomiting, diarrhea or poor appetite. The two herbs are commonly used together to address symptoms of disharmony of the Liver, Spleen and Stomach. However, there are other important similarities and differences. The qi-regulating function of *Qing Pi* is strong and descending in nature to treat stagnation of the Liver and Gallbladder channels. Clinical manifestations of this stagnation include hypochondriac, breast and hernial distention and pain. *Qing Pi* can be used to break up palpable masses and nodules. *Chen Pi* is weaker in strength than *Qing Pi*, but regulates qi as well as causing it to descend. It is mainly used for Spleen and Lung qi stagnation. It regulates qi, harmonizes the middle *jiao*, dries dampness and resolves phlegm. It is used for cough with profuse sputum, chest congestion or poor appetite, and diarrhea due to Spleen qi deficiency with qi stagnation.

References

1. *Xian Dai Zhong Yao Yao Li Xue* (*Contemporary Pharmacology of Chinese Herbs*), 1997; 642-643
2. *Zhong Yao Zhi* (*Chinese Herbology Journal*), 1984; 37
3. *Zhong Yao Yao Li Yu Ying Yong* (*Pharmacology and Applications of Chinese Herbs*), 1983; 586
4. Ibid.
5. *Shang Hai Zhong Yi Yao Za Zhi* (*Shanghai Journal of Chinese Medicine and Herbology*), 1987; 2:21
6. *Zhong Yi Za Zhi* (*Journal of Chinese Medicine*), 1987; 3:38

Zhi Shi (Fructus Aurantii Immaturus)

枳實 枳实

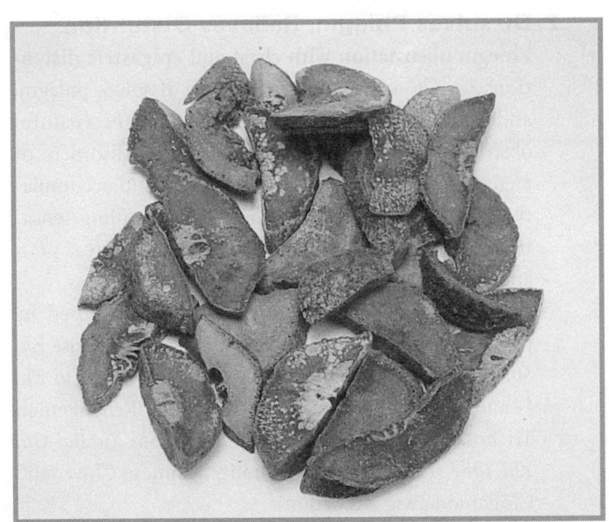

Pinyin Name: *Zhi Shi*
Alternate Chinese Names: *Jiang Zhi Shi, Chao Zhi Shi*
Original Source: *Shen Nong Ben Cao Jing* (Divine Husbandman's Classic of the Materia Medica) in the second century
English Name: aurantium immaturus, immature bitter orange, immature sweet orange
Botanical Name: *Citrus aurantium* L. (*Suan Cheng*); *Citrus wilsonii* Tanaka. (*Xiang Yuan*); *Poncirus trifoliata* (L.) Raf. (*Gou Ju*)
Pharmaceutical Name: Fructus Aurantii Immaturus
Properties: bitter, acrid, cool
Channels Entered: Large Intestine, Spleen, Stomach

Zhi Shi (Fructus Aurantii Immaturus)

CHINESE THERAPEUTIC ACTIONS

1. Breaks Up Stagnant Qi, Resolves Accumulation

Gastrointestinal disorders: Gastrointestinal disorders caused by stagnant qi in the middle *jiao* is characterized by indigestion, epigastric and abdominal fullness, distention, belching, and foul breath. *Zhi Shi* (Fructus Aurantii Immaturus) is one of the most potent qi-regulating herbs. It breaks up stagnant qi to treat food accumulation, abdominal hardness, distention and pain, constipation, dysentery and rectal tenesmus.

- Food accumulation: use *Zhi Shi* with *Shan Zha* (Fructus Crataegi), *Mai Ya* (Fructus Hordei Germinatus) and *Shen Qu* (Massa Fermentata).
- Constipation with abdominal fullness and pain: combine it with *Hou Po* (Cortex Magnoliae Officinalis) and *Da Huang* (Radix et Rhizoma Rhei). **Exemplar Formula:** *Xiao Cheng Qi Tang* (Minor Order the Qi Decoction).
- Diarrhea, feeling of incomplete evacuation after defecation, and rectal tenesmus caused by damp-heat: use this herb with *Da Huang* (Radix et Rhizoma Rhei), *Huang Lian* (Rhizoma Coptidis) and *Huang Qin* (Radix Scutellariae).

Spleen and Stomach deficiencies: Qi stagnation may occur in patients who have an underlying deficiency. In cases of Spleen and Stomach deficiencies with compromised transformation and transportation functions, epigastric and abdominal fullness and distention will often develop after meals. If the underlying cause is deficiency and cold of the Spleen, the patient will express fatigue with preference for warm drinks and food.

- Epigastric and abdominal fullness and distention secondary to Spleen and Stomach deficiencies: use *Zhi Shi* with *Bai Zhu* (Rhizoma Atractylodis Macrocephalae) and *Su Geng* (Caulis Perillae).

2. Dissolves Phlegm, Relieves Distention

Phlegm obstruction with chest and epigastric distention: *Zhi Shi* activates qi circulation, dissolves phlegm, and relieves distention. It treats *xiong bi* (painful obstruction of the chest), coronary heart disorders or angina caused by Heart yang deficiency and accumulation of cold phlegm. Symptoms include stifling sensations and pain in the chest and epigastric area, poor appetite, shortness of breath, fatigue and weakness.

- *Xiong bi* (painful obstruction of the chest) caused by phlegm accumulation and Heart yang deficiency: use *Zhi Shi* with *Xie Bai* (Bulbus Allii Macrostemonis), *Gui Zhi* (Ramulus Cinnamomi) and *Gua Lou Ren* (Semen Trichosanthis). **Exemplar Formula:** *Zhi Shi Xie Bai Gui Zhi Tang* (Immature Bitter Orange, Chinese Chive, and Cinnamon Twig Decoction).
- Epigastric fullness and distention, lack of appetite, and fatigue: combine this herb with *Hou Po* (Cortex Magnoliae Officinalis), *Ban Xia* (Rhizoma Pinelliae), and *Bai Zhu* (Rhizoma Atractylodis Macrocephalae).
- For patients recovering from chronic illness, with epigastric fullness and distention: add *Hou Po* (Cortex Magnoliae Officinalis).
- Feelings of heat in the body: use it with *Zhi Zi* (Fructus Gardeniae) and *Dan Dou Chi* (Semen Sojae Praeparatum).
- Abdominal fullness, pain, gas, and irregular bowel movements: combine it with *Mu Xiang* (Radix Aucklandiae), *Bing Lang* (Semen Arecae) and *Shen Qu* (Massa Fermentata).

Cholecystitis: *Zhi Shi* is one of the best herbs to relieve distention and hardness of the epigastric area caused by cholecystitis.

- Cholecystitis: combine *Zhi Shi* with *Chai Hu* (Radix Bupleuri), *Huang Qin* (Radix Scutellariae) and *Ban Xia* (Rhizoma Pinelliae). **Exemplar Formula:** *Xiao Chai Hu Tang* (Minor Bupleurum Decoction).

DOSAGE

3 to 10 grams in decoction. The maximum dosage of *Zhi Shi* is 15 grams. Apply as powder for topical use. Unprocessed *Zhi Shi* has a potent ability to break up stagnant qi and resolve accumulation. However, such impact is often associated with consumption of qi and irritation of the Spleen and Stomach. Dry-frying increases the warmth and moderates the harsh nature of *Zhi Shi*, therefore minimizing potential side effects.

CAUTIONS / CONTRAINDICATIONS

- Use *Zhi Shi* with caution during pregnancy.
- *Zhi Shi* should not be used as a single remedy when treating patients with Spleen and Stomach deficiencies, since its qi-regulating potency may disperse and consume qi. Patients with Spleen and Stomach deficiencies should be treated with both qi-tonics and qi-regulating herbs.
- *Zhi Shi* should be used with caution in patients who have gastric or duodenal peptic ulcers, because the acidity of the herb may irritate the gastrointestinal tract.[1]

CHEMICAL COMPOSITION

Synephrine, N-methyltyramine, hesperidin, neohesperidin, nobiletin, desmethyl nobiletin, quinoline, narcotine, noradrenaline, quinoline, tryptamine, tyramine, naringin, rhoifolin, tengeretin, and lonicerin.[2,3]

Zhi Shi (Fructus Aurantii Immaturus)

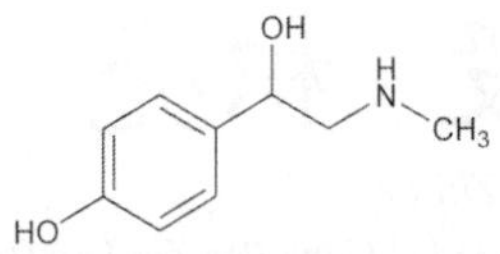

Synephrine

PHARMACOLOGICAL EFFECTS

- **Cardiovascular:** Oral administration of *Zhi Shi* decoction in dogs and rabbits stimulates the heart to increase contractility, blood pressure, and cardiac output. Intravenous injection of *Zhi Shi* solution at dosage of 1.5 g/kg is similar to 0.1 mg/kg of epinephrine in its effect to raise blood pressure. *Zhi Shi*, however, has a prolonged influence on raising blood pressure and does not affect heart rate or respiration.[4]
- **Circulatory:** Intravenous injection of *Zhi Shi* decreases peripheral vascular resistance and enhances microcirculation to the heart, brain and kidneys. Studies in dogs have demonstrated an increase of 82.6 +/- 20.56 ml/100g of blood to the brain, and 64.5 +/- 9.4 ml/100g of blood to the kidneys.[5]
- **Diuretic:** Intravenous injection of *Zhi Shi* has shown marked diuretic effect in dogs.[6]
- **Gastrointestinal:** Oral administration of *Zhi Shi* decoction in dogs stimulates smooth muscle and increases intestinal peristalsis.[7]
- **Effects on the uterus:** Oral administration of *Zhi Shi* decoction has a marked stimulating effect on the uterus of rabbits, but it has an inhibitory effect in rats.[8]

CLINICAL STUDIES AND RESEARCH

- **Shock:** Seventy-five patients experiencing a state of shock were treated with intravenous administration of *Zhi Shi*, with 96% efficacy.[9]
- **Cardiac failure:** Intravenous infusion of *Zhi Shi* injection with D10W demonstrated marked cardiotonic and diuretic effects in 20 patients.[10]
- **Uterine prolapse:** In one study, 924 patients with uterine prolapse were given an herbal decoction of 15 grams of *Zhi Shi* and 15 grams of *Chong Wei Zi* (Semen Leonuri) once daily for 30 days with an 83.87% rate of effectiveness.[11]

HERB-DRUG INTERACTION

- **Diuretics:** *Zhi Shi* has a diuretic effect. Though this potential interaction has not been documented, concurrent use with diuretic drugs may lead to increased elimination of water and/or electrolytes.[12] [Note: Examples of diuretics include chlorothiazide, hydrochlorothiazide, furosemide (Lasix), bumetanide (Bumex), and torsemide (Demadex).]

TOXICOLOGY

Zhi Shi has minimal toxicity. In anesthetized dogs, no significant adverse reactions were observed following intravenous injections at 2 g/kg. The only side effects noted were abdominal distention and salivation. In mice, the LD_{50} is 71.8 g/kg via intravenous injection.[13]

AUTHORS' COMMENTS

Zhi Shi is one of the best herbs to treat gastrointestinal disorders characterized by stagnation and accumulation. Diagnostic keys are as follows:

- If *dampness* is pronounced, there may be abdominal fullness with no desire to eat or drink.
- If *damp-heat* is the cause, there may be nausea, thirst with no desire to drink, a thick, and yellow tongue coating. The individual may also experience feelings of incomplete defecation after bowel movement.
- If *food stagnation* is severe, there may be a foul stench to the stool and acid regurgitation with a rotten, sour, undigested smell.

References

1. Brinker, Francis. *Herb Contraindications and Drug Interactions*, 1997; 24
2. *Xian Dai Zhong Yao Yao Li Xue* (Contemporary Pharmacology of Chinese Herbs), 1997; 636
3. *The Merck Index* 12th edition, Chapman & Hall/CRCnetBASE/Merck, 2000
4. *Zhong Yao Yao Li Yu Ying Yong* (Pharmacology and Applications of Chinese Herbs), 1983; 737
5. *Ke Xue Tong Bao* (Journal of Science), 1978; (I):58
6. *Liao Ning Zhong Yi Za Zhi* (Liaoning Journal of Chinese Medicine), 1984; 10:32
7. *Zhong Guo Yi Yao Xue Bao* (Chinese Journal of Medicine and Herbology), 1991; 6(1):39
8. Ibid.
9. *Hu Nan Yi Yao Za Zhi* (Hunan Journal of Medicine and Herbology), 1974; 6:15
10. *Zhong Cao Yao* (Chinese Herbal Medicine), 1980; 4:171
11. *Zhong Xi Yi Jie He Za Zhi* (Journal of Integrated Chinese and Western Medicine), 1984; 4:238
12. *Liao Ning Zhong Yi Za Zhi* (Liaoning Journal of Chinese Medicine), 1984; 10:32
13. *Zhong Yao Yao Li Yu Ying Yong* (Pharmacology and Applications of Chinese Herbs), 1983: 737

Zhi Ke (Fructus Aurantii)

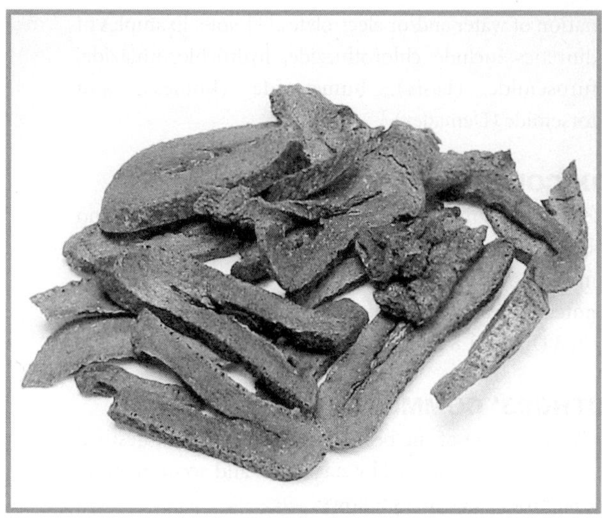

枳殼 枳壳

Pinyin Name: *Zhi Ke*

Original Source: *Lei Gong Pao Zhi Lun* (Grandfather Lei's Discussions of Herb Preparation) by Lei Xiao in 470 A.D.

English Name: aurantium fruit, bitter orange

Botanical Name: *Citrus aurantium* L. (*Suan Cheng*); *Citrus wilsonii* Tanaka. (*Xiang Yuan*); *Poncirus trifoliata* (L.) Raf. (*Gou Ju*)

Pharmaceutical Name: Fructus Aurantii

Properties: bitter, acrid, cool

Channels Entered: Spleen, Stomach, Large Intestine

CHINESE THERAPEUTIC ACTIONS

1. Relieves Distention

Zhi Ke (Fructus Aurantii) activates qi circulation to relieve abdominal distention and pressure. The qi-regulating function of *Zhi Ke* is mild, and is most helpful for patients who are weak or deficient.

2. Breaks Up Stagnant Qi, Resolves Accumulation

Although *Zhi Ke* is mild in action, it breaks up stagnant qi in mild-to-moderate cases of stagnation and accumulation, and expands the chest to relieve congestion.

- Chest congestion: use *Zhi Ke* with *Jie Geng* (Radix Platycodonis).
- Itching of the skin: combine this herb with *Jing Jie* (Herba Schizonepetae), *Fang Feng* (Radix Saposhnikoviae), *Hong Hua* (Flos Carthami) and *Chi Shao* (Radix Paeoniae Rubrae).

DOSAGE

3 to 10 grams. Dry-frying *Zhi Ke* reduces its drying tendencies.

CAUTIONS / CONTRAINDICATIONS

- *Zhi Ke* should be used with caution during pregnancy.
- *Zhi Ke* should be used with caution in cases of Spleen and Stomach deficiencies.
- *Zhi Ke* should be used with caution in patients who have gastric or duodenal ulcers, because the acidity of this herb may irritate the gastrointestinal tract.[1]

CHEMICAL COMPOSITION

Synephrine, N-methyltyramine, hesperidin, neohesperidin, nobiletin, desmethyl nobiletin, quinoline, narcotine, noradrenaline, quinoline, narcotine, tryptamine, tyramine, synephrine, N-methyltyramine, naringin, rhoifolin, and lonicerin.[2,3]

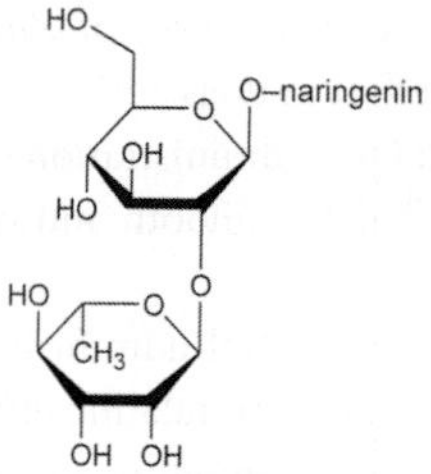

Naringin

PHARMACOLOGICAL EFFECTS

- **Cardiovascular:** Administration of *Zhi Ke* via intravenous injection showed a marked ability to increase blood pressure, lower the oxygen requirement of cardiac muscle, and promote diuresis.[4]
- **Respiratory:** Synephrine demonstrated a moderate effect to relax and dilate the airways.[5]
- **Antiplatelet**: *Zhi Ke* has antiplatelet action, and inhibits thrombus formation in rats.[6]
- **Antineoplastic:** Nobiletin has demonstrated antineoplastic action in nose and throat cancer with ED_{50} of 3 to 28 μg/ml.[7]

HERB-DRUG INTERACTION

- **Anticoagulant or antiplatelet drugs:** *Zhi Ke* has antiplatelet action, and should be used with caution in patients who take anticoagulant or antiplatelet medications. Though this potential interaction has not been documented, this herb may potentiate the effect of drugs such as warfarin. [Note: Examples of anticoagulants include heparin, warfarin (Coumadin) and enoxaparin

Zhi Ke (Fructus Aurantii)

(Lovenox); and examples of antiplatelets include aspirin, dipyridamole (Persantine), and clopidogrel (Plavix).][8]

AUTHORS' COMMENTS

Zhi Ke (Fructus Aurantii) and *Zhi Shi* (Fructus Aurantii Immaturus) have similar functions, but they are not interchangeable. While *Zhi Ke* relieves distention, it is gentle in resolving stagnation and accumulation or chest congestion. *Zhi Shi* is more potent and breaks up stagnation and masses. In cases of severe accumulation or constipation, *Zhi Shi* is more suitable since it is more potent.

References

1. Brinker, Francis. *Herb Contraindications and Drug Interactions*, 1997; 24
2. *Xian Dai Zhong Yao Yao Li Xue* (Contemporary Pharmacology of Chinese Herbs); 1997; 639-640
3. *The Merck Index* 12th edition, Chapman & Hall/CRCnetBASE/Merck, 2000
4. *Zhi Wu Yao You Xiao Cheng Fen Shou Ce* (Manual of Plant Medicinals and Their Active Constituents), 1986; 725
5. Ibid., 1012
6. Ibid., 774
7. Ibid., 774
8. Chen, J. Recognition & prevention of herb-drug interactions, *Medical Acupuncture*, Fall/Winter 1998/1999; volume 10/number 2; 9-13

Xiang Yuan (Fructus Citri)

香橼 香櫞

Pinyin Name: *Xiang Yuan*
Alternate Chinese Names: *Chen Xiang Yuan, Xiang Yuan Pi*
Original Source: *Ming Yi Za Zhu* (Miscellaneous Records of Famous Physicians) by Tao Hong-Jing in 500 A.D.
English Name: citrus fruit, citron fruit
Botanical Name: *Citrus medica* L. (*Gou Yuan*); *Citrus wilsonii* Tanaka (*Xiang Yuan*)
Pharmaceutical Name: Fructus Citri
Properties: acrid, slightly bitter, sour, warm
Channels Entered: Liver, Spleen, Lung

CHINESE THERAPEUTIC ACTIONS

Spreads Liver Qi, Regulates Qi, Harmonizes the Middle and Dissolves Phlegm

Qi stagnation of the Liver, Spleen and Stomach: Common manifestations of this type of qi stagnation include chest congestion, hypochondriac pain, belching, decreased food intake and vomiting. *Xiang Yuan* (Fructus Citri) is acrid and has a dispersing influence. The bitter taste of the herb helps to properly redirect the rising Stomach qi that manifests in belching or vomiting. *Xiang Yuan* is relatively mild and should be combined with other qi-regulating herbs for maximum effectiveness.

- Chest congestion, hypochondriac pain: use *Xiang Yuan* with *Gua Lou Pi* (Pericarpium Trichosanthis), *Yu Jin* (Radix Curcumae), and *Xiang Fu* (Rhizoma Cyperi).
- Epigastric pain and abdominal distention: add *Mu Xiang* (Radix Aucklandiae), *Chuan Lian Zi* (Fructus Toosendan) and *Wu Zhu Yu* (Fructus Evodiae).
- A bitter taste in the mouth or acid regurgitation: combine *Xiang Yuan* with *Huang Lian* (Rhizoma Coptidis).

Phlegm and damp accumulation, cough with profuse sputum: *Xiang Yuan* has similar potency to *Chen Pi* (Pericarpium Citri Reticulatae) in relieving cough and dissolving phlegm. Other manifestations of phlegm and damp accumulation may include chest congestion and dyspnea.

- Cough with profuse sputum: use this herb with *Ban Xia* (Rhizoma Pinelliae), *Fu Ling* (Poria), *Gua Lou Shi* (Fructus Trichosanthis), *Su Zi* (Fructus Perillae) and *Lai Fu Zi* (Semen Raphani).

DOSAGE

3 to 10 grams in decoction or in pills.

CAUTIONS / CONTRAINDICATIONS

- Use *Xiang Yuan* with caution during pregnancy, or in patients with yin or blood deficiencies.

Xiang Yuan (Fructus Citri)

CHEMICAL COMPOSITION

Citrusin, essential oils.[1]

AUTHORS' COMMENTS

Both *Xiang Yuan* and *Fo Shou* (Fructus Citri Sarcodactylis) share similar traits in resolving phlegm and relieving chest congestion, hypochondriac pain, epigastric and abdominal fullness and pain, belching, poor appetite, and vomiting. *Xiang Yuan* regulates Lung and Spleen qi and more effectively relieves cough and resolves phlegm. *Fo Shou* enters the Stomach and has a stronger function to treat nausea and vomiting.

References

1. *Chang Yong Zhong Yao Cheng Fen Yu Yao Li Shou Ce* (A Handbook of the Composition and Pharmacology of Common Chinese Drugs), 1994; 1434-1435

Fo Shou (Fructus Citri Sarcodactylis)

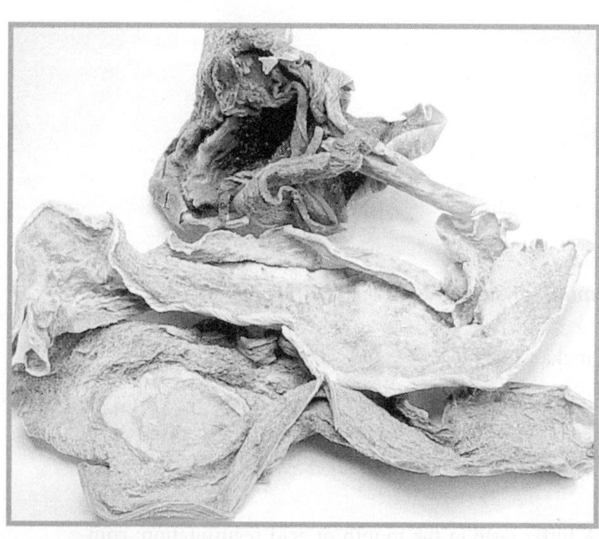

佛手

Pinyin Name: *Fo Shou*
Literal Name: "Buddha's hand"
Alternate Chinese Names: *Fo Shou Ju, Fo Shou Xiang Yuan, Fo Shou Pian*
Original Source: *Tu Jing Ben Cao* (Illustrated Classic of the Materia Medica) by Su Song in 1061
English Name: citrus sarcodactylus, finger citron
Botanical Name: *Citrus medica* L. var. *sarcodactylis* Swingle (*Fo Shou*)
Pharmaceutical Name: Fructus Citri Sarcodactylis
Properties: acrid, bitter, warm
Channels Entered: Liver, Lung, Stomach, Spleen

CHINESE THERAPEUTIC ACTIONS

1. Spreads Liver Qi and Regulates Qi

Liver qi stagnation: Clinical manifestations of Liver qi stagnation include hypochondriac and abdominal distention and fullness, belching, hiccups and vomiting. *Fo Shou* (Fructus Citri Sarcodactylis), acrid yet not drying in action, is an excellent herb to promote circulation of qi and relieve Liver qi stagnation. Overall, it effectively activates and regulates qi circulation without drying or consuming yin. However, it only has a mild function to relieve pain.

- Liver qi stagnation: use *Fo Shou* with *Xiang Fu* (Rhizoma Cyperi) and *Yu Jin* (Radix Curcumae).
- Epigastric pain from Liver qi stagnation: combine it with *Qing Pi* (Pericarpium Citri Reticulatae Viride) and *Chuan Lian Zi* (Fructus Toosendan).

Spleen and Stomach qi stagnation: This condition is characterized by poor appetite, epigastric and abdominal fullness and distention, belching, and vomiting. This pattern of symptoms usually reveals the Wood element (Liver) overacting on the Earth element (Spleen/Stomach).

- Spleen and Stomach qi stagnation: use *Fo Shou* with *Xiang Yuan* (Fructus Citri), *Xiang Fu* (Rhizoma Cyperi), *Mu Xiang* (Radix Aucklandiae) and *Zhi Ke* (Fructus Aurantii).
- Vomiting and nausea: combine it with *Sheng Jiang* (Rhizoma Zingiberis Recens), *Chen Xiang* (Lignum Aquilariae Resinatum) and *Jiang Xiang* (Lignum Dalbergiae Odoriferae).
- Nausea and vomiting in pregnant women: use it with *Zhu Ru* (Caulis Bambusae in Taenia), *Zi Su Ye* (Folium Perillae) and *Huang Qin* (Radix Scutellariae).

Fo Shou (Fructus Citri Sarcodactylis)

2. Harmonizes the Middle *Jiao*, Dissolves Phlegm and Relieves Cough

Cough with profuse sputum: *Fo Shou* serves to mildly dissolve phlegm. It is commonly used to treat chronic and persistent cough with profuse sputum and chest pain. It is not, however, suitable for the initial stage of cough characteristic of an exterior condition.

- Persistent cough with profuse sputum and chest pain: use *Fo Shou* with *Si Gua Luo* (Retinervus Luffae Fructus), *Yu Jin* (Radix Curcumae) and *Pi Pa Ye* (Folium Eriobotryae).

DOSAGE

3 to 10 grams in decoction. *Fo Shou* is commonly used as an herbal decoction or tea.

CAUTIONS / CONTRAINDICATIONS

Use *Fo Shou* with caution for patients who have yin-deficient fire, or do not have qi stagnation.

CHEMICAL COMPOSITION

Bergapten, limettin, diosmin, hesperidin.[1,2]

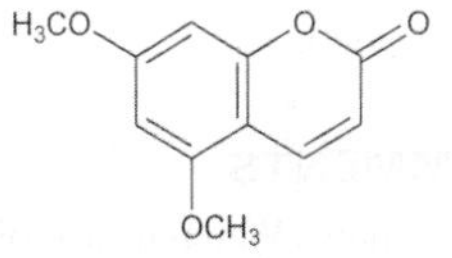

H_3CO … O … O … OCH_3

Limettin

PHARMACOLOGICAL EFFECTS

- **Cardiovascular:** Administration of *Fo Shou* increases blood perfusion to the coronary arteries, reduces the risk of cardiac ischemia, prevents arrhythmia, and lowers blood pressure.[3]
- **Antiasthmatic:** Administration of *Fo Shou* via intravenous injection inhibits constriction of bronchi and facilitates breathing.[4]
- **Gastrointestinal:** Administration of *Fo Shou* in rats, cats and rabbits via intravenous injection has demonstrated a marked inhibitory effect on the smooth muscles of the gastrointestinal system. It inhibits contractions, relaxes muscle, and prevents spasms and cramps.[5]
- **CNS suppressant:** Administration of *Fo Shou* in mice via intraperitoneal injection has demonstrated a sedative influence on the central nervous system (CNS) for up to two hours. Furthermore, it exerts a protective effect against metrazol- or caffeine-induced seizures.[6]

CLINICAL STUDIES AND RESEARCH

- **Infectious hepatitis in children:** According to one study, 64 children of various ages were given *Fo Shou* and *Bai Jiang Cao* (Herba cum Radice Patriniae) for treatment of infectious hepatitis and jaundice. All children received the herbs on a daily basis for 7 to 10 days per course of treatment. The daily dosage of *Fo Shou* was 10 to 15 grams for children between 1 and 3 years of age, 15 to 20 grams for those between 3 and 5 years, 20 to 25 grams for those between 5 and 7 years, and 30 grams for those between 7 and 10 years. The daily dosage of *Bai Jiang Cao* was 1 gram per day for children under 10 years of age, with 1 additional gram for every 2 years over 10 years of age. Most children reported an increase in energy and appetite, and resolution of jaundice within 4 to 5 days.[7]

TOXICOLOGY

The LD_{50} for limettin in mice is 10.0 g/kg via oral administration, and 4 g/kg via intraperitoneal injection.[8]

SUPPLEMENT

- 佛手花 *Fo Shou Hua* (Flos Citri Sarcodactylis) is derived from the flower of the same plant as *Fo Shou*. The function of *Fo Shou* is more focused on the middle *jiao* in relieving nausea, vomiting and epigastric pain. *Fo Shou Hua* has a similar but weaker function, and is better at relieving qi stagnation in the chest, that manifests in congestion and pain. The recommended dosage of *Fo Shou Hua* is 3 to 6 grams in decoction.

AUTHORS' COMMENTS

Fo Shou is relatively mild in nature and is most suitable for minor cases of qi stagnation. It is also useful in patients who have concurrent qi stagnation and qi deficiency, and cannot tolerate the use of strong qi-regulating herbs. However, because its effect is rather mild, *Fo Shou* must be combined with other qi-regulating herbs to achieve maximum effectiveness in cases of severe qi stagnation.

While *Fo Shou* has pain-relieving characteristics, it is weaker in potency than *Chuan Lian Zi* (Fructus Toosendan), *Zhi Shi* (Fructus Aurantii Immaturus) or *Qing Pi* (Pericarpium Citri Reticulatae Viride).

References

1. *Xian Dai Zhong Yao Yao Li Xue* (Contemporary Pharmacology of Chinese Herbs), 1997; 664
2. *The Merck Index* 12th edition, Chapman & Hall/CRCnetBASE/Merck, 2000
3. *Zhong Yao Yao Li Yu Ying Yong* (Pharmacology and Applications of Chinese Herbs), 1983; 538
4. Ibid.
5. Ibid.
6. Ibid.
7. *Zhong Yi Za Zhi* (Journal of Chinese Medicine),1957; 7:361
8. *Zhi Wu Yao You Xiao Cheng Fen Shou Ce* (Manual of Plant Medicinals and Their Active Constituents), 1986; 123, 359, 561

Po Bu Zi Ye (Folium Cordia Dichotoma)

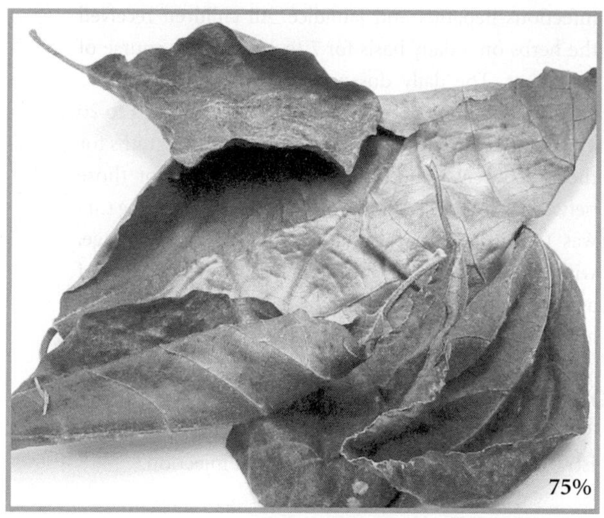
75%

破布子葉
破布子叶

Pinyin Name: *Po Bu Zi Ye*
Literal Name: "leaves from broken fabric"
Alternate Chinese Names: *Qing Tong Tsui Mu*
English Name: sebastan plum cordia
Botanical Name: *Cordia dichotoma* Forst. F.
Pharmaceutical Name: Folium Cordia Dichotoma
Properties: bitter, slightly astringent, cool
Channels Entered: Liver, Kidney, Stomach

CHINESE THERAPEUTIC ACTIONS

1. Regulates Qi, Relieves Pain

Bone spurs: *Po Bu Zi Ye* (Folium Cordia Dichotoma) relieves pain by regulating qi and blood circulation in the body. It is best to treat the pain associated with bone spurs.

- Bone spurs: use *Po Bu Zi Ye* with *Huang Jin Gui* (Caulis Vanieriae), *Mo Gu Xiao* (Caulis Hyptis Capitatae) and *Liu Zhi Huang* (Herba Solidaginis).

Epigastric pain: Unlike most qi-regulating herbs that may irritate the stomach, *Po Bu Zi Ye* benefits the stomach and relieves pain.

- Epigastric pain: combine it with *Yan Hu Suo* (Rhizoma Corydalis) and *Mu Xiang* (Radix Aucklandiae).

2. Dispels Phlegm and Relieves Coughing

Cough: Though this herb can relieve cough, it is not commonly used for this function.

- Cough with yellow phlegm: add *Chen Pi* (Pericarpium Citri Reticulatae).

DOSAGE

5 to 20 grams in decoction.

AUTHORS' COMMENTS

According to Dr. Chang Wei-Yen, use of *Po Bu Zi Ye* is most effective to relieve pain associated with bone spurs. While some patients may experience immediate relief, others may require approximately half a year of treatment to achieve relief of the pain. Furthermore, use of *Po Bu Zi Ye* usually has an all-or-none response when treating bone spurs. Approximately 20 to 30% of patients experience long-term resolution of pain, but others may only notice symptomatic reduction of pain and inflammation.

Da Fu Pi (Pericarpium Arecae)

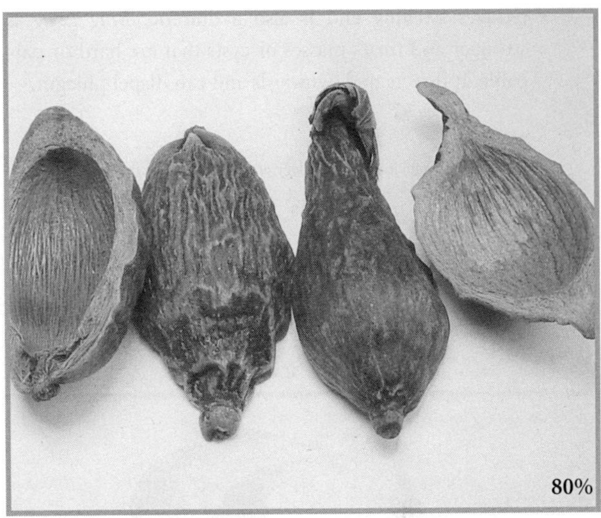

大腹皮

Pinyin Name: *Da Fu Pi*
Literal Name: "big abdomen peel"
Alternate Chinese Names: *Bing Lang Pi, Da Fu Mao, Bing Lang Yi*
Original Source: *Ri Hua Zi Ben Cao* (Materia Medica of Ri Hua-Zi) by Ri Hua-Zi in 713 A.D.
English Name: areca husk, areca peel, betel nut peel
Botanical Name: *Areca catechu* L. (*Bing Lang*)
Pharmaceutical Name: Pericarpium Arecae
Properties: acrid, slightly warm
Channels Entered: Large Intestine, Small Intestine, Spleen, Stomach

CHINESE THERAPEUTIC ACTIONS

1. Directs Qi Downward, Expands the Middle *Jiao*

Da Fu Pi (Pericarpium Arecae) regulates qi and expands the middle *jiao* to treat sensations of oppression, distention and fullness in the abdomen and epigastrium, and feelings of incomplete evacuation after defecation.

- Accumulation of dampness and qi stagnation: use *Da Fu Pi* with *Hou Po* (Cortex Magnoliae Officinalis) and *Chen Pi* (Pericarpium Citri Reticulatae).

2. Promotes Diuresis, Relieves Edema

Da Fu Pi helps to reduce accumulation of water to treat edema and leg *qi*.

- Edema or leg *qi*: combine this herb with *Fu Ling Pi* (Cortex Poria) and *Sheng Jiang Pi* (Pericarpium Zingiberis Recens).

DOSAGE

3 to 10 grams.

CAUTIONS / CONTRAINDICATIONS

- Use *Da Fu Pi* with caution during pregnancy, because of its teratogenic and fetotoxic effects, as shown in mice.[1]

CHEMICAL COMPOSITION

α-catechin, tannoids.[2]

PHARMACOLOGICAL EFFECTS

- **Gastrointestinal:** Administration of *Da Fu Pi* via herbal decoction increased intestinal contraction and tension. This effect is reversed by atropine.[3]

HERB-DRUG INTERACTION

- **Antipsychotics:** It has been suggested that an exacerbation of extrapyramidal effects may occur with concurrent use of neuroleptic drugs and betel nuts. Two cases of severe extrapyramidal symptoms were reported, when patients with chronic schizophrenic disorders treated with depot neuroleptics also consumed a heavy dose of betel nuts for a long period of time. [Note: Examples of antipsychotics include chlorpromazine (Thorazine), fluphenazine (Prolixin), thioridazine (Mellaril), and haloperidol (Haldol).][4,5]

TOXICOLOGY

One instance of anaphylactic shock was reported in a 16-year-old patient following the ingestion of a Chinese herbal decoction containing 12 grams of *Da Fu Pi* and other herbs. Ten minutes after ingestion, the patient reported chest congestion and tightness, nausea, palpitations, itching, irritability, pale face and lips, cold sweats, and cold extremities. She had a thready, rapid and weak pulse, a heart rate of 122 beats/minute, and blood pressure of 74/50 mmHg. The patient was treated for anaphylactic shock and recovered shortly thereafter. She had no prior history of allergy to drugs or to other herbs in the decoction.[6] [Note: Anaphylactic shock is the most severe type of allergic reaction. Unfortunately, it is very difficult, if not impossible, to predict when patients will have such serious reactions. Despite this one reported case, use of *Da Fu Pi* does not necessarily have a higher risk of allergy than other herbs.]

AUTHORS' COMMENTS

Da Fu Pi (Pericarpium Arecae) and *Bing Lang* (Semen Arecae) are derived from the same plant, commonly known as betel nuts. They both treat accumulations of water such as edema and leg *qi*. *Da Fu Pi* treats qi stagnation with no visible or palpable masses present. It

Da Fu Pi (Pericarpium Arecae)

reduces swelling and is also a diuretic. *Bing Lang* is stronger and treats masses or cysts that are hard or palpable. It directs qi downwards and can dispel phlegm.

References

1. Brinker, Francis. *The Toxicology of Botanical Medicines*, rev. 2nd ed., 1996
2. *Xian Dai Zhong Yao Yao Li Xue* (Contemporary Pharmacology of Chinese Herbs), 1997; 654
3. *Xin Yi Yao Xue Za Zhi* (New Journal of Medicine and Herbology), 1974; 12:39
4. *Lancet* 355(9198):134-8, 2000 Jan 8
5. *Movement Disorders*. 4(4):330-2, 1989
6. *Zhong Yi Yao Xue Bao* (Report of Chinese Medicine and Herbology), 1989; 2:37

Wan Dian Jin (Radix Ilicis Asprellae)

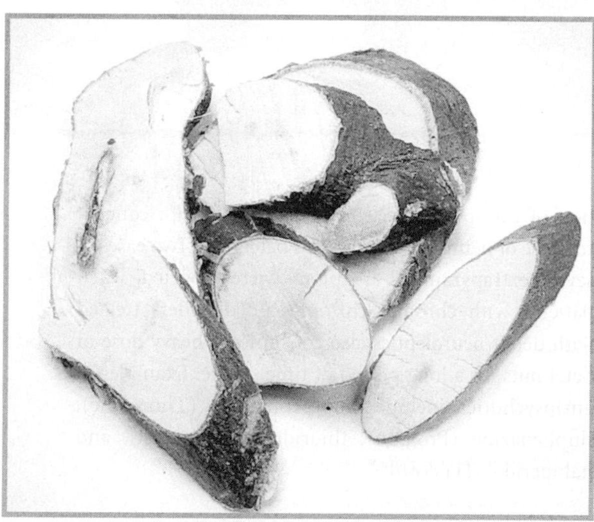

萬點金 万点金

Pinyin Name: *Wan Dian Jin*
Literal Name: "ten thousand golds"
Alternate Chinese Names: *Ding Ping Gen, Ding Ping Zi Tou, Bai Gan Cao, Gang Mei Gen*
English Name: ilex
Botanical Name: *Ilex asprella* (Hook. et Am.) Champ.
Pharmaceutical Name: Radix Ilicis Asprellae
Properties: bland, cool
Channels Entered: Lung

CHINESE THERAPEUTIC ACTIONS

1. Regulates and Tonifies Lung Qi

Chest congestion from traumatic injuries: *Wan Dian Jin* (Radix Ilicis Asprellae) treats chest obstruction and labored respiration caused by blood and qi stagnation in the chest.

- Chest congestion: use *Wan Dian Jin* with *Zheng Gu Zi Jin Dan* (Purple and Gold Pill for Righteous Bones) or *Xue Fu Zhu Yu Tang* (Drive Out Stasis in the Mansion of Blood Decoction).

Feelings of chest congestion from Lung qi deficiency: *Wan Dian Jin* also benefits Lung qi and treats chest congestion arising from Lung qi deficiency. Symptoms may include feeble cough, low voice and fatigue.

- Feeble cough: use this herb with *Ren Shen* (Radix Ginseng), *Huang Qi* (Radix Astragali), *Zi Wan* (Radix Asteris), *Kuan Dong Hua* (Flos Farfarae), *Bai Zhu* (Rhizoma Atractylodis Macrocephalae) and *Jie Geng* (Radix Platycodonis).
- *Zhong* (central) *qi* deficiency with difficult respiration: combine it with *Ren Shen* (Radix Ginseng), *Dang Shen* (Radix Codonopsis), *Huang Qi* (Radix Astragali), *Chai Hu* (Radix Bupleuri) and *Sheng Ma* (Rhizoma Cimicifugae).

2. Clears Heat and Eliminates Toxins

Wan Dian Jin can be used to clear heat, eliminate toxins, and promote the generation of body fluids. Clinical applications include lung infection and breast abscess.

- Pneumonia: add *Da Qing Ye* (Folium Isatidis), *Yi Zhi Xiang* (Herba Vernoniae Cinereae) and *Mai Men Dong* (Radix Ophiopogonis).
- Lung abscess: use *Wan Dian Jin* with *Lu Gen* (Rhizoma Phragmitis), *Bai Ji* (Rhizoma Bletillae), *Yu Xing Cao* (Herba Houttuyniae), *Dong Gua Zi* (Semen Benincasae), *Yi Yi Ren* (Semen Coicis), *Zi Hua Di Ding* (Herba Violae) and *Jin Yin Hua* (Flos Lonicerae).
- Breast abscess: use this herb with *Chuan Shan Jia* (Squama Manis), *Wang Bu Liu Xing* (Semen Vaccariae), *Ji Xue Cao* (Herba Centella) and *Pu Gong Ying* (Herba Taraxaci).

3. Regulates Qi and Promotes Diuresis

Gout, edema: combine *Wan Dian Jin* with *Shan Pu Tao* (Radix Vitis Amurensis), *Shui Ding Xiang* (Herba Ludwigiae Prostratae) and *Ding Shu Xiu* (Herba Elephantopus Scaber).

DOSAGE

3 to 15 grams in decoction.

Mu Xiang (Radix Aucklandiae)

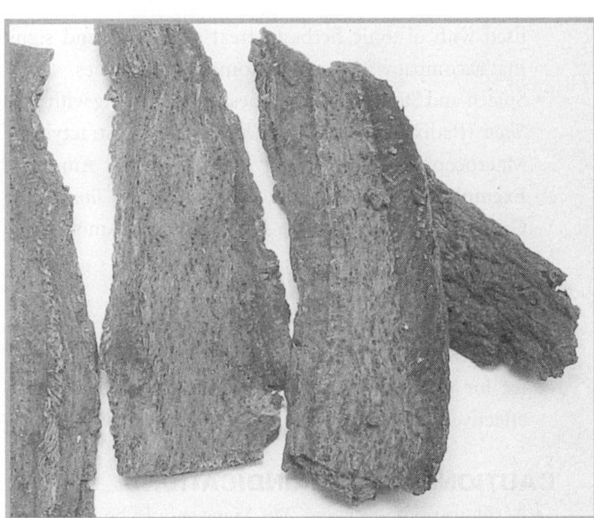

木香

Pinyin Name: *Mu Xiang*
Literal Name: "fragrant wood," "wood aroma," "wood fragrance"
Alternate Chinese Names: *Guang Mu Xiang, Yun Mu Xiang, Wei Mu Xiang*
Original Source: *Shen Nong Ben Cao Jing* (Divine Husbandman's Classic of the Materia Medica) in the second century
English Name: saussurea, aucklandia, costus root
Botanical Name: *Aucklandiae Lappa* Decne. (*Saussurea lappa* Clarke) (*Yun Mu Xiang*); *Vladimiria souliei* (Franch.) Ling. (*Chuan Mu Xiang*)
Pharmaceutical Name: Radix Aucklandiae
Properties: acrid, bitter, warm
Channels Entered: Gallbladder, Large Intestine, Spleen, Stomach

CHINESE THERAPEUTIC ACTIONS

1. Unblocks Qi Stagnation, Regulates the Middle *Jiao* and Relieves Pain

Qi stagnation of the Spleen and Stomach: This condition is characterized by poor appetite, indigestion, food stagnation, epigastric and abdominal fullness, bloating, distention and pain, diarrhea and/or rectal tenesmus. The warm, acrid, bitter properties of *Mu Xiang* (Radix Aucklandiae) help to move and clear stagnation, restore appropriate functioning of the middle *jiao*, and relieve pain.

- Epigastric and abdominal fullness and pain: combine *Mu Xiang* with *Zhi Ke* (Fructus Aurantii), *Chuan Lian Zi* (Fructus Toosendan), *Lai Fu Zi* (Semen Raphani) and *Yan Hu Suo* (Rhizoma Corydalis).
- Damp-heat diarrhea: use it with *Huang Lian* (Rhizoma Coptidis) and *Huo Xiang* (Herba Agastache).
- Diarrhea with profuse pus and blood: use *Mu Xiang* with a large dose of *Bai Shao* (Radix Paeoniae Alba).
- Dysentery and rectal tenesmus due to damp-heat: add *Huang Lian* (Rhizoma Coptidis).
- Dysentery with severe heat: use this herb with *Huang Bai* (Cortex Phellodendri), *Bai Tou Weng* (Radix Pulsatillae), and *Ma Chi Xian* (Herba Portulacae).
- Dysentery with severe dampness: add *Yi Yi Ren* (Semen Coicis), *Fu Ling* (Poria), *Cang Zhu* (Rhizoma Atractylodis) and *Che Qian Zi* (Semen Plantaginis).
- Food stagnation, qi stagnation, diarrhea and rectal tenesmus because of damp-heat: combine it with *Bing Lang* (Semen Arecae), *Zhi Ke* (Fructus Aurantii), *Ge Gen* (Radix Puerariae), *Da Huang* (Radix et Rhizoma Rhei) and *Huang Lian* (Rhizoma Coptidis). **Exemplar Formula:** *Mu Xiang Bing Lang Wan* (Aucklandia and Betel Nut Pill).
- Lower abdominal coldness and pain: add *Wu Yao* (Radix Linderae).

2. Dispels Damp-Heat, Harmonizes the Liver and Spleen

Liver qi stagnation: Disharmony between the Liver and Spleen interferes with the normal transformation and transportation functions of the Spleen. When the flow of water becomes stagnant, damp-heat begins to accumulate, leading to distention and pain in the hypochondriac region, a bitter taste in the mouth, a yellow tongue coat, and possibly jaundice.

- Disharmony of Liver and Spleen: use *Mu Xiang* with *Chai Hu* (Radix Bupleuri), *Yu Jin* (Radix Curcumae), and *Zhi Ke* (Fructus Aurantii).
- Damp-heat accumulation: use it with *Da Huang* (Radix et Rhizoma Rhei), *Yin Chen Hao* (Herba Artemisiae Scopariae) and *Jin Qian Cao* (Herba Lysimachiae).

3. Regulates Qi Circulation, Prevents Stagnation

Spleen qi deficiency: The chief manifestations of Spleen qi deficiency include epigastric and abdominal fullness, distention, bloating, pain, poor appetite, vomiting, diarrhea, preference for warmth and pressure applied to the abdomen, and white, greasy, tongue coating. *Mu Xiang* also activates and regulates qi circulation to prevent stagnation and the bloating sensations associated with the use of herbs that tonify qi. Qi-activating herbs are commonly

Mu Xiang (Radix Aucklandiae)

used with qi-tonic herbs to treat symptoms and signs that accompany Spleen and Stomach deficiencies.

- Spleen and Stomach deficiencies: use *Mu Xiang* with *Ren Shen* (Radix Ginseng), *Bai Zhu* (Rhizoma Atractylodis Macrocephalae), and *Sha Ren* (Fructus Amomi). **Exemplar Formula:** *Xiang Sha Liu Jun Zi Tang* (Six-Gentleman Decoction with Aucklandia and Amomum).

DOSAGE

3 to 10 grams. *Mu Xiang* may be used in herbal decoction, powder or pill forms. The unprocessed herb is better for treating qi stagnation. The roasted herb more effectively treats diarrhea and rectal tenesmus.

CAUTIONS / CONTRAINDICATIONS

- Acrid, warm and drying, *Mu Xiang* should be used with caution for patients experiencing yin deficiency, fluid deficiency, or excess fire.

CHEMICAL COMPOSITION

Saussurine, costus lactone, dihydrocostus lactone, dehydrocostus lactone, costunolide, dihydrocostunolide, 12-methoxydihydro-costunolide, α-costol, α-costic acid, saussurea lactone, α-costene, β-costene.[1]

PHARMACOLOGICAL EFFECTS

- **Respiratory:** Administration of *Mu Xiang* has demonstrated ability to relax spasms of the trachea and bronchi.[2]
- **Effects on smooth muscles:** Components of *Mu Xiang* have various effects on the smooth muscle of the intestines: some stimulate the intestines and increase peristalsis, some relax intestinal spasms, and some have an inhibitory action.[3]
- **Cardiovascular:** Laboratory studies of frogs, dogs and rats have demonstrated that administration of *Mu Xiang* has different effects on the cardiovascular system depending on the dosage. At a small dosage, there is a stimulating effect on the heart, and dilation of blood vessels. At a large dosage, there is an inhibiting effect on the heart, and constriction of blood vessels.[4]
- **Antibiotic:** The essential oil of *Mu Xiang* has an inhibitory effect on streptococcus, staphylococcus, *E. coli*, and *Corynebacterium diphtheriae*.[5]

CLINICAL STUDIES AND RESEARCH

- **Flatulence:** Intramuscular injection of 100% *Mu Xiang* solution twice daily was 93% effective in treating 29 patients with flatulence caused by indigestion, acute gastroenteritis, gastric nervosa, and post-surgical complications.[6]
- **Gallbladder pain:** *Mu Xiang* demonstrated promising effects in 8 patients with pain related to gallbladder disorders.[7]
- **Peptic ulcer disease:** Two formulas with herbs such as *Mu Xiang*, *Wu Yao* (Radix Linderae), *Hong Teng* (Caulis Sargentodoxae), *Gan Jiang* (Rhizoma Zingiberis), *Gou Teng* (Ramulus Uncariae cum Uncis), and *Chen Pi* (Pericarpium Citri Reticulatae) were combined to treat 217 patients with gastric or duodenal ulcers. The treatment protocol was to administer the herbs in decoction twice daily for 20 days. The study reported that 90.3% of patients had complete recovery, with 15.8% recurrence in follow-up visits.[8]

TOXICOLOGY

Oral administration of *Mu Xiang* at a dosage of 1.77 mg/kg in male rats and 2.17 mg/kg in female rats over a 90-day period did not reveal any adverse effects. Examination showed that blood, urine, and the function of internal organs all remained normal throughout the entire study. The LD_{50} for costuslactone in rats via intraperitoneal administration is 300 mg/kg.[9]

AUTHORS' COMMENTS

Mu Xiang is acrid, bitter, dispersing, descending, warming and drying. It can raise qi or cause it to descend, to open all three *jiaos*. The strongest function of this herb is its ability to relieve qi stagnation of the gastrointestinal tract. The chief manifestations of this stagnation are bloating, gas, fullness, distention and pain. Secondary disorders that are also treated with *Mu Xiang* include diarrhea, dysentery with rectal tenesmus, food accumulation and poor appetite. It is one of the strongest, most essential and effective herbs in regulating abdominal qi and relieving pain.

References

1. *Xian Dai Zhong Yao Yao Li Xue* (Contemporary Pharmacology of Chinese Herbs), 1997; 655
2. *Zhong Yao Yao Li Yu Ying Yong* (Pharmacology and Applications of Chinese Herbs), 1983: 169
3. Ibid.
4. Ibid.
5. Ibid.
6. *Zhong Cao Yao Tong Xun* (Journal of Chinese Herbal Medicine), 1979; 3:37
7. *Zhong Hua Wai Ke Za Zhi* (Chinese Journal of External Medicine), 1958; 1:24
8. *Xin Yi Xue* (New Medicine), 1976; 5:214
9. *Zhong Yao Yao Li Yu Ying Yong* (Pharmacology and Applications of Chinese Herbs), 1983: 169

Xiang Fu (Rhizoma Cyperi)

香附

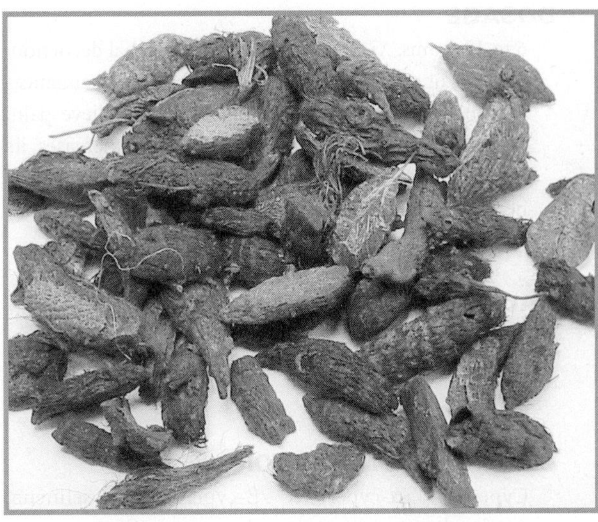

Pinyin Name: *Xiang Fu*
Literal Name: "aromatic appendage"
Original Source: *Ming Yi Za Zhu* (Miscellaneous Records of Famous Physicians) by Tao Hong-Jing in 500 A.D.
English Name: cyperus, nutgrass rhizome
Botanical Name: *Cyperus rotundus* L. (*Sha Cao*)
Pharmaceutical Name: Rhizoma Cyperi
Properties: acrid, slightly bitter, slightly sweet, neutral
Channels Entered: Liver, *San Jiao*

CHINESE THERAPEUTIC ACTIONS

1. Spreads the Liver, Regulates Qi

Liver qi stagnation: Clinically, *Xiang Fu* (Rhizoma Cyperi) is commonly used to treat Liver qi stagnation characterized by hypochondriac pain and epigastric and abdominal fullness and pain. Secondary symptoms include emotional disturbances and poor appetite, chest congestion and frequent sighing. This herb is also excellent in relieving stomach pain caused by stress, as is seen in patients with peptic or duodenal ulcers.

- Hypochondriac pain: use *Xiang Fu* with *Chai Hu* (Radix Bupleuri), *Bai Shao* (Radix Paeoniae Alba) and *Zhi Ke* (Fructus Aurantii).
- Liver and Stomach disharmony with poor appetite: use it with *Mu Xiang* (Radix Aucklandiae), *Fo Shou* (Fructus Citri Sarcodactylis), *Sha Ren* (Fructus Amomi) and *Shen Qu* (Massa Fermentata).
- Epigastric and abdominal pain caused by cold: combine it with *Gao Liang Jiang* (Rhizoma Alpiniae Officinarum).
- Stress and emotional disturbances: add it to *Bai Shao* (Radix Paeoniae Alba), *Yu Jin* (Radix Curcumae), *Chai Hu* (Radix Bupleuri), *Mu Xiang* (Radix Aucklandiae) and *Hou Po* (Cortex Magnoliae Officinalis).
- Stomach pain caused by stress: use this herb with *Gao Liang Jiang* (Rhizoma Alpiniae Officinarum), *Mu Xiang* (Radix Aucklandiae), *Chuan Lian Zi* (Fructus Toosendan), *Yan Hu Suo* (Rhizoma Corydalis) and *Bai Shao* (Radix Paeoniae Alba).
- Abdominal pain that worsens with cold: combine *Xiang Fu* with *Gao Liang Jiang* (Rhizoma Alpiniae Officinarum).
- Epigastric pain due to alternating cold and heat: add *Gao Liang Jiang* (Rhizoma Alpiniae Officinarum), *Bai He* (Bulbus Lilii), *Wu Yao* (Radix Linderae), *Dan Shen* (Radix Salviae Miltiorrhizae), *Tan Xiang* (Lignum Santali Albi) and *Sha Ren* (Fructus Amomi).
- Acid regurgitation: use *Xiang Fu* with *Wa Leng Zi* (Concha Arcae), *Hai Piao Xiao* (Endoconcha Sepiae) and *Bei Mu* (Bulbus Fritillaria).

Hernial pain: *Xiang Fu* can also be used to treat cold stagnation along the Liver channel that manifests in abdominal and hernial pain.

- Hernial pain due to cold: use *Xiang Fu* with *Xiao Hui Xiang* (Fructus Foeniculi) and *Wu Yao* (Radix Linderae).

2. Regulates Menstruation, Relieves Pain

Irregular menstruation, dysmenorrhea and breast distention: *Xiang Fu* is commonly used to treat menstrual disorders or pre-menstrual syndrome arising from Liver qi stagnation. This is an herb that regulates qi in the *xue* (blood) level and can also lead blood to the *qi* (energy) level to help generate blood. Because of this unique trait, it is often used in pregnant and postpartum women who are blood-deficient. *Xiang Fu* is considered one of the most important herbs for treatment of obstetric/gynecologic disorders.

- Irregular menstruation with breast distention and abdominal pain: use *Xiang Fu* with *Dang Gui* (Radicis Angelicae Sinensis), *Chuan Xiong* (Rhizoma Ligustici Chuanxiong), *Bai Shao* (Radix Paeoniae Alba) and *Chai Hu* (Radix Bupleuri).
- Breast distention or breast nodules: add *Chai Hu* (Radix Bupleuri), *Qing Pi* (Pericarpium Citri Reticulatae Viride), *Wang Bu Liu Xing* (Semen Vaccariae) and *Gua Lou Shi* (Fructus Trichosanthis).
- Dysmenorrhea: combine *Xiang Fu* with *Wu Ling Zhi* (Excrementum Trogopteri seu Pteromi), *Pu Huang* (Pollen Typhae) and *Yan Hu Suo* (Rhizoma Corydalis).

Xiang Fu (Rhizoma Cyperi)

DOSAGE

6 to 12 grams. *Xiang Fu* can be used as herbal decoction, powder, or pills. Frying the herb with vinegar enhances its function to reduce accumulations and relieve pain. Frying the herb with grain-based liquor increases its function to open channels and collaterals. Frying the herb with ginger potentiates its action to dissolve phlegm stagnation and unblock Liver qi stagnation.

CAUTIONS / CONTRAINDICATIONS

- Use *Xiang Fu* with caution for patients experiencing qi deficiency in the absence of stagnation, or yin deficiency with heat in the blood.

CHEMICAL COMPOSITION

Cyperene, α-cyperone, β-cyperone, β-selinene, patchoulenone, limonene, limonene, β-pinene, p-cymene, camphene, cyperol, isocyperol, cyperolone, cyperotundone, sugenolacetate, α-rotunol, β-rotunol.[1,2]

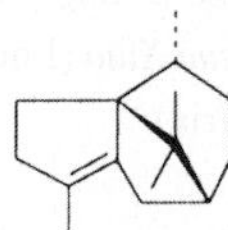

Cyperene

PHARMACOLOGICAL EFFECTS

- **Sedative:** Intraperitoneal administration of the essential oils of *Xiang Fu* in mice at a dose of 0.10 ml/kg demonstrated a sedative effect similar to that of pentobarbital sodium solution with $p<0.01$. The sedative effect was also observed when the essential oil was given to rabbits via intravenous administration.[3]
- **Uterine relaxant:** Oral administration of a 5% solution of *Xiang Fu* showed an inhibitory effect on the uterus in rats, rabbits, dogs and cats.[4]
- **Analgesic:** Administration of a 20% *Xiang Fu* injection in mice showed marked analgesic effects.[5]
- **Antipyretic:** The antipyretic effect of *Xiang Fu* is approximately 6 times stronger than sodium salicylate in experiments conducted in rats.[6]
- **Cardiovascular:** Administration of *Xiang Fu* via subcutaneous injection has demonstrated positive inotropic and negative chronotropic effects in frogs, rabbits and cats. Administration of *Xiang Fu* at a dosage of 0.1 ml/kg via intravenous injection lowered blood pressure in cats and dogs for a duration of 5 to 8 minutes.[7]
- **Antibiotic:** *Xiang Fu* has demonstrated an inhibitory effect against *Staphylococcus aureus*, but with little or no effect against other pathogens.[8]

CLINICAL STUDIES AND RESEARCH

- **Gastrointestinal disorders:** Thirty patients with stomach cramps and pain characterized by cold and qi stagnation were treated with an herbal preparation, with an 80% rate of effectiveness. The herbal preparation was made by grounding into powder 120 grams of *Xiang Fu* and 90 grams of *Gao Liang Jiang* (Rhizoma Alpiniae Officinarum). The treatment protocol was to administer 2 grams of powder twice daily.[9]
- **Flat warts:** For 15 patients with flat warts, 4 ml of *Xiang Fu* (equivalent to 12 grams of bulk herb), administered via intramuscular injection for 10 to 15 doses per treatment course, was 85.7% effective.[10] Furthermore, oral administration of *Xiang Fu* (10 grams of powder stir fried with one egg), was 85.7% effective in 14 patients with flat warts when given every 2 to 4 days for a total of 5 to 8 doses.[11]

TOXICOLOGY

Xiang Fu is well-tolerated by animals. No significant adverse reactions were observed in rats when *Xiang Fu* was incorporated to supply up to 25% of their daily diet. The LD_{50} in mice for cyperone via intraperitoneal administration is approximately 1500 mg/kg; and the LD_{50} for the essential oil of *Xiang Fu* via intraperitoneal administration is 0.297 +/- 0.019 ml/kg.[12]

AUTHORS' COMMENTS

Xiang Fu is one of the most commonly used qi-regulating herbs. Some records state that this herb enters all twelve channels, and relieves stagnation of all six factors (qi, blood, phlegm, food, fire, and dampness).

Both *Xiang Fu* and *Chai Hu* (Radix Bupleuri) smooth Liver qi, and enter the Liver to regulate Liver qi and menstruation. Both are excellent for hypochondriac pain, irregular menstruation, breast distention and dysmenorrhea. However, there are some important differences. *Xiang Fu* is neutral and aromatic, and is mainly used to relieve qi stagnation and pain, primarily epigastric or abdominal distention and pain caused by Liver qi stagnation. *Chai Hu* is cool and most effective for Liver qi stagnation, in addition to clearing heat and resolving *shaoyang* disorders. It also raises the yang and treats symptoms of prolapse, when combined with other Spleen tonics.

According to Dr. Ding Guang-Di, *Xiang Fu* and *Xuan Fu Hua* (Flos Inulae) most effectively address right-sided hypochondriac pain, while *Chuan Lian Zi* (Fructus Toosendan) and *Yan Hu Suo* (Rhizoma Corydalis) are better for left-sided hypochondriac pain.

Xiang Fu (Rhizoma Cyperi)

References

1. *Xian Dai Zhong Yao Yao Li Xue* (Contemporary Pharmacology of Chinese Herbs), 1997; 645
2. Yan X, Zhou J, Xie G, *Traditional Chinese Medicines Molecular Structures, Natural Sources and Applications*; Ashgate, 1999; 1437
3. *Zhong Guo Yao Ke Da Xue Xue Bao* (Journal of University of Chinese Herbology), 1989; 20(1):48
4. *Zhong Hua Yi Xue Za Zhi* (Chinese Journal of Medicine), 1935; 12:1351
5. *Gui Yang Yi Xue Yuan Xue Bao* (Journal of Guiyang Medical University), 1959:113
6. *Indian J Med Res; 1971; 59(1):76*
7. *Zhong Guo Yao Ke Da Xue Xue Bao* (Journal of University of Chinese Herbology), 1989; 20(1):48
8. Ibid.
9. *Zhong Cao Yao Fang Ji De Ying Yong* (Applications of Chinese Herbal Formulas), 1976; 101
10. *Zhong Yi Za Zhi* (Journal of Chinese Medicine), 1984; 6:58
11. *Fu Jian Yi Yao Za Zhi* (Fujian Journal of Medicine and Herbology), 1980; 1:51
12. *Zhong Guo Yao Ke Da Xue Xue Bao* (Journal of University of Chinese Herbology), 1989; 20(1):48

Wu Yao (Radix Linderae)

烏藥 乌药

Pinyin Name: *Wu Yao*
Literal Name: "black medicine"
Alternate Chinese Names: *Tai Wu Yao*
Original Source: *Ben Cao Gang Mu Shi Yi* (Omissions from the Grand Materia Medica) by Zhao Xue-Min in 1765
English Name: lindera root
Botanical Name: *Lindera strychnifolia* (Sieb. et Zucc.) Villar (*Wu Yao*)
Pharmaceutical Name: Radix Linderae
Properties: acrid, warm
Channels Entered: Urinary Bladder, Kidney, Lung, Spleen

CHINESE THERAPEUTIC ACTIONS

1. Regulates Qi and Relieves Pain

Qi stagnation and cold accumulation: *Wu Yao* (Radix Linderae) activates qi circulation, disperses cold, and relieves pain in the chest, abdomen, hypochondriac and epigastric areas.

- Hypochondriac pain with feelings of oppression in the chest: use *Wu Yao* with *Xie Bai* (Bulbus Allii Macrostemonis), *Gua Lou Pi* (Pericarpium Trichosanthis), *Yu Jin* (Radix Curcumae), and *Yan Hu Suo* (Rhizoma Corydalis).
- Epigastric and abdominal fullness and pain: combine it with *Mu Xiang* (Radix Aucklandiae), *Wu Zhu Yu* (Fructus Evodiae) and *Zhi Ke* (Fructus Aurantii).
- Lower abdominal pain, hernial pain, and testicular pain caused by cold: use it with *Xiao Hui Xiang* (Fructus Foeniculi), *Mu Xiang* (Radix Aucklandiae), and *Qing Pi* (Pericarpium Citri Reticulatae Viride).
- Menstrual pain: add *Xiang Fu* (Rhizoma Cyperi), *Dang Gui* (Radicis Angelicae Sinensis) and *Mu Xiang* (Radix Aucklandiae).
- Stroke caused by wind-cold attacking the channels and collaterals: combine it with *Chen Pi* (Pericarpium Citri Reticulatae), *Jiang Can* (Bombyx Batryticatus), *Ma Huang* (Herba Ephedrae) and *Chuan Xiong* (Rhizoma Ligustici Chuanxiong). **Exemplar Formula**: *Wu Yao Shun Qi San* (Lindera Powder to Smooth the Flow of Qi).

2. Warms the Kidney, Disperses Cold

Enuresis caused by Kidney yang deficiency, or by deficiency and cold of the Urinary Bladder: With deficiency of the Kidney and Urinary Bladder, the bladder cannot

Wu Yao (Radix Linderae)

retain urine, resulting in enuresis. There may be accompanying soreness, coldness and weakness of the low back and knees, pale complexion, frequent urination during the night, fatigue, spermatorrhea in men, and profuse, clear, vaginal discharge in women.

- Frequent urination and enuresis: use *Wu Yao* with *Yi Zhi Ren* (Fructus Alpiniae Oxyphyllae) and *Shan Yao* (Rhizoma Dioscoreae). **Exemplar Formula:** *Suo Quan Wan* (Shut the Sluice Pill).

DOSAGE

3 to 10 grams. *Wu Yao* may be used in herbal decoction or pills.

CAUTIONS / CONTRAINDICATIONS

- The use of this acrid, warm and drying herb may consume qi and blood. Thus, *Wu Yao* is not recommended in cases of qi and blood deficiencies or in patients who have interior heat.

CHEMICAL COMPOSITION

Lindeneol, lindenene, linderoxide, isolinderoxide, isofuranogermacrene, lindestrene, lindestrenolide, linderalactone, isolinderalactone, linderane, neolinderalactone, laurolitsine, linderol, linderic acid.[1]

PHARMACOLOGICAL EFFECTS

- **Gastrointestinal:** It has been reported that *Wu Yao* increases the secretion of gastric acid. Furthermore, it has a dual effect on the intestines; it may cause either contraction or relaxation of smooth muscle. Contraction increases intestinal peristalsis and expulsion of gas, and relaxation relieves spasms and cramps.[2]
- **Metabolic:** Long-term use of *Wu Yao* as food led to an increase in body weight in rats.[3]
- **Hemostatic:** The powder of *Wu Yao* shortens coagulation time in rabbits and may be used to stop bleeding.[4]

SUPPLEMENT

- 烏藤 / 乌藤 *Wu Teng* (Ramulus Linderae) is derived from the branches and leaves of the same plant as *Wu Yao*. It harmonizes the middle *jiao*, benefits qi, and treats frequent urination.

AUTHORS' COMMENTS

Wu Yao, *Mu Xiang* (Radix Aucklandiae) and *Xiang Fu* (Rhizoma Cyperi) all regulate qi and relieve pain.

- *Wu Yao* enters the Kidney to treat hernial pain.
- *Mu Xiang* is best for qi stagnation of the Spleen and Stomach to treat bloating, distention, and abdominal pain. It is one of the strongest herbs to relieve the pain associated with qi stagnation.
- *Xiang Fu* is neutral and dispersing in nature. It is one of the best herbs for treating hypochondriac pain and gynecological disorders such as pre-menstrual syndrome, irregular menstruation, dysmenorrhea, bloating and breast distention.

References

1. *Xian Dai Zhong Yao Yao Li Xue* (Contemporary Pharmacology of Chinese Herbs), 1997; 650
2. *Zhong Yao Yao Li Yu Ying Yong* (Pharmacology and Applications of Chinese Herbs), 1983; 217
3. *Zhong Cao Yao Cheng Fen Hua Xue* (Composition and Chemistry of Chinese Herbs), 1977; 493
4. *Zhong Yao Xue* (Chinese Herbology), 1998; 413:414

Xie Bai (Bulbus Allii Macrostemonis)

薤白 薤白

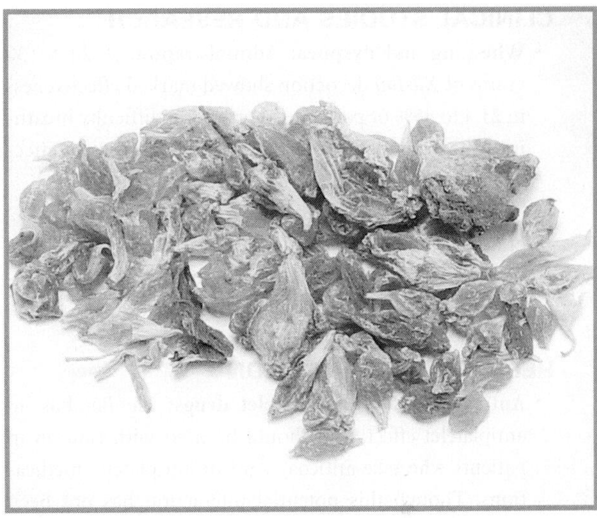

Pinyin Name: *Xie Bai*
Alternate Chinese Names: *Xie Gen*
Original Source: *Shen Nong Ben Cao Jing* (Divine Husbandman's Classic of the Materia Medica) in the second century
English Name: bakeri, long-stamen onion bulb
Botanical Name: *Allium macrostemon* Bge. (*Xiao Gen Suan*); *Allium chinense* G. Don. (*Xie*)
Pharmaceutical Name: Bulbus Allii Macrostemonis
Properties: acrid, bitter, warm
Channels Entered: Large Intestine, Stomach, Lung

CHINESE THERAPEUTIC ACTIONS

1. Opens Yang Qi, Disperses Stagnation due to Cold Phlegm

Chest pain: *Xiong bi* (painful obstruction of the chest), or angina, often occurs as a result of cold phlegm in the chest obstructing the flow and smooth circulation of yang qi. Clinically, *xiong bi* is characterized by feelings of oppression and pain in the chest, shortness of breath, coughing and wheezing. *Xie Bai* (Bulbus Allii Macrostemonis) is one of the best herbs to treat *xiong bi* as it opens yang qi and disperses stagnation.

- *Xiong bi* (painful obstruction of the chest) with profuse phlegm: use *Xie Bai* with *Gua Lou Shi* (Fructus Trichosanthis).
- *Xiong bi* (painful obstruction of the chest) with stabbing pain from blood stagnation: combine it with *Dan Shen* (Radix Salviae Miltiorrhizae), *Hong Hua* (Flos Carthami), *Chuan Xiong* (Rhizoma Ligustici Chuanxiong), and *Chi Shao* (Radix Paeoniae Rubrae).

2. Moves Qi and Eliminates Stagnation

Diarrhea or dysentery with rectal tenesmus: Rectal tenesmus is usually caused by qi stagnation. Comparatively speaking, if there is more qi stagnation than heat, the prominent signs would be diarrhea with gas, and bloating and pain that are relieved by defecation. If damp-heat is more prominent than qi stagnation, there would be burning sensations of the anus, along with a feeling of incomplete evacuation.

- Diarrhea and dysentery with rectal tenesmus because of Liver and Stomach qi stagnation: use *Xie Bai* with *Chai Hu* (Radix Bupleuri), *Bai Shao* (Radix Paeoniae Alba) and *Zhi Shi* (Fructus Aurantii Immaturus).
- Diarrhea and dysentery with rectal tenesmus from damp-heat: add *Huang Bai* (Cortex Phellodendri) and *Qin Pi* (Cortex Fraxini).

DOSAGE

5 to 10 grams in decoction, powder, or pills. *Xie Bai* may be used either internally or topically.

CAUTIONS / CONTRAINDICATIONS

- Use of *Xie Bai* is not recommended in cases where there is qi deficiency but no stagnation, or for patients with poor appetite.
- Those who are hypersensitive to *Xie Bai* should avoid using it.

CHEMICAL COMPOSITION

Alliin, scorodoes, diallyl sulfide, diallyl disulfide, methyl allyl trisulfide (MATS), $A_1(PGA_1)$, $B_1(PGB_1)$.[1]

[Structure: H_2C=CH–CH$_2$–S(=O)–CH$_2$–CH(NH$_2$)–COOH]

Alliin

PHARMACOLOGICAL EFFECTS

- **Antibiotic:** *Xie Bai* has demonstrated inhibitory effects against *Bacillus dysenteriae, Staphylococcus aureus,* and *pneumococci*.[2]
- **Cardiovascular:** PGA_1 lowers blood pressure and induces diuresis while PGB_1 constricts blood vessels.[3]
- **Antiplatelet:** Essential oil of *Xie Bai* markedly inhibits the aggregation of platelets and prolongs clotting time.[4]
- **Antihyperlipidemic:** *Xie Bai* has shown marked effectiveness to lower plasma cholesterol and triglyceride levels.[5]

Xie Bai (Bulbus Allii Macrostemonis)

CLINICAL STUDIES AND RESEARCH

- **Wheezing and dyspnea:** Administration of 20 to 30 grams of *Xie Bai* decoction showed marked effectiveness in 21.4 to 45% of patients experiencing difficulty breathing. The onset of effect is rapid. This herb is most effective when there is loud wheezing.[6]
- **Atherosclerosis:** Extract of *Xie Bai* (equivalent to 12.2 grams of bulk herb) given three times daily for 4 weeks demonstrated marked usefulness to lower plasma cholesterol levels and inhibit platelet aggregation.[7]

HERB-DRUG INTERACTION

- **Anticoagulant or antiplatelet drugs:** *Xie Bai* has an antiplatelet effect, and should be used with caution in patients who take anticoagulant or antiplatelet medications. Though this potential interaction has not been documented, this herb may potentiate the effect of drugs such as warfarin. [Note: Examples of anticoagulants include heparin, warfarin (Coumadin) and enoxaparin (Lovenox); and examples of antiplatelets include aspirin, dipyridamole (Persantine), and clopidogrel (Plavix).][8]

References

1. *Xian Dai Zhong Yao Yao Li Xue* (Contemporary Pharmacology of Chinese Herbs), 1997; 657
2. *Zhong Cao Yao Xue* (Study of Chinese Herbal Medicine), 1980; 1280
3. *Zhong Cao Yao* (Chinese Herbal Medicine), 1991; 1280
4. *Bai Qiu En Yi Ke Da Xue Xue Bao* (Journal of Baiqiuen University of Medicine), 1984; 10(16):609
5. *Prostaglandins*, 1976; 12:685
6. *Nan Jing Zhong Yi Xue Yuan Xue Bao* (Journal of Nanjing University of Traditional Chinese Medicine), 1984; 2:40
7. *Zhong Xi Yi Jie He Za Zhi* (Journal of Integrated Chinese and Western Medicine), 1988; 5:266
8. Chen, J. Recognition & prevention of herb-drug interactions, *Medical Acupuncture*, Fall/Winter 1998/1999; volume 10/number 2; 9-13

Tan Xiang (Lignum Santali Albi)

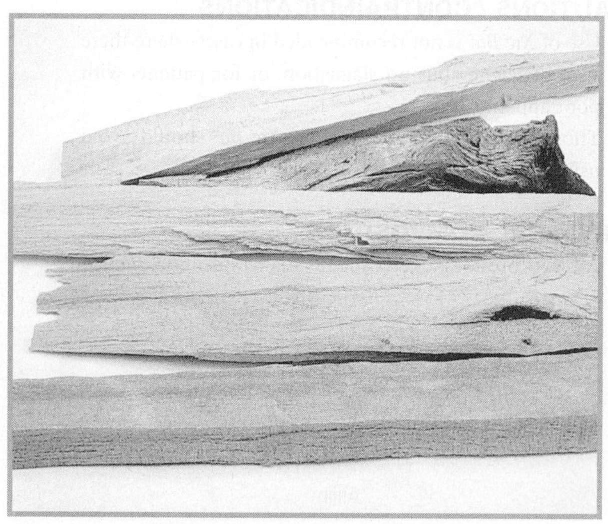

檀香 檀香

Pinyin Name: *Tan Xiang*
Alternate Chinese Names: *Bai Tan Xiang, Huang Tan Xiang*
Original Source: *Ming Yi Za Zhu* (Miscellaneous Records of Famous Physicians) by Tao Hong-Jing in 500 A.D.
English Name: santalum, sandalwood
Botanical Name: *Santalum album* L. (*Mu Tan Xiang*)
Pharmaceutical Name: Lignum Santali Albi
Properties: acrid, warm, aromatic
Channels Entered: Spleen, Stomach, Lung

CHINESE THERAPEUTIC ACTIONS

1. Regulates Qi, Harmonizes the Middle *Jiao*

Abdominal pain due to cold and qi stagnation: Acrid and dispersing, *Tan Xiang* (Lignum Santali Albi) regulates qi in the diaphragm and aromatically wakes up the Spleen to treat epigastric or abdominal coldness and pain, and vomiting of clear fluids. Secondary symptoms may include poor appetite and hiccups.

- Abdominal pain with vomiting of clear fluids: use *Tan Xiang* with *Sha Ren* (Fructus Amomi), *Bai Dou Kou* (Fructus Amomi Rotundus), *Ding Xiang* (Flos Caryophylli) and *Wu Yao* (Radix Linderae).
- Hiccups: combine it with *Ren Shen* (Radix Ginseng) and *Ju Hong* (Exocarpium Citri Rubrum).
- Epigastric distention and bloating: use this herb with *Dan Shen* (Radix Salviae Miltiorrhizae), *Sha Ren* (Fructus Amomi), *Wu Yao* (Radix Linderae) and *Bai He* (Bulbus Lilii).

Tan Xiang (Lignum Santali Albi)

- Poor appetite: combine it with *Chen Pi* (Pericarpium Citri Reticulatae), *Mai Ya* (Fructus Hordei Germinatus), *Sha Shen* (Radix Glehniae seu Adenophorae) and *Mai Men Dong* (Radix Ophiopogonis).

2. Disperses Cold and Relieves Pain

Chest pain from cold and qi stagnation: Cold and qi stagnation constrict the chest and manifest in symptoms of angina, dyspnea and feelings of oppression in the chest. *Tan Xiang* disperses cold, and relieves chest constriction, oppression and pain.

- Chest pain: use *Tan Xiang* with *Yan Hu Suo* (Rhizoma Corydalis), *Bi Ba* (Fructus Piperis Longi), *Gao Liang Jiang* (Rhizoma Alpiniae Officinarum) and *Bing Pian* (Borneolum Syntheticum).

DOSAGE

1 to 3 grams in decoction. *Tan Xiang* is also taken in pill form.

CAUTIONS / CONTRAINDICATIONS

- *Tan Xiang* should be used with caution for patients who have yin-deficient heat or are vomiting because of heat.
- Use *Tan Xiang* with caution during pregnancy, due to its abortifacient effect.[1]

CHEMICAL COMPOSITION

α-santalol, β-santalol, santene, α-santalene, β-santalene, santenone, santenone alcohol, santalic acid, teresantalic acid, santal aldehyde.[2]

AUTHORS' COMMENTS

Tan Xiang and *Mu Xiang* (Radix Aucklandiae) have similar qi-regulating functions. *Tan Xiang* is stronger in relieving chest pain arising from cold and qi stagnation in the chest. *Mu Xiang* is more effective for relieving abdominal pain caused by cold and qi stagnation in the Stomach and Spleen.

References

1. Brinker, Francis. *The Toxicology of Botanical Medicines,* rev. 2nd ed., 1996
2. *Xian Dai Zhong Yao Yao Li Xue* (Contemporary Pharmacology of Chinese Herbs), 1997; 666

Chen Xiang (Lignum Aquilariae Resinatum)

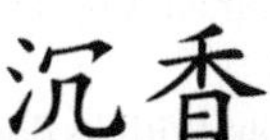

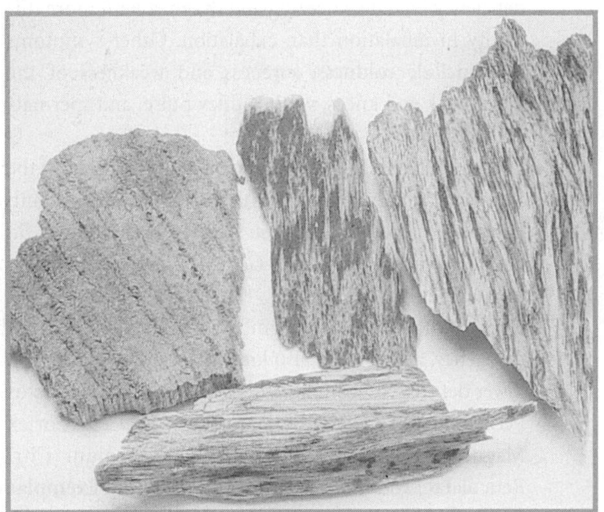

Pinyin Name: *Chen Xiang*
Literal Name: "sinking aroma," "sinking fragrance"
Alternate Chinese Names: *Chen Sui Xiang*
Original Source: *Ming Yi Za Zhu* (Miscellaneous Records of Famous Physicians) by Tao Hong-Jing in 500 A.D.
English Name: aquilaria, Chinese eaglewood
Botanical Name: *Aquilaria agallocha* Roxb. (*Chen Xiang*); *Aquilaria sinensis* (Lour.) Gilg. (*Bai Mu Xiang*)
Pharmaceutical Name: Lignum Aquilariae Resinatum
Properties: acrid, bitter, warm, aromatic
Channels Entered: Kidney, Spleen, Stomach

CHINESE THERAPEUTIC ACTIONS

1. Moves Qi, Relieves Pain

Qi stagnation and cold accumulation with chest and abdominal distention and pain: *Chen Xiang* (Lignum Aquilariae Resinatum) warms the body, dispels cold, and moves qi to relieve pain in the chest and abdominal

Chen Xiang (Lignum Aquilariae Resinatum)

regions. It is commonly used to treat pain characterized by cold and stagnation.

- Chest and abdominal distention and pain caused by accumulation of cold and stagnation of qi: use *Chen Xiang* with *Wu Yao* (Radix Linderae), *Bing Lang* (Semen Arecae), and *Mu Xiang* (Radix Aucklandiae).
- Epigastric, hypochondriac, and/or abdominal fullness and pain accompanied by deficiency and cold of the Spleen and Stomach: add *Rou Gui* (Cortex Cinnamomi), *Fu Zi* (Radix Aconiti Lateralis Praeparata) and *Gan Jiang* (Rhizoma Zingiberis).
- Extreme coldness of the hands and feet, pain in the abdomen and umbilical area due to lack of fire in the *ming men* (life gate): incorporate *Chen Xiang* with *Fu Zi* (Radix Aconiti Lateralis Praeparata), *Ding Xiang* (Flos Caryophylli), and *She Xiang* (Moschus).

2. Warms the Middle *Jiao*, Relieves Vomiting

Stomach qi reversal due to cold: *Chen Xiang* warms and harmonizes the middle *jiao* to treat chronic nausea, hiccups and vomiting from deficiency and cold of the Spleen and Stomach.

- Nausea and vomiting: combine *Chen Xiang* with *Ding Xiang* (Flos Caryophylli), *Bai Dou Kou* (Fructus Amomi Rotundus), *Zi Su Ye* (Folium Perillae) and *Sheng Jiang* (Rhizoma Zingiberis Recens).

3. Warms the Kidney, Grasps Qi Downwards

Kidney yang deficiency with inability to grasp qi downwards: The chief clinical manifestations of this deficiency include wheezing and dyspnea with more difficulty in inhalation than exhalation. Other symptoms may include coldness, soreness and weakness of the lower back and knees, weak Kidney pulse, and spermatorrhea in men.

- Difficult inhalation because of deficiency and cold of the Kidney: use *Chen Xiang* with *Fu Zi* (Radix Aconiti Lateralis Praeparata), *Rou Gui* (Cortex Cinnamomi), *Bu Gu Zhi* (Fructus Psoraleae), *Ge Jie* (Gecko) and *Bai Guo* (Semen Ginkgo).
- Cough with profuse phlegm accompanied by Kidney deficiency, a syndrome also known as "upper excess and lower deficiency:" combine this herb with *Su Zi* (Fructus Perillae), *Qian Hu* (Radix Peucedani), *Hou Po* (Cortex Magnoliae Officinalis), *Chen Pi* (Pericarpium Citri Reticulatae) and *Ban Xia* (Rhizoma Pinelliae). **Exemplar Formula:** *Su Zi Jiang Qi Tang* (Perilla Fruit Decoction for Directing Qi Downward).
- Premature ejaculation: use it with *Fu Zi* (Radix Aconiti Lateralis Praeparata), *Yang Qi Shi* (Actinolitum) and *Bu Gu Zhi* (Fructus Psoraleae).

DOSAGE

1.0 to 1.5 grams. *Chen Xiang* should be post-decocted to ensure its effectiveness. It is also taken in powder concurrently with a decoction, or made into pills.

CAUTIONS / CONTRAINDICATIONS

- Use *Chen Xiang* with caution in the presence of yin-deficient fire, or organ prolapse due to qi deficiency.

CHEMICAL COMPOSITION

Baimuxinic acid, baimuxinal, agarospirol, baimuxinol, dehydrobaimuxinol, isobaimuxinol, benzylacetone, p-methoxybenzylacetone, anisic acid, β-agarofuran, sinenofuranal, sinenofuranol, dihydrokaranone, β-agarofuran.[1]

PHARMACOLOGICAL EFFECTS

- **Smooth muscle relaxant**: Administration of *Chen Xiang* via intraperitoneal injection relaxes the smooth muscle of the intestines and decreases intestinal peristalsis.[2]

CLINICAL STUDIES AND RESEARCH

- **Respiratory disorders:** Administration of an herbal formula containing 1.5 grams of *Chen Xiang* and 3 grams of *Ce Bai Ye* (Cacumen Platycladi) in powder form showed marked effectiveness for treatment of bronchial wheezing and dyspnea. The herbal formula was given once daily, before bedtime.[3]

AUTHORS' COMMENTS

Chen Xiang, *Jiang Xiang* (Lignum Dalbergiae Odoriferae) and *Tan Xiang* (Lignum Santali Albi) are all aromatic herbs that move qi.

- *Chen Xiang* enters the Spleen and Kidney. With its downward-moving tendency, it works to help the Kidney pull qi downwards to treat dyspnea and asthma due to Kidney deficiency, with or without the accumulation of phlegm in the Lung.
- *Tan Xiang* enters the Lung, Spleen and Stomach. It is best for regulating qi stagnation in the upper and middle *jiaos* that manifests in symptoms of angina, hiccups, and chest and epigastric pain.
- *Jiang Xiang* enters the Liver, Spleen and Heart. It regulates qi in the chest and hypochondrium to relieve pain, and redirects rebellious qi downwards to relieve nausea and vomiting.

References

1. *Xian Dai Zhong Yao Yao Li Xue* (Contemporary Pharmacology of Chinese Herbs), 1997; 649
2. *Zhong Yao Cai* (Study of Chinese Herbal Material), 1989; 12(12):40
3. *Zhe Jiang Zhong Yi Za Zhi* (Zhejiang Journal of Chinese Medicine), 1957; 8:10

Chuan Lian Zi (Fructus Toosendan)

川楝子 川栋子

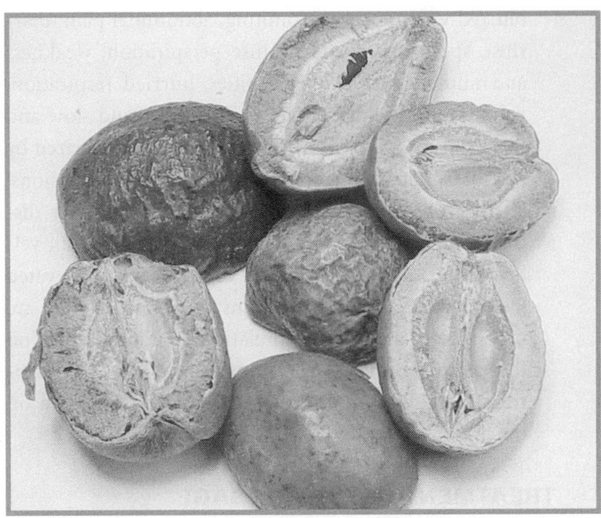

Pinyin Name: *Chuan Lian Zi*
Alternate Chinese Names: *Jin Ling Zi, Lian Shi*
Original Source: *Shen Nong Ben Cao Jing* (Divine Husbandman's Classic of the Materia Medica) in the second century
English Name: melia, Sichuan chinaberry fruit
Botanical Name: *Melia toosendan* Sieb. et. Zucc. (*Chuan Lian*)
Pharmaceutical Name: Fructus Toosendan
Properties: bitter, cold
Channels Entered: Liver, Small Intestine, Stomach, Urinary Bladder
Safety Index: slightly toxic

CHINESE THERAPEUTIC ACTIONS

1. Moves Qi and Relieves Pain

Liver qi stagnation: With bitter taste and cold thermal property, *Chuan Lian Zi* (Fructus Toosendan) regulates Liver qi and relieves stagnation to treat hypochondriac distention and pain, and abdominal pain with heat signs of irritability, insomnia, red face and eyes, and short temper.

- Hypochondriac and abdominal pain: use *Chuan Lian Zi* with *Yan Hu Suo* (Rhizoma Corydalis) and *Xiang Fu* (Rhizoma Cyperi).

Disharmony of Liver and Stomach: When Wood overacts on Earth, the Spleen and Stomach are affected. Typical symptoms include poor appetite, bloating, distention and pain.

- Bloating: use *Chuan Lian Zi* with *Mu Xiang* (Radix Aucklandiae) and *Xiang Fu* (Rhizoma Cyperi).

Hernial pain with lower abdominal coldness and distention:

- Hernial disorders with hypochondriac, epigastric, or abdominal pain caused by Liver qi stagnation with heat: use this herb with *Yan Hu Suo* (Rhizoma Corydalis).
- Hernial disorders with lower abdominal distention and pain caused by cold: use it with *Xiao Hui Xiang* (Fructus Foeniculi), *Wu Zhu Yu* (Fructus Evodiae) and *Mu Xiang* (Radix Aucklandiae). **Exemplar Formula:** *Dao Qi Tang* (Conduct the Qi Decoction).

2. Kills Parasites

Chuan Lian Zi kills intestinal parasites and relieves pain. It is most effective for roundworms and hookworms.

- Parasitic infection: use *Chuan Lian Zi* with *Bing Lang* (Semen Arecae) and *Shi Jun Zi* (Fructus Quisqualis).

3. Kills Fungus

Chuan Lian Zi kills fungi, and is used topically as an herbal paste to treat fungal infections of the scalp. The herbal paste is prepared by roasting the herb, grinding it to powder, and mixing the powder with sesame oil. The affected area should be cleaned with salt water prior to application of the herbal paste.

DOSAGE

3 to 10 grams. *Chuan Lian Zi* is commonly used in herbal decoctions, pills, and topical creams/ointments. Bitter and cold, the unprocessed herb is slightly toxic. Dry-frying increases its warmth, minimizes toxicity, and reduces irritation to the Spleen and Stomach. Dry-frying with salt enhances its ability to enter the Kidney, and this form is commonly used to relieve pain in the lower *jiao*, such as hernial pain.

CAUTIONS / CONTRAINDICATIONS

- Use *Chuan Lian Zi* with caution in cases of deficiency and cold of the Spleen and Stomach.
- Large dosages of *Chuan Lian Zi* are not recommended as it is slightly toxic.

OVERDOSAGE

The entire melia plant is toxic, with the fruit being the most toxic part and the leaves the least. Eating 6 to 8 fresh *Chuan Lian Zi* fruits can cause dizziness, vomiting, diarrhea, respiratory difficulties, palpitations, tremors, spasms, and in severe cases, numbness and unconsciousness.

Adverse reactions to *Chuan Lian Zi* usually occur 4 to 6 hours after ingestion, but may begin as rapidly as 30 minutes. Early, mild symptoms of toxicity include dizziness,

Chuan Lian Zi (Fructus Toosendan)

blurred vision, nausea, vomiting, abdominal pain, diarrhea, spontaneous and profuse perspiration, weakness and numbness of the extremities, hurried respiration, palpitations, feelings of chest oppression, and slow and weak pulse. Severe cases of toxicity are characterized by tremor, spasms and cramps of the muscles, convulsions, altered consciousness, arrhythmia, and respiratory distress. Some patients also show hepatotoxicity, with yellow urine, yellow discoloration of the skin, and elevated liver enzymes. Adverse reactions to *Chuan Lian Zi* are usually attributed to its stimulating (irritating) effect on the gastrointestinal system, stimulating effect on the central nervous system, and toxic effect of toosendanin on the liver.

TREATMENT OF OVERDOSAGE

The early stage of overdose (4 to 5 hours after ingestion) may be treated with emetic methods followed by intake of 4 to 5 egg whites. The egg whites minimize irritation and damage caused by the herb. If overdose of the herb occurred 5 hours prior to treatment, the patient should be treated with a purgative method by dissolving 10 grams of *Mang Xiao* (Natrii Sulfas) in warm water as a drink to induce diarrhea and minimize absorption of the toxins.[1]

Acute liver damage with such symptoms as yellow urination, yellow discoloration of the skin and eyes, yellow and greasy tongue coat, and slippery pulse can be treated with an herbal formula in decoction that contains *Hu Zhang* (Rhizoma Polygoni Cuspidati) 12g, *Sheng Ma* (Rhizoma Cimicifugae) 12g, *Yin Chen Hao* (Herba Artemisiae Scopariae) 15g, *Hou Po* (Cortex Magnoliae Officinalis) 15g, *Che Qian Cao* (Herba Plantaginis) 15g, *Chui Peng Cao* 18g, and *Dan Shen* (Radix Salviae Miltiorrhizae) 15g.[2]

CHEMICAL COMPOSITION

Toosendanin, mergsine, melianone, melianol, melianediol, melialactone, azadirachtin, 21-o-acetyltoosendatriol, lipomelianol.[3,4]

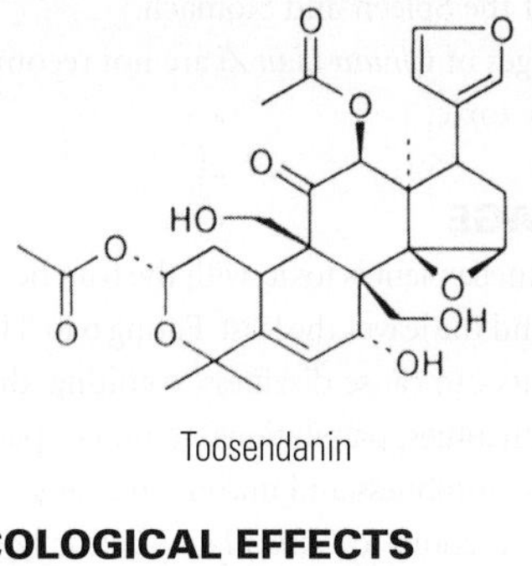

Toosendanin

PHARMACOLOGICAL EFFECTS

- **Antiparasitic:** *Chuan Lian Zi* has demonstrated marked effectiveness against intestinal parasites. It has been proposed that toosendanin causes constant muscle contraction in the parasites, leading to muscle fatigue, inability to adhere to the intestines, and eventual expulsion of the parasites. The expulsion of parasites generally occurs 24 to 48 hours after administration of *Chuan Lian Zi*. When compared to santonin, *Chuan Lian Zi* has slower onset but more prolonged duration of effect.[5]
- **Respiratory:** Administration of *Chuan Lian Zi* in rats via intravenous or intramuscular injection leads to dyspnea, a reaction attributed to its inhibiting influence on the central nervous system. Dyspnea may be reversed with administration of nicotine.[6]
- **Antitoxin**: The survival rate is over 80% in rats when toosendanin is administered within 6 hours of exposure to botulism, and approximately 50% in monkeys when administered within 24 hours.[7]

CLINICAL STUDIES AND RESEARCH

- **Acute mastitis:** In one study, 43 patients with acute mastitis were treated with an herbal formula one to two times daily for 2 to 5 days. The herbal formula was composed of 9 grams of *Chuan Lian Zi*, 30 grams of brown sugar, and 100 to 200 ml of grain-based liquor or boiling water. Patients without suppuration (34 out of 43) reported complete recovery, after 2 to 4 doses within 3 days. Patients with suppuration (9 out of 43), after removal or draining of pus, reported complete recovery after 6 to 12 doses within 4 to 8 days.[8]

TOXICOLOGY

The LD_{50} for toosendanin in mice is 13.8 +/- 1.2 mg/kg via intraperitoneal injection, 14.6 +/- 0.9 mg/kg via intravenous injection, 14.3 +/- 1.5 mg/kg via subcutaneous injection, and 244.2 +/- 44.0 mg/kg via oral administration. Adverse reactions included an elevated SGPT and muscle fatigue.[9]

SUPPLEMENT

- 苦楝子 / 苦栋子 *Ku Lian Zi* (Fructus Meliae), derived from *Melia azedarach L.*, is sometimes used inappropriately in place of *Chuan Lian Zi* (Fructus Toosendan). In some other regions in China, *Ku Lian Zi* is used as a substitute when *Chuan Lian Zi* is unavailable. In others, such as Xian and Jinan, *Ku Lian Zi* is used interchangeably as *Chuan Lian Zi*. *Ku Lian Zi* is bitter and more toxic than *Chuan Lian Zi*. Overdose of *Ku Lian Zi* can result from the ingestion of approximately 10 to 70 pieces, and can cause toxic side effects within 4 to 8 hours. Signs of toxicity include vomiting, nausea, diarrhea, difficulty breathing, numbness of limbs, paroxysmal convulsions and elevated blood pressure. Therefore, extreme caution should be exercised when *Ku Lian Zi* is used.

Chuan Lian Zi (Fructus Toosendan)

AUTHORS' COMMENTS

Chuan Lian Zi and *Wu Yao* (Radix Linderae) both have excellent abilities to regulate qi and relieve hernial pain. *Chuan Lian Zi* is bitter, cold, has a descending nature, and slightly toxic. It enters the Liver, Stomach, Small Intestine and Urinary Bladder. It sedates Liver heat and damp-heat found in hernial pain and redness and swelling of the testicles. *Wu Yao* is warm, dispersing, and enters the Lung, Spleen, Kidney and Urinary Bladder. It warms the Kidney and is more suitable for hernial pain arising from cold.

According to Dr. Ding Guang-Di, *Chuan Lian Zi* and *Yan Hu Suo* (Rhizoma Corydalis) are specific for left-sided hypochondriac pain. *Xuan Fu Hua* (Flos Inulae) and *Xiang Fu* (Rhizoma Cyperi) effectively address right-sided hypochondriac pain.

According to Jang Meng-Chau, *Chuan Lian Zi* increases duct peristalsis and facilitates the passage of stones. Thus, it is an essential herb for treatment of gall-stones and kidney stones.

References

1. *Zhong Yao Du Li Xue* (Toxicology of Chinese Herbs); 33-35, 1989
2. Ibid.
3. *Xian Dai Zhong Yao Yao Li Xue* (Contemporary Pharmacology of Chinese Herbs), 1997; 651
4. Yan X, Zhou J, Xie G, *Traditional Chinese Medicines Molecular Structures, Natural Sources and Applications*; Ashgate, 1999; 6325
5. *Zhong Yao Yao Li Yu Lin Chuan* (Pharmacology and Clinical Applications of Chinese Herbs), 1983: 648
6. *Sheng Li Xue Bao* (Physiology News), 1980; 32(4):338
7. Ibid.
8. *Zhong Ji Yi Kan* (Medium Medical Journal), 1965; 7:454
9. *Zhong Cao Yao* (Chinese Herbal Medicine), 1982; 13(7):29

Qing Mu Xiang (Radix Aristolochiae)

青木香

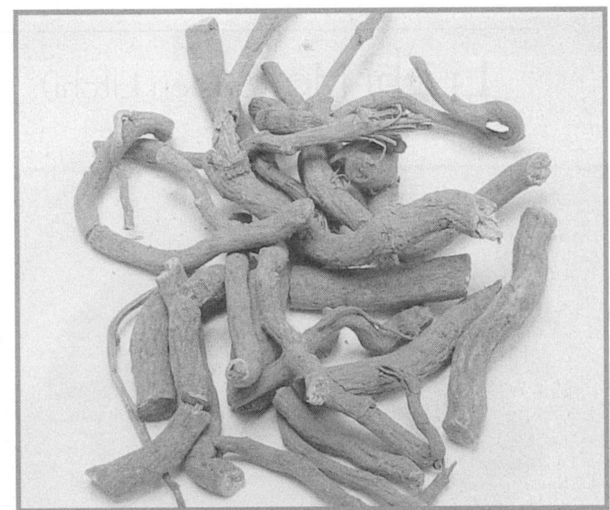

Pinyin Name: *Qing Mu Xiang*

Alternate Chinese Names: *Bei Ma Dou Ling, Ma Dou Ling Gen, Tu Qing Mu Xiang*

Original Source: *Xin Xiu Ben Cao* (Newly Revised Materia Medica) by Su Jing in 657-659 A.D.

English Name: aristolochia root, slender Dutchman's pipe root

Botanical Name: *Aristolochia debilis* Sieb. et Zucc. (*Ma Dou Ling*); *Aristolochia contorta* Bge. (*Bei Ma Dou Ling*)

Pharmaceutical Name: Radix Aristolochiae

Properties: acrid, bitter, cool

Channels Entered: Liver, Stomach

Safety Index: toxic

CHINESE THERAPEUTIC ACTIONS

1. Regulates Qi and Relieves Pain

Liver and Stomach qi stagnation: *Qing Mu Xiang* (Radix Aristolochiae) treats Liver and Stomach qi stagnation, a condition characterized by distention and pain of the chest, hypochondriac, epigastric and abdominal regions.

- Liver and Stomach qi stagnation: use this herb with *Xiang Fu* (Rhizoma Cyperi) and *Chuan Lian Zi* (Fructus Toosendan).

2. Eliminates Toxins and Reduces Swelling

Qing Mu Xiang treats abdominal pain and diarrhea caused by food poisoning or improper food intake.

- Diarrhea and abdominal pain: use it with *Huang Lian* (Rhizoma Coptidis) and *Bing Lang* (Semen Arecae).

Snake bites: *Qing Mu Xiang,* used topically, relieves swelling and pain caused by snake bites.

- Snake bites: use this herb with *Bai Zhi* (Radix Angelicae Dahuricae) and apply topically or take internally.

Qing Mu Xiang (Radix Aristolochiae)

DOSAGE

3 to 10 grams in decoction, 1.5 to 2 grams as powder.

CAUTIONS / CONTRAINDICATIONS

- Because *Qing Mu Xiang* is toxic, high doses are contraindicated. Potential side effects include nausea and vomiting.
- *Qing Mu Xiang* should be used with caution in patients experiencing deficiency and cold conditions.

CHEMICAL COMPOSITION

Aristolochic acid A, B, C; aristolochia lactan, debilic acid, allantoin, magnoflorine, cyclanoline, aristolone, debilone, aristolenone, isoaristolone, aristolin, α-pinene, β-pinene.[1]

TOXICOLOGY

Qing Mu Xiang contains a trace amount of aristolochic acid. For more information on the toxicology of this compound, please refer to *Guang Fang Ji* (Radix Aristolochiae Fangchi) or *Guan Mu Tong* (Caulis Aristolochiae Manshuriensis).

No fatalities were reported following oral ingestion of 20 to 40 grams of *Qing Mu Xiang* in cats weighing 2 kg. The LD_{50} for aristolochic acid in mice was 48.7 mg/kg via oral ingestion and 22.4 mg/kg via intravenous injection.[2]

AUTHORS' COMMENTS

Qing Mu Xiang (Radix Aristolochiae) is also known as "*Ma Dou Ling Gen*." Like *Ma Dou Ling* (Fructus Aristolochiae), *Qing Mu Xiang* is toxic and should be used with extreme caution.

Mu Xiang (Radix Aucklandiae) and *Qing Mu Xiang* (Radix Aristolochiae) have similar names, but have completely different functions and safety profiles. They should never be confused, or used interchangeably.

References

1. *Xian Dai Zhong Yao Yao Li Xue* (Contemporary Pharmacology of Chinese Herbs), 1997; 646
2. *Zhong Yao Yao Li Yu Ying Yong* (Pharmacology and Applications of Chinese Herbs), 1983; 604

Li Zhi He (Semen Litchi)

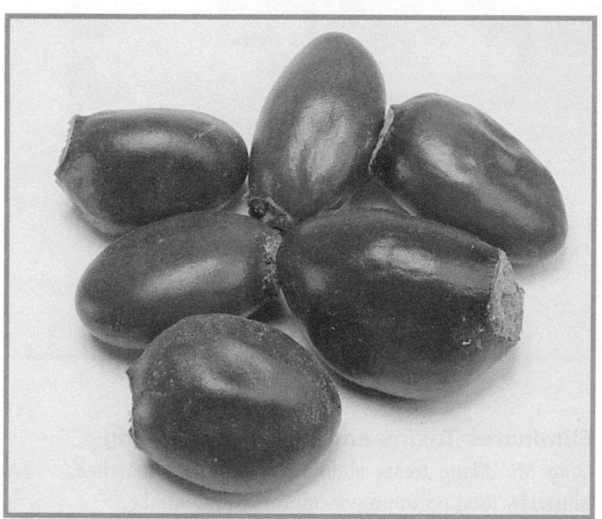

荔枝核 荔枝核

Pinyin Name: *Li Zhi He*
Literal Name: "litchi seed"
Alternate Chinese Names: *Da Li He, Li Ren*
Original Source: *Ben Cao Yan Yi* (Extension of the Materia Medica) by Kou Zong-Shi in 1116
English Name: litchi seed, lychee seed
Botanical Name: *Litchi chinensis* Sonn. (*Li Zhi Shu*)
Pharmaceutical Name: Semen Litchi
Properties: sweet, astringent, warm
Channels Entered: Liver, Stomach

CHINESE THERAPEUTIC ACTIONS

1. Moves Qi, Relieves Pain, Disperses Cold

Hernial pain: *Li Zhi He* (Semen Litchi) is an excellent herb to treat cold hernial disorders with testicular swelling and pain.

- Hernial disorders with swelling and pain in the testicles caused by cold stagnation in the Liver channel: use *Li Zhi He* with *Xiao Hui Xiang* (Fructus Foeniculi), *Wu Zhu Yu* (Fructus Evodiae) and *Ju He* (Semen Citri Rubrum).
- Redness, swelling and pain in the testicles due to damp-

Li Zhi He (Semen Litchi)

heat and fire in the Liver channel: use this herb with *Long Dan Cao* (Radix Gentianae), *Zhi Zi* (Fructus Gardeniae), *Da Huang* (Radix et Rhizoma Rhei) and *Chuan Lian Zi* (Fructus Toosendan).

***Ben tun* (running piglet) sensation:** This is an upward shooting sensation of qi from the lower abdomen to the epigastric or chest region, causing pain.

- *Ben tun* sensation: use *Li Zhi He* with *Mu Xiang* (Radix Aucklandiae), *Wu Zhu Yu* (Fructus Evodiae) and *Rou Gui* (Cortex Cinnamomi). Use *Rou Gui* only if there are signs of cold.

2. Regulates Liver Qi

Chronic epigastric pain: *Li Zhi He* regulates Liver qi, dispels cold, and relieves chronic epigastric pain.

- Chronic epigastric pain from Liver qi stagnation: use *Li Zhi He* with *Mu Xiang* (Radix Aucklandiae), *Yan Hu Suo* (Rhizoma Corydalis) and *Chuan Lian Zi* (Fructus Toosendan).

Pre-menstrual or postpartum abdominal pain because of qi and blood stagnation.

- Abdominal pain: add *Xiang Fu* (Rhizoma Cyperi).

DOSAGE

10 to 15 grams. *Li Zhi He* may be used in decoction or pills. Frying with salt directs the function of the herb downwards to the lower *jiao* and potentiates its ability to treat hernia and pain.

CAUTIONS / CONTRAINDICATIONS

- *Li Zhi He* is contraindicated in patients who do not exhibit cold and damp accumulation.

CHEMICAL COMPOSITION

3-acetoin, 2,3-butanediol, copaene, cis-caryophyllene, alloaromadendrene, humulene, 6-cadinene, α-curcumene, calamenene, ledol, quaiazulene, xanthorrhizol, palmatic acid.[1]

PHARMACOLOGICAL EFFECTS

- **Antidiabetic:** Administration of *Li Zhi He* to mice via subcutaneous injection lowered blood glucose levels.[2]

HERB-DRUG INTERACTION

- **Antidiabetics:** Herbs that lower the plasma glucose levels, such as *Li Zhi He,* should be used with caution with insulin, sulfonylureas, and other antidiabetic medications, as the combination may have a synergistic effect, leading to hypoglycemia.[3] [Note: Examples of antidiabetic drugs include insulin, tolbutamide (Orinase), glipizide (Glucotrol), and glyburide (DiaBeta/Micronase).]

TOXICOLOGY

Li Zhi He is very well-tolerated. There are no fatalities following administration of 20 g/kg in mice via oral ingestion.[4]

AUTHORS' COMMENTS

According to Jang Meng-Chau, *Li Zhi He* and *Ju He* (Semen Citri Rubrum) guide other herbs through the channels to the testicles and ovaries. They are indispensable herbs when treating hernias, infertility, ovarian cysts, polycystic ovaries and other disorders specific to those regions.

References

1. *Xian Dai Zhong Yao Yao Li Xue* (Contemporary Pharmacology of Chinese Herbs), 1997; 653
2. *Experientia*, 1985; 4(12):1622
3. Chen, J. Recognition & prevention of herb-drug interactions, *Medical Acupuncture*, Fall/Winter 1998/1999; volume 10/number 2; 9-13
4. *Zhe Jiang Yao Xue* (Zhejiang Journal of Chinese Herbology), 1986; 3(4):8

Suo Luo Zi (Semen Aesculi)

娑羅子 娑罗子

Pinyin Name: *Suo Luo Zi*
Alternate Chinese Names: *Kai Xin Guo*
Original Source: *Ben Cao Gang Mu* (Materia Medica) by Li Shi-Zhen in 1578
English Name: aesculus seed, Chinese buckeye seed, Wilson buckeye seed
Botanical Name: *Aesculus chinensis* Bge. (*Chi Ye Shu*); *Aesculus wilsonii* Rehd. (*Tian Shi Li*)
Pharmaceutical Name: Semen Aesculi
Properties: sweet, warm
Channels Entered: Liver, Stomach

CHINESE THERAPEUTIC ACTIONS

Regulates Liver Qi, Expands the Middle *Jiao* and Harmonizes the Stomach

Liver and Stomach qi stagnation: *Suo Luo Zi* (Semen Aesculi) relieves Liver qi stagnation and treats epigastric, abdominal and hypochondriac distention, bloating and pain. It also treats breast distention that occurs prior to menstruation.

- Epigastric, abdominal and hypochondriac distention and pain: use *Suo Luo Zi* with *Ba Yue Zha* (Fructus Akebiae) and *Fo Shou* (Fructus Citri Sarcodactylis).
- Breast distention: use it with *Lu Lu Tong* (Fructus Liquidambaris), *Xiang Fu* (Rhizoma Cyperi) and *Yu Jin* (Radix Curcumae).

DOSAGE

3 to 10 grams in decoction.

CAUTIONS / CONTRAINDICATIONS

- *Suo Luo Zi* is contraindicated in cases of qi or yin deficiency.

CHEMICAL COMPOSITION

Aescin, eslin.[1]

References

1. *Xian Dai Zhong Yao Yao Li Xue* (Contemporary Pharmacology of Chinese Herbs), 1997; 670

Ba Yue Zha (Fructus Akebiae)

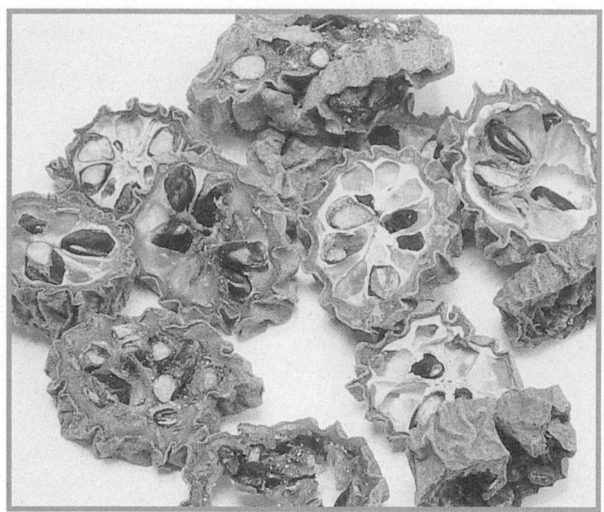

八月札

Pinyin Name: *Ba Yue Zha*
Alternate Chinese Names: *San Ye Mu Tong, Bai Mu Tong, Mu Tong Zi*
Original Source: *Ben Cao Shi Yi* (Omissions from the [Classic of the] Materia Medica) by Chen Cang-Qi in 741 A.D.
English Name: akebia fruit
Botanical Name: *Akebia quinata* (Thunb.) Decne. (*Mu Tong*); *Akebia trifoliata* (Thunb.) Koidz. (*San Ye Mu Tong*); *Akebia trifoliata* (Thunb.) Koidz. var. *australis* (Diels) Rehd. (*Bai Mu Tong*)
Pharmaceutical Name: Fructus Akebiae
Properties: bitter, neutral
Channels Entered: Liver, Stomach

Ba Yue Zha (Fructus Akebiae)

CHINESE THERAPEUTIC ACTIONS

1. Spreads Liver Qi

Liver qi stagnation: *Ba Yue Zha* (Fructus Akebiae) treats Liver qi stagnation manifesting in chest, hypochondriac, epigastric and hernial pain.

- Pain caused by Liver qi stagnation: use *Ba Yue Zha* with *Xiang Fu* (Rhizoma Cyperi), *Zhi Ke* (Fructus Aurantii), *Chuan Lian Zi* (Fructus Toosendan) and *Yan Hu Suo* (Rhizoma Corydalis).

2. Disperses Masses

Nodules and tumors: Masses, nodules and tumors represent the result of qi stagnation and phlegm accumulation.

- Fibrocystic breast disorder: use *Ba Yue Zha* with *Lu Feng Fang* (Nidus Vespae), *Qing Pi* (Pericarpium Citri Reticulatae Viride), and *Wang Bu Liu Xing* (Semen Vaccariae).

DOSAGE

6 to 12 grams in decoction.

CHEMICAL COMPOSITION

Sugars, saponins. [1]

References

1. *Zhong Yao Xue* (Chinese Herbology), 1998; 426-427

Gan Song (Radix seu Rhizoma Nardostachys)

甘松

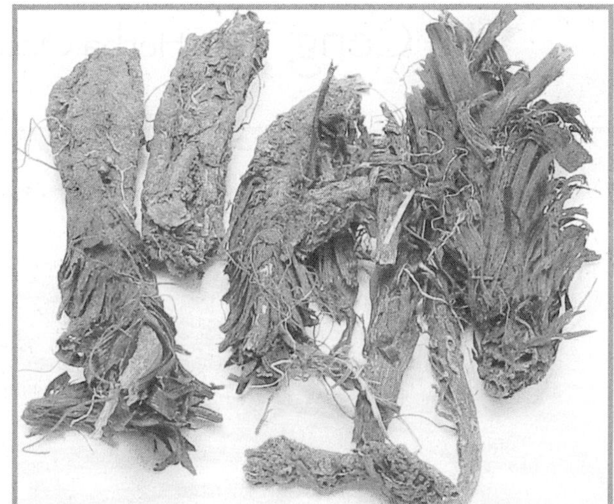

Pinyin Name: *Gan Song*
Literal Name: "sweet pine"
Alternate Chinese Names: *Gan Song Xiang, Kuan Ye Gan Song, Xiang Song*
Original Source: *Ben Cao Shi Yi* (Omissions from the [Classic of the] Materia Medica) by Chen Cang-Qi in 741 A.D.
English Name: nardostachys, Chinese nardostachys rhizome, spoon-leaf nardostachys rhizome
Botanical Name: *Nardostachys chinensis* Batal. (*Gan Song Xiang*); *Nardostachys jatamanse* DC. (*Kuan Ye Gan Song*)
Pharmaceutical Name: Radix seu Rhizoma Nardostachys
Properties: acrid, sweet, warm
Channels Entered: Spleen, Stomach

CHINESE THERAPEUTIC ACTIONS

Regulates Qi, Relieves Pain, Opens Stagnation and Awakens the Spleen

Qi stagnation in the chest and abdomen: *Gan Song* (Radix seu Rhizoma Nardostachys), warm but not hot, sweet but not stagnating, and acrid yet not drying, regulates qi in the chest and abdomen and awakens the Spleen. It is mainly used to treat patients who have damaged their Spleen by excessive worrying, which manifests as a feeling of oppression in the chest, with epigastric and abdominal distention and pain, and poor appetite.

- Qi stagnation in the chest and abdomen: use *Gan Song* with *Mu Xiang* (Radix Aucklandiae), and *Xiang Yuan* (Fructus Citri).
- Qi stagnation with yang deficiency and coldness: use this herb with *Sha Ren* (Fructus Amomi), *Ding Xiang* (Flos Caryophylli) and *Rou Gui* (Cortex Cinnamomi).

DOSAGE

3 to 6 grams in decoction.

Gan Song (Radix seu Rhizoma Nardostachys)

CAUTIONS / CONTRAINDICATIONS

- *Gan Song* is contraindicated in patients with qi deficiency or heat in the blood.

CHEMICAL COMPOSITION

Nardosinone, valeranone, aristolene, maaliol, β-maaliene, nardostachone, dibelon.[1]

PHARMACOLOGICAL EFFECTS

- **Antiarrhythmic:** Intravenous injection of alcohol extract of *Gan Song* was effective in treating chemically-induced arrhythmia in mice and rats. Though the mechanism is unclear, it has been suggested that *Gan Song* acts directly on the cardiac muscle to exert its antiarrhythmic effect.[2]

CLINICAL STUDIES AND RESEARCH

- **Arrhythmia:** In one study, 55 patients with various arrhythmia disorders were treated with an herbal formula with an 83.6% rate of effectiveness. The herbal formula included *Gan Song*, *Da Qing Ye* (Folium Isatidis), *Dang Shen* (Radix Codonopsis), *Ren Shen* (Radix Ginseng), *Gui Zhi* (Ramulus Cinnamomi), *Gan Cao* (Radix Glycyrrhizae) and *Zhi Ke* (Fructus Aurantii).[3]

AUTHORS' COMMENTS

Gan Song treats leg *qi* when combined with *Gao Ben* (Rhizoma Ligustici) and *He Ye* (Folium Nelumbinis) as an external wash or soak. It also serves as a gargle to treat toothache caused by Kidney deficiency.

References

1. *Xian Dai Zhong Yao Yao Li Xue* (Contemporary Pharmacology of Chinese Herbs), 1997; 666-667
2. *An Yi Xue Bao* (Anyi Medical Journal), 1980; (4):2
3. *Zhe Jiang Yi Xue* (Zhejiang Journal of Medicine), 1982; (1):49

Jiu Ceng Ta (Herba Ocimi Basilici)

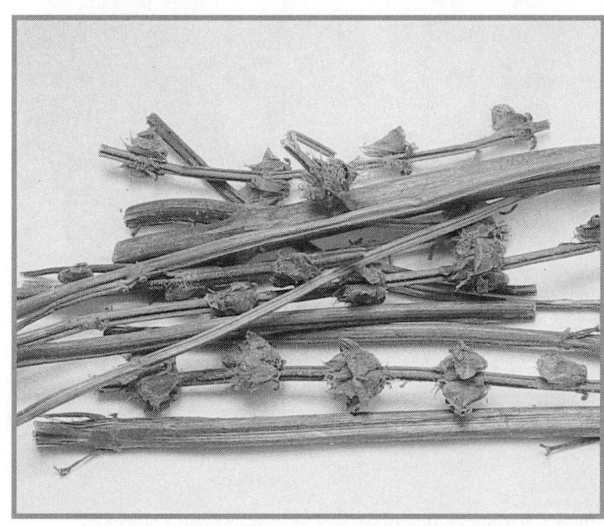

九層塔 九层塔

Pinyin Name: *Jiu Ceng Ta*
Literal Name: "nine-layered temple"
Alternate Chinese Names: *Lou Le, Xiang Cai, Lan Xiang, Shen Zi Cao, Guang Ming Zi*
English Name: basil
Botanical Name: *Ocimum basilicum* L.
Pharmaceutical Name: Herba Ocimi Basilici
Properties: acrid, pungent, warm
Channels Entered: Stomach, Liver, Kidney

CHINESE THERAPEUTIC ACTIONS

1. Regulates the Middle *Jiao*, Promotes Digestion

Stomach cramps, poor appetite in children: *Jiu Ceng Ta* (Herba Ocimi Basilici) treats Stomach cold with qi stagnation. This type of pain may be relieved or lessened by warmth, and aggravated by cold drinks, cold food or pressure.

- Stomach cramps: use *Jiu Ceng Ta* with *Chuan Lian Zi* (Fructus Toosendan), *Yan Hu Suo* (Rhizoma Corydalis), *Bai Shao* (Radix Paeoniae Alba) and *Gan Cao* (Radix Glycyrrhizae).
- Poor appetite in children: use this herb with *Shen Qu* (Massa Fermentata) and *Mai Ya* (Fructus Hordei Germinatus).

Jiu Ceng Ta (Herba Ocimi Basilici)

2. Invigorates Blood Circulation, Dispels Water

Irregular menstruation, postpartum blood stagnation: *Jiu Ceng Ta* treats obstetric/gynecological disorders arising from blood and qi stagnation.

- Irregular menstruation and postpartum blood stagnation: use this herb with *Dan Shen* (Radix Salviae Miltiorrhizae) and *Yi Mu Cao* (Herba Leonuri).

3. Opens Channels and Collaterals

Soreness and pain in the tendons and bones: The aromatic property of *Jiu Ceng Ta* disperses stagnation in the channels and collaterals to relieve pain.

- Soreness and pain in the tendons and bones: combine it with *Ji Xiang Teng* (Caulis Paederiae), *Yi Tiao Gen* (Radix Moghaniae) and *Chuan Shan Long* (Rhizoma Dioscoreae Nipponicae).

4. Eliminates Toxins and Disperses Wind

Toothache, eye swelling and pain: *Jiu Ceng Ta* treats toothache and eye disorders when combined with herbs with heat-clearing and toxin-eliminating functions.

- Toothache: use it with *Shui Ding Xiang* (Herba Ludwigiae Prostratae) and *Shi Gao* (Gypsum Fibrosum).
- Redness, pain and swelling of the eyes: combine it with *Ye Ju Hua* (Flos Chrysanthemi Indici), *Xia Ku Cao* (Spica Prunellae) and *Qian Li Guang* (Herba Senecionis Scandens).
- Superficial visual obstruction: use this herb with *Chan Tui* (Periostracum Cicadae) and *Qian Li Guang* (Herba Senecionis Scandens).

DOSAGE

5 to 12 grams in decoction.

CAUTIONS / CONTRAINDICATIONS

- *Jiu Ceng Ta* is contraindicated during pregnancy.

AUTHORS' COMMENTS

Jiu Ceng Ta has functions similar to those of *Ze Lan* (Herba Lycopi) to invigorate blood circulation and dispel water.

8 QI-REGULATING HERBS

Tian Xian Teng (Herba Aristolochiae)

天仙藤 天仙藤

Pinyin Name: *Tian Xian Teng*
Literal Name: "heavenly vine from the sky"
Alternate Chinese Names: *Ma Dou Ling Teng, Xiang Teng, Tian Xian Gen, Qing Mu Xiang*
English Name: aristolochia herb, Dutchman's pipe herb
Botanical Name: *Aristolochia debilis* Sieb. et Zucc.; *Aristolochia contorta* Bge.; *Aristolochia shimadi* Hay
Pharmaceutical Name: Herba Aristolochiae
Properties: bitter, warm
Channels Entered: Heart, Lung, Spleen, Kidney
Safety Index: toxic

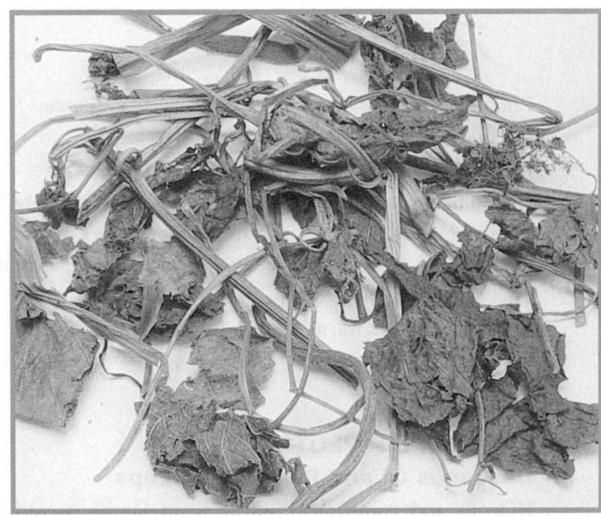

CHINESE THERAPEUTIC ACTIONS

1. Regulates Qi, Invigorates Blood and Relieves Pain

Pain due to qi and blood stagnation: *Tian Xian Teng* (Herba Aristolochiae) treats various kinds of pain, including hernial pain, chest and abdominal pain, and neuralgia.

- Hernial pain: use *Tian Xian Teng* with *Wu Yao* (Radix Linderae) and *Xiao Hui Xiang* (Fructus Foeniculi).

Tian Xian Teng (Herba Aristolochiae)

- Chest and abdominal pain: use this herb with *Xi Xin* (Herba Asari) and *Pao Zai Cao* (Herba Physalis Angulatae).
- Neuralgia: combine it with *Huang Jin Gui* (Caulis Vanieriae), *Mo Gu Xiao* (Caulis Hyptis Capitatae) and *Huang Teng* (Caulis Fibraurea).

2. Clears Heat, Eliminates Toxins, Promotes Urination

Toxic heat: *Tian Xian Teng* treats toxic heat infections, including snake bites, sexually-transmitted diseases and liver cancer.

- Toxic snake bite: use *Tian Xian Teng* with *Ku Shen Gen* (Radix Sophorae Flavescentis), *Da Huang* (Radix et Rhizoma Rhei), *Mu Xiang* (Radix Aucklandiae), *Ban Xia* (Rhizoma Pinelliae), *Tong Cao* (Medulla Tetrapanacis), *Bai Bu* (Radix Stemonae), *Du Huo* (Radix Angelicae Pubescentis) and *Shu Wei Huang* (Herba Rostellulariae).
- Sexually-transmitted diseases: use *Tian Xian Teng* with *Tu Fu Ling* (Rhizoma Smilacis Glabrae), *Xian Feng Cao* (Herba Bidentis), *Shan Pu Tao* (Radix Vitis Amurensis) and *Che Qian Zi* (Semen Plantaginis).
- Liver cancer: combine this herb with *Huang Shui Qie* (Herba Solani), *Hu Zhang* (Rhizoma Polygoni Cuspidati), *Xue Fu Zhu Yu Tang* (Drive Out Stasis in the Mansion of Blood Decoction) and *Ren Shen Yang Ying Tang* (Ginseng Decoction to Nourish the Nutritive Qi).

DOSAGE

5 to 20 grams.

CAUTIONS / CONTRAINDICATIONS

Tian Xian Teng is contraindicated during pregnancy.

CHEMICAL COMPOSITION

Aristolochic acid.

TOXICOLOGY

Tian Xian Teng contains a trace amount of aristolochic acid. For more information on the toxicology of this compound, please refer to *Guang Fang Ji* (Radix Aristolochiae Fangchi) or *Guan Mu Tong* (Caulis Aristolochiae Manshuriensis).

Dao Dou (Semen Canavaliae)

刀豆

Pinyin Name: *Dao Dou*
Literal Name: "knife bean"
Alternate Chinese Names: *Jia Jian Dou, Dao Dou Zi*
Original Source: *Jiu Huang Ben Cao* (Materia Medica to Rescue Emergencies)
English Name: canavalia, jack bean, sword bean
Botanical Name: *Canavalia gladiata* (Jacq.) DC. (*Dao Dou*)
Pharmaceutical Name: Semen Canavaliae
Properties: sweet, warm
Channels Entered: Stomach, Kidney

CHINESE THERAPEUTIC ACTIONS

Descends Qi and Relieves Hiccups

Hiccups and vomiting resulting from Stomach cold and deficiency: In the case of Stomach cold and deficiency, the sound of the hiccups is weak, and low in tone and volume. Excessive reversal or rebellion of qi will often cause these patients to have respiratory difficulties. Other symptoms may include poor appetite, pale complexion, fatigue and cold extremities. *Dao Dou* (Semen Canavaliae) is mild and must be combined with other herbs for maximum effectiveness.

- Hiccups and vomiting: use *Dao Dou* with *Ding Xiang* (Flos Caryophylli) and *Shi Di* (Calyx Kaki).

Dao Dou has a mild effect to tonify Kidney to warm yang. It is combined with other herbs to treat low back pain caused by Kidney yang deficiency.

Dao Dou (Semen Canavaliae)

DOSAGE

10 to 15 grams in decoction. *Dao Dou* can also be used in powder form.

CAUTIONS / CONTRAINDICATIONS

- *Dao Dou* is contraindicated when the hiccups are caused by Stomach heat.

CHEMICAL COMPOSITION

Urease, hemogglutinin, canavanine, arginase, concanavalin A, stachyose, spermidine, spermine, putrescine.[1]

References

1. *Chang Yong Zhong Yao Cheng Fen Yu Yao Li Shou Ce* (A Handbook of the Composition and Pharmacology of Common Chinese Drugs), 1994; 123-124

Shi Di (Calyx Kaki)

柿蒂 柿蒂

Pinyin Name: *Shi Di*
Alternate Chinese Names: *Shi Qian, Shi Zi Ba, Shi Ding*
Original Source: *Ming Yi Za Zhu* (Miscellaneous Records of Famous Physicians) by Tao Hong-Jing in 500 A.D.
English Name: kaki calyx, persimmon calyx and receptacle
Botanical Name: *Diospyros kaki* L. f. (*Shi Shu*)
Pharmaceutical Name: Calyx Kaki
Properties: bitter, neutral
Channels Entered: Stomach

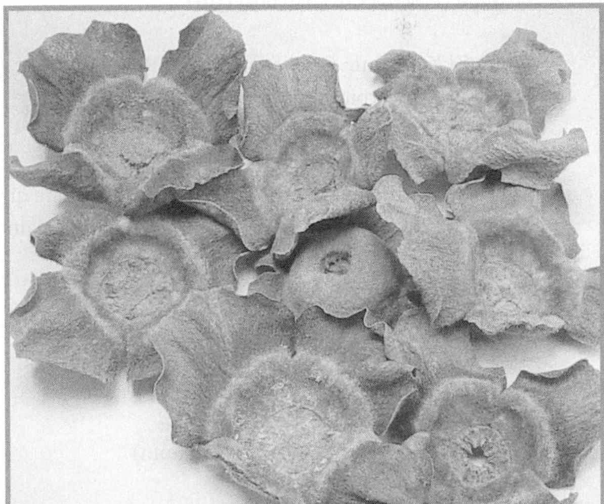

CHINESE THERAPEUTIC ACTIONS

Descends Qi, Stops Hiccups

Hiccups are caused when disharmony of the Stomach leads qi that would otherwise descend to rise in an abnormal manner. *Shi Di* (Calyx Kaki) is a neutral herb that addresses this problem in both hot or cold conditions.

- Hiccups due to cold in the Stomach: use *Shi Di* with *Ding Xiang* (Flos Caryophylli) and *Sheng Jiang* (Rhizoma Zingiberis Recens).
- Hiccups because of heat in the Stomach: use it with *Lu Gen* (Rhizoma Phragmitis) and *Zhu Ru* (Caulis Bambusae in Taenia).
- Hiccups due to deficiency or in the elderly: combine it with *Dang Shen* (Radix Codonopsis), *Ren Shen* (Radix Ginseng) and *Bai Zhu* (Rhizoma Atractylodis Macrocephalae).

DOSAGE

3 to 12 grams. *Shi Di* may be used as herbal decoction or pills.

CHEMICAL COMPOSITION

Oleanolic acid, ursolic acid, trifolin, β-sitosteryl-β-D-glucoside, stearic acid, palmitic acid, succinic acid, syringic acid, vanillin acid, gallic acid, kaempferol, frifolin, hyperin, hydroxytripterpenic acid.[1]

PHARMACOLOGICAL EFFECTS

- **Antiarrhythmic:** Administration of 0.5% *Shi Di* in mice at the dosage of 50 mg/kg has demonstrated a marked effect against chlorine- or aconitine-induced arrhythmia.[2]
- **Antifertility:** Administration of *Shi Di* is 79.6% successful as an antifertility agent in rabbits.[3]

References

1. *Xian Dai Zhong Yao Yao Li Xue* (Contemporary Pharmacology of Chinese Herbs), 1997; 659
2. *Zhong Cheng Yao* (Study of Chinese Patent Medicine), 1987; (3):28
3. Ibid., 1983; (7):27

Chapter 8 summary — Qi-Regulating Herbs

Herb	Similarities	Differences
Chen Pi (Pericarpium Citri Reticulatae)	Regulate qi, dissolve phlegm	Regulates Spleen and Stomach qi, dries dampness and dissolves phlegm
Qing Pi (Pericarpium Citri Reticulatae Viride)		Regulates Liver qi, breaks up qi stagnation and accumulation
Zhi Shi (Fructus Aurantii Immaturus)		Breaks qi stagnation and accumulation, dissolves phlegm and relieves distention
Zhi Ke (Fructus Aurantii)		Regulates qi and spreads the middle *jiao*
Xiang Yuan (Fructus Citri)		Regulates Spleen, Stomach and Liver qi
Fo Shou (Fructus Citri Sarcodactylis)		Relieves Liver qi stagnation and cough with profuse phlegm
Po Bu Zi Ye (Folium Cordia Dichotoma)		Dispels phlegm and relieves coughing
Da Fu Pi (Pericarpium Arecae)		Promotes diuresis and relieves edema
Wan Dian Jin (Radix Ilicis Asprellae)		Redirects Lung qi to treat cough, chest congestion, and lung abscess
Mu Xiang (Radix Aucklandiae)	Regulate qi, relieve pain	Regulates Spleen, Stomach and Large Intestine qi
Xiang Fu (Rhizoma Cyperi)		Regulates Liver qi, regulates menstruation; used mainly for obstetric/gynecologic disorders
Wu Yao (Radix Linderae)		Enters the lower *jiao;* used for lower abdominal pain and frequent urination
Xie Bai (Bulbus Allii Macrostemonis)		Redirects qi, opens yang qi and treats *xiong bi* (painful obstruction of the chest) syndrome
Tan Xiang (Lignum Santali Albi)		Alleviates chest pain caused by cold
Chen Xiang (Lignum Aquilariae Resinatum)		Redirects qi to relieve nausea, cough, dyspnea and vomiting
Chuan Lian Zi (Fructus Toosendan)		Regulates Liver qi, more for pain from heat, kills parasites
Qing Mu Xiang (Radix Aristolochiae)		Eliminates toxins, reduces swelling
Li Zhi He (Semen Litchi)		Alleviates hernial or abdominal pain caused by cold
Suo Luo Zi (Semen Aesculi)		Harmonizes the Liver and Stomach
Ba Yue Zha (Fructus Akebiae)		Relieves hypochondriac and hernial pain, disperses stagnation to treat nodules
Gan Song (Radix seu Rhizoma Nardostachys)		Relieves Liver qi stagnation and awakens the Spleen
Jiu Ceng Ta (Herba Ocimi Basilici)		Regulates qi in the middle *jiao*, promotes digestion
Tian Xian Teng (Herba Aristolochiae)		Clears heat and eliminates toxins
Dao Dou (Semen Canavaliae)	Re-direct Stomach qi to relieve vomiting and nausea	Treats nausea and vomiting in deficient, cold individuals
Shi Di (Calyx Kaki)		Stops hiccups

Chapter 8 summary

General Characteristics of Qi-Regulating Herbs:

Taste: acrid, bitter
Thermal property: warm and drying
Channels entered: Lung, Liver, Spleen/Stomach
Therapeutic actions: invigorates qi circulation, relieves qi stagnation, relieves pain

Qi-regulating herbs regulate qi, promote the normal circulation of qi, correct reversed flow of qi, and relieve qi stagnation. These herbs are usually acrid, warm and drying, and may consume yin and body fluids. Therefore, they should be used with caution for patients who have qi and yin deficiencies. Clinical presentation varies depending on the organ affected.

Spleen and Stomach: nausea, vomiting, hiccups, epigastric and abdominal bloating, fullness and pain, acid regurgitation, belching, poor appetite and irregular bowel movement.

Lung: stifling sensations in the chest, cough, dyspnea and wheezing.

Liver: emotional disturbances, stress, irritability, anger, hypochondriac distention or pain, hernial pain, breast distention and tenderness (with or without palpable masses), irregular menstruation and loss of appetite.

Chen Pi (Pericarpium Citri Reticulatae) and ***Qing Pi*** (Pericarpium Citri Reticulatae Viride) are from the same fruit. *Chen Pi* is the peel of ripe oranges, and *Qing Pi* is the peel of green or unripe oranges. Both are warm and regulate qi and dissolve stagnation, treating food and phlegm stagnation that cause epigastric and abdominal fullness, distention and pain.

Chen Pi more specifically influences the upper and middle *jiaos* to relieve qi stagnation of the Lung, Spleen and Stomach. This herb helps to dry dampness, dissolve phlegm, regulate qi, and harmonize the middle *jiao*. Chief applications of *Chen Pi* include cough with profuse sputum, stifling sensations of the chest, and diarrhea with abdominal pain and gas due to the Liver overacting on the Spleen.

Qing Pi is more potent in its effect to regulate qi and break up qi stagnation. *Qing Pi* enters the Liver and Gallbladder and has a descending nature. It is commonly used to treat Liver qi stagnation affecting upper, middle and lower *jiaos*. Clinical indications include palpable masses in the breast, chest and hypochondriac fullness, distention and pain; hernial pain or any palpable masses due to phlegm and qi stagnation.

Chen Pi and *Qing Pi* are often used together to treat disharmony of Wood (Liver) and Earth (Spleen/Stomach).

Zhi Shi (Fructus Aurantii Immaturus) and ***Zhi Ke*** (Fructus Aurantii) have been used interchangeably since ancient times. The smaller, immature fruits are designated as *Zhi Shi*, and the larger, mature fruits are designated *Zhi Ke*. Both are cool and have similar functions.

Zhi Shi and *Zhi Ke* are used together in conjunction with tonic herbs that have yang raising functions to treat organ prolapse.

Zhi Shi is bitter, has descending tendencies, and strongly functions to break qi stagnation, dissolve phlegm and relieve fullness. It is often used in acute cases of food stagnation, abdominal pain, constipation, rectal tenesmus, feelings of stagnation or stifling sensations in the epigastric and chest areas.

Zhi Ke, milder in potency, is more suitable for deficient patients or chronic cases of qi stagnation. It regulates qi, opens the middle *jiao*, relieves distention, and is often used in less severe cases of chest and epigastric fullness and distention.

Zhi Shi (Fructus Aurantii Immaturus) and ***Qing Pi*** (Pericarpium Citri Reticulatae Viride) are potent herbs to regulate qi.

Zhi Shi more strongly opens the chest and diaphragm to relieve stagnation associated with the Stomach and intestines.

Qing Pi, warming and descending in nature, breaks qi stagnation and treats hypochondriac pain.

Chapter 8 summary

Xiang Yuan (Fructus Citri) and ***Fo Shou*** (Fructus Citri Sarcodactylis), acrid, aromatic, bitter and warm, regulate Liver qi, harmonize the middle *jiao* and dissolve phlegm. Since both are relatively mild in nature, they are often combined with other herbs to treat chest and hypochondriac pain and distention, epigastric fullness and poor appetite, belching, and vomiting and cough with profuse sputum.

Xiang Yuan more strongly regulates Spleen and Lung qi to relieve cough.

Fo Shou regulates Liver qi and more effectively relieves pain.

Po Bu Zi Ye (Folium Cordia Dichotoma) regulates qi, relieves pain, dispels phlegm, and eases cough. It has shown promise in treatment of bone spurs.

Da Fu Pi (Pericarpium Arecae) promotes movement of qi, dissipates stagnation, promotes diuresis, and treats edema.

Wan Dian Jin (Radix Ilicis Asprellae) regulates qi and treats Lung disorders, such as cough, chest congestion, pneumonia, and lung abscess.

Mu Xiang (Radix Aucklandiae), ***Xiang Fu*** (Rhizoma Cyperi) and ***Wu Yao*** (Radix Linderae), acrid and aromatic, regulate qi and relieve pain.

Mu Xiang is acrid, aromatic, warm and drying, and is commonly said to open all three *jiaos*. In addition, since it promotes digestion and strengthens the Spleen, it is one of the best herbs to relieve qi stagnation of Spleen and Stomach involving food accumulation. Common clinical manifestations include epigastric and abdominal distention, pain, rectal tenesmus and poor appetite. *Mu Xiang* also helps in treatment of jaundice caused by damp-heat, gallstones and other hepatic or gallbladder disorders secondary to impairment of the Spleen's function in transportation and transformation.

Xiang Fu is aromatic and penetrating in nature. It is mild, and is often used to regulate Liver qi and relieve irritability, regulate menstrual cycles and relieve pain to treat irregular menstruation and dysmenorrhea. It also treats chest, hypochondriac, epigastric and abdominal distention and pain, breast tenderness and hernial pain.

Wu Yao is acrid, warm and less aromatic than the other two herbs. It is milder in nature and enters the Spleen, Lung, Kidney and Urinary Bladder. It effectively regulates qi, disperses cold, and relieves pain. It is often used to treat chest, hypochondriac, epigastric, abdominal, hernial and menstrual pain caused by cold. It also warms the Urinary Bladder and Kidney to treat polyuria and enuresis caused by deficiency and cold.

Xiang Fu (Rhizoma Cyperi) and ***Qing Pi*** (Pericarpium Citri Reticulatae Viride) are potent qi-regulating herbs.

Xiang Fu invigorates qi circulation in all twelve channels, and regulates menstruation and blood.

Qing Pi enters the Liver and strongly breaks up qi stagnation and relieves hernial pain.

Xie Bai (Bulbus Allii Macrostemonis) is warm and enters the upper *jiao* to open the yang and disperse stagnation. It is essential for treatment of *xiong bi* (painful obstruction of the chest) caused by cardiovascular disorders, such as angina and coronary artery disorder. *Xie Bai* also enters the lower *jiao* to relieve rectal tenesmus caused by qi stagnation.

Tan Xiang (Lignum Santali Albi) and ***Chen Xiang*** (Lignum Aquilariae Resinatum) are aromatic, acrid and warm. They regulate qi, disperse cold and relieve pain, and treat cold stagnation in the body.

Tan Xiang more strongly regulates Spleen and Lung qi. It opens the chest and the diaphragm to regulate the middle *jiao* to relieve chest and abdominal pain, angina, and hiccups caused by cold and qi stagnation.

Chapter 8 summary

Chen Xiang is bitter and dense, and descending in nature. It brings down abnormal qi reversal of the Stomach to treat hiccups and vomiting caused by deficiency and cold. It warms the Kidney to help grasp the qi downward to treat asthma characterized by short inhalation and long exhalation. *Chen Xiang* is warm but not drying, moving yet does not cause qi loss. It is one of the best qi-regulating herbs.

Chuan Lian Zi (Fructus Toosendan), cold and bitter, is essential for treatment of Liver-related disorders, such as the pain of Liver qi stagnation, or disharmony of Liver and Spleen involving heat. It also kills parasites and sedates Liver fire. Clinical applications include parasites with abdominal pain, Liver yang rising, dizziness, blurred vision and dermatological disorders of the head. *Chuan Lian Zi* is slightly toxic and should not be prescribed at high dosages.

Qing Mu Xiang (Radix Aristolochiae), cold in nature, regulates qi, relieves pain, eliminates toxins, reduces swelling and lowers blood pressure. It treats Liver and Stomach qi stagnation with heat, abdominal pain, and fever, or heat sensations from toxic snake bite, or high blood pressure. Large dosages of this herb are not recommended, as nausea and vomiting may occur.

Li Zhi He (Semen Litchi) is warm, regulates qi, relieves pain, dispels cold and stagnation. It is essential for treatment of hernial pain, swelling and testicular pain. It treats abdominal pain caused by the Liver overacting on the Spleen and Stomach, and dysmenorrhea or postpartum pain due to blood stagnation.

Suo Luo Zi (Semen Aesculi) and ***Ba Yue Zha*** (Fructus Akebiae) regulate qi and harmonize the middle *jiao* to relieve various kinds of pain caused by qi stagnation of the Stomach, Liver, or both.

Suo Luo Zi more strongly regulates qi and harmonizes the middle *jiao*, and is often used to treat disharmony of Wood and Earth elements.

Ba Yue Zha disperses stagnation, promotes diuresis, and treats scrofulae, urinary stones and dysuria.

Gan Song (Radix seu Rhizoma Nardostachys) is warm but not hot, tonifying but not cloying, aromatic yet not drying. It is a good herb to remedy Spleen and Stomach disharmony with qi stagnation of the chest.

Jiu Ceng Ta (Herba Ocimi Basilici) regulates the middle *jiao*, promotes digestion, invigorates blood circulation, and opens channels and collaterals.

Tian Xian Teng (Herba Aristolochiae) regulates qi and blood circulation to relieve pain, and dispels heat and toxins to promote normal urination.

Dao Dou (Semen Canavaliae) and ***Shi Di*** (Calyx Kaki) are excellent for treatment of hiccups and vomiting, as they lower abnormally rising qi of the Stomach.

Dao Dou warms and tonifies the Kidney yang, and is suitable for deficiency and cold-related cases of hiccups and vomiting.

Shi Di is neutral in thermal property, and appropriate for both heat- and cold-related cases of hiccups and vomiting.

Chapter 8 summary

HERBS FROM OTHER FUNCTIONAL CATEGORIES WITH QI-REGULATING FUNCTIONS

Name	Functional Category
Bai Dou Kou (Fructus Amomi Rotundus)	Aromatic Damp-Dissolving Herbs (Chapter 5)
Bai Jie Zi (Semen Sinapis)	Phlegm-Resolving and Coughing- and Wheezing-Relieving Herbs (Chapter 13)
Bing Lang (Semen Arecae)	Antiparasitic Herbs (Chapter 10)
Chai Hu (Radix Bupleuri)	Exterior-Releasing Herbs (Chapter 1)
Chuan Xiong (Rhizoma Ligustici Chuanxiong)	Blood-Invigorating and Stasis-Removing Herbs (Chapter 12)
E Zhu (Rhizoma Curcumae)	Blood-Invigorating and Stasis-Removing Herbs (Chapter 12)
Hou Po (Cortex Magnoliae Officinalis)	Aromatic Damp-Dissolving Herbs (Chapter 5)
Jiang Huang (Rhizoma Curcumae Longae)	Blood-Invigorating and Stasis-Removing Herbs (Chapter 12)
Lai Fu Zi (Semen Raphani)	Digestive Herbs (Chapter 9)
San Leng (Rhizoma Sparganii)	Blood-Invigorating and Stasis-Removing Herbs (Chapter 12)
Sha Ren (Fructus Amomi)	Aromatic Damp-Dissolving Herbs (Chapter 5)
Su Zi (Fructus Perillae)	Phlegm-Resolving and Coughing- and Wheezing-Relieving Herbs (Chapter 13)
Xiao Hui Xiang (Fructus Foeniculi)	Interior-Warming Herbs (Chapter 7)
Yan Hu Suo (Rhizoma Corydalis)	Blood-Invigorating and Stasis-Removing Herbs (Chapter 12)
Yu Jin (Radix Curcumae)	Blood-Invigorating and Stasis-Removing Herbs (Chapter 12)
Zi Su Ye (Folium Perillae)	Exterior-Releasing Herbs (Chapter 1)

Chapter 9

— Digestive Herbs

消食药

Chapter 9 — Digestive Herbs

Chapter 9

消食药 — Digestive Herbs

Definition: Herbs that promote digestion function to strengthen the Spleen, enhance the appetite, promote digestion, and relieve food stagnation.

Digestive herbs promote digestion, disperse stagnation, relieve abdominal fullness, harmonize the digestive system, and strengthen the Spleen and Stomach. Signs and symptoms of digestive disorders include epigastric and abdominal fullness and distention, belching, acid regurgitation, irregular bowel movement, indigestion and weak digestion.

SUBCATEGORIES OF ACTION

Herbs that promote digestion are usually sweet, and neutral or warm. They enter the Spleen and Stomach channels to strengthen the organs, harmonize the middle *jiao*, promote digestion, and eliminate food stagnation. While some herbs have a general influence to promote digestion, and others more specifically facilitate the breakdown of certain foods, they are not usually separated into subcategories beyond the designation of 'digestive.'

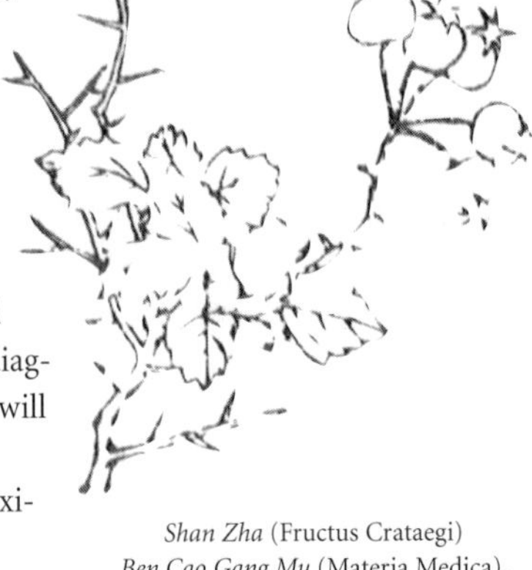

Shan Zha (Fructus Crataegi)
Ben Cao Gang Mu (Materia Medica), by Li Shi-Zhen, 1578 A.D.

DIFFERENTIAL DIAGNOSIS AND TREATMENT

Treatment of digestive problems must always include assessment of the Spleen and Stomach. However, these disorders are often accompanied by complications. While diagnosis of a digestive disorder is relatively simple, maximum treatment effectiveness will not be achieved unless one recognizes and treats the complicating factors.

- With *food stagnation* in the middle *jiao*, qi-regulating herbs should be added for maximum effectiveness.
- For *heat* secondary to food stagnation, incorporate heat-clearing herbs.
- For *damp* accumulation secondary to food stagnation, add aromatic herbs to dissolve dampness and awaken the Spleen.
- If there is accumulation of *coldness*, include interior-warming herbs.
- If Spleen or Stomach *deficiency* is causing indigestion, combine digestive herbs with qi tonics.
- In *severe cases of food stagnation*, purgative herbs can be added.

CAUTIONS/CONTRAINDICATIONS

Most digestive herbs are mild in nature. However, some could exhaust qi with their strong moving influence. Therefore, those herbs should be used with caution in cases of qi deficiency, weakness of the middle *jiao*, accumulation of dampness, and in the absence of food stagnation.

~
Maximum effectiveness in treatment of digestive disorders requires simultaneous treatment of complicating factors.
~

PHARMACOLOGICAL EFFECTS

- **Gastrointestinal**: Herbs in this category promote digestion, stimulate the production of gastric acid, increase intestinal peristalsis, and stop the formation of gas to relieve bloating. *Shan Zha* (Fructus Crataegi) contains lipase, that promotes digestion of fat. *Mai Ya* (Fructus Hordei Germinatus), *Gu Ya* (Fructus Setariae Germinatus) and *Shen Qu* (Massa Fermentata) contain amylase, that promotes digestion of carbohydrates. *Shen Qu* also contains pancreatin, protease, yeast and vitamin B, all of which help with digestion and promote a healthier appetite. *Shen Qu* helps digest food and minimizes production of gas. *Ji Nei Jin* (Endothelium Corneum Gigeriae Galli) increases the production of gastric acid by approximately 30 to 70%. Even though *Ji Nei Jin* has a delayed onset (approximately 2 to 3 hours after ingestion), it has a prolonged duration of

Chapter 9 — Digestive Herbs

action. Administration of *Ji Nei Jin* is also associated with increased intestinal peristalsis.

- **Cardiovascular***:* Some digestives have a significant impact on the cardiovascular system. *Shan Zha* (Fructus Crataegi) dilates blood vessels, increases blood perfusion to the coronary arteries, controls arrhythmia, and reduces blood cholesterol and blood pressure. Sublingual administration of *Shan Zha* extract is sometimes used to treat mild to moderate cases of angina.
- **Antibiotic***:* Many of these herbs, like *Shan Zha* (Fructus Crataegi) and *Lai Fu Zi* (Semen Raphani), inhibit the activities of bacteria and dermatophytes.

POTENTIAL HERB-DRUG INTERACTIONS

- **Antiulcer agents**: Many digestive herbs stimulate the gastrointestinal system to increase the production of gastric acid. Therefore, these herbs may counter the effect of certain drugs, specifically histamine-2 receptor antagonists (such as ranitidine or famotidine) and proton-pump inhibitors (such as omeprazole or lansoprazole).

Shan Zha (Fructus Crataegi)

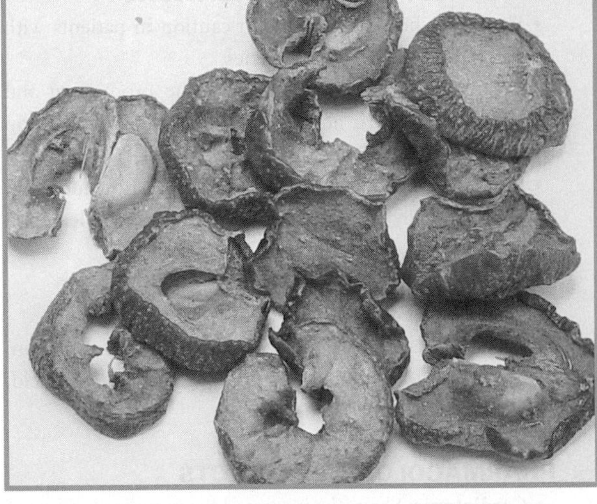

山楂

Pinyin Name: *Shan Zha*
Literal Name: "mountain hawthorn"
Alternate Chinese Names: *Jiao Shan Zha, Shan Zha Tan*
Original Source: *Ben Cao Jing Ji Zhu* (Collection of Commentaries on the Classic of the Materia Medica) by Tao Hong-Jing in 480-498 A.D.
English Name: crataegus, hawthorn berry, hawthorn fruit
Botanical Name: *Crataegus cuneata* Sieb. et Zucc. (*Ye Shan Zha*); *Crataegus pinnatifida* Bge. var. *major* N. E. Br. (*Shan Zha*)
Pharmaceutical Name: Fructus Crataegi
Properties: sweet, sour, slightly warm
Channels Entered: Liver, Spleen, Stomach

CHINESE THERAPEUTIC ACTIONS

1. Promotes Digestion, Eliminates Stagnation

Food stagnation: Sweet and sour, *Shan Zha* (Fructus Crataegi) stimulates the Spleen and Stomach to promote digestion and eliminate food stagnation, and is particularly useful against manifestations of epigastric and abdominal fullness, distention, pain and diarrhea. It is especially effective to promote digestion of red meat or oily, greasy, and fatty foods.

- Difficulty digesting meat products: use *Shan Zha* individually.
- General indigestion and food stagnation: use it with *Shen Qu* (Massa Fermentata). **Exemplar Formula:** *Bao He Wan* (Preserve Harmony Pill from the Precious Mirror).
- Indigestion with abdominal distention and pain: combine it with *Mu Xiang* (Radix Aucklandiae) and *Zhi Ke* (Fructus Aurantii).
- Indigestion with abdominal pain and diarrhea: use 10 grams of charred *Shan Zha* as herbal powder.
- Phlegm and food stagnation with palpable masses in the abdomen: add *Zhi Shi* (Fructus Aurantii Immaturus), *San Leng* (Rhizoma Sparganii), *E Zhu* (Rhizoma Curcumae), *Shen Qu* (Massa Fermentata) and *Hong Hua* (Flos Carthami).

2. Activates Blood Circulation, Disperses Blood Stagnation

Shan Zha enters the *xue* (blood) level to activate blood circulation, reduce swelling and disperse blood stagnation. It is commonly used to treat spotting or severe abdominal pain associated with amenorrhea, and postpartum abdominal pain. It also effectively treats pain associated with hernial disorders.

- Abdominal pain associated with postpartum sequelae or amenorrhea: use *Shan Zha* with *Dang Gui* (Radicis Angelicae Sinensis), *Chuan Xiong* (Rhizoma Ligustici Chuanxiong), and *Yi Mu Cao* (Herba Leonuri).
- Pain associated with hernial disorders: use this herb with *Xiao Hui Xiang* (Fructus Foeniculi) and *Ju He* (Semen Citri Rubrum).

3. Treats Cardiovascular Disorders

In combination with herbs that activate blood circulation and remove blood stagnation, *Shan Zha* has been used recently to treat hypertension, coronary artery disorders, angina, and hypercholesterolemia.

- Hypertension: use *Shan Zha* with *Tian Ma* (Rhizoma Gastrodiae) and *Ge Gen* (Radix Puerariae).
- Coronary artery disorder: use this herb with *Dan Shen* (Radix Salviae Miltiorrhizae), and *Mao Dong Qing* (Radix Ilicis Pubescentis).
- Angina: combine this herb with *Dan Shen* (Radix Salviae Miltiorrhizae), *San Qi* (Radix Notoginseng), and *Yan Hu Suo* (Rhizoma Corydalis).
- Hypercholesterolemia: use it with *Jue Ming Zi* (Semen Cassiae) and *Jiao Gu Lan* (Rhizoma seu Herba Gynostemmatis).

DOSAGE

10 to 15 grams in decoction. The maximum dosage of *Shan Zha* is 30 grams. The unprocessed herb dissolves food stagnation and activates blood circulation. Dry-frying the herb reduces the sour taste and astringent property of the herb, thereby harmonizing the overall effect. Blackening the herb increases the bitter taste, which potentiates its effect to reduce abdominal distention and relieve diarrhea. Charring, that is, burning the herb to ash, enhances its influence to stop bleeding.

Shan Zha (Fructus Crataegi)

CAUTIONS / CONTRAINDICATIONS

- *Shan Zha* should be used with caution in patients with Spleen and Stomach deficiencies.
- Because *Shan Zha* may stimulate the production and secretion of gastric acid, it should be used with caution in patients who have gastritis or peptic ulcers.
- Prolonged intake of *Shan Zha* is not recommended as it will eventually interrupt the normal flow of Spleen and Stomach qi.

CHEMICAL COMPOSITION

Crataegolic acid, maslinic acid, chlorogenic acid, vitexin, hyperin, epicatechin, amygdalin, quercetin, ursolic acid, tartaric acid, caffeic acid.[1]

PHARMACOLOGICAL EFFECTS

- **Cardiotonic:** *Shan Zha* increased the contractile force of the heart by approximately 20 to 30% in studies of laboratory animals.[2]
- **Vasodilating:** Extract of *Shan Zha* has shown marked influence in dilating the coronary artery, decreasing oxygen consumption by the cardiac muscle, and reversing cardiac ischemia.[3]
- **Antihypertensive:** Injection of *Shan Zha* has been shown to decrease blood pressure by 20 to 25% in rabbits and cats, with a duration of effect of over three hours.[4]
- **Antihyperlipidemic:** *Shan Zha* has marked effectiveness for reduction of plasma cholesterol levels in laboratory animals. A preparation containing a 15% extract of *Shan Zha* reduced the plasma cholesterol levels by 18.06% with $p<0.01$, while 30% extract reduced plasma cholesterol levels by 30.80% with $p<0.005$. Its mechanism of action included enhancement of LDL-receptor activity, increased hepatic breakdown and decreased synthesis of cholesterol.[5,6]
- **Gastrointestinal:** *Shan Zha* given as herbal decoction and intramuscular injection showed marked stimulating effects on gastric acid in rats. By comparison, subjects who received the herbal decoction produced 2.9 times more gastric acid than those who received intramuscular injection.[7]
- **Antibiotic:** *Shan Zha* has demonstrated an inhibitory effect against *Staphylococcus aureus*, *Staphylococcus albus*, *Salmonella typhi*, *Pseudomonas aeruginosa*, *E. coli*, and hemolytic streptococcus.[8]

CLINICAL STUDIES AND RESEARCH

- **Angina:** Patients with angina related to coronary artery disease were treated with a preparation of *Shan Zha* three times daily, for 4 weeks per treatment course. Out of 219 patients, the study reported an overall effective rate of 92.2%, with 47.1% showing improvement based on ECG evaluation.[9]
- **Hyperlipidemia:** In one study, 127 patients were treated with powdered extract of *Shan Zha* and *Mai Ya* (Fructus Hordei Germinatus) (equivalent to 30 grams of bulk herb) twice daily for 2 weeks per treatment course. The study reported that 92% of the participants experienced a reduction of their cholesterol levels.[10] In another study, 130 patients with hyperlipidemia were treated with an herbal formulation of *Shan Zha* and other herbs, and the serum cholesterol and triglyceride levels were lowered in 87% and 80.8% of the patients, respectively.[11]
- **Acute bacterial enteritis:** Administration of *Shan Zha* once daily showed satisfactory results in treating 100 patients with acute bacterial enteritis. The herbal remedy was prepared by stir-frying 60 grams of *Shan Zha* with 30 ml of grain-based liquor, cooking the herbs for 15 minutes in 200 ml of boiling water, and adding 30 grams of brown sugar to the decoction prior to consumption.[12]
- **Infantile diarrhea:** In one report, 5 to 10 ml of *Shan Zha* syrup was given three times daily for treatment of infantile diarrhea. Out of 212 patients, 176 recovered within 2 to 3 days.[13]
- **Nephritis:** Patients with acute and chronic nephritis were treated with an herbal decoction containing 90 grams of *Shan Zha*, with 14 days per treatment course. The study reported a 91.1% rate of effectiveness in 45 patients with acute nephritis, and a 88.3% rate of effectiveness in 60 patients with chronic nephritis.[14]
- **Nausea:** Chronic nausea in 85 patients was treated with 15 ml of fresh *Shan Zha* juice three times daily. There were excellent results in most patients within one day.[15]
- **Polyps of the vocal cords:** Ten patients were treated with an herbal decoction of *Shan Zha*, with marked success. The herbal decoction was prepared by cooking 24 to 30 grams of *Shan Zha* twice, to yield 1500 ml of decoction, which was taken slowly after it cooled to room temperature.[16]

HERB-DRUG INTERACTION

- **Digoxin (Lanoxin):** Both *Shan Zha* and digoxin have marked cardiotonic effects. Therefore, concurrent use of *Shan Zha* and digoxin (Lanoxin) should be monitored carefully to avoid possible side effects.[17]

TOXICOLOGY

The LD_{50} for mice is 1.042 ml/kg, based on intravenous injectables of 100% *Shan Zha* preparation.[18]

AUTHORS' COMMENTS

Jiao San Xian (Three Charred Miracles) is the shorthand name for the combination of *Shan Zha* (Fructus Crataegi), *Shen Qu* (Massa Fermentata), and *Mai Ya* (Fructus Hordei Germinatus), all charred. When charred *Bing Lang* (Semen Arecae) is added, the combination is

Shan Zha (Fructus Crataegi)

called *Jiao Si Xian* (Four Charred Miracles). These herbs are often used together because they have excellent synergy to promote digestion and eliminate food stagnation.

According to Dr. Liu Hong-Xiang, *Shan Zha*, when used in high doses for postpartum pain, constricts the uterus and helps to dispel residual blood clots that cause continued bleeding.

According to Dr. Zhang Xiao-Ping, *Shan Zha* effectively lowers cholesterol, but is not suitable for individuals who have stomach ulcers. *Shan Zha, Zi Su Ye* (Folium Perillae), *Shi Chang Pu* (Rhizoma Acori), and *Ze Xie* (Rhizoma Alismatis) taken as tea on a daily basis are effective to reduce body weight and lower cholesterol. For patients who have stomach ulcers or gastric hyperacidity with high cholesterol, the practitioner should opt for other cholesterol-reducing herbs that are not sour, such as *Jue Ming Zi* (Semen Cassiae).

Shan Zha and *Lai Fu Zi* (Semen Raphani) share similar actions to promote digestion and eliminate stagnation. *Shan Zha* more effectively promotes the digestion of meat. It also invigorates blood circulation and eliminates blood stasis. *Lai Fu Zi* treats abdominal fullness and distention caused by food stagnation and accumulation. It also eliminates phlegm and directs abnormally rising qi downwards.

Shan Zha, Mai Ya (Fructus Hordei Germinatus) and *Shen Qu* (Massa Fermentata) have similar yet different functions to promote digestion. Clinically, they are commonly charred and used together to treat food stagnation and indigestion.

- *Shan Zha* is best for food stagnation due to excess intake of meat. It is also good for palpable masses and blood stagnation in the abdomen.
- *Mai Ya* is best for food stagnation caused by inability to digest starch.
- *Shen Qu* is the most strategic choice to counter hard-to-digest foods.

References

1. *Xian Dai Zhong Yao Yao Li Xue* (Contemporary Pharmacology of Chinese Herbs); 1997; 683
2. *Guang Xi Zhong Yi Yao* (Guangxi Chinese Medicine and Herbology), 1990; 13(3):45
3. Ibid.
4. *Qing Dao Yi Xue Yuan Bao Dao* (Medical Journal of Qingdao Institution), 1957; 1:14
5. *Zhong Yi Yao Xue Bao* (Report of Chinese Medicine and Herbology), 1989; 2:45
6. Rajendran, S. et al. Effect of tincture of crataegus on the LDL-receptor activity of the hepatic plasma membrane of rats fed on atherogenic diet. *Atherosclerosis*. 123(1-2):235-41, June 1997
7. *Ying Yang Xue Bao* (Report of Nutrition), 1984; 6(2):109
8. *Guang Xi Zhong Yi Yao* (Guangxi Chinese Medicine and Herbology), 1990; 13(3):45
9. *Bei Jing Yi Xue* (Beijing Medicine), 1986; 2:101
10. *Liao Ning Zhong Yi* (Liaoning Chinese Medicine), 1979; 5:23
11. Guan, Y. et al. Yishou Jiangshi (de-blood-lipid) tablets in the treatment of hyperlipidemia. *Journal of Traditional Chinese Medicine*. 15(3):178-9, Sep. 1995
12. *Xin Yi Xue* (New Medicine), 1975; 2:111
13. *Zhong Cao Yao Tong Xun* (Journal of Chinese Herbal Medicine); 1973; 3:31
14. *Shan Xi Xin Yi Yao* (New Medicine and Herbology of Shanxi), 1975; 1:35
15. *Zhong Xi Yi Jie He Za Zhi* (Journal of Integrated Chinese and Western Medicine), 1984; 5:315
16. *Tian Jing Yi Yao* (Tianjing Medicine and Herbology); 1977; 6:281
17. *Archives of Internal Medicine*, v.158, n.20, Nov. 9, 1998: 2200-2211
18. *Chang Yong Zhong Yao Cheng Fen Yu Yao Li Shou Ce* (A Handbook of the Composition and Pharmacology of Common Chinese Drugs), 1994; 387

Shen Qu (Massa Fermentata)

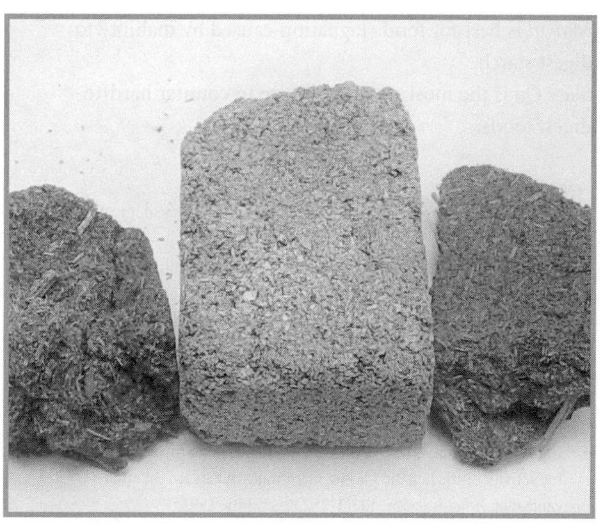

神麴 神曲

Pinyin Name: *Shen Qu*
Alternate Chinese Names: *Liu Shen Qu, Jiao Shen Qu*
Original Source: *Yao Xing Ben Cao* (Materia Medica of Medicinal Properties) by Zhen Quan in 600 A.D.
English Name: massa fermentata, medicated leaven
Pharmaceutical Name: Massa Fermentata
Properties: sweet, acrid, warm
Channels Entered: Spleen, Stomach

CHINESE THERAPEUTIC ACTIONS

Dissolves Food Stagnation, Promotes Digestion and Harmonizes the Stomach

Shen Qu (Massa Fermentata) treats poor digestion, food stagnation, poor appetite, borborygmus, diarrhea, abdominal fullness and distention. It is useful when trying to dissolve hard-to-digest food.

- Indigestion: use *Shen Qu* with *Shan Zha* (Fructus Crataegi) and *Mai Ya* (Fructus Hordei Germinatus).
- Food stagnation and diarrhea due to Spleen deficiency: add *Bai Zhu* (Rhizoma Atractylodis Macrocephalae) and *Dang Shen* (Radix Codonopsis).
- Food stagnation with abdominal pain: combine it with *Mu Xiang* (Radix Aucklandiae) and *Sha Ren* (Fructus Amomi).
- Chronic food stagnation with palpable masses: use it with *San Leng* (Rhizoma Sparganii), *E Zhu* (Rhizoma Curcumae), *Mu Li* (Concha Ostreae) and *Bie Jia* (Carapax Trionycis).

DOSAGE

6 to 15 grams. *Shen Qu* is used in herbal decoctions, pills, and powder. Unprocessed, it treats food stagnation. Dry-fried, it strengthens the Spleen and Stomach and promotes digestion. Dry-fried *Shen Qu* is the preferred form of this herb.

CAUTIONS / CONTRAINDICATIONS

- *Shen Qu* should be used with caution during pregnancy.

CHEMICAL COMPOSITION

Yeast, amylase, vitamin B, ergosterol, protein.[1]

PHARMACOLOGICAL EFFECTS

- **Gastrointestinal:** *Shen Qu* contains many different enzymes to facilitate digestion of starches and carbohydrates.[2]

CLINICAL STUDIES AND RESEARCH

- **Infantile indigestion:** In one study, 129 infants with indigestion were treated with a 50% *Shen Qu* decoction. The decoction was given in two equally-divided portions, with the daily dosage of 5 to 10 ml for infants over one year of age, 10 to 20 ml for children between 2 and 3 years old, and other dosages adjusted accordingly for those over three years of age. The study reported an overall rate of effectiveness of 91.5%, which was better than the results for the group receiving pharmaceuticals.[3]

SUPPLEMENT

- 建神麴 / 建神曲 *Jian Shen Qu* (Massa Fermentata Preparata) is a combination of over 40 herbs fermented together, including *Zi Su Ye* (Folium Perillae), *Jing Jie* (Herba Schizonepetae), *Fang Feng* (Radix Saposhnikoviae), *Hou Po* (Cortex Magnoliae Officinalis), *Bai Zhu* (Rhizoma Atractylodis Macrocephalae), *Mu Xiang* (Radix Aucklandiae), *Zhi Shi* (Fructus Aurantii Immaturus) and others. Quite different from *Shen Qu*, *Jian Shen Qu* is bitter and warm, and functions to dissolve food stagnation, expel wind-cold, regulate qi, dissolve dampness and strengthen the Spleen. It is often used for patients with food stagnation, with or without the presence of wind-cold. The recommended dosage of *Jian Shen Qu* is 6 to 15 grams.

AUTHORS' COMMENTS

Shen Qu has a unique function to protect the stomach and promote digestion of hard-to-digest substances. It is commonly added to herbal formulas that contain hard-to-digest minerals such as *Ci Shi* (Magnetitum) and *Dai*

Shen Qu (Massa Fermentata)

Zhe Shi (Haematitum). It is helpful for patients who take drugs that are harsh to the stomach, such as non-steroidal-anti-inflammatory drugs (NSAIDS).

Shen Qu (Massa Fermentata), *Mai Ya* (Fructus Hordei Germinatus) and *Gu Ya* (Fructus Setariae Germinatus) all aid in the digestion of food.

- *Shen Qu* is specifically good for stagnation of dietary starches and is commonly used for epigastric and abdominal distention and pain, poor appetite and diarrhea. It can also help with the digestion of mineral medicinal substances.
- *Mai Ya* is best for digesting starch and fruits. It strengthens the Spleen to build the appetite. It treats indigestion, poor appetite and deficiencies of the Spleen and Stomach. It inhibits lactation and relieves Liver qi stagnation.
- *Gu Ya* has functions similar to *Mai Ya* but is milder in nature. It is more suitable to help deficiency patients with food stagnation.

References

1. *Xian Dai Zhong Yao Yao Li Xue* (Contemporary Pharmacology of Chinese Herbs), 1997; 681
2. *Zhong Yao Xue* (Chinese Herbology), 1998; 436:437
3. *Zhong Hua Er Ke Za Zhi* (Chinese Journal of Pediatrics), 1960; 3:231

Hong Qu (Monascus)

紅麴 红曲

Pinyin Name: *Hong Qu*
Alternate Chinese Names: *Hong Mi, Chi Qu*
Original Source: *Yin Shan Zheng Yao* (Correct Guide to Eating and Drinking)
English Name: red yeast rice
Botanical Name: *Monascus purpureus* Went.
Pharmaceutical Name: Monascus
Properties: sweet, acrid, warm
Channels Entered: Spleen, Liver, Large Intestine

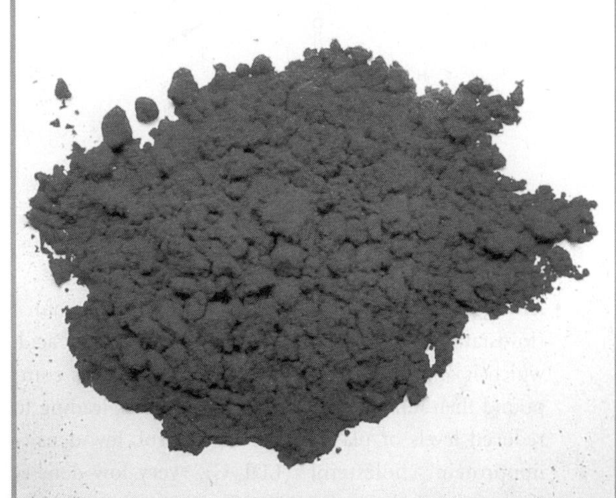

CHINESE THERAPEUTIC ACTIONS

1. Strengthens the Spleen and Stomach, Promotes Digestion

Indigestion: *Hong Qu* (Monascus) strengthens the Spleen and Stomach and promotes digestion to treat indigestion in which there is undigested food in the stool.

- Indigestion: use *Hong Qu* with *Shan Zha* (Fructus Crataegi) and *Mai Ya* (Fructus Hordei Germinatus).
- Food stagnation due to Spleen deficiency: add *Bai Zhu* (Rhizoma Atractylodis Macrocephalae) and *Dang Shen* (Radix Codonopsis).

2. Invigorates Blood Circulation, Eliminates Blood Stasis

Blood stasis: *Hong Qu* activates blood circulation to treat blood stasis in postpartum women, individuals with traumatic injuries, external injuries, and abdominal pain caused by blood stasis.

- Blood stasis in the upper body: use this herb with *Jiang Xiang* (Lignum Dalbergiae Odoriferae), *Tong Cao* (Medulla Tetrapanacis), and *Mo Yao* (Myrrha).
- Pain due to trauma and injuries: combine it with *Yan Hu Suo* (Rhizoma Corydalis), *Dang Gui* (Radicis Angelicae Sinensis), *Hong Hua* (Flos Carthami), *Niu Xi* (Radix Cyathulae seu Achyranthis), *Mo Yao* (Myrrha) and *Ru Xiang* (Gummi Olibanum).
- Abdominal pain or postpartum blood stasis: incorporate *Hong Qu* with *Ze Lan* (Herba Lycopi), *Niu Xi* (Radix Cyathulae seu Achyranthis), *Sheng Di Huang* (Radix Rehmanniae), *Xu Duan* (Radix Dipsaci), *Pu Huang*

Hong Qu (Monascus)

(Pollen Typhae), and *Chi Shao* (Radix Paeoniae Rubrae).

DOSAGE

6 to 12 grams in decoction. *Hong Qu* is also used in powder and pill forms. It is ground into powder for topical application.

CAUTIONS / CONTRAINDICATIONS

- Use *Hong Qu* with caution in cases of Spleen and Stomach deficiency, or individuals who do not have any food stagnation or blood stasis.
- *Hong Qu* is contraindicated in individuals with active liver disease.

CHEMICAL COMPOSITION

Monascidin, monascolin I (lovastatin, mevinolin), monascolin II (β-hydroxy acid), monascin, starch, fatty acids, phytosterols, isoflavones.[1,2]

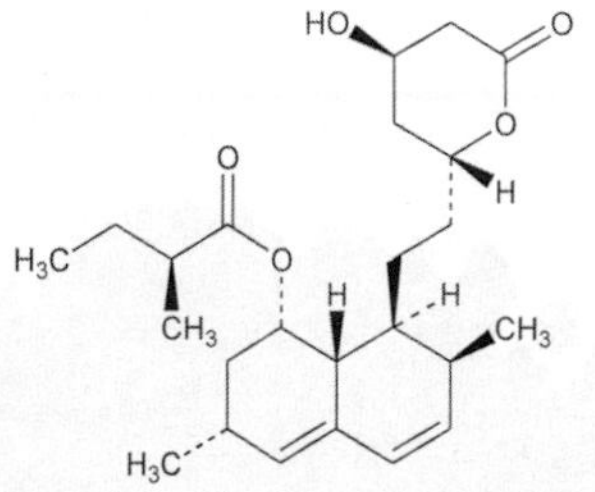

Lovastatin

PHARMACOLOGICAL EFFECTS

- **Antihyperlipidemic:** Following ingestion, monascolin I (lovastatin) is converted in the body to β-hydroxy acid, which is an HMG-CoA reductase inhibitor. This compound then inhibits cholesterol biosynthesis, leading to reduced levels of plasma total cholesterol, low-density lipoprotein cholesterol (LDL-C), very-low-density lipoprotein cholesterol (VLDL-C), and triglycerides. In addition, it may produce a slight increase in high-density lipoprotein (HDL-C).[3]

CLINICAL STUDIES AND RESEARCH

- **Hyperlipidemia:** In one multi-center, randomized, single-blind trial, 502 patients with hyperlipidemia were treated with 600 mg of *Hong Qu* twice daily (1200 mg total per day). After four weeks of treatment, the study reported 17% reduction in total cholesterol levels, 24.6% reduction in LDL-cholesterol, 19.8% decrease in triglycerides, and a 12.8% increase in HDL-cholesterol. After 8 weeks of treatment, the study reported 22.7% reduction in total cholesterol levels, 30.9% reduction in LDL-cholesterol, 34.1% decrease in triglycerides, and a 19.9% increase in HDL-cholesterol.[4]

HERB-DRUG INTERACTION

Listed below are interactions that have been documented between pharmaceuticals and lovastatin, a constituent of *Hong Qu*.[5]

- **Liver metabolism:** Lovastatin is metabolized primarily by CYP3A4, and may interact with CYP3A4 inhibitors.
- **Azole antifungals:** Concurrent use of itraconazole and ketoconazole increased lovastatin levels twenty fold in health volunteers, as well as increased the risk of myopathy.
- **Bile acid sequestrants:** Co-administration of cholestyramine decreases the bioavailability of lovastatin. To avoid this interaction, lovastatin should be taken 1 hour before or 4 hours after bile acid sequestrants.
- **Fibric acid derivatives:** Avoid concurrent use of gemfibrozil and lovastatin, as severe myopathy and rhabdomyolysis have been reported.
- **Isradipine:** Isradipine increases hepatic blood flow, and may increase the clearance of lovastatin and its metabolites.
- **Warfarin:** Bleeding and increased prothrombin time have been reported with concomitant use of lovastatin and warfarin.

AUTHORS' COMMENTS

Hong Qu is rice that has been fermented with yeast *Monascus purpureus*. The fermentation process changes the color of rice from white to red, thereby giving it the name "red yeast rice." For centuries, *Hong Qu* has been used in China as both food and herbal medicine. It has also been used as a coloring agent to prepare fish, fish sauce, fish paste, rice wine, and red soybean curd. In the late 1990s, it was introduced and used in the US as a dietary supplement to promote healthy cholesterol levels.

Most medical journals attribute the hypolipidemic effect of *Hong Qu* to one single component, lovastatin. This explanation, however, is not sufficient nor entirely accurate. The therapeutic dose of *Hong Qu* delivers approximately 7.2 mg of lovastatin, while the synthetic drug lovastatin (Mevacor) contains from 10 to 40 mg of lovastatin. Yet, despite the lower dose of the supposed active component, the hypolipidemic effects of *Hong Qu* are much greater than the synthetic drug lovastatin. Thus, it is clear that lovastatin is not the only active component, and more research needs to be done on *Hong Qu* as an herbal medicine, not just on lovastatin as a single compound.

References

1. *Plant Physiol*, 1977; 60(4):578) (*J Food Sci*, 1981; 46(2):589
2. *The Merck Index* 12th edition, Chapman & Hall/CRCnetBASE/Merck, 2000
3. *PDR for Nutritional Supplements 1st Edition*, Medical Economics, 2001
4. Ibid.
5. Facts and Comparison, Jan. 2000. *Drug Facts and Comparison*. A Wolters Kluwer Company.

Mai Ya (Fructus Hordei Germinatus)

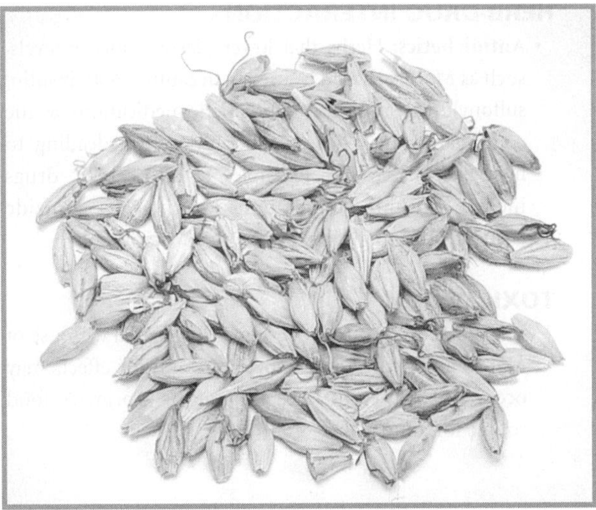

麥芽 麦芽

Pinyin Name: *Mai Ya*
Alternate Chinese Names: *Sheng Mai Ya, Chao Mai Ya, Jiao Mai Ya*
Original Source: *Yao Xing Ben Cao* (Materia Medica of Medicinal Properties) by Zhen Quan in 600 A.D.
English Name: barley sprouts
Botanical Name: *Hordeum vulgare* L. (*Da Mai*)
Pharmaceutical Name: Fructus Hordei Germinatus
Properties: sweet, neutral
Channels Entered: Liver, Spleen, Stomach

CHINESE THERAPEUTIC ACTIONS

1. Dissolves Food Stagnation, Promotes Digestion and Strengthens the Middle *Jiao*

Mai Ya (Fructus Hordei Germinatus) strengthens the Spleen and Stomach to enhance their functions of transformation and transportation. It is especially effective to promote digestion of starches, such as rice, noodles, wheat, yams and potatoes.

- Indigestion and food stagnation: use *Mai Ya* with *Shan Zha* (Fructus Crataegi), *Shen Qu* (Massa Fermentata), and *Ji Nei Jin* (Endothelium Corneum Gigeriae Galli).

2. Inhibits Lactation

Mai Ya has a definite effect on lactation. Large dosages of *Mai Ya* inhibit lactation, while a small dosage may promote it.

- To inhibit or cease lactation: use 30 to 60 grams each of fresh *Mai Ya* and dry-fried *Mai Ya* on a daily basis.

3. Regulates Liver Qi

Liver qi stagnation: *Mai Ya* enters the Liver to promote the smooth flow of Liver qi and relieve qi stagnation. It treats the condition of the Liver overacting on the Spleen and Stomach, which causes feelings of distention and oppression in the hypochondriac and epigastric regions, breast distention, belching, and loss of appetite.

DOSAGE

10 to 15 grams. Up to 30 to 120 grams may be used. *Mai Ya* is commonly used in herbal decoctions, pills or powder. Use larger dosages to stop lactation.

CAUTIONS / CONTRAINDICATIONS

- Use *Mai Ya* cautiously for patients who do not have food stagnation. Prolonged usage of it may injure qi.
- For nursing mothers who desire to continue nursing their infants, large dosages of this herb are contraindicated because production of milk may be terminated.

CHEMICAL COMPOSITION

Amylase, invertase, esterase, proteinase, oxidase, catalyticase, cellobiosase, gentiobiosase, lichenase, emulsin, peroxidisomerase, hordenine, maltoxin.[1]

PHARMACOLOGICAL EFFECTS

- **Gastrointestinal:** *Mai Ya* contains many different enzymes to facilitate digestion of starches and carbohydrates.[2]
- **Antidiabetic:** Oral ingestion of *Mai Ya* lowers blood glucose levels in human and rabbits. Furthermore, 5% intravenous injection may lower blood glucose levels by 40% or more, for up to 7 hours, in rabbits.[3]

CLINICAL STUDIES AND RESEARCH

- **Chronic hepatitis:** In one study, 161 patients with hepatitis were treated with 10 ml *Mai Ya* syrup three times daily after meals, for 30 days per treatment course. Marked improvement was reported in 48 out of 56 patients with acute hepatitis, and 60 out of 105 patients with chronic hepatitis. The study reported an overall rate of effectiveness of 67.1%. Improvements included decreased hypochondriac pain, increased appetite, elevated energy levels, and reduced liver enzymes.[4]
- **Galactorrhea:** Patients with galactorrhea were treated with 100 to 200 grams of *Mai Ya* daily in decoction or pills. The study reported that 13 of 15 patients showed complete recovery or marked improvement, while 2 reported no change.[5]

Mai Ya (Fructus Hordei Germinatus)

HERB-DRUG INTERACTION

- **Antidiabetics:** Herbs that lower plasma glucose levels, such as *Mai Ya,* should be used with caution with insulin, sulfonylureas, and other antidiabetic medications, as the combination may have a synergistic effect, leading to hypoglycemia. [Note: Examples of antidiabetic drugs include insulin, tolbutamide (Orinase), glipizide (Glucotrol), and glyburide (DiaBeta/Micronase).][6]

TOXICOLOGY

The incidence of adverse reactions associated with use of *Mai Ya* is extremely rare. However, mild side effects may occur if it is used in large amounts as a primary food source for animals.[7]

AUTHORS' COMMENTS

Mai Ya (Fructus Hordei Germinatus) and *Gu Ya* (Fructus Setariae Germinatus) have similar functions to promote digestion and strengthen the middle *jiao. Mai Ya* more effectively promotes digestion, while *Gu Ya* more strongly nourishes the Stomach.

References

1. *Xian Dai Zhong Yao Yao Li Xue* (Contemporary Pharmacology of Chinese Herbs), 1997; 675
2. *Zhong Yao Yao Li Yu Ying Yong* (Pharmacology and Applications of Chinese Herbs), 1983; 473
3. Ibid.
4. *Xin Yi Yao Tong Xun* (Journal of New Medicine and Herbology), 1972; 1:21
5. *Zhong Xi Yi Jie He Za Zhi* (Journal of Integrated Chinese and Western Medicine), 1984; 3:134
6. Chen, J. Recognition & prevention of herb-drug interactions, *Medical Acupuncture,* Fall/Winter 1998/1999; volume 10/number 2; 9-13
7. *Zhong Yao Yao Li Yu Ying Yong* (Pharmacology and Applications of Chinese Herbs), 1983; 473

Gu Ya (Fructus Setariae Germinatus)

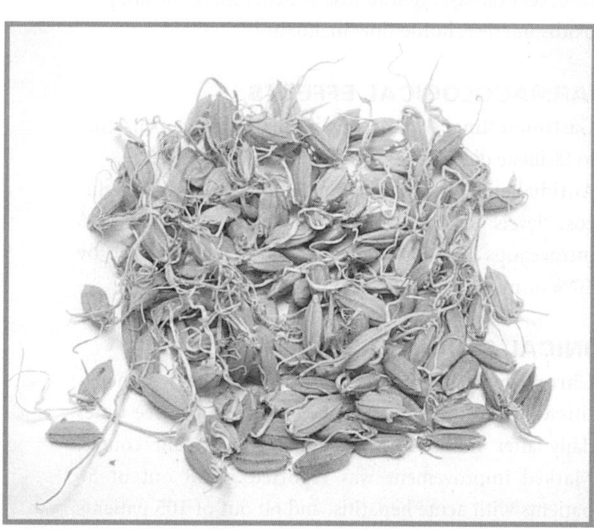

谷芽 谷芽

Pinyin Name: *Gu Ya*

Alternate Chinese Names: *Sheng Gu Ya, Chao Gu Ya, Jiao Gu Ya*

Original Source: *Ming Yi Za Zhu* (Miscellaneous Records of Famous Physicians) by Tao Hong-Jing in 500 A.D.

English Name: sprouted setaria, sprouted oryza, sprouted millet

Botanical Name: *Setaria italica* (L.) Beauv.; *Oryza sativa* L.

Pharmaceutical Name: Fructus Setariae Germinatus

Properties: sweet, neutral

Channels Entered: Spleen, Stomach

CHINESE THERAPEUTIC ACTIONS

1. Dissolves Food Stagnation, Promotes Digestion and Harmonizes the Middle *Jiao*

Gu Ya (Fructus Setariae Germinatus) has a mild digestive function. It does not damage the normal qi and thus is preferred for patients with indigestion and poor appetite caused by deficiency. Clinical manifestations of this weakened state include slow digestion, decreased dietary intake, and diarrhea.

- Poor digestion due to Spleen and Stomach deficiencies: use *Gu Ya* with *Dang Shen* (Radix Codonopsis), *Bai Zhu* (Rhizoma Atractylodis Macrocephalae), *Sha Ren* (Fructus Amomi), *Gan Cao* (Radix Glycyrrhizae) and *Chen Pi* (Pericarpium Citri Reticulatae).

Gu Ya (Fructus Setariae Germinatus)

2. Strengthens the Spleen and Encourages Appetite

Spleen deficiency with poor appetite: *Gu Ya* strengthens the middle *jiao* to enhance the functions of transformation and transportation.

- Poor digestion with decreased food intake and diarrhea from Spleen and Stomach deficiencies: combine this herb with *Shen Qu* (Massa Fermentata), *Shan Zha* (Fructus Crataegi), *Bian Dou* (Semen Lablab Album), *Ze Xie* (Rhizoma Alismatis), *Fu Ling* (Poria), and *Qian Shi* (Semen Euryales).

DOSAGE

10 to 15 grams. Use up to 30 grams of this herb for severe cases. Fresh *Gu Ya* strengthens the middle *jiao*; dry-fried *Gu Ya* promotes digestion; and charred *Gu Ya* eliminates stagnation.

CHEMICAL COMPOSITION

Amylase, maltose, adenine, choline, polyamine oxidase, B vitamins, and dipeptides containing D-alanine.[1]

PHARMACOLOGICAL EFFECTS

- **Gastrointestinal:** *Gu Ya* contains many different enzymes to facilitate digestion of starches and carbohydrates.[2]

AUTHORS' COMMENTS

Gu Ya (Fructus Setariae Germinatus) and *Mai Ya* (Fructus Hordei Germinatus) have similar functions to promote digestion and strengthen the middle *jiao*. *Gu Ya* more strongly nourishes the Stomach, while *Mai Ya* more effectively promotes digestion.

Gu Ya, *Dang Shen* (Radix Codonopsis) and *Bai Zhu* (Rhizoma Atractylodis Macrocephalae) all tonify and strengthen the middle *jiao*. *Gu Ya* promotes digestion, and indirectly strengthens the middle *jiao* by decreasing the burden on the Spleen and Stomach. *Dang Shen* and *Bai Zhu*, on the other hand, tonify the Spleen and Stomach to enhance digestive functions.

References

1. *Xian Dai Zhong Yao Yao Li Xue* (Contemporary Pharmacology of Chinese Herbs), 1997; 676
2. *CA*, 1991; 114:3923

Lai Fu Zi (Semen Raphani)

萊菔子 莱菔子

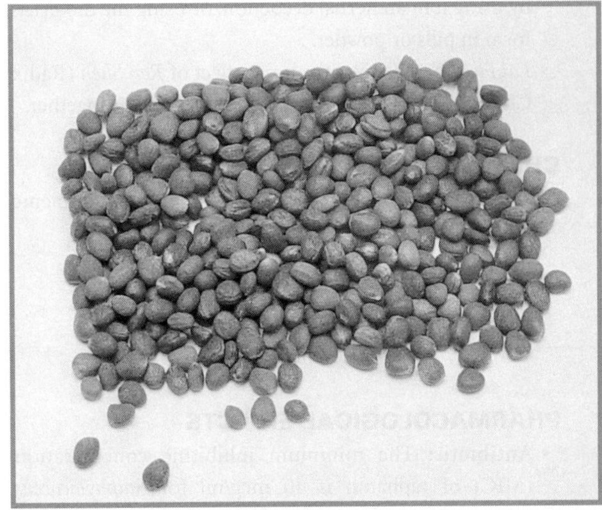

Pinyin Name: *Lai Fu Zi*
Alternate Chinese Names: *Luo Bo Zi*
Original Source: *Ri Hua Zi Ben Cao* (Materia Medica of Ri Hua-Zi) by Ri Hua-Zi in 713 A.D.
English Name: raphanus, radish seed
Botanical Name: *Raphanus sativus* L. (*Lai Fu*)
Pharmaceutical Name: Semen Raphani
Properties: acrid, sweet, neutral
Channels Entered: Spleen, Stomach, Lung

CHINESE THERAPEUTIC ACTIONS

1. Dissolves Food Stagnation, Promotes Digestion and Reduces Distention

Lai Fu Zi (Semen Raphani) promotes digestion by treating food stagnation and indigestion typified by epigastric and abdominal fullness and distention, belching, acid reflux, and diarrhea.

- Indigestion and food stagnation: use *Lai Fu Zi* with *Shan Zha* (Fructus Crataegi), *Shen Qu* (Massa Fermentata), and *Chen Pi* (Pericarpium Citri Reticulatae).

Lai Fu Zi (Semen Raphani)

- Food stagnation with Spleen deficiency: use it with *Bai Zhu* (Rhizoma Atractylodis Macrocephalae).
- Abdominal distention: use *Lai Fu Zi* as a single remedy.

2. Descends Qi, Dissolves Phlegm

Lai Fu Zi treats coughing and wheezing resulting from phlegm stagnation and abnormal upward circulation of Lung qi. This herb is excellent for patients with profuse phlegm and food stagnation.

- Cough and wheezing due to phlegm stagnation: add *Su Zi* (Fructus Perillae) and *Bai Jie Zi* (Semen Sinapis). **Exemplar Formula:** *San Zi Yang Qin Tang* (Three-Seed Decoction to Nourish One's Parents).

DOSAGE

6 to 10 grams. *Lai Fu Zi* is used in herbal decoctions, pills, or powder. Unprocessed, this herb has stronger ascending and dispersing actions, and is commonly used to eliminate phlegm. Dry-fried, the herb has a better function to counter adverse rising qi, dissolve phlegm, promote digestion, and reduce distention. In addition, dry-frying the herb enhances the extraction of active constituents.

CAUTIONS / CONTRAINDICATIONS

- *Lai Fu Zi* is contraindicated in patients with qi and blood deficiencies, or in those who do not have food stagnation.
- Use *Lai Fu Zi* with caution, as prolonged use or overdose may consume qi.
- Fresh *Lai Fu Zi* may cause nausea. This can be minimized by using it in an herbal decoction, or using the dry-fried form in pills or powder.
- *Lai Fu Zi* antagonizes the tonic effect of *Ren Shen* (Radix Ginseng); these two herbs should not be used together.

CHEMICAL COMPOSITION

Erucic acid, raphanin, β-sitosterol, oleic acid, linolenic acid, linoleic acid, glycerol sinapate.[1,2]

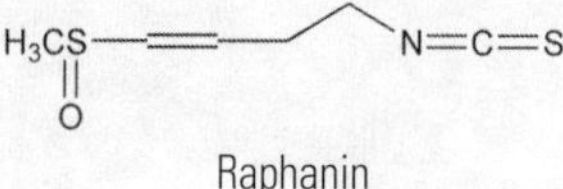

Raphanin

PHARMACOLOGICAL EFFECTS

- **Antibiotic:** The minimum inhibiting concentration (MIC) of raphanin is 40 mcg/ml for *Staphylococcus aureus*, 125 mcg/ml for *Bacillus dysenteriae*, 125 mcg/ml for *Salmonella typhi*, and 200 mcg/ml for *E. coli*.[3]
- **Antihypertensive:** Intravenous injection of *Lai Fu Zi* extract has demonstrated a slow but prolonged antihypertensive effect in rabbits, cats and dogs.[4]

CLINICAL STUDIES AND RESEARCH

- **Habitual constipation:** In one report, 32 elderly patients over 60 years of age with chronic habitual constipation were treated with 30 to 40 grams of *Lai Fu Zi* powder, given with warm water two to three times daily. The herb was prepared by dry-frying it until it became golden yellow. Out of 32 patients, 20 had a bowel movement within 12 hours, 9 within 24 hours, and 3 had no bowel movement after 24 hours. The overall rate of effectiveness was 90.6%.[5]
- **Hypertension:** A study evaluating the effectiveness of *Lai Fu Zi* for treatment of hypertension in 467 patients reported reduction of blood pressure in 92% of all subjects, with 49.8% demonstrating marked effectiveness. The antihypertensive effect was attributed to either dilation of blood vessels and/or sedation of the central nervous system.[6]

TOXICOLOGY

The LD_{50} of *Lai Fu Zi* via intraperitoneal injection is 127.4 g/kg in mice, with fatality occurring within 1 hour.[7]

AUTHORS' COMMENTS

Lai Fu Zi strongly disperses qi. Thus, it antagonizes the effect of *Ren Shen* (Radix Ginseng) to build qi. These two herbs are generally not used together, as each will cancel the effect of the other. However, in cases of overdose of *Ren Shen*, use of *Lai Fu Zi* is actually beneficial, as it will alleviate many side effects and adverse reactions.

According to Dr. Wei Jia, *Lai Fu Zi* is an excellent herb to treat *bi zheng* (painful obstruction syndrome) and alleviate pain caused by excessive damp blocking the channels.

References

1. *Xian Dai Zhong Yao Yao Li Xue* (Contemporary Pharmacology of Chinese Herbs), 1997; 676-677
2. *The Merck Index* 12th edition, Chapman & Hall/CRCnetBASE/Merck, 2000
3. *Zhong Yao Yao Li Yu Ying Yong* (Pharmacology and Applications of Chinese Herbs), 1983; 867
4. *Zhong Cao Yao* (Chinese Herbal Medicine), 1990; 21(10):25
5. *Chong Qing Yi Yao* (Chongching Medicine and Herbology), 1986; 6:46
6. *Yi Xue Yan Jiu Tong Xun* (Report of Medical Studies), 1986; 6:46
7. *Zhong Yi Yao Xue Bao* (Report of Chinese Medicine and Herbology), 1990;(1)48

Ji Nei Jin (Endothelium Corneum Gigeriae Galli)

雞内金 鸡内金

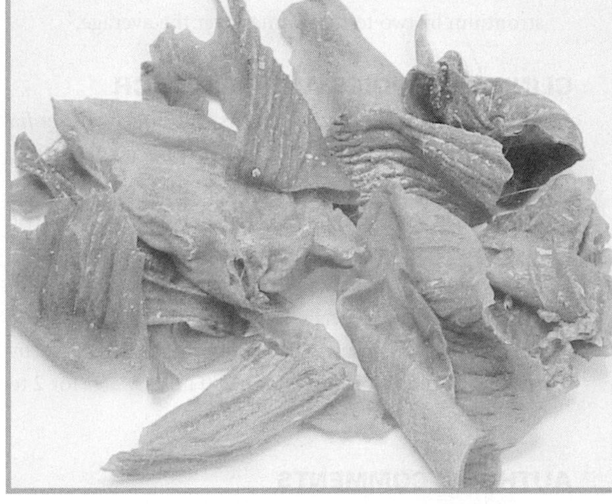

Pinyin Name: *Ji Nei Jin*
Literal Name: "chicken inner gold"
Alternate Chinese Names: *Ji Su Zi, Ji Pi Zi*
Original Source: *Shen Nong Ben Cao Jing* (Divine Husbandman's Classic of the Materia Medica) in the second century
English Name: gallus, chicken gizzard
Zoological Name: *Gallus gallus* domesticus Brisson. (*Ji*)
Pharmaceutical Name: Endothelium Corneum Gigeriae Galli
Properties: sweet, neutral
Channels Entered: Urinary Bladder, Small Intestine, Spleen, Stomach

CHINESE THERAPEUTIC ACTIONS

1. Promotes Digestion, Stimulates the Spleen

Indigestion, food stagnation, *gan ji* (infantile malnutrition): *Ji Nei Jin* (Endothelium Corneum Gigeriae Galli) stimulates the Spleen and Stomach, and strongly promotes digestion. It is effective for indigestion and food stagnation, including stagnation resulting from consuming meat, dairy, and starch. *Gan ji* is nutritional impairment in children, characterized by a sallow complexion, thin body appearance, abdominal distention, thinning hair, poor digestion, weakness and improper growth.

- Poor digestion, nausea and vomiting after food intake: use the dry-fried form of *Ji Nei Jin*.
- Severe indigestion and food stagnation: use this herb with *Shan Zha* (Fructus Crataegi) and *Mai Ya* (Fructus Hordei Germinatus).
- Decreased food intake, diarrhea, and stools containing undigested food due to Spleen deficiency: use *Ji Nei Jin* with *Bai Zhu* (Rhizoma Atractylodis Macrocephalae), *Da Zao* (Fructus Jujubae) and *Gan Jiang* (Rhizoma Zingiberis).
- *Gan ji* (infantile malnutrition): combine it with *Bai Zhu* (Rhizoma Atractylodis Macrocephalae), *Shan Yao* (Rhizoma Dioscoreae) and *Fu Ling* (Poria). These herbs can be made into pastries to improve patient compliance.

2. Consolidates *Jing* (Essence) and Prevents Leakage

Enuresis, spermatorrhea: *Ji Nei Jin* has a restraining property and is commonly used to treat leakage of body fluids, namely enuresis and spermatorrhea, caused by deficiency and cold of the Urinary Bladder.

- Enuresis or spermatorrhea caused by deficiency and cold of the Urinary Bladder: use *Ji Nei Jin* with *Sang Piao Xiao* (Ootheca Mantidis), *Tu Si Zi* (Semen Cuscutae), *Long Gu* (Os Draconis), and *Lu Rong* (Cornu Cervi Pantotrichum).
- Urinary incontinence, frequent urination, and cloudy urine from Urinary Bladder and Kidney deficiencies: use this herb with *Tu Si Zi* (Semen Cuscutae) and *Wu Wei Zi* (Fructus Schisandrae Chinensis).
- Spermatorrhea: use *Ji Nei Jin* individually with grain-based liquor, or in combination with *Lian Zi* (Semen Nelumbinis) and *Tu Si Zi* (Semen Cuscutae).

3. Softens Hardness, Dissolves Stones

Ji Nei Jin is commonly used to dissolve kidney or gallstones.

- Kidney stones or gallstones: add *Ji Nei Jin* to *Jin Qian Cao* (Herba Lysimachiae), *Yu Jin* (Radix Curcumae), *Hai Jin Sha* (Herba Lygodii) and *Shi Wei* (Folium Pyrrosiae).

DOSAGE

3 to 10 grams in decoction, 1.5 to 3.0 grams in powder. Powdered *Ji Nei Jin* is more effective than decoction. Dry-frying enhances its effect to strengthen the Spleen and promote digestion. Vinegar-frying does the same, and eliminates the odor.

CAUTIONS / CONTRAINDICATIONS

- Because *Ji Nei Jin* has a strong stimulant effect on the Spleen and Stomach, it should be used with caution in Spleen-deficient patients, or in those without food stagnation.

CHEMICAL COMPOSITION

Ventriculin, pepsin, protein, amylase, amino acids (lysine, arginine, threonine, glutamic acid, valine, leucine, isoleucine, and phenylalanine).[1]

PHARMACOLOGICAL EFFECTS

- **Effect on elimination of strontium:** Oral ingestion of *Ji*

Ji Nei Jin (Endothelium Corneum Gigeriae Galli)

Nei Jin in decoction increases the urinary excretion of strontium by two to three times over the average.[2]

CLINICAL STUDIES AND RESEARCH

- **Indigestion:** In healthy volunteers, 5 grams of *Ji Nei Jin* powder taken orally showed an increase in peristalsis, and gastric emptying time, and a 30 to 37% increase in gastric acid production after 45 to 60 minutes. Gastric acid levels returned to normal after 2 hours.[3]
- **Flat warts:** Ten patients were treated with a *Ji Nei Jin* solution applied topically five to six times daily for 10 days, with good results. The solution was prepared by soaking 20 grams of *Ji Nei Jin* in 200 ml of water for 2 to 3 days.[4]

AUTHORS' COMMENTS

Ji Nei Jin, Shan Zha (Fructus Crataegi), and *Lai Fu Zi* (Semen Raphani) all dissolve food stagnation and promote digestion.

- *Ji Nei Jin,* besides treating food stagnation, helps to dissolve urinary stones and gallstones.
- *Shan Zha* is strongest to assist digestion of meat, and oily or greasy foods. It also activates blood circulation and treats palpable masses in the abdomen. Recently, it has been used to lower cholesterol and treat cardiovascular disorders.
- *Lai Fu Zi* is stronger for relief of abdominal fullness and distention. It also dissolves phlegm and relieves cough and dyspnea.

References

1. *Xian Dai Zhong Yao Yao Li Xue* (Contemporary Pharmacology of Chinese Herbs), 1997; 679
2. *Zhong Yao Cai* (Study of Chinese Herbal Material), 1990; 13(11):30
3. *Zhong Yao Yao Li Yu Ying Yong* (Pharmacology and Applications of Chinese Herbs), 1983; 581
4. *Zhe Jiang Zhong Yi Za Zhi* (Zhejiang Journal of Chinese Medicine), 1987; 1:45

Chapter 9 summary — Digestive Herbs

Name	Similarities	Differences
Shan Zha (Fructus Crataegi)	Dissolve food, strengthen the Stomach	Digests meat, disperses blood stagnation
Shen Qu (Massa Fermentata)		Breaks down hard-to-digest foods, protects the Stomach
Hong Qu (Monascus)		Invigorates blood circulation, eliminates blood stasis
Mai Ya (Fructus Hordei Germinatus)		Digests starch, inhibits lactation
Gu Ya (Fructus Setariae Germinatus)		Digests starch, best for weak patients
Lai Fu Zi (Semen Raphani)		Relieves fullness and distention, lowers Lung qi and dispels phlegm
Ji Nei Jin (Endothelium Corneum Gigeriae Galli)		Strong digestive function, consolidates *jing* (essence), dissolves stones

General Characteristics of Digestive Herbs:

Taste: sweet
Thermal property: neutral or warm
Channels entered: Spleen, Stomach
Therapeutic actions: promote digestion, strengthen the middle *jiao*

Digestive herbs treat food stagnation and indigestion in cases of either excess or deficiency. Some have direct effect to digest food, others strengthen the Spleen and Stomach to indirectly promote digestion.

Sweet, sour and slightly warm, ***Shan Zha*** (Fructus Crataegi) strengthens the Spleen, improves appetite, promotes digestion of meat and breaks blood stagnation. It is used for postpartum pain and bleeding, hernial pain and food stagnation. It also has good effect to lower blood cholesterol levels and treat cardiovascular diseases.

Shen Qu (Massa Fermentata), ***Mai Ya*** (Fructus Hordei Germinatus) and ***Gu Ya*** (Fructus Setariae Germinatus) enter the Spleen and Stomach channels to dissolve food, harmonize the middle *jiao* and treat food stagnation. Generally speaking, unprocessed digestive herbs harmonize the middle *jiao*, dry-fried herbs facilitate digestion of food, and when charred, they resolve stagnation.

Shen Qu is best for food stagnation that is hard to digest. It is often used in formulas containing minerals, to facilitate digestion.

Mai Ya is weaker in action but focuses on digesting rice, starch and noodles. Interestingly, small doses of *Mai Ya* promote lactation while large doses inhibit it.

Gu Ya is the mildest and most suitable for Spleen and Stomach deficient patients.

Shen Qu (Massa Fermentata) and ***Hong Qu*** (Monascus) are both fermented herbs with similar functions to promote digestion.

Shen Qu promotes digestion to treat food stagnation. It also protects the stomach from hard-to-digest substances.

Hong Qu invigorates blood circulation to resolve blood stasis. It also is excellent to treat hyperlipidemia.

Lai Fu Zi (Semen Raphani) more effectively addresses epigastric and abdominal fullness and distention. It redirects Lung qi downwards to treat cough, dyspnea and profuse phlegm.

Chapter 9 summary

Ji Nei Jin (Endothelium Corneum Gigeriae Galli) is sweet and neutral. It strengthens the Spleen, dissolves food, and dissolves urinary stones and gallstones.

HERBS FROM OTHER FUNCTIONAL CATEGORIES WITH DIGESTIVE FUNCTIONS

Name	Functional Category
Bing Lang (Semen Arecae)	Antiparasitic Herbs (Chapter 10)
Chen Pi (Pericarpium Citri Reticulatae)	Qi-Regulating Herbs (Chapter 8)
E Zhu (Rhizoma Curcumae)	Blood-Invigorating and Stasis-Removing Herbs (Chapter 12)
Hou Po (Cortex Magnoliae Officinalis)	Aromatic Damp-Dissolving Herbs (Chapter 5)
Jiu Ceng Ta (Herba Ocimi Basilici)	Qi-Regulating Herbs (Chapter 8)
Mu Gua (Fructus Chaenomelis)	Wind-Damp Dispelling Herbs (Chapter 4)
Qing Pi (Pericarpium Citri Reticulatae Viride)	Qi-Regulating Herbs (Chapter 8)
Wu Long Cha (Folium Camellia Sinensis Fermentata)	Heat-Clearing Herbs (Chapter 2)
Zhi Shi (Fructus Aurantii Immaturus)	Qi-Regulating Herbs (Chapter 8)

Chapter 10

— Antiparasitic Herbs

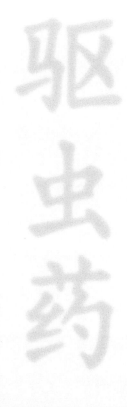

Chapter 10 — Antiparasitic Herbs

Chapter 10

驱虫药 — Antiparasitic Herbs

Definition: These herbs act to kill and expel parasites, relieve pain, and reduce stagnation. Applications for these herbs include treatment of internal and external parasites, such as roundworm, hookworm, tapeworm, and ringworm.

Causes of parasitic infestations include accumulation of damp-heat, and ingestion of parasites or parasite eggs. Clinical manifestations include poor appetite, frequent intake of food without satisfying hunger, emaciation, intermittent para-umbilical pain, vomiting of clear fluids, pale or cyanotic facial complexion, a peeled tongue, and an alternating forceful and weak pulse. When a parasitic condition goes untreated or is not treated properly, one sees sallow complexion, emaciation, and abdominal enlargement with obvious visible veins: expressions of the malnutrition that results from the infestation.

SUBCATEGORIES OF ACTION

Herbs that expel parasites usually enter the Spleen, Stomach, and Large Intestine channels. They should be administered on an empty stomach. In addition, patients must avoid oily or greasy food during treatments. Purgative herbs are often added to help with the expulsion of parasites. There are no subcategories of action in this instance, but optimal treatment of parasitic infestations requires awareness of specific indications, possible toxicity, and dosage adjustment for patients of different ages.

DIFFERENTIAL DIAGNOSIS AND TREATMENT

Different parasites may have different clinical presentations. Historically, diagnosis of parasitic infection was based primarily on presentation of signs and symptoms. Today, diagnosis can be additionally confirmed by stool examination for the presence of parasites or eggs.

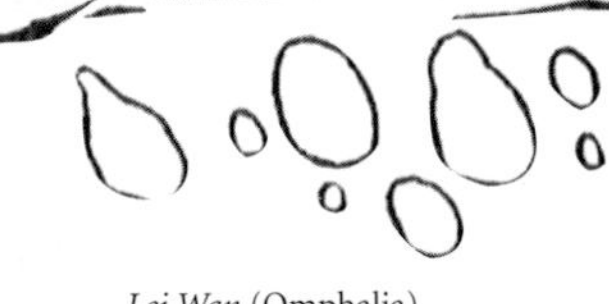

Lei Wan (Omphalia)
Ben Cao Gang Mu (Materia Medica), by Li Shi-Zhen, 1578 A.D.

Unique Symptomology of Parasitic Infestations

Parasite	Clinical Presentation
Roundworm	Red and white dots on the mucous membranes of the mouth; white flakes and segments appearing in the stools
Pinworm	Anal itching, often worse at night
Hookworm	Sallow facial appearance, cravings for unusual foods, a marked change in appetite, and uncharacteristic weakness and swelling

When using antiparasitic herbs, one should take into consideration the type of parasite, the patient's constitution, the severity of the disorder, and what other herbs are appropriate. Antiparasitic herbs are often combined with interior-warming herbs in cold conditions. For patients with fever or heat sensations, heat-clearing herbs should be used. If the patient has alternating chills and fever, both interior-warming and heat-clearing herbs should be used. If the condition is acute and severe, purgative herbs are added. If the condition is chronic, the addition of tonic herbs may be helpful.

When a parasitic condition goes untreated . . . malnutrition results.

Chapter 10 — Antiparasitic Herbs

CAUTIONS/CONTRAINDICATIONS

- Antiparasitic herbs should be used with caution during pregnancy, in elderly patients, or in individuals with Spleen and Stomach deficiencies.
- Many antiparasitic herbs have some degree of toxicity. They must be used with caution to avoid damaging the qi or causing toxic side effects.

PHARMACOLOGICAL EFFECTS

Antiparasitic herbs should be used with caution, as many have some degree of toxicity.

- **Antiparasitic**: These herbs have marked effectiveness to kill and expel intestinal parasites. Most exert their effect via paralyzing the muscles of the parasites, leading to the death or expulsion of the parasites (paralyzed muscle would mean the parasites cannot physically attach to the intestines to remain inside the host). Some herbs are also effective for topical parasitic infestations, such as ringworm. Individual herb monographs include details on the sensitivity of various parasites to the herbs.
- **Effects on smooth muscle**: Some herbs have a pronounced effect on the smooth muscle of the lungs or uterus. *Bing Lang* (Semen Arecae) increases peristalsis of the intestines, constricts bronchi, dilates blood vessels, and lowers blood pressure. *Fei Zi* (Semen Torreyae) and *Guan Zhong* (Rhizoma Dryopteridis) stimulate smooth muscle, leading to uterine contraction. Use of these herbs during pregnancy increases the risk of miscarriage.
- **Antibiotic**: Some herbs show excellent inhibitory effects against dermatophytes, such as *Shi Jun Zi* (Fructus Quisqualis), *Ku Lian Pi* (Cortex Meliae), *Bing Lang* (Semen Arecae) and *Wu Yi* (Fructus Ulmi Praeparatus).
- **Antineoplastic**: Some antiparasitics inhibit the growth of cancer cells, especially in uterine cancer.
- **Toxicity**: Many of these herbs have some degree of toxicity and may cause adverse reactions such as nausea, vomiting, edema, inflammation, abscess, ulceration, internal bleeding, sedation, diarrhea, visual disturbance, tremor, or seizures. Herbs that are to be used with caution include *Ku Lian Pi* (Cortex Meliae), *Bing Lang* (Semen Arecae), and *Guan Zhong* (Rhizoma Dryopteridis).

POTENTIAL HERB-DRUG INTERACTIONS

Herbs that expel parasites are generally used only if necessary, and only for a short period of time. Because of this relatively infrequent usage, there are no known or documented herb-drug interactions. However, because many antiparasitic herbs are toxic to both the parasite and the host (humans), those herbs should always be used with caution.

Shi Jun Zi (Fructus Quisqualis)

使君子

Pinyin Name: *Shi Jun Zi*
Literal Name: "envoy seeds"
Alternate Chinese Names: *Jun Zi*
Original Source: *Kai Bao Ben Cao* (Materia Medica of the Kai Bao Era) by Ma Zhi in 973-974 A.D.
English Name: quisqualis, rangoon creeper fruit
Botanical Name: *Quisqualis indica* L. (*Shi Jun Zi*)
Pharmaceutical Name: Fructus Quisqualis
Properties: sweet, warm
Channels Entered: Spleen, Stomach
Safety Index: slightly toxic

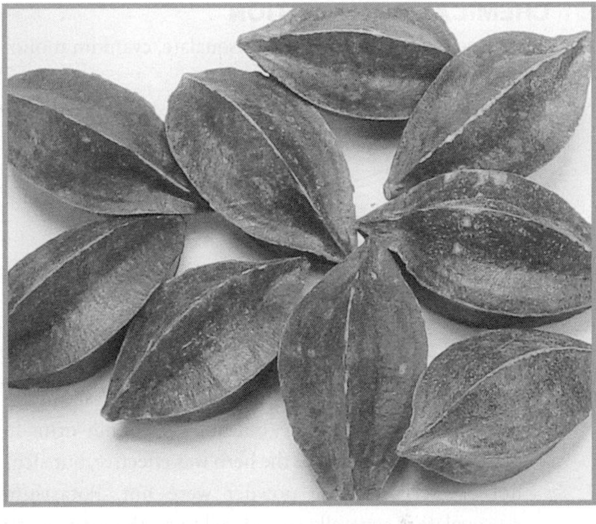

CHINESE THERAPEUTIC ACTIONS

1. Kills Parasites

Roundworms: *Shi Jun Zi* (Fructus Quisqualis) is sweet, aromatic and moistening. It gently lubricates the intestines and kills parasites. It is mild in action and especially suitable for weaker patients or children, to dispel parasites and relieve abdominal pain.

- Roundworms: remove the shell and crush the contents into a fine powder. Mix it with rice water and serve on an empty stomach at 5 a.m. or in the early morning.

2. Strengthens the Spleen and Relieves Stagnation

***Gan ji* (infantile malnutrition):** *Shi Jun Zi* kills intestinal parasites, strengthens the middle *jiao,* and improves the overall health of children with malnutrition caused by parasitic infection.

- *Gan ji* with food stagnation: use *Shi Jun Zi* with *Ji Nei Jin* (Endothelium Corneum Gigeriae Galli) and *Shen Qu* (Massa Fermentata).
- *Gan ji* accompanied by Spleen qi deficiency and weakness: use this herb with *Ren Shen* (Radix Ginseng) and *Bai Zhu* (Rhizoma Atractylodis Macrocephalae).
- *Gan ji* and abdominal bloating: use it with *Zhi Ke* (Fructus Aurantii) and *Bing Lang* (Semen Arecae).
- *Gan ji* with constipation: add *Da Huang* (Radix et Rhizoma Rhei).

DOSAGE

6 to 10 grams. Take *Shi Jun Zi* on an empty stomach for at least 2 to 3 days. Crush *Shi Jun Zi* before decocting, to enhance extraction of active constituents. Traditionally, the dosage used is one seed of *Shi Jun Zi* for a one-year-old, adding one seed for each additional year of age. However, do not exceed 20 seeds a day.

CAUTIONS / CONTRAINDICATIONS

- Use of *Shi Jun Zi* is contraindicated with all teas, including black tea, green tea, oolong tea and others. Serving this herb with hot tea will cause vomiting, nausea and diarrhea. Nausea, hiccups and vomiting can usually be resolved by stopping the intake of this herb. When necessary, one can chew *Ding Xiang* (Flos Caryophylli) or *Gan Cao* (Radix Glycyrrhizae) to clear those unwanted side effects.
- Allergic reactions are sometimes associated with the use of *Shi Jun Zi.* Characteristic symptoms include purple and red skin rashes, with or without itching and pain, ankle swelling and pain, lethargy, poor appetite, slight increase in body temperature, and possibly hematochezia.

OVERDOSAGE

Gross overdose of *Shi Jun Zi* is characterized by headache, dizziness, vertigo, nausea, vomiting, diarrhea, abdominal pain, perspiration, and cold extremities. In severe cases, there may be seizures, convulsions, dyspnea, and decreased blood pressure. To avoid overdose, keep dosages under 20 seeds per day.[1]

TREATMENT OF OVERDOSAGE

Overdose of *Shi Jun Zi* is treated with a decoction of *Ding Xiang* (Flos Caryophylli) and *Gan Cao* (Radix Glycyrrhizae).

Shi Jun Zi (Fructus Quisqualis)

CHEMICAL COMPOSITION

Quisqualic acid, potassium quisqualate, cyanidin monoglycoside, trigonelline.[2,3]

Quisqualic Acid

PHARMACOLOGICAL EFFECTS

- **Antiparasitic**: Administration of *Shi Jun Zi* showed a marked ability to paralyze, but not kill, roundworms in pigs. The water extract of the herb was effective, but alcohol extract or crude powder were not. Potassium quisqualate is generally considered to be the main active constituent. The powder of *Shi Jun Zi* is also effective against pinworm.[4,5]
- **Antibiotic:** *Shi Jun Zi* has an inhibitory effect *in vitro* against various pathogenic fungi and dermatophytes.[6]

CLINICAL STUDIES AND RESEARCH

- **Roundworm infestation:** In a clinical study, 194 patients with roundworms were divided into two groups and treated with separate preparations of *Shi Jun Zi*. The first group of 10 patients received the dry-fried form twice daily for 2 days. Roundworms were expelled in 100% of the patients. A second group of 184 patients received pills (prepared by mixing the crude powder with honey) twice daily for 3 days. Roundworms were expelled in 80.89% of the patients.[7]
- **Pinworm infestation:** Patients with pinworm infestations were successfully treated using a *Shi Jun Zi* preparation. The treatment protocol was to dry fry the herb until it turned yellowish. The patients were instructed to take the herb 30 minutes before meals, three times daily, for 15 days per course of treatment, followed by one month of rest, and continue for another course of treatment if necessary. Daily dosage of *Shi Jun Zi* used in this study was 15 to 30 seeds for adults, and 3 to 15 seeds for children. Patients were instructed to avoid tea before and after ingestion of herbs.[8]
- **Trichomoniasis:** According to one study, 7 patients with intestinal trichomoniasis were treated with dry-fried *Shi Jun Zi* with good results. The daily dosage was 3 grams in infants under 1 year of age, 1.5 grams for infants between 1 and 3 years old, and 15 grams for adults. The herbs were given in 1 or 2 equally-divided doses. The duration of treatment was 3 to 5 days, followed by 3 to 5 days of rest, for a total of 1 or 2 courses of treatments. The study reported complete recovery in all 3 adults after 1 course of treatment, and in all 4 infants after 2 to 3 courses of treatment.[9]

TOXICOLOGY

Shi Jun Zi has little toxicity when given orally in therapeutic doses. Toxicity, however, has been observed following overdose and in non-oral administrations. In one study, subcutaneous injection of water extract of *Shi Jun Zi* in mice was associated with convulsions, respiratory depression and fatality within several minutes. With overdose at 26.6 g/kg of crude powder in dogs, side effects such as nausea, vomiting, diarrhea and gastrointestinal disturbances were observed.[10]

AUTHORS' COMMENTS

There are numerous herbs with antiparasitic activities, such as *Bing Lang* (Semen Arecae), *Chuan Lian Zi* (Fructus Toosendan), *Lei Wan* (Omphalia), and *Wu Zhu Yu* (Fructus Evodiae). *Shi Jun Zi* is considered the strongest and most potent of the group.

Shi Jun Zi and *Ku Lian Pi* (Cortex Meliae) are both commonly used to kill parasites. *Shi Jun Zi* is sweet, less toxic, and tonifies the Spleen while killing parasites. For that reason, it is more suitable for children. *Ku Lian Pi* is stronger in killing parasites, especially the fresh form. However, it is more toxic and slight overdose may result in problems. See *Ku Lian Pi* monograph for additional information.

References

1. *Zhong Yao Bu Liang Fan Ying Yu Zhi Liao* (Adverse Reactions and Treatment of Chinese Herbal Medicine), 1996; 218:220, 1996; 153:155
2. *Xian Dai Zhong Yao Yao Li Xue* (Contemporary Pharmacology of Chinese Herbs), 1997; 703
3. *The Merck Index* 12th edition, Chapman & Hall/CRCnetBASE/Merck, 2000
4. *Zhong Yao Yao Li Yu Ying Yong* (Pharmacology and Applications of Chinese Herbs), 1983:686
5. *Zhong Cao Yao Xue* (Study of Chinese Herbal Medicine), 1976; 701
6. Ibid.
7. *Jiang Su Zhong Yi* (Jiangsu Chinese Medicine), 1960; 2:34
8. Ibid., 1960; 2:34
9. Ibid., 1964; 10:16
10. *Chang Yong Zhong Yao Cheng Fen Yu Yao Li Shou Ce* (A Handbook of the Composition and Pharmacology of Common Chinese Drugs), 1994; 1248:1249

Ku Lian Pi (Cortex Meliae)

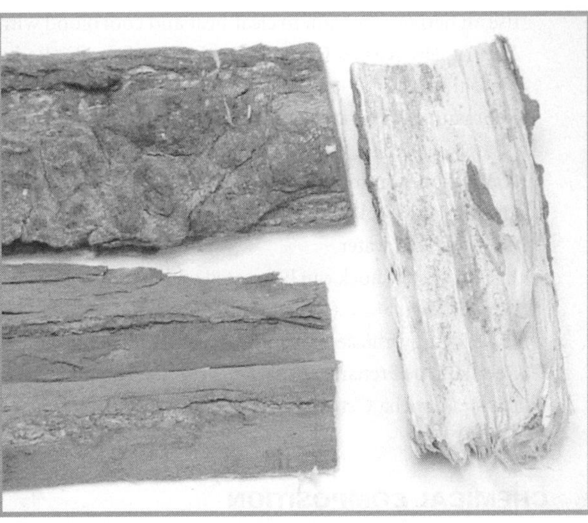

苦楝皮 苦楝皮

Pinyin Name: *Ku Lian Pi*
Literal Name: "bitter Chinaberry tree bark"
Alternate Chinese Names: *Ku Lian Gen Pi*
Original Source: *Ming Yi Za Zhu* (Miscellaneous Records of Famous Physicians) by Tao Hong-Jing in 500 A.D.
English Name: melia bark, Sichuan chinaberry bark, chinaberry tree bark
Botanical Name: *Melia toosendan* Sieb. et Zucc. (*Chuan Lian Shu*); *Melia azedarach* L.(*Lian Shu*)
Pharmaceutical Name: Cortex Meliae
Properties: bitter, cold
Channels Entered: Liver, Spleen, Stomach
Safety Index: toxic

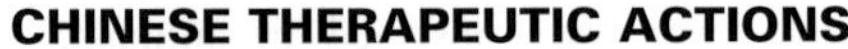

CHINESE THERAPEUTIC ACTIONS

1. Kills Parasites

Ku Lian Pi (Cortex Meliae) exerts good antiparasitic action against infestations of hookworms, pinworms, and roundworms.

- Hookworm: use this herb with *Bing Lang* (Semen Arecae) and serve with honey before bedtime, on an empty stomach, for two days.
- Pinworm: use it with *Bai Bu* (Radix Stemonae) and *Wu Mei* (Fructus Mume) as an enema one time every night for two to four nights.
- Parasites: the combination of powdered *Ku Lian Pi*, *Ku Shen Gen* (Radix Sophorae Flavescentis), *She Chuang Zi* (Fructus Cnidii) and *Zao Jiao* (Fructus Gleditsiae) can be inserted into the rectum or vagina to kill parasites.

2. Trichomonas Infection

Ku Lian Pi is used as an external wash or douche to treat trichomonas infection.

3. Treats Tinea Infections and Sores

Ku Lian Pi is commonly used topically to treat various infections.

- Tinea and sores: use *Ku Lian Pi* alone as a powder and mix with vinegar or tea tree oil for topical applications. Use every other day for three to four applications, to relieve itching.

Toothache and painful gums can be treated with administration of *Ku Lian Pi* decoction as a mouthwash.

DOSAGE

6 to 15 grams, up to 60 grams when used alone. *Ku Lian Pi* can be used in decoction, pill or powder forms. The dose for the fresh herb is 15 to 30 grams. Dosage should be adjusted appropriately for children of different ages.

CAUTIONS / CONTRAINDICATIONS

- *Ku Lian Pi* is toxic and should not be administered in large dosages.
- Those with deficiency and cold of the Spleen and Stomach should only use *Ku Lian Pi* with caution.
- *Ku Lian Pi* should be used with extreme caution in patients with pre-existing cardiovascular disease, hepatic disease, or peptic ulcers.

OVERDOSAGE

Overdose of *Ku Lian Pi* is characterized by dizziness, headache, desire for sleep, nausea, vomiting, abdominal distention and pain, diarrhea, palpitations, tachycardia, perspiration, pale face, cyanotic lips, and a weak pulse. In severe cases, there may be gastrointestinal bleeding, jaundice, hepatomegaly, elevated liver enzymes, toxic hepatitis, disorientation, and visual impairment. *Ku Lian Pi* has a narrow range of safety index, as adverse reactions may occur at therapeutic doses.[1]

TREATMENT OF OVERDOSAGE

In cases of *Ku Lian Pi* overdose, immediately induce vomiting and perform gastrolavage. When necessary, administer a heavy dose of purgative herbs, egg whites, activated charcoal, or flour. Intravenous infusion of glucose or dextrose are also beneficial to replenish lost fluids.

Mild cases of overdose can be treated with an herbal formula with 120 grams of *Lu Dou* (Semen Phaseoli Radiati), 60 grams of *Long Yan Rou* (Arillus Longan), and 15 grams of *Gan Cao* (Radix Glycyrrhizae).

For cases of bleeding (hematochezia and hematuria),

Ku Lian Pi (Cortex Meliae)

use an herbal decoction to clear heat and cool blood with *Xue Yu Tan* (Crinis Carbonisatus) 6-9g, *San Qi* (Radix Notoginseng) 3-6g, *Sheng Di Huang* (Radix Rehmanniae) 30g, and *Mu Dan Pi* (Cortex Moutan) 15g.

If adverse reaction is characterized by spasms and convulsion, administer 1.5 grams of *Quan Xie* (Scorpio) and 2 pieces of *Wu Gong* (Scolopendra) by mixing the powders with water.

Patients in shock can be treated with an herbal decoction of *Ren Shen* (Radix Ginseng) 9g, *Zhi Gan Cao* (Radix Glycyrrhizae Preparata) 9g, *Shu Di Huang* (Radix Rehmanniae Preparata) 12g, *Long Gu* (Os Draconis) 15g, *Mu Li* (Concha Ostreae) 15g, and *Shan Zhu Yu* (Fructus Corni) 15g.

CHEMICAL COMPOSITION

Toosendanin.[2]

PHARMACOLOGICAL EFFECTS

- **Antiparasitic:** Toosendanin has a marked antiparasitic effect. At high concentrations, it effectively paralyzes the muscles of intestinal parasites, leading to their expulsion.[3]
- **Respiratory:** Toosendanin has an inhibiting influence on the respiratory system in animal studies. Following intramuscular injection, respiration slowed down in 60 minutes and stopped in 120 minutes. Following intravenous injection, respiration slowed down in 10 minutes and stopped in 30 minutes. The respiratory depression is attributed to the action of toosendanin on the central nervous system in the brain.[4]
- **Gastrointestinal:** Administration of toosendanin is associated with an increase in intestinal peristalsis and contraction. In large doses, it may lead to spasms and cramps.[5]

CLINICAL STUDIES AND RESEARCH

- **Roundworm infestation:** In a comprehensive study of the treatment of intestinal parasitic infestation, 4,757 patients with roundworm infestation were treated with two different preparations of *Ku Lian Pi* for 2 to 3 days with an overall rate of effectiveness of 93.6%. Patients received either decoction or pills. The decoction was prepared by cooking the herb to yield a 50% solution. Patients were instructed to take 40 to 60 ml of the decoction on an empty stomach before bedtime and in the morning. The pills were prepared from powdered extract with each pill containing 0.45 grams of herb. Patients were instructed to take 4 to 8 pills on an empty stomach before bedtime and in the morning. Though the treatment was effective, side effects were reported in 35.2% of the patients. Side effects included dizziness, headache, abdominal pain, diarrhea, nausea, vomiting, blurred vision, lethargy, and numbness of the extremities.[6]
- **Vaginal trichomoniasis:** Patients with vaginal trichomoniasis were treated with a topical application of *Ku Lian Pi* with great success. In the first study, 200 grams of the herb were cooked in 1,000 to 1,500 ml of water for 20 minutes. The treatment protocol was to first instill 5 ml of the solution into the vagina, followed by insertion into the vagina of a gauze ball soaked with the solution, that was removed the following day. Out of 27 patients, most reported improvement after 5 to 10 treatments.[7]

TOXICOLOGY

Overdose of toosendanin is associated with edema, ulceration, nausea, vomiting, elevated liver enzymes and liver damage in dogs, rabbits, mice and monkeys. With gross overdose, decreased blood pressure, internal bleeding, and fatality have been observed in animals. Sensitivity varies depending on the animals studied. The LD_{50} for oral ingestion of toosendanin is 244 mg/kg in mice, 120 mg/kg in rats, and 3 to 4 mg/kg in cats.[8]

AUTHORS' COMMENTS

Ku Lian Pi and *Shi Jun Zi* (Fructus Quisqualis) are both commonly used to kill parasites. The fresh form of *Ku Lian Pi* is markedly stronger in killing parasites. However, *Ku Lian Pi* is more toxic and must be used with extreme caution. Slight overdose of *Ku Lian Pi* may result in dizziness, headache, desire to sleep, nausea or abdominal pain. In severe cases, side effects may include internal bleeding, toxic hepatitis, disorientation, and visual impairment. *Shi Jun Zi* is sweet, less toxic than *Ku Lian Pi* and tonifies the Spleen while killing parasites. For that reason, *Shi Jun Zi* is more suitable for children.

References

1. *Zhong Yao Bu Liang Fan Ying Yu Zhi Liao* (Adverse Reactions and Treatment of Chinese Herbal Medicine), 1996; 218:220, 1996; 205:206
2. *Xian Dai Zhong Yao Yao Li Xue* (Contemporary Pharmacology of Chinese Herbs), 1997; 707
3. *Sheng Li Xue Bao* (Physiology News), 1958; 22(1):18
4. Ibid., 1980; 32(4):338
5. *Zhong Yao Yao Li Yu Ying Yong* (Pharmacology and Applications of Chinese Herbs), 1983; 648
6. *Zhong Hua Nei Ke Za Zhi* (Chinese Journal of Internal Medicine), 1962; 8:491
7. *Zhong Hua Fu Chan Ke Za Zhi* (Chinese Journal of OB/GYN), 1959; 3:193
8. *Zhong Cao Yao* (Chinese Herbal Medicine), 1982; 13(7):29

Bing Lang (Semen Arecae)

檳榔 槟榔

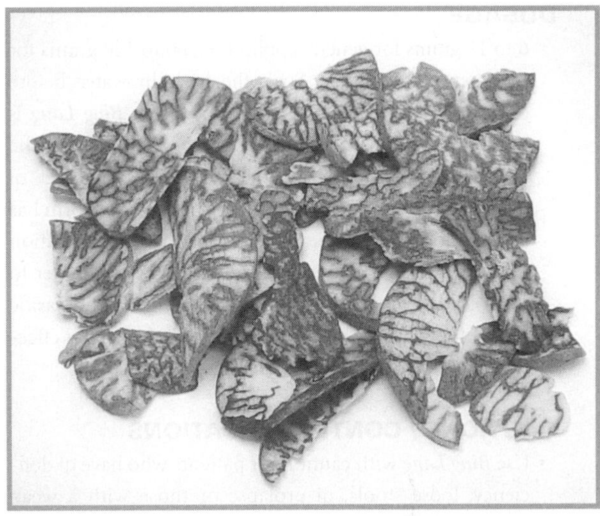

Pinyin Name: *Bing Lang*
Alternate Chinese Names: *Jian Bing, Da Fu Zi, Hai Nan Zi*
Original Source: *Ming Yi Za Zhu* (Miscellaneous Records of Famous Physicians) by Tao Hong-Jing in 500 A.D.
English Name: areca seed, betel nut
Botanical Name: *Areca catechu* L. (*Bing Lang*)
Pharmaceutical Name: Semen Arecae
Properties: acrid, bitter, warm
Channels Entered: Large Intestine, Stomach

CHINESE THERAPEUTIC ACTIONS

1. Kills Parasites

Bing Lang (Semen Arecae) treats various types of intestinal parasites, such as tapeworms, pinworms, fasciolopsis, roundworms and blood flukes. It is especially effective in treatment of tapeworms. *Bing Lang* is a very effective herb because it has both antiparasitic and purgative effects.

- Intestinal parasites: use *Bing Lang* with *Nan Gua Zi* (Semen Cucurbitae Moschatae), *Shi Jun Zi* (Fructus Quisqualis) and *Da Huang* (Radix et Rhizoma Rhei).
- Fasciolopsiasis: use it with *Wu Mei* (Fructus Mume) and *Gan Cao* (Radix Glycyrrhizae).
- Intestinal obstruction due to parasites: combine this herb with *Hu Jiao* (Fructus Piper), *Ku Lian Pi* (Cortex Meliae) and *Ming Fan* (Alumen).

2. Dissipates Stagnation and Promotes the Movement of Qi

Qi and food stagnation: Dampness accumulation secondary to qi and food stagnation may cause abdominal fullness and distention, constipation or diarrhea, rectal tenesmus, dysentery, chest congestion, fullness and stifling sensations, wheezing with phlegm, belching, organomegaly, benign masses, cysts, and muscle tension and ascites in severe cases. *Bing Lang* functions to send stagnant qi downward from the highest part of the body to the lowest. It is at its best when used to treat qi reversal or stagnation in the upper *jiao*.

- Chest congestion: use *Bing Lang* with *Zhi Ke* (Fructus Aurantii), *Su Geng* (Caulis Perillae), *Huo Xiang* (Herba Agastache) and *Hou Po* (Cortex Magnoliae Officinalis).
- Wheezing with phlegm: use it with *Ting Li Zi* (Semen Descurainiae seu Lepidii).
- Belching and nausea: combine it with *Dai Zhe Shi* (Haematitum) (pre-decoct), *Xuan Fu Hua* (Flos Inulae), *Su Zi* (Fructus Perillae), *Zhu Ru* (Caulis Bambusae in Taenia) and *Ban Xia* (Rhizoma Pinelliae).
- Abdominal distention with constipation: use this herb with *Hou Po* (Cortex Magnoliae Officinalis), *Zhi Shi* (Fructus Aurantii Immaturus) and *Da Huang* (Radix et Rhizoma Rhei).
- Rectal tenesmus: add *Mu Xiang* (Radix Aucklandiae) and *Hou Po* (Cortex Magnoliae Officinalis).
- Organomegaly, masses and cysts: use *Bing Lang* with *Mu Li* (Concha Ostreae), *Lai Fu Zi* (Semen Raphani), *San Leng* (Rhizoma Sparganii), *E Zhu* (Rhizoma Curcumae) and *Yu Jin* (Radix Curcumae).
- Ascites: use this herb with *Fu Ling* (Poria), *Zhu Ling* (Polyporus), *Ze Xie* (Rhizoma Alismatis) and *Dong Gua Pi* (Exocarpium Benincasae).
- Dysentery: use this herb with *Huang Lian* (Rhizoma Coptidis), *Mu Xiang* (Radix Aucklandiae) and *Chi Shao* (Radix Paeoniae Rubrae).

3. Promotes Urination

Bing Lang promotes normal urination to eliminate water stagnation. It treats edema and leg *qi*.

- Edema of the lower limbs, leg *qi*: use it with *Zi Su Ye* (Folium Perillae), *Chen Pi* (Pericarpium Citri Reticulatae), *Mu Gua* (Fructus Chaenomelis) and *Fen Fang Ji* (Radix Stephaniae Tetandrae).

4. Relieves Nausea

Bing Lang is often combined with *Chang Shan* (Radix Dichroae) for treatment of malaria. *Bing Lang* relieves nausea and vomiting to improve patient compliance in taking herbal medicines, and to enhance overall effectiveness. *Chang Shan* has antimalarial action, but may cause nausea and vomiting if administered alone.

Bing Lang (Semen Arecae)

DOSAGE

6 to 15 grams for general application, 60 to 120 grams for treatment of parasites. Soak the herb in water before decocting, for best results against parasites. *Bing Lang* is usually used in decoctions, pills or powder. The unprocessed herb has a better function to redirect qi downwards and reduce stagnation. The dry-fried form has a more moderate action, and is less likely to cause irritation to the Spleen and Stomach. The charred herb is better to stop bleeding and treat bloody dysentery. The antiparasitic effect of *Bing Lang* against roundworms becomes less effective when the herb is cooked in hot water.[1]

CAUTIONS / CONTRAINDICATIONS

- Use *Bing Lang* with caution for patients who have qi deficiency, loose stools, qi prolapse or those with a weak Spleen and Stomach.
- *Bing Lang* should be used with caution during pregnancy, due to its teratogenic and fetotoxic effects, as shown in mice.[2]

CHEMICAL COMPOSITION

Areca red, arecoline, arecaine, guracine, guvacoline, arecolidine, homoarecoline.[3,4]

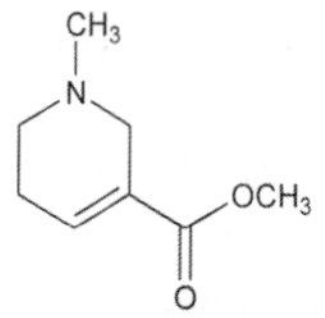

Arecoline

PHARMACOLOGICAL EFFECTS

- **Antiparasitic:** Both water and alcohol extracts of *Bing Lang* have demonstrated marked impact in paralyzing liver flukes. Therapeutic effects vary depending on the concentration of the final solution. Concentrations of $1x10^{-2}$ and $1x10^{-3}$ were determined to be the most effective.[5]
- **Antiparasitic:** *Bing Lang* has a strong antiparasitic effect against various intestinal parasites, including but not limited to tapeworm, roundworm, and hookworm. According to one study, a 30% solution of *Bing Lang* can kill tapeworms in dogs within 40 minutes. In another study, a preparation of *Bing Lang* effectively paralyzed tapeworms in cows and pigs.[6,7]
- **Antihypertensive:** According to studies by Inokuchi, administration of Areca II-5-C acts as an angiotensin-converting enzyme (ACE) inhibitor that shows marked antihypertensive functions. Direct comparison between Areca II-5-C and captopril showed that both substances have comparable effects in reducing blood pressure.[8]
- **Gastrointestinal:** Arecoline increases production of gastric acid, increases intestinal peristalsis, and increases appetite. In one study, decoction of *Bing Lang* at 9.98 g/kg induced diarrhea within 65 minutes to expel parasites. In another study, a 20% injection of *Bing Lang* was associated with stimulation of and increased contractility of the gallbladder, in cats and dogs. When used with *Da Huang* (Radix et Rhizoma Rhei), the combination stimulated the expulsion of gallstones. Lastly, arecoline stimulated smooth muscle and led to uterine contraction in rabbits.[9,10,11]

CLINICAL STUDIES AND RESEARCH

- **Roundworm infestation:** Patients with roundworms were treated with an herbal formula containing 9 grams each of *Bing Lang* and *Lei Wan* (Omphalia). The herbs were cooked in 200 ml of water to yield 40 ml of the final solution. Patients were instructed to take the decoction in the morning on an empty stomach followed by breakfast two hours later. All patients received 3 days of treatment, followed by 5 to 7 days of rest, and concluded by 3 more days of treatment. The study reported successful expulsion of roundworms in 22 out of 36 patients.[12]
- **Blood flukes:** An herbal decoction was used effectively to treat 400 patients with blood flukes. The herbal formula contained 45 grams of *Bing Lang* and 45 grams of *Cang Er Cao* (Herba Xanthii), cooked to yield 60 ml of the final decoction. The patients were instructed to take the herbs twice daily for 20 days per course of treatment.[13]
- **Hookworm infestation:** In one study, 24 patients with hookworm were successfully treated with a formula consisting of 30 grams of *Bing Lang*, 15 grams of *Nan Gua Zi* (Semen Cucurbitae Moschatae), and 30 grams of brown sugar. The patients were instructed to take the herbal decoction in the morning on an empty stomach for 3 days, followed by 1 week of rest, and conclude with another 3 days of treatment.[14]
- **Fasciolopsiasis:** Treatment of 370 patients with an herbal formula resulted in an 87.03% rate of effectiveness. The herbal formula contained arecoline, pharbitin, and crude powder of *Bing Lang*.[15]

HERB-DRUG INTERACTION

- **Antipsychotics:** It has been suggested that an exacerbation of extrapyramidal effects may occur with concurrent use of neuroleptic drugs and betel nuts. Two cases of severe extrapyramidal symptoms were reported when patients with chronic schizophrenic disorders treated with depot neuroleptics also consumed a heavy dose of betel nuts for a long period of time.[16,17] [Note: Examples of antipsychotics include chlorpromazine (Thorazine), fluphenazine (Prolixin), thioridazine (Mellaril), and haloperidol (Haldol).]

Bing Lang (Semen Arecae)

TOXICOLOGY

Administration of *Bing Lang* in animals is associated with such side effects as salivation, diarrhea, increased respiration, restlessness and seizures. The LD_{50} for oral ingestion of *Bing Lang* decoction in mice is 120 g/kg.[18,19]

AUTHORS' COMMENTS

Bing Lang has both antiparasitic and purgative functions. Because it kills several kinds of parasites, it is one of the most commonly-used antiparasitic herbs. It also breaks up or moves qi to relieve stagnation. It has recently been used to treat post-surgical bloating and distention of the abdomen with good results.

References

1. *Guo Wai Yi Xue Zhong Yi Zhong Yao Fen Ce* (Monograph of Chinese Herbology from Foreign Medicine), 1988; 10(6):29
2. Brinker, Francis. *The Toxicology of Botanical Medicines,* rev. 2nd ed., 1996
3. *Xian Dai Zhong Yao Yao Li Xue* (Contemporary Pharmacology of Chinese Herbs), 1997; 711
4. *The Merck Index* 12th edition, Chapman & Hall/CRCnetBASE/Merck, 2000
5. *Nan Jing Zhong Yi Xue Yuan Xue Bao* (Journal of Nanjing University of Traditional Chinese Medicine), 1990; 6(4):34
6. *Zhe Jiang Yi Ke Da Xue Xue Bao* (Journal of Zhejiang Province School of Medicine), 1980; 9(1):1
7. *Zhong Hua Yi Xue Za Zhi* (Chinese Journal of Medicine), 1956; 42(2):138
8. *CA*, 1986; 104:218801z
9. *Tai Wan Yi Xue Hui Za Zhi* (Journal of Taiwan Medical Association), 1933; 36(6):857
10. *Xin Yi Yao Xue Za Zhi* (New Journal of Medicine and Herbology), 1979; (6):26
11. CA, 1969; 70:113690p
12. *Jiang Su Zhong Yi Za Zhi* (Jiangsu Journal of Chinese Medicine), 1960; (5):30
13. *Guang Dong Zhong Yi* (Guangdong Chinese Medicine), 1959; 4(7):307
14. *Zhong Hua Yi Xue Za Zhi* (Chinese Journal of Medicine), 1957; 43(5):371
15. *Zhong Cheng Yao Yan Jiu* (Research of Chinese Patent Medicine), 1981; 5:13
16. *Lancet* 355(9198):134-8, 2000 Jan 8
17. *Movement Disorders.* 4(4):330-2, 1989
18. *J Parasitology*, 1946; 37:185
19. *Jiang Su Yi Ke Da Xue Xue Bao* (Journal of Jiangsu Universidy of Medicine), 1980; 9(1):1

Nan Gua Zi (Semen Cucurbitae Moschatae)

南瓜子

Pinyin Name: *Nan Gua Zi*
Literal Name: "southern fruit seed," "southern melon seeds"
Alternate Chinese Names: *Nan Gua Ren, Bai Gua Zi*
Original Source: *Ben Cao Shi Yi* (Omissions from the [Classic of the] Materia Medica) by Chen Cang-Qi in 741 A.D.
English Name: pumpkin seed, cushaw seed
Botanical Name: *Cucurbita moschata* Duch. (*Nan Gua*)
Pharmaceutical Name: Semen Cucurbitae Moschatae
Properties: sweet, neutral
Channels Entered: Stomach, Large Intestine

CHINESE THERAPEUTIC ACTIONS

1. Kills Parasites

Nan Gua Zi (Semen Cucurbitae Moschatae) has a proven, reliable antiparasitic effect, especially against tapeworms and roundworms. Furthermore, it is safe and has minimal side effects. It may be used individually or in combination with other herbs.

- Tapeworm (especially from beef): use *Nan Gua Zi* with *Bing Lang* (Semen Arecae). The treatment protocol is to first give 60 to 120 grams of *Nan Gua Zi* in powder with cold water, followed in 2 hours by 60 to 120 grams of *Bing Lang* in decoction, and finish with 15 grams of *Mang Xiao* (Natrii Sulfas) with hot water, to purge the parasites.
- Schistosomiasis: use 120 to 200 grams of *Nan Gua Zi* daily on a long-term basis.

Nan Gua Zi (Semen Cucurbitae Moschatae)

- Parasites in patients showing signs of malnutrition and sallow complexion: use this herb with peanuts and walnuts.

2. Promotes Lactation

Nan Gua Zi also promotes lactation in women who have difficulty nursing.

DOSAGE

60 to 120 grams. *Nan Gua Zi* is often taken in powder form with cold water. The outer shells of the seeds are often removed prior to crushing *Nan Gua Zi* into powder. This herb is generally taken with cold water because heat significantly decreases its effects.

CAUTIONS / CONTRAINDICATIONS

- Use of *Nan Gua Zi* is sometimes associated with mild gastrointestinal side effects, such as nausea, poor appetite, and diarrhea. These reactions are mild and self-limiting.

OVERDOSAGE

In one report, two rare cases of jaundice and hepatic coma were associated with overdose and prolonged use of *Nan Gua Zi* for treatment of schistosomiasis. Specific information on the dosage and the duration of treatment were unavailable.[1]

CHEMICAL COMPOSITION

Cucurbitine, m-carboxyphenylalanine, N-methylasparagine, minhychrin.[2]

PHARMACOLOGICAL EFFECTS

- **Antiparasitic:** According to *in vitro* studies, *Nan Gua Zi* paralyzed tapeworms in cattle and roundworms in pigs. *Nan Gua Zi* also inhibited and killed young schistosomes. Lastly, synergistic action was observed when *Nan Gua Zi* was combined with *Bing Lang* (Semen Arecae).[3]

CLINICAL STUDIES AND RESEARCH

- **Tapeworm:** In one study, 70 patients with tapeworm infestations were treated with a protocol that incorporated *Nan Gua Zi*, *Bing Lang* (Semen Arecae) and magnesium sulfate. Patients were given *Nan Gua Zi* in powder on an empty stomach in the morning, followed 2 hours later by a decoction of *Bing Lang*, and in another 30 minutes, a 50% magnesium sulfate solution. The dosage for *Nan Gua Zi* was 60 to 80 grams for adults, and 30 to 50 grams for children under 15 years of age; the dosage of *Bing Lang* was 60 to 80 grams for adults, and 30 to 60 grams for children under 15 years of age; and the dosage for magnesium sulfate was 60 ml for adults, and 20 to 40 ml for children under 15 years of age. Out of 70 patients, 68 who returned for follow-up showed a 97.06% rate of successful treatment. Two patients did not return for the follow-up exam.[4]
- **Nursing:** Nursing women with inadequate milk production were treated with 150 to 180 grams of *Nan Gua Zi* given in powder form twice daily on an empty stomach. Treatment lasted for 3 to 5 days, with patients showing marked improvement. The herb was prepared by removing the outer shells, and crushing the inside seeds into powder. *Nan Gua Zi* was ineffective if dry-fried or cooked.[5]

TOXICOLOGY

No significant side effects were observed in mice following oral administration of *Nan Gua Zi* at the dosage of 2 to 10 g/kg.[6]

References

1. *Chang Yong Zhong Yao Xian Dai Yan Jiu Yu Lin Chuan* (Recent Study & Clinical Application of Common Traditional Chinese Medicine), 1995; 347:348
2. *Xian Dai Zhong Yao Yao Li Xue* (Contemporary Pharmacology of Chinese Herbs), 1997; 700
3. *Zhong Yao Xue* (Chinese Herbology), 1998; 451:452
4. *Zhong Hua Ji Sheng Chong Chuan Ran Bing Za Zhi* (Chinese Journal of Infectious Parasitic Diseases), 1958; 3:188
5. *Zhong Yi Za Zhi* (Journal of Chinese Medicine), 1966; 3:25
6. *Chang Yong Zhong Yao Xian Dai Yan Jiu Yu Lin Chuan* (Recent Study & Clinical Application of Common Traditional Chinese Medicine), 1995; 347:348

Fei Zi (Semen Torreyae)

榧子

Pinyin Name: *Fei Zi*
Alternate Chinese Names: *Bi Zi, Xie Shi, Xiang Fei Zi*
Original Source: *Shen Nong Ben Cao Jing* (Divine Husbandman's Classic of the Materia Medica) in the second century
English Name: torreya seeds, grand torreya seed, Chinese torreya seed, tall torreya seed
Botanical Name: *Torreya grandis* Fort. (*Fei Shu*)
Pharmaceutical Name: Semen Torreyae
Properties: sweet, neutral
Channels Entered: Lung, Large Intestine

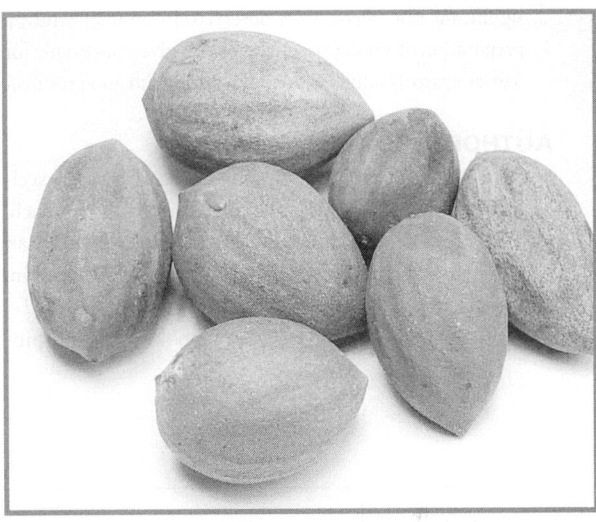

CHINESE THERAPEUTIC ACTIONS

1. Kills Parasites

Fei Zi (Semen Torreyae) is one of the most important herbs for treatment of parasites. It kills parasites, purges them from the intestines, and does not injure the stomach. Furthermore, it is sweet and encourages patient compliance. It may be used individually or in an herbal formula; it may either be used fresh or in decoction; and it is effective against a variety of intestinal parasites, including roundworm, tapeworm, hookworm and pinworm.

- Tapeworm proglottid: use *Fei Zi* as a single herb. Bake the herb and take seven seeds daily for seven days.
- Tapeworm: use it with *Bing Lang* (Semen Arecae) and *Wu Yi* (Fructus Ulmi Praeparatus). It is commonly recommended that the patient ingest beef before taking the herbs, to bait and kill the tapeworms.
- Hookworm: take 30 to 40 seeds of *Fei Zi* in the morning on an empty stomach, daily, until hookworms are expelled from the body.
- Parasitic infestation with roundworm, tapeworm, hookworm or pinworm: combine this herb with *Shi Jun Zi* (Fructus Quisqualis) and *Da Suan* (Bulbus Alli Sativi) as a decoction, three times daily on an empty stomach.

2. Moistens the Lung and Large Intestine, Stops Cough

Oily in nature, *Fei Zi* moistens the Lung and Large Intestine. Clinically, it treats dryness of the Lung characterized by dry, non-productive cough, or cough with thick, scanty sputum. It also promotes bowel movement and relieves constipation.

- Cough from Lung dryness: use *Fei Zi* with *Xuan Shen* (Radix Scrophulariae), *Sha Shen* (Radix Glehniae seu Adenophorae), *Mai Men Dong* (Radix Ophiopogonis), *E Jiao* (Colla Corii Asini) and *Sang Ye* (Folium Mori).
- Constipation due to dryness of the Large Intestine: combine it with *Huo Ma Ren* (Fructus Cannabis), *Hei Zhi Ma* (Semen Sesami Nigrum), *Yu Li Ren* (Semen Pruni) and *Dang Gui* (Radicis Angelicae Sinensis).

DOSAGE

30 to 50 grams. Dry fry *Fei Zi* and remove the shell to eat the fruit inside. *Fei Zi* should be crushed prior to cooking to increase surface area and facilitate the extraction of active constituents.

CAUTIONS / CONTRAINDICATIONS

- The outer peel of *Fei Zi* is incompatible with *Lu Dou* (Semen Phaseoli Radiati).
- *Fei Zi* is contraindicated during pregnancy as it may cause contraction of the uterus.[1]
- Overdose may cause diarrhea.

CHEMICAL COMPOSITION

Gliadin, sterol, palmitic acid, linoleic acid, stearic acid, oleic acid, oxalic acid, tannin.[2]

PHARMACOLOGICAL EFFECTS

- **Antiparasitic:** Extract of *Fei Zi* has demonstrated antiparasitic effects against tapeworm in cats and roundworm in pigs. The essential oil was effective against hookworm.[3]
- **Abortifacient:** Administration of *Fei Zi* is associated with uterine contractions. Overdose may lead to miscarriage.[4]

CLINICAL STUDIES AND RESEARCH

- **Hookworm:** Five patients with hookworm ingested 90 to 150 grams of dry-fried *Fei Zi* daily for 1 month, with a 100% success rate in eliminating the infestation.[5] No

Fei Zi (Semen Torreyae)

significant side effects were observed. In another study, a preparation of *Fei Zi* (essential oils) was given once daily for 3 to 4 days to 94 adults with hookworms, with good results.[6]

AUTHORS' COMMENTS

Both *Fei Zi* and *Shi Jun Zi* (Fructus Quisqualis) have excellent abilities to kill parasites without injuring the stomach. They are sweet and thus more tolerable for patients than bitter substances. Because they both promote defecation, there is no need to add purgative herbs to the formula. *Fei Zi* is more effective for tapeworm, hookworm, and pinworm and moistens the Lung to relieve dry cough; *Shi Jun Zi* is more effective for roundworm, and functions to strengthen the Spleen and Stomach.

References

1. *Zhong Yao Xue* (Chinese Herbology), 1998; 456:458
2. *Xian Dai Zhong Yao Yao Li Xue* (Contemporary Pharmacology of Chinese Herbs), 1997; 731
3. *Zhong Yao Zhi* (Chinese Herbology Journal), 1984; 657
4. *Zhong Yao Xue* (Chinese Herbology), 1998; 456:458
5. *Ha Yi Da Xue Bao* (Journal of Ha Medical University), 1957; 1:73
6. *Zhong Ji Yi Kan* (Medium Medical Journal), 1959; 5:18

He Shi (Fructus Carpesii)

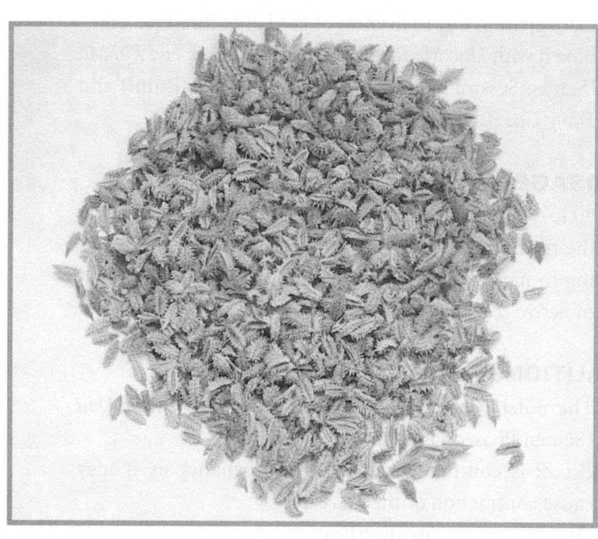

鶴虱 鹤虱

Pinyin Name: *He Shi*
Literal Name: "crane's louse"
Alternate Chinese Names: *Gui Shi, Hu Shi*
Original Source: *Xin Xiu Ben Cao* (Newly Revised Materia Medica) by Su Jing in 657-659 A.D.
English Name: carpesium fruit, common carpesium fruit
Botanical Name: *Carpesium abrotanoides* L. (*Bei He Shi*); *Daucus carota* L. (*Nan He Shi*); *Torilis japonica* (Houtt.) DC. (*Hua Nan He Shi*); *Lappula echinata* Gilib. (*Dong Bei He Shi*)
Pharmaceutical Name: Fructus Carpesii
Properties: bitter, acrid, neutral
Channels Entered: Spleen, Stomach
Safety Index: slightly toxic

CHINESE THERAPEUTIC ACTIONS

Kills Parasites

He Shi (Fructus Carpesii) kills numerous intestinal parasites, such as roundworm, pinworm, hookworm, and tapeworm.

- Abdominal pain from intestinal parasites: use *He Shi* as a single remedy.
- Roundworm: use it with *Chuan Lian Zi* (Fructus Toosendan), *Bing Lang* (Semen Arecae), and *Ming Fan* (Alumen).
- Tapeworm: combine it with *Bing Lang* (Semen Arecae), *Nan Gua Zi* (Semen Cucurbitae Moschatae), and *Lei Wan* (Omphalia).

DOSAGE

5 to 15 grams in decoction, pill or powder form.

OVERDOSAGE

He Shi is slightly toxic. Reactions such as dizziness, nausea, tinnitus, and abdominal pain generally occur within the first few hours, or the next day, following oral ingestion. These reactions are self-limiting and will subside within a short period of time after discontinuation of the herb.

CHEMICAL COMPOSITION

Essential oils 0.25 to 0.65% (carabrone, carpe-sia-lactone).[1]

He Shi (Fructus Carpesii)

PHARMACOLOGICAL EFFECTS

- **Antiparasitic:** According to *in vitro* studies, preparations of *He Shi* were effective against roundworms and tapeworms.[2]

CLINICAL STUDIES AND RESEARCH

- **Hookworm:** In one study, 57 patients with hookworm were treated effectively using an herbal decoction. The treatment protocol was to wash and cook 90 grams of *He Shi* two times to yield 60 ml of final decoction. A small amount of sugar was added to the decoction. Patients were instructed to drink 30 ml at bedtime for 2 days. The dosage was adjusted appropriately for children and elderly patients. Stool exam for hookworms was negative in 45 out of 57 patients who returned for follow-up exams 15 days later. Some patients reported side effects, such as dizziness, nausea, tinnitus, and abdominal pain. The side effects were self-limiting and were relieved upon discontinuation of the herb.[3]

References

1. *Xian Dai Zhong Yao Yao Li Xue* (Contemporary Pharmacology of Chinese Herbs), 1997; 719-720
2. *Zhong Yao Da Ci Dien* (Dictionary of Chinese Herbs), 1977; 2629
3. *Xin Yi Yao Tong Xun* (Journal of New Medicine and Herbology), 1972; 5:45

Wu Yi (Fructus Ulmi Praeparatus)

蕪荑 芜荑

Pinyin Name: *Wu Yi*
Alternate Chinese Names: *Bai Wu Yi, Chou Wu Yi*
Original Source: *Shen Nong Ben Cao Jing* (Divine Husbandman's Classic of the Materia Medica) in the second century
English Name: ulmus
Botanical Name: *Ulmus macroparpa* Hance. (*Da Guo Yu*)
Pharmaceutical Name: Fructus Ulmi Praeparatus
Properties: acrid, bitter, warm
Channels Entered: Spleen, Stomach

CHINESE THERAPEUTIC ACTIONS

Kills Parasites and Reduces Stagnation

Wu Yi (Fructus Ulmi Praeparatus) kills various intestinal parasites. It may be used individually, or in combination with other herbs. Clinical applications include treatment of roundworm, tapeworm, tinea infection, and malnutrition caused by parasitic infestation.

- General parasitic infestation: use *Wu Yi* with *Ku Lian Pi* (Cortex Meliae), *Shi Jun Zi* (Fructus Quisqualis), *Bing Lang* (Semen Arecae), *Lei Wan* (Omphalia) and *He Shi* (Fructus Carpesii).
- Intestinal parasitic infestation with pale/sallow facial appearance and abdominal pain when eating: use *Wu Yi* individually.
- Roundworm infestation with severe pain and vomiting of clear fluids or saliva: use it with *Lei Wan* (Omphalia) and *Gan Qi* (Resina Toxicodendri), as powder, with warm water.
- Parasitic infestation with prolapse of rectum: combine this herb with *Huang Lian* (Rhizoma Coptidis).
- Parasitic infestation with cold in the abdomen: use this herb with *Da Hui Xiang* (Fructus Anisi Stellati) and *Mu Xiang* (Radix Aucklandiae).
- Parasitic infestation with malnutrition, sallow facial appearance, or constant diarrhea: use *Wu Yi* with *Bai Zhu* (Rhizoma Atractylodis Macrocephalae), *Ji Nei Jin* (Endothelium Corneum Gigeriae Galli), *Mu Xiang* (Radix Aucklandiae) and *Shan Yao* (Rhizoma Dioscoreae).

DOSAGE

3 to 10 grams in pills.

CAUTIONS / CONTRAINDICATIONS

- *Wu Yi* is contraindicated for patients who have Spleen and Stomach deficiencies.

PHARMACOLOGICAL EFFECTS

- **Antiparasitic:** Extract of *Wu Yi* kills roundworms in pigs.[1]
- **Antifungal:** Extract of *Wu Yi* inhibits the growth of many pathogenic fungi.[2]

References

1. *Zhong Yao Xue* (Chinese Herbology), 1998; 458:459
2. Ibid

Lei Wan (Omphalia)

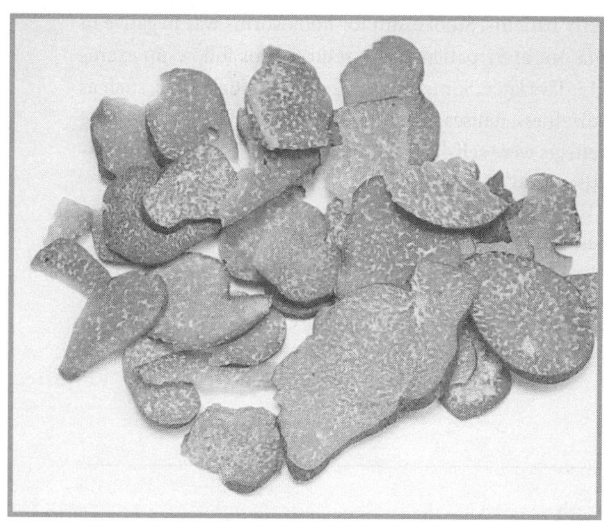

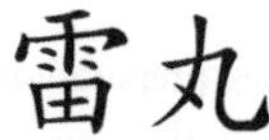

雷丸

Pinyin Name: *Lei Wan*
Literal Name: "thunder ball"
Alternate Chinese Names: *Lei Shi, Bai Lei Wan, Zhu Ling*
Original Source: *Shen Nong Ben Cao Jing* (Divine Husbandman's Classic of the Materia Medica) in the second century
English Name: omphalia, stone-like omphalia
Botanical Name: *Omphalia lapidescens* Schhroet. (*Zhen Jun Lei Wan*); *Polyporus mylittae* Cook. et Mass. (*Lei Wan Jun*)
Pharmaceutical Name: Omphalia
Properties: bitter, cold
Channels Entered: Stomach, Large Intestine
Safety Index: slightly toxic

CHINESE THERAPEUTIC ACTIONS

Kills Parasites

Lei Wan (Omphalia) effectively kills intestinal parasites, including tapeworm, hookworm, and roundworm. It may be used individually, or in combination with other herbs.

- Intestinal parasites: use *Lei Wan* with *Bing Lang* (Semen Arecae), *Qian Niu Zi* (Semen Pharbitidis), *Mu Xiang* (Radix Aucklandiae), and *Ku Lian Pi* (Cortex Meliae).
- Parasitic infestation with malnutrition: combine it with *Shi Jun Zi* (Fructus Quisqualis), *He Shi* (Fructus Carpesii), *Bing Lang* (Semen Arecae) and *Fei Zi* (Semen Torreyae), as powder, taken before meals with warm rice water.

DOSAGE

6 to 15 grams. It is best to use *Lei Wan* in pill or powder form, as heat may decrease the effectiveness of the herb. The recommended therapy is 12 to 18 grams with rice water, three times daily after meals, for 3 days.

CAUTIONS / CONTRAINDICATIONS

- *Lei Wan* should be used with caution for patients with deficiency and cold of the Spleen and Stomach. Side effects, such as nausea and abdominal discomfort, are generally self-limiting and do not require treatment.[1]
- Heat (greater than 60° C) and acidity deactivate *Lei Wan*. Therefore, it should not be cooked in decoctions. For enhanced effectiveness, it may be taken with an alkaline solution (such as rice water) to neutralize gastric acid.[2]

CHEMICAL COMPOSITION

Proteolytic enzyme, β-glucan.[3]

PHARMACOLOGICAL EFFECTS

- **Antiparasitic (tapeworm):** Tapeworms were placed into three environments at 37° C: 30% *Lei Wan* solution, normal saline, and distilled water. In the *Lei Wan* solution, all tapeworms died in between 2.5 and 9 hours. In normal saline, all tapeworms appeared normal after 9 hours, and continued to live for up to 62 hours. In distilled water, tapeworms lived for 24 to 30 hours. It was also noted that *Lei Wan* solution was most effective at pH 8, and was ineffective in an acidic environment.[4]
- **Antiparasitic (roundworm):** In *in vitro* studies, alcohol extract of *Lei Wan* showed a marked inhibitory influence against roundworms while the water extract was ineffective. The ineffectiveness of the water extract was attributed to destruction of the active constituents when the substance was cooked at high temperatures.[5]

CLINICAL STUDIES AND RESEARCH

- **Tapeworm infestation:** Patients with tapeworm infestations were effectively treated using 20 grams of *Lei Wan* powder with cool water, three times daily, for 3 days.[6]
- **Hookworm infestation:** In one study, 20 patients with hookworm infestations were treated with an 85% rate of effectiveness using 40 grams of *Lei Wan* powder each day for 3 days.[7] In another study, 188 patients were treated with 100% effectiveness with an herbal formula which contained 3.2 grams of *Lei Wan*, 11.2 grams of *Da Huang* (Radix et Rhizoma Rhei) and 11.2 grams of *Qian Niu Zi* (Semen Pharbitidis). The herbal formulas were given as powder daily in the morning, on an empty stomach with cold water. Hookworms were expelled by all patients within 1 to 2 doses.[8]

Lei Wan (Omphalia)

References

1. *Zhong Yao Yao Li Yu Ying Yong* (Pharmacology and Applications of Chinese Herbs), 1983; 1184
2. Ibid.
3. *Xian Dai Zhong Yao Yao Li Xue* (Contemporary Pharmacology of Chinese Herbs), 1997; 724
4. *Zhong Yao Yao Li Yu Ying Yong* (Pharmacology and Applications of Chinese Herbs), 1983; 1184
5. Ibid.
6. *Zhong Hua Yi Xue Za Zhi* (Chinese Journal of Medicine), 1956; 6:556
7. *Shang Hai Zhong Yi Yao Za Zhi* (Shanghai Journal of Chinese Medicine and Herbology), 1957; 5:22
8. *Zhong Ji Yi Kan* (Medium Medical Journal), 1960; 7:35

He Cao Ya (Gemma Agrimoniae)

鶴草芽 鹤草芽

Pinyin Name: *He Cao Ya*
Literal Name: "crane herb bud"
Alternate Chinese Names: *Lang Ya Cao Gen Ya, Xian He Cao Gen Ya*
English Name: agrimonia, hairy-vein agrimonia bud
Botanical Name: *Agrimonia pilosa* Ledeb. (*Xian He Cao; Long Ya Cao*)
Pharmaceutical Name: Gemma Agrimoniae
Properties: bitter, astringent, cool
Channels Entered: Liver, Small Intestine, Large Intestine

CHINESE THERAPEUTIC ACTIONS

Kills Parasites

He Cao Ya (Gemma Agrimoniae) kills parasites and promotes bowel movement. It is generally used in powder form against tapeworms. *He Cao Ya* is also used with other herbs to treat trichomonas vaginalis.

DOSAGE

30 to 50 grams in powder for adults. The dosage should be calculated carefully in children: use 0.7 to 0.8 gram of *He Cao Ya* per kilogram of body weight. According to classic texts, *He Cao Ya* should not be decocted.

CAUTIONS / CONTRAINDICATIONS

- In comparison with other antiparasitic herbs, *He Cao Ya* is a safe herb that has few or no toxic effects. However, mild gastrointestinal disturbances, such as nausea and vomiting, may still occur following oral ingestion.

CHEMICAL COMPOSITION

Phenolic compounds.[1]

TOXICOLOGY

The LD_{50} for oral ingestion of phenolic compounds of *He Cao Ya* in mice is 599.8 mg/kg.[2]

References

1. *Xian Dai Zhong Yao Yao Li Xue* (Contemporary Pharmacology of Chinese Herbs), 1997; 717
2. *Zhong Cao Yao Tong Xun* (Journal of Chinese Herbal Medicine), 1978; 9(1):32

Guan Zhong (Rhizoma Dryopteridis)

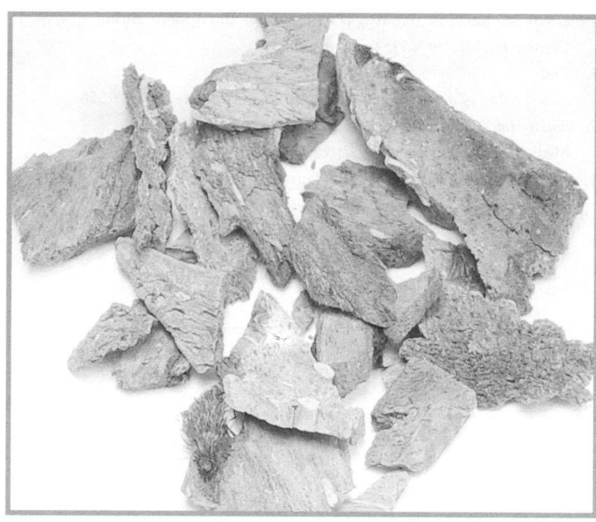

貫衆 贯众

Pinyin Name: *Guan Zhong*
Literal Name: "link the multitude"
Alternate Chinese Names: *Guan Jie*
Original Source: *Shen Nong Ben Cao Jing* (Divine Husbandman's Classic of the Materia Medica) in the second century
English Name: dryopteris root
Botanical Name: *Dryopteris crassirhizoma* Nakai. (*Cu Jing Lin Mao Jue*). Other sources include *Lunathyrium acrostichoides* (Sw.) Ching (*E Mei Jue*); *Woodwardia unigemmata* (Makino) Nakai. (*Dan Ya Gou Ji*); and *Osmunda japonica* Thunb. (*Zi Ji*)
Pharmaceutical Name: Rhizoma Dryopteridis
Properties: bitter, cool
Channels Entered: Liver, Spleen
Safety Index: slightly toxic

CHINESE THERAPEUTIC ACTIONS

1. Kills Parasites

Guan Zhong (Rhizoma Dryopteridis) effectively kills various intestinal parasites, such as hookworm, pinworm and ringworm. It is generally used in an herbal combination formula, and rarely by itself.

- Parasitic infestation: use *Guan Zhong* with *Lei Wan* (Omphalia), *Bing Lang* (Semen Arecae), *Wu Yi* (Fructus Ulmi Praeparatus), *He Shi* (Fructus Carpesii), and *Shi Jun Zi* (Fructus Quisqualis).

2. Clears Heat, Removes Toxins

Bitter and cold, *Guan Zhong* clears heat and eliminates toxins to treat and prevent viral and bacterial infections. Clinical applications include the common cold, influenza, measles, epidemic encephalitis, parotitis, and viral pneumonia.

- Prevention of common colds and influenza: use this herb with *Sang Ye* (Folium Mori).
- Treatment of viral infection, parotitis, infectious bronchitis: combine it with *Jin Yin Hua* (Flos Lonicerae), *Ban Lan Gen* (Radix Isatidis), *Da Qing Ye* (Folium Isatidis) and *Lian Qiao* (Fructus Forsythiae).

3. Stops Bleeding

Charred *Guan Zhong* clears heat and stops bleeding. It is commonly used to treat bleeding characterized by heat in the blood, such as hematemesis, epistaxis, hematochezia, and profuse uterine bleeding.

- Epistaxis: use *Guan Zhong* powder alone.
- Bleeding in postpartum women: ingest 6 grams of vinegar-processed *Guan Zhong* with rice water.
- Hematemesis: use powdered *Guan Zhong* with *Huang Lian* (Rhizoma Coptidis), serve with sticky rice.
- Severe and persistent hematemesis: combine it with *Xue Yu Tan* (Crinis Carbonisatus), the juice of fresh *Ce Bai Ye* (Cacumen Platycladi), *Tong Bian* (urine from children) and grain-based liquor.
- Hematochezia due to lower gastrointestinal bleeding: use this herb with *She Xiang* (Moschus).
- Uterine bleeding that is purple, with blood clots, abdominal pain and a deep pulse: use it with *Wu Ling Zhi* (Excrementum Trogopteri seu Pteromi).

DOSAGE

10 to 15 grams. Unprocessed *Guan Zhong* is used to clear heat, eliminate toxins, and kill parasites. The charred form stops bleeding.

CAUTIONS / CONTRAINDICATIONS

- *Guan Zhong* is not recommended for use in cases of yin-deficient heat, or in deficiency and cold of the Spleen and Stomach.
- Avoid concurrent ingestion of *Guan Zhong* with fatty or greasy food.
- *Guan Zhong* is slightly toxic, and its use is contraindicated in infants, and those who have weak constitutions, or ulceration of the gastrointestinal tract.
- *Guan Zhong* should be used with caution during pregnancy, as it is slightly toxic and also stimulates the contraction of uterus.

Guan Zhong (Rhizoma Dryopteridis)

OVERDOSAGE

Adverse reactions reported include nausea, vomiting, abdominal pain, diarrhea, hematochezia, headache, tremor, seizures, and miscarriage. Filmarone, one of the components of *Guan Zhong*, has a poor absorption rate and is responsible for gastrointestinal irritation. Ingestion of *Guan Zhong* with fatty or greasy food increases the absorption rate and may cause disturbance to the central nervous system.[1]

CHEMICAL COMPOSITION

Filmarone, dryocrassin, filic acids, flavaspidic acids, fibaspidins, aspidinol, filicinic acid, ferene, diploptene, diplopterol.[2]

PHARMACOLOGICAL EFFECTS

- **Antiparasitic:** Filmarone, one active component of *Guan Zhong*, has a marked antiparasitic effect against tapeworm. In *in vitro* studies, a preparation of *Guan Zhong* was effective against roundworms in pigs. Decoction of *Guan Zhong* was effective against liver flukes.[3]
- **Antibiotic:** *Guan Zhong* has a mild to moderate inhibitory action against *Bacillus dysenteriae, Salmonella typhi, E. coli, Pseudomonas aeruginosa, Diplococcus meningitidis,* and *Staphylococcus aureus*. It has a strong inhibiting influence on influenza virus, adenovirus, encephalitis B, and herpes simplex virus. It also has an antineoplastic effect.[4]
- **Uterine stimulant:** Decoction of *Guan Zhong* is associated with contraction of the uterus. It increases both the frequency and strength of uterine contractions in rabbits. Similar characteristics were observed in use of the alcohol extract.[5]

CLINICAL STUDIES AND RESEARCH

- **Common colds and influenza:** Through observation of over 1,000 cases, the decoction of *Guan Zhong* and *Sang Ye* (Folium Mori) given twice weekly was found effective in prevention of common colds and influenza.[6]
- **Cerebrospinal meningitis:** To prevent cerebrospinal meningitis during an epidemic, the powder of *Guan Zhong* was given once a week for 2 weeks as one course of treatment. The treatment protocol was to administer 2 grams of the herb to adults, 1 gram to children under 10 years of age, and 0.5 gram to infants under 1 year of age. Out of 28 cases, the study concluded that the preventative effect of *Guan Zhong* was similar to that of penicillin.[7] [Note: Penicillin was an effective antibiotic in China in the 1960s, when there was still little or no bacterial resistance.]
- **Hookworm:** In one study, 30 patients with hookworm infestations were treated with 8 to 15 grams of *Guan Zhong* powder twice daily for 5 to 7 days per course of treatment. Six months later, 26 patients who returned for follow-up tested negative for hookworm. Four patients did not return for follow-up tests.[8]
- **Intestinal parasitic infestation:** In one report, 262 patients with intestinal parasitic infestations, such as hookworm, roundworm and whipworm, were treated with a preparation of *Guan Zhong* (equivalent to 25 grams of herb) daily for 2 days, with marked effectiveness.[9]
- **Acute orchitis:** Decoctions of *Guan Zhong* were used with good results in treating 45 patients with acute orchitis. The treatment protocol was to cook 60 grams of the herb in water, and drink the decoction in two equally-divided doses daily. The duration of treatment was between 3 and 5 days.[10]
- **Uterine bleeding:** In one report, 15 women with profuse uterine bleeding after abortion or delivery were treated with 2 to 4 ml of intramuscular injection of *Guan Zhong* solution (each 2 ml contains 5 grams of dried herb). The study reported 100% effectiveness with contraction of the uterus, and diminished bleeding within 3 to 5 minutes.[11]

TOXICOLOGY

The LD_{50} for filmarone in mice via intraperitoneal injection is 34 ml/kg.[12]

References

1. *Zhong Yao Xue* (Chinese Herbology), 1998; 459:462
2. *Xian Dai Zhong Yao Yao Li Xue* (Contemporary Pharmacology of Chinese Herbs), 1997; 736
3. *Chang Yong Zhong Yao Xian Dai Yan Jiu Yu Lin Chuan* (Recent Study & Clinical Application of Common Traditional Chinese Medicine), 1995; 351:353
4. *Zhong Yao Xue* (Chinese Herbology), 1998; 459:462
5. *Chang Yong Zhong Yao Xian Dai Yan Jiu Yu Lin Chuan* (Recent Study & Clinical Application of Common Traditional Chinese Medicine), 1995; 351:353
6. *Zhong Cao Yao Tong Xun* (Journal of Chinese Herbal Medicine), 1973; 6:40
7. *Jiang Xi Yi Yao* (Jiangxi Medicine and Herbology), 1962; 1:8
8. *Zhong Yi Han Shou Tong Xun* (Reports of Chinese Medicine), 1987; 6:38
9. *Jiang Su Zhong Yi* (Jiangsu Chinese Medicine), 1962; 10:14
10. *Zhong Yi Za Zhi* (Journal of Chinese Medicine), 1981; 8:13
11. *Zhong Cao Yao Tong Xun* (Journal of Chinese Herbal Medicine), 1970; 5,6:35
12. *Chang Yong Zhong Yao Xian Dai Yan Jiu Yu Lin Chuan* (Recent Study & Clinical Application of Common Traditional Chinese Medicine), 1995; 351:353

Chapter 10 summary — Antiparasitic Herbs

Name	Similarities				Differences
	Round-Worm	Tape-Worm	Hook-Worm	Others	
Shi Jun Zi (Fructus Quisqualis)	x			Pinworm, trichomonas	Lubricates the intestines
Ku Lian Pi (Cortex Meliae)	x		x	Pinworm, trichomonas	Kills tinea
Bing Lang (Semen Arecae)	x	x		Pinworm, fasciolopsis, blood flukes	Promotes movement of qi
Nan Gua Zi (Semen Cucurbitae Moschatae)	x	x		Schistomiasis	Promotes lactation
Fei Zi (Semen Torreyae)		x	x	Pinworm	Moistens the bowel
He Shi (Fructus Carpesii)	x	x	x	Pinworm	
Wu Yi (Fructus Ulmi Praeparatus)	x	x			Kills tinea
Lei Wan (Omphalia)	x	x	x		
He Cao Ya (Gemma Agrimoniae)		x		Trichomonas	
Guan Zhong (Rhizoma Dryopteridis)			x	Pinworm, ringworm	Clears heat and toxins, stops bleeding

General Characteristics of Antiparasitic Herbs:

Taste: varies
Thermal property: varies
Channels entered: Spleen, Stomach, Large Intestine
Therapeutic actions: kills internal and external parasites
Safety index: some are toxic

Herbs that expel parasites are mainly used to kill intestinal parasites, with some being effective for dermatological disorders such as tinea.

Shi Jun Zi (Fructus Quisqualis) is warm, and kills parasites, especially roundworms and tapeworms. It strengthens the middle *jiao* and reduces stagnation. Sweet and aromatic, this is the herb of choice for children with parasites or malnutrition, as the taste improves patient compliance. *Shi Jun Zi* is effective as a single-herb remedy because it has both antiparasitic and purgative effects. Serving the herb with hot tea or in large dosages are both contraindicated to avoid side effects such as nausea, dizziness, vomiting and diarrhea.

Ku Lian Pi (Cortex Meliae), cold and toxic, is stronger than *Shi Jun Zi* to kill internal and external parasites. It is contraindicated in patients with deficiency and cold of the Spleen and Stomach.

Bing Lang (Semen Arecae) is warm and most effective against tapeworm, but also treats roundworm, fasciolopsis, and blood flukes. Dispelling dampness, it reduces abdominal distention from food and qi stagnation, and relieves feelings of incomplete evacuation. *Bing Lang* is also used for edema and leg *qi*.

Nan Gua Zi (Semen Cucurbitae Moschatae), sweet and neutral, dispels parasites without injuring the body. It is most suitable for deficient patients. *Nan Gua Zi* should never be cooked or fried, as

Chapter 10 summary

heat significantly decreases its effectiveness. The combination of *Nan Gua Zi* and *Bing Lang* (Semen Arecae) is very effective to treat pinworms.

Fei Zi (Semen Torreyae), sweet and neutral, is not toxic. It is a safe herb, but has only mild potency to kill and dispel parasites. Because it is rich in oil, this herb also treats constipation.

He Shi (Fructus Carpesii), slightly toxic, relieves abdominal pain caused by parasites.

Wu Yi (Fructus Ulmi Praeparatus) is warm in thermal property, kills parasites and treats abdominal pain and diarrhea.

Lei Wan (Omphalia) and ***He Cao Ya*** (Gemma Agrimoniae) kill parasites, and have active components that are destroyed by heat, and thus should be taken in pill or powder form.

Lei Wan is slightly toxic, but has a broad spectrum of antiparasitic action against all kinds of intestinal parasites.

He Cao Ya is not toxic, and is most effective against tapeworms.

Guan Zhong (Rhizoma Dryopteridis), cool in thermal property, kills parasites and clears heat to eliminate toxins. It treats infectious diseases such as parasites, measles, flu and encephalitis. Charred to ash, this herb stops hematemesis, epistaxis, uterine bleeding and rectal bleeding.

HERBS FROM OTHER FUNCTIONAL CATEGORIES WITH ANTIPARASITIC FUNCTIONS

Name	Functional Category
Bai Bu (Radix Stemonae)	Phlegm-Resolving and Coughing- and Wheezing-Relieving Herbs (Chapter 13)
Chuan Lian Zi (Fructus Toosendan)	Qi-Regulating Herbs (Chapter 8)
Chun Gen Pi (Cortex Ailanthi)	Astringent Herbs (Chapter 18)
Cong Bai (Bulbus Allii Fistulosi)	Exterior-Releasing Herbs (Chapter 1)
Gan Qi (Resina Toxicodendri)	Blood-Invigorating and Stasis-Removing Herbs (Chapter 12)
Qian Niu Zi (Semen Pharbitidis)	Downward Draining Herbs (Chapter 3)
Shi Liu Pi (Pericarpium Granati)	Astringent Herbs (Chapter 18)
Wu Mei (Fructus Mume)	Astringent Herbs (Chapter 18)
Xiong Huang (Realgar)	Substances for Topical Application (Chapter 20)

Chapter 11

— Stop-Bleeding Herbs

止血药

Chapter 11 — Stop-Bleeding Herbs

Chapter 11

止血药 — Stop-Bleeding Herbs

Definition: These herbs stop bleeding, both internally and externally.

Bleeding occurs when normal blood flow in the vessels is interrupted by injury or leakage so that the blood leaves the vessels. Bleeding can occur in various parts of the body, including tissues, organs, channels and collaterals. Common instances of bleeding include epistaxis and hemoptysis in the upper *jiao*, hematemesis in the middle *jiao*, and hematochezia, hematuria, abnormal uterine bleeding, and bleeding hemorrhoids in the lower *jiao*. Subcutaneous bleeding results in purpura, while traumatic injury to musculoskeletal tissues causes bleeding and bruising.

SUBCATEGORIES OF ACTION

1. ***Cool the blood and stop bleeding***: Herbs in this category are cool or cold. They cool the blood, dispel heat, and stop bleeding, and are often combined with heat-clearing herbs for maximum effectiveness. Clinical manifestations of heat in the blood include bleeding of bright red blood, irritability, thirst, redness of the face, red tongue, and a slippery, rapid pulse.
2. ***Restrain blood and stop bleeding***: These herbs are bitter, astringent and neutral in thermal property. They have a restraining function and are most suitable for bleeding from deficiency, where there is continuous bleeding with fatigue, pale tongue and a weak pulse. This type of bleeding can be seen in patients who have recently suffered traumatic injuries with profuse bleeding. Deficiency bleeding usually involves the Spleen, the organ responsible for keeping blood circulating within the vessels, or the Liver, the organ responsible for storing blood. Herbs that restrain blood are often combined with tonic herbs for best results.
3. ***Invigorate blood and stop bleeding***: These herbs have a unique influence to invigorate blood circulation, eliminate blood stasis, and stop bleeding. In other words, they achieve homeostasis of the blood. These herbs are best for bleeding related to blood stagnation, in which blood cannot properly circulate within the vessels and channels. Bleeding in this case is usually dark with clots, with sharp pain in a fixed location. Qi- and blood-activating herbs are sometimes added to achieve maximum effectiveness.
4. ***Warm the body and stop bleeding***: These herbs warm the body and the channels, relieve pain, and stop bleeding. They are mostly used for patients suffering from bleeding due to deficiency and cold, characterized by chronic, pale bleeding that is light in texture. Clinical manifestations may include sallow facial complexion, a pale tongue, fatigue, cold extremities, intolerance to cold, and a thready, slow pulse. Interior-warming, qi-tonifying, Spleen-strengthening and blood-nourishing herbs are often added for best results. Note: These symptoms also would be present in an individual for whom excessive bleeding has caused deficiency and cold and has changed to chronic, light bleeding.

Bai Mao Gen (Rhizoma Imperatae)
Ben Cao Gang Mu (Materia Medica), by Li Shi-Zhen, 1578 A.D.

Differential Diagnosis of Bleeding

Subcategories	TCM Diagnosis	Key Symptoms
Cool the blood and stop bleeding	Heat in the blood	Bright red blood
Restrain blood and stop bleeding	Spleen qi or Liver deficiency	Continuous bleeding
Invigorate blood and stop bleeding	Blood stasis	Dark blood with clots, pain in a fixed location
Warm the body and stop bleeding	Deficiency and cold	Chronic, pale bleeding with light texture

Chapter 11 — Stop-Bleeding Herbs

DIFFERENTIAL DIAGNOSIS AND TREATMENT

Bleeding is a *symptom* that represents an *underlying condition*. While it is important to treat symptomatically and stop the bleeding, it is equally important to identify the underlying cause and treat accordingly. ***Heat in the blood*** pushes it outwards, leading to a condition referred to as "reckless movement of blood" with bleeding from various openings of the body. Such conditions must be treated both with herbs that cool blood and herbs that stop bleeding.

Deficiency of the Spleen or the Liver may also cause bleeding. Qi is considered to be the leader that guides the movement of blood. Therefore, ***deficiency of Spleen qi*** allows bleeding and "aimless movement of blood." The Liver stores blood; therefore, ***deficiency of the Liver*** compromises its ability to store blood, allowing blood to leak out of the body. Bleeding due to deficiency of the Spleen and Liver must be treated with herbs that stop bleeding and tonify these organs.

~

Bleeding is a symptom. ...While it is important to stop the bleeding, it is equally important to identify and treat the underlying cause.

~

In addition to treating the symptoms and cause of a bleeding disorder, one must recognize that blood loss is often accompanied by complications. Bleeding due to trauma is often accompanied by ***qi and blood stagnation***. While the use of hemostatic herbs stops bleeding, it also causes more qi and blood stasis. Therefore, optimal treatment requires concurrent use of herbs that stop bleeding with herbs that activate qi and blood circulation. Prolonged or profuse bleeding may lead to ***deficiency and cold*** (as well as vice-versa, mentioned in #4, above), in which case qi tonic herbs are indicated to prevent qi collapse.

CAUTIONS/CONTRAINDICATIONS

- When using herbs that are cool or astringent in property, one should first rule out the possibility of blood stagnation to avoid making the situation worse.
- If blood stagnation is present, blood-activating herbs should be used to stop bleeding and remove stasis at the same time.
- If profuse bleeding occurs over a long period of time, instead of using only herbs from this category, qi tonics should also be added to prevent collapse.

PROCESSING

Many herbs are charred to ash to enhance their potency to stop bleeding.

PHARMACOLOGICAL EFFECTS

- **Hemostatic**: These herbs shorten coagulation and clotting time to stop bleeding.

  Herbs that affect earlier steps of the clotting cascade to facilitate clotting include *San Qi* (Radix Notoginseng), *Pu Huang* (Pollen Typhae), *Bai Ji* (Rhizoma Bletillae), *Xian He Cao* (Herba Agrimoniae) and *Bai Mao Gen* (Rhizoma Imperatae).

  Herbs that affect later steps of the clotting cascade are *Bai Ji* (Rhizoma Bletillae), *Di Yu* (Radix Sanguisorbae), *Ai Ye* (Folium Artemisiae Argyi), *Da Ji* (Herba seu Radix Cirsii Japonici), *Xiao Ji* (Herba Cirisii) and *Fu Long Gan* (Terra Flava Usta).

  Herbs that increase the number of platelets include *Zi Zhu* (Folium Callicarpae).

~

Charring herbs to ash enhances potency to stop bleeding.

~

- **Hematological**: While most herbs that stop bleeding have a marked hemostatic effect, some have a more dynamic effect on the chemistry of blood. Herbs such as *San Qi* (Radix Notoginseng), *Pu Huang* (Pollen Typhae) and *Qian Cao* (Radix Rubiae) have the unique abilities to stop bleeding, dissolve blood clots and inhibit the aggregation of platelets. In other words, these herbs help to restore normal homeostasis of blood.
- **Cardiovascular**: Many of these herbs dilate blood vessels, increase blood perfusion to the coronary artery, and decrease oxygen consumption by the cardiac muscle, as exemplified by *San Qi* (Radix Notoginseng).
- **Antineoplastic**: Some inhibit the growth of cancer cells, as does *Xian He Cao* (Herba Agrimoniae).

Chapter 11 — Stop-Bleeding Herbs

- **Respiratory**: Some stop-bleeding herbs have expectorant and antiasthmatic effects, including *Ce Bai Ye* (Cacumen Platycladi) and *Ai Ye* (Folium Artemisiae Argyi).

POTENTIAL HERB-DRUG INTERACTIONS

- **Antiplatelets and anticoagulants**: Herbs that stop bleeding have inherent hemostatic effects. These herbs are generally used only when necessary to stop bleeding, and are to be discontinued when the bleeding stops. Because of their effect on the hemodynamics of circulation, these herbs should be used with caution in patients who have clotting disorders. The use of hemostatic herbs may increase the risk of clotting. Thus, these herbs should be prescribed with caution for patients taking antiplatelet or anticoagulant medications, as they may counteract the beneficial effect of such medications.

Da Ji (Herba seu Radix Cirsii Japonici)

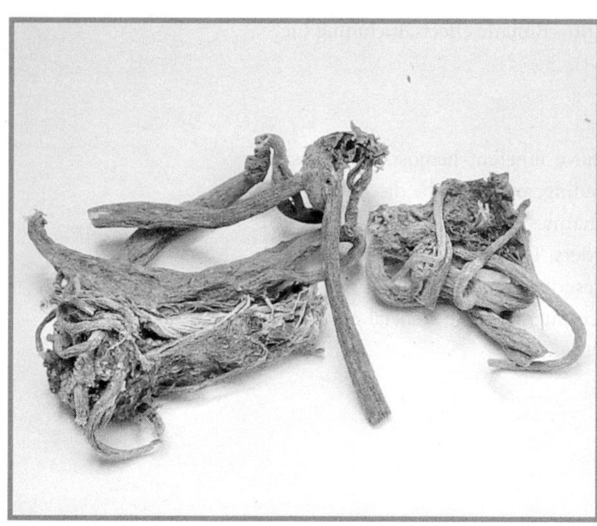

大蓟 大薊

Pinyin Name: *Da Ji*
Literal Name: "big thistle"
Alternate Chinese Names: *Hu Ji, Ma Ji*
Original Source: *Ming Yi Za Zhu* (Miscellaneous Records of Famous Physicians) by Tao Hong-Jing in 500 A.D.
English Name: cirsium, Japanese thistle
Botanical Name: *Cirsium japonicum* DC. (*Ji*)
Pharmaceutical Name: Herba seu Radix Cirsii Japonici
Properties: sweet, bitter, cool
Channels Entered: Liver, Heart

CHINESE THERAPEUTIC ACTIONS

1. Cools Blood, Stops Bleeding

Da Ji (Herba seu Radix Cirsii Japonici) treats various types of bleeding caused by heat in the blood, including hemoptysis, epistaxis, metrorrhagia, and hematuria. In this type of bleeding, the blood appears bright red in color, because of heat. Fresh *Da Ji* has the strongest action to cool blood and stop bleeding. Charred *Da Ji* has a stronger astringent and restraining property to enter the *xue* (blood) level in order to stop bleeding.

- Hematemesis, epistaxis, profuse menstrual bleeding: use the juice from the fresh form of this herb individually.
- Hematemesis: use it with *Sheng Di Huang* (Radix Rehmanniae), *Sheng Jiang* (Rhizoma Zingiberis Recens), and light-colored honey.
- Hematemesis and hemoptysis: use the charred forms of *Da Ji*, *Xiao Ji* (Herba Cirisii), *Ce Bai Ye* (Cacumen Platycladi), *Bai Mao Gen* (Rhizoma Imperatae), and *Qian Cao* (Radix Rubiae).

2. Disperses Blood Stasis, Reduces Swelling

Abscess and toxic swelling: *Da Ji* treats abscess, whether internally or on the skin. Swelling and abscess are caused by toxicity and blood stagnation. The fresh herb is preferred for stronger potency in this case. It can be used both internally and topically.

- Intestinal abscess: use the leaf of *Da Ji* in powder form, with grain-based liquor, and *Ren Zhong Bai* (Urinae Hominis Sedimen).
- Intestinal abscess and cellulitis: combine this herb with *Di Yu* (Radix Sanguisorbae), *Niu Xi* (Radix Cyathulae seu Achyranthis), *Jin Yin Hua* (Flos Lonicerae) and warm grain-based liquor.
- Lung abscess: use *Da Ji* alone.
- Sores and carbuncles: mix fresh *Da Ji* with salt and apply topically.

3. Treats Jaundice

Da Ji treats jaundice arising from damp-heat in the Liver and Gallbladder.

- Jaundice: use this herb with *Yin Chen Hao* (Herba Artemisiae Scopariae) and *Hu Zhang* (Rhizoma Polygoni Cuspidati).

4. Lowers Blood Pressure

Hypertension: *Da Ji* has been used recently to reduce blood pressure caused by Liver heat or Liver fire.

- Hypertension: use alone or with *Xia Ku Cao* (Spica Prunellae) and *Xi Xian Cao* (Herba Siegesbeckiae). The root of *Da Ji* is preferred for this function.

DOSAGE

10 to 15 grams, with a maximum of 30 grams, for dried *Da Ji*. Use up to 60 grams of the fresh form. The unprocessed herb is stronger to cool the blood, stop bleeding, and reduce swelling. The charred herb is stronger in retaining the blood and stopping bleeding. The aerial parts of the plant have stronger functions to drain abscesses, while the root has better attributes to lower blood pressure.

CAUTIONS / CONTRAINDICATIONS

- Because of its blood-invigorating function, *Da Ji* should be used with caution during pregnancy, or for patients who do not have signs or symptoms of blood stagnation.
- Bitter and cold in nature, *Da Ji* is contraindicated in deficiency and cold of the Spleen and Stomach.
- Oral administration of *Da Ji* has been associated with nausea, vomiting and other gastrointestinal disturbances.[1]

Da Ji (Herba seu Radix Cirsii Japonici)

CHEMICAL COMPOSITION

Cirsimarin, pectolinarin, luleclin-7-glucoside, acacetin rhamnoglucoside, vitamin K.[2]

PHARMACOLOGICAL EFFECTS

- **Hemostatic:** Charred *Da Ji* has demonstrated hemostatic properties, and shortens bleeding time.[3]
- **Antibiotic:** An alcohol tincture of *Da Ji* at a concentration of 1:30,000 demonstrated an inhibitory effect on *Mycobacterium tuberculosis*, based on *in vitro* tests.[4]
- **Cardiovascular:** Administration of water or alcohol extract of *Da Ji* decreased heart rate and lowered blood pressure in experiments with dogs, cats and rabbits.[5]

CLINICAL STUDIES AND RESEARCH

- **Hematuria:** According to one report, 35 patients were treated with 15 to 20 grams of *Da Ji* powder given three times daily for 2 weeks with an overall effective rate of 74.3%. The hemostatic action was assessed as being more effective than that of vitamin K.[6]
- **Upper gastrointestinal bleeding:** In one study, 369 patients with gastric ulcers, duodenal ulcers, and various other upper-gastrointestinal bleeding problems were treated with an herbal preparation containing *Da Ji*, *Ji Mu Ye* (Folium Loropetali), and *Bai Ji* (Rhizoma Bletillae) as the main ingredients. The study reported an overall effective rate of 84.3%, with an average of 5 days to achieve hemostasis.[7]
- **Hypertension:** *Da Ji Gen* (Radix Cirsii Japonici) and *Da Ji Ye* (Folium Cirsii Japonici) were used to treat patients at various stages of hypertension. Out of 72 patients treated with *Da Ji Gen*, 17 showed marked response, 45 showed moderate effects, 10 showed no response, and the overall rate of effectiveness was 86.1%. Out of 30 patients treated with *Da Ji Ye*, 5 showed marked effects, 10 showed moderate effects, 15 showed no response, and the overall rate of effectiveness was 50%.[8]
- **Intramuscular nodules:** Fibrous nodules in 500 patients were treated with an herbal paste applied to the affected area for 6 to 8 hours, one to two times daily, for an average of 3 to 5 treatments. The herbal paste contained equal amounts of *Da Ji* and starch, mixed with hot water. The study reported satisfactory results in all patients in softening of the nodules and reduction of pain.[9]
- **Pulmonary tuberculosis:** In one study, 18 patients with pulmonary tuberculosis were treated with preparations of *Da Ji*, for 15 to 72 days. Evaluation based on chest x-ray showed 3 patients with significant improvement, 8 with slight improvement and 7 with no change. Symptomatic evaluation, such as cough, chest pain, fever and amount of sputum, also showed varying degrees of improvement.[10]
- **Nephritis:** Daily administration of 15 to 30 grams of *Da Ji* has been shown to reduce edema and the quantity of white blood cells present in the urine in patients with nephritis.[11]

HERB-DRUG INTERACTION

- **Anticoagulant drugs:** *Da Ji* contains vitamin K, which may reduce the anticoagulant effect of warfarin. While use of the herb is not contraindicated, it should be used with caution to prevent the formation of clots.[12]

SUPPLEMENT

Da Ji (Herba seu Radix Cirsii Japonici) is the collective name that includes both the root and the aerial parts of the plant, though the parts have slightly different functions.

- 大薊葉 / 大蓟叶 *Da Ji Ye* (Herba Cirsii Japonici), the aerial part of the herb (primarily the leaf), drains abscesses.
- 大薊根 / 大蓟根 *Da Ji Gen* (Radix Cirsii Japonici), the root, lowers blood pressure.

AUTHORS' COMMENTS

大薊 / 大蓟 *Da Ji* (Herba seu Radix Cirsii Japonici) and 大戟 *Da Ji* (Radix Euphorbiae seu Knoxiae) have identical pinyin names, but are two distinct herbs with completely different functions. *Da Ji* (Herba seu Radix Cirsii Japonici) has hemostatic actions and stops bleeding. *Da Ji* (Radix Euphorbiae seu Knoxiae) has cathartic properties and treats excess conditions. To avoid errors and confusion, one must always specify which "*Da Ji*" is to be used, whether in written or verbal communication.

References

1. *Hu Nan Sheng Jie He Bing Yan Jiu Yuan* (Hunan Treatment and Research Center of Tuberculosis), 1971; 37
2. *Xian Dai Zhong Yao Yao Li Xue* (Contemporary Pharmacology of Chinese Herbs), 1997; 780-781
3. *Zhong Yao Xue* (Chinese Herbology), 1998; 465:466
4. *Zhong Guo Fang Lao Za Zhi* (Chinese Journal on Prevention of Tuberculosis), 1964; 5(3):481
5. *Cardiovas Res*, 1982; 16:11
6. *Zhong Hua Mi Niao Wai Ke* (Chinese Journal of Urology and External Medicine), 1982; 3(4):287
7. *Zhong Cao Yao Tong Xun* (Journal of Chinese Herbal Medicine), 1973; 2:45
8. *Zhong Cheng Yao Yan Jiu* (Research of Chinese Patent Medicine), 1982; 8:36
9. *Shi Yong Yi Xue Za Zhi* (Practical Journal of Medicine), 1985; 1(2):40
10. *Hu Nan Sheng Jie He Bing Yan Jiu Yuan* (Hunan Treatment and Research Center of Tuberculosis), 1971; 37
11. *Zhong Cao Yao Xue* (Study of Chinese Herbal Medicine), 1979; 378
12. Chen, J. Recognition & prevention of herb-drug interactions, *Medical Acupuncture*, Fall/Winter 1998/1999; volume 10/number 2; 9-13

Xiao Ji (Herba Cirisii)

小薊 小蓟

Pinyin Name: *Xiao Ji*
Literal Name: "small thistle"
Alternate Chinese Names: *Mao Ji, Ci Ji Cai, Ci Er Cai, Qian Zhen Cao*
Original Source: *Ming Yi Za Zhu* (Miscellaneous Records of Famous Physicians) by Tao Hong-Jing in 500 A.D.
English Name: cirsium, cephalano, common cephalanoplos, field thistle, setose cephalanoplos
Botanical Name: *Cirsium setosum* (Willd) MB; *Cephalanoplos setosum* (Willd.) Kitam. (*Ke Ye Ci Er Cai*) and *Cephalanoplos segetum* (Bge.) Kitam. (*Ci Er Cai*) are also listed.
Pharmaceutical Name: Herba Cirisii
Properties: sweet, cool
Channels Entered: Liver, Heart

CHINESE THERAPEUTIC ACTIONS

1. Cools Blood, Stops Bleeding

Bleeding caused by heat in the blood: *Xiao Ji* (Herba Cirisii) cools blood, promotes urination and treats *lin zheng* (dysuria syndrome). It also cools blood in the *ren* (conception) and *chong* (thoroughfare) channels to treat metrorrhagia or abnormal spotting between periods. It treats bleeding disorders caused by heat, with the blood appearing bright red. Clinical applications include hemoptysis, epistaxis, metrorrhagia, hematuria and hemorrhoidal bleeding.

- Hematemesis and hemoptysis: use charred *Xiao Ji, Da Ji* (Herba seu Radix Cirsii Japonici), *Ce Bai Ye* (Cacumen Platycladi), *Bai Mao Gen* (Rhizoma Imperatae), and *Qian Cao* (Radix Rubiae).
- Heart fire with hematemesis and thirst: use fresh juices of *Xiao Ji, Ou Jie* (Nodus Nelumbinis Rhizomatis), *Niu Bang Zi* (Fructus Arctii) and *Sheng Di Huang* (Radix Rehmanniae) with light-colored honey.
- Deficiency heat with blood in the sputum: use *Xiao Ji* with *Bai Mao Gen* (Rhizoma Imperatae) and the juice of *Ou Jie* (Nodus Nelumbinis Rhizomatis).
- Bleeding of the tongue related to Heart fire: use the juice of *Xiao Ji* individually.
- Hematuria with dysuria: use *Xiao Ji* individually, or with *Sheng Di Huang* (Radix Rehmanniae), *Hua Shi* (Talcum), *Zhi Zi* (Fructus Gardeniae) and *Dan Zhu Ye* (Herba Lophatheri). **Exemplar Formula:** *Xiao Ji Yin Zi* (Cephalanoplos Decoction).
- Metrorrhagia: combine *Xiao Ji* with *Bai Zhu* (Rhizoma Atractylodis Macrocephalae) and fresh juice of *Sheng Di Huang* (Radix Rehmanniae).
- Bleeding after abortion: use it with *Yi Mu Cao* (Herba Leonuri).
- Hemorrhoidal or rectal bleeding: drink the juice of *Xiao Ji*. Serve warm.
- Bleeding from knife wounds: crush young sprouts of *Xiao Ji* into a paste, and apply topically.

2. Disperses Blood Stasis, Reduces Swelling

Abscess and toxic swelling: *Xiao Ji* can be used internally or externally to relieve abscesses and swelling accompanied by toxicity and heat.

- Abscess and swelling: mix the powder of *Xiao Ji* leaves with water, and apply topically.
- Itch and rash: use *Xiao Ji* with *Ru Xiang* (Gummi Olibanum) and *Ming Fan* (Alumen). Serve with grain-based liquor.

3. Clears Damp-Heat from the Liver and Gallbladder

Damp-heat in the Liver and Gallbladder: *Xiao Ji* treats jaundice, hypertension, high cholesterol and hepatitis.

- Jaundice: use it with *Yin Chen Hao* (Herba Artemisiae Scopariae) and *Hu Zhang* (Rhizoma Polygoni Cuspidati).

DOSAGE

10 to 30 grams for the dried herb, 30 to 60 grams for fresh. Fresh *Xiao Ji* is stronger to eliminate toxins and is often used topically to treat toxic swellings. Dried *Xiao Ji* is best for clearing heat and stopping bleeding. Charred *Xiao Ji* is used only to stop bleeding.

CAUTIONS / CONTRAINDICATIONS

- Use *Xiao Ji* with caution in patients with loose stools or deficiency and cold of the Spleen and Stomach.

CHEMICAL COMPOSITION

Acacetin-7-rhamnogluioside, rutin, protocatechuic acid, caffeic acid, chlorogenic acid.[1]

SUPPLEMENT

- 大小薊 / 大小蓟 *Da Xiao Ji* is the collective name for the combination of *Da Ji* (Herba seu Radix Cirsii Japonici) and *Xiao Ji* (Herba Cirisii). These herbs are commonly used together because they have synergistic action to clear heat and stop bleeding.

Xiao Ji (Herba Cirisii)

AUTHORS' COMMENTS

Many practitioners use *Xiao Ji* (Herba Cirisii) and *Da Ji* (Herba seu Radix Cirsii Japonici) interchangeably. Both have a blood-cooling quality to stop bleeding, and both can be used for swelling and abscesses. *Xiao Ji* is stronger in treating hematuria and dysuria. It is best for acute urinary infection when used with other diuretic herbs to clear heat. *Da Ji* has a stronger effect to reduce swelling and disperse blood stagnation.

References

1. *Xian Dai Zhong Yao Yao Li Xue* (Contemporary Pharmacology of Chinese Herbs), 1997; 783

Di Yu (Radix Sanguisorbae)

地榆

Pinyin Name: *Di Yu*
Alternate Chinese Names: *Yu Chi, Suan Zhi*
Original Source: *Shen Nong Ben Cao Jing* (Divine Husbandman's Classic of the Materia Medica) in the second century
English Name: sanguisorba, garden burnet root, long-leaf garden burnet root
Botanical Name: *Sanguisorba officinalis* L. (*Di Yu*); *Sanguisorba officinalis* var. *longifolia* (Bert.) *Yu et Li* (*Chang Ye Di Yu*)
Pharmaceutical Name: Radix Sanguisorbae
Properties: bitter, sour, cool
Channels Entered: Liver, Large Intestine, Stomach

CHINESE THERAPEUTIC ACTIONS

1. Cools Blood and Stops Bleeding

Various patterns of bleeding caused by heat: *Di Yu* (Radix Sanguisorbae) treats hemoptysis, epistaxis, hematemesis, hematuria, hematochezia, hemorrhoidal bleeding, bleeding dysentery, metrorrhagia and abnormal uterine bleeding between periods. With its descending nature and its excellent action to cool the blood, clear heat, and retain blood inside the body, it is mostly used to treat bleeding in the lower *jiao* caused by heat in the blood or damp-heat. Bleeding due to heat is usually characterized by a profuse flow of bright, red blood.

Hematochezia, bleeding hemorrhoids: Toxic heat accumulation in the Large Intestine causes bleeding that appears either in the accompanying stool, or preceding the evacuation of stools.

- Bleeding hemorrhoids, hematochezia, or bleeding preceding the evacuation of stools, with bright red blood because of heat in the blood, or damp-heat in the lower *jiao*: use *Di Yu* with *Gan Cao* (Radix Glycyrrhizae) and *Sha Ren* (Fructus Amomi).
- Large amounts of blood in the stools and abdominal pain from heat in the *xue* (blood) level: use *Di Yu* with *Sheng Di Huang* (Radix Rehmanniae), *Bai Shao* (Radix Paeoniae Alba), *Huang Qin* (Radix Scutellariae) and *Huai Hua* (Flos Sophorae).
- Bleeding hemorrhoids: use it with *Huai Jiao* (Fructus Sophorae), *Fang Feng* (Radix Saposhnikoviae), *Huang Qin* (Radix Scutellariae), and *Zhi Ke* (Fructus Aurantii).
- Bleeding dysentery with rectal tenesmus, mucus, and lower abdominal pain: combine this herb with *Gan Cao* (Radix Glycyrrhizae).

Dysentery: Damp-heat in the intestines manifests as dysentery, abdominal pain, rectal tenesmus, or diarrhea with pus and blood.

- Chronic and non-healing bleeding dysentery: use *Di Yu*

Di Yu (Radix Sanguisorbae)

with *Huang Lian* (Rhizoma Coptidis), *Mu Xiang* (Radix Aucklandiae), *Wu Mei* (Fructus Mume), and *He Zi* (Fructus Chebulae).
- Hematemesis or metrorrhagia due to heat in the blood: cook *Di Yu* with rice vinegar.

Metrorrhagia or abnormal bleeding between periods:
- Profuse menstrual bleeding with bright red blood, and dry mouth and lips due to heat in the blood: use *Di Yu* with *Huang Qin* (Radix Scutellariae), *Sheng Di Huang* (Radix Rehmanniae), *Mu Dan Pi* (Cortex Moutan) and *Lian Xu* (Stamen Nelumbinis).
- Profuse bleeding and abdominal pain after miscarriage or abortion: combine this herb with *Ai Ye* (Folium Artemisiae Argyi), *E Jiao* (Colla Corii Asini), *Bai Zhu* (Rhizoma Atractylodis Macrocephalae) and *Dang Gui* (Radicis Angelicae Sinensis).

2. Clears Toxic Heat and Generates Flesh

Di Yu addresses dermatological disorders characterized by heat and toxins, such as burns, sores, ulcers and eczema. In addition to clearing heat and eliminating toxins, it promotes healing with its restraining function to prevent spreading of the wound and the oozing of fluids. It also relieves pain and promotes generation of flesh.
- Burns: mix *Di Yu* powder with sesame oil and apply topically for burns (first- through fourth- degree). See Cautions below.
- Carbuncles and sores without pus: apply the juice of *Di Yu* topically.
- Eczema or ulcerations with itching, redness, swelling and discharge: the herbs are applied topically. For topical application as an herbal wash, cook *Di Yu* and *Ku Shen Gen* (Radix Sophorae Flavescentis). For topical application using powder, mix *Di Yu*, *Shi Gao* (Gypsum Fibrosum) and *Ming Fan* (Alumen).

DOSAGE

10 to 15 grams, with a maximum of 30 grams, in herbal decoctions; or 1.5 to 3.0 grams per dose of *Di Yu*, one to three times daily as an herbal powder or pills. *Di Yu* is commonly used both internally and topically. Bitter, sour and cold, the unprocessed herb has a stronger function to cool the blood and eliminate toxins. Bitter, sour and astringent, the charred herb functions more effectively to stop bleeding.

CAUTIONS / CONTRAINDICATIONS

- Cold, sour and restraining in nature, *Di Yu* should be used with caution in cases of bleeding caused by deficiency, cold, or blood stasis.
- External use of *Di Yu* is generally considered safe. However, topical application of *Di Yu* is not recommended for burns that have affected a large area of the skin surface. In this case, excessive absorption of the herb (water-soluble tannins) may lead to overdose and liver toxicity, such as toxic hepatitis.
- Do not use *Di Yu* as a single herb treatment in the early stages of dysentery caused by heat.

CHEMICAL COMPOSITION

Ziyuglycoside I, ziyuglycoside II, sanguisorbin, sanguisorbigenin tannins.[1]

PHARMACOLOGICAL EFFECTS

- **Hemostatic:** Oral administration of unprocessed *Di Yu* powder and charred *Di Yu* powder to mice, at the dosage of 5 g/kg, reduced bleeding time by 31.9% and 45.5%, respectively. Oral administration of unprocessed *Di Yu* powder and charred *Di Yu* powder to rabbits, at the dosage of 2 g/kg, reduced bleeding time by 25% in both groups.[2]
- **Effect on relief of burns:** Topical application of *Di Yu* powder in dogs and rabbits with second and third degree burns showed marked effectiveness in reducing swelling and inflammation by decreasing vascular permeability. Furthermore, it lowered the risk of infection, shortened recovery time, and minimized the risk of shock.[3]
- **Antibiotic:** Water extract of *Di Yu* exhibits an inhibitory influence on *Salmonella typhi*, *Diplococcus meningitidis*, β-hemolytic streptococcus, *Staphylococcus aureus*, and *Diplococcus pneumoniae*; and alcohol extract of *Di Yu* exerts an inhibitory effect on *E. coli* and *Bacillus subtilis*.[4]
- **Antiemetic:** Administration of *Di Yu* decoction, at the dosage of 3 g/kg given orally twice daily for 2 days, was effective in controlling vomiting in pigeons induced by digitalis tincture, but ineffective for vomiting in dogs induced by apomorphine. The antiemetic effect of *Di Yu* is similar to 0.25 mg/kg of intramuscular injection of chlorpromazine.[5]
- **Anti-inflammatory:** Both water and alcohol extracts of *Di Yu* have demonstrated marked anti-inflammatory effects.[6]

CLINICAL STUDIES AND RESEARCH

- **Upper gastrointestinal bleeding:** According to one report, 100 patients with upper-gastrointestinal bleeding were treated with an herbal formula containing equal portions of *Di Yu*, *Bai Ji* (Rhizoma Bletillae) and *Yun Nan Bai Yao*. All patients received 3 grams of the herbal formula three to four times daily; effectiveness was evaluated by the absence of blood in the stools. The study reported a 95% rate of effectiveness. Of 5 cases that did not respond, three had stomach cancer and two had duodenal ulcers.[7]
- **Hemostasis:** Bleeding following tooth extraction in 40 patients was treated topically with an herbal formula. The study reported that bleeding stopped 3 to 5 minutes

Di Yu (Radix Sanguisorbae)

after application of the herbs. The herbal formula contained the following: charred *Di Yu* 2g, *Xi Xin* (Herba Asari) 1g, *Xue Yu Tan* (Crinis Carbonisatus) 1g, and *Bing Pian* (Borneolum Syntheticum) 0.1g.[8]

- **Pulmonary tuberculosis:** An herbal formula based on *Di Yu* showed satisfactory results in relieving hemoptysis secondary to pulmonary tuberculosis. The herbal formula contained 12 grams of dry-fried *Di Yu*, 60 grams of *Bai Mao Gen* (Rhizoma Imperatae), 6 grams of *Gan Cao* (Radix Glycyrrhizae) and others.[9]
- **Profuse menstrual bleeding:** One patient with functional uterine bleeding refractory to western medical treatment was healed after taking an herbal formula once daily for 4 days. The herbal formula contained 45 grams of *Di Yu* cooked in equal parts of water and vinegar.[10]
- **Burns:** Topical treatment of 216 burn patients with an herbal gel resulted in tremendous improvement in speed of recovery and pain relief. The herbal gel dressing was changed every 6 to 7 days for burns without infection, and every 2 to 3 days for infected burns. The study reported growth of new skin after 3 applications, and complete recovery after 6 to 8 applications. The herbal gel contained *Di Yu* 30g, *Zi Cao Gen* (Radix Lithospermi) 30g, *Dang Gui* (Radicis Angelicae Sinensis) 30g, *Bing Pian* (Borneolum Syntheticum) 15g, and *Gan Cao* (Radix Glycyrrhizae) 6g. In another study, 55 patients with second or third degree burns treated topically with *Di Yu* gel recovered within 5 to 7 days.[11] The herbal gel was prepared by mixing equal amounts of *Di Yu* powder and sesame oil.[12]
- **Bacterial dysentery:** In one study, 91 patients with acute bacterial dysentery were treated with a preparation of *Di Yu* three times daily with 95.6% effectiveness.[13]
- **Cervical erosion:** In one report, 573 patients were treated every other day with an herbal formula as vaginal suppository. The herbal formula contained *Di Yu*, *Huai Hua* (Flos Sophorae), *Ming Fan* (Alumen), and *Long Gu* (Os Draconis). The treatment protocol was to first wash the genital region with 0.1% potassium permanganate, followed by insertion of two vaginal suppositories. This procedure is repeated every other day, with four applications per course of treatment. The total duration of treatment was 1 to 3 months, with 5 days of rest between each course of treatment. Patients were advised not to use herbs for the 5 days prior to menstruation. Out of 573 patients, 212 had complete recovery, 62 showed significant improvement, 191 made slight improvement, and 78 had no response.[14]
- **Dermatological disorders:** Various dermatological disorders in 109 patients were treated with 30% charred *Di Yu* in petroleum jelly, with good results. Of the 109 cases, 47 individuals experienced complete recovery, 50 showed improvement, and 12 had no response. The average time to resolution was 8.3 days. The dermatological disorders treated include a rash, eczema, and dermatitis.[15]

HERB-DRUG INTERACTION

- **Ciprofloxacin:** It has been suggested that the absorption and disposition of ciprofloxacin may be affected when given concurrently with *Di Yu*. In one study, rats were divided into two groups, with one receiving ciprofloxacin only, and the other receiving both ciprofloxacin and *Di Yu*. Blood and urine samples were collected after 6 and 24 hours and analyzed by HPLC. Compared with the control group, the group receiving *Di Yu* showed a decrease of maximum plasma concentration by 94%, area under the curve by 78%, and urinary recovery by 79%. Furthermore, the apparent volume of distribution and terminal half-life were both increased, by eight-fold and two-fold, respectively. The mechanism of the interaction was attributed to the high content of minerals present in the herb. To avoid drug-herb interaction and interference with the bioavailability of ciprofloxacin, the researchers concluded that an adequate time should be allowed between the intake of the drug and the herb to ensure efficacy of ciprofloxacin if the two agents were to be used concurrently.[16]

TOXICOLOGY

Continuous oral administration of *Di Yu* herbal extract solution (3:1 concentration) to rats, at the dosage of 20 ml/kg, for 10 days did not demonstrate any significant adverse reactions or toxicities. However, liver biopsy at 5 and 10 days after the initiation of administration of herbs showed an increase in the lipid content of liver cells.[17]

AUTHORS' COMMENTS

Di Yu is cold and has a downward-moving nature, and most effectively addresses various types of bleeding in the lower *jiao* that are caused by toxic heat or damp-heat accumulation. For hematochezia, the charred form is usually used. When using the fresh form of *Di Yu* in decoction for hematochezia, dosage should be increased to 15 to 30 grams.

References

1. *Xian Dai Zhong Yao Yao Li Xue* (Contemporary Pharmacology of Chinese Herbs), 1997; 785
2. *Zhong Yao Yao Li Yu Ying Yong* (Pharmacology and Applications of Chinese Herbs), 1983; 406
3. Ibid.
4. *Zhong Yao Zhi* (Chinese Herbology Journal), 1993; 343
5. *Zhong Yao Yao Li Yu Ying Yong* (Pharmacology and Applications of Chinese Herbs), 1983; 406
6. *Zhong Yao Xue* (Chinese Herbology), 1998; 469-472
7. *Zhe Jiang Zhong Yi Xue Yuan Xue Bao* (Journal of Zhejiang University of Chinese Medicine), 1985; 9(4):26
8. *Zhong Yao Xue* (Chinese Herbology), 1988; 469-473

Dí Yu (Radix Sanguisorbae)

9. *Zhong Yi Za Zhi* (Journal of Chinese Medicine), 1966; 4:31
10. *Zhe Jiang Zhong Yi Za Zhi* (Zhejiang Journal of Chinese Medicine), 1965; 8(3):4
11. *Zhong Yi Za Zhi* (Journal of Chinese Medicine), 1963; 9:21
12. *Jiang Su Xin Yi Xue Yuan* (New Jiangsu University of Medicine), 1970
13. *Hu Nan Yi Yao Za Zhi* (Hunan Journal of Medicine and Herbology), 1978; 3:18
14. *Xin Zhong Yi* (New Chinese Medicine), 1978; 3:25
15. *Zhong Hua Pi Fu Ke Xue Za Zhi* (Chinese Journal of Dermatology), 1963; 9(5):324
16. *Journal of Antimicrob Chemother*, 1999 July; 44(1):125-8
17. *Yun Nan Zhong Yao Zhi* (Yunan Journal of Chinese Herbal Medicine), 1990; 241

Bai Mao Gen (Rhizoma Imperatae)

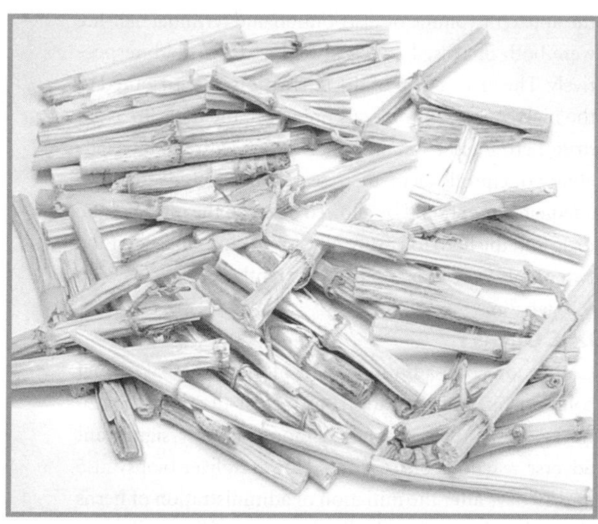

白茅根 白茅根

Pinyin Name: *Bai Mao Gen*
Alternate Chinese Names: *Mao Gen, Ru Gen, Mao Cao Gen*
Original Source: *Shen Nong Ben Cao Jing* (Divine Husbandman's Classic of the Materia Medica) in the second century
English Name: imperata, lalang grass rhizome
Botanical Name: *Imperata cylindrica* (L.) Beauv. var. *major* (Nees.) C.E. Hubb. (*Bai Mao*)
Pharmaceutical Name: Rhizoma Imperatae
Properties: sweet, cold
Channels Entered: Lung, Stomach, Urinary Bladder

CHINESE THERAPEUTIC ACTIONS

1. Cools Blood and Stops Bleeding

Bleeding: Neither drying nor stagnating in nature, *Bai Mao Gen* (Rhizoma Imperatae) addresses various bleeding disorders caused by heat in the blood. Clinical applications include epistaxis, hemoptysis or hematemesis.

- Epistaxis, hemoptysis or hematemesis from Lung or Stomach heat: drink the juice of fresh *Bai Mao Gen*. It may be combined with *Ou Jie* (Nodus Nelumbinis Rhizomatis) and *Xiao Ji* (Herba Cirisii) for synergistic effect.

2. Clears Heat and Promotes Urination

Dysuria: *Bai Mao Gen* treats *re lin* (heat dysuria), edema, and damp-heat jaundice by draining heat through urination.

- Hematuria due to Urinary Bladder heat: use *Bai Mao Gen* individually.
- Hematuria with deficiency heat: combine it with *Ren Shen* (Radix Ginseng), *Sheng Di Huang* (Radix Rehmanniae) and *Fu Ling* (Poria).
- Chronic presence of red blood cells in the urine, with back ache: pair *Bai Mao Gen* with either *Xu Duan* (Radix Dipsaci) or *Sang Ji Sheng* (Herba Taxilli).
- Edema and decreased volume of urine: use it individually.
- Dysuria: use it with *Shi Wei* (Folium Pyrrosiae), *Chuan Mu Tong* (Caulis Clematidis Armandii) and *Dong Kui Zi* (Semen Malvae).
- Damp-heat jaundice: combine this herb with *Yin Chen Hao* (Herba Artemisiae Scopariae) and *Zhi Zi* (Fructus Gardeniae).

3. Clears Heat from Lung and Stomach

Febrile disorders affecting the Lung and Stomach: Clinical manifestations include irritability, thirst, cough, wheezing, nausea and vomiting.

- Nausea and vomiting caused by Stomach heat: use *Bai Mao Gen* with *Lu Gen* (Rhizoma Phragmitis).
- Asthma and wheezing from Lung heat: combine it with *Sang Bai Pi* (Cortex Mori).

Bai Mao Gen (Rhizoma Imperatae)

DOSAGE

15 to 30 grams in herbal decoction. The dosage for fresh *Bai Mao Gen* is 30 to 60 grams, with a maximum of 250 to 500 grams. The fresh or the unprocessed herb has a stronger function to clear heat, cool blood, and promote urination. The charred herb functions more effectively to stop bleeding, but is unable to clear heat or cool blood.

CAUTIONS / CONTRAINDICATIONS

- Use *Bai Mao Gen* with caution in patients with deficiency and cold of the Spleen and Stomach.
- *Bai Mao Gen* is contraindicated in vomiting caused by cold in the middle *jiao*.

CHEMICAL COMPOSITION

Arundoin, cylindrin, ferneol, simiarenol, coixol.[1,2]

PHARMACOLOGICAL EFFECTS

- **Hemostatic:** Topical application of *Bai Mao Gen* powder showed marked hemostatic action in rabbits.[3]
- **Diuretic:** Decoction of *Bai Mao Gen* has demonstrated a diuretic effect in rabbits, with maximum effectiveness evident 5 to 10 days after the initiation of treatment.[4]
- **Antibiotic:** It has a strong inhibitory influence *in vitro* against *Shigella flexneri* and *Shigella sonnei*.[5]

CLINICAL STUDIES AND RESEARCH

- **Epidemic hemorrhagic fever:** Of 60 hemorrhagic fever patients treated one to three times daily with an herbal decoction, 58 patients recovered completely, but 2 died. The herbal decoction contained *Bai Mao Gen* 50 to 100g, *Dan Shen* (Radix Salviae Miltiorrhizae) 20 to 30g, *Lu Gen* (Rhizoma Phragmitis) 30 to 40g, *Huang Bai* (Cortex Phellodendri) 10 to 15g, *Mu Dan Pi* (Cortex Moutan) 10 to 15g, *Pei Lan* (Herba Eupatorii) 15 to 30g, and other herbs according to the condition of each individual patient.[6]
- **Epistaxis:** An herbal decoction containing 18 grams of *Zhi Zi* (Fructus Gardeniae) and 120 grams of fresh *Bai Mao Gen* (or 36 grams of dried *Bai Mao Gen*) given after meals or before bedtime was effective in stopping epistaxis characterized by excess heat of the Lung and Stomach within 1 to 3 doses.[7]
- **Nephritis:** Children with acute nephritis were treated with 32 to 59 doses of an herbal decoction, with marked reduction in edema, lowered blood pressure, absence of protein and blood cells in the urine, and normalization of urine. Out of 11 patients, there was complete recovery in 9 patients and moderate improvement in 2 patients. The herbal decoction was prepared by cooking 250 grams of *Bai Mao Gen* in 500 ml of water to yield a final solution that was taken in 2 to 3 equally-divided doses.[8]

HERB-DRUG INTERACTION

- **Diuretics:** *Bai Mao Gen* has a diuretic effect. Though this potential interaction has not been documented, concurrent use with diuretic drugs may lead to increased elimination of water and/or electrolytes. [Note: Examples of diuretics include chlorothiazide, hydrochlorothiazide, furosemide (Lasix), bumetanide (Bumex), and torsemide (Demadex).][9]

TOXICOLOGY

Herbal decoction at the dosage of 25 g/kg decreased motor activity and increased respiration rate in rabbits 36 hours after administration. Intravenous injection at the dosage of 10 to 15 g/kg showed the same effect. Intravenous injection at the dosage of 25 g/kg induced fatality in one rabbit 6 hours after injection.[10]

SUPPLEMENT

- 白茅花/白茅花 *Bai Mao Hua* (Flos Imperatae), also known as *Guan Hua*, was first cited in the *Xin Xiu Ben Cao* (Newly Revised Materia Medica) by Su Jing in 657-659 A.D. *Bai Mao Hua* is the flower of the same plant as *Bai Mao Gen*. Sweet and neutral, *Bai Mao Hua* is commonly used to stop bleeding. Clinical applications include treatment of internal and external bleeding, such as epistaxis, hemoptysis and hematemesis, and bleeding due to trauma. By comparison, *Bai Mao Hua* is more effective for bleeding in the upper *jiao*, as seen in hematemesis and epistaxis, while *Bai Mao Gen* is more effective for bleeding in the lower *jiao*, as in hematuria. The recommended dosage of *Bai Mao Hua* is 10 to 15 grams.

References

1. *Xian Dai Zhong Yao Yao Li Xue* (Contemporary Pharmacology of Chinese Herbs), 1997; 790
2. *Chang Yong Zhong Yao Cheng Fen Yu Yao Li Shou Ce* (A Handbook of the Composition and Pharmacology of Common Chinese Drugs), 1994; 754
3. *Yun Nan Zhong Yi Za Zhi* (Yunan Journal of Chinese Medicine), 1987; 8(5):43
4. *Ren Min Wei Sheng Chu Ban She* (Journal of People's Public Health), 1983; 327
5. Ibid.
6. *Zhong Xi Yi Jie He Za Zhi* (Journal of Integrated Chinese and Western Medicine), 1986; 6(4):212
7. *Zhong Yi Za Zhi* (Journal of Chinese Medicine), 1984; 5:64
8. *Guang Dong Yi Xue* (Guangdong Medicine), 1965; 3:28
9. Chen, J. Recognition & prevention of herb-drug interactions, *Medical Acupuncture*, Fall/Winter 1998/1999; volume 10/number 2; 9-13
10. *Xian Dai Zhong Yao Yao Li Xue* (Contemporary Pharmacology of Chinese Herbs), 1997; 282-283, 1997; 790-792

Huai Hua (Flos Sophorae)

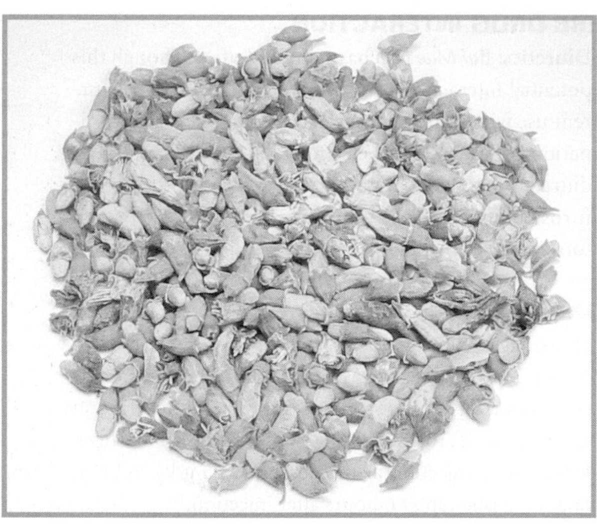

槐花 槐花

Pinyin Name: *Huai Hua*
Literal Name: "pagoda flower"
Alternate Chinese Names: *Huai Mi, Huai Rui, Huai Hua Mi*
Original Source: *Ri Hua Zi Ben Cao* (Materia Medica of Ri Hua-Zi) by Ri Hua-Zi in 713 A.D.
English Name: sophora, Japanese pagoda tree flower
Botanical Name: *Sophora japonica* L. (*Huai*)
Pharmaceutical Name: Flos Sophorae
Properties: bitter, cool
Channels Entered: Liver, Large Intestine

CHINESE THERAPEUTIC ACTIONS

1. Cools Blood and Stops Bleeding

Bleeding: *Huai Hua* (Flos Sophorae) treats various bleeding disorders characterized by heat in the blood. Because it enters the Liver and Large Intestine, *Huai Hua* is most effective and most commonly used to treat bleeding in the lower *jiao*, such as hematochezia, bleeding hemorrhoids, hematuria and profuse menstrual bleeding.

- Hematochezia with bright red blood, caused by damp-heat in the Large Intestine: add *Huai Hua* to *Ce Bai Ye* (Cacumen Platycladi), *Jing Jie* (Herba Schizonepetae), and *Zhi Ke* (Fructus Aurantii). **Exemplar Formula:** *Huai Hua San* (Sophora Japonica Flower Powder).
- Hematochezia with bright red blood, caused by excess heat and fire: use this herb with *Zhi Zi* (Fructus Gardeniae).
- Bleeding hemorrhoids: combine it with *Di Yu* (Radix Sanguisorbae), *Cang Zhu* (Rhizoma Atractylodis) and *Gan Cao* (Radix Glycyrrhizae).
- Hematuria caused by heat in the Urinary Bladder: use charred *Huai Hua* and *Yu Jin* (Radix Curcumae).
- Metrorrhagia or abnormal uterine bleeding: mix the powder of *Huai Hua* and *Gan Cao* (Radix Glycyrrhizae) with warm liquor.
- Persistent hematemesis: mix charred *Huai Hua* with a small amount of *She Xiang* (Moschus), and serve it with sticky rice soup.
- Persistent epistaxis: mix equal portions of *Huai Hua* and *Hai Piao Xiao* (Endoconcha Sepiae) powder and apply the powder directly into the nostrils.
- Bleeding of the tongue: apply *Huai Hua* powder topically.

2. Clears Liver Heat and Sedates Fire

Huai Hua treats red eyes, headache, dizziness and vertigo associated with Liver heat and fire.

- Liver heat and fire: combine *Huai Hua* with *Ju Hua* (Flos Chrysanthemi) and *Xia Ku Cao* (Spica Prunellae), and serve as tea.

DOSAGE

10 to 15 grams for decoction, reduce the dosage for *Huai Hua* powder. The fresh herb has a stronger function to cool blood, purge fire, and lower blood pressure. The dry-fried form is warmer, and is less likely to cause irritation to the Spleen and Stomach. The charred herb is better to stop bleeding.

CAUTIONS / CONTRAINDICATIONS

- *Huai Hua* should be used with caution in deficiency and cold of the Spleen and Stomach.

CHEMICAL COMPOSITION

Rutin, betulin, sophoradiol, sophorin A, sophorin B, sophorin C, quercetin, and rutoside.[1,2,3]

HO, OH, OH, O–rutinose, OH, O

Rutin

HO, OH, OH, OH, OH, O

Quercetin

Huai Hua (Flos Sophorae)

PHARMACOLOGICAL EFFECTS

- **Hemostatic:** Both unprocessed and charred *Huai Hua* may shorten bleeding time. Charred *Huai Hua* is stronger than the unprocessed herb in this hemostatic function.[4]
- **Effect on blood vessels:** Rutin and quercetin have been shown to maintain the integrity of the capillaries by decreasing permeability and increasing flexibility.[5]
- **Cardiovascular:** Administration of rutin and quercetin to frogs has demonstrated positive inotropic and negative chronotropic effects, leading to increased cardiac output and decreased heart rate. These substances also improve blood perfusion to the cardiac muscle by dilating the coronary artery. Lastly, administration of water and alcohol extracts of *Huai Hua* have marked antihypertensive effects, as demonstrated in anesthetized dogs.[6]
- **Antihyperlipidemic:** Administration of quercetin has been associated with reduction of liver and plasma cholesterol levels. It has demonstrated promising protective and therapeutic effects for atherosclerosis treatment.[7]
- **Anti-inflammatory:** Administration of rutin and quercetin via the intraperitoneal route has demonstrated marked anti-inflammatory effects in mice and rats with arthritis.[8]
- **Antispasmodic and antiulcer:** Rutin and quercetin have been shown to reduce the contractility of the intestines and decrease the secretion of gastric acid. Quercetin is five times more potent than rutin in its antispasmodic effect.[9]
- **Protective effect against radiation:** Administration of rutin reduced the severity of adverse effects and the incidence of fatality in mice exposed to x-ray radiation.[10]
- **Preventative effect against frostbite:** Rutin has a protective effect against frostbite, and is most effective in treating cases of third-degree frostbite.[11]

CLINICAL STUDIES AND RESEARCH

- **Menstrual bleeding:** Patients with profuse menstrual bleeding were treated with an herbal decoction once or twice daily, for up to 7 days, with 83.6% effectiveness. The herbal decoction contained charred *Huai Hua* 30g, *Ji Cai* (Herba Capsellae Bursapastoris) 30g, *Ma Chi Xian* (Herba Portulacae) 30g, charred *Hai Piao Xiao* (Endoconcha Sepiae) 15g, charred *Qian Cao* (Radix Rubiae) 15g, charred *Di Yu* (Radix Sanguisorbae) 15g, *Ji Mu* (Radix Loropetali) 15g, charred *Pu Huang* (Pollen Typhae) 10g, *Gan Cao* (Radix Glycyrrhizae) 5g, and others (based on the condition of each patient). Patients were advised to take the herbs once daily, or twice daily if there was profuse bleeding. Out of 140 patients, 64 patients stopped bleeding within 1 to 3 days, 53 stopped within 4 to 6 days, and 23 continued to bleed after 7 days.[12]
- **Hemorrhoids:** In one study, 400 patients with hemorrhoids were treated with an herbal decoction once daily with good success. The study reported that 61% showed significant improvement, 31% showed moderate improvement and 8% experienced no improvement. The formula contained *Huai Hua* 15g, *Huai Jiao* (Fructus Sophorae) 15g, *Hua Shi* (Talcum) 15g, *Sheng Di Huang* (Radix Rehmanniae) 12g, *Jin Yin Hua* (Flos Lonicerae) 12g, *Dang Gui* (Radicis Angelicae Sinensis) 12g, *Huang Lian* (Rhizoma Coptidis) 12g, *Huang Bai* (Cortex Phellodendri) 10g, *Huang Qin* (Radix Scutellariae) 10g, *Sheng Ma* (Rhizoma Cimicifugae) 6g, *Chai Hu* (Radix Bupleuri) 6g, *Zhi Ke* (Fructus Aurantii) 6g, *Gan Cao* (Radix Glycyrrhizae) 3g, and others (based on the condition of each patient).[13]
- **Psoriasis:** Sufferers of psoriasis were treated with 3 grams of dry-fried *Huai Hua* in powder, taken twice daily with warm water after meals. Out of 53 patients, 6 showed significant improvement, 22 made moderate progress, 19 had slight improvement, and 6 showed no response. The herbal remedy was prepared by dry-frying *Huai Hua* until it turned yellow, grinding it to powder, and mixing it with honey to make pills.
- **Summer boil:** Application of a *Huai Hua* solution topically two to three times daily, followed by application of *Huai Hua* paste, showed marked effectiveness within 1 to 2 days. The herbal solution was prepared by cooking 30 to 60 grams of the herb in 1,500 ml of water.[14]

TOXICOLOGY

The LD_{50} for quercetin in mice is 160 mg/kg via oral ingestion.[15]

SUPPLEMENT

- 槐角 / 槐角 *Huai Jiao* (Fructus Sophorae), first cited in *Shen Nong Ben Cao Jing* (Divine Husbandman's Classic of the Materia Medica) in the second century, is derived from the fruit of the same plant as *Huai Hua* (Flos Sophorae). *Huai Jiao* is bitter, cold, and enters the Liver and Large Intestine. In comparison with *Huai Hua, Huai Jiao* has weaker action to stop bleeding, and stronger effect to sedate heat. It can also lubricate the intestines. For treatment of hemorrhoidal bleeding, hematochezia or bleeding caused by abscesses or swelling with pain, *Huai Jiao* is often combined with *Di Yu* (Radix Sanguisorbae), *Huang Qin* (Radix Scutellariae) and *Dang Gui* (Radicis Angelicae Sinensis). To sedate Liver fire to lower blood pressure and treat red eyes, headache and dizziness, *Huai Jiao* is commonly combined with *Huang Qin, Jue Ming Zi* (Semen Cassiae) and *Xia Ku Cao* (Spica Prunellae). *Huai Jiao* is contraindicated in pregnant women, or patients with deficiency and cold of the Spleen and Stomach. The recommended dosage of *Huai Jiao* is 10 to 15 grams in decoction.

Huai Hua (Flos Sophorae)

References

1. *Xian Dai Zhong Yao Yao Li Xue* (Contemporary Pharmacology of Chinese Herbs), 1997; 792-793
2. *The Merck Index* 12th edition, Chapman & Hall/CRCnetBASE/Merck, 2000.
3. Ibid.
4. *Guang Xi Zhong Yi Yao* (Guangxi Chinese Medicine and Herbology), 1990; 13(1):44
5. *Zhong Yao Xue* (Chinese Herbology), 1998; 478:481
6. Ibid., 478-480
7. *Zhi Wu Yao You Xiao Cheng Fen Shou Ce* (Manual of Plant Medicinals and Their Active Constituents), 1986; 902:876
8. Ibid.
9. *Zhong Yao Xue* (Chinese Herbology), 1998; 478-480
10. Ibid.
11. Ibid.
12. *Zhong Yi Za Zhi* (Journal of Chinese Medicine), 1982; 3(6):28
13. *Si Chuan Zhong Yi* (Sichuan Chinese Medicine), 1985; 3(5):49
14. *Zhe Jiang Zhong Yi Za Zhi* (Zhejiang Journal of Chinese Medicine), 1966; 9(7):40
15. *Zhi Wu Yao You Xiao Cheng Fen Shou Ce* (Manual of Plant Medicinals and Their Active Constituents), 1986: 902,876

Ce Bai Ye (Cacumen Platycladi)

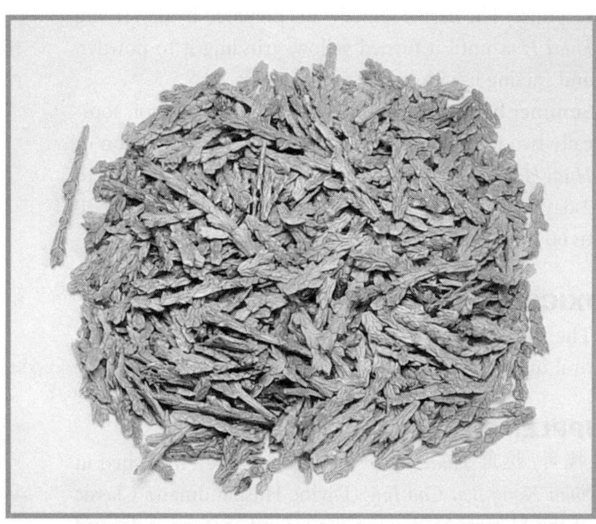

側柏葉 侧柏叶

Pinyin Name: *Ce Bai Ye*
Literal Name: "flat fir leaves"
Alternate Chinese Names: *Ce Bai, Bai Ye, Bian Bai*
Original Source: *Ming Yi Za Zhu* (Miscellaneous Records of Famous Physicians) by Tao Hong-Jing in 500 A.D.
English Name: platycladus leaves, leafy twigs of Chinese arborvitae, leafy twigs of oriental arborvitae
Botanical Name: *Platycladus orientalis* (L.) Franco; *Biota orientalis* (L.) Endl.
Pharmaceutical Name: Cacumen Platycladi
Properties: bitter, astringent, cool
Channels Entered: Lung, Liver, Large Intestine

CHINESE THERAPEUTIC ACTIONS

1. Cools Blood and Stops Bleeding

Bleeding due to heat: *Ce Bai Ye* (Cacumen Platycladi) treats various bleeding disorders, including epistaxis, hematemesis, hemoptysis, profuse menstrual bleeding, hematochezia, hematuria and external bleeding caused by trauma. It can also treat bleeding from deficiency and cold, when combined with interior-warming herbs.

- Hematemesis or epistaxis with bright red blood: use *Ce Bai Ye* with *Da Ji* (Herba seu Radix Cirsii Japonici), *Xiao Ji* (Herba Cirisii) and *Bai Mao Gen* (Rhizoma Imperatae).
- Persistent hematemesis with sallow facial appearance, pale tongue, and a weak pulse from deficiency and cold: combine it with *Gan Jiang* (Rhizoma Zingiberis) and *Ai Ye* (Folium Artemisiae Argyi).
- Hematuria caused by heat in the Urinary Bladder: use it with *Da Ji* (Herba seu Radix Cirsii Japonici), *Xiao Ji* (Herba Cirisii), and *Bai Mao Gen* (Rhizoma Imperatae).
- Hematochezia: add *Huai Hua* (Flos Sophorae) and *Di Yu* (Radix Sanguisorbae) to this herb.
- Profuse menstrual bleeding: add *Bai Shao* (Radix Paeoniae Alba).
- Profuse menstrual bleeding with qi and blood deficiencies: use it with *Dang Shen* (Radix Codonopsis), *Dang Gui* (Radicis Angelicae Sinensis), *Sheng Di Huang* (Radix Rehmanniae) and *Xian He Cao* (Herba Agrimoniae).
- Burns: use *Ce Bai Ye* topically as herbal powder.
- External bleeding: use it topically as herbal paste.

2. Dispels Phlegm and Stops Cough

Cough with profuse sputum: *Ce Bai Ye* is most effective

Ce Bai Ye (Cacumen Platycladi)

for treating cough caused by accumulation of hot phlegm that is difficult to expectorate.

- Cough with hot phlegm: use this herb with *Ban Xia* (Rhizoma Pinelliae).

3. Treats Hair Loss

Hair loss and itchy scalp from oily hair:

- Hair loss: cook *Ce Bai Ye* with *Fu Zi* (Radix Aconiti Lateralis Praeparata) and lard, and use the herbal decoction as herbal wash.
- Hair loss and/or itchy scalp: soak *Ce Bai Ye* in 60% alcohol for 7 days and apply the tincture to the scalp as herbal wash.

DOSAGE

10 to 15 grams, maximum 30 grams, in herbal decoction. *Ce Bai Ye* is commonly used as herbal decoction, herbal powder, and topically as herbal paste or wash. The unprocessed herb has a stronger function to cool the blood, while the charred form is better to stop bleeding.

CAUTIONS / CONTRAINDICATIONS

- Bitter and cold in nature, *Ce Bai Ye* should be prescribed with caution for patients experiencing deficiency and cold of the Spleen and Stomach, as it may cause diarrhea.
- Because of its cold and astringent nature, use *Ce Bai Ye* with caution in patients with bleeding and blood stasis, as the stasis may become more difficult to disperse.
- Overdose or prolonged use of *Ce Bai Ye* may cause dizziness, nausea, and decreased appetite.

CHEMICAL COMPOSITION

Volatile oil, juniperic acid, sabinic acid.[1]

PHARMACOLOGICAL EFFECTS

- **Hemostatic:** Herbal decoction of *Ce Bai Ye* has demonstrated marked influence to shorten bleeding time in mice and rabbits. Interestingly, the fresh herb was found to be slightly more effective than the charred herb.[2]
- **Antitussive:** Oral administration of water and alcohol extracts of *Ce Bai Ye* in mice at the dosage of 250 mg/kg demonstrated marked ability to relieve artificially-induced cough.[3]
- **Expectorant:** Extract of *Ce Bai Ye* demonstrated marked expectorant effects in mice.[4]
- **Respiratory:** Extract of *Ce Bai Ye* demonstrated marked potency to relax smooth muscle of the respiratory tract in mice and guinea pigs. It did not, however, exhibit significant protective effect against asthma in guinea pigs.[5]
- **Sedative:** Herbal decoction of *Ce Bai Ye* showed sedative action on the central nervous system as it prolonged phenobarbital-induced sleeping time, decreased motor activities, and prevented caffeine-induced seizures in mice.[6]
- **Antihypertensive:** Intravenous or oral administration of *Ce Bai Ye* lowered blood pressure in rabbits through vasodilation.[7]
- **Antibiotic:** *Ce Bai Ye* shows inhibitory activity against *Staphylococcus aureus, Neisseria catarrhalis, Salmonella typhi, Corynebacterium diphtheriae,* β-hemolytic streptococcus, and *Bacillus anthracis.*[8]

CLINICAL STUDIES AND RESEARCH

- **Bleeding ulcers:** In one study, 100 patients with bleeding ulcers were divided into two groups, with 50 patients receiving herbal treatment and 50 receiving a placebo substance. The treatment group received an herbal decoction with 15 grams of *Ce Bai Ye.* Negative hemoccult tests were reported in the treatment group after an average of 2.8 days, and in the placebo group after 4.5 days.[9]
- **Bleeding hemorrhoids:** Eight patients were treated with rectal instillation of 200 ml of herbal solution once daily, with satisfactory results. The herbal solution was prepared by mixing 30 grams of charred *Ce Bai Ye,* 15 grams of charred *Jing Jie* (Herba Schizonepetae), and 20 grams of charred *Da Huang* (Radix et Rhizoma Rhei) with warm water.[10]
- **Whooping cough:** Children with whooping cough were treated with a preparation of *Ce Bai Ye* for 4 to 10 days with good success. Children under two years of age received 15 to 25 ml of herbal decoction three times daily; and dosages for children over two years of age were adjusted accordingly. Out of 56 children, 41 made complete recovery, 9 showed moderate improvement, and 6 had no response.[11]
- **Pulmonary tuberculosis:** Daily administration of 120 grams of *Ce Bai Ye* via intravenous and oral routes for 3 to 5 months showed excellent results in 153 patients with pulmonary tuberculosis. There was marked improvement in coughing, sputum, night sweats, hemoptysis, fatigue and other symptoms.[12]
- **Hair loss:** In one study, 160 patients with hair loss were treated with a topical herbal preparation with a 77.5% rate of effectiveness. The herbal formula was prepared by soaking 25 to 35 grams of *Ce Bai Ye* in 100 ml of 60 to 75% rubbing alcohol for 7 days. The treatment protocol was to apply the herbal preparation three to four times daily.[13]
- **Parotitis:** Topical application of *Ce Bai Ye* paste was effective in reducing pain and swelling within 1 to 2 days in 48 out of 50 patients with parotitis. The herbal paste was prepared by grinding 200 to 300 grams of fresh *Ce Bai Ye,* and combining it with egg whites. The herbal paste was applied externally to the affected area seven to eight times daily.[14]

Ce Bai Ye (Cacumen Platycladi)

TOXICOLOGY

Oral administration of *Ce Bai Ye* decoction to mice at the dosage of 60 g/kg did not show any significant toxicity or cause any fatalities. There were no significant changes in the growth, liver function and blood panel of mice who received high dosages of the herb for 6 weeks. The LD_{50} for intraperitoneal administration of *Ce Bai Ye* injectable in mice is 15.2 g/kg.[15]

AUTHORS' COMMENTS

Platycladus orientalis is the standard name and official source for *Ce Bai Ye*.[16] The previous name, *Biota orientalis*, is no longer used.

Ce Bai Ye has a strong function to stop bleeding, and is one of the most commonly-used herbs for this purpose. Clinical applications vary depending on the herbal combination:

- For bleeding caused by heat, it is combined with *Da Ji* (Herba seu Radix Cirsii Japonici) or *Xiao Ji* (Herba Cirisii).
- For persistent bleeding, it is used with *Xian He Cao* (Herba Agrimoniae), *Ou Jie* (Nodus Nelumbinis Rhizomatis) and *Pu Huang* (Pollen Typhae).
- If bleeding is from deficiency and cold, this herb is added to charred *Ai Ye* (Folium Artemisiae Argyi) and charred *Pao Jiang* (Rhizoma Zingiberis Preparatum).

References

1. Yen, KY. *The Illustrated Chinese Materia Medica Crude and Prepared*, SMC Publishing Inc. Taipei, 1992; 100
2. *Zhong Yi Yao Yang Jiu Zi Liao* (Research and Resource of Chinese Medicine and Herbology), 1965; (3):48
3. *Zhe Jiang Wei Sheng Shi Yan Yuan* (Zhejiang Department of Health Research), 1973: 175
4. *Ke Ji Zi Liao* (Scientific Techniques and Knowledge), 1976; 3:21
5. *Zhe Jiang Wei Sheng Shi Yan Yuan* (Zhejiang Department of Health Research), 1973: 175
6. Ibid.
7. Ibid.
8. *Hu Nan Wei Sheng Fang Yi Tong Xun* (Hunan Journal of Preventative Health), 1974; (1):112
9. *Zhong Hua Nei Ke Xue Za Zhi* (Journal of Chinese Internal Medicine), 1960; 8(3):249
10. *Zhong Guo Gang Chang Bing Za Zhi* (Chinese Journal of Proctology), 1985; 4:5
11. *Zhong Yi Er Ke Za Zhi* (Chinese Medical Journal of Pediatrics), 1960; 11(2):146
12. *Ren Min Jun Yi* (Military Reserve Medicine), 1976; 7:57
13. *Zhong Hua Yi Xue Za Zhi* (Chinese Journal of Medicine), 1973; 53(8):459
14. *He Bei Zhong Yi* (Hebei Chinese Medicine), 1985; 4:31
15. *Zhe Jiang Wei Sheng Shi Yan Yuan* (Zhejiang Department of Health Research), 1973: 175
16. *Zhong Hua Ren Min Gong He Guo Yao Dian* (Chinese Herbal Pharmacopoeia by People's Republic of China), 2000

Zi Zhu (Folium Callicarpae)

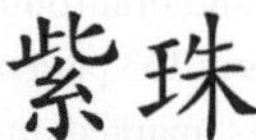

Pinyin Name: *Zi Zhu*
Literal Name: "purple beads," "purple pearl"
Alternate Chinese Names: *Zi Jing, Zhi Xue Cao, Zi Jing Cao*
Original Source: *Ben Cao Shi Yi* (Omissions from the [Classic of the] Materia Medica) by Chen Cang-Qi in 741 A.D.
English Name: callicarp leaf
Botanical Name: *Callicarpa pedunculata* R. Br. (*Du Hong Hua*); *Callicarpa macrophylla* Vahl. (*Da Ye Zi Zhu*); *Callicarpa nudiflora* Hook. et. Arn. (*Luo Hua Zi Zhu*); *Callicarpa dichotamoa* (Lour.) K. Koch (*Bai Tang Zi Shu*); *Callicarpa loureiri* Hook. et Arn (*Chang Ye Zi Zhu*); *Callicarpa arborea* Roxb. (*Da Ye Zi Zhu*); *Callicarpa kwangtungensis* Chun. (*Guang Dong Zi Zhu*); *Callicarpa rubella* Lindl. (*Hong Zi Zhu*); *Callicarpa cathayana* H. T. Chang (*Hua Zi Zhu*)
Pharmaceutical Name: Folium Callicarpae
Properties: bitter, astringent, cool
Channels Entered: Liver, Lung, Stomach

Zi Zhu (Folium Callicarpae)

CHINESE THERAPEUTIC ACTIONS

1. Retains Blood and Stops Bleeding

Gastrointestinal or respiratory bleeding: *Zi Zhu* (Folium Callicarpae) is one of the best herbs to stop bleeding, especially in the digestive and respiratory tracts. It may be used alone in powder form with cold or warm water. It can also be used as tea to treat gastrointestinal bleeding. This herb has been made into injectable form or topical gauze to stop bleeding. It is also used during surgery to stop bleeding. Clinical applications of *Zi Zhu* include hemoptysis, hematemesis, hematuria, hematochezia, uterine bleeding or bleeding from external injuries.

- Hemoptysis, epistaxis: mix the powder of *Zi Zhu* with egg whites.
- Bleeding caused by external injuries: crush fresh *Zi Zhu*, or use the powder, and apply the herb to the affected sites.
- Incessant bleeding from a tooth extraction: apply *Zi Zhu* powder to the affected area and cover it with sterilized cotton.
- Various types of bleeding: use it with *Xian He Cao* (Herba Agrimoniae), *Qian Cao* (Radix Rubiae) and *Han Lian Cao* (Herba Ecliptae).

2. Eliminates Toxins and Treats Toxic Sores

Toxic sores, abscesses, carbuncles, burns:

- Burns: apply *Zi Zhu* decoction topically. It can also be used topically with *Da Huang* (Radix et Rhizoma Rhei), *Huang Qin* (Radix Scutellariae) and *Huang Bai* (Cortex Phellodendri) to prevent infection for first- and second-degree burns with oozing fluids.
- Toxic sores, abscesses, carbuncles: use it with *Jin Yin Hua* (Flos Lonicerae) and *Pu Gong Ying* (Herba Taraxaci) as decoction. Apply topically as powder.
- Sore throat, redness and eye pain: use *Zi Zhu* alone as a decoction.

DOSAGE

As decoction, 10 to 15 grams for the dried herb, and 30 to 60 grams for the fresh herb. As a powder, 1.5 to 3 grams per dose.

CAUTIONS / CONTRAINDICATIONS

- Use *Zi Zhu* with caution in patients who are bleeding because of deficiency and cold.

CHEMICAL COMPOSITION

Calliterpenone, luteolin, apigenin, flavones, tannins, calcium, iron, magnesium.[1]

PHARMACOLOGICAL EFFECTS

- **Hemostatic:** In both *in vitro* and *in vivo* studies, injection of *Zi Zhu* stops bleeding by increasing the number of platelets.[2]
- **Antibiotic:** *Zi Zhu* inhibits *Staphylococcus aureus*, *Staphylococcus albus*, *Pseudomonas aeruginosa*, *Salmonella typhi*, *Bacillus dysenteriae*, *E. coli*, *Diplococcus meningitidis*, and *Bacillus proteus*.[3]

CLINICAL STUDIES AND RESEARCH

- **Bleeding:** In one study, 500 patients who required invasive procedures for tooth extraction were treated with topical application of *Zi Zhu* to stop bleeding. In cases of moderate bleeding, topical application of *Zi Zhu* powder stopped bleeding within 2 to 3 minutes. In cases of severe bleeding, topical application of *Zi Zhu* powder under cotton with light pressure was effective to stop bleeding within 2 to 3 minutes. The study reported approximately a 99% rate of effectiveness.[4]
- **Bleeding during surgery:** Gauze soaked in a 10 to 15% *Zi Zhu* solution was used topically to stop bleeding during 53 surgical procedures, with good results. Upon application of the herb-soaked gauze, bleeding generally stopped within 1 to 2 minutes.[5]
- **Upper gastrointestinal bleeding:** In one clinical study, 12 patients with duodenal bleeding, 2 patients with gastric bleeding, and 1 patient with hematochezia and hematemesis caused by liver cirrhosis, were treated with two preparations of *Zi Zhu*. Preparation I was 30 to 60 grams of *Zi Zhu* as herbal decoction, taken once daily. Preparation II was 2 to 4 ml of a 2% *Zi Zhu* preparation, injected intramuscularly twice daily. Patients with severe bleeding were treated with both methods. The study reported that most patients stopped bleeding within 3 to 5 days.[6]
- **Epistaxis:** Four patients with nosebleeds were treated by topical instillation of 2% *Zi Zhu* drops with the immediate effect of stopping bleeding.[7]
- **Burns:** In one study, 21 burn patients were treated with external and internal administrations of *Zi Zhu*, with good results. The treatment protocol was to deliver *Zi Zhu* to the burnt area via vapor daily, and then cover with gauze. If necessary, intramuscular injection of 2% *Zi Zhu* or oral ingestion of 50% *Zi Zhu* were given three to four times daily. Complete recovery was reported in 20 out of 21 patients. The length of hospitalization was 5 to 35 days. The one patient who did not respond suffered from severe burns, that subsequently turned into septicemia, renal failure, and eventually fatality.[8]
- **Skin ulceration:** Patients with skin ulceration with abscesses and pus were treated with a topical wash of *Zi Zhu* solution, with excellent results. The average time to complete recovery was 9.87 days. The treatment protocol was to wash the affected area with normal saline, then

Zi Zhu (Folium Callicarpae)

wash with a solution of *Zi Zhu*, and cover with gauze. This protocol was repeated on a daily basis. Out of 232 patients, there was complete recovery in 228 cases and significant improvement in the remaining 4 cases.[9]

- **Gynecological uses:** Topical application of *Zi Zhu* was used to treat cervicitis and vaginitis from various causes. The treatment protocol was to first cleanse the affected area, then apply *Zi Zhu* as powder, suppository, or via cotton ball soaked with herbal solution. The patients were treated one time daily for 5 days. Out of 78 patients, there was complete recovery in 38 cases, and moderate improvement in 33 cases, with an overall rate of effectiveness of 91%.[10]

TOXICOLOGY

No toxic effect was observed following intraperitoneal injection of 10% *Zi Zhu* at 200 mg/kg in rabbits. The LD_{50} for mice is 237.5 mg/kg via intravenous injection.[11]

AUTHORS' COMMENTS

Zi Zhu was originally cited by Chen Cang-Qi, in *Ben Cao Shi Yi* (Omissions from the [Classic of the] Materia Medica), 741 A.D. However, little information was provided. Most knowledge of *Zi Zhu* has been documented relatively recently, leading to increased use of this herb.

References

1. *Xian Dai Zhong Yao Yao Li Xue* (Contemporary Pharmacology of Chinese Herbs), 1997; 852
2. *Zhong Yao Xue* (Chinese Herbology), 1998; 487:490
3. Ibid.
4. *Xin Yi Xue* (New Medicine), 1971; 10:45
5. *Zhong Cao Yao Tong Xun* (Journal of Chinese Herbal Medicine), 1971; 1:21
6. Ibid., 1970; (5-6):39
7. Ibid., 1970; (5-6):39
8. *Xin Yi Xue* (New Medicine), 1971; 3:12
9. *Zhong Cao Yao Tong Xun* (Journal of Chinese Herbal Medicine), 1972; 2:42
10. *Xin Yi Xue* (New Medicine), 1971; 6-7:45
11. *Zhong Yao Xue* (Chinese Herbology), 1998; 487:490

Xian He Cao (Herba Agrimoniae)

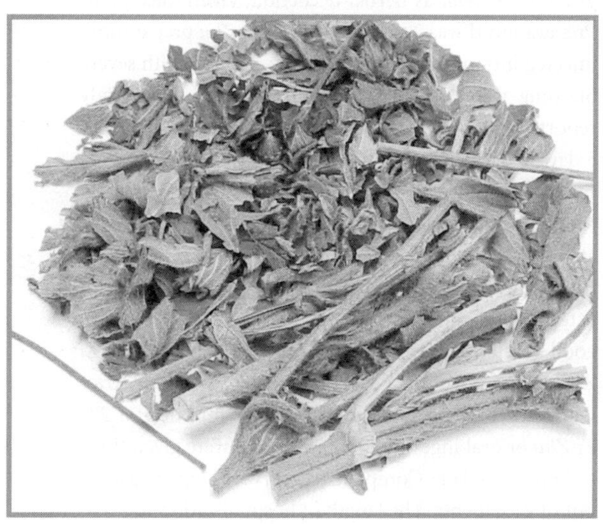

仙鶴草 仙鹤草

Pinyin Name: *Xian He Cao*

Literal Name: "red-crowned crane plant," "immortal crane herb"

Alternate Chinese Names: *Long Ya Cao, Jin Ding Long Ya, Tou Li Cao, Lang Ya Cao*

Original Source: *Tu Jing Ben Cao* (Illustrated Classic of the Materia Medica) by Su Song in 1061

English Name: agrimony, hairy-vein agrimonia

Botanical Name: *Agrimonia pilosa* Ledeb. (*Long Ya Cao*)

Pharmaceutical Name: Herba Agrimoniae

Properties: bitter, astringent, neutral

Channels Entered: Lung, Liver, Spleen

CHINESE THERAPEUTIC ACTIONS

1. Stops Bleeding

Bleeding due to damage of the Lung and Stomach channels: *Xian He Cao* (Herba Agrimoniae) has a good restraining function and is commonly used to treat bleeding, including epistaxis, hemoptysis, hematemesis, hematuria, hematochezia, and abnormal uterine bleeding.

- Hemoptysis and hematemesis from heat injuring the Lung or Stomach: use *Xian He Cao* individually.
- Epistaxis, hemoptysis or hematemesis due to yin deficiency with heat: combine it with *Ce Bai Ye* (Cacumen Platycladi), *Ou Jie* (Nodus Nelumbinis Rhizomatis), *Bai*

Xian He Cao (Herba Agrimoniae)

Mao Gen (Rhizoma Imperatae) and *Sheng Di Huang* (Radix Rehmanniae).
- Hematochezia: use it with *Pu Huang* (Pollen Typhae) and *Da Ji* (Herba seu Radix Cirsii Japonici).
- Profuse menstrual bleeding with sallow yellow appearance, pale tongue, thready and weak pulse: add this herb to *Dang Shen* (Radix Codonopsis), *Huang Qi* (Radix Astragali), *Shu Di Huang* (Radix Rehmanniae Preparata) and *Pao Jiang* (Rhizoma Zingiberis Preparatum).
- Thrombocytopenic purpura: use 30 to 60 grams of *Xian He Cao* with *Sheng Di Huang* (Radix Rehmanniae), *Xuan Shen* (Radix Scrophulariae), *Bai Shao* (Radix Paeoniae Alba), *Dang Gui* (Radicis Angelicae Sinensis), *Bai Mao Gen* (Rhizoma Imperatae), *E Jiao* (Colla Corii Asini), charred *Qian Cao* (Radix Rubiae), and charred *Mu Dan Pi* (Cortex Moutan).

2. Relieves Diarrhea

Diarrhea and dysentery: *Xian He Cao* relieves diarrhea and dysentery with pus and/or blood. It is especially effective if the condition is accompanied by gastrointestinal bleeding or by white mucus.
- Chronic diarrhea or dysentery with mucus and blood: use *Xian He Cao* individually.
- Bloody diarrhea or dysentery: use it with *Di Yu* (Radix Sanguisorbae).

3. Kills Parasites

Xian He Cao treats various parasitic infections, including malaria, tapeworm, roundworm, and trichomonas vaginitis.
- Malaria: administer 9 grams of *Xian He Cao* in powder with warm grain-based liquor and a large quantity of water, one time per day for 3 days.
- Trichomonas vaginitis: use *Xian He Cao* topically.

4. Tonifies Qi and Blood

In patients with qi and blood deficiencies caused by overexertion, *Xian He Cao* prevents the further loss of qi and blood by its stabilizing and binding effects, thereby enhancing the overall tonic effect of other herbs in a formula.
- Fatigue and lack of energy with normal appetite: use 50 grams of *Xian He Cao* with 50 to 100 grams of *Da Zao* (Fructus Jujubae). Drink the decoction and eat the *Da Zao*.
- Qi and blood deficiencies with fatigue, dizziness, lightheadedness, weak knees and low back: combine it with *Long Yan Rou* (Arillus Longan), *Ren Shen* (Radix Ginseng), *Shu Di Huang* (Radix Rehmanniae Preparata), and *Gou Qi Zi* (Fructus Lycii).

5. Reduces Swelling, Eliminates Pus

Xian He Cao, used externally or internally, treats breast abscesses, swellings and ulcerations. Clinical manifestations include sores, swellings, hemorrhoids and breast nodules. The vine of this plant is usually used for this function.

DOSAGE

10 to 15 grams in decoction. The maximum dosage of *Xian He Cao* is 30 to 60 grams. It may be taken internally or applied topically. Topical application is commonly administered as an herbal wash or herbal paste.

CAUTIONS / CONTRAINDICATIONS

- Use of *Xian He Cao* may cause palpitations and flushing.
- *Xian He Cao* is astringent in nature, and should not be used in acute diarrhea or dysentery, as it may contribute to retention of pathogens.

CHEMICAL COMPOSITION

Agrimol, agrimonolide, agrimonine A, B, C, D, E; vanillic acid, ellagic acid, L-taxifoine, cosmosilin, vitamin K.[1]

PHARMACOLOGICAL EFFECTS

- **Hemostatic:** Administration of *Xian He Cao* in rabbits and dogs via intravenous injection, at a dosage of 2 mg/kg, demonstrated an increase in platelets and a reduction in bleeding time.[2]
- **Cardiovascular:** Administration of *Xian He Cao* has varying effects on the cardiovascular system in rabbits and frogs. Water extract of the herb decreases blood pressure and has an inhibiting effect on the heart; alcohol extract increases blood pressure and has a stimulating effect on the heart.[3]
- **Gastrointestinal:** Water extract of *Xian He Cao* has a direct effect on the smooth muscles of the gastrointestinal tract. At low dosages, it has a stimulating effect; at high dosages, it has an inhibiting effect.[4]
- **Antibiotic:** *Xian He Cao* has an inhibitory effect against *Staphylococcus aureus, E. coli, Pseudomonas aeruginosa, Salmonella typhi,* and *Mycobacterium tuberculosis.*[5]
- **Antiparasitic:** Administration of *Xian He Cao* at the dosage of 300 mg/kg has demonstrated marked effectiveness within for treatment of schistosomiasis 3 to 5 days.[6]
- **Antiparasitic:** Administration of *Xian He Cao* has demonstrated marked antiparasitic effect against roundworm, tapeworm and others.[7]
- **Spermicidal**: Sperm samples from both humans and animals were obtained and placed in containers: some were diluted and some were not. Extract of *Xian He Cao* was added to all sample containers, and killed all sperm in all samples within 1 to 5 minutes.[8]
- **Antineoplastic:** Extract of *Xian He Cao* has demonstrated preliminary effectiveness against tumor cells in mice.[9]

Xían He Cao (Herba Agrimoniae)

CLINICAL STUDIES AND RESEARCH

- **Upper gastrointestinal bleeding:** In one study, 100 patients with upper gastrointestinal bleeding were treated with ingestion of an herbal decoction [30 grams of *Xian He Cao* and 10 grams of *Da Zao* (Fructus Jujubae)] once daily and an herbal powder [6 grams of *Bai Ji* (Rhizoma Bletillae)] three times daily. *Bu Zhong Yi Qi Tang* (Tonify the Middle and Augment the Qi Decoction) was also given if indicated. The study reported 70% effectiveness overall, with bleeding stopping in 70 of the 100 patients within 7 days.[10]
- **Menstrual bleeding:** Profuse menstrual bleeding in 147 patients was treated with an herbal decoction consisting of *Xian He Cao* 30g, *Han Lian Cao* (Herba Ecliptae) 20g, *Di Yu* (Radix Sanguisorbae) 20g, charred *Guan Zhong* (Rhizoma Dryopteridis) 15g, *Yi Mu Cao* (Herba Leonuri) 12g, *Zhi Ke* (Fructus Aurantii) 12g, *E Jiao* (Colla Corii Asini) 12g, charred *Xi Xian Cao* (Herba Siegesbeckiae) 10g, and others as needed. The treatment protocol was to administer the herbs in decoction one time daily (two times daily in severe cases), for 8 to 12 doses per treatment course. This process was repeated in the next menstrual cycle. The study reported recovery in most patients within two to three courses of treatment. The overall rate of effectiveness was 96.4%.[11]
- **Trichomonas vaginitis:** According to one report, 37 of 40 patients (92.5%) with trichomonas vaginitis reported complete recovery following topical treatment with *Xian He Cao*. The treatment protocol was to first use the herbal solution as a topical wash, followed by insertion of a cotton ball saturated with the herbal solution into the vagina, with the cotton ball retained for 3 to 4 hours. The procedure was performed once daily for 7 days per treatment course.[12]

HERB-DRUG INTERACTION

- **Anticoagulant drugs:** *Xian He Cao* contains vitamin K, which may reduce the anticoagulant effect of warfarin (Coumadin). While use of the herb is not contraindicated, it should be used with caution, in order to prevent formation of clots.[13]

TOXICOLOGY

The LD_{50} for *Xian He Cao* in mice via intraperitoneal injection is 90.7 +/- 4.9 mg/kg. Toxic reactions included increased movement, followed by a lack of activity, closed eyes, muscle stiffness, and in severe cases, fatality within 1 to 24 hours.[14]

References

1. *Xian Dai Zhong Yao Yao Li Xue* (Contemporary Pharmacology of Chinese Herbs), 1997; 795
2. *Zhong Yao Yao Li Yu Ying Yong* (Pharmacology and Applications of Chinese Herbs), 1983:323
3. Ibid.
4. Ibid.
5. Ibid.
6. *Xi Xue Xue Bao* (Academic Journal of Medicine), 1982; 17(9):663
7. *Zhong Yao Xue* (Chinese Herbology), 1998; 491:492
8. *Shen Yang Yi Xue Yuan Xue Bao* (Journal of Shenyang University of Medicine), 1980; (12):11
9. Ibid., (12):6
10. *Shang Hai Zhong Yi Yao Za Zhi* (Shanghai Journal of Chinese Medicine and Herbology), 1979; 4:28
11. *Shan Xi Zhong Yi* (Shanxi Chinese Medicine), 1985; 6(7):323
12. *Zhong Cao Yao Tong Xun* (Journal of Chinese Herbal Medicine), 1972; 1:37
13. Chen, J. Recognition & prevention of herb-drug interactions, *Medical Acupuncture*, Fall/Winter 1998/1999; volume 10/number 2; 9-13
14. *Shen Yang Yi Xue Yuan Xue Bao* (Journal of Shenyang University of Medicine), 1987; 4(4):123

Bai Ji (Rhizoma Bletillae)

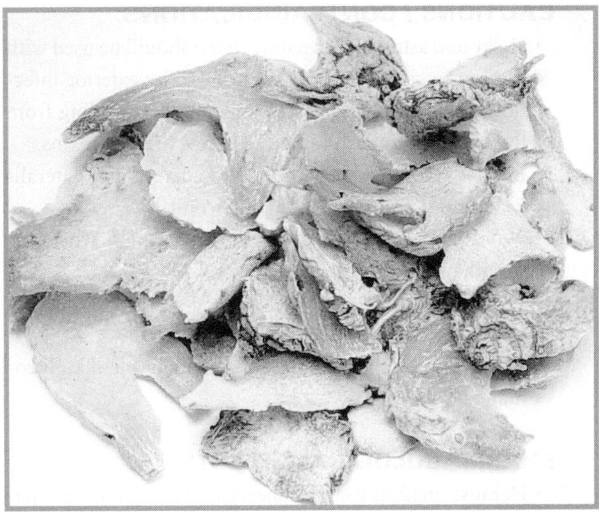

白芨 白及

Pinyin Name: *Bai Ji*
Literal Name: "white orchid"
Alternate Chinese Names: *Bai Gen, Gan Gen, Lian Ji Cao*
Original Source: *Shen Nong Ben Cao Jing* (Divine Husbandman's Classic of the Materia Medica) in the second century
English Name: bletilla, common bletilla tuber, hyacinth bletilla tuber
Botanical Name: *Bletilla striata* (Thunb.) Reichb. f. (*Bai Ji*)
Pharmaceutical Name: Rhizoma Bletillae
Properties: bitter, sweet, astringent, cool
Channels Entered: Lung, Stomach, Liver

CHINESE THERAPEUTIC ACTIONS

1. Restrains Leakage of Blood, Stops Bleeding

Hemoptysis and hematemesis, bleeding due to trauma, lung abscess: *Bai Ji* (Rhizoma Bletillae) cools heat, nourishes yin, and retains body fluids. It is most effective for bleeding from the lung and stomach, such as hemoptysis, hematemesis, and epistaxis. Cool in property, this herb is good to stop hemoptysis due to Lung heat or Lung yin deficiency. Topical application is effective to stop bleeding and treat wounds.

- Hemoptysis due to Lung heat damaging yin: use *Bai Ji* individually; or combine it with *Pi Pa Ye* (Folium Eriobotryae), *E Jiao* (Colla Corii Asini), *Ou Jie* (Nodus Nelumbinis Rhizomatis), and *Sheng Di Huang* (Radix Rehmanniae).
- Hemoptysis from pulmonary tuberculosis: use this herb with *Bai Bu* (Radix Stemonae) and *Chuan Xin Lian* (Herba Andrographis).
- Hematemesis because of Stomach heat damaging yin: use it with *Hai Piao Xiao* (Endoconcha Sepiae).
- Bleeding peptic or duodenal ulcers due to Stomach heat: combine this herb with *Hai Piao Xiao* (Endoconcha Sepiae), and *Bei Mu* (Bulbus Fritillaria).
- Hematemesis due to damp-heat: add *Yi Yi Ren* (Semen Coicis) and *Huang Lian* (Rhizoma Coptidis).
- External bleeding due to cuts: apply *Bai Ji* powder topically.
- Profuse external bleeding with deep cuts: use powdered *Bai Ji* with calcined *Shi Gao* (Gypsum Fibrosum) and calcined *Long Gu* (Os Draconis) in powder form.

2. Reduces Swelling, Promotes Generation of Flesh

Bai Ji is commonly used topically to treat sores and swellings with or without ulceration. It is especially effective for chronic, non-healing sores. This herb should be used in powder form, as its astringent property helps the closing of sores and wounds. It also promotes the generation of flesh.

- Sores with or without ulceration: apply *Bai Ji* powder topically.
- Erysipelas: use it with *Huang Bai* (Cortex Phellodendri) and *Cong Bai* (Bulbus Allii Fistulosi).
- Carbuncles, furuncles, sores and general dermatological disorders: combine this herb with *Fu Rong Ye* (Folium Hibisci), *Da Huang* (Radix et Rhizoma Rhei), *Huang Bai* (Cortex Phellodendri) and *Wu Bei Zi* (Galla Chinensis), and apply topically. Another source recommends mixing *Bai Ji*, *Jin Yin Hua* (Flos Lonicerae), *Zao Jiao* (Fructus Gleditsiae), *Ru Xiang* (Gummi Olibanum) and *Bei Mu* (Bulbus Fritillaria) with equal portions of water and rubbing alcohol, and applying it topically.
- Chronic non-healing wounds: use *Bai Ji* powder individually to promote healing.
- Chronic non-healing wounds with pus: use it with *Huang Lian* (Rhizoma Coptidis), *Bei Mu* (Bulbus Fritillaria), and *Wu Bei Zi* (Galla Chinensis).
- Chapped skin, fingers, toes, or anus, and burns: apply *Bai Ji* powder topically.

DOSAGE

3 to 10 grams in decoction, with a maximum dose of 30 grams. 1.5 to 3.0 grams of *Bai Ji* powder per dose, taken one to three times daily. *Bai Ji* is commonly used as herbal decoction, powder, and topical powder. When treating internal bleeding, this herb is not usually decocted with the others, as its sticky nature will easily burn on the sides and bottom of the pot. Therefore, the powdered herb is usually mixed with the strained decoction before administration.

Bai Ji (Rhizoma Bletillae)

CAUTIONS / CONTRAINDICATIONS

- Sticky and astringent in nature, *Bai Ji* should be used with caution in cases of hemoptysis caused by exterior infection, early-stage lung abscess or excessive bleeding from the Lung or Stomach caused by excess fire and toxins.
- *Bai Ji* is incompatible with *Fu Zi* (Radix Aconiti Lateralis Praeparata) and *Wu Tou* (Radix Aconiti).
- Avoid using heat-clearing herbs with *Bai Ji* when the sores have already ulcerated.

CHEMICAL COMPOSITION

Acacia gum, tragacanth, bletilla mannan, bletilla-glucomannan, starch.[1]

PHARMACOLOGICAL EFFECTS

- **Hemostatic:** Intravenous injection of a 2% *Bai Ji* preparation at the dosage of 1.5 ml/kg demonstrated a significant reduction in both bleeding and thrombin time in rabbits. Furthermore, it showed excellent hemostatic action when applied topically.[2]
- **Antiulcer:** In anesthetized dogs with a perforation one millimeter in diameter in the stomach and duodenum, administration of 9 grams of *Bai Ji* powder closed the perforation in the stomach after 15 seconds, and in the duodenum after 40 seconds. However, *Bai Ji* had no effect when the stomach was full or if the perforation was larger. Unlike most antiulcer medications that inhibit or neutralize gastric acid, *Bai Ji* does not affect the production of gastric acid nor the acidity of the stomach. It has been proposed that *Bai Ji* stimulates the production of prostaglandin and the stomach lining to exert its antiulcer effect.[3,4]
- **Antibiotic:** *Bai Ji* has an inhibitory influence on *Mycobacterium tuberculosis, Microsporum audouini*, and gram-positive bacterium.[5]

CLINICAL STUDIES AND RESEARCH

- **Hemoptysis in pulmonary tuberculosis:** Administration of 9 grams of *Bai Ji* powder in three equally-divided doses demonstrated satisfactory effects within 1 to 3 days in stopping the coughing of blood.[6]
- **Hemoptysis due to bronchiectasis:** According to one report, 2 to 4 grams of *Bai Ji* powder given three times daily for 3 to 6 months showed marked effectiveness in 21 patients: decreasing the amount of sputum, reducing the frequency and severity of coughing, and relieving hemoptysis.[7]
- **Upper gastrointestinal bleeding:** Bleeding ulcers in 108 patients were treated with 2 grams each of powdered *Bai Ji* and *Hai Piao Xiao* (Endoconcha Sepiae) three to four times daily. Based on hemoccult examination, 20.6% tested negative for presence of blood in the stools within 3 days, and 76.4% after 7 days.[8]
- **Bleeding due to ruptured rectum:** Eleven patients were treated with powdered *Bai Ji* and *Shi Gao* (Gypsum Fibrosum) applied topically once daily for 10 to 15 days. All patients reported excellent results.[9]
- **Peptic ulcers:** Patients with acute perforating gastric or duodenal ulcers were treated first with gastric lavage to empty the stomach, followed by ingestion of 9 grams of *Bai Ji* powder with 90 ml or less of water, repeated again in one hour. The dosage of *Bai Ji* was then reduced to 3 grams, with the same procedure performed three times daily, starting on day two. Strict diet guidelines were implemented as follows: nothing given orally on day one, water and a small portion of liquid food given on day two, and moderate portions of liquid food on day three. The study reported complete recovery in 23 out of 29 patients.[10]
- **Pulmonary tuberculosis:** Patients with chronic pulmonary tuberculosis were treated with 6 grams of *Bai Ji* daily for 3 months. Out of 60 patients, the study reported excellent results in 42, marked improvement in 13, and no response in 2 cases. Reports from the last three patients were not available.[11]
- **Whooping cough:** Patients were treated with oral administration of *Bai Ji* powder with the dosages of 0.1 to 0.15 g/kg in infants under one year of age, and 0.2 to 0.25 g/kg in infants over one year of age. Out of 89 patients, 37 demonstrated marked improvement within 5 days, 15 demonstrated moderate improvement within 10 days, 6 showed no response, and 31 discontinued treatment.[12]
- **Silicosis:** According to one report, 44 patients were treated with 1.5 grams of *Bai Ji* three times daily for anywhere from three months to one year. Most patients reported a reduction in the frequency and severity of chest pain, shortness of breath, cough, black sputum, and hemoptysis. Overall, there was an improvement in pulmonary function and an increase in body weight. X-ray results, however, were inconclusive.[13]
- **Burns and cuts:** Patients with external injuries were treated topically with a paste of *Bai Ji*, with excellent results. Dressings were changed every 5 to 7 days in cases not showing infection, and daily when infection was present. Nine patients with burns (covering less than 8% of total body surface area) and 38 patients with cuts reported complete recovery after 1 to 3 treatments.[14]
- **Plasma substitute:** A 2% *Bai Ji* preparation was used as a plasma substitute in patients with profuse blood loss, such as in surgery, bleeding ulcers, and liver cirrhosis with bleeding, with satisfactory results. The volume of *Bai Ji* preparation used was between 250 and 500 ml.[15]
- **Chapped skin:** Thirteen patients with chapped hands and feet were treated topically with an herbal paste, three times daily. Complete recovery was reported within 2 to

Bai Ji (Rhizoma Bletillae)

3 days in mild cases, and 5 to 7 days for those with more severe chapping. The herbal paste was composed of 30 grams of *Bai Ji*, 50 grams of *Da Huang* (Radix et Rhizoma Rhei), 3 grams of *Bing Pian* (Borneolum Syntheticum), and a small amount of honey.[16]

TOXICOLOGY

According to the classic list of *Shi Ba Fan* (Eighteen Incompatibles), *Bai Ji* is incompatible with *Chuan Wu* (Radix Aconiti Preparata), *Cao Wu* (Radix Aconiti Kusnezoffii) and *Fu Zi* (Radix Aconiti Lateralis Praeparata). In one toxicology study, this hypothesis was tested by dividing frogs into two groups: one group received *Chuan Wu*, *Cao Wu* or *Fu Zi* with *Bai Ji*, and the other group received the same base group of herbs without *Bai Ji*. With identical dosage, preparation and administration, no significant difference in toxicity was observed between the two groups.[17]

AUTHORS' COMMENTS

According to Dr. Zhang Xiao-Ping, *Bai Ji* is one of the most effective herbs to stop gastrointestinal bleeding. *Bai Ji* has a strong binding effect. When ingested, this herb will attach itself to the ulcer to stop bleeding and promote healing. However, because of this strong binding effect, its use is sometimes associated with constipation.

References

1. *Xian Dai Zhong Yao Yao Li Xue* (Contemporary Pharmacology of Chinese Herbs), 1997; 802
2. *Zhong Yao Zhi* (Chinese Herbology Journal), 1993; 384
3. *Zhong Yao Xue* (Chinese Herbology), 1998; 493:497
4. *Zhong Cao Yao* (Chinese Herbal Medicine), 1990; 21(2):312
5. *Zhong Hua Pi Fu Ke Xue Za Zhi* (Chinese Journal of Dermatology), 1957; (4):286
6. *Fu Jian Zhong Yi Yao* (Fujian Chinese Medicine and Herbology), 1964; 9(4):32
7. *Shan Dong Yi Kan* (Shandong Medical Journal), 1960; 10:9
8. *Jiang Su Zhong Yi* (Jiangsu Chinese Medicine), 1965; 11:3
9. *Zhong Hua Wai Ke Za Zhi* (Chinese Journal of External Medicine), 1959; 7(7):661
10. Ibid., 1963; 11(7):511
11. *Zhong Guo Fang Lao* (Chinese Prevention of Tuberculosis), 1960; 2:106
12. *Shan Xi Yi Kan* (Shanxi Journal of Medicine), 1957; 2:53
13. *Zhong Hua Jie He Bing Ke Za Zhi* (Chinese Journal of Tuberculosis), 1959; 7(2):149
14. *Zhong Yi Za Zhi* (Journal of Chinese Medicine), 1965;(7):37
15. *Zhong Cao Tong Xun* (Journal of Chinese Herbs), 1973; 1:34
16. *He Nan Zhong Yi* (Henan Chinese Medicine), 1985; 2:21
17. *Zhong Yao Xue* (Chinese Herbology), 1998; 493:497

Zong Lu Pi (Fibra Stipulae Trachycarpi)

棕櫚皮 棕榈皮

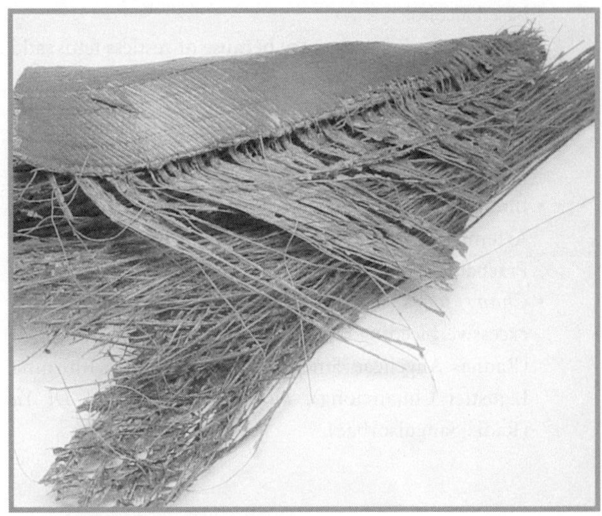

Pinyin Name: *Zong Lu Pi*
Literal Name: "palm stipule"
Alternate Chinese Names: *Zong Lu Tan, Zong Lu*
Original Source: *Ben Cao Shi Yi* (Omissions from the [Classic of the] Materia Medica) by Chen Cang-Qi in 741 A.D.
English Name: trachycarpus stiple fiber
Botanical Name: *Trachycarpus fortunei* H. Wendl. (*Zong Lu Shu*)
Pharmaceutical Name: Fibra Stipulae Trachycarpi
Properties: bitter, sour, neutral
Channels Entered: Liver, Lung, Large Intestine

Zong Lu Pi (Fibra Stipulae Trachycarpi)

CHINESE THERAPEUTIC ACTIONS

Restrains Leakage and Stops Bleeding

Zong Lu Pi (Fibra Stipulae Trachycarpi) is a mild and essential herb in stopping bleeding such as epistaxis, hemoptysis, hematemesis, hematuria, uterine bleeding, hematochezia and hemorrhoidal bleeding. It has a strong astringent function and is best for bleeding in the absence of blood stagnation.

- Epistaxis: combine *Zong Lu Pi* with *Xiao Ji* (Herba Cirisii), *Long Gu* (Os Draconis) and *San Qi* (Radix Notoginseng), taken internally. For external use, apply the powder directly to the nostrils.
- Hemoptysis and hematemesis: use it with *Da Ji* (Herba seu Radix Cirsii Japonici), *Xiao Ji* (Herba Cirisii), *Ce Bai Ye* (Cacumen Platycladi), *Qian Cao* (Radix Rubiae) and *Bai Mao Gen* (Rhizoma Imperatae). **Exemplar Formula:** *Shi Hui San* (Ten Partially-charred Substance Powder).
- Uterine bleeding or excessive menstrual bleeding: use *Zong Lu Pi* alone internally. It can also be combined with *Fu Long Gan* (Terra Flava Usta) and *She Xiang* (Moschus).
- Excessive menstrual bleeding caused by heat in the blood: add *Ce Bai Ye* (Cacumen Platycladi).
- Excessive menstrual bleeding from blood stagnation: use *Zong Lu Pi* with *Pu Huang* (Pollen Typhae) and *San Qi* (Radix Notoginseng).
- Excessive menstrual bleeding from deficiency: combine it with *Huang Qi* (Radix Astragali), *Bai Zhu* (Rhizoma Atractylodis Macrocephalae), *Shan Zhu Yu* (Fructus Corni) and *Qian Cao* (Radix Rubiae).
- Continuous light-colored uterine bleeding with no blood clots: use this herb with *Wu Mei* (Fructus Mume), *Pao Jiang* (Rhizoma Zingiberis Preparatum) and grain-based alcohol.
- Bleeding during pregnancy because of restless fetus: add *E Jiao* (Colla Corii Asini).
- Intestinal bleeding, hemorrhoidal bleeding: combine *Zong Lu Pi* with *Huai Jiao* (Fructus Sophorae) and *Ku Lian Pi* (Cortex Meliae).
- Intestinal bleeding due to cold: use it with *Ai Ye* (Folium Artemisiae Argyi), *Fu Zi* (Radix Aconiti Lateralis Praeparata) and egg yolk.
- *Chang feng* (intestinal wind) with hemorrhoids, excessive bleeding: combine this herb with *Dang Gui* (Radicis Angelicae Sinensis), *Chuan Xiong* (Rhizoma Ligustici Chuanxiong), *Fu Ling* (Poria) and *Di Yu* (Radix Sanguisorbae).
- Chronic bleeding hemorrhoids: use it with *Gan Jiang* (Rhizoma Zingiberis), *Wu Mei* (Fructus Mume) and *Gui Xin* (Cortex Rasus Cinnamomi).

DOSAGE

3 to 10 grams in decoction. *Zong Lu Pi* can also be made into pill or powder form (1.5 grams per dose, three times daily). The unprocessed herb does not stop bleeding. It must be charred to ashes to exert its ability to restrain the leakage of blood and stop bleeding.

CAUTIONS / CONTRAINDICATIONS

- Do not use *Zong Lu Pi* as a single-herb remedy in patients experiencing bleeding with blood stagnation. It must be combined with other herbs to invigorate blood and stop bleeding.
- It is contraindicated for patients who have intestinal bleeding and dysentery caused by damp-heat.

CHEMICAL COMPOSITION

Glucoluteolin, luteolin-7-O-rutinoside, dioscin, methyl protodioscin, tannins.[1,2]

PHARMACOLOGICAL EFFECTS

- **Hemostatic:** Decoction of charred *Zong Lu Pi* is associated with marked action to stop bleeding in mice.[3] Decoction of fresh *Zong Lu Pi*, however, did not have any hemostatic effect.[4]

SUPPLEMENT

- 棕櫚子 / 棕榈子 *Zong Lu Zi* (Fructus Trachycarpi) is derived from the fruit of the same plant as *Zong Lu Pi*. Both herbs have very similar functions and indications. However, *Zong Lu Zi* is more effective in treating hypertension, insomnia, or excessive dreaming. The dosage of *Zong Lu Zi* is 6 to 30 grams.

References

1. *Xian Dai Zhong Yao Yao Li Xue* (Contemporary Pharmacology of Chinese Herbs), 1997; 867
2. *Chang Yong Zhong Yao Cheng Fen Yu Yao Li Shou Ce* (A Handbook of the Composition and Pharmacology of Common Chinese Drugs), *1994*; 1657-1658
3. *Zhong Yao Tong Bao* (Journal of Chinese Herbology), 1983; 8(2):23
4. *Zhong Yao Xue* (Chinese Herbology), 1998; 498:500

Ou Jie (Nodus Nelumbinis Rhizomatis)

藕節 藕节

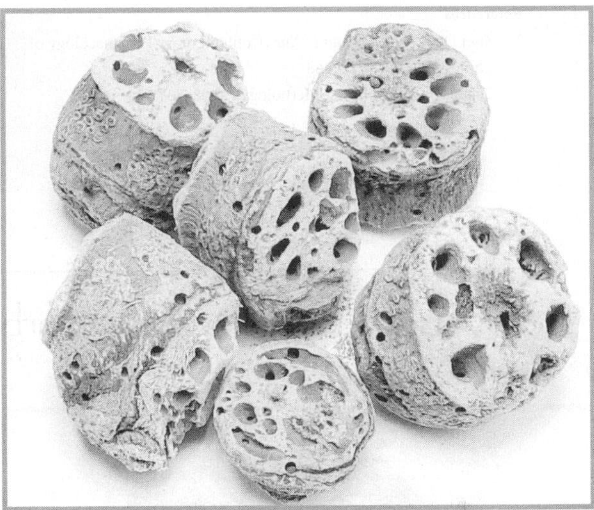

Pinyin Name: *Ou Jie*
Literal Name: "lotus joint"
Alternate Chinese Names: *Guang Ou Jie, Ou Jie Ba*
Original Source: *Yao Xing Ben Cao* (Materia Medica of Medicinal Properties) by Zhen Quan in 600 A.D.
English Name: lotus node, lotus rhizome node
Botanical Name: *Nelumbo nucifera* Gaertn. (*Lian*)
Pharmaceutical Name: Nodus Nelumbinis Rhizomatis
Properties: sweet, astringent, neutral
Channels Entered: Lung, Stomach, Liver

CHINESE THERAPEUTIC ACTIONS

Stops Bleeding

Ou Jie (Nodus Nelumbinis Rhizomatis) treats various bleeding disorders, but is especially effective for hemoptysis and hematemesis. It restrains leakage, stops bleeding, and disperses blood stasis. This herb is preferred for treatment of bleeding caused by blood stagnation. It has dual actions to both move the blood and stop bleeding.

- Hematemesis: drink the juice of fresh *Ou Jie*. It may also be used with *He Di* (Calyx Nelumbinis).
- Hemoptysis: combine *Ou Jie* with *E Jiao* (Colla Corii Asini), *Bai Ji* (Rhizoma Bletillae), and *Pi Pa Ye* (Folium Eriobotryae).
- Hemoptysis with bright red blood from Lung heat: use it with *Ce Bai Ye* (Cacumen Platycladi), *Bai Mao Gen* (Rhizoma Imperatae), and *E Jiao* (Colla Corii Asini).
- Epistaxis: instill the juice of *Ou Jie* into the nostrils.
- Hematuria, hematochezia because of heat in the lower *jiao*: use it with *Xiao Ji* (Herba Cirisii), *Tong Cao* (Medulla Tetrapanacis), *Hua Shi* (Talcum), and *Dan Zhu Ye* (Herba Lophatheri).
- Hematuria, hematochezia from deficiency: mix with *Ren Shen* (Radix Ginseng) and honey.

DOSAGE

10 to 15 grams, with a maximum of 30 grams, in herbal decoction. The dosage for fresh *Ou Jie* is 30 to 60 grams. It is commonly used as herbal decoction, herbal juice, or incorporated into pills and powders. The unprocessed herb clears heat and cools blood, and is most effective in treating bleeding caused by heat. The charred herb has a neutral or slightly warm property, and stops bleeding from deficiency and cold.

CHEMICAL COMPOSITION

Asparagine, tannins, vitamin C, starch.[1]

PHARMACOLOGICAL EFFECTS

- **Hemostatic:** Both fresh and charred *Ou Jie* have demonstrated hemostatic effects. The charred herb is stronger than the fresh form for this application.[2]

CLINICAL STUDIES AND RESEARCH

- **Bleeding hemorrhoids:** An herbal decoction containing 9 grams of *Ou Jie* and 15 grams of *Bai Guo* (Semen Ginkgo), taken twice daily, showed marked effectiveness in treatment of chronic bleeding hemorrhoids. After recovery, patients were advised to take *Shi Quan Da Bu Tang* (All-Inclusive Great Tonifying Decoction) to tonify the constitution.[3]
- **Ocular bleeding:** Two patients with chronic bleeding and blood stasis in the anterior chamber of the eyes (refractory to western medical treatment) received an herbal decoction with 40 grams of *Ou Jie* twice daily, with significant improvement.[4]
- **Nasal polyps:** In one study, patients were treated with an herbal powder applied topically to the affected area once every hour for 5 days per course of treatment. Of 35 patients, the study reported complete recovery in 27 patients, marked improvement in 5 patients, and no response in 3 patients. The herbal powder contained *Ou Jie* 60g, *Wu Mei* (Fructus Mume) 30g, *Ming Fan* (Alumen) 15g, and *Bing Pian* (Borneolum Syntheticum) 3g.[5]

AUTHORS' COMMENTS

There are eight parts of the lotus plant that are used as medicines. Please refer to the monograph on *Lian Zi* (Semen Nelumbinis) for a complete description of each of them.

Ou Jie (Nodus Nelumbinis Rhizomatis)

References
1. *Xian Dai Zhong Yao Yao Li Xue* (Contemporary Pharmacology of Chinese Herbs), 1997; 868
2. *Zhong Yao Xue* (Chinese Herbology), 1998; 504:505
3. *Shan Dong Zhong Yi Za Zhi* (Shandong Journal of Chinese Medicine), 1982; 6:363
4. *Jiang Su Zhong Yi Za Zhi* (Jiangsu Journal of Chinese Medicine), 1987; 8(7):46
5. *Zhong Yi Za Zhi* (Journal of Chinese Medicine), 1987; 6:412

Xue Yu Tan (Crinis Carbonisatus)

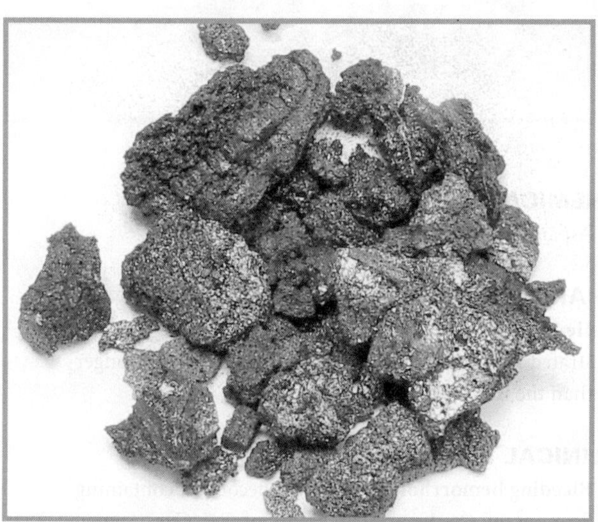

血餘炭 血余炭

Pinyin Name: *Xue Yu Tan*
Literal Name: "charred excess of the blood"
Alternate Chinese Names: *Luan Fa, Ren Tui, Du Xue Yu*
Original Source: *Shen Nong Ben Cao Jing* (Divine Husbandman's Classic of the Materia Medica) in the second century
English Name: charred human hair
Zoological Name: *Homo sapiens* L. (*Ren Tou Fa*)
Pharmaceutical Name: Crinis Carbonisatus
Properties: bitter, neutral
Channels Entered: Liver, Stomach

CHINESE THERAPEUTIC ACTIONS

1. Stops Bleeding and Disperses Stagnation

Xue Yu Tan (Crinis Carbonisatus) treats bleeding disorders including epistaxis, hematemesis, hemoptysis, hematuria, hematochezia and uterine bleeding. It stops bleeding and yet does not have the side effect of creating stagnation, because it disperses obstruction. It can be used externally or internally to stop bleeding.

- Bleeding gums: apply *Xue Yu Tan* topically in powder form.
- Epistaxis: apply it topically in the nostrils, and drink the fresh juice of *Ou Jie* (Nodus Nelumbinis Rhizomatis).
- Hematemesis and hemoptysis: use this substance with *Hua Rui Shi* (Ophicalcitum) and *San Qi* (Radix Notoginseng).
- Hematuria: use it with vinegar.
- Burning dysuria with blood: add it to *Xiao Ji* (Herba Cirisii), *Bai Mao Gen* (Rhizoma Imperatae) and *Chuan Mu Tong* (Caulis Clematidis Armandii).
- Hematochezia: combine it with *Di Yu* (Radix Sanguisorbae) and *Huai Hua* (Flos Sophorae).
- Hematochezia with middle *jiao* deficiency and cold: use *Xue Yu Tan* with *Gan Jiang* (Rhizoma Zingiberis).
- Hemorrhoidal bleeding of bright red blood: use it with *Huai Jiao* (Fructus Sophorae) and *Ku Lian Pi* (Cortex Meliae).

2. Tonifies Yin and Promotes Urination

Dysuria: *Xue Yu Tan* enters the *xue* (blood) level in the lower *jiao* to stop bleeding.

- Dysuria in women: serve *Xue Yu Tan* with warm liquor.
- Burning sensations during urination: use this substance with *Hua Shi* (Talcum) and *Che Qian Zi* (Semen Plantaginis).
- Urinary stones: combine it with *Che Qian Cao* (Herba Plantaginis), *Hai Jin Sha* (Herba Lygodii), *Ji Nei Jin* (Endothelium Corneum Gigeriae Galli) and *Jin Qian Cao* (Herba Lysimachiae).

DOSAGE

6 to 10 grams in decoction. *Xue Yu Tan* is also given in powder form, 1.5 to 3 grams three times daily. *Xue Yu Tan* can be made into pills. *Xue Yu Tan* is ineffective to stop bleeding if not properly processed. It must be charred to ashes to stop bleeding and disperse stagnation.

Xue Yu Tan (Crinis Carbonisatus)

CAUTIONS / CONTRAINDICATIONS

- Use *Xue Yu Tan* with caution for patients with weak digestive systems, as nausea and vomiting may occur.

CHEMICAL COMPOSITION

Eukeratin, melanin.[1]

PHARMACOLOGICAL EFFECTS

- **Hemostatic:** In animal studies, administration of water and alcohol extracts of *Xue Yu Tan* is associated with marked effectiveness to stop bleeding. Without charring, however, it has no effect on clotting.[2]
- **Antibiotic:** *Xue Yu Tan* has an inhibitory effect against *Staphylococcus aureus*, *Salmonella typhi*, and *Bacillus dysenteriae*.[3]

CLINICAL STUDIES AND RESEARCH

- **Peptic ulcer disease:** Gastric or duodenal ulcerations and bleeding in 34 patients were treated with an herbal formula, with marked success. The study reported stabilization in most patients within 3 to 5 days, and in all patients within 10 days. The herbal formula was given in powder form, and contained *Xue Yu Tan* 2 parts, *San Qi* (Radix Notoginseng) 2.5 parts, and *Bai Ji* (Rhizoma Bletillae) 3 parts.[4]
- **Upper gastrointestinal bleeding:** An herbal formula containing 3 to 9 grams of *Xue Yu Tan* added to 20 to 40 ml of fresh juice of *Ou Jie* (Nodus Nelumbinis Rhizomatis) was given three times daily for treatment of upper gastrointestinal bleeding. The study reported complete recovery in 23 of 25 patients.[5]
- **External bleeding:** In one clinical study, 61 patients who were bleeding because of various external and traumatic injuries were treated topically with an herbal formula, with marked effectiveness. The herbal formula was given in powder, and contained *Xue Yu Tan* 25g, charred *Zhu Zong Cao* (Herba Adianti) 25g, roasted *Chuan Shan Jia* (Squama Manis) 40g, charred *Bai Ji* (Rhizoma Bletillae) 20g, *Hai Piao Xiao* (Endoconcha Sepiae) 40g, *Ming Fan* (Alumen) 20g, *Bing Pian* (Borneolum Syntheticum) 10g, and *Lu Gan Shi* (Galamina) 20g.[6]

References

1. *Xian Dai Zhong Yao Yao Li Xue* (Contemporary Pharmacology of Chinese Herbs), 1997; 845
2. *Zhong Yao Xue* (Chinese Herbology), 1998; 513:516
3. Ibid.
4. *Hu Nan Yi Yao Za Zhi* (Hunan Journal of Medicine and Herbology), 1979; 2:20
5. *Xin Zhong Yi* (New Chinese Medicine), 5:35
6. Ibid., 1985; 17(8):31

San Qi (Radix Notoginseng)

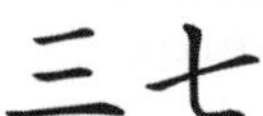

Pinyin Name: *San Qi*
Literal Name: "three-seven"
Alternate Chinese Names: *Tian Qi, Shen San Qi, Shen Qi, Jin Bu Huan*
English Name: pseudoginseng, notoginseng
Botanical Name: *Panax notoginseng* (Burk.) F. H. Chen. (*San Qi*)
Pharmaceutical Name: Radix Notoginseng
Properties: sweet, slightly bitter, warm
Channels Entered: Liver, Stomach

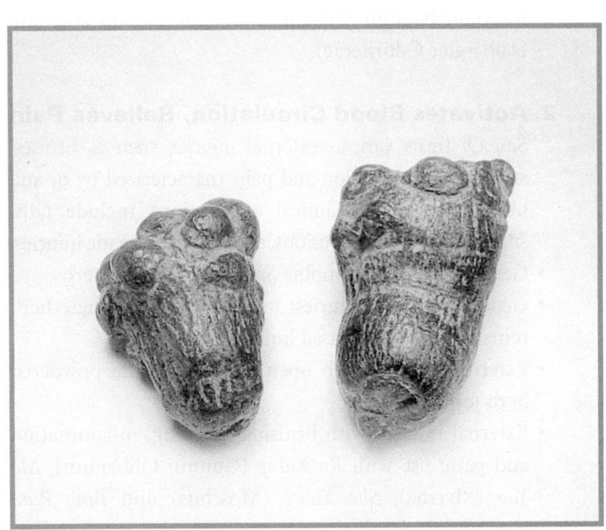

San Qi (Radix Notoginseng)

CHINESE THERAPEUTIC ACTIONS

1. Disperses Blood Stasis, Stops Bleeding

Internal and external bleeding: *San Qi* (Radix Notoginseng) has a unique ability to stop bleeding without causing blood stasis, and can be taken internally or applied topically. Clinically, it treats hematemesis, hemoptysis, epistaxis, hematochezia, profuse menstrual bleeding, profuse postpartum bleeding, and external bleeding arising from trauma.

- Epistaxis or hematemesis: use *San Qi* individually.
- Epistaxis, hemoptysis, hematemesis, or hematuria: combine this herb with *Hua Rui Shi* (Ophicalcitum) and *Xue Yu Tan* (Crinis Carbonisatus).
- Qi deficiency caused by profuse hematemesis: use it with *Dang Shen* (Radix Codonopsis), *Shan Yao* (Rhizoma Dioscoreae), *Sheng Di Huang* (Radix Rehmanniae) and *Zhi Mu* (Radix Anemarrhenae).
- Hemoptysis with chest pain because of dryness and heat attacking the Lung: use this herb with *Bai Mao Gen* (Rhizoma Imperatae), *Da Huang* (Radix et Rhizoma Rhei), and *Long Gu* (Os Draconis).
- Chronic hemoptysis and hematemesis: combine it with *Long Gu* (Os Draconis), *Mu Li* (Concha Ostreae) and *Shan Zhu Yu* (Fructus Corni).
- Uterine bleeding: use *San Qi* alone internally.
- Hematochezia: mix it with a small portion of grain-based liquor.
- Profuse postpartum or menstrual bleeding: add it to *Si Wu Tang* (Four-Substance Decoction).
- External bleeding with pus and ulceration: use it alone topically as powder.
- External bleeding due to cuts: use it with *Long Gu* (Os Draconis), *Xue Jie* (Sanguis Draconis), *Mo Yao* (Myrrha), *Ru Xiang* (Gummi Olibanum) and *Jiang Xiang* (Lignum Dalbergiae Odoriferae).

2. Activates Blood Circulation, Relieves Pain

San Qi treats various external injuries such as bruises, swelling, inflammation and pain characterized by qi and blood stagnation. Clinical applications include falls, sprains, fractures, contusions, and other traumatic injuries.

- General bleeding: combine *San Qi* with other herbs.
- General external injuries: use *San Qi* as a single-herb remedy with grain-based liquor or hot water.
- External injuries with open cuts: apply the powdered herb topically.
- External injuries with bruising, swelling, inflammation and pain: use with *Ru Xiang* (Gummi Olibanum), *Mo Yao* (Myrrha), *She Xiang* (Moschus) and *Bing Pian* (Borneolum Syntheticum).
- Muscle and tendon injuries with pain: combine it with *Xiang Fu* (Rhizoma Cyperi) and *Gan Cao* (Radix Glycyrrhizae).
- External injuries with severe bruises and pain: use it with *Cao Wu* (Radix Aconiti Kusnezoffii), *Chi Shao* (Radix Paeoniae Rubrae) and *Hong Hua* (Flos Carthami).
- Angina: use it with *Dan Shen* (Radix Salviae Miltiorrhizae) and *Mao Dong Qing* (Radix Ilicis Pubescentis).

3. Reduces Swelling and Pain

External injuries are often accompanied by infection, suppuration and pus formation.

- Early-stage external injuries with no complications: use *San Qi* internally with grain-based liquor, or topically as powder.
- External injuries with suppuration: mix *San Qi* powder with vinegar and apply it topically.
- External injuries with open sores and suppuration: apply *San Qi* without vinegar
- External injuries with sores, lesions, and ulcerations: use it with *Ru Xiang* (Gummi Olibanum), *Mo Yao* (Myrrha), *Xue Jie* (Sanguis Draconis) and *Er Cha* (Catechu).

DOSAGE

3 to 10 grams as herbal decoction. 1.0 to 1.5 grams per dose as powder, one to three times daily. In severe cases of bleeding, the dosage of *San Qi* is increased to 3 to 6 grams of powder orally, two to three times daily. This herb is often used as powder or pills instead of decoction, because of its high cost.

CAUTIONS / CONTRAINDICATIONS

- Use *San Qi* with caution during pregnancy.
- Use of *San Qi* is sometimes associated with the following side effects: nausea, vomiting, loss of appetite, dizziness, headache, toothache, fatigue, and restlessness.

OVERDOSAGE

In rare cases, *San Qi* may cause bleeding, such as in epistaxis, bleeding gums, and increased menstrual bleeding. This occurs because *San Qi* has the dual effect to invigorate blood circulation and stop bleeding.

Allergic reactions associated with use of *San Qi* have also been reported. These adverse reactions are self-limiting, and generally subside with reduction of dosage or discontinuation of herbal therapy.[1]

CHEMICAL COMPOSITION

Saponins 3 to 12% (ginsenoside R_{b1}, R_d, R_e, R_{g1}, R_{g2}, R_{h2}; notoginsenoside R_1, R_2, R_3, R_4, R_6; 20-glucoginsenoside Rf, gypenoside XVII), dencichine, essential oils (α-copaene, β-cubebene, caryophyllene, guaiene, α-cedrene).[2,3,4]

San Qi (Radix Notoginseng)

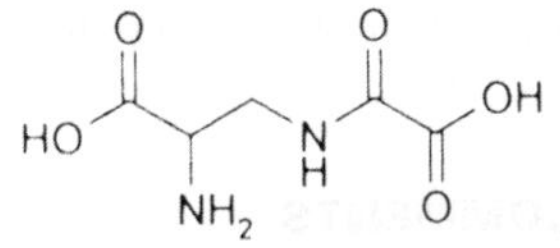

Dencichine

PHARMACOLOGICAL EFFECTS

- **Hemostatic:** Administration of *San Qi* in powder or water extract is associated with marked effects to decrease prothrombin time and stop bleeding. This hemostatic function is attributed mainly to dencichine.[5]
- **Antiplatelet:** Saponins of *San Qi* has been shown to inhibit the aggregation of platelets. [6]
- **CNS stimulant and suppressant:** Administration of *San Qi* has demonstrated both stimulating and sedative effects on the central nervous system (CNS). Aerial parts of this plant are rich in ginsenoside Rb, and are characterized by sedative, tranquilizing and hypnotic effects. The roots are rich in ginsenoside Rg, and are characterized by stimulating and adaptogenic effects. [7]
- **Cardiovascular:** Administration of *San Qi* in dogs via intravenous injection decreases blood pressure, decreases heart rate, increases blood perfusion to the coronary artery, and decreases oxygen consumption by the cardiac muscle. It is commonly used to treat arrhythmia secondary to decreased cardiac output. [8]
- **Immunostimulant:** *San Qi* has an immune-enhancing effect similar to that of *Ren Shen* (Radix Ginseng), as both herbs have overlapping active compounds. Please refer to the monograph on *Ren Shen* for additional details.

CLINICAL STUDIES AND RESEARCH

- **Upper gastrointestinal bleeding:** Patients with upper gastrointestinal bleeding were treated once daily with an intravenous infusion of 8 to 16 ml of *San Qi* injectable (equivalent to 4 to 6 grams of dried herb) mixed with 500 ml of D5W. The study reported an absence of blood in the stools after an average of 5.98 days, with an average of 15.02 days of hospitalization. [9]
- **Stomach bleeding:** In one study, 1.5 grams of *San Qi* powder with warm water were given three times daily to patients with stomach bleeding. Oral ingestion of food was allowed, except for patients with hematemesis. Patients were instructed to continue taking the herbs for 2 days after a stool exam confirmed the absence of blood. The study reported that bleeding stopped in 58 of the 60 patients. [10]
- **Hemoptysis:** According to one report, administration of *San Qi* powder was used to treat 10 patients with coughing of blood due to bronchiectasis, pulmonary tuberculosis or pulmonary abscess. The treatment protocol was to administer 6 to 9 grams of *San Qi* powder per dose, two to three times daily. The study reported that bleeding stopped in 8 patients after 5 days, and 2 patients continued to have coughing of blood for 1 to 2 weeks.[11]
- **Hematuria:** According to one report, administration of 0.9 to 1.5 grams of *San Qi* powder every 4 to 8 hours was effective to stop hematuria after 3 days in 39 patients.[12]
- **Hyphema:** In one study, 21 patients were treated with a 2% *San Qi* ophthalmic solution six times daily with excellent results.[13]
- **Craniocerebral trauma:** Forty patients were treated with 3 grams of *San Qi* powder two to three times daily via oral administration if the patients were conscious, or intranasal administration if unconscious. The duration of treatment ranged from 3 to 10 days, with a maximum of 21 days. Patients with severe craniocerebral trauma were also treated with intravenous fluids, diuretics, antibiotics and sedatives. The study reported an overall rate of effectiveness of 75%, with marked success in mild to moderate conditions.[14]
- **Coronary artery disease:** In a multi-center study of 778 patients, administration of 0.6 to 1.2 grams of *San Qi* demonstrated a 70.2% effective rate in treatment of angina.[15]
- **Hypercholesterolemia:** Ten patients with hypercholesterolemia, atherosclerosis, and coronary artery disease were treated with 0.6 grams of *San Qi* powder three times daily. The average cholesterol level was reduced from 272.6 to 185 mg/dL after one month of continuous herbal therapy.[16]
- **Liver disorders:** One gram of *San Qi* powder given three times daily for 1 month was administered to patients with elevated liver enzyme levels from unknown causes. The study reported a reduction of these enzyme levels in 44 out of 45 patients.[17]
- **Chronic hepatitis:** According to one report, 65 patients with chronic hepatitis due to blood stasis were treated with a *San Qi* injectable one time each day for 3 to 4 months. Daily dosages varied between 2 to 6 ml of the injectable (equivalent to 1 to 3 grams of dried herb). Out of 65 patients, 47 reported marked improvement, 5 reported moderate improvement, and 13 reported no response. The overall rate of effectiveness was 80%.[18]

HERB-DRUG INTERACTION

- **Anticoagulant or antiplatelet drugs:** *San Qi* has an unique action to regulate the blood, with action to invigorate blood circulation and stop bleeding. Though this potential interaction has not been documented, use of this herb may interfere with anticoagulant or antiplatelet medications.[19] [Note: Examples of anticoagulants include heparin, warfarin (Coumadin) and enoxaparin (Lovenox); and examples of antiplatelets include aspirin, dipyridamole (Persantine), and clopidogrel (Plavix).]

San Qi (Radix Notoginseng)

TOXICOLOGY

Oral administration of *San Qi* powder in mice at 15 g/kg did not cause any significant adverse reactions. Biopsy of the heart, liver, kidney, spleen and intestinal tissues did not reveal any abnormalities 2 weeks after termination of herbal therapy. The lethal dose of *San Qi* through intravenous injection is 2.5 to 3.0 g/kg for rabbits, 0.5 to 0.75 g/kg for rats, and 0.075 to 0.1 g/kg for mice.[20]

SUPPLEMENT

- 菊葉三七 / 菊叶三七 *Ju Ye San Qi* (Herba seu Radix Gynura Segetum), first cited in the *Zhen Nan Ben Cao* (Materia Medica of South Yunnan) by Lan Mao in the Qing Dynasty, is used for its functions to disperse blood stagnation, stop bleeding, eliminate toxins, and reduce swelling. Sweet, slightly bitter and neutral, *Ju Ye San Qi* is used both internally and topically. Clinical applications include epistaxis, hematemesis, traumatic injuries with bleeding and bruises, sores and swelling, and breast abscesses. The dosage of *Ju Ye San Qi* is 1.5 to 3.0 grams of powder, given one to three times daily. The powder is to be mixed with the decoction prior to ingestion. The fresh form can be applied topically as a paste. It is contraindicated during pregnancy.
- 景天三七 *Jing Tian San Qi* (Herba seu Radix Sedum Aizoom), first cited in the *Zhi Wu Ming Shi Tu Kao* (Illustrated Guide for Nomenclature and Identification of Botanical Products), stops bleeding, disperses stagnation, nourishes blood, and calms the *shen* (spirit). Sweet, sour and neutral, the clinical applications of *Jing Tian San Qi* include epistaxis, hemoptysis, hematemesis, hematuria, hematochezia, profuse menstrual bleeding, purpura, palpitations, insomnia, restlessness, and neurosis. It can also be used topically to treat external bleeding from trauma. *Jing Tian San Qi* incorporates the entire plant (both the aerial part and the root) as the medicinal herb. The dosage is 15 to 30 grams for the aerial part, and 6 to 10 grams for the root.

AUTHORS' COMMENTS

San Qi should be used with herbs that cool the blood, if bleeding is caused by heat in the blood. It should be used with yin tonics if bleeding is accompanied by dry mouth due to yin deficiency.

References

1. *Xian Dai Zhong Yao Yao Li Xue* (Contemporary Pharmacology of Chinese Herbs), 1997; 282-283, 1997; 807:824
2. Ibid., 807
3. *Chang Yong Zhong Yao Cheng Fen Yu Yao Li Shou Ce* (A Handbook of the Composition and Pharmacology of Common Chinese Drugs), 1994; 127-129
4. Yan X, Zhou J, Xie G, *Traditional Chinese Medicines Molecular Structures, Natural Sources and Applications*; Ashgate, 1999; 1621
5. *Zhong Cao Yao* (Chinese Herbal Medicine), 1986; 17(6):34
6. *Zhong Yao Xue* (Chinese Herbology), 1998; 507:512
7. *Zhong Cao Yao* (Chinese Herbal Medicine), 1986; 17(1):15
8. *Zhong Yao Xue* (Chinese Herbology), 1998; 507:512
9. *Shang Hai Zhong Yi Yao Za Zhi* (Shanghai Journal of Chinese Medicine and Herbology), 1983; 9:15
10. *Yun Nan Zhong Yi Za Zhi* (Yunan Journal of Chinese Medicine), 1985; 1:28
11. *Zhong Yi Za Zhi* (Journal of Chinese Medicine), 1965; 11:29
12. *Ha Yi Da Xue Bao* (Journal of Ha Medical University), 1974; 7(2):51
13. *Shang Hai Yi Xue* (Shanghai Medicine), 1978; 3:16
14. *Xin Yi Xue* (New Medicine), 1979; 10(7):330
15. *Zhong Cao Yao* (Chinese Herbal Medicine), 1980; 11(10):439
16. *Xin Yi Yao Xue Za Zhi* (New Journal of Medicine and Herbology), 1973; 10:13
17. *Zhong Yi Za Zhi* (Journal of Chinese Medicine), 1980; 8:12
18. *Shang Hai Zhong Yi Yao Za Zhi* (Shanghai Journal of Chinese Medicine and Herbology), 1983; 8:12
19. *Shen Yang Yi Xue Yuan Xue Bao* (Journal of Shenyang University of Medicine)
20. *Xian Dai Zhong Yao Yao Li Xue* (Contemporary Pharmacology of Chinese Herbs), 1997; 282-283, 1997; 807:824

Qian Cao (Radix Rubiae)

茜草 茜草

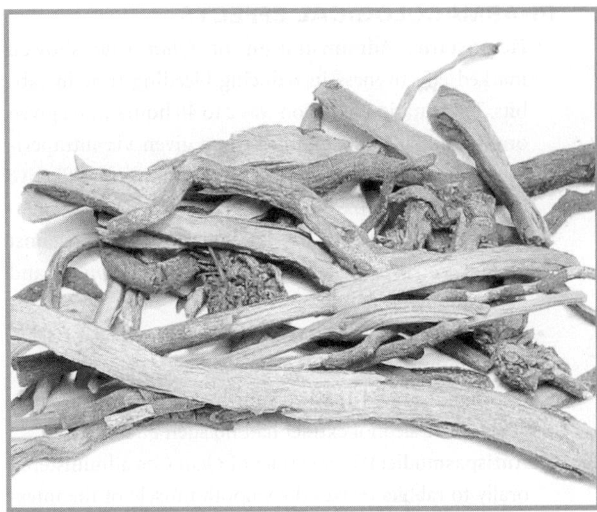

Pinyin Name: *Qian Cao*
Alternate Chinese Names: *Qian Cao Gen, Qian Gen, Xue Jian Chou, Huo Xue Dan, Di Xue, Ru Lu, Ran Fei Cao*
Original Source: *Shen Nong Ben Cao Jing* (Divine Husbandman's Classic of the Materia Medica) in the second century
English Name: madder, India madder root
Botanical Name: *Rubia cordifolia* L. (*Qian Cao*)
Pharmaceutical Name: Radix Rubiae
Properties: bitter, cold
Channels Entered: Liver

CHINESE THERAPEUTIC ACTIONS

1. Cools the Blood, Stops Bleeding

Qian Cao (Radix Rubiae) cools blood, balances yin, sedates fire, and thus stops bleeding caused by heat in the blood. Manifestations of heat in the blood include epistaxis, hematemesis, profuse menstrual bleeding, and hematochezia.

- Epistaxis because of heat and fire rising upwards: combine *Qian Cao* with *Ai Ye* (Folium Artemisiae Argyi) and *Wu Mei* (Fructus Mume).
- Persistent hematemesis: use it with *Hei Dou* (Semen Glycine Max) and *Gan Cao* (Radix Glycyrrhizae).
- Profuse hematemesis: use it with *San Qi* (Radix Notoginseng) and *Ji Xue Teng* (Caulis Spatholobi).
- Hematemesis due to heat in the Lung and Stomach, with underlying deficiency and weakness: combine this herb with *Huang Qin* (Radix Scutellariae), *Ce Bai Ye* (Cacumen Platycladi), *Huang Qi* (Radix Astragali), and *Dang Gui* (Radicis Angelicae Sinensis).
- Hematemesis due to heat: use *Qian Cao* individually.
- Profuse uterine bleeding from qi deficiency: use this herb with *Huang Qi* (Radix Astragali), *Bai Zhu* (Rhizoma Atractylodis Macrocephalae), *Shan Zhu Yu* (Fructus Corni) and *Long Gu* (Os Draconis).
- Hematochezia due to accumulation of damp-heat in the Large Intestine: combine it with *Huang Lian* (Rhizoma Coptidis), *Sheng Ma* (Rhizoma Cimicifugae), *Bai Shao* (Radix Paeoniae Alba) and *Di Yu* (Radix Sanguisorbae).

2. Activates Blood Circulation, Dispels Blood Stasis

Amenorrhea, traumatic injuries, musculoskeletal pain: In addition to stopping bleeding, *Qian Cao* has a unique function to move blood and dispel blood stasis. Clinically, it is commonly used to treat amenorrhea, traumatic injuries, sports injuries, and musculoskeletal pain caused by blood stasis.

- Amenorrhea caused by blood stasis: use *Qian Cao* with *Dang Gui* (Radicis Angelicae Sinensis), *Xiang Fu* (Rhizoma Cyperi) and *Chi Shao* (Radix Paeoniae Rubrae).
- Traumatic or sports injuries: combine it with *Hong Hua* (Flos Carthami), *Dang Gui* (Radicis Angelicae Sinensis), and *Chuan Xiong* (Rhizoma Ligustici Chuanxiong).
- Musculoskeletal or arthritic pain: use with *Ji Xue Teng* (Caulis Spatholobi), *Hai Feng Teng* (Caulis Piperis Kadsurae) and *Yan Hu Suo* (Rhizoma Corydalis), as a medicinal tincture.

DOSAGE

10 to 15 grams, with a maximum of 30 grams, for herbal decoction. *Qian Cao* is commonly used as both decoction and powder. The fresh herb has a stronger function to activate blood circulation and dispel blood stasis. The charred form more effectively stops bleeding.

CAUTIONS / CONTRAINDICATIONS

- Bitter, cold and draining in nature, *Qian Cao* should be used with caution in cases of weakness and deficiency of the Spleen and Stomach, deficiency of *jing* (essence) or blood, or yin-deficient fire.
- Because of its hemostatic effect, *Qian Cao* should be used with caution in the absence of blood stasis.

CHEMICAL COMPOSITION

Purpurin, purpuroxanthin, alizarin, munjistin, pseudopurpurin, physcion, quinizarin, rubian, rubimaillin.[1]

Qian Cao (Radix Rubiae)

PHARMACOLOGICAL EFFECTS

- **Hemostatic:** Administration of *Qian Cao* showed marked effectiveness in reducing bleeding time in rabbits. The duration of action was 2 to 48 hours when given orally, and 30 to 60 minutes when given via intraperitoneal injection. The charred herb was more effective than the fresh herb.[2]
- **Antibiotic:** *Qian Cao* has an inhibitory effect against *Staphylococcus aureus, Diplococcus pneumoniae,* and dermatophytes.[3]
- **Antitussive and expectorant:** A water extract of *Qian Cao*, administered orally to mice at the dosage of 75 g/kg, has demonstrated marked antitussive and expectorant effects. The alcohol extract had no such effect.[4]
- **Antispasmodic:** Water extract of *Qian Cao* administered orally to rabbits relaxes the smooth muscle of the intestines to treat intestinal spasms and cramps.[5]
- **Effect on kidney stones:** A diet regimen containing 20% *Qian Cao* showed promise in preventing or minimizing the formation of kidney stones in mice.[6]
- **Immunostimulant:** Administration of *Qian Cao* to mice and dogs is associated with a 151.9% rise in the white blood cell count, compared to a placebo.[7]

CLINICAL STUDIES AND RESEARCH

- **Bleeding:** In one report, 41 patients with profuse bleeding after tooth extraction were treated with topical application of powdered extract of *Qian Cao*. Bleeding stopped in all patients within 1 to 2 minutes.[8]
- **Chronic tracheitis:** According to one study, 123 patients with chronic tracheitis were treated with an herbal formula containing *Qian Cao* and *Chen Pi* (Pericarpium Citri Reticulatae) for 20 days. The rate of effectiveness was 69.1%.[9]

TOXICOLOGY

No significant toxicity or fatalities were reported when *Qian Cao* decoction was given at a dosage of 150 g/kg in mice. At 175 g/kg, 1 out of 5 mice died.[10]

AUTHORS' COMMENTS

According to Dr. Gan Zhu-Wang, *Qian Cao* (Radix Rubiae), *Zi Cao Gen* (Radix Lithospermi), and *Han Lian Cao* (Herba Ecliptae) cool blood and treat various dermatological disorders characterized by itching. The same combination relieves nasal itching associated with allergic rhinitis or sinusitis.

References

1. *Chang Yong Zhong Yao Cheng Fen Yu Yao Li Shou Ce* (A Handbook of the Composition and Pharmacology of Common Chinese Drugs), 1994; 1355-1356
2. *Zhong Yi Yao Yan Jiu* (Research of Chinese Medicine and Herbology), 1991; (3):54
3. *Zhong Yao Yao Li Yu Ying Yong* (Pharmacology and Applications of Chinese Herbs), 1989; 3:751
4. Ibid.
5. *Zhong Yao Xue* (Chinese Herbology), 1998; 516:519
6. Ibid.
7. *Zhong Yi Yao Yan Jiu* (Research of Chinese Medicine and Herbology), 1991; (3):54
8. *Yi Xue Wei Sheng Tong Xun* (Journal of Medicine and Sanitation), 1974; 1:54
9. *Fu Jian Jun Qu Wei Sheng Bu* (Health Department of Fujian Military), 1972; 3:10
10. *Zhong Yi Yao Yan Jiu* (Research of Chinese Medicine and Herbology), 1991; (3):54

Pu Huang (Pollen Typhae)

蒲黄 蒲黄

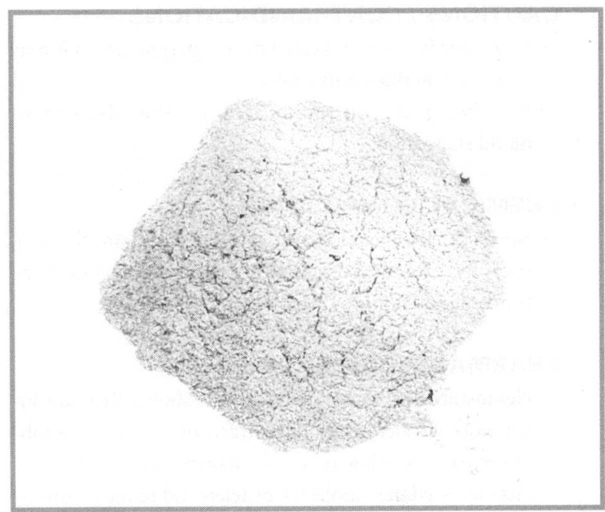

Pinyin Name: *Pu Huang*
Literal Name: "cattail pollen"
Alternate Chinese Names: *Pu Li Hua Fen, Pu Peng Hua Fen, Pu Cao Huang, Pu Hua*
Original Source: *Shen Nong Ben Cao Jing* (Divine Husbandman's Classic of the Materia Medica) in the second century
English Name: bulrush, cattail pollen
Botanical Name: *Typha angustifolia* L. (*Shui Zu Xiang Pu*); *Typha orientalis* Presl. (*Dong Fang Xiang Pu*)
Pharmaceutical Name: Pollen Typhae
Properties: sweet, neutral
Channels Entered: Liver, Pericardium

CHINESE THERAPEUTIC ACTIONS

1. Retains Blood and Stops Bleeding

Pu Huang (Pollen Typhae) has a dual function to simultaneously move the blood and stop bleeding. It treats various types of bleeding without causing blood stagnation. Clinical applications include uterine bleeding, epistaxis, hemoptysis, hematemesis, hematuria, hematochezia, profuse menstrual bleeding, and excessive bleeding from traumatic injuries.

- Hemoptysis or hematemesis resulting from improperly ascending qi: use *Pu Huang* as a single remedy.
- Hemoptysis or hematemesis because of heat in the blood: combine it with *Da Ji* (Herba seu Radix Cirsii Japonici), *Xiao Ji* (Herba Cirisii), and *Bai Mao Gen* (Rhizoma Imperatae).
- Epistaxis due to Lung heat: add *Qing Dai* (Indigo Naturalis).
- External bleeding: use *Pu Huang* topically.

Abnormal uterine bleeding: Recent research has shown that *Pu Huang* promotes contraction of the uterus. It is best for stopping abnormal uterine bleeding.

- Chronic uterine bleeding from deficiency of the *ren* (conception) and *chong* (thoroughfare) channels: combine this herb with *Lu Rong* (Cornu Cervi Pantotrichum) and *Dang Gui* (Radicis Angelicae Sinensis).
- Profuse menstrual bleeding: use *Pu Huang* with *Long Gu* (Os Draconis), *Ai Ye* (Folium Artemisiae Argyi) and *Yi Mu Cao* (Herba Leonuri).

2. Activates Blood Circulation, Eliminates Stagnation

Pu Huang is commonly used to treat pain caused by blood stagnation.

- Severe abdominal pain due to blood stagnation during the postpartum period or accompanying irregular menstruation: use *Pu Huang* with *Wu Ling Zhi* (Excrementum Trogopteri seu Pteromi).
- Dysmenorrhea: use this herb with *Yan Hu Suo* (Rhizoma Corydalis) and *Wu Ling Zhi* (Excrementum Trogopteri seu Pteromi). **Exemplar Formula:** *Shi Xiao San* (Sudden Smile Powder).
- Postpartum abdominal pain with blood deficiency, blood stagnation or cold: combine *Pu Huang* with *Rou Gui* (Cortex Cinnamomi), *Pao Jiang* (Rhizoma Zingiberis Preparatum), *Dang Gui* (Radicis Angelicae Sinensis) and *Shu Di Huang* (Radix Rehmanniae Preparata).
- Profuse postpartum bleeding with irritability, distention, pain and a feeling of oppression because of blood stagnation and heat: use this herb with *He Ye* (Folium Nelumbinis), *Mu Dan Pi* (Cortex Moutan), *Sheng Di Huang* (Radix Rehmanniae) and *Yan Hu Suo* (Rhizoma Corydalis).

3. Promotes Urination

Dysuria or hematuria: *Pu Huang* promotes urination and treats *xue lin* (bloody dysuria).

- Hematuria caused by heat in the Urinary Bladder: use it with *Yu Jin* (Radix Curcumae).
- Burning dysuria: combine this herb with *Sheng Di Huang* (Radix Rehmanniae) and *Dong Kui Zi* (Semen Malvae).

DOSAGE

3 to 10 grams in decoction. Wrap *Pu Huang* in cheesecloth during decoction. It may be used internally or topically. The unprocessed herb activates blood circulation, removes blood stasis, and relieves pain, while the charred herb stops bleeding.

Pu Huang (Pollen Typhae)

CAUTIONS / CONTRAINDICATIONS

- *Pu Huang* is contraindicated during pregnancy, as it may stimulate uterine contractions.
- *Pu Huang* is contraindicated in the absence of blood stagnation.

CHEMICAL COMPOSITION

Isorhamnetin, pentacosane, α-sitosterol, palmitic acid, α-typhasterol, quercetin, kaempferol 3-glucosires, hentriacontanol, nonacosanediol, arachidonic acid.[1]

PHARMACOLOGICAL EFFECTS

- **Hemostatic:** Laboratory studies have shown that administration of water or alcohol extracts of *Pu Huang* in rabbits reduced bleeding time; subcutaneous injection in rabbits increased the number of platelets and reduced thrombin time; and topical application stopped bleeding. Furthermore, charred *Pu Huang* showed a hemostatic effect better than that of unprocessed *Pu Huang*. Conversely, administration of *Pu Huang* demonstrated antiplatelet effects in 31 patients with coronary artery disease and atherosclerosis. In fact, the antiplatelet effect of *Pu Huang* was comparable to 300 mg/day of aspirin.[2,3,4]
- **Cardiovascular:** Administration of *Pu Huang* is associated with increased contractility of the heart, increased blood perfusion to the coronary arteries, decreased blood pressure, and decreased peripheral vascular resistance.[5]
- **Antihypertensive:** Administration of water or alcohol extracts of *Pu Huang* via injection demonstrated a marked effectiveness in reduction of heart rate and blood pressure in cats, rabbits, and dogs. Oral intake of *Pu Huang*, however, showed little or no effect on blood pressure.[6]
- **Antihyperlipidemic:** Administration of *Pu Huang* has demonstrated a marked effect to elevate high density lipoprotein (HDL) and lower total cholesterol (TC) levels. The proposed mechanisms of action include a decrease in absorption and an increase in utilization of cholesterols.[7]
- **Effects on the uterus:** Administration of water or alcohol extract of *Pu Huang* has a stimulating effect on the uterus at small dosages. At larger dosages, however, overstimulation may lead to spasms and cramps. Injection of *Pu Huang* during the third trimester of pregnancy induces labor in mice and rats.[8]
- **Gastrointestinal:** Administration of *Pu Huang* extract in rabbits demonstrated increased intestinal peristalsis and relieved intestinal cramps. Water extract of *Pu Huang* was especially effective for treatment of peptic ulcer and enteritis.[9]
- **Anti-inflammatory:** Administration of *Pu Huang* decoction showed marked anti-inflammatory action, especially for treatment of burns and arthritis. The proposed mechanisms of action include improved circulation and decreased permeability of blood vessels.[10]
- **Immunologic:** Administration of *Pu Huang* may affect both cellular and humoral immunity. At small dosages, it has little or no effect; at moderate dosages, it inhibits the immune system; and at large dosages, it stimulates the immune system. Its immune-enhancing effect is associated with increased phagocytic activity by macrophages.[11]

CLINICAL STUDIES AND RESEARCH

- **Abnormal uterine bleeding in postpartum women:** Continuous bleeding with blood clots in 31 women was treated with 3 grams of *Pu Huang*, three times daily for 3 consecutive days. Most women reported satisfactory results, with a gradual decrease in bleeding and clots.[12]
- **Coronary artery disorder:** One report described 66 patients who were treated with *Pu Huang* for 2 months. According to this report, 89% of the patients reported symptomatic improvement, 89% reported a decrease in angina, 48% showed improvement based on echocardiogram, 58% had a decrease in blood pressure, 60% had a decrease in total cholesterol levels, and 94% had a reduction in triglycerides.[13]
- **Hypercholesterolemia:** In one study, 200 patients were treated with 30 grams of *Pu Huang* in three equally-divided doses daily, with marked reduction in total cholesterol and triglyceride levels.[14]
- **Angiocardiopathy:** In one clinical study, 400 patients with angiocardiopathy were treated with an herbal formula consisting of *Pu Huang*, *Dang Shen* (Radix Codonopsis), *Hong Hua* (Flos Carthami), *Jiang Huang* (Rhizoma Curcumae Longae), *E Zhu* (Rhizoma Curcumae) and *Jiang Xiang* (Lignum Dalbergiae Odoriferae). The effect of the formula was similar to that of *Pu Huang* alone in managing coronary artery disorder and reducing blood cholesterol levels. The herbal formula, however, was 90% effective in reducing blood pressure, especially in stage I and II hypertensive patients.[15]
- **Eczema:** Thirty eczema patients were treated by sprinkling *Pu Huang* powder on the affected area. All 30 patients reported complete recovery in between 6 and 15 days. In addition, 25 of 30 patients reported relief from itching on the same day.[16]
- **Colitis:** Patients suffering from varying degrees of colitis were given three doses of 1.5 grams of an enteric-coated *Pu Huang* preparation. In addition, a rectal instillation of 100 ml of a 5% *Pu Huang* solution was given daily. Out of 17 patients, 2 reported complete recovery, 4 reported satisfactory results, 10 reported slight improvement, and 1 had no response. The rate of effectiveness was 94.12%.[17]

HERB-DRUG INTERACTION

- **Anticoagulant or antiplatelet drugs:** *Pu Huang* has a

Pu Huang (Pollen Typhae)

unique action to regulate the blood, with both hemostatic and antiplatelet effects. Though this potential interaction has not been documented, use of this herb may interfere with anticoagulant or antiplatelet medications.[18] [Note: Examples of anticoagulants include heparin, warfarin (Coumadin) and enoxaparin (Lovenox); and examples of antiplatelets include aspirin, dipyridamole (Persantine), and clopidogrel (Plavix).]

TOXICOLOGY

Pu Huang is generally well-tolerated. The LD_{50} for mice via intraperitoneal administration is 35.57 g/kg. Allergic reactions have been observed in guinea pigs, and reduction of red and white blood cells has been observed in mice.[19]

References

1. *Chang Yong Zhong Yao Cheng Fen Yu Yao Li Shou Ce* (A Handbook of the Composition and Pharmacology of Common Chinese Drugs), 1994; 1715
2. *Zhong Yao Da Ci Dien* (Dictionary of Chinese Herbs), 1977; 2457
3. *Su Zhou Yi Xue Yuan Xue Bao* (Journal of Suzhou University of Medicine), 1988; 8(4):267
4. *Shang Hai Yi Xue* (Shanghai Medicine), 1980; 8:53
5. *Zhong Xi Yi Jie He Za Zhi* (Journal of Integrated Chinese and Western Medicine), 1985; 5(5):299
6. *Zhong Yao Xue* (Chinese Herbology), 1998; 519:522
7. *Zhong Yi Za Zhi* (Journal of Chinese Medicine), 1981; 7:69
8. *Zhong Xi Yi Jie He Za Zhi* (Journal of Integrated Chinese and Western Medicine), 1985; 5(5):299
9. *Hu Nan Yi Yao Za Zhi* (Hunan Journal of Medicine and Herbology), 1984; 11(6):56
10. *Zhong Yao Xue* (Chinese Herbology), 1998; 519:522
11. *Zhong Yi Za Zhi* (Journal of Chinese Medicine), 1990; 25(5):259
12. *Shang Hai Zhong Yi Yao Za Zhi* (Shanghai Journal of Chinese Medicine and Herbology), 1963; 9:1
13. *Hu Nan Yi Yao Za Zhi* (Hunan Journal of Medicine and Herbology), 1982; 9:(3):6
14. *Zhong Xi Yi Jie He Za Zhi* (Journal of Integrated Chinese and Western Medicine), 1985; 5(3):141
15. *Hu Nan Yi Yao Za Zhi* (Hunan Journal of Medicine and Herbology), 1977; 4:20
16. *Xin Yi Yao Xue Za Zhi* (New Journal of Medicine and Herbology), 1977; 9:22
17. *Zhong Yao Tong Bao* (Journal of Chinese Herbology), 1987; 12(8):48
18. Chen, J. Recognition & prevention of herb-drug interactions, *Medical Acupuncture*, Fall/Winter 1998/1999; volume 10/number 2; 9-13
19. *Zhong Xi Yi Jie He Za Zhi* (Journal of Integrated Chinese and Western Medicine), 1985; 5(5):296

Hua Rui Shi (Ophicalcitum)

花蕊石 花蕊石

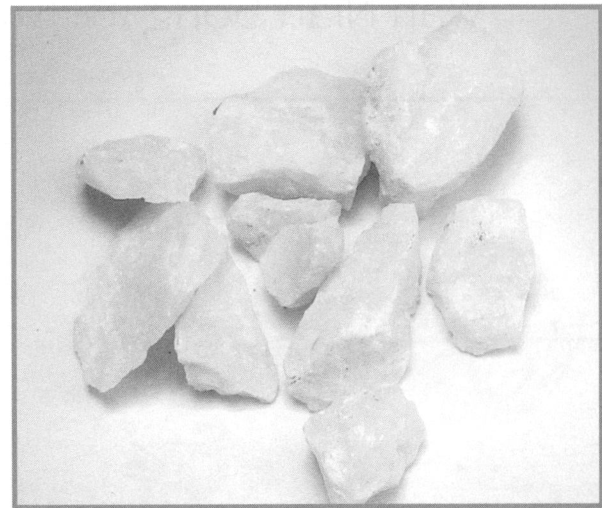

Pinyin Name: *Hua Rui Shi*
Alternate Chinese Names: *Hua Ru Shi*
Original Source: *Jia You Ben Cao* (Materia Medica of the Jia You Era) by Zhang Yu-Xi and Su Song in 1057-1060
English Name: ophicalcite
Pharmaceutical Name: Ophicalcitum
Properties: sour, astringent, neutral
Channels Entered: Liver

CHINESE THERAPEUTIC ACTIONS

Disperses Blood Stasis, Stops Bleeding

Hemoptysis and hematemesis: *Hua Rui Shi* (Ophicalcitum) treats bleeding problems that are complicated by internal blood stasis. Clinical applications include hemoptysis and hematemesis. The powder may be applied topically to stop trauma-related bleeding. When applied topically, *Hua Rui Shi* acts to dry oozing fluids and promote healing.

Hua Rui Shi (Ophicalcitum)

- Hematemesis with blood stasis: use charred *Hua Rui Shi* with alcohol or vinegar.
- Gastric or intestinal bleeding: combine this herb with *San Qi* (Radix Notoginseng) and *Xue Yu Tan* (Crinis Carbonisatus).
- Bleeding with bruises from traumatic injuries or animal bites: mix charred *Hua Rui Shi* and charred *Liu Huang* (Sulfur) and apply topically.
- Cuts: use *Hua Rui Shi* with *Mi Tuo Seng* (Lithargyrum), *Long Gu* (Os Draconis), *Ru Xiang* (Gummi Olibanum) and *Qing Fen* (Calomelas) topically to promote generation of flesh and facilitate recovery.

DOSAGE

10 to 15 grams in decoction, 1.0 to 1.5 grams in powder. *Hua Rui Shi* is commonly used both internally and topically. The fresh form is stronger in dispersing blood stasis and stopping internal bleeding. The charred form is stronger in restraining the leakage of blood and is used to stop external bleeding.

CAUTIONS / CONTRAINDICATIONS

- *Hua Rui Shi* should be used with extreme caution during pregnancy.

PHARMACOLOGICAL EFFECTS

- **Hemostatic:** Topical application of *Hua Rui Shi* powder was more effective than a placebo in reducing bleeding time in mice with external bleeding.[1]

CLINICAL STUDIES AND RESEARCH

- **Bleeding disorders:** Oral administration of 4 to 8 grams of *Hua Rui Shi* powder three times daily was approximately 70% effective in treating various bleeding disorders, including gastric ulcers, duodenal ulcers, and hemoptysis due to pulmonary tuberculosis. Patients with gastrointestinal bleeding were most responsive to the treatment with a 98.1% rate of effectiveness.[2] In another study, patients with hematemesis, epistaxis and profuse uterine bleeding were treated with *Hua Rui Shi* powder with marked hemostatic results. *Hua Rui Shi* powder was calcined with vinegar. Patients were also given *Ba Zhen Tang* (Eight-Treasure Decoction) after bleeding stopped.[3]

References

1. *Zhong Yao Xue* (Chinese Herbology), 1998; 523:524
2. *Zhong Cheng Yao* (Study of Chinese Patent Medicine), 1985; 8:42
3. *Zhe Jiang Zhong Yi Za Zhi* (Zhejiang Journal of Chinese Medicine), 1965; 8(7):21

Wan Nian Song (Herba Selaginellae)

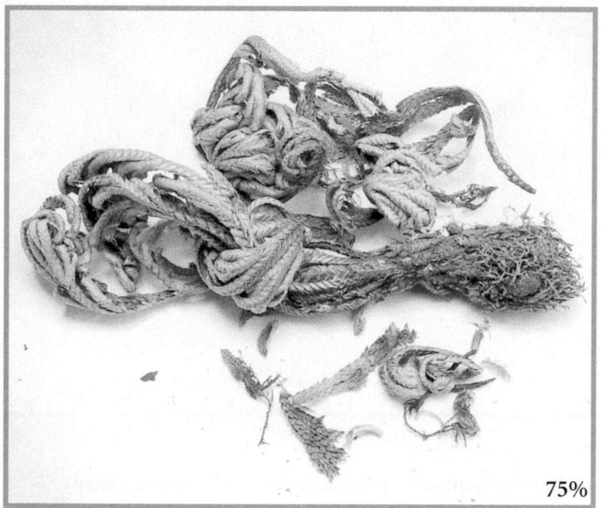

萬年松 万年松

Pinyin Name: *Wan Nian Song*
Alternate Chinese Names: *Juan Bo, Wan Sui, Sui Fu Rong, Huai Hun Cao*
English Name: selaginella
Botanical Name: *Selaginella tamariscina* (Beauv.) Spring
Pharmaceutical Name: Herba Selaginellae
Properties: acrid, neutral
Channels Entered: Lung, Large Intestine

Wan Nian Song (Herba Selaginellae)

CHINESE THERAPEUTIC ACTIONS

1. Stops Bleeding and Disperses Wind

Various bleeding: *Wan Nian Song* (Herba Selaginellae) treats various patterns of bleeding such as hemoptysis, rectal bleeding, intestinal bleeding, hemorrhoidal bleeding and hematuria.

- Hemoptysis: use *Wan Nian Song* with *Ce Bai Ye* (Cacumen Platycladi), *Sha Shen* (Radix Glehniae seu Adenophorae), *Wu Tian* (Radix et Folium Viticis Quinatae), *Bai He* (Bulbus Lilii), *Pi Pa Ye* (Folium Eriobotryae), *Ou Jie* (Nodus Nelumbinis Rhizomatis), *Mu Xiang* (Radix Aucklandiae), *Gua Lou Shi* (Fructus Trichosanthis) and *Gan Cao* (Radix Glycyrrhizae).
- Rectal bleeding, intestinal bleeding or hemorrhoidal bleeding: combine this herb with *Huai Hua* (Flos Sophorae) and *Di Yu* (Radix Sanguisorbae).
- Hematuria: use it with *Bai Mao Gen* (Rhizoma Imperatae), *Da Ji* (Herba seu Radix Cirsii Japonici) and *Xiao Ji* (Herba Cirisii).

2. Invigorates Blood Circulation and Expands the Chest to Regulate Lung Qi

Post-traumatic cough: *Wan Nian Song* is excellent to treat coughing that occurs after traumatic injuries to the chest area. Because this herb also invigorates blood circulation, it can be used to treat back sprain and strain.

- Post-traumatic cough: use this herb with *Wan Dian Jin* (Radix Ilicis Asprellae) or *Xue Fu Zhu Yu Tang* (Drive Out Stasis in the Mansion of Blood Decoction).
- Sprain and strain of the back: use it with *Chun Gen* (Radix Ailanthi).

DOSAGE

3 to 12 grams

CAUTIONS / CONTRAINDICATIONS

- Use *Wan Nian Song* with caution in patients with cold and deficiency.

Xiao Jin Ying (Fructus Rosae Cymosae)

小金樱 小金樱

Pinyin Name: *Xiao Jin Ying*
Literal Name: "little golden cherry"
English Name: rosa cymosa, small fruit rose
Botanical Name: *Rosa cymosa* Tratt.
Pharmaceutical Name: Fructus Rosae Cymosae
Properties: bitter, neutral
Channels Entered: Liver

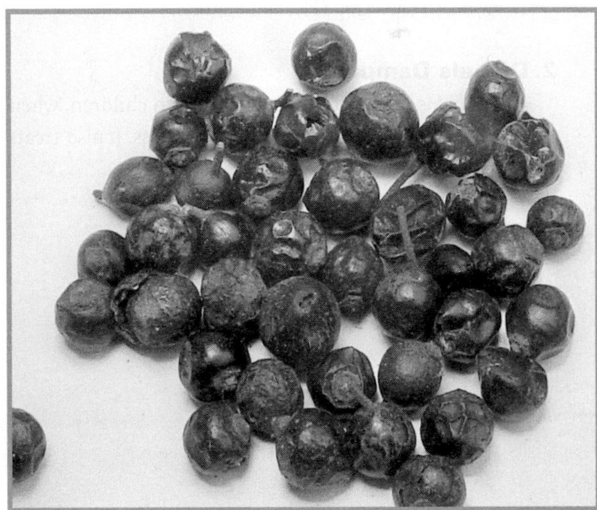

CHINESE THERAPEUTIC ACTIONS

Disperses Stagnation, Stops Bleeding

Xiao Jin Ying (Fructus Rosae Cymosae) stops bleeding that is accompanied by blood clots. Clinical applications include irregular menstruation, bleeding disorders, and traumatic injuries. It also clears heat and eliminates toxins, for topical treatment of sores and lesions.

DOSAGE

15 to 60 grams

Lian Fang (Receptaculum Nelumbinis)

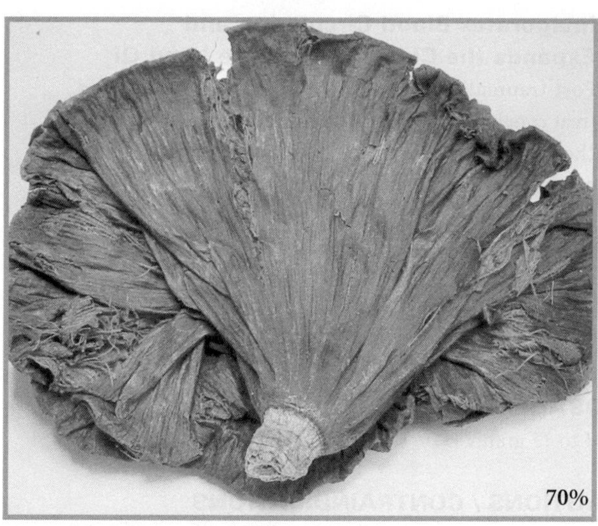
70%

蓮房 莲房

Pinyin Name: *Lian Fang*
Literal Name: "lotus mansion"
Alternate Chinese Names: *Lian Peng Ke*
Original Source: *Shi Liao Ben Cao* (Materia Medica of Diet Therapy) by Meng Shan in the seventh century
English Name: lotus receptacle
Botanical Name: *Nelumbo nucifera* Gaertn. (*Lian*)
Pharmaceutical Name: Receptaculum Nelumbinis
Properties: bitter, astringent, warm
Channels Entered: Liver, Spleen, Kidney

CHINESE THERAPEUTIC ACTIONS

1. Disperses Blood Stasis, Stops Bleeding

Lian Fang (Receptaculum Nelumbinis) treats a variety of bleeding disorders, and is most commonly used for profuse menstrual bleeding and hematuria. It is often used in cases of hemorrhoidal bleeding or rectal prolapse. *Lian Fang* is often charred to ashes to enhance its hemostatic effect.

- Profuse menstrual bleeding and hematuria: use *Lian Fang* with *Yi Mu Cao* (Herba Leonuri).

2. Dispels Dampness

Lian Fang is useful to address diarrhea in children, when it is caused by summer-heat and dampness. It also treats rash and eczema due to dampness.

DOSAGE

5 to 10 grams. The charred herb has stronger hemostatic action than the fresh herb.

CHEMICAL COMPOSITION

Roemerine, nornuciferine, meratin, hyperoside, vitamins.[1]

AUTHORS' COMMENTS

There are eight parts of the lotus plant that are used as medicines. Please refer to the monograph on *Lian Zi* (Semen Nelumbinis) for a complete description.

References

1. *An Hui Zhong Yi Xue Yuan Xue Bao* (Journal of Anhui University School of Medicine)

Zhu Fan Hua Tou (Rhizoma Mirabilidis)

煮飯花頭
煮饭花头

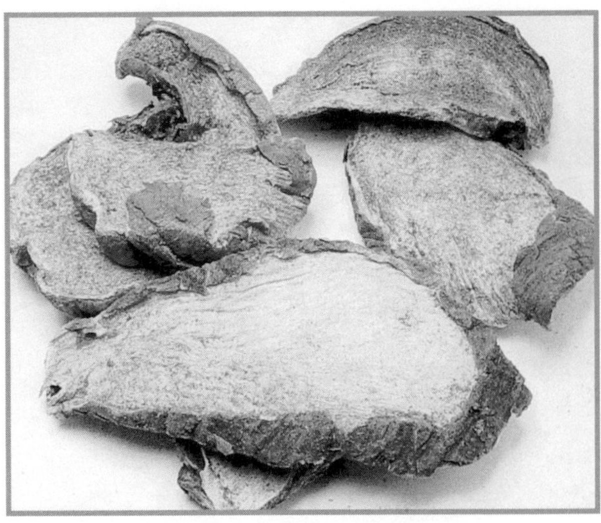

Pinyin Name: *Zhu Fan Hua Tou*
Alternate Chinese Names: *Zi Mo Li, Su Xiang, Yan Zhi Hua, Wan Xiang Hua*
English Name: mirabilis
Botanical Name: *Mirabilis jalapa* Linn.
Pharmaceutical Name: Rhizoma Mirabilidis
Properties: sweet, bitter, astringent
Channels Entered: Lung, Stomach, Urinary Bladder

CHINESE THERAPEUTIC ACTIONS

1. Invigorates Blood and Disperses Stasis

Zhu Fan Hua Tou (Rhizoma Mirabilidis) effectively treats disorders of the digestive system, such as peptic ulcer and bleeding ulcer.

- Peptic ulcer: use *Zhu Fan Hua Tou* with *Bai Ji* (Rhizoma Bletillae), *Wu Bei Zi* (Galla Chinensis), *Huang Lian* (Rhizoma Coptidis) and *Hai Piao Xiao* (Endoconcha Sepiae).
- Gastric bleeding: combine this herb with *Hua Rui Shi* (Ophicalcitum), *Chi Shi Zhi* (Halloysitum Rubrum) and *Wu Bei Zi* (Galla Chinensis).
- Hemorrhoids: add it to *Zhen Ren Huo Ming Yin* (True Man Decoction to Revitalize Life).
- Carbuncles and cellulitis: apply this herb topically.
- Tonsillitis and inflammation: use it with *Da Qing Ye* (Folium Isatidis), *Ban Lan Gen* (Radix Isatidis) and *Zao Jiao Ci* (Spina Gleditsiae).

2. Sedates Heat and Promotes Urination

- Turbid urine: use *Zhu Fan Hua Tou* with *Da Huang* (Radix et Rhizoma Rhei), *Hua Shi* (Talcum), *Gan Cao* (Radix Glycyrrhizae), *Bian Xu* (Herba Polygoni Avicularis), *Qu Mai* (Herba Dianthi), *Che Qian Zi* (Semen Plantaginis) and *Ze Xie* (Rhizoma Alismatis).
- Leukorrhea: combine it with *Ji Guan Hua* (Flos Celosiae Cristatae) and *Ya She Huang* (Herba Lippiae).

DOSAGE

3 to 9 grams in decoction.

CAUTIONS / CONTRAINDICATIONS

- *Zhu Fan Hua Tou* is contraindicated during pregnancy.

AUTHORS' COMMENTS

Zhu Fan Hua Tou is excellent for treatment of gastric disorders such as peptic ulcers or gastritis. When *Zhu Fan Hua Tou* is combined with blood-invigorating herbs, a much better effect can be achieved.

Ai Ye (Folium Artemisiae Argyi)

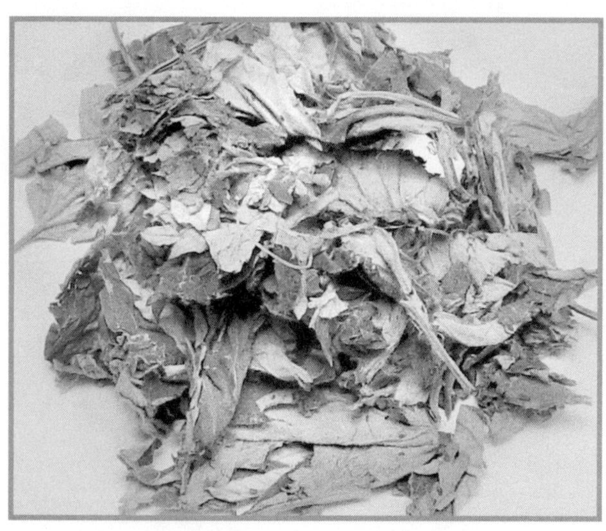

艾葉 艾叶

Pinyin Name: *Ai Ye*
Original Source: *Ming Yi Za Zhu* (Miscellaneous Records of Famous Physicians) by Tao Hong-Jing in 500 A.D.
English Name: artemisia argyi, argy wormwood leaf
Botanical Name: *Artemisia argyi* Levl. et Vant. (*Ai*)
Pharmaceutical Name: Folium Artemisiae Argyi
Properties: bitter, acrid, warm
Channels Entered: Spleen, Liver, Kidney

CHINESE THERAPEUTIC ACTIONS

1. Warms the Channels, Stops Bleeding

Ai Ye (Folium Artemisiae Argyi) warms the channels and collaterals and treats a variety of bleeding disorders. It is especially effective to stop gynecological bleeding caused by deficiency and cold. Clinical applications include profuse menstrual bleeding, vaginal bleeding in unstable pregnancy, epistaxis, and hemoptysis.

- Profuse menstrual bleeding from deficiency and cold: combine *Ai Ye* with *Gan Jiang* (Rhizoma Zingiberis) and *E Jiao* (Colla Corii Asini).
- Excessive loss of blood and profuse bleeding because of deficiency and cold: use this herb with *E Jiao* (Colla Corii Asini), *Bai Shao* (Radix Paeoniae Alba), *Dang Gui* (Radicis Angelicae Sinensis) and *Shu Di Huang* (Radix Rehmanniae Preparata).
- Unstable pregnancy with vaginal bleeding caused by deficiency and cold: use it with *E Jiao* (Colla Corii Asini), *Dang Gui* (Radicis Angelicae Sinensis), *Bai Shao* (Radix Paeoniae Alba), *Sheng Di Huang* (Radix Rehmanniae), *Gan Cao* (Radix Glycyrrhizae) and *Chuan Xiong* (Rhizoma Ligustici Chuanxiong).
- Epistaxis, hemoptysis and hematemesis: combine *Ai Ye* with *Sheng Di Huang* (Radix Rehmanniae), *Ce Bai Ye* (Cacumen Platycladi) and *He Ye* (Folium Nelumbinis).

2. Dispels Cold, Relieves Pain

Ai Ye warms the Liver, Spleen and Stomach channels to dispel cold and relieve pain. It is commonly used to treat deficiency and cold of the middle and lower *jiaos* manifesting in lower abdominal coldness and pain, irregular menses, dysmenorrhea, infertility, and profuse clear menstrual discharge.

- Deficiency and cold of the middle *jiao* with epigastric and abdominal cold and pain: add *Gan Jiang* (Rhizoma Zingiberis).
- Deficiency and cold of the lower *jiao* with abdominal cold and pain, and irregular menstruation with pain: use *Ai Ye* with *Xiang Fu* (Rhizoma Cyperi), *Chuan Xiong* (Rhizoma Ligustici Chuanxiong), *Dang Gui* (Radicis Angelicae Sinensis), and *Bai Shao* (Radix Paeoniae Alba). If there is severe deficiency and cold, also add *Wu Zhu Yu* (Fructus Evodiae), *Rou Gui* (Cortex Cinnamomi), *Huang Qi* (Radix Astragali) and *Xu Duan* (Radix Dipsaci).
- Lower abdominal coldness and pain: dry fry *Ai Ye* and apply it warm to the umbilicus. This treatment is also effective for postpartum women with abdominal coldness and pain.

3. Dispels Dampness, Relieves Itching

Ai Ye may be used topically to treat various dermatological disorders. As an herbal wash, it is commonly used to treat eczema and itching.

- Eczema: use it with *Di Fu Zi* (Fructus Kochiae) and *Bai Xian Pi* (Cortex Dictamni).

4. Dispels Phlegm, Stops Cough, Relieves Wheezing

Essential oil of *Ai Ye* has good properties for treatment of respiratory disorders such as cough and wheezing with phlegm.

DOSAGE

3 to 10 grams as herbal decoction. *Ai Ye* is also ingested orally as essential oil, 0.1 ml of per dose three times daily. It is commonly used topically as an herbal wash or as moxa. The unprocessed herb functions more effectively to dispel cold and dry dampness. Vinegar-processed *Ai Ye* has

Ai Ye (Folium Artemisiae Argyi)

a potent action to dispel cold and relieve pain. The charred herb has a stronger characteristic to stop bleeding. Processing this herb will reduce irritation to the stomach.

CAUTIONS / CONTRAINDICATIONS

- Warm and drying, *Ai Ye* should be used with caution for patients with yin deficiency or heat in the blood.
- Topical application of this herb's essential oil may irritate the skin and cause local redness and warmth.
- Oral administration of the essential oil of *Ai Ye* may stimulate the gastrointestinal tract and lead to increase in both appetite and consumption of food.

OVERDOSAGE

Adverse reactions to *Ai Ye* can be divided into acute and chronic types:

- **Acute** reaction is caused by overdose and may begin to develop within 1 to 4 hours following ingestion of the herb. Clinical presentation will include dry mouth and throat, thirst, nausea, vomiting, dizziness, and tinnitus, followed by abdominal pain, diarrhea, tremor, generalized spasms and convulsions for 20 to 30 minutes, and altered consciousness. If the overdose is not treated properly, it may lead to jaundice and possibly liver damage.
- **Chronic** reaction occurs because of prolonged exposure to the herb at large dosages. Clinical presentation includes hypersensitivity reactions, numbness of the extremities, neuritis, hallucination, and muscle spasms and cramps. Even with treatment and recovery, forgetfulness is noted as a lingering effect in some patients.[1]

The normal dose of *Ai Ye* is 3 to 10 grams. Adverse reactions may be noted at doses of 20 to 30 grams, and fatality may occur at doses above 100 grams. There has been one fatality associated with overdose of *Ai Ye*, in which a 32-year-old female ingested 500 ml of unknown concentration of *Ai Ye*.

TREATMENT OF OVERDOSAGE

Early stage *Ai Ye* overdose can be treated via emesis within 4 hours of ingestion of the herb. Following vomiting of the offending agent, the patient should be given 250 ml of milk or 6 egg whites to protect the stomach and neutralize any remaining toxin.

If the response to overdose of *Ai Ye* is characterized by seizures and convulsions, 0.6 gram of *Niu Huang* (Calculus Bovis) should be given, to clear heat, eliminate toxins, and stop seizure and epilepsy.

If overdose of *Ai Ye* is characterized by jaundice, yellow urine, a bitter taste in the mouth, and a wiry pulse, herbs should be prescribed to relieve jaundice and hepatitis. An herbal decoction used with good success consists of *Hu Zhang* (Rhizoma Polygoni Cuspidati) 15g, *Yin Chen Hao* (Herba Artemisiae Scopariae) 15g, *Sheng Ma* (Rhizoma Cimicifugae) 15g, *Huang Bai* (Cortex Phellodendri) 12g, *Che Qian Zi* (Semen Plantaginis) 15g, and *She Xiang* (Moschus) 0.06g [60mg]. The formula is taken in decoction twice daily, in the morning and at night.

Hepatitis associated with overdose of *Ai Ye* has been treated with a formula that includes *Yin Chen Hao* (Herba Artemisiae Scopariae) 30g, *Ban Lan Gen* (Radix Isatidis) 30g, *Zhi Zi* (Fructus Gardeniae) 9g, *Long Dan Cao* (Radix Gentianae) 9g, *Gan Cao* (Radix Glycyrrhizae) 9g, and *Che Qian Zi* (Semen Plantaginis) 15g.

Dermatological reactions caused by direct contact with the herb can be relieved by a topical solution of herbs made from 60 grams each of *Hu Zhang* (Rhizoma Polygoni Cuspidati) and *Lei Gong Teng* (Radix Tripterygii Wilfordii). Soak a towel in the decoction and apply to the affected area.

CHEMICAL COMPOSITION

D-α-phellandrene, α-cadinene, 1,8-cineole, camphene, trans-carveol, borneol acetate, elemol, isoborneol, α-terpineol, carvone.[2]

PHARMACOLOGICAL EFFECTS

- **Hemostatic:** Both fresh and charred forms of *Ai Ye* have demonstrated marked effectiveness to stop bleeding. The charred form was found to be more effective than the fresh herb.[3]
- **Antibiotic:** It has an inhibitory effect against *Bacillus anthracis*, α-hemolytic streptococcus, β-hemolytic streptococcus, *Corynebacterium diphtheriae, Diplococcus pneumoniae, Staphylococcus aureus, Staphylococcus citreus, Staphylococcus albus*, and *Bacillus subtilis*.[4]
- **Antiasthmatic:** Essential oil of *Ai Ye* has demonstrated antiasthmatic effects in animal studies.[5]
- **Antitussive and expectorant:** Intraperitoneal or oral administration of essential oil of *Ai Ye* has demonstrated marked antitussive and expectorant effects in cats, dogs and guinea pigs.[6]
- **Cholagogic:** Administration of a 2% solution of *Ai Ye* has marked effectiveness to increase the production and excretion of bile.[7]

CLINICAL STUDIES AND RESEARCH

- **Unstable pregnancy:** According to one report, 45 pregnant women experiencing profuse uterine bleeding were treated with an herbal decoction with marked effectiveness in 26 patients, moderate results in 16 patients, and no response in 3 patients. The herbal formula contained *Ai Ye* 6g, *Sha Ren* (Fructus Amomi) 6g, *E Jiao* (Colla Corii Asini) 15g, *Bai Zhu* (Rhizoma Atractylodis Macrocephalae) 15g, *Huang Qin*

Ai Ye (Folium Artemisiae Argyi)

(Radix Scutellariae) 12g, *Su Geng* (Caulis Perillae) 12g, *Sang Ji Sheng* (Herba Taxilli) 24g, *Du Zhong* (Cortex Eucommiae) 24g, and others as deemed necessary.[8]

- **Chronic tracheitis:** Essential oil of *Ai Ye* administered daily for 10 days per course of treatment, for two courses, was 86.4 to 96.7% effective in 544 patients with chronic tracheitis; and 82% effective in 319 patients when given via oral inhalation. It has antiasthmatic effect, onset of action, and duration of action similar to isoproterenol.[9]
- **Allergy:** In one study, 0.15 ml of essential oil of *Ai Ye* administered orally three times daily was 77.3% effective in treating patients with various allergies, including bronchial asthma, allergic dermatitis (treated with both oral and topical application of *Ai Ye*), eczema, allergic rhinitis, chemical allergies, and drug allergies.[10]
- **Liver disorders:** Intramuscular injection of *Ai Ye* one time daily for 1 to 2 months was 92% effective in 100 patients with chronic hepatitis or liver cirrhosis. The study noted that *Ai Ye* was much more effective for chronic hepatitis than liver cirrhosis.[11]
- **Burns:** Application of moxa (*Ai Ye* used as the main ingredient of moxa) to burns in children is associated with a reduction of secretions from the burned area, decreased risk of infection, and shortened healing time.[12]
- **Bacterial dysentery:** One study reported that 40 ml of 20% *Ai Ye* decoction given four times daily was very effective in treating 21 patients with acute bacterial dysentery.[13]
- **Malaria:** Administration of 15 to 30 grams of *Ai Ye* as herbal decoction 2 hours before the onset of malarial symptoms for 2 days was 56.2% effective in treating 53 patients with malaria.[14]
- **Skin ulcer:** Twelve patients with skin ulcers were treated topically with an herbal wash three times daily with a 100% success rate. The herbal wash was prepared by cooking 15 grams each of *Ai Ye*, *Lu Cha* (Folium Camellia Sinensis), *Nu Zhen Zi* (Fructus Ligustri Lucidi) and *Zao Jiao* (Fructus Gleditsiae) in 250 ml of water to yield 100 to 150 ml of the final solution.[15]

TOXICOLOGY

The LD_{50} in mice for the essential oil of *Ai Ye* is 2.47 ml/kg via oral routes, and 1.12 mg/kg via intraperitoneal routes. The LD_{50} in mice for the decoction of *Ai Ye* is 23 g/kg via intraperitoneal injection.[16]

AUTHORS' COMMENTS

Ai Ye is the main ingredient compressed into moxa sticks. When burned, the heat penetrates into the muscles, tendons and bones to activate qi and blood circulation, and warms peripheral channels and collaterals.

References

1. *Zhong Yao Du Li Xue* (Toxicology of Chinese Herbs); 1989, 70-71
2. *Xian Dai Zhong Yao Yao Li Xue* (Contemporary Pharmacology of Chinese Herbs), 1997; 839
3. *Zhong Yao Cai* (Study of Chinese Herbal Material), 1992; 15(2):22
4. *China Med J*, 1949; 67(12):648
5. *Zhong Cao Yao* (Chinese Herbal Medicine), 1981; 12(12):58
6. *Zhong Yao Xue* (Chinese Herbology), 1998; 526:529
7. *Gui Yang Yi Xue Yuan Xue Bao* (Journal of Guiyang Medical University), 1988; (3):52
8. *He Bei Zhong Yi Za Zhi* (Hebei Journal of Chinese Medicine), 1985; 5:31
9. *Yi Yao Gong Ye* (Pharmaceutical Industry), 1977;(4-5):51
10. *Zhong Cao Yao Tong Xun* (Journal of Chinese Herbal Medicine), 1975; 1:43
11. *Xin Yi Xue* (New Medicine), 1974; 2:83
12. *Zhong Hua Wai Ke Za Zhi* (Chinese Journal of External Medicine), 1960; 13(9):787
13. *Zhe Jiang Yi Xue* (Zhejiang Journal of Medicine), 1960; 13(9):787
14. *Shan Dong Yi Kan* (Shandong Medical Journal), 1962; 5:22
15. *Guang Xi Zhong Yi Yao* (Guangxi Chinese Medicine and Herbology), 1982; 4:35
16. *Zhong Cao Yao Tong Xun* (Journal of Chinese Herbal Medicine), 1976; (9):26

Fu Long Gan (Terra Flava Usta)

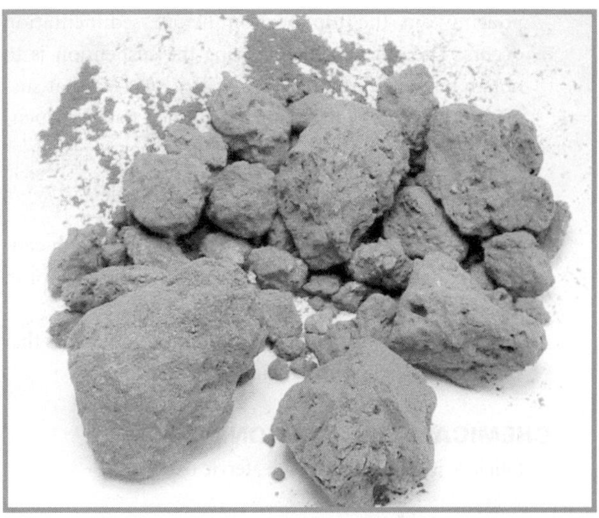

伏龍干 伏龙干

Pinyin Name: *Fu Long Gan*
Literal Name: "hidden dragon liver"
Alternate Chinese Names: *Zao Xin Tu*
Original Source: *Ming Yi Za Zhu* (Miscellaneous Records of Famous Physicians) by Tao Hong-Jing in 500 A.D.
English Name: soot and ash from an enclosed fire pit
Pharmaceutical Name: Terra Flava Usta
Properties: acrid, warm
Channels Entered: Spleen, Stomach

CHINESE THERAPEUTIC ACTIONS

1. Warms the Middle *Jiao,* Stops Bleeding

Fu Long Gan (Terra Flava Usta) treats various bleeding disorders characterized by deficiency and cold of the Spleen, and its inability to hold blood within the vessels. Clinical applications include hematemesis, epistaxis, hematochezia, and profuse, dark menstrual bleeding. The other signs and symptoms of Spleen deficiency and cold include sallow facial appearance, cold extremities, pale tongue, and a thready pulse.

- General bleeding: use *Fu Long Gan* as a single-herb remedy.
- Hematemesis or epistaxis: mix it with honey.
- Hematochezia with cold in the lower *jiao*: combine this substance with *Gan Jiang* (Rhizoma Zingiberis), *E Jiao* (Colla Corii Asini), and *Huang Qin* (Radix Scutellariae).
- Bloody dysentery with abdominal pain, irritability, and dry mouth: use it with *Huang Lian* (Rhizoma Coptidis), *E Jiao* (Colla Corii Asini) and *Ai Ye* (Folium Artemisiae Argyi).
- Profuse menstrual bleeding: combine it with *E Jiao* (Colla Corii Asini) and *Jiang Can* (Bombyx Batryticatus), and take with grain-based liquor.
- Bloody leukorrhea: combine it with *Zong Lu Pi* (Fibra Stipulae Trachycarpi) and *She Xiang* (Moschus), and take with warm alcohol or vinegar.
- Hematochezia, hematemesis, epistaxis, and profuse menstrual bleeding caused by deficiency of Spleen qi: use this substance with *E Jiao* (Colla Corii Asini), *Fu Zi* (Radix Aconiti Lateralis Praeparata), *Bai Zhu* (Rhizoma Atractylodis Macrocephalae) and *Shu Di Huang* (Radix Rehmanniae Preparata).

2. Relieves Nausea

Fu Long Gan warms the middle *jiao*, redirects rebellious qi, and relieves nausea.

- Nausea and vomiting: take this substance as powder with rice water.
- Nausea and vomiting from Stomach deficiency: use it with *Ren Shen* (Radix Ginseng), *Bai Zhu* (Rhizoma Atractylodis Macrocephalae), *Sha Ren* (Fructus Amomi), and *Chen Pi* (Pericarpium Citri Reticulatae).
- Nausea and vomiting during pregnancy: use *Fu Long Gan* individually, or with *Su Geng* (Caulis Perillae), *Sha Ren* (Fructus Amomi), and *Zhu Ru* (Caulis Bambusae in Taenia).

3. Stops Diarrhea

Fu Long Gan warms the middle *jiao*, strengthens the Spleen, and stops diarrhea.

- Chronic diarrhea caused by Spleen deficiency: combine it with *Fu Zi* (Radix Aconiti Lateralis Praeparata), *Gan Jiang* (Rhizoma Zingiberis), and *Bai Zhu* (Rhizoma Atractylodis Macrocephalae).
- Postpartum diarrhea: mix it with *Shan Zha* (Fructus Crataegi) and sugar.

4. Treats Skin Disorders

Topical application of *Fu Long Gan* treats sores, swelling, erysipelas, ulcers, and other skin disorders characterized by dampness. It should always be combined with herbs that clear heat and eliminate toxins, for optimal effect.

DOSAGE

15 to 30 grams of *Fu Long Gan* should be wrapped in cheesecloth and pre-decocted for herbal decoction. Powder of this substance is used both internally and topically.

The 'suspension' of *Fu Long Gan* is sometimes used in place of water to cook herbs. The suspension is made by mixing 60 to 120 grams of this substance with water and

Fu Long Gan (Terra Flava Usta)

pouring out the top portion before sedimentation occurs. The purpose of preparing the suspension is to obtain only the finest particles of *Fu Long Gan* that suspend in water. The herbs are then added to the suspension, cooked, and the final decoction is then ingested.

CAUTIONS / CONTRAINDICATIONS

- Warm in nature, *Fu Long Gan* should be used with caution in cases of bleeding arising from yin deficiency, or in nausea and vomiting caused by heat.
- To treat sores and skin ulcers, combine it with herbs that clear heat and eliminate toxins.

CHEMICAL COMPOSITION

Silicic acid, aluminum oxide, ferric oxide.[1]

PHARMACOLOGICAL EFFECTS

- **Antiemetic:** Intravenous or oral administration of *Fu Long Gan* in pigeons was effective in treating nausea and vomiting induced by digitalis tincture. However, it was ineffective in suppressing apomorphine-induced vomiting in dogs.[2]

CLINICAL STUDIES AND RESEARCH

- **Bleeding disorders:** Bleeding problems characterized by deficiency and cold were treated with an herbal decoction. Of 108 patients, there was marked improvement in 81 patients, moderate improvement in 24 patients and no improvement in 3 patients. The herbal formula was cooked in a suspension of *Fu Long Gan* instead of water. It contained *E Jiao* (Colla Corii Asini) 15g, *Bai Zhu* (Rhizoma Atractylodis Macrocephalae) 15g, *Fu Zi* (Radix Aconiti Lateralis Praeparata) 12g, *Sheng Di Huang* (Radix Rehmanniae) 12g, *Huang Qin* (Radix Scutellariae) 10g, and *Zhi Gan Cao* (Radix Glycyrrhizae Preparata) 10g. Modifications were made if necessary by adding *Dang Shen* (Radix Codonopsis) 15g in cases of qi deficiency, and *Hai Piao Xiao* (Endoconcha Sepiae) 12g and *Qian Cao* (Radix Rubiae) 12g if bleeding was profuse. The formula was cooked in a suspension of *Fu Long Gan* instead of water. The suspension was made by mixing 300 grams of *Fu Long Gan* in water, with the top portion of the water poured out prior to sedimentation to obtain the fine particles of *Fu Long Gan*.[3]
- **Bacterial dysentery:** In one study, 90 children with bacterial dysentery were treated with 30 to 60 ml of an herbal decoction one time daily with marked effectiveness in 17 patients after 1 dose, in 34 patients after 2 doses, in 19 patients after 3 doses, in 8 patients after 5 doses, and with no response in 7 patients. Reports for the last 5 patients were unavailable. The formula contained 100 grams of *Huang Lian* (Rhizoma Coptidis), 200 grams of *Da Huang* (Radix et Rhizoma Rhei), 200 grams of *Bai Shao* (Radix Paeoniae Alba), 250 grams of *Huang Qin* (Radix Scutellariae), 150 grams of *Chuan Lian Zi* (Fructus Toosendan), 150 grams of charred *Jing Jie* (Herba Schizonepetae), and 50 grams of *Yan Hu Suo* (Rhizoma Corydalis). The herbs were cooked in the suspension of *Fu Long Gan*, which was made by mixing 500 grams of *Fu Long Gan* in 5,000 ml of water, with the top portion of the water poured out prior to sedimentation to obtain the fine particles of *Fu Long Gan*.[4]

References

1. *Xian Dai Zhong Yao Yao Li Xue* (Contemporary Pharmacology of Chinese Herbs), 1997; 833
2. *Zhong Yao Xue* (Chinese Herbology), 1998; 530-532
3. *Zhong Yuan Yi Kan* (Resource Journal of Chinese Medicine), 1985; 4:26
4. *He Nan Zhong Yi* (Henan Chinese Medicine), 1985; 3:42

Chapter 11 summary

— Stop-Bleeding Herbs

Name	Similarities	Differences
Da Ji (Herba seu Radix Cirsii Japonici)	Cool blood to stop bleeding	Stops bleeding, removes blood stasis, reduces swelling
Xiao Ji (Herba Cirisii)		Stops bleeding, alleviates dysuria
Di Yu (Radix Sanguisorbae)		Stops lower *jiao* bleeding
Bai Mao Gen (Rhizoma Imperatae)		Clears heat in the Lung and Stomach, promotes urination
Huai Hua (Flos Sophorae)		Clears Liver heat, lowers blood pressure
Ce Bai Ye (Cacumen Platycladi)		Dispels phlegm and relieves cough
Zi Zhu (Folium Callicarpae)	Stabilize and bind to consolidate blood and stop bleeding	Stops bleeding and eliminates toxins to treat sores, carbuncles and burns
Xian He Cao (Herba Agrimoniae)		Kills parasites
Bai Ji (Rhizoma Bletillae)		Stops bleeding of the Lung and Stomach; used externally, reduces swelling and promotes generation of flesh
Zong Lu Pi (Fibra Stipulae Trachycarpi)		Stops bleeding, especially metrorrhagia
Ou Jie (Nodus Nelumbinis Rhizomatis)		Removes blood stasis when used in unprocessed form
Xue Yu Tan (Crinis Carbonisatus)	Activate blood circulation, remove blood stasis, stop bleeding	Promotes urination, treats bloody dysuria
San Qi (Radix Notoginseng)		Strongly stops bleeding and relieves pain
Qian Cao (Radix Rubiae)		Invigorates blood and promotes normal menstruation
Pu Huang (Pollen Typhae)		Promotes urination, removes abdominal blood stasis
Hua Rui Shi (Ophicalcitum)		Consolidates leakage of blood
Wan Nian Song (Herba Selaginellae)		Regulates Lung qi and relieves cough
Xiao Jin Ying (Fructus Rosae Cymosae)		Disperses stagnation and stops bleeding
Lian Fang (Receptaculum Nelumbinis)		Treats abnormal menstrual bleeding and hematuria
Zhu Fan Hua Tou (Rhizoma Mirabilidis)		Sedates heat and promotes urination
Ai Ye (Folium Artemisiae Argyi)	Warm the body to stop bleeding	Warms the channels to stop bleeding, disperses cold and relieves pain
Fu Long Gan (Terra Flava Usta)		Warms the Spleen to stop bleeding, relieves nausea and vomiting

General Characteristics of Stop-Bleeding Herbs:

Taste: varies
Thermal property: varies
Channels entered: Heart, Spleen, Liver
Therapeutic actions: stop bleeding

These herbs stop internal and external bleeding, and are administered orally or topically. Stop-bleeding herbs have four primary therapeutic effects:

To cool blood to stop bleeding
To stabilize and bind to consolidate blood and stop bleeding
To remove blood stasis to stop bleeding
To warm the body to stop bleeding

Chapter 11 summary

Herbs that cool blood to stop bleeding include ***Da Ji*** (Herba seu Radix Cirsii Japonici), ***Xiao Ji*** (Herba Cirisii), ***Di Yu*** (Radix Sanguisorbae), ***Bai Mao Gen*** (Rhizoma Imperatae), ***Huai Hua*** (Flos Sophorae), and ***Ce Bai Ye*** (Cacumen Platycladi). They are the herbs of choice when treating bleeding due to heat in the blood.

Da Ji invigorates blood circulation, removes blood stasis, eliminates toxins, reduces swelling and lowers blood pressure.

Xiao Ji has essentially the same functions as *Da Ji*, except that *Xiao Ji* treats dysuria or hematuria, but does not invigorate blood or remove stasis.

Di Yu sedates fire, eliminates toxins, treats sores, and stops bleeding of the lower *jiao* such as hematochezia, hemorrhoidal bleeding, metrorrhagia and bloody dysentery.

Bai Mao Gen clears heat, promotes urination and is the most effective herb for heat in the Lung and Stomach.

Huai Hua treats bleeding from the lower *jiao* and lowers blood pressure.

Ce Bai Ye dispels phlegm and stops cough.

Herbs that stabilize and bind to consolidate blood and stop bleeding include ***Zi Zhu*** (Folium Callicarpae), ***Xian He Cao*** (Herba Agrimoniae), ***Bai Ji*** (Rhizoma Bletillae), ***Zong Lu Pi*** (Fibra Stipulae Trachycarpi), and ***Ou Jie*** (Nodus Nelumbinis Rhizomatis). They are most suitable for bleeding that does not involve blood stasis.

Zi Zhu eliminates toxins and treats sores.

Xian He Cao stops diarrhea and dysentery, kills parasites, and treats malaria and over-exhaustion.

Bai Ji more effectively stops bleeding, promotes generation of flesh, and reduces swelling.

Zong Lu Pi stops bleeding.

Ou Jie, when used fresh, stops bleeding and removes blood stasis. When charred, it consolidates blood and stops bleeding.

Herbs that invigorate blood, remove blood stasis and stop bleeding include ***Xue Yu Tan*** (Crinis Carbonisatus), ***San Qi*** (Radix Notoginseng), ***Qian Cao*** (Radix Rubiae), ***Pu Huang*** (Pollen Typhae), ***Hua Rui Shi*** (Ophicalcitum), ***Wan Nian Song*** (Herba Selaginellae), ***Xiao Jin Ying*** (Fructus Rosae Cymosae), ***Lian Fang*** (Receptaculum Nelumbinis), and ***Zhu Fan Hua Tou*** (Rhizoma Mirabilidis). They are most effective to stop bleeding involving blood stagnation.

Xue Yu Tan tonifies yin and promotes urination.

San Qi strongly invigorates the blood and relieves pain.

Qian Cao cools the blood and stops bleeding.

Pu Huang stops bleeding and simultaneously invigorates blood circulation.

Hua Rui Shi stabilizes and binds to stop bleeding.

Wan Nian Song invigorates blood circulation to treat sprains and strains, and treats rectal bleeding, hemoptysis, and hematuria.

Xiao Jin Ying and *Lian Fang* both disperse blood stagnation and stop bleeding.

Zhu Fan Hua Tou invigorates blood circulation, clears heat, and stops bleeding.

Herbs that warm the body to stop bleeding include ***Ai Ye*** (Folium Artemisiae Argyi) and ***Fu Long Gan*** (Terra Flava Usta).

Ai Ye warms the channels to stop bleeding, and disperses cold to relieve pain. Charred *Ai Ye* should be used when there is bleeding.

Fu Long Gan warms the middle *jiao* and stops bleeding caused by cold and deficiency.

Chapter 11 summary

HERBS FROM OTHER FUNCTIONAL CATEGORIES WITH STOP-BLEEDING FUNCTIONS

Name	Functional Category
Da Huang (Radix et Rhizoma Rhei)	Downward Draining Herbs (Chapter 3)
Dai Zhe Shi (Haematitum)	Liver-Calming and Wind-Extinguishing Herbs (Chapter 15)
E Jiao (Colla Corii Asini)	Tonic Herbs (Chapter 17)
Er Cha (Catechu)	Substances for Topical Application (Chapter 20)
Guan Zhong (Rhizoma Dryopteridis)	Antiparasitic Herbs (Chapter 10)
Hai Piao Xiao (Endoconcha Sepiae)	Astringent Herbs (Chapter 18)
Han Lian Cao (Herba Ecliptae)	Tonic Herbs (Chapter 17)
Jing Jie (Herba Schizonepetae), charred	Exterior-Releasing Herbs (Chapter 1)
Long Gu (Os Draconis)	*Shen*-Calming Herbs (Chapter 14)
Mu Dan Pi (Cortex Moutan)	Heat-Clearing Herbs (Chapter 2)
Mu Zei (Herba Equiseti Hiemalis)	Exterior-Releasing Herbs (Chapter 1)
Pao Jiang (Rhizoma Zingiberis Preparatum)	Interior-Warming Herbs (Chapter 7)
Qing Dai (Indigo Naturalis)	Heat-Clearing Herbs (Chapter 2)
Sheng Di Huang (Radix Rehmanniae)	Heat-Clearing Herbs (Chapter 2)
Wu Ling Zhi (Excrementum Trogopteri seu Pteromi)	Blood-Invigorating and Stasis-Removing Herbs (Chapter 12)
Wu Mei (Fructus Mume), charred	Astringent Herbs (Chapter 18)
Zhi Zi (Fructus Gardeniae), charred	Heat-Clearing Herbs (Chapter 2)

Chapter 12

— Blood-Invigorating and Stasis-Removing Herbs

活血化瘀药

Chapter 12 – Blood-Invigorating and Stasis-Removing Herbs

Chapter 12

— Blood-Invigorating and Stasis-Removing Herbs

Definition: Herbs that invigorate blood circulation and eliminate blood stasis function to open blood vessels, activate blood circulation, disperse blood stagnation, and break blood stasis.

Blood-invigorating and stasis-removing herbs are mostly ***acrid, bitter*** and ***warm***. The ***acrid*** taste promotes movement of blood and disperses stagnation, the ***bitter*** taste descends and drains stagnation, and the ***warm*** property helps to invigorate and facilitate the movement of blood. All of these herbs are 'moving' by nature, and function to activate blood circulation, disperse stasis, regulate menstruation, and open channels and collaterals, as well as help to heal wounds, relieve *bi zheng* (painful obstruction syndrome), and reduce swelling and pain. Clinical manifestations of blood stagnation include: stabbing pain in a fixed location or all over the body, numbness of the limbs and extremities, lumps found on the skin or internal palpable masses, swelling caused by traumatic injuries or internal bleeding, internal bleeding with visible blotches of bruises, purpura of the skin, and purple spots on the tongue.

The complex causes and complications of blood stagnation make it imperative that treatment incorporate herbs to address the overall condition of the patient.

SUBCATEGORIES OF ACTION

Although blood-invigorating herbs are generally not broken into subcategories, they do form a range of potencies and indications. These herbs may exert

- mild action to *invigorate blood circulation,*
- moderate action to *eliminate blood stagnation,* or
- potent action to *break blood stasis.*

DIFFERENTIAL DIAGNOSIS AND TREATMENT

Blood stagnation often involves a wide range of potential causes and complications. Many of these causes and complications are opposites, such as deficiency and excess, cold and hot, and interior and exterior. Due to the complex array of causes and complications of blood stagnation, it is imperative that the treatment plan incorporate herbs to address the overall condition of the patient, in addition to using herbs that eliminate blood stagnation.

Potential causes of blood stagnation include:

- *wei* (defensive) *qi* deficiency with exterior invasion of wind-cold or wind-damp
- *bi zheng* (painful obstruction syndrome) with obstruction of channels and collaterals
- febrile disorders
- excess heat consuming *ying* (nutritive) and *xue* (blood)
- stagnation of phlegm and dampness
- traumatic injuries leading to obstructed qi and blood circulation

Potential complications of blood stagnation are:

- amenorrhea
- postpartum abdominal pain
- cardiovascular disorders including (but not limited to) angina
- hypochondriac pain
- paralysis
- ulcers
- swellings

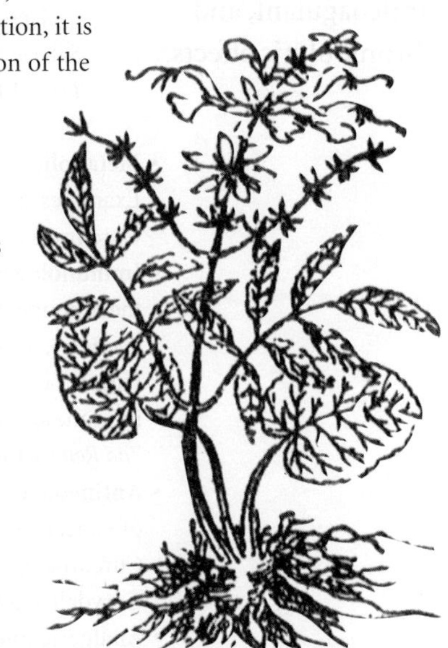

Dan Shen (Radix Salviae Miltiorrhizae)
Ben Cao Gang Mu (Materia Medica),
by Li Shi-Zhen, 1578 A.D.

Chapter 12 – Blood-Invigorating and Stasis-Removing Herbs

CAUTIONS/CONTRAINDICATIONS

- Blood-invigorating herbs should be used with extreme caution for women with hypermenorrhea.
- During pregnancy, mild to moderate herbs that invigorate blood circulation may be used *only* if necessary; while herbs that eliminate and break up blood stasis are ***contraindicated***.

PHARMACOLOGICAL EFFECTS

- **Cardiovascular**: Many of these herbs exert profound influence on the cardiovascular system. They dilate blood vessels, increase blood perfusion to smaller blood vessels, inhibit platelet aggregation, delay coagulation, and treat angina and ischemia.

  Herbs that dilate coronary arteries include *Hong Hua* (Flos Carthami), *Dan Shen* (Radix Salviae Miltiorrhizae), *Chuan Xiong* (Rhizoma Ligustici Chuanxiong), *San Qi* (Radix Notoginseng), *Yan Hu Suo* (Rhizoma Corydalis), *Chi Shao* (Radix Paeoniae Rubrae), and *Ji Xue Teng* (Caulis Spatholobi).

  Herbs that dilate veins include *Chi Shao* (Radix Paeoniae Rubrae), *Tao Ren* (Semen Persicae), and *Dan Shen* (Radix Salviae Miltiorrhizae).

  Herbs that dilate arteries include *Chuan Shan Jia* (Squama Manis), *Shui Zhi* (Hirudo), *E Zhu* (Rhizoma Curcumae), *Tao Ren* (Semen Persicae), and *Yi Mu Cao* (Herba Leonuri).

  Herbs that improve micro-circulation include *Chuan Xiong* (Rhizoma Ligustici Chuanxiong), *Dan Shen* (Radix Salviae Miltiorrhizae), *Pu Huang* (Pollen Typhae), *Jiang Huang* (Rhizoma Curcumae Longae), *Hong Hua* (Flos Carthami), *Dang Gui* (Radicis Angelicae Sinensis) and *Yi Mu Cao* (Herba Leonuri).

Blood-moving herbs offer great therapeutic value as they exert profound influence on the cardiovascular system.

- **Hematological**: Many herbs have anticoagulant and antiplatelet effects. Blood clots form in the veins mainly due to coagulation, while blood clots form in the arteries mainly due to aggregation of platelets. Therefore, anticoagulant substances are prescribed to stop formation of clots in veins, and antiplatelet medicines are prescribed to stop formation of clots in arteries. Many herbs have excellent inhibitory influence on thrombus formation, and are used in treatment of angina, stroke and embolism.

  Herbs with anticoagulant properties include *Dan Shen* (Radix Salviae Miltiorrhizae) and *Chi Shao* (Radix Paeoniae Rubrae).

  Herbs exerting antiplatelet activity include *Dan Shen* (Radix Salviae Miltiorrhizae), *Chuan Xiong* (Rhizoma Ligustici Chuanxiong) and *Hong Hua* (Flos Carthami).

  Herbs with thrombolytic effects include *Chi Shao* (Radix Paeoniae Rubrae), *Dan Shen* (Radix Salviae Miltiorrhizae), *Yi Mu Cao* (Herba Leonuri), *Dang Gui* (Radicis Angelicae Sinensis), *San Leng* (Rhizoma Sparganii), *E Zhu* (Rhizoma Curcumae), and *Hong Hua* (Flos Carthami).

These herbs may have antiplatelet, anticoagulant, and thrombolytic effects.

- **Metabolic**: Some blood-invigorating herbs lower plasma cholesterol levels to various degrees. Examples are *Yu Jin* (Radix Curcumae), *Hong Hua* (Flos Carthami), *Jiang Huang* (Rhizoma Curcumae Longae), *Dan Shen* (Radix Salviae Miltiorrhizae) and *Pu Huang* (Pollen Typhae).
- **Immunologic**: Blood-moving herbs act on the immune system in a number of ways. Some inhibit the immune system to treat allergy or hyperactivity of the immune system, such as *Yi Mu Cao* (Herba Leonuri), *Dang Gui Wei* (Extremitas Radicis Angelicae Sinensis), and *Chuan Xiong* (Rhizoma Ligustici Chuanxiong). Others enhance the immune system to treat patients who have compromised immune systems, such as *Dan Shen* (Radix Salviae Miltiorrhizae), *Chi Shao* (Radix Paeoniae Rubrae), *Tao Ren* (Semen Persicae), *San Leng* (Rhizoma Sparganii), and *E Zhu* (Rhizoma Curcumae).
- **Antineoplastic**: Herbs that address blood stagnation have shown promise in inhibiting the growth of cancer cells *in vitro*, such as *Chuan Xiong* (Rhizoma Ligustici Chuanxiong), *E Zhu* (Rhizoma Curcumae), *Hong Hua* (Flos Carthami), *Yu Jin* (Radix Curcumae), *Yan Hu Suo* (Rhizoma Corydalis), *Ru Xiang* (Gummi Olibanum), *Mo Yao* (Myrrha) and *San Leng* (Rhizoma Sparganii).
- **Analgesic and anti-inflammatory**: Many blood-moving substances have an analgesic action via their effect on the central nervous system, including *Dan Shen* (Radix Salviae Miltiorrhizae), *Dang Gui* (Radicis Angelicae Sinensis), *Chi Shao* (Radix Paeoniae Rubrae), *Ru Xiang* (Gummi

Olibanum), *Mo Yao* (Myrrha), *Yan Hu Suo* (Rhizoma Corydalis), *Yu Jin* (Radix Curcumae) and *Wu Ling Zhi* (Excrementum Trogopteri seu Pteromi).

Others reduce inflammation by reducing the permeability of the capillaries.

- **Antibiotic**: Many herbs inhibit the growth of bacteria, such as *Chi Shao* (Radix Paeoniae Rubrae), *Mu Dan Pi* (Cortex Moutan), and *Chuan Xiong* (Rhizoma Ligustici Chuanxiong).

POTENTIAL HERB-DRUG INTERACTIONS

- **Antihypertensives:** Herbs that dilate the blood vessels may potentiate the effect of antihypertensive drugs and cause hypotension.
- **Antiplatelets and anticoagulants:** Herbs that treat blood stasis may enhance the actions of antiplatelet and anticoagulant medications, and prolong bleeding or increase bruising.
- **Analgesics:** Herbs with analgesic effects may cause drowsiness, therefore accentuating the sedative effect of many drugs and of alcohol.

As described above, herbs that invigorate blood circulation and eliminate blood stasis have a wide variety of pharmacological effects. This also implies possibilities for theoretical or actual clinical herb-drug interactions. Additional information on possible interactions is given in individual herb monographs.

Note: Blood-invigorating and stasis-removing herbs are tremendously important and effective substances in the Chinese materia medica. Practitioners ought not to shy away from using them for fear of their potency or of herb-drug interactions. Instead, being well-informed about the nature of each of these substances and aware of the pharmaceuticals each patient is taking will allow practitioners the confident exercise of superior herbal care.

Chuan Xiong (Rhizoma Ligustici Chuanxiong)

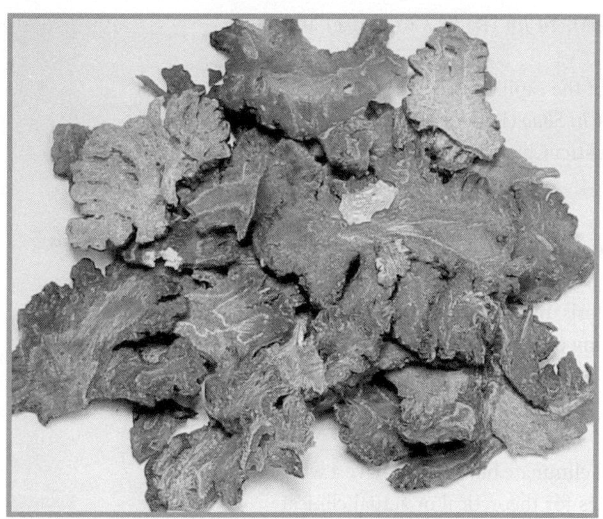

川芎 川芎

Pinyin Name: *Chuan Xiong*

Alternate Chinese Names: *Xiong Xiong, Fu Xiong, Jing Xiong, Shan Ju Xiong*

Original Source: *Shen Nong Ben Cao Jing* (Divine Husbandman's Classic of the Materia Medica) in the second century

English Name: cnidium, Sichuan lovage rhizome, Szechwan lovage rhizome

Botanical Name: *Ligusticum chuanxiong* Hort. (*Chuan Xiong*)

Pharmaceutical Name: Rhizoma Ligustici Chuanxiong

Properties: acrid, warm

Channels Entered: Liver, Gallbladder, Pericardium

CHINESE THERAPEUTIC ACTIONS

1. Activates Qi and Blood Circulation

Acrid and warm, *Chuan Xiong* (Rhizoma Ligustici Chuanxiong) is one of the most effective and commonly used herbs to activate qi and blood circulation. It has excellent ascending, descending and dispersing functions and reaches every part of the body. *Chuan Xiong* is one of the best herbs to treat gynecological disorders. It is also added to blood-tonic herbs to prevent any stagnating side effects.

Obstetric/gynecological disorders: *Chuan Xiong* has an excellent function to regulate blood circulation and is commonly used to treat gynecological disorders such as irregular menstruation, amenorrhea, dysmenorrhea, difficult labor, and postpartum abdominal pain caused by residual blood stagnation. Menstruation is closely related to the *chong* (thoroughfare) channel, which is the point from which all twelve channels emerge and is thus considered the "sea of blood." *Chuan Xiong*, with its descending influence, enters the *chong* channel to regulate qi and blood circulation and normalize menstruation.

Irregular Menstruation:

- Irregular menstruation, with either early or delayed onset: use *Chuan Xiong* with *Dang Gui* (Radicis Angelicae Sinensis), *Bai Shao* (Radix Paeoniae Alba), *Chong Wei Zi* (Semen Leonuri), and *Yi Mu Cao* (Herba Leonuri).
- Irregular menstruation with heat in the blood, usually seen as shortened periods between cycles: use this herb with *Mu Dan Pi* (Cortex Moutan) and *Sheng Di Huang* (Radix Rehmanniae).
- Irregular menstruation with cold in the blood, usually seen as prolonged periods between cycles: use it with *Rou Gui* (Cortex Cinnamomi).
- Epistaxis during menstruation: combine *Chuan Xiong* with *Niu Xi* (Radix Cyathulae seu Achyranthis) and *Bai Mao Gen* (Rhizoma Imperatae).

Amenorrhea:

- Amenorrhea: use *Chuan Xiong* with *Hong Hua* (Flos Carthami) and *Ze Lan* (Herba Lycopi).
- Amenorrhea due to accumulation of phlegm and dampness, in cases of obesity: combine it with *Dang Gui* (Radicis Angelicae Sinensis), *Xiang Fu* (Rhizoma Cyperi), *Cang Zhu* (Rhizoma Atractylodis), *Ban Xia* (Rhizoma Pinelliae), *Ju Hong* (Exocarpium Citri Rubrum), *Chi Fu Ling* (Poria Rubrae), *Tian Nan Xing* (Rhizoma Arisaematis), *Zhi Shi* (Fructus Aurantii Immaturus), *Zhi Gan Cao* (Radix Glycyrrhizae Preparata) and *Sheng Jiang* (Rhizoma Zingiberis Recens).

Dysmenorrhea:

- Dysmenorrhea caused by blood stasis, with dark, purplish clots: use *Chuan Xiong* with *Tao Ren* (Semen Persicae), *Hong Hua* (Flos Carthami), *Dang Gui* (Radicis Angelicae Sinensis) and *Bai Shao* (Radix Paeoniae Alba). **Exemplar Formula:** *Tao Hong Si Wu Tang* (Four-Substance Decoction with Safflower and Peach Pit).
- Dysmenorrhea with a scanty flow of blood and cold sensations in the abdomen caused by deficiency and cold in the *ren* (conception) and *chong* (thoroughfare) channels: use this herb with *Gui Zhi* (Ramulus Cinnamomi), *Wu Zhu Yu* (Fructus Evodiae), *Mu Dan Pi* (Cortex Moutan), and *Dang Gui* (Radicis Angelicae Sinensis).

Childbirth-related disorders:

- Difficult labor: combine *Chuan Xiong* with *Dang Gui* (Radicis Angelicae Sinensis), *Niu Xi* (Radix Cyathulae

Chuan Xiong (Rhizoma Ligustici Chuanxiong)

seu Achyranthis), and *Gui Ban* (Plastrum Testudinis).

- Continuous postpartum bleeding caused by blood stasis with blood deficiency and cold: use this herb with *Dang Gui* (Radicis Angelicae Sinensis), *Tao Ren* (Semen Persicae), *Pao Jiang* (Rhizoma Zingiberis Preparatum), and *Zhi Gan Cao* (Radix Glycyrrhizae Preparata). **Exemplar Formula:** *Sheng Hua Tang* (Generation and Transformation Decoction).

Pain due to blood and qi stagnation: *Chuan Xiong* has an excellent function to regulate qi and blood circulation to alleviate pain. Clinical manifestations include hypochondriac and chest pain, numbness of the limbs and extremities, paralysis, and pain from traumatic injuries.

- Hypochondriac pain with chest and epigastric distention from Liver qi stagnation: use *Chuan Xiong* with *Chai Hu* (Radix Bupleuri), *Xiang Fu* (Rhizoma Cyperi), *Bai Shao* (Radix Paeoniae Alba) and *Zhi Ke* (Fructus Aurantii). **Exemplar Formula:** *Chai Hu Shu Gan Tang* (Bupleurum Powder to Spread the Liver).
- Sharp, stabbing pain in the chest and hypochondriac area due to blood stagnation: add this herb to *Tao Ren* (Semen Persicae), *Hong Hua* (Flos Carthami), *Dang Gui* (Radicis Angelicae Sinensis), and *Chai Hu* (Radix Bupleuri). **Exemplar Formula:** *Xue Fu Zhu Yu Tang* (Drive Out Stasis in the Mansion of Blood Decoction).
- Numbness of the extremities and paralysis: use this herb with *Huang Qi* (Radix Astragali), *Dang Gui* (Radicis Angelicae Sinensis), *Hong Hua* (Flos Carthami), and *Di Long* (Pheretima). **Exemplar Formula:** *Bu Yang Huan Wu Tang* (Tonify the Yang to Restore Five Decoction).
- Pain due to traumatic injuries: combine it with *Dang Gui* (Radicis Angelicae Sinensis), *Chi Shao* (Radix Paeoniae Rubrae) and *Hong Hua* (Flos Carthami).
- Chronic non-healing sores, with or without pus, in deficient patients: add *Chuan Xiong* to *Huang Qi* (Radix Astragali), *Dang Gui* (Radicis Angelicae Sinensis), and *Zao Jiao Ci* (Spina Gleditsiae). **Exemplar Formula:** *Tuo Li Xiao Du Yin* (Drain the Interior and Detoxify Decoction).

2. Dispels Wind and Relieves Pain

Acrid and aromatic, ascending and dispersing, *Chuan Xiong* dispels wind and relieves pain. *Chuan Xiong* is an essential herb in relieving all kinds of aches and pains, when combined with other herbs.

Headaches:

- Headache caused by wind-cold: use *Chuan Xiong* with *Bai Zhi* (Radix Angelicae Dahuricae), *Fang Feng* (Radix Saposhnikoviae), and *Xi Xin* (Herba Asari). **Exemplar Formula:** *Chuan Xiong Cha Tiao San* (Ligusticum Chuanxiong Powder to be Taken with Green Tea).
- Headache from wind-heat: combine this herb with *Ju Hua* (Flos Chrysanthemi), *Shi Gao* (Gypsum Fibrosum), and *Jiang Can* (Bombyx Batryticatus).
- Headache caused by wind and dampness: use it with *Qiang Huo* (Rhizoma et Radix Notopterygii), *Gao Ben* (Rhizoma Ligustici), and *Fang Feng* (Radix Saposhnikoviae). **Exemplar Formula:** *Qiang Huo Sheng Shi Tang* (Notopterygium Decoction to Overcome Dampness).
- Headache from blood stasis: use this herb with *Dang Gui* (Radicis Angelicae Sinensis), *Tao Ren* (Semen Persicae), and *Hong Hua* (Flos Carthami). **Exemplar Formula:** *Xue Fu Zhu Yu Tang* (Drive Out Stasis in the Mansion of Blood Decoction).
- Headache from blood deficiency: use it with *Dang Gui* (Radicis Angelicae Sinensis), *Shu Di Huang* (Radix Rehmanniae Preparata), and *Bai Shao* (Radix Paeoniae Alba).
- Severe headache without interior fire: combine this herb with *Gao Ben* (Rhizoma Ligustici).

***Bi zheng* (painful obstruction syndrome):**

- Musculoskeletal and joint pain caused by the accumulation of wind, cold and dampness: add *Chuan Xiong* to *Dang Gui* (Radicis Angelicae Sinensis), *Du Huo* (Radix Angelicae Pubescentis) and *Hai Feng Teng* (Caulis Piperis Kadsurae). **Exemplar Formula:** *Juan Bi Tang* (Remove Painful Obstruction Decoction).

DOSAGE

3 to 10 grams in herbal decoction, 1.0 to 1.5 grams as powder. Frying *Chuan Xiong* with grain-based liquor enhances its potency to activate qi and blood circulation, dispel wind, and relieve pain.

CAUTIONS / CONTRAINDICATIONS

- Acrid, warm and dispersing in nature, *Chuan Xiong* should not be used in cases of yin-deficient fire, red tongue, and dry mouth.
- *Chuan Xiong* should be used with caution in cases of hypermenorrhea due to its strong function to activate qi and blood circulation.

CHEMICAL COMPOSITION

Alkaloids (chuanxiongzine, tetramethylprazine, L-isoleucine-L-valine anhydride, L-valine-L-valine anhydride, trimethylamine, choline, perlolyrine, cnidiumlactone, chuanxingol, 4-hydroxy-3-butyl-phathalide, ligustilide, neocnidilide); organic acids (ferulic acid, sedanonic acid, folic acid, vanillic, caffeic acid, protocatechuic acid, palmitic acid, linolenic acid, chrysophanol, methyl phenylacetate, sedanoic acid lactone, methyl pentadecanoate); essential oils (ethyl pentadecanoate, ethyl

12

BLOOD-INVIGORATING AND STASIS-REMOVING HERBS

Chuan Xiong (Rhizoma Ligustici Chuanxiong)

palmitate, ethyl heptadecanoate, ethyl isoheptadecanoate, ethyl octadecanoate, ethyl isoctadecanoate, methyl palmitate, methyl linolenate).[1,2]

Ligustilide

PHARMACOLOGICAL EFFECTS

- **Cardiovascular:** *Chuan Xiong* dilates blood vessels to lower blood pressure, increases blood perfusion to coronary arteries, and decreases oxygen consumption by the cardiac muscle. The effect of *Chuan Xiong* on the cardiovascular system varies depending on the dosage given, as demonstrated in frog studies. At 20 to 30 g/kg via oral route, there is a positive inotropic and negative chronotropic effect on the heart; at 40 g/kg, the heart may exert little or no contraction.[3]
- **Antiplatelet and anticoagulant:** Administration of *Chuan Xiong* has demonstrated marked antiplatelet and anticoagulant effects in various animal studies.[4]
- **Circulatory:** Administration of *Chuan Xiong* is associated with increased blood perfusion to and reduced swelling of the brain, and is commonly used to treat disorders such as cerebral ischemia, Alzheimer's disease, and migraine headache.[5]
- **Sedative:** Oral administration of *Chuan Xiong* decoction to mice and rats has a sedative effect on the central nervous system, as it decreases motor activities, prolongs phenobarbital-induced sleeping time, and counteracts the stimulating effects produced by caffeine.[6]
- **Effects on the smooth muscle:** Administration of *Chuan Xiong* has marked influences on the smooth muscle of the uterus and intestines. At small dosages, it leads to mild contraction and/or spasms of the smooth muscle. At large dosages, it causes numbness and inhibits contraction of smooth muscle. Subcutaneous administration of a 20% *Chuan Xiong* injection at the dosage of 4 ml/100g may cause fatality of the fetus in pregnant mice or rabbits, presumably due to severe contraction of the muscles shutting off blood circulation.[7]
- **Protective effect against radiation:** Intramuscular, oral and intraperitoneal administration of *Chuan Xiong* have all been associated with a protective effect against radiation in dogs, mice and rats.[8]

CLINICAL STUDIES AND RESEARCH

- **Headache:** In one study, 50 patients with headaches were treated with herbal formulas with great success. The base formula contained *Chuan Xiong*, *Shi Gao* (Gypsum Fibrosum), *Xi Xin* (Herba Asari) and *Ju Hua* (Flos Chrysanthemi). Modifications were made if necessary, depending on the differential diagnosis. For wind-cold headache, larger dosages of *Chuan Xiong*, *Bai Zhi* (Radix Angelicae Dahuricae) *Xi Xin* (Herba Asari), and regular dosages of *Qiang Huo* (Rhizoma et Radix Notopterygii) and *Fang Feng* (Radix Saposhnikoviae) were used. For wind-heat headache, larger dosages of *Ju Hua* (Flos Chrysanthemi), and *Shi Gao* (Gypsum Fibrosum), and regular dosages of *Bo He* (Herba Menthae) and *Lian Qiao* (Fructus Forsythiae) were used. For wind-damp headache, larger dosages of *Xi Xin* (Herba Asari), *Chuan Xiong* (Rhizoma Ligustici Chuanxiong), and *Bai Zhi* (Radix Angelicae Dahuricae), and regular dosages of *Qiang Huo* (Rhizoma et Radix Notopterygii), *Cang Zhu* (Rhizoma Atractylodis) and *Gao Ben* (Rhizoma Ligustici) were used. For headaches caused by blood stasis, large dosage of *Chuan Xiong* and regular dosages of *She Xiang* (Moschus), *Tao Ren* (Semen Persicae), *Hong Hua* (Flos Carthami) and *Dang Gui* (Radicis Angelicae Sinensis) were used.[9]
- **Angina:** Eight patients with angina were treated with 20 mg of ferulic acid in 250 ml of D5W, administered via intravenous infusion once daily, for 10 days. The study reported an overall improvement of chest pain, ECG evaluation, and reduction of cholesterol levels.[10] In another study, preparation of a *Chuan Xiong* injectable was used to treat 30 angina patients, with relief of pain observed in 92.5% of patients and improvement of ECG seen in 40% of patients.[11]
- **Hypertrophic myelitis and bone spurs of the heels:** Patients with these conditions were treated with *Chuan Xiong* powder placed in a small cloth bag and taped directly onto the affected area. A fresh batch of herbs was placed in the cloth bag on a weekly basis. The study reported moderate to significant reduction of pain within 5 to 10 days. The patients were treated with the same method if the condition recurred in 2 or 3 months.[12]
- **Cerebral thrombosis:** An herbal injectable was used to treat 400 cerebral thrombosis patients, with an overall 94.5% rate of effectiveness, based on both subjective and objective evaluations. The herbal injectable contained *Chuan Xiong*, *Chi Shao* (Radix Paeoniae Rubrae), *Dan Shen* (Radix Salviae Miltiorrhizae) and *Dang Gui* (Radicis Angelicae Sinensis).[13]
- **Cerebral embolism:** In one report, 50 patients with acute cerebral embolisms were treated with a preparation of *Chuan Xiong* injectable for 14 days, with an overall effective rate of 90%. Most patients showed significant improvement in motor functions, with up to 66% regaining the ability to walk. There was a 6% mortality rate.[14]
- **Trigeminal nerve pain:** Twenty-one patients were treated

Chuan Xiong (Rhizoma Ligustici Chuanxiong)

with an herbal decoction daily for 1 month with a 90.6% rate of effectiveness. The herbal formula contained 30 grams of *Chuan Xiong*, and 9 grams each of *Dang Gui* (Radicis Angelicae Sinensis), *Dan Shen* (Radix Salviae Miltiorrhizae), *Bai Shao* (Radix Paeoniae Alba), *Chai Hu* (Radix Bupleuri), *Huang Qin* (Radix Scutellariae), *Bai Zhi* (Radix Angelicae Dahuricae), *Quan Xie* (Scorpio), *Chan Tui* (Periostracum Cicadae) and *Di Long* (Pheretima).[15]

HERB-DRUG INTERACTION

- **Anticoagulant or antiplatelet drugs:** *Chuan Xiong* should be used with caution in patients receiving anticoagulant or antiplatelet medications, as combining these substances may have additive or synergistic effects. Though this potential interaction has not been documented, the use of *Chuan Xiong* may potentiate the effect of such drugs as warfarin.[16] [Note: Examples of anticoagulants include heparin, warfarin (Coumadin) and enoxaparin (Lovenox); and examples of antiplatelets include aspirin, dipyridamole (Persantine), and clopidogrel (Plavix).]

TOXICOLOGY

No abnormalities of liver, kidney and blood exams were observed in mice following continuous oral administration of chuanxingzine at 5 to 10 mg/kg, for 4 weeks. The LD_{50} for a *Chuan Xiong* preparation in mice was 65.86 g/kg with intraperitoneal injection and 66.42 g/kg with intravenous injection.[17]

AUTHORS' COMMENTS

Chuan Xiong (Rhizoma Ligustici Chuanxiong), *Qiang Huo* (Rhizoma et Radix Notopterygii), *Bai Zhi* (Radix Angelicae Dahuricae), *Chai Hu* (Radix Bupleuri) and *Gao Ben* (Rhizoma Ligustici) all treat headaches. According to Dr. Li Shou-Shan, the differences between these herbs are as follows:

- *Chuan Xiong* is most effective for headaches related to menstruation.
- *Qiang Huo* is more specific to occipital headaches.
- *Bai Zhi* focuses on frontal headaches.
- *Chai Hu* treats temporal headaches.
- *Gao Ben* is best for vertex headaches.

According to Dr. Liu Feng-Wu, the following sets of herbs are listed in order of their potency to invigorate blood:

- For slow blood flow with no actual stasis: *Dang Gui* (Radicis Angelicae Sinensis), *Chuan Xiong* (Rhizoma Ligustici Chuanxiong), and *Yi Mu Cao* (Herba Leonuri).
- For blood clots that are not very apparent, or are moderate in severity: *Tao Ren* (Semen Persicae), *Hong Hua* (Flos Carthami), *Liu Ji Nu* (Herba Artemisiae Anomalae), *Pu Huang* (Pollen Typhae), and *Wu Ling Zhi* (Excrementum Trogopteri seu Pteromi).
- For blood clots that are palpable or causing obstruction: *San Leng* (Rhizoma Sparganii), *E Zhu* (Rhizoma Curcumae), *Dan Shen* (Radix Salviae Miltiorrhizae), *Xue Jie* (Sanguis Draconis), and *Su Mu* (Lignum Sappan).
- For severe blood stasis: *Shui Zhi* (Hirudo), *Meng Chong* (Tabanus), and *Da Huang* (Radix et Rhizoma Rhei).

References

1. *Zhong Yi Yao Li* (Pharmacology of Chinese Herbs), 1997; 890
2. Yan X, Zhou J, Xie G, *Traditional Chinese Medicines Molecular Structures, Natural Sources and Applications*; Ashgate, 1999; 3883
3. *Zhong Yao Yao Li Yu Ying Yong* (Pharmacology and Applications of Chinese Herbs), 1989;(2):40
4. *Hua Xi Yi Xue Za Zhi* (Huaxi Medical Journal), 1993; 8(3):170
5. *Zhong Yao Xue* (Chinese Herbology), 1989; 535:539
6. *Zhong Yao Yao Li Yu Ying Yong* (Pharmacology and Applications of Chinese Herbs), 1983:123
7. *Hua Xue Xue Bao* (Journal of Chemistry), 1957; 23:246
8. *Zhong Yao Yao Li Yu Ying Yong* (Pharmacology and Applications of Chinese Herbs), 1983:123
9. *Shan Xi Zhong Yi Za Zhi* (Shanxi Journal Chinese Medicine), 1985; 10:447
10. *Chong Qing Yi Yao* (Chongching Medicine and Herbology), 1978; 1:23
11. *Xin Yi Yao Xue Za Zhi* (New Journal of Medicine and Herbology), 1977; 1:15
12. *Xin Yi Xue* (New Medicine), 1975; 6(1):50
13. *Zhong Xi Yi Jie He Za Zhi* (Journal of Integrated Chinese and Western Medicine), 1986; 6(4):234
14. *Zhong Yi Yan Jiu Yuan* (Research Hospital of Chinese Medicine), 1976; 4(4):261
15. *He Bei Zhong Yi Za Zhi* (Hebei Journal of Chinese Medicine), 1982; 4:34
16. Chen, J. Recognition & prevention of herb-drug interactions, *Medical Acupuncture*, Fall/Winter 1998/1999; volume 10/number 2; 9-13
17. *Zhong Yao Yao Li Yu Ying Yong* (Pharmacology and Applications of Chinese Herbs), 1983; 123

Yan Hu Suo (Rhizoma Corydalis)

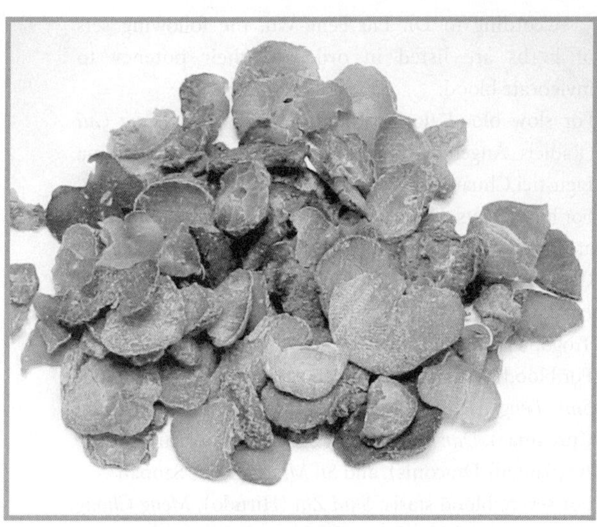

延胡索

Pinyin Name: *Yan Hu Suo*

Alternate Chinese Names: *Yan Hu, Yuan Hu, Xuan Hu, Xuan Hu Suo*

Original Source: *Ben Cao Shi Yi* (Omissions From the [Classic of the] Materia Medica) by Chen Cang-Qi in 741 A.D.

English Name: corydalis

Botanical Name: *Corydalis turtschaninovii* Bess. f. yanhusuo Y.H. Chou et C.C. Hsu (*Yan Hu Suo*)

Pharmaceutical Name: Rhizoma Corydalis

Properties: acrid, bitter, warm

Channels Entered: Heart, Liver, Spleen

CHINESE THERAPEUTIC ACTIONS

Activates Qi and Blood Circulation to Relieve Pain

Pain in the chest, abdomen and limbs: In traditional Chinese medicine, pain is a manifestation of qi stagnation, blood stagnation, or both. It is often said that where there is pain, there is stagnation; where there is stagnation, there is pain. *Yan Hu Suo* (Rhizoma Corydalis) is one of the most commonly used and the most effective herbs to relieve pain because it has an excellent ability to activate qi in the *qi* (energy) level and invigorate blood circulation in the *xue* (blood) level. It is used to treat pain from a variety of causes in all parts of the body.

Chest pain:

- Severe epigastric and chest pain: use *Yan Hu Suo* individually.
- Angina, coronary artery disease, chest pain: combine it with *Dan Shen* (Radix Salviae Miltiorrhizae), *Hong Hua* (Flos Carthami), and *Chuan Xiong* (Rhizoma Ligustici Chuanxiong).
- Chest and hypochondriac pain: add this herb to *Gua Lou Shi* (Fructus Trichosanthis), *Xie Bai* (Bulbus Allii Macrostemonis), and *Yu Jin* (Radix Curcumae).
- Arrhythmia: use it with *Shan Zha* (Fructus Crataegi), *Yu Zhu* (Rhizoma Polygonati Odorati), and *Dan Shen* (Radix Salviae Miltiorrhizae).

Epigastric and abdominal pain:

- Epigastric and abdominal pain caused by qi and blood stagnation: add *Yan Hu Suo* to *Chuan Lian Zi* (Fructus Toosendan).
- Abdominal pain caused by cold and blood stagnation: combine it with *Gao Liang Jiang* (Rhizoma Alpiniae Officinarum), *Pao Jiang* (Rhizoma Zingiberis Preparatum), *Xiang Fu* (Rhizoma Cyperi), and *Sha Ren* (Fructus Amomi).
- Abdominal fullness and pain from qi stagnation: use it with *Mu Xiang* (Radix Aucklandiae), *Qing Pi* (Pericarpium Citri Reticulatae Viride), *Sha Ren* (Fructus Amomi) and *Yu Jin* (Radix Curcumae).
- Hernial pain: add it to *Xiao Hui Xiang* (Fructus Foeniculi) and *Wu Yao* (Radix Linderae).

Gynecological pain:

- Amenorrhea or menstrual pain caused by qi and blood stagnation: use *Yan Hu Suo* with *Dang Gui* (Radicis Angelicae Sinensis), *Chuan Xiong* (Rhizoma Ligustici Chuanxiong), *Bai Shao* (Radix Paeoniae Alba), and *Xiang Fu* (Rhizoma Cyperi).
- Amenorrhea and menstrual pain because of cold and blood stagnation: combine this herb with *Gan Jiang* (Rhizoma Zingiberis), *Rou Gui* (Cortex Cinnamomi), *Dang Gui* (Radicis Angelicae Sinensis), *Wu Ling Zhi* (Excrementum Trogopteri seu Pteromi), *Pu Huang* (Pollen Typhae) and *Chuan Xiong* (Rhizoma Ligustici Chuanxiong).

Pain in the extremities:

- Pain of the upper extremities: use *Yan Hu Suo* with *Dang Gui* (Radicis Angelicae Sinensis), *Gui Zhi* (Ramulus Cinnamomi), and *Chi Shao* (Radix Paeoniae Rubrae).
- Pain in the lower extremities: combine this herb with *Sang Ji Sheng* (Herba Taxilli), *Chuan Niu Xi* (Radix Cyathulae), *Xu Duan* (Radix Dipsaci) and *Du Huo* (Radix Angelicae Pubescentis).
- Traumatic injuries and pain: use it with *Dang Gui* (Radicis Angelicae Sinensis), *Chuan Xiong* (Rhizoma Ligustici Chuanxiong), *Ru Xiang* (Gummi Olibanum), and *Mo Yao* (Myrrha).

Yan Hu Suo (Rhizoma Corydalis)

Masses:

Prolonged stagnation of qi and blood in the abdomen can result in palpable masses, which may be fixed and varied in size depending on the severity of the condition. The masses may be present one day but not another, and more palpable and painful when there is a flare-up of disease. *Yan Hu Suo* enters the *xue* (blood) level to invigorate circulation, dispel stagnation and reduce masses.

- Palpable masses in the abdomen: combine *Yan Hu Suo* with *Dang Gui* (Radicis Angelicae Sinensis), *Hong Hua* (Flos Carthami), *Tao Ren* (Semen Persicae), *Chuan Niu Xi* (Radix Cyathulae), *Ze Lan* (Herba Lycopi), *Chuan Shan Jia* (Squama Manis), *E Zhu* (Rhizoma Curcumae), *San Leng* (Rhizoma Sparganii), *Da Huang* (Radix et Rhizoma Rhei), *Wu Yao* (Radix Linderae) and *Qing Pi* (Pericarpium Citri Reticulatae Viride).

DOSAGE

Use 3 to 10 grams in decoction, with maximum dosage of 20 grams. Use 1 to 1.5 grams of *Yan Hu Suo* powder, served with warm water. Frying this herb with grain-based liquor enhances its blood-activating function. Frying it with vinegar enhances the analgesic function.

CAUTIONS / CONTRAINDICATIONS

- *Yan Hu Suo* is contraindicated in pregnant women, because of its strong function to move qi and blood.
- *Yan Hu Suo* should be used with caution in patients who have pain with an underlying deficiency, as the herb may consume qi and blood.

CHEMICAL COMPOSITION

D-corydaline, dl-tetrahydropalmatine, corydalis L, protopine, 1-tetrahydrocoptisine, l-tetrahydrocolumbamine, corydalis H, corydalis I, corybulbine, B-homochelidonine, coptisine, dehydrocorydaline, corydalmine, dehydrocorydalmine, and columbamine.[1,2,3,4]

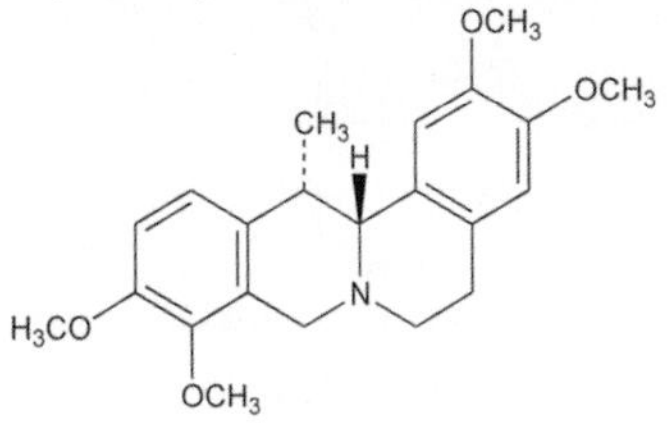

Corydaline

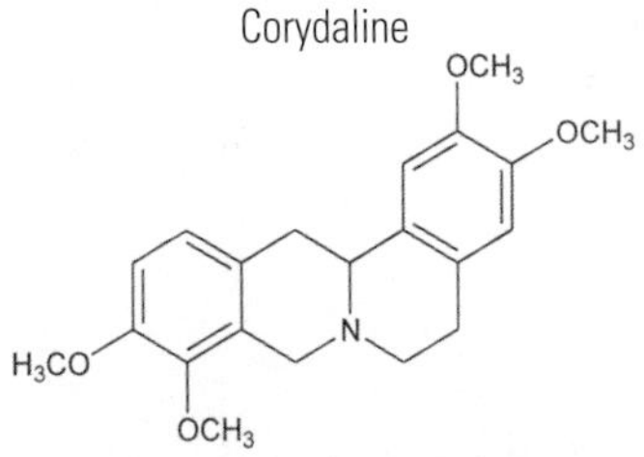

Tetrahydropalmatine

PHARMACOLOGICAL EFFECTS

- **Analgesic:** *Yan Hu Suo* has demonstrated a strong analgesic effect, with dl-tetrahydropalmatine and corydalis I as the strongest components. When compared to morphine, *Yan Hu Suo* has shown a slower onset and weaker analgesic effect when given by injection. Evaluation of analgesic effect based on weight showed *Yan Hu Suo* to be approximately 100:1 in effect by comparison to morphine. *Yan Hu Suo*, however, has not been associated with any signs or symptoms related to dependence. In addition, development of tolerance occurs approximately 100% faster with morphine than with *Yan Hu Suo*.[5]
- **Analgesic:** It was demonstrated in a research study that, combined with *Yan Hu Suo*, the analgesic effect of electroacupuncture increased significantly, when compared to a control group that received electro-acupuncture only.[6]
- **Sedative and tranquilizing:** *Yan Hu Suo* has demonstrated sedative and tranquilizing effects in rabbits, mice, dogs and monkeys.[7]
- **Effects on the central nervous system:** Tetrahydropalmatine has demonstrated marked analgesic, sedative, tranquilizing and hypnotic actions on the central nervous system.[8]
- **Anti-inflammatory:** Extract of *Yan Hu Suo* has demonstrated marked anti-inflammatory effect by inhibiting histamine release and formation of edema in arthritic rats. The extract was found to be effective in both acute and chronic phases of inflammation.[9]
- **Antiulcer:** *Yan Hu Suo* suppresses the secretion of gastric acid when given at the dosage of 80 mg/kg in rabbits and mice.[10]
- **Cardiovascular:** *Yan Hu Suo* has been shown to decrease resistance of blood flow and increase blood perfusion to coronary arteries in cats. It decreases oxygen consumption of the cardiac muscle and increases contractility of the heart.[11]
- **Adrenocortical:** *Yan Hu Suo* has been shown to increase hormone secretion from adrenal glands when given via injection to mice at a dosage of 70 mg/kg.[12]
- **Muscle relaxant:** *Yan Hu Suo* has demonstrated a muscle-relaxant effect in rabbits and mice.[13]

CLINICAL STUDIES AND RESEARCH

- **Coronary artery disorder:** In one clinical trial, *Yan Hu Suo* extract was used for treatment of coronary artery disorder in 575 patients (424 diagnosed with angina and 148 with myocardial infarction). For 424 patients with angina, improvement was reported in both symptomatic evaluation and EKG monitoring. For symptomatic evaluation, the study stated that there was significant symptomatic improvement in 44.4% and moderate improvement in 38.8% of the patients. For EKG monitoring,

Yan Hu Suo (Rhizoma Corydalis)

there was significant improvement in 26.8% and moderate improvement in 26.1% of the patients. For 148 patients with myocardial infarction, the fatality rate was 14.1% for patients treated with *Yan Hu Suo*, and 32.3% for patients who did not receive any treatment.[14]

- **Local anesthetic:** Local injection of a *Yan Hu Suo* preparation demonstrated satisfactory anesthetic effects in 98 out of 105 patients (93.4%) who underwent surgery. Only 6 patients (5.7%) experienced mild pain.[15]
- **Arrhythmia:** In one report, 48 patients with arrhythmia and 27 patients with pre-ventricular arrhythmia were treated with 5 to 10 grams of *Yan Hu Suo* three times daily, with good results.[16]

TOXICOLOGY

The LD_{50} for oral administration of *Yan Hu Suo* in mice is 100 +/- 4.53 g/kg. Side effects included lowered blood pressure, decreased heart rate, mild respiratory depression, sedation, and tremor.[17]

AUTHORS' COMMENTS

According to Dr. Ding Guang-Di, *Yan Hu Suo* and *Chuan Lian Zi* (Fructus Toosendan) are better for left-sided hypochondriac pain. *Xuan Fu Hua* (Flos Inulae) and *Xiang Fu* (Rhizoma Cyperi) are more effective to address right-sided hypochondriac pain.

According to Dr. Chen Ke-Fen, *Yan Hu Suo* and *Chuan Xiong* (Rhizoma Ligustici Chuanxiong) are an effective pair to relieve angina and *xiong bi* (painful obstruction of the chest).

Yan Hu Suo, Ru Xiang (Gummi Olibanum), *Mo Yao* (Myrrha) and *Fen Fang Ji* (Radix Stephaniae Tetandrae) all have marked pain-relief action.

- *Yan Hu Suo* has the strongest analgesic effect, and is used for all kinds of pain in the chest, abdomen and limbs caused by qi and blood stagnation.
- *Ru Xiang* and *Mo Yao* are commonly used together to treat pain related to traumatic injuries and external injuries.
- *Fen Fang Ji* is most effective for *bi zheng* (painful obstruction syndrome) in the extremities.

References

1. *Xian Dai Zhong Yao Yao Li Xue* (Contemporary Pharmacology of Chinese Herbs), 1997; 894-895
2. *Chang Yong Zhong Yao Cheng Fen Yu Yao Li Shou Ce* (A Handbook of the Composition and Pharmacology of Common Chinese Drugs), 1994; 874-875
3. *The Merck Index* 12th edition, Chapman & Hall/CRCnetBASE/Merck, 2000
4. Ibid.
5. *Zhong Yao Yao Li Yu Ying Yong* (Pharmacology and Applications of Chinese Herbs), 1983; 447
6. *Chen Tzu Yen Chiu* (Acupuncture Research), 1994; 19(1):55-8
7. *Zhong Cao Yao Xue* (Study of Chinese Herbal Medicine), 1976; 340
8. *Memorias do Instituto Oswaldo Cruz.* 1991; 86 suppl 2:173-5
9. *Biol Pharm Bull*, 1994:Feb; 17(2):262-5
10. *Zhong Cao Yao Xue* (Study of Chinese Herbal Medicine), 1976; 340
11. *Zhong Yao Yao Li Yu Ying Yong* (Pharmacology and Applications of Chinese Herbs), 1983; 447
12. *Xi Xue Xue Bao* (Academic Journal of Medicine), 1988; 23(10)721
13. *Zhong Guo Yao Li Xue Tong Bao* (Journal of Chinese Herbal Pharmacology), 1990; 6(3):179
14. *Zhong Yao Tong Bao* (Journal of Chinese Herbology), 1980; 4:192
15. *He Bei Xin Yi Yao* (Hebei New Medicine and Herbology), 1973; 4:34
16. *Zhong Hua Xin Xue Guan Bing Za Zhi* (Chinese Journal of Cardiology), 1983
17. *Zhong Yao Yao Li Yu Ying Yong* (Pharmacology and Applications of Chinese Herbs), 1983; 447

Yu Jin (Radix Curcumae)

鬱金 郁金

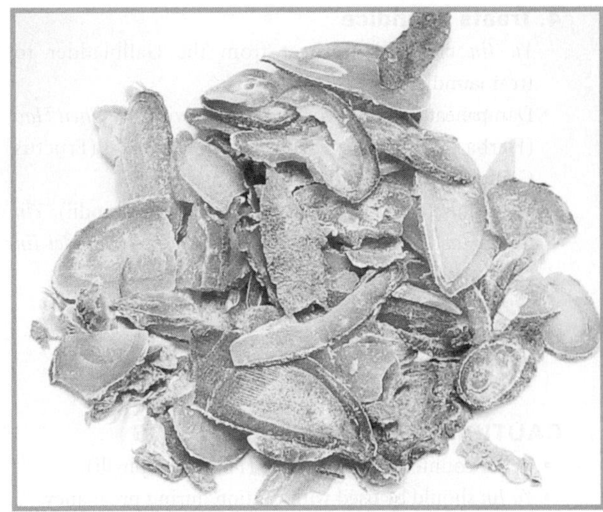

Pinyin Name: *Yu Jin*
Literal Name: "constrained metal"
Alternate Chinese Names: *Chuan Yu Jin, Guang Yu Jin*
Original Source: *Yao Xing Ben Cao* (Materia Medica of Medicinal Properties) by Zhen Quan in 600 A.D.
English Name: curcuma, aromatic turmeric tuber, aromatic kwangsi turmeric tuber, zedoary turmeric tuber
Botanical Name: *Curcuma aromatica* Salisb. (*Yu Jin*); *Curcuma kwangsiensis* S. Lee et C. F. Liang. (*Guang Xi E Zhu*); *Curcuma longa* L. (*Jiang Huang*); *Curcuma zedoaria* (Berg.) Rosc. (*E Zhu*)
Pharmaceutical Name: Radix Curcumae
Properties: acrid, bitter, cold
Channels Entered: Heart, Liver, Gallbladder

CHINESE THERAPEUTIC ACTIONS

1. Activates Qi and Blood Circulation, Relieves Pain

Hypochondriac pain, irregular menstruation, masses caused by blood stagnation: *Yu Jin* (Radix Curcumae) is most effective for treating pain due to qi and blood stagnation. It resolves Liver qi stagnation and regulates qi in the *xue* (blood) level. Hypochondriac pain is the chief manifestation of Liver qi stagnation. The Liver stores blood, therefore, irregular menstruation denotes stagnation in the Liver and irregularity of the *ren* (conception) and *chong* (thoroughfare) channels. Accompanying symptoms may include bloating and dysmenorrhea during menstruation. Masses due to blood stagnation can appear anywhere in the abdomen. *Yu Jin* is best for masses in the hypochondriac region. It treats disorders such as liver cirrhosis, or enlargement of the liver or spleen.

- Hypochondriac pain due to Liver qi stagnation: use *Yu Jin* with *Chai Hu* (Radix Bupleuri), *Xiang Fu* (Rhizoma Cyperi), *Bai Shao* (Radix Paeoniae Alba), and *Dan Shen* (Radix Salviae Miltiorrhizae).
- Irregular menstruation with pain and cramps caused by stagnation of qi and blood and disharmony of *chong* (thoroughfare) and *ren* (conception) channels: use this herb with *Dang Gui* (Radicis Angelicae Sinensis), *Bai Shao* (Radix Paeoniae Alba) and *Xiang Fu* (Rhizoma Cyperi).
- Pain due to masses in the hypochondriac area: combine it with *Bie Jia* (Carapax Trionycis), *Dan Shen* (Radix Salviae Miltiorrhizae) and *Ze Lan* (Herba Lycopi).

2. Clears Heat and Cools Blood

Bleeding: *Yu Jin* treats various bleeding disorders caused by heat in the blood. Clinical applications include hematemesis, epistaxis, hematuria, and epistaxis during menstruation.

- Bleeding due to heat in the blood: combine *Yu Jin* with *Sheng Di Huang* (Radix Rehmanniae), *Mu Dan Pi* (Cortex Moutan), *Zhi Zi* (Fructus Gardeniae) and *Niu Xi* (Radix Cyathulae seu Achyranthis).

3. Clears the Heart, Opens Orifices and Promotes Consciousness

Disorientation, epilepsy, mania and other disorders with disturbed *shen* (spirit): *Yu Jin* strongly clears heat from the Heart and mildly promotes consciousness. It is commonly used to treat cases of heat, dampness and phlegm covering the Heart leading to anxiety, irritability, disorientation, seizures, convulsions, and in severe cases, epilepsy, mania, and semi-consciousness or unconsciousness.

- Psychological disorders with feelings of oppression in the chest due to accumulation of dampness: use *Yu Jin* with *Shi Chang Pu* (Rhizoma Acori), *Zhu Li* (Succus Bambusae), *Huang Lian* (Rhizoma Coptidis), *Tian Zhu Huang* (Concretio Silicea Bambusae), *Niu Huang* (Calculus Bovis) and *Zhi Zi* (Fructus Gardeniae).
- Mania and delirium due to phlegm covering the Heart: use this herb with *Ming Fan* (Alumen).
- Schizophrenia and other psychological disorders with insomnia and alternating spells of laughter and anger: use *Yu Jin* with *Xiang Fu* (Rhizoma Cyperi), *Bai Shao* (Radix Paeoniae Alba), *Dai Zhe Shi* (Haematitum), *Zhen Zhu Mu* (Concha Margaritaferae), *Tian Zhu Huang* (Concretio Silicea Bambusae), *Dan Nan Xing* (Arisaema cum Bile), *Yuan Zhi* (Radix Polygalae), *Shi Chang Pu* (Rhizoma Acori), *Ban Xia* (Rhizoma Pinelliae), *Fu Ling* (Poria), *Huang Lian* (Rhizoma Coptidis), *Sheng Tie Luo* (Frusta Ferri) and *Da Huang* (Radix et Rhizoma Rhei).

Yu Jin (Radix Curcumae)

4. Treats Jaundice

Yu Jin clears damp-heat from the Gallbladder to treat jaundice.

- Damp-heat jaundice: combine *Yu Jin* with *Yin Chen Hao* (Herba Artemisiae Scopariae), *Zhi Zi* (Fructus Gardeniae), and *Zhi Ke* (Fructus Aurantii).
- Gallstones: use it with *Hai Jin Sha* (Herba Lygodii), *Yin Chen Hao* (Herba Artemisiae Scopariae), and *Ji Nei Jin* (Endothelium Corneum Gigeriae Galli).

DOSAGE

6 to 12 grams in decoction.

CAUTIONS / CONTRAINDICATIONS

- *Yu Jin* counteracts *Ding Xiang* (Flos Caryophylli).
- *Yu Jin* should be used with caution during pregnancy.
- *Yu Jin* is contraindicated in patients without qi and blood stagnation, or those with underlying yin deficiency and bleeding.

CHEMICAL COMPOSITION

Essential oils, d-camphene, d-camphor, l-α-curcumene, l-β-curcumene, curcumin, demethoxycurcumin, bis-demethoxycurcumin, turmerone, starch, lipids, carvone.[1]

PHARMACOLOGICAL EFFECTS

- **Hepatoprotective:** Compared with a placebo group, administration of *Yu Jin* was associated with a 10% greater reduction of SGOT and SGPT in mice and rats with carbon tetrachloride-induced liver damage. In addition, essential oil of *Yu Jin* has shown promising effects in treatment of viral hepatitis, by altering the immune system.[2]
- **Antihyperlipidemic:** Administration of a *Yu Jin* preparation in animals once daily for 40 days has demonstrated a marked reduction in both plasma and liver content of cholesterol and triglycerides.[3]
- **Gastrointestinal:** According to an animal study, oral administration of *Yu Jin* decoction increases the secretion of gastric acid, lowers the pH in the stomach and duodenum, and promotes the production and excretion of bile.[4]

CLINICAL STUDIES AND RESEARCH

- **Coronary artery disease:** Administration of an herbal formula containing *Yu Jin*, *San Qi* (Radix Notoginseng) and *Chi Shao* (Radix Paeoniae Rubrae) demonstrated marked antiplatelet effect in 40 patients with coronary artery disease.[5]
- **Gastric bleeding:** Twenty patients with bleeding ulcers were treated with an herbal decoction with marked effectiveness, especially in patients who were otherwise healthy. The chief complaints among the patients before treatment were hematemesis and hematochezia. The herbal formula contained *Yu Jin*, *San Qi* (Radix Notoginseng), *Da Huang* (Radix et Rhizoma Rhei), *Niu Xi* (Radix Cyathulae seu Achyranthis), and other herbs depending on the individual condition of the patient.[6] [*Da Huang* should be cooked to minimize gastrointestinal irritation and prevent diarrhea.]
- **Pre-ventricular contraction (PVC):** Patients with PVCs were treated with *Yu Jin* powder daily for 3 months, with approximately 75% effectiveness. Patients began taking 5 to 10 grams of *Yu Jin* powder three times daily for 3 days, with the dosage increased to 10 to 15 grams three times daily if no side effects were reported. Out of 52 patients, 14 had complete recovery, 11 showed significant improvement, 9 showed moderate improvement, and 18 showed no response. None of these patients received drug treatment during the entire 3 month period.[7]

HERB-DRUG INTERACTION

Anticoagulant or antiplatelet drugs: *Yu Jin* has antiplatelet effects, and should be used with caution in patients who take anticoagulant or antiplatelet medications. Though this potential interaction has not been documented, this herb may potentiate the effect of drugs such as warfarin.[8] [Note: Examples of anticoagulants include heparin, warfarin (Coumadin) and enoxaparin (Lovenox); and examples of antiplatelets include aspirin, dipyridamole (Persantine), and clopidogrel (Plavix).]

TOXICOLOGY

In an acute toxicology study in rats, oral administration of *Yu Jin* did not demonstrate any significant changes in body weight, blood exam, or functioning of the internal organs.[9]

References

1. *Chang Yong Zhong Yao Xian Dai Yan Jiu Yu Lin Chuan* (Recent Study & Clinical Application of Common Traditional Chinese Medicine), 1995; 392-393
2. *Zhong Guo Mian Yi Xue Za Zhi* (Chinese Journal of Immunology), 1989; 5(2):121
3. *Xin Yi Yao Xue Za Zhi* (New Journal of Medicine and Herbology), 1978; (9):540
4. *Zhong Cheng Yao Yan Jiu* (Research of Chinese Patent Medicine), 1987; (5):44
5. *Shang Hai Zhong Yi Yao Za Zhi* (Shanghai Journal of Chinese Medicine and Herbology), 1986; 12:40
6. *Zhong Yi Za Zhi* (Journal of Chinese Medicine), 1982; 12:14
7. *Bei Jing Zhong Yi* (Beijing Chinese Medicine), 1984; 3:18
8. Chen, J. Recognition & prevention of herb-drug interactions, *Medical Acupuncture*, Fall/Winter 1998/1999; volume 10/number 2; 9-13
9. *Zhong Cheng Yao Yan Jiu* (Research of Chinese Patent Medicine), 1987; (5):44

Jiang Huang (Rhizoma Curcumae Longae)

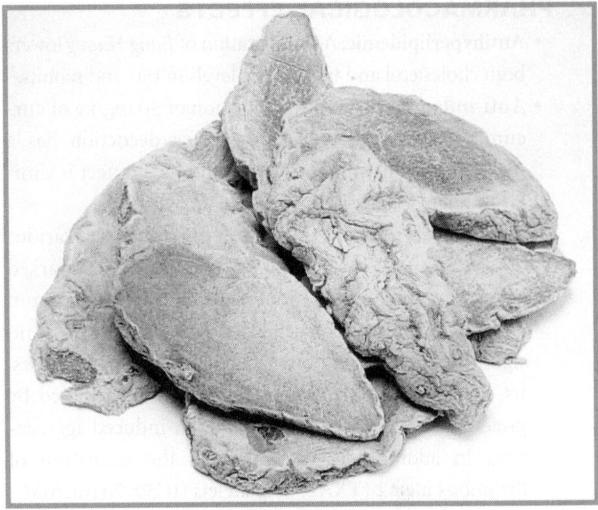

薑黄 姜黄

Pinyin Name: *Jiang Huang*
Literal Name: "ginger yellow"
Alternate Chinese Names: *Pian Zi Jiang Huang*
Original Source: *Xin Xiu Ben Cao* (Newly Revised Materia Medica) by Su Jing in 657-659 A.D.
English Name: turmeric
Botanical Name: *Curcuma longa* L. (*Jiang Huang*)
Pharmaceutical Name: Rhizoma Curcumae Longae
Properties: acrid, bitter, warm
Channels Entered: Spleen, Liver

CHINESE THERAPEUTIC ACTIONS

1. Activates Blood Circulation, Eliminates Blood Stasis

Pain due to blood stasis: *Jiang Huang* (Rhizoma Curcumae Longae) is commonly said to "break" blood stasis to activate qi and blood circulation. It has been described to invigorate circulation and eliminate stasis for qi and blood in both *qi* (energy) and *xue* (blood) levels.

- Hypochondriac pain due to Liver qi stagnation, amenorrhea or abdominal pain due to blood stagnation in the Liver channel: use *Jiang Huang* with *Bai Shao* (Radix Paeoniae Alba), *Dang Gui* (Radicis Angelicae Sinensis), *Yan Hu Suo* (Rhizoma Corydalis) and *Hong Hua* (Flos Carthami).
- Chest and hypochondriac pain: combine this herb with *Zhi Ke* (Fructus Aurantii), *Su Geng* (Caulis Perillae), *Jie Geng* (Radix Platycodonis), *Chuan Lian Zi* (Fructus Toosendan), *Xiang Fu* (Rhizoma Cyperi) and *Yan Hu Suo* (Rhizoma Corydalis).
- Epigastric pain: use it with *Gao Liang Jiang* (Rhizoma Alpiniae Officinarum), *Xiang Fu* (Rhizoma Cyperi), *Sha Ren* (Fructus Amomi), *Mu Xiang* (Radix Aucklandiae), *Gan Jiang* (Rhizoma Zingiberis), *Wu Yao* (Radix Linderae) and *Yan Hu Suo* (Rhizoma Corydalis).
- Dysmenorrhea: add *Jiang Huang* to *Wu Ling Zhi* (Excrementum Trogopteri seu Pteromi), *Xiang Fu* (Rhizoma Cyperi), and *Bai Shao* (Radix Paeoniae Alba).
- Hepatitis with hypochondriac pain: use it with *Zhi Ke* (Fructus Aurantii), *Bai Ji Li* (Fructus Tribuli) and *Chuan Lian Zi* (Fructus Toosendan).

2. Opens Channels and Collaterals to Relieve Pain

Bi zheng **(painful obstruction syndrome):** *Jiang Huang* is commonly used to treat *bi zheng* caused by wind, cold or dampness. It is better for the upper limbs.

- *Bi zheng*: use this herb with *Hai Tong Pi* (Cortex Erythrinae), *Qiang Huo* (Rhizoma et Radix Notopterygii) and *Dang Gui* (Radicis Angelicae Sinensis).

3. Reduces Swelling

In addition to activating qi and blood circulation, *Jiang Huang* treats swelling and pain from sores and lesions caused by toxic heat accumulation with blood and qi stagnation.

- Sores and lesions: combine *Jiang Huang* with *Da Huang* (Radix et Rhizoma Rhei), *Bai Zhi* (Radix Angelicae Dahuricae) and *Tian Hua Fen* (Radix Trichosanthis).

DOSAGE

3 to 10 grams in decoction.

CAUTIONS / CONTRAINDICATIONS

- Use *Jiang Huang* with caution in deficiency patients, or those who have no symptoms of blood stagnation.
- *Jiang Huang* is contraindicated during pregnancy.

CHEMICAL COMPOSITION

Curcumin, demethoxycurcumin, bisdemethoxycurcumin, curcuminoids, turmerone, zingiberene, phellandrene, cineole, sabinene, borneo, arturmerone, caryophyllene.[1,2]

Curcumin

Jiang Huang (Rhizoma Curcumae Longae)

PHARMACOLOGICAL EFFECTS

- **Antihyperlipidemic:** Administration of *Jiang Huang* lowers both cholesterol and triglyceride levels in rats and rabbits.[3]
- **Anti-inflammatory:** Administration of 30 mg/kg of curcumin or 60 mg/kg of *Jiang Huang* decoction has a marked anti-inflammatory effect in rats. It effect is similar to phenylbutazone.[4]
- **Antiplatelet:** Administration of curcumin at various doses (20, 40, 60, and 80 mg/kg/day) has shown marked action to inhibit aggregation of platelets. The maximum antiplatelet effect was reached at 40 mg/kg/day, with no significant increase in potency linked to the higher doses. Its effect to inhibit platelet aggregation is mediated by preferential inhibition of PAF- and AA-induced aggregation. In addition, it also inhibited the formation of thromboxane A2 (TXA2) by platelets (IC50; 70 microM). It is suggested that the curcumin-mediated preferential inhibition of PAF- and AA-induced platelet aggregation involves inhibitory action on TXA2 synthesis and Ca^{2+} signaling, but without the involvement of PKC.[5,6]
- **Cholagogic:** Many components of *Jiang Huang*, including, but not limited to, curcumin and the essential oils, have demonstrated marked effectiveness to increase the production and excretion of bile.[7]
- **Uterine stimulant:** Administration of *Jiang Huang* decoction via intraperitoneal or subcutaneous routes at the dosage of 10 g/kg terminated pregnancy in 90 to 100% of mice between 6 and 18 days of pregnancy. The dosage of 5 g/kg did not terminate pregnancy. The proposed mechanism of action is stimulation and contraction of the uterus.[8]

HERB-DRUG INTERACTION

- **Anticoagulant or antiplatelet drugs:** *Jiang Huang* has antiplatelet effects, and should be used with caution in patients who take anticoagulant or antiplatelet medications. Though this potential interaction has not been documented, this herb may potentiate the effect of drugs such as warfarin.[9] [Note: Examples of anticoagulants include heparin, warfarin (Coumadin) and enoxaparin (Lovenox); and examples of antiplatelets include aspirin, dipyridamole (Persantine), and clopidogrel (Plavix).]

TOXICOLOGY

Consumption of *Jiang Huang* is relatively safe. There are very few reports of adverse reactions. Administration of 40 to 100 grams of herb daily for 3 days did not lead to any fatalities in mice. Furthermore, administration of *Jiang Huang* to rats at dosages up to 50 times the normal dosage range for humans for 30 days did not demonstrate any significant change in body weight, dietary habits, physical activities, or functioning of internal organs.[10]

References

1. *Xian Dai Zhong Yao Yao Li Xue* (Contemporary Pharmacology of Chinese Herbs), 1997; 909
2. *The Merck Index* 12th edition, Chapman & Hall/CRCnetBASE/Merck, 2000
3. *Zhong Yao Yao Li Yu Ying Yong* (Pharmacology and Applications of Chinese Herbs), 1983; 846
4. *Zhong Cao Yao* (Chinese Herbal Medicine), 1991; 22(3):141
5. *Di Yi Jun Yi Da Xue Xue Bao* (Journal of First Military University of Medicine), 1990; 10(4):364
6. *Biochemical Pharmacology*. 58(7):1167-72, 1999 Oct 1
7. *Zhong Yao Yao Li Yu Ying Yong* (Pharmacology and Applications of Chinese Herbs), 1983; 846
8. *Yao Xue Tong Bao* (Report of Herbology), 1980; 15(10):40
9. Chen, J. Recognition & prevention of herb-drug interactions, *Medical Acupuncture*, Fall/Winter 1998/1999; volume 10/number 2; 9-13
10. *Zhong Yao Yao Li Yu Ying Yong (Pharmacology and Applications of* Chinese Herbs), 1983: 846

Lu Lu Tong (Fructus Liquidambaris)

路路通

Pinyin Name: *Lu Lu Tong*
Literal Name: "all roads open"
English Name: liquidambar, beautiful sweetgum fruit
Botanical Name: *Liquidambar taiwaniana* Hance.
Pharmaceutical Name: Fructus Liquidambaris
Properties: bitter, neutral
Channels Entered: Liver, Stomach

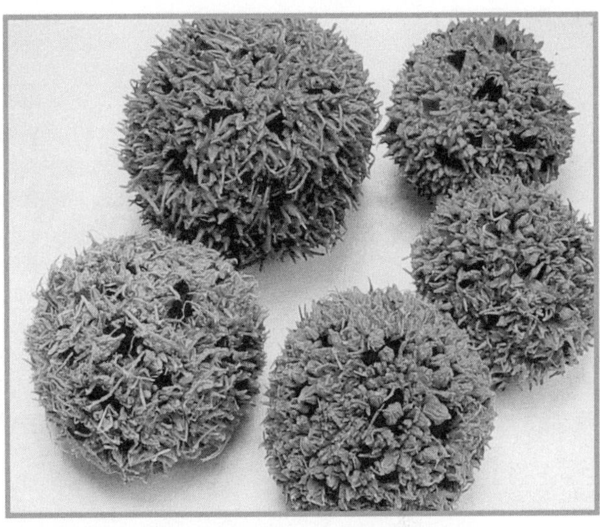

CHINESE THERAPEUTIC ACTIONS

1. Activates Qi and Blood Circulation, Opens Channels

Lu Lu Tong (Fructus Liquidambaris) treats various kinds of pain characterized by stagnation of qi and blood in the peripheral channels and collaterals. It is especially effective for pain in the lower back and extremities.

- Joint pain: combine *Lu Lu Tong* with *Qiang Huo* (Rhizoma et Radix Notopterygii), *Du Huo* (Radix Angelicae Pubescentis) and *Ji Xue Teng* (Caulis Spatholobi).
- External or traumatic injuries: use this herb with *Chi Shao* (Radix Paeoniae Rubrae) and *Dan Shen* (Radix Salviae Miltiorrhizae).

2. Promotes Urination

Lu Lu Tong treats dysuria and edema by draining water downwards.

- Edema: add it to *Fu Ling Pi* (Cortex Poria) and *Sang Bai Pi* (Cortex Mori).
- Angioneurotic edema: combine it with *Wu Pi Yin* (Five-Peel Decoction).

3. Treats Allergy

Lu Lu Tong treats both skin and nasal allergies, such as itching, urticaria, and allergic rhinitis.

- Itching and urticaria: use this herb with *Fang Feng* (Radix Saposhnikoviae) and *Chan Tui* (Periostracum Cicadae).
- Allergic rhinitis: combine *Lu Lu Tong* with *Cang Er Zi* (Fructus Xanthii), *Bai Zhi* (Radix Angelicae Dahuricae), and *Xin Yi Hua* (Flos Magnoliae).

DOSAGE

3 to 9 grams in herbal decoction.

CAUTIONS / CONTRAINDICATIONS

Lu Lu Tong is contraindicated during pregnancy and in cases of hypermenorrhea.

CHEMICAL COMPOSITION

Bornyl cinnamate, styracin epoxide, isostyracin epoxide, betulonic acid, liquidambaronic acid, caryophyllene oxide, styracin, cinnamyl cinnamate, liquidambaric acid.[1]

PHARMACOLOGICAL EFFECTS

- **Hepatoprotective:** Betulonic acid and liquidambaronic acid have demonstrated marked hepatoprotective effects in rats, especially against carbon tetrachloride-induced liver toxicity.[2]
- **Others:** *Lu Lu Tong* has been observed to have anti-inflammatory, diuretic, and antibiotic effects.

AUTHORS' COMMENTS

According to Dr. Gan Zhu-Wang, *Lu Lu Tong* and *Shi Chang Pu* (Rhizoma Acori) treat nasal obstruction with loss of smell.

According to Dr. Wang Zi-Yu, *Lu Lu Tong* opens fallopian tube blockage caused by dampness, chronic or acute pelvic inflammatory disease, endometriosis or post-surgical adhesions.

References

1. *Chang Yong Zhong Yao Cheng Fen Yu Yao Li Shou Ce* (A Handbook of the Composition and Pharmacology of Common Chinese Drugs), 1994; 1712
2. *Planta Med*, 1988; 54(5):417

Ru Xiang (Gummi Olibanum)

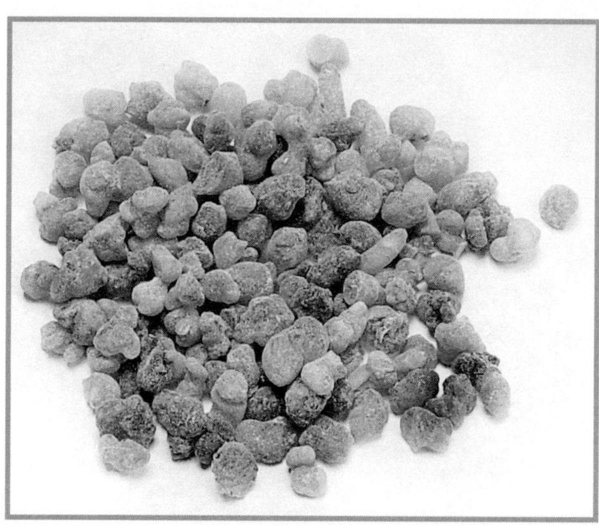

乳香

Pinyin Name: *Ru Xiang*
Literal Name: "fragrant breast," "fragrant milk"
Alternate Chinese Names: *Xun Lu Xiang, Ta Xiang, Tian Ze Xiang, Di Ru Xiang*
Original Source: *Ming Yi Za Zhu* (Miscellaneous Records of Famous Physicians) by Tao Hong-Jing in 500 A.D.
English Name: mastic, frankincense, olibanum
Botanical Name: *Boswellia carterii* Birdw. (*Ru Xiang Shu*)
Pharmaceutical Name: Gummi Olibanum
Properties: acrid, bitter, warm
Channels Entered: Heart, Liver, Spleen

CHINESE THERAPEUTIC ACTIONS

1. Activates Blood Circulation and Relieves Pain

Pain: *Ru Xiang* (Gummi Olibanum) has an excellent effect to relieve aches and pain caused by stagnation of qi and blood circulation. Clinical manifestations may include dysmenorrhea, amenorrhea, epigastric pain, *bi zheng* (painful obstruction syndrome), and traumatic injuries.

- Amenorrhea and dysmenorrhea: combine *Ru Xiang* with *Dang Gui* (Radicis Angelicae Sinensis), *Hong Hua* (Flos Carthami) and *Tao Ren* (Semen Persicae).
- Stomach and epigastric pain from qi and blood stagnation: use this herb with *Chuan Lian Zi* (Fructus Toosendan), *Xiang Fu* (Rhizoma Cyperi) and *Mu Xiang* (Radix Aucklandiae).
- Chest and abdominal pain: use it with *Yan Hu Suo* (Rhizoma Corydalis).
- *Bi zheng* (painful obstruction syndrome) due to wind and dampness: combine it with *Qiang Huo* (Rhizoma et Radix Notopterygii), *Qin Jiao* (Radix Gentianae Macrophyllae), *Dang Gui* (Radicis Angelicae Sinensis) and *Hai Feng Teng* (Caulis Piperis Kadsurae). **Exemplar Formula:** *Juan Bi Tang* (Remove Painful Obstruction Decoction).
- Traumatic injuries with severe pain and bruising: use it with *Mo Yao* (Myrrha), *Hong Hua* (Flos Carthami), *She Xiang* (Moschus), *Bing Pian* (Borneolum Syntheticum), *Xue Jie* (Sanguis Draconis) and *Tao Ren* (Semen Persicae). **Exemplar Formula:** *Qi Li San* (Seven-Thousandths of a Tael Powder).

2. Reduces Swelling and Promotes Generation of Flesh

Skin lesions and ulcerations: *Ru Xiang* has an excellent ability to reduce swelling, relieve pain, promote generation of flesh, and enhance healing of skin lesions and ulcerations. Heat-clearing and blood-cooling herbs are usually added to reduce inflammation.

- Initial stages of abscess or sores with redness, swelling and pain: use *Ru Xiang* with *Jin Yin Hua* (Flos Lonicerae), *Lian Qiao* (Fructus Forsythiae), *Chi Shao* (Radix Paeoniae Rubrae), *Hong Hua* (Flos Carthami), *Tian Hua Fen* (Radix Trichosanthis), *Zao Jiao Ci* (Spina Gleditsiae), *Chuan Shan Jia* (Squama Manis), *Bai Zhi* (Radix Angelicae Dahuricae) and *Fang Feng* (Radix Saposhnikoviae).
- If the sore has ulcerated, use the herbs listed above but remove *Zao Jiao Ci* (Spina Gleditsiae) and *Chuan Shan Jia* (Squama Manis).
- If pus has been completely cleared, apply the powders of *Ru Xiang, Mo Yao* (Myrrha), *Bing Pian* (Borneolum Syntheticum), *Long Gu* (Os Draconis), *Xue Jie* (Sanguis Draconis) and *Er Cha* (Catechu) topically.
- Sores that are flat without redness or pain: add this herb to *Dang Gui* (Radicis Angelicae Sinensis), *Huang Qi* (Radix Astragali), *Lian Qiao* (Fructus Forsythiae), *Mu Xiang* (Radix Aucklandiae), *Mo Yao* (Myrrha), *Gui Xin* (Cortex Rasus Cinnamomi), *Jie Geng* (Radix Platycodonis), *Dang Shen* (Radix Codonopsis) and *Gan Cao* (Radix Glycyrrhizae).
- Skin lesions and ulcerations: apply *Ru Xiang* and *Mo Yao* (Myrrha) as powder topically.

Intestinal abscess: *Ru Xiang* treats intestinal abscess that results from the accumulation of blood stagnation with heat and toxicity.

- Intestinal abscess: use *Ru Xiang* with *Zi Hua Di Ding* (Herba Violae), *Hong Teng* (Caulis Sargentodoxae), *Lian Qiao* (Fructus Forsythiae), *Yi Yi Ren* (Semen Coicis) and *Mu Dan Pi* (Cortex Moutan).

Ru Xiang (Gummi Olibanum)

DOSAGE

3 to 10 grams in decoction. Unprocessed *Ru Xiang* has a pungent smell, and is often irritating to the stomach. Dry-frying or frying it with vinegar minimizes both the odor and side effects such as nausea and vomiting. In addition, both methods of preparation facilitate the crushing and extraction of active components. Lastly, frying *Ru Xiang* with vinegar will enhance its potency to activate blood circulation, relieve pain, and promote generation of flesh.

CAUTIONS / CONTRAINDICATIONS

- Patients with a sensitive stomach should take *Ru Xiang* with caution as the bitter taste may cause nausea and vomiting.
- *Ru Xiang* is contraindicated during pregnancy, and for individuals who do not have blood stagnation.

CHEMICAL COMPOSITION

α-boswellic acid, β-boswellic acid, olibanoresene, arabic acid, bassorin, pinene, dipentene, α-phellandrene, β-phellandrene.[1,2]

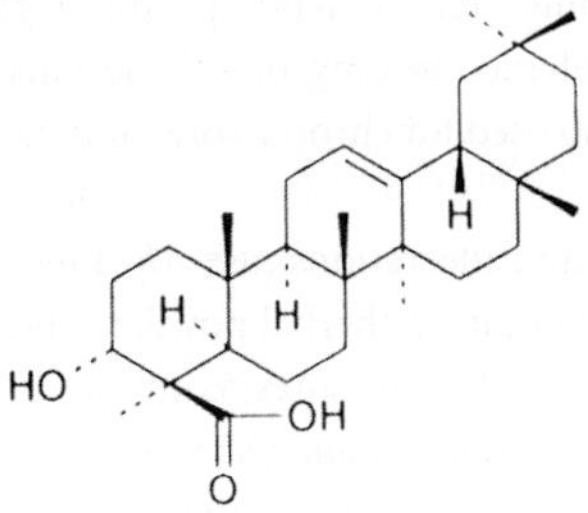

α-Boswellic Acid

PHARMACOLOGICAL EFFECTS

- **Analgesic:** *Ru Xiang* has demonstrated a marked analgesic effect in humans and in laboratory animals.[3]

CLINICAL STUDIES AND RESEARCH

- **Hypochondriac pain in hepatitis patients:** According to one report, 32 patients with hypochondriac pain were treated topically with herbs with marked success. The treatment protocol was to soak a towel in the herbal decoction, place the towel on the affected area and cover with paraffin on top of the towel to keep the temperature between 15° and 55° C. The body should also be covered with a blanket, and the herbs kept in place for half an hour. Out of 32 patients, 21 showed marked improvement, 6 showed moderate improvement, 3 showed slight improvement, and 2 showed no response. The herbs used in the herbal formulation included *Ru Xiang, Mo Yao* (Myrrha), *Bie Jia* (Carapax Trionycis) and *Wu Ling Zhi* (Excrementum Trogopteri seu Pteromi).[4]
- **Pain:** The combination of *Ru Xiang* and *Mo Yao* (Myrrha) has demonstrated analgesic action in treating chest pain, and colicky or sharp pain.[5]
- **External injury:** Topical application of *Ru Xiang* and *Mo Yao* (Myrrha) one to two times daily for 3 to 5 days showed satisfactory results in patients suffering from acute sprain of the lower back and legs.[6]

AUTHORS' COMMENTS

Ru Xiang and *Mo Yao* (Myrrha) have very similar functions and are commonly used together to enhance their effects. *Ru Xiang* is stronger in activating blood circulation and relaxing the tendons. It is more commonly used to treat musculoskeletal aches and pains, and *bi zheng* (painful obstruction syndrome) caused by wind and dampness. On the other hand, *Mo Yao* is stronger in dispersing blood and eliminating blood stasis. It is more commonly used to treat epigastric pain with qi stagnation and blood stasis.

References

1. *Zhong Yao Xue* (Chinese Herbology), 1998; 539:540
2. Yan X, Zhou J, Xie G, *Traditional Chinese Medicines Molecular Structures, Natural Sources and Applications*; Ashgate, 1999; 5404
3. *Zhong Yao Xue* (Chinese Herbology), 1998; 539:540
4. *Jiang Su Zhong Yi* (Jiangsu Chinese Medicine), 1962; 3:39
5. *Zhong Yao Xue* (Chinese Herbology), 1998; 539:540
6. *He Nan Zhong Yi Xue Yuan Xue Bao* (Journal of University of Henan School of Medicine), 1980; 3:38

Mo Yao (Myrrha)

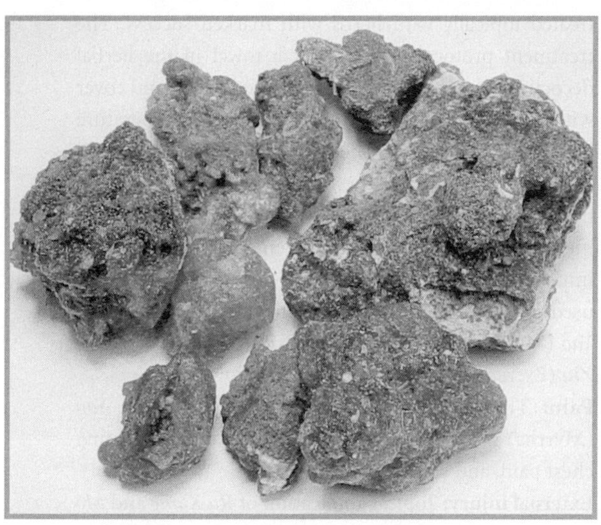

沒藥 没药

Pinyin Name: *Mo Yao*
Original Source: *Yao Xing Ben Cao* (Materia Medica of Medicinal Properties) by Zhen Quan in 600 A.D.
English Name: myrrh
Botanical Name: *Commiphora myrrha* Engl. (*Mo Yao Shu*); *Balsamodendron ehrenbergianum* Berg. (*Mo Yao Shu*)
Pharmaceutical Name: Myrrha
Properties: bitter, neutral
Channels Entered: Heart, Liver, Spleen

CHINESE THERAPEUTIC ACTIONS

1. Activates Blood Circulation and Relieves Pain

Pain: *Mo Yao* (Myrrha) activates blood circulation and relieves pain. Clinically, it is commonly combined with *Ru Xiang* (Gummi Olibanum) to treat a wide variety of aches and pains, such as amenorrhea, menstrual pain and cramps, stomach and epigastric pain, musculoskeletal pain from wind and dampness, traumatic injuries with pain and bruising, and intestinal abscesses.

- Traumatic injuries with bruising: use *Mo Yao* with *Ru Xiang* (Gummi Olibanum), *Dang Gui* (Radicis Angelicae Sinensis), *Chuan Xiong* (Rhizoma Ligustici Chuanxiong), *Niu Xi* (Radix Cyathulae seu Achyranthis), and *Hong Hua* (Flos Carthami).
- Abdominal masses with pain and dysmenorrhea: combine this herb with *Ru Xiang* (Gummi Olibanum), *Dang Gui* (Radicis Angelicae Sinensis), *Tao Ren* (Semen Persicae), *Hong Hua* (Flos Carthami), *Chuan Xiong* (Rhizoma Ligustici Chuanxiong), *San Leng* (Rhizoma Sparganii), *E Zhu* (Rhizoma Curcumae), *Yan Hu Suo* (Rhizoma Corydalis), *Shui Zhi* (Hirudo), *Meng Chong* (Tabanus) and *Da Huang* (Radix et Rhizoma Rhei).
- Postpartum abdominal pain with spotting: add *Mo Yao* to *Dang Gui* (Radicis Angelicae Sinensis), *Hong Hua* (Flos Carthami), *Chuan Xiong* (Rhizoma Ligustici Chuanxiong), *Yan Hu Suo* (Rhizoma Corydalis), *Pao Jiang* (Rhizoma Zingiberis Preparatum) and *Yi Mu Cao* (Herba Leonuri).
- *Bi zheng* (painful obstruction syndrome): use it with *Qiang Huo* (Rhizoma et Radix Notopterygii), *Du Huo* (Radix Angelicae Pubescentis), *Fang Feng* (Radix Saposhnikoviae), *Sang Ji Sheng* (Herba Taxilli), *Wei Ling Xian* (Radix Clematidis), *Xi Xin* (Herba Asari), *Chi Shao* (Radix Paeoniae Rubrae) and *Hong Hua* (Flos Carthami).

2. Reduces Swelling and Promotes Generation of Flesh

When used externally, *Mo Yao* has excellent functions to reduce swelling, relieve pain, promote generation of flesh, and enhance healing of skin lesions and ulcerations. It is also used for chronic sores and ulcerations that do not heal.

- Skin lesions and ulcerations: use *Mo Yao* and *Ru Xiang* (Gummi Olibanum) as herbal powder topically.
- Redness and swelling of sores: combine it with *Jin Yin Hua* (Flos Lonicerae), *Lian Qiao* (Fructus Forsythiae), *Chi Shao* (Radix Paeoniae Rubrae), *Hong Hua* (Flos Carthami), *Fang Feng* (Radix Saposhnikoviae), *Bai Zhi* (Radix Angelicae Dahuricae), *Dang Gui Wei* (Extremitas Radicis Angelicae Sinensis), *Chuan Shan Jia* (Squama Manis) and *Zao Jiao Ci* (Spina Gleditsiae).

DOSAGE

3 to 10 grams in decoction.

CAUTIONS / CONTRAINDICATIONS

- *Mo Yao* should be used with caution in patients who have sensitive stomachs because the bitter taste may induce nausea and vomiting.
- The dosage of *Mo Yao* should be lowered if it is combined with *Ru Xiang* (Gummi Olibanum).
- Use of *Mo Yao* is contraindicated in pregnant women.

CHEMICAL COMPOSITION

Heerabomyrrholic acid, commiphoric acid, commiphorinic acid, heerabomyrrhol, heeraborescene, commiferin, ergenol, m-cresol, cumin aldehyde, pinene, dipentene, limonene, cinnamic aldehyde, heerabolene.[1]

Mo Yao (Myrrha)

PHARMACOLOGICAL EFFECTS

- **Antihyperlipidemic:** *Mo Yao* has demonstrated a marked effect in reducing blood cholesterol in humans and rabbits.[2]

CLINICAL STUDIES AND RESEARCH

- **Hyperlipidemia:** Concentrated extract of *Mo Yao*, given in two to three 0.1 mg capsules three times daily for 2 months, resulted in reduction of cholesterol at a 65.7% rate of effectiveness. [3]
- **Pain:** The combination of *Mo Yao* and *Ru Xiang* (Gummi Olibanum) has demonstrated analgesic properties in treating chest pain, and colicky or sharp pain.[4]
- **External injury:** Topical application of *Mo Yao* and *Ru Xiang* (Gummi Olibanum) one to two times daily for 3 to 5 days showed satisfactory results in patients suffering from acute sprain of the lower back and legs. The topical herbal paste was made by mixing equal portions of *Mo Yao* and *Ru Xiang* with 30% rubbing alcohol.[5]

AUTHORS' COMMENTS

Mo Yao and *Ru Xiang* (Gummi Olibanum) have very similar functions and are commonly used together for their synergistic strength, especially in treating pain associated with blood stagnation. *Mo Yao*, stronger in dispersing blood stagnation and eliminating blood stasis, is more commonly used to treat epigastric pain from qi and blood stasis. *Ru Xiang*, stronger in activating blood circulation and relaxing the tendons, is more commonly used to treat musculoskeletal aches and pain, and *bi zheng* (painful obstruction syndrome) due to wind and dampness.

References

1. *Chang Yong Zhong Yao Xian Dai Yan Jiu Yu Lin Chuan* (Recent Study & Clinical Application of Common Traditional Chinese Medicine), 1995; 387-388
2. *Zhong Yao Xue* (Chinese Herbology), 1998; 541:542
3. *Zhong Yi Za Zhi* (Journal of Chinese Medicine), 1988; 6:36
4. *Zhong Yao Xue* (Chinese Herbology), 1998; 541:542
5. *He Nan Zhong Yi Xue Yuan Xue Bao* (Journal of University of Henan School of Medicine), 1980; 3:38

Hu Zhang (Rhizoma Polygoni Cuspidati)

虎杖 虎杖

Pinyin Name: *Hu Zhang*
Literal Name: "tiger's cane"
Alternate Chinese Names: *Ban Zhang*
Original Source: *Ming Yi Za Zhu* (Miscellaneous Records of Famous Physicians) by Tao Hong-Jing in 500 A.D.
English Name: polygonum cuspidatum
Botanical Name: *Polygonum cuspidatum* Sieb. et. Zucc. (*Hu Zhang*)
Pharmaceutical Name: Rhizoma Polygoni Cuspidati
Properties: bitter, cold
Channels Entered: Liver, Gallbladder, Lung

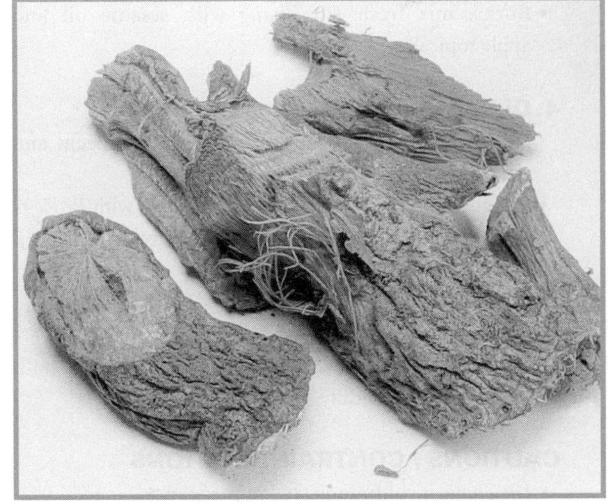

CHINESE THERAPEUTIC ACTIONS

1. Activates Blood Circulation, Stops Pain

Pain: *Hu Zhang* (Rhizoma Polygoni Cuspidati) has an excellent ability to relieve pain, such as menstrual pain, abdominal pain with amenorrhea, *bi zheng* (painful obstruction syndrome), and sports and traumatic injuries.

- Menstrual pain from blood stasis: combine *Hu Zhang* with *Yi Mu Cao* (Herba Leonuri) and *Dan Shen* (Radix Salviae Miltiorrhizae).
- *Bi zheng* (painful obstruction syndrome) due to wind and dampness: add it to *Ji Xue Teng* (Caulis Spatholobi).
- Sports and traumatic injuries: use this herb with *Ru*

Hu Zhang (Rhizoma Polygoni Cuspidati)

Xiang (Gummi Olibanum), *Mo Yao* (Myrrha), and *Hong Hua* (Flos Carthami).

2. Clears Damp-Heat

Damp-heat in the Liver: Clinical manifestations include jaundice, gallstones, and foul-smelling leukorrhea.

- Damp-heat jaundice: use *Hu Zhang* with *Yin Chen Hao* (Herba Artemisiae Scopariae), *Zhi Zi* (Fructus Gardeniae), and *Da Huang* (Radix et Rhizoma Rhei).
- Gallstones: use this herb with *Yu Jin* (Radix Curcumae), *Ji Nei Jin* (Endothelium Corneum Gigeriae Galli), *Hai Jin Sha* (Herba Lygodii), *Jin Qian Cao* (Herba Lysimachiae), *Chuan Lian Zi* (Fructus Toosendan), and *Yan Hu Suo* (Rhizoma Corydalis).
- Foul-smelling leukorrhea: combine it with *Yi Yi Ren* (Semen Coicis) and *Bi Xie* (Rhizoma Dioscoreae Hypoglaucae).

3. Clears Heat and Eliminates Toxins

Abscesses, swellings caused by heat toxins, snake bites: *Hu Zhang* treats both internal and external heat toxins, and can be used both internally and topically.

- Abscess of internal organs: use *Hu Zhang* with *Jin Yin Hua* (Flos Lonicerae), *Lian Qiao* (Fructus Forsythiae), and *Pu Gong Ying* (Herba Taraxaci).
- Snake bites: apply herbal paste topically by combining *Hu Zhang* with *Jin Yin Hua* (Flos Lonicerae), *Lian Qiao* (Fructus Forsythiae) and *Pu Gong Ying* (Herba Taraxaci).
- Burns: mix fresh *Hu Zhang* with sesame oil and apply topically.

4. Dissolves Phlegm, Stops Cough

Hu Zhang treats coughing by eliminating phlegm and clearing heat.

- Cough with yellow phlegm: use *Hu Zhang* with *Pi Pa Ye* (Folium Eriobotryae), *Huang Qin* (Radix Scutellariae), and *Jin Yin Hua* (Flos Lonicerae).

DOSAGE

10 to 30 grams in decoction. *Hu Zhang* is used both internally and topically.

CAUTIONS / CONTRAINDICATIONS

- *Hu Zhang* is contraindicated in pregnancy.

CHEMICAL COMPOSITION

Resveratrol, emodin, physide, chrysophanol, physcion-8-D-glucoside, polydatin.[1,2]

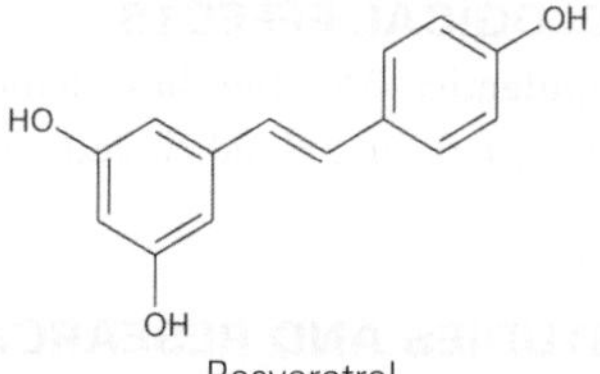

Resveratrol

PHARMACOLOGICAL EFFECTS

- **Cardiovascular:** Intravenous injection of *Hu Zhang* lowers the heart rate and blood pressure in rabbits. *Hu Zhang* also increases blood perfusion to the cardiac muscle, although this effect is negated by propranolol.[3,4]
- **Antibiotic:** *Hu Zhang* exhibits inhibitory action against *Staphylococcus aureus*, *Staphylococcus albus*, β-hemolytic streptococcus, *Neisseria catarrhalis*, *E. coli*, *Bacillus proteus*, some viruses, and leptospira.[5]
- **Respiratory:** According to one report, a 7.5% *Hu Zhang* decoction demonstrated marked antitussive and antiasthmatic effects in guinea pigs. The antiasthmatic effect is weaker than aminophyllin, and the decoction is ineffective in reversing bronchospasm induced by acetylcholine.[6]
- **Analgesic and anti-inflammatory:** Extract of *Hu Zhang* has been shown to have antipyretic, analgesic and anti-inflammatory effects.[7]
- **Antidiabetic:** Intravenous administration of *Hu Zhang* lowers blood glucose, and at large doses, may cause hypoglycemic shock. Oral administration has demonstrated promising effects in treatment of diabetes mellitus.[8]
- **Antihyperlipidemic:** Administration of resveratrol at the dosage of 200 mg/kg for 7 days lowered the plasma level of total cholesterol in rats. Herbal decoction of *Hu Zhang*, however, did not demonstrate significant changes. Lack of effectiveness of the herbal decoction is attributed to the low concentration of resveratrol present in *Hu Zhang*.[9]
- **Hemostatic:** Oral administration of *Hu Zhang* has marked effectiveness to stop upper gastrointestinal bleeding and external bleeding.[10]
- **Hepatoprotective:** Resveratrol has demonstrated a hepatoprotective effect by lowering the liver enzymes SGOT and SGPT.[11]
- **Antineoplastic:** Components of *Hu Zhang* have shown antineoplastic effects by inhibiting the synthesis of DNA and RNA.[12]

CLINICAL STUDIES AND RESEARCH

- **Bile duct infection:** In one study, 113 patients with infection of the bile duct were treated with an herbal formula

Hu Zhang (Rhizoma Polygoni Cuspidati)

with an 88.14% rate of effectiveness. The formula contained *Hu Zhang, Yin Chen Hao* (Herba Artemisiae Scopariae) and *Da Huang* (Radix et Rhizoma Rhei).[13]

- **Psoriasis:** According to one report, 25 patients with psoriasis refractory to aminopterin or other drug remedies were treated with an herbal formula containing *Hu Zhang, Jin Yin Hua* (Flos Lonicerae), *Dan Shen* (Radix Salviae Miltiorrhizae), and others. Out of 25 patients, 8 were treated successfully, 8 showed moderate improvement, and 9 showed slight improvement.[14]
- **Infectious icteric jaundice:** Administration of an herbal formula one time each day for 10 to 15 days in 115 patients with acute infectious icteric jaundice showed excellent results. Improvements included stabilization of liver function and the absence of adverse clinical signs or symptoms. The herbal formula included 30 grams of fresh *Hu Zhang*, 15 grams of fresh *Liu Ye* (Folium Salicis Babylonicae) and 60 grams of fresh *Di Jin Cao* (Herba Euphorbiae Humifusae).[15]
- **Chronic hepatitis:** In one study, 27 patients with chronic hepatitis were treated daily with an herbal decoction for 50 days. Most patients reported marked improvement, with increased appetite, increased energy levels, diminished pain in the hypochondriac region, relief of diarrhea and abdominal fullness, and increased body weight. The herbal decoction included 30 grams of *Hu Zhang* and 30 grams of *Da Zao* (Fructus Jujubae).[16]
- **Chronic hepatitis:** In another study, 32 patients with chronic hepatitis and positive HBsAg were treated daily with an herbal formula with 90.63% effectiveness, based on symptomatic evaluation. Most patients reported an improvement in energy levels and appetite, and a reduction in abdominal fullness and hypochondriac pain.[17]

HERB-DRUG INTERACTION

- **Antidiabetics:** It is prudent to use *Hu Zhang* with caution with insulin, sulfonylureas, and other antidiabetic medications as the combination may have a synergistic effect, leading to hypoglycemia.[18] [Note: Examples of antidiabetic drugs include insulin, tolbutamide (Orinase), glipizide (Glucotrol), and glyburide (DiaBeta/Micronase).]

TOXICOLOGY

Oral administration in mice of a *Hu Zhang* preparation at the dosage of 9 g/kg was determined to be safe with no fatality reported. The LD_{50} of polygonin in mice is 1363.9 +/- 199.4 mg/kg, and of polydatin is 1,000 +/- 57.3 mg/kg, via intraperitoneal injection.[19]

References

1. *Xian Dai Zhong Yao Yao Li Xue* (Contemporary Pharmacology of Chinese Herbs), 1997; 915
2. *The Merck Index* 12th edition, Chapman & Hall/CRCnetBASE/Merck, 2000
3. *Xi An Yi Ke Da Xue Xue Bao* (Journal of Xian University School of Medicine), 1982; 3(4):941
4. *Di Yi Jun Yi Da Xue Xue Bao* (Journal of First Military University of Medicine), 1983; 3(3):231
5. *Zhong Yao Xue* (Chinese Herbology), 1998; 556-558
6. *Xin Yi Yao Xue Za Zhi* (New Journal of Medicine and Herbology), 1973; (12):31
7. *Zhong Guo Yi Yuan Yao Xue Za Zhi* (Chinese Hospital Journal of Herbology), 1988; 8(5)214
8. *Yao Yong Zi Wu Da Ci Dien* (Encyclopedia of Medicinal Herbs), 1976; 28
9. *Zhong Yao Yao Li Yu Ying Yong* (Pharmacology and Applications of Chinese Herbs), 1983; 653:654
10. *Yao Yong Zi Wu Da Ci Dien* (Encyclopedia of Medicinal Herbs), 1976; 28
11. *Chem Pharm Bull*, 1982; 30(5):1766
12. *Planta Med*, 1988; 54(5):413
13. *Xin Jiang Zhong Yi Yao* (Xinjiang Chinese Medicine and Herbology), 1986; 3:49
14. *Zhe Jiang Zhong Yi Za Zhi* (Zhejiang Journal of Chinese Medicine), 1982; 4:187
15. *Xin Jiang Zhong Yi Yao* (Xinjiang Chinese Medicine and Herbology), 1986; 3:49
16. *Jiang Su Zhong Yi* (Jiangsu Chinese Medicine), 1965; 5:40
17. *Shan Dong Zhong Yi Za Zhi* (Shandong Journal of Chinese Medicine), 1982; 2:84
18. Chen, J. Recognition & prevention of herb-drug interactions, *Medical Acupuncture*, Fall/Winter 1998/1999; volume 10/number 2; 9-13
19. *Xin Yi Yao Xue Za Zhi* (New Journal of Medicine and Herbology), 1973; (12):31

Wu Ling Zhi (Excrementum Trogopteri seu Pteromi)

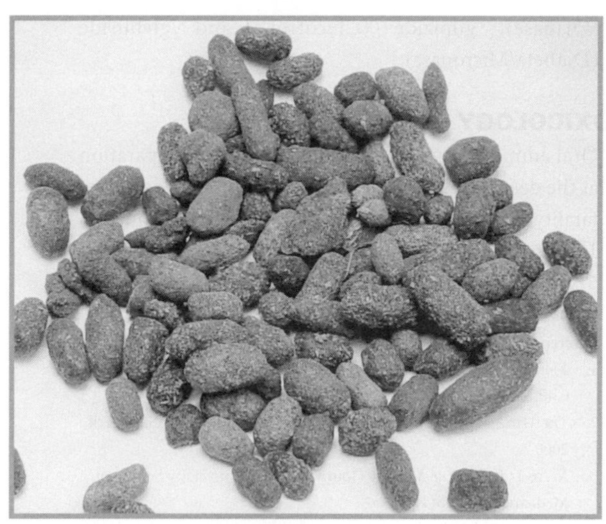

五靈脂 五灵脂

Pinyin Name: *Wu Ling Zhi*
Literal Name: "fat of the five spirits"
Original Source: *Kai Bao Ben Cao* (Materia Medica of the Kai Bao Era) by Ma Zhi in 973-974 A.D.
English Name: pteropus feces, trogopterus dung
Zoological Name: *Trogopterus xanthipes* Milne-Edwards; *Pteromys volans* L.
Pharmaceutical Name: Excrementum Trogopteri seu Pteromi
Properties: bitter, sweet, warm
Channels Entered: Liver

CHINESE THERAPEUTIC ACTIONS

1. Activates Blood Circulation, Relieves Pain

Wu Ling Zhi (Excrementum Trogopteri seu Pteromi) treats various internal disorders characterized by blood stasis and pain. It enters the *xue* (blood) level and eliminates blood stasis to relieve menstrual pain, amenorrhea and postpartum abdominal pain. It is also effective for chest and epigastric pain arising from blood stasis.

- Menstrual pain, amenorrhea and postpartum abdominal pain: combine *Wu Ling Zhi* with *Pu Huang* (Pollen Typhae) to dispel blood stasis and relieve pain. **Exemplar Formula:** *Shi Xiao San* (Sudden Smile Powder).
- Chest and epigastric pain due to blood stasis: add this herb to *Yan Hu Suo* (Rhizoma Corydalis), *Mo Yao* (Myrrha) and *Ru Xiang* (Gummi Olibanum).
- Chest and epigastric pain due to blood and qi stagnation: combine it with *Xiang Fu* (Rhizoma Cyperi) and *Yan Hu Suo* (Rhizoma Corydalis).
- Abdominal pain: use it with *Dang Gui* (Radicis Angelicae Sinensis), *Bai Shao* (Radix Paeoniae Alba), *Chuan Xiong* (Rhizoma Ligustici Chuanxiong), and *Gui Zhi* (Ramulus Cinnamomi).
- Lower abdominal pain: use it with *Xiao Hui Xiang* (Fructus Foeniculi) and *Chuan Lian Zi* (Fructus Toosendan).
- Hypochondriac pain: combine it with *Chai Hu* (Radix Bupleuri), *Zhi Ke* (Fructus Aurantii), *Qing Pi* (Pericarpium Citri Reticulatae Viride), *Bai Ji Li* (Fructus Tribuli), *Jiang Huang* (Rhizoma Curcumae Longae), *Chi Shao* (Radix Paeoniae Rubrae) and *Xiang Fu* (Rhizoma Cyperi).

2. Dispels Blood Stasis, Stops Bleeding

Uterine bleeding: *Wu Ling Zhi* treats bleeding disorders characterized by the presence of blood stasis blocking the normal flow of blood and forcing it outwards. In patients with uterine bleeding of this kind, the blood will be dark purple with clots. Patients would also experience needling or stabbing pain. The treatment principle in this case is to move the blood. Once the clots are resolved, uterine bleeding will stop. Charred *Wu Ling Zhi* is usually used for this purpose, as it can activate blood circulation and stop bleeding concurrently.

- Profuse uterine bleeding with dark purplish blood, clots, and sharp abdominal pain: use *Wu Ling Zhi* with *San Qi* (Radix Notoginseng), *Sheng Di Huang* (Radix Rehmanniae) and *Mu Dan Pi* (Cortex Moutan).

3. Eliminates Toxins

Wu Ling Zhi is used internally or topically to treat various snake and insect bites.

DOSAGE

3 to 10 grams in decoction or pills. *Wu Ling Zhi* should be wrapped in cheesecloth prior to cooking in decoctions. It is used both internally and topically. Unprocessed *Wu Ling Zhi* has a distinct odor that may decrease patient compliance. The odor may be eliminated by frying this substance with vinegar or grain-based liquor. Vinegar-fried *Wu Ling Zhi* has a stronger function to disperse stagnation. Liquor-fried (with grain-based liquor) *Wu Ling Zhi* has a stronger function to move the blood and open the channels. Charred *Wu Ling Zhi* stops bleeding.

CAUTIONS / CONTRAINDICATIONS

- *Wu Ling Zhi* is contraindicated during pregnancy, or for patients with blood deficiency or no blood stasis.
- *Wu Ling Zhi* antagonizes *Ren Shen* (Radix Ginseng).

Wu Ling Zhi (Excrementum Trogopteri seu Pteromi)

CHEMICAL COMPOSITION

Urea, uric acid, vitamin A.[1]

PHARMACOLOGICAL EFFECTS

- **Antibiotic:** *Wu Ling Zhi* has an inhibitory effect against *Mycobacterium tuberculosis* and dermatophytes.[2]
- **Antispasmodic:** It has a marked effect to relieve spasms and cramps of the smooth muscle.[3]

CLINICAL STUDIES AND RESEARCH

- **Viral hepatitis:** In one study, 200 patients with viral hepatitis (139 with acute hepatitis, 61 with chronic hepatitis) were treated with an herbal preparation with significant improvement in 140 patients, moderate improvement in 50 patients, and no change in 10 patients. The herbal formula contained *Wu Ling Zhi, Yin Chen Hao* (Herba Artemisiae Scopariae), *Pu Huang* (Pollen Typhae), and others as needed.[4]
- **Infertility:** Patients with infertility due to endometrial hyperplasia were treated with modified *Shi Xiao San* (Sudden Smile Powder) with marked effectiveness.[5]

AUTHORS' COMMENTS

According to Dr. Liu Hong-Xiang, *Wu Ling Zhi, Pu Huang* (Pollen Typhae), *Dang Gui* (Radicis Angelicae Sinensis), *Shan Zha* (Fructus Crataegi), and *Chuan Xiong* (Rhizoma Ligustici Chuanxiong) are used together to treat dysfunctional uterine bleeding or bleeding and abdominal pain following miscarriage or delivery.

References

1. *Zhong Yao Xue* (Chinese Herbology), 1998; 566-567
2. *Dong Wu Xue Za Zhi* (Journal of Zoology), 1977; (4):20
3. Ibid.
4. *Hu Bei Zhong Yi Za Zhi* (Hubei Journal of Chinese Medicine), 1985; 1985; 5:17
5. *Zhe Jiang Zhong Yi Za Zhi* (Zhejiang Journal of Chinese Medicine), 1985; 9(4):24

Jiang Xiang (Lignum Dalbergiae Odoriferae)

降香

Pinyin Name: *Jiang Xiang*
Literal Name: "descending fragrance"
Alternate Chinese Names: *Jiang Zhen Xiang*
Original Source: *Hai Yao Ben Cao* (Materia Medica of Herbs from [Across the] Seas) by Li Xun in 907-960 A.D.
English Name: dalbergia, rosewood
Botanical Name: *Dalbergia odorifera* T. Chen (*Jiang Xiang Tan*)
Pharmaceutical Name: Lignum Dalbergiae Odoriferae
Properties: acrid, warm
Channels Entered: Liver, Spleen, Heart

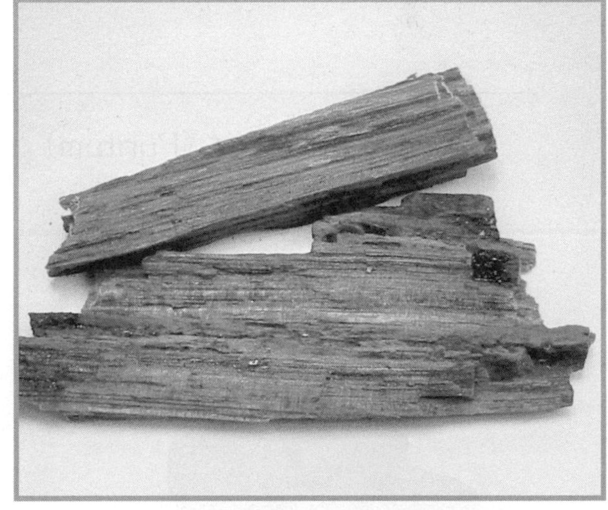

CHINESE THERAPEUTIC ACTIONS

1. Activates Blood Circulation, Dispels Stasis, Stops Bleeding, Relieves Pain

Chest pain, trauma-related pain, bleeding from cuts: *Jiang Xiang* (Lignum Dalbergiae Odoriferae) has a unique function to both move the blood and stop bleeding. It is commonly used for pain characterized by the presence of bleeding with blood stasis, such as chest and hypochondriac pain, sports or traumatic injuries, and external injuries. It may be used both internally and topically.

- Chest or hypochondriac pain from blood and qi stasis: combine *Jiang Xiang* with *Yu Jin* (Radix Curcumae), *Tao Ren* (Semen Persicae), and *Gua Lou Shi* (Fructus Trichosanthis).

Jiang Xiang (Lignum Dalbergiae Odoriferae)

- Sports or traumatic injuries: use this herb with *Ru Xiang* (Gummi Olibanum) and *Mo Yao* (Myrrha).
- Bleeding from cuts: apply *Jiang Xiang* as powder, topically.

2. Harmonizes the Middle *Jiao,* Relieves Nausea

Nausea, vomiting and abdominal pain: *Jiang Xiang* clears accumulation of dampness and turbidity in the middle *jiao*.

- Nausea and vomiting: use it with *Huo Xiang* (Herba Agastache) and *Mu Xiang* (Radix Aucklandiae).

DOSAGE

3 to 6 grams in decoction, 1 to 2 grams in powder. *Jiang Xiang* is used both internally and topically.

CAUTIONS / CONTRAINDICATIONS

- Acrid and warm in nature, *Jiang Xiang* should not be used in cases of bleeding caused by heat in the blood.
- Similarly, *Jiang Xiang* should not be used in cases of yin deficiency with excess fire.

CHEMICAL COMPOSITION

β-bisalolene, β-farnesen, nerolidol, dalbergin, nordalbergin, isodalbergin, o-methydalbergin, dalbergenone, dalbergichromene.[1]

PHARMACOLOGICAL EFFECTS

- **Hemostatic:** Oral administration of *Jiang Xiang* lengthened thrombin time.[2]
- **Anti-inflammatory:** Oral administration of *Jiang Xiang* has demonstrated an anti-inflammatory effect.[3]

CLINICAL STUDIES AND RESEARCH

- **Traumatic injuries:** An herbal formula containing *Jiang Xiang*, *San Qi* (Radix Notoginseng), *Su Mu* (Lignum Sappan), *Zi Ran Tong* (Pyritum), *Hong Hua* (Flos Carthami), *Ru Xiang* (Gummi Olibanum), *Mo Yao* (Myrrha) and others showed marked effectiveness in treatment of acute pain and inflammation of traumatic injuries. In four patients with acute pain, marked analgesic effect was observed 1 to 2 hours after administration.[4]

References

1. *Chang Yong Zhong Yao Cheng Fen Yu Yao Li Shou Ce* (A Handbook of the Composition and Pharmacology of Common Chinese Drugs), 1994; 1303
2. *Zhong Yao Xue* (Chinese Herbology), 1998; 576:577
3. Ibid.
4. *Guang Dong Zhong Yi* (Guangdong Chinese Medicine), 1959; 4(9):391

Zi Ran Tong (Pyritum)

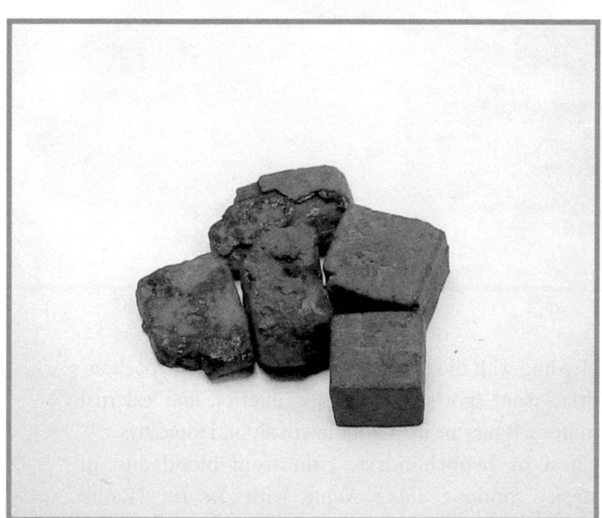

自然铜 自然铜

Pinyin Name: *Zi Ran Tong*
Literal Name: "natural copper"
Original Source: *Lei Gong Pao Zhi Lun* (Grandfather Lei's Discussions of Herb Preparation) by Lei Xiao in 470 A.D.
English Name: pyrite
Pharmaceutical Name: Pyritum
Properties: acrid, neutral
Channels Entered: Liver

Zi Ran Tong (Pyritum)

CHINESE THERAPEUTIC ACTIONS

Disperses Blood Stasis, Relieves Pain, Connects Bones and Facilitates Healing

Fractured bones, traumatic injuries with swelling and pain: *Zi Ran Tong* (Pyritum) is used for the treatment of external and traumatic injuries with swelling, pain, inflammation and bruises. Clinical applications include sprains, strains, contusions, and bone fractures. This is one of the most important substances in the trauma departments of hospitals in China.

- Traumatic injuries and external injuries: use *Zi Ran Tong* with *Su Mu* (Lignum Sappan), *Ru Xiang* (Gummi Olibanum), *Mo Yao* (Myrrha) and *Xue Jie* (Sanguis Draconis).
- Bone fractures with severe pain and swelling: use this substance with *Dang Gui* (Radicis Angelicae Sinensis), *Qiang Huo* (Rhizoma et Radix Notopterygii), *Gu Sui Bu* (Rhizoma Drynariae) and *Ru Xiang* (Gummi Olibanum).

DOSAGE

10 to 15 grams in decoction, 0.3 grams in powder or pills. *Zi Ran Tong* is used both internally and topically. *Zi Ran Tong* is calcined to facilitate crushing and extraction of active constituents. The calcined form also has a stronger effect to disperse stagnation and relieve pain.

CAUTIONS / CONTRAINDICATIONS

- *Zi Ran Tong* is contraindicated in blood deficiency or when there is no blood stasis.

CHEMICAL COMPOSITION

Ferrous disulfide (FeS_2), copper, nickel, arsenic.[1]

CLINICAL STUDIES AND RESEARCH

- **Bone fracture:** In one study, 106 patients with fractured bones were treated with an herbal preparation with marked improvement in 79 patients, moderate improvement in 15 patients, and minimal improvement in 9 patients. Three patients discontinued treatment prior to the end of the study. The herbal preparation included *Zi Ran Tong*, *Gu Sui Bu* (Rhizoma Drynariae), *Jiang Huang* (Rhizoma Curcumae Longae), *Dang Gui* (Radicis Angelicae Sinensis), *Bai Zhi* (Radix Angelicae Dahuricae), *Ban Xia* (Rhizoma Pinelliae), *Shi Gao* (Gypsum Fibrosum), *Da Huang* (Radix et Rhizoma Rhei) and other herbs as needed.[2]

AUTHORS' COMMENTS

Zi Ran Tong is commonly used to treat external and traumatic injuries. Not only does it have excellent effects to reduce swelling and relieve pain, it also facilitates and speeds recovery from broken bones.

References

1. *Zhong Yao Xue* (Chinese Herbology), 1998; 581
2. *Jiang Su Zhong Yi* (Jiangsu Chinese Medicine), 1958; 7:33

Niao Bu Su (Ramus Kalopanax Pictus)

鳥不宿 乌不宿

Pinyin Name: *Niao Bu Su*
Alternate Chinese Names: *Yan Jiao, Shuang Mian Ci, Hu Gen, Xing Ke Chi*
English Name: kalopanacis
Botanical Name: *Kalopanax septemlobus (pictus)* (Thunb.) Koidz.
Pharmaceutical Name: Ramus Kalopanax Pictus
Properties: acrid, bitter, warm
Channels Entered: Liver, Kidney
Safety Index: slightly toxic

Niao Bu Su (Ramus Kalopanax Pictus)

CHINESE THERAPEUTIC ACTIONS

Eliminates Toxins, Invigorates Blood and Relieves Pain

Niao Bu Su (Ramus Kalopanax Pictus) promotes the normal circulation of blood to relieve pain throughout the body.

- *Bi zheng* (painful obstruction syndrome): combine *Niao Bu Su* with *Wang Bu Liu Xing* (Semen Vaccariae), *Yi Wu Gen* (Radix Elaeagni) and *Xi Xian Cao* (Herba Siegesbeckiae).
- Involuntary spasms, or tremors or hemiplegia: add this herb to *Yi Wu Gen* (Radix Elaeagni), *San Qi* (Radix Notoginseng), *Gui Zhi* (Ramulus Cinnamomi), *Hong Gu She* (Radix Kadsura Japonicae), *Da Feng Teng* (Caulis Sinomenii) and *Yi Tiao Gen* (Radix Moghaniae).
- Sexually-transmitted diseases (STDs): use *Niao Bu Su* with *Mo Gu Xiao* (Caulis Hyptis Capitatae), *Ren Dong Teng* (Caulis Lonicerae), *Tu Fu Ling* (Rhizoma Smilacis Glabrae), *Fu Rong* (Radix Hibisci) and *Jin Yin Hua* (Flos Lonicerae).
- Toothache: use it with *Shui Ding Xiang* (Herba Ludwigiae Prostratae), *Hong Gu She* (Radix Kadsura Japonicae), *Shu Wei Huang* (Herba Rostellulariae) and *Yi Zhi Xiang* (Herba Vernoniae Cinereae).
- Metroendometritis, inflammation of the ovaries: combine this herb with *Yi Zhi Xiang* (Herba Vernoniae Cinereae), *Xiang Si Cao* (Herba Eupatorii Formosani), *Ma Bian Cao* (Herba Verbenae), *Gao Liang Jiang* (Rhizoma Alpiniae Officinarum), *Dang Gui* (Radicis Angelicae Sinensis), *Xiang Fu* (Rhizoma Cyperi), *Feng Wei Cao* (Herba Pteris) and *Ya She Huang* (Herba Lippiae).

DOSAGE

9 to 15 grams.

CAUTIONS / CONTRAINDICATIONS

- Overdose of *Niao Bu Su* may cause side effects such as dizziness, blurred vision and vomiting.
- *Niao Bu Su* should be used with caution during pregnancy.

CHEMICAL COMPOSITION

Akeboside, kalopanax-genin.[1]

References

1. *Chem Pharm Bull*, 1989; 37(12):3251

Dan Shen (Radix Salviae Miltiorrhizae)

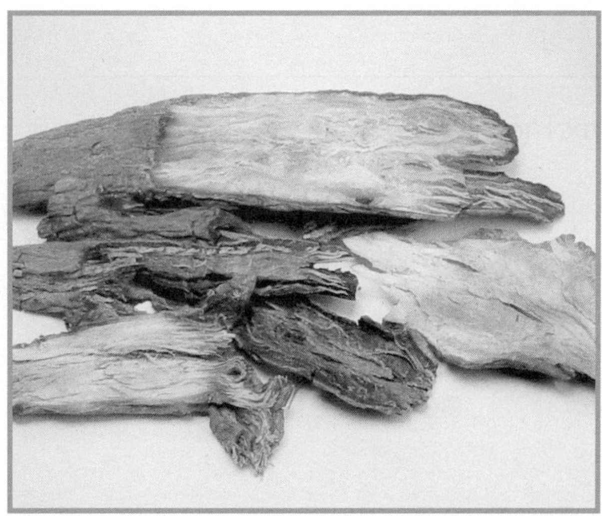

丹參 丹参

Pinyin Name: *Dan Shen*
Literal Name: "red ginseng"
Alternate Chinese Names: *Chi Shen*, *Zi Dan Shen*
Original Source: *Shen Nong Ben Cao Jing* (Divine Husbandman's Classic of the Materia Medica) in the second century
English Name: salvia root
Botanical Name: *Salvia miltiorrhiza* Bge. (*Dan Shen*)
Pharmaceutical Name: Radix Salviae Miltiorrhizae
Properties: bitter, cool
Channels Entered: Heart, Pericardium, Liver

CHINESE THERAPEUTIC ACTIONS

1. Activates Blood Circulation, Dispels Blood Stasis

Dan Shen (Radix Salviae Miltiorrhizae) regulates blood circulation and addresses various disorders caused by blood stagnation, including gynecological or cardiovascular disorders, and the formation of nodules of blood stagnation.

Dan Shen (Radix Salviae Miltiorrhizae)

Gynecology: *Dan Shen* is an excellent herb to treat various gynecological disorders caused by blood stagnation, such as irregular menstruation, amenorrhea and postpartum abdominal pain.

- Abdominal pain with irregular menstruation because of blood stasis or during the postpartum period: use this herb with *Hong Hua* (Flos Carthami), *Tao Ren* (Semen Persicae) and *Yi Mu Cao* (Herba Leonuri).
- Abdominal pain with blood stasis due to cold: combine it with *Wu Zhu Yu* (Fructus Evodiae) and *Rou Gui* (Cortex Cinnamomi).

Chest, epigastric and abdominal pain: *Dan Shen* treats pain and stifling sensations in the chest and epigastric areas caused by qi and blood stagnation.

- Chest pain: use *Dan Shen* with *Gua Lou Pi* (Pericarpium Trichosanthis) and *Ban Xia* (Rhizoma Pinelliae).
- Epigastric and abdominal pain due to qi and blood stagnation: use it with *Tan Xiang* (Lignum Santali Albi) and *Sha Ren* (Fructus Amomi).

Palpable masses and accumulations due to blood stagnation: *Dan Shen* has a strong dispersing action that can be used with other blood- and qi-invigorating herbs to treat masses in the abdomen.

- Palpable masses: use this herb with *San Leng* (Rhizoma Sparganii), *E Zhu* (Rhizoma Curcumae), *Ze Lan* (Herba Lycopi) and *Bie Jia* (Carapax Trionycis).
- Hepatomegaly or splenomegaly: combine this herb with *Bie Jia* (Carapax Trionycis), *Mu Li* (Concha Ostreae), *Zhi Ke* (Fructus Aurantii), *Dang Gui Wei* (Extremitas Radicis Angelicae Sinensis), *Tao Ren* (Semen Persicae), *Hong Hua* (Flos Carthami), *Bai Zhu* (Rhizoma Atractylodis Macrocephalae), *Fu Ling* (Poria), *San Leng* (Rhizoma Sparganii), *E Zhu* (Rhizoma Curcumae), and *Xiang Fu* (Rhizoma Cyperi).

Traumatic injuries and *bi zheng* (painful obstruction syndrome): *Dan Shen* invigorates blood circulation in the channels and collaterals to treat arthritis or traumatic injury.

- External or traumatic injuries with pain and bruising: use this herb with *Dang Gui* (Radicis Angelicae Sinensis), *Hong Hua* (Flos Carthami), and *Chuan Xiong* (Rhizoma Ligustici Chuanxiong).
- Redness, swelling and pain due to heat-type *bi zheng* (painful obstruction syndrome): combine *Dan Shen* with *Ren Dong Teng* (Caulis Lonicerae), *Chi Shao* (Radix Paeoniae Rubrae), *Qin Jiao* (Radix Gentianae Macrophyllae), and *Sang Zhi* (Ramulus Mori).

2. Cools the Blood, Reduces Swelling of Sores and Abscesses

Heat in the *ying* (nutritive) and *xue* (blood) levels: Manifestations include delirium, high fever, unconsciousness, irritability, insomnia, purpura or subcutaneous bleeding, with a dark, purplish-red tongue. *Dan Shen* cools the blood to treat febrile disorders or the presence of heat in the *ying* or *xue* levels.

- Heat in the *ying* or *xue* levels: use *Dan Shen* with *Sheng Di Huang* (Radix Rehmanniae), *Xuan Shen* (Radix Scrophulariae), and *Zhu Ye* (Herba Phyllostachys).

Sores and abscesses: *Dan Shen* has potent action to reduce swelling in toxic sores and breast abscesses.

- Initial stage of breast abscess: use this herb with *Jin Yin Hua* (Flos Lonicerae) and *Lian Qiao* (Fructus Forsythiae).
- Erysipelas: use it with *Mu Dan Pi* (Cortex Moutan), *Chi Shao* (Radix Paeoniae Rubrae), *Tian Hua Fen* (Radix Trichosanthis), *Jin Yin Hua* (Flos Lonicerae), *Lian Qiao* (Fructus Forsythiae), and *Pu Gong Ying* (Herba Taraxaci).

3. Nourishes Blood, Calms the *Shen* (Spirit)

Palpitations and insomnia related to heat in the blood or Heart blood deficiency: Cool in nature, *Dan Shen* dispels heat from the Heart and nourishes blood, to treat insomnia and palpitations.

- Palpitations and insomnia due to heat: use it with *Xuan Shen* (Radix Scrophulariae), *Lian Qiao* (Fructus Forsythiae) and *Jin Yin Hua* (Flos Lonicerae). **Exemplar Formula:** *Qing Ying Tang* (Clear the Nutrition Level Decoction).
- Palpitations and insomnia from Heart blood deficiency: combine this herb with *Sheng Di Huang* (Radix Rehmanniae), *Bai Zi Ren* (Semen Platycladi), and *Suan Zao Ren* (Semen Zizyphi Spinosae). **Exemplar Formula:** *Tian Wang Bu Xin Dan* (Emperor of Heaven's Special Pill to Tonify the Heart).

DOSAGE

5 to 10 grams in decoction, up to a maximum of 30 grams. Liquor-fried *Dan Shen* (with grain-based liquor) has a stronger function to activate blood circulation, remove blood stasis, and relieve pain.

CAUTIONS / CONTRAINDICATIONS

- *Dan Shen* is incompatible with *Li Lu* (Radix et Rhizoma Veratri).
- Patients with hypermenorrhea, hemoptysis or hematuria should use *Dan Shen* with caution.

CHEMICAL COMPOSITION

Tanshinone I, II_A, II_B; hydroxytanshionone, methyltanshinonate, methylenetanshinquinone, przewatanshin-

Dan Shen (Radix Salviae Miltiorrhizae)

quinone A, miltirone, dihydrotanshinone I, tanshinol A, tanshinol B, tanshinol C, nortanshinone, 1,2,15,16-tetrahydrotanshiquinone, isotanshinone I, II; isocryptotanshinone, tanshiquinone A, B, C.[1]

PHARMACOLOGICAL EFFECTS

- **Cardiovascular:** Administration of *Dan Shen* in various laboratory animals is associated with negative chronotropic and inotropic effects, and reduction of blood pressure.[2] *Dan Shen* dilates and increases blood perfusion to the coronary arteries to reduce the damage of cardiac ischemia and prevent or diminish death of cardiac muscle.[3]
- **Antiplatelet:** Injection of *Dan Shen* is associated with antiplatelet effects in healthy rabbits, rats and mice. The antiplatelet effect reaches its peak 30 minutes after intravenous injection, and lasted for approximately 2 hours.
- **Anticoagulant and thrombolytic:** Administration of *Dan Shen* is also associated with anticoagulant and thrombolytic effects.[4,5]
- **Antibiotic:** It has an inhibitory influence on *Staphylococcus aureus*.[6]
- **Hepatoprotective:** Administration of *Dan Shen* is associated with a marked hepatoprotective effect by lowering liver enzyme levels in mice exposed to carbon tetrachloride. It is also beneficial in treating mice with liver cirrhosis. The hepatoprotective function of *Dan Shen* is due in part to its effect at improving blood circulation and promoting regeneration of liver cells.[7,8,9]
- **Antineoplastic:** In mice with lung cancer, intraperitoneal injection of a *Dan Shen* preparation at the dosage of 9.0 g/kg showed marked inhibitory action on the growth of cancer cells with $p<0.05$ to 0.02. In mice with ascites carcinoma, intraperitoneal injection of a *Dan Shen* preparation was effective in inhibiting the growth and spread of tumor cells.[10,11]
- **CNS suppressant:** Administration of *Dan Shen* has a marked sedative effect, as it prolongs the hypnotic influence of phenobarbital and negates the stimulating effects of caffeine.[12]

CLINICAL STUDIES AND RESEARCH

- **Acute viral hepatitis:** One report covered 104 patients who were treated with intravenous injection of a *Dan Shen* preparation with an effective rate of 97%. The effectiveness is attributed to the ability of *Dan Shen* to promote regeneration of liver cells.[13]
- **Chronic nephritis:** According to another report, 48 patients were treated with an intravenous infusion of 16 to 20 ml of a *Dan Shen* preparation in 500 ml of D5W (2 ml of injectable contain 3 grams of dried herb) for 14 days per treatment course. Depending on the severity of illness, the effective rate ranged from 62.5 to 80%. Patients with hematuria were treated with extreme caution, as *Dan Shen* has both antiplatelet and anticoagulant effects.[14]
- **Oral leukoplakia:** Presence in the oral cavity of abnormal growths with white discoloration and distinct borders was diagnosed as oral leukoplakia and treated with *Dan Shen* injectable. After application of anesthetic to the affected area, 2 to 4 ml of the preparation were injected at the base of the abnormal growth every other day for a total of 7 injections per treatment course. The study reported good patient response with shrinkage and disappearance of the abnormal white growth.[15]
- **Chronic hepatitis:** According to one report, 22 patients with chronic active hepatitis (characterized as blood stasis) were divided into two groups. Patients in group one received 4 ml of *Dan Shen* via intramuscular injection. Patients in group two received 100 ml of individually-customized herbal decoctions twice daily plus 250mg of glucurolactone three times daily. The study reported normal liver function in 11 out of 11 patients in the *Dan Shen* injectable group after just 2 months, and in only 6 out of 11 patients in the herbal decoction group after 3 months.[16]
- **Cervical erosion:** In one study, 11 patients with cervical erosion were treated topically with a *Dan Shen* preparation, with up to a 57.66% success rate. Additional benefits included good patient compliance and lack of toxicity, adverse effects and/or allergic reactions.[17]
- **Epidemic hemorrhagic fever:** Oral or intravenous administration of *Dan Shen* showed marked effectiveness in treatment of epidemic hemorrhagic fever by reducing the length of illness, decreasing the duration of oliguria, and minimizing the amount of blood lost.[18]
- **Whooping cough:** In one study, 28 patients with whooping cough were treated with 2 ml of an intravenous infusion of *Dan Shen* (2 ml of injectable contained 2 grams of dried herb) one or two times daily. Marked improvement was reported in 21 out of 28 patients.[19]
- **Schistosomal hepatomegaly:** Administration of a 30 to 50% *Dan Shen* decoction (equivalent to 18 to 45 grams of dried herb daily) for 30 to 42 days showed a reduction in size of the liver in 44.4% of the patients, softening of the liver in 55.5%, a reduction in size of the spleen in 48.8%, and softening of the spleen in 53.6%.[20]
- **Coronary artery disease:** In one study, 323 patients with coronary artery disease were treated with oral administration of a *Dan Shen* preparation given three times daily (equivalent to daily dose of 60 grams of dried herbs). The study reported improvement based on symptomatic evaluation in 80.9% of the patients, and improvement based on ECG reading in 57.3% of the patients. That study noted that patients without previous incidence of myocardial infarction were most responsive to the treatment.

Dan Shen (Radix Salviae Miltiorrhizae)

Furthermore, a reduction of total cholesterol levels was reported in many patients. [21] In another study, 108 patients with angina were treated with an injectable of a *Dan Shen* preparation with improvement in 86% of the patients based on symptomatic evaluation, and in 54.7% of the patients based on an ECG evaluation.[22]

- **Shock:** Two patients with cardiogenic shock and sudden arrest of heartbeat were successfully rescued by intravenous injection of a *Dan Shen* preparation. The therapeutic effect was described as being similar to that of phentolamine or dobutamine.[23]
- **Scleroderma:** Sixteen patients with scleroderma were treated by intravenous infusion of a *Dan Shen* preparation for an average of 43.3 days. The study reported marked improvement in 37.6%, slight improvement in 31.2%, and no improvement in 31.2%.[24]
- **Ischemic stroke:** Intravenous administration of *Dan Shen* was 83.42% effective in treating 43 patients with stroke due to cerebral ischemia. The group that received Chinese herbs responded better than the group that received drugs.[25]
- **Cerebral thrombosis:** Intravenous administration of *Dan Shen* was 93.5% effective in treating 46 patients with cerebral thrombosis.[26]
- **Insomnia:** Injection of *Dan Shen* into *Zusanli* (ST 36) bilaterally was 61% effective in treating 100 patients diagnosed with insomnia.[27]
- **Allergic rhinitis:** Bilaterally injection of *Dan Shen* into inferior nasal concha of the nose was 86% effective in treating 50 patients diagnosed with allergic rhinitis.[28]
- **Glaucoma:** Intramuscular injection of *Dan Shen* in 94 patients for treatment of mid- to late-stage glaucoma showed good overall results. Out of 116 affected eyes, the study reported vision improvement in 58 eyes, no change in 49 eyes, and deterioration in 9 eyes.[29]

HERB-DRUG INTERACTION

- **Anticoagulant or antiplatelet drugs:** *Dan Shen* has a significant impact on the pharmacodynamics and pharmacokinetics of warfarin, according to studies conducted in rats. After a single dose of warfarin, use of *Dan Shen* orally for three days increased the absorption rate constant, plasma concentration, prothrombin time, steady-state plasma level, area under plasma-concentration-time curves, maximum concentrations and elimination half-lives of warfarin. However, there was a decrease of clearances and apparent volume of distribution of warfarin. The researchers concluded that this herb-drug interaction explains the exaggerated warfarin effect when herbs such as *Dan Shen* and *Dang Gui* (Radicis Angelicae Sinensis) were administered concurrently.[30] [Note: Examples of anticoagulants include heparin, warfarin (Coumadin) and enoxaparin (Lovenox); and examples of antiplatelets include aspirin, dipyridamole (Persantine), and clopidogrel (Plavix).]
- **Digoxin:** In an *in vitro* study, it was demonstrated that *Dan Shen* has digoxin-like immunoreactivity. Concurrent use of both digoxin and *Dan Shen* may result in falsely elevated serum digoxin concentrations (positive interference) as measured by the fluorescence polarization immunoassay, and a falsely lowered level (negative interference) when measured by the microparticle enzyme immunoassay. A more reliable assay can be obtained by monitoring the free digoxin concentration.[31]

TOXICOLOGY

No fatalities were reported following bolus intraperitoneal injection of *Dan Shen* decoction at 43 g/kg in mice. No abnormalities were observed following daily intraperitoneal injection of a *Dan Shen* preparation at 2.4 g/kg for 14 days.[32,33]

AUTHORS' COMMENTS

Of all blood-invigorating and stasis-removing herbs, *Dan Shen* is one of the most commonly used. It markedly lowers the viscosity of blood and improves perfusion of blood to various vital organs of the body, including, but not limited to, the brain, the heart, and the kidneys. Because it dilates coronary arteries and improves blood perfusion to the heart, *Dan Shen* is one of the most important herbs in the treatment of cardiac ischemia and angina.

Some traditional texts consider using the single herb *Dan Shen* to be equivalent to the function of the formula *Si Wu Tang* (Four-Substance Decoction). But this herb is cool and is mainly used to dispel blood stagnation. Although it can calm the *shen* (spirit) to treat palpitations and insomnia, this is not its primary function. Some believe that with only a minor function to tonify blood, the effect of using *Dan Shen* will be significantly lower than that of using blood-tonic herbs. Therefore the theory of *Dan Shen* being equivalent to *Si Wu Tang* does not meet with unanimous agreement among scholars and clinicians.

Dan Shen, *Dang Gui* (Radicis Angelicae Sinensis) and *Dang Gui Wei* (Extremitas Radicis Angelicae Sinensis) all invigorate and tonify the blood. The differences are as follows:

- *Dan Shen* is cool and has a stronger function to dispel blood stagnation.
- *Dang Gui* is warm and functions more effectively to tonify blood.
- *Dang Gui Wei* is warm, and is used primarily to invigorate blood circulation.

Dan Shen (Radix Salviae Miltiorrhizae)

References

1. *Xian Dai Zhong Yao Yao Li Xue* (Contemporary Pharmacology of Chinese Herbs), 1997; 881
2. *Shang Hai Di Yi Xue Yuan Xue Bao* (Journal of First Shanghai Medical College), 1980; 7(5):347
3. *Guo Wai Yi Xue Zhong Yi Zhong Yao Fen Ce* (Monograph of Chinese Herbology from Foreign Medicine), 1991; 13(3):41
4. *Shang Hai Di Yi Xue Yuan Xue Bao* (Journal of First Shanghai Medical College), 1979; 6(3):144
5. Ibid., 1982; 9(1):14
6. *Yao Xue Xue Bao* (Journal of Herbology), 1979; 14(2):75
7. *Zhong Yi Za Zhi* (Journal of Chinese Medicine), 1982; (1):67
8. *Zhong Xi Yi Jie He Za Zhi* (Journal of Integrated Chinese and Western Medicine), 1988; 8(3):161
9. Ibid., 1983; 3(3):180
10. *Zhong Cao Yao* (Chinese Herbal Medicine), 1981; 12(10):22
11. *Xi An Yi Ke Da Xue Xue Bao* (Journal of Xian University School of Medicine), 1986; 7(4):403
12. *Yao Xue Xue Bao* (Journal of Herbology), 1979; 14(5):288
13. *Shan Xi Zhong Yi* (Shanxi Chinese Medicine), 1980; 6:15
14. *Shang Hai Yi Yao Za Zhi* (Shanghai Journal of Medicine and Herbology), 1981; 1:17
15. *He Nan Yi Yao* (Henan Medicine and Herbology), 1982; 4:19
16. *Zhong Xi Yi Jie He Za Zhi* (Journal of Integrated Chinese and Western Medicine), 1984; 2:86
17. *Shan Xi Xin Zhong Yi* (New Shanxi Chinese Medicine), 1984; 3:61
18. *Shan Xi Zhong Yi* (Shanxi Chinese Medicine), 1984; 2:13
19. *Jiang Su Yi Yao* (Jiangsu Journal of Medicine and Herbology), 1978; 1:30
20. *Zhong Hua Yi Xue Za Zhi* (Chinese Journal of Medicine), 1958; 44(6):542
21. *Xin Zhang Xue Guan Ji Bing* (Cardiovascular Diseases), 1974; 2(1):5
22. *Zhong Cao Yao Tong Xun* (Journal of Chinese Herbal Medicine), 1978; 1:37
23. *Zhong Xi Yi Jie He Za Zhi* (Journal of Integrated Chinese and Western Medicine), 1986; 6(6):368
24. *Xin Yi Yao Xue Za Zhi* (New Journal of Medicine and Herbology), 1978; 8:48
25. *Shang Hai Yi Xue* (Shanghai Medicine), 1978; 1(2):64
26. *An Hui Zhong Yi Xue Yuan Xue Bao* (Journal of Anhui University School of Medicine), 1986; 5(4):45
27. *Si Chuan Zhong Yi* (Sichuan Chinese Medicine), 1986; 4:42
28. *Zhong Yi Za Zhi* (Journal of Chinese Medicine), 1984; 9:43
29. *Zhong Cao Yao* (Chinese Herbal Medicine), 1980; 11(12):553
30. Chan-K. Lo-AC, Yeung-JH, and Woo-KS. *Journal of Pharmacy and Pharmacology*, (1995, May) vol. 47(5):402-6
31. Wahed A. Dasgupta A., Positive and negative in vitro interference of Chinese medicine dan shen in serum digoxin measurement. Elimination of interference by monitoring free digoxin concentration. *American Journal of Clinical Pathology.* 116(3):403-8, 2001 Sep.
32. *Liao Ning Yi Yao* (Liaoning Medicine and Herbology), 1975; (1):25
33. *Zhe Jiang Yi Xue* (Zhejiang Journal of Medicine), 1979; 1(1):25

Hong Hua (Flos Carthami)

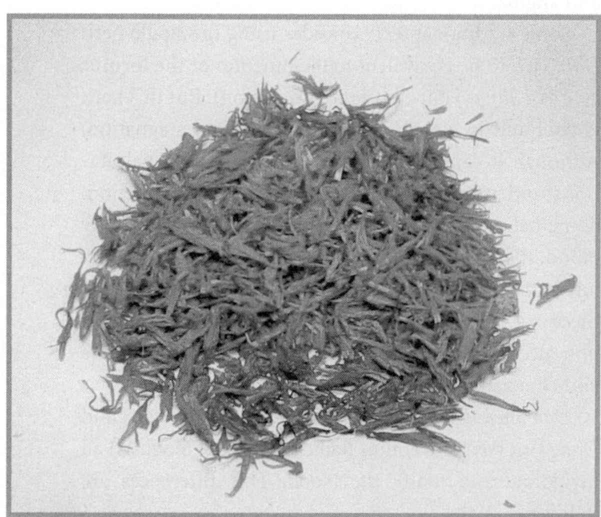

紅花 红花

Pinyin Name: *Hong Hua*
Literal Name: "red flower"
Alternate Chinese Names: *Hong Lan Hua*
Original Source: *Xin Xiu Ben Cao* (Newly Revised Materia Medica) by Su Jing in 657-659 A.D.
English Name: carthamus, safflower
Botanical Name: *Carthamus tinctorius* L. (*Hong Hua*)
Pharmaceutical Name: Flos Carthami
Properties: acrid, warm
Channels Entered: Heart, Liver

CHINESE THERAPEUTIC ACTIONS

Activates Blood Circulation, Eliminates Blood Stasis, Opens Channels, Regulates Menstruation

Hong Hua (Flos Carthami) functions extremely well to activate blood circulation and eliminate blood stasis. It has a broad range of clinical applications including menstrual pain, amenorrhea, postpartum abdominal pain, external and sports injuries, joint pain, and macular skin eruptions.

Hong Hua (Flos Carthami)

Obstetric/gynecological disorders: *Hong Hua* is one of the most commonly-used herbs in the obstetric and gynecologic departments in China. When used in small dosages, it activates and nourishes blood. When used in large dosages, it breaks blood stagnation.

- Menstrual pain or amenorrhea: combine *Hong Hua* with *Tao Ren* (Semen Persicae), *Dang Gui* (Radicis Angelicae Sinensis), *Chuan Xiong* (Rhizoma Ligustici Chuanxiong), and *Chi Shao* (Radix Paeoniae Rubrae). **Exemplar Formula:** *Tao Hong Si Wu Tang* (Four-Substance Decoction with Safflower and Peach Pit).
- Postpartum dizziness or abdominal pain from blood stasis: add this herb to *He Ye* (Folium Nelumbinis), *Pu Huang* (Pollen Typhae), *Dang Gui* (Radicis Angelicae Sinensis), and *Mu Dan Pi* (Cortex Moutan).
- Stillbirth or difficult labor: use it with *Niu Xi* (Radix Cyathulae seu Achyranthis), *Chuan Xiong* (Rhizoma Ligustici Chuanxiong), and *Dang Gui* (Radicis Angelicae Sinensis).

Abdominal masses or accumulations: Clinical manifestations may include palpable masses, abdominal pain or enlarged spleen or liver. These are usually chronic cases, and the tongue is often dark with purple spots.

- Abdominal masses due to blood stasis: use *Hong Hua* with *San Leng* (Rhizoma Sparganii) and *E Zhu* (Rhizoma Curcumae).
- Epigastric or abdominal pain: use it with *Gao Liang Jiang* (Rhizoma Alpiniae Officinarum), *Xiang Fu* (Rhizoma Cyperi), *Wu Ling Zhi* (Excrementum Trogopteri seu Pteromi), *Pu Huang* (Pollen Typhae) and *Sha Ren* (Fructus Amomi).
- Abdominal pain: combine this herb with *Dang Gui* (Radicis Angelicae Sinensis), *Yan Hu Suo* (Rhizoma Corydalis), and *Mu Xiang* (Radix Aucklandiae).
- Hepatomegaly: add *Hong Hua* to *Chai Hu* (Radix Bupleuri), *Zao Jiao Ci* (Spina Gleditsiae), *Bai Ji Li* (Fructus Tribuli), *Chuan Lian Zi* (Fructus Toosendan), *Bing Lang* (Semen Arecae), *E Zhu* (Rhizoma Curcumae), *Chuan Shan Jia* (Squama Manis), *Mu Li* (Concha Ostreae) and *Jiang Huang* (Rhizoma Curcumae Longae).

Joint pain: *Hong Hua* invigorates the circulation of blood in the channels and collaterals. Clinical manifestations include *bi zheng* (painful obstruction syndrome), hemiplegia or paralysis.

- *Bi zheng*: use it with *Di Long* (Pheretima) and *Di Bie Chong* (Eupolyphaga).
- Hemiplegia: combine this herb with *Sang Zhi* (Ramulus Mori), *Di Long* (Pheretima), *Chuan Shan Jia* (Squama Manis), *Chuan Xiong* (Rhizoma Ligustici Chuanxiong), *Chi Shao* (Radix Paeoniae Rubrae), *Niu Xi* (Radix Cyathulae seu Achyranthis) and *Huang Qi* (Radix Astragali).

Dermatological disorders: Macular eruptions are usually caused by heat in the blood forcing it out of the vessels. The eruptive patch is usually dark purplish.

- Macular eruption: use *Hong Hua* with *Dang Gui* (Radicis Angelicae Sinensis), *Zi Cao Gen* (Radix Lithospermi) and *Da Qing Ye* (Folium Isatidis).

Chest pain: *Hong Hua* enters the Lung to activate qi and blood circulation to relieve pain.

- Chest pain, angina: use this herb with *Tan Xiang* (Lignum Santali Albi), *Gua Lou Shi* (Fructus Trichosanthis), *Xie Bai* (Bulbus Allii Macrostemonis), *Gui Zhi* (Ramulus Cinnamomi), and *Wu Ling Zhi* (Excrementum Trogopteri seu Pteromi).

DOSAGE

3 to 10 grams in decoction.

CAUTIONS / CONTRAINDICATIONS

- Use of *Hong Hua* is contraindicated during pregnancy.
- Do not exceed the recommended dose of *Hong Hua*: doing so may cause incessant bleeding.

CHEMICAL COMPOSITION

Carthamin, neocarthamin, carthamone, carthamidin, neocarthamin.[1,2]

Carthamin

PHARMACOLOGICAL EFFECTS

- **Cardiovascular:** A small dose of *Hong Hua* decoction has positive inotropic effects as it stimulates the heart; however, a large dose has negative inotropic and chronotropic effects as it inhibits the heart and decreases overall cardiac output.[3]
- **Antiplatelet:** *Hong Hua* has demonstrated marked effectiveness to inhibit the aggregation of platelets and formation of thrombi. It was reported in one study that *Hong Hua* is 73.4% effective in preventing the formation of thrombi in rats.
- **CNS suppressant:** Intraperitoneal administration of *Hong Hua* has a sedative effect on the central nervous system, as demonstrated in mice. It also has a preventative effect against drug-induced seizures.[4]
- **Adaptogenic:** Intraperitoneal administration of *Hong Hua* at the dosage of 1,100 mg/kg increased the total

Hong Hua (Flos Carthami)

swimming time of mice by up to 117%.[5]

- **Uterine stimulant:** Decoction of *Hong Hua* has a stimulating effect on the smooth muscle of the uterus to increase muscle contraction, as demonstrated in various animal studies.[6]

CLINICAL STUDIES AND RESEARCH

- **Cerebral thrombosis:** Intravenous infusion of 15 ml of a 50% *Hong Hua* solution (equivalent to 75 grams of dried herb) in 500 ml of D10W once daily for 15 days was 94.7% effective in treating 137 patients with cerebral thrombosis. Side effects reported include skin allergy, hypermenorrhea, and fatigue.[7]
- **Coronary artery disease:** In one study, 100 patients treated with intravenous injection or infusion of 50% *Hong Hua* solution showed chest pain relief in 80.8% of the study group, marked ECG improvement in 26%, and moderate ECG improvement in 40%. Most patients also reported reduction of headaches, dizziness, and palpitations.[8]
- **Duodenal ulcer:** Twelve patients with duodenal ulcers were treated with an herbal decoction once daily for 20 days with a 100% success rate. The herbal decoction was prepared by cooking 60 grams of *Hong Hua* and 12 pieces of *Da Zao* (Fructus Jujubae) in 300 ml of water to yield 150 ml of the final decoction. The decoction was mixed with 60 grams of honey. The patients were instructed to drink 150 ml of the decoction and ingest the *Da Zao* on an empty stomach one time daily.[9]
- **Flat warts:** According to one report, 36 patients with flat warts were treated with 9 grams of *Hong Hua* soaked in hot water and taken by mouth several times daily for 10 days per treatment course. Out of 36 patients, 2 patients were successfully treated after 1 course of treatment, 18 patients after 2 courses, 12 patients after 3 courses, 1 patient after 4 courses, and 3 patients showed no response. The overall rate of effectiveness was 91.6%.[10]

HERB-DRUG INTERACTION

- **Anticoagulant or antiplatelet drugs:** *Hong Hua* should be used with caution in patients receiving anticoagulant or antiplatelet medications, as the combination may lead to additive or synergistic effects. Though this potential interaction has not been documented, the use of *Hong Hua* may potentiate the effect of such drugs as warfarin.[11] [Note: Examples of anticoagulants include heparin, warfarin (Coumadin) and enoxaparin (Lovenox); and examples of antiplatelets include aspirin, dipyridamole (Persantine), and clopidogrel (Plavix).]

TOXICOLOGY

The maximum safe dosage for oral administration of *Hong Hua* is 8 g/kg, as determined by animal studies. The LD_{50} for carthamin via intravenous injection is 2.35 +/- 0.14 g/kg. Daily administration of *Hong Hua* at the dosage up to 1.5 g/kg for 3 months showed no abnormality in liver, kidney, heart, stomach or intestinal functions in rats.[12]

SUPPLEMENT

- 藏紅花 / 藏红花 *Zhang Hong Hua* (Flos Crocus Sativus), first cited in the *Yin Shan Zheng Yao* (Correct Guide to Eating and Drinking), is grown and harvested in Tibet, India and some European countries. It is sweet and cold, and enters the Heart and Liver. In comparison with *Hong Hua*, *Zhang Hong Hua* has a similar but much stronger overall ability to invigorate blood circulation, eliminate blood stasis, cool blood and eliminate heat toxins. It is commonly used when heat is attacking the *ying* (nutritive) and *xue* (blood) stages, leading to symptoms such as macula and high fever. As *Zhang Hong Hua* is an expensive herb, it is seldom used. The dosage for *Zhang Hong Hua* is 1.5 to 3.0 grams.

AUTHORS' COMMENTS

Hong Hua and *Tao Ren* (Semen Persicae) are commonly used together for their synergistic actions. *Hong Hua* is better at dispersing blood stagnation to open the channels and collaterals. It is also used to treat pain in the extremities. *Tao Ren* is better for treatment of abdominal blood stagnation. It is also effective to treat lung and intestinal abscesses.

References

1. *Xian Dai Zhong Yao Yao Li Xue* (Contemporary Pharmacology of Chinese Herbs), 1997; 900
2. *The Merck Index* 12th edition, Chapman & Hall/CRCnetBASE/Merck, 2000
3. *Zhong Cheng Yao Yan Jiu* (Research of Chinese Patent Medicine), 1983; 12:31
4. *Zhong Cao Yao* (Chinese Herbal Medicine), 1984; 15(5):21
5. Ibid., 1985; 16(10):27
6. *Zhong Yao Yao Li Yu Ying Yong* (Pharmacology and Applications of Chinese Herbs), 1983:462
7. *Shan Xi Yi Yao Za Zhi* (Shanxi Journal of Medicine and Herbology), 1983; 5:297
8. *Xin Zhang Xue Guan Ji Bing* (Cardiovascular Diseases), 1976; 4(4):265
9. *Shan Dong Zhong Yi Za Zhi* (Shandong Journal of Chinese Medicine), 1985; 4:20
10. *Chong Qing Yi Yao* (Chongching Medicine and Herbology), 1976; 5:49
11. Chen, J. Recognition & prevention of herb-drug interactions, *Medical Acupuncture*, Fall/Winter 1998/1999; volume 10/number 2; 9-13
12. *Zhong Yao Yao Li Yu Ying Yong* (Pharmacology and Applications of Chinese Herbs), 1983:462

Tao Ren (Semen Persicae)

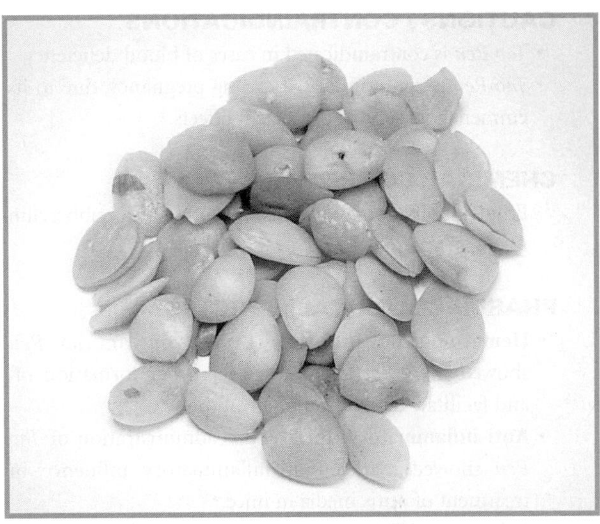

桃仁

Pinyin Name: *Tao Ren*
Literal Name: "persica seed," "peach pit"
Original Source: *Shen Nong Ben Cao Jing* (Divine Husbandman's Classic of the Materia Medica) in the second century
English Name: persica, peach seed
Botanical Name: *Prunus persica* (Linn) Batsch. (*Tao*); *Prunus davidana* (Carr.) Franch. (*Shan Tao*)
Pharmaceutical Name: Semen Persicae
Properties: bitter, neutral
Channels Entered: Heart, Large Intestine, Liver, Lung

CHINESE THERAPEUTIC ACTIONS

1. Activates Blood Circulation, Removes Blood Stasis

Obstetric/gynecological disorders: *Tao Ren* (Semen Persicae) has a potent function to activate blood circulation and eliminate blood stasis that makes it useful for a broad range of clinical applications. It is commonly used to treat menstrual pain, amenorrhea and postpartum abdominal pain.

- Postpartum abdominal pain with profuse uterine bleeding: combine *Tao Ren* with *Dang Gui* (Radicis Angelicae Sinensis), *Chuan Xiong* (Rhizoma Ligustici Chuanxiong), *Pao Jiang* (Rhizoma Zingiberis Preparatum) and *Gan Cao* (Radix Glycyrrhizae). **Exemplar Formula:** *Sheng Hua Tang* (Generation and Transformation Decoction).
- Menstrual pain, amenorrhea, or irregular menstruation caused by blood stasis: add it to *Hong Hua* (Flos Carthami), *Dang Gui* (Radicis Angelicae Sinensis), *Chuan Xiong* (Rhizoma Ligustici Chuanxiong) and *Chi Shao* (Radix Paeoniae Rubrae). **Exemplar Formula:** *Tao Hong Si Wu Tang* (Four-Substance Decoction with Safflower and Peach Pit).

External and sports injuries: Entering and invigorating blood in the channels and collaterals, *Tao Ren* treats traumatic injuries and related symptoms caused by blood stagnation.

- External and sports injuries with bruising and pain: add this herb to *Hong Hua* (Flos Carthami), *Da Huang* (Radix et Rhizoma Rhei), and *Chuan Shan Jia* (Squama Manis). **Exemplar Formula:** *Fu Yuan Huo Xue Tang* (Revive Health by Invigorating the Blood Decoction).
- Blood stasis in the abdomen from traumatic injuries: combine *Tao Ren* with *Meng Chong* (Tabanus), *Pu Huang* (Pollen Typhae), *Chuan Xiong* (Rhizoma Ligustici Chuanxiong), *Da Huang* (Radix et Rhizoma Rhei), and *Gui Zhi* (Ramulus Cinnamomi).

2. Drains Abscesses

Lung and intestinal abscesses:

- Lung abscess: add *Tao Ren* to *Lu Gen* (Rhizoma Phragmitis), *Dong Gua Zi* (Semen Benincasae), and *Yi Yi Ren* (Semen Coicis).
- Intestinal abscess: combine it with *Da Huang* (Radix et Rhizoma Rhei), *Mu Dan Pi* (Cortex Moutan) and *Mang Xiao* (Natrii Sulfas). **Exemplar Formula:** *Da Huang Mu Dan Tang* (Rhubarb and Moutan Decoction).
- Sores and abscesses: use this herb with *Jin Yin Hua* (Flos Lonicerae), *Lian Qiao* (Fructus Forsythiae), *Chi Shao* (Radix Paeoniae Rubrae), *Tian Hua Fen* (Radix Trichosanthis), *Ru Xiang* (Gummi Olibanum) and *Mo Yao* (Myrrha).

3. Moistens the Intestines, Relieves Constipation

Chronic constipation: *Tao Ren* is commonly used with other seeds to moisten the intestines and relieve constipation caused by dryness from chronic illness, yin deficiency, or blood deficiency.

- Constipation: use this herb with *Huo Ma Ren* (Fructus Cannabis), *Xing Ren* (Semen Armeniacae Amarum), and *Yu Li Ren* (Semen Pruni).

DOSAGE

6 to 10 grams in decoction. *Tao Ren* seeds should be crushed prior to decoction. The unprocessed herb has a strong effect to move the blood and eliminate blood stasis. The dry-fried herb has a strong effect to moisten dryness and treat constipation.

Tao Ren (Semen Persicae)

CAUTIONS / CONTRAINDICATIONS

- *Tao Ren* is contraindicated in cases of blood deficiency.
- *Tao Ren* is contraindicated during pregnancy, due to its emmenagogic and abortifacient effects.[1]

CHEMICAL COMPOSITION

Emulsin, allantoinase, lipids, essential oils (gibberellin A_5, A_{33}); vitamin B_1.[2]

PHARMACOLOGICAL EFFECTS

- **Hematological:** Intravenous injection of *Tao Ren* showed marked effectiveness to prevent formation of, and facilitate dissolution of, thrombi.[3]
- **Anti-inflammatory:** Intravenous administration of *Tao Ren* showed marked anti-inflammatory influence in treatment of otitis media in mice.[4]
- **Others:** *Tao Ren* has also demonstrated antiallergic, antitussive, and antiparasitic effects in various animal studies.[5]

CLINICAL STUDIES AND RESEARCH

- **Schistosomal cirrhosis:** Intravenous infusion of *Tao Ren* in D5W once every other day for 90 days produced marked improvement based on symptom assessment and hematological evaluation.[6]
- **Angiitis:** In one study, 50 patients with angiitis were treated with an herbal injectable with good results. The herbal injectable contained *Tao Ren, Hong Hua* (Flos Carthami) and *Dan Shen* (Radix Salviae Miltiorrhizae).[7]

HERB-DRUG INTERACTION

- **Anticoagulant or antiplatelet drugs:** *Tao Ren* should be used with caution in patients receiving anticoagulant or antiplatelet medications as the combination may lead to additive or synergistic effects. Though this interaction has not been documented, the use of *Tao Ren* may potentiate the effect of drugs such as warfarin.[8] [Note: Examples of anticoagulants include heparin, warfarin (Coumadin) and enoxaparin (Lovenox); and examples of antiplatelets include aspirin, dipyridamole (Persantine), and clopidogrel (Plavix).]

TOXICOLOGY

In toxicology studies in mice, intramuscular injection of a water extract of *Tao Ren* at 3.5 g/kg leads to reactions such as flaccid muscles, irregular muscle movement, and constriction of the skin pores. The LD_{50} via injection in mice is approximately 222 g/kg.[9]

References

1. Brinker, Francis. *The Toxicology of Botanical Medicines,* rev. 2nd ed., 1996
2. *Xian Dai Zhong Yao Yao Li Xue* (Contemporary Pharmacology of Chinese Herbs), 1997; 903
3. *Shang Hai Zhong Yi Yao Za Zhi* (Shanghai Journal of Chinese Medicine and Herbology), 1985; 7:45
4. *Zhong Yao Tong Bao* (Journal of Chinese Herbology), 1986; 11(11):37
5. *Zhong Yao Zhi* (Chinese Herbology Journal), 1984:89
6. Ibid., 1986; 6:24
7. *Liao Ning Zhong Ji Yi Kan* (Liaoning Journal of Medium Medicine), 1979; 2:43
8. Chen, J. Recognition & prevention of herb-drug interactions, *Medical Acupuncture*, Fall/Winter 1998/1999; volume 10/number 2; 9-13
9. *Xian Dai Zhong Yao Yao Li Xue* (Contemporary Pharmacology of Chinese Herbs), 1997; 282-283, 1997; 903-9041.

Yi Mu Cao (Herba Leonuri)

益母草 益母草

Pinyin Name: *Yi Mu Cao*
Literal Name: "mother's herb," "good for mother herb," "benefit mother herb"
Alternate Chinese Names: *Cong Wei, Yi Ming*
Original Source: *Shen Nong Ben Cao Jing* (Divine Husbandman's Classic of the Materia Medica) in the second century
English Name: leonurus, motherwort herb
Botanical Name: *Leonurus heterophyllus* Sweet (*Yi Mu Cao*)
Pharmaceutical Name: Herba Leonuri
Properties: acrid, bitter, cool
Channels Entered: Heart, Liver, Urinary Bladder

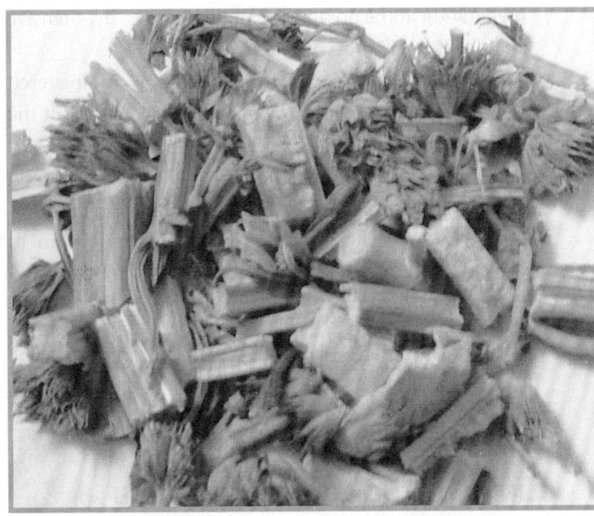

CHINESE THERAPEUTIC ACTIONS

1. Activates Blood Circulation, Dispels Blood Stasis

Irregular menstruation, amenorrhea, postpartum abdominal pain: *Yi Mu Cao* (Herba Leonuri) is one of the best and most-commonly used herbs for treatment of various gynecological disorders caused by blood stagnation. It is essential in regulating blood circulation in the *chong* (thoroughfare) channel without damaging qi or blood. It regenerates blood without causing stagnation. In postpartum women with spotting, *Yi Mu Cao* helps to contract the uterus to expel residual stagnation.

- Abdominal pain because of irregular menstruation or amenorrhea: use *Yi Mu Cao* with *Dang Gui* (Radicis Angelicae Sinensis), *Bai Shao* (Radix Paeoniae Alba), and *Dan Shen* (Radix Salviae Miltiorrhizae).
- Severe postpartum abdominal pain and uterine bleeding: use *Yi Mu Cao* as a single herb remedy.

2. Promotes Urination, Reduces Swelling and Edema

Edema and dysuria: In cases of Kidney qi deficiency, *Yi Mu Cao* treats symptoms of dysuria, scanty urine, chronic edema, heavy sensations of the back and legs, abdominal distention and fullness after meals, sallow complexion, movement difficulties, fatigue and listlessness. This herb can also treat edema due to chronic nephritis.

- Edema and dysuria: add *Bai Mao Gen* (Rhizoma Imperatae).

3. Clears Heat and Eliminates Toxins

Dermatological disorders: *Yi Mu Cao* clears heat and eliminates toxins from both the interior and the exterior. Clinical applications include eczema, sores, lesions, and ulcers. It may be used internally and topically.

DOSAGE

10 to 15 grams, with a maximum of 30 grams, in herbal decoction. *Yi Mu Cao* is commonly used internally and topically.

CAUTIONS / CONTRAINDICATIONS

- *Yi Mu Cao* is contraindicated in cases of yin deficiency, blood deficiency, or yang deficiency with prolapse.
- *Yi Mu Cao* must be used with extreme caution during pregnancy because of its stimulating effect on the uterus.

CHEMICAL COMPOSITION

Leonurine, stachydrine, leonuridien, leonurinine, lauric acid, linolenic acid, sterol, prehispanolone, 4-guanidino-1-butanol, vitamin A.[1,2]

H_3CO, HO, OCH_3, O, H N, NH_2, NH

Leonurine

PHARMACOLOGICAL EFFECTS

- **Uterine stimulant:** Administration of water or alcohol extracts of *Yi Mu Cao* has demonstrated a stimulating effect on the uterus of rabbits, cats, dogs, and guinea pigs. The onset of action is approximately 15 to 20 minutes following oral administration of the decoction. The stimulating effect is observed whether or not animals are pregnant, and in both early and late pregnancy. In regard to the medicinal parts of the plant, the leaf has the strongest stimulating effect, the root has milder influence, and the stem has none.[3]
- **Cardiovascular:** A small dose of *Yi Mu Cao* has a stimulating effect on cardiac contraction, while a large dose has an inhibiting effect. Intravenous injection of *Yi Mu Cao*

Yi Mu Cao (Herba Leonuri)

preparation at the dosage of 2 mg/kg exerts a hypotensive effect with a duration of only a few minutes.[4]

- **Antiplatelet:** Alcohol extract of *Yi Mu Cao* administered via injection demonstrated a marked effect to inhibit the aggregation of platelets.[5]
- **Respiratory:** A small dose of *Yi Mu Cao* stimulates the respiratory system to increase the frequency and depth of respiration. A large dose inhibits the respiratory system to weaken the strength and disrupt the rhythm of respiration.[6]
- **Renal:** In one study, 20 ml of an *Yi Mu Cao* preparation (equivalent to 60 grams of bulk herb) administered via intravenous injection showed marked effectiveness in treatment of acute renal failure in dogs, using such evaluating criteria as BUN, FE_{Na} and renal blood flow.[7]

CLINICAL STUDIES AND RESEARCH

- **Acute nephritis:** Herbal decoction of *Yi Mu Cao* administered three times daily had marked effectiveness in reducing edema in patients with acute nephritis. The herbal decoction was prepared by cooking 90 to 120 grams of dried *Yi Mu Cao* in 700 ml of water to yield 300 ml of final decoction. Fresh *Yi Mu Cao* at double the dosage was shown to be more effective than the dried herb.[8]
- **Coronary artery disease (CAD):** Patients with CAD were treated with an intravenous drip of an *Yi Mu Cao* preparation. Of 100 patients, the study reported an 84% effective rate based on symptom evaluation, and a 61% effective rate based on ECG evaluation.[9]
- **Hypertension:** According to one report, 56 patients with elevated blood pressure were treated with an herbal pill that contained *Yi Mu Cao*, *Chou Wu Tong* (Folium Clerodendri Trichotomi), *Xi Xian Cao* (Herba Siegesbeckiae), and *Xia Ku Cao* (Spica Prunellae). The herbs started to lower blood pressure on day one, and reached maximum impact on day ten.[10]
- **Irregular menstruation:** Herbal decoction or extract of *Yi Mu Cao* at 15 to 20 grams per dose, given three times daily, was effective in the treatment of irregular menstruation, hypermenorrhea, and postpartum bleeding. After ingestion, uterine contraction was observed in 16.4% of patients after one hour, and 25% of patients after two hours. The strength of contraction did not depend on the dose of the herbs.[11]

HERB-DRUG INTERACTION

- **Anticoagulant or antiplatelet drugs:** *Yi Mu Cao* has antiplatelet action, and should be used with caution in patients who take anticoagulant or antiplatelet medications. Though this potential interaction has not been documented, this herb may potentiate the effect of drugs such as warfarin.[12] [Note: Examples of anticoagulants include heparin, warfarin (Coumadin) and enoxaparin (Lovenox); and examples of antiplatelets include aspirin, dipyridamole (Persantine), and clopidogrel (Plavix).]

TOXICOLOGY

The LD_{50} for intravenous administration of an *Yi Mu Cao* preparation was 30 to 60 g/kg in mice.[13]

SUPPLEMENT

- 茺蔚子 / 茺蔚子 *Chong Wei Zi* (Semen Leonuri), first cited in *Shen Nong Ben Cao Jing* (Divine Husbandman's Classic of the Materia Medica) in the second century, is derived from the seed of the same plant as *Yi Mu Cao*. *Chong Wei Zi* is sweet and cool. It activates blood circulation, regulates menstruation, clears the Liver and brightens the eyes. Clinical manifestations include irregular menstruation, dysmenorrhea, amenorrhea, postpartum abdominal pain, headache, and red, swollen or painful eyes due to Liver heat. Recommended dosage of *Chong Wei Zi* is 6 to 15 grams in decoction.

AUTHORS' COMMENTS

Yi Mu Cao was used in the Tang dynasty by the famous Tai-Ping princess as a body wash, to retain beautiful, soft skin.

According to Dr. Shu Run-San, the combination of *Yi Mu Cao*, *Zhi Ke* (Fructus Aurantii), and *Pu Huang* (Pollen Typhae) has a stimulating effect to induce uterine contraction. These three herbs are commonly used to dispel blood stasis in postpartum patients with retention of lochia, or the pain associated with endometriosis.

According to Dr. Zhu Lang-Chun, when using *Yi Mu Cao* for diuretic purposes, the dosage for adults must be as high as 60-120 grams (lower dosages for children). High dosages are especially necessary in cases involving blood stasis and edema.

References

1. *Xian Dai Zhong Yao Yao Li Xue* (*Contemporary Pharmacology of Chinese Herbs*), 1997; 898
2. *The Merck Index* 12th edition, Chapman & Hall/CRCnetBASE/Merck, 2000
3. *Zhong Yao Yan Jiu* (*Research of Chinese Herbology*), 1979; 581
4. Ibid.
5. *Zhong Xi Yi Jie He Za Zhi* (*Journal of Integrated Chinese and Western Medicine*), 1986; 6(1):39
6. *Zhong Yao Yan Jiu* (*Research of Chinese Herbology*), 1979; 581
7. *Shang Hai Di Er Yi Ke Da Xue Xue Bao* (*Journal of Second Shanghai University College of Medicine*), 1988; 8(3):219
8. *Yun Nan Zhong Yi Za Zhi* (*Yunan Journal of Chinese Medicine*), 1984; 2:48
9. *Zhong Yi Za Zhi* (*Journal of Chinese Medicine*), 1985; 26(3):29
10. *Fu Jian Sheng Yi Yao Yan Jiu Suo* (*Fujian Province Institute of Medicine and Herbal Research*), 1977; 3:23
11. *Zhong Hua Fu Chan Ke Za Zhi* (*Chinese Journal of OB/GYN*), 1958; 1:1
12. Chen, J. Recognition & prevention of herb-drug interactions, *Medical Acupuncture*, Fall/Winter 1998/1999; volume 10/number 2; 9-13
13. *Shan Xi Yi Yao Za Zhi* (*Shanxi Journal of Medicine and Herbology*), 1978; (4):21

Ze Lan (Herba Lycopi)

澤蘭 泽兰

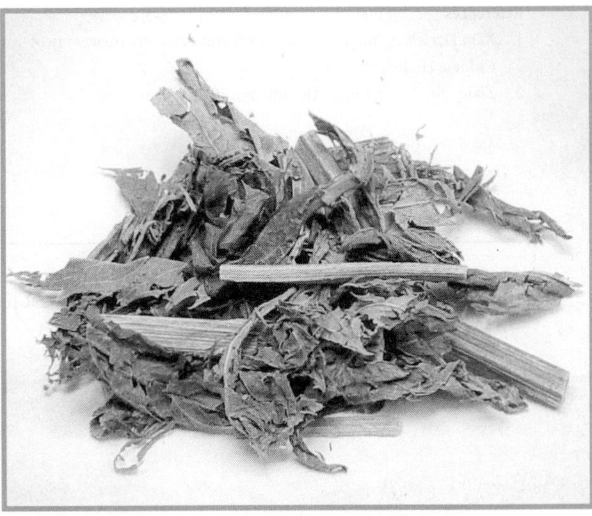

Pinyin Name: *Ze Lan*
Literal Name: "marsh orchid"
Original Source: *Shen Nong Ben Cao Jing* (Divine Husbandman's Classic of the Materia Medica) in the second century
English Name: lycopus, hirsute shiny bugleweed
Botanical Name: *Lycopus lucidus* Turcz. (*Di Gua Er Miao*); *Lycopus lucidus* Turcz. var. *hirtus* Regel. (*Mao Ye Di Gua Er Miao*)
Pharmaceutical Name: Herba Lycopi
Properties: bitter, acrid, slightly warm
Channels Entered: Liver, Spleen

CHINESE THERAPEUTIC ACTIONS

1. Activates Blood Circulation, Dispels Blood Stasis

Gynecological disorders: *Ze Lan* (Herba Lycopi) activates blood circulation by warming the channels. It is a mild herb, regulates menstruation and treats various gynecological disorders characterized by qi and blood stagnation. Clinical applications include menstrual pain, irregular menstruation, and postpartum abdominal pain.

- Menstrual pain, irregular menstruation, and postpartum abdominal pain: combine *Ze Lan* with *Dang Gui* (Radicis Angelicae Sinensis), *Dan Shen* (Radix Salviae Miltiorrhizae), and *Bai Shao* (Radix Paeoniae Alba).
- Amenorrhea caused by blood deficiency with fire: add this herb to *Dang Gui* (Radicis Angelicae Sinensis), *Bai Shao* (Radix Paeoniae Alba) and *Zhi Gan Cao* (Radix Glycyrrhizae Preparata).

Pain and bruises due to external and sports injuries, and chest and hypochondriac pain:

- Pain and bruises: combine *Ze Lan* with *Dang Gui* (Radicis Angelicae Sinensis), *Chuan Xiong* (Rhizoma Ligustici Chuanxiong), *Hong Hua* (Flos Carthami) and *Tao Ren* (Semen Persicae).
- Sores and swellings on the skin: use this herb with *Jin Yin Hua* (Flos Lonicerae), *Gan Cao* (Radix Glycyrrhizae) and *Dang Gui* (Radicis Angelicae Sinensis).
- Chest and hypochondriac pain from qi and blood stagnation: use this herb with *Dan Shen* (Radix Salviae Miltiorrhizae) and *Yu Jin* (Radix Curcumae).
- Back pain due to blood stagnation from traumatic injuries: add *Chuan Niu Xi* (Radix Cyathulae).

2. Regulates Water Circulation, Reduces Swelling

Dysuria, edema: *Ze Lan* has a very mild function to regulate water circulation, and is used with diuretic herbs to treat edema.

- Edema: add *Fen Fang Ji* (Radix Stephaniae Tetandrae).

DOSAGE

10 to 15 grams in decoction.

CAUTIONS / CONTRAINDICATIONS

- *Ze Lan* should be used with caution in patients with blood deficiency, and in the absence of blood stasis.

CHEMICAL COMPOSITION

Glycosides, flavones, saponins, lycopose, raffinose, stachyose, guaianolides, eurecuivin.[1]

PHARMACOLOGICAL EFFECTS

- **Cardiotonic:** *Ze Lan* has been shown to have a cardiotonic effect.[2]

CLINICAL STUDIES AND RESEARCH

- **Disseminated intravascular coagulation (DIC):** Administration of a *Ze Lan* preparation via intravenous injection was effective in prevention of DIC.[3]

HERB-DRUG INTERACTION

- **Diuretics:** *Ze Lan* has diuretic action. Though this potential interaction has not been documented, concurrent use with diuretic drugs may lead to increased elimination of water and/or electrolytes.[4] [Note: Examples of diuretics include chlorothiazide, hydrochlorothiazide, furosemide (Lasix), bumetanide (Bumex), and torsemide (Demadex).]

Ze Lan (Herba Lycopi)

References

1. *Xian Dai Zhong Yao Yao Li Xue* (Contemporary Pharmacology of Chinese Herbs), 1997; 934
2. *Zhong Yao Xue* (Chinese Herbology), 1998; 578:579
3. *Zhong Yi Za Zhi* (Journal of Chinese Medicine), 1981; 1:17
4. Chen, J. Recognition & prevention of herb-drug interactions, *Medical Acupuncture*, Fall/Winter 1998/1999; volume 10/number 2; 9-13

Chuan Niu Xi (Radix Cyathulae)

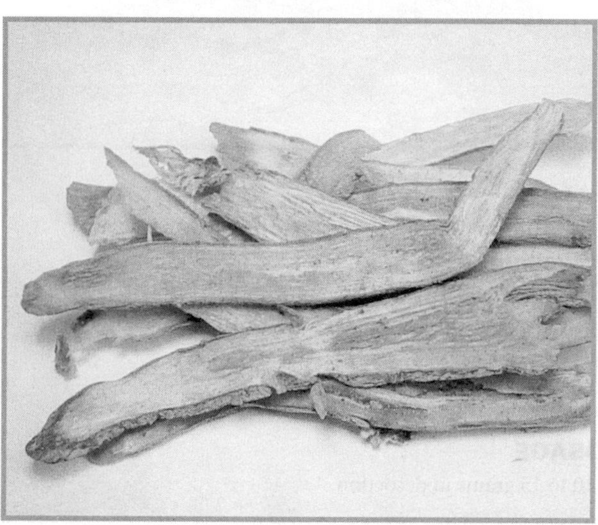

川牛膝

Pinyin Name: *Chuan Niu Xi*
Literal Name: "ox knee from Sichuan," "cow's knee from Sichuan"
Alternate Chinese Names: *Niu Xi, Ma Niu Xi*
Original Source: *Shen Nong Ben Cao Jing* (Divine Husbandman's Classic of the Materia Medica) in the second century
English Name: cyathula, medicinal cyathula root
Botanical Name: *Cyathula officinalis* Kuan. (*Chuan Niu Xi*); *Cyathula capitata* (Wall.) Moq. (*Ma Niu Xi*)
Pharmaceutical Name: Radix Cyathulae
Properties: bitter, sour, neutral
Channels Entered: Liver, Kidney

CHINESE THERAPEUTIC ACTIONS

1. Activates Blood Circulation, Dispels Blood Stasis

Gynecological disorders: *Chuan Niu Xi* (Radix Cyathulae) is one of the stronger blood-activating herbs for treatment of disorders characterized by blood stasis, such as menstrual pain, irregular menstruation, amenorrhea, and postpartum abdominal pain.

- Gynecological disorders: *Chuan Niu Xi* is often combined with *Hong Hua* (Flos Carthami), *Dang Gui* (Radicis Angelicae Sinensis) and *Tao Ren* (Semen Persicae).
- Difficult labor: use this herb with *Dang Gui* (Radicis Angelicae Sinensis), *Chuan Xiong* (Rhizoma Ligustici Chuanxiong) and *Gui Ban* (Plastrum Testudinis).

Musculoskeletal pain due to external and sports injuries: *Chuan Niu Xi* dispels stasis and is commonly used for musculoskeletal pain.

- Musculoskeletal pain: use this herb with *Hong Hua* (Flos Carthami), *Ru Xiang* (Gummi Olibanum) and *Mo Yao* (Myrrha).

2. Promotes Urination, Treats Dysuria

Hematuria, dysuria: *Chuan Niu Xi* dispels damp-heat and eliminates blood stasis in the lower *jiao* to treat burning sensations and pain on urination.

- Hematuria with burning sensations and pain during urination: combine this herb with *Dang Gui* (Radicis Angelicae Sinensis), *Qu Mai* (Herba Dianthi), and *Hua Shi* (Talcum).

3. Directs Fire and Blood Downwards

Abnormal bleeding caused by fire flaring upwards: Clinical applications include hematemesis, epistaxis, toothache, ulceration of the mouth and tongue, headache and dizziness. Furthermore, *Chuan Niu Xi* tonifies the Liver and Kidney yin to help anchor Liver yang and prevent Liver wind from rising upwards.

- Hematemesis and epistaxis: add this herb to *Xiao Ji* (Herba Cirisii), *Bai Mao Gen* (Rhizoma Imperatae), and *Zhi Zi* (Fructus Gardeniae).
- Toothache or ulcerations of the tongue and mouth from yin-deficient fire: use *Chuan Niu Xi* with *Shu Di Huang* (Radix Rehmanniae Preparata), *Zhi Mu* (Radix Anemarrhenae) and *Shi Gao* (Gypsum Fibrosum).

Chuan Niu Xi (Radix Cyathulae)

Exemplar Formula: *Yu Nu Jian* (Jade Woman Decoction).

- Liver yang and Liver wind rising: use it with *Dai Zhe Shi* (Haematitum), *Mu Li* (Concha Ostreae) and *Gui Ban* (Plastrum Testudinis). **Exemplar Formula:** *Zhen Gan Xi Feng Tang* (Sedate the Liver and Extinguish Wind Decoction).

4. Tonifies the Liver and Kidney, Strengthens Tendons and Bones

Lower back and knee soreness, weakness and pain: Tendons and bones are tissues controlled by the Liver and the Kidney, respectively. *Chuan Niu Xi* treats soreness and pain in the muscles and joints by tonifying both Liver and Kidney and strengthening their respective tissues. It is one of the most important and effective herbs for chronic pain in the lower body, such as lumbago and weak knees.

- Weakness of the low back and knees: combine *Chuan Niu Xi* with *Shu Di Huang* (Radix Rehmanniae Preparata), *Gui Ban* (Plastrum Testudinis), *Du Zhong* (Cortex Eucommiae) and *Suo Yang* (Herba Cynomorii).
- Redness, swelling and pain in lower body joints because of damp-heat: use this herb with *Cang Zhu* (Rhizoma Atractylodis), *Huang Bai* (Cortex Phellodendri) and *Yi Yi Ren* (Semen Coicis). **Exemplar Formula:** *Er Miao San* (Two-Marvel Powder).
- Joint pain in the lower body from wind and dampness: use it with *Mu Gua* (Fructus Chaenomelis), *Fen Fang Ji* (Radix Stephaniae Tetandrae), and *Bi Xie* (Rhizoma Dioscoreae Hypoglaucae).

DOSAGE

10 to 15 grams in herbal decoction.

CAUTIONS / CONTRAINDICATIONS

- *Chuan Niu Xi* is contraindicated during pregnancy and in cases of profuse menstrual bleeding.

CHEMICAL COMPOSITION

Cyasterone, isocyasterone, 5-epicyasterone, sengosterone, amerasterone A, amerasterone B, capitasterone, poststerone, ecdysterone, crustecdysone, and precyasterone.[1]

PHARMACOLOGICAL EFFECTS

- **Effect on pregnancy:** Administration of *Chuan Niu Xi* in mice at the dosage of 250 to 500 mg/kg for up to 20 days is associated with a decreased percentage of fertilization and an increased risk of miscarriage.[2]

CLINICAL STUDIES AND RESEARCH

- **Uterine bleeding:** According to one report, 23 patients with profuse uterine bleeding were treated with a decoction of *Chuan Niu Xi* at a dosage of 30 to 45 grams. Bleeding stopped in most patients after 2 to 4 days. Patients continued to take the herbs at a lower dose for 5 to 10 more days as maintenance.[3]
- **Acute epistaxis:** Acute nosebleeds in 110 patients were treated with an herbal preparation for up to 10 doses with 100% effectiveness. The herbal preparation contained *Niu Xi* (Radix Cyathulae seu Achyranthis), *Dai Zhe Shi* (Haematitum), and *Xian He Cao* (Herba Agrimoniae).[4]

SUPPLEMENT

- 牛膝 / 牛膝 *Niu Xi* (Radix Cyathulae seu Achyranthis) is the collective name that refers to *Chuan Niu Xi* (Radix Cyathulae) and *Huai Niu Xi* (Radix Achyranthis Bidentatae), since many classic texts did not make any specific differentiation of these two herbs.

AUTHORS' COMMENTS

Chuan Niu Xi (Radix Cyathulae) and *Huai Niu Xi* (Radix Achyranthis Bidentatae) have very similar functions and indications. *Chuan Niu Xi* is stronger in activating blood circulation, eliminating blood stasis, promoting urination, and draining heat downwards. Therefore, *Chuan Niu Xi* is commonly used to treat pain disorders characterized by blood stasis, gynecological disorders, dysuria, and various bleeding disorders caused by heat and fire. *Huai Niu Xi*, on the other hand, is stronger in tonifying the Liver and Kidney and strengthening the tendons and bones. Therefore, *Huai Niu Xi* is commonly used to treat pain disorders of the lower body characterized by weakness and deficiency, especially of the lower back and knees.

As stated above, many classic texts use the term "*Niu Xi*" without specifying either *Chuan Niu Xi* (Radix Cyathulae) or *Huai Niu Xi* (Radix Achyranthis Bidentatae). Thus, although the two herbs are presented in separate monographs in this text, some generic information on "*Niu Xi*" is duplicated in both monographs. The distinction between the two is to be found in the relative potencies of their individual therapeutic actions, which are listed from most potent to least, in each case.

According to Dr. Zhang Liang-Lin, *Chuan Niu Xi* and *Fen Fang Ji* (Radix Stephaniae Tetandrae) treat the lower back soreness and pain associated with dysmenorrhea.

References

1. *Chang Yong Zhong Yao Cheng Fen Yu Yao Li Shou Ce* (A Handbook of the Composition and Pharmacology of Common Chinese Drugs), 1994; 411-412
2. *Xi An Yi Ke Da Xue Xue Bao* (Journal of Xian University School of Medicine), 1990; 11(1):27
3. *Zhe Jiang Zhong Yi Za Zhi* (Zhejiang Journal of Chinese Medicine), 1982; 17(2):86
4. Ibid., 1984; 19(7):305

Huai Niu Xi (Radix Achyranthis Bidentatae)

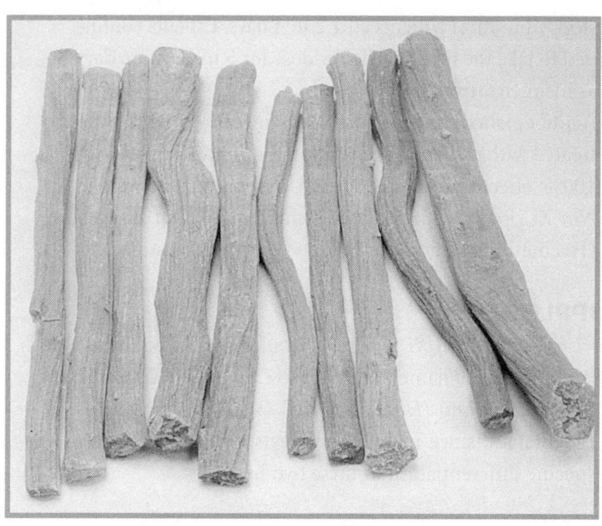

淮牛膝 淮牛膝

Pinyin Name: *Huai Niu Xi*
Literal Name: "ox knee from Huai," "cow's knee from Huai"
Alternate Chinese Names: *Niu Xi*
Original Source: *Shen Nong Ben Cao Jing* (Divine Husbandman's Classic of the Materia Medica) in the second century
English Name: achyranthes root
Botanical Name: *Achyranthes bidentata* Blume (*Huai Niu Xi*)
Pharmaceutical Name: Radix Achyranthis Bidentatae
Properties: bitter, sour, neutral
Channels Entered: Liver, Kidney

CHINESE THERAPEUTIC ACTIONS

1. Tonifies the Liver and Kidney, Strengthens Tendons and Bones

Lower back and knee soreness, weakness and pain: The tendons and bones are tissues controlled by the Liver and the Kidney, respectively. *Huai Niu Xi* (Radix Achyranthis Bidentatae) treats soreness and pain in the muscles and joints by tonifying both the Liver and Kidney and strengthening their respective tissues. It is one of the most important and effective herbs for chronic pain in the lower body, such as lumbago and weak knees.

- Weakness of the low back and knees: use *Huai Niu Xi* with *Shu Di Huang* (Radix Rehmanniae Preparata), *Gui Ban* (Plastrum Testudinis), *Du Zhong* (Cortex Eucommiae) and *Suo Yang* (Herba Cynomorii).
- Redness, swelling and pain of lower body joints caused by damp-heat: combine this herb with *Cang Zhu* (Rhizoma Atractylodis), *Huang Bai* (Cortex Phellodendri) and *Yi Yi Ren* (Semen Coicis). **Exemplar Formula:** *Er Miao San* (Two-Marvel Powder).
- Joint pain in lower body due to wind and dampness: add *Mu Gua* (Fructus Chaenomelis), *Fen Fang Ji* (Radix Stephaniae Tetandrae), and *Bi Xie* (Rhizoma Dioscoreae Hypoglaucae).

2. Activates Blood Circulation, Dispels Blood Stasis

Gynecological disorders: *Huai Niu Xi* is one of the stronger blood-activating herbs, treating various disorders characterized by blood stasis, such as menstrual pain, irregular menstruation, amenorrhea and postpartum abdominal pain.

- Gynecological disorders such as menstrual pain, irregular menstruation, amenorrhea, and postpartum abdominal pain: use *Huai Niu Xi* with *Hong Hua* (Flos Carthami), *Dang Gui* (Radicis Angelicae Sinensis) and *Tao Ren* (Semen Persicae).

Difficult labor: combine *Huai Niu Xi* with *Dang Gui* (Radicis Angelicae Sinensis), *Chuan Xiong* (Rhizoma Ligustici Chuanxiong) and *Gui Ban* (Plastrum Testudinis).

Musculoskeletal pain due to external and sports injuries: *Huai Niu Xi* dispels stasis and is commonly used for musculoskeletal pain.

- Musculoskeletal pain due to external and sports injuries: use this herb with *Hong Hua* (Flos Carthami), *Ru Xiang* (Gummi Olibanum) and *Mo Yao* (Myrrha).

3. Promotes Urination, Treats Dysuria

Hematuria, dysuria: *Huai Niu Xi* dispels damp-heat and eliminates blood stasis in the lower *jiao,* to treat burning sensations and pain on urination.

- Hematuria with burning sensations and pain during urination: use *Huai Niu Xi* with *Dang Gui* (Radicis Angelicae Sinensis), *Qu Mai* (Herba Dianthi), and *Hua Shi* (Talcum).

4. Directs Fire and Blood Downwards

Abnormal bleeding because of fire flaring upwards: Clinical applications include hematemesis, epistaxis, toothache, ulcerations of the mouth and tongue, headache and dizziness. Furthermore, *Huai Niu Xi* tonifies Liver and Kidney yin help to anchor Liver yang and prevent Liver wind from rising upwards.

- Hematemesis and epistaxis: use this herb with *Xiao Ji* (Herba Cirisii), *Bai Mao Gen* (Rhizoma Imperatae), and *Zhi Zi* (Fructus Gardeniae).

Huai Niu Xi (Radix Achyranthis Bidentatae)

- Toothache or ulcerations of the tongue and mouth from yin-deficient fire: combine *Huai Niu Xi* with *Shu Di Huang* (Radix Rehmanniae Preparata), *Zhi Mu* (Radix Anemarrhenae) and *Shi Gao* (Gypsum Fibrosum). **Exemplar Formula:** *Yu Nu Jian* (Jade Woman Decoction).
- Liver yang and Liver wind rising: use it with *Dai Zhe Shi* (Haematitum), *Mu Li* (Concha Ostreae) and *Gui Ban* (Plastrum Testudinis) to nourish yin and anchor yang. **Exemplar Formula:** *Zhen Gan Xi Feng Tang* (Sedate the Liver and Extinguish Wind Decoction).

DOSAGE

10 to 15 grams in herbal decoction. Frying *Huai Niu Xi* with grain-based liquor enhances its effectiveness to invigorate blood circulation and open the channels and collaterals. Frying the herb with salt enables it to more readily enter the Kidney, and increases its potency to strengthen bones and tendons.

CAUTIONS / CONTRAINDICATIONS

- *Huai Niu Xi* is contraindicated during pregnancy, and in cases of profuse menstrual bleeding.

CHEMICAL COMPOSITION

Ecdysterone, inoteosterone, inokosterone, α-aminobutyric acid, betaine.[1,2]

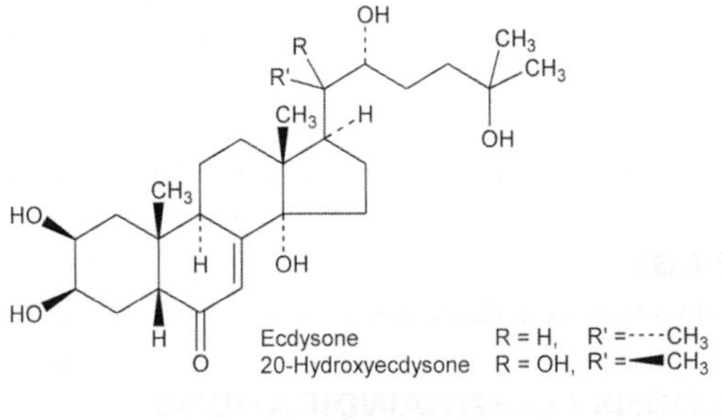

Ecdysone R = H, R' = ----CH3
20-Hydroxyecdysone R = OH, R' = ◄CH3

Ecdysteroids

PHARMACOLOGICAL EFFECTS

- **Analgesic and anti-inflammatory:** Administration of *Huai Niu Xi* via intravenous, intraperitoneal, subcutaneous and oral routes have all demonstrated marked analgesic and anti-inflammatory effects in laboratory animals.[3]
- **Cardiovascular:** Decoction of *Huai Niu Xi* is associated with a mild hypotensive effect with a short duration of action.[4]
- **Uterine stimulant:** It has a stimulating effect on smooth muscle and leads to uterine contraction in rats and rabbits.[5]
- **Effect on pregnancy:** Administration of *Huai Niu Xi* in mice at the dosage of 250 to 500 mg/kg for up to 20 days is associated with a decreased percentage of fertilization and an increased risk of miscarriage.[6]

CLINICAL STUDIES AND RESEARCH

- **Dilation of cervical os:** Use of *Huai Niu Xi* was associated with marked dilation of the cervical os in 78 women who had abortions.[7]
- **Galacturia:** According to one report, 21 patients with galacturia were treated with a *Huai Niu Xi* preparation two to three times daily for 6 doses with marked improvement in 14, moderate improvement in 4, and no response in 3 patients. After the initial treatment, patients were placed on general tonic formulas for maintenance.[8]

TOXICOLOGY

The LD_{50} via intraperitoneal injection in mice is 6.4 g/kg for ecdysterone and 7.8 g/kg for inoteosterone. The LD_{50} in mice via oral administration for the combination of ecdysterone and inoteosterone is 9 g/kg. Oral administration of *Huai Niu Xi* decoction at the dosage of 60 g/kg/day for 30 days did not result in any abnormalities on examination of the blood, or of the liver, kidney, or other internal organs.[9,10]

SUPPLEMENT

- 土牛膝 / 土牛膝 *Tu Niu Xi* (Radix Achyranthes Longifolia), first cited in *Tu Jing Ben Cao* (Illustrated Classic of the Materia Medica) by Su Song in 1061, is bitter, sour and neutral. The botanical names for this herb are *Achyranthes longifolia* Mak. or *Achyranthes aspera* L. It activates blood circulation, dispels blood stasis, clears heat, eliminates toxins and promotes urination. Common applications include amenorrhea, arthritis, throat swelling and pain, diphtheria, edema of the lower extremities, hematuria and trauma-related pain. The dosage for *Tu Niu Xi* is 10 to 15 grams.

AUTHORS' COMMENTS

Please refer to *Chuan Niu Xi* (Radix Cyathulae) for a description of similarities and differences between *Huai Niu Xi* (Radix Achyranthis Bidentatae).

References

1. *Xian Dai Zhong Yao Yao Li Xue* (Contemporary Pharmacology of Chinese Herbs), 1997; 905
2. *The Merck Index* 12th edition, Chapman & Hall/CRCnetBASE/Merck, 2000
3. *Zhong Yao Tong Bao* (Journal of Chinese Herbology), 1988; 13(7):43
4. *Shang Hai Zhong Yi Yao Za Zhi* (Shanghai Journal of Chinese Medicine and Herbology), 1965; (3):31
5. *Zhong Cao Yao* (Chinese Herbal Medicine), 1987; 18(4):17
6. *Xi An Yi Ke Da Xue Xue Bao* (Journal of Xian University School of Medicine), 1987; 8(3):246
7. *Jiang Su Zhong Yi* (Jiangsu Chinese Medicine), 1963; 1:23
8. *Shan Dong Zhong Yi Za Zhi* (Shandong Journal of Chinese Medicine), 1989; 6:40
9. *Zhong Yao Yao Li Yu Ying Yong* (Pharmacology and Applications of Chinese Herbs), 1983:198
10. *Yao Xue Tong Bao* (Report of Herbology), 1988; 23(11):666

Ma Bian Cao (Herba Verbenae)

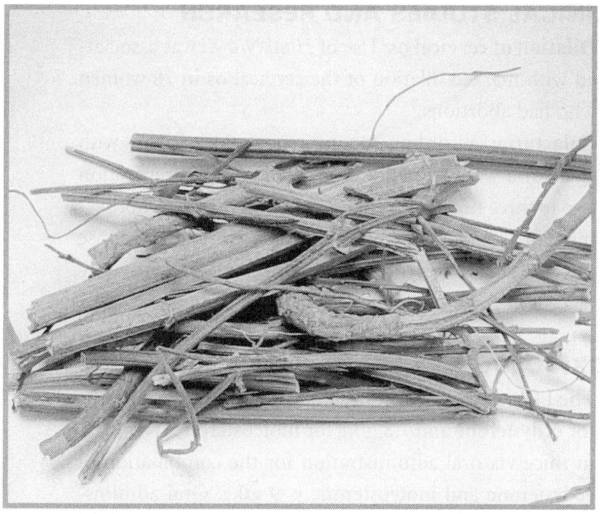

馬鞭草 马鞭草

Pinyin Name: *Ma Bian Cao*
Literal Name: "horse whip herb"
Alternate Chinese Names: *Long Ya Cao, Feng Jing Cao, Zi Ding Long Ya*
Original Source: *Ming Yi Za Zhu* (Miscellaneous Records of Famous Physicians) by Tao Hong-Jing in 500 A.D.
English Name: verbena, European verbena
Botanical Name: *Verbena officinalis* L. (*Ma Bian Cao*)
Pharmaceutical Name: Herba Verbenae
Properties: bitter, cool
Channels Entered: Liver, Spleen

CHINESE THERAPEUTIC ACTIONS

1. Activates Blood Circulation, Disperses Blood Stagnation

Blood stagnation: *Ma Bian Cao* (Herba Verbenae) enters *xue* (blood) level to treat amenorrhea, dysmenorrhea, abdominal masses, joint soreness and pain, pain from traumatic injuries, mass accumulation, and other disorders involving blood stagnation.

- Amenorrhea and dysmenorrhea: use this herb with *Xiang Fu* (Rhizoma Cyperi) and *Yi Mu Cao* (Herba Leonuri).
- Abdominal masses: combine it with *San Leng* (Rhizoma Sparganii) and *E Zhu* (Rhizoma Curcumae).
- Joint pain and traumatic injuries: add it to *Ru Xiang* (Gummi Olibanum), *Mo Yao* (Myrrha), *Hong Hua* (Flos Carthami) and *Yan Hu Suo* (Rhizoma Corydalis).

2. Clears Heat and Eliminates Toxins

Toxic heat: *Ma Bian Cao* treats various presentations of toxic heat, such as sores and carbuncles, swollen and painful gums, sore throat, and diarrhea due to damp-heat. Fresh *Ma Bian Cao* is often used topically for this purpose.

- Carbuncles and sores: use *Ma Bian Cao* with *Pu Gong Ying* (Herba Taraxaci), *Zi Hua Di Ding* (Herba Violae) and *Ye Ju Hua* (Flos Chrysanthemi Indici).
- Swollen and painful gums: combine it with *Shi Gao* (Gypsum Fibrosum) and *Zhi Mu* (Radix Anemarrhenae).
- Sore throat: use with *She Gan* (Rhizoma Belamcandae), *Shan Dou Gen* (Radix Sophorae Tonkinensis) and *Ma Bo* (Lasiosphaera seu Calvatia).
- Diarrhea or dysentery: add this herb to *Bai Tou Weng* (Radix Pulsatillae) and *Qin Pi* (Cortex Fraxini).

3. Treats Malaria

Use 30 grams of *Ma Bian Cao* 2 to 4 hours before the onset of malaria symptoms.

4. Promotes Diuresis and Reduces Edema

Ma Bian Cao is also used for treatment of edema, ascites and water accumulation during the late stages of parasitic infections.

- Edema and leg *qi*: use this herb with *Mu Gua* (Fructus Chaenomelis) and *Niu Xi* (Radix Cyathulae seu Achyranthis).
- Ascites: combine it with *Liu Ji Nu* (Herba Artemisiae Anomalae) and *Ban Bian Lian* (Herba Lobeliae Chinensis).

DOSAGE

15 to 30 grams in decoction.

CAUTIONS / CONTRAINDICATIONS

- *Ma Bian Cao* should be used with caution during pregnancy.

CHEMICAL COMPOSITION

Verbenalin, cornin, verbenol, stachyose, adenosine.[1,2]

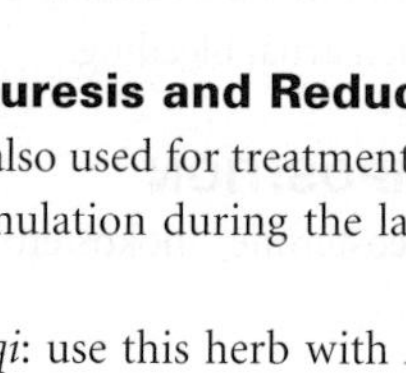

Verbenalin

References

1. *Xian Dai Zhong Yao Yao Li Xue* (Contemporary Pharmacology of Chinese Herbs), 1997; 721
2. *The Merck Index* 12th edition, Chapman & Hall/CRCnetBASE/Merck, 2000

Jin Bu Huan (Herba Lycopodii Serrati)

金不換 金不换

Pinyin Name: *Jin Bu Huan*
Literal Name: "will not exchange for gold"
Alternate Chinese Names: *Qian Ceng Ta, Qi Chun Jin*
English Name: lycopodium
Botanical Name: *Lycopodium serratum* Thunb.
Pharmaceutical Name: Herba Lycopodii Serrati
Properties: acrid, sweet, neutral
Channels Entered: Lung, Liver, Large Intestine

CHINESE THERAPEUTIC ACTIONS

1. Disperses Blood Stagnation, Invigorates Blood Circulation and Stops Bleeding

Blood stagnation: *Jin Bu Huan* (Herba Lycopodii Serrati) treats blood-stagnation disorders including traumatic injuries, tendon pain and irregular menstruation due to blood stagnation.

- Traumatic injuries: use *Jin Bu Huan* with *Hong Hua* (Flos Carthami), *Ze Lan* (Herba Lycopi), *Dang Gui* (Radicis Angelicae Sinensis), *San Qi* (Radix Notoginseng), *Xiang Fu* (Rhizoma Cyperi), *Su Mu* (Lignum Sappan), *Yu Jin* (Radix Curcumae), *Yan Hu Suo* (Rhizoma Corydalis), and *Bai Shao* (Radix Paeoniae Alba).
- Tendon and bone pain: combine *Jin Bu Huan* with *Tao Ren* (Semen Persicae), *Sheng Di Huang* (Radix Rehmanniae), *Dang Gui* (Radicis Angelicae Sinensis), *Bai Zhi* (Radix Angelicae Dahuricae), *Shen Jin Cao* (Herba Lycopodii) and *Hong Hua* (Flos Carthami).
- Irregular menstruation: add this herb to *Ma Bian Cao* (Herba Verbenae), *Hong Hua* (Flos Carthami), *Tao Ren* (Semen Persicae), *Chi Shao* (Radix Paeoniae Rubrae), *Dang Gui* (Radicis Angelicae Sinensis) and *Xiang Fu* (Rhizoma Cyperi).

2. Regulates Qi, Relieves Pain and Reduces Swelling and Abscess

- Lung abscess: use *Jin Bu Huan* with *Yu Xing Cao* (Herba Houttuyniae), *Yi Yi Ren* (Semen Coicis), *Lu Gen* (Rhizoma Phragmitis), *Da Qing Ye* (Folium Isatidis), *Yi Zhi Xiang* (Herba Vernoniae Cinereae) and *Bai Ji* (Rhizoma Bletillae).
- Hemorrhoids or hemorrhoidal bleeding: use this herb with *Huai Hua* (Flos Sophorae) and *Zao Jiao Ci* (Spina Gleditsiae).

DOSAGE

3 to 9 grams in decoction.

CAUTIONS / CONTRAINDICATIONS

- Use of *Jin Bu Huan* at a large dose may cause dizziness.

AUTHORS' COMMENTS

Jin Bu Huan literally means "will not exchange for gold," implying that the substance is so valuable that it is worth even more than gold. Because it has such a positive image and connotation, this name has been used for both the single herb and a patent product with multiple ingredients. Therefore, it is sometimes necessary to clarify whether the name "*Jin Bu Huan*" is used in reference to the single herb or the patent product.

Ye Ming Sha (Excrementum Vespertilionis Murini)

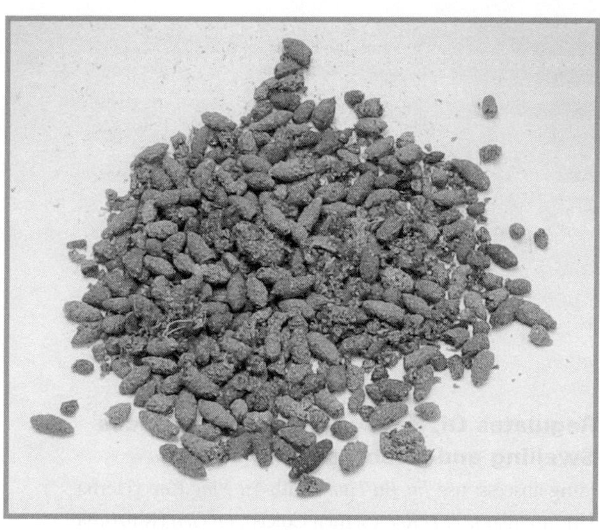

夜明砂

Pinyin Name: *Ye Ming Sha*
Literal Name: "night brightness sand"
Alternate Chinese Names: *Hei Sha Xing*
Original Source: *Shen Nong Ben Cao Jing* (Divine Husbandman's Classic of the Materia Medica) in the second century
English Name: bat droppings, bat dung
Zoological Name: *Vesperlitis superans* Thomas (*Bian Fu*)
Pharmaceutical Name: Excrementum Vespertilionis Murini
Properties: acrid, cold
Channels Entered: Liver

CHINESE THERAPEUTIC ACTIONS

1. Disperses Bruises and Resolves Stasis

Traumatic injuries: *Ye Ming Sha* (Excrementum Vespertilionis Murini) disperse bruises and removes stasis. It is commonly combined with qi- and blood-activating herbs to treat musculoskeletal injuries.

2. Clears Liver Heat and Benefits the Eyes

Redness, pain and blood suffusion in the eyes: *Ye Ming Sha* treats eye disorders characterized by Liver heat and blood stasis. Clinical applications include redness and pain in the eyes, night blindness, visual obstruction and cataracts.

- Eye disorders characterized by Liver heat and blood stasis: use 1.5 grams of *Ye Ming Sha* two times per day. It can also be used with other herbs that clear the Liver and benefit the eyes.
- Blurred vision: use this herb with *Shi Jue Ming* (Concha Haliotidis) and *Gou Qi Zi* (Fructus Lycii).
- Redness and pain in the eyes: add *Jue Ming Zi* (Semen Cassiae).

DOSAGE

3 to 10 grams in decoction, 1 to 2 grams in powder. *Ye Ming Sha* should be wrapped in cheesecloth before decoction.

CAUTIONS / CONTRAINDICATIONS

- *Ye Ming Sha* should be used with caution in patients who have eye disorders but no blood stasis.

CHEMICAL COMPOSITION

Urea, uric acid, cholesterol.[1]

CLINICAL STUDIES AND RESEARCH

- **Ocular blood suffusion:** Oral ingestion of 1.5 grams of *Ye Ming Sha* powder one to two times daily with warm water showed effectiveness in treating patients with ocular blood suffusion. It is especially effective in patients with recurrent conditions that do not respond to standard treatment.[2]

References

1. *Zhong Yao Xue* (Chinese Herbology), 1998; 595:596
2. *Zhong Yi Za Zhi* (Journal of Chinese Medicine), 1985; 8:24

Chuan Shan Jia (Squama Manis)

穿山甲

Pinyin Name: *Chuan Shan Jia*
Literal Name: "penetrate mountain scale"
Alternate Chinese Names: *Lin Li*
Original Source: *Ming Yi Za Zhu* (Miscellaneous Records of Famous Physicians) by Tao Hong-Jing in 500 A.D.
English Name: pangolin scales, anteater scales
Zoological Name: *Manis pentadactyia* L. (*Lin Li*)
Pharmaceutical Name: Squama Manis
Properties: salty, cool
Channels Entered: Liver, Stomach

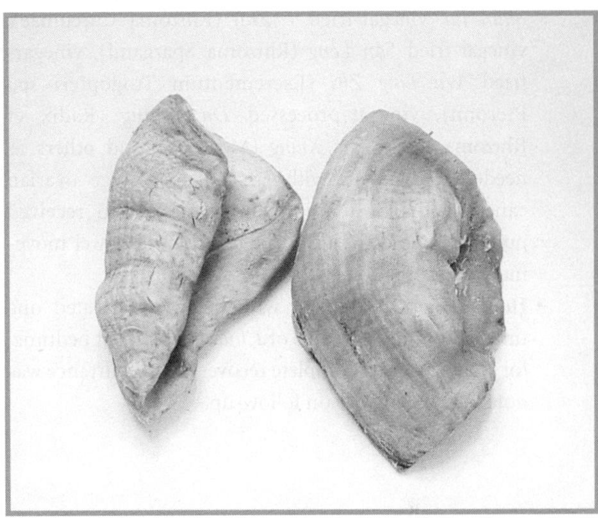

CHINESE THERAPEUTIC ACTIONS

1. Activates Blood Circulation, Opens Channels

Blood Stasis: *Chuan Shan Jia* (Squama Manis) has excellent penetrating and dispersing functions as its effects reach every organ and open every channel and collateral. Clinical applications include amenorrhea, abdominal masses, and *bi zheng* (painful obstruction syndrome).

- Amenorrhea due to blood stasis: *Chuan Shan Jia* is commonly used with *Dang Gui* (Radicis Angelicae Sinensis), *Hong Hua* (Flos Carthami) and *Chuan Xiong* (Rhizoma Ligustici Chuanxiong).
- Abdominal masses: use it with *San Leng* (Rhizoma Sparganii) and *E Zhu* (Rhizoma Curcumae).
- *Bi zheng* (painful obstruction syndrome): combine this substance with *Dang Gui* (Radicis Angelicae Sinensis), *Du Huo* (Radix Angelicae Pubescentis) and *Qiang Huo* (Rhizoma et Radix Notopterygii).

2. Promotes Lactation

Insufficient lactation: *Chuan Shan Jia* aids lactation in cases in which blood stagnation is causing insufficient flow.

- Lack of or insufficient lactation: use this herb with *Wang Bu Liu Xing* (Semen Vaccariae).

3. Reduces Swelling, Drains Pus

Sores, scrofula, goiter: *Chuan Shan Jia* is commonly used to treat various types of sores, nodules, swellings, and hardness. It is effective for sores and nodules with or without pus formation. Sores with pus are treated with herbs that drain pus and eliminate toxins. Sores without pus are treated with herbs that clear heat and eliminate toxins. Ulcerated sores with pus should not be treated with this herb. Scrofula and goiter are treated with this and other herbs that eliminate stagnation of qi and blood.

- Sores with pus: combine *Chuan Shan Jia* with *Huang Qi* (Radix Astragali), *Zao Jiao Ci* (Spina Gleditsiae) and *Dang Gui* (Radicis Angelicae Sinensis).
- Sores without pus: use this substance with *Bai Zhi* (Radix Angelicae Dahuricae), *Pu Gong Ying* (Herba Taraxaci), and *Zi Hua Di Ding* (Herba Violae).
- Scrofula or goiter due to stagnation of phlegm and qi: use it with *Xuan Shen* (Radix Scrophulariae), *Zhe Bei Mu* (Bulbus Fritillariae Thunbergii) and *Xia Ku Cao* (Spica Prunellae).

DOSAGE

3 to 10 grams in decoction, 1.0 to 1.5 grams in powder. The unprocessed form of *Chuan Shan Jia* is not suitable for decoction, as it is a hard substance and has a distinct odor. Dry-frying or vinegar-frying will eliminate the odor and facilitate the extraction of active constituents. In addition, frying the scales with vinegar facilitates the effect of dispersing stasis and relieving pain.

PHARMACOLOGICAL EFFECTS

- **Immunostimulant:** *Chuan Shan Jia* has been shown to increase the number of white blood cells.[1]
- **Hematological:** Oral administration of *Chuan Shan Jia* as decoction for 3 days significantly prolonged bleeding time in mice.[2]
- **Anti-inflammatory:** Oral administration of *Chuan Shan Jia* as decoction for one week showed significant reduction of ear inflammation in mice.[3]

CLINICAL STUDIES AND RESEARCH

- **Ovarian cancer:** Eight patients with ovarian cancer were treated with an herbal formula with satisfactory results. The formula contained herbs such as dry-fried *Chuan*

Chuan Shan Jia (Squama Manis)

Shan Jia, vinegar-fried *E Zhu* (Rhizoma Curcumae), vinegar-fried *San Leng* (Rhizoma Sparganii), vinegar-fried *Wu Ling Zhi* (Excrementum Trogopteri seu Pteromi), vinegar-processed *Da Huang* (Radix et Rhizoma Rhei), *She Xiang* (Moschus), and others as needed. Individuals with larger-than-average ovarian cancer with constipation and dysuria also received purgative and cathartic herbs to promote bowel movement and urination.[4]

- **Hematuria:** One patient with hematuria treated one time daily with 1.5 grams of *Chuan Shan Jia* at bedtime, for 3 days, showed complete recovery. No recurrence was noted for over 1 year on follow-up.[5]

TOXICOLOGY

Abdominal fullness, lack of appetite, and yellow discoloration of the eyes and body, with normal liver function, was reported in one person after ingestion of 15 to 20 grams of *Chuan Shan Jia*. The patient promptly returned to normal after symptomatic treatment with Chinese herbs.[6]

References

1. *Zhong Yao Xue* (Chinese Herbology), 1998; 570:571
2. *Chang Yong Zhong Yao Cheng Fen Yu Yao Li Shou Ce* (A Handbook of the Composition and Pharmacology of Common Chinese Drugs), 1994; 1459:1462
3. Ibid.
4. *Shan Xi Yi Yao* (Shanxi Medicine and Herbology), 1981; 3:35
5. *Ha Er Bing Zhong Yi* (Haerbing Chinese Medicine), 1964; 6:35
6. *Zhe Jiang Zhong Yi Za Zhi* (Zhejiang Journal of Chinese Medicine), 1989; 24(12):550

Wang Bu Liu Xing (Semen Vaccariae)

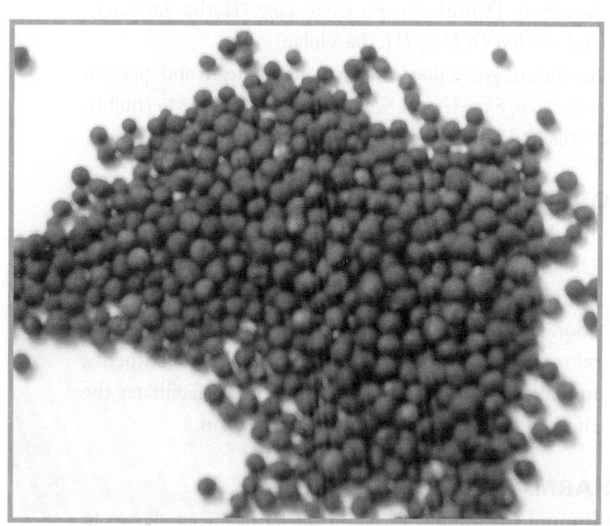

王不留行

Pinyin Name: *Wang Bu Liu Xing*
Literal Name: "king who does not stay but departs"
Alternate Chinese Names: *Liu Xing Zi, Wang Bu Liu*
Original Source: *Shen Nong Ben Cao Jing* (Divine Husbandman's Classic of the Materia Medica) in the second century
English Name: vaccaria seed, cow-herb seed, cow-fat seed, cow soapwort seed
Botanical Name: *Vaccaria segetalis* (neck.) Garcke (*Mai Lan Cai*)
Pharmaceutical Name: Semen Vaccariae
Properties: bitter, neutral
Channels Entered: Liver, Stomach

CHINESE THERAPEUTIC ACTIONS

1. Activates Blood Circulation, Opens Channels

Dysmenorrhea, amenorrhea: *Wang Bu Liu Xing* (Semen Vaccariae) has a dispersing action that treats menstrual disorders with pain and swelling caused by blood stasis and obstruction of the channels.

- Irregular menstruation, menstrual pain, and amenorrhea arising from blood stasis: use *Wang Bu Liu Xing* with *Dang Gui* (Radicis Angelicae Sinensis), *Xiang Fu* (Rhizoma Cyperi), *Hong Hua* (Flos Carthami) and *Chuan Xiong* (Rhizoma Ligustici Chuanxiong).

***Bi zheng* (painful obstruction syndrome):** *Wang Bu Liu Xing* also promotes blood circulation to open blockages in the channels and collaterals, to relieve arthritis.

- *Bi zheng*: use this herb with *Qiang Huo* (Rhizoma et Radix Notopterygii), *Du Huo* (Radix Angelicae Pubescentis), *Fang Feng* (Radix Saposhnikoviae), *Gui Zhi* (Ramulus Cinnamomi), *Hong Hua* (Flos Carthami), *Wei*

Wang Bu Liu Xing (Semen Vaccariae)

Ling Xian (Radix Clematidis), *Chi Shao* (Radix Paeoniae Rubrae) and *Ji Xue Teng* (Caulis Spatholobi).

2. Promotes Lactation, Drains Abscesses

Insufficient lactation, breast abscess: *Wang Bu Liu Xing* is commonly used to treat breast disorders. It has a dispersing function to promote lactation, and a draining action to treat abscesses and swelling of the breasts.

- Absence of lactation: use this herb with *Chuan Shan Jia* (Squama Manis).
- Insufficient lactation caused by emotional disturbances: use it with *Chuan Shan Jia* (Squama Manis), *Long Gu* (Os Draconis), *Qu Mai* (Herba Dianthi), and *Mai Men Dong* (Radix Ophiopogonis).
- Insufficient lactation from qi and blood deficiency: combine *Wang Bu Liu Xing* with *Huang Qi* (Radix Astragali) and *Dang Gui* (Radicis Angelicae Sinensis).
- Swelling and abscess of the breast: use it with *Pu Gong Ying* (Herba Taraxaci), *Lian Qiao* (Fructus Forsythiae), *Xia Ku Cao* (Spica Prunellae) and *Gua Lou Shi* (Fructus Trichosanthis).

DOSAGE

6 to 10 grams in herbal decoction. *Wang Bu Liu Xing* should be dry-fried and crushed to facilitate extraction of active constituents.

CAUTIONS / CONTRAINDICATIONS

- *Wang Bu Liu Xing* is contraindicated in pregnancy, as it stimulates contraction of the uterus.

CHEMICAL COMPOSITION

Vacsegoside, gypsogenin, vaccaroside, isosaponarin, saponaretin, vitexin, glucoronic acid, glucose, arabinose, xylose, fructose, rhamnose.[1,2]

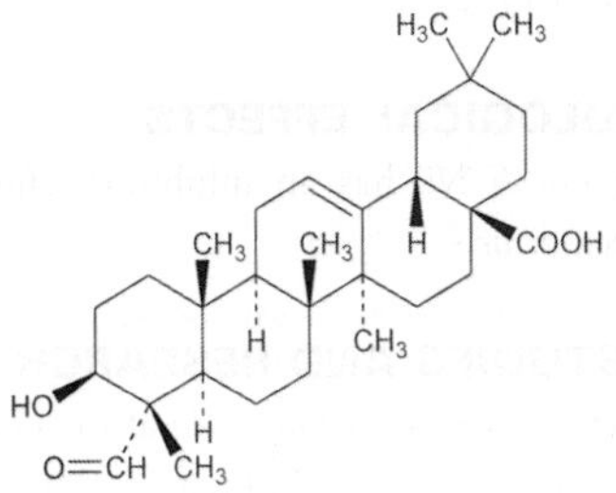

Gypsogenin

PHARMACOLOGICAL EFFECTS

- **Uterine stimulant**: Administration of *Wang Bu Liu Xing* has a stimulating effect on the uterus, as demonstrated in animal studies. The alcohol extract of the herb had a stronger effect than the water extract.[3]

CLINICAL STUDIES AND RESEARCH

- **Induction of labor:** Decoction of large dosages of *Wang Bu Liu Xing* and *Ji Xing Zi* (Semen Impatientis) was used to induce labor in 4 women with varying degrees of success. Once the desired effect was achieved, ingestion of the decoction was immediately stopped, to prevent over-stimulation of the uterus and thus minimize the possibility of adverse effects.[4]
- **Stones in the urinary tract:** In one study, 95 patients with stones in various parts of the urinary tract (from the kidneys to the bladder) were treated with an herbal decoction for an average of 89 doses, with an 88.4% rate of effectiveness. The herbal formula contained *Wang Bu Liu Xing*, *Ji Xing Zi* (Semen Impatientis), *Chuan Niu Xi* (Radix Cyathulae), *Zhi Ke* (Fructus Aurantii), *Ji Nei Jin* (Endothelium Corneum Gigeriae Galli), *Shi Wei* (Folium Pyrrosiae), and *Bian Xu* (Herba Polygoni Avicularis).

TOXICOLOGY

Administration of *Wang Bu Liu Xing* was associated with one incident of increased photosensitivity in which the patient reported dermatitis, and swelling and edema and of the skin after prolonged exposure to the sun.[5]

References

1. *Xian Dai Zhong Yao Yao Li Xue* (Contemporary Pharmacology of Chinese Herbs), 1997; 933
2. *The Merck Index* 12th edition, Chapman & Hall/CRCnetBASE/Merck, 2000
3. *Zhong Yao Xue* (Chinese Herbology), 1998; 582:584
4. *An Hui Zhong Yi Xue Yuan Xue Bao* (Journal of Anhui University School of Medicine), 1986; 5(3):33
5. *Zhong Hua Pi Fu Ke Xue Za Zhi* (Chinese Journal of Dermatology), 1991; (4):281

Liu Ji Nu (Herba Artemisiae Anomalae)

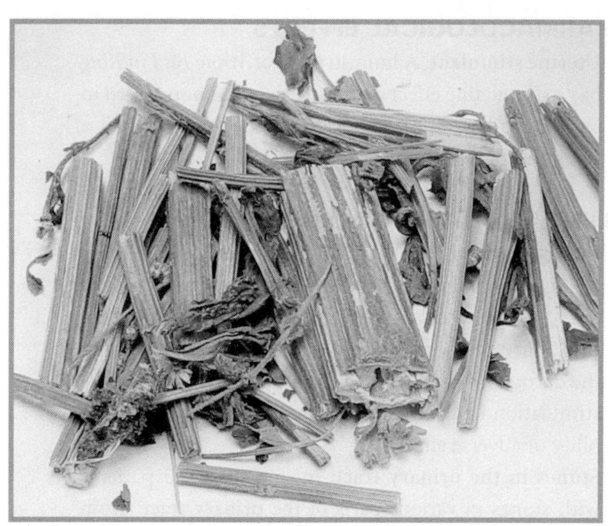

劉寄奴 刘寄奴

Pinyin Name: *Liu Ji Nu*
Literal Name: "Liu's resident slave"
Alternate Chinese Names: *Hua Shi Dan, Nan Liu Ji Nu*
Original Source: *Xin Xiu Ben Cao* (Newly Revised Materia Medica) by Su Jing in 657-659 A.D.
English Name: artemisiae anomalae
Botanical Name: *Artemisia anomala* S. Moore (*Qi Hao*)
Pharmaceutical Name: Herba Artemisiae Anomalae
Properties: bitter, warm
Channels Entered: Heart, Spleen

CHINESE THERAPEUTIC ACTIONS

1. Breaks Up Blood Stasis, Opens Channels

Amenorrhea, postpartum abdominal pain: *Liu Ji Nu* (Herba Artemisiae Anomalae) treats severe cases of blood stasis. Clinical applications include amenorrhea and abdominal pain.

- Amenorrhea or postpartum abdominal pain: use *Liu Ji Nu* with *Dang Gui* (Radicis Angelicae Sinensis), *Chuan Xiong* (Rhizoma Ligustici Chuanxiong), *Chi Shao* (Radix Paeoniae Rubrae) and *Hong Hua* (Flos Carthami).

2. Disperses Blood Stagnation and Relieves Pain

Liu Ji Nu treats blood stagnation both externally and internally.

- External and traumatic injuries: use *Liu Ji Nu* with *Dang Gui* (Radicis Angelicae Sinensis), *Tao Ren* (Semen Persicae) and *Hong Hua* (Flos Carthami).
- External or traumatic injuries with severe pain and blood stasis: use this herb with *Yan Hu Suo* (Rhizoma Corydalis) and *Gu Sui Bu* (Rhizoma Drynariae).
- Bleeding due to cuts: apply powdered *Liu Ji Nu* topically.
- Hepatomegaly or hepatitis: use it with *Chai Hu* (Radix Bupleuri), *Huang Qin* (Radix Scutellariae), *Zao Jiao Ci* (Spina Gleditsiae), *Hu Zhang* (Rhizoma Polygoni Cuspidati), *Bai Ji Li* (Fructus Tribuli), *Hong Hua* (Flos Carthami), *Ze Xie* (Rhizoma Alismatis), *Bing Lang* (Semen Arecae) and *Qian Cao* (Radix Rubiae).

3. Promotes Digestion, Eliminates Food Stagnation

Abdominal pain due to food stagnation: Aromatic in nature, *Liu Ji Nu* awakens the Spleen and Stomach to promote digestion and eliminate food stagnation. It treats the epigastric and abdominal distention and pain of indigestion.

- Indigestion: use *Liu Ji Nu* individually.
- Indigestion with food stasis: use this herb with *Shan Zha* (Fructus Crataegi), *Mai Ya* (Fructus Hordei Germinatus), *Ji Nei Jin* (Endothelium Corneum Gigeriae Galli), *Zhi Shi* (Fructus Aurantii Immaturus) and *Hou Po* (Cortex Magnoliae Officinalis).

DOSAGE

3 to 10 grams in herbal decoction.

CAUTIONS / CONTRAINDICATIONS

- *Liu Ji Nu* is contraindicated during pregnancy.

CHEMICAL COMPOSITION

Essential oils 0.45%.[1]

PHARMACOLOGICAL EFFECTS

- **Antibiotic:** *Liu Ji Nu* has an inhibitory effect against *Bacillus dysenteriae*.[2]

CLINICAL STUDIES AND RESEARCH

- **Heat stroke:** Decoction of *Liu Ji Nu* at the dosage of 50 to 100 grams was successful in treating 16 patients with mild, moderate or severe heat stroke.[3]
- **Bacterial dysentery:** Administration of *Liu Ji Nu* as pills four times daily for 5 days was effective in treating 34 patients with bacterial dysentery. The pills were made from water extract of the herb, with each dose containing 6 grams of dried herb. There was no recurrence of symptoms after one to three months of follow up.[4]

Liu Ji Nu (Herba Artemisiae Anomalae)

References
1. *Chang Yong Zhong Yao Xian Dai Yan Jiu Yu Lin Chuan* (Recent Study & Clinical Application of Common Traditional Chinese Medicine), 1995; 427-428
2. *Lin Chuan Zhong Yao Xue* (Clinical Chinese Pharmacology), 1989; 81:82
3. *Jiang Xi Zhong Yi Yao* (Jiangxi Chinese Medicine and Herbology), 1982; 3:23
4. *Shang Hai Zhong Yi Yao Za Zhi* (Shanghai Journal of Chinese Medicine and Herbology), 1983; 1:21

Su Mu (Lignum Sappan)

蘇木 苏木

Pinyin Name: *Su Mu*
Alternate Chinese Names: *Su Fang Mu*
Original Source: *Xin Xiu Ben Cao* (Newly Revised Materia Medica) by Su Jing in 657-659 A.D.
English Name: sappan wood
Botanical Name: *Caesalpinia sappan* L. (*Su Mu*)
Pharmaceutical Name: Lignum Sappan
Properties: sweet, salty, slightly acrid, neutral
Channels Entered: Heart, Liver, Spleen

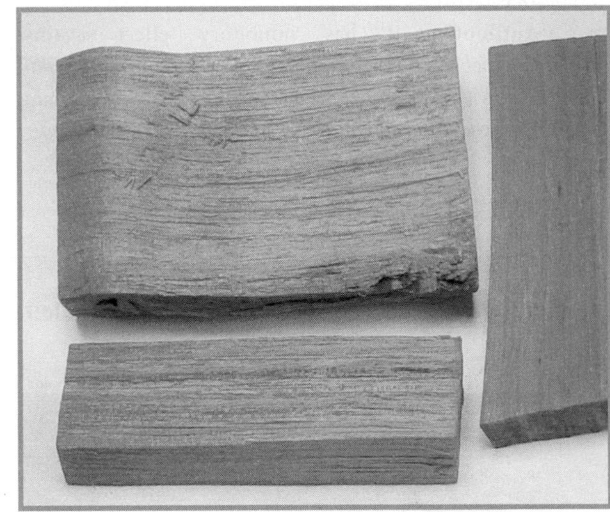

CHINESE THERAPEUTIC ACTIONS

1. Activates Blood Circulation, Dispels Blood Stasis, Opens Channels and Relieves Pain

Amenorrhea, postpartum abdominal pain: *Su Mu* (Lignum Sappan) treats various disorders characterized by blood stasis and pain. It enters the *xue* (blood) level and eliminates blood stasis to relieve amenorrhea and postpartum abdominal pain.

- Amenorrhea and postpartum abdominal pain: use *Su Mu* with *Hong Hua* (Flos Carthami), *Dang Gui* (Radicis Angelicae Sinensis) and *Chi Shao* (Radix Paeoniae Rubrae).

Traumatic injuries, paralysis, chest and abdominal pain: *Su Mu* opens the peripheral channels and collaterals to relieve pain associated with paralysis, and with external or traumatic injuries.

- External or traumatic injuries: combine it with *Ru Xiang* (Gummi Olibanum), *Mo Yao* (Myrrha), and *Xue Jie* (Sanguis Draconis).
- Paralysis, hemiplegia: use this herb with *Fang Feng* (Radix Saposhnikoviae), *Sang Zhi* (Ramulus Mori), *Hong Hua* (Flos Carthami), *Chi Shao* (Radix Paeoniae Rubrae), *Di Long* (Pheretima), *Jiang Huang* (Rhizoma Curcumae Longae), and *Dan Nan Xing* (Arisaema cum Bile).
- Chest and abdominal pain: use it with *Gua Lou Shi* (Fructus Trichosanthis), *Xie Bai* (Bulbus Allii Macrostemonis), *Tan Xiang* (Lignum Santali Albi), *Wu Ling Zhi* (Excrementum Trogopteri seu Pteromi), *Hong Hua* (Flos Carthami), *Pu Huang* (Pollen Typhae), *Yuan Zhi* (Radix Polygalae) and *Bing Lang* (Semen Arecae).

DOSAGE

3 to 10 grams in decoction. The maximum dose of *Su Mu* is 15 grams.

CAUTIONS / CONTRAINDICATIONS

- *Su Mu* is contraindicated during pregnancy.

CHEMICAL COMPOSITION

Brazilin, brasilein, sappanin, a-1-phellandrene, ocimene.[1]

Su Mu (Lignum Sappan)

PHARMACOLOGICAL EFFECTS

- **Anti-inflammatory:** Brazilin has an anti-inflammatory effect, as demonstrated in animal studies.[2]
- **Cardiovascular:** Decoction of *Su Mu* has a positive inotropic effect on frog heart specimens.[3]
- **CNS suppressant:** *Su Mu* has sedative and hypnotic effects when administered via oral routes to mice, rabbits and guinea pigs. It counteracts seizures induced by strychnine.[4]
- **Antineoplastic:** Extract of *Su Mu* has demonstrated marked effectiveness in killing cancer cells in mice and prolonging life expectancy of those with cancer by 185%.[5]
- **Antibiotic:** It has inhibitory effect against *Corynebacterium diphtheriae*, *Salmonella typhi*, *Staphylococcus aureus*, β-hemolytic streptococcus, and *Diplococcus pneumoniae*.[6]

TOXICOLOGY

The LD_{50} for water extract of *Su Mu* in mice via intraperitoneal injection is 18.9 ml/kg.[7]

References

1. *Xian Dai Zhong Yao Yao Li Xue* (Contemporary Pharmacology of Chinese Herbs), 1997; 935-936
2. *Zhi Wu Yao You Xiao Cheng Fen Shou Ce* (Manual of Plant Medicinals and Their Active Constituents), 1986; 137
3. *Phytochemistry*, 1985; 33(8):3545
4. *Zhong Cao Yao Xue* (Study of Chinese Herbal Medicine), 1976; 483
5. *Zhong Guo Zhong Yao Za Zhi* (People's Republic of China Journal of Chinese Herbology), 1990; 15(5):50
6. *Zhong Yao Xue* (Chinese Herbology), 1998; 586-587
7. *Zhong Guo Zhong Yao Za Zhi* (People's Republic of China Journal of Chinese Herbology), 1990; 15(5):50

Gan Qi (Resina Toxicodendri)

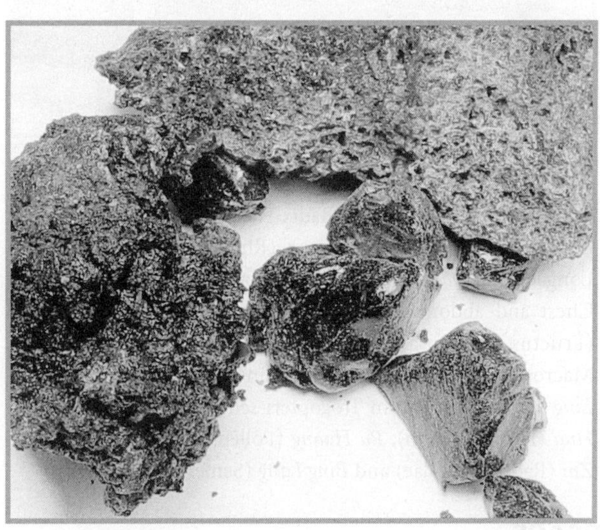

干漆

Pinyin Name: *Gan Qi*
Literal Name: "dried lacquer"
Alternate Chinese Names: *Gan Qi Tan*
Original Source: *Shen Nong Ben Cao Jing* (Divine Husbandman's Classic of the Materia Medica) in the second century
English Name: dried lacquer
Botanical Name: *Toxicodendron verniciflluum* (Stokes) F.A. Barkl. (*Qi Shu*)
Pharmaceutical Name: Resina Toxicodendri
Properties: acrid, bitter, warm
Channels Entered: Liver, Stomach
Safety Index: slightly toxic

CHINESE THERAPEUTIC ACTIONS

1. Breaks Blood Stagnation, Eliminates Blood Stasis, and Opens Channels

Blood stasis: Acrid, bitter, and dispersing, *Gan Qi* (Resina Toxicodendri) has a potent function to break down and eliminate blood stasis to treat severe cases of hardness, mass accumulation, and amenorrhea.

- For amenorrhea caused by blood stasis: use *Gan Qi* with *Da Huang* (Radix et Rhizoma Rhei), *Shui Zhi* (Hirudo), and *Tao Ren* (Semen Persicae).

2. Kills Parasites

Gan Qi has antiparasitic action and treats parasitic infestation accompanied by abdominal pain. However, it is rarely used for this now, as there are other more effective herbs.

DOSAGE

Gan Qi should be used only in pill or powder form, with a maximum of 0.06 to 0.1 gram [60 to 100mg] per dose. It should not be used in herbal decoctions. The unprocessed herb is slightly toxic and may damage *ying* (nutritive) and

Gan Qi (Resina Toxicodendri)

xue (blood) levels, and injure the Spleen and Stomach. Charring will reduce the toxicity of the herb.

CAUTIONS / CONTRAINDICATIONS

- *Gan Qi* is contraindicated in cases of pregnancy, and in the absence of blood stasis.
- *Gan Qi* is not recommended for use in cases of Stomach deficiency.

CHEMICAL COMPOSITION

Laccase.[1]

References

1. *Chang Yong Zhong Yao Cheng Fen Yu Yao Li Shou Ce* (A Handbook of the Composition and Pharmacology of Common Chinese Drugs), 1994; 178

Mao Dong Qing (Radix Ilicis Pubescentis)

毛冬青

Pinyin Name: *Mao Dong Qing*
Original Source: *Guangxi Zhong Yao Zhi* (Guangxi Journal of Chinese Herbal Medicines)
English Name: ilex pubescentis
Botanical Name: *Ilex pubescens* Hook. et Arn. (*Mao Dong Qing*)
Pharmaceutical Name: Radix Ilicis Pubescentis
Properties: bitter, astringent, neutral
Channels Entered: Heart

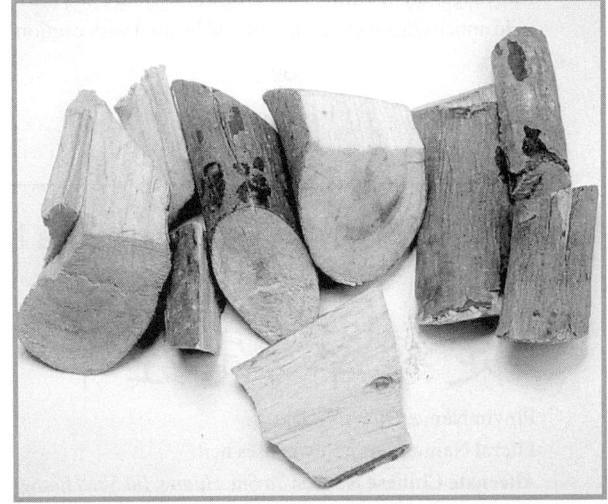

CHINESE THERAPEUTIC ACTIONS

1. Activates Blood Circulation, Opens Channels

***Xiong bi* (painful obstruction of the chest), paralysis:** *Mao Dong Qing* (Radix Ilicis Pubescentis) enters the *xue* (blood) level and disperses blood stagnation secondary to stroke or heart disorders.

- *Xiong bi*, paralysis: combine *Mao Dong Qing* with *Dan Shen* (Radix Salviae Miltiorrhizae), *Hong Hua* (Flos Carthami), *Tao Ren* (Semen Persicae) and *Chuan Xiong* (Rhizoma Ligustici Chuanxiong).

2. Clears Heat and Eliminates Toxins

Mao Dong Qing treats coughing and sore and swollen throat caused by Lung heat. When applied topically in powder form, this herb also treats burns.

- Cough: use this herb with *Huang Qin* (Radix Scutellariae) and *Gua Lou Shi* (Fructus Trichosanthis).
- Sore and swollen throat: use it with *Ma Bo* (Lasiosphaera seu Calvatia) and *She Gan* (Rhizoma Belamcandae).

DOSAGE

30 to 60 grams in decoction.

CAUTIONS / CONTRAINDICATIONS

- Use of *Mao Dong Qing* is not recommended for deficiency patients.

CHEMICAL COMPOSITION

Ilexolide A, ilexsaponin A.[1]

PHARMACOLOGICAL EFFECTS

- **Cardiovascular:** Preparations of *Mao Dong Qing* have shown marked effectiveness to dilate blood vessels and increase blood perfusion to the coronary arteries. It has positive inotropic and antiarrhythmic effects in rabbits. It also has anticoagulant effects.[2]

Mao Dong Qing (Radix Ilicis Pubescentis)

- **Others:** *Mao Dong Qing* has antitussive, expectorant, antiasthmatic and antibiotic effects.[3]

CLINICAL STUDIES AND RESEARCH

- **Coronary artery disease:** In one study, 274 patients with coronary artery disease were treated with a preparation of *Mao Dong Qing*. After the treatment, the study reported significant relief of chest pain in 60.7% of the patients, and moderate relief in 28.6%. The overall rate of effectiveness was 89.3%. No abnormalities were noted in liver and kidney function or shown by blood tests.[4]
- **Ischemic stroke:** A preparation of *Mao Dong Qing* was used to treat 20 patients with ischemic stroke, with a 95% rate of effectiveness.[5]

HERB-DRUG INTERACTION

- **Anticoagulant or antiplatelet drugs:** *Mao Dong Qing* has a mild anticoagulant effect, and should be used with caution in patients who take anticoagulant or antiplatelet medications. Though this potential interaction has not been documented, this herb may potentiate the effect of drugs such as warfarin.[6] [Note: Examples of anticoagulants include heparin, warfarin (Coumadin) and enoxaparin (Lovenox); and examples of antiplatelets include aspirin, dipyridamole (Persantine), and clopidogrel (Plavix).]

References

1. *Xian Dai Zhong Yao Yao Li Xue* (Contemporary Pharmacology of Chinese Herbs), 1997; 919
2. *Zhong Yao Xue* (Chinese Herbology), 1998; 588:589
3. Ibid.
4. *Xin Yi Yao Xue Za Zhi* (New Journal of Medicine and Herbology), 1979; 11:48
5. *Guang Dong Yi Xue* (Guangdong Medicine), 1983; 4(8):28
6. Chen, J. Recognition & prevention of herb-drug interactions, *Medical Acupuncture*, Fall/Winter 1998/1999; volume 10/number 2; 9-13

Ding Jing Cao (Herba Linderniae)

定經草 定经草

Pinyin Name: *Ding Jing Cao*
Literal Name: "settle the menses herb"
Alternate Chinese Names: *Ya She Huang, Jia She Huang, Long Jiao Cao*
English Name: lindernia
Botanical Name: *Lindernia anagallis* (Burm.f.) Pennell
Pharmaceutical Name: Herba Linderniae
Properties: sweet, slightly bitter, neutral
Channels Entered: Liver, Kidney

CHINESE THERAPEUTIC ACTIONS

1. Invigorates Blood Circulation, Nourishes Blood and Regulates Menses

Irregular menstruation: *Ding Jing Cao* (Herba Linderniae) treats irregular menstruation that arises from blood stagnation secondary to blood deficiency. Lack of nourishment of blood, and stagnation in the *ren* (conception) and *chong* (thoroughfare) channels, will manifest in irregular menstruation with pale blood and clots.

- Irregular menstruation: use *Ding Jing Cao* with *Xiang Fu* (Rhizoma Cyperi), *Tao Ren* (Semen Persicae), *Chuan Xiong* (Rhizoma Ligustici Chuanxiong) and *Dang Gui* (Radicis Angelicae Sinensis).

2. Tonifies the Kidney

White vaginal discharge: *Ding Jing Cao* treats Kidney qi deficiency manifesting in clear or white vaginal discharge.

- White vaginal discharge: use this herb with *Bai Long Chuan Hua Tou* (Radix Clerodendron Paniculatum).

DOSAGE

5 to 15 grams in decoction.

CAUTIONS / CONTRAINDICATIONS

- Use of *Ding Jing Cao* is contraindicated during pregnancy.

Ji Xue Teng (Caulis Spatholobi)

雞血藤 鸡血藤

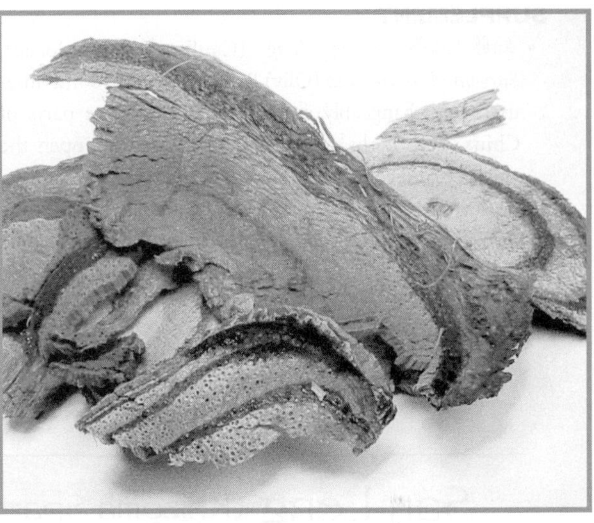

Pinyin Name: *Ji Xue Teng*
Literal Name: "chicken blood vine"
Alternate Chinese Names: *Shan Ji Xue Teng*
Original Source: *Ben Cao Shi Yi* (Omissions from the [Classic of the] Materia Medica) by Chen Cang-Qi in 741 A.D.
English Name: spatholobus, sub-erect spatholobus stem
Botanical Name: *Spatholobus suberectus* Dunn. (*San Ye Ji Xue Teng*). *Milletia dielsiana* Harms. (*Shan Ji Xue Teng*) and *Millettia reticulata* Benth. (*Kun Ming Ji Xue Teng*) are sometimes used as substitutes.
Pharmaceutical Name: Caulis Spatholobi
Properties: bitter, slightly sweet, warm
Channels Entered: Liver

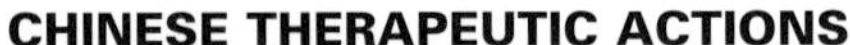

CHINESE THERAPEUTIC ACTIONS

1. Activates Blood Circulation, Tonifies Blood

Menstrual disorders: *Ji Xue Teng* (Caulis Spatholobi) treats gynecological disorders such as irregular menstruation, menstrual pain, cramps, and amenorrhea from either blood stagnation or deficiency.

- Menstrual disorders: combine this herb with *Dang Gui* (Radicis Angelicae Sinensis), *Chuan Xiong* (Rhizoma Ligustici Chuanxiong), and *Bai Shao* (Radix Paeoniae Alba).

2. Relaxes the Tendons, Opens the Channels and Collaterals

***Bi zheng* (painful obstruction syndrome):** *Ji Xue Teng* treats musculoskeletal pain by unblocking stagnation in peripheral channels and collaterals. Usually the cause of this stagnation is either blood stagnation or blood deficiency.

- *Bi zheng* arising from blood deficiency: add *Ji Xue Teng* to *Niu Xi* (Radix Cyathulae seu Achyranthis), *Sang Ji Sheng* (Herba Taxilli) and *Du Huo* (Radix Angelicae Pubescentis).
- *Bi zheng* caused by blood stasis: use it with *Qiang Huo* (Rhizoma et Radix Notopterygii), *Wei Ling Xian* (Radix Clematidis), *Luo Shi Teng* (Caulis Trachelospermi), and *Dang Gui* (Radicis Angelicae Sinensis).

DOSAGE

10 to 15 grams. The maximum dose of *Ji Xue Teng* is 30 grams.

CAUTIONS / CONTRAINDICATIONS

- Use *Ji Xue Teng* with caution in cases of hypermenorrhea. *Ji Xue Teng* is contraindicated during pregnancy because of its stimulating effect on the uterus.

CHEMICAL COMPOSITION

Formononetin, ononin, prunetin, afromosin, cajinin, licochalcone A, isoliquiritigenin, 2,4-tetrahydroxychalcone, procatechuic acid, (-) epicatechin, 3,7-dihydroxy-6-methoxyflavanonol, daucosterol, 7-carbonyl-β-sitosterol.[1]

PHARMACOLOGICAL EFFECTS

- **Sedative and hypnotic:** Intraperitoneal injections of *Ji Xue Teng* have demonstrated both sedative and hypnotic influences in rats.[2]
- **Cardiovascular:** Administration of herbal decoction at the dosage of 0.5 g/kg in rabbits or 0.3 g/kg in dogs lowered blood pressure.[3]
- **Uterine stimulant:** Administration of *Ji Xue Teng* decoction has a stimulating effect on the uterus in both pregnant and non-pregnant laboratory animals.[4]

CLINICAL STUDIES AND RESEARCH

- **Coronary artery disease:** In one double-blind study, 38 patients with coronary artery disease were randomly divided into two groups. Group one received 2 weeks of dipyridamole followed by 2 weeks of an herbal remedy containing *Ji Xue Teng* and *Chuan Xiong* (Rhizoma Ligustici Chuanxiong). Group two received the same herbal and dipyridamole treatments, but in reversed order. Both groups showed improvement based on symptomatic and ECG evaluations, with no statistically-significant difference between them.[5]
- **Neutropenia:** In one clinical study, administration of *Ji Xue Teng* in syrup or pills three times daily for 3 to 5 days showed a marked increase in neutrophils and some increase in red blood cells starting on the third day.[6]

Ji Xue Teng (Caulis Spatholobi)

SUPPLEMENT

- 紅藤 / 红藤 *Hong Teng* (Caulis Sargentodoxae), *Sargentodoxa cuneata* (Oliv) Rehd. et. Wils., is sometimes used interchangeably as *Ji Xue Teng* in some parts of China. Both herbs activate blood circulation, open the channels and collaterals, and relieve pain. The difference, however, is that *Hong Teng* treats intestinal abscess while *Ji Xue Teng* tonifies blood. These two herbs have some similarities yet significantly distinct functions, and should not be confused, or substituted for each other.

References

1. *Chang Yong Zhong Yao Cheng Fen Yu Yao Li Shou Ce* (A Handbook of the Composition and Pharmacology of Common Chinese Drugs), 1994; 1146-1147
2. *Zhong Yao Xue* (Chinese Herbology), 1988; 560:561
3. *Zhong Cao Yao Yao Li Xue* (Herbology of Chinese Medicinals), 1983; 200
4. *Zhong Yao Xue* (Chinese Herbology), 1988; 560:561
5. *Xin Yi Xue* (New Medicine), 1978; 9(4):176
6. *Shang Hai Zhong Yi Yao Za Zhi* (Shanghai Journal of Chinese Medicine and Herbology), 1965; 9:16

San Leng (Rhizoma Sparganii)

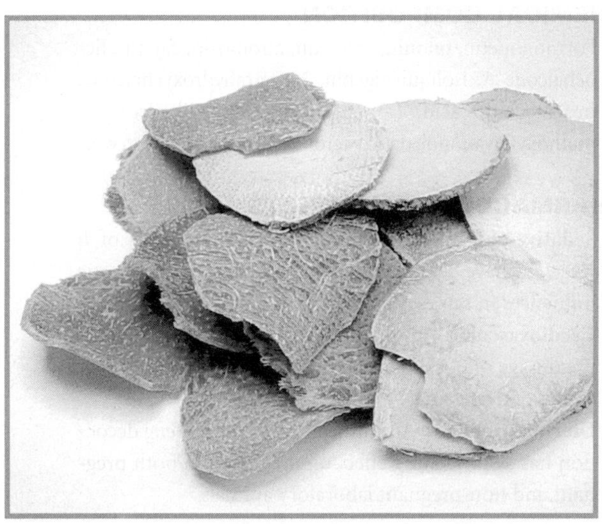

三稜 三棱

Pinyin Name: *San Leng*
Literal Name: "three edges"
Alternate Chinese Names: *Jing San Leng, Hei San Leng*
Original Source: *Ben Cao Shi Yi* (Omissions from the [Classic of the] Materia Medica) by Chen Cang-Qi in 741 A.D.
English Name: sparganium, common bur-reed rhizome
Botanical Name: *Sparganium stoloniferum* Buch.-Ham. (*Hei San Leng*); *Scirpus flaviatilis* (*Jing San Leng*) is sometimes used as a substitute in Northern China.
Pharmaceutical Name: Rhizoma Sparganii
Properties: bitter, neutral
Channels Entered: Liver, Spleen

CHINESE THERAPEUTIC ACTIONS

1. Breaks and Dispels Blood Stasis

Amenorrhea, abdominal pain, masses: *San Leng* (Rhizoma Sparganii) breaks up severe blood stasis, a condition characterized by palpable masses and severe pain. This is one of the strongest blood-moving herbs and is often reserved for the most serious conditions. It enters the *xue* (blood) level and strongly invigorates circulation to break open any stagnation.

- Abdominal pain, amenorrhea or abdominal masses due to blood stasis: use *San Leng* with *E Zhu* (Rhizoma Curcumae), *Niu Xi* (Radix Cyathulae seu Achyranthis) and *Yan Hu Suo* (Rhizoma Corydalis).

2. Activates Qi Circulation and Relieves Pain

Epigastric and abdominal distention and pain: In addition to breaking up blood stasis, *San Leng* disperses qi and relieves pain. Clinical applications include epigastric and abdominal distention and pain due to qi stagnation and indigestion.

- Epigastric and abdominal distention and pain due to qi stagnation and indigestion: use *San Leng* with *E Zhu* (Rhizoma Curcumae), *Qing Pi* (Pericarpium Citri Reticulatae Viride) and *Shan Zha* (Fructus Crataegi).
- Epigastric and abdominal pain from Spleen deficiency: use this herb with *Dang Shen* (Radix Codonopsis) and *Bai Zhu* (Rhizoma Atractylodis Macrocephalae).
- Splenomegaly or hepatomegaly: add *San Leng* to *E Zhu* (Rhizoma Curcumae), *Mu Li* (Concha Ostreae), *Bie Jia* (Carapax Trionycis), *Chuan Shan Jia* (Squama Manis), *Hong Hua* (Flos Carthami) and *Tao Ren* (Semen Persicae).

San Leng (Rhizoma Sparganii)

DOSAGE

3 to 10 grams in herbal decoction. Frying *San Leng* with vinegar enhances its effect to invigorate blood circulation, eliminate blood stasis, and relieve pain.

CAUTIONS / CONTRAINDICATIONS

- *San Leng* is contraindicated during pregnancy or in cases of hypermenorrhea.

CHEMICAL COMPOSITION

Essential oils, starch.[1]

PHARMACOLOGICAL EFFECTS

- **Antineoplastic:** *San Leng* has demonstrated an inhibitory effect on cancer cells.[2]
- **Gastrointestinal:** Decoction of *San Leng* has repeatedly demonstrated a stimulating effect on the smooth muscle of the intestines, leading to muscle contractions. This effect is negated by atropine.[3]
- **Hematological:** In one report, 10 grams of *San Leng* administered via herbal decoction demonstrated marked effectiveness to inhibit aggregation of platelets and prolong thrombin time.[4]

CLINICAL STUDIES AND RESEARCH

- **Ectopic pregnancy:** According to one report, 25 patients with ectopic pregnancies were treated with up to 92% effectiveness using an herbal formula containing *San Leng*, *E Zhu* (Rhizoma Curcumae), *Shui Zhi* (Hirudo), *Mu Li* (Concha Ostreae), *Dan Shen* (Radix Salviae Miltiorrhizae) and other herbs as deemed necessary.[5]
- **Hepatic carcinoma:** Patients with hepatic carcinoma were treated with both herbal injection and powder with a 43.3% rate of effectiveness. Out of 30 patients, the study reported marked improvement in 3 patients, slight improvement in 10 patients, and no response in 17 patients. The herbal injection contained *San Leng* and *E Zhu* (Rhizoma Curcumae); the herbal powder contained *San Leng*, *E Zhu*, *Shui Zhi* (Hirudo), *Wa Leng Zi* (Concha Arcae), *Su Mu* (Lignum Sappan), *Hong Hua* (Flos Carthami), *Yan Hu Suo* (Rhizoma Corydalis), *Xiang Fu* (Rhizoma Cyperi), *Mu Xiang* (Radix Aucklandiae), *Sha Ren* (Fructus Amomi), *Chen Pi* (Pericarpium Citri Reticulatae), *Ban Xia* (Rhizoma Pinelliae), *Hou Po* (Cortex Magnoliae Officinalis), *Zhi Shi* (Fructus Aurantii Immaturus), *Da Huang* (Radix et Rhizoma Rhei) and *Chuan Mu Tong* (Caulis Clematidis Armandii). No significant side effects were reported.[6]
- **Malignant tumor:** In one study, 31 patients at terminal stages of malignant cancers were treated with an herbal formula, including *San Leng*, with marked improvement in 5 patients, slight improvement in 19 patients, and no response in 7 patients. The types of cancer treated included stomach, liver, esophageal, cervical, breast, rectal, lung, and lymphatic.[7]

HERB-DRUG INTERACTION

Anticoagulant or antiplatelet drugs: *San Leng* should be used with caution in patients receiving anticoagulant or antiplatelet medications as the combination may lead to additive or synergistic effects. Though this potential interaction has not been documented, the use of *San Leng* may potentiate the effect of drugs such as warfarin.[8] [Note: Examples of anticoagulants include heparin, warfarin (Coumadin) and enoxaparin (Lovenox); and examples of antiplatelets include aspirin, dipyridamole (Persantine), and clopidogrel (Plavix).]

TOXICOLOGY

The LD_{50} for oral administration of *San Leng* in mice is 233.9 +/- 9.9 g/kg. At the lethal level, there were seizures, convulsions and respiratory suppression prior to fatality.[9]

AUTHORS' COMMENTS

It is important to remember the basic concept that "it takes qi to move qi, and it takes blood to move blood." Therefore, when herbs are prescribed to move the blood and break up blood stasis, it is important to ensure that the fundamental constitution of the patient is strong enough to tolerate such aggressive treatment. *San Leng* and *E Zhu* (Rhizoma Curcumae) are two of the strongest herbs and are commonly used synergistically to break open stagnation. *San Leng* has a stronger function to break blood stasis while *E Zhu* is stronger in breaking qi stagnation. In patients with deficient conditions, these two should be used with tonic herbs to strengthen the Spleen, to ensure that the herbs do not damage the body.

References

1. *Chang Yong Zhong Yao Cheng Fen Yu Yao Li Shou Ce* (A Handbook of the Composition and Pharmacology of Common Chinese Drugs), 1994; 175
2. *Zhong Yao Xue* (Chinese Herbology), 1988; 549:550
3. *Xin Yi Yao Xue Za Zhi* (New Journal of Medicine and Herbology), 1975; (10):36
4. *Chang Yong Zhong Yao Cheng Fen Yu Yao Li Shou Ce* (A Handbook of the Composition and Pharmacology of Common Chinese Drugs), 1994; 175:176
5. *Fu Jian Yi Yao Za Zhi* (Fujian Journal of Medicine and Herbology), 1981; 2:23
6. *Zhong Liu Yu Fang Yan Jiu* (Tumor Prevention and Research), 1973; 1:31
7. *Zhe Jiang Zhong Yi Xue Yuan Xue Bao* (Journal of Zhejiang University of Chinese Medicine), 1983; 3:31
8. Chen, J. Recognition & prevention of herb-drug interactions, *Medical Acupuncture*, Fall/Winter 1998/1999; volume 10/number 2; 9-13
9. *Chang Yong Zhong Yao Cheng Fen Yu Yao Li Shou Ce* (A Handbook of the Composition and Pharmacology of Common Chinese Drugs), 1994; 175:176

E Zhu (Rhizoma Curcumae)

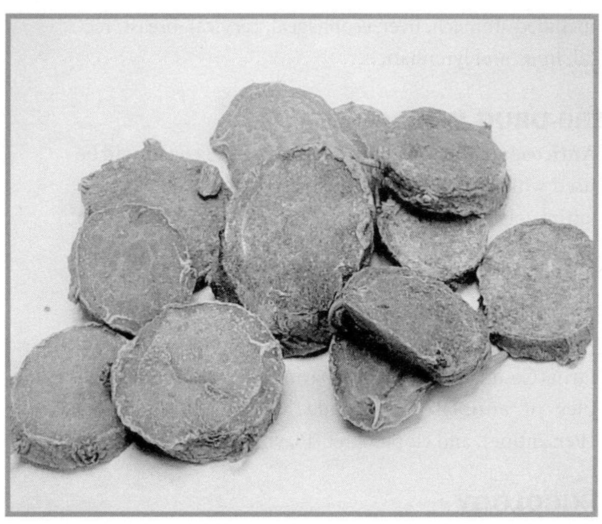

莪朮 莪术

Pinyin Name: *E Zhu*
Original Source: *Yao Xing Ben Cao* (Materia Medica of Medicinal Properties) by Zhen Quan in 600 A.D.
English Name: curcuma zedoaria
Botanical Name: *Curcuma zedoaria* (Berg.) Rosc. (*E Zhu*); *Curcuma aromatica* Salisb. (*Yu Yin*); *Curcuma kwangsiensis* S. Lee et. C.F. Liang. (*Guang Xi E Zhu*)
Pharmaceutical Name: Rhizoma Curcumae
Properties: bitter, acrid, warm
Channels Entered: Spleen, Liver

CHINESE THERAPEUTIC ACTIONS

1. Invigorates Blood Circulation and Breaks Up Blood Stasis

Amenorrhea, abdominal pain: *E Zhu* (Rhizoma Curcumae) strongly works to break up chronic or severe blood stasis. It is usually used in cases where all other blood-invigorating herbs have failed to show satisfactory results. Most commonly, this herb treats blood stagnation in the *chong* (thoroughfare) channel that has resulted in amenorrhea and/or lower abdominal pain, a condition often characterized by palpable masses and severe pain.

- Amenorrhea due to blood stasis: use *E Zhu* with *San Leng* (Rhizoma Sparganii), *Chuan Xiong* (Rhizoma Ligustici Chuanxiong), and *Niu Xi* (Radix Cyathulae seu Achyranthis).

Palpable masses: *E Zhu* is used when a prolonged period of blood stagnation results in palpable abdominal masses.

- Palpable masses in the abdomen due to blood stasis: combine *E Zhu* with *Bie Jia* (Carapax Trionycis), *Dan Shen* (Radix Salviae Miltiorrhizae) and *San Leng* (Rhizoma Sparganii).
- Epigastric distention and hardness: use this herb with *Shen Qu* (Massa Fermentata), *Mai Ya* (Fructus Hordei Germinatus), *Lai Fu Zi* (Semen Raphani), *Ban Xia* (Rhizoma Pinelliae), *Huang Lian* (Rhizoma Coptidis) and *Zhi Shi* (Fructus Aurantii Immaturus).
- Hypochondriac distention and hardness of the right rib cage: use *E Zhu* with *Chai Hu* (Radix Bupleuri), *Zhi Ke* (Fructus Aurantii), *Mu Li* (Concha Ostreae) and *Jiang Huang* (Rhizoma Curcumae Longae).
- Hypochondriac distention and hardness of the left rib cage: use it with *Chai Hu* (Radix Bupleuri), *Bie Jia* (Carapax Trionycis) and *She Gan* (Rhizoma Belamcandae).
- Periumbilical or lower abdominal masses: combine it with *Xiang Fu* (Rhizoma Cyperi), *Qing Pi* (Pericarpium Citri Reticulatae Viride), *Dan Shen* (Radix Salviae Miltiorrhizae) and *Yu Jin* (Radix Curcumae).
- Palpable masses in the abdomen: add this herb to *Yan Hu Suo* (Rhizoma Corydalis), *Niu Xi* (Radix Cyathulae seu Achyranthis), *Ze Lan* (Herba Lycopi), *Wu Ling Zhi* (Excrementum Trogopteri seu Pteromi) and *Meng Chong* (Tabanus).

2. Activates Qi Circulation and Relieves Pain

Epigastric and abdominal fullness, distention and pain: *E Zhu* treats abdominal distention and pain secondary to indigestion, and qi stagnation due to deficiency of the Spleen and Stomach. It is often used to promote digestion by increasing the circulation of qi and blood.

- Abdominal pain due to qi stagnation and indigestion: use *E Zhu* with *San Leng* (Rhizoma Sparganii), *Mu Xiang* (Radix Aucklandiae), and *Zhi Shi* (Fructus Aurantii Immaturus).
- Abdominal fullness and pain due to Spleen deficiency: combine this herb with *Dang Shen* (Radix Codonopsis) and *Bai Zhu* (Rhizoma Atractylodis Macrocephalae).

DOSAGE

3 to 10 grams in herbal decoction. Frying *E Zhu* with vinegar enhances its potency to disperse stasis and relieve pain.

CAUTIONS / CONTRAINDICATIONS

- *E Zhu* is contraindicated in deficiency patients, or those with hypermenorrhea.
- *E Zhu* is contraindicated during pregnancy.

CHEMICAL COMPOSITION

Zederone, zedoarone, furanodine, curzerene, furano-

E Zhu (Rhizoma Curcumae)

dienone, isofuranodienone, curzerenone, epicurzerenone, curdione, curcolone, curcumenol, procurcumenol, isocurmenol, curcumol, curcumadiol, curcumin.[1,2,3]

PHARMACOLOGICAL EFFECTS

- **Antineoplastic:** Intraperitoneal injection of a 100% *E Zhu* solution showed satisfactory results in treatment of sarcoma and cervical carcinoma in mice.[4]
- **Antibiotic:** It has an inhibitory effect on *Staphylococcus aureus*, β-hemolytic streptococcus, *E. coli*, *Salmonella typhi*, and *Vibrio cholerae*.[5]
- **Hematological:** The essential oil of *E Zhu* prolongs the aggregation of platelets and prevents the formation of thrombi.[6]

CLINICAL STUDIES AND RESEARCH

- **Coronary artery disease (CAD):** Patients with CAD were treated with intramuscular injection of an herbal preparation twice daily for 14 days per treatment course for a total of two courses. Each dose of the herbal injectable contained 2 grams each of *E Zhu*, *San Leng* (Rhizoma Sparganii), *An Ye* (Folium Eucalypti Globuli), *Xiang Fu* (Rhizoma Cyperi) and *Jiang Xiang* (Lignum Dalbergiae Odoriferae). Out of 35 patients, the study reported 82.8% effectiveness based on symptom evaluation, and 66.7% effectiveness based on ECG evaluation. [7]
- **Chronic obstructive pulmonary disease (COPD):** In one study, 37 patients with COPD were treated with herbal formulas, with significant improvement in 16 patients, moderate improvement in 16 patients, and no response in 5 patients. The herbal formula contained *E Zhu*, *Fen Fang Ji* (Radix Stephaniae Tetandrae), and *Ma Bian Cao* (Herba Verbenae), with modifications to treat qi deficiency, yang deficiency, and *wei* (defensive) *qi* deficiency.[8]
- **Malignant cancer:** Patients with malignant cancers, including stomach, lung, liver, and esophageal cancers, were treated with intravenous infusion of an herbal solution daily. The herbal injection was prepared by mixing 60 to 100 ml of 150% *E Zhu* solution with 500 ml of D5W. Out of 19 patients, the study reported complete recovery in 1 case, marked effectiveness in 4 cases, slight improvement in 3 case, and no response in 11 cases.[9]
- **Neurodermatitis:** Intramuscular injection of an herbal solution to acupuncture points was used to treat patients with neurodermatitis. The herbal injectable contained *E Zhu* and *San Leng* (Rhizoma Sparganii). The acupuncture points selected included *Quchi* (LI 11) and *Xuehai* (SP 10). Out of 48 patients, the study reported marked improvement in 21 patients, moderate improvement in 9 patients, slight improvement in 9 patients, and no response in 9 patients.[10]
- **Psychiatric disorders with blood stasis:** In one report, 71 patients with schizophrenia or mania, characterized by excess yang and blood stagnation, were treated with 6 to 8 pills of an herbal formula three times daily for 30 days, with a 59.1% rate of effectiveness. Most patients responded within 2 to 4 weeks of therapy. Each pill of the herbal formula was equivalent to 8 grams of bulk herbs, with a 10:3:3 ratio of *E Zhu*, *Chi Shao* (Radix Paeoniae Rubrae), and *Da Huang* (Radix et Rhizoma Rhei), respectively.[11]

HERB-DRUG INTERACTION

- **Anticoagulant or antiplatelet drugs:** *E Zhu* should be used with caution in patients receiving anticoagulant or antiplatelet medications, as the combination may lead to additive or synergistic effect. Though this potential interaction has not been documented, the use of *E Zhu* may potentiate the effect of drugs such as warfarin.[12] [Note: Examples of anticoagulants include heparin, warfarin (Coumadin) and enoxaparin (Lovenox); and examples of antiplatelets include aspirin, dipyridamole (Persantine), and clopidogrel (Plavix).]

TOXICOLOGY

The LD_{50} of *E Zhu* extract in mice is 147.0 g/kg via oral ingestion and 55 g/kg via intramuscular injection.[13]

AUTHORS' COMMENTS

Traditionally, *E Zhu* has been used as one of the stronger herbs to break blood stagnation. It is used today to break masses in cases of tumors or cancer. From animal testing and actual case reports, this herb seems to be most effective against cervical cancer.

E Zhu and *San Leng* (Rhizoma Sparganii) are often used together synergistically to break blood stagnation. *E Zhu* enters *qi* (energy) level and is stronger in breaking qi stagnation. *San Leng* enters *xue* (blood) level and has a stronger function to break blood stasis.

According to Dr. Lu Zhi-Zheng, the combination of *E Zhu* and *Jiang Can* (Bombyx Batryticatus) can treat intestinal polyps.

References

1. *Chem Pharm Bull*; 1972;20:987
2. *Chang Yong Zhong Yao Cheng Fen Yu Yao Li Shou Ce* (A Handbook of the Composition and Pharmacology of Common Chinese Drugs), 1994; 1494-1495
3. *Xian Dai Ben Cao Gang Mu* (Contemporary Materia Medica), 2000; 2910
4. *Xin Yi Yao Xue Za Zhi* (New Journal of Medicine and Herbology), 1976; 12:28
5. *CA*, 1970;73:6354n
6. *Zhong Xi Yi Jie He Fang Zhi Yan Jiu Xue Guan Zhi Liao* (Research on Prevention and Treatment of Cardiovascular Disorders Using Integrated Chinese and Western Medicines), 1977; (3):47,50
7. *Zhong Cao Yao Tong Xun* (Journal of Chinese Herbal Medicine), 1979; 8:27

E Zhu (Rhizoma Curcumae)

8. *Zhong Yi Za Zhi* (Journal of Chinese Medicine), 1983; 4:74
9. *Shan Dong Zhong Yi Xue Yuan Xue Bao* (Journal of Shandong University School of Chinese Medicine), 1980; 1:30
10. *Pi Fu Bing Fang Zhi Yan Jiu Tong Xun* (Research Journal on Prevention and Treatment of Dermatological Disorders), 1979; 3:152
11. *Zhong Xi Yi Jie He Za Zhi* (Journal of Integrated Chinese and Western Medicine), 1988; 10:638
12. Chen, J. Recognition & prevention of herb-drug interactions, *Medical Acupuncture*, Fall/Winter 1998/1999; volume 10/number 2; 9-13
13. *Xian Dai Zhong Yao Yao Li Xue* (Contemporary Pharmacology of Chinese Herbs), 1997; 282-283, 1997; 907:908

Shui Zhi (Hirudo)

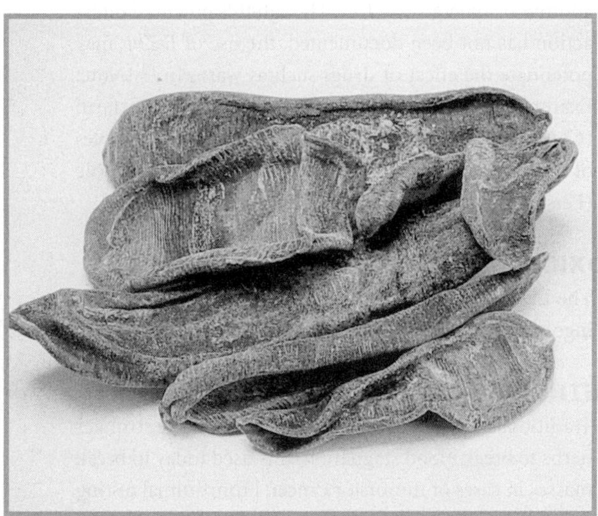

水蛭

Pinyin Name: *Shui Zhi*
Literal Name: "leech"
Alternate Chinese Names: *Ma Huang*
Original Source: *Shen Nong Ben Cao Jing* (Divine Husbandman's Classic of the Materia Medica) in the second century
English Name: medicinal leech
Zoological Name: *Hirudo nipponica* Whitman (*Shui Zhi*); *Whitmania pigra* Whitman (*Ma Huang*); *Whitmania acranulata* Whitman. (*Liu Ye Ma Huang*)
Pharmaceutical Name: Hirudo
Properties: salty, bitter, neutral
Channels Entered: Liver
Safety Index: slightly toxic

CHINESE THERAPEUTIC ACTIONS

Breaks Up and Eliminates Blood Stasis

Amenorrhea, palpable masses, traumatic injuries: *Shui Zhi* (Hirudo) is one of the strongest medicinal substances to treat disorders characterized by severe blood stasis. Clinical applications include amenorrhea, immobile abdominal masses, and external and traumatic injuries. *Shui Zhi* is not suitable for amenorrhea caused by deficiency and other cases of deficiency, as its action may damage the patient's constitution.

- Amenorrhea and immobile abdominal masses due to blood stasis: use *Shui Zhi* with *Tao Ren* (Semen Persicae), *Da Huang* (Radix et Rhizoma Rhei) and *Meng Chong* (Tabanus).
- Amenorrhea due to blood stasis in deficiency: combine it with *Ren Shen* (Radix Ginseng) and *Shu Di Huang* (Radix Rehmanniae Preparata) to prevent injury to *zheng* (upright) *qi*.
- External and traumatic injuries with severe pain, bruises, chest and abdominal pain, anuria and constipation: use it with *Da Huang* (Radix et Rhizoma Rhei) and *Qian Niu Zi* (Semen Pharbitidis).
- Abdominal pain and hardness with black, tarry stool: add *Shui Zhi* to *Meng Chong* (Tabanus) and *Tao Ren* (Semen Persicae).

DOSAGE

3 to 6 grams in decoction, 0.3 to 0.6 grams in powder. Dry-frying *Shui Zhi* minimizes its toxicity, reduces odor, and facilitates extraction of active components.

CAUTIONS / CONTRAINDICATIONS

- *Shui Zhi* is contraindicated during pregnancy, and for those who do not have blood stagnation.

CHEMICAL COMPOSITION

Hirudin.[1]

PHARMACOLOGICAL EFFECTS

- **Anticoagulant:** Hirudin is generally considered to be

Shui Zhi (Hirudo)

one of the most effective anticoagulant substances. It interferes with the effect of thrombin to prevent fibrinogen formation and therefore, prevents coagulation.[2]

- **Antihyperlipidemic:** Administration of *Shui Zhi* powder is associated with a marked reduction of total cholesterol and triglyceride levels.[3]
- **Effect on pregnancy:** Administration of a 40% *Shui Zhi* preparation terminated pregnancy in a positive dose-effect relationship in mice. This effect is observed in the first, second and third trimesters of pregnancy.[4]

CLINICAL STUDIES AND RESEARCH

- **Cor pulmonale:** According to one report, 130 patients with cor pulmonale were divided into two groups, with 63 patients receiving 1 gram of *Shui Zhi* powder three times daily and 67 patients receiving a placebo. Patients in both groups were of similar age and presentation of "blood stasis." After 2 weeks, the treatment group showed 90.5% improvement while the placebo group showed 77.6% improvement. Patients in the treatment group also showed more improvement than the placebo group in symptoms such as chest oppression and dyspnea.[5]
- **Thrombotic phlebitis:** Twenty patients with thrombotic phlebitis in the lower extremities or trunk were treated with an herbal formula for 25 to 33 doses with a 100% success rate; with no recurrence during the 6 month follow-up. The herbal formula contained *Shui Zhi*, *Dang Gui* (Radicis Angelicae Sinensis), *Chi Shao* (Radix Paeoniae Rubrae), *Chuan Xiong* (Rhizoma Ligustici Chuanxiong), *Hong Hua* (Flos Carthami), *Chuan Niu Xi* (Radix Cyathulae), and *Huang Qi* (Radix Astragali). Herbal paste was used topically to reduce swelling and relieve pain.[6]
- **Thrombocytosis:** An herbal decoction was used to treat 18 patients with thrombocytosis 5 to 8 days post-splenectomy, with marked effectiveness. The herbal decoction contained *Shui Zhi*, *Meng Chong* (Tabanus), *Di Bie Chong* (Eupolyphaga), *Tao Ren* (Semen Persicae), *Mu Dan Pi* (Cortex Moutan), *Chi Shao* (Radix Paeoniae Rubrae), *Sheng Di Huang* (Radix Rehmanniae), *Pu Huang* (Pollen Typhae), and *Wu Ling Zhi* (Excrementum Trogopteri seu Pteromi).[7]
- **Hypercholesterolemia:** In one study, 25 patients with high cholesterol levels were treated with 3 to 5 grams of *Shui Zhi* powder once daily at bedtime for 30 days. The study reported an average reduction of 23.24 mg/dL in cholesterol and 144.52 mg/dL in triglycerides. No adverse reactions were observed in regards to liver function, red blood cells, or coagulation time. The rate of effectiveness was 91%.[8]

HERB-DRUG INTERACTION

- **Anticoagulant or antiplatelet drugs:** *Shui Zhi* should be used with caution for patients receiving anticoagulant or antiplatelet medications, as the combination may lead to additive or synergistic effect. Though this potential interaction has not been documented, the use of *Shui Zhi* may potentiate the effect of drugs such as warfarin.[9] [Note: Examples of anticoagulants include heparin, warfarin (Coumadin) and enoxaparin (Lovenox); and examples of antiplatelets include aspirin, dipyridamole (Persantine), and clopidogrel (Plavix).]

TOXICOLOGY

No significant side effects have been associated with intravenous or subcutaneous injection of hirudin. Administration of hirudin in mice at the dosage of 1 mg/kg for four weeks did not show any adverse effect to liver or kidney functions. The LD_{50} in mice for subcutaneous injection of decoction of *Shui Zhi* is 15.24 +/- 2.04 g/kg.[10]

AUTHORS' COMMENTS

The use of *Shui Zhi* as a medicinal substance is well-documented in many countries and many cultures. Hirudin, a natural substance present in *Shui Zhi*, is one of the components responsible for its anticoagulant effect. The therapeutic effect of hirudin is also the foundation for approval of a new pharmaceutical drug, lepirudin (Refludan). Structurally, lepirudin is identical to hirudin except for a few minor chemical changes. In 1998, lepirudin was patented and approved by the Food and Drug Administration as an anticoagulant medication for the treatment of thromboembolic disease.[11]

Meng Chong (Tabanus), *Di Bie Chong* (Eupolyphaga) and *Shui Zhi* (Hirudo) are all very strong substances to break open severe blood stasis. They can easily injure qi if not used properly. When necessary, tonic herbs should be added to prevent damage. Of the three substances, *Meng Chong* is the strongest, followed by *Shui Zhi*, and then *Di Bie Chong*. Practitioners should select these substances in accordance with the patient's constitution and condition.

References

1. *Xian Dai Zhong Yao Yao Li Xue* (Contemporary Pharmacology of Chinese Herbs), 1997; 927
2. *Pharmazie*, 1988; 43:737
3. *Zhong Hua Nei Ke Xue Za Zhi* (Journal of Chinese Internal Medicine), 1988; 27(8):472
4. *Zhong Cao Yao* (Chinese Herbal Medicine), 1984; 15(3):19
5. *Zhe Jiang Zhong Yi Za Zhi* (Zhejiang Journal of Chinese Medicine), 1982; 17(3):101
6. Ibid., 1981; 16(10):417
7. *Shang Hai Zhong Yi Yao Za Zhi* (Shanghai Journal of Chinese Medicine and Herbology), 1963; 5:15
8. *Xin Zhong Yi* (New Chinese Medicine), 1985; 2:36
9. Chen, J. Recognition & prevention of herb-drug interactions, *Medical Acupuncture*, Fall/Winter 1998/1999; volume 10/number 2; 9-13
10. *Zhong Cao Yao* (Chinese Herbal Medicine), 1984; 15(3):19
11. *Drug Topics*, February 1, 1999; 64

Meng Chong (Tabanus)

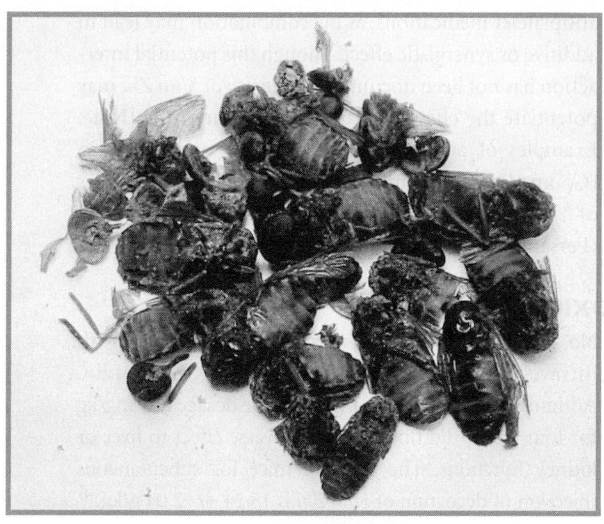

蛀蟲 虻虫

Pinyin Name: *Meng Chong*

Original Source: *Shen Nong Ben Cao Jing* (Divine Husbandman's Classic of the Materia Medica) in the second century

English Name: tabanus, gadfly

Zoological Name: *Tabanus bivttatus* Matsumura (*Fu Dai Mang*)

Pharmaceutical Name: Tabanus

Properties: bitter, cool

Channels Entered: Liver

Safety Index: slightly toxic

CHINESE THERAPEUTIC ACTIONS

Breaks Up and Eliminates Blood Stasis

Amenorrhea, palpable masses, traumatic injuries: *Meng Chong* (Tabanus) enters the *xue* (blood) level in the Liver channel. It has a potent effect to treat disorders characterized by severe blood stasis. Clinical applications include amenorrhea, irregular menstruation, traumatic injuries and external injuries.

- Amenorrhea due to blood stagnation, palpable masses: use *Meng Chong* with *Shui Zhi* (Hirudo), *Di Bie Chong* (Eupolyphaga) and *Da Huang* (Radix et Rhizoma Rhei).
- Irregular menstruation or postpartum bleeding and pain: use this herb with *Shu Di Huang* (Radix Rehmanniae Preparata), *Shui Zhi* (Hirudo) and *Tao Ren* (Semen Persicae).
- Pain from traumatic injuries: combine *Meng Chong* with *Ru Xiang* (Gummi Olibanum) and *Mo Yao* (Myrrha).

DOSAGE

1 to 1.5 grams in decoction, 0.3 gram in powder.

CAUTIONS / CONTRAINDICATIONS

- *Meng Chong* is contraindicated during pregnancy.

PHARMACOLOGICAL EFFECTS

- **Cardiovascular:** Administration of *Meng Chong* is associated with increased resistance to hypoxia in mice. In rabbits, it has a positive inotropic effect, and increased blood perfusion to peripheral parts of the body.[1]

CLINICAL STUDIES AND RESEARCH

- **Angina:** In a clinical study, 18 patients with angina were treated with an herbal formula containing *Meng Chong* and *Chen Pi* (Pericarpium Citri Reticulatae). The treatment protocol was daily administration of herbs for 30 consecutive days. Out of 18 patients, the study reported marked improvement in 12 and mild improvement in 6 patients. ECG was improved in 72.2% of patients. No significant changes were reported with plasma cholesterol levels.[2]

AUTHORS' COMMENTS

Meng Chong, Di Bie Chong (Eupolyphaga) and *Shui Zhi* (Hirudo) are all very strong substances to break open severe blood stasis. They can easily injure qi if not used properly. When necessary, tonic herbs should be added to prevent damage. Of the three substances, *Meng Chong* is the strongest, followed by *Shui Zhi*, and then *Di Bie Chong*. Practitioners should select these substances in accordance with the patient's constitution and condition.

References

1. *Zhong Yao Xue* (Chinese Herbology), 1998; 575-576
2. *Bei Jing Zhong Yi Xue Yuan Xue Bao* (Journal of Beijing University School of Medicine), 1982; 4:31

Di Bie Chong (Eupolyphaga)

地鱉蟲 地鳖虫

Pinyin Name: *Di Bie Chong*
Alternate Chinese Names: *Di Bie, Zhe Chong, Tu Bie Chong, Tu Bie, Bo Ji Chong*
Original Source: *Shen Nong Ben Cao Jing* (Divine Husbandman's Classic of the Materia Medica) in the second century
English Name: eupolyphaga
Zoological Name: *Eupolyphaga sinensis* Walk. (*Di Bie*); *Steleophaga plancyi* (Bol.) (*Ji Di Bie*)
Pharmaceutical Name: Eupolyphaga
Properties: salty, cold
Channels Entered: Liver
Safety Index: slightly toxic

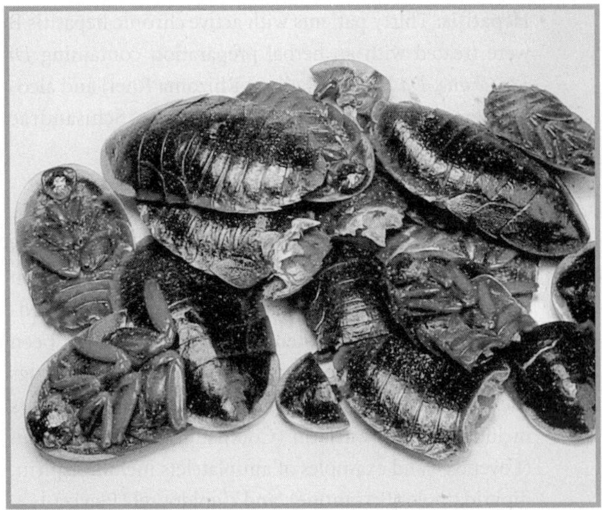

CHINESE THERAPEUTIC ACTIONS

1. Breaks and Eliminates Blood Stasis

Amenorrhea, postpartum abdominal pain, palpable masses in the abdomen: *Di Bie Chong* (Eupolyphaga) treats various disorders characterized by severe blood stasis, such as amenorrhea, immobile abdominal masses, dry skin, afternoon fevers, traumatic injuries, and external injuries. It is a strong and indispensable herb for breaking masses due to blood stagnation.

- Amenorrhea caused by blood stasis: combine *Di Bie Chong* with *Da Huang* (Radix et Rhizoma Rhei), *Shui Zhi* (Hirudo) and *Meng Chong* (Tabanus).
- Menstrual pain or postpartum abdominal pain from blood stasis: use this herb with *Da Huang* (Radix et Rhizoma Rhei) and *Tao Ren* (Semen Persicae).
- Immobile abdominal masses due to blood stasis: add it to *Bie Jia* (Carapax Trionycis), *San Leng* (Rhizoma Sparganii) and *Mu Dan Pi* (Cortex Moutan).

2. Connects Tendons, Fuses Bones

Traumatic injuries, bone fractures: *Di Bie Chong* treats traumatic injuries and external injuries, including torn tendons and ligaments, and bone fractures.

- Injuries to tendons, ligaments and bones: use *Di Bie Chong* with *Zi Ran Tong* (Pyritum), *Ru Xiang* (Gummi Olibanum) and *Mo Yao* (Myrrha).
- External or traumatic injuries with bruises and pain: combine this herb with *Dang Gui* (Radicis Angelicae Sinensis) and *Chuan Xiong* (Rhizoma Ligustici Chuanxiong).

DOSAGE

3 to 10 grams in decoction, 1.0 to 1.5 grams in powder.

CAUTIONS / CONTRAINDICATIONS

- *Di Bie Chong* is contraindicated during pregnancy.
- *Di Bie Chong* should be used with caution in the absence of blood stasis.

PHARMACOLOGICAL EFFECTS

- **Antiplatelet:** Water extract of *Di Bie Chong* has an inhibiting effect on the aggregation of platelets in rats.[1]

CLINICAL STUDIES AND RESEARCH

- **Placental remnants:** Administration of *Di Bie Chong* at the dosage of 30 to 45 grams was extremely effective in treating amenorrhea or menstrual pain caused by placental remnants following abortion, miscarriage or delivery. Other herbs commonly used with *Di Bie Chong* to enhance its effectiveness included *Tao Ren* (Semen Persicae), *Hong Hua* (Flos Carthami), *Yi Mu Cao* (Herba Leonuri) and *Pao Jiang* (Rhizoma Zingiberis Preparatum). Complete elimination of placental remnants was achieved within 3 to 4 days. No significant side effects were observed.[2]
- **Coronary artery disease:** In one study, 127 patients with coronary artery disease were divided into three groups. The first group of 47 patients received *Di Bie Chong, Dan Shen* (Radix Salviae Miltiorrhizae), *Chuan Xiong* (Rhizoma Ligustici Chuanxiong), *Hong Hua* (Flos Carthami), *Chi Shao* (Radix Paeoniae Rubrae), *Jiang Xiang* (Lignum Dalbergiae Odoriferae), *Ge Gen* (Radix Puerariae), *Gua Lou Shi* (Fructus Trichosanthis) and others. The second group of 18 patients received *Di Bie Chong*. The third group of 52 patients received 50 mg of dipyridamole three times daily. Based on ECG evaluation, the first group showed a 71.08% rate of effectiveness, the second group showed 50% effectiveness, and the third group showed 43.44%.[3]

Di Bie Chong (Eupolyphaga)

- **Hepatitis:** Thirty patients with active chronic hepatitis B were treated with an herbal preparation containing *Di Bie Chong, Da Huang* (Radix et Rhizoma Rhei) and alcohol extract of *Wu Wei Zi* (Fructus Schisandrae Chinensis) with satisfactory results.[4]

HERB-DRUG INTERACTION

- **Anticoagulant or antiplatelet drugs:** *Di Bie Chong* has an antiplatelet action, and should be used with caution in patients who take anticoagulant or antiplatelet medications. Though this potential interaction has not been documented, this herb may potentiate the effect of drugs such as warfarin.[5] [Note: Examples of anticoagulants include heparin, warfarin (Coumadin) and enoxaparin (Lovenox); and examples of antiplatelets include aspirin, dipyridamole (Persantine), and clopidogrel (Plavix).]

TOXICOLOGY

The LD_{50} for intraperitoneal injection of *Di Bie Chong* in mice is 136.45 +/- 7.98 mg/kg. Fatality occurred within 10 to 20 minutes.[6]

AUTHORS' COMMENTS

According to Dr. Jiao Shu-De, *Di Bie Chong* treats one-sided stiffness, swelling, hardening and pain of the tongue caused by extreme accumulation of heat toxins in cases of erysipelas and scarlet fever. Secondary symptoms include involuntary salivation, and difficulty swallowing. Use 6 grams of *Di Bie Chong* with 3 grams of salt to make a decoction. The instruction is to gargle first before swallowing, and repeat twice daily.

Meng Chong (Tabanus), *Di Bie Chong* (Eupolyphaga) and *Shui Zhi* (Hirudo) are all very strong substances to break open severe blood stasis. They can easily injure qi if not used properly. When necessary, tonic herbs should be added to prevent damage. Of the three substances, *Meng Chong* is the strongest, followed by *Shui Zhi*, and then *Di Bie Chong*. Practitioners should select these substances in accordance with the patient's constitution and condition.

References

1. *Chang Yong Zhong Yao Cheng Fen Yu Yao Li Shou Ce* (A Handbook of the Composition and Pharmacology of Common Chinese Drugs), 1994; 208:213
2. *Zhe Jiang Zhong Yi Za Zhi* (Zhejiang Journal of Chinese Medicine), 1983; 4:177
3. *Shan Xi Yi Yao Za Zhi* (Shanxi Journal of Medicine and Herbology), 1985; 14(1):49
4. *Zhong Xi Yi Jie He Za Zhi* (Journal of Integrated Chinese and Western Medicine), 1983; 3(5):277
5. Chen, J. Recognition & prevention of herb-drug interactions, *Medical Acupuncture*, Fall/Winter 1998/1999; volume 10/number 2; 9-13
6. *Zhong Cao Yao* (Chinese Herbal Medicine), 1989; 20(6):20

Chapter 12 summary

— Blood-Invigorating and Stasis-Removing Herbs

Name	Similarities	Differences
Chuan Xiong (Rhizoma Ligustici Chuanxiong)	Activate qi and blood circulation	Actives blood circulation, dispels wind, relieves pain
Yan Hu Suo (Rhizoma Corydalis)		Strongly activates qi and blood circulation, effectively relieves pain throughout the entire body
Yu Jin (Radix Curcumae)		Soothes the Liver, regulates the Gallbladder, dissolves phlegm, cools blood
Jiang Huang (Rhizoma Curcumae Longae)		Breaks up blood stasis, eliminates blood stasis
Lu Lu Tong (Fructus Liquidambaris)		Promotes normal urination, relieves pain
Ru Xiang (Gummi Olibanum)	Activate blood circulation, relieve pain	Treats traumatic injuries with qi stagnation
Mo Yao (Myrrha)		Treats traumatic injuries with blood stagnation
Hu Zhang (Rhizoma Polygoni Cuspidati)		Eliminates blood stasis, clears heat and toxins, dispels damp-heat
Wu Ling Zhi (Excrementum Trogopteri seu Pteromi)		Eliminates blood stasis, relieves pain due to blood stasis, treats obstetric and gynecologic disorders
Jiang Xiang (Lignum Dalbergiae Odoriferae)		Disperses turbid obstruction, relieves abdominal pain and vomiting
Zi Ran Tong (Pyritum)		Eliminates blood stasis, treats trauma-related pain
Niao Bu Su (Ramus Kalopanax Pictus)		Eliminates toxins and relieves pain
Dan Shen (Radix Salviae Miltiorrhizae)	Activate blood circulation, eliminate blood stasis	Treats cardiovascular disorders, gynecological disorders, masses and accumulations, traumatic injuries, disturbed *shen* (spirit)
Hong Hua (Flos Carthami)		Treats gynecological disorders, masses or accumulations, joint pain, and dermatological disorders
Tao Ren (Semen Persicae)		Treats gynecological disorders, external and sports injuries, Lung and intestinal abscesses, and chronic constipation
Yi Mu Cao (Herba Leonuri)		Promotes diuresis, treats gynecological disorders
Ze Lan (Herba Lycopi)		Promotes diuresis
Chuan Niu Xi (Radix Cyathulae)		Moves blood and sedates heat
Huai Niu Xi (Radix Achyranthis Bidentatae)		Tonifies Kidney
Ma Bian Cao (Herba Verbenae)		Clears heat, eliminates toxins, treats malaria, promotes diuresis, reduces swelling
Jin Bu Huan (Herba Lycopodii Serrati)		Reduces swelling and inflammation, relieves pain
Ye Ming Sha (Excrementum Vespertilionis Murini)		Clears the Liver, brightens the eyes
Chuan Shan Jia (Squama Manis)	Activate blood circulation, open channels and collaterals	Promotes lactation, treats dermatological disorders
Wang Bu Liu Xing (Semen Vaccariae)		Promotes lactation
Liu Ji Nu (Herba Artemisiae Anomalae)		Regulates menstruation
Su Mu (Lignum Sappan)		Treats gynecological disorders, addresses trauma-related disorders
Gan Qi (Resina Toxicodendri)		Opens channels, kills parasites
Mao Dong Qing (Radix Ilicis Pubescentis)		Clears heat and toxins, treats cough or sore throat due to heat, relieves pain
Ding Jing Cao (Herba Linderniae)		Nourishes the blood, regulates menses
Ji Xue Teng (Caulis Spatholobi)		Activates blood circulation and tonifies blood, treats *bi zheng* (painful obstruction syndrome)

Chapter 12 summary

Name	Similarities	Differences
San Leng (Rhizoma Sparganii)	Break up blood stasis, eliminate blood stasis	Breaks blood stagnation better
E Zhu (Rhizoma Curcumae)		Breaks qi stagnation better
Shui Zhi (Hirudo)		Strongly breaks up blood stasis
Meng Chong (Tabanus)		Breaks up blood stasis
Di Bie Chong (Eupolyphaga)		Treats chronic traumatic injuries

General Characteristics of Blood-Invigorating and Stasis-Removing Herbs:

Taste: acrid, bitter
Thermal property: warm
Channels entered: varies
Therapeutic actions: invigorate blood circulation, remove blood stasis, break blood stasis.

Blood-invigorating and stasis-removing herbs function to treat abnormal circulation of blood, and related complications such as qi stagnation, obstruction of the channels and collaterals, and pain. Clinical applications of these herbs include stabbing pain in a fixed location, numbness and pain of the limbs and extremities, lumps found on the skin or internal palpable masses, traumatic injuries, internal bleeding, purpura of the skin, and purple spots on the tongue.

Chuan Xiong (Rhizoma Ligustici Chuanxiong), ***Yan Hu Suo*** (Rhizoma Corydalis), ***Yu Jin*** (Radix Curcumae), ***Jiang Huang*** (Rhizoma Curcumae Longae), and ***Lu Lu Tong*** (Fructus Liquidambaris) all have dual effects to activate qi and blood circulation.

Chuan Xiong is one of the most commonly used herbs to invigorate qi and blood circulation. It treats headaches and regulates menstruation.

Yan Hu Suo is one of the most potent herbs to relieve pain. It alleviates both traumatic and/or visceral pain.

Yu Jin disperses Liver qi stagnation and cools blood to clear heat in the Heart.

Jiang Huang strongly breaks up stagnation, regulates qi, and is best for *bi zheng* (painful obstruction syndrome) of the upper limbs.

Lu Lu Tong, in addition to activating qi and blood circulation, also promotes normal urination and relieves allergies.

Ru Xiang (Gummi Olibanum), ***Mo Yao*** (Myrrha), ***Hu Zhang*** (Rhizoma Polygoni Cuspidati), ***Wu Ling Zhi*** (Excrementum Trogopteri seu Pteromi), ***Jiang Xiang*** (Lignum Dalbergiae Odoriferae), ***Zi Ran Tong*** (Pyritum) and ***Niao Bu Su*** (Ramus Kalopanax Pictus) have similar functions to activate qi and blood circulation to relieve pain.

Ru Xiang and *Mo Yao* have excellent effects to relieve pain and disperse blood stagnation caused by traumatic injuries. When used externally, this pair has the effect to reduce swelling and generate flesh.

Hu Zhang opens channels and collaterals, clears heat, drains dampness, eliminates toxins, dispels phlegm and relieves cough. It is also effective to detoxify the Liver for treatment of hepatitis.

Wu Ling Zhi has a strong analgesic function, removes stasis and stops bleeding simultaneously.

Jiang Xiang treats pain in the chest and hypochondriac area caused by traumatic injuries. It also separates the clear from the turbid to harmonize the middle *jiao* and relieve nausea.

Zi Ran Tong promotes healing of bones and sinews in cases of fracture.

Niao Bu Su activates qi and blood circulation, eliminates toxins, and effectively treats infection and inflammations.

Dan Shen (Radix Salviae Miltiorrhizae), ***Hong Hua*** (Flos Carthami) and ***Tao Ren*** (Semen Persicae) invigorate blood circulation, remove stasis and are used on a wide variety of disorders due to blood stagnation.

Dan Shen is cool in thermal property and thus cools blood, reduces abscesses, nourishes blood and calms the *shen* (spirit).

Chapter 12 summary

Hong Hua disperses blood stagnation to open the channels and collaterals and relieves pain in the extremities.

Tao Ren (Semen Persicae) disperses blood stagnation in the body to treat lung and intestinal abscesses. In addition, it is rich in oil and lubricates the Large Intestine to relieve constipation.

Yi Mu Cao (Herba Leonuri) and ***Ze Lan*** (Herba Lycopi) invigorate blood and remove stasis, especially in gynecological disorders. In addition, they have diuretic functions.

Chuan Niu Xi (Radix Cyathulae) and ***Huai Niu Xi*** (Radix Achyranthis Bidentatae) have descending characteristics and direct the effect of a formula downwards. Used fresh, they lead heat or blood downwards to treat disorders of the lower body, such as irregular menstruation or knee pain. Used in processed form, they tonify the Kidney and Liver to strengthen tendons and bones.

Chuan Niu Xi more strongly moves blood and sedates heat.

Huai Niu Xi more effectively tonifies the Liver and Kidney.

Ma Bian Cao (Herba Verbenae) invigorates blood, removes masses, and clears heat and toxins. It is most commonly used to promote diuresis, reduce swelling, and treat dysentery and malaria.

Jin Bu Huan (Herba Lycopodii Serrati) invigorates qi and blood circulation, removes stasis, stops bleeding, and relieves pain.

Ye Ming Sha (Excrementum Vespertilionis Murini) treats traumatic injuries to disperse bruising and remove stasis. It also clears the Liver and brightens the eyes.

Chuan Shan Jia (Squama Manis), ***Wang Bu Liu Xing*** (Semen Vaccariae), ***Liu Ji Nu*** (Herba Artemisiae Anomalae), ***Su Mu*** (Lignum Sappan), ***Gan Qi*** (Resina Toxicodendri), ***Mao Dong Qing*** (Radix Ilicis Pubescentis), ***Ding Jing Cao*** (Herba Linderniae) and ***Ji Xue Teng*** (Caulis Spatholobi) all invigorate blood circulation and open channels and collaterals.

Chuan Shan Jia and *Wang Bu Liu Xing* have very similar effects to invigorate blood, open channels and promote lactation. They are commonly used for irregular menstruation, amenorrhea or insufficient milk production in nursing women.

Liu Ji Nu regulates menstruation, dispels stasis, relieves pain and relieves food stagnation.

Su Mu relieves pain in gynecological disorders or cases of trauma.

Gan Qi strongly breaks blood stagnation, reduces accumulations and masses, and kills parasites.

Mao Dong Qing mainly treats cardiovascular disorders involving blood stagnation.

Ding Jing Cao treats menstrual disorders by invigorating blood circulation and nourishing the blood.

Ji Xue Teng effectively treats *bi zheng* (painful obstruction syndrome), activates blood circulation, eliminates blood stasis, and opens the channels and collaterals. It is excellent for blood-deficient patients who also need blood-invigorating effects.

San Leng (Rhizoma Sparganii), ***E Zhu*** (Rhizoma Curcumae), ***Shui Zhi*** (Hirudo), ***Meng Chong*** (Tabanus), and ***Di Bie Chong*** (Eupolyphaga) have the most potent influence on the blood to break up and eliminate blood stasis.

San Leng and *E Zhu* break up blood stagnation and activate qi to reduce masses or accumulations.

Shui Zhi and *Meng Chong* break up blood stagnation in patients experiencing an excess condition, who have not yet been weakened by the disease.

Di Bie Chong has a purgative function and also attacks toxins and treats convulsions.

Chapter 12 summary

HERBS FROM OTHER FUNCTIONAL CATEGORIES WITH BLOOD-INVIGORATING AND STASIS-REMOVING FUNCTIONS

Name	Functional Category
Chi Shao (Radix Paeoniae Rubrae)	Heat-Clearing Herbs (Chapter 2)
Da Huang (Radix et Rhizoma Rhei)	Downward Draining Herbs (Chapter 3)
Dang Gui (Radicis Angelicae Sinensis)	Tonic Herbs (Chapter 17)
Gui Zhi (Ramulus Cinnamomi)	Exterior-Releasing Herbs (Chapter 1)
Mu Dan Pi (Cortex Moutan)	Heat-Clearing Herbs (Chapter 2)
Pu Huang (Pollen Typhae)	Stop-Bleeding Herbs (Chapter 11)
Qian Cao (Radix Rubiae)	Stop-Bleeding Herbs (Chapter 11)
San Qi (Radix Notoginseng)	Stop-Bleeding Herbs (Chapter 11)
Shan Zha (Fructus Crataegi)	Digestive Herbs (Chapter 9)
She Xiang (Moschus)	Orifice-Opening Herbs (Chapter 16)
Xue Jie (Sanguis Draconis)	Substances for Topical Application (Chapter 20)

Chapter 13 — Phlegm-Resolving and Coughing- and Wheezing- Relieving Herbs

化痰止咳平喘药

Chapter 13 — Phlegm-Resolving and Coughing- and Wheezing- Relieving Herbs

Section 1 Phlegm-Resolving Herbs

Section 2 Coughing- and Wheezing- Relieving Herbs

Chapter 13

— Phlegm-Resolving and Coughing- and Wheezing- Relieving Herbs

Definition: Herbs in this category, as the name implies, function to resolve phlegm, arrest coughing, and relieve wheezing and dyspnea. In other words, they have expectorant, antitussive, and antiasthmatic functions.

The pathological factor ***phlegm*** forms as a result of poor water metabolism. After ingestion of food or liquids, if water is not properly absorbed and metabolized, it begins to accumulate and stagnate, leading to the formation of dampness and phlegm. This inability to absorb and metabolize water often results from Spleen qi and Spleen yang deficiencies. Phlegm can be present in the respiratory or gastrointestinal systems, or in the channels, collaterals and muscles. But most often, it is present in the Lung. Therefore, it is commonly noted that the Spleen is the organ that *produces* phlegm, and the Lung is the organ that *stores* phlegm.

In TCM, the Spleen *produces* phlegm, the Lung *stores* phlegm.

Phlegm, ***cough*** and ***dyspnea*** are closely related pathological conditions. Poor circulation of qi, such as found in cough or dyspnea, creates stagnation and allows the consequent formation of phlegm. Obstruction by phlegm, on the other hand, may irritate the respiratory tract and cause more coughing or dyspnea. Together, they create a vicious cycle for the patient, with the presence of one contributing to the formation of the other. For that reason, herbs that dissolve phlegm, stop coughing, and relieve wheezing are classified and used together. In general, herbs in this category treat the type of phlegm associated with common colds or chronic respiratory disorders. Other applications include sores, carbuncles, masses, nodules, epilepsy, seizures, convulsions and phlegm-related stroke.

SUBCATEGORIES OF ACTION

1. ***Warm herbs that dispel cold phlegm*** warm the Lung, dispel cold, dry dampness, and dissolve phlegm. They are most useful for clear or white phlegm caused by cold attacking the Lung. Accompanying symptoms may include chest tightness, aversion to cold, weak limbs, and dyspnea. Other symptoms of cold phlegm include sore limbs, yin sores, and palpable masses. In these cases, treatment should include specific herbs with interior-warming, Spleen-strengthening or dampness-drying functions.
2. ***Cold herbs that clear hot phlegm*** clear heat and eliminate phlegm. They are most useful to address yellow, sticky phlegm caused by heat. These herbs treat epilepsy, convulsions, seizures and nodules. In addition, since heat may consume yin and body fluids, heat-clearing herbs and yin-tonic herbs are often combined to simultaneously clear heat and moisten dryness.
3. ***Herbs that stop coughing and relieve wheezing*** ventilate the lungs to dispel phlegm, moisten the lungs to stop coughing, and redirect rebellious qi to relieve cough and wheezing.

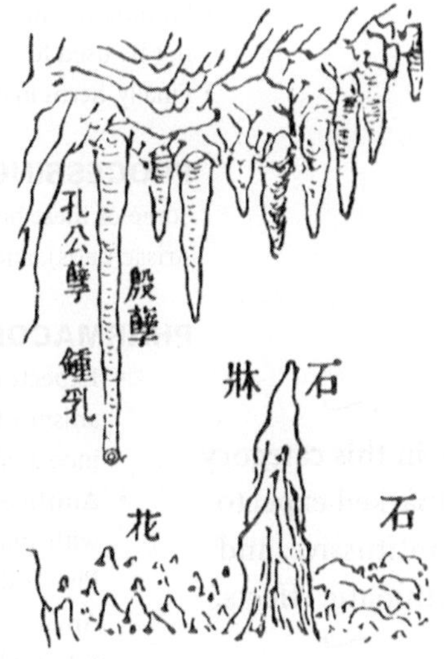

Zhong Ru Shi (Stalactitum)
Ben Cao Gang Mu (Materia Medica),
by Li Shi-Zhen, 1578 A.D.

Chapter 13

DIFFERENTIAL DIAGNOSIS AND TREATMENT

Phlegm is a component or cause of many diseases. During the Yuan Dynasty, Dr. Wang Gui-Cheng stated: "Phlegm is the mother of hundreds of disorders." Thus, differential diagnosis of causes and complications in phlegm-related illness is extremely important for optimal treatment. The following is a list of imbalances caused or complicated by the presence of phlegm:

- Coughing with profuse phlegm caused by wind-cold or wind-heat must be treated with herbs that dispel exterior wind.
  - Cases of phlegm with interior heat must be addressed with addition of heat-clearing herbs, and conditions of phlegm with interior cold must be treated with concomitant use of interior-warming herbs.
  - Chronic cough and wheezing must be treated with concurrent use of herbs to resolve phlegm and tonify underlying deficiency.
  - Seizures or convulsions must be treated with herbs that extinguish Liver wind.
  - Nodules or palpable masses require herbs that soften hardness and dissipate nodules.
  - Yin sores with oozing fluids are addressed by the addition of yang-tonic herbs.
  - Dyspnea with phlegm requires addition of qi-regulating herbs with phlegm-resolving herbs.

Differential diagnosis is extremely important, as phlegm is considered to be the "mother of hundreds of disorders."

Wheezing and dyspnea are *symptoms* that affect the lungs. However, the *causes* of these lung disorders may be imbalance of the Lung and/or Kidney. ***Reversal of Lung qi*** results in coughing, wheezing and dyspnea. ***Deficiency of Kidney qi*** leaves the Kidney unable to pull Lung qi downwards, leading to shortness of breath and shallow inhalation (compared to exhalation).

CAUTIONS/CONTRAINDICATIONS

- Substances from this category should not be used for treatment of coughing or phlegm during the initial stages of rashes or measles. Instead, use herbs that release the exterior.
- In order to prevent trapping pathogenic factors (phlegm, excess heat or cold) in the Lung, herbs such as *Bai Guo* (Semen Ginkgo), *Kuan Dong Hua* (Flos Farfarae), *Zi Wan* (Radix Asteris) and *Wu Wei Zi* (Fructus Schisandrae Chinensis), that exert astringent or restraining influences, should not be used.
- Stimulating herbs such as *Bai Fu Zi* (Rhizoma Typhonii) and *Bai Jie Zi* (Semen Sinapis) should not be used for treatment of patients who are coughing blood, as they may aggravate bleeding.
- Finally, herbs in this category should not be used for prolonged periods of time, as they consume qi.

PROCESSING

Some of these herbs are toxic, such as *Ban Xia* (Rhizoma Pinelliae) and *Tian Nan Xing* (Rhizoma Arisaematis), and must be processed accordingly to remove toxins and insure safe use.

PHARMACOLOGICAL EFFECTS

Herbs in this category have marked expectorant, antitussive, and antiasthmatic effects.

- **Expectorant**: Most phlegm-resolving herbs have a marked expectorant effect. The mechanism of action includes increased production of mucus by the respiratory tract, and increased ciliary action to push phlegm out of the lungs.
- **Antitussive**: Many herbs exert a suppressant effect on the cough reflex in the brain. Herbs with marked antitussive action include *Ban Xia* (Rhizoma Pinelliae), *Jie Geng* (Radix Platycodonis), *Kuan Dong Hua* (Flos Farfarae), and *Xing Ren* (Semen Armeniacae Amarum). Of these herbs, *Ban Xia* has a longer duration of influence, with antitussive action observed for up to 5 hours after ingestion.
- **Antiasthmatic**: Many of these herbs dilate the smooth muscle of the bronchi, relieve spasms and cramps of the bronchial muscle, and relieve wheezing and dyspnea. Herbs with marked antiasthmatic effect include *Zhe Bei Mu* (Bulbus Fritillariae Thunbergii) and *Kuan Dong Hua* (Flos Farfarae). The effect of *Zhe Bei Mu* is similar to atropine, as demonstrated in rabbits and cats. The antiasthmatic effect of *Kuan Dong Hua* is dose-related, with small doses dilating the lungs and large doses constricting them.

- **Antiepileptics**: Some herbs in this category exert marked effectiveness in the treatment of convulsions, seizures, and epilepsy. Water-based decoction of *Tian Nan Xing* (Rhizoma Arisaematis) has been shown to effectively treat drug-induced seizures and epilepsy. *Bai Fu Zi* (Rhizoma Typhonii) has shown excellent preventative and treatment action against tetanus and muscle contractions. The mechanisms of action of both herbs have been attributed to their effect on the central nervous system.
- **Others**: *Ban Xia* (Rhizoma Pinelliae) has an antiemetic effect. *Ting Li Zi* (Semen Descurainiae seu Lepidii) has a cardiotonic effect, and can be used to treat cardiovascular disorders. *Yin Guo Ye* (Folium Ginkgo) and *Gua Lou Shi* (Fructus Trichosanthis) increase blood perfusion to the coronary arteries and reduce the consumption of oxygen by cardiac muscles. *Tian Nan Xing* (Rhizoma Arisaematis), *Gua Lou Shi* (Fructus Trichosanthis) and *Zi Wan* (Radix Asteris) have antineoplastic activity. *Hai Zao* (Sargassum) and *Kun Bu* (Thallus Laminariae seu Eckloniae) are rich in iodine, and are beneficial in treatment of thyroid disorders. *Gua Lou Shi* (Fructus Trichosanthis), *Zao Jiao* (Fructus Gleditsiae), *Zi Wan* (Radix Asteris) and *Bai Bu* (Radix Stemonae) have antibiotic effects, and treat respiratory tract infections.

POTENTIAL HERB-DRUG INTERACTIONS

Herbs that transform phlegm, stop cough and relieve wheezing are used for their expectorant, antitussive, and antiasthmatic effects. Though these herbs are used commonly and frequently, there are no reported or documented cases of herb-drug interactions involving this group of herbs.

Section 1

— Phlegm-Resolving Herbs

Ban Xia (Rhizoma Pinelliae)

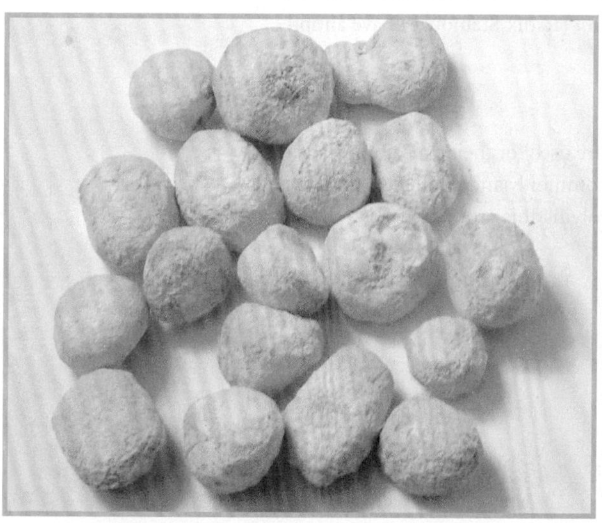

半夏

Pinyin Name: *Ban Xia*
Literal Name: "middle summer," "half summer"
Original Source: *Shen Nong Ben Cao Jing* (Divine Husbandman's Classic of the Materia Medica) in the second century
English Name: pinellia, pinellia tuber
Botanical Name: *Pinellia ternata* (Thunb.) Breit. (*Ban Xia*)
Pharmaceutical Name: Rhizoma Pinelliae
Properties: acrid, warm
Channels Entered: Spleen, Stomach, Lung
Safety Index: toxic

CHINESE THERAPEUTIC ACTIONS

1. Dries Dampness, Dissolves Phlegm

Accumulation of damp and phlegm: According to theories of traditional Chinese medicine, the Spleen produces phlegm and the Lung stores phlegm. When the Spleen does not properly dissolve dampness, symptoms such as cough, profuse sputum and Lung qi reversal will occur. Acrid, warm and drying, *Ban Xia* (Rhizoma Pinelliae) enters the Spleen and Lung to eliminate phlegm both from its source and from wherever it has accumulated. *Ban Xia* is commonly used to treat various phlegm accumulations and complications.

- Profuse sputum, cough and dyspnea from accumulation of phlegm in the lungs: use *Ban Xia* with *Chen Pi* (Pericarpium Citri Reticulatae) and *Fu Ling* (Poria). **Exemplar Formula:** *Er Chen Tang* (Two-Cured Decoction).
- Watery sputum with nausea and vomiting from accumulation of cold phlegm: use this herb with *Xi Xin* (Herba Asari) and *Gan Jiang* (Rhizoma Zingiberis) to warm the Lung and dissolve phlegm.
- Copious yellow sputum indicating an accumulation of hot phlegm: combine it with *Huang Qin* (Radix Scutellariae), *Zhi Mu* (Radix Anemarrhenae) and *Gua Lou Shi* (Fructus Trichosanthis) to clear heat and dissolve phlegm.
- Liver wind rising with phlegm stagnation leading to headache, dizziness, vertigo, feelings of congestion and oppression in the chest, a white greasy tongue coat, and a wiry, slippery pulse: add this herb to *Tian Ma* (Rhizoma Gastrodiae), *Fu Ling* (Poria) and *Bai Zhu* (Rhizoma Atractylodis Macrocephalae) to calm Liver wind, strengthen the Spleen, and dispel phlegm and dampness. **Exemplar Formula:** *Ban Xia Bai Zhu Tian Ma Tang* (Pinellia, Atractylodes Macrocephala, and Gastrodia Decoction).
- *Xiong bi* (painful obstruction of the chest) with yang deficiency and accumulated cold and phlegm leading to shortness of breath and chest pain: use *Ban Xia* with *Gua Lou Shi* (Fructus Trichosanthis) and *Xie Bai* (Bulbus Allii Macrostemonis) to dissolve phlegm and relieve pain. **Exemplar Formula:** *Gua Lou Xie Bai Ban Xia Tang* (Trichosanthes Fruit, Chinese Chive, and Pinellia Decoction).

Ban Xia (Rhizoma Pinelliae)

2. Redirects Abnormally Rising Stomach Qi, Relieves Nausea and Vomiting

Nausea and vomiting: *Ban Xia* relieves nausea and vomiting caused by phlegm obstruction, Stomach deficiency, Stomach heat, or pregnancy. The normal direction of Stomach qi is downward. When it is obstructed by phlegm, the blockage and upward reversal of Stomach qi results in nausea and vomiting. *Ban Xia* has an excellent effect to treat nausea and vomiting: it dries dampness, dissolves phlegm, harmonizes the Stomach and redirects abnormal qi flow.

- Nausea and vomiting due to cold and phlegm: combine *Ban Xia* and *Sheng Jiang* (Rhizoma Zingiberis Recens) to dry dampness, dissolve phlegm, warm the middle *jiao*, and stop vomiting.
- Nausea and vomiting with generalized deficiency: use this herb with *Ren Shen* (Radix Ginseng) to tonify qi.
- Nausea and vomiting with excess cold in the interior: combine it with *Gan Jiang* (Rhizoma Zingiberis) and *Wu Zhu Yu* (Fructus Evodiae).
- Nausea and vomiting due to Stomach heat: add *Ban Xia* to *Huang Lian* (Rhizoma Coptidis) and *Zhu Ru* (Caulis Bambusae in Taenia), to clear heat.
- Nausea and vomiting caused by heat and cold: add this herb to *Huang Lian* (Rhizoma Coptidis), *Huang Qin* (Radix Scutellariae), *Gan Jiang* (Rhizoma Zingiberis) and *Ren Shen* (Radix Ginseng). **Exemplar Formula:** *Ban Xia Xie Xin Tang* (Pinellia Decoction to Drain the Epigastrium).
- Nausea and vomiting during pregnancy: use it with *Su Geng* (Caulis Perillae) and *Sha Ren* (Fructus Amomi) to regulate qi and calm the fetus.
- Chronic neurogenic vomiting: combine it with *Dai Zhe Shi* (Haematitum), *Xuan Fu Hua* (Flos Inulae), *Da Huang* (Radix et Rhizoma Rhei), *Gan Cao* (Radix Glycyrrhizae), *Gua Lou Shi* (Fructus Trichosanthis), *Bing Lang* (Semen Arecae) and *Tao Ren* (Semen Persicae).

3. Dissipates Nodules and Disperses Stagnation

Phlegm accumulation: Acrid and warm, *Ban Xia* dissolves phlegm and dissipates nodules to treat swelling, plum pit (globus hystericus) syndrome, goiter, scrofula, chest and epigastric congestion or obstruction that worsens with pressure.

- Accumulation of hot phlegm with feelings of chest congestion and oppression, tenderness upon palpation, copious yellow sputum, greasy yellow tongue coat, and slippery, rapid pulse: use *Ban Xia* with *Gua Lou Shi* (Fructus Trichosanthis) and *Huang Lian* (Rhizoma Coptidis) to clear heat and dissolve phlegm. **Exemplar Formula:** *Xiao Xian Xiong Tang* (Minor Sinking into the Chest Decoction).
- Plum pit syndrome: use this herb with *Hou Po* (Cortex Magnoliae Officinalis), *Zi Su Ye* (Folium Perillae) and *Fu Ling* (Poria). **Exemplar Formula:** *Ban Xia Hou Po Tang* (Pinellia and Magnolia Bark Decoction).
- Scrofula or thyroid nodules: combine *Ban Xia* with *Kun Bu* (Thallus Laminariae seu Eckloniae), *Hai Zao* (Sargassum) and *Zhe Bei Mu* (Bulbus Fritillariae Thunbergii) to soften hardness and dissipate nodules.

4. Treats Sores, Skin Ulcerations and Carbuncles

Topical application of *Ban Xia* powder treats sores, ulcerations, and carbuncles on the skin. When combined with egg white, the mixture can be used to reduce breast abscesses. To alleviate a swollen tongue, cook *Ban Xia* with vinegar and gargle with the herbal decoction.

DOSAGE

5 to 10 grams in decoction. According to some scholars, the maximum dosage for *Ban Xia* is 60 grams in special circumstances. *Ban Xia* is often used in decoction to maximize therapeutic effect and minimize potential side effects. The component of *Ban Xia* responsible for antitussive and antiemetic effects has high water solubility, and the component responsible for the toxicity has a low water solubility. Furthermore, *Ban Xia* is processed with ginger and alumen to deactivate the constituents responsible for adverse reactions. Thus, processed *Ban Xia* will have greater effectiveness and fewer side effects.[1]

Ban Xia is available in many different forms:

- "*Sheng Ban Xia*," in its original form without any processing, is toxic and therefore generally used externally for treatment of sores, ulcerations and carbuncles.
- "*Qing Ban Xia*," soaked in water and cooked with alumen to reduce its acrid and drying nature, is more suitable for infants, the elderly, and weak patients who have accumulations of dampness and phlegm.
- "*Fa Ban Xia*," processed in water, alumen, calcium oxide, and *Gan Cao* (Radix Glycyrrhizae), is the standard dosage form of *Ban Xia* and is commonly used to treat accumulations of phlegm and dampness in the Spleen and Stomach.
- "*Zhu Li Ban Xia*," processed with *Zhu Li* (Succus Bambusae) to greatly reduce its warm and drying nature, is most suitable for nausea caused by Stomach heat, cough with yellow copious sputum from Lung heat, or post-stroke conditions with hot phlegm.
- "*Jiang Ban Xia*," processed with ginger juice, has a stronger function than the others to warm the Stomach and relieve nausea and vomiting.

While there are many who strongly stress the importance of processing *Ban Xia* to remove its toxicity, it is also important to keep in mind that over-processing the

Ban Xia (Rhizoma Pinelliae)

herb destroys its clinical effectiveness. For decoction, cooking fresh *Ban Xia* in hot water with *Sheng Jiang* (Rhizoma Zingiberis Recens) for 30 minutes will be sufficient to remove any toxicity.[2]

CAUTIONS / CONTRAINDICATIONS

- Warm and drying in nature, *Ban Xia* should be avoided, or used with extreme caution, for patients who have dry coughing from yin deficiency, sore throat caused by heat and fire, and for those experiencing bleeding or who have hot phlegm.
- *Ban Xia* is incompatible with *Wu Tou* (Radix Aconiti).
- Fresh or unprocessed *Ban Xia* is toxic, and its use should be reserved for topical applications only. For internal use, it should be processed to minimize toxicity.
- Allergic reactions have been reported following the use of *Ban Xia*. Symptoms include redness and an excruciating itch throughout the entire body.

OVERDOSAGE

Overdose of *Ban Xia* is characterized by numbness, swelling and pain of the tongue and throat, dry mouth, upper abdominal discomfort, involuntary salivation, slowed respiration, hoarse voice, slurred speech, difficulty swallowing, nausea, vomiting, abdominal pain, diarrhea, dizziness, headache, palpitations, perspiration, pale face, weak and forceless pulse, irregular breathing, and in severe cases, respiratory depression.

TREATMENT OF OVERDOSAGE

Treatment of overdose includes immediate ingestion of egg whites, diluted vinegar, tea, fresh ginger juice or other supportive methods. If fresh ginger is not available, dried ginger can be used as a substitute. Grind 250 grams of *Sheng Jiang* (Rhizoma Zingiberis Recens) and mix with 250 ml of hot water to make tea. Administer 20 to 25 ml of tea every 3 to 4 hours, until the symptoms are resolved.

Two herbal formulas are also beneficial for overdose management. Formula one includes *Fang Feng* (Radix Saposhnikoviae) 60g, *Lu Dou* (Semen Phaseoli Radiati) 30g, and *Gan Cao* (Radix Glycyrrhizae) 15g. Formula two includes *Lu Dou* (Semen Phaseoli Radiati) 15g, *Jin Yin Hua* (Flos Lonicerae) 30g, *Lian Qiao* (Fructus Forsythiae) 30g, *Sheng Jiang* (Rhizoma Zingiberis Recens) 15g, and *Gan Cao* (Radix Glycyrrhizae) 9g. The formulas are taken in decoction until the patient stabilizes.[3]

CHEMICAL COMPOSITION

Homogentisic acid, homogentisic acid glucoside, 3,4-dihydroxybenzaldehyde, 3,4-dihydroyxybenzaldehyde diglucoside, choline.[4]

PHARMACOLOGICAL EFFECTS

- **Antitussive:** Oral or intravenous administration of *Ban Xia* has marked and prolonged antitussive effects in cats. The duration of action is approximately 5 hours.[5]
- **Antiemetic:** Administration of *Ban Xia* processed with ginger or alumen has demonstrated marked antiemetic effects. Such preparations were especially effective in relieving nausea and vomiting induced by chemicals. Though the exact mechanism of action is unclear, it is probably due to the effect of the herb on the central nervous system.[6]
- **Antineoplastic:** Administration of *Ban Xia* in rats is associated with an inhibitory effect on the growth of cancer cells in the liver.[7]

CLINICAL STUDIES AND RESEARCH

- **Cervical carcinoma:** In one study, 247 cervical cancer patients at various stages were treated with oral and vaginal applications of a *Ban Xia* preparation, with complete recovery in 63 cases, marked improvement in 84 cases, and slight improvement in 44 cases. The dosage for the oral preparation is equivalent to 60 grams of the herb given daily in three equally-divided doses. The dosage for the topical preparation is equivalent to 50 grams of the herb, applied into and around the cervix.[8]
- **Nausea and vomiting during pregnancy:** Eighteen women in their third month of pregnancy who experienced severe nausea and vomiting, feelings of chest discomfort and oppression, heavy sensations of the head, and vertigo were given 1 dose of an herbal decoction daily with great success. The formula was prepared by cooking 30 grams of "*Qing Ban Xia*" for 45 minutes, filtering out *Ban Xia* residues, adding in 30 grams of powdered *Shan Yao* (Rhizoma Dioscoreae), then adding white sugar prior to serving.[9]
- **Cervical erosion:** Topical application of *Ban Xia* was used to treat 1,347 patients with cervical erosion, with a 97.18% effective rate and a 44.77% recovery rate. The treatment protocol was to grind the herb into a fine powder, and apply it to the affected area with a cotton ball, leaving it in place for 24 hours. This application was carried out one to two times per week, for 8 applications per course of treatment.[10]
- **Chronic lymphadenitis:** According to one report, 30 patients with chronic lymphadenitis were treated with topical application of *Ban Xia,* with satisfactory results. The herb was prepared by roasting 50 grams of the herb and grinding it into a powder. Vinegar and hot water were added to 3 parts of the herb and 1 part flour to make an herbal paste. The treatment protocol was to apply the paste to the affected area at night, and remove it in the morning, for 5 to 7 applications per course of treatment.[11]

TOXICOLOGY

For unprocessed *Ban Xia*, the LD_{50} in mice is 325 mg/kg

Ban Xia (Rhizoma Pinelliae)

via intraperitoneal injection and 42.7 g/kg via oral ingestion. For processed *Ban Xia*, oral administration of 16 g/kg every 3 hours for 5 doses showed no toxicity. In another toxicology study, administration of unprocessed *Ban Xia* in mice at $^1/_5$ to $^1/_{20th}$ the lethal dose for three weeks resulted in a significant decrease in body weight, compromised liver and kidney functions, and some fatalities. By comparison, the group of mice that received processed *Ban Xia* at the same dose showed no signs or symptoms of toxicity.[12,13,14]

AUTHORS' COMMENTS

Classic texts advised that unprocessed *Ban Xia* should only be used externally, due to its toxicity. More recent studies, however, indicate that if unprocessed *Ban Xia* is cooked for an extended period of time, or if *Sheng Jiang* (Rhizoma Zingiberis Recens) is incorporated into an herbal formula with unprocessed *Ban Xia*, the toxicity is minimized. Therefore, when the benefits of usage outweigh the risks, most authorities agree that the use of unprocessed *Ban Xia* internally is not contraindicated.

Shi Ba Fan (Eighteen Incompatibles) stated that *Wu Tou* (Radix Aconiti) is incompatible with *Ban Xia*. However, the combination of these two have not demonstrated an increase in toxicity or adverse reactions in recent studies. Thus, the validity of this incompatibility is currently under more challenge and investigation.

One classic text mentions that *Ban Xia* may cause miscarriage; however, this concern has been invalidated since many doctors commonly incorporate *Ban Xia* to treat nausea and vomiting during pregnancy. Furthermore, according to *Ming Yi Bie Lun* (*Theories of Famous Doctors*), this herb can be used safely, specifically to treat nausea and vomiting during pregnancy.

References

1. *Zhong Yao Xue* (Chinese Herbology), 1998; 600:604
2. *Zhe Jiang Zhong Yi Za Zhi* (Zhejiang Journal of Chinese Medicine), 1985; 5:196
3. *Zhong Yao Bu Liang Fan Ying Yu Zhi Liao* (Adverse Reactions and Treatment of Chinese Herbal Medicine), 1996; 218:220, 1996; 144:147
4. *Xian Dai Zhong Yao Yao Li Xue* (Contemporary Pharmacology of Chinese Herbs), 1997; 941
5. *Zhong Yao Yao Li Yu Ying Yong* (Pharmacology and Applications of Chinese Herbs), 1983: 383
6. Ibid.
7. *Sheng Wu Hua Xue Yu Sheng Wu Wu Li Xue Bao* (Journal of Biochemistry and Biophysiology), 1983; 15(4):333
8. *Shang Hai Yi Xue* (Shanghai Medicine), 1978; 1:13
9. *Jiang Su Zhong Yi Za Zhi* (Jiangsu Journal of Chinese Medicine), 1987; 3:16
10. *Shan Xi Zhong Yi* (Shanxi Chinese Medicine), 1984; 5:11
11. *Da Zhong Yi Xue* (Public Medicine), 1984; 8:43
12. *Zhong Yao Yao Li Yu Ying Yong* (Pharmacology and Applications of Chinese Herbs), 1983: 383
13. *Zhong Cheng Yao* (Study of Chinese Patent Medicine), 1988; (7):18
14. Ibid.

Tian Nan Xing (Rhizoma Arisaematis)

天南星

Pinyin Name: *Tian Nan Xing*
Literal Name: "sky's southern star," "star of the southern heavens"
Alternate Chinese Names: *She Liu Gu*
Original Source: *Shen Nong Ben Cao Jing* (Divine Husbandman's Classic of the Materia Medica) in the second century
English Name: arisaema, jack-in-the-pulpit tuber
Botanical Name: *Arisaema consanguineum* Schott. (*Tian Nan Xing*); *Arisaema heterophyllum* Bl. (*Yi Ye Tian Nan Xing*); *Arisaema amurense* Maxim. (*Dong Bei Tian Nan Xing*)
Pharmaceutical Name: Rhizoma Arisaematis
Properties: bitter, acrid, warm
Channels Entered: Liver, Lung, Spleen
Safety Index: toxic

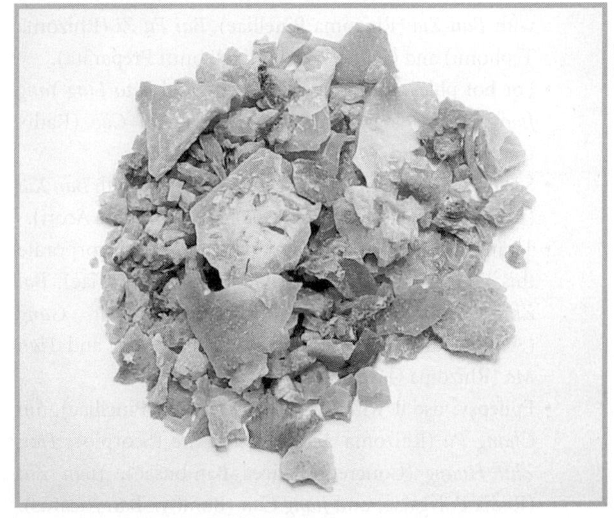

Tian Nan Xing (Rhizoma Arisaematis)

CHINESE THERAPEUTIC ACTIONS

1. Dries Dampness, Dissolves Phlegm

Accumulation of hot phlegm: Bitter, warm and acrid, *Tian Nan Xing* (Rhizoma Arisaematis) is extremely potent in its function to dry dampness and dissolve phlegm. It is commonly used to treat various types of phlegm accumulation and complications. When combined with the proper heat-clearing herbs, it can also be used to treat coughing caused by hot phlegm.

- Accumulation of dampness and phlegm leading to cough, profuse white sputum, feelings of coldness on the back, chest oppression, and a greasy tongue coat: use *Tian Nan Xing* with *Chen Pi* (Pericarpium Citri Reticulatae), *Ban Xia* (Rhizoma Pinelliae), *Fu Ling* (Poria) and *Zhi Shi* (Fructus Aurantii Immaturus) to regulate qi and dissolve phlegm.
- Cough with copious yellow sputum from Lung heat: combine this herb with *Huang Qin* (Radix Scutellariae) and *Gua Lou Shi* (Fructus Trichosanthis).

2. Dispels Wind to Relieve Convulsions

Liver wind rising, with phlegm stagnation: Clinical manifestations include dizziness, vertigo, facial paralysis, seizures, convulsions, tetanus, epilepsy, opisthotonos and stroke. *Tian Nan Xing* dispels wind and phlegm from the channels and collaterals to relieve muscle spasms and cramps. Other manifestations of Liver wind rising and phlegm stagnation include chest congestion, nausea, poor appetite and a preference for sleep.

- Dizziness and vertigo because of phlegm obstruction: use *Tian Nan Xing* with *Ban Xia* (Rhizoma Pinelliae) and *Tian Ma* (Rhizoma Gastrodiae).
- Numbness of the hands and feet, hemiplegia, or deviation of the eyes and mouth caused by phlegm obstruction in the channels and collaterals: combine this herb with *Ban Xia* (Rhizoma Pinelliae), *Bai Fu Zi* (Rhizoma Typhonii) and *Chuan Wu* (Radix Aconiti Preparata).
- For hot phlegm and blockage of qi: add it to *Ling Yang Jiao* (Cornu Saigae Tataricae), *Long Dan Cao* (Radix Gentianae), and *Zhu Li* (Succus Bambusae).
- Seizures and convulsions: use *Tian Nan Xing* with *Ban Xia* (Rhizoma Pinelliae) and *Shi Chang Pu* (Rhizoma Acori).
- Tetany, clenched fist and jaws, opisthotonos: incorporate this herb with *Fang Feng* (Radix Saposhnikoviae), *Bai Zhi* (Radix Angelicae Dahuricae), *Wu Gong* (Scolopendra), *Bai Fu Zi* (Rhizoma Typhonii) and *Tian Ma* (Rhizoma Gastrodiae).
- Epilepsy: use it with *Ban Xia* (Rhizoma Pinelliae), *Shi Chang Pu* (Rhizoma Acori), *Quan Xie* (Scorpio), *Tian Zhu Huang* (Concretio Silicea Bambusae), *Yuan Zhi* (Radix Polygalae) and *Jiang Can* (Bombyx Batryticatus).

3. Dissipates Nodules, Relieves Pain

Topical use of *Tian Nan Xing* reduces swelling and dissipates nodules. It treats various traumatic and sports injuries, muscle and joint pain, and nodules caused by phlegm accumulation.

- Joint pain and swelling: add this herb to *Gan Jiang* (Rhizoma Zingiberis) and *Shi Chang Pu* (Rhizoma Acori), and apply topically.
- Nodules caused by phlegm accumulation: mix *Tian Nan Xing* powder with vinegar, and apply topically.
- Cervical or uterine cancer: use a larger dose of *Tian Nan Xing* orally or topically (as powder or suppository).
- Facial paralysis: crush *Tian Nan Xing* and *Sheng Jiang* (Rhizoma Zingiberis Recens) into a paste, and apply topically.

DOSAGE

5 to 10 grams for general application. The unprocessed form of *Tian Nan Xing* is toxic and not suitable for internal use: it must always be pre-processed, usually with ginger, to make it safe for internal consumption. For treatment of tumors, processed *Tian Nan Xing* is used internally at dosage of up to 15 grams.

CAUTIONS / CONTRAINDICATIONS

- Bitter, acrid, warm and toxic, *Tian Nan Xing* must be used with caution for patients with dry cough from yin deficiency, and rising of Liver wind caused by excess fire or blood deficiency. Use of this herb is contraindicated in treating dry phlegm caused by yin deficiency.
- *Tian Nan Xing* should be used with extreme caution in pregnant women.
- Unprocessed *Tian Nan Xing* is toxic and is not suitable for internal use.
- Allergic reaction may occur when the skin comes in direct contact with *Tian Nan Xing*. Swelling, itching, and pain are the main symptoms, and may be alleviated by topical washing with vinegar.
- Use of *Tian Nan Xing* may be associated with drowsiness and sedation. Therefore, individuals who take this herb should exercise caution if driving or operating heavy machinery.

OVERDOSAGE

The entire plant of *Tian Nan Xing*, from leaves to the root, is toxic. Overdose and adverse reactions associated with ingestion of this plant include numbness of the tongue and mouth, itching, burning sensations, swelling, involuntary salivation, loss of the sense of taste, difficulty opening the mouth, swelling and pain in the tongue and oral cavity, headache, dizziness, palpitations, nausea, vomiting, slurred speech, and hoarse voice. In severe

Tian Nan Xing (Rhizoma Arisaematis)

cases, there may be muscle spasms and convulsions of the extremities, dyspnea and respiratory depression. Adverse reactions may occur at dosages as low as 10 grams, and may last between 15 minutes and several hours.

TREATMENT OF OVERDOSAGE

Overdose of *Tian Nan Xing* can be treated with an herbal decoction of 30 grams of *Sheng Jiang* (Rhizoma Zingiberis Recens), 60 grams of *Fang Feng* (Radix Saposhnikoviae), and 15 grams of *Gan Cao* (Radix Glycyrrhizae). However, if the herbs are not available, administration of 30 to 60 ml of vinegar and a small quantity of fresh ginger juice is also helpful. In both cases, the treatment is most effective if the patient holds the solution in his/her mouth prior to swallowing it.[1] [Note: Holding the solution in the mouth facilitates the sublingual absorption of the herbs, to speed up the treatment].

CHEMICAL COMPOSITION

γ-aminobutyric acid, ornithine, citrulline, arginine, glutamic acid, aspartic acid, leucine, saponins, starch, alkaloids.[2,3]

PHARMACOLOGICAL EFFECTS

- **Antiseizure and anticonvulsant:** Intraperitoneal injection of water extract of *Tian Nan Xing* in mice has preventative effects against seizures and convulsions induced by strychnine and caffeine. Other studies indicated that while *Tian Nan Xing* had questionable antiseizure action, it did effectively control tremor.[4,5]
- **Sedative:** Intraperitoneal injection of water extract of *Tian Nan Xing* is associated with marked sedative effects in mice. Clinical effects included a decrease in spontaneous physical activities, delayed reflexes, and prolonged sleeping time induced by barbiturates.[6]
- **Antineoplastic:** Water extract of unprocessed *Tian Nan Xing* has an inhibitory effect on the growth of cancer cells in mice with sarcoma.[7]

CLINICAL STUDIES AND RESEARCH

- **Cervical cancer:** In one study, 105 patients with cervical cancer were treated with a 78% rate of effectiveness using both oral and topical applications of *Tian Nan Xing*. The treatment protocol was to use a decoction of the herb, starting with 15 g/day and gradually increasing to 45 g/day. In addition to oral administration, local application was given, utilizing various dosage forms such as powder, suppository, and local injection.[8]
- **Parotitis:** Six patients with parotitis were treated with topical application of *Tian Nan Xing*, with satisfactory results. The topical form was prepared by soaking powdered *Tian Nan Xing* in vinegar for 5 days. The herbal paste was applied topically three to four times daily, for 3 to 4 days. The fever usually subsided within the first day, while decrease in swelling required up to 4 days.[9]

HERB-DRUG INTERACTION

- **Sedatives:** *Tian Nan Xing* is associated with marked sedative and analgesic effects. It also potentiates the sedative effect of barbiturates.[10] [Note: Many categories of drugs induce sedation, such as antihistamines, narcotic analgesics, barbiturates, benzodiazepines and many others.]

TOXICOLOGY

Decoction of processed *Tian Nan Xing* given orally at 150 g/kg showed no significant toxicity in mice. The LD_{50} for intraperitoneal injection in mice is 13.5 g/kg.[11,12]

AUTHORS' COMMENTS

Tian Nan Xing and *Ban Xia* (Rhizoma Pinelliae), both belonging to the araceae family, have similar functions and levels of toxicity. *Tian Nan Xing* mainly treats wind and phlegm. It reduces swelling, relieves pain and enters the peripheral channels and collaterals to treat musculoskeletal disorders. *Ban Xia* mainly treats dampness and phlegm. It enters the Spleen and Stomach to relieve nausea and vomiting.

Tian Nan Xing and *Dan Nan Xing* (Arisaema cum Bile) also share similarities but differ slightly in function. *Tian Nan Xing* is bitter, warm and dry. It more strongly dries dampness, dissolves phlegm, and subdues wind. *Dan Nan Xing* is bitter, cool and moistening. It more effectively clears hot phlegm and relieves convulsions.

References

1. *Zhong Yao Bu Liang Fan Ying Yu Zhi Liao* (Adverse Reactions and Treatment of Chinese Herbal Medicine), 1996; 218:220, 1996; 130:132
2. *Xian Dai Zhong Yao Yao Li Xue* (Contemporary Pharmacology of Chinese Herbs), 1997; 945
3. *Chang Yong Zhong Yao Cheng Fen Yu Yao Li Shou Ce* (A Handbook of the Composition and Pharmacology of Common Chinese Drugs), 1994; 482-483
4. *Zhong Yao Zhi* (Chinese Herbology Journal), 1984: 32
5. *Zhong Yao Yao Li Yu Ying Yong* (Pharmacology and Applications of Chinese Herbs), 1983: 162
6. Ibid.
7. Ibid.
8. *Zhong Yao Xue* (Chinese Herbology), 1998; 1972; 17:8
9. *Xin Yi Xue* (New Medicine), 1972; 10:49
10. *Zhong Yao Yao Li Yu Ying Yong* (Pharmacology and Applications of Chinese Herbs), 1983: 162
11. Ibid.
12. *Chang Yong Zhong Yao Xian Dai Yan Jiu Yu Lin Chuan* (Recent Study & Clinical Application of Common Traditional Chinese Medicine), 1995; 437:439

Dan Nan Xing (Arisaema cum Bile)

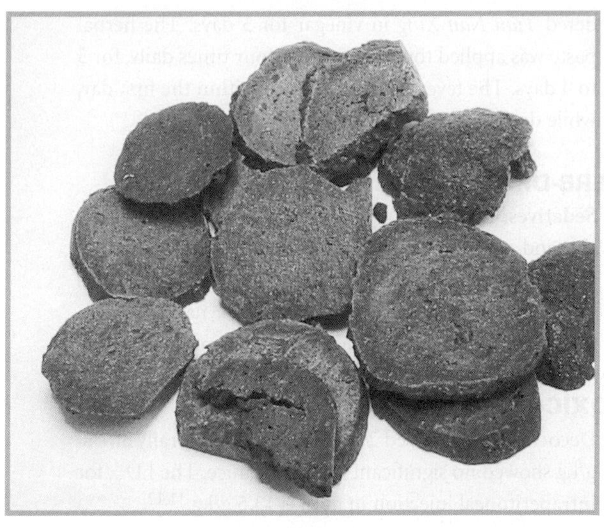

膽南星 胆南星

Pinyin Name: *Dan Nan Xing*
Literal Name: "gallbladder southern star"
Original Source: *Ben Cao Gang Mu* (Materia Medica) by Li Shi-Zhen in 1578
English Name: arisaema pulvis
Botanical Name: *Arisaema consanguineum* Schott. (*Tian Nan Xing*); *Arisaema heterophyllum* Bl. (*Yi Ye Tian Nan Xing*); *Arisaema amurense* Maxim. (*Dong Bei Tian Nan Xing*)
Pharmaceutical Name: Arisaema cum Bile
Properties: bitter, cool
Channels Entered: Liver, Lung, Spleen
Safety Index: slightly toxic

CHINESE THERAPEUTIC ACTIONS

Clears Heat, Dissolves Phlegm, Calms Wind, Stops Convulsions

Dan Nan Xing (Arisaema cum Bile) dispels wind and phlegm obstruction from the channels and collaterals to relieve muscle spasms and cramps. Clinical applications include infantile convulsions, seizures, facial paralysis, tetanus, and stroke.

- Seizures and convulsions in infants: combine *Dan Nan Xing* with *Niu Huang* (Calculus Bovis), *Huang Lian* (Rhizoma Coptidis), *Tian Ma* (Rhizoma Gastrodiae), and *Quan Xie* (Scorpio) to clear heat and calm wind.

DOSAGE

2 to 5 grams. *Dan Nan Xing* is made from the powder of *Tian Nan Xing* (Rhizoma Arisaematis) mixed with bovine bile. Processing with bovine bile (or, in some regions, pig or goat bile) reduces the drying nature of the herb and makes it more suitable for patients with underlying yin deficiency.

CAUTIONS / CONTRAINDICATIONS

- *Dan Nan Xing* must be used with caution for patients who have dry cough due to rising Liver wind from excess fire or blood deficiency.
- *Dan Nan Xing* should be used with extreme caution in pregnant women.
- Allergic reaction may occur when the skin comes in direct contact with *Dan Nan Xing*. Swelling and itching are the main symptoms, and may be alleviated by topical washing with vinegar.

OVERDOSAGE

Dan Nan Xing is slightly toxic. Adverse reactions and potential side effects include numbness of the tongue and mouth, itching, burning sensations, swelling, involuntary salivation, nausea, vomiting, slurred speech, and hoarseness. In severe cases, reactions include muscle spasms and convulsions of the four limbs, and dyspnea.

TREATMENT OF OVERDOSAGE

Overdose of *Dan Nan Xing* can be treated by one or more of the following methods:

- Administration of 30 to 60 ml vinegar and a small amount of ginger juice.
- Administration of an herbal decoction containing 30 grams of *Sheng Jiang* (Rhizoma Zingiberis Recens), 60 grams of *Fang Feng* (Radix Saposhnikoviae), and 15 grams of *Gan Cao* (Radix Glycyrrhizae).

AUTHORS' COMMENTS

Please refer to *Tian Nan Xing* (Rhizoma Arisaematis).

Bai Fu Zi (Rhizoma Typhonii)

白附子

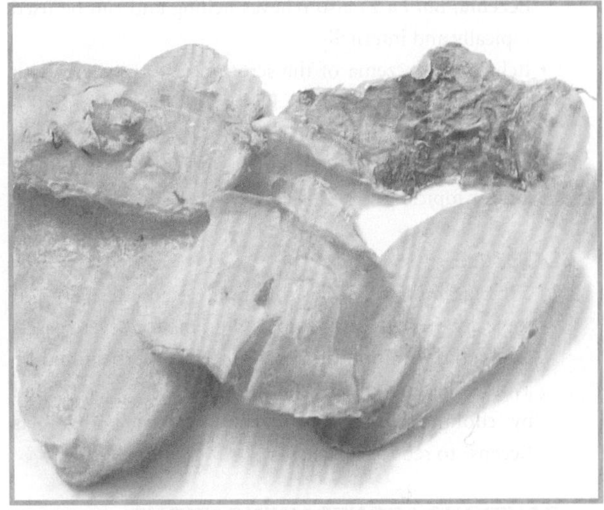

Pinyin Name: *Bai Fu Zi*
Literal Name: "white appendage"
Alternate Chinese Names: *Yu Bai Fu, Guan Bai Fu, Niu Nai Bai Fu, Ji Xin Bai Fu*
Original Source: *Zhong Guo Zhi Wu Zi* (Chinese Journal of Botany)
English Name: typhonium, giant typhonium rhizome
Botanical Name: *Typhonium giganteum* Engl. (*Yu Bai Fu*); *Aconitum coreanum* (Levl.) Raipaics. (*Guan Bai Fu*)
Pharmaceutical Name: Rhizoma Typhonii
Properties: acrid, sweet, warm
Channels Entered: Spleen, Stomach
Safety Index: toxic

CHINESE THERAPEUTIC ACTIONS

1. Dries Dampness, Dissolves Phlegm, Dispels Wind, Stops Convulsions

Accumulation of wind-phlegm: Acrid and warm, *Bai Fu Zi* (Rhizoma Typhonii) dispels wind and phlegm obstruction from the channels and collaterals to relieve muscle spasms and cramps. It is one of the most commonly used herbs to treat convulsions, tremors, paralysis and deviation of the mouth and eyes. Clinical applications include infantile convulsions, seizures, facial paralysis, tetanus, and stroke.

- Post-stroke deviation of the eyes and mouth: combine *Bai Fu Zi* with *Jiang Can* (Bombyx Batryticatus) and *Quan Xie* (Scorpio). **Exemplar Formula:** *Qian Zheng San* (Lead to Symmetry Powder).
- Tetanus, muscle spasms and stiffness of the neck, opisthotonos, clenched jaws: use this herb with *Tian Nan Xing* (Rhizoma Arisaematis), *Tian Ma* (Rhizoma Gastrodiae), and *Fang Feng* (Radix Saposhnikoviae). **Exemplar Formula:** *Yu Zhen San* (True Jade Powder).
- Facial paralysis: incorporate *Bai Fu Zi* for internal use with *Jiang Can* (Bombyx Batryticatus), *Quan Xie* (Scorpio), *Bai Zhi* (Radix Angelicae Dahuricae), *Jing Jie* (Herba Schizonepetae), *Fang Feng* (Radix Saposhnikoviae), *Hong Hua* (Flos Carthami), *Tian Nan Xing* (Rhizoma Arisaematis), *Bai Jie Zi* (Semen Sinapis), *Zao Jiao Ci* (Spina Gleditsiae), *Tao Ren* (Semen Persicae) and *Su Mu* (Lignum Sappan). This same formula can be used topically by applying a towel saturated with the warm decoction to the affected area.

Headache and migraine: Acrid, warm and dispersing, *Bai Fu Zi* enters the *yangming* channel to treat headache and migraine characterized by cold-damp and wind-phlegm. This type of headache and migraine usually has an abrupt onset and the pain is very severe either on one or both sides of the head. The patient usually feels heavy and the tongue coating is white and greasy.

- Headache and migraine: use *Bai Fu Zi* with *Bai Zhi* (Radix Angelicae Dahuricae), *Chuan Xiong* (Rhizoma Ligustici Chuanxiong), *Man Jing Zi* (Fructus Viticis) and *Ju Hua* (Flos Chrysanthemi). If the patient is deficient in qi and blood, tonics should be added accordingly.

2. Eliminates Toxins and Dissipates Nodules

Scrofula, phlegm masses, toxic snake bites: *Bai Fu Zi* softens hardness and dissipates nodules to treat scrofula and thyroid nodules. It can be used internally and topically. This herb also treats snake bites by clearing toxicity and reducing swelling.

- Scrofula or thyroid nodules: crush fresh *Bai Fu Zi* and use topically as a paste.
- Snake bite: use this herb with *Bai Zhi* (Radix Angelicae Dahuricae), *Jin Yin Hua* (Flos Lonicerae) and *Zhe Bei Mu* (Bulbus Fritillariae Thunbergii), and apply topically.
- Fungal skin diseases (such as tinea versicolor): mix this herb with *Xiong Huang* (Realgar) and water or grain-based alcohol, and apply topically.

3. Dries Dampness, Relieves Pain, Stops Itching

***Bi zheng* (painful obstruction syndrome):** *Bai Fu Zi* treats *bi zheng* characterized by muscle and joint aches and pains, that worsen with rainy or cold weather. It also treats difficulty with flexion and extension.

- *Bi zheng*: combine it with *Wei Ling Xian* (Radix Clematidis) and *Du Huo* (Radix Angelicae Pubescentis).

Bai Fu Zi (Rhizoma Typhonii)

Eczema: *Bai Fu Zi* also relieves itching and can be used topically and internally.

- Itching and eczema of the scrotum: use this herb with *Qiang Huo* (Rhizoma et Radix Notopterygii), *Bai Ji Li* (Fructus Tribuli), and *Huang Qi* (Radix Astragali) in powder form. These herbs can be used internally and/or topically.

DOSAGE

3 to 5 grams. *Bai Fu Zi* is commonly used internally and topically. Dosage can be up to 9 grams for severe cases. Oral administration of the unprocessed herb should be avoided because of its toxicity. *Bai Fu Zi* may be treated by cooking with *Sheng Jiang* (Rhizoma Zingiberis Recens) to reduce toxicity.

CAUTIONS / CONTRAINDICATIONS

- Fresh or unprocessed *Bai Fu Zi* is toxic and should only be used topically.
- Since *Bai Fu Zi* is toxic, do not exceed appropriate dosage of the herb or give it for an extended period of time.
- *Bai Fu Zi* is contraindicated during pregnancy.
- *Bai Fu Zi* is also contraindicated in cases of wind-stroke from Liver fire.

CHEMICAL COMPOSITION

Saponin, alkaloid, β-sitosterol, lectin.[1]

PHARMACOLOGICAL EFFECTS

- **Antibiotic:** Injection of *Bai Fu Zi* was effective in treatment of guinea pigs infected with tuberculosis.[2]
- **Antiarrhythmic:** A preparation of *Bai Fu Zi* has been shown to have an antiarrhythmic effect.[3]

CLINICAL STUDIES AND RESEARCH

- **Numbness of facial nerves:** In one clinical study, 418 patients with numbness of the face were treated by injection of an herbal formula into acupuncture points, with 90% reporting complete recovery. The herbal formula was modified from *Qian Zheng San* (Lead to Symmetry Powder), and contained *Bai Fu Zi* 60g, *Dang Gui* (Radicis Angelicae Sinensis) 60g, *Quan Xie* (Scorpio) 60g, *Jiang Can* (Bombyx Batryticatus) 60g and *Wu Gong* (Scolopendra) 40 pieces. Acupuncture points selected included *Dicang* (ST 4), *Jiache* (ST 6), *Yangbai* (GB 14), *Taiyang* (Extra), and *Hegu* (LI 4).[4]

SUPPLEMENT

Bai Fu Zi (Rhizoma Typhonii) is derived from two sources: *Yu Bai Fu* (Rhizoma Typhonium Giganteum) and *Guan Bai Fu* (Rhizoma Aconitum Coreanum). Both herbs dispel wind and phlegm.

- 禹白附 *Yu Bai Fu* (Rhizoma Typhonium Giganteum) is the standard source of *Bai Fu Zi*. It is more effective to clear toxins and disperse stagnation. It is better to treat arthritis and relieve pain.
- 關白附 / 关白附 *Guan Bai Fu* (Rhizoma Aconitum Coreanum) is sometimes used as a substitute for *Bai Fu Zi*.

AUTHORS' COMMENTS

Bai Fu Zi (Rhizoma Typhonii) and *Fu Zi* (Radix Aconiti Lateralis Praeparata) have a similar physical appearance, and thus share a similar name. These two herbs, however, have completely different natures and functions, and should not be confused or used interchangeably. *Bai Fu Zi* is used primarily to eliminate wind-phlegm and cold. *Fu Zi* (Radix Aconiti Lateralis Praeparata) warms both the interior and Kidney yang.

References

1. *Zhong Yao Da Ci Dien* (Dictionary of Chinese Herbs), 1977;1689
2. *Zhong Yao Xue* (Chinese Herbology), 1998; 607:608
3. Ibid.
4. *Hu Bei Zhong Yi Za Zhi* (Hubei Journal of Chinese Medicine), 1982; 1:33

Bai Jie Zi (Semen Sinapis)

白芥子 白芥子

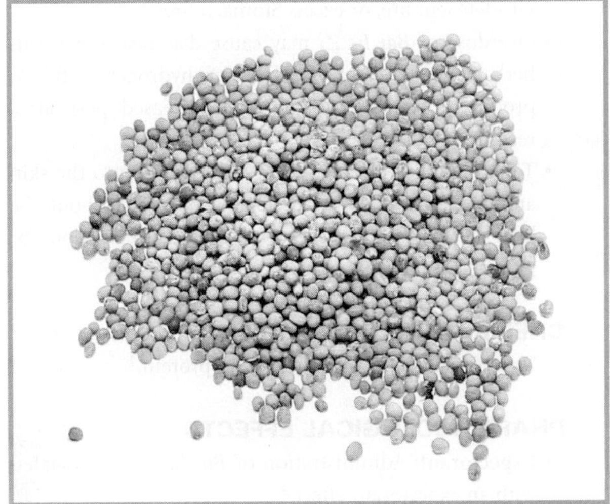

Pinyin Name: *Bai Jie Zi*
Literal Name: "white mustard seed"
Alternate Chinese Names: *Huang Jie Zi*
Original Source: *Ming Yi Za Zhu* (Miscellaneous Records of Famous Physicians) by Tao Hong-Jing in 500 A.D.
English Name: mustard seed, white mustard seed
Botanical Name: *Sinapis alba* (L.) Boiss. (*Bai Jie Zi*); *Brassica juncea* (L.) Czern. et Coss. (*Huang Jie Zi*)
Pharmaceutical Name: Semen Sinapis
Properties: acrid, warm
Channels Entered: Lung

CHINESE THERAPEUTIC ACTIONS

1. Warms the Lung, Dispels Phlegm

Phlegm stagnation: Acrid, warm and dispersing in nature, *Bai Jie Zi* (Semen Sinapis) warms the Lung, ventilates Lung qi and dispels phlegm. Cold phlegm obstruction in the Lung causes cough, wheezing and dyspnea, while obstruction of phlegm at the diaphragm causes sudden sharp pain in the thorax and neck, profuse clear or white sputum, greasy tongue coat and wiry, slippery pulse.

- Cough, wheezing and chest pain due to accumulation of phlegm and water in the chest and diaphragm: combine *Bai Jie Zi* with *Su Zi* (Fructus Perillae) and *Lai Fu Zi* (Semen Raphani). **Exemplar Formula:** *San Zi Yang Qin Tang* (Three-Seed Decoction to Nourish One's Parents).
- Obstruction of phlegm above and below the diaphragm with sharp pain in the thorax and neck (an excess condition): use *Bai Jie Zi* with *Gan Sui* (Radix Euphorbiae Kansui) and *Da Ji* (Radix Euphorbiae seu Knoxiae).

Lung qi reversal caused by phlegm stagnation: *Bai Jie Zi* is commonly used to treat accumulation of dampness and phlegm in the Lung that causes profuse, clear sputum, cough, dyspnea, and wheezing.

- Wheezing and dyspnea due to cold phlegm: combine *Bai Jie Zi* with *Su Zi* (Fructus Perillae) and *Lai Fu Zi* (Semen Raphani) to warm the Lung and dispel phlegm.

2. Regulates Qi, Dissipates Nodules, Opens Channels and Collaterals, Relieves Pain

Phlegm obstruction of the channels and collaterals: Phlegm obstruction in the peripheral channels and collaterals causes severe numbness and pain, especially around the waist and back.

- Phlegm obstruction in the peripheral channels and collaterals: add *Bai Jie Zi* to *Mo Yao* (Myrrha), *Gui Zhi* (Ramulus Cinnamomi) and *Mu Xiang* (Radix Aucklandiae), for use as herbal powder. Serve with grain-based liquor.

Scrofula, phlegm masses: These masses are caused when phlegm obstruction hardens into masses or nodules. Treatment involves mixing *Bai Jie Zi* powder with vinegar and applying topically.

Yin sores: This type of cellulitis or sore is caused by phlegm obstruction of the channels and collaterals. Treatment requires warming the yang, dissolving phlegm and dispersing nodules.

- Yin sores: use *Bai Jie Zi* with *Lu Jiao Jiao* (Gelatinum Cornu Cervi), *Rou Gui* (Cortex Cinnamomi), *Pao Jiang* (Rhizoma Zingiberis Preparatum) and *Shu Di Huang* (Radix Rehmanniae Preparata). **Exemplar Formula:** *Yang He Tang* (Yang-Heartening Decoction).

DOSAGE

3 to 10 grams as herbal decoction. Mix *Bai Jie Zi* powder with vinegar for topical application. Use of unprocessed *Bai Jie Zi*, which is acrid and warm, is sometimes associated with excessive consumption of qi and yin in the body. To minimize this side effect, the herb should be dry-fried. In addition, dry-frying facilitates the extraction of active components. *Bai Jie Zi* should be decocted towards the end or at the close of cooking, to avoid deactivation of its active constituents.

CAUTIONS / CONTRAINDICATIONS

- Acrid and dispersing, *Bai Jie Zi* is contraindicated in patients with chronic coughing from Lung deficiency,

Bai Jie Zi (Semen Sinapis)

yin-deficient fire, or excess Stomach fire.

- Overdose of *Bai Jie Zi* may cause diarrhea. When this herb comes in contact with water, hydrogen sulfide is produced, which can stimulate increased peristalsis, resulting in diarrhea.
- Topical application of *Bai Jie Zi* is irritating to the skin and may cause allergic reactions or blisters. It should be kept away from the eyes and used with caution for patients with sensitive skin.

CHEMICAL COMPOSITION

Sinalbin, sinapine, myrosin, lipids, protein.[1]

PHARMACOLOGICAL EFFECTS

- **Expectorant:** Administration of *Bai Jie Zi* is associated with an expectorant effect.[2]
- **Dermatological:** Direct contact with *Bai Jie Zi* has a stimulating effect on the skin, causing redness, swelling, and formation of blisters. When used as a topical application, it should not be left on the skin for more than 15 to 30 minutes.[3]
- **Antibiotic:** Water extract of *Bai Jie Zi* has an inhibitory influence against some pathogenic fungi and dermatophytes.[4]

CLINICAL STUDIES AND RESEARCH

- **Tracheitis in children:** According to one study, 50 children with acute or chronic tracheitis were treated with topical application of *Bai Jie Zi*, with good results. The herb paste was prepared by mixing 33 grams of *Bai Jie Zi* and 90 grams of flour with water. The paste was applied on the upper back at bedtime, removed in the morning, for a total of 2 or 3 treatments.[5]
- **Pneumonia in children:** Topical application of *Bai Jie Zi* on the chest had a beneficial effect in treating 100 children with pneumonia.[6]
- **Numbness in the facial region:** In one clinical study, patients with numbness of the face were treated with topical application of *Bai Jie Zi*. The paste was prepared by mixing 5 to 10 grams of *Bai Jie Zi* powder with water, and was applied topically to the affected area between *Dicang* (ST 4), *Xiguan* (LR 7) and *Jiache* (ST 6). After application, the herbal paste was covered with gauze, and removed 3 to 12 hours later. The same treatment was repeated in 10 to 14 days if necessary. Out of 1,052 patients, 137 dropped out of the study. Of the 915 patients who stayed throughout the study, there was a 97.7% rate of effectiveness.[7]

AUTHORS' COMMENTS

Chronic asthma can be treated with topical application of an herbal paste to acupuncture points *Feishu* (BL 13), *Xinshu* (BL 15) and *Geshu* (BL 17). The herbal paste is made by mixing fresh ginger juice with powdered *Bai Jie Zi*, *Gan Sui* (Radix Euphorbiae Kansui), *Yan Hu Suo* (Rhizoma Corydalis) and *Xi Xin* (Herba Asari).

Bai Jie Zi, *Zi Su Zi* (Fructus Perillae), and *Lai Fu Zi* (Semen Raphani) are commonly used together to treat wheezing and dyspnea with phlegm, such as in *San Zi Yang Qin Tang* (Three-Seed Decoction to Nourish One's Parents).

- *Bai Jie Zi* warms and dispels the accumulation of phlegm in the Lung.
- *Zi Su Zi* descends qi and dissolves phlegm.
- *Lai Fu Zi* regulates Spleen qi to stop the production of phlegm.

References

1. *Xian Dai Zhong Yao Yao Li Xue* (Contemporary Pharmacology of Chinese Herbs), 1997; 964
2. *Zhong Yao Xue* (Chinese Herbology), 1998; 608:610
3. *Chang Yong Zhong Yao Xian Dai Yan Jiu Yu Lin Chuan* (Recent Study & Clinical Application of Common Traditional Chinese Medicine), 1995; 439:441
4. Ibid.
5. *Hei Long Jiang Zhong Yi Yao* (Heilongjiang Chinese Medicine and Herbology), 1988; 1:29
6. *Zhong Xi Yi Jie He Za Zhi* (Journal of Integrated Chinese and Western Medicine), 1986; 2:124
7. *Shan Dong Zhong Yi Za Zhi* (Shandong Journal of Chinese Medicine), 1986; 5:25

Zao Jiao (Fructus Gleditsiae)

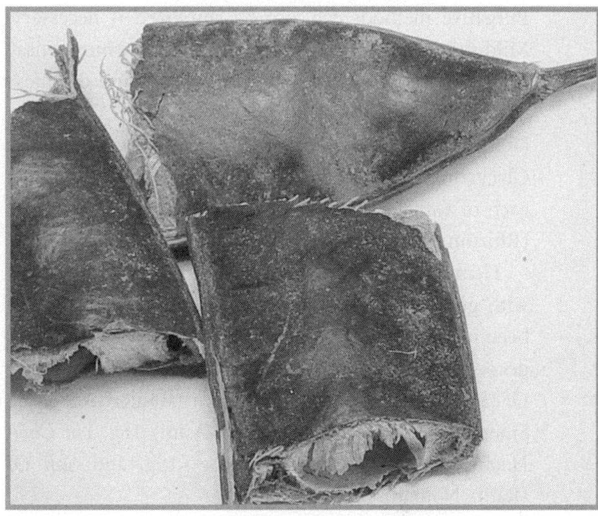

皂角 皂角

Pinyin Name: *Zao Jiao*
Literal Name: "soap thorn"
Alternate Chinese Names: *Zao Jia, Zhu Ya Zao*
Original Source: *Shen Nong Ben Cao Jing* (Divine Husbandman's Classic of the Materia Medica) in the second century
English Name: gleditsia fruit, Chinese honey locust
Botanical Name: *Gleditsia sinensis* Lam. (*Zao Jiao*)
Pharmaceutical Name: Fructus Gleditsiae
Properties: acrid, warm
Channels Entered: Large Intestine, Lung
Safety Index: slightly toxic

CHINESE THERAPEUTIC ACTIONS

1. Dispels Phlegm

Acrid and dispersing, *Zao Jiao* (Fructus Gleditsiae) strongly breaks up and dispels phlegm. It treats chronic and stubborn accumulations of phlegm in the Lung that lead to chest congestion, cough, dyspnea, and sputum that is difficult to expectorate.

- Phlegm accumulation in the chest, with cough: use *Zao Jiao* to dispel the phlegm and *Da Zao* (Fructus Jujubae) to protect the Stomach.
- Chronic pulmonary infection with cough, wheezing, chest congestion, and copious, difficult-to-expectorate sputum: use this herb with *Ma Huang* (Herba Ephedrae) and pig bile.
- Consumptive lung disorders, lung abscesses with cough: combine *Zao Jiao* with *Da Zao* (Fructus Jujubae) and honey.

2. Opens Sensory Orifices

Zao Jiao opens the sensory orifices to resuscitate patients who are unconscious, with foaming of the mouth, locked jaw, difficulty breathing, and a pale face. This herb is most suitable for symptoms of excess-type *bi zheng* (closed disorder).

- Sudden loss of consciousness: blow powdered *Zao Jiao* and *Xi Xin* (Herba Asari) into the nostrils to induce sneezing and restore consciousness.
- Stroke with clenched jaw: mix *Zao Jiao* with warm water and *Ming Fan* (Alumen) to induce vomiting.

3. Reduces Swelling and Abscesses

Zao Jiao reduces swelling and drains abscesses that have not ulcerated. It treats initial stages of boils, clumping, and abscesses.

- Abscesses and boils: cook *Zao Jiao* with vinegar and apply topically as a paste.

4. Relieves Constipation

Zao Jiao stimulates peristalsis and induces bowel movement.

- Constipation: mix *Zao Jiao*, *Xi Xin* (Herba Asari) and honey to make suppositories and insert rectally. For oral ingestion, combine *Zao Jiao* with *Tao Ren* (Semen Persicae) and *Gua Lou Shi* (Fructus Trichosanthis).

DOSAGE

1.5 to 5 grams in decoction. *Zao Jiao* powder may be used in dosages of 0.6 to 1.5 grams daily for internal use.

CAUTIONS / CONTRAINDICATIONS

- Use of *Zao Jiao* is contraindicated for patients who are coughing blood, or for those with deficiencies of qi and yin.
- *Zao Jiao* is contraindicated during pregnancy.
- Ingestion of a large dose of *Zao Jiao* may cause nausea or diarrhea.

OVERDOSAGE

Overdose of *Zao Jiao* may cause nausea, vomiting, diarrhea, irritability, weak extremities, and fullness in the epigastric region. It stimulates, then inhibits, the central nervous system. In severe cases, respiratory depression may occur. In rare cases, hemolytic anemia has been associated with gross overdose of *Zao Jiao* (dosages in excess of 30 grams).

TREATMENT OF OVERDOSAGE

Early-stage overdose can be treated with emetic methods, followed by ingestion of egg whites or milk.

Zao Jiao (Fructus Gleditsiae)

Purgative methods can also be employed if necessary. Mild systemic reactions characterized by burning sensations and pain of the throat, palpitations, and dizziness can be treated with an herbal decoction of *Xuan Shen* (Radix Scrophulariae) 30g, *Gan Cao* (Radix Glycyrrhizae) 15g, and honey 60g. Decoction of 9 grams each of *Gan Cao* (Radix Glycyrrhizae) and *Sheng Jiang* (Rhizoma Zingiberis Recens) is also beneficial.[1]

Hemolytic anemia, a rare adverse reaction associated with gross overdose of over 30 grams of *Zao Jiao*, has been noted. This condition can be treated with an herbal decoction of *Hei Dou* (Semen Glycine Max) 30g, *Huang Qi* (Radix Astragali) 30g, *Dang Gui* (Radicis Angelicae Sinensis) 15g, *E Jiao* (Colla Corii Asini) 15g, *Yin Chen Hao* (Herba Artemisiae Scopariae) 15g, and *San Qi* (Radix Notoginseng) 3g.[2]

CHEMICAL COMPOSITION

Gledinin, gledigenin, gleditschiasaponin, gleditschiasapogenin, arabinose, ceryl alcohol, nonacosane, stigmasterol, sitosterol.[3]

PHARMACOLOGICAL EFFECTS

- **Expectorant:** The expectorant action of *Zao Jiao* is associated with stimulation and increased secretion of the respiratory tract.[4]
- **Gastrointestinal:** *Zao Jiao* has a stimulating effect on the stomach and intestines and may cause nausea, vomiting or diarrhea. Nausea and vomiting usually occur within 10 minutes of ingestion.[5]
- **Antibiotic:** It has an inhibitory effect against *E. coli*, *Bacillus dysenteriae*, *Pseudomonas aeruginosa*, *Vibrio cholerae*, and some dermatophytes.[6]

CLINICAL STUDIES AND RESEARCH

- **Expectorant:** *Zao Jiao* was used successfully in treating 103 patients with various respiratory disorders characterized by accumulation of sputum. The herbal formula was prepared by mixing *Zao Jiao* powder with honey to make pills. The dosage was 0.4 to 0.6 gram of the herb, three times daily. The average duration of treatment was 16.5 days. This treatment was contraindicated for individuals with deficiencies or at risk of bleeding.[7]
- **Acute postpartum mastitis:** In one study, 36 patients with acute postpartum mastitis were treated with intranasal administration of *Zao Jiao* with good success. The treatment protocol was to grind the herb into powder, mix it with 75% alcohol, wrap the paste in a piece of cloth, and insert it into the nostril on the same side as the mastitis. The nasal insert was retained for 12 hours.[8]
- **Anorexia:** A *Zao Jiao* preparation was used with 94.5% effectiveness in treating 110 children with anorexia. The herb was calcined, dry-fried, and then ground into powder. Children were given 1 gram of the herb mixed with sugar twice daily, for 3 to 10 days. Most children responded within 5 days.[9]

HERB-DRUG INTERACTION

- **Absorption:** According to Dr. Zhang Xiao-Ping, *Zao Jiao* has a "detergent" effect which enables it to bind to other substances to form a large and insoluble complex that cannot be absorbed. Though this potential interaction with pharmaceuticals has not been documented, it is wise to instruct the patient not to take *Zao Jiao* and drugs concurrently, as there may be a decrease in absorption and blood concentration of the drug.

AUTHORS' COMMENTS

Zao Jiao (Fructus Gleditsiae) and *Zao Jiao Ci* (Spina Gleditsiae) have similar functions. *Zao Jiao* more strongly dispels phlegm. *Zao Jiao Ci* more effectively activates blood circulation and disperses stagnation, and is used for sores and carbuncles that have not yet ulcerated.

According to Dr. Zhang Xiao-Ping, both *Zao Jiao* (Fructus Gleditsiae) and *Zao Jiao Ci* (Spina Gleditsiae) can be used for treatment of obesity, elevated cholesterol level, and lipoma. Both of these herbs have a "detergent" effects with both lipophilic and hydrophilic properties, enabling the flushing of fatty substances from the body. The recommended dose for this application is 3 to 5 grams in decoction.

References

1. *Zhong Yao Du Li Xue* (Toxicology of Chinese Herbs), 99-101, 1989
2. *Lin Chuan Shou Ce You Du Zhong Yao Shi Yong* (Clinical Handbook on Applications of Toxic Chinese Herbs), 1992; 131-132
3. *Chang Yong Zhong Yao Xian Dai Yan Jiu Yu Lin Chuan* (Recent Study & Clinical Application of Common Traditional Chinese Medicine), 1995; 442
4. *Zhong Yao Xue* (Chinese Herbology), 1998; 610:612
5. Ibid.
6. Ibid.
7. *Zhong Hua Nei Ke Xue Za Zhi* (Journal of Chinese Internal Medicine), 1982; 12:783
8. *Zhong Hua Yi Xue Za Zhi* (Chinese Journal of Medicine), 1973; 11:685
9. *Hu Bei Zhong Yi Za Zhi* (Hubei Journal of Chinese Medicine), 1987; 1:25

Zao Jiao Ci (Spina Gleditsiae)

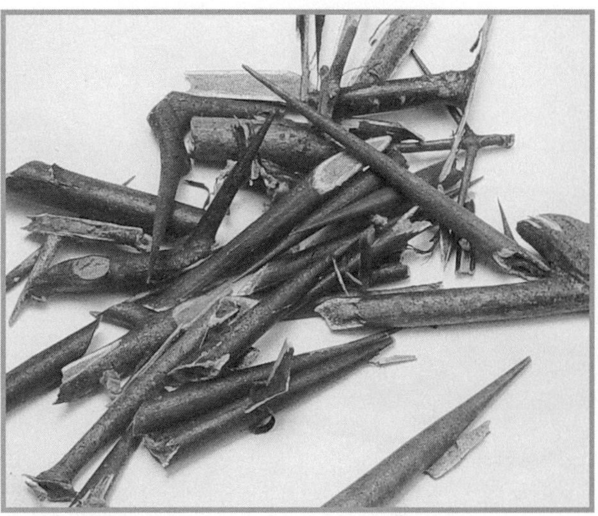

皂角刺 皂角刺

Pinyin Name: *Zao Jiao Ci*
Literal Name: "soap thorn spine"
Alternate Chinese Names: *Zao Jiao Zhen*
Original Source: *Tu Jing Ben Cao* (Illustrated Classic of the Materia Medica) by Su Song in 1061
English Name: gleditsia spine, Chinese honey locust spine
Botanical Name: *Gleditsia sinensis* Lam. (*Zao Jiao*)
Pharmaceutical Name: Spina Gleditsiae
Properties: acrid, warm
Channels Entered: Liver, Stomach

CHINESE THERAPEUTIC ACTIONS

Eliminates Toxicity, Drains Pus, Activates Blood Circulation, Reduces Swelling

Sores, carbuncles, masses with pus, that have not suppurated: Acrid and warm, *Zao Jiao Ci* (Spina Gleditsiae) reduces swelling and drains sores with accumulated heat and toxins. It is commonly used in the early stages of sores to encourage suppuration, or to induce the drainage of sores with pus.

- Acute mastitis: take 30 grams of herbal powder (1:10 ratio of *Zao Jiao Ci* to *Hai Ge Fen* (Concha Meretricis seu Cyclinae)) followed by warm grain-based liquor.
- Scrofula, sores: mix *Zao Jiao Ci* and *Bai Ji* (Rhizoma Bletillae) and apply topically.
- Tonsillitis: use this herb individually.

DOSAGE

3 to 10 grams.

CAUTIONS / CONTRAINDICATIONS

- *Zao Jiao Ci* is contraindicated during pregnancy.
- It is also contraindicated if the sores have already ruptured.

CHEMICAL COMPOSITION

Flavonoids, phenols, amino acids.[1]

CLINICAL STUDIES AND RESEARCH

- **Tonsillitis:** In one study, 9 out of 10 patients with tonsillitis showed complete recovery following treatment with *Zao Jiao Ci*. The treatment protocol was to cook 9 grams of the herb in water, and drink the decoction in 2 equally-divided doses daily for 2 to 6 days. Therapeutic benefits included reduced swelling, pain relief, reduced fever, and normal white blood cell count.[2]

HERB-DRUG INTERACTION

- **Absorption:** According to Dr. Zhang Xiao-Ping, *Zao Jiao Ci* has a "detergent" effect that enables it to bind to other substances to form a large and insoluble complex that cannot be absorbed. Though this potential interaction with pharmaceuticals has not been documented, it is wise to instruct the patient not to take *Zao Jiao Ci* and drugs concurrently, as there may be a decrease in absorption and blood concentration of the drug.

AUTHORS' COMMENTS

According to Dr. Long Pang-Chi, *Zao Jiao Ci* reduces swelling and dispels pus. It is excellent for treatment of obstruction or adhesions of the fallopian tubes secondary to pelvic inflammatory disease. *Zao Jiao Ci* is commonly combined with *Tao Ren* (Semen Persicae) and *Bai Jiang Cao* (Herba cum Radice Patriniae) for maximum effectiveness in this action.

References

1. *Zhong Yao Xue* (Chinese Herbology), 1998; 612
2. *Zhong Hua Er Bi Hou Ke Za Zhi* (Chinese Journal of ENT), 1959; 2:159

Jie Geng (Radix Platycodonis)

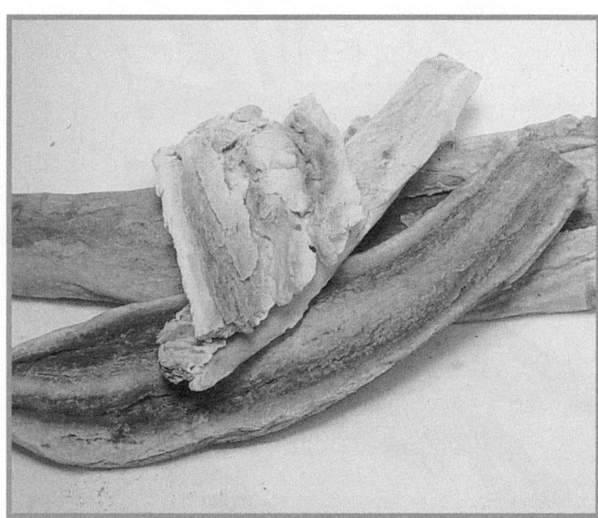

桔梗

Pinyin Name: *Jie Geng*
Literal Name: "solid and straight root"
Alternate Chinese Names: *Ku Jie Geng, Bai Jie Geng, Yu Jie Geng*
Original Source: *Shen Nong Ben Cao Jing* (Divine Husbandman's Classic of the Materia Medica) in the second century
English Name: platycodon, platycodon root, balloon-flower root
Botanical Name: *Platycodon grandiflorum* (Jacq.) A. DC. (*Jie Geng*)
Pharmaceutical Name: Radix Platycodonis
Properties: bitter, acrid, neutral
Channels Entered: Lung

CHINESE THERAPEUTIC ACTIONS

1. Ventilates the Lung, Dispels Phlegm, and Benefits the Throat

Cough with profuse phlegm, sore throat with hoarse voice: Acrid, bitter and dispersing in nature, *Jie Geng* (Radix Platycodonis) enters the Lung to ventilate Lung qi, dispel phlegm, and benefit the throat. It is one of the most essential herbs for treatment of Lung disorders. *Jie Geng* can be used for phlegm caused by wind-heat or wind-cold invasions. Common clinical manifestations include cough with profuse sputum, sore throat and hoarse voice.

- Cough, stuffy nose, sputum, aversion to cold, and headache caused by wind-cold: combine *Jie Geng* with *Zi Su Ye* (Folium Perillae), *Xing Ren* (Semen Armeniacae Amarum) and *Chen Pi* (Pericarpium Citri Reticulatae). **Exemplar Formula:** *Xing Su San* (Apricot Kernel and Perilla Leaf Powder).
- Cough, fever, thirst, stuffy nose and headache from wind-heat or febrile disorders: use this herb with *Sang Ye* (Folium Mori), *Ju Hua* (Flos Chrysanthemi), and *Xing Ren* (Semen Armeniacae Amarum). **Exemplar Formula:** *Sang Ju Yin* (Mulberry Leaf and Chrysanthemum Decoction).
- Sore throat and hoarse voice: add *Jie Geng* to *Gan Cao* (Radix Glycyrrhizae).
- Severe sore throat and loss of voice: use it with *Gan Cao* (Radix Glycyrrhizae), *Huang Qin* (Radix Scutellariae) and *Gu Zhi Hua* (Semen Oroxyli).
- Sore throat and loss of voice due to wind-heat: add this herb to *Bo He* (Herba Menthae), *Niu Bang Zi* (Fructus Arctii) and *Chan Tui* (Periostracum Cicadae).
- Chest congestion and discomfort with phlegm stagnation: use it with *Zhi Ke* (Fructus Aurantii) and *Gua Lou Pi* (Pericarpium Trichosanthis).

2. Dispels Pus

Lung abscess: *Jie Geng* is one of the strongest herbs to dispel phlegm and pus. It clears heat and eliminates toxins to treat formation of pus and abscesses. Secondary symptoms include chest pain, fever, cough with blood and pus, and thick, yellow sputum with a putrid stench.

- Lung abscess with chest pain, fever, cough with foul-smelling, yellow, sticky sputum: combine this herb with *Gan Cao* (Radix Glycyrrhizae) and *Yi Yi Ren* (Semen Coicis).
- Lung abscess with profuse phlegm and pus accumulation: use *Jie Geng* with *Bei Mu* (Bulbus Fritillaria), *Yi Yi Ren* (Semen Coicis) and *Ba Dou* (Fructus Crotonis).
- Lobar pneumonia and bronchitis caused by heat and toxins: use this herb with *Yu Xing Cao* (Herba Houttuyniae), *Yi Yi Ren* (Semen Coicis) and *Dong Gua Zi* (Semen Benincasae).
- Formation of pus and abscesses: use it with *Bai Shao* (Radix Paeoniae Alba) and *Zhi Shi* (Fructus Aurantii Immaturus). **Exemplar Formula:** *Pai Nong San* (Drain the Pus Powder).

3. Raises Qi

Jie Geng raises the qi of the Lung and Large Intestine, two organs connected by their *zang fu* relationship. It is commonly used to lift sunken qi, for treatment of diarrhea, rectal tenesmus, anuria, and edema.

DOSAGE

3 to 9 grams. Honey-baked *Jie Geng* is stronger for moistening the Lung and dispelling phlegm.

Jie Geng (Radix Platycodonis)

CAUTIONS / CONTRAINDICATIONS

- Bitter, dispersing and draining, *Jie Geng* should be used with caution for patients experiencing chronic cough from yin deficiency, or cough with blood-streaked sputum.

CHEMICAL COMPOSITION

Platycodigenin, polygalacic acid, platycogenic acid A, B, C; glucose, amino acids.[1]

PHARMACOLOGICAL EFFECTS

- **Expectorant and antitussive:** Decoction of *Jie Geng* at 1 g/kg has a marked expectorant effect in anesthetized dogs and cats. Intraperitoneal injection of *Jie Geng* was effective in suppressing cough in guinea pigs.[2]
- **Cardiovascular:** Intravenous injection of a *Jie Geng* preparation was associated with a decrease in blood pressure, heart rate, and respiratory rate in rats. It also dilated blood vessels and increased blood perfusion to peripheral parts of the body.[3]
- **Anti-inflammatory:** Administration of *Jie Geng* is associated with a suppressed sensitivity for allergic reaction and decreased capillary permeability.[4]
- **Gastrointestinal:** Administration of *Jie Geng* is beneficial in treatment of stomach and duodenal ulcers. At $1/5^{th}$ the LD_{50}, *Jie Geng* exerts close to 100% inhibition of the secretion of gastric acid in mice.[5]
- **Antidiabetic:** Oral administration of water or alcohol extract of *Jie Geng* in rabbits may lower plasma glucose levels and prevent sharp increases in levels following meals. The alcohol extract was more effective than the water extract.[6]
- **Others:** It has analgesic, antihyperlipidemic, sedative, and antipyretic effects.[7]

CLINICAL STUDIES AND RESEARCH

- **Pulmonary abscess:** Ten patients with pulmonary abscesses were treated with an herbal decoction with satisfactory results. The initial treatment used 60 grams of *Jie Geng* and 30 grams of *Gan Cao* (Radix Glycyrrhizae). The dosage of both herbs was reduced by two-thirds after the condition improved.[8]

TOXICOLOGY

The LD_{50} for decoction of *Jie Geng* is 24 g/kg in mice. No fatalities were reported in rabbits that received the decoction at 20 g/kg. However, at 40 g/kg, there was a 100% fatality in 5 out of 5 rabbits within 24 hours of administration.[9,10]

SUPPLEMENT

- 疏花沙参 / 疏花沙参 *Shu Hua Sha Shen* (Radix Adenophora Remotiflora) was mentioned in some classic texts as a substitute for *Jie Geng*. However, they are two separate entities and should not be used interchangeably.

AUTHORS' COMMENTS

Jie Geng and *Xing Ren* (Semen Armeniacae Amarum) are commonly used to treat improperly rising Lung qi. *Jie Geng* is neutral, and can be used in patients with Lung disorders caused by either cold or heat. It causes Lung qi to descend, expands the chest and dispels phlegm and pus. *Xing Ren* directs Lung qi downward, and is effective to treat cough, wheezing and dyspnea. It also dissolves turbidity and phlegm.

References

1. *Xian Dai Zhong Yao Yao Li Xue* (Contemporary Pharmacology of Chinese Herbs), 1997; 949
2. *Zhong Yao Yao Li Yu Ying Yong* (Pharmacology and Applications of Chinese Herbs), 1983; 866
3. Ibid.
4. Ibid.
5. Ibid.
6. Ibid.
7. *Chang Yong Zhong Yao Cheng Fen Yu Yao Li Shou Ce* (A Handbook of the Composition and Pharmacology of Common Chinese Drugs), 1994; 1488;1491
8. *Jiang Su Zhong Yi Za Zhi* (Jiangsu Journal of Chinese Medicine), 1981; 3:35
9. *Zhong Yao Yao Li Yu Ying Yong* (Pharmacology and Applications of Chinese Herbs), 1983: 866
10. *Zhong Cao Yao* (Chinese Herbal Medicine), 1991; 22(7):324

Xuan Fu Hua (Flos Inulae)

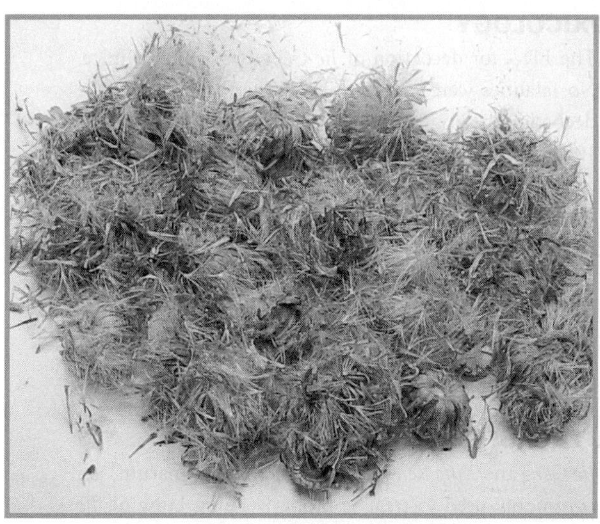

旋覆花 旋覆花

Pinyin Name: *Xuan Fu Hua*
Literal Name: "revolved, upturned flower"
Alternate Chinese Names: *Jin Fei Hua, Jin Fei Cao, Xuan Fu Geng*
Original Source: *Shen Nong Ben Cao Jing* (Divine Husbandman's Classic of the Materia Medica) in the second century
English Name: inula flowers
Botanical Name: *Inula japonica* Thunb. (*Xuan Fu Hua*); *Inula britannica* L. (*Ou Ya Xuan Fu Hua*)
Pharmaceutical Name: Flos Inulae
Properties: bitter, acrid, salty, slightly warm
Channels Entered: Large Intestine, Lung, Stomach, Spleen

CHINESE THERAPEUTIC ACTIONS

1. Dissolves Phlegm, Regulates Water Circulation

Excess phlegm accumulation in the Lung: *Xuan Fu Hua* (Flos Inulae) dissolves phlegm, regulates qi, and activates water circulation. The salty nature of these flowers softens hardness and treats stubborn phlegm. The slightly warm property unblocks stagnation caused by cold and facilitates water circulation. *Xuan Fu Hua* treats accumulation of phlegm and fluids in the Lung.

- Accumulation of cold phlegm in the Lung with cough, wheezing, and white or clear sputum: combine *Xuan Fu Hua* with *Ban Xia* (Rhizoma Pinelliae) and *Xing Ren* (Semen Armeniacae Amarum).
- Accumulation of hot phlegm in the Lung with cough, wheezing, and yellow sputum: use this herb with *Jie Geng* (Radix Platycodonis), *Sang Bai Pi* (Cortex Mori), *Huang Qin* (Radix Scutellariae) and *Da Huang* (Radix et Rhizoma Rhei).
- Accumulation of phlegm with exterior conditions: add it to *Sheng Jiang* (Rhizoma Zingiberis Recens), *Ban Xia* (Rhizoma Pinelliae) and *Ma Huang* (Herba Ephedrae). **Exemplar Formula:** *Jin Fei Cao San* (Inula Powder).
- Accumulation of phlegm with Stomach qi deficiency: combine it with *Dai Zhe Shi* (Haematitum), *Ban Xia* (Rhizoma Pinelliae) and *Ren Shen* (Radix Ginseng). **Exemplar Formula:** *Xuan Fu Dai Zhe Shi Tang* (Inula and Hematite Decoction).

2. Descends Qi and Stops Vomiting

Stomach qi reversal: *Xuan Fu Hua* has an excellent function to redirect abnormally-rising qi downward, to relieve nausea, vomiting, and hiccups. When the Spleen and Stomach are deficient, phlegm accumulates in the middle *jiao* and causes Stomach qi to rise.

- Nausea and vomiting caused by phlegm accumulation and Stomach deficiency: *Xuan Fu Hua* is combined with *Ren Shen* (Radix Ginseng), *Ban Xia* (Rhizoma Pinelliae), *Sheng Jiang* (Rhizoma Zingiberis Recens) and *Dai Zhe Shi* (Haematitum).
- Nausea and vomiting because of Stomach heat: use this herb with *Huang Lian* (Rhizoma Coptidis) and *Zhu Ru* (Caulis Bambusae in Taenia).
- Indigestion with feelings of congestion and oppression in the abdomen and epigastrium: combine it with *Mu Xiang* (Radix Aucklandiae), *Shen Qu* (Massa Fermentata) and *Bai Zhu* (Rhizoma Atractylodis Macrocephalae).

DOSAGE

3 to 10 grams as decoction. *Xuan Fu Hua* should be wrapped in cheesecloth prior to decoction to avoid irritation to the throat or digestive tract by the fuzz on the flowers. The unprocessed herb more strongly lowers qi, dissolves phlegm, and stops nausea. The honey-fried herb more effectively moistens the Lung, dispels phlegm, and relieves cough and wheezing.

CAUTIONS / CONTRAINDICATIONS

- Bitter, warm and dispersing in nature, *Xuan Fu Hua* should be used with caution for patients experiencing dry cough due to yin deficiency, or loose stools because of Spleen deficiency.
- Allergic dermatitis and diarrhea have been reported following the use of *Xuan Fu Hua*.[1,2,3]

CHEMICAL COMPOSITION

Quercetin, isoquercetin, caffeic acid, chlorogenic acid, taraxasterol, britannin, inulicin.[4]

Xuan Fu Hua (Flos Inulae)

PHARMACOLOGICAL EFFECTS

- **Antiasthmatic and antitussive:** Intraperitoneal injection of water extract of *Xuan Fu Hua* is associated with marked antiasthmatic and antitussive effects. It has been proposed that *Xuan Fu Hua* relieves wheezing and asthma by relaxing the bronchioli. No expectorant effect was observed.[5]
- **Diuretic:** It has a mild diuretic effect.[6]
- **Antibiotic:** Decoction of *Xuan Fu Hua* has an inhibitory effect against *Staphylococcus aureus, Bacillus anthracis,* and *Bacillus dysenteriae*.[7]

HERB-DRUG INTERACTION

- **Diuretics:** *Xuan Fu Hua* has a mild diuretic action. Though this potential interaction has not been documented, concurrent use with diuretic drugs may lead to increased elimination of water and/or electrolytes.[8] [Note: Examples of diuretics include chlorothiazide, hydrochlorothiazide, furosemide (Lasix), bumetanide (Bumex), and torsemide (Demadex).]

TOXICOLOGY

The LD_{50} for intraperitoneal injection of a 15% *Xuan Fu Hua* decoction is 22.5 g/kg in mice. Adverse reactions due to overdose included increased respiration rate, excitation, tremor, and convulsions.[9]

SUPPLEMENT

- 金沸草 / 金沸草 *Jin Fei Cao* (Herba Inulae), first cited in the *Shen Nong Ben Cao Jing* (Divine Husbandman's Classic of the Materia Medica) in the second century, is derived from the aerial parts of the same plant as *Xuan Fu Hua*. Salty, slightly bitter and warm, *Jin Fei Cao* has actions similar to *Xuan Fu Hua* in dissolving phlegm, stopping cough and raising qi. Toxic swellings and sores can be treated with topical application of fresh *Jin Fei Cao*. The dosage for *Jin Fei Cao* is 8 to 12 grams.

AUTHORS' COMMENTS

According to Dr. Ding Guang-Di, *Xuan Fu Hua* and *Xiang Fu* (Rhizoma Cyperi) are more effective to address right-sided hypochondriac pain, while *Chuan Lian Zi* (Fructus Toosendan) and *Yan Hu Suo* (Rhizoma Corydalis) are better for left-sided hypochondriac pain.

References

1. *Zhong Cheng Yao Yan Jiu* (Research of Chinese Patent Medicine), 1986; 7:47
2. *Zhe Jiang Zhong Yi Xue Yuan Xue Bao* (Journal of Zhejiang University of Chinese Medicine), 1980; 2:55
3. *Zhong Guo Zhong Yao Za Zhi* (People's Republic of China Journal of Chinese Herbology), 1989; 14(1):56
4. *Xian Dai Zhong Yao Yao Li Xue* (Contemporary Pharmacology of Chinese Herbs), 1997; 947-948
5. *Zhong Yao Yao Li Yu Ying Yong* (Pharmacology and Applications of Chinese Herbs), 1983: 1080
6. *Zhong Yao Xue* (Chinese Herbology), 1998; 614:616
7. *Zhong Yao Yao Li Yu Ying Yong* (Pharmacology and Applications of Chinese Herbs), 1983: 1080
8. Chen, J., Recognition and Prevention of Herb-Drug Interactions, Medical Acupuncture, Fall/Winter 1998/1999; volume 10, number 2; 9-13
9. *Zhong Yao Yao Li Yu Ying Yong* (Pharmacology and Applications of Chinese Herbs), 1983: 1080

Qian Hu (Radix Peucedani)

前胡

Pinyin Name: *Qian Hu*
Literal Name: "before barbarians"
Alternate Chinese Names: *Yan Feng, Xin Qian Hu*
Original Source: *Ming Yi Za Zhu* (Miscellaneous Records of Famous Physicians) by Tao Hong-Jing in 500 A.D.
English Name: peucedanum, white-flowered hog-fennel root, common hog-fennel root
Botanical Name: *Peucedanum praeruptorum* Dunn. (*Bai Hua Qian Hu*); *Peucedanum decursivum* Maxim. (*Zi Hua Qian Hu*)
Pharmaceutical Name: Radix Peucedani
Properties: bitter, acrid, cool
Channels Entered: Lung

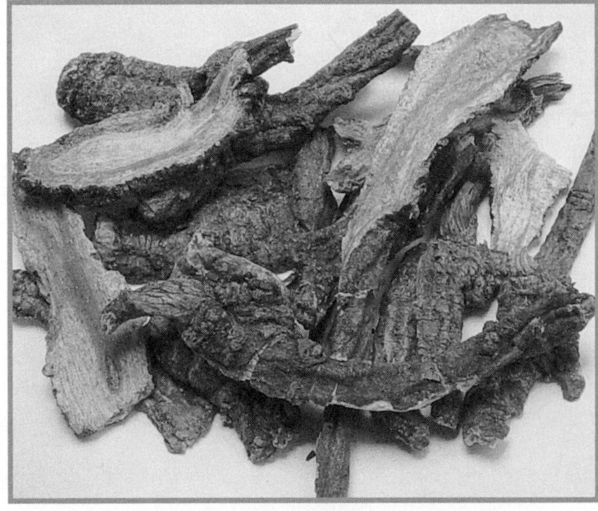

Qian Hu (Radix Peucedani)

CHINESE THERAPEUTIC ACTIONS

1. Redirects Qi Downward and Dispels Phlegm

Excess accumulation of phlegm in the Lung causing cough and dyspnea: *Qian Hu* (Radix Peucedani) has dispersing and draining properties to redirect rebellious Lung qi and dispel phlegm. Clinical applications of *Qian Hu* include accumulation of phlegm in the Lung, abnormally rising Lung qi, copious, difficult-to-expectorate sputum, cough, wheezing and chest oppression. This herb is often combined with other herbs with descending properties to relieve cough and dispel phlegm.

- Accumulation of heat and phlegm in the chest: combine *Qian Hu* with *Sang Bai Pi* (Cortex Mori), *Bei Mu* (Bulbus Fritillaria) and *Xing Ren* (Semen Armeniacae Amarum).

2. Disperses and Dispels Wind-Heat

Qian Hu dispels wind-heat from the exterior. It is commonly used to treat wind-heat syndrome with headache, cough, and/or Lung heat.

- Wind-heat: use this herb with *Bo He* (Herba Menthae), *Niu Bang Zi* (Fructus Arctii), and *Jie Geng* (Radix Platycodonis).

DOSAGE

6 to 10 grams in decoction. Honey-frying *Qian Hu* neutralizes its cold thermal property and enhances its moistening effect on the Lung. Honey-fried *Qian Hu* is more suitable for treating chronic cough caused by Lung deficiency or dry cough with little sputum.

CHEMICAL COMPOSITION

Nodakenin and nodakenetin.[1,2]

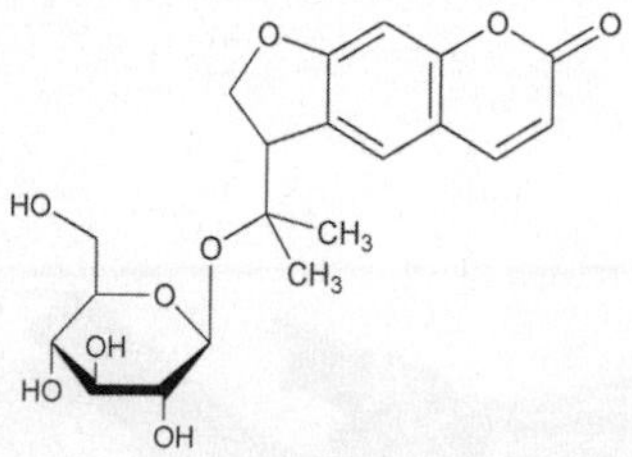

Nodakenin

PHARMACOLOGICAL EFFECTS

- **Expectorant:** Decoction of *Qian Hu* at 1 g/kg showed marked expectorant effects in anesthetized cats. It also had a long duration of action.[3]
- **Antiplatelet:** Nodakenin and nodakenetin have marked inhibitory effects on platelet aggregation *in vivo*.[4]
- **Antibiotic:** *Qian Hu* has an inhibitory effect against some influenza viruses and dermatophytes.[5]
- **Cardiovascular:** Administration of a preparation of *Qian Hu* is associated with increased blood perfusion to the coronary artery and increased resistance to hypoxia. It has no effect on the rhythm and contractility of the heart.[6,7]

HERB-DRUG INTERACTION

- **Anticoagulant or antiplatelet drugs:** *Qian Hu* has antiplatelet action, and should be used with caution in patients who take anticoagulant or antiplatelet medications. Though this potential interaction has not been documented, this herb may potentiate the effect of drugs such as warfarin.[8] [Note: Examples of anticoagulants include heparin, warfarin (Coumadin) and enoxaparin (Lovenox); and examples of antiplatelets include aspirin, dipyridamole (Persantine), and clopidogrel (Plavix).]

AUTHORS' COMMENTS

Qian Hu (Radix Peucedani) and *Chai Hu* (Radix Bupleuri) are often known as "*Er Hu*," meaning "two *Hu*." *Qian Hu* enters the Lung to descend qi and dispel phlegm while *Chai Hu* enters the Liver to lift qi and harmonize pathogenic factors in the *shaoyang* level. Together, they can treat *shaoyang* disorders that reside between disease stages (half exterior, half interior). Chief manifestations include alternating chills and fever, and chest congestion with coughing.

References

1. *Planta Med*, 1986; 52(2):132
2. *The Merck Index* 12th edition, Chapman & Hall/CRCnetBASE/Merck, 2000
3. *Zhong Yao Yao Li Yu Ying Yong* (Pharmacology and Applications of Chinese Herbs), 1983: 815
4. *Planta Med*, 1986; 52(2):132
5. *Zhong Yao Xue* (Chinese Herbology), 1998; 617:618
6. *Yao Xue Xue Bao* (Journal of Herbology), 1982; 17(6):431
7. *Zhong Yao Yao Li Yu Ying Yong* (Pharmacology and Applications of Chinese Herbs), 1983; 815
8. Chen, J. Recognition & prevention of herb-drug interactions, *Medical Acupuncture*, Fall/Winter 1998/1999; volume 10/number 2; 9-13

Bai Qian (Rhizoma Cynanchi Stauntonii)

白前

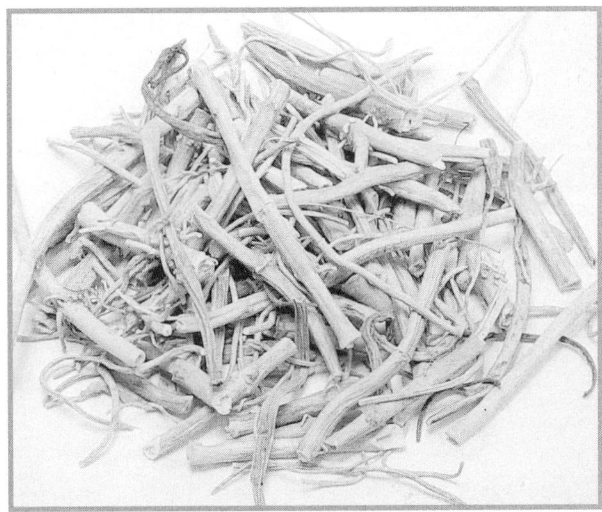

Pinyin Name: *Bai Qian*
Literal Name: "white before"
Alternate Chinese Names: *E Guan Bai Qian*
Original Source: *Ming Yi Za Zhu* (Miscellaneous Records of Famous Physicians) by Tao Hong-Jing in 500 A.D.
English Name: cynanchum rhizome, willow leaf swallow wort rhizome, glaucescent swallow wort rhizome
Botanical Name: *Cynanchum stauntoni* (Decne.) Schltr. ex Levl. (*Liu Ye Bai Qian*); *Cynanchum glaucescens* (Decne.) (*Yuan Hua Ye Bai Qian*)
Pharmaceutical Name: Rhizoma Cynanchi Stauntonii
Properties: acrid, sweet, neutral
Channels Entered: Lung

CHINESE THERAPEUTIC ACTIONS

Descends Qi, Dispels Phlegm, Stops Cough

Excess condition of the Lung, cough with profuse sputum, wind-cold invasion: Acrid and warm, yet not drying, *Bai Qian* (Rhizoma Cynanchi Stauntonii) is an excellent herb to treat cough and wheezing secondary to the accumulation of phlegm in the Lung. It is a key herb used to treat any respiratory disorders manifesting in cough and dyspnea. When combined with appropriate herbs, *Bai Qian* can treat cough, wheezing and sputum caused by either hot or cold phlegm.

- Cough and dyspnea due to cold phlegm: combine *Bai Qian* with *Zi Wan* (Radix Asteris) and *Ban Xia* (Rhizoma Pinelliae).
- Cough and dyspnea due to hot phlegm: use it with *Sang Bai Pi* (Cortex Mori) and *Di Gu Pi* (Cortex Lycii).

Exterior wind-cold syndrome: *Bai Qian* dispels wind-cold and is commonly used in combination with appropriate herbs to treat cough caused by externally-contracted wind-cold syndrome.

- Cough due to wind-cold: use *Bai Qian* with *Jie Geng* (Radix Platycodonis), *Jing Jie* (Herba Schizonepetae), and *Chen Pi* (Pericarpium Citri Reticulatae). **Exemplar Formula:** *Zhi Sou San* (Stop Coughing Powder).

DOSAGE

3 to 10 grams in decoction. Unprocessed *Bai Qian* may irritate the stomach, leading to nausea and vomiting. Frying the herb with honey will minimize this irritation. In addition, honey-frying enhances the moistening effect of this herb and makes it more suitable for patients with dry cough and dyspnea from Lung yin deficiency.

CAUTIONS / CONTRAINDICATIONS

- Acrid and warm, *Bai Qian* should be used with caution for patients having dry cough from Lung yin deficiency.
- *Bai Qian* should be used with caution in patients with peptic ulcers or bleeding ulcers, because of the irritating effect it has on the gastrointestinal system.

Chuan Bei Mu (Bulbus Fritillariae Cirrhosae)

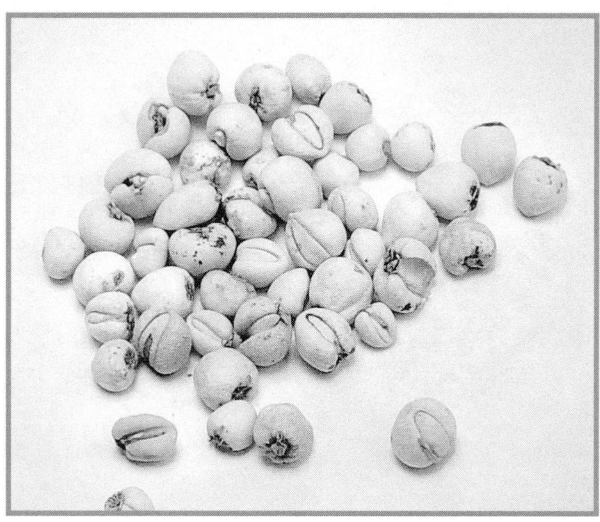

川貝母 川贝母

Pinyin Name: *Chuan Bei Mu*
Literal Name: "shell mother from Sichuan"
Original Source: *Shen Nong Ben Cao Jing* (Divine Husbandman's Classic of the Materia Medica) in the second century
English Name: fritillaria cirrhosae, fritillary bulb from several species: tendril-leaf, unibract, przewalsk, and delavay
Botanical Name: *Fritillaria cirrhosa* D. Don. (*Chuan Bei Mu*); *Fritillaria unibracteata* Hsiao et K.C. Hsia. (*An Zi Bei Mu*); *Fritillaria przewalskii* Maxim. (*Gan Su Bei Mu*); *Fritillaria delavayi* Franch. (*Leng Sha Bei Mu*)
Pharmaceutical Name: Bulbus Fritillariae Cirrhosae
Properties: bitter, sweet, cool
Channels Entered: Heart, Lung

CHINESE THERAPEUTIC ACTIONS

1. Dissolves Phlegm and Stops Cough

Chuan Bei Mu (Bulbus Fritillariae Cirrhosae) is cool and sweet, moistens the Lung and dissolves phlegm. It is mostly used for chronic dry cough with scanty, difficult-to-expectorate sputum, either with or without blood.

- Chronic cough with Lung deficiency, dry cough with little sputum, or cough with blood-streaked sputum: use *Chuan Bei Mu* with *Xing Ren* (Semen Armeniacae Amarum), *Zi Wan* (Radix Asteris), and *Kuan Dong Hua* (Flos Farfarae).
- Cough with phlegm and dryness in the Lung: use this herb with *Gua Lou Ren* (Semen Trichosanthis) and *Tian Hua Fen* (Radix Trichosanthis). **Exemplar Formula:** *Bei Mu Gua Lou San* (Fritillaria and Trichosanthes Fruit Powder).
- Cough with excess phlegm and heat: use it with snake bile.
- Cough due to exterior wind-cold attacking the body: use *Chuan Bei Mu* with *Bo He* (Herba Menthae), *Xing Ren* (Semen Armeniacae Amarum), *Su Zi* (Fructus Perillae), and *Jie Geng* (Radix Platycodonis). **Exemplar Formula:** *Ning Sou Wan* (Quiet the Cough Pills).

2. Clears Heat and Disperses Nodules

Bitter and cold in nature, *Chuan Bei Mu* clears heat and disperses nodules and hardness. It is commonly used to treat sores, nodules, scrofula, goiter, and lung or breast abscesses.

- Scrofula: combine *Chuan Bei Mu* and *Zhe Bei Mu* (Bulbus Fritillariae Thunbergii).

DOSAGE

3 to 10 grams in decoction, 1.0 to 1.5 grams in powder.

CAUTIONS / CONTRAINDICATIONS

- *Chuan Bei Mu* is not suitable if phlegm is characterized by cold or dampness.
- *Chuan Bei Mu* is incompatible with *Wu Tou* (Radix Aconiti).

CHEMICAL COMPOSITION

Chinpeimine, fritiminine, beilupeimine, sonpeimine, sipeimine, minpeimine, minpeiminine, verticine, verticinine, fritillarine, fritimine.[1]

PHARMACOLOGICAL EFFECTS

- **Antitussive:** *Chuan Bei Mu* has a marked antitussive effect in rats. The maximum effect was reached 30 minutes after oral administration of herbs, and the effect lasted up to 2 hours.[2]
- **Expectorant:** *Chuan Bei Mu* has a marked expectorant effect in mice. The maximum effect was reached 60 minutes after oral administration of herbs, and lasted up to 2 hours.[3]
- **Others:** It has mild antihypertensive, spasmolytic, and muscle-relaxant effects.[4]

CLINICAL STUDIES AND RESEARCH

- **Whooping cough:** Equal portions of *Chuan Bei Mu*, *Bai Ji* (Rhizoma Bletillae) and *Kuan Dong Hua* (Flos Farfarae) were ground into powder and given to children for treatment of whooping cough. The dosage was 1 gram per day for infants under 1 year of age, and adjusted accordingly for children over 1 year of age. Out of 56 cases, 51 showed complete recovery, 4 showed moderate improvement, and 1 had no response.[5]
- **Chapped nipples:** Good results were reported for

Chuan Bei Mu (Bulbus Fritillariae Cirrhosae)

treatment of chapped nipples using topical application of an herbal paste containing 10 grams of *Chuan Bei Mu*, 20 grams of white sesame seeds and 20 grams of black sesame seeds.[6]

TOXICOLOGY

No fatalities were reported following an oral bolus dose of *Chuan Bei Mu* (at the dosage of 8.0 g/kg in mice). No abnormalities were noted in a follow-up examination one week later.[7]

SUPPLEMENT

- 貝母 / 贝母 *Bei Mu* (Bulbus Fritillaria) is the generic name that refers to both *Chuan Bei Mu* (Bulbus Fritillariae Cirrhosae) and *Zhe Bei Mu* (Bulbus Fritillariae Thunbergii). Many classic texts do not distinguish between *Chuan Bei Mu* and *Zhe Bei Mu* as these two herbs have similar functions, and have been used interchangeably.

AUTHORS' COMMENTS

Chuan Bei Mu (Bulbus Fritillariae Cirrhosae) and *Zhe Bei Mu* (Bulbus Fritillariae Thunbergii) both clear the Lung, dissolve phlegm and arrest cough. They are commonly used to treat cough with yellow sputum caused by heat in the Lung.

Chuan Bei Mu and *Mai Men Dong* (Radix Ophiopogonis) both moisten the Lung and arrest cough. However, *Chuan Bei Mu* is best used to disperse stagnation in the Lung that manifests in cough with sputum. *Mai Men Dong* more strongly nourishes Lung yin and clears heat.

References

1. *Xian Dai Zhong Yao Yao Li Xue* (Contemporary Pharmacology of Chinese Herbs), 1997; 951
2. *Zhong Guo Yi Ke Da Xue Xue Bao* (Journal of University of Chinese Medicine), 1992; 23(2):118
3. *Si Chuan Yi Xue Yuan Xue Bao* (Journal of Sichuan School of Medicine), *1978*; (2):30
4. *Zhong Yao Xue* (Chinese Herbology), 1998; 620:622
5. *Zhong Yi Yao Xue Bao* (Report of Chinese Medicine and Herbology), 1988; (6):23
6. *Zhe Jiang Zhong Yi Za Zhi* (Zhejiang Journal of Chinese Medicine), 1984; 19(7):309
7. *Zhong Yao Yao Li Xue* (Study of Chinese Herbology), 1986; 222

Zhe Bei Mu (Bulbus Fritillariae Thunbergii)

浙貝母 浙贝母

Pinyin Name: *Zhe Bei Mu*
Literal Name: "shell mother from Zhejiang"
Alternate Chinese Names: *Xiang Bei Mu, Da Bei Mu*
Original Source: *Shen Nong Ben Cao Jing* (Divine Husbandman's Classic of the Materia Medica) in the second century
English Name: fritillaria thunbergii, thunbergy fritillary bulb
Botanical Name: *Fritillaria verticillata* Willd. var. *thunbergii* Bak. (*Zhe Bei Mu*)
Pharmaceutical Name: Bulbus Fritillariae Thunbergii
Properties: bitter, cold
Channels Entered: Heart, Lung

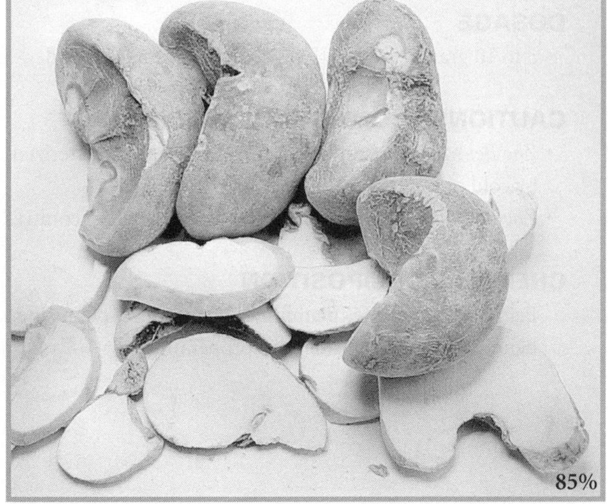
85%

CHINESE THERAPEUTIC ACTIONS

1. Dissolves Phlegm and Stops Cough

Zhe Bei Mu (Bulbus Fritillariae Thunbergii) is one of the most effective herbs for stopping coughing caused by either exterior pathogenic factors or interior disharmony. *Zhe Bei Mu* is cold and bitter and has a strong sedating function that is most suitable for beginning stages of coughing caused by excess conditions such as Lung heat or wind-heat.

Zhe Bei Mu (Bulbus Fritillariae Thunbergii)

- Cough caused by wind-heat or accumulation of phlegm and heat: use *Zhe Bei Mu* with *Sang Ye* (Folium Mori), *Niu Bang Zi* (Fructus Arctii), *Qian Hu* (Radix Peucedani) and *Xing Ren* (Semen Armeniacae Amarum).
- Dry cough arising from Lung yin deficiency: use this herb with *Xing Ren* (Semen Armeniacae Amarum), *Zi Wan* (Radix Asteris), *Kuan Dong Hua* (Flos Farfarae) and *Mai Men Dong* (Radix Ophiopogonis).

2. Clears Heat and Disperses Nodules

Scrofula, sores, carbuncles, goiter, breast and lung abscesses: *Zhe Bei Mu* disperses stagnation and clears heat. For sores and abscess that have not ulcerated, *Zhe Bei Mu* is often used with herbs that clear heat, cool blood, and eliminate toxins.

- Nodules without abscesses: combine *Zhe Bei Mu* with *Xuan Shen* (Radix Scrophulariae) and *Mu Li* (Concha Ostreae).
- Thyroid nodules, goiter, tumor: use this herb with *Hai Zao* (Sargassum), *Kun Bu* (Thallus Laminariae seu Eckloniae), *Xia Ku Cao* (Spica Prunellae), and *E Zhu* (Rhizoma Curcumae). **Exemplar Formula:** *Hai Zao Yu Hu Tang* (Sargassum Decoction for the Jade Flask).
- Cough with pus or blood: add *Zhe Bei Mu* to *Jie Geng* (Radix Platycodonis) and *Zi Wan* (Radix Asteris).
- Lung abscess with copious pus, sputum and blood: use this herb with *Yu Xing Cao* (Herba Houttuyniae), *Lu Gen* (Rhizoma Phragmitis), and *Yi Yi Ren* (Semen Coicis).
- Carbuncles, abscesses and breast lumps: combine it with *Pu Gong Ying* (Herba Taraxaci), *Tian Hua Fen* (Radix Trichosanthis) and *Lian Qiao* (Fructus Forsythiae).

DOSAGE

3 to 10 grams in decoction, 1.0 to 1.5 grams in powder.

CAUTIONS / CONTRAINDICATIONS

- *Zhe Bei Mu* is not suitable if the phlegm is characterized by cold or dampness.
- *Zhe Bei Mu* is incompatible with *Wu Tou* (Radix Aconiti).

CHEMICAL COMPOSITION

Peimine, peiminine, peimidine, peimiphine, peimisine, peimitidine, peiminoside, and propeimine.[1,2]

Peimine

PHARMACOLOGICAL EFFECTS

- **Antitussive:** Peimine and peiminine have marked antitussive effects in rats.[3]
- **Effects on smooth muscle:** In laboratory studies, a low concentration of *Zhe Bei Mu* has been associated with relaxation of bronchial muscles, while a high concentration is associated with contraction.[4]

CLINICAL STUDIES AND RESEARCH

- **Upper respiratory tract infection and cough from chronic bronchitis:** Extract of the flowers of *Zhe Bei Mu* was made into liquid and pills for treatment of respiratory disorders. For the 245 patients in the clinical trial, the rate of effectiveness was 76.5% for treatment of upper respiratory tract infection and 68.2% for cough from chronic bronchitis.[5]

TOXICOLOGY

The LD_{50} for intravenous injection of peiminine is 10 to 12 mg/kg in rabbits and 8 to 10 mg/kg in cats. Adverse reaction caused by overdose included respiratory depression, dilation of pupils, tremor, muscle spasms, incontinence, and in severe cases, fatality.[6]

SUPPLEMENT

- 土貝母/土贝母 *Tu Bei Mu* (Bulbus Bolbostemma Paniculatum) clears heat, disperses stagnation and reduces sores and swelling. It is mainly used externally. It is not the same as *Zhe Bei Mu* or *Chuan Bei Mu* (Bulbus Fritillariae Cirrhosae) and should not be confused or substituted for them.

AUTHORS' COMMENTS

Zhe Bei Mu (Bulbus Fritillariae Thunbergii) and *Chuan Bei Mu* (Bulbus Fritillariae Cirrhosae) share many similarities, and some small differences. *Zhe Bei Mu* is bitter and cold. It has greater effectiveness to clear heat, and treats cough arising from Lung heat or heat and phlegm. *Zhe Bei Mu* more strongly disperses and softens nodules to treat abscesses, scrofula, and thyroid nodules. *Chuan Bei Mu* is bitter, sweet and cool. It acts to moisten the Lung, dissolve phlegm, and treat chronic or deficient coughing.

References

1. *Xian Dai Zhong Yao Yao Li Xue* (Contemporary Pharmacology of Chinese Herbs), 1997; 952
2. *The Merck Index* 12th edition, Chapman & Hall/CRCnetBASE/Merck, 2000
3. *Chang Yong Zhong Yao Cheng Fen Yu Yao Li Shou Ce* (A Handbook of the Composition and Pharmacology of Common Chinese Drugs), 1994; 1523:1524
4. *Zhong Yao Xue* (Chinese Herbology), 1998; 620:622
5. *Zhe Jiang Zhong Yi Za Zhi* (Zhejiang Journal of Chinese Medicine), 1977; 2:31
6. *Chang Yong Zhong Yao Xian Dai Yan Jiu Yu Lin Chuan* (Recent Study & Clinical Application of Common Traditional Chinese Medicine), 1995; 455:457

Gua Lou Shi (Fructus Trichosanthis)

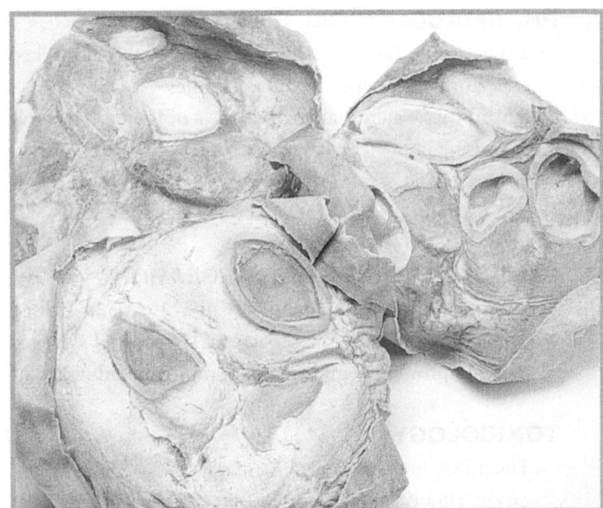

瓜蔞實 瓜蒌实

Pinyin Name: *Gua Lou Shi*
Alternate Chinese Names: *Gua Lou, Yao Gua*
Original Source: *Ming Yi Za Zhu* (Miscellaneous Records of Famous Physicians) by Tao Hong-Jing in 500 A.D.
English Name: trichosanthes fruit, snake gourd fruit
Botanical Name: *Trichosanthes kirilowii* Maxim. (*Gua Lou*); *Trichosanthes rosthornii* Harms. (*Xuan Bian Gua Lou*)
Pharmaceutical Name: Fructus Trichosanthis
Properties: sweet, cold
Channels Entered: Large Intestine, Lung, Stomach

CHINESE THERAPEUTIC ACTIONS

1. Clears the Lungs, Dissolves Phlegm

Sweet and cold, *Gua Lou Shi* (Fructus Trichosanthis) moistens dryness, clears the Lung, and dissolves phlegm. It is commonly used to treat Lung heat with cough and copious, difficult-to-expectorate sputum.

- In infants, wheezing caused by phlegm: use *Gua Lou Shi* as a single-herb remedy.
- Productive cough with yellow, sticky phlegm, chest congestion and hard stools because of heat in the Lung and Large Intestine: combine this herb with *Ban Xia* (Rhizoma Pinelliae), *Huang Qin* (Radix Scutellariae), *Zhi Shi* (Fructus Aurantii Immaturus) and *Dan Nan Xing* (Arisaema cum Bile). **Exemplar Formula:** *Qing Qi Hua Tan Wan* (Clear the Qi and Transform Phlegm Pill).
- Productive cough with phlegm due to Lung heat: use *Gua Lou Shi* with *Zhi Mu* (Radix Anemarrhenae) and *Bei Mu* (Bulbus Fritillaria).

2. Regulates Qi and Expands the Chest

***Xiong bi* (painful obstruction of the chest):** In addition to clearing the Lung and dissolving phlegm, *Gua Lou Shi* regulates qi circulation in the chest to relieve feelings of chest oppression and pain. Clinically, it treats *xiong bi* caused by accumulation of heat and phlegm beneath the Heart leading to congestion and oppression in the chest, increased pain upon pressure, and yellow, copious, sticky sputum. *Xiong bi* may also be caused by stagnation of cold with yang deficiency manifesting in severe pain with an inability to lie down, as well as in wheezing, dyspnea, and cough.

- *Xiong bi* due to accumulation of heat and phlegm beneath the Heart: use *Gua Lou Shi* with *Ban Xia* (Rhizoma Pinelliae) and *Huang Lian* (Rhizoma Coptidis) to clear heat, dissolve phlegm and regulate qi in the chest. **Exemplar Formula:** *Xiao Xian Xiong Tang* (Minor Sinking into the Chest Decoction).
- *Xiong bi* due to stagnation of cold with yang deficiency: combine this herb with *Xie Bai* (Bulbus Allii Macrostemonis) and *Ban Xia* (Rhizoma Pinelliae). **Exemplar Formula:** *Gua Lou Xie Bai Ban Xia Tang* (Trichosanthes Fruit, Chinese Chive, and Pinellia Decoction).

3. Dissipates Nodules and Eliminates Pus

Abscess: *Gua Lou Shi* dissipates nodules and eliminates pus to treat abscesses of the lungs, intestines or breasts.

- Productive cough with sputum and blood, with chest congestion: use *Gua Lou Shi* with *Gan Cao* (Radix Glycyrrhizae), *Ru Xiang* (Gummi Olibanum) and *Mo Yao* (Myrrha).
- Intestinal abscess with deficiency of qi and blood: combine this herb with *Jin Yin Hua* (Flos Lonicerae), *Lian Qiao* (Fructus Forsythiae), *Dang Gui* (Radicis Angelicae Sinensis), and *Huang Qi* (Radix Astragali).

DOSAGE

10 to 20 grams in decoction.

CAUTIONS / CONTRAINDICATIONS

- *Gua Lou Shi* should be used with caution for patients with deficiency and weakness of the Spleen and Stomach.
- *Gua Lou Shi* is incompatible with *Wu Tou* (Radix Aconiti).

CHEMICAL COMPOSITION

Trichosanic acid, fatty oil, organic acids.[1]

Gua Lou Shi (Fructus Trichosanthis)

PHARMACOLOGICAL EFFECTS

- **Expectorant:** Trichosanic acid has demonstrated marked expectorant influence in animal studies.[2]
- **Antibiotic:** Water or alcohol extracts of the herb have an inhibiting influence *in vitro* against *E. coli, Staphylococcus aureus, Diplococcus pneumoniae,* α-hemolytic streptococcus, and *Bacillus dysenteriae.*[3]

CLINICAL STUDIES AND RESEARCH

- **Coronary artery disease:** A study of 413 patients treated by *Gua Lou Shi* injection reports 78.1% showed symptomatic improvement and 56% had improvement in ECG.[4]

TOXICOLOGY

The LD_{50} for *Gua Lou Shi* in mice was 363 g/kg via intraperitoneal injection and 306 g/kg via intravenous injection. In anesthetized dogs, a bolus dose of 100 g/kg (approximately 100 times the therapeutic human dose) led to a small decrease in blood pressure, but no significant adverse reactions.[5]

AUTHORS' COMMENTS

In the earlier history of traditional Chinese medicine, *Gua Lou* (Trichosanthes) was always used as a whole fruit. As more experiential information became available, the use became more sophisticated, as different uses were found for different parts of the plant. The differences are as follows:

- *Gua Lou Pi* (Pericarpium Trichosanthis), the peel, strongly clears Lung heat, dissolves phlegm, regulates qi and expands the chest. Clinical applications include cough and phlegm caused by Lung heat, and *xiong bi* (painful obstruction of the chest).
- *Gua Lou Ren* (Semen Trichosanthis), the seeds, are used mainly to moisten the intestines and promote bowel movement.
- *Gua Lou Shi* (Fructus Trichosanthis), the entire fruit, shares the functions of both the peel and seeds.

References

1. *Xian Dai Zhong Yao Yao Li Xue* (Contemporary Pharmacology of Chinese Herbs), 1997; 955
2. *Chang Yong Zhong Yao Cheng Fen Yu Yao Li Shou Ce* (A Handbook of the Composition and Pharmacology of Common Chinese Drugs), 1994; 765:767
3. Ibid.
4. *Zhong Cao Yao Tong Xun* (Journal of Chinese Herbal Medicine), 1976; 9:47
5. *Lao Nian Xue Za Zhi* (Journal of Geriatrics), 1991; 11(2):115

Gua Lou Ren (Semen Trichosanthis)

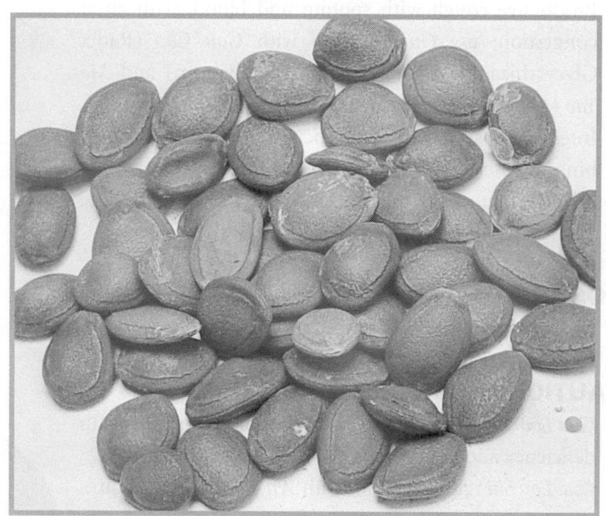

瓜蔞仁 瓜蒌仁

Pinyin Name: *Gua Lou Ren*
English Name: trichosanthes seed, snake gourd seed
Botanical Name: *Trichosanthes kirilowii* Maxim. (*Gua Lou*); *Trichosanthes rosthornii* Harms. (*Xuan Bian Gua Lou*)
Pharmaceutical Name: Semen Trichosanthis
Properties: sweet, cold
Channels Entered: Large Intestine, Lung, Stomach

Gua Lou Ren (Semen Trichosanthis)

CHINESE THERAPEUTIC ACTIONS

1. Moistens the Lungs, Dissolves Phlegm

Dry cough with scanty sputum that is difficult to expectorate: Sweet and cold, *Gua Lou Ren* (Fructus Trichosanthis) moistens dryness, clears Lung heat, and dissolves phlegm. It is commonly used to treat Lung heat with cough and copious, difficult-to-expectorate sputum.

- Accumulation of heat and phlegm with copious yellow sputum, chest oppression, and constipation: use *Gua Lou Ren* with *Huang Qin* (Radix Scutellariae), *Zhi Shi* (Fructus Aurantii Immaturus) and *Dan Nan Xing* (Arisaema cum Bile). **Exemplar Formula:** *Qing Qi Hua Tan Wan* (Clear the Qi and Transform Phlegm Pill).

2. Lubricates the Intestines to Promote Bowel Movement

Dry stools, constipation: *Gua Lou Ren*, rich in oil, is both moistening and lubricating. It is commonly used to treat constipation caused by dryness and heat in the Stomach and Large Intestine.

- Constipation: combine *Gua Lou Ren* with *Huo Ma Ren* (Fructus Cannabis), *Yu Li Ren* (Semen Pruni) and *Zhi Ke* (Fructus Aurantii).

3. Dissipates Nodules and Eliminates Pus

Breast and intestinal abscesses, sores and carbuncles: *Gua Lou Ren* dissipates nodules and eliminates pus to treat lung, intestinal, and breast abscesses.

- Productive cough with sputum and blood, accompanied by feelings of congestion and oppression in the chest: use *Gua Lou Ren* with *Gan Cao* (Radix Glycyrrhizae), *Ru Xiang* (Gummi Olibanum) and *Mo Yao* (Myrrha).
- Intestinal abscess with deficiency of qi and blood: use this herb with *Jin Yin Hua* (Flos Lonicerae), *Lian Qiao* (Fructus Forsythiae), *Dang Gui* (Radicis Angelicae Sinensis), and *Huang Qi* (Radix Astragali).

DOSAGE

10 to 15 grams. *Gua Lou Ren* should be crushed to increase available surface area and facilitate extraction of active ingredients. Unprocessed *Gua Lou Ren* is cold, and can sometimes cause nausea. Dry-frying the herb increases its warmth, reduces the frequency of nausea, and facilitates the extraction of active constituents.

CAUTIONS / CONTRAINDICATIONS

- *Gua Lou Ren* should be used with caution in patients experiencing deficiency and weakness of the Spleen and Stomach.
- *Gua Lou Ren* is incompatible with *Wu Tou* (Radix Aconiti).

CHEMICAL COMPOSITION

Trichosanic acid, karounidiol, 7-oxodihydrokarounidiol, bryonolic acid, fatty oil, organic acids.[1,2]

PHARMACOLOGICAL EFFECTS

- **Laxative:** Various parts of this plant have laxative actions, with *Gua Lou Ren* being the strongest and *Gua Lou Pi* (Pericarpium Trichosanthis) being the weakest.[3]

AUTHORS' COMMENTS

Please refer to *Gua Lou Shi* (Fructus Trichosanthis) for comparative information on *Gua Lou Pi* (Pericarpium Trichosanthis), *Gua Lou Ren* (Semen Trichosanthis) and *Gua Lou Shi* (Fructus Trichosanthis).

References

1. *Xian Dai Zhong Yao Yao Li Xue* (Contemporary Pharmacology of Chinese Herbs), 1997; 955
2. *Chang Yong Zhong Yao Cheng Fen Yu Yao Li Shou Ce* (A Handbook of the Composition and Pharmacology of Common Chinese Drugs), 1994; 768-769
3. Ibid., 765:767

Gua Lou Pi (Pericarpium Trichosanthis)

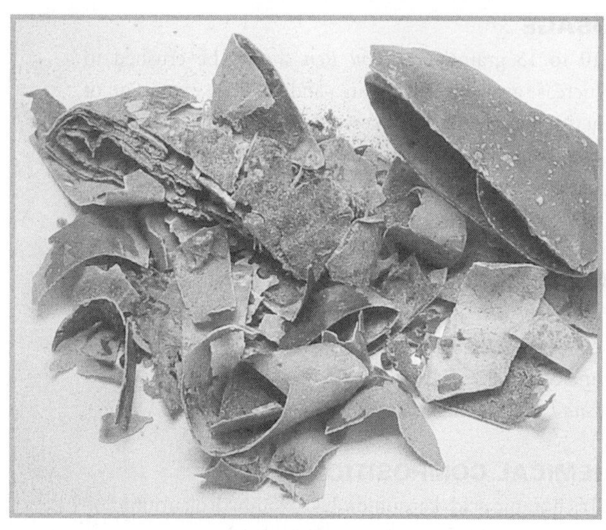

瓜蔞皮 瓜蒌皮

Pinyin Name: *Gua Lou Pi*
Alternate Chinese Names: *Yao Gua*
English Name: trichosanthes peel, snake gourd peel
Botanical Name: *Trichosanthes kirilowii* Maxim. (*Gua Lou*); *Trichosanthes rosthornii* Harms. (*Xuan Bian Gua Lou*)
Pharmaceutical Name: Pericarpium Trichosanthis
Properties: sweet, cold
Channels Entered: Large Intestine, Lung, Stomach

CHINESE THERAPEUTIC ACTIONS

Clears the Lungs, Dissolves Phlegm, Regulates Qi and Expands the Chest

Cough due to Lung heat, chest congestion: Sweet and cold, *Gua Lou Pi* (Pericarpium Trichosanthis) clears Lung heat and helps with difficult-to-expectorate sputum. Other manifestations may include cough, dyspnea, chest congestion, chest pain that worsens with pressure, yellow sputum and wheezing.

- Cough with phlegm due to Lung qi stagnation: use *Gua Lou Pi* with *Bei Mu* (Bulbus Fritillaria), *Jie Geng* (Radix Platycodonis), and *Xing Ren* (Semen Armeniacae Amarum).

***Xiong bi* (painful obstruction of the chest):** *Gua Lou Pi* clears Lung and Stomach heat to dissolve phlegm and also regulates upper *jiao* qi to relieve chest pain.

- *Xiong bi* with cough and yellow sputum: use *Gua Lou Pi* with *Huang Lian* (Rhizoma Coptidis) and *Ban Xia* (Rhizoma Pinelliae). **Exemplar Formula:** *Xiao Xian Xiong Tang* (Minor Sinking into the Chest Decoction).
- *Xiong bi* due to cold and damp accumulation in the upper *jiao*: use this herb with *Xie Bai* (Bulbus Allii Macrostemonis) and *Ban Xia* (Rhizoma Pinelliae). **Exemplar Formula:** *Gua Lou Xie Bai Ban Xia Tang* (Trichosanthes Fruit, Chinese Chive, and Pinellia Decoction).

DOSAGE

6 to 12 grams in decoction.

CAUTIONS / CONTRAINDICATIONS

- *Gua Lou Pi* should be used with caution in patients experiencing deficiency and weakness of the Spleen and Stomach
- *Gua Lou Pi* is incompatible with *Wu Tou* (Radix Aconiti).

CHEMICAL COMPOSITION

Fatty oil, organic acids.[1]

PHARMACOLOGICAL EFFECTS

- **Cardiovascular:** According to laboratory studies, the extract of *Gua Lou Shi* (Fructus Trichosanthis) dilates the coronary arteries, increases blood perfusion, and reduces the oxygen requirement of cardiac muscle. Upon more detailed study, it was determined that *Gua Lou Pi* (Pericarpium Trichosanthis) has the strongest effect on the cardiovascular system, followed by *Gua Lou Ren* (Semen Trichosanthis), and then *Gua Lou Shi* (Fructus Trichosanthis).[2]

AUTHORS' COMMENTS

Please refer to *Gua Lou Shi* (Fructus Trichosanthis) for comparative information on *Gua Lou Pi* (Pericarpium Trichosanthis), *Gua Lou Ren* (Semen Trichosanthis) and *Gua Lou Shi* (Fructus Trichosanthis).

References

1. *Xian Dai Zhong Yao Yao Li Xue* (Contemporary Pharmacology of Chinese Herbs), 1997; 955
2. *Chang Yong Zhong Yao Cheng Fen Yu Yao Li Shou Ce* (A Handbook of the Composition and Pharmacology of Common Chinese Drugs), 1994; 765:767

Tian Zhu Huang (Concretio Silicea Bambusae)

天竺黄 天竺黄

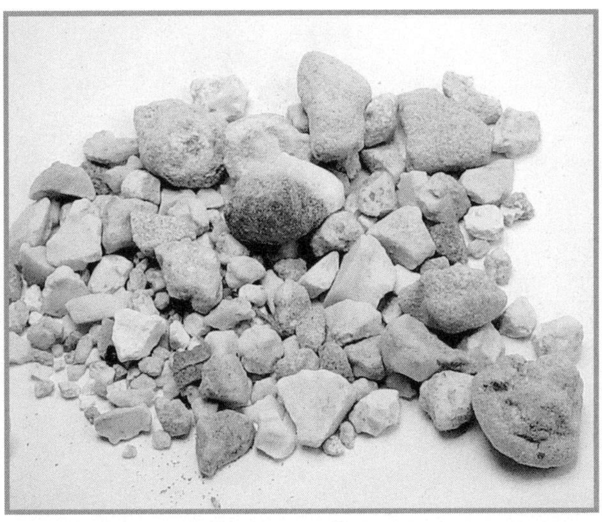

Pinyin Name: *Tian Zhu Huang*
Literal Name: "heavenly bamboo yellow"
Alternate Chinese Names: *Zhu Gao*
Original Source: *Ri Hua Zi Ben Cao* (Materia Medica of Ri Hua-Zi) by Ri Hua-Zi in 713 A.D.
English Name: bamboo silicea, tabasheer
Botanical Name: *Bambusa textilis* Mc-Clure (*Qing Pi Zhu*); *Schizostachyum chinense* Rendle (*Hua Si Lao Zhu*)
Pharmaceutical Name: Concretio Silicea Bambusae
Properties: sweet, cold
Channels Entered: Gallbladder, Heart, Liver

CHINESE THERAPEUTIC ACTIONS

Clears Heat, Dissolves Phlegm, Cools the Heart and Stops Convulsions

Convulsions due to heat, stroke from phlegm accumulation, infantile convulsions: *Tian Zhu Huang* (Concretio Silicea Bambusae) is commonly used to treat convulsions secondary to heat and phlegm obstructing the Heart *shen* (spirit). Clinically, symptoms are fever, red face, labored breathing and profuse sputum. In severe cases, patients may exhibit spasms, epilepsy, convulsions, and loss of consciousness.

- Infantile seizure and convulsions: use *Tian Zhu Huang* with *Zhi Zi* (Fructus Gardeniae), *Jiang Can* (Bombyx Batryticatus) and *Yu Jin* (Radix Curcumae).
- Stroke due to phlegm stagnation: combine this herb with *Dan Nan Xing* (Arisaema cum Bile), *Shi Chang Pu* (Rhizoma Acori), *Tian Ma* (Rhizoma Gastrodiae), and *Quan Xie* (Scorpio).

DOSAGE

3 to 6 grams in decoction, 0.6 to 1.0 gram as powder.

CHEMICAL COMPOSITION

Silica, potassium hydroxide.[1]

PHARMACOLOGICAL EFFECTS

- **Analgesic:** Administration of *Tian Zhu Huang* at 2 to 3 g/kg has an analgesic effect in mice.[2]
- **Cardiovascular:** *Tian Zhu Huang* has negative inotropic and chronotropic effects in frog heart specimens. It dilates blood vessels in anesthetized rabbits.[3]

AUTHORS' COMMENTS

Tian Zhu Huang (Concretio Silicea Bambusae), *Chuan Mu Tong* (Caulis Clematidis Armandii), *Mai Men Dong* (Radix Ophiopogonis), and *Huang Lian* (Rhizoma Coptidis) all clear the Heart and eliminate irritability.

- *Tian Zhu Huang* dissolves hot phlegm and is most effective for irritability with spasms and convulsions.
- *Chuan Mu Tong* is a diuretic that clears damp-heat to relieve irritability accompanied by oral ulcers and yellow urine.
- *Mai Men Dong* is a tonic used to relieve deficient Heart yin and heat that manifests as irritability and insomnia.
- *Huang Lian* treats febrile disease with excess fire in the Heart that is disturbing the *shen* (spirit), and manifesting in irritability and insomnia.

References

1. *Xian Dai Zhong Yao Yao Li Xue* (Contemporary Pharmacology of Chinese Herbs), 1997; 968
2. *Zhong Yao Tong Bao* (Journal of Chinese Herbology), 1982; 7(5):31
3. Ibid.

Zhu Ru (Caulis Bambusae in Taenia)

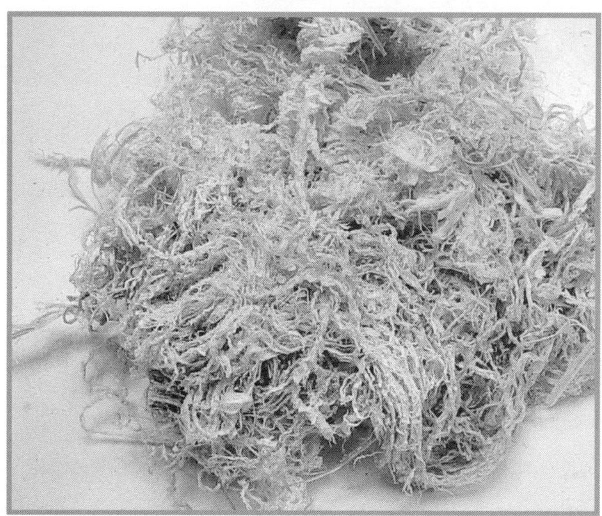

竹茹 竹茹

Pinyin Name: *Zhu Ru*

Alternate Chinese Names: *Zhu Er Qing, Dan Zhu Ru, Zhu Jing, Er Qing*

Original Source: *Ming Yi Za Zhu* (Miscellaneous Records of Famous Physicians) by Tao Hong-Jing in 500 A.D.

English Name: bamboo shavings

Botanical Name: *Bambusa breviflora* Munro (*Qing Gan Zhu*); *Phyllostachys nigra* (Lodd.) Munro var. *henonis* (Mitf.) Stapf ex Rendl (*Dan Zhu*)

Pharmaceutical Name: Caulis Bambusae in Taenia

Properties: sweet, cool

Channels Entered: Lung, Stomach, Gallbladder

CHINESE THERAPEUTIC ACTIONS

1. Clears Heat, Dissolves Phlegm

Cough due to Lung heat: Cool and moistening, *Zhu Ru* (Caulis Bambusae in Taenia) clears heat and dissolves thick yellow phlegm to treat various disorders characterized by Lung heat. The fresh form of this herb is the strongest in sedating Lung heat and relieving irritability.

- Cough with yellow copious sputum from Lung heat: combine *Zhu Ru* with *Huang Qin* (Radix Scutellariae) and *Gua Lou Shi* (Fructus Trichosanthis), or use a large dosage of fresh *Zhu Ru.*

Gallbladder fire with phlegm: When Gallbladder fire invades the Stomach and causes disharmony of the middle *jiao*, in addition to phlegm fire there may be symptoms of irritability, insomnia, nausea, chest congestion, hypochondriac distention, and a bitter taste in the mouth with profuse phlegm. If the patient vomits, the vomitus will appear sticky, much like the texture of phlegm.

- Gallbladder fire with phlegm: add *Zhu Ru* to *Ban Xia* (Rhizoma Pinelliae), *Chen Pi* (Pericarpium Citri Reticulatae), *Zhi Shi* (Fructus Aurantii Immaturus) and *Fu Ling* (Poria). **Exemplar Formula:** *Wen Dan Tang* (Warm the Gallbladder Decoction).

2. Relieves Nausea and Irritability

Vomiting due to Stomach heat, morning sickness: *Zhu Ru* is an excellent herb to treat nausea and vomiting. It clears excess heat, deficiency heat, or hot phlegm from the Stomach to relieve nausea, vomiting and acid regurgitation.

- Nausea, vomiting, thirst and epigastric discomfort with yellow greasy tongue coating due to hot phlegm in the Stomach: use *Zhu Ru* with *Chen Pi* (Pericarpium Citri Reticulatae), *Ban Xia* (Rhizoma Pinelliae), and *Huang Lian* (Rhizoma Coptidis).
- Nausea and vomiting because of deficiency heat in the Stomach: combine this herb with *Ren Shen* (Radix Ginseng), *Chen Pi* (Pericarpium Citri Reticulatae), and *Sheng Jiang* (Rhizoma Zingiberis Recens). **Exemplar Formula:** *Ju Pi Zhu Ru Tang* (Tangerine Peel and Bamboo Shaving Decoction).
- Nausea and vomiting during pregnancy: process *Zhu Ru* with *Sheng Jiang* (Rhizoma Zingiberis Recens), and use it with *Bai Zhu* (Rhizoma Atractylodis Macrocephalae) and *Su Geng* (Caulis Perillae). *Sheng Jiang* neutralizes the cold nature of *Zhu Ru* and makes it more suitable for use during pregnancy.

DOSAGE

6 to 10 grams in decoction. Fresh or unprocessed *Zhu Ru* is colder in nature and functions more effectively to clear heat, and is commonly used to treat Lung heat with coughing and thick sputum, or accumulation of hot phlegm causing irritability, mania and disorientation. The ginger-processed herb is warmer, and is more effective to relieve nausea and vomiting.

CHEMICAL COMPOSITION

2,5-dimethoxy-p-benzoguinone, p-hydroxy benzaldehyde, syringa-aldehyde.[1]

PHARMACOLOGICAL EFFECTS

- **Antibiotic:** *Zhu Ru* has an inhibitory effect against *Staphylococcus albus, Bacillus subtilis, E. coli*, and *Salmonella typhi.*[2]

References

1. *Chang Yong Zhong Yao Cheng Fen Yu Yao Li Shou Ce* (A Handbook of the Composition and Pharmacology of Common Chinese Drugs), 1994; 869
2. *Zhong Yao Xue* (Chinese Herbology), 1998; 623:625

Zhu Li (Succus Bambusae)

竹瀝 竹沥

Pinyin Name: *Zhu Li*
Alternate Chinese Names: *Dan Zhu Li, Zhu Yiu*
Original Source: *Ming Yi Za Zhu* (Miscellaneous Records of Famous Physicians) by Tao Hong-Jing in 500 A.D.
English Name: dried bamboo sap
Botanical Name: *Bambusa breviflora* Munro (*Qing Gan Zhu*); *Phyllostachys nigra* (Lodd.) Munro var. *henonis* (Mitf.) Stapf ex Rendl (*Dan Zhu*)
Pharmaceutical Name: Succus Bambusae
Properties: sweet, cold
Channels Entered: Heart, Lung, Stomach

CHINESE THERAPEUTIC ACTIONS

Clears Heat, Dissolves Phlegm

Lung heat with phlegm, stroke caused by phlegm, epilepsy due to phlegm and fire: *Zhu Li* (Succus Bambusae) is commonly used to eliminate phlegm accumulations in the body. It is described in classic texts as being able to reach everywhere, including the head, internal organs, interior and exterior aspects of the body. It is often considered the king of phlegm-dispelling herbs. For that reason, it can treat various disorders such as stroke, aphasia, paralysis, sudden unconsciousness, clenched jaws, difficulty with speech and *bi zheng* (closed disorder).

- Yellow copious sputum, cough, and chest congestion due to Lung heat: combine *Zhu Li* with *Gua Lou Shi* (Fructus Trichosanthis) and *Pi Pa Ye* (Folium Eriobotryae).
- Stroke patients with excessive sputum and a throttling sound in the throat: use the fresh juice of *Zhu Li* and *Sheng Jiang* (Rhizoma Zingiberis Recens). Force feed these juices through the nose if necessary.
- Infantile convulsions, with rolling of the eyes and foaming of the mouth: use 3 to 6 grams *Zhu Li* twice daily.
- Epilepsy and *bi zheng* (closed disorder) caused by phlegm: use it with heat-clearing and other resuscitating herbs.
- Meningitis or epidemic cerebrospinal meningitis with high fever, nausea, and vomiting: use *Zhu Li* with 0.6 to 1.2 grams of *An Gong Niu Huang Wan* (Calm the Palace Pill with Cattle Gallstone).
- Hemiplegia due to cerebral embolism: use this substance with *Sheng Jiang* (Rhizoma Zingiberis Recens), *Sang Zhi* (Ramulus Mori), *Hong Hua* (Flos Carthami), *Chi Shao* (Radix Paeoniae Rubrae), *Chuan Xiong* (Rhizoma Ligustici Chuanxiong), *Dang Gui Wei* (Extremitas Radicis Angelicae Sinensis), *Tao Ren* (Semen Persicae), *Chuan Shan Jia* (Squama Manis), *Di Long* (Pheretima), *Dan Nan Xing* (Arisaema cum Bile), *Gou Teng* (Ramulus Uncariae cum Uncis), *Gua Lou Shi* (Fructus Trichosanthis) and *Ban Xia* (Rhizoma Pinelliae).
- Liver qi stagnation with heat manifesting in disorientation, shouting or aggressive behavior, crying and laughing spells, unusual behavior, and talking to oneself: add *Zhu Li* to *Yu Jin* (Radix Curcumae), *Tian Zhu Huang* (Concretio Silicea Bambusae), *Shi Chang Pu* (Rhizoma Acori), *Yuan Zhi* (Radix Polygalae), *Xiang Fu* (Rhizoma Cyperi), *Dai Zhe Shi* (Haematitum), *Meng Shi* (Lapis Micae seu Chloriti), *Dan Nan Xing* (Arisaema cum Bile), *Sheng Tie Luo* (Frusta Ferri), *Huang Lian* (Rhizoma Coptidis), *Huang Qin* (Radix Scutellariae) and *Da Huang* (Radix et Rhizoma Rhei).

DOSAGE

30 to 50 grams. Do not decoct *Zhu Li* with other herbs. Instead, it is to be dissolved in the decoction immediately prior to ingestion.

CAUTIONS / CONTRAINDICATIONS

- Cold in nature, *Zhu Li* is contraindicated in cases of cough due to cold, or with loose stools from Spleen deficiency.

CHEMICAL COMPOSITION

Asparagine, methionine, salicylic acid, leucine, amino acids, sugars.[1]

CLINICAL STUDIES AND RESEARCH

- **Cough:** Administration of *Zhu Li* showed marked antitussive and expectorant effects in 125 patients. The overall rate of effectiveness was 88.8%.[2]

References

1. *Xian Dai Zhong Yao Yao Li Xue* (Contemporary Pharmacology of Chinese Herbs), 1997; 983
2. *Zhong Guo Yi Yuan Yao Xue Za Zhi* (Chinese Hospital Journal of Herbology), 1988; 11:519

Fu Hai Shi (Pumice)

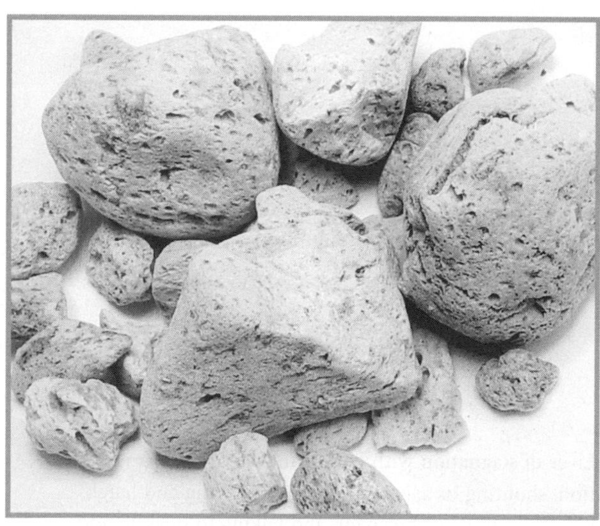

浮海石

Pinyin Name: *Fu Hai Shi*
Literal Name: "float on the sea stone"
Alternate Chinese Names: *Hai Fu Shi, Sui Hua*
Original Source: *Ben Cao Shi Yi* (Omissions from the [Classic of the] Materia Medica) by Chen Cang-Qi in 741 A.D.
English Name: pumice
Zoological Name: *Costazia aculeata* Canu et. Bassler (*Ji Tu Tai Chong*)
Pharmaceutical Name: Pumice
Properties: salty, cold
Channels Entered: Lung

CHINESE THERAPEUTIC ACTIONS

1. Clears the Lung, Dissolves Phlegm

Phlegm stagnation in the Lung: *Fu Hai Shi* (Pumice) is most effective for treating chronic and stubborn phlegm stagnation, usually found in lumps that are difficult to expectorate or swallow. Blood-streaked sputum is often seen in chronic respiratory disorders caused by Lung yin deficiency.

- Chronic and stubborn phlegm stagnation: use *Fu Hai Shi* with *Dan Nan Xing* (Arisaema cum Bile), *Bei Mu* (Bulbus Fritillaria) and *Bai Jie Zi* (Semen Sinapis).
- Chronic cough with blood-streaked sputum from Lung heat: combine this substance with *Hai Ge Fen* (Concha Meretricis seu Cyclinae), *Gua Lou Shi* (Fructus Trichosanthis), and *Zhi Zi* (Fructus Gardeniae).

2. Softens Hardness and Dissipates Nodules

Scrofula and thyroid nodules: In addition to clearing heat and dissolving phlegm, *Fu Hai Shi* softens hardness and dissipates nodules.

- Scrofula or nodules: use it with *Mu Li* (Concha Ostreae), *Zhe Bei Mu* (Bulbus Fritillariae Thunbergii), *Kun Bu* (Thallus Laminariae seu Eckloniae) and *Hai Zao* (Sargassum).

3. Regulates Water Circulation to Treat Dysuria

***Lin zheng* (dysuria syndrome):** *Fu Hai Shi* regulates water circulation, promotes urination, and treats dysuria, hematuria or stones.

- *Xue lin* (bloody dysuria): combine *Fu Hai Shi* with *Chuan Mu Tong* (Caulis Clematidis Armandii), *Hua Shi* (Talcum) and *Che Qian Zi* (Semen Plantaginis).
- *Shi lin* (stone dysuria): use this substance with *Gan Cao* (Radix Glycyrrhizae), *Hai Jin Sha* (Herba Lygodii), *Ji Nei Jin* (Endothelium Corneum Gigeriae Galli), and *Jin Qian Cao* (Herba Lysimachiae).

DOSAGE

6 to 10 grams in decoction. Crush *Fu Hai Shi* into a powder and use in decoction, pills, or powder.

CAUTIONS / CONTRAINDICATIONS

- *Fu Hai Shi* should be used with caution in cases of cough caused by deficiency and cold.

CHEMICAL COMPOSITION

Silicon dioxide, aluminum, potassium, calcium, sodium, iron.[1,2]

References

1. *Zhong Yao Xue* (Chinese Herbology), 1998; 626-627
2. *Chang Yong Zhong Yao Xian Dai Yan Jiu Yu Lin Chuan* (Recent Study & Clinical Application of Common Traditional Chinese Medicine), 1995; 458-459

Hai Ge Fen (Concha Meretricis seu Cyclinae)

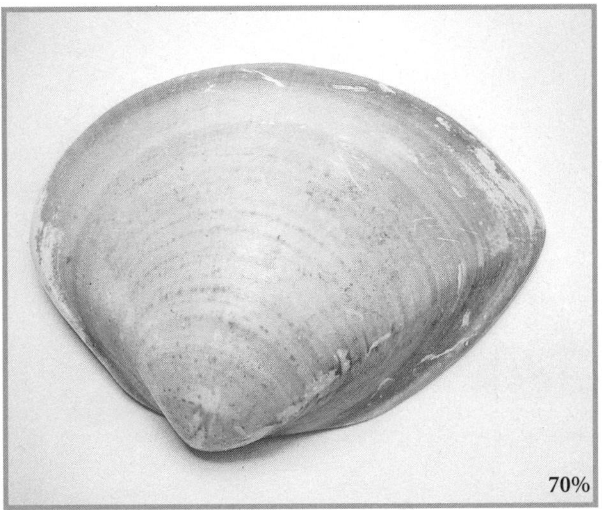

海蛤粉

Pinyin Name: *Hai Ge Fen*
Alternate Chinese Names: *Hai Ge Ke*
Original Source: *Shen Nong Ben Cao Jing* (Divine Husbandman's Classic of the Materia Medica) in the second century
English Name: clam shell
Zoological Name: *Meretrix meretrix* L. (*Wen Ge*); *Cyclina sinensis* Gmelin (*Qing Ge*)
Pharmaceutical Name: Concha Meretricis seu Cyclinae
Properties: bitter, salty, cold
Channels Entered: Lung, Stomach

CHINESE THERAPEUTIC ACTIONS

1. Clears the Lung, Dissolves Phlegm

Hai Ge Fen (Concha Meretricis seu Cyclinae) clears Lung heat and dissolves sticky, copious phlegm. It treats accumulation of hot phlegm in the chest that has led to feelings of oppression in the chest, wheezing, dyspnea, cough and copious, yellow sputum. It also treats accumulation of phlegm and fire that has caused chest and hypochondriac pain, cough and wheezing.

- Accumulation of hot phlegm in the chest: use *Hai Ge Fen* with *Huang Qin* (Radix Scutellariae), *Gua Lou Ren* (Semen Trichosanthis) and *Jie Geng* (Radix Platycodonis).
- Accumulation of phlegm and fire in the chest: combine this substance with *Gua Lou Shi* (Fructus Trichosanthis), *Zhi Zi* (Fructus Gardeniae) and *Qing Dai* (Indigo Naturalis).
- Productive cough and dyspnea from Lung heat: add it to *Fu Hai Shi* (Pumice), *Bai Qian* (Rhizoma Cynanchi Stauntonii) and *Sang Bai Pi* (Cortex Mori).

2. Softens Hardness and Dissipates Nodules

Bitter and salty in nature, *Hai Ge Fen* softens hardness and dissipates nodules. Clinical applications include treatment of scrofula and thyroid nodules.

- Scrofula or thyroid nodules: use *Hai Ge Fen* with *Hai Zao* (Sargassum), *Kun Bu* (Thallus Laminariae seu Eckloniae) and *Wa Leng Zi* (Concha Arcae).

3. Neutralizes Gastric Acid to Relieve Pain

Hai Ge Fen neutralizes gastric acid to treat stomach pain, acid reflux, and gastric and duodenal ulcers.

- Gastric and duodenal ulcers: combine it with *Hai Piao Xiao* (Endoconcha Sepiae), *Gan Cao* (Radix Glycyrrhizae) and *Yan Hu Suo* (Rhizoma Corydalis).

4. Promotes Urination

Hai Ge Fen has a mild action to promote urination to treat edema and dysuria.

- Edema and dysuria: add it to *Fu Ling* (Poria), *Zhu Ling* (Polyporus) and *Hua Shi* (Talcum).

5. Topical Uses

When applied topically, *Hai Ge Fen* aids healing of wounds, burns and eczema. Mix the calcined form of *Hai Ge Fen* with oil for topical application.

DOSAGE

10 to 15 grams in decoction. *Hai Ge Fen* should be wrapped in cheesecloth prior to decocting. It is used primarily in powder or pill form. The fresh form functions more effectively to clear heat and dissolve phlegm, while the calcined form has a stronger astringent function to heal wounds.

CAUTIONS / CONTRAINDICATIONS

- *Hai Ge Fen* is contraindicated in patients who have middle *jiao* yang deficiency, or deficiency and cold of the Lung.

CHEMICAL COMPOSITION

Calcium carbonate, chitin.[1]

References

1. *Xian Dai Zhong Yao Yao Li Xue* (Contemporary Pharmacology of Chinese Herbs), 1997; 970

Meng Shi (Lapis Micae seu Chloriti)

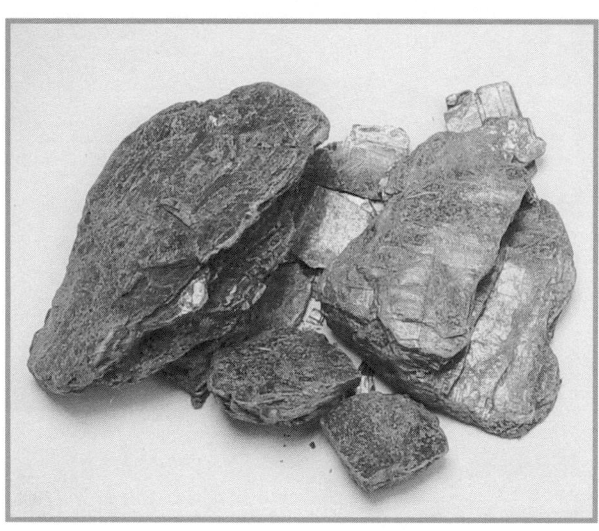

礞石 礞石

Pinyin Name: *Meng Shi*
Alternate Chinese Names: *Qing Meng Shi, Jin Meng Shi*
Original Source: *Jia You Ben Cao* (Materia Medica of the Jia You Era) by Zhang Yu-Xi and Su Song in 1057-1060
Mineral Name: Lapis Micae (*Jin Meng Shi*), Lapis Choriti (*Qing Meng Shi*)
Pharmaceutical Name: Lapis Micae seu Chloriti
Properties: salty, sweet, neutral
Channels Entered: Lung, Liver

CHINESE THERAPEUTIC ACTIONS

1. Redirects Qi Downwards and Dissolves Phlegm

Stubborn phlegm with cough and dyspnea: *Meng Shi* (Lapis Micae seu Chloriti) is strong and heavy in nature. It has a descending property that directs qi downwards to treat abnormally-rising Lung and Liver qi. It treats stubborn, difficult-to-expel phlegm in the Lung. It is also good for excess-type cough and dyspnea caused by phlegm stagnation in the upper and middle *jiaos*.

- Chronic cough with phlegm: use *Meng Shi* with *Da Huang* (Radix et Rhizoma Rhei), *Huang Qin* (Radix Scutellariae) and *Chen Xiang* (Lignum Aquilariae Resinatum).

2. Anchors the Liver and Stops Seizures

Seizures: *Meng Shi* treats seizures and convulsions caused by hot phlegm in the Liver and misting the orifices. Clinical presentations include high fever, delirium, unconsciousness, palpitations, seizures and convulsions.

- Seizures and convulsions with constipation: use *Meng Shi* powder and mix it with *Bo He* (Herba Menthae) juice and honey.

DOSAGE

6 to 10 grams in decoction, 1.5 to 3 grams in the powdered form.

CAUTIONS / CONTRAINDICATIONS

- Use of *Meng Shi* is contraindicated in children, pregnant women, or patients who have qi deficiency or weak digestive systems.

CHEMICAL COMPOSITION

Potassium, iron, aluminum, magnesium, silicon, silicic acid.[1]

CLINICAL STUDIES AND RESEARCH

- **Epilepsy:** In one study, 139 patients with seizure disorders were treated with an herbal formula, with 93 cases of complete recovery, 34 cases of marked improvement, and 12 cases showing no effect. The rate of effectiveness was 91.4%. The herbal formula contained processed *Meng Shi*, ginger-processed *Ban Xia* (Rhizoma Pinelliae), *Tian Nan Xing* (Rhizoma Arisaematis), *Fu Hai Shi* (Pumice), *Chen Xiang* (Lignum Aquilariae Resinatum), fresh *Qian Niu Zi* (Semen Pharbitidis), cooked *Qian Niu Zi* (Semen Pharbitidis), dry-fried *Shen Qu* (Massa Fermentata) and others, based on the condition of the patient.[2]

References

1. *Zhong Yao Xue* (Chinese Herbology), 1998; 628-629
2. *Zhong Yi Za Zhi* (Journal of Chinese Medicine), 1965; 6:21

Hai Zao (Sargassum)

海藻 海藻

Pinyin Name: *Hai Zao*

Original Source: *Shen Nong Ben Cao Jing* (Divine Husbandman's Classic of the Materia Medica) in the second century

English Name: sargassum, seaweed

Botanical Name: *Sargassum pallidum* (Turn.) C. Ag. (*Hai Hao Zi*); *Sargassum fusiforme* (Harv.) Setch. (*Yang Qi Cai*)

Pharmaceutical Name: Sargassum

Properties: bitter, salty, cold

Channels Entered: Liver, Stomach, Kidney

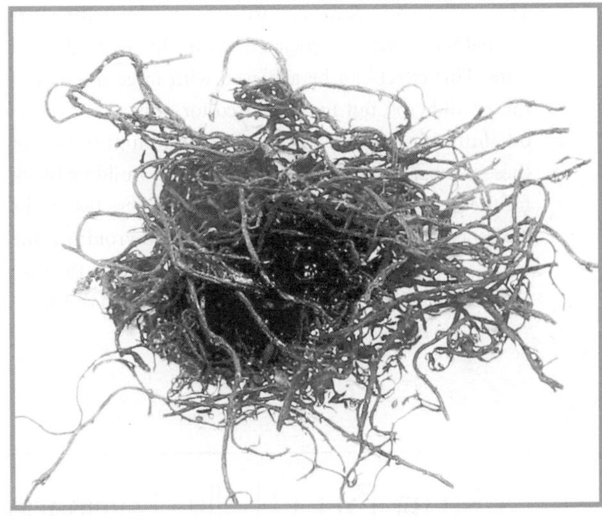

CHINESE THERAPEUTIC ACTIONS

1. Dissolves Phlegm, Softens Hardnesses

Scrofula, goiters, nodules: Scrofula is characterized by Liver fire drying body fluids and phlegm and transforming them into a solid obstruction. Goiter is caused by accumulation of phlegm secondary to blood and qi stagnation of the Liver and Gallbladder. *Hai Zao* (Sargassum) is commonly used to soften hardness, dissipate nodules, and treat scrofula and goiter. This herb has been recently used to treat thyroid enlargement, thyroiditis, lymphadenitis, hernia and enlargement of the scrotum.

- Scrofula: use *Hai Zao* with *Xia Ku Cao* (Spica Prunellae), *Lian Qiao* (Fructus Forsythiae), and *Xuan Shen* (Radix Scrophulariae).
- Goiter: use this substance with *Kun Bu* (Thallus Laminariae seu Eckloniae), *Bei Mu* (Bulbus Fritillaria) and *Qing Pi* (Pericarpium Citri Reticulatae Viride). **Exemplar Formula:** *Hai Zao Yu Hu Tang* (Sargassum Decoction for the Jade Flask).
- Hyperthyroidism: use large doses of *Hai Zao* and *Kun Bu* (Thallus Laminariae seu Eckloniae) for only a short period of time.
- Hypothyroidism: use the normal doses of *Hai Zao* and *Kun Bu* (Thallus Laminariae seu Eckloniae) for long-term treatment.

2. Regulates Water Circulation and Reduces Swelling

Leg *qi*, edema: *Hai Zao* regulates water circulation to treat edema, beriberi, and dysuria. It is rather mild and must be combined with other diuretic herbs, such as *Ze Xie* (Rhizoma Alismatis), *Zhu Ling* (Polyporus), and *Che Qian Zi* (Semen Plantaginis).

DOSAGE

10 to 15 grams in decoction.

CAUTIONS / CONTRAINDICATIONS

- *Hai Zao* is incompatible with *Gan Cao* (Radix Glycyrrhizae).
- *Hai Zao* should be used cautiously for patients having Spleen and Stomach qi deficiency.

CHEMICAL COMPOSITION

Alginic acid, mannitol, potassium, iodine, laminine, sargassan, fucosterol, protein, lipids, vitamin C.[1,2]

PHARMACOLOGICAL EFFECTS

- **Effects on the thyroid gland:** *Hai Zao* has a high iodine content and may be used to treat thyroid disorders.[3]
- **Immunostimulant:** Intraperitoneal injection of a *Hai Zao* preparation increased phagocytic activities in mice.[4]

CLINICAL STUDIES AND RESEARCH

- **Ischemic cerebral vascular accident:** PSS, a substance isolated from *Hai Zao*, has marked effectiveness to reduce blood viscosity, slow coagulation, and lower cholesterol levels in blood. It has been reported to be 92% effective in treating 288 patients with cerebral thrombosis and 92% effective in treating 251 patients with cerebral emboli.[5]

AUTHORS' COMMENTS

The use of *Hai Zao* and *Kun Bu* (Thallus Laminariae seu Eckloniae) is beneficial in treating both hyperthyroid and hypothyroid conditions. In hyperthyroid conditions, administration of these two herbs is associated with a negative feedback inhibition effect on the endocrine system to stop the release of additional thyroid hormone.

Hai Zao (Sargassum)

This approach is beneficial to temporarily counter the sympathetic excess associated with the hyperthyroid state. This effect can be achieved with large dosages of these two herbs, but must be used for only a short period of time. In hypothyroid conditions, administration of these two herbs supply iodine, a necessary building block for the production of thyroid hormone. These two herbs are especially beneficial in cases of hypothyroidism due to lack of iodine in the diet. For this application, they are used at normal dosages for a prolonged period of time.

References

1. *Xian Dai Zhong Yao Yao Li Xue* (Contemporary Pharmacology of Chinese Herbs), 1997; 971
2. *Chang Yong Zhong Yao Cheng Fen Yu Yao Li Shou Ce* (A Handbook of the Composition and Pharmacology of Common Chinese Drugs), 1994; 1533
3. *Zhong Yao Xue* (Chinese Herbology), 1998; 629:631
4. *Zhong Guo Yao Ke Da Xue Xue Bao* (Journal of University of Chinese Herbology), 1988; 19(4):279
5. *Shi Yong Nei Ke Za Zhi* (Practical Journal of Internal Medicine), 1987; 11:580

Kun Bu (Thallus Laminariae seu Eckloniae)

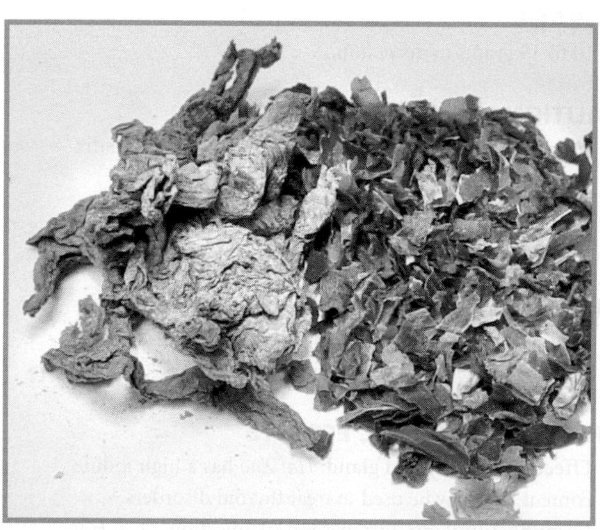

昆布 昆布

Pinyin Name: *Kun Bu*

Original Source: *Ming Yi Za Zhu* (Miscellaneous Records of Famous Physicians) by Tao Hong-Jing in 500 A.D.

English Name: laminaria, kelp, tangle

Botanical Name: *Laminaria japonica* Aresch. (*Hai Dai*); *Ecklonia kurome* Okam. (*Kun Bu*)

Pharmaceutical Name: Thallus Laminariae seu Eckloniae

Properties: salty, cold

Channels Entered: Liver, Stomach, Kidney

CHINESE THERAPEUTIC ACTIONS

1. Dissolves Phlegm, Softens Hardness

Scrofula, goiters, nodules: *Kun Bu* (Thallus Laminariae seu Eckloniae) dissolves phlegm, softens hardness, and dissipates nodules. It treats enlargement of the thyroid gland, goiter due to iodine deficiency, hyperthyroidism, palpable abdominal masses such as liver and spleen enlargement, and swelling and pain in the scrotum.

- Scrofula, goiter, and other nodules: use *Kun Bu* with *Hai Zao* (Sargassum), *Xia Ku Cao* (Spica Prunellae), *Bei Mu* (Bulbus Fritillaria), *Xuan Shen* (Radix Scrophulariae) and *Hai Ge Fen* (Concha Meretricis seu Cyclinae).
- Palpable abdominal masses, splenomegaly, hepatomegaly: *Kun Bu* is combined with *Bie Jia* (Carapax Trionycis), *Mu Li* (Concha Ostreae), *Xiang Fu* (Rhizoma Cyperi), *Hong Hua* (Flos Carthami), *Chuan Shan Jia* (Squama Manis), *San Leng* (Rhizoma Sparganii) and *E Zhu* (Rhizoma Curcumae).
- Hyperthyroidism: use large doses of *Kun Bu* and *Hai Zao* (Sargassum) for only a short period of time.
- Hypothyroidism: use normal doses of *Kun Bu* and *Hai Zao* (Sargassum) for long-term treatment.

2. Regulates Water Circulation

Leg *qi*, edema: *Kun Bu* regulates water circulation and reduces accumulation of water to treat edema and dysuria. This function, however, is rather mild and *Kun Bu* must be combined with other diuretic herbs for maximum effectiveness.

DOSAGE

10 to 15 grams in decoction.

Kun Bu (Thallus Laminariae seu Eckloniae)

CAUTIONS / CONTRAINDICATIONS

- Use *Kun Bu* with caution for patients who have deficiency and cold of the Spleen and Stomach.
- *Kun Bu* should be used with caution in patients with phlegm due to cold.

CHEMICAL COMPOSITION

Laminine, laminarin, alginic acid, algin, potassium, iodine, iron, calcium.[1]

PHARMACOLOGICAL EFFECTS

- **Cardiovascular:** According to *in vitro* studies, administration of laminine is associated with reduction in blood pressure.[2]
- **Hypoglycemic:** Administration of laminarin is associated with reduction of blood glucose levels in mice with normal or elevated levels.[3]
- **Metabolic:** Continuous administration of a *Kun Bu* preparation inhibits the elevation of serum cholesterol and triglyceride levels.[4]

CLINICAL STUDIES AND RESEARCH

- **Hypertension:** According to one study, *Kun Bu* powder was 76.4% effective in treating 110 patients with hypertension.[5]

HERB-DRUG INTERACTION

- **Antidiabetics:** Herbs that lower plasma glucose levels, such as *Kun Bu,* should be used with caution with insulin, sulfonylureas, and other antidiabetic medications, as the combination may have a synergistic effect, leading to hypoglycemia. [Note: Examples of antidiabetic drugs include insulin, tolbutamide (Orinase), glipizide (Glucotrol), and glyburide (DiaBeta/Micronase).][6]

SUPPLEMENT

- 海帶 / 海带 *Hai Dai* (Thallus Laminariae) is commonly used as another source for *Kun Bu.* They can be used interchangeably, as they have essentially the same taste, properties, functions, indications, and chemical composition.

AUTHORS' COMMENTS

According to Dr. Jiao Shu-De, use of *Kun Bu* and *Hai Zao* (Sargassum) is effective for treatment of obesity, arteriosclerosis and hyperlipidemia.

Hai Zao (Sargassum), *Kun Bu* (Thallus Laminariae seu Eckloniae) and *Hai Dai* (Thallus Laminariae) are all from the ocean and have similar composition and functions. Generally speaking, *Kun Bu* has the strongest potency, followed by *Hai Zao*, and then *Hai Dai.* Please refer to *Hai Zao* for more discussion on treatment of thyroid disorders using these herbs.

References

1. *Xian Dai Zhong Yao Yao Li Xue* (Contemporary Pharmacology of Chinese Herbs), 1997; 974
2. *Yao Xue Za Zhi* (Journal of Medicinals), 1983; 103(6):683
3. *Zhong Cao Yao* (Chinese Herbal Medicine), 1987; 18(2):15
4. Ibid.
5. *Zhong Cao Yao Tong Xun* (Journal of Chinese Herbal Medicine), 1974; 3:39
6. Chen, J. Recognition & prevention of herb-drug interactions, *Medical Acupuncture*, Fall/Winter 1998/1999; volume 10/number 2; 9-13

Huang Yao Zi (Herba Dioscoreae Bulbiferae)

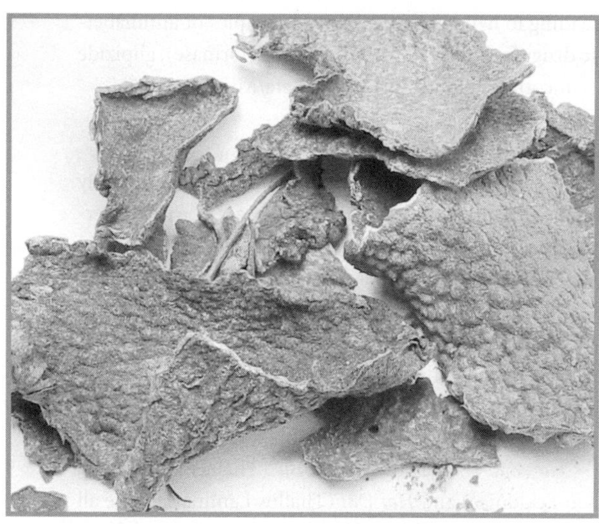

黄藥子 黄药子

Pinyin Name: *Huang Yao Zi*
Literal Name: "yellow medicine seed"
Alternate Chinese Names: *Huang Yao Zhi, Jin Qian Diao Ha Ma, Ling Xu Shu*
Original Source: *Kai Bao Ben Cao* (Materia Medica of the Kai Bao Era) by Ma Zhi in 973-974 A.D.
English Name: dioscorea bulbifera root, airpotato yam rhizome
Botanical Name: *Dioscorea bulbifera* L. (*Huang Du*)
Pharmaceutical Name: Herba Dioscoreae Bulbiferae
Properties: bitter, cold
Channels Entered: Lung, Liver
Safety Index: toxic

CHINESE THERAPEUTIC ACTIONS

1. Disperses Stagnation and Reduces Masses

Masses, nodules and goiters: *Huang Yao Zi* (Herba Dioscoreae Bulbiferae) strongly dissolves phlegm and disperses palpable nodules.

- Goiter: use *Huang Yao Zi* alone as medicinal tincture, or use with *Hai Zao* (Sargassum), *Mu Li* (Concha Ostreae) and *Kun Bu* (Thallus Laminariae seu Eckloniae).

2. Clears Heat and Toxins

Ulcers, toxic swellings with redness, sore throat, snake bites, tumors and cancer: *Huang Yao Zi* has an excellent function to clear heat and toxins. It is often used with other heat-clearing, toxin-eliminating herbs to enhance the overall effect.

- Snake bite: use the fresh form of *Huang Yao Zi* topically as a paste. Because there are various kinds of snake venom, combine with other herbs according to the patient's immediate symptoms.
- Sore throat: use the herb with *Shan Dou Gen* (Radix Sophorae Tonkinensis), *She Gan* (Rhizoma Belamcandae) and *Ban Lan Gen* (Radix Isatidis).
- Cancer of the esophagus, stomach, liver, colon or thyroid: add this herb to *Bai Hua She She Cao* (Herba Oldenlandia), *Ban Zhi Lian* (Herba Scutellariae Barbatae), *Yi Yi Ren* (Semen Coicis), *Hai Zao* (Sargassum) and *Shan Ci Gu* (Pseudobulbus Cremastrae).

3. Cools Blood and Stops Bleeding

Epistaxis, hematemesis, hemoptysis: *Huang Yao Zi* is cold in thermal property and treats bleeding caused by heat in the blood.

- Bleeding: use it with charred *Pu Huang* (Pollen Typhae), charred *Zong Lu Pi* (Fibra Stipulae Trachycarpi) and charred *Qian Cao* (Radix Rubiae).

In addition, *Huang Yao Zi* stops cough and relieves dyspnea. It is suitable for acute and chronic bronchitis, asthma and whooping cough. It may be used as a single-herb remedy for this application.

DOSAGE

10 to 15 grams. The fresh form of *Huang Yao Zi* can be crushed into a paste and applied topically.

CAUTIONS / CONTRAINDICATIONS

- Long-term use of *Huang Yao Zi* may cause vomiting, diarrhea, abdominal pain and other gastrointestinal discomforts.
- Though rare, the use of *Huang Yao Zi* has been associated with potential liver damage. Therefore, liver functions must be monitored when prescribing *Huang Yao Zi.*
- *Huang Yao Zi* is contraindicated in patients with pre-existing liver disorders, such as hepatitis and cirrhosis.

OVERDOSAGE

Overdose reactions associated with the use of this herb often occur 1 to 2 hours after ingestion, with a very gradual onset and progression. Early reaction is characterized by burning sensations of the mouth, tongue and throat, followed by dizziness, headache, nausea, vomiting, salivation, diarrhea and constricted pupils. Six to seven days after ingestion, the patient may experience fatigue, lack of appetite, upper abdominal discomfort, yellow discoloration of the eyes and skin, itching skin, and possibly liver damage.[1]

Huang Yao Zi (Herba Dioscoreae Bulbiferae)

TREATMENT OF OVERDOSAGE

Early overdose can be treated with emetic methods, followed by ingestion of 5 to 6 egg whites, or 250 grams of *Lu Dou* (Semen Phaseoli Radiati) in decoction. Another proposed antidote contains fresh *Sheng Jiang* (Rhizoma Zingiberis Recens) juices (squeezed from 30g of herb), 60 ml of white vinegar, and 9 grams of *Gan Cao* (Radix Glycyrrhizae). The patients are instructed to first gargle with, and then swallow the decoction.

Huang Yao Zi must be discontinued immediately if symptoms and signs of liver damage are noted, such as yellow discoloration of the eyes and skin and elevated liver enzymes.

CHEMICAL COMPOSITION

Disgenin, yamogenin, diosbulbins A, B, C, D; iodine.[2]

PHARMACOLOGICAL EFFECTS

- **Effect on the thyroid gland:** In rats with normal thyroid glands, oral administration of *Huang Yao Zi* did not affect body weight, basal metabolic rate, or weight of the thyroid gland. In subjects with hypertrophy of the thyroid gland caused by a small amount of potassium thiocyanate or by lack of iodine in diet, *Huang Yao Zi* had a marked therapeutic effect to reduce the enlargement and increase the content of serum protein-bound iodine.[3,4]
- **Cardiovascular:** Water and alcohol preparations of *Huang Yao Zi* show an inhibitory action on frog heart specimens.[5]
- **Effects on smooth muscle:** Water and alcohol preparations of *Huang Yao Zi* inhibit the smooth muscle of the intestines in rabbits, but stimulate the smooth muscle of the uterus in rabbits and rats. The alcohol preparation has a faster onset of action and a more potent effect.[6]
- **Antibiotic:** A preparation of *Huang Yao Zi* had an inhibitory action on various pathogenic fungi.[7]

CLINICAL STUDIES AND RESEARCH

- **Thyroid tumor:** Daily administration of *Huang Yao Zi* in decoction for 5 to 8 weeks had an 80% overall rate of effectiveness for 25 patients with thyroid tumors.[8]
- **Enlargement of the thyroid gland:** Decoction or powder of *Huang Yao Zi* was used to treat 127 patients with enlargement of the thyroid gland, with good results.[9]
- **Thyroid adenoma:** In one study, 37 out of 42 patients experienced complete recovery using an herbal formula containing *Huang Yao Zi* 6g, *Mu Li* (Concha Ostreae) 30g, *Hai Zao* (Sargassum) 30g, *Kun Bu* (Thallus Laminariae seu Eckloniae) 30g, *Shan Ci Gu* (Pseudobulbus Cremastrae) 10g, *Xia Ku Cao* (Spica Prunellae) 10g, *Yu Jin* (Radix Curcumae) 10g, *Chuan Shan Jia* (Squama Manis) 10g, *Jiang Can* (Bombyx Batryticatus) 10g, *Tian Hua Fen* (Radix Trichosanthis) 12g, and *Xuan Shen* (Radix Scrophulariae) 15g. The herbal decoction was given once daily.[10]

TOXICOLOGY

With regard to the dosage form, decoction of *Huang Yao Zi* is sometimes associated with dry mouth, and tincture of this herb is sometimes associated with severe nausea and gastrointestinal discomfort. In addition, a large dose or prolonged use may damage the liver and cause jaundice.[11]

AUTHORS' COMMENTS

According to Dr. Zhang Xiao-Ping, *Huang Yao Zi* is one of the most effective herbs for treatment of hyperthyroidism and goiter. However, it is generally used as the last alternative in patients who do not respond to other herbs, and do not wish to have surgery or radioactive iodine treatment. Though it is effective, use of this herb should be monitored closely, as it has been linked with rare cases of liver toxicity.

References

1. *Zhong Yao Du Li Xue* (Toxicology of Chinese Herbs), 1989; 134-135
2. *Xian Dai Zhong Yao Yao Li Xue* (Contemporary Pharmacology of Chinese Herbs), 1997; 984
3. *Chang Yong Zhong Yao Xian Dai Yan Jiu Yu Lin Chuan* (Recent Study & Clinical Application of Common Traditional Chinese Medicine), 1995; 464:465
4. *Zhong Yao Xue* (Chinese Herbology), 1998; 632:633
5. *Chang Yong Zhong Yao Xian Dai Yan Jiu Yu Lin Chuan* (Recent Study & Clinical Application of Common Traditional Chinese Medicine), 1995; 464:465
6. Ibid.
7. Ibid.
8. *Fu Jian Yi Xue Yuan Xue Bao* (Journal of Fujian University of Medicine), 1964; 2:21
9. *Zhong Hua Yi Xue Za Zhi* (Chinese Journal of Medicine), 1961; 4:223
10. *Ji Lin Zhong Yi Yao* (Jilin Chinese Medicine and Herbology), 1991; (3):29
11. *Chang Yong Zhong Yao Xian Dai Yan Jiu Yu Lin Chuan* (Recent Study & Clinical Application of Common Traditional Chinese Medicine), 1995; 464:465

Pang Da Hai (Semen Sterculiae Lychnophorae)

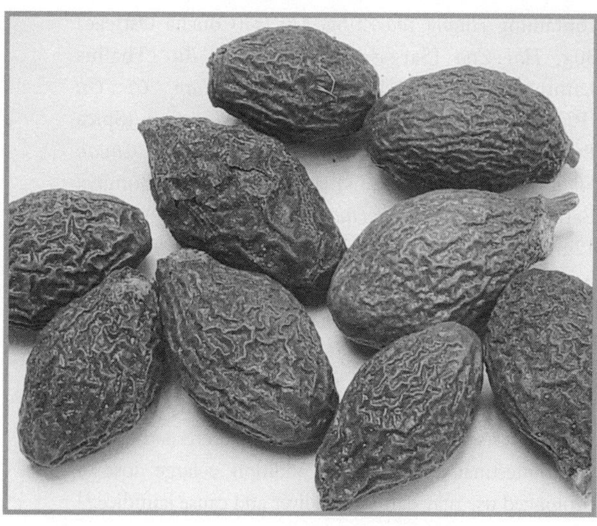

胖大海

Pinyin Name: *Pang Da Hai*
Literal Name: "fat big ocean," "fat big sea"
Alternate Chinese Names: *An Nan Zi, Da Dong Guo, Hu Da Fa*
Original Source: *Ben Cao Shi Yi* (Omissions from the [Classic of the] Materia Medica) by Chen Cang-Qi in 741 A.D.
English Name: sterculia, boat-fruited sterculia seed
Botanical Name: *Sterculia lychnophora* Hance.; *Sterculia scaphigera* Wall.
Pharmaceutical Name: Semen Sterculiae Lychnophorae
Properties: sweet, cold
Channels Entered: Lung, Large Intestine

CHINESE THERAPEUTIC ACTIONS

1. Clears and Ventilates Lung Qi

Cough due to hot phlegm: *Pang Da Hai* (Semen Sterculiae Lychnophorae) is commonly used to treat accumulations of phlegm and heat in the Lung, characterized by a throttling sound in the throat, profuse yellow sticky sputum, a bitter taste in the mouth, and dry throat. In addition, it can also be used when Lung heat is damaging Lung qi, leading to hoarseness and loss of voice. This herb is mild and can be used daily as a tea. It is often combined with other herbs in this category to expel phlegm.

- Phlegm and heat in the Lung: combine *Pang Da Hai* with *Jie Geng* (Radix Platycodonis), *Chan Tui* (Periostracum Cicadae) and *Bei Mu* (Bulbus Fritillaria).

Hoarse voice due to Lung heat or yin deficiency: *Pang Da Hai* is good for hoarse voice caused by influenza or from excessive talking, singing or shouting.

- Hoarseness and loss of voice: use *Pang Da Hai* with *Sha Shen* (Radix Glehniae seu Adenophorae), *Sheng Di Huang* (Radix Rehmanniae), *Gan Cao* (Radix Glycyrrhizae) and *Gu Zhi Hua* (Semen Oroxyli).

2. Lubricates the Bowels to Relieve Constipation

Constipation due to heat: Cold and moist in nature, *Pang Da Hai* lubricates the bowels and purges heat in the intestines to relieve constipation or dry stools.

- Mild constipation: combine this herb with *Huo Ma Ren* (Fructus Cannabis) and *Yu Li Ren* (Semen Pruni).
- Severe constipation: use it with purgative herbs.

DOSAGE

3 to 5 seeds in decoction. Halve the dosage of *Pang Da Hai* when serving it as powder. *Pang Da Hai* is also taken as tea as needed.

CHEMICAL COMPOSITION

Bassorin, arabinose, galactose.[1]

PHARMACOLOGICAL EFFECTS

- **Gastrointestinal:** Oral administration of *Pang Da Hai* is associated with an increase in water content of the intestines, thereby simulating peristalsis and promoting bowel movement. This effect is negated by atropine.[2]
- **Antihypertensive:** Oral or intramuscular administration of *Pang Da Hai* is associated with a reduction of blood pressure in anesthetized dogs and cats. The exact mechanism of action is unclear, but is thought to be related to its effect on the central nervous system.[3]

CLINICAL STUDIES AND RESEARCH

- **Acute tonsillitis:** In one study, 100 patients with acute tonsillitis were treated with *Pang Da Hai* tea with complete recovery in 68 patients, marked improvement in 21 patients, and no response in 11 patients. The tea was prepared by soaking 4 to 8 seeds in hot water for 30 minutes prior to consumption. Patients were advised to drink one dose of tea every 4 hours for 2 to 3 days. The same herbs may be re-used up to three to four times to make tea.[4]

TOXICOLOGY

The LD_{50} for oral administration of *Pang Da Hai* in mice is 12.96 g/kg. Adverse reactions due to overdose included poor balance and respiratory depression.[5]

AUTHORS' COMMENTS

Pang Da Hai and *Gu Zhi Hua* (Semen Oroxyli) are two of

Pang Da Hai (Semen Sterculiae Lychnophorae)

the best herbs to restore loss of voice. They can be taken as tea throughout the day for those who need to speak or sing for a prolonged period of time.

References

1. *Xian Dai Zhong Yao Yao Li Xue* (Contemporary Pharmacology of Chinese Herbs), 1997; 986
2. *Chang Yong Zhong Yao Xian Dai Yan Jiu Yu Lin Chuan* (Recent Study & Clinical Application of Common Traditional Chinese Medicine), 1995; 468:469
3. Ibid.
4. *Zhe Jiang Zhong Yi Za Zhi* (Zhejiang Journal of Chinese Medicine), 1966; 5:180
5. *Chang Yong Zhong Yao Xian Dai Yan Jiu Yu Lin Chuan* (Recent Study & Clinical Application of Common Traditional Chinese Medicine), 1995; 468:469

Luo Han Guo (Fructus Momordicae)

羅漢果 罗汉果

Pinyin Name: *Luo Han Guo*
Literal Name: "big fellow's fruit," "arhat fruit"
Alternate Chinese Names: *La Han Guo, Jia Ku Gua*
Original Source: *Ling Nan Cai Yao Lu* (Records of Picking Herbs in Guangdong)
English Name: momordica fruit, grosvenor momordica fruit
Botanical Name: *Momordica grosvenori* Swingle (*Luo Han Guo*)
Pharmaceutical Name: Fructus Momordicae
Properties: sweet, cool
Channels Entered: Lung, Large Intestine

CHINESE THERAPEUTIC ACTIONS

1. Moistens the Lung and Stops Cough

Coughing due to Lung heat or dryness: Chronic dry cough with or without sputum that may be scanty, blood-streaked and/or difficult to expectorate. Other symptoms may include dryness of the throat and tongue. *Luo Han Guo* (Fructus Momordicae), nourishing in nature, is most suitable for weak patients with chronic respiratory disorders.

- Dry cough: combine *Luo Han Guo* with *Bei Sha Shen* (Radix Glehniae), *Mai Men Dong* (Radix Ophiopogonis) and *Bai He* (Bulbus Lilii).
- Acute or chronic tonsillitis, pharyngitis, bronchitis and pertussis: use *Luo Han Guo* as tea twice daily.

2. Generates Body Fluids and Relieves Thirst

Summer-heat injuring the body fluids: *Luo Han Guo* is excellent to relieve thirst during the summer. It is usually used as a daily beverage to cool the body.

- Summer-time thirst: decoct it alone and serve as tea.

Recently, *Luo Han Guo* has been used to address acute gastritis and constipation.

DOSAGE

15 to 30 grams, or 1 to 2 pieces of the entire fruit, in decoction. The fruit should be crushed to enhance the extraction of active constituents.

CHEMICAL COMPOSITION

Mogroside V, VI.[1]

PHARMACOLOGICAL EFFECTS

- **Antitussive:** Preparations of *Luo Han Guo* have shown mild antitussive effects.[2]

Luo Han Guo (Fructus Momordicae)

TOXICOLOGY

Luo Han Guo has shown very little toxicity when consumed as tea over a period of time.[3]

SUPPLEMENT

- 羅漢果葉 / 罗汉果叶 *Luo Han Guo Ye* (Folium Momordicae) is derived from the leaves of the same plant. Both herbs have similar properties. *Luo Han Guo Ye* is used for chronic throat disorders.

AUTHORS' COMMENTS

Because mogroside VI is approximately 256 to 344 times sweeter than cane sugar, it is commonly used as a sweetening agent in drinks. It is also used as a sugar substitute by obese individuals or those with diabetes mellitus.[4]

References

1. *Xian Dai Zhong Yao Yao Li Xue* (Contemporary Pharmacology of Chinese Herbs), 1997; 982
2. *Guang Xi Zhi Wu* (Guangxi Plants), 1990; 10(3):254
3. *Guang Xi Zhong Yi Yao* (Guangxi Chinese Medicine and Herbology), 1989; 12(3):37
4. *Guang Xi Zhi Wu* (Guangxi Plants), 1987; 7(3):285

Section 2

— Coughing- and Wheezing-Relieving Herbs

Xing Ren (Semen Armeniacae Amarum)

杏仁

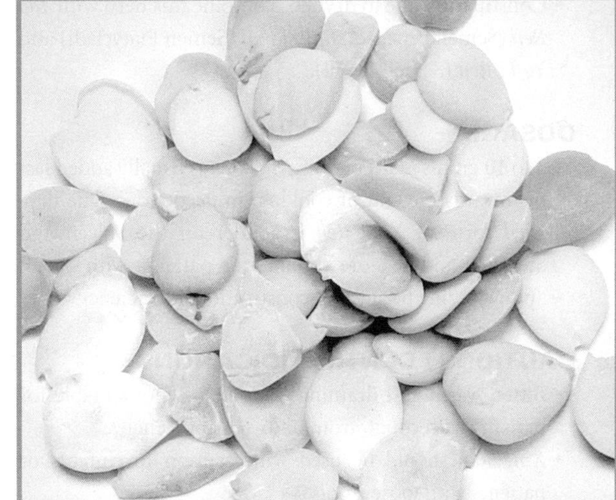

Pinyin Name: *Xing Ren*
Literal Name: "apricot seed"
Alternate Chinese Names: *Ku Xing Ren, Tian Xing Ren, Guang Xing Ren, Bei Xing Ren*
Original Source: *Shen Nong Ben Cao Jing* (Divine Husbandman's Classic of the Materia Medica) in the second century
English Name: apricot seed, sweet apricot seed, bitter apricot kernel
Botanical Name: *Prunus armeniaca* L. (*Xing*); *Prunus armeniaca* L. var. *ansu* Maxim. (*Shan Xing*); *Prunus sibirica* L. (*Xi Bo Li Ya Xing*); *Prunus mandshurica* (Maxim.) Koehne (*Dong Bei Xing*)
Pharmaceutical Name: Semen Armeniacae Amarum
Properties: bitter, slightly warm
Channels Entered: Lung, Large Intestine
Safety Index: slightly toxic

CHINESE THERAPEUTIC ACTIONS

1. Arrests Cough and Relieves Wheezing

Cough due to wind-heat, wind-cold, dryness or Lung heat: *Xing Ren* (Semen Armeniacae Amarum) is bitter, draining and lubricating in nature. It enters the *qi* (energy) level of the Lung to redirect adverse rising qi in the form of coughing, dyspnea and wheezing. It is one of the most essential herbs in treating coughing, as it can treat the initial, acute and chronic stages of cough, depending on the prescription.

- Cough due to wind-cold: use *Xing Ren* with *Zi Su Ye* (Folium Perillae), *Ban Xia* (Rhizoma Pinelliae) and *Fu Ling* (Poria). **Exemplar Formula:** *Xing Su San* (Apricot Kernel and Perilla Leaf Powder).
- Cough due to wind-heat: combine this herb with *Sang Ye* (Folium Mori) and *Ju Hua* (Flos Chrysanthemi). **Exemplar Formula:** *Sang Ju Yin* (Mulberry Leaf and Chrysanthemum Decoction).
- Cough with profuse sputum, nasal obstruction, and hoarse voice: add it to *Ma Huang* (Herba Ephedrae) and *Gan Cao* (Radix Glycyrrhizae).
- Cough due to heat and dryness consuming Lung yin: use it with *Sang Ye* (Folium Mori), *Bei Mu* (Bulbus Fritillaria), and *Sha Shen* (Radix Glehniae seu Adenophorae). **Exemplar Formula:** *Sang Xing Tang* (Mulberry Leaf and Apricot Kernel Decoction).
- Cough, wheezing and thirst due to Lung heat: combine this herb with *Ma Huang* (Herba Ephedrae) and *Shi Gao* (Gypsum Fibrosum). **Exemplar Formula:** *Ma Xing Gan Shi Tang* (Ephedra, Apricot Kernel, Licorice, and Gypsum Decoction).

Xing Ren (Semen Armeniacae Amarum)

2. Lubricates the Bowels and Promotes Bowel Movements

Constipation, dry stools: *Xing Ren*, lubricating, moistening and descending in nature, is commonly used to treat constipation secondary to dryness and heat in the Large Intestine and Stomach. It may also be used for elderly or deficient patients who have constipation caused by deficiency of qi, blood, and/or body fluids.

- Constipation due to deficiency of qi, blood, and/or body fluids: use *Xing Ren* with *Huo Ma Ren* (Fructus Cannabis), *Da Huang* (Radix et Rhizoma Rhei), and *Zhi Ke* (Fructus Aurantii). **Exemplar Formula:** *Ma Zi Ren Wan* (Hemp Seed Pill).
- Constipation due to dryness: combine this herb with *Tao Ren* (Semen Persicae), *Bai Zi Ren* (Semen Platycladi) and *Yu Li Ren* (Semen Pruni).

DOSAGE

3 to 10 grams in decoction. *Xing Ren* is usually added last or towards the end of cooking, in decoctions. The dry-fried form of *Xing Ren* is gentler on the Spleen and Stomach and is more suitable for patients with cough and wheezing because of constitutional deficiency.

CAUTIONS / CONTRAINDICATIONS

- Bitter, warm and draining, *Xing Ren* is not suitable for patients with cough from qi or yin deficiencies.
- *Xing Ren* should be used with caution for infants or patients with loose stools.
- *Xing Ren* is slightly toxic. However, the toxicity can be reduced by cooking, removing the outer coating, and mixing the seed with sugar.

OVERDOSAGE

Xing Ren is slightly toxic. Adverse reactions have been reported following the consumption of 40 to 60 kernels by adults, and 10 to 20 kernels by children.

Symptoms of overdose of *Xing Ren* usually occur within 30 minutes to 5 hours after excessive ingestion. Moderate overdose of *Xing Ren* causes dizziness, weakness, nausea, vomiting, abdominal pain, burning sensations in the upper abdominal region, increased blood pressure and increased respiration. Severe overdose of *Xing Ren* causes slow, shallow respiration, coma, convulsions, pupil dilation, decreased blood pressure, and possibly respiratory or cardiovascular collapse. Adverse reactions are summarized by disturbances of the respiratory system (dyspnea, itchy throat, soreness and burning sensations in the throat, excessive salivation, increased or irregular respiration, chest congestion and pain), gastrointestinal system (nausea, vomiting, diarrhea, and burning sensations in the stomach), and central nervous system (dizziness, headache, fatigue, tachycardia, increased blood pressure, and semiconsciousness). In severe cases, there may be urinary and bowel incontinence, dilated pupils, muscle convulsions, locked jaw, increased body temperature, hepatomegaly, labored breath, cold extremities, unconsciousness, shock, and respiratory depression.[1]

TREATMENT OF OVERDOSAGE

Overdose of *Xing Ren* can be treated with emetic methods within the first four (4) hours following ingestion of *Xing Ren*. Once systemic reactions occur, it must be treated accordingly. There are two published methods for treatment of overdose of *Xing Ren:*

1. Herbal decoction of *Xing Ren Shu Pi* (Cortex Pruni Armeniacae). The standard protocol is to cook 60 grams of this tree bark in 300 ml of water for 20 minutes, and have the affected individual drink the decoction. Their condition should improve within approximately two (2) hours.[2]
2. Herbal decoction with *Gui Zhi* (Ramulus Cinnamomi) 9g, *Wu Yao* (Radix Linderae) 9g, *Chi Shao* (Radix Paeoniae Rubrae) 9g, *Hong Hua* (Flos Carthami) 15g, and *Tao Ren* (Semen Persicae) 15g. This formula is taken as a decoction twice daily.[3] [Note: The original formula also contained 1.5 gm of *Zhu Sha* (Cinnabaris) added to the decoction immediately prior to ingestion. However, use of *Zhu Sha* is no longer recommended.]

CHEMICAL COMPOSITION

Amygdalin, emulsin, hydroxynitrile lyase, amygdalase, punnase, cholesterol, estrone, α-estradiol.[4,5]

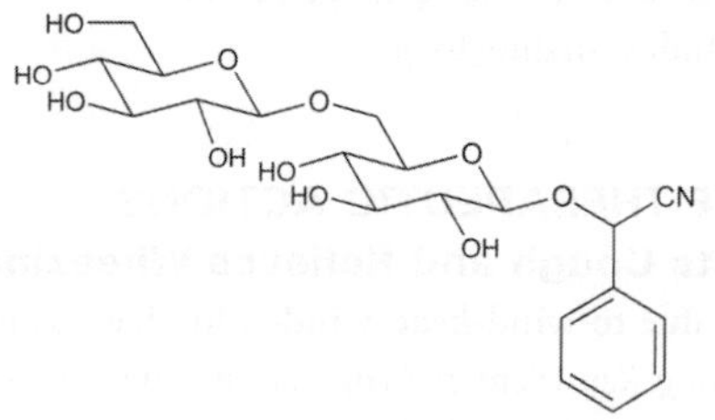

Amygdalin

PHARMACOLOGICAL EFFECTS

- **Antihypertensive:** Intravenous injection of 20% water extract of *Xing Ren* has a marked and sustained antihypertensive effect.[6]
- **Antitussive and antiasthmatic:** After ingestion, amygdalin and emulsin are metabolized in the presence of gastric acid to hydrocyanic acid. In small doses, hydrocyanic acid has a mild inhibitory effect on the respiratory center in the brain, thereby exerting its antitussive and antiasthmatic effects.[7]
- **Antineoplastic:** Oral administration of a *Xing Ren*

Xing Ren (Semen Armeniacae Amarum)

preparation has a marked inhibitory effect on liver cancer cells in mice.[8]

CLINICAL STUDIES AND RESEARCH

- **Chronic tracheitis:** An herbal preparation containing equal portions of *Xing Ren* (with outer shell intact) and rock sugar was given for treatment of chronic tracheitis. The treatment protocol was to administer 9.375 grams of the preparation twice daily for 10 days per course of treatment. Out of 124 patients, 23 reported complete recovery, 66 reported marked effectiveness, 31 experienced some improvement, and 4 had no response. The rate of effectiveness was 96.8%. This treatment was reported to be effective in relieving cough, wheezing and sputum. Most patients began to notice improvement after 3 to 4 days of treatment.[9]

TOXICOLOGY

After oral ingestion in humans, amygdalin and emulsin are metabolized in the presence of gastric acid to hydrocyanic acid and benzaldehyde. Amygdalin is a component of *Xing Ren*, and hydrocyanic acid is a derivative of amygdalin. One gram of *Xing Ren* yields approximately 0.03g [30 mg] of amygdalin and 2.5 mg of hydrocyanic acid. Hydrocyanic acid is a toxic substance, and can be lethal at 0.05g [50 mg]. The LD_{50} for amygdalin in rats is 25 g/kg via intravenous injection, 8 g/kg via intraperitoneal injection and 0.6 g/kg via oral administration. Because hydrocyanic acid is produced from amygdalin in the presence of gastric acid, the toxicity is higher when given via oral administration. The lethal dose of *Xing Ren* has been reported to be as low as 60 grams, or 50 to 60 kernels, in adults. However, small doses of the herb are unlikely to cause toxicity as there will be a gradual and continuous metabolism and excretion of the herb.[10,11,12]

SUPPLEMENT

- 杏仁樹皮 / 杏仁树皮 *Xing Ren Shu Pi* (Cortex Pruni Armeniacae), the bark of the same tree from which *Xing Ren* is harvested, treats overdose of *Xing Ren* (Semen Armeniacae Amarum). Cook 60 grams of *Xing Ren Shu Pi* in 300 ml of water for 20 minutes, and administer the decoction to the affected individual. Improvement should be observed within approximately two (2) hours.[13]

References

1. *Zhong Yao Bu Liang Fan Ying Yu Zhi Liao* (Adverse Reactions and Treatment of Chinese Herbal Medicine), 1996; 218:220, 1996; 213:217
2. *Zhong Yi Za Zhi* (Journal of Chinese Medicine), 2:20; 1965
3. *Lin Chuan Shou Ce You Du Zhong Yao Shi Yong* (Clinical Handbook on Applications of Toxic Chinese Herbs), 1992; 106-107
4. *Zhong Yi Yao Li* (Pharmacology of Chinese Herbs), 1997; 1005
5. *Chang Yong Zhong Yao Cheng Fen Yu Yao Li Shou Ce* (A Handbook of the Composition and Pharmacology of Common Chinese Drugs), 1994; 1198-1199
6. *Zhong Cao Yao Xue* (Study of Chinese Herbal Medicine), 1976; 411
7. *Life Sci*, 1980; 27(8):659
8. *Chang Yong Zhong Yao Cheng Fen Yu Yao Li Shou Ce* (A Handbook of the Composition and Pharmacology of Common Chinese Drugs), 1994; 1198:1201
9. *Zhong Yi Yan Jiu Yuan* (Research Hospital of Chinese Medicine), 1971; 34
10. *Zhong Yao Da Ci Dien* (Dictionary of Chinese Herbs), 1977: 509
11. *Arzneim-Forsch*, 1972; 22(8):1347
12. *Zhong Yao Da Ci Dien* (Dictionary of Chinese Herbs), 1977: 509
13. *Zhong Yi Za Zhi* (Journal of Chinese Medicine), 2:20; 1965

Bai Bu (Radix Stemonae)

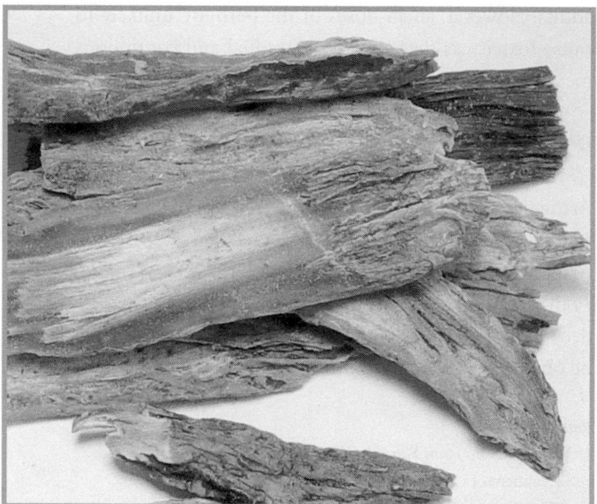

百部

Pinyin Name: *Bai Bu*
Literal Name: "hundred parts"
Alternate Chinese Names: *Fei Bai Bu, Zhi Bai Bu, Zheng Bai Bu*
Original Source: *Ming Yi Za Zhu* (Miscellaneous Records of Famous Physicians) by Tao Hong-Jing in 500 A.D.
English Name: stemona, sessile stemona root, Japanese stemona root, tuber stemona root
Botanical Name: *Stemona sessilifolia* (Miq.) Franch. et. Sav. (*Zhi Li Bai Bu*); *Stemona japonica* (*Bl.*) Miq.; *Stemona tuberosa* Lour. (*Man Sheng Bai Bu*)
Pharmaceutical Name: Radix Stemonae
Properties: sweet, bitter, neutral
Channels Entered: Lung

CHINESE THERAPEUTIC ACTIONS

1. Moistens the Lung and Stops Cough

Cough: Sweet, bitter and moistening, *Bai Bu* (Radix Stemonae) enters the Lung to relieve cough. Traditionally, it is one of the most essential herbs used in treating tuberculosis. Today, it treats a wide range of cough disorders, including acute or chronic, cold or hot, and excess or deficient conditions. When used alone, this herb is most suitable for the feeble cough associated with chronic respiratory disorders.

- Cough due to wind: use *Bai Bu* with *Jing Jie* (Herba Schizonepetae), *Jie Geng* (Radix Platycodonis), and *Zi Wan* (Radix Asteris). **Exemplar Formula:** *Zhi Sou San* (Stop Coughing Powder).
- Whooping cough, spasmodic cough in children: use this herb with *Sha Shen* (Radix Glehniae seu Adenophorae), *Chuan Bei Mu* (Bulbus Fritillariae Cirrhosae), *Wu Wei Zi* (Fructus Schisandrae Chinensis), *Ma Huang* (Herba Ephedrae), *Sheng Jiang* (Rhizoma Zingiberis Recens) and *Bai Qian* (Rhizoma Cynanchi Stauntonii).
- Cough in tuberculosis, possibly with blood-streaked sputum: combine *Bai Bu* with *Mai Men Dong* (Radix Ophiopogonis), *Sheng Di Huang* (Radix Rehmanniae), *Bai Ji* (Rhizoma Bletillae), and *San Qi* (Radix Notoginseng).
- Tuberculosis with afternoon fever, night sweats, flushed cheeks, *wu xin re* (five-center heat): use this herb with *Bie Jia* (Carapax Trionycis), *Mu Dan Pi* (Cortex Moutan), *Di Gu Pi* (Cortex Lycii), *Sheng Di Huang* (Radix Rehmanniae), *Xuan Shen* (Radix Scrophulariae) and *Qin Jiao* (Radix Gentianae Macrophyllae).

2. Kills Parasites

Parasites: *Bai Bu* has antiparasitic action and is commonly used internally or topically to treat pinworm, head or body lice, and other itching dermatological disorders.

- Pinworms: 30 grams of *Bai Bu* is cooked to obtain 30 ml of herbal solution, then used as a rectal enema each night for 5 nights.
- Intestinal parasites: combine this herb with *Wu Mei* (Fructus Mume), *Bing Lang* (Semen Arecae), and *Shi Jun Zi* (Fructus Quisqualis).
- Vaginal trichomonas: use it as a topical wash.
- Head and body lice: apply 50% *Bai Bu* solution topically.

DOSAGE

5 to 10 grams in decoction. Unprocessed *Bai Bu* is irritating to the gastrointestinal tract and may cause stomach discomfort and diarrhea. Frying it with honey enhances the moistening influence and makes it more suitable for treatment of cough due to deficiency, dryness, or weakness. Steaming the herb will prolong the overall therapeutic function, but weaken the initial peak effect.

CAUTIONS / CONTRAINDICATIONS

- *Bai Bu* is contraindicated in patients with loose stools or Spleen deficiency.

CHEMICAL COMPOSITION

Stemonine, stemonidine, isostemonidine, protostemonine, paipunine, sinostemonine.[1,2]

Stemonine

Bai Bu (Radix Stemonae)

PHARMACOLOGICAL EFFECTS

- **Respiratory:** According to *in vitro* studies, the alkaloids of *Bai Bu* demonstrated a mild inhibitory influence on the respiratory center of the brain to suppress cough.[3]
- **Antibiotic:** *Bai Bu* shows inhibitory activity against *Staphylococcus aureus, Mycobacterium tuberculosis hominis, Diplococcus pneumoniae, Bacillus dysenteriae, Salmonella typhi, Pseudomonas aeruginosa, E. coli,* and some influenza viruses and dermatophytes.[4]
- **Others:** Water and alcohol extracts of *Bai Bu* are both effective in killing lice, and bedbugs. The alcohol extract was stronger than the water extract for this purpose.[5]

CLINICAL STUDIES AND RESEARCH

- **Pulmonary tuberculosis:** Chinese herbal formulas were used successfully in treating 93 patients with pulmonary tuberculosis. The herbal formula contained *Bai Bu* 18g, *Huang Qin* (Radix Scutellariae) 9g, *Dan Shen* (Radix Salviae Miltiorrhizae) 9g, and *Tao Ren* (Semen Persicae) 9g, cooked in water to yield 60 ml of decoction. The herbal formula was modified as necessary to best treat each patient. The treatment protocol was to administer the decoction once daily for 3 months.[6]
- **Whooping cough:** According to one report, 10 to 15 ml of *Bai Bu* syrup given three times daily was 85.2% effective in treating 95 patients with whooping cough. Each ml of syrup contained 1.5g of the herb.[7]
- **Chronic tracheitis:** An herbal preparation was used with an 87.2% rate of effectiveness in treating 110 patients with chronic tracheitis. Response was better for those with uncomplicated tracheitis, as compared with those with wheezing and dyspnea. The herbal preparation was made by cooking 20 grams of *Bai Bu* in water twice to yield 60 ml of the final decoction. The dosage was 60 ml of decoction twice daily. If necessary, a small amount of sugar or honey was added to improve taste and compliance.[8]
- **Rosacea:** Topical application of a *Bai Bu* preparation was 92% effective in treating 13 patients with rosacea. The topical preparation was made by soaking *Bai Bu* in 95% alcohol for 5 to 7 days, then diluting it to make a 50% tincture. The tincture was applied to the affected area two or three times daily for 1 month per course of treatment.[9]

TOXICOLOGY

Gross overdose of alkaloids of *Bai Bu* may cause respiratory depression by blocking the stimulation of the respiratory center in the brain.[10]

References

1. *Xian Dai Zhong Yao Yao Li Xue* (Contemporary Pharmacology of Chinese Herbs), 1997; 1011
2. Yan X, Zhou J, Xie G, *Traditional Chinese Medicines Molecular Structures, Natural Sources and Applications*; Ashgate, 1999; 5983
3. *Zhong Yao Yao Li Yu Ying Yong* (Pharmacology and Applications of Chinese Herbs), 1983: 419
4. *Zhong Yao Xue* (Chinese Herbology), 1998; 643:645
5. *Zhong Yao Yao Li Yu Ying Yong* (Pharmacology and Applications of Chinese Herbs), 1983: 419
6. *Zhong Guo Fang Lao Za Zhi* (Chinese Journal on Prevention of Tuberculosis), 1966; 1:27
7. *Shang Hai Zhong Yi Yao Za Zhi* (Shanghai Journal of Chinese Medicine and Herbology), 1959; 4:39
8. *Shan Xi Zhong Yi* (Shanxi Chinese Medicine), 1986; 10:439
9. *Zhong Yi Za Zhi* (Journal of Chinese Medicine), 1981; 4:273
10. *Zhong Yao Yao Li Du Li Yu Lin Chuan* (Pharmacology, Toxicology and Clinical Applications of Chinese Herbs), 1992; 285

Zi Wan (Radix Asteris)

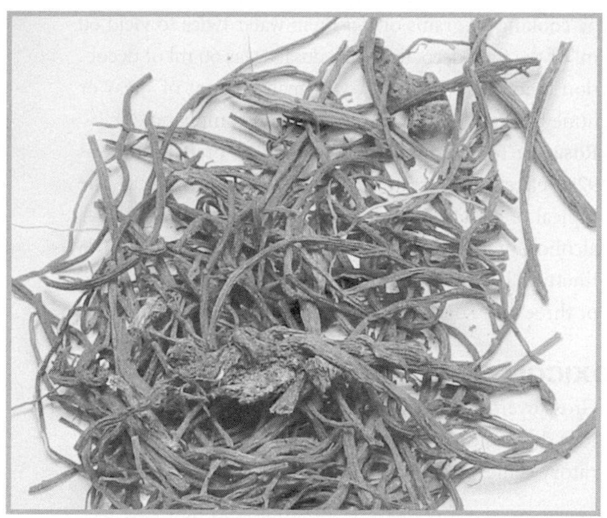

紫菀 紫菀

Pinyin Name: *Zi Wan*
Literal Name: "purple-soft roots"
Original Source: *Shen Nong Ben Cao Jing* (Divine Husbandman's Classic of the Materia Medica) in the second century
English Name: aster, tatarian aster root
Botanical Name: *Aster tataricus* L. f. (*Zi Wan*)
Pharmaceutical Name: Radix Asteris
Properties: bitter, sweet, slightly warm
Channels Entered: Lung

CHINESE THERAPEUTIC ACTIONS

Dissolves Phlegm and Stops Cough

Cough due to wind-cold, wind-heat or Lung deficiency: *Zi Wan* (Radix Asteris) is warm but not hot, moistening, not drying. Mild in nature, it treats coughing caused by numerous factors, including exterior invasion, interior imbalance, and excess or deficient conditions. *Zi Wan* has a wide range of clinical applications, as it can be combined with various herbs to treat different patterns of coughing.

- Cough due to wind-cold: use fresh *Zi Wan*.
- Cough caused by profuse phlegm and sputum: use this herb with *Jie Geng* (Radix Platycodonis), *Jing Jie* (Herba Schizonepetae), *Bai Bu* (Radix Stemonae) and *Bai Qian* (Rhizoma Cynanchi Stauntonii). **Exemplar Formula:** *Zhi Sou San* (Stop Coughing Powder).
- Cough due to Lung heat with copious yellow sputum: combine it with *Huang Qin* (Radix Scutellariae) and *Bei Mu* (Bulbus Fritillaria).
- Chronic cough due to Lung heat and yin deficiency: use *Zi Wan* with *Jie Geng* (Radix Platycodonis), *Zhi Mu* (Radix Anemarrhenae), *E Jiao* (Colla Corii Asini), and *Bei Mu* (Bulbus Fritillaria). **Exemplar Formula:** *Zi Wan Tang* (Aster Decoction).
- Chronic cough with blood-streaked sputum from Lung deficiency: add this herb to *Zhi Mu* (Radix Anemarrhenae), *Bei Mu* (Bulbus Fritillaria) and *E Jiao* (Colla Corii Asini).
- Chronic cough due to Lung deficiency: use with *Ren Shen* (Radix Ginseng), *Huang Qi* (Radix Astragali), and *Wu Wei Zi* (Fructus Schisandrae Chinensis). **Exemplar Formula:** *Bu Fei Tang* (Tonify the Lungs Decoction).
- Tuberculosis or late-stage lung abscess: use it with *Zhi Mu* (Radix Anemarrhenae), *Bei Mu* (Bulbus Fritillaria), *E Jiao* (Colla Corii Asini), *Ren Shen* (Radix Ginseng), *Fu Ling* (Poria), *Gan Cao* (Radix Glycyrrhizae), *Jie Geng* (Radix Platycodonis) and *Wu Wei Zi* (Fructus Schisandrae Chinensis).

DOSAGE

5 to 10 grams in decoction. Frying *Zi Wan* with honey enhances the moistening influence and makes it more suitable for treatment of chronic dry or feeble coughing due to Lung deficiency.

CAUTIONS / CONTRAINDICATIONS

- *Zi Wan* is not suitable for cough due to excess heat or yin-deficient fire as a single-herb remedy.

CHEMICAL COMPOSITION

Astersaponin, shionone, quercetin, friedelin, epifriedelinol, shionoside A, B, astersaponins A, B, C, D, E, F; phytosterol glucosides, lachnophyllol, lachnophyllol acetate, anethole, butyl-D-ribuloside, cyclopeptide.[1]

PHARMACOLOGICAL EFFECTS

- **Respiratory:** Oral administration of *Zi Wan* in rabbits was associated with a marked expectorant effect that lasted for approximately 4 hours. It did not, however, show significant antitussive or antiasthmatic effects.[2]
- **Antibiotic:** *Zi Wan* has an inhibitory influence against *E. coli, Bacillus dysenteriae, Bacillus proteus, Salmonella typhi, Bacillus paratyphosus, Pseudomonas aeruginosa, Vibrio cholerae,* and some dermatophytes and influenza viruses.[3]
- **Antineoplastic:** *Zi Wan* has shown preliminary inhibitory effects on the growth of cancer cells in mice.[4]

Zi Wan (Radix Asteris)

References

1. *Xian Dai Zhong Yao Yao Li Xue* (Contemporary Pharmacology of Chinese Herbs), 1997; 019
2. *Chang Yong Zhong Yao Cheng Fen Yu Yao Li Shou Ce* (A Handbook of the Composition and Pharmacology of Common Chinese Drugs), 1994; 1678:1681
3. Ibid.
4. *Guo Wai Yi Xue Zhong Yi Zhong Yao Fen Ce* (Monograph of Chinese Herbology from Foreign Medicine), 1987; 9(1):57

Kuan Dong Hua (Flos Farfarae)

款冬花 款冬花

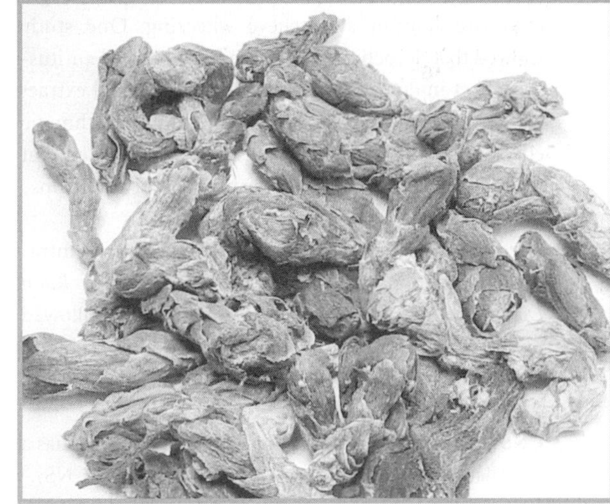

Pinyin Name: *Kuan Dong Hua*
Literal Name: "welcome winter flower"
Original Source: *Shen Nong Ben Cao Jing* (Divine Husbandman's Classic of the Materia Medica) in the second century
English Name: tussilago
Botanical Name: *Tussilago farfara* L. (*Kuan Dong*)
Pharmaceutical Name: Flos Farfarae
Properties: acrid, warm
Channels Entered: Lung, Heart

CHINESE THERAPEUTIC ACTIONS

Moistens the Lung, Descends Qi, Dissolves Phlegm, Stops Cough

Cough due to Lung cold, Lung heat or Lung yin deficiency: Dispersing yet not draining, warm yet not drying, *Kuan Dong Hua* (Flos Farfarae) moistens the Lung, dissolves phlegm and relieves cough. It is most effective for treating cough due to cold attacking the Lung, or chronic cough with blood-streaked sputum. However, when combined with appropriate herbs, *Kuan Dong Hua* treats upper respiratory infection, influenza and a wide range of coughing disorders, including cold or hot, exterior or interior, and excess or deficient conditions.

- Chronic cough with blood-streaked sputum from Lung yin deficiency: use *Kuan Dong Hua* with *Bai He* (Bulbus Lilii) and take it as powder.
- Cough caused by wind and Lung heat: use this herb with *Zhi Mu* (Radix Anemarrhenae), *Sang Ye* (Folium Mori), *Bei Mu* (Bulbus Fritillaria) and *Xing Ren* (Semen Armeniacae Amarum).
- Cough and wheezing due to phlegm obstruction: combine it with *Xing Ren* (Semen Armeniacae Amarum).
- Cough and wheezing due to water accumulation: add *Kuan Dong Hua* to *Ban Xia* (Rhizoma Pinelliae) and *Wu Wei Zi* (Fructus Schisandrae Chinensis).
- Cough due to qi and phlegm obstruction: combine it with *Bai Qian* (Rhizoma Cynanchi Stauntonii).

DOSAGE

5 to 10 grams. Frying *Kuan Dong Hua* with honey enhances the moistening action and makes it more suitable for treatment of chronic cough from Lung deficiency.

CAUTIONS / CONTRAINDICATIONS

- Acrid and warm, *Kuan Dong Hua* should be used with caution for patients who have coughing caused by heat.
- *Kuan Dong Hua* should be used with caution for patients with lung abscesses, or pus and blood in the sputum.

Kuan Dong Hua (Flos Farfarae)

OVERDOSAGE

Overdose of *Kuan Dong Hua* may cause restlessness, excitation, irritability, and increased respiration.[1]

CHEMICAL COMPOSITION

Faradiol, arnidiol, taraxanthin, phytosterine, senkirkine, rutin, hyperin, essential oils, farfaratin, tussilagin, tussilagone. Pyrrolidizine alkaloids are present in the plant *Tussilago farfara*, but their presence in the flower has not been confirmed.[2]

PHARMACOLOGICAL EFFECTS

- **Respiratory:** Administration of *Kuan Dong Hua* has a marked effect on the respiratory tract to suppress cough, eliminate sputum and relieve wheezing. One study showed that decoction of the herb has a marked antitussive effect in dogs. Another showed that alcohol extract of the herb has marked expectorant and antiasthmatic effects in rabbits and guinea pigs. It was also noted that while a small dose may dilate the bronchioli, a large dose may actually constrict them.[3]
- **Cardiovascular:** In cats, rabbits, dogs and rats, intravenous injection of water or alcohol extract of *Kuan Dong Hua* is associated with an initial decline, followed by a prolonged rise, of blood pressure. The rise in blood pressure is attributed to the rise in sympathetic tone and constriction of blood vessels.[4]
- **CNS stimulant:** Administration of *Kuan Dong Hua* has a stimulating effect on the central nervous system (CNS).[5]

CLINICAL STUDIES AND RESEARCH

- **Asthma:** Extract of *Kuan Dong Hua* (equivalent to 6 grams of herb) given three times daily provided marked relief in treating 36 asthma patients. The preparation, however, was ineffective for treating the acute and severe onset of an asthma attack.[6]

TOXICOLOGY

The LD_{50} for *Kuan Dong Hua* preparations in mice is 124 g/kg via oral ingestion for decoction, 112 g/kg via intraperitoneal injection for alcohol extract, and 43 g/kg via intraperitoneal injection for ether extract. Adverse reactions due to overdose included restlessness, excitation, mania, increased respiration, muscle stiffness, tremor, and muscle spasms.[7]

References

1. *Zhong Yao Xue* (Chinese Herbology), 1998; 646:647
2. *Xian Dai Zhong Yao Yao Li Xue* (Contemporary Pharmacology of Chinese Herbs), 1997; 1008-1009
3. *Zhong Yao Yao Li Yu Ying Yong* (Pharmacology and Applications of Chinese Herbs), 1983: 1132
4. *Zhong Guo Yao Li Xue Bao* (Chinese Herbal Pharmacology Journal), 1986; 7(4):333
5. *Zhong Yao Xue* (Chinese Herbology), 1998; 646:647
6. *Shang Hai Zhong Yi Yao Za Zhi* (Shanghai Journal of Chinese Medicine and Herbology), 1964; 10:12
7. *Zhong Yao Yao Li Yu Ying Yong* (Pharmacology and Applications of Chinese Herbs), 1983: 1132

Su Zi (Fructus Perillae)

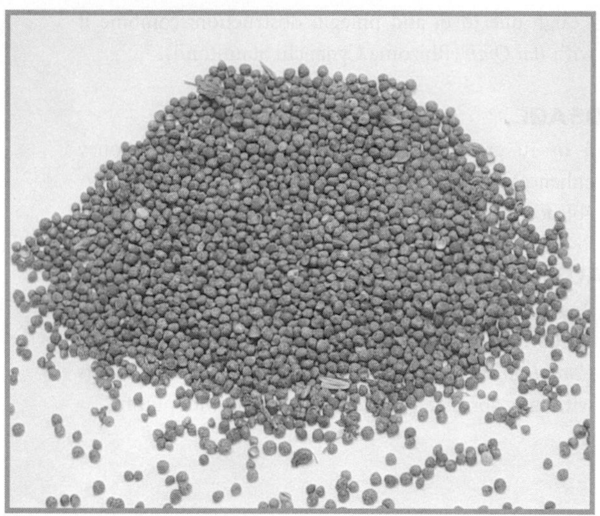

蘇子 苏子

Pinyin Name: *Su Zi*
Literal Name: "perilla seed"
Alternate Chinese Names: *Zi Su Zi, Hei Su Zi, Du Su Zi*
English Name: perilla fruit
Botanical Name: *Perilla frutescens* (L.) Britt. var. *acuta* (Thunb.) Kudo (*Zi Su*)
Pharmaceutical Name: Fructus Perillae
Properties: acrid, warm
Channels Entered: Lung, Large Intestine

Su Zi (Fructus Perillae)

CHINESE THERAPEUTIC ACTIONS

1. Stops Cough, Relieves Wheezing

Cough, dyspnea and wheezing due to excess accumulation of phlegm: Acrid and warm but not drying, *Su Zi* (Fructus Perillae) directs qi downward and benefits the diaphragm to relieve cough and wheezing. It treats cough and wheezing accompanied by profuse sputum, and feelings of fullness and oppression in the chest and diaphragm regions.

- Cough and wheezing due to phlegm obstruction and food stagnation: use *Su Zi* with *Bai Jie Zi* (Semen Sinapis) and *Lai Fu Zi* (Semen Raphani). **Exemplar Formula:** *San Zi Yang Qin Tang* (Three-Seed Decoction to Nourish One's Parents).
- Cough, wheezing and shortness of breath due to cold phlegm obstruction and Lung qi stagnation: combine this herb with *Ban Xia* (Rhizoma Pinelliae), *Hou Po* (Cortex Magnoliae Officinalis) and *Qian Hu* (Radix Peucedani). **Exemplar Formula:** *Su Zi Jiang Qi Tang* (Perilla Fruit Decoction for Directing Qi Downward).

2. Lubricates the Intestines to Promote Bowel Movement

Constipation with dry stools: *Su Zi* has moistening and lubricating effects to treat constipation caused by dryness in the intestines.

- Constipation: use *Su Zi* with *Huo Ma Ren* (Fructus Cannabis), *Gua Lou Ren* (Semen Trichosanthis) and *Xing Ren* (Semen Armeniacae Amarum).

DOSAGE

5 to 10 grams in decoction. Unprocessed *Su Zi* functions more effectively to lower qi downwards and relieve coughing and wheezing. Dry-frying the herb moderates the overall effect, but increases the extraction of active constituents. Honey-baked, the herb has a better effect to moisten the Lung and relieve dry coughing.

CAUTIONS / CONTRAINDICATIONS

- *Su Zi* is contraindicated for patients with loose stools or Spleen qi deficiency.

CHEMICAL COMPOSITION

Fatty oil 45.3%, linoleic acid 14.1%, flavonoids, β-sitosterol, stigmasterol, tannins, vitamin B_1.[1]

CLINICAL STUDIES AND RESEARCH

- **Cough:** An extract of *Su Zi*, *Bai Jie Zi* (Semen Sinapis) and *Lai Fu Zi* (Semen Raphani) was given twice daily for 7 days per course of treatment, and was effective for treatment of chronic and stubborn coughs. Out of 40 patients, the study reported marked improvement in 62.5%, and moderate improvement in 37.5%.[2]
- **Ascariasis:** According to one report, 92 out of 100 patients with ascariasis were treated successfully with ingestion of fresh *Su Zi* on an empty stomach two to three times daily for 3 days (or more if necessary). The dosage was 50 to 70 grams for adults, and 20 to 50 grams for children between 4 and 10 years of age.[3]

AUTHORS' COMMENTS

Su Zi (Fructus Perillae), *Zi Su Ye* (Folium Perillae), and *Su Geng* (Caulis Perillae) are different parts of the same plant, but they each have different functions:

- *Su Zi* is used for its effect to redirect rebellious qi to relieve coughing and wheezing.
- *Zi Su Ye* is used primarily for its ability to release the exterior.
- *Su Geng* regulates qi and expands the chest.

References

1. *Xian Dai Zhong Yao Yao Li Xue* (Contemporary Pharmacology of Chinese Herbs), 1997; 1023
2. *Zhong Yao Tong Bao* (Journal of Chinese Herbology), 1986; 8:56
3. *Si Chuan Zhong Yi* (Sichuan Chinese Medicine), 1986; 8; 47

Zhong Ru Shi (Stalactitum)

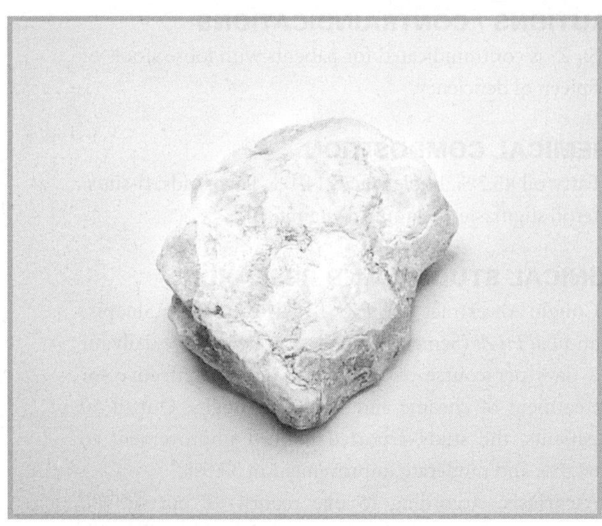

鐘乳石 钟乳石

Pinyin Name: *Zhong Ru Shi*
Literal Name: "breast rocks"
Alternate Chinese Names: *Shi Zhong Ru, Di Ru Shi, E Guan Shi*
Original Source: *Shen Nong Ben Cao Jing* (Divine Husbandman's Classic of the Materia Medica) in the second century
English Name: stalactitum
Pharmaceutical Name: Stalactitum
Properties: sweet, warm
Channels Entered: Lung, Kidney, Stomach

CHINESE THERAPEUTIC ACTIONS

1. Warms the Lung to Relieve Wheezing

Sweet and warm, *Zhong Ru Shi* (Stalactitum) warms the Lung and dispels cold. Clinically, it is commonly used for respiratory disorders characterized by cold, such as cough or wheezing with white phlegm.

- Cough and wheezing caused by Lung cold: use *Zhong Ru Shi* with *Ma Huang* (Herba Ephedrae) and *Xing Ren* (Semen Armeniacae Amarum).
- Wheezing and shortness of breath due to deficiency: use this substance with *Shan Yao* (Rhizoma Dioscoreae) and *Yi Yi Ren* (Semen Coicis).

2. Tonifies Kidney Yang to Relieve Wheezing

Zhong Ru Shi tonifies Kidney yang to relieve wheezing characterized by the inability of the Kidney to grasp Lung qi downwards, which leads to labored inhalation. In addition, *Zhong Ru Shi* is also effective for treatment of impotence, spermatorrhea, and coldness and pain in the feet.

- Wheezing with labored inhalation: use *Zhong Ru Shi* with *Hu Tao Ren* (Semen Juglandis), *Wu Wei Zi* (Fructus Schisandrae Chinensis) and *Ge Jie* (Gecko).
- Impotence and spermatorrhea due to Kidney yang deficiency: combine this substance with *Rou Cong Rong* (Herba Cistanches), *Ba Ji Tian* (Radix Morindae Officinalis), *Bu Gu Zhi* (Fructus Psoraleae) and *Dong Chong Xia Cao* (Cordyceps).

3. Promotes Lactation

Zhong Ru Shi tonifies the Stomach to promote lactation and milk production.

- Difficult lactation due to stagnation: use *Zhong Ru Shi* with *Lou Lu* (Radix Rhapontici), *Tong Cao* (Medulla Tetrapanacis), and *Tian Hua Fen* (Radix Trichosanthis).
- Insufficient milk production due to deficiency of qi and blood: add it to *Huang Qi* (Radix Astragali) and *Dang Gui* (Radicis Angelicae Sinensis).

Zhong Ru Shi is also used as calcium supplement for pregnant women with hypocalcemia.

DOSAGE

9 to 15 grams. *Zhong Ru Shi* is sometimes calcined first to warm the herb and improve its function to treat respiratory tract disorders.

CAUTIONS / CONTRAINDICATIONS

- *Zhong Ru Shi* should be used with caution for patients with interior heat, such as fever, hemoptysis or hematemesis.

CHEMICAL COMPOSITION

Calcium carbonate, magnesium, iron, aluminum, and other minerals.[1]

References

1. *Zhong Yao Xue* (Chinese Herbology), 1998; 660-661

Ma Dou Ling (Fructus Aristolochiae)

馬兜鈴 马兜铃

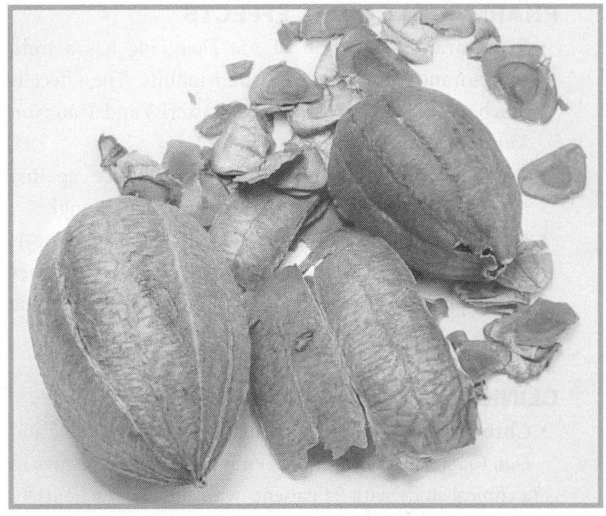

Pinyin Name: *Ma Dou Ling*
Literal Name: "bell of a horse's hat"
Original Source: *Yao Xing Ben Cao* (Materia Medica of Medicinal Properties) by Zhen Quan in 600 A.D.
English Name: aristolochia fruit, dutchman's pipe fruit
Botanical Name: *Aristolochia contorta* Bge. (*Bei Ma Dou Ling*); *Aristolochia debilis* S. et. Z. (*Ma Dou Ling*)
Pharmaceutical Name: Fructus Aristolochiae
Properties: bitter, slightly acrid, cold
Channels Entered: Lung, Large Intestine
Safety Index: slightly toxic

CHINESE THERAPEUTIC ACTIONS

1. Clears the Lung, Dissolves Phlegm, Stops Cough and Wheezing

Coughing and wheezing caused by accumulation of phlegm or Lung heat: All types of cough and dyspnea due to Lung heat can be treated with *Ma Dou Ling* (Fructus Aristolochiae). Clinical manifestations include labored respiration, profuse yellow phlegm and cough.

- Coughing and wheezing due to accumulation of phlegm or Lung heat: use *Ma Dou Ling* with *Sang Bai Pi* (Cortex Mori), *Huang Qin* (Radix Scutellariae) and *Xing Ren* (Semen Armeniacae Amarum).

Chronic cough: *Ma Dou Ling* treats chronic cough from Lung deficiency characterized by scanty or blood-streaked sputum, and dry mouth and throat.

- Chronic cough due to Lung deficiency: combine this herb with *E Jiao* (Colla Corii Asini), *Xing Ren* (Semen Armeniacae Amarum), and *Niu Bang Zi* (Fructus Arctii).

2. Clears Heat from the Large Intestine and Treats Hemorrhoids

Hemorrhoidal pain: The Lung and Large Intestine are paired organs. By sedating Lung heat, Large Intestine fire can also be cleared. *Ma Dou Ling* treats excess accumulation of fire in the Large Intestine that is causing hemorrhoids, swelling and bleeding.

- Hemorrhoids: use this herb with *Zao Jiao Ci* (Spina Gleditsiae), *Shao Yao Tang* (Peony Decoction) or *Zhen Ren Huo Ming Yin* (True Man Decoction to Revitalize Life).

3. Lowers Blood Pressure

Hypertension: *Ma Dou Ling* has shown marked and prolonged antihypertensive effects. It is commonly used for early-stage primary hypertension, characterized by Liver yang rising with dizziness and a red face.

- Hypertension: use this herb with *Xia Ku Cao* (Spica Prunellae), *Gou Teng* (Ramulus Uncariae cum Uncis), and *Huang Qin* (Radix Scutellariae).

DOSAGE

3 to 10 grams in decoction. Because it is bitter, cold and slightly toxic, use of unprocessed *Ma Dou Ling* may cause numerous side effects. This herb should be fried with honey to neutralize the bitter taste, cold property, and toxic component. In addition, frying it with honey enhances the moistening effect and makes it more suitable for treatment of cough and wheezing caused by Lung deficiency and heat. Frying with honey minimizes the frequency of nausea and vomiting associated with this herb.

CAUTIONS / CONTRAINDICATIONS

- Large dosages of *Ma Dou Ling* may cause nausea and vomiting.
- Bitter and cold, *Ma Dou Ling* should not be used if the coughing and/or wheezing is caused by deficiency or cold, or if the patient has loose stools due to Spleen deficiency.

OVERDOSAGE

Gross overdose of 30 grams *Ma Dou Ling* in decoction may cause side effects such as nausea, vomiting, irritability, dizziness, shortness of breath and hematemesis.[1]

CHEMICAL COMPOSITION

Magnoflorine, aristolochic acid, aristolochinic acid, allantoin, diblic acid.[2]

Ma Dou Ling (Fructus Aristolochiae)

PHARMACOLOGICAL EFFECTS

- **Expectorant:** Decoction of *Ma Dou Ling* has a mild expectorant effect in anesthetized rabbits. The effect is much weaker than *Zi Wan* (Radix Asteris) and *Tian Nan Xing* (Rhizoma Arisaematis).[3]
- **Antibiotic:** It has an inhibiting influence against *Diplococcus pneumoniae* and some pathogenic fungi.[4]
- **Antihypertensive:** Administration of *Ma Dou Ling* is associated with a mild and prolonged effect to lower blood pressure. However, some subjects reported side effects such as nausea, diarrhea, and loss of appetite.[5]

CLINICAL STUDIES AND RESEARCH

- **Chronic tracheitis:** The combination of *Ma Dou Ling* and *Gan Cao* (Radix Glycyrrhizae) was found to be effective in a clinical study with 94 patients with chronic tracheitis.[6]
- **Infection:** Intramuscular injection of a *Ma Dou Ling* preparation one to two times daily was 88.8% effective in 1,202 patients with various infectious diseases, such as pneumonia, tracheitis, gastroenteritis, bacterial dysentery, and upper respiratory infection.[7]

TOXICOLOGY

The LD_{50} for alcohol extract of *Ma Dou Ling* in mice via oral ingestion is 22.02 g/kg.[8]

The alkaloids of *Ma Dou Ling* have been associated with nephritis when given as injection in rabbits at 7.5 mg/kg. When the dose was increased to 20 mg/kg, anuria, hematuria, numbness of the extremities, respiratory depression and fatality were reported in rabbits.[9]

Ma Dou Ling contains a trace amount of aristolochic acid. For more information on the toxicology of this compound, please refer to *Guang Fang Ji* (Radix Aristolochiae Fangchi) or *Guan Mu Tong* (Caulis Aristolochiae Manshuriensis).

References

1. *Yao Xue Xue Bao* (Journal of Herbology), 1958; (5):316
2. *Xian Dai Zhong Yao Yao Li Xue* (Contemporary Pharmacology of Chinese Herbs), 1997; 1002
3. *Zhong Yao Xue* (Chinese Herbology), 1998; 653:654
4. Ibid.
5. Ibid.
6. *Hu Nan Yi Cao Gong Ye Yan Jiu* (Hunan Research and Industry of Medicine and Medicinals), 1978; 5:4
7. *Zhong Cao Yao Tong Xun* (Journal of Chinese Herbal Medicine), 1979; 2:26
8. *Zhong Yao Yao Li Yu Ying Yong* (Pharmacology and Applications of Chinese Herbs), 1989; 5(4):34
9. Ibid., 1958; 165

Pí Pa Ye (Folium Eriobotryae)

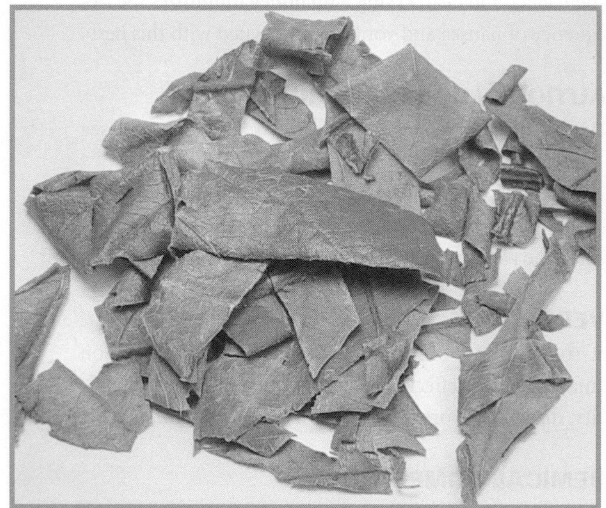

枇杷葉 枇杷叶

Pinyin Name: *Pi Pa Ye*

Original Source: *Ming Yi Za Zhu* (Miscellaneous Records of Famous Physicians) by Tao Hong-Jing in 500 A.D.

English Name: eriobotrya, loquat leaf

Botanical Name: *Eriobotrya japonica* (Thunb.) Lindl. (*Pi Pa*)

Pharmaceutical Name: Folium Eriobotryae

Properties: bitter, cool

Channels Entered: Lung, Stomach

Pi Pa Ye (Folium Eriobotryae)

CHINESE THERAPEUTIC ACTIONS

1. Dissolves Phlegm, Stops Cough

Cough due to Lung heat: Bitter and cool, *Pi Pa Ye* (Folium Eriobotryae) sedates Lung heat, dissolves phlegm and stops cough. It is commonly used to treat coughing with copious yellow sputum, bitter taste, and dry mouth from Lung heat.

- Cough with copious yellow phlegm due to Lung heat: combine *Pi Pa Ye* with *Huang Lian* (Rhizoma Coptidis), *Zhi Zi* (Fructus Gardeniae), and *Sang Bai Pi* (Cortex Mori).

Cough caused by dryness and heat: This is characterized by a dry cough, or coughing with a feeling that phlegm remains in the chest after expectoration, along with dry mouth and red tongue. This herb is commonly served with honey.

- Cough due to dryness and heat: use *Pi Pa Ye* with *Sang Bai Pi* (Cortex Mori), *Jie Geng* (Radix Platycodonis) and *Bai Bu* (Radix Stemonae).

2. Harmonizes the Stomach, Directs Qi Downwards

Stomach qi reversal: *Pi Pa Ye* relieves nausea and vomiting by clearing Stomach heat and directing the abnormal rising qi downwards. Secondary symptoms may include vomitus with sour smell, acid regurgitation and thirst.

- Nausea and vomiting: use this herb with *Mai Men Dong* (Radix Ophiopogonis), *Zhu Ru* (Caulis Bambusae in Taenia) and *Lu Gen* (Rhizoma Phragmitis).

DOSAGE

10 to 15 grams of dried herb, 15 to 30 grams of fresh herb, in decoction. *Pi Pa Ye* should be wrapped in cheesecloth prior to decoction to prevent the hair-like components from irritating the throat during ingestion. *Pi Pa Ye* fried with honey enhances the moistening effect and makes it more suitable for treatment of coughing or wheezing caused by heat and dryness. The unprocessed herb treats nausea and vomiting, while honey-fried *Pi Pa Ye* dissolves phlegm and relieves cough.

CAUTIONS / CONTRAINDICATIONS

- *Pi Pa Ye* is not suitable for treatment of cough due to cold, or for nausea and vomiting due to Stomach cold.
- *Pi Pa Ye* leaves have fine hair-like components that may irritate the throat if ingested. To prevent this irritation, the leaves should be scrubbed clean, or wrapped in cheesecloth, prior to decoction.

CHEMICAL COMPOSITION

Neiolidol, farnesol, amygdalin, ursolic acid, oleanolic acid, trans-nerolidol, trans-farnesol.[1,2]

PHARMACOLOGICAL EFFECTS

- **Antitussive:** Administration of *Pi Pa Ye* is associated with good antitussive, but poor expectorant effects.[3]
- **Antibiotic:** Decoction of *Pi Pa Ye* has an inhibitory effect *in vitro* against *Staphylococcus aureus*.[4]

CLINICAL STUDIES AND RESEARCH

- **Chronic tracheitis:** In one study, 167 patients with chronic tracheitis were treated with an herbal preparation with 42 showing significant improvement, 60 showing moderate improvement, 35 showing slight improvement, and 30 showing none. The herbal formula was prepared by cooking 90 grams of *Pi Pa Ye* and 150 grams of *Su Geng* (Caulis Perillae) in water to yield a final decoction of 2,000 ml. To make the final preparation, 240 ml of syrup was added to the decoction. The treatment protocol was to administer 10 ml of the preparation, three times daily, for 20 days per course of treatment. It was noted that the preparation had strong antitussive, but mild expectorant effects.[5]
- **Pinworm:** An herbal preparation was used to treat 122 children with pinworm infestations with a 78.85% success rate. The herbal preparation was made by cooking 100 grams of *Pi Pa Ye* at boiling temperature for 1 hour to yield 200 ml of the decoction. The treatment protocol was to administer 100 ml of decoction on an empty stomach twice daily in the morning and at night for 15 days.[6]

References

1. *Xian Dai Zhong Yao Yao Li Xue* (Contemporary Pharmacology of Chinese Herbs), 1997; 1014-1015
2. *Chang Yong Zhong Yao Cheng Fen Yu Yao Li Shou Ce* (A Handbook of the Composition and Pharmacology of Common Chinese Drugs), 1994; 1178-1179
3. *Zhong Yao Xue* (Chinese Herbology), 1998; 651:653
4. *Chang Yong Zhong Yao Cheng Fen Yu Yao Li Shou Ce* (A Handbook of the Composition and Pharmacology of Common Chinese Drugs), 1994; 1970: 10
5. *Yi Yao Wei Sheng* (Medicine, Medicinals, and Sanitation), 1972; 3:29
6. *Jiang Su Zhong Yi Za Zhi* (Jiangsu Journal of Chinese Medicine), 1990; 2:48

Gu Zhi Hua (Semen Oroxyli)

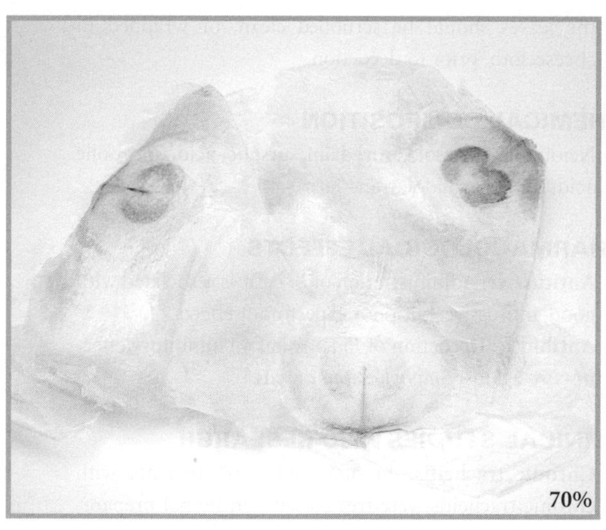
70%

故紙花 故纸花

Pinyin Name: *Gu Zhi Hua*
Alternate Chinese Names: *Mu Hu Die, Yu Hu Die*
English Name: oroxylum
Botanical Name: *Oroxylum indicum* (L.) Ventenat
Pharmaceutical Name: Semen Oroxyli
Properties: sweet, bland, cool
Channels Entered: Liver, Lung

CHINESE THERAPEUTIC ACTIONS

1. Moistens the Lung, Relieves Cough, Restores Voice

Gu Zhi Hua (Semen Oroxyli) moistens the Lung and relieves dryness. It is commonly used to treat cough and loss of voice caused by heat and dryness.

- Loss of voice: combine *Gu Zhi Hua* with *Pang Da Hai* (Semen Sterculiae Lychnophorae) and *Chan Tui* (Periostracum Cicadae).

2. Eliminates Heat and Dampness from the Skin

Gu Zhi Hua is used topically to promote healing of ulcerated suppurative sores characterized by damp-heat.

DOSAGE

3 to 6 grams.

CAUTIONS / CONTRAINDICATIONS

- *Gu Zhi Hua* should be used with caution in patients with loss of voice caused by wind-cold.

CHEMICAL COMPOSITION

Baicalein, tetuin, oroxin A, B; chrysin, baicalein-7-O-β-gentiobioside, oroxindin.[1]

AUTHORS' COMMENTS

Gu Zhi Hua and *Pang Da Hai* (Semen Sterculiae Lychnophorae) are two of the best herbs to restore loss of voice. They can be taken as tea throughout the day for those who need to speak or sing for a prolonged period of time.

References

1. *Xian Dai Zhong Yao Yao Li Xue* (Contemporary Pharmacology of Chinese Herbs), 1997; 1064-1065

Bai Guo (Semen Ginkgo)

白果

Pinyin Name: *Bai Guo*
Literal Name: "white fruit seed"
Alternate Chinese Names: *Bai Guo Ren, Yin Xing, Yin Guo*
Original Source: *Yin Shan Zheng Yao* (Correct Guide to Eating and Drinking)
English Name: ginkgo nut, ginkgo seed
Botanical Name: *Ginkgo biloba* L. (*Yin Xing*)
Pharmaceutical Name: Semen Ginkgo
Properties: sweet, bitter, astringent, neutral
Channels Entered: Lung
Safety Index: slightly toxic

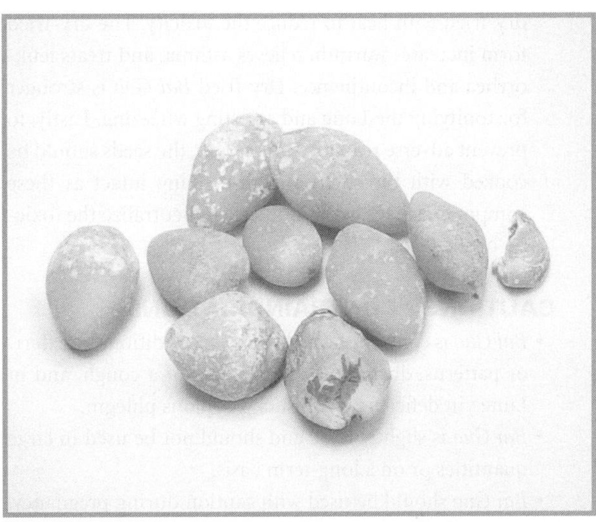

CHINESE THERAPEUTIC ACTIONS

1. Arrests Wheezing and Dispels Phlegm

Asthma due to phlegm, heat or Lung deficiency: Astringent and restraining in property, *Bai Guo* (Semen Ginkgo) treats dyspnea, wheezing, asthma, chronic cough, and loss of voice characterized by Lung qi deficiency. Most texts state that this herb is used in chronic respiratory disorders no longer involving any external pathogenic factor or internal excess accumulation. However, it can also be combined with herbs in the heat-clearing and phlegm-eliminating categories to treat excess conditions.

- Asthma, dyspnea or cough: use *Bai Guo* with *Ma Huang* (Herba Ephedrae), *Su Zi* (Fructus Perillae), *Kuan Dong Hua* (Flos Farfarae), *Ban Xia* (Rhizoma Pinelliae), *Sang Bai Pi* (Cortex Mori) and *Xing Ren* (Semen Armeniacae Amarum).
- Chronic cough with loss of voice: combine this herb with *Sang Bai Pi* (Cortex Mori), *Chan Tui* (Periostracum Cicadae) and *Mai Men Dong* (Radix Ophiopogonis).
- Chronic wheezing due to Kidney and Lung qi deficiencies: add *Ge Jie* (Gecko).
- Accelerated respiration with yellow phlegm: use *Bai Guo* with *Huang Qin* (Radix Scutellariae) and *Sang Bai Pi* (Cortex Mori). **Exemplar Formula:** *Ding Chuan Tang* (Arrest Wheezing Decoction).
- Feeble, dry cough: combine this herb with *E Jiao* (Colla Corii Asini), *Sha Shen* (Radix Glehniae seu Adenophorae) and *Dang Shen* (Radix Codonopsis).
- Chronic loss of voice and dryness: add it to *Chan Tui* (Periostracum Cicadae), *Mai Men Dong* (Radix Ophiopogonis), *Sang Bai Pi* (Cortex Mori) and *Xuan Shen* (Radix Scrophulariae).

2. Restrains the Leakage of Fluids from the Lower *Jiao*

Leakage of body fluids: *Bai Guo* dispels dampness and restrains the leakage of body fluids to treat spermatorrhea, clear or yellow leukorrhea and other disorders characterized by leakage of fluid from the lower *jiao.*

- Spermatorrhea: combine it with *Shan Yao* (Rhizoma Dioscoreae).
- Clear and watery vaginal discharge due to Spleen deficiency: *Bai Guo* is combined with *Shan Yao* (Rhizoma Dioscoreae) and *Qian Shi* (Semen Euryales).
- Yellow vaginal discharge with foul odor due to damp-heat: add it to *Huang Bai* (Cortex Phellodendri) and *Che Qian Zi* (Semen Plantaginis).
- White vaginal discharge due to Kidney deficiency: use this herb with *Bai Ji Guan Hua* (Flos Celosiae Cristatae).

Cloudy urine: When combined with other diuretic herbs, *Bai Guo* can dispel dampness to treat cloudy urine and polyuria.

- Cloudy urine or frequent urination: use this herb with *Bi Xie* (Rhizoma Dioscoreae Hypoglaucae) and *Yi Zhi Ren* (Fructus Alpiniae Oxyphyllae).
- Frequent urination or enuresis: use it with *Wu Yao* (Radix Linderae), *Yi Zhi Ren* (Fructus Alpiniae Oxyphyllae), *Fu Pen Zi* (Fructus Rubi), *Shan Yao* (Rhizoma Dioscoreae) and *Shan Zhu Yu* (Fructus Corni).

DOSAGE

1.5 to 9 grams in decoction. Unprocessed *Bai Guo* is sometimes used to dispel phlegm. However, the unprocessed herb is slightly toxic, and is generally not used, even though it has a stronger effect to eliminate phlegm. Most commercial forms of *Bai Guo* have been

Bai Guo (Semen Ginkgo)

dry-fried with heat to reduce the toxicity. The dry-fried form increases warmth, relieves asthma, and treats leukorrhea and incontinence. Dry-fried *Bai Guo* is stronger for tonifying the Lung and arresting wheezing. Lastly, to prevent adverse reactions to *Bai Guo*, the seeds should be cooked with the shells and thin lining intact as these components have good influence to neutralize the toxicity of the seeds.

CAUTIONS / CONTRAINDICATIONS

- *Bai Guo* is contraindicated in excess conditions or exterior patterns, during the initial stages of a cough, and in Lung yin deficiency with sticky, copious phlegm.
- *Bai Guo* is slightly toxic and should not be used in large quantities or on a long-term basis.
- *Bai Guo* should be used with caution during pregnancy, as it stimulates contraction of the uterus.

OVERDOSAGE

Overdose of or side effects from use of *Bai Guo* generally occur within 2 to 3 hours after ingestion of excessive amounts of the offending agent. However, reactions have been observed within 1 hour, or delayed by up to 14 hours. The reactions are characterized by headache, vomiting (usually without nausea), dyspnea, spasms, tremor, fever (38° to 39° C), irrational fear, muscle stiffness, and pupil dilation. Many patients experiencing overdose also exhibit increased sensitivity to outside stimuli such as light and sound, with continued stimulation leading to convulsions. In severe cases, there may be altered consciousness, foaming at the mouth, dyspnea, accelerated respiration, purple lips, and respiratory depression.

One study reported that overdose of *Bai Guo* may occur following ingestion of 7 to 150 seeds in children and 40 to 300 seeds in adults. Adverse reactions included nausea, vomiting, sedation, stupor, abdominal pain, diarrhea, irritability, restlessness, dyspnea, seizures, convulsions and other symptoms related to disturbance of the central nervous system. An increase in white blood cells has been reported in some cases. Muscle weakness, paralysis, and loss of feeling in the lower extremities have also been reported in a small number of patients. In severe cases, fatalities have been reported following gross overdose and lack of emergency treatment. Use of *Bai Guo* preparations is also associated with dermatitis and increased risk of bleeding, as ginnol has a hemolytic effect.[1]

TREATMENT OF OVERDOSAGE

Acute overdose of *Bai Guo* may be treated initially by gastric lavage or purgative methods. Ingestion of activated charcoal or egg whites will decrease absorption of the toxin. A decoction of 30 grams of *Gan Cao* (Radix Glycyrrhizae) is also helpful in treating overdose. Those who exhibit dyspnea, seizures and convulsions require immediate emergency treatment.[2]

CHEMICAL COMPOSITION

Ginnol, bilobol, ginkgolic acid, hydroginkgolic acid, ginkgolinic acid, ginkgol, anacardic acid, protein, lipids, carbohydrates.[3,4]

Bilobol

PHARMACOLOGICAL EFFECTS

- **Antibiotic:** Preparations of *Bai Guo* have an inhibitory influence against gram-positive and gram-negative bacteria, and various pathogenic fungi.[5]
- **Respiratory:** Intraperitoneal injection of a *Bai Guo* preparation showed expectorant and bronchodilating effects.[6]
- **Cardiovascular:** According to one report, 500 mg/kg of bilobol lowered blood pressure in rabbits, rats, and guinea pigs. It increases vascular permeability, and may cause edema.[7]
- **Uterine stimulant:** Administration of bilobol is associated with contraction of the uterus in rabbits.[8]

CLINICAL STUDIES AND RESEARCH

- **Meniere's syndrome:** One case report describes a patient who had Meniere's syndrome for over 10 years but was treated successfully with an herbal formula containing 30 grams of *Bai Guo*, with 6 grams of *Gan Jiang* (Rhizoma Zingiberis) added if there was nausea. The herbal formula was crushed into fine powder, divided into four doses and administered twice daily over 2 days. A five-year follow-up showed no recurrence since the initial treatment.[9]
- **Headache:** Ten patients with headaches caused by tension or stress were treated with an herbal decoction twice daily with complete recovery within 3 days. The herbal decoction was prepared by cooking 60 grams of *Bai Guo* in 500 ml of water to yield 300 ml of the final solution.[10]

TOXICOLOGY

In mice, gross overdose of *Bai Guo* for 60 days was associated with poor appetite, weight loss, various degrees of liver damage, glomerulonephritis, and in severe cases, fatality. Intravenous injection of a *Bai Guo* preparation led to an initial increase of blood pressure, followed by a decrease, then dyspnea, seizures and death.[11,12]

Bai Guo (Semen Ginkgo)

AUTHORS' COMMENTS

Bai Guo is often used with herbs such as *Jie Geng* (Radix Platycodonis) and *Ma Huang* (Herba Ephedrae) that can open the Lung qi so that lingering pathogenic factors can be dispelled and not further trapped.

This herb is not the same as the ginkgo product that is commonly sold over the counter for memory enhancement. The ginkgo product for memory enhancement uses the leaves, *Yin Guo Ye* (Folium Ginkgo), not the nut, *Bai Guo* (Semen Ginkgo). These two herbs are not to be used interchangeably as they have different therapeutic effects and safety profiles.

References

1. *Chang Yong Zhong Yao Xian Dai Yan Jiu Yu Lin Chuan* (Recent Study & Clinical Application of Common Traditional Chinese Medicine), 1995; 479:482
2. *Zhong Yao Xue* (Chinese Herbology), 1998; 655:656
3. *Xian Dai Zhong Yao Yao Li Xue* (Contemporary Pharmacology of Chinese Herbs), 1997; 1056
4. Yan X, Zhou J, Xie G, *Traditional Chinese Medicines Molecular Structures, Natural Sources and Applications*; Ashgate, 1999; 2587
5. *Zhong Cao Yao Xue* (Study of Chinese Herbal Medicine), 1976; 66
6. *Zhong Yao Yao Li Yu Ying Yong* (Pharmacology and Applications of Chinese Herbs), 1983:1054
7. Ibid.
8. *Chang Yong Zhong Yao Cheng Fen Yu Yao Li Shou Ce* (A Handbook of the Composition and Pharmacology of Common Chinese Drugs), 1994; 756:758
9. *Zhong Yi Za Zhi* (Journal of Chinese Medicine), 1982; (4):50
10. Ibid.
11. *Jiang Su Zhong Yi* (Jiangsu Chinese Medicine), 1989; 10(8):32
12. *Chang Yong Zhong Yao Xian Dai Yan Jiu Yu Lin Chuan* (Recent Study & Clinical Application of Common Traditional Chinese Medicine), 1995; 479:482

Yin Guo Ye (Folium Ginkgo)

銀果葉 银果叶

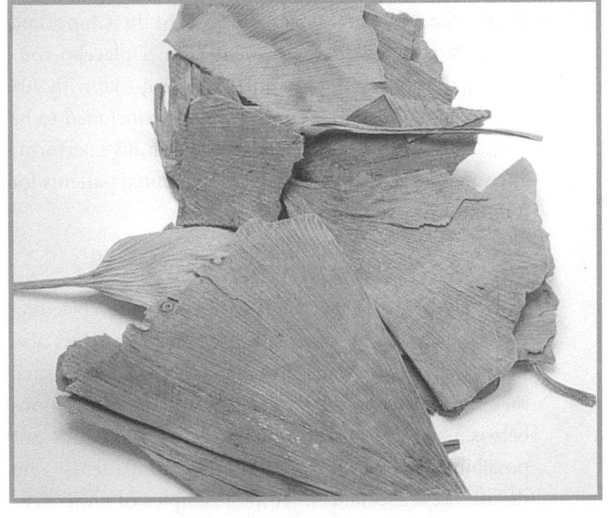

Pinyin Name: *Yin Guo Ye*
Literal Name: "silver fruit leaf"
Alternate Chinese Names: *Yin Xing Ye, Bai Guo Ye*
Original Source: *Ben Cao Pin Hui Jing Yao* (Essentials of Materia Medica) by Liu Wen-Tai in 1505
English Name: ginkgo leaf
Botanical Name: *Ginkgo biloba* L. (*Yin Xing*)
Pharmaceutical Name: Folium Ginkgo
Properties: sweet, bitter, astringent, neutral
Channels Entered: Lung

CHINESE THERAPEUTIC ACTIONS

1. Astringes the Lung, Calms Wheezing and Stops Pain

Yin Guo Ye (Folium Ginkgo) relieves wheezing, and alleviates the shortness of breath and dyspnea characteristic of Lung deficiency.

2. Relieves Chest Oppression and Pain

Yin Guo Ye improves circulation in the chest to relieve feelings of chest oppression and pain. Current applications of this herb include coronary artery disease, angina, hypertension and hyperlipidemia.

DOSAGE

3 to 6 grams.

CHEMICAL COMPOSITION

Ginkgetin, isoginkegetin, bilobetin, isorhamnetin,

Yín Guo Ye (Folium Ginkgo)

kaempferol, quercetin, rutin, ginkgolide A, B, C; bilobalide A, shikimic acid, D-glucaric acid, anacardic acids, ginkgolic acid, girmol, ginnone.[1,2]

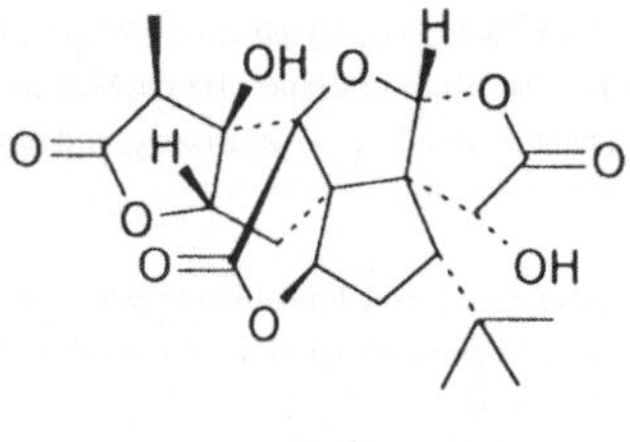

Ginkgolide A

PHARMACOLOGICAL EFFECTS

- **Cardiovascular:** Intravenous injection of *Yin Guo Ye* in rabbits and rats was associated with vasodilation, decreased blood pressure and increased perfusion of blood to peripheral parts of the body.[3]
- **Metabolic:** Administration of water extract of *Yin Guo Ye* has been associated with a mild decrease in plasma cholesterol levels.[4]
- **Respiratory:** Administration of alcohol extract of *Yin Guo Ye* has been associated with an antispasmodic effect on the respiratory tract in mice and guinea pigs.[5]

CLINICAL STUDIES AND RESEARCH

- **Dementia:** *Yin Guo Ye* has been used in China and Europe for treatment of dementia. In a placebo-controlled, double-blind, randomized clinical trial with 309 patients over 52 weeks, *Yin Guo Ye* was concluded to be "safe" and capable of "improving the cognitive performance and the social functioning of demented patients for 6 months to 1 year."[6]

HERB-DRUG INTERACTION

- **Anticoagulant drugs:** *Yin Guo Ye* may alter bleeding time and should be used with caution for patients also taking anticoagulant and antiplatelet medications, such as warfarin. Actual reports of problematic interactions between *Yin Guo Ye* and warfarin remain rare, but this possibility should be monitored in all patients who receive these substances. [Note: Examples of anticoagulants include heparin, warfarin (Coumadin) and enoxaparin (Lovenox)][7]
- **Antiplatelet drugs:** It was suggested in one animal study that the use of *Yin Guo Ye* extract may potentiate the antiplatelet and antithrombotic effects of ticlopidine. [Note: Examples of antiplatelets include aspirin, dipyridamole (Persantine), and clopidogrel (Plavix).][8]
- **Surgery:** It has been recommended that the use of *Yin Guo Ye* should be discontinued for two to three weeks prior to surgery, to avoid potential interaction with anesthetics and/or increased risk of bleeding.[9]

TOXICOLOGY

Side effects such as salivation, nausea, vomiting, poor appetite and diarrhea were reported in a toxicology study in dogs who received intravenous injections of alcohol extract of *Yin Guo Ye* in dogs at 40 times the normal human dose, one injection daily for 7 days.[10]

AUTHORS' COMMENTS

Yin Guo Ye (Folium Ginkgo) is the same as the ginkgo product that is commonly sold over the counter for memory enhancement. While ginkgo leaf is quite popular among the general public, it is not frequently used in traditional Chinese medicine.

References

1. *Xian Dai Zhong Yao Yao Li Xue* (Contemporary Pharmacology of Chinese Herbs), 1997; 922
2. Yan X, Zhou J, Xie G, *Traditional Chinese Medicines Molecular Structures, Natural Sources and Applications*; Ashgate, 1999; 2588
3. *Guo Wai Yi Xue Zhong Yi Zhong Yao Fen Ce* (Monograph of Chinese Herbology from Foreign Medicine), 1979; 4:200
4. *Xian Dai Zhong Yao Yao Li Xue* (Contemporary Pharmacology of Chinese Herbs), 1997; 922-923
5. *Curr Sci*, 1970; 39(23):533
6. Le Bars, P. et al. A placebo-controlled, double-blind, randomized trial of an extract of ginkgo biloba for dementia. *Journal of American Medical Association;* 278:1327-1332. October 22, 1997
7. *Archives of Internal Medicine*, v.158, n.20, Nov. 9, 1998: 2200-2211
8. *Thromb Res*, 1998 Jul, 1;(91):1; 33-38
9. *JAMA*, 281(20) May 26, 1999
10. *Xian Dai Zhong Yao Yao Li Xue* (Contemporary Pharmacology of Chinese Herbs), 1997; 922-923

Sang Bai Pi (Cortex Mori)

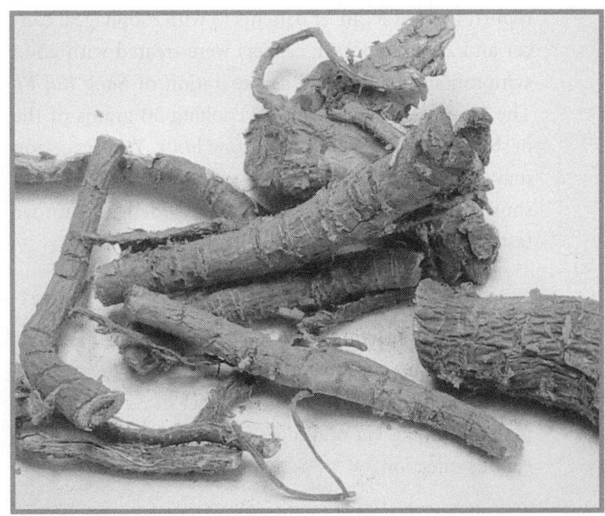

桑白皮

Pinyin Name: *Sang Bai Pi*
Literal Name: "mulberry white bark"
Original Source: *Shen Nong Ben Cao Jing* (Divine Husbandman's Classic of the Materia Medica) in the second century
English Name: mulberry bark, white mulberry root bark
Botanical Name: *Morus alba* L. (*Sang Shu*)
Pharmaceutical Name: Cortex Mori
Properties: sweet, cold
Channels Entered: Lung

CHINESE THERAPEUTIC ACTIONS

1. Sedates Lung Heat, Relieves Wheezing

Cough and dyspnea caused by Lung heat: Sweet, cold and downward-moving in nature, *Sang Bai Pi* (Cortex Mori) is the best herb to sedate Lung heat and the accompanying misdirection of Lung qi. Clinically, *Sang Bai Pi* treats coughing and wheezing with yellow copious sputum caused by excess heat in the Lung.

- Cough due to Lung heat: combine *Sang Bai Pi* with *Di Gu Pi* (Cortex Lycii) and *Gan Cao* (Radix Glycyrrhizae). **Exemplar Formula:** *Xie Bai San* (Drain the White Powder).

2. Promotes Urination, Reduces Swelling

Edema: *Sang Bai Pi* regulates water circulation to treat excess types of facial or generalized edema, dysuria, and dyspnea with fullness of the chest. It promotes normal urination and reduces swelling.

- Edema: combine this herb with *Da Fu Pi* (Pericarpium Arecae) and *Fu Ling Pi* (Cortex Poria). **Exemplar Formula:** *Wu Pi Yin* (Five-Peel Decoction).

3. Reduces Blood Pressure

Sang Bai Pi treats hypertension characterized by Liver yang rising.

- Hypertension due to Liver yang rising: use *Sang Bai Pi* with *Huang Qin* (Radix Scutellariae), *Jue Ming Zi* (Semen Cassiae) and *Xia Ku Cao* (Spica Prunellae).

DOSAGE

10 to 15 grams in decoction. Unprocessed *Sang Bai Pi* is cold, and more strongly sedates the Lung and regulates water circulation. The honey-fried herb is warmer, and more effectively moistens the Lung and relieves dry cough and wheezing.

CAUTIONS / CONTRAINDICATIONS

- *Sang Bai Pi* is contraindicated for patients who are coughing due to cold in the Lung.

CHEMICAL COMPOSITION

Morusin, mulberrin, mulberrochromene, cyclomulberrin, cyclomuberrochromene, mulberrofuran A, kuwanon, sanggenon, moracenin, betulinic acid, α-amyrin, β-amyrin.[1]

PHARMACOLOGICAL EFFECTS

- **Diuretic:** Water and alcohol extracts of *Sang Bai Pi* given via oral or intraperitoneal administration had a marked diuretic effect by increasing the excretion of water, sodium, chloride and potassium.[2]
- **Cardiovascular:** Water and alcohol extracts of *Sang Bai Pi* have moderate and prolonged antihypertensive effects in dogs, rabbits, and rats. The antihypertensive effect was negated by administration of atropine.[3]
- **Gastrointestinal:** Intravenous injection of alcohol extract of *Sang Bai Pi* in dogs stimulated intestinal smooth muscle to increase peristalsis. Water extract did not have the same effect.[4]
- **Analgesic:** Water extract of *Sang Bai Pi* has an analgesic effect in mice. At 2 g/kg, *Sang Bai Pi* is comparable in effect to 0.5 g/kg of aspirin.[5]
- **Antibiotic:** *Sang Bai Pi* has an inhibitory effect against *Staphylococcus aureus, Salmonella typhi,* and *Bacillus dysenteriae.*[6]
- **Others:** *Sang Bai Pi* has antitussive, sedative, hypnotic, and antipyretic effects.[7]

CLINICAL STUDIES AND RESEARCH

- **Esophageal and stomach cancers:** According to one

Sang Bai Pi (Cortex Mori)

report, 4 out of 5 cancer patients (3 with esophageal cancer and 2 with stomach cancer) were treated with good symptomatic relief using a preparation of *Sang Bai Pi*. The preparation was made by cooking 30 grams of the herb with 90 ml of vinegar for one hour. The decoction may be taken all at once, or in smaller portions over a short period of time. Sugar may be added to improve taste and patient compliance.[8]

TOXICOLOGY

Few adverse reactions were observed following bolus or continuous administration of *Sang Bai Pi* in mice. The LD_{50} for water or alcohol extract of *Sang Bai Pi* in mice is 10 g/kg via oral ingestion, and 5 g/kg via intravenous injection.[9]

References

1. *Xian Dai Zhong Yao Yao Li Xue* (Contemporary Pharmacology of Chinese Herbs), 1997; 1017
2. *Chang Yong Zhong Yao Cheng Fen Yu Yao Li Shou Ce* (A Handbook of the Composition and Pharmacology of Common Chinese Drugs), 1994; 1551:1554
3. Ibid.
4. Ibid.
5. Ibid.
6. *Zhong Yao Xue* (Chinese Herbology), 1998; 648:650
7. Ibid.
8. *Fu Jian Zhong Yi Yao* (Fujian Chinese Medicine and Herbology), 1965; 3:23
9. *Zhong Yao Yao Li Yu Ying Yong* (Pharmacology and Applications of Chinese Herbs), 1983: 927

Ting Li Zi (Semen Descurainiae seu Lepidii)

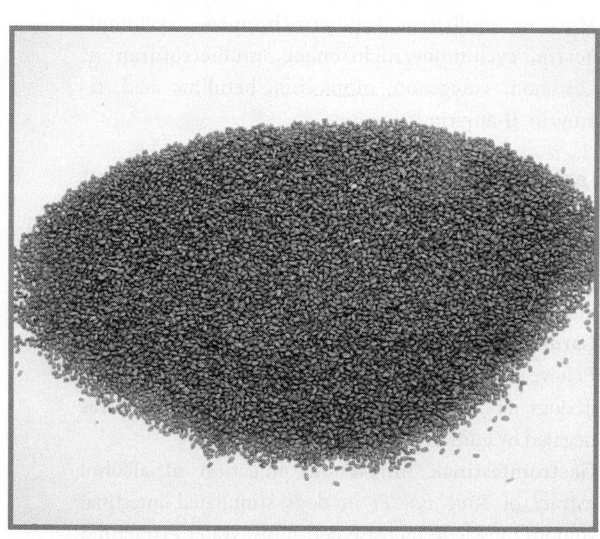

葶藶子 葶苈子

Pinyin Name: *Ting Li Zi*
Original Source: *Shen Nong Ben Cao Jing* (Divine Husbandman's Classic of the Materia Medica) in the second century
English Name: descurainia, lepidium
Botanical Name: *Descurainia sophia* (L.) Schur. (*Bo Niang Hao*); *Lepidium apetalum* Willd. (*Du Xing Cai*)
Pharmaceutical Name: Semen Descurainiae seu Lepidii
Properties: acrid, bitter, very cold
Channels Entered: Lung, Urinary Bladder

CHINESE THERAPEUTIC ACTIONS

1. Sedates the Lung, Relieves Wheezing

Wheezing, dyspnea and cough due to profuse phlegm accumulation: *Ting Li Zi* (Semen Descurainiae seu Lepidii) sedates the Lung, dissolves phlegm and relieves wheezing. It is most effective for excess-type coughing and wheezing, gurgling sounds in the throat, and chest fullness and congestion with discomfort when lying down, caused by accumulation of phlegm in the lungs. *Ting Li Zi* has recently been used to treat pleurisy and water retention in the thoracic cavity.

- Accumulation of phlegm in the lungs: combine *Ting Li Zi* with *Da Zao* (Fructus Jujubae). **Exemplar Formula:** *Ting Li Da Zao Xie Fei Tang* (Descurainia and Jujube Decoction to Drain the Lungs).
- Lung abscess: add this herb to *Yi Yi Ren* (Semen Coicis), *Dong Gua Zi* (Semen Benincasae), *Tao Ren* (Semen Persicae), *Jin Yin Hua* (Flos Lonicerae), and *Lu Gen* (Rhizoma Phragmitis).

Ting Li Zi (Semen Descurainiae seu Lepidii)

2. Reduces Swelling, Promotes Diuresis

Edema and water retention in the chest and abdomen: The Lung is the organ in the upper *jiao* that regulates water circulation. When there is qi stagnation obstructing water passages, edema and water retention will result. *Ting Li Zi* treats edema, dysuria, and water accumulation caused by the inability of Lung qi to disperse water to peripheral parts of the body.

- Dysuria: use *Ting Li Zi* with *Fen Fang Ji* (Radix Stephaniae Tetandrae), *Jiao Mu* (Semen Zanthoxyli Bungeani), and *Da Huang* (Radix et Rhizoma Rhei).
- Congestion in the chest with hardness, fullness and pain: combine it with *Xing Ren* (Semen Armeniacae Amarum), *Da Huang* (Radix et Rhizoma Rhei), and *Mang Xiao* (Natrii Sulfas). **Exemplar Formula:** *Da Xian Xiong Tang* (Major Sinking into the Chest Decoction).
- Congestive heart failure with edema, or pulmonary heart disease, dyspnea, generalized swelling, or cardiac failure: use *Ting Li Zi* with *Fu Zi* (Radix Aconiti Lateralis Praeparata) and *Huang Qi* (Radix Astragali).

DOSAGE

3 to 10 grams in decoction. *Ting Li Zi* can be used at 1 to 2 grams per dose, as powder, three times daily. Bitter, cold and downward-moving, unprocessed seeds are sometimes associated with consumption of Lung qi. Therefore, *Ting Li Zi* is dry-fried to increase its warmth and to minimize the frequency and severity of side effects.

CAUTIONS / CONTRAINDICATIONS

- Strong in its sedating function, *Ting Li Zi* should be reserved for use in cases of accumulation of phlegm or water characterized by excess conditions. It should not be used in deficient conditions.
- *Ting Li Zi* should be used with caution for patients with constitutional deficiency or weakness. If *Ting Li Zi* must be used, it should be taken in combination with Spleen-tonic or qi-tonic herbs to neutralize its cold and sedating properties.
- Use of *Ting Li Zi* is contraindicated during pregnancy.

CHEMICAL COMPOSITION

Strophanthidine, evomonoside, helveticoside, evobioside, erysimoside, benzylisothiocyanate, allyl isothiocyanate, allyl disulfide, linolenic acid, linoleic acid, oleic acid, erucic acid, palmitic acid, stearic acid, sitosterol, sinapic acid, 3-butenyl isothiocyanate, 2-phenylethyl isothiocyanate, 4-methylthiobutyl isothiocyanate, epithiobutane derivatives.[1]

PHARMACOLOGICAL EFFECTS

- **Cardiotonic:** Administration of *Ting Li Zi* is associated with positive inotropic and negative chronotropic effects in frogs, rabbits and cats.[2]
- **Diuretic:** *Ting Li Zi* has a mild diuretic effect.[3]

CLINICAL STUDIES AND RESEARCH

- **Chronic congestive heart failure:** Administration of 1 to 2 grams of *Bei Ting Li Zi* (Semen Lepidii) in powder three times daily after meals had a good therapeutic effect in 10 cases of congestive heart failure.[4]
- **Respiratory disorders:** Thirty children with cough and dyspnea from bronchitis were treated with a preparation of *Ting Li Zi* (6 to 15 grams) with a 96.7% success rate.[5]

HERB-DRUG INTERACTION

- **Diuretics:** *Ting Li Zi* has a mild diuretic effect. Though not documented, concurrent use with diuretic drugs may lead to increased elimination of water and/or electrolytes. [Note: Examples of diuretics include chlorothiazide, hydrochlorothiazide, furosemide (Lasix), bumetanide (Bumex), and torsemide (Demadex).][6]

SUPPLEMENT

- 南葶藶子/南葶苈子 *Nan Ting Li Zi* (Semen Descurainiae), derived from *Descurainia sophia* (L.) Schur., is also known as the "sweet *Ting Li Zi*." Bland and milder in potency than Lepidium, it is used primarily to sedate the Lung and relieve wheezing.
- 北葶藶子/北葶苈子 *Bei Ting Li Zi* (Semen Lepidii), derived from *Lepidium apetalum* Willd., is known as the "bitter *Ting Li Zi*." It is used primarily to reduce swelling and promote diuresis. Because of its potency, *Bei Ting Li Zi* is more likely to injure the Stomach. Therefore, *Da Zao* (Fructus Jujubae) should be added to minimize potential side effects, and use of the herbs discontinued immediately when the desired effect is achieved.

AUTHORS' COMMENTS

The use of *Ting Li Zi* is generally reserved for disorders found in excess conditions because of its acrid, bitter, cold and draining properties. One of its recent clinical applications is for congestive heart failure with dyspnea and edema, a condition characterized by Lung and Spleen deficiencies. The use of *Ting Li Zi* here is appropriate only because it has a strong cardiotonic function, and tonic herbs should be added to prevent side effects.

According to Dr. Chen Yuan-Da, *Ting Li Zi* is one of the best and most effective herbs for treatment of acute asthma. *Ting Li Zi* has an excellent and immediate action to eliminate visible phlegm (the sputum in the lungs) and invisible phlegm (the inflammation and the swelling in the lungs).

Ting Li Zi (Semen Descurainiae seu Lepidii)

References

1. *Xian Dai Zhong Yao Yao Li Xue* (Contemporary Pharmacology of Chinese Herbs), 1997; 1062
2. *Wu Han Yi Xue Yuan Xue Bao* (Journal of Wuhan University School of Medicine), 1963; (20):9
3. *Zhong Yao Zhi* (Chinese Herbology Journal), 1984: 625
4. *Zhong Yi Za Zhi* (Journal of Chinese Medicine), 1961; 4:27
5. Ibid., 1984; 10:43
6. Chen, J. Recognition & prevention of herb-drug interactions, *Medical Acupuncture*, Fall/Winter 1998/1999; volume 10/number 2; 9-13

Chapter 13 summary — Phlegm-Resolving and Coughing- and Wheezing- Relieving Herbs

SECTION 1: PHLEGM-RESOLVING HERBS

Name	Similarities	Differences
Ban Xia (Rhizoma Pinelliae)	Dry dampness, resolve phlegm	Relieves nausea and vomiting
Tian Nan Xing (Rhizoma Arisaematis)		Dispels wind and relieves spasms
Dan Nan Xing (Arisaema cum Bile)		Dispels wind and relieves spasms, cool in thermal property
Bai Fu Zi (Rhizoma Typhonii)		Eliminates toxins and disperses nodules
Bai Jie Zi (Semen Sinapis)		Warms the Lung to dispel phlegm, disperses qi, opens channels to relieve pain
Zao Jiao (Fructus Gleditsiae)		Opens orifices, disperses nodules and masses
Zao Jiao Ci (Spina Gleditsiae)		Eliminates toxins, dispels pus, invigorates blood circulation, reduces swelling
Jie Geng (Radix Platycodonis)	Dissolve phlegm, arrest cough	Ventilates the Lung, benefits the throat, dispels pus
Xuan Fu Hua (Flos Inulae)		Descends Lung and Stomach qi
Qian Hu (Radix Peucedani)		Disperses wind-heat
Bai Qian (Rhizoma Cynanchi Stauntonii)		Sedates the Lung, disperses wind-cold
Chuan Bei Mu (Bulbus Fritillariae Cirrhosae)		Arrests chronic cough, moistens the Lung
Zhe Bei Mu (Bulbus Fritillariae Thunbergii)		Clears heat, eliminates toxins, disperses stagnation
Gua Lou Shi (Fructus Trichosanthis)	Clear heat, dissolve phlegm	Regulates Lung qi, expands the chest, lubricates the bowels
Gua Lou Ren (Semen Trichosanthis)		Lubricates the bowels
Gua Lou Pi (Pericarpium Trichosanthis)		Regulates Lung qi, expands the chest
Tian Zhu Huang (Concretio Silicea Bambusae)		Stops convulsions
Zhu Ru (Caulis Bambusae in Taenia)		Clears heat and phlegm from the Lung and Stomach
Zhu Li (Succus Bambusae)		Clears heat and phlegm from the Heart, Lung, and Stomach
Fu Hai Shi (Pumice)		Softens hardness, dissipates nodules
Hai Ge Fen (Concha Meretricis seu Cyclinae)		Softens hardness, neutralizes stomach acid
Meng Shi (Lapis Micae seu Chloriti)		Dispels stubborn phlegm, anchors the Liver, stops tremors
Hai Zao (Sargassum)		Softens hardness and masses
Kun Bu (Thallus Laminariae seu Eckloniae)		Softens hardness and masses
Huang Yao Zi (Herba Dioscoreae Bulbiferae)		Disperses stagnation, treats goiter, clears heat, reduces swelling, cools blood to stop bleeding
Pang Da Hai (Semen Sterculiae Lychnophorae)	Benefit the Lung	Clears and ventilates the Lung, lubricates the bowels, restores voice
Luo Han Guo (Fructus Momordicae)		Moistens the Lung, arrests cough, generates body fluids, relieves thirst

General Characteristics of Phlegm-Resolving Herbs:

Taste: bitter
Thermal property: warm or cold
Channels entered: Spleen, Lung
Therapeutic actions: resolve phlegm, treat phlegm-related disorders

Chapter 13 summary

The main functions of phlegm-resolving herbs are to dispel phlegm and relieve phlegm-related disorders, such as cough, dyspnea, mania, epilepsy, convulsions, spasms, scrofula, nodules, goiters and other masses.

Ban Xia (Rhizoma Pinelliae), ***Tian Nan Xing*** (Rhizoma Arisaematis) and ***Dan Nan Xing*** (Arisaema cum Bile), warm and drying, are essential herbs in drying dampness and phlegm.

Ban Xia most effectively dispels dampness in the middle *jiao* with symptoms of cough, nausea and vomiting, especially when characterized by reversed flow of Stomach qi. *Ban Xia* is one of the best, most effective, herbs to treat dampness and phlegm.

Tian Nan Xing, warmer and drier than *Ban Xia*, more directly dispels wind and phlegm in the channels to relieve spasms, vertigo, dizziness, stroke, convulsions, tetany and other symptoms created by wind and phlegm.

Dan Nan Xing, cool and bitter, exerts a stronger influence to clear heat, dissolve phlegm, arrest wind and relieve convulsions.

Bai Fu Zi (Rhizoma Typhonii), toxic, warm and drying, dispels abundant accumulation of wind and phlegm causing symptoms of stroke, facial paralysis and tetany.

Bai Jie Zi (Semen Sinapis), warm and acrid, warms the Lung to dissolve phlegm, benefit qi and disperse stagnation in cold-type coughing with white sputum, chest congestion and fullness, and soreness of the limbs and joints, pus, and yin-type swellings or nodules caused by cold.

Zao Jiao (Fructus Gleditsiae) and ***Zao Jiao Ci*** (Spina Gleditsiae) are derived from the same plant and have similar functions.

Zao Jiao dispels phlegm, opens orifices, and effectively resuscitates unconscious patients who are foaming at the mouth, have locked jaw, epilepsy or convulsions due to profuse phlegm obstruction.

Zao Jiao Ci functions better to eliminate toxins, invigorate blood circulation and reduce swelling.

Jie Geng (Radix Platycodonis) has ascending and descending functions. It ventilates the Lung to relieve cough, dissolves sputum, benefits the throat, and dispels pus and abscesses.

Xuan Fu Hua (Flos Inulae) dispels phlegm, moves water and treats cough involving profuse sputum. It redirects abnormally-rising Stomach qi to relieve nausea, vomiting and hiccups caused by phlegm accumulation.

Qian Hu (Radix Peucedani) and ***Bai Qian*** (Rhizoma Cynanchi Stauntonii) dispel phlegm and descend qi.

Qian Hu is used more in wind-heat conditions because it is stronger in its ventilating and dispersing effects.

Bai Qian descends qi and relieves coughing characterized by excess heat or phlegm conditions in the Lung.

There are two varieties of ***Bei Mu*** (Bulbus Fritillaria): ***Chuan Bei Mu*** (Bulbus Fritillariae Cirrhosae) and ***Zhe Bei Mu*** (Bulbus Fritillariae Thunbergii).

Chuan Bei Mu, sweet and cool, moistens the Lung, relieves dry cough, and treats yin-deficient chronic cough with scanty sputum and dry throat.

Zhe Bei Mu, bitter and cold, more strongly sedates the Lung in excess conditions and thus treats wind-heat or phlegm-heat in the Lung.

Chapter 13 summary

Gua Lou Pi (Pericarpium Trichosanthis), ***Gua Lou Ren*** (Semen Trichosanthis), and ***Gua Lou Shi*** (Fructus Trichosanthis) are derived from the same plant and have similar functions.

Gua Lou Pi strongly clears the Lung, dissolves phlegm and expands the chest.

Gua Lou Ren moistens the Lung, dissolves phlegm and moistens the Large Intestine to promote bowel movement.

Gua Lou Shi has all of the above functions.

Tian Zhu Huang (Concretio Silicea Bambusae), ***Zhu Ru*** (Caulis Bambusae in Taenia) and ***Zhu Li*** (Succus Bambusae) are all from the bamboo plant, but have different functions.

Tian Zhu Huang clears the Heart, dissolves phlegm, and treats phlegm obstructing the Heart (epilepsy, convulsions, or unconsciousness).

Zhu Ru clears Lung and Stomach heat, and treats cough due to Lung heat, or vomiting and nausea due to Stomach heat and phlegm.

Zhu Li, sweet and cold, treats stroke, epilepsy and mania caused by heat and phlegm.

Fu Hai Shi (Pumice) and ***Hai Ge Fen*** (Concha Meretricis seu Cyclinae) are salty and cold, clear the Lung, dissolve phlegm, soften hardness and disperse stagnation.

Fu Hai Shi also promotes urination.

Hai Ge Fen reduces swelling via diuresis, and neutralizes gastric acid to relieve pain.

Meng Shi (Lapis Micae seu Chloriti) descends qi, anchors the Liver and treats excess conditions involving chronic, difficult-to-expectorate phlegm.

Hai Zao (Sargassum) and ***Kun Bu*** (Thallus Laminariae seu Eckloniae) dispel phlegm, soften hardness and are essential to disperse and soften masses, nodules, scrofula and goiter. These herbs are taken steadily over a long period of time to gain results.

Huang Yao Zi (Herba Dioscoreae Bulbiferae) clears heat, eliminates toxins, cools the blood, reduces swelling, and dissipates nodules, goiter and masses. *Huang Yao Zi* may be toxic to the liver, and must only be used with caution.

Pang Da Hai (Semen Sterculiae Lychnophorae) and ***Luo Han Guo*** (Fructus Momordicae) address Lung disorders characterized by yin deficiency and dryness.

Pang Da Hai is sweet and cold, and treats hoarseness or loss of voice from Lung heat.

Luo Han Guo moistens the Lung and treats symptoms associated with Lung yin deficiency.

Chapter 13 summary

SECTION 2: COUGHING- AND WHEEZING-RELIEVING HERBS

Name	Similarities	Differences
Xing Ren (Semen Armeniacae Amarum)	Arrest cough	Relieves wheezing, moistens the Lung, lubricates the bowels
Bai Bu (Radix Stemonae)		Kills parasites
Zi Wan (Radix Asteris)		Moistens dryness, dissolves phlegm
Kuan Dong Hua (Flos Farfarae)		Moistens dryness, dissolves phlegm
Su Zi (Fructus Perillae)		Descends qi, dissolves phlegm, relieves dyspnea
Zhong Ru Shi (Stalactitum)		Warms the Lung and Kidney to relieve wheezing, promotes lactation
Ma Dou Ling (Fructus Aristolochiae)		Clears the Lung, dissolves phlegm
Pi Pa Ye (Folium Eriobotryae)		Dissolves phlegm, descends Stomach qi
Gu Zhi Hua (Semen Oroxyli)		Restores voice
Bai Guo (Semen Ginkgo)		Relieves wheezing, consolidates *jing* (essence)
Yin Guo Ye (Folium Ginkgo)		Relieves chest oppression and pain, improves cognitive functions
Sang Bai Pi (Cortex Mori)	Sedate the Lung, arrest dyspnea, promote urination and reduce swelling	Clears the Lung more strongly
Ting Li Zi (Semen Descurainiae seu Lepidii)		Sedates water in the Lung more effectively

General Characteristics of Coughing- and Wheezing-Relieving Herbs:

Taste: sweet, bitter
Thermal property: warm or cold
Channels entered: Lung
Therapeutic actions: arrest cough, relieve wheezing and dyspnea

Herbs in this category ventilate the Lung to dispel phlegm, moisten the Lung to stop coughing, and redirect rebellious qi downwards to relieve cough, wheezing and dyspnea.

Xing Ren (Semen Armeniacae Amarum), bitter and descending in nature, drains downwards and is essential to stop cough and relieve wheezing. Used with other herbs, it treats all types of cough and dyspnea. *Xing Ren* also lubricates the intestines and treats dry stools or constipation.

Bai Bu (Radix Stemonae) moistens the Lung and arrests both acute and chronic coughing.

Zi Wan (Radix Asteris) and ***Kuan Dong Hua*** (Flos Farfarae), commonly used together, are both warm and moistening. They are most suitable for cold-type cough involving profuse sputum or chronic cough with blood-streaked sputum.
Zi Wan more strongly dissolves phlegm.
Kuan Dong Hua more strongly relieves cough.

Su Zi (Fructus Perillae) descends qi and dissolves phlegm, for profuse phlegm accumulation in the chest with Lung qi reversal.

Zhong Ru Shi (Stalactitum) warms the Lung and Kidney to relieve coughing and wheezing, and promotes lactation.

Ma Dou Ling (Fructus Aristolochiae), bitter and cold, clears the Lung to dissolve phlegm in cough due to heat with profuse phlegm and accelerated respiration. *Ma Dou Ling* also sedates Large Intestine heat to treat hemorrhoids with swelling, bleeding and pain.

Chapter 13 summary

Pi Pa Ye (Folium Eriobotryae) moistens the Lung, dissolves phlegm, relieves cough, harmonizes the Stomach, and reverses rising Stomach qi caused by heat. It is one of the best herbs for sticky, difficult-to-expectorate sputum.

Gu Zhi Hua (Semen Oroxyli) moistens the Lung, relieves cough, restores voice, and releases damp-heat from the skin.

Bai Guo (Semen Ginkgo) and ***Yin Guo Ye*** (Folium Ginkgo) are derived from the same plant with similar functions to relieve coughing and wheezing.

Bai Guo is sweet, astringent and moves downwards. It stabilizes and binds the Lung to relieve wheezing, stops leukorrhea and retains urine.

Yin Guo Ye relieves chest oppression disorders such as coronary artery disease, angina, hypertension, and hyperlipidemia. It also increases blood perfusion to the brain to treat dementia and Alzheimer's disease.

Sang Bai Pi (Cortex Mori) and ***Ting Li Zi*** (Semen Descurainiae seu Lepidii) are excellent in sedating the Lung to regulate the water passages in the body. They treat phlegm accumulation in the Lung with Lung qi reversal manifesting as cough and dyspnea.

Sang Bai Pi is sweet and cold, and mild in potency to clear Lung heat.

Ting Li Zi is bitter and cold, and strong in potency to sedate the Lung to dispel phlegm and water.

HERBS FROM OTHER FUNCTIONAL CATEGORIES WITH PHLEGM-RESOLVING AND COUGHING- AND WHEEZING-RELIEVING FUNCTIONS

Name	Functional Category
Chen Pi (Pericarpium Citri Reticulatae)	Qi-Regulating Herbs (Chapter 8)
Gan Cao (Radix Glycyrrhizae)	Tonic Herbs (Chapter 17)
Gan Jiang (Rhizoma Zingiberis)	Interior-Warming Herbs (Chapter 7)
Ge Jie (Gecko)	Tonic Herbs (Chapter 17)
He Zi (Fructus Chebulae)	Astringent Herbs (Chapter 18)
Hu Tao Ren (Semen Juglandis)	Tonic Herbs (Chapter 17)
Lai Fu Zi (Semen Raphani)	Digestive Herbs (Chapter 9)
Ma Huang (Herba Ephedrae)	Exterior-Releasing Herbs (Chapter 1)
Nan Sha Shen (Radix Adenophorae)	Tonic Herbs (Chapter 17)
Wu Mei (Fructus Mume)	Astringent Herbs (Chapter 18)
Wu Wei Zi (Fructus Schisandrae Chinensis)	Astringent Herbs (Chapter 18)
Xi Xin (Herba Asari)	Interior-Warming Herbs (Chapter 7)
Yuan Zhi (Radix Polygalae)	*Shen*-Calming Herbs (Chapter 14)

Chapter 14

— Shen-Calming Herbs

安神药

Chapter 14 — Shen-Calming Herbs

Chapter 14

安神药 — Shen-Calming Herbs

Definition: When dealing with imbalances of *shen* (spirit) and emotions, the medicinal substances that tranquilize and calm the mind and emotions are said to calm the *shen*.

Shen (spirit) disturbance is an emotional disorder that interferes with the proper health and functioning of the mind. In traditional Chinese medicine, the Heart controls *shen* and the Liver controls emotions. Characteristic clinical presentations of *shen* disturbance are signs and symptoms such as restlessness, anxiety, irritability, and insomnia.

SUBCATEGORIES OF ACTION

Shen-calming herbs are divided into two types: sedative herbs that treat excess-type *shen* disturbance, and nourishing herbs that calm deficient-type *shen* disturbance.

1. ***Sedative herbs that calm the shen***: Most of these are minerals and shells whose heavy nature is said to sedate and calm the *shen*. Thus, they are more suitable for excess-type *shen* disturbances.
2. ***Nourishing herbs that calm the shen***: Most of these are plant parts with nourishing and tonifying properties, and are most effective for deficient-type *shen* disturbances.

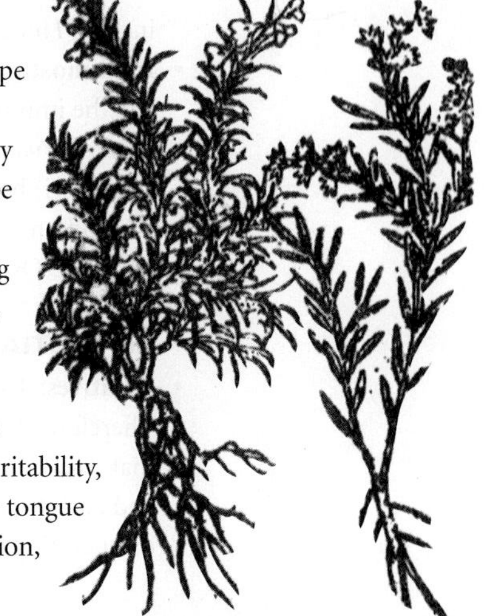

Yuan Zhi (Radix Polygalae)
Ben Cao Gang Mu (Materia Medica), by Li Shi-Zhen, 1578 A.D.

DIFFERENTIAL DIAGNOSIS AND TREATMENT

Shen disturbances are usually classified as being either deficient or excess in nature:

- ***Excess-type*** *shen* disturbances are characterized by irritability, anxiety, restlessness, irritability, insomnia, headache, chest congestion, red eyes, a bitter taste in the mouth, yellow tongue coating, and a slippery, rapid pulse. Liver qi stagnation, Liver fire rising, food stagnation, and phlegm accumulation are ***excess*** conditions in this disease pattern.
- ***Deficient-type*** *shen* disturbances are characterized by dizziness, light-headedness, palpitations, restlessness, fearfulness, forgetfulness, night sweats, a pale tongue, and thready pulse. The Heart, Spleen, Liver, Kidney, yin and blood may be ***deficient***.

In traditional Chinese medicine, the Heart controls *shen* and the Liver controls emotions. Thus, most herbs that treat disturbances of *shen* and emotion enter the ***Heart*** and ***Liver.*** However, many other factors may contribute to or complicate *shen* disturbance disorders:

- Liver Qi stagnation with emotional disturbances
- Disharmony of the Heart and Spleen, in which the deficient Spleen fails to produce blood to nourish the Heart
- Heart yin deficiency characterized by deficient fire
- Disharmony of the Heart and Kidney, in which Kidney yin deficiency allows heat to rise upwards and disturb the Heart
- Heat and phlegm interfering with the free flow of *shen* and emotions

Shen **(spirit) disturbance is an emotional disorder that interferes with the proper health and functioning of the mind.**

CAUTIONS/CONTRAINDICATIONS

Herbs that calm the *shen* (spirit) are used for symptomatic treatment. They should be used only as needed, and are not to be used for prolonged periods of time. Optimal treatment requires assessment of the cause and severity of the disturbance, and should address both the cause and the symptoms.

Chapter 14 — Shen-Calming Herbs

- Mineral substances used individually consume qi and damage the Stomach. Therefore, they should be used with herbs that nourish and protect the Stomach.
- Some *shen*-calming herbs are toxic, and must be used only when necessary, with extreme caution.

PHARMACOLOGICAL EFFECTS

~ *Shen*-calming herbs are used in symptomatic treatment. Optimal treatment should address both the cause and the symptoms of *shen* disturbance. ~

- **Effects on the central nervous system**: The pharmacological effects of herbs on the central nervous system include sedative, hypnotic, analgesic and antiepileptic effects.

  Herbs that decrease spontaneous physical activity include *Suan Zao Ren* (Semen Zizyphi Spinosae), *Ling Zhi* (Ganoderma), *Xie Cao* (Radix et Rhizoma Valerianae) and *He Huan Hua* (Flos Albiziae).

  Herbs that potentiate the effect of hypnotics by prolonging sleeping time include *Suan Zao Ren* (Semen Zizyphi Spinosae), *Xie Cao* (Radix et Rhizoma Valerianae), *Yuan Zhi* (Radix Polygalae) and *Ling Zhi* (Ganoderma).

  Herbs that diminish reactivity to external stimuli include *Suan Zao Ren* (Semen Zizyphi Spinosae) and *Xie Cao* (Radix et Rhizoma Valerianae).

  Herbs that prevent and/or treat seizures and epilepsy by inhibiting the central nervous system include *Ling Zhi* (Ganoderma) and *Xie Cao* (Radix et Rhizoma Valerianae).
- **Immunostimulant**: *Ling Zhi* (Ganoderma) and *Suan Zao Ren* (Semen Zizyphi Spinosae) stimulate the immune system by increasing the phagocytic activities of the macrophages.
- **Others**: *Yuan Zhi* (Radix Polygalae) has expectorant properties. *Ye Jiao Teng* (Caulis Polygoni Multiflori) has an antihyperlipidemic effect. *Xie Cao* (Radix et Rhizoma Valerianae) and *Ling Zhi* (Ganoderma) are hepatoprotective. *Bai Zi Ren* (Semen Platycladi) has a mild laxative effect, and *Long Gu* (Os Draconis) acts as a hemostatic.

POTENTIAL HERB-DRUG INTERACTIONS

- **Sedatives**: Herbs that calm the *shen* (spirit) have marked sedative and tranquilizing effects. Therefore, they should be used with caution when prescribed for a patient also taking other agents that may cause drowsiness, such as alcohol, antihistamines, benzodiazepines, opioid analgesics, and barbiturates. Individuals who take such herbs and/or drugs should exercise caution if driving or operating heavy machinery.

Section 1

— Sedative Herbs that Calm the Shen (Spirit)

Zhu Sha (Cinnabaris)

硃砂 朱砂

Pinyin Name: *Zhu Sha*
Literal Name: "dull red sand," "vermillion sand"
Alternate Chinese Names: *Jing Mian Sha, Dou Bian Sha, Zhu Bao Sha, Chen Sha*
Original Source: *Shen Nong Ben Cao Jing* (Divine Husbandman's Classic of the Materia Medica) in the second century
English Name: cinnabar
Pharmaceutical Name: Cinnabaris
Properties: sweet, cold
Channels Entered: Heart
Safety Index: toxic

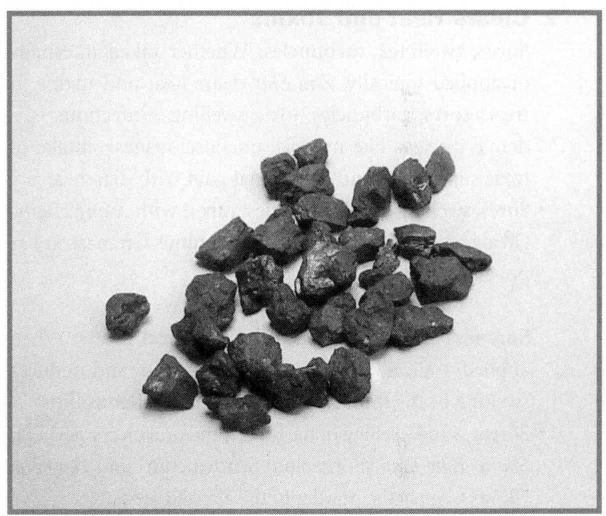

CHINESE THERAPEUTIC ACTIONS

1. Sedates the Heart and Calms the *Shen* (Spirit)

Sinking, heavy and cold in nature, *Zhu Sha* (Cinnabaris) enters the Heart channel to sedate Heart fire, arrest fright, and calm the *shen*. It is one of the most essential medicinal substances when treating excess fire conditions associated with the Heart. The Heart houses the *shen*: when fire accumulates, symptoms of restlessness, irritability, and insomnia occur. In more severe cases of phlegm and heat misting the Heart, epilepsy, delirium, convulsions, mania, schizophrenia and seizures may occur.

Restless *shen*: Disturbed *shen* can be caused either by excess or deficient conditions. In excess conditions, usually fire attacking the Heart, typical manifestations are restlessness, irritability, insomnia, anger, constipation and a scarlet tongue. In cases involving deficiency, usually blood deficiency unable to nourish the Heart, manifestations include palpitations, dream-disturbed sleep, a sallow complexion, sadness, a desire to cry, and fearfulness. *Zhu Sha*, when combined with heat-clearing herbs, treats excess conditions, and in combination with blood-tonic herbs, treats deficiency. Depending on the other herbs combined with it, *Zhu Sha* can address *shen* disturbances caused by excess fire, yin-deficient fire, blood deficiency and hot phlegm.

- Restlessness, irritability, insomnia: add *Zhu Sha* to *Huang Lian* (Rhizoma Coptidis) and *Ci Shi* (Magnetitum).
- Heart blood deficiency with irritability, palpitations, fright, dizziness and vertigo: combine this substance with *Dang Gui* (Radicis Angelicae Sinensis), *Sheng Di Huang* (Radix Rehmanniae) and *Zhi Gan Cao* (Radix Glycyrrhizae Preparata). **Exemplar Formula:** *Zhu Sha An Shen Wan* (Cinnabar Pills to Tranquilize the Spirit).
- Patients who are weak and easily frightened: combine this substance with *Ci Shi* (Magnetitum) to calm the *shen*, and with *Shen Qu* (Massa Fermentata) to protect the stomach from the harsh effects of the mineral substances.
- Epilepsy in children: combine it with *Xiong Huang* (Realgar) and *Zhen Zhu* (Margarita) as powder.
- Febrile disorders with hot phlegm or *bi zheng* (closed

Zhu Sha (Cinnabaris)

disorder) with high fever, delirium and incoherent speech: use *An Gong Niu Huang Wan* (Calm the Palace Pill with Cattle Gallstone) or *Niu Huang Qing Xin Dan* (Cattle Gallstone Pill to Clear the Heart), both of which contain *Zhu Sha*.

- Schizophrenia: combine *Zhu Sha* with *Xiang Fu* (Rhizoma Cyperi), *Bai Shao* (Radix Paeoniae Alba), *Huang Qin* (Radix Scutellariae), *Huang Lian* (Rhizoma Coptidis), *Tian Zhu Huang* (Concretio Silicea Bambusae), *Shi Chang Pu* (Rhizoma Acori), *Yuan Zhi* (Radix Polygalae), *Yu Jin* (Radix Curcumae), *Dai Zhe Shi* (Haematitum), *Mu Li* (Concha Ostreae) and *Sheng Tie Luo* (Frusta Ferri).

2. Clears Heat and Toxins

Sores, swellings, carbuncles: Whether taken internally or applied topically, *Zhu Sha* clears heat and toxins. It treats sores, carbuncles, toxic swellings, infectious epidemic diseases like malaria, unconsciousness, intake of toxic substances, and abdominal pain with diarrhea.

- Sores, swellings and carbuncles: mix it with *Xiong Huang* (Realgar) and *Shan Ci Gu* (Pseudobulbus Cremastrae) as powder for topical use.

Soreness and swelling of the throat, oral ulcers: When applied topically, *Zhu Sha* relieves pain and reduces swelling of the throat associated with acute tonsillitis.

- Soreness and swelling of the throat, and oral ulcers: add *Zhu Sha* to *Bing Pian* (Borneolum Syntheticum) and *Peng Sha* (Borax). Apply the powder to the affected area.

DOSAGE

0.3 to 1.0 gram. Internally, *Zhu Sha* is taken in pill form ***only***. The toxicity of *Zhu Sha* increases significantly when processed with heat (such as in decoction).

CAUTIONS / CONTRAINDICATIONS

- To prevent cumulative toxicity, *Zhu Sha* should not be used at a large dosage or for a long period of time.
- *Zhu Sha* should be used with extreme caution for those with compromised liver and kidney functions.
- Do not process *Zhu Sha* with heat, as this increases the risk of mercury poisoning.

OVERDOSAGE

Acute overdose of *Zhu Sha* is characterized by disturbance of the central nervous system, with nervousness, a metallic taste in the mouth, swollen gums, poor appetite, abdominal pain, diarrhea, tremor, sexual dysfunction, and liver and kidney damage.

TREATMENT OF OVERDOSAGE

Toxicity of *Zhu Sha* may be treated by gastric lavage with warm water or sodium bicarbonate, ingestion of milk, egg whites, or *Lu Dou* (Semen Phaseoli Radiati) soup. *Huang Lian Jie Du Tang* (Coptis Decoction to Relieve Toxicity) plus *Jin Yin Hua* (Flos Lonicerae) and *Tu Fu Ling* (Rhizoma Smilacis Glabrae) may also be used for detoxification.

Chronic overdose due to long-term consumption can be treated with the following two methods:

1. Ingestion of 10 to 15 grams of tea (green, oolong or black) one or two times daily. Tea clears heat, promotes urination, and facilitates the elimination of mercury.
2. Ingestion of one dose of an herbal decoction at room temperature containing 250 grams of *Tu Fu Ling* (Rhizoma Smilacis Glabrae), for 10 days (this process can be repeated after 3 to 4 days of rest).

Lastly, adverse reactions characterized by nausea, vomiting, salivation, moist tongue coat, and slow pulse can be treated with 15 grams of *Hua Jiao* (Pericarpium Zanthoxyli) and 30 grams of *Yi Tang* (Saccharum Granorum).[1]

CHEMICAL COMPOSITION

Mercuric sulfide.[2]

TOXICOLOGY

According to an acute toxicology study, the LD_{50} for *Zhu Sha* in mice is 12.10 g/kg.[3]

AUTHORS' COMMENTS

Zhu Sha is sometimes used to coat tablets and pills. It has tranquilizing functions to calm the *shen* (spirit). It also seals the pills against moisture to prolong shelf life.

Zhu Sha should be used with caution, as mineral substances may injure the Spleen and Stomach. To minimize side effects and adverse reactions, *Shen Qu* (Massa Fermentata), *Ji Nei Jin* (Endothelium Corneum Gigeriae Galli) and other digestive herbs may be added for protection of the middle *jiao*.

Fu Ling (Poria), *Mai Men Dong* (Radix Ophiopogonis) and *Deng Xin Cao* (Medulla Junci) can be added to *Zhu Sha* to enhance tranquilizing functions.

Zhu Sha is rarely used as a medicinal substance now. Its discussion here is included primarily for academic purposes, to reflect the historical use of this substance. Interestingly, western culture also used mercury in the past, for treatment of syphilis.

References

1. *Zhong Yao Du Li Xue* (Toxicology of Chinese Herbs), 1989; 188-191
2. *Xian Dai Zhong Yao Yao Li Xue* (Contemporary Pharmacology of Chinese Herbs), 1997; 1096
3. *Lin Chuan Shou Ce You Du Zhong Yao Shi Yong* (Clinical Handbook on Applications of Toxic Chinese Herbs), 1992; 350-351

Ci Shi (Magnetitum)

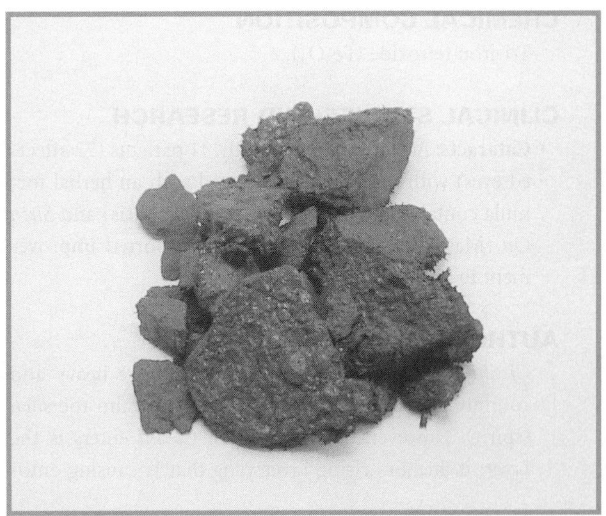

磁石

Pinyin Name: *Ci Shi*
Literal Name: "magnetic stone"
Alternate Chinese Names: *Sheng Ci Shi, Ling Ci Shi*
Original Source: *Shen Nong Ben Cao Jing* (Divine Husbandman's Classic of the Materia Medica) in the second century
English Name: lodestone, magnetite
Pharmaceutical Name: Magnetitum
Properties: acrid, salty, cold
Channels Entered: Liver, Kidney, Heart

CHINESE THERAPEUTIC ACTIONS

1. Anchors Liver Yang and Calms the *Shen* (Spirit)

Ci Shi (Magnetitum) is salty and heavy, to anchor rising Liver yang, protect the yin, and nourish the *shen.* Tinnitus, impaired hearing, deafness, dizziness, blurred vision, palpitations, forgetfulness, irritability, insomnia, epilepsy, infantile convulsions, restlessness, visual disturbances, vertigo and headaches are signs of Liver yang rising and disturbing the Heart, secondary to Liver yin and Kidney *jing* (essence) deficiencies.

- Blurred vision due to cataracts, disorders of the retina or optic nerves: add this substance to *Shu Di Huang* (Radix Rehmanniae Preparata), *Gou Qi Zi* (Fructus Lycii), *Chan Tui* (Periostracum Cicadae), *Ye Ming Sha* (Excrementum Vespertilionis Murini), *Qing Xiang Zi* (Semen Celosiae), *Shi Hu* (Herba Dendrobii) or *Ju Hua* (Flos Chrysanthemi).
- Heart *shen* disturbance with irritability, palpitations, insomnia or epilepsy: *Ci Shi* has historically been combined with *Zhu Sha* (Cinnabaris) for this purpose.
- Anemia, palpitations, insomnia, anxiety and neurasthenia: use it with *Shu Di Huang* (Radix Rehmanniae Preparata), *Dang Gui* (Radicis Angelicae Sinensis), *Bai Shao* (Radix Paeoniae Alba) and *Suan Zao Ren* (Semen Zizyphi Spinosae).

2. Improves Hearing and Brightens Eyes

The Liver opens to the eyes and the Kidney opens to the ears. If there is yin deficiency of either, deficiency fire will flare and manifest in symptoms of tinnitus, hearing loss, dizziness and blurred vision. *Ci Shi* can nourish Liver and Kidney yin and cool deficient fire.

- Tinnitus, hearing loss: combine *Ci Shi* with *Shu Di Huang* (Radix Rehmanniae Preparata), *Shan Zhu Yu* (Fructus Corni) and *Shan Yao* (Rhizoma Dioscoreae).
Exemplar Formula: *Er Long Zuo Ci Wan* (Pill for Deafness that Is Kind to the Left [Kidney]).
- Cataracts and disorders of the retina: use it with *Shu Di Huang* (Radix Rehmanniae Preparata), *Gou Qi Zi* (Fructus Lycii) and *Ju Hua* (Flos Chrysanthemi).

3. Stops Wheezing and Helps Kidney in Grasping Lung Qi

Respiratory difficulties: Chronic coughing or wheezing is the result of Kidney qi deficiency associated with constitutional weakness. Accompanying symptoms include shortness of breath that grows worse with exertion, difficulty with inhalation as compared to exhalation, shallow respiration, a dark, lusterless complexion, and a weak Kidney pulse.

- Respiratory difficulties: use *Ci Shi* with *Shu Di Huang* (Radix Rehmanniae Preparata), *Shan Zhu Yu* (Fructus Corni), *Wu Wei Zi* (Fructus Schisandrae Chinensis), *Xing Ren* (Semen Armeniacae Amarum), *Chen Xiang* (Lignum Aquilariae Resinatum) and *Hu Tao Ren* (Semen Juglandis).

DOSAGE

10 to 30 grams in decoction, 1 to 3 grams of *Ci Shi* when taken as powder or pills. Crush and pre-decoct it to maximize the extraction of active components. The calcined form prepared by fire and vinegar is preferred, as it is easier to extract the active constituents from this than from the unprocessed form.

CAUTIONS / CONTRAINDICATIONS

- Because *Ci Shi* is difficult to digest when taken as powder or pills, excessive or prolonged intake in these forms is contraindicated.

Ci Shi (Magnetitum)

CHEMICAL COMPOSITION

Tri-iron tetroxide (Fe_3O_4).

CLINICAL STUDIES AND RESEARCH

- **Cataracts:** According to one study, 41 patients (72 affected eyes) with cataracts were treated with an herbal formula containing *Ci Shi*, *Zhu Sha* (Cinnabaris) and *Shen Qu* (Massa Fermentata). The study reported improvement in vision in 55.6% of patients.[1]

AUTHORS' COMMENTS

Ci Shi and *Zhu Sha* (Cinnabaris) both are heavy and commonly used to pacify the Heart and calm the *shen* (spirit). However, the main organ *Ci Shi* enters is the Liver: it anchors rising Liver yang that is causing emotional, ocular or aural disorders. It tonifies the Kidney and helps grasp Lung qi to treat asthma. *Zhu Sha*, mainly entering the Heart channel, is strongest in pacifying Heart fire that manifests in symptoms of restless *shen*, palpitations, anxiety and insomnia.

Ci Shi and other mineral substances should be used with caution as they may injure the Spleen and Stomach. To minimize side effects and adverse reactions, *Shen Qu* (Massa Fermentata), *Ji Nei Jin* (Endothelium Corneum Gigeriae Galli) and other digestive herbs may be added for protection of the middle *jiao*.

References

1. *Zhong Hua Yan Ke Za Zhi* (Chinese Journal of Ophthalmology), 1957; 1:1

Long Gu (Os Draconis)

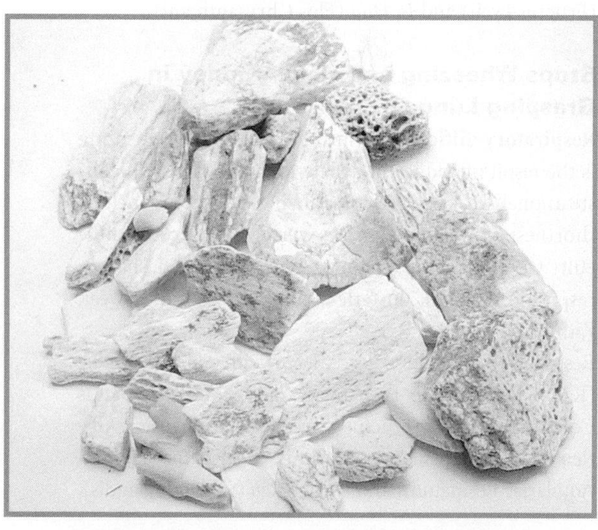

龍骨 龙骨

Pinyin Name: *Long Gu*
Literal Name: "dragon bone"
Original Source: *Shen Nong Ben Cao Jing* (Divine Husbandman's Classic of the Materia Medica) in the second century
English Name: dragon bone (fossil), fossilized animal bones
Pharmaceutical Name: Os Draconis
Properties: sweet, astringent, cool
Channels Entered: Heart, Liver

CHINESE THERAPEUTIC ACTIONS

1. Calms the Liver and Anchors Rising Yang

Liver yin deficiency with rising yang or Liver wind: *Long Gu* (Os Draconis) treats symptoms such as dizziness, vertigo, irritability, short temper, muscular rigidity, facial paralysis, and deviation of the mouth and eyes. Use the unprocessed form of this herb for this purpose.

- Dizziness, vertigo, irritability and short temper: use *Long Gu* with *Dai Zhe Shi* (Haematitum), *Mu Li* (Concha Ostreae), *Bai Shao* (Radix Paeoniae Alba) and *Bai Ji Li* (Fructus Tribuli). **Exemplar Formula:** *Zhen Gan Xi Feng Tang* (Sedate the Liver and Extinguish Wind Decoction).

2. Calms the *Shen* (Spirit)

Restless *shen* from external agitation: Signs of this disorder include insomnia, restlessness, forgetfulness, anxiety, palpitations, and mania. The unprocessed form of *Long Gu* is best for this application.

- Restless *shen*: use this substance with *Shi Chang Pu* (Rhizoma Acori) and *Yuan Zhi* (Radix Polygalae).
- *Shen* disturbance: combine *Long Gu* with *Mu Li* (Concha Ostreae). **Exemplar Formula:** *Chai Hu Jia Long*

Long Gu (Os Draconis)

Mu Tang (Bupleurum plus Dragon Bone and Oyster Shell Decoction).

- Schizophrenia: combine it with *Zhi Gan Cao* (Radix Glycyrrhizae Preparata), *Xiao Mai* (Fructus Tritici), and *Da Zao* (Fructus Jujubae).

Restless *shen* (spirit) from Heart deficiency. Signs include palpitations, insomnia, easily becoming frightened or awakened by dreams, dizziness and forgetfulness.

- Restless *shen* due to Heart deficiency: add *Long Gu* to *Suan Zao Ren* (Semen Zizyphi Spinosae), *Bai Zi Ren* (Semen Platycladi), *Fu Shen* (Poria Paradicis) and *Zhen Zhu Mu* (Concha Margaritaferae).

3. Prevents and Consolidates Leakage of Fluids

Leakage of body fluids due to deficiency: Clinical manifestations include spermatorrhea, vaginal discharge, spontaneous sweating, night sweating, uterine bleeding, epistaxis, enuresis, chronic diarrhea or dysentery, hematemesis and hematochezia. Secondary symptoms include soreness and weakness of the back and knees, and tinnitus. The calcined form of *Long Gu* is best for addressing these symptoms.

- Spermatorrhea, low back pain or tinnitus: combine *Long Gu* with *Mu Li* (Concha Ostreae), *Sha Yuan Zi* (Semen Astragali Complanati) and *Qian Shi* (Semen Euryales). **Exemplar Formula:** *Jin Suo Gu Jing Wan* (Metal Lock Pill to Stabilize the Essence).
- Spermatorrhea with Kidney yin deficiency: add *Long Gu* and *Mu Li* (Concha Ostreae) to *Liu Wei Di Huang Wan* (Six-Ingredient Pill with Rehmannia).
- Hypermenorrhea or uterine bleeding: use this substance with *Mu Li* (Concha Ostreae), charred *Xu Duan* (Radix Dipsaci), *Bai Zhu* (Rhizoma Atractylodis Macrocephalae) and *E Jiao* (Colla Corii Asini).
- White vaginal discharge: use it with *Cang Zhu* (Rhizoma Atractylodis), *Yi Yi Ren* (Semen Coicis) and *Fu Ling* (Poria).
- Enuresis: add it to *Sang Piao Xiao* (Ootheca Mantidis), *Fu Pen Zi* (Fructus Rubi), *Yi Zhi Ren* (Fructus Alpiniae Oxyphyllae), *Wu Yao* (Radix Linderae) and *Shan Zhu Yu* (Fructus Corni).
- Chronic diarrhea or dysentery: use *Long Gu* with *Chi Shi Zhi* (Halloysitum Rubrum), *Mu Xiang* (Radix Aucklandiae) and *Wu Mei* (Fructus Mume).
- Spontaneous or night sweating: combine it with *Huang Qi* (Radix Astragali), *Mu Li* (Concha Ostreae) and *Wu Wei Zi* (Fructus Schisandrae Chinensis).
- Profuse sweating with icy cold extremities and feeble pulse due to yang collapse: use it with *Ren Shen* (Radix Ginseng), *Fu Zi* (Radix Aconiti Lateralis Praeparata) and *Mu Li* (Concha Ostreae).

4. Promotes Healing of Sores and Helps Generate Flesh

The calcined form of *Long Gu* is most effective to promote the generation of flesh and healing of wounds.

- Non-healing ulcerations or sores, eczema or rashes: apply it topically as powder.

DOSAGE

15 to 30 grams for unprocessed *Long Gu*; 9 to 15 grams for the calcined form. Crush and pre-decoct this substance to enhance the extraction of active components. Calcine processing enhances its binding effect to prevent the loss of body fluids, as in treatment of spermatorrhea, diarrhea, and excessive vaginal discharge. Use unprocessed *Long Gu* for all the other functions.

CAUTIONS / CONTRAINDICATIONS

- Use of *Long Gu* is contraindicated in nocturnal emissions caused by fire.
- It is contraindicated for those who have damp-heat or externally-contracted disorders. Inappropriate use of *Long Gu* may lead to burning dysuria.

CHEMICAL COMPOSITION

Calcium carbonate, calcium phosphate, oxides of silicone, iron, aluminum, manganese, calcium, magnesium, titanium, phosphorus, sodium, potassium, zinc.[1]

CLINICAL STUDIES AND RESEARCH

- **Schizophrenia:** In one clinical study, 79 schizophrenic patients were treated with an herbal decoction containing *Long Gu* 30g, *Mu Li* (Concha Ostreae) 30g, *Zhi Gan Cao* (Radix Glycyrrhizae Preparata) 10g, *Xiao Mai* (Fructus Tritici) 30g, *Da Zao* (Fructus Jujubae) 5 pieces, and other herbs, according to the condition of each patient. Out of 79 patients, the study reported significant improvement in 5 cases, moderate improvement in 23 cases, slight improvement in 34 cases, and no response in 17 cases. The rate of effectiveness was 78.5%.[2]

SUPPLEMENT

- 龍齒 / 龙齿 *Long Chi* (Dens Draconis), sweet, astringent and cool, is fossilized animal teeth. Use of *Long Chi* was first cited in the *Shen Nong Ben Cao Jing* (Divine Husbandman's Classic of the Materia Medica) in the second century. It has functions similar to those of *Long Gu* but is stronger in calming the *shen* (spirit), and is often used to treat palpitations, anxiety, insomnia, dream-disturbed sleep and mania. For restlessness or crying in babies or children during the night, this substance can be used with *Bai Shao* (Radix Paeoniae Alba), *Mai Men Dong* (Radix Ophiopogonis), *Da Huang* (Radix et

Long Gu (Os Draconis)

Rhizoma Rhei) and *Sheng Ma* (Rhizoma Cimicifugae). Unprocessed *Long Chi* is preferred for this application.

AUTHORS' COMMENTS

Derived from the same source, *Long Gu* (Os Draconis) is fossilized animal bones and *Long Chi* (Dens Draconis) is fossilized animal teeth. Both pacify restless *shen* (spirit), and have common application such as restlessness, palpitations, insomnia, anxiety, and seizures or mania in severe cases. *Long Gu* is used as an astringent to stop spermatorrhea, vaginal discharge, uterine bleeding or sweating. In addition, calcined forms of *Long Gu* treat non-healing ulcers and sores. *Long Chi* is sweet, astringent and cool. It is used mainly to pacify the *shen* and treat psychological disorders.

References

1. *Xian Dai Zhong Yao Yao Li Xue* (Contemporary Pharmacology of Chinese Herbs), 1997; 1098-1099
2. *Zhe Jiang Zhong Yi Za Zhi* (Zhejiang Journal of Chinese Medicine), 1982; 6:273

Hu Po (Succinum)

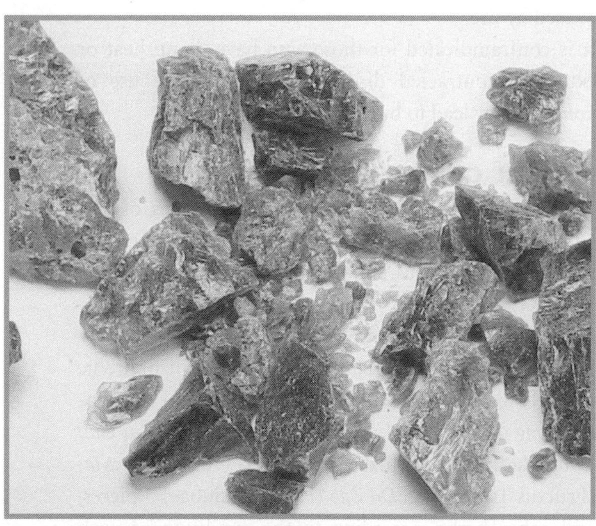

琥珀 琥珀

Pinyin Name: *Hu Po*
Alternate Chinese Names: *Xue Hu Po, Hong Hu Po, Hu Po Xie*
Original Source: *Ming Yi Za Zhu* (Miscellaneous Records of Famous Physicians) by Tao Hong-Jing in 500 A.D.
English Name: amber
Pharmaceutical Name: Succinum
Properties: sweet, neutral
Channels Entered: Heart, Liver, Urinary Bladder

CHINESE THERAPEUTIC ACTIONS

1. Arrests Tremors and Calms the *Shen* (Spirit)

***Shen* disturbance causing restlessness, insomnia, palpitations, forgetfulness, tremors, seizures, infantile convulsions:** Depending on the other herbs with which it is combined, *Hu Po* (Succinum) treats a variety of *shen* disturbance problems caused by fire or hot phlegm misting the Heart.

- Restlessness, insomnia, palpitations: use *Hu Po* with *Ren Shen* (Radix Ginseng), *Fu Shen* (Poria Paradicis), *Yuan Zhi* (Radix Polygalae) and *Shi Chang Pu* (Rhizoma Acori).
- Infantile convulsions: combine it with *Tian Zhu Huang* (Concretio Silicea Bambusae), *Fu Ling* (Poria) and *Dan Nan Xing* (Arisaema cum Bile).
- Epilepsy or trance: use this substance with *Zhu Sha* (Cinnabaris), *Niu Huang* (Calculus Bovis), *Quan Xie* (Scorpio), *Tian Zhu Huang* (Concretio Silicea Bambusae) and *Dan Nan Xing* (Arisaema cum Bile).

2. Invigorates Blood Circulation and Dissipates Stasis

Menstrual disorders, amenorrhea: Blood and qi stagnation in the lower *jiao* results in menstrual disorders such as amenorrhea. Other symptoms of blood and qi stagnation may include palpable masses in the abdomen.

- Palpable masses and pain: use *Hu Po* with *San Leng* (Rhizoma Sparganii), *E Zhu* (Rhizoma Curcumae), and *Yan Hu Suo* (Rhizoma Corydalis).
- Amenorrhea or postpartum bleeding due to qi and blood stagnation: combine this substance with *Bie Jia*

Hu Po (Succinum)

(Carapax Trionycis), *Hong Hua* (Flos Carthami), *Tao Ren* (Semen Persicae) and *Wu Ling Zhi* (Excrementum Trogopteri seu Pteromi).

Coronary heart disorders:
- Blood stagnation causing angina: use *Hu Po* with *San Qi* (Radix Notoginseng) as powder for internal use.

Hematoma of the scrotum:
- Blood stagnation in the lower *jiao*: use *Hu Po* alone as a powder. Administer 0.9 grams of powder, taken internally twice daily with water, for 9 to 10 days.
- Traumatic injury to the scrotum: use *Hu Po* with *Ru Xiang* (Gummi Olibanum) and *Mo Yao* (Myrrha).

3. Promotes Urination

***Lin zheng* (dysuria syndrome):** Urinary dysfunction such as hematuria, burning dysuria, urinary retention and urinary stones can be treated with *Hu Po*.
- Hematuria: use it with *Deng Xin Cao* (Medulla Junci) and *Da Ji* (Herba seu Radix Cirsii Japonici).
- Urinary stone: add it to *Hai Jin Sha* (Herba Lygodii), *Jin Qian Cao* (Herba Lysimachiae), *Pu Huang* (Pollen Typhae), *Mo Yao* (Myrrha) and *Tong Cao* (Medulla Tetrapanacis).
- Kidney stones with hematuria: use *Hu Po* alone in powder form.
- Burning dysuria: combine it with *Chuan Mu Tong* (Caulis Clematidis Armandii), *Bian Xu* (Herba Polygoni Avicularis) and *Ze Xie* (Rhizoma Alismatis).

4. Reduces Swelling and Promotes Healing

Non-healing ulcerated sores: use *Hu Po* topically with *Zhen Zhu* (Margarita), *Xue Jie* (Sanguis Draconis) and *Chi Shi Zhi* (Halloysitum Rubrum).

DOSAGE

1.5 to 3 grams in powder form. *Hu Po* is usually taken as powder or pills. It is <u>not</u> to be processed with fire and heat, as processing at high temperature decreases its effectiveness.

CAUTIONS / CONTRAINDICATIONS

- *Hu Po* is contraindicated for patients with yin-deficient heat and/or frequent urination.
- Use of this herb may be associated with drowsiness and sedation. Therefore, individuals who take this herb should exercise caution if driving or operating heavy machinery.

CHEMICAL COMPOSITION

Diabietinolic acid, succinic acid, succoxyabietic acid, succinoabietinolic acid, succinosilvic acid, succinoresinol, succinoabietol, succinic acid, benzine, resin, essential oils, trace amounts of Mg, Ca, Fe, Al, Pb, Zn, Ni, Sn, Ti, Mn, Sr.[1,2]

PHARMACOLOGICAL EFFECTS

- **CNS suppressant:** Administration of *Hu Po* in mice reduced spontaneous movement and prolonged sleeping time induced by barbiturates.[3]

CLINICAL STUDIES AND RESEARCH

- **Scrotal hematoma:** Oral ingestion of 0.9 grams of powdered *Hu Po* twice daily (1.8 grams daily dose) for 8 to 10 days showed marked effectiveness in 3 patients with scrotal hematoma.[4]

HERB-DRUG INTERACTION

- **Sedatives:** *Hu Po* potentiates the sedative effect of barbiturates. [Note: Many categories of drugs induce sedation, such as antihistamines, narcotic analgesics, barbiturates, benzodiazepines and many others.][5]

References

1. *Zhong Yao Xue* (Chinese Herbology), 1998; 670-671
2. *Xian Dai Ben Cao Gang Mu* (Contemporary Materia Medica), 2000; 2709
3. *Zhong Yao Xue* (Chinese Herbology), 1998; 670-671
4. *Shang Hai Zhong Yi Yao Za Zhi* (Shanghai Journal of Chinese Medicine and Herbology), 1958; 11:33
5. *Zhong Yao Xue* (Chinese Herbology), 1998; 670-671

Section 2

— Nourishing Herbs that Calm the Shen (Spirit)

Suan Zao Ren (Semen Zizyphi Spinosae)

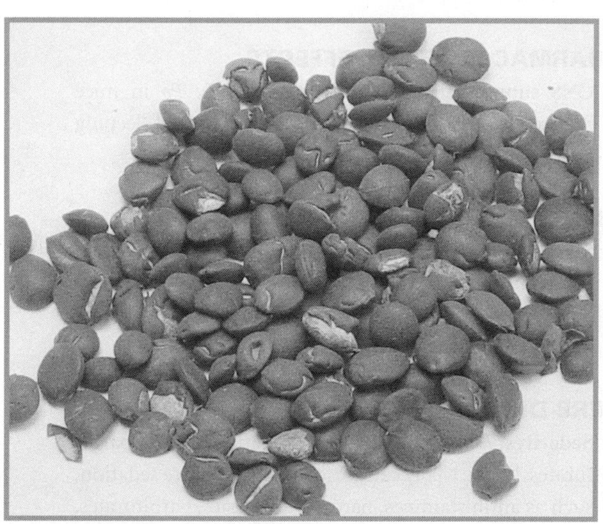

酸棗仁 酸枣仁

Pinyin Name: *Suan Zao Ren*
Literal Name: "sour date seed"
Original Source: *Shen Nong Ben Cao Jing* (Divine Husbandman's Classic of the Materia Medica) in the second century
English Name: zizyphus, spiny date seed
Botanical Name: *Ziziphus jujuba* Mill. var. *spinosa* (Bunge) Hu ex H.F. Chou (*Suan Zao*)
Pharmaceutical Name: Semen Zizyphi Spinosae
Properties: sweet, neutral
Channels Entered: Heart, Liver

CHINESE THERAPEUTIC ACTIONS

1. Nourishes the Heart and Calms the *Shen* (Spirit)

***Shen* disturbance due to Spleen and Heart deficiencies:** The Heart dominates blood and the Spleen produces blood. Insomnia or difficulty falling or staying asleep, palpitations, excessive dreaming, shallow sleep with a tendency to wake easily, fatigue, poor appetite, forgetfulness, and sallow complexion are all symptoms of a deficient Spleen not producing sufficient blood to nourish the Heart and *shen.*

- *Shen* disturbance due to Spleen and Heart deficiencies: use *Suan Zao Ren* with *Ren Shen* (Radix Ginseng), *Huang Qi* (Radix Astragali), *Dang Gui* (Radicis Angelicae Sinensis) and *Long Yan Rou* (Arillus Longan). **Exemplar Formula:** *Gui Pi Tang* (Restore the Spleen Decoction).

***Shen* disturbance due to Liver yin deficiency:** The Liver stores the blood necessary to nourish the *shen* of the Heart. When Liver yin is deficient, the patient may experience irritability, bad temper, insomnia, palpitations, dizziness, tinnitus and vertigo, night sweating, thirst, dry mouth and a wiry, thready pulse.

- *Shen* disturbance due to Liver yin deficiency: combine *Suan Zao Ren* with *Bai Shao* (Radix Paeoniae Alba), *Ye Jiao Teng* (Caulis Polygoni Multiflori), *Shi Jue Ming* (Concha Haliotidis), *Sheng Di Huang* (Radix Rehmanniae), *Fu Shen* (Poria Paradicis), *Mu Li* (Concha Ostreae) and *Long Chi* (Dens Draconis). **Exemplar Formula:** *Suan Zao Ren Tang* (Sour Jujube Decoction).

***Shen* disturbance due to Heart and Kidney deficiencies:** This condition is characterized by insomnia, palpitations, thirst with dry mouth and throat due to Kidney yin deficiency, with inability to nourish the Heart. Other symptoms may include nocturnal emissions in men, forgetfulness, dry stools, ulcers on the tongue, a red tongue with scanty coating, and a thready, rapid pulse.

- *Shen* disturbance due to Heart and Kidney deficiencies: use *Suan Zao Ren* with *Sheng Di Huang* (Radix Rehmanniae), *Wu Wei Zi* (Fructus Schisandrae Chinensis), *Dang Gui* (Radicis Angelicae Sinensis) and

Suan Zao Ren (Semen Zizyphi Spinosae)

Bai Zi Ren (Semen Platycladi). **Exemplar Formula:** *Tian Wang Bu Xin Dan* (Emperor of Heaven's Special Pill to Tonify the Heart).

Neurasthenia is often associated with blood deficiency and lack of nourishment to the *shen.*

- Neurasthenia: use *Suan Zao Ren* alone as powder and ingest before bedtime.

2. Prevents Sweating

Spontaneous or night sweating due to qi deficiency or yin deficiency: *Suan Zao Ren* is used as symptomatic treatment to stop sweating.

- Spontaneous sweating: combine *Suan Zao Ren* with *Huang Qi* (Radix Astragali), *Dang Shen* (Radix Codonopsis) and *Wu Wei Zi* (Fructus Schisandrae Chinensis).
- Night sweating: use this herb with *Shan Zhu Yu* (Fructus Corni), *Mu Li* (Concha Ostreae) and *Wu Wei Zi* (Fructus Schisandrae Chinensis).

DOSAGE

10 to 18 grams in decoction. The maximum dose for *Suan Zao Ren* is 30 grams. Crush before decocting to increase the surface area and enhance the extraction of active constituents. As a powder, take 1.5 to 3 grams before bedtime. Unprepared *Suan Zao Ren* is cooler and better for insomnia with heat signs. The dry-fried form is warmer, and better for Heart and Spleen deficiencies with palpitations, poor appetite and spontaneous sweating. The dry-fried form has a more potent effect to calm the *shen* and relieve insomnia. Dry frying is done by cooking the herb at a low temperature until the seeds turn dark in color, expand in size, or burst. The dry-fried herb should also be crushed prior to decoction. Once dry fried, it should be used as quickly as possible to prevent loss of efficacy.

CAUTIONS / CONTRAINDICATIONS

- *Suan Zao Ren* is contraindicated in patients with insomnia caused by excess heat or by hot phlegm accumulation.
- Use it with caution for patients who have diarrhea or an exterior condition.
- Use of this herb may be associated with drowsiness and sedation. Therefore, individuals who take this herb should exercise caution if driving or operating heavy machinery.
- *Suan Zao Ren* should be used with caution during pregnancy, as it stimulates contraction of the uterus.

CHEMICAL COMPOSITION

Jujuboside, betulin, betulinic acid, jujubogenin, ebetinlaetone, zivulgarin, spinosin, swertisin, ceanothic acid, alphitolic acid.[1,2]

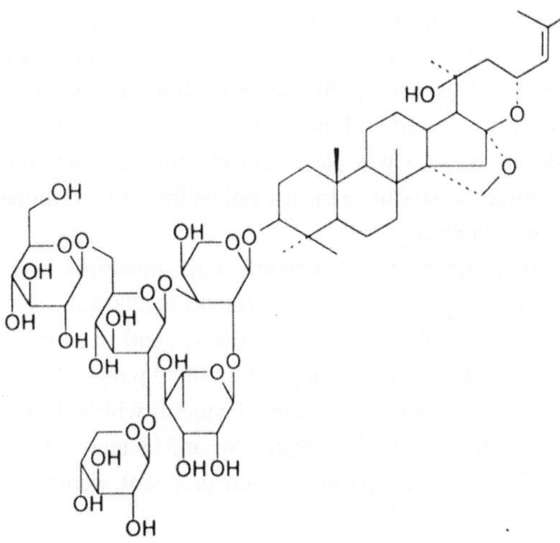

Jujuboside A

PHARMACOLOGICAL EFFECTS

- **Sedative and hypnotic:** Administration of *Suan Zao Ren* is associated with a sedative and hypnotic effect in mice, rats, cats, rabbits, dogs, and guinea pigs. It reduces spontaneous activities in a dose-dependent fashion, prolongs sleeping time induced by barbiturates, reverses excitation caused by caffeine, and inhibits hyperactivity induced by morphine. Both fresh and fried forms of the herb have demonstrated sedative and hypnotic effects with no statistically-significant differences between the two. Jujuboside is considered by many to be the main component responsible for the sedative and hypnotic effects.[3]
- **Cardiovascular:** Decoction of *Suan Zao Ren* has negative chronotropic, positive inotropic and positive cardiotonic effects in frog heart specimens. Clinically, it treats arrhythmia caused by aconitine, chloroform, and barium chloride.[4,5]
- **Uterine stimulant:** Water extract of *Suan Zao Ren* has a stimulating effect on smooth muscle and causes contraction of the uterus.[6]
- **Analgesic:** Decoction of *Suan Zao Ren* at 5 g/kg has a marked analgesic effect in mice.[7]
- **Antipyretic:** A reduction in body temperature has been observed following oral ingestion of decoction of *Suan Zao Ren* at 40 g/kg in cats or 2.5 to 5.0 g/kg via intraperitoneal injection in rats.[8]

CLINICAL STUDIES AND RESEARCH

- **Insomnia:** According to one report, 30 patients with insomnia were treated with *Suan Zao Ren*, with significant improvement in 9 cases, moderate improvement in 19 cases, and no response in 2 cases. The treatment protocol was to incorporate *Suan Zao Ren* as ear seeds, applied to ear points such as *Shenmen*, Endocrine, Heart, Kidney, and Brain, using 1 to 2 points per treatment. Ear

Suan Zao Ren (Semen Zizyphi Spinosae)

seeds and points were changed every 5 days, with a total of 4 sessions per course of treatment. Prior to application, *Suan Zao Ren* was first soaked in hot water, then the skin was removed and the seeds split in halves. The flat side of the seed was placed on the ear. Patients were instructed to stimulate the ear points for 3 to 5 minutes prior to bedtime.[9]

In another study, patients with insomnia were allowed to drink 15 grams of green tea at 8:00 a.m., with no other stimulants throughout the day, and 10 grams of *Suan Zao Ren* powder at night. Out of 39 patients, complete recovery was reported in 34 patients within 3 to 10 days. Patients who had hypertension, increased heart rate, habitual constipation, or were pregnant, were treated with caution.[10]

- **Neurasthenia:** Administration of *Suan Zao Ren Tang* (Sour Jujube Decoction) showed satisfactory effects in treating 129 patients with neurasthenia characterized by insomnia, irritability, and fidgeting.[11]
- **Altitude stress:** In one clinical study, 76 people traveling to Tibet were divided into two groups, with one group receiving *Suan Zao Ren* and the other group receiving a placebo. All patients were instructed to take the herbs for 11 days, starting 3 days prior to departure, and continue for 3 days after arrival in Tibet. At the end of the study, it was concluded that the patients who received *Suan Zao Ren* experienced significantly less altitude sickness, including symptoms such as headache, dizziness, palpitations, nausea, dyspnea, and poor appetite. The incidence of vomiting was approximately the same between both groups.[12]

HERB-DRUG INTERACTION

- **Sedatives:** *Suan Zao Ren* has sedative and hypnotic effects. It potentiates the sedative effect of barbiturates, and reverses the stimulating effect of caffeine. Jujuboside is considered by many to be the main component responsible for the sedative and hypnotic effects.[13] [Note: Many categories of drugs induce sedation, such as antihistamines, narcotic analgesics, barbiturates, benzodiazepines and many others.]

TOXICOLOGY

Suan Zao Ren is a very safe herb. Up to 70 grams may be used in clinical application without toxic reactions. In animal toxicology studies, decoction of *Suan Zao Ren* at 150 g/kg did not show any toxicity. The LD_{50} for intraperitoneal injection of *Suan Zao Ren* is 14.3 g/kg in mice.[14]

AUTHORS' COMMENTS

Suan Zao Ren and *Bai Zi Ren* (Semen Platycladi) are both used for treating irritability, insomnia, anxiety and palpitations arising from deficient blood reserves failing to nourish the Heart. *Suan Zao Ren* is stronger to calm the *shen* (spirit) and also has an astringent action to stop spontaneous or night sweating. *Bai Zi Ren* is rich in oil and functions to lubricate the intestines.

References

1. *Xian Dai Zhong Yao Yao Li Xue* (Contemporary Pharmacology of Chinese Herbs), 1997; 1073
2. Yan X, Zhou J, Xie G, *Traditional Chinese Medicines Molecular Structures, Natural Sources and Applications*; Ashgate, 1999; 3664
3. *Chang Yong Zhong Yao Xian Dai Yan Jiu Yu Lin Chuan* (Recent Study & Clinical Application of Common Traditional Chinese Medicine), 1995; 489:491
4. *Zhong Guo Shou Yi Za Zhi* (Chinese Journal of Husbandry), 1988; 14(6):44
5. *Di Yi Jun Yi Da Xue Xue Bao* (Journal of First Military University of Medicine), 1985; 5(1):31
6. *Zhong Yao Xue* (Chinese Herbology), 1998; 671:673
7. *Chang Yong Zhong Yao Xian Dai Yan Jiu Yu Lin Chuan* (Recent Study & Clinical Application of Common Traditional Chinese Medicine), 1995; 489:491
8. Ibid.
9. *Xin Zhong Yi* (New Chinese Medicine), 1982; (11):35
10. *Shang Hai Zhong Yi Yao Za Zhi* (Shanghai Journal of Chinese Medicine and Herbology), 1984; (10):30
11. *Zhong Xi Yi Jie He Za Zhi* (Journal of Integrated Chinese and Western Medicine), 1982; 2:97
12. *Zhong Yao Yao Li Yu Lin Chuan* (Pharmacology and Clinical Applications of Chinese Herbs), 1986; 2(1):44
13. *Chang Yong Zhong Yao Xian Dai Yan Jiu Yu Lin Chuan* (Recent Study & Clinical Application of Common Traditional Chinese Medicine), 1995; 489:491
14. *Zhong Yao Tong Bao* (Journal of Chinese Herbology), 1987; 12(8):51

Bai Zi Ren (Semen Platycladi)

柏子仁

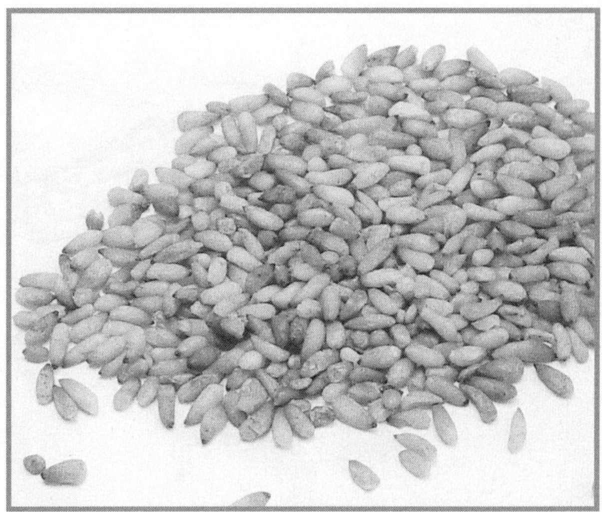

Pinyin Name: *Bai Zi Ren*
Literal Name: "lateral cypress kernel," "oriental arborvitae seed"
Original Source: *Shen Nong Ben Cao Jing* (Divine Husbandman's Classic of the Materia Medica) in the second century
English Name: platycladus seed, biota seed, Chinese arborvitae seed, Oriental arborvitae seed
Botanical Name: *Platycladus orientalis* (L.) Franco; [also known as *Biota orientalis* (L.) Endl.]
Pharmaceutical Name: Semen Platycladi
Properties: sweet, neutral
Channels Entered: Heart, Kidney, Large Intestine

CHINESE THERAPEUTIC ACTIONS

1. Nourishes the Heart and Calms the *Shen* (Spirit)

Insomnia due to Heart blood deficiency: *Bai Zi Ren* (Semen Platycladi) is rich in oil and is best for blood-deficient insomnia with dry stools or constipation. It is most suitable for feelings of insecurity, insomnia, palpitations, night sweats, anxiety, and forgetfulness caused by excessive worrying damaging the Spleen and Heart.

- Insomnia, palpitations, dizziness and forgetfulness: combine *Bai Zi Ren* with *Ren Shen* (Radix Ginseng), *Wu Wei Zi* (Fructus Schisandrae Chinensis), *Fu Shen* (Poria Paradicis), *Suan Zao Ren* (Semen Zizyphi Spinosae) and *Dang Gui* (Radicis Angelicae Sinensis).

2. Moistens the Intestines and Unblocks the Bowels

Constipation or dry stools in elderly, anemic or postpartum patients, due to yin or blood deficiencies.

- Dry stools or constipation: combine *Bai Zi Ren* with *Tao Ren* (Semen Persicae), *Xing Ren* (Semen Armeniacae Amarum), *Dang Gui* (Radicis Angelicae Sinensis), *Huo Ma Ren* (Fructus Cannabis) and *Gua Lou Ren* (Semen Trichosanthis).

DOSAGE

10 to 18 grams. Crush *Bai Zi Ren* seeds before decocting, to facilitate the extraction of active constituents.

CAUTIONS / CONTRAINDICATIONS

- *Bai Zi Ren* should be used with caution for patients with loose stools or excess phlegm.

CHEMICAL COMPOSITION

Saponins, lipids, essential oils.[1]

PHARMACOLOGICAL EFFECTS

- **Gastrointestinal:** *Bai Zi Ren* has mild effect to lubricate the bowel and relieve constipation.[2]

AUTHORS' COMMENTS

Bai Zi Ren and *Suan Zao Ren* (Semen Zizyphi Spinosae) are both used for treating irritability, insomnia, anxiety, palpitations, and other symptoms caused by inability of blood to nourish the Heart. The herbs differ in that *Bai Zi Ren* is rich in oil and functions to lubricate the intestines, while *Suan Zao Ren* is stronger to calm the *shen* and also has an astringent function to stop spontaneous or night sweating.

References

1. *Zhong Yao Xue* (Chinese Herbology), 1998; 674
2. Ibid., 673:674

14 SHEN-CALMING HERBS

Yuan Zhi (Radix Polygalae)

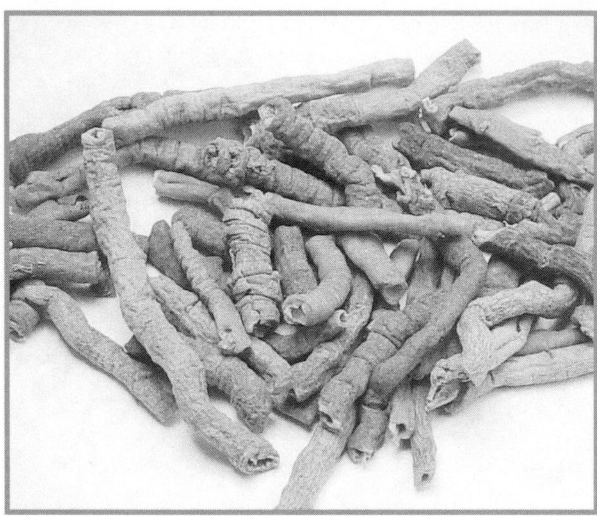

遠志 远志

Pinyin Name: *Yuan Zhi*
Literal Name: "profound will," "long determination"
Alternate Chinese Names: *Yuan Zhi Tong, Yuan Zhi Rou, Guan Yuan Zhi*
Original Source: *Shen Nong Ben Cao Jing* (Divine Husbandman's Classic of the Materia Medica) in the second century
English Name: polygala, thin-leaf milkwort root, Siberian milkwort root
Botanical Name: *Polygala tenuifolia* Willd. (*Yuan Zhi*), *Polygala sibirica* L. (*Ruan Ye Yuan Zhi*)
Pharmaceutical Name: Radix Polygalae
Properties: acrid, bitter, slightly warm
Channels Entered: Lung, Heart

CHINESE THERAPEUTIC ACTIONS

1. Pacifies the Heart and Calms the *Shen* (Spirit)

Disturbed *shen* with insomnia, Heart and Kidney deficiencies: *Yuan Zhi* (Radix Polygalae) strengthens Heart qi, and disperses stagnation in the Heart. It is mostly used for restlessness, palpitations, insomnia, or weakness of the Kidney and Heart that result in symptoms of nocturnal emissions, spermatorrhea and forgetfulness. Honey-fried *Yuan Zhi* more strongly nourishes the Heart and calms the *shen.*

- Insomnia, palpitations with anxiety, restlessness and disorientation, nocturnal emissions and spermatorrhea: combine *Yuan Zhi* with *Fu Shen* (Poria Paradicis), *Long Chi* (Dens Draconis) or *Zhu Sha* (Cinnabaris).
- Forgetfulness, memory loss or inability to concentrate: use this herb with *Ren Shen* (Radix Ginseng), *Fu Ling* (Poria), *Yin Guo Ye* (Folium Ginkgo) and *Shi Chang Pu* (Rhizoma Acori).
- Insomnia, excessive dreaming: use honey-fried *Yuan Zhi* as a single-herb remedy.

2. Expels Phlegm and Clears the Orifices

Phlegm obstructing the Heart and orifices, seizures: *Yuan Zhi* has an excellent ability to dispel phlegm in the Heart that manifests in mental or emotional disorientation, seizures, or hearing loss from phlegm blocking the orifices.

- Disorientation, seizures: combine it with *Shi Chang Pu* (Rhizoma Acori), *Yu Jin* (Radix Curcumae), *Tian Zhu Huang* (Concretio Silicea Bambusae) and *Dan Nan Xing* (Arisaema cum Bile).

3. Expels Phlegm from the Lung

Phlegm stagnation in the Lung: *Yuan Zhi* dispels phlegm in the Lung to treat cough with white sputum. Clinical applications include bronchitis, pneumonia and other respiratory disorders.

- Cough with white sputum arising from cold: add this herb to *Xing Ren* (Semen Armeniacae Amarum), *Jie Geng* (Radix Platycodonis) and *Gan Cao* (Radix Glycyrrhizae).

4. Reduces Abscesses and Dissipates Swellings

This herb is commonly used to treat boils, abscesses, sores, or swollen and painful breasts caused by phlegm obstructing the channels and collaterals. *Yuan Zhi* can be taken internally as powder with liquor, or made into a paste to be applied topically.

DOSAGE

3 to 9 grams. Fresh *Yuan Zhi* more strongly dispels phlegm and opens orifices, while honey-processed *Yuan Zhi* more effectively calms the *shen* (spirit) and tranquilizes the mind. However, fresh or unprocessed *Yuan Zhi* is sometimes irritating to the throat. This irritation can be eliminated by dry frying *Yuan Zhi*, or by boiling it with *Gan Cao* (Radix Glycyrrhizae) in hot water.

To enhance its effect to eliminate phlegm and stop coughing, the herb may be processed with honey.

CAUTIONS / CONTRAINDICATIONS

- Because *Yuan Zhi* is drying in nature, use it with caution in patients experiencing heat symptoms or hot phlegm.
- Use *Yuan Zhi* with caution in patients who have gastritis, peptic or duodenal ulcers. *Gan Cao* (Radix Glycyrrhizae) can be added to ease the irritating effect *Yuan Zhi* has on the stomach and to prevent nausea and vomiting.

Yuan Zhi (Radix Polygalae)

- *Yuan Zhi* should be used with caution during pregnancy, as it stimulates uterine contraction.

CHEMICAL COMPOSITION

Onjisaponin A, B, C, D, E, F, G; tenuigenin A, B; tenuifolin, presenegenin, tenuidine, polygalitol, xanthones, 3,4,5-trimethoxycinnamic acid, 6-hydroxy-1,2,3,7-tetramethoxyxanthone.[1]

PHARMACOLOGICAL EFFECTS

- **Expectorant:** *Yuan Zhi* has demonstrated a marked expectorant effect in mice and dogs. Its potency is similar to that of *Jie Geng* (Radix Platycodonis).[2]
- **CNS suppressant:** The root, bark and entire plant of *Polygala tenuifolia* have all demonstrated sedative effects in mice. It may also prevent seizures and convulsions.[3]
- **Diuretic:** A 50% alcohol extract of *Yuan Zhi* has demonstrated marked diuretic effects in treating edema.[4]
- **Antibiotic:** Water extract of *Yuan Zhi* has an inhibitory effect against *Diplococcus pneumoniae.* Alcohol extract has an inhibitory effect against *Bacillus dysenteriae*, *Salmonella typhi*, and *Mycobacterium tuberculosis hominis.*[5]
- **Uterine stimulant:** Administration of both water and alcohol extracts of *Yuan Zhi* has a stimulating effect on the uterus in both pregnant and non-pregnant laboratory animals such as rabbits, cats, and dogs.[6]

CLINICAL STUDIES AND RESEARCH

- **Acute mastitis:** In one study, 62 patients with acute mastitis were treated with satisfactory results using *Yuan Zhi.* The herbal decoction was prepared by soaking 12 grams of the herb in 15 ml of grain-based liquor, then cooking it with a bowl of water for 15 to 20 minutes. In another study, patients with acute mastitis were treated with topical applications of an herbal paste. The paste was prepared by cooking 500 grams of *Yuan Zhi* in 1,500 ml of water for 5 to 6 hours to yield a paste-like preparation. It is most effective during early-stage acute mastitis without pus formation.[7,8]
- **Trichomonal vaginitis:** According to one report, 36 out of 37 patients with trichomonal vaginitis reported complete recovery following herbal treatment with vaginal suppository. The herbal suppository contained 1 part *Yuan Zhi*, 2 parts *Bu Gu Zhi* (Fructus Psoraleae) and 2 parts *Da Huang* (Radix et Rhizoma Rhei).[9]

HERB-DRUG INTERACTION

- **Ethanol:** In an *in vitro* study, a traditional Chinese medicinal preparation (composed of *Yuan Zhi*, *Ren Shen* (Radix Ginseng), *Shi Chang Pu* (Rhizoma Acori) and *Fu Ling* (Poria)) reduced the ethanol-induced impairment of memory registration. It also ameliorated the scopolamine-induced memory registration deficit. These results suggest that the herbal preparation ameliorates the impairment effect of ethanol on learning and memory processes.[10]
- **Diuretics:** *Yuan Zhi* has a diuretic effect. Though this potential interaction has not been documented, concurrent use with diuretic drugs may lead to increased elimination of water and/or electrolytes.[11] [Note: Examples of diuretics include chlorothiazide, hydrochlorothiazide, furosemide (Lasix), bumetanide (Bumex), and torsemide (Demadex).]

AUTHORS' COMMENTS

Yuan Zhi and *Shi Chang Pu* (Rhizoma Acori) both dissolve phlegm, open the orifices, and calm the *shen.* They both treat delirium, mania, stupor, insomnia, forgetfulness or restless *shen* caused by the accumulation of turbid phlegm in the Heart. *Yuan Zhi* is mainly used to dissolve phlegm and stop coughing. It is used for patients with cough and profuse sputum that is difficult to expectorate. *Yuan Zhi* also disperses nodules or abscesses and relieves pain. *Shi Chang Pu* dissolves dampness and is stronger in harmonizing the Stomach to treat feelings of congestion or pain in the chest and abdomen.

References

1. *Xian Dai Zhong Yao Yao Li Xue* (Contemporary Pharmacology of Chinese Herbs), 1997; 1077
2. *Zhong Yao Yao Li Yu Ying Yong* (Pharmacology and Applications of Chinese Herbs), 1983; 477
3. Ibid.
4. *Chem Pharm Bull*, 1979; 27(6):1464
5. *Zhong Yao Yao Li Yu Ying Yong* (Pharmacology and Applications of Chinese Herbs), 1983; 477
6. *Xian Dai Zhong Yao Yao Li Xue* (Contemporary Pharmacology of Chinese Herbs), 1997; 1077-78.
7. *Xin Yi Yao Tong Xun* (Journal of New Medicine and Herbology), 1973; 6:5
8. *Zhong Yi Za Zhi* (Journal of Chinese Medicine), 1981; 22(4):78
9. *Tian Jing Yi Yao* (Tianjing Medicine and Herbology), 1982; 10(7):436
10. *Biological and Pharmaceutical Bulletin.* 17(11):1472-6, Nov 1994
11. Chen, J. Recognition & prevention of Herb-drug interactions, *Medical Acupuncture*, Fall/Winter 1998/1999; volume 10/number 2; 9-13

He Huan Pi (Cortex Albiziae)

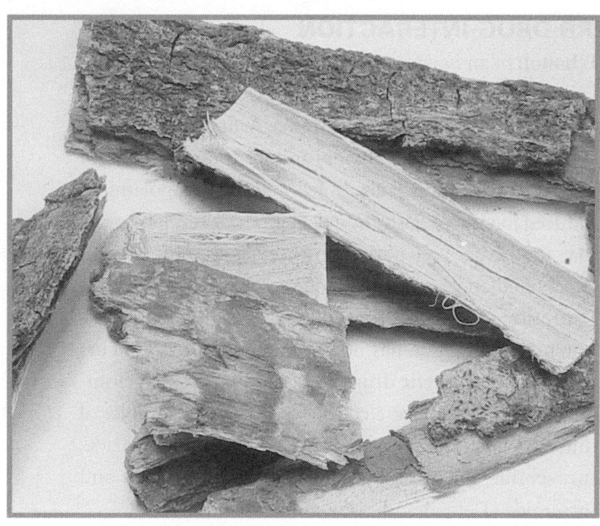

合歡皮 合欢皮

Pinyin Name: *He Huan Pi*
Literal Name: "collective happiness bark"
Original Source: *Shen Nong Ben Cao Jing* (Divine Husbandman's Classic of the Materia Medica) in the second century
English Name: albizia bark, silk tree albizia bark
Botanical Name: *Albizia julibrissin* Durazz. (*He Huan*); *Albizia kalkora* (Roxb) (*Shan He Huan*)
Pharmaceutical Name: Cortex Albiziae
Properties: sweet, neutral
Channels Entered: Heart, Liver

CHINESE THERAPEUTIC ACTIONS

1. Calms the *Shen* (Spirit) and Relieves Constraint

Emotional constraint due to Liver qi stagnation: *He Huan Pi* (Cortex Albiziae) treats short temper, depression, insomnia, irritability, pre-menstrual syndrome and forgetfulness. *He Huan Pi* is mild and is usually used as an adjunct to other tranquilizing herbs.

- Emotional disturbance: combine *He Huan Pi* with *Suan Zao Ren* (Semen Zizyphi Spinosae), *Bai Zi Ren* (Semen Platycladi), *Long Chi* (Dens Draconis) and *Hu Po* (Succinum).

2. Invigorates the Blood and Reduces Swelling

Pain and swelling due to traumatic injury, including bone fractures: *He Huan Pi* invigorates blood circulation, reduces swelling, promotes generation of flesh, and facilitates healing of bone fractures. It is one of the most important herbs for treatment of external trauma and injuries.

- Pain and swelling: combine *He Huan Pi* with *Dang Gui* (Radicis Angelicae Sinensis), *Chi Shao* (Radix Paeoniae Rubrae), *Tao Ren* (Semen Persicae) and *Su Mu* (Lignum Sappan).

He Huan Pi is also effective to treat vomiting of sputum and blood.

- Lung abscesses with chest pain and coughing of sputum and blood: use this herb with *Yu Xing Cao* (Herba Houttuyniae), *Dong Gua Zi* (Semen Benincasae), *Tao Ren* (Semen Persicae) and *Lu Gen* (Rhizoma Phragmitis).
- Abscess and swellings: use *He Huan Pi* with *Pu Gong Ying* (Herba Taraxaci Mongolici cum Radice), *Zi Hua Di Ding* (Herba Violae) and *Ye Ju Hua* (Flos Chrysanthemi Indici).

DOSAGE

10 to 15 grams.

CAUTIONS / CONTRAINDICATIONS

- *He Huan Pi* should be used with caution during pregnancy, as it stimulates contraction of the uterus.

CHEMICAL COMPOSITION

Albitocin, β-sitosterol, α-amyrin, 3,4,7-trihydroxyflavone, α-spinasterylglucoside, machaerinic acid lactone, machaerinic acid, methyl ester, acacic acid lactone.[1]

PHARMACOLOGICAL EFFECTS

- **CNS suppressant:** *He Huan Pi* has sedative and hypnotic actions. Administration of *He Huan Pi* in mice is associated with a reduction of spontaneous movement.[2]
- **Uterine stimulant:** It has a stimulating effect on smooth muscle and causes contraction of the uterus.[3]

TOXICOLOGY

Gross overdose of albitocin is linked with fatality in mice between 12 hours and 7 days following ingestion. The exact reason of fatality is unknown, but is attributed to necrosis of liver and kidney cells.[4]

SUPPLEMENT

- 合歡花 / 合欢花 *He Huan Hua* (Flos Albiziae), first cited in *Ben Cao Yan Yi* (Extension of the Materia Medica) by Kou Zong-Shi in 1116, is derived from the flower of the same plant as *He Huan Pi*. It is also known as *Ye He Hua* or *Ye He Mi*. It calms the *shen*, relieves Liver constraint, regulates qi and harmonizes the Stomach. *He Huan Hua* is primarily used for chest and epigastric fullness and

He Huan Pi (Cortex Albiziae)

pain with irritability, restlessness, forgetfulness and insomnia from deficiency. Its effect is mild, thus, it should be used with other herbs for maximum effectiveness.

AUTHORS' COMMENTS

He Huan Hua (Flos Albiziae), *Ye Jiao Teng* (Caulis Polygoni Multiflori) and *Bai Zi Ren* (Semen Platycladi) all treat insomnia. *He Huan Hua* is best for insomnia due to Liver qi stagnation. *Ye Jiao Teng* is for insomnia due to general blood deficiency and *Bai Zi Ren* is for insomnia due to Heart deficiency.

References

1. *Xian Dai Zhong Yao Yao Li Xue* (Contemporary Pharmacology of Chinese Herbs), 1997; 1097
2. *Zhong Yao Xue* (Chinese Herbology), 1998; 676:677
3. *Chang Yong Zhong Yao Cheng Fen Yu Yao Li Shou Ce* (A Handbook of the Composition and Pharmacology of Common Chinese Drugs), 1994; 886:887
4. *Chang Yong Zhong Yao Xian Dai Yan Jiu Yu Lin Chuan* (Recent Study & Clinical Application of Common Traditional Chinese Medicine), 1995; 495:496

Ye Jiao Teng (Caulis Polygoni Multiflori)

夜交藤 夜交藤

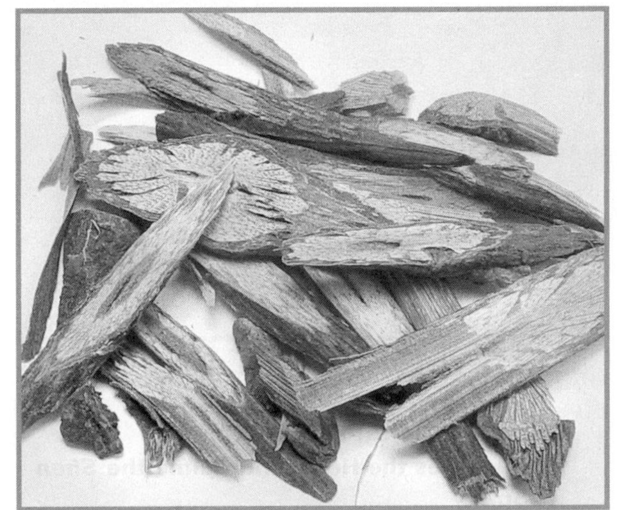

Pinyin Name: *Ye Jiao Teng*
Literal Name: "vine of the night," "vine to pass through the night"
Alternate Chinese Names: *Jiao Teng, Shou Wu Teng*
English Name: polygonum vine
Botanical Name: *Polygonum multiflorum* Thunb.
Pharmaceutical Name: Caulis Polygoni Multiflori
Properties: sweet, slightly bitter, neutral
Channels Entered: Heart, Liver

CHINESE THERAPEUTIC ACTIONS

1. Nourishes the Heart and Calms the *Shen* (Spirit)

Heart blood deficiency: *Ye Jiao Teng* (Caulis Polygoni Multiflori) treats the lack of nourishment to the Heart that causes sleep disorders such as insomnia, difficulty falling asleep or staying asleep, and excessive dreams.

- Insomnia: use *Ye Jiao Teng* with *Suan Zao Ren* (Semen Zizyphi Spinosae), *He Huan Hua* (Flos Albiziae), and *Bai Zi Ren* (Semen Platycladi).

2. Opens the Channels and Collaterals and Dispels Wind

- Soreness and pain in the limbs from blood deficiency: add this herb to *Ren Dong Teng* (Caulis Lonicerae) and *Wu Jia Pi* (Cortex Acanthopanacis).
- Eczema, rash and itching of the skin: use 15 to 30 grams of *Ye Jiao Teng* externally as a wash.
- *Bi zheng* (painful obstruction syndrome) due to yin or blood deficiencies: add this herb to *Wei Ling Xian* (Radix Clematidis), *Du Huo* (Radix Angelicae Pubescentis), and *Qiang Huo* (Rhizoma et Radix Notopterygii).

DOSAGE

15 to 30 grams in decoction. *Ye Jiao Teng* is also used as an external herbal paste, to relieve itching.

CHEMICAL COMPOSITION

Emodin, physcion, β-sitosterol, emodin-8-O-β-D-monoglucoside.[1]

Ye Jiao Teng (Caulis Polygoni Multiflori)

AUTHORS' COMMENTS

Ye Jiao Teng, He Huan Hua (Flos Albiziae) and *Bai Zi Ren* (Semen Platycladi) all treat insomnia. The difference is that *Ye Jiao Teng* corrects insomnia due to general blood deficiency, *He Huan Hua* is best for insomnia caused by Liver qi stagnation, and *Bai Zi Ren* addresses insomnia from Heart deficiency.

References

1. *Xian Dai Zhong Yao Yao Li Xue* (Contemporary Pharmacology of Chinese Herbs), 1997; 1095

Ling Zhi (Ganoderma)

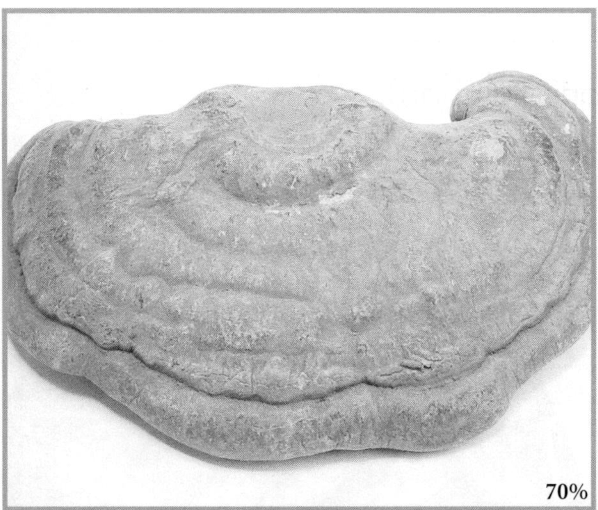

70%

靈芝 灵芝

Pinyin Name: *Ling Zhi*
Literal Name: "spiritual mushroom"
Alternate Chinese Names: *Mu Ling Zhi, Zi Ling Zhi*
Original Source: *Shen Nong Ben Cao Jing* (Divine Husbandman's Classic of the Materia Medica) in the second century
English Name: ganoderma, lucid ganoderma, reishi mushroom
Botanical Name: *Ganoderma lucidum* (Leyss. Ex. Fr.) Karst. (*Chi Zhi*); *Ganoderma japonicum* (Fr.) Lloyd. (*Zi Zhi*)
Pharmaceutical Name: Ganoderma
Properties: sweet, neutral
Channels Entered: Heart, Liver, Lung

CHINESE THERAPEUTIC ACTIONS

1. Nourishes the Heart and Calms the *Shen* (Spirit)

Restless *shen*: *Ling Zhi* (Ganoderma) nourishes the Heart and strengthens qi and blood to treat Heart and Spleen deficiencies that manifest in insomnia, forgetfulness, fatigue, listlessness and poor appetite.

- Insomnia: combine *Ling Zhi* with *Dang Gui* (Radicis Angelicae Sinensis), *Bai Shao* (Radix Paeoniae Alba), *Suan Zao Ren* (Semen Zizyphi Spinosae) and *Long Yan Rou* (Arillus Longan).

2. Stops Coughing and Arrests Wheezing

Cough and asthma: *Ling Zhi* dispels phlegm, stops cough and arrests wheezing. Symptoms include coughing caused by cold, coughing with profuse sputum, accelerated respiration, chronic asthma and difficulty sleeping due to dyspnea.

- Asthma and coughing: add it to *Dang Shen* (Radix Codonopsis), *Wu Wei Zi* (Fructus Schisandrae Chinensis), *Gan Jiang* (Rhizoma Zingiberis) and *Ban Xia* (Rhizoma Pinelliae).

3. Tonifies Qi and Nourishes Blood

Qi and blood deficiencies, weak digestion: *Ling Zhi* has traditionally been used to strengthen the body and tonify qi. It treats qi and blood deficiencies with weak digestion, poor appetite, listlessness, loose stools, fatigue, dizziness and soreness of the lower back.

- Qi and blood deficiencies: use *Ling Zhi* alone.

DOSAGE

3 to 15 grams in decoction, 1.5 to 3 grams in powder.

CHEMICAL COMPOSITION

Ganoderic acid, lucidenic acid, ganoderma acid, ganodosterone oleic acid.[1]

Ling Zhi (Ganoderma)

PHARMACOLOGICAL EFFECTS

- **Antineoplastic:** *Ling Zhi* has been shown to have antineoplastic activity due to its immune-enhancing properties. The specific effects of *Ling Zhi* include an increase in monocytes, macrophages and T-lymphocytes. In addition, there is also an increased production of cytokine, interleukin, tumor-necrosis-factor and interferon.[2]
- **Cardiovascular:** *Ling Zhi* has been shown to increase cardiac contractility, lower blood pressure, and increase resistance to hypoxia in the cardiac muscles.
- **Antibiotic:** *Ling Zhi* has a broad spectrum of antibacterial activity, and inhibits the growth of *E. coli, B. dysenteriae, Pseudomonas* spp., pneumococci, streptococci (type A), staphylococci, and others.[3]
- **Others:** *Ling Zhi* exerts hepatoprotective, antidiabetic, antitussive, expectorant, sedative, analgesic, and antiasthmatic effects.

CLINICAL STUDIES AND RESEARCH

- **Neurasthenia:** Administration of *Ling Zhi* (3 grams three times daily for 10 to 60 days) showed 83.5 to 86.3% effectiveness in treating 225 patients with neurasthenia. The therapeutic effects of *Ling Zhi* include sedation, hypnosis, regulation of the nervous system, and enhancement of the immune system.[4]
- **Hyperlipidemia:** In one study, 120 patients with high cholesterol levels were treated with 4 to 6 ml of *Ling Zhi* syrup two to three times daily for 1 to 3 months with 86% rate of effectiveness.[5]
- **Leukopenia:** Administration of *Ganoderma japonicum* was associated with a rise in leukocyte counts in 72.57% of 175 patients with leukopenia.[6]
- **Chronic hepatic diseases:** In one study, 367 patients with chronic hepatic diseases, such as chronic hepatitis, and chronic infectious hepatitis, and liver cirrhosis, were treated with *Ling Zhi* extract as tea, with good results. Most patients reported subjective symptomatic improvement. In addition, the study reported a reduction in liver enzymes in 67.7% of patients.[7]
- **Dermatological disorders:** Concurrent administration of *Ling Zhi* via intramuscular injection and oral tablets was 79.1% effective in treating 173 patients with scleroderma, 95% effective in 40 patients with dermatomyositis, 90% effective in 84 patients with lupus erythematosus, and 78.88% effective in 232 patients with alopecia areata.[8]
- **Frostbite:** According to one report, 428 patients with frostbite were treated with *Ling Zhi* topically with a 89.5% rate of effectiveness after 3 or 4 days.[9]

AUTHORS' COMMENTS

Because wild-crafted *Ling Zhi* is rare and difficult to collect, the cultivated mushroom is generally used commercially.

Ling Zhi has recently been used to treat angina pectoris, hepatitis, high cholesterol, hypertension and leukopenia.

References

1. *Xian Dai Zhong Yao Yao Li Xue* (Contemporary Pharmacology of Chinese Herbs), 1997; 1079
2. *International Journal of Cancer*, 1997 Mar 17; 70(6):699-705
3. *Handbook Of Chinese Herbs. Institute of Chinese Medicine*, 1996
4. *Xin Yi Xue* (New Medicine), 1976; 3:140
5. *Zhong Cao Tong Xun* (Journal of Chinese Herbs), 1973; 1:31
6. *Zhong Hua Xue Yi Za Zhi* (Chinese Journal of Hematology), 1985; 7:428
7. *Lin Chuan Gan Dan Bing Za Zhi* (Clinical Journal of Hepatic and Gallbladder Diseases), 1985; 4:242
8. *Xi Yao Yan Jiu Tong Xun* (Research Journal of Medicine and Herbology), 1984; 12:22
9. *Lin Chuan Pi Fu Ke Za Zhi* (Clinical Journal of Dermatology), 1986; 6:296

Xie Cao (Radix et Rhizoma Valerianae)

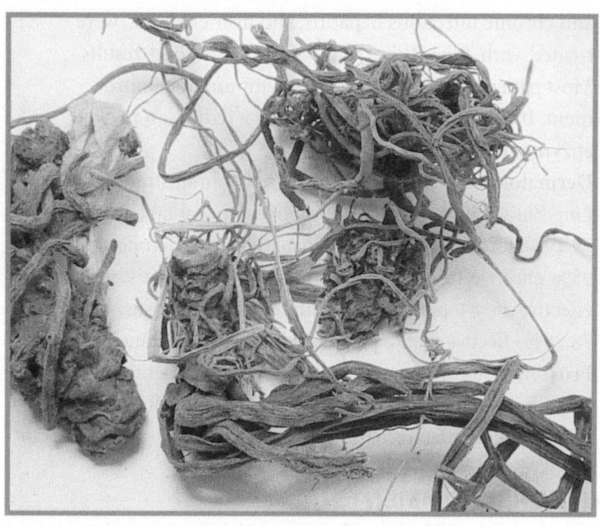

纈草 缬草

Pinyin Name: *Xie Cao*
Alternate Chinese Names: *Guang Ye Ba Di Ma, Jie Cao*
English Name: valerian root, valerian
Botanical Name: *Valeriana officinalis; Valeriana fauriei* Briquet
Pharmaceutical Name: Radix et Rhizoma Valerianae
Properties: bitter, sweet, neutral
Channels Entered: Heart, Liver

CHINESE THERAPEUTIC ACTIONS

1. Tranquilizes the *Shen* (Spirit)

***Shen* disturbance:** Clinical applications of *Xie Cao* (Radix et Rhizoma Valerianae) include insomnia, emotional stress and excessive worrying.

- Neurasthenia: use *Xie Cao* with *Wu Wei Zi* (Fructus Schisandrae Chinensis) in decoction or as herbal tincture.

2. Relieves Spasms and Pain

Liver qi stagnation: Clinical manifestations include muscle tightness and spasms, stomach cramps, dysmenorrhea and pre-menstrual syndrome.

- Muscle aches and pains: use this herb with *Bai Shao* (Radix Paeoniae Alba) and *Gan Cao* (Radix Glycyrrhizae).

DOSAGE

2 to 5 grams.

CAUTIONS / CONTRAINDICATIONS

Use of *Xie Cao* may be associated with drowsiness and sedation. Therefore, individuals who take this herb should exercise caution if driving or operating heavy machinery.

CHEMICAL COMPOSITION

Essential oils 0.5-2.0% (bornyl isovalerate, borneol, l-camphene, α-pinene, d-terpineol, l-limonene); flavonoids (quercetin, diosmelin, acacetin, apigenie); alkaloids (β-valerine, chatinine, alkaloid A, B, actinidine, valeriamine); terpenoids (valepotriate, isovaleroxy-hydroxy-dihydrovaltrate, valechlorine, 7-epideacetyl-isovaltrate, valeridine, valerosidatum, acevaltrate); and organic acids (valerenic acid, valerenolic acid, behenic acid, hesperitinic acid, β-bisabolene, curcumene, ledol, maaliol).[1,2]

Valerenic acid

PHARMACOLOGICAL EFFECTS

- **Sedative:** Essential oil of *Xie Cao* administered orally at 2 ml/kg effectively prolonged the sleeping time induced by barbiturates.[3]
- **Antispasmodic and analgesic:** Administration of *Xie Cao* is associated with an antispasmodic effect, and valerenic acid is associated with an analgesic effect.[4,5]
- **Cardiovascular:** Administration of *Xie Cao* is associated with a decrease in blood pressure, dilation of blood vessels, and increased blood perfusion to the cardiac muscle. Following studies on dogs, cats, and rabbits, it was proposed that the antihypertensive effect of *Xie Cao* is due in part to its inhibitory effect on the sympathetic nervous system. It was also noted that following injection of a *Xie Cao* preparation, there is an immediate and prolonged dilation of blood vessels, which, in turn, significantly increases blood perfusion to peripheral parts of the body. Specifically for the heart, there is a 5.7 time increase in blood perfusion to the cardiac muscles. Lastly, intravenous injection of *Xie Cao* has a preventative effect against arrhythmia induced by adrenalin, aconitine and other chemicals.[6,7,8]

CLINICAL STUDIES AND RESEARCH

- **Insomnia:** In a randomized, placebo-controlled, multicenter study, 121 patients were divided into either an

Xie Cao (Radix et Rhizoma Valerianae)

herb group or a placebo group. Both groups received pills one hour before bedtime for 28 consecutive days. The subjects in the herb group received 600 mg of 70% alcohol extract of *Xie Cao* standardized to 0.4 to 0.6% valerenic acid. At the end of the trial, the study reported good or very good results in 66% of subjects in the herb group, compared to only 29% in the placebo group.[9]

HERB-DRUG INTERACTION

- **Sedatives:** *Xie Cao* potentiates the sedative effect of barbiturates.[10] [Note: Many categories of drugs induce sedation, such as antihistamines, narcotic analgesics, barbiturates, benzodiazepines and many others.]

TOXICOLOGY

The LD_{50} for essential oil of *Xie Cao* in mice is 2,950 mg/kg for intravenous injection, 4,760 mg/kg via intraperitoneal injection, and 7.14 ml/kg via oral administration.[11]

References

1. *Xian Dai Zhong Yao Yao Li Xue* (Contemporary Pharmacology of Chinese Herbs), 1997; 1092
2. Yan X, Zhou J, Xie G, *Traditional Chinese Medicines Molecular Structures, Natural Sources and Applications*; Ashgate, 1999; 6573
3. *Xian Dai Zhong Yao Yao Li Xue* (Contemporary Pharmacology of Chinese Herbs), 1997; 1092
4. *Zhi Wu Yao You Xiao Cheng Fen Shou Ce* (Manual of Plant Medicinals and Their Active Constituents), 1986; 1107
5. *Xian Dai Zhong Yao Yao Li Xue* (Contemporary Pharmacology of Chinese Herbs), 1997; 1093
6. *Guo Wai Yao Xue Zhi Wu Yao Fen Ce* (Foreign Study of Medicine: Herbology), 1982; (3): 24
7. *Yao Xue Xue Bao* (Journal of Herbology), 1982; (5): 382
8. *Zhong Yao Yao Li Yu Lin Chuan* (Pharmacology and Clinical Applications of Chinese Herbs), 1989; 5(6):15
9. *PDR for Herbal Medicine*, 2nd Edition, Medical Economics Company, 2000; 783-786
10. *Xian Dai Zhong Yao Yao Li Xue* (Contemporary Pharmacology of Chinese Herbs), 1997; 1092
11. *Zhong Yao Yao Li Yu Lin Chuan* (Pharmacology and Clinical Applications of Chinese Herbs), 1989; 5(6):15

Xiao Mai (Fructus Tritici)

小麥 小麦

Pinyin Name: *Xiao Mai*
Literal Name: "little wheat"
Alternate Chinese Names: *Huai Xiao Mai, Jing Xiao Mai*
English Name: wheat
Botanical Name: *Triticum aestivum* L. (*Xiao Mai*)
Pharmaceutical Name: Fructus Tritici
Properties: sweet, cool
Channels Entered: Heart

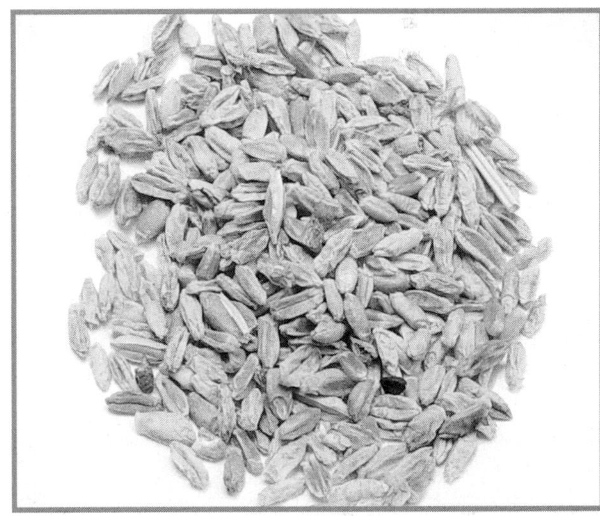

CHINESE THERAPEUTIC ACTIONS

1. Nourishes the Heart and Relieves Irritability

***Zang zao* (dry organ) disorder:** *Xiao Mai* (Fructus Tritici) treats patients who suffer from *zang zao* disorder with symptoms such as excessive worrying, anxiety, pensiveness, disorientation, frequent melancholy and crying spells, dream-disturbed sleep and depression. The cause of this disorder is Liver qi stagnation along with qi and blood deficiencies.

- *Zang zao* disorder: use *Xiao Mai* with *Da Zao* (Fructus Jujubae) and *Gan Cao* (Radix Glycyrrhizae). **Exemplar Formula:** *Gan Mai Da Zao Tang* (Licorice, Wheat, and Jujube Decoction).
- Severe emotional disturbance: combine this herb with *Chai*

Xiao Mai (Fructus Tritici)

Hu (Radix Bupleuri), *Xiang Fu* (Rhizoma Cyperi), *Bai Shao* (Radix Paeoniae Alba), *Yuan Zhi* (Radix Polygalae), *Fu Shen* (Poria Paradicis), *Zhen Zhu Mu* (Concha Margaritaferae) and *Long Chi* (Dens Draconis). **Exemplar Formula:** *Chai Hu Jia Long Mu Tang* (Bupleurum plus Dragon Bone and Oyster Shell Decoction).

2. Promotes Urination

Dysuria: *Xiao Mai* treats difficult, painful urination due to heat accumulation in the Urinary Bladder.

- Dysuria: use *Xiao Mai* with *Tong Cao* (Medulla Tetrapanacis) and *Che Qian Cao* (Herba Plantaginis).

DOSAGE

15 to 30 grams in decoction.

CHEMICAL COMPOSITION

Starch, proteins, carbohydrates, lipids, fiber, enzymes, vitamins.[1]

AUTHORS' COMMENTS

Xiao Mai (Fructus Tritici) and *Fu Xiao Mai* (Semen Tritici Aestivi Levis) are derived from the same plant, but have different characteristics and functions. When *Xiao Mai* and *Fu Xiao Mai* are both placed in water, *Xiao Mai* sinks and *Fu Xiao Mai* floats. *Xiao Mai* can nourish the Heart and calm *shen* (spirit), while *Fu Xiao Mai* has astringent functions to stop sweating.

References

1. *Xian Dai Ben Cao Gang Mu* (Contemporary Materia Medica), 2000; 200

Chapter 14 summary

— Shen-Calming Herbs

SECTION 1: SEDATIVE HERBS THAT CALM THE *SHEN* (SPIRIT)

Name	Similarities	Differences
Zhu Sha (Cinnabaris)	Sedate the Heart, calm the *shen*	Treats sores and abscesses when used externally, toxic when taken internally
Ci Shi (Magnetitum)		Anchors Liver yang, stops wheezing
Long Gu (Os Draconis)		Anchors Liver yang, prevents leakage of fluids
Hu Po (Succinum)		Treats seizures and convulsions due to hot phlegm obstructing the Heart, activates blood circulation, treats dysuria

General Characteristics of Sedative Herbs that Calm the *Shen* (Spirit):

Taste: sweet
Thermal property: neutral, cold
Channels entered: Heart, Liver
Therapeutic actions: sedate the Heart, calm the *shen*

These are usually mineral or shell substances that anchor the *shen* of the Heart, relieving insomnia, palpitations, anger, irritability, restlessness, and in severe cases, mania and epilepsy.

Zhu Sha (Cinnabaris), ***Ci Shi*** (Magnetitum), ***Long Gu*** (Os Draconis) and ***Hu Po*** (Succinum) all tranquilize the *shen.*

Zhu Sha clears Heart fire disturbing the *shen*. It is rarely used today because of its toxicity.

Ci Shi clears rising yang secondary to yin deficiency.

Long Gu anchors Liver yang to calm the *shen*. It has astringent effects to stop leakage of body fluids, such as spontaneous sweating, night sweating, leukorrhea, and chronic dysentery.

Hu Po dispels hot phlegm to calm the *shen*. It also invigorates blood circulation, disperses stasis, promotes urination, and treats *lin zheng* (dysuria syndrome).

SECTION 2: NOURISHING HERBS THAT CALM THE *SHEN* (SPIRIT)

Name	Similarities	Differences
Suan Zao Ren (Semen Zizyphi Spinosae)	Nourish the Heart, calm the *shen*	Nourishes Spleen, Liver, and Kidney to calm deficiency-type *shen* disturbances, stops perspiration
Bai Zi Ren (Semen Platycladi)		Eases excessive worrying that has caused Heart blood deficiency, relieves constipation
Yuan Zhi (Radix Polygalae)		Eliminates phlegm obstructing the Heart
He Huan Pi (Cortex Albiziae)		Soothes Liver qi stagnation, activates blood circulation and reduces swelling
Ye Jiao Teng (Caulis Polygoni Multiflori)		Opens channels and collaterals, dispels wind
Ling Zhi (Ganoderma)		Arrests cough, tonifies qi and blood
Xie Cao (Radix et Rhizoma Valerianae)		Soothes Liver to relieve spasms and pain
Xiao Mai (Fructus Tritici)		Relieves irritability, promotes urination

Chapter 14 summary

General Characteristics of Nourishing Herbs that Calm the *Shen* (Spirit):

Taste: sweet
Thermal property: neutral
Channels entered: Heart, Spleen, Liver
Therapeutic actions: nourish the Heart, calm the *shen*

Nourishing herbs that calm the *shen* are plant substances used for *shen*-disturbance characterized by deficiency, with such signs and symptoms as palpitations, insomnia, excessive dreaming and memory loss.

Suan Zao Ren (Semen Zizyphi Spinosae) and ***Bai Zi Ren*** (Semen Platycladi) are the most frequently used herbs in this category.

Suan Zao Ren tonifies the Liver, tranquilizes the *shen* and is essential in treatment of insomnia caused by deficiency heat.

Bai Zi Ren nourishes the Heart and calms the *shen* and is used for insomnia and palpitations from blood deficiency. It also lubricates the Large Intestine and treats dry stools or constipation.

Yuan Zhi (Radix Polygalae) tranquilizes the Heart, dispels phlegm and reduces abscesses. It disperses phlegm that is misting the Heart, thus relieves palpitations, insomnia and manic behaviors. *Yuan Zhi* treats insomnia and excessive dreaming arising from disharmony between the Heart and Kidney.

He Huan Pi (Cortex Albiziae) and ***Ye Jiao Teng*** (Caulis Polygoni Multiflori) tranquilize the *shen* and relieve insomnia.

He Huan Pi is best for insomnia caused by Liver qi stagnation.

Ye Jiao Teng corrects insomnia due to general blood deficiency.

Ling Zhi (Ganoderma) calms the *shen* and nourishes and strengthens the constitution. It also stops coughing.

Xie Cao (Radix et Rhizoma Valerianae) has excellent effects to calm the *shen* and relieve Liver qi stagnation.

Xiao Mai (Fructus Tritici) nourishes the Heart, relieves irritability, promotes normal urination, and treats *zang zao* (dry organ) disorder caused by Heart yin deficiency.

HERBS FROM OTHER FUNCTIONAL CATEGORIES WITH *SHEN*-CALMING FUNCTIONS

Name	Functional Category
Bai He (Bulbus Lilii)	Tonic Herbs (Chapter 17)
Da Zao (Fructus Jujubae)	Tonic Herbs (Chapter 17)
Dan Shen (Radix Salviae Miltiorrhizae)	Blood-Invigorating and Stasis-Removing Herbs (Chapter 12)
Fu Shen (Poria Paradicis)	Water-Regulating and Damp-Resolving Herbs (Chapter 6)
Fu Xiao Mai (Semen Tritici Aestivi Levis)	Astringent Herbs (Chapter 18)
Lian Zi (Semen Nelumbinis)	Astringent Herbs (Chapter 18)
Long Yan Rou (Arillus Longan)	Tonic Herbs (Chapter 17)
Mai Men Dong (Radix Ophiopogonis)	Tonic Herbs (Chapter 17)
Mu Li (Concha Ostreae)	Liver-Calming and Wind-Extinguishing Herbs (Chapter 15)
Ren Shen (Radix Ginseng)	Tonic Herbs (Chapter 17)
Shi Chang Pu (Rhizoma Acori)	Orifice-Opening Herbs (Chapter 16)
Wu Wei Zi (Fructus Schisandrae Chinensis)	Astringent Herbs (Chapter 18)
Zhen Zhu (Margarita)	Liver-Calming and Wind-Extinguishing Herbs (Chapter 15)
Zhen Zhu Mu (Concha Margaritaferae)	Liver-Calming and Wind-Extinguishing Herbs (Chapter 15)

Chapter 15

— Liver-Calming and Wind-Extinguishing Herbs

平肝息风药

Chapter 15

— Liver-Calming and Wind-Extinguishing Herbs

Chapter 15 — Liver-Calming and Wind-Extinguishing Herbs

平肝息风药

Definition: Substances said to calm Liver wind and sedate Liver yang address a complex range of disorders involving the need to regulate or sedate mild-to-severe spontaneous movement or seizures, heat and mood disturbances, and problems in the head, face and eyes.

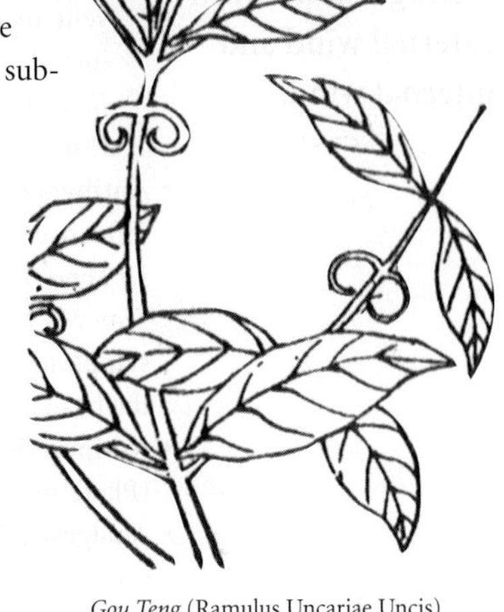

Gou Teng (Ramulus Uncariae Uncis)
Ben Cao Gang Mu (Materia Medica),
by Li Shi-Zhen, 1578 A.D.

W***ind*** disorders may attack via both exterior and interior routes. As discussed in chapter 1, **external** wind is dispelled by herbs that release the exterior. **Internal** wind, though, must be addressed by incorporating substances that calm the Liver and extinguish pathogenic wind.

SUBCATEGORIES OF ACTION

Substances that calm Liver wind and sedate Liver yang are not generally divided into subcategories, although,

- some *calm Liver wind,*
- some *sedate Liver yang,* and
- some *purge Liver fire.*

Most of these herbs are cool to cold in temperature, and enter the Liver channel. Many substances in this section are animal medicinals.

DIFFERENTIAL DIAGNOSIS AND TREATMENT

Liver disorders may arise from either deficient or excess conditions.

- ***Deficiency conditions*** develop from Liver yin deficiency.
- ***Excess conditions*** involve the presence of Liver wind, Liver yang rising, or Liver fire. All three excess conditions have the same origin, but have different presentations and implications.

Differential Diagnosis of Liver Excess

Diagnosis	Characteristics	Symptoms
Liver wind	movement, mobile in nature	dizziness, vertigo, headache, seizures, tremors, convulsions, sudden unconsciousness, deviation of the eyes and mouth, and hemiplegia
Liver yang	internal heat surging upwards	dizziness, vertigo, restlessness, irritability, anger, insomnia, and excessive dreaming
Liver fire	internal fire surging upwards	pain, redness and swelling of the eyes, and numerous other eye disorders

Optimal treatment depends heavily on correct differential diagnosis and treatment. Liver-based disorders may be primarily deficient, primarily excess, or a combination of both. Dysfunction arising from *Liver yin deficiency* requires treatment with yin-tonifying herbs (see Chapter 17 for herbs appropriate for treatment of Liver yin deficiency). Patients with excess conditions, such as *Liver wind, Liver yang rising* or *Liver fire,* must be treated, respectively, with herbs that calm Liver wind, sedate Liver yang, and purge Liver fire. If complications include phlegm, herbs that dissolve and dispel phlegm must be prescribed. If there are excessive dreams and emotional disturbance, herbs that calm the *shen* (spirit) must be included.

Chapter 15 – Liver-Calming and Wind-Extinguishing Herbs

CAUTIONS/CONTRAINDICATIONS

Herbs that are *cold* should be used with caution in cases of deficiency and cold of the Spleen and Stomach. Herbs that are *hot* should be used with caution in cases of yin or blood deficiency.

PROCESSING

Where indicated, requirements for pre-processing individual herbs should be followed carefully.

PHARMACOLOGICAL EFFECTS

For effective treatment, one must distinguish between external wind and internal wind.

- **Antiseizure and antiepileptic**: Many of these herbs are excellent for prevention and treatment of seizures and epilepsy. In clinical studies, single-herb treatment has been less than satisfactory. Combination therapy is needed in most cases to effectively control seizures and epilepsy. In animal studies, many herbs exert an inhibitory influence on the central nervous system to decrease spontaneous physical activity, prolong sleeping time induced by barbiturates, and prevent drug-induced seizures. Examples of herbs with antiseizure and antiepileptic actions include *Tian Ma* (Rhizoma Gastrodiae), *Gou Teng* (Ramulus Uncariae cum Uncis), *Ling Yang Jiao* (Cornu Saigae Tataricae), *Quan Xie* (Scorpio), *Wu Gong* (Scolopendra), *Di Long* (Pheretima), and *Bai Jiang Cao* (Herba cum Radice Patriniae).
- **Antihypertensive**: Liver-calming and wind-extinguishing herbs can have moderate and sustained influence to lower blood pressure, as demonstrated by *Gou Teng* (Ramulus Uncariae cum Uncis), *Di Long* (Pheretima), *Ling Yang Jiao* (Cornu Saigae Tataricae), *Jue Ming Zi* (Semen Cassiae) and *Tian Ma* (Rhizoma Gastrodiae). In addition, many of them effectively treat hypertension-related symptoms. For example, *Tian Ma* (Rhizoma Gastrodiae) and *Jue Ming Zi* (Semen Cassiae) relieve the headache and dizziness that often accompany hypertension.
- **Antipyretic**: Some herbs, including *Ling Yang Jiao* (Cornu Saigae Tataricae), and *Di Long* (Pheretima), lower body temperature in animals with artificially-induced fevers.
- **Analgesic**: There are strong pain relievers in this category, including *Tian Ma* (Rhizoma Gastrodiae), *Gou Teng* (Ramulus Uncariae cum Uncis), *Ling Yang Jiao* (Cornu Saigae Tataricae), and *Jiang Can* (Bombyx Batryticatus).

POTENTIAL HERB-DRUG INTERACTIONS

- **Sedatives**: Herbs with antiseizure and antiepileptic action may induce drowsiness, and should be used with caution by patients concurrently taking drugs that also have sedative properties, such as alcohol, benzodiazepines, opioid analgesics, and barbiturates.
- **Antihypertensives**: Herbs with antihypertensive action may lower blood pressure. To avoid inducing hypotension, they should not be used aggressively by patients already taking antihypertensive medications.

Ling Yang Jiao (Cornu Saigae Tataricae)

羚羊角 羚羊角

Pinyin Name: *Ling Yang Jiao*
Literal Name: "antelope horn"
Original Source: *Shen Nong Ben Cao Jing* (Divine Husbandman's Classic of the Materia Medica) in the second century
English Name: antelope horn
Zoological Name: *Saiga tatarica* L. (*Ling Yang*)
Pharmaceutical Name: Cornu Saigae Tataricae
Properties: salty, cold
Channels Entered: Liver, Heart

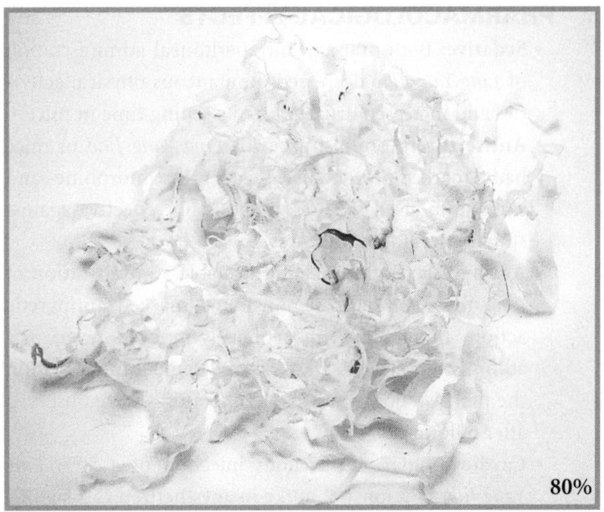

CHINESE THERAPEUTIC ACTIONS

1. Calms the Liver and Extinguishes Wind

Liver wind: Clinical manifestations of this condition include convulsions in adults and children, spasms, tremors, epilepsy and seizures. *Ling Yang Jiao* (Cornu Saigae Tataricae) clears heat and extinguishes wind simultaneously. It is most suitable for patients who suffer from Liver wind disorders that have arisen with or following high fever caused by Liver yang rising.

- Dizziness, vertigo: incorporate *Ling Yang Jiao* with *Sheng Di Huang* (Radix Rehmanniae), *Gou Teng* (Ramulus Uncariae cum Uncis), *Bai Shao* (Radix Paeoniae Alba) and *Ju Hua* (Flos Chrysanthemi).
- Epilepsy: use this substance with *Fang Feng* (Radix Saposhnikoviae), *Du Huo* (Radix Angelicae Pubescentis) and *Fu Shen* (Poria Paradicis).
- Epilepsy, palpitations and fear: combine it with *Gou Teng* (Ramulus Uncariae cum Uncis), *Tian Zhu Huang* (Concretio Silicea Bambusae), *Yu Jin* (Radix Curcumae) and *Zhu Sha* (Cinnabaris).

2. Calms the Liver and Anchors Liver Yang

Rising Liver yang: Hypertension, red eyes, dizziness, vertigo, irritability, insomnia, a bitter taste in the mouth, short temper, nightmares, and sensations of burning and pain in the hypochondrium, are all symptoms associated with Liver yang rising.

- Hypertension and associated symptoms: use *Ling Yang Jiao* with *Shi Jue Ming* (Concha Haliotidis), *Ju Hua* (Flos Chrysanthemi) and *Huang Qin* (Radix Scutellariae).

3. Clears the Liver and Brightens the Eyes

Eye disorders caused by Liver fire: Red, swollen and painful eyes, headache, photophobia, feelings of pressure and pain in the eyeballs, and blurred vision. The Liver is said to open to the eyes; thus heat rising in the Liver channel results in eye disorders.

- Eye disorders: add *Ling Yang Jiao* to *Jue Ming Zi* (Semen Cassiae), *Long Dan Cao* (Radix Gentianae), *Ju Hua* (Flos Chrysanthemi) and *Huang Qin* (Radix Scutellariae).

4. Clears Heat and Eliminates Toxins

Febrile disorders or heat in the Pericardium: *Ling Yang Jiao* treats high fever, dizziness, delirium, manic behavior, tremors and loss of consciousness.

- High fever, delirium, convulsions: combine this substance with *Shi Gao* (Gypsum Fibrosum), *Han Shui Shi* (Mirabilite), and *She Xiang* (Moschus).
- High fever, delirium and subcutaneous bleeding: use it with *Bai Hu Tang* (White Tiger Decoction).
- End stage of exanthema variolosum with residual toxic heat: add *Ling Yang Jiao* to *Huang Qi* (Radix Astragali) and *Jin Yin Hua* (Flos Lonicerae).

DOSAGE

The dosage of *Ling Yang Jiao* is 1 to 3 grams in decoction, and 0.3 to 0.5 gram when taken in powder or pill form. For decoction, *Ling Yang Jiao* is cooked separately from the rest of the ingredients, then combined with the separate decoction, before ingestion.

CAUTIONS / CONTRAINDICATIONS

- *Ling Yang Jiao* is contraindicated in patients with Spleen deficiency.

CHEMICAL COMPOSITION

Calcium phosphate, protein, cholesterol, keratin.[1]

Ling Yang Jiao (Cornu Saigae Tataricae)

PHARMACOLOGICAL EFFECTS

- **Sedative:** Both oral and intraperitoneal administration of *Ling Yang Jiao* decreased spontaneous physical activities and increased drug-induced sleeping time in mice.[2]
- **Antiseizure:** Administration of *Ling Yang Jiao* in mice had a marked preventative effect against morphine- and caffeine-induced seizures, but was not effective against strychnine-induced seizures.[3]
- **Antipyretic:** Both oral and injectable administration of *Ling Yang Jiao* have demonstrated marked antipyretic action. In rabbits with artificially-induced fever, oral administration at 4 g/kg lowered temperatures within the first two hours; normal temperatures were observed after 6 hours.[4]
- **Cardiovascular:** Intravenous injection of a 50% *Ling Yang Jiao* solution at 2 ml/kg in anesthetized cats significantly lowered blood pressure.[5]

CLINICAL STUDIES AND RESEARCH

- **Fever:** Patients with fevers of various etiologies were treated with intramuscular injection of *Ling Yang Jiao* two to three times daily. Out of 100 patients, there was significant reduction of temperature in 41 cases, moderate reduction in 45 cases, and no change in 14 patients. The rate of effectiveness was 86%.[6]

TOXICOLOGY

No abnormalities were observed following an intravenous bolus dose of 4% *Ling Yang Jiao* preparation at 8 ml/kg (equivalent to 100 times the therapeutic dose in human) in mice. In another study, mice were given a 10% solution at 2 g/kg/day continuously for 7 days. Other than slight weight gain, no abnormalities were observed.[7]

SUPPLEMENT

- 山羊角/山羊角 *Shan Yang Jiao* (Cornu Naemorhedis), the horn of mountain goats, has functions similar to those of *Ling Yang Jiao* (Cornu Saigae Tataricae). However, the effect of *Shan Yang Jiao* is milder and the dosage needs to be larger to achieve the same result. It is cold, salty and enters the Liver channel. It pacifies the Liver and treats Liver yang or Liver fire rising with dizziness, vertigo or convulsions, spasms, and redness, pain and swelling of the eyes. It is combined with *Gou Teng* (Ramulus Uncariae cum Uncis), *Tian Ma* (Rhizoma Gastrodiae), *Shi Jue Ming* (Concha Haliotidis) and *Zao Xiu* (Rhizoma Paridis) for Liver yang rising. It is used with *Long Dan Cao* (Radix Gentianae) and *Huang Lian* (Rhizoma Coptidis) for high fever with tremors and convulsions. Lastly, it is combined with *Sang Ye* (Folium Mori), *Ju Hua* (Flos Chrysanthemi) and *Xia Ku Cao* (Spica Prunellae) for redness and pain of the eyes caused by Liver yang rising. The dosage of *Shan Yang Jiao* is 10 to 15 grams.
- 黄羊角/黄羊角 *Huang Yang Jiao* (Cornu Procapra Gutturosa), the horn of yellow goats, is also used as a substitute for *Ling Yang Jiao*. It is used mainly to treat fever by lowering body temperature.

References

1. *Xian Dai Zhong Yao Yao Li Xue* (Contemporary Pharmacology of Chinese Herbs), 1997; 1102-1103
2. *Zhong Cheng Yao Yan Jiu* (Research of Chinese Patent Medicine), 1981; (4):36
3. *Zhong Yao Yao Li Yu Ying Yong* (Pharmacology and Applications of Chinese Herbs), 1983; 1110
4. Ibid.
5. Ibid.
6. *Zhong Cao Yao Tong Xun* (Journal of Chinese Herbal Medicine), 1977; 1:1
7. *Zhong Yao Yao Li Yu Ying Yong* (Pharmacology and Applications of Chinese Herbs), 1983; 1110

Gou Teng (Ramulus Uncariae cum Uncis)

鉤藤 钩藤

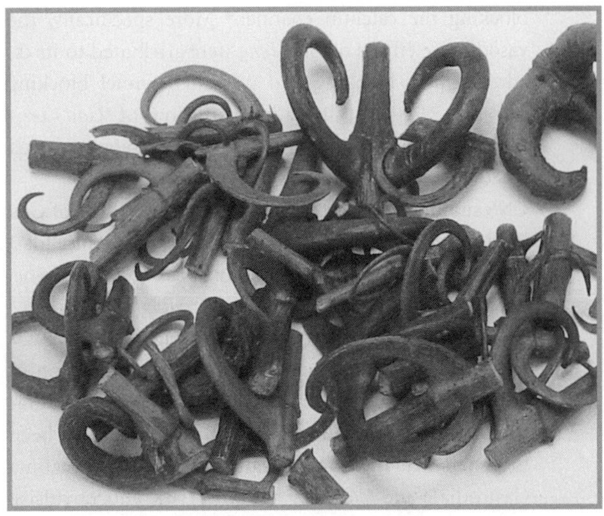

Pinyin Name: *Gou Teng*
Literal Name: "hook vine," "hooky branches"
Alternate Chinese Names: *Shuang Gou Teng, Nen Gou Teng, Shuang Gou Gou*
Original Source: *Ming Yi Za Zhu* (Miscellaneous Records of Famous Physicians) by Tao Hong-Jing in 500 A.D.
English Name: gambir
Botanical Name: *Uncaria rhynchophylla* (Miq.) Jacks. (*Gou Teng*); *Uncaria macrophylla* Wall. (*Da Ye Gou Teng*); *Uncaria hirsuta* Havil. (*Mao Gou Teng*); *Uncaria sinensis* (Oliv.) Havil. (*Hua Gou Teng*); *Uncaria sessifructus* Roxb. (*Wu Bing Ye Gou Teng*)
Pharmaceutical Name: Ramulus Uncariae cum Uncis
Properties: sweet, cool
Channels Entered: Liver, Pericardium

CHINESE THERAPEUTIC ACTIONS

1. Extinguishes Wind and Alleviates Spasms

Liver wind: *Gou Teng* (Ramulus Uncariae cum Uncis) is essential in extinguishing wind and sedating fire. It is commonly used to treat presentations of Liver wind, such as convulsions, tremors, infantile convulsions, high fever, spasms, seizures, eclampsia, clenching of teeth, rolling of eyes, tetany, irritability and restlessness.

- Childhood convulsions, clenching of jaws, tremors: use *Gou Teng* with *Tian Ma* (Rhizoma Gastrodiae) and *Quan Xie* (Scorpio).
- Liver wind: combine this herb with *Quan Xie* (Scorpio), *Wu Gong* (Scolopendra), *Tian Zhu Huang* (Concretio Silicea Bambusae), *Ju Hua* (Flos Chrysanthemi) and *Dan Nan Xing* (Arisaema cum Bile).
- High fever in Liver yang rising: use *Gou Teng* with *Ling Yang Jiao* (Cornu Saigae Tataricae), *Long Dan Cao* (Radix Gentianae), and *Ju Hua* (Flos Chrysanthemi).
- Headache, red and painful eyes, or incomplete eruption of rashes caused by wind-heat: add this herb to *Bo He* (Herba Menthae), *Chan Tui* (Periostracum Cicadae) and *Jing Jie* (Herba Schizonepetae).

Stroke: Liver wind in combination with phlegm may result in sudden stroke, fainting, facial paralysis, hemiplegia or loss of the ability to speak.

- Stroke: combine *Gou Teng* with *Ban Xia* (Rhizoma Pinelliae), *Chen Pi* (Pericarpium Citri Reticulatae), *Bai Ji Li* (Fructus Tribuli), *Chi Shao* (Radix Paeoniae Rubrae), *Di Long* (Pheretima) and *Chuan Shan Jia* (Squama Manis).

2. Clears Heat and Pacifies Liver Yang

Rising Liver yang: Headache, feelings of distention in the head, dizziness, vertigo and hypertension, tinnitus, insomnia, heavy-headed sensations, and involuntary muscle twitching.

- Hypertension with headache, feelings of distention in the head: use *Gou Teng* with *Xia Ku Cao* (Spica Prunellae) and *Huang Qin* (Radix Scutellariae).
- Dizziness and vertigo: add it to *Ju Hua* (Flos Chrysanthemi) and *Shi Jue Ming* (Concha Haliotidis).
- Hypertension: use it with *Tian Ma* (Rhizoma Gastrodiae) and *Bai Ji Li* (Fructus Tribuli).

DOSAGE

10 to 15 grams. The maximum dosage of *Gou Teng* is 30 grams. Post-decoction for no more than ten minutes is recommended. The antihypertensive effect of *Gou Teng* is greatly reduced if cooked for more than 20 minutes.[1]

CHEMICAL COMPOSITION

Rhynchophylline, isorhynchophylline, corynoxeine, isocorynoxeine, corynantheine, dihydrocorynatheine, hirsutine, hirsuteine, hyperin, trifolin.[2]

PHARMACOLOGICAL EFFECTS

- **Antihypertensive:** Administration of *Gou Teng* is associated with moderate and prolonged antihypertensive effects. The decrease in blood pressure is attributed to decreased heart rate and a reduced peripheral vascular resistance. This is observed with normal or anesthetized animals, normotensive or hypertensive animals, and via intravenous or oral routes.[3] Another study characterized *Gou Teng* as a potent and long-lasting vasodilator that relaxes the aorta and thereby reduces blood pressure. *Gou Teng* has demonstrated an effect similar to verapamil in

Gou Teng (Ramulus Uncariae cum Uncis)

blocking the calcium channel.[4] More specifically, the vasodilative effects of *Gou Teng* were attributed to its α-adrenoceptor blocking and calcium channel blocking activities.[5,6] Clinically, administration of *Gou Teng* reduces both systolic and diastolic blood pressure as well as slowing the heart rate.[7,8]

- **CNS suppressant:** Both water and alcohol extracts of *Gou Teng* decrease spontaneous physical activities in mice for 3 to 4 hours. They reverse the stimulating effect of caffeine, but do not prolong sleeping time induced by barbiturates.[9]
- **Antiseizure:** Alcohol extract of *Gou Teng* has a preventative effect in management of seizures. The duration of action was approximately three days following subcutaneous injection in guinea pigs.[10] In addition, it has been indicated that the combination of *Tian Ma* (Rhizoma Gastrodiae) and *Gou Teng* has synergistic anticonvulsive and free-radical scavenging actions, as demonstrated in laboratory studies in rats.[11]
- **Uterine suppressant:** *Gou Teng* inhibits uterine contraction in rats.[12]

CLINICAL STUDIES AND RESEARCH

- **Hypertension:** In one study, 245 patients with hypertension were treated with a preparation of *Gou Teng*, with marked effectiveness in 38.2%, and an overall rate of effectiveness of 77.2%. Effectiveness was defined as significant and prolonged reduction of blood pressure. Patients with hypertension characterized by yin deficiency and yang excess were most responsive to the treatments. Some mild side effects were observed.[13]
- **Infantile night crying:** An herbal decoction was effective in treating 17 out of 18 infants exhibiting constant crying at night. The formula contains *Gou Teng* 3g, *Chan Tui* (Periostracum Cicadae) 3g, and *Bo He* (Herba Menthae) 1g. The decoction was given one time each day for 2 to 3 doses.[14]

HERB-DRUG INTERACTION

- **Caffeine:** *Gou Teng* reverses the stimulating effect of caffeine, but does not potentiate the sedative effect of barbiturates.[15]

TOXICOLOGY

No abnormalities were observed in rabbits following injection of a *Gou Teng* preparation at 5 g/kg twice daily for 10 days. The LD_{50} for intraperitoneal injection of *Gou Teng* decoction was 29.05 g/kg.[16]

AUTHORS' COMMENTS

Gou Teng has a sedative function but not a tranquilizing one. It helps to calm the *shen* (spirit) but does not treat insomnia.

Gou Teng and *Ren Dong Teng* (Caulis Lonicerae) both treat wind. *Gou Teng* is stronger in treating twitching and spasms caused by Liver wind and Liver heat. *Ren Dong Teng* relieves pain due to wind-heat in the channels and collaterals.

Gou Teng and *Tian Ma* (Rhizoma Gastrodiae) both pacify the Liver, extinguish wind and treat twitching, spasms, convulsions, dizziness and headaches caused by Liver wind. These herbs are frequently used together in clinical settings.

- *Gou Teng* is cold and has a stronger effect to extinguish Liver wind by clearing rising Liver yang. It is often used for Liver wind secondary to rising Liver yang in cases such as convulsions with high fever.
- *Tian Ma* is neutral and rich in oil. It does not clear heat as strongly as *Gou Teng*, but is stronger in relieving pain, as the oil moistens dryness and helps to extinguish wind. It is more commonly used to stop pain associated with headache, vertigo, twitching and spasms caused by Liver wind.

References

1. *Zhong Yao Xue* (Chinese Herbology), 1998; 694:696
2. *Xian Dai Zhong Yao Yao Li Xue* (Contemporary Pharmacology of Chinese Herbs), 1997; 1107
3. *Chang Yong Zhong Yao Cheng Fen Yu Yao Li Shou Ce* (A Handbook of the Composition and Pharmacology of Common Chinese Drugs), 1994; 1419:1423
4. Kuramochi, T. et al. *Gou-Teng* (from uncaria rhynchophylla miquel)-induced endothelium-dependent and independent relaxation in the isolated rat aorta. *Life Science*, 54(26):2061-9 1994
5. Ozaki, Y. Vasodilative effects of indole alkaloids obtained from domestic plants uncaria rhynchophylla miq. and amsonia elliptica roem. et schult. *Nippon Yakurigaku Zasshi*, 95(2):47-54 Feb. 1990
6. Horie, S. et al. Effects of hirsutine and antihypertensive indol alkaloid from uncaria rhynchophylla on intracellular calcium in rat thoracic aorta. *Life Science*, 50(7):491-8 1992
7. Yano, S. et al. Calcium channel blocking effects of hirsutine and indol alkaloid from uncaria genus in the isolated rat aorta. *Planta Med*, 57(5):403-5 Oct. 1991
8. Mok, SJ. et al. Cardiovascular responses in the normotensive rat produced by intravenous injection of gambirine isolated from uncariae bl. ex korth.
9. *Zhong Yao Yao Li Yu Ying Yong* (Pharmacology and Applications of Chinese Herbs), 1983; 786
10. *Pharm Pharmacol*, 1985; 37; 401
11. *Life Sci* 1999; 65(20):2071-82
12. *Zhong Guo Yao Li Xue Yu Du Li Xue Za Zhi* (Journal of Herbology and Toxicology), 1988; 2(2):93
13. *Zhong Cao Yao Tong Xun* (Journal of Chinese Herbal Medicine), 1976; 7:45
14. Ibid., 1979; 3:38
15. *Zhong Yao Yao Li Yu Ying Yong* (Pharmacology and Applications of Chinese Herbs), 1983; 786
16. Ibid.

Tian Ma (Rhizoma Gastrodiae)

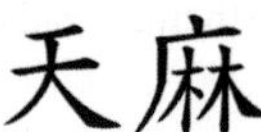

Pinyin Name: *Tian Ma*
Literal Name: "heavenly hemp," "sky hemp"
Alternate Chinese Names: *Ming Tian Ma, Chi Jian, Ding Feng Cao*
Original Source: *Shen Nong Ben Cao Jing* (Divine Husbandman's Classic of the Materia Medica) in the second century
English Name: gastrodia, tall gastrodia tuber
Botanical Name: *Gastrodia elata* Bl. (*Tian Ma*)
Pharmaceutical Name: Rhizoma Gastrodiae
Properties: sweet, neutral
Channels Entered: Liver

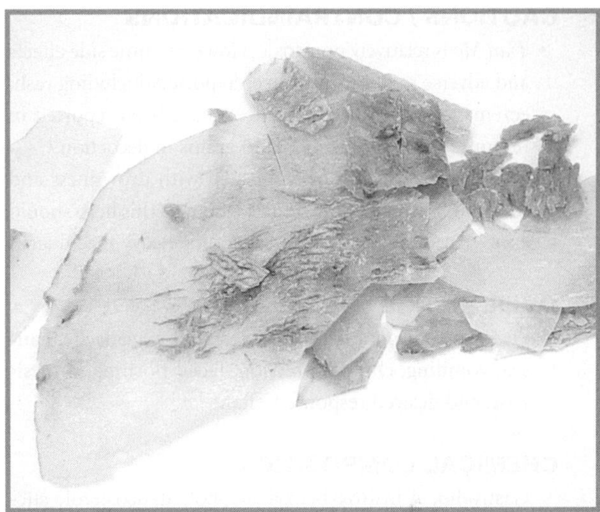

CHINESE THERAPEUTIC ACTIONS

1. Extinguishes Wind and Stops Spasms and Tremors

Convulsions, tremors, spasms, tetany: *Tian Ma* (Rhizoma Gastrodiae), rich in oil, is unique in that it extinguishes Liver wind and fire, and dispels phlegm, without drying yin. It is useful in both excess and deficient conditions. *Tian Ma* has excellent therapeutic functions to dispel Liver wind with an underlying deficiency, presenting tremors, spasms, tonic-clonic convulsions, opisthotonos, tetany, high fever, infantile and childhood seizures, and epilepsy.

- Acute infantile or childhood convulsions: combine *Tian Ma* with *Gou Teng* (Ramulus Uncariae cum Uncis) and *Quan Xie* (Scorpio).
- Chronic infantile convulsions: add this herb to *Ren Shen* (Radix Ginseng), *Bai Zhu* (Rhizoma Atractylodis Macrocephalae) and *Quan Xie* (Scorpio).
- Tetany with spasms, twitching and opisthotonos: use it with *Dan Nan Xing* (Arisaema cum Bile), *Fang Feng* (Radix Saposhnikoviae) and *Bai Fu Zi* (Rhizoma Typhonii). **Exemplar Formula:** *Yu Zhen San* (True Jade Powder).
- Stroke with facial paralysis and drooling of saliva: incorporate this herb with *Quan Xie* (Scorpio), *Bai Fu Zi* (Rhizoma Typhonii), *Jiang Can* (Bombyx Batryticatus), *Ban Xia* (Rhizoma Pinelliae), *Bai Zhi* (Radix Angelicae Dahuricae), *Jing Jie* (Herba Schizonepetae) and *Dan Nan Xing* (Arisaema cum Bile).
- Stroke with hemiplegia, numbness and slurred speech: use *Tian Ma* with *Dan Nan Xing* (Arisaema cum Bile), *Bai Ji Li* (Fructus Tribuli), *Gou Teng* (Ramulus Uncariae cum Uncis), *Ji Xue Teng* (Caulis Spatholobi), *Chuan Xiong* (Rhizoma Ligustici Chuanxiong), *Chi Shao* (Radix Paeoniae Rubrae) and *Di Long* (Pheretima).

2. Pacifies the Liver and Anchors Yang

Rising Liver yang with headache, vertigo, dizziness: *Tian Ma* is used for hypertension caused by either excess or deficient conditions.

- Headache, dizziness, hypertension: use *Tian Ma* with *Gou Teng* (Ramulus Uncariae cum Uncis), *Huang Qin* (Radix Scutellariae) and *Niu Xi* (Radix Cyathulae seu Achyranthis). **Exemplar Formula:** *Tian Ma Gou Teng Yin* (Gastrodia and Uncaria Decoction).
- Migraine headache, blurred vision: combine this herb with *Chuan Xiong* (Rhizoma Ligustici Chuanxiong), *Bai Ji Li* (Fructus Tribuli) and *Jing Jie* (Herba Schizonepetae).
- Heavy feeling, congested headache: use *Tian Ma* with *Bai Zhu* (Rhizoma Atractylodis Macrocephalae), *Ban Xia* (Rhizoma Pinelliae) and *Fu Ling* (Poria). **Exemplar Formula:** *Ban Xia Bai Zhu Tian Ma Tang* (Pinellia, Atractylodes Macrocephala, and Gastrodia Decoction).
- Migraine, temporal or frontal headache: add this herb to *Chuan Xiong* (Rhizoma Ligustici Chuanxiong), *Bai Ji Li* (Fructus Tribuli), *Bai Zhi* (Radix Angelicae Dahuricae) and *Jing Jie* (Herba Schizonepetae).

3. Relieves *Bi Zheng* (Painful Obstruction Syndrome) and Alleviates Pain

***Bi zheng* due to wind-damp:** *Tian Ma* treats joint pain, numbness of muscles and limbs, arthritic pain, and decreased agility.

- *Bi zheng*: use *Tian Ma* with *Cao Wu* (Radix Aconiti Kusnezoffii) and *Ma Huang* (Herba Ephedrae).

DOSAGE

3 to 10 grams of *Tian Ma* in decoction, 1 to 1.5 grams in powder.

Tian Ma (Rhizoma Gastrodiae)

CAUTIONS / CONTRAINDICATIONS

- *Tian Ma* is relatively non-toxic. However, some side effects and adverse reactions have been reported, including rash, eczema, and hair loss. Side effects have been reported in response to dosages as low as 10 grams in decoction.[1]
- Use of *Tian Ma* may be associated with drowsiness and sedation. Therefore, individuals who take this herb should exercise caution if driving or operating heavy machinery.

OVERDOSAGE

Overdose of *Tian Ma* is characterized by headache, nausea, vomiting, chest oppression, facial flushing, drowsiness, and delayed response to light.[2]

CHEMICAL COMPOSITION

Gastrodin, 4-hydroxybenzyl alcohol, daucosterol, succinic acid, vanillin, vanillyl alcohol, β-sitosterol.[3,4]

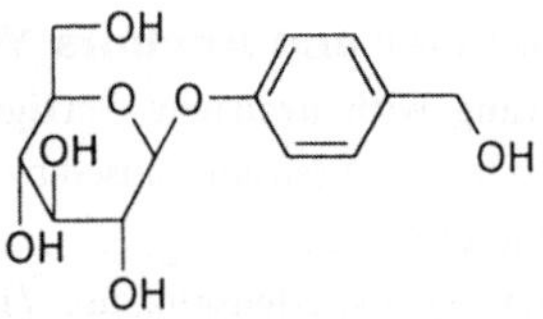

Gastrodin

PHARMACOLOGICAL EFFECTS

- **Sedative:** Decoction of *Tian Ma* significantly reduced the amount of spontaneous physical activity in mice. It also prolonged sleeping time induced by barbiturates.[5,6]
- **Antiseizure and anticonvulsant:** Intraperitoneal or intravenous injection of *Tian Ma* decoction has marked effectiveness in treating seizures and convulsions.[7] Studies have shown *Tian Ma* to have a positive effect in treatment of seizures, cranial-cerebral injury, cervical spondylosis and cerebrovascular diseases.[8,9] Lastly, it has been shown that the combination of *Tian Ma* and *Gou Teng* (Ramulus Uncariae cum Uncis) has a synergistic anticonvulsive and free-radical scavenging action, as demonstrated in laboratory studies in rats.[10]
- **Cardiovascular:** Multiple studies reveal that *Tian Ma* has positive cardiovascular effects.[11] It increases the volume of blood flow to the cardiac muscle and increases resistance to hypoxia. Additionally, by increasing blood flow to the cardiac muscle, *Tian Ma* decreases the risks of myocardial ischemia and myocardial infarct. It was demonstrated that *Tian Ma* reduced the size of myocardial ischemia and myocardial infarct by 23.5% and 34.5%, respectively.[12] In another study, injection of *Tian Ma* increased resistance to hypoxia in mice.[13]

CLINICAL STUDIES AND RESEARCH

- **Headache:** Gastrodin has demonstrated good results in treatment of 156 patients with neurasthenic headache and 72 patients with vascular headache.[14]
- **Seizures:** Administration of vanillin three times daily for 3 to 6 months was 73.9% effective in treating 291 patients with seizures.[15]
- **Nerve pain:** Intramuscular injection of *Tian Ma* was 91 to 95% effective in treating 162 patients with vascular headache, 130 patients with trigeminal pain, 148 patients with sciatica, and 20 patients with toxic polyneuritis. The treatment protocol was 2 to 4 ml of a *Tian Ma* preparation two to three times daily for 20 days per course of treatment, for a total of 1 to 2 courses.[16]

HERB-DRUG INTERACTION

- **Sedatives:** *Tian Ma* potentiates the sedative effect of barbiturates.[17] [Note: Many categories of drugs induce sedation, such as antihistamines, narcotic analgesics, barbiturates, benzodiazepines and many others.]

TOXICOLOGY

The LD_{50} for gastrodin in mice is 337 mg/kg via intravenous injection, and 1,000 mg/kg via oral ingestion. With gross overdose, adverse reactions and fatalities were observed in rabbits following intraperitoneal injection at 12 g/kg. Adverse reactions included lethargy, reduced deep-tendon reflexes, loss of appetite, and tachycardia up to 300 beats per minutes. Most rabbit fatalities occurred within 48 hours.[18,19]

AUTHORS' COMMENTS

Most herbs that extinguish Liver wind and purge Liver fire are bitter and cold, and have the potential to injure yin by being too drying. *Tian Ma* is the herb of choice to treat Liver yang imbalance and Liver wind conditions because it treats excess without creating deficiency.

Tian Ma is also known as "*Ding Feng Cao*," literally meaning "settle the wind herb." This name marks it as one of the most essential herbs for treatment of Liver wind conditions.

References

1. *Chang Yong Zhong Yao Cheng Fen Yu Yao Li Shou Ce* (A Handbook of the Composition and Pharmacology of Common Chinese Drugs), 1994; 486:502
2. *Zhong Yao Bu Liang Fan Ying Yu Zhi Liao* (Adverse Reactions and Treatment of Chinese Herbal Medicine), 1996; 218:220, 1996; 134:135
3. *Xian Dai Zhong Yao Yao Li Xue* (Contemporary Pharmacology of Chinese Herbs), 1997; 1110-1111
4. Yan X, Zhou J, Xie G, *Traditional Chinese Medicines Molecular Structures, Natural Sources and Applications*; Ashgate, 1999; 2505
5. *Zhong Hua Yi Xue Za Zhi* (Chinese Journal of Medicine), 1977; 57(8)470)
6. *Zhong Guo Yi Xue Ke Xue Xue Bao* (Journal of Chinese Medical Science University), 1989; 11(2):147

Tian Ma (Rhizoma Gastrodiae)

7. *Zhong Yao Yao Li Yu Ying Yong* (Pharmacology and Applications of Chinese Herbs), 1983:164
8. Wu, HQ. et al. The effect of vanillin on the fully amygdala-kindled seizures in the rat. *Acta Pharmaceutica Sinica.* 24(7):482-6, 1989
9. Lu, SL. et al. The development of *nao li shen* and its clinical application. *J Pharm Pharmacol* 1997 Nov; 49(11):1162-4
10. *Life Sci* 1999; 65(20):2071-82
11. Huang, JH. Comparison studies on the pharmacological properties of injected gastrodia elata, gastrodin-free fraction and gastrodin. *Acta Academiae Medicinae Sinicae.* 11(2):147-50, Apr. 1989
12. Luo, H. et al. Effects of tian-ma injection on myocardial ischemia and lipid peroxidation in rabbits. *Journal of West China University of Medical Sciences.* 23(1):53-6, Mar. 1992
13. *Zhong Yao Yao Li Yu Ying Yong* (Pharmacology and Applications of Chinese Herbs), 1983:164
14. *Zhong Guo Shen Jing Jing Shen Ke Za Zhi* (Chinese Journal of Psychiatric Disorders), 1986; 5:265
15. Ibid., 1985; 3:139
16. *Ji Lin Yi Xue Yuan Xue Bao* (Journal of Jilin University of Medicine), 1982; 1:28
17. *Zhong Guo Yi Xue Ke Xue Xue Bao* (Journal of Chinese Medical Science University), 1989; 11(2):147
18. *Zhong Cao Yao* (Chinese Herbal Medicine), 1985; 16(9):40
19. *Zhong Yao Yao Li Yu Ying Yong* (Pharmacology and Applications of Chinese Herbs), 1983; 164

Quan Xie (Scorpio)

全蠍 全蝎

Pinyin Name: *Quan Xie*
Literal Name: "whole scorpion"
Alternate Chinese Names: *Quan Cong, Xie Wei*
Original Source: *Ri Hua Zi Ben Cao* (Materia Medica of Ri Hua-Zi) by Ri Hua-Zi in 713 A.D.
English Name: scorpion
Zoological Name: *Buthus martensi* Karsch. (*Dong Ya Qian Xie*)
Pharmaceutical Name: Scorpio
Properties: acrid, neutral
Channels Entered: Liver
Safety Index: toxic

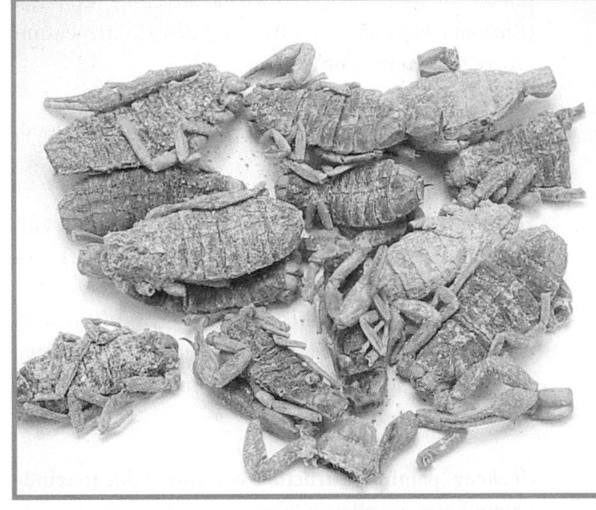

CHINESE THERAPEUTIC ACTIONS

1. Extinguishes Wind and Stops Tremors and Convulsions

Liver wind: Applicable conditions include acute or chronic convulsions, childhood convulsions, facial paralysis, stroke, involuntary twitching of facial muscles, tetanus, spasms, cramps, opisthotonos, slurred speech, tightness of the tongue, tics and seizures. Penetrating in nature, *Quan Xie* (Scorpio) is a key component to extinguish wind and relieve spasms.

- Facial paralysis, involuntary facial twitching due to wind and phlegm: combine *Quan Xie* with *Bai Fu Zi* (Rhizoma Typhonii) and *Jiang Can* (Bombyx Batryticatus). **Exemplar Formula:** *Qian Zheng San* (Lead to Symmetry Powder).
- Stroke: use this substance with *Chuan Shan Jia* (Squama Manis) and *Di Long* (Pheretima).
- Childhood convulsions, high fever: use it with *Ling Yang Jiao* (Cornu Saigae Tataricae), *Da Qing Ye* (Folium Isatidis), and *Gou Teng* (Ramulus Uncariae cum Uncis).
- Chronic childhood convulsions with Spleen deficiency (convulsions after vomiting and diarrhea): add it to *Dang Shen* (Radix Codonopsis), *Bai Zhu* (Rhizoma Atractylodis Macrocephalae) and *Tian Ma* (Rhizoma Gastrodiae).
- Seizure and epilepsy: use this substance with *Jiang Can* (Bombyx Batryticatus), *Tian Ma* (Rhizoma Gastrodiae), *Hu Po* (Succinum), and *Deng Xin Cao* (Medulla Junci). **Exemplar Formula:** *Ding Xian Wan* (Arrest Seizures Pill).
- Tetany, opisthotonos, spasms and cramps: combine it

Quan Xie (Scorpio)

with *Gou Teng* (Ramulus Uncariae cum Uncis), *Wu Gong* (Scolopendra) and *Zhu Sha* (Cinnabaris).

- Tetanus: use *Quan Xie* with *Tian Nan Xing* (Rhizoma Arisaematis), *Chan Tui* (Periostracum Cicadae), *Jiang Can* (Bombyx Batryticatus) and *Tian Ma* (Rhizoma Gastrodiae).

2. Eliminates Toxins and Disperses Toxic Fire Nodules

Toxic heat accumulations, painful swellings, nodules and masses: *Quan Xie* is used topically to treat toxic sores, mastitis, mumps, swellings and scrofula. It is often made into an ointment with sesame oil and beeswax. Traditionally, when all else fails, one of the last strategies to be tried is "use toxins to attack toxins."

- Toxic sores, swellings: cook *Quan Xie* with sesame oil and *Zhi Zi* (Fructus Gardeniae), and mix with beeswax to make an ointment. Apply topically.
- Scrofula and fibrocystic breast disorders: use this substance with *Ma Qian Zi* (Semen Strychni), *Ban Xia* (Rhizoma Pinelliae) and *Wu Ling Zhi* (Excrementum Trogopteri seu Pteromi) as powders.
- Mastitis: apply powdered *Quan Xie* topically.
- Mumps in children: deep fry two scorpions and eat as food.

3. Opens Channels and Stops Pain

Headache: *Quan Xie* treats frontal, temporal and migraine headaches due to heat in the Liver channel with internal wind.

- Headache: use *Quan Xie* with *Tian Ma* (Rhizoma Gastrodiae), *Wu Gong* (Scolopendra), *Gou Teng* (Ramulus Uncariae cum Uncis) and *Jiang Can* (Bombyx Batryticatus). Serve as powder.

***Bi zheng* (painful obstruction syndrome) due to wind-damp:** *Quan Xie* effectively opens the channels and collaterals to relieve pain. It is primarily used for severe pain, numbness and decreased joint mobility.

- Arthritis: use it with *She Xiang* (Moschus), and serve with grain-based liquor.

DOSAGE

2 to 5 grams in decoction, 0.6 to 1.0 grams as powder. When treating chronic childhood convulsions, use 0.06 to 0.09 grams [60 to 90 mg] of *Quan Xie* as powder for children under two years of age. The tail segment is believed to be the strongest, approximately 2.5 to 3 times more potent than the body. However, the tail is no longer sold separately. The whole scorpion is the most commonly available form.

CAUTIONS / CONTRAINDICATIONS

- Use of *Quan Xie* is contraindicated during pregnancy, and in blood-deficient patients with internal wind.
- This substance is toxic and should never be prescribed at a high dose. No apparent side effects or toxicity occurs when it is used at normal dosages.

OVERDOSAGE

Overdose may occur with intake of 30 to 60 grams of *Quan Xie*. Signs and symptoms of overdose include dizziness, fever, spontaneous perspiration, increased sensitivity to light, tearing, runny nose, salivation, nausea, vomiting, stiff tongue, decreased body temperature, convulsions, dyspnea, and bleeding from the gastrointestinal tract, nose or lungs. In severe cases, there may be increased or decreased heart rate, weak pulse, hypertension or hypotension, seizures, unconsciousness, dyspnea, cyanosis, pulmonary edema, and respiratory depression. The presence of blood, protein and glucose in the urine have also been reported following overdose.[1]

TREATMENT OF OVERDOSAGE

Overdose of *Quan Xie* may be treated with one or more of the following approaches:

- Ingestion of 20 grams of *Yuan Ming Fen* (Natrii Sulfas Praeparata) to facilitate the elimination of toxins through defecation.
- A decoction containing *Jin Yin Hua* (Flos Lonicerae) 30g, *Ban Bian Lian* (Herba Lobeliae Chinensis) 10g, *Tu Fu Ling* (Rhizoma Smilacis Glabrae) 15g, *Lu Dou* (Semen Phaseoli Radiati) 15g, and *Gan Cao* (Radix Glycyrrhizae) 10g.
- A decoction of *Da Huang* (Radix et Rhizoma Rhei) 15g and *Mang Xiao* (Natrii Sulfas) 6g, taken in three equally-divided doses.
- A decoction of *Wu Ling Zhi* (Excrementum Trogopteri seu Pteromi) 10g, *Pu Huang* (Pollen Typhae) 9g, and *Xiong Huang* (Realgar) 3g, mixed and ground into powder and taken in three equally-divided doses with vinegar every 4 hours.
- A decoction of *Jin Yin Hua* (Flos Lonicerae) 30g, *Ban Bian Lian* (Herba Lobeliae Chinensis) 9g, *Tu Fu Ling* (Rhizoma Smilacis Glabrae) 15g, *Lu Dou* (Semen Phaseoli Radiati) 15g, and *Gan Cao* (Radix Glycyrrhizae) 9g, taken as herbal decoction twice daily.[2]

CHEMICAL COMPOSITION

Buthatoxin, trimethylamine, taurine, betaine.[3]

PHARMACOLOGICAL EFFECTS

- **Antiseizure:** Administration of *Quan Xie* in mice showed marked effectiveness in treating seizures artificially induced by caffeine and megimide.[4]

Quan Xie (Scorpio)

- **Antiepileptic:** In rats with artificially-induced epilepsy, intravenous injection of *Quan Xie* was effective in reducing the severity and duration of epileptic episodes, and preventing recurrent incidences.[5]
- **Cardiovascular:** Administration of *Quan Xie* is associated with a positive inotropic effect and negative chronotropic effect. It also has a prolonged effect to reduce blood pressure.[6]
- **Antineoplastic:** *Quan Xie* has demonstrated preliminary preventative and treatment effectiveness against sarcoma in mice.[7]

CLINICAL STUDIES AND RESEARCH

- **Mastitis:** In one study, 308 patients having mastitis for 1 to 7 days were treated with two *Quan Xie* daily, with a 99.9% rate of effectiveness.[8] In another study, 10 patients with acute mastitis were treated with 3 grams of *Quan Xie* daily with good results.[9]
- **Whooping cough:** According to one report, 74 patients with whooping cough were treated with *Quan Xie* twice daily, with complete recovery reported in all patients. The treatment protocol was to cook and ingest one *Quan Xie* (from head to tail) with one egg, twice daily for 4 to 7 days. The average duration of treatment was 5 days.[10]
- **Cerebral embolism:** Patients with first episodes of cerebral embolism were treated with intravenous infusion of *Quan Xie*, *Bai Hua She* (Bungarus Parvus) and *Wu Gong* (Scolopendra) one time each day. Out of 47 patients, 24 showed complete recovery, 17 showed some improvement, and 6 showed no response. The average duration of treatment was 14 days, with a range of 10 to 30 days.[11]
- **Migraine:** An herbal preparation was used to treat 26 patients with migraine. Most patients reported significant pain relief within the first 12 hours and complete recovery in 48 hours. The herbal preparation contained equal portions of *Quan Xie*, *Gou Teng* (Ramulus Uncariae cum Uncis), and *Zi He Che* (Placenta Hominis). The patients were instructed to take 0.9 grams of the powder three times daily.[12]
- **Epilepsy:** In one study, 104 patients with epilepsy were treated with a *Quan Xie* preparation for 6 months to 1 year, with marked improvement in 78 cases, moderate improvement in 17 cases, and no response in 9 cases. The overall rate of effectiveness was 95%.[13]

TOXICOLOGY

The LD_{50} for intraperitoneal injection of *Quan Xie* in mice is 2.4 mg/kg.[14]

AUTHORS' COMMENTS

Traditionally, the tail of *Quan Xie* is considered to be the most potent, but also the most toxic part of the scorpion. Dosage when prescribing only the tail should be ***one-third*** of the regular recommended dosage. Historically, the tail was used for tetany, convulsions and high fever, while the whole body was used for paralysis and hemiplegia. However, the tail is no longer sold separately. The whole body is the most commonly available form.

Quan Xie, *Wu Gong* (Scolopendra) and *Jiang Can* (Bombyx Batryticatus) are commonly used to treat wind. *Quan Xie* and *Wu Gong* are much stronger than *Jiang Can* to extinguish wind. When treating convulsions, *Jiang Can* is selected only in less severe cases or for those patients who also have phlegm accumulation.

References

1. *Zhong Yao Bu Liang Fan Ying Yu Zhi Liao* (Adverse Reactions and Treatment of Chinese Herbal Medicine), 1996; 218:220, 1996; 241:244
2. Ibid.
3. *Xian Dai Zhong Yao Yao Li Xue* (Contemporary Pharmacology of Chinese Herbs), 1997; 1119
4. *Shen Yang Yi Xue Yuan Xue Bao* (Journal of Shenyang University of Medicine), 1988; 5(2):110
5. Ibid., 1989; 6(2):95
6. Ibid., 1987; 4(2):109
7. *Jiang Su Yi Yao* (Jiangsu Journal of Medicine and Herbology), 1990; 16(9):513
8. *Zhong Yi Za Zhi* (Journal of Chinese Medicine), 1986; 1:40
9. *Hei Long Jiang Zhong Yi Yao* (Heilongjiang Chinese Medicine and Herbology), 1988; 1:23
10. *Zhe Jiang Zhong Yi Za Zhi* (Zhejiang Journal of Chinese Medicine), 1990; (3):114
11. *Ji Lin Zhong Yi Yao* (Jilin Chinese Medicine and Herbology), 1989; (4):15
12. *Jiang Su Zhong Yi* (Jiangsu Chinese Medicine), 1988; 9(4):10
13. *Si Chuan Zhong Yi* (Sichuan Chinese Medicine), 1991; 9(11):12
14. *Sheng Wu Hua Xue Yu Sheng Wu Wu Li Xue Bao* (Journal of Biochemistry and Biophysiology), 1983; 15(6):517

Wu Gong (Scolopendra)

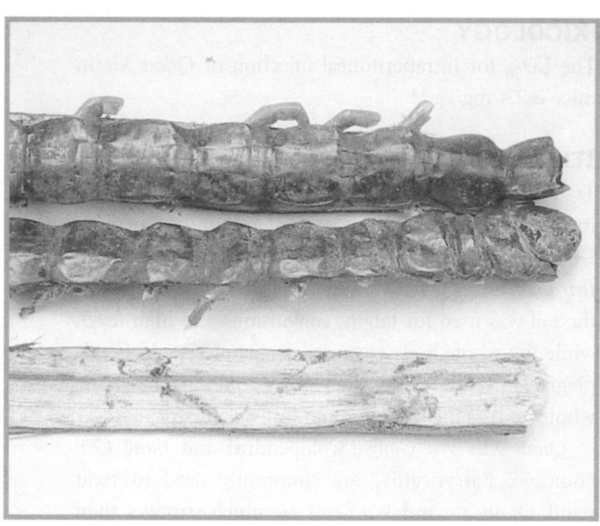

蜈蚣 蜈蚣

Pinyin Name: *Wu Gong*
Literal Name: "centipede"
Alternate Chinese Names: *Tian Long, Chi Zu Wu Gong, Chuan Zu, Bai Zu*
Original Source: *Shen Nong Ben Cao Jing* (Divine Husbandman's Classic of the Materia Medica) in the second century
English Name: centipede
Zoological Name: *Scolopendra mutilans* L. Koch.
Pharmaceutical Name: Scolopendra
Properties: acrid, warm
Channels Entered: Liver
Safety Index: toxic

CHINESE THERAPEUTIC ACTIONS

1. Extinguishes Wind, Stops Tremors and Convulsions

Liver wind: Clinical manifestations of Liver wind include acute or chronic convulsions, childhood convulsions, stroke, tetanus, spasms, cramps, opisthotonos, epilepsy, and seizures. *Wu Gong* (Scolopendra) has strong penetrating functions, and is effective to extinguish wind and stop tremors. It is an essential substance when treating symptoms associated with Liver wind.

- Twitching, tetany and opisthotonos: use *Wu Gong* with *Quan Xie* (Scorpio).
- Stroke: use it with *Chuan Shan Jia* (Squama Manis) and *Di Long* (Pheretima).
- Childhood convulsions, high fever: combine this substance with *Ling Yang Jiao* (Cornu Saigae Tataricae), *Da Qing Ye* (Folium Isatidis), and *Gou Teng* (Ramulus Uncariae cum Uncis).
- Epilepsy: use it with *Tian Ma* (Rhizoma Gastrodiae), *Gou Teng* (Ramulus Uncariae cum Uncis), *Quan Xie* (Scorpio), *Tian Zhu Huang* (Concretio Silicea Bambusae) and *Shi Chang Pu* (Rhizoma Acori).
- Tetanus: add it to *Tian Nan Xing* (Rhizoma Arisaematis), *Quan Xie* (Scorpio), *Bai Fu Zi* (Rhizoma Typhonii), *Jiang Can* (Bombyx Batryticatus), and *Gou Teng* (Ramulus Uncariae cum Uncis).
- Delirium associated with high fever, spasms, convulsions or clenched teeth: use *Wu Gong* with *Tian Zhu Huang* (Concretio Silicea Bambusae), *Ling Yang Jiao* (Cornu Saigae Tataricae), *Quan Xie* (Scorpio), *Jiang Can* (Bombyx Batryticatus), *Gou Teng* (Ramulus Uncariae cum Uncis), *Fang Feng* (Radix Saposhnikoviae) and *Bai Ji Li* (Fructus Tribuli).

2. Eliminates Toxins and Disperses Toxic Fire Nodules

Toxic nodules: *Wu Gong* is used internally or externally to relieve toxicity. Clinical applications include sores, carbuncles, neck lumps, snake bites, ulcerated sores and scrofula.

- Toxic nodules: mix it with *Xiong Huang* (Realgar) and tea leaves as powder. Apply topically.
- Tuberculosis of the bone: combine *Wu Gong* with *Quan Xie* (Scorpio) and *Di Bie Chong* (Eupolyphaga) as powder for internal use.
- Snake bite with dizziness, blurred vision, spasms: *Wu Gong* is given with *Huang Lian* (Rhizoma Coptidis), *Da Huang* (Radix et Rhizoma Rhei) and *Gan Cao* (Radix Glycyrrhizae).
- Submandibular lymphadenitis: use *Wu Gong* topically.

3. Opens Channels and Stops Pain

***Bi zheng* (painful obstruction syndrome):** *Wu Gong* treats *bi zheng* caused by wind, a condition characterized by pain that travels from one joint to another.

- *Bi zheng*: use this substance with *Fang Feng* (Radix Saposhnikoviae), *Du Huo* (Radix Angelicae Pubescentis) and *Wei Ling Xian* (Radix Clematidis).

Chronic headache with severe intolerable pain

- Chronic stubborn headache: add *Wu Gong* to *Tian Ma* (Rhizoma Gastrodiae), *Chuan Xiong* (Rhizoma Ligustici Chuanxiong), *Jiang Can* (Bombyx Batryticatus) and *Dang Gui* (Radicis Angelicae Sinensis).

DOSAGE

1 to 3 grams in decoction, 0.6 to 1.0 gram in powder. Mix *Wu Gong* powder with sesame oil for external applications.

Wu Gong (Scolopendra)

CAUTIONS / CONTRAINDICATIONS

- Use of *Wu Gong* is contraindicated during pregnancy, for patients with blood deficiency, or in cases of chronic childhood convulsion.
- *Wu Gong* is toxic and should be used with extreme caution. It should not be administered at higher than recommended dosages.

OVERDOSAGE

Overdose of *Wu Gong* may result in symptoms of nausea, vomiting, abdominal pain, diarrhea, lethargy, slow heartbeat, palpitations, dyspnea, a sudden drop in body temperature and blood pressure, and unconsciousness. Oral ingestion of *Wu Gong* has a dose-dependant effect. At small doses, it stimulates the cardiac tissue. At large doses, it paralyzes the cardiac muscle and inhibits respiration. Lastly, use of *Wu Gong* is also associated with rare cases of allergic shock. [1]

TREATMENT OF OVERDOSAGE

Overdose of *Wu Gong* may be treated by one or more of the following methods:

- For general overdose of *Wu Gong*, use *Feng Wei Cao* (Herba Pteris) 100g, *Jin Yin Hua* (Flos Lonicerae) 100g, and *Gan Cao* (Radix Glycyrrhizae) 20g. Serve decoction twice daily, separating the doses by 4 hours.
- For slow pulse with dyspnea, use *Ren Shen* (Radix Ginseng) 10g, *Fu Zi* (Radix Aconiti Lateralis Praeparata) 10g, *Wu Wei Zi* (Fructus Schisandrae Chinensis) 10g, and *Gan Cao* (Radix Glycyrrhizae) 10g. Serve decoction twice daily, separating the doses by 4 hours.
- For centipede bites, grind fresh *Ban Bian Lian* (Herba Lobeliae Chinensis) and *Bai Hua She She Cao* (Herba Oldenlandia) into paste and apply topically. This can also be treated internally with an herbal decoction of *Feng Wei Cao* (Herba Pteris) 120g, *Jin Yin Hua* (Flos Lonicerae) 90g, and *Gan Cao* (Radix Glycyrrhizae) 60g, taken twice daily.
- For severe allergic reaction, use corticosteroids.[2]

CHEMICAL COMPOSITION

235-hydroxylysine, taurine, hydroxylysine, chitin, chitosan, glucosamine.[3]

PHARMACOLOGICAL EFFECTS

- **Antineoplastic:** *Wu Gong* has demonstrated antineoplastic effects *in vitro*.[4]
- **Antibiotic:** It has an inhibitory effect against *Staphylococcus aureus*, *Pseudomonas aeruginosa*, *Candida albicans*, and dermatophytes.[5]
- **Antiseizure:** It has marked preventative and treatment actions against seizures induced by various drugs. The effect of *Wu Gong* is slightly stronger than that of *Quan Xie* (Scorpio).[6]

CLINICAL STUDIES AND RESEARCH

- **Dermatological use:** Topical application of herbs was used to successfully treat 600 patients with various skin disorders characterized by sores, swelling, ulceration and pus. The herbal tincture was prepared by soaking 2 pieces of *Wu Gong* and 5 grams of *Hong Hua* (Flos Carthami) in 500 ml of 75% alcohol for 7 days.[7]
- **Submandibular lymphadenitis:** In one study, 226 adults with submandibular lymphadenitis were treated with 3 to 9 grams of *Wu Gong* in decoction, with good results. *Wu Gong* was roasted until it turned yellow/brown in color, then decocted. The dosage for children was adjusted appropriately.[8]
- **Tuberculosis of the bone:** Ten patients with tuberculosis of the bone were treated with an herbal formula, with complete recovery in 8 cases and moderate improvement in 1 case (information was not available on one patient). The herbal formula is prepared by grinding 40 grams of *Wu Gong*, 40 grams of *Quan Xie* (Scorpio), and 50 grams of *Di Bie Chong* (Eupolyphaga) into fine powder and divided equally into 40 doses. The patients were instructed to cook 1 dose of the formula with one egg. Take the herb and the egg twice daily for 20 days per course of treatment, for a total of 3 to 6 courses.[9]

AUTHORS' COMMENTS

Some texts suggest that the head and tail of *Wu Gong* must be removed, as they are toxic. Some other records suggest that the head and tail have the strongest functions. Clinical findings, however, have revealed that *Wu Gong* is at its strongest when used as a whole. Thus, there is no need to remove the head or the tail.

Wu Gong and *Quan Xie* (Scorpio) both extinguish wind and arrest tremors. *Wu Gong* has stronger functions to extinguish wind and relieve spasms, disperse stagnation, and dissipate toxic nodules. *Quan Xie* is neutral, and is more suitable for twitching and tremors. *Wu Gong* is more often used topically, while *Quan Xie* is more frequently used internally.

Dr. Li Shou-Shan states that 2 to 3 pieces of *Wu Gong* (Scolopendra) added to *Chuan Xiong* (Rhizoma Ligustici Chuanxiong), *Dang Gui* (Radicis Angelicae Sinensis) and *Xi Xin* (Herba Asari) enhance the effectiveness of treating chronic headache caused by blood stasis. It is best to use *Wu Gong* in powder form, added to the decoction prior to serving. This combination is commonly used for trigeminal neuralgia, angioneurotic headaches, and migraines.

Wu Gong (Scolopendra)

References

1. *Zhong Yao Bu Liang Fan Ying Yu Zhi Liao* (Adverse Reactions and Treatment of Chinese Herbal Medicine), 1996; 218:220, 1996; 258:259
2. Ibid.
3. *Xian Dai Zhong Yao Yao Li Xue* (Contemporary Pharmacology of Chinese Herbs), 1997; 1120
4. *Chang Yong Zhong Yao Cheng Fen Yu Yao Li Shou Ce* (A Handbook of the Composition and Pharmacology of Common Chinese Drugs), 1994; 1725:1728
5. Ibid.
6. *Zhong Yao Xue* (Chinese Herbology), 1998; 704:706
7. *Zhong Xi Yi Jie He Za Zhi* (Journal of Integrated Chinese and Western Medicine), 1988; 9:566
8. *Chi Jiao Yi Shi Za Zhi* (Journal of Barefoot Doctors), 1979; 10:16
9. *Zhong Xi Yi Jie He Za Zhi* (Journal of Integrated Chinese and Western Medicine), 1988; 6:379

Jiang Can (Bombyx Batryticatus)

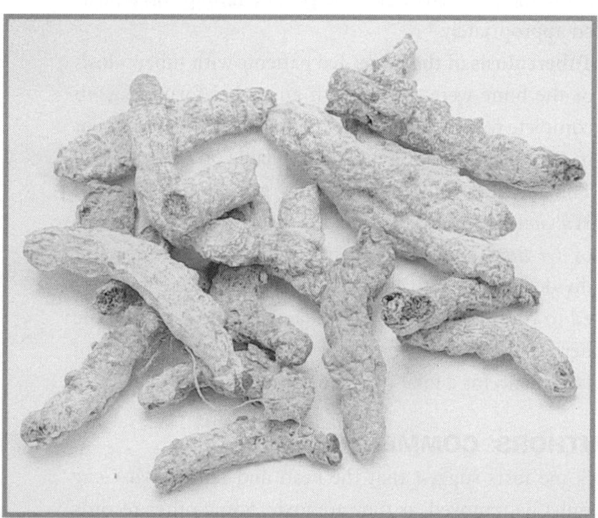

殭蠶 僵蚕

Pinyin Name: *Jiang Can*
Literal Name: "stiff silkworm"
Alternate Chinese Names: *Bai Jiang Can, Tian Cong*
Original Source: *Shen Nong Ben Cao Jing* (Divine Husbandman's Classic of the Materia Medica) in the second century
English Name: sick silkworm, silkworm with batrytis
Zoological Name: *Bombyx mori* Linnaeus (*Jia Can*) infected with *Beauveria bassiana* (Bals.) Vuillant
Pharmaceutical Name: Bombyx Batryticatus
Properties: salty, acrid, neutral
Channels Entered: Liver, Lung

CHINESE THERAPEUTIC ACTIONS

1. Extinguishes Wind, Dispels Phlegm, Stops Tremors and Convulsions

Liver wind with phlegm accumulation: *Jiang Can* (Bombyx Batryticatus) is most suitable for Liver wind with phlegm heat stagnation, causing high fever, convulsions, chronic childhood convulsions, facial paralysis, and involuntary twitching of facial muscles.

- High fever, convulsions and muscle twitching: combine *Jiang Can* with *Chan Tui* (Periostracum Cicadae), *Gou Teng* (Ramulus Uncariae cum Uncis) and *Ju Hua* (Flos Chrysanthemi).
- Convulsions with phlegm and fire: use this substance with *Quan Xie* (Scorpio), *Tian Ma* (Rhizoma Gastrodiae) and *Dan Nan Xing* (Arisaema cum Bile).
- Childhood convulsions with night crying and fear: add it to *Fang Feng* (Radix Saposhnikoviae), *Quan Xie* (Scorpio), *Wu Gong* (Scolopendra), *Dan Nan Xing* (Arisaema cum Bile), *Tian Zhu Huang* (Concretio Silicea Bambusae) and *Chan Tui* (Periostracum Cicadae).
- Chronic childhood convulsions after chronic diarrhea and Spleen deficiency: use with *Bai Zhu* (Rhizoma Atractylodis Macrocephalae), *Dang Shen* (Radix Codonopsis) and *Tian Ma* (Rhizoma Gastrodiae).
- Paralysis, involuntary facial twitching or facial paralysis: combine *Jiang Can* with *Quan Xie* (Scorpio), *Bai Zhi* (Radix Angelicae Dahuricae) and *Bai Fu Zi* (Rhizoma Typhonii). **Exemplar Formula:** *Qian Zheng San* (Lead to Symmetry Powder).
- Headache due to Liver yang rising: use it with *Tian Ma* (Rhizoma Gastrodiae), *Ju Hua* (Flos Chrysanthemi), *Gou Teng* (Ramulus Uncariae cum Uncis), *Bai Ji Li* (Fructus Tribuli) and *Bai Shao* (Radix Paeoniae Alba).

2. Dispels Wind and Stops Pain

Headache, red eyes, sore and swollen throat, toothache:

Jiang Can (Bombyx Batryticatus)

These symptoms are caused by wind-heat attacking the head. Secondary symptoms may include excessive tearing and hoarse voice.

- Headache, red eyes and excessive tearing: use *Jiang Can* with *Sang Ye* (Folium Mori), *Mu Zei* (Herba Equiseti Hiemalis) and *Jing Jie* (Herba Schizonepetae).
- Sore throat, hoarse voice: use it with *Jing Jie* (Herba Schizonepetae), *Fang Feng* (Radix Saposhnikoviae), *Jie Geng* (Radix Platycodonis), *Xuan Shen* (Radix Scrophulariae), *Pang Da Hai* (Semen Sterculiae Lychnophorae), *Gu Zhi Hua* (Semen Oroxyli) and *Ban Lan Gen* (Radix Isatidis).

3. Eliminates Toxins and Dissipates Nodules

Toxic phlegm heat nodules: *Jiang Can* treats scrofula, toxic sores, swellings, erysipelas, mastitis and parotitis caused by phlegm.

- Toxic nodules: use it with *Zhe Bei Mu* (Bulbus Fritillariae Thunbergii), *Xia Ku Cao* (Spica Prunellae), *Lian Qiao* (Fructus Forsythiae), *Jin Yin Hua* (Flos Lonicerae), *Jie Geng* (Radix Platycodonis), *Gan Cao* (Radix Glycyrrhizae), *Ma Bo* (Lasiosphaera seu Calvatia), *Qing Dai* (Indigo Naturalis), *Bei Mu* (Bulbus Fritillaria), and *Xuan Shen* (Radix Scrophulariae).

4. Dispels Wind and Relieves Itching

In addition to extinguishing internal Liver wind, *Jiang Can* expels external wind to relieve rashes and itching.

- **Eczema or rash due to wind:** combine it with *Chan Tui* (Periostracum Cicadae) and *Bo He* (Herba Menthae).

DOSAGE

3 to 10 grams in decoction, 1 to 1.5 grams in powder. Unprocessed *Jiang Can* is sometimes used to treat rashes. However, the unprocessed form has a distinct odor that may significantly reduce patient compliance. Therefore, the standard preparation is to dry fry *Jiang Can* to reduce its odor.

CHEMICAL COMPOSITION

Protein, lipids, ammonium oxalate.[1]

PHARMACOLOGICAL EFFECTS

- **Antiseizure:** Administration of a 10% *Jiang Can* decoction at the dose of 2 g/kg has marked effectiveness in treating mice with drug-induced seizures.[2]
- **Sedative:** Alcohol extract of *Jiang Can* potentiates the sedative effect of phenobarbital in mice.[3]
- **Antibiotic:** *Jiang Can* has a mild inhibitory action against *Staphylococcus aureus*, *E. coli*, *Pseudomonas aeruginosa*.[4]

CLINICAL STUDIES AND RESEARCH

- **Epilepsy:** According to one report, 100 patients with epileptic disorders were treated with a preparation of *Jiang Can* for 2 months to 2 years. Patients were given 0.9 to 1.5 grams of *Jiang Can* powder per dose three times daily. Dosage for children was adjusted accordingly. Based on reduced frequency of epilepsy, the study reported an overall effective rate of 77%.[5]
- **High fever with seizure:** Significant improvement was reported in 30 of 32 patients with high fevers and seizures after herbal treatment. The formula was prepared by soaking 6 grams of *Jiang Can* in a fresh cow gallbladder for one month. *Jiang Can* is then removed, mixed with *Huang Lian* (Rhizoma Coptidis), and ground into fine powder. *Huang Qin* (Radix Scutellariae) may be used in place of *Huang Lian* if necessary.[6]

TOXICOLOGY

Administration of *Jiang Can* at 35 g/kg caused death in 1 out of 10 mouse subjects.[7]

AUTHORS' COMMENTS

Dr. Li Shou-Shan stated that the combination of *Jiang Can*, *Shi Gao* (Gypsum Fibrosum) and *Wu Gong* (Scolopendra) treats stubborn, pounding headaches that resemble a hammer striking the head. Administer this combination in powder form.

References

1. *Xian Dai Zhong Yao Yao Li Xue* (Contemporary Pharmacology of Chinese Herbs), 1997; 1126
2. *Zhong Cao Yao Xue* (Study of Chinese Herbal Medicine), 1980: 1423
3. *Chang Yong Zhong Yao Cheng Fen Yu Yao Li Shou Ce* (A Handbook of the Composition and Pharmacology of Common Chinese Drugs), 1994; 1810:1812
4. *Zhong Yao Xue* (Chinese Herbology), 1998; 706:708
5. *Jiang Su Yi Yao* (Jiangsu Journal of Medicine and Herbology), 1976; 2:33
6. *Zhong Guo Nong Cun Yi Xue* (Chinese Agricultural Medicine), 1984; (2):20
7. *Chang Yong Zhong Yao Cheng Fen Yu Yao Li Shou Ce* (A Handbook of the Composition and Pharmacology of Common Chinese Drugs), 1994; 1810:18131.

Dí Long (Pheretima)

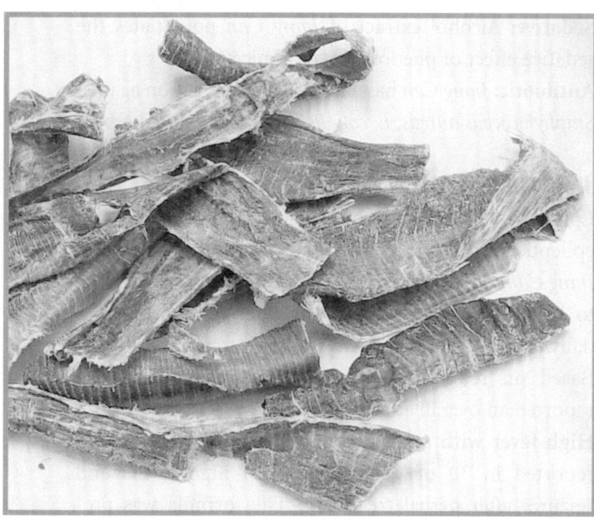

地龍 地龙

Pinyin Name: *Di Long*
Literal Name: "earth dragon"
Alternate Chinese Names: *Chiu Jin, Chu Tan, Zhuo Jin, Guang Di Long, Gan Di Long*
Original Source: *Shen Nong Ben Cao Jing* (Divine Husbandman's Classic of the Materia Medica) in the second century
English Name: earthworm
Zoological Name: *Pheretima aspergillum* (Eperrier) (*Guang Di Long*); *Allalobophora caliginosa* (Savigny) *trapezoides* (Ant. Duges) (*Tu Di Long*)
Pharmaceutical Name: Pheretima
Properties: salty, cold
Channels Entered: Liver, Spleen, Urinary Bladder, Lung

CHINESE THERAPEUTIC ACTIONS

1. Clears Heat and Extinguishes Wind

Febrile disorders: *Di Long* (Pheretima) is penetrating in nature and extinguishes wind and heat to treat high fever, mania, convulsions, seizures, and epilepsy. It is used alone or in combination with other herbs.

- High fever, epilepsy: use this substance alone with salt water.
- Convulsions: pair *Di Long* with *Zhu Sha* (Cinnabaris). Grind both into powder and serve as pills.
- Seizures, twitching, spasms or meningitis with unremitting fever, unconsciousness: use it with *Gou Teng* (Ramulus Uncariae cum Uncis), *Shi Gao* (Gypsum Fibrosum), *Quan Xie* (Scorpio) and *Zao Xiu* (Rhizoma Paridis).
- Schizophrenia or mania with high fever: wash fresh *Di Long* and serve with white sugar and water.

2. Arrests Wheezing

Asthma, bronchial wheezing, whooping cough in children and respiratory disorders due to heat: *Di Long* dilates the bronchial muscles and arrests wheezing. It has been used recently as an injectable to treat asthma.

- Lung heat with dyspnea and cough: use this substance with *Shi Gao* (Gypsum Fibrosum), *Zhi Mu* (Radix Anemarrhenae) and *Xing Ren* (Semen Armeniacae Amarum).
- Whooping cough or bronchial spasms with phlegm: use *Di Long* alone.

3. Opens the Channels

***Bi zheng* (painful obstruction syndrome):** *Di Long* unblocks channels, relieves pain and treats various disorders related to blockage in the channels and collaterals.

- *Bi zheng* caused by heat with red and swollen joints that are hot to the touch, and pain that worsens with exposure to heat: use *Di Long* with *Sang Zhi* (Ramulus Mori), *Ren Dong Teng* (Caulis Lonicerae), *Luo Shi Teng* (Caulis Trachelospermi) and *Chi Shao* (Radix Paeoniae Rubrae).
- *Bi zheng* caused by cold, with coldness in the joints, reduced mobility, and pain that worsens with exposure to cold: combine this substance with *Cao Wu* (Radix Aconiti Kusnezoffii), *Chuan Wu* (Radix Aconiti Preparata), *Tian Nan Xing* (Rhizoma Arisaematis) and *Ru Xiang* (Gummi Olibanum). **Exemplar Formula:** *Xiao Huo Luo Dan* (Minor Invigorate the Collaterals Special Pill).
- Post-stroke hemiplegia, paralysis with qi and blood stagnation: use it with *Huang Qi* (Radix Astragali), *Dang Gui* (Radicis Angelicae Sinensis), *Chuan Xiong* (Rhizoma Ligustici Chuanxiong), and *Hong Hua* (Flos Carthami). **Exemplar Formula:** *Bu Yang Huan Wu Tang* (Tonify the Yang to Restore Five Decoction).
- Bone fractures with swelling and pain: combine this substance with *Dang Gui Wei* (Extremitas Radicis Angelicae Sinensis), *Su Mu* (Lignum Sappan), *Tao Ren* (Semen Persicae) and *Xue Jie* (Sanguis Draconis).

4. Promotes Urination

Heat in the Urinary Bladder: *Di Long* is salty and enters the Kidney to clear heat and promote diuresis. It is best for urinary difficulties with dysuria, urinary stones or the inability to urinate. It is used alone or in combination with other herbs.

- Dysuria: use *Di Long* with *Che Qian Zi* (Semen Plantaginis), *Chuan Mu Tong* (Caulis Clematidis Armandii), *Dong Kui Zi* (Semen Malvae).
- Urinary stones: combine it with *Jin Qian Cao* (Herba Lysimachiae) and *Hai Jin Sha* (Herba Lygodii).

Di Long (Pheretima)

Dampness accumulation in the lower limbs: Edema of the lower extremities, with itching between the toes, and numb, weak feet.

- Edema of the lower extremities: use *Di Long* with *Mu Gua* (Fructus Chaenomelis), *Fen Fang Ji* (Radix Stephaniae Tetandrae), and *Bing Lang* (Semen Arecae).

5. Anchors Liver Yang and Lowers Blood Pressure

Rising Liver yang: *Di Long* has a mild but lasting effect to lower blood pressure. It effectively treats hypertension caused by Liver yang rising with red eyes, headache, dizziness or a bitter taste in the mouth.

- Hypertension: add *Di Long* to *Tian Ma* (Rhizoma Gastrodiae), *Shi Jue Ming* (Concha Haliotidis) and *Xia Ku Cao* (Spica Prunellae).

6. Used Topically to Promote Healing

Di Long is also effective for treatment of acute parotitis, chronic ulcers of the lower limbs, burns, boils or carbuncles. It should be crushed into powder, mixed with sugar, and applied topically.

DOSAGE

5 to 15 grams in decoction, 1 to 2 grams in powder. When using fresh *Di Long* in decoction, the dosage is 10 to 20 grams.

CAUTIONS / CONTRAINDICATIONS

- Use of *Di Long* is contraindicated in patients with Spleen and Stomach deficiencies, or those who do not show excess heat symptoms.
- *Di Long* should be used with caution during pregnancy, as it stimulates contraction of the uterus.

CHEMICAL COMPOSITION

Lumbrofebrine, lumbritin, terrestrolumbrolysin, adenine, hypoxanthine, choline, guanine, guanidine, arachidonic acid.[1]

PHARMACOLOGICAL EFFECTS

- **Antiasthmatic:** Alcohol extract of *Di Long* has significant impact to dilate the bronchi and relieve asthma in rats and rabbits.[2]
- **Cardiovascular:** Both water and alcohol extracts of *Di Long* in mice have a marked effect to lower blood pressure, with the peak effect observed 90 minutes after ingestion and duration of action lasting 2 to 3 hours. The exact mechanism of action is unclear, but is thought to be related to the central nervous system. Probanthine reverses the hypotensive effect of *Di Long*, but atropine does not.[3]
- **Uterine stimulant:** Injection of a *Di Long* preparation has a strong stimulating effect on the smooth muscle of the uterus, leading to contraction and spasms in rabbits and rats.[4]
- **Antiseizure:** Intraperitoneal injection of alcohol extract of *Di Long* at 20 g/kg to treat seizures in mice has an effect comparable to that of 20 mg/kg of phenobarbital.[5]
- **Antipyretic:** It reduces body temperature in rabbits with artificially-induced fever. Its antipyretic effect is slightly weaker than that of aspirin.[6]
- **Hematological:** Administration of *Di Long* via oral or intravenous injection inhibits the formation of thrombi and facilitates their dissolution.[7]

CLINICAL STUDIES AND RESEARCH

- **Hypertension:** According to one report, 34 patients with hypertension were treated with a preparation of *Di Long* three times daily for 6 to 64 days with good results. The average duration of treatment was 27.9 days.[8]
- **Epilepsy:** An herbal treatment of epilepsy was effective for 16 out of 20 patients. The treatment protocol was to administer 3 to 6 grams of *Di Long* as decoction for 2 to 12 months. The average duration of treatment was 5.5 months.[9]
- **Schizophrenia:** In one clinical study, 110 patients with schizophrenia were divided into three groups for treatment: group one received decoction of *Di Long* with antipsychotic medications, group two received injection of *Di Long* with antipsychotic medications, and group three received only decoction of *Di Long*. Patients in all three groups reported improvement, with groups one and two being most noticeable. In addition, those with schizophrenia characterized by blood stagnation showed the most improvement.[10]
- **Asthma:** A preparation of *Di Long* given three times daily was effective in treating asthma in 37 out of 44 patients.[11]

TOXICOLOGY

Allergic reactions have been reported following the injection of *Di Long*. The frequency and severity of allergic reactions are unavailable at the time of publication.[12]

References

1. *Xian Dai Zhong Yao Yao Li Xue* (Contemporary Pharmacology of Chinese Herbs), 1997; 1104
2. *Chang Yong Zhong Yao Cheng Fen Yu Yao Li Shou Ce* (A Handbook of the Composition and Pharmacology of Common Chinese Drugs), 1994; 185:789
3. *Zhong Yao Yao Li Yu Ying Yong* (Pharmacology and Applications of Chinese Herbs); 1983; 35
4. *Zhong Cheng Yao Yan Jiu* (Research of Chinese Patent Medicine); 1984; (3):42
5. *Zhong Yao Yao Li Yu Ying Yong* (Pharmacology and Applications of Chinese Herbs); 1983; 35
6. Ibid.

Di Long (Pheretima)

7. *Zhe Jiang Zhong Yi Za Zhi* (Zhejiang Journal of Chinese Medicine), 1991; 26(11):512
8. *Shang Hai Zhong Yi Yao Za Zhi* (Shanghai Journal of Chinese Medicine and Herbology), 1959; 4:39
9. *He Bei Yi Yao* (Hebei Medicine and Herbology), 1983; 3:48
10. *Zhe Jiang Yi Xue* (Zhejiang Journal of Medicine), 1979; 11:440
11. *Zhong Cao Yao Tong Xun* (Journal of Chinese Herbal Medicine), 1970; 1:14
12. *Xian Dai Zhong Yao Yao Li Xue* (Contemporary Pharmacology of Chinese Herbs), 1997; 1104

Shi Jue Ming (Concha Haliotidis)

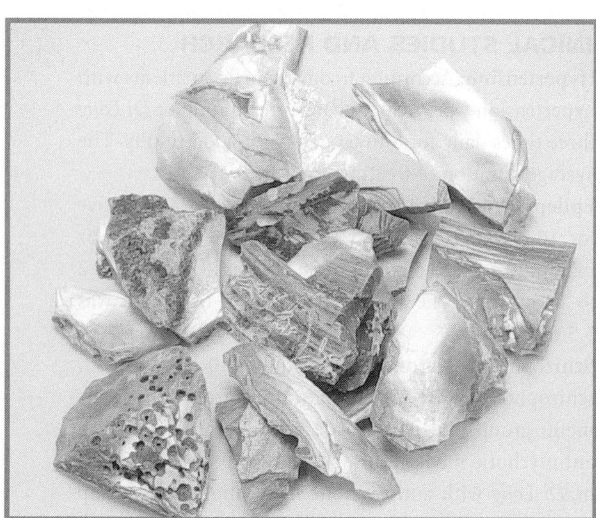

石决明 石决明

Pinyin Name: *Shi Jue Ming*
Literal Name: "stone sense brightness"
Alternate Chinese Names: *Jiu Kong Shi Jue*
Original Source: *Shen Nong Ben Cao Jing* (Divine Husbandman's Classic of the Materia Medica) in the second century
English Name: haliotis, sea-ear shell, abalone shell
Zoological Name: *Haliotis diversicolor* Reeve. (*She Bao*); *Haliotis gigantea discus* Reeve (*Pan Da Bao*); *Haliotis discus hannai* Ino (*Zhou Wen Pan Bao*); *Haliotis ovina* Gmelin (*Yang Bao*); *Haliotis ruler* (Leach) (*Ao Zhou Bao*); *Haliotis asinina* L. (*Er Bao*); *Haliotis laevigata* (Donovan) (*Bai Bao*)
Pharmaceutical Name: Concha Haliotidis
Properties: salty, cold
Channels Entered: Liver

CHINESE THERAPEUTIC ACTIONS

1. Pacifies the Liver and Anchors Yang

Liver yang rising (excess) or Liver yang rising with yin deficiency (excess with deficiency): The sinking nature of *Shi Jue Ming* (Concha Haliotidis) anchors the rising yang of the Liver. Chief manifestations include hypertension with dizziness, vertigo, tinnitus, headache or migraine, flushed face, a bitter taste in the mouth, dry mouth, irritability, short temper, insomnia, tidal fever, palpitations, forgetfulness, sore and weak lower back and knees, constipation and dark, yellow urine. Patients may also feel spells of heat in the body. *Shi Jue Ming* nourishes Liver yin and is suitable to treat yang rising with deficient signs such as dizziness, and weakness of the back. The unprocessed form is stronger for this function.

- Liver yang rising without yin deficiency: combine *Shi Jue Ming* with *Xia Ku Cao* (Spica Prunellae), *Gou Teng* (Ramulus Uncariae cum Uncis), *Tian Ma* (Rhizoma Gastrodiae) and *Ju Hua* (Flos Chrysanthemi).
- Liver yang rising with Kidney and Liver yin deficiencies: use this substance with *Sheng Di Huang* (Radix Rehmanniae), *Bai Shao* (Radix Paeoniae Alba) and *Mu Li* (Concha Ostreae).
- Neurasthenia: add it to *Dai Zhe Shi* (Haematitum), *Sheng Di Huang* (Radix Rehmanniae), *Bai Shao* (Radix Paeoniae Alba), *Xiang Fu* (Rhizoma Cyperi), *Huang Qin* (Radix Scutellariae), *Bai Ji Li* (Fructus Tribuli), *Ju Hua* (Flos Chrysanthemi), *Yuan Zhi* (Radix Polygalae) and *Ye Jiao Teng* (Caulis Polygoni Multiflori).

2. Clears the Liver and Brightens the Eyes

Eye disorders: The Liver opens to the eyes. Heat in the Liver channel results in symptoms of red, swollen and painful eyes, photophobia, glaucoma, cataract, headache, dizziness, vertigo and a bitter taste in the mouth. *Shi Jue Ming* is one of the most essential substances in treating eye disorders caused by Liver yang rising, Liver fire or Liver yin deficiency with heat. The unprocessed form is

Shi Jue Ming (Concha Haliotidis)

stronger for this function.

- Eye disorders caused by Liver yang rising: use *Shi Jue Ming* with *Bai Ji Li* (Fructus Tribuli), *Long Dan Cao* (Radix Gentianae), *Huang Lian* (Rhizoma Coptidis), and *Ye Ming Sha* (Excrementum Vespertilionis Murini).
- Red eyes, superficial visual obstruction because of Liver yang rising and wind-heat invasion: use it with *Mi Meng Hua* (Flos Buddlejae), *Jue Ming Zi* (Semen Cassiae) and *Ju Hua* (Flos Chrysanthemi).
- Dry eyes, blurred vision, and diminished visual acuity caused by Liver blood deficiency: combine this substance with *Shu Di Huang* (Radix Rehmanniae Preparata), *Shi Hu* (Herba Dendrobii), *Shan Yao* (Rhizoma Dioscoreae), *Gou Qi Zi* (Fructus Lycii) and pig or goat liver.

3. Clears Stomach Fire, Stops Pain and Bleeding

Stomach fire: *Shi Jue Ming* neutralizes acid and treats acid reflux, heartburn, bleeding ulcers and stomach pain. The calcined form is stronger.

- Stomach fire: combine *Shi Jue Ming* with *Hai Piao Xiao* (Endoconcha Sepiae), *Huang Lian* (Rhizoma Coptidis) and *Wu Zhu Yu* (Fructus Evodiae).

Shi Jue Ming can be applied as powder topically to treat trauma and cuts or bleeding resulting from injury.

DOSAGE

15 to 30 grams. Crush and pre-decoct *Shi Jue Ming* to maximize extraction of active components. The unprocessed form is stronger to anchor the yang and clear heat. The calcined form is not as cold, and stronger in its astringent function.

CAUTIONS / CONTRAINDICATIONS

Shi Jue Ming is salty and cold and can easily injure the Spleen and Stomach. *Shi Jue Ming* is contraindicated for patients with deficiency and cold of the Spleen and Stomach, or those with poor appetite and loose stools.

CHEMICAL COMPOSITION

Calcium carbonate, small amounts of magnesium, iron, silica, phosphate, and 17 different amino acids.[1]

References

1. *Chang Yong Zhong Yao Cheng Fen Yu Yao Li Shou Ce* (A Handbook of the Composition and Pharmacology of Common Chinese Drugs), 1994; 685-686

Mu Li (Concha Ostreae)

牡蠣 牡蛎

Pinyin Name: *Mu Li*
Alternate Chinese Names: *Mu Li Ke, Zuo Mu Li*
Original Source: *Shen Nong Ben Cao Jing* (Divine Husbandman's Classic of the Materia Medica) in the second century
English Name: oyster shell
Zoological Name: *Ostrea gigas* Thunb. (*Chang Mu Li*); *Ostrea talienwhanensis* Crosse. (*Da Lian Wan Mu Li*); *Ostrea rivularis* Gould. (*Jin Jiang Mu Li*)
Pharmaceutical Name: Concha Ostreae
Properties: salty, astringent, cool
Channels Entered: Liver, Kidney

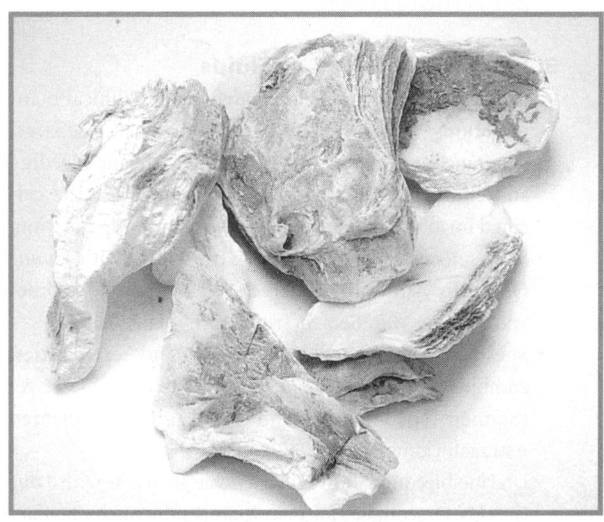

Mu Li (Concha Ostreae)

CHINESE THERAPEUTIC ACTIONS

1. Calms the Liver and Anchors Rising Yang

Liver yang rising due to Liver yin deficiency: Signs and symptoms of this condition include dizziness, vertigo, palpitations, insomnia, irritability, short temper, restlessness and tinnitus. The unprocessed form of *Mu Li* (Concha Ostreae) is best for this function.

- Liver yang rising: use *Mu Li* with *Long Gu* (Os Draconis), *Gui Ban* (Plastrum Testudinis) and *Bai Shao* (Radix Paeoniae Alba).
- Insomnia: pair it with *Ye Jiao Teng* (Caulis Polygoni Multiflori).

Liver wind caused by post-febrile disorder injuring the yin: *Mu Li* treats convulsions and muscle twitches.

- Liver wind: use it with *Gui Ban* (Plastrum Testudinis), *Bie Jia* (Carapax Trionycis), and *Bai Shao* (Radix Paeoniae Alba).

2. Softens Hardness and Dissipates Nodules

Hardness and nodules: The vinegar-processed form of *Mu Li* is often used to treat hot phlegm with lumps or palpable masses such as scrofula, goiter, lymphogranuloma, splenomegaly and hepatomegaly.

- Scrofula, goiter and lymphogranuloma: use *Mu Li* with *Zhe Bei Mu* (Bulbus Fritillariae Thunbergii) and *Xuan Shen* (Radix Scrophulariae).
- Splenomegaly, hepatomegaly: add it to *Dan Shen* (Radix Salviae Miltiorrhizae), *Bie Jia* (Carapax Trionycis), *San Leng* (Rhizoma Sparganii), *E Zhu* (Rhizoma Curcumae), *Yu Jin* (Radix Curcumae), *Chai Hu* (Radix Bupleuri) and *Ze Lan* (Herba Lycopi).

3. Prevents Leakage of Fluids

Leakage of body fluids due to deficiency: Clinical manifestations include spermatorrhea, vaginal discharge, spontaneous sweating, night sweating, uterine bleeding and enuresis. For maximum effectiveness, use the calcined form of *Mu Li* to enhance the restraining function.

- Spontaneous or night sweating: use *Mu Li* with *Huang Qi* (Radix Astragali), *Ma Huang Gen* (Radix Ephedrae) and *Fu Xiao Mai* (Semen Tritici Aestivi Levis).
- Spermatorrhea, sore lower back and extremities: combine it with *Qian Shi* (Semen Euryales), *Lian Xu* (Stamen Nelumbinis) and *Sha Yuan Zi* (Semen Astragali Complanati).
- Uterine bleeding and vaginal discharge: use it with *Long Gu* (Os Draconis), *Hai Piao Xiao* (Endoconcha Sepiae) and *Shan Yao* (Rhizoma Dioscoreae).
- Enuresis: add it to *Fu Pen Zi* (Fructus Rubi) and *Yi Zhi Ren* (Fructus Alpiniae Oxyphyllae).

4. Neutralizes Acid and Relieves Stomach Pain

Stomach fire with acid regurgitation, heartburn, stomach pain: *Mu Li* is alkaline and neutralizes acid and stops bleeding. The calcined form, powdered, is usually used for this purpose.

- Duodenal or peptic ulcer: use *Mu Li* with *Hai Piao Xiao* (Endoconcha Sepiae), *Bai Ji* (Rhizoma Bletillae), *Yan Hu Suo* (Rhizoma Corydalis), *Pu Gong Ying* (Herba Taraxaci) and *Bai Hua She She Cao* (Herba Oldenlandia).
- Acid reflux: use it with *Wu Zhu Yu* (Fructus Evodiae), *Huang Lian* (Rhizoma Coptidis) and *Zhe Bei Mu* (Bulbus Fritillariae Thunbergii).

DOSAGE

15 to 30 grams in unprocessed form. Crush and predecoct *Mu Li* to maximize extraction of active constituents. The recommended dosage for the calcined form is slightly lower, due to increased rate of extraction. The unprocessed form more strongly calms Liver wind and anchors Liver yang. The calcined form more effectively neutralizes stomach acid and relieves pain.

CAUTIONS / CONTRAINDICATIONS

- Due to its restraining property, *Mu Li* is contraindicated in patients with damp-heat or excess conditions.
- Overdose of *Mu Li* may cause indigestion or constipation.

PHARMACOLOGICAL EFFECTS

- **Gastrointestinal:** *Mu Li* is commonly used to treat gastric and duodenal ulcers.[1]

CLINICAL STUDIES AND RESEARCH

- **Perspiration associated with pulmonary tuberculosis:** A reduction of perspiration was reported in 7 out of 10 patients who received a decoction containing *Mu Li*. The decoction was prepared by cooking 15 grams of *Mu Li* in 500 ml of water to yield 200 ml of the final decoction. The patients were instructed to drink the decoction in two equally-divided doses (100 ml per dose) twice daily. The herbal treatment continued for 2 to 3 days after perspiration stopped.[2]
- **Gastric and duodenal ulcer:** According to one study, two patients with gastric ulcers and 18 patients with duodenal ulcers were treated with a decoction, with complete recovery in 6 cases, marked improvement in 5 cases, slight improvement in 6 cases, and no effect in 3 cases. The decoction contained 30 to 50 grams each of *Long Gu* (Os Draconis) and *Mu Li*. Furthermore, 10 grams of *Yan Hu Suo* (Rhizoma Corydalis) were added for severe pain, and 15 grams of *Ye Jiao Teng* (Caulis Polygoni Multiflori) were added for insomnia. The patients were instructed to take

Mu Li (Concha Ostreae)

the decoction twice daily for 10 to 20 days per course of treatment.[3]

AUTHORS' COMMENTS

Mu Li and *Shi Jue Ming* (Concha Haliotidis) both anchor Liver yang and treat hypertension. *Mu Li* also disperses stagnation, softens hardness and consolidates body fluids. *Shi Jue Ming* treats eye disorders caused by heat in the Liver channel.

Mu Li and *Long Gu* (Os Draconis) both anchor Liver yang, calm the *shen* (spirit), and stop loss of bodily fluids. *Mu Li* enters the Liver, and more strongly anchors Liver yang, clears heat, and nourishes yin. *Long Gu* enters the Heart, and more effectively calms the *shen* and astringes body fluids.

According to Dr. Wang Shi-Xiang, *Mu Li*, *Bai Ji Li* (Fructus Tribuli), and *Xia Ku Cao* (Spica Prunellae) should be combined for hyperthyroid patients who have bulging eyes. The three herbs function to soften hardness, clear toxins and bring down Liver fire.

References

1. *Zhong Yao Xue* (Chinese Herbology), 1998; 686:688
2. *Jiang Su Zhong Yi* (Jiangsu Chinese Medicine), 1964; 2:39
3. *Zhong Yi Za Zhi* (Journal of Chinese Medicine), 1983; 3:36

Dai Zhe Shi (Haematitum)

代赭石

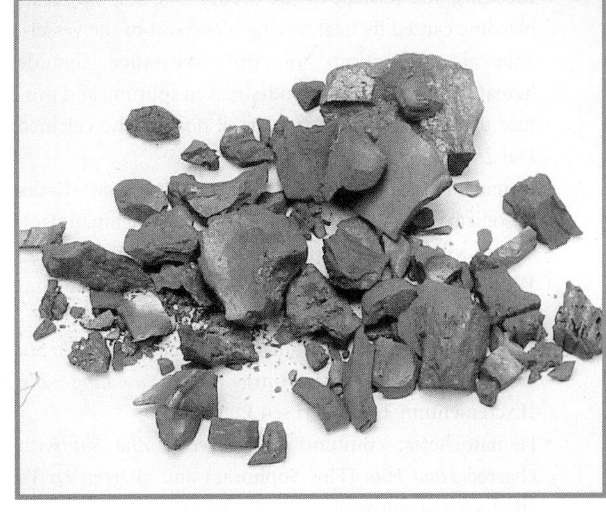

Pinyin Name: *Dai Zhe Shi*
Literal Name: "red stone from Dai county"
Original Source: *Shen Nong Ben Cao Jing* (Divine Husbandman's Classic of the Materia Medica) in the second century
English Name: hematite
Pharmaceutical Name: Haematitum
Properties: bitter, cold
Channels Entered: Heart, Liver

CHINESE THERAPEUTIC ACTIONS

1. Calms the Liver and Anchors Rising Yang

Liver yang rising with yin deficiency: Heavy and sinking in nature, *Dai Zhe Shi* (Haematitum) anchors rising Liver yang that manifests in symptoms such as dizziness, vertigo, headache and distention, tinnitus, short temper, irritability, insomnia, increased pressure in the eyes, high blood pressure, palpitations and constipation. The unprocessed form should be used for maximum effectiveness.

- Dizziness, vertigo, headache and distention: use *Dai Zhe Shi* with *Long Gu* (Os Draconis) and *Mu Li* (Concha Ostreae).
- Hypertension with irritability, dizziness, and constipation: combine it with *Long Gu* (Os Draconis), *Mu Li* (Concha Ostreae), *Bai Shao* (Radix Paeoniae Alba) and *Chuan Niu Xi* (Radix Cyathulae).
- Anger, irritability, headache, insomnia: use it with *Huang Qin* (Radix Scutellariae), *Huang Lian* (Rhizoma Coptidis), *Tian Zhu Huang* (Concretio Silicea Bambusae), *Dan Nan Xing* (Arisaema cum Bile), *Xiang Fu* (Rhizoma Cyperi) and *Mu Li* (Concha Ostreae).

2. Redirects Rebellious Qi Downwards

Hiccups, vomiting and nausea: *Dai Zhe Shi* reverses the ascending Stomach qi to relieve hiccups, vomiting and nausea. Ascending qi is often caused by Stomach qi deficiency or damp accumulating in the middle *jiao*, leading

Dai Zhe Shi (Haematitum)

to the Stomach's inability to direct the qi downwards. Use the unprocessed form of *Dai Zhe Shi* for this function.

- Hiccups, vomiting and nausea due to Stomach qi deficiency: combine *Dai Zhe Shi* with *Dang Shen* (Radix Codonopsis), *Xuan Fu Hua* (Flos Inulae) and *Ban Xia* (Rhizoma Pinelliae).
- Nausea due to cold: use it with *Fu Zi* (Radix Aconiti Lateralis Praeparata), *Rou Gui* (Cortex Cinnamomi) and *Dao Dou* (Semen Canavaliae).

Asthma: *Dai Zhe Shi* directs Lung qi downwards, treating asthma, wheezing, dyspnea, and cough.

- Asthma due to deficiency of the Kidney and Lung: use this mineral with *Dang Shen* (Radix Codonopsis) and *Shan Zhu Yu* (Fructus Corni) to tonify the Kidney and Lung.
- Cough and dyspnea with fever and yellow sputum from Lung heat: use *Dai Zhe Shi* with *Sang Bai Pi* (Cortex Mori), *Su Zi* (Fructus Perillae) and *Xuan Fu Hua* (Flos Inulae).

3. Cools the Blood and Stops Bleeding

Bleeding due to heat in the blood: *Dai Zhe Shi* treats bleeding caused by heat forcing blood out of the vessels. Clinical applications of this substance include hematemesis, epistaxis, blood-streaked sputum, and profuse uterine bleeding. Use a small dose of the calcined *Dai Zhe Shi* for this function.

- Hematemesis, epistaxis: use it with *Bai Shao* (Radix Paeoniae Alba) and *Sheng Di Huang* (Radix Rehmanniae).
- Cough with blood or bloody sputum: combine it with *Zi Wan* (Radix Asteris), *Kuan Dong Hua* (Flos Farfarae) and *Pi Pa Ye* (Folium Eriobotryae).
- Chronic uterine bleeding and dizziness: add it to *Chi Shi Zhi* (Halloysitum Rubrum) and *Wu Ling Zhi* (Excrementum Trogopteri seu Pteromi).
- Hematochezia: combine calcined *Dai Zhe Shi* with charred *Huai Hua* (Flos Sophorae) and charred *Di Yu* (Radix Sanguisorbae).

DOSAGE

10 to 30 grams of the unprocessed form, 6 to 15 grams of the calcined form, in decoction. In severe cases, the highest dose for the unprocessed form is 60 to 90 grams. Crush and pre-decoct *Dai Zhe Shi* to maximize extraction of active constituents. The unprocessed form anchors rising Liver yang. The calcined form stops bleeding.

CAUTIONS / CONTRAINDICATIONS

- Because *Dai Zhe Shi* is cold, heavy and descending in nature, it should be used with caution during pregnancy and in patients with cold conditions.
- Do not use a large dose of *Dai Zhe Shi* or for a prolonged period of time, as this substance contains a trace amount of arsenic.

CHEMICAL COMPOSITION

Aluminum, silicon, magnesium, tin, calcium, diferric trioxide, and arsenic.[1]

PHARMACOLOGICAL EFFECTS

- **Smooth muscle stimulant:** Injection of *Dai Zhe Shi* has a stimulating effect on the smooth muscle of the intestines to increase peristalsis.[2]

CLINICAL STUDIES AND RESEARCH

- **Auditory vertigo:** In one study, 86 patients with vertigo were treated with 95.3% effectiveness using an herbal formula as decoction once daily. The formula contained *Dai Zhe Shi* 45g, *Ban Xia* (Rhizoma Pinelliae) 18g, *Che Qian Cao* (Herba Plantaginis) 18g, and *Xia Ku Cao* (Spica Prunellae) 18g.[3]

AUTHORS' COMMENTS

Dai Zhe Shi and *Chi Shi Zhi* (Halloysitum Rubrum) both treat bleeding. *Dai Zhe Shi* is bitter and cold, and treats upper and lower *jiao* bleeding such as epistaxis and uterine bleeding. *Chi Shi Zhi* is warm and is used mainly for lower *jiao* bleeding such as hematochezia, bleeding dysentery, or uterine bleeding.

References

1. *Chang Yong Zhong Yao Xian Dai Yan Jiu Yu Lin Chuan* (Recent Study & Clinical Application of Common Traditional Chinese Medicine), 1995; 502
2. Ibid., 502:503
3. *Zhong Cao Yao Tong Xun* (Journal of Chinese Herbal Medicine), 1972; 4:57

Bai Ji Li (Fructus Tribuli)

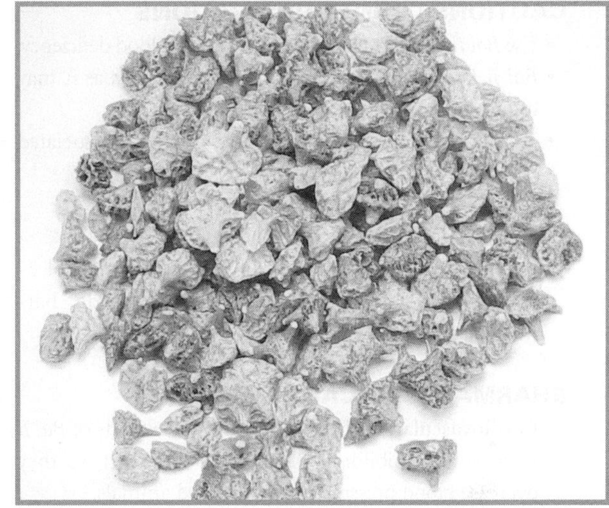

白蒺藜 白蒺藜

Pinyin Name: *Bai Ji Li*
Alternate Chinese Names: *Ci Ji Li, Ji Li*
Original Source: *Shen Nong Ben Cao Jing* (Divine Husbandman's Classic of the Materia Medica) in the second century
English Name: tribulus, puncture vine caltrop fruit
Botanical Name: *Tribulus terrestris* L. (*Ji Li*)
Pharmaceutical Name: Fructus Tribuli
Properties: bitter, acrid, neutral
Channels Entered: Liver

CHINESE THERAPEUTIC ACTIONS

1. Pacifies the Liver and Anchors Yang

Liver yang rising: *Bai Ji Li* (Fructus Tribuli) enters the Liver channel to treat disorders of the head caused by rising Liver yang. Symptoms may include blurred vision, a bitter taste in the mouth, headache, dizziness, vertigo or hypertension.

- Dizziness, blurred vision: use *Bai Ji Li* with *Ju Hua* (Flos Chrysanthemi) and *Bai Shao* (Radix Paeoniae Alba).
- Hypertension with vertigo: add it to *Gou Teng* (Ramulus Uncariae cum Uncis), *Mu Li* (Concha Ostreae), *Tian Ma* (Rhizoma Gastrodiae) and *Niu Xi* (Radix Cyathulae seu Achyranthis).

2. Facilitates the Flow of Liver Qi and Disperses Stagnation

Liver qi stagnation: Liver qi stagnation may result in symptoms of chest and hypochondriac fullness, distention and pain, irregular menstruation, and breast nodules and insufficient milk in women, caused by obstruction of the Liver channel.

- Chest and hypochondriac pain: combine *Bai Ji Li* with *Chai Hu* (Radix Bupleuri), *Zhi Ke* (Fructus Aurantii), *Xiang Fu* (Rhizoma Cyperi), *Yu Jin* (Radix Curcumae), *Chuan Lian Zi* (Fructus Toosendan), and *Yan Hu Suo* (Rhizoma Corydalis).
- Hypochondriac pain related to hepatitis: use it with *Zao Jiao Ci* (Spina Gleditsiae), *Jiang Huang* (Rhizoma Curcumae Longae) and *Bai Hua She She Cao* (Herba Oldenlandia).
- Palpable masses associated with Liver qi stagnation: use it with *Bie Jia* (Carapax Trionycis), *Dan Shen* (Radix Salviae Miltiorrhizae), *Mu Li* (Concha Ostreae), *Zao Jiao Ci* (Spina Gleditsiae), *Hong Hua* (Flos Carthami) and *Tao Ren* (Semen Persicae).

3. Dispels Wind and Brightens the Eyes

Eye disorders: *Bai Ji Li* is commonly used to treat eye disorders caused by heat in the Liver channel, with such symptoms as redness, itching, swelling, pain, superficial visual obstruction, increased tears and photophobia.

- Red and painful eyes, increased tears, photophobia: use *Bai Ji Li* with *Jue Ming Zi* (Semen Cassiae), *Zhi Zi* (Fructus Gardeniae), *Mu Zei* (Herba Equiseti Hiemalis), *Sang Ye* (Folium Mori), *Ju Hua* (Flos Chrysanthemi), *Shi Jue Ming* (Concha Haliotidis) and *Mi Meng Hua* (Flos Buddlejae).
- Superficial visual obstruction: add it to *Ju Hua* (Flos Chrysanthemi), *Man Jing Zi* (Fructus Viticis), *Jue Ming Zi* (Semen Cassiae) and *Lian Qiao* (Fructus Forsythiae).

4. Dispels Wind and Stops Itching

Eczema, skin lesions with significant itching, vitiligo, or neurodermatitis arising from wind with blood deficiency.

- Skin lesions, chronic eczema or neurodermatitis: use *Bai Ji Li* with *Dang Gui* (Radicis Angelicae Sinensis), *He Shou Wu* (Radix Polygoni Multiflori), and *Fen Fang Ji* (Radix Stephaniae Tetandrae).
- Vitiligo: use 15 grams of *Bai Ji Li* alone in decoction, twice daily.
- Eczema with itching: use this herb with *Dang Gui* (Radicis Angelicae Sinensis), *Jing Jie* (Herba Schizonepetae) and *Chan Tui* (Periostracum Cicadae).

DOSAGE

6 to 10 grams. Dry-frying increases the warmth of *Bai Ji Li* and facilitates extraction of the active components. Dry-frying with salt facilitates its entry to the Kidney and Liver channels, and treatment of related disorders.

Bai Ji Li (Fructus Tribuli)

CAUTIONS / CONTRAINDICATIONS

- Use *Bai Ji Li* with caution in patients with blood deficiency.
- *Bai Ji Li* is contraindicated during pregnancy, as it may induce miscarriage.
- Topical application of *Bai Ji Li* is sometimes associated with rash and itching.

CHEMICAL COMPOSITION

Kaempferol, kaempferol-3-glucoside, kaempferol-3-rutinoside, tribuloside, furostanol bisglycoside, harmane, harmine.[1]

PHARMACOLOGICAL EFFECTS

- **Cardiovascular:** Both water and alcohol extracts of *Bai Ji Li* have an inhibitory influence on the heart, as they decrease blood pressure in anesthetized animals.[2]
- **Diuretic:** *Bai Ji Li* has a mild diuretic effect in rats.[3]

CLINICAL STUDIES AND RESEARCH

- **Warts:** In one study, 123 patients with warts were treated with a success rate close to 100% using topical application of tribulus. The treatment protocol was to grind the fresh herb into paste, and rub it on the affected area until the patients feel a slight burning sensation and pain. The herbal paste should not be wiped off immediately. This process is performed one time each day or every other day, for a total of 1 to 4 treatments. [4]
- **Vitiligo:** One report describes that 27 patients with vitiligo were treated with an 87% rate of effectiveness using 15 grams of *Bai Ji Li* in tea twice daily.[5]

HERB-DRUG INTERACTION

- **Diuretics:** *Bai Ji Li* has a mild diuretic effect. Though this potential interaction has not been documented, concurrent use with diuretic drugs may lead to increased elimination of water and/or electrolytes.[6] [Note: Examples of diuretics include chlorothiazide, hydrochlorothiazide, furosemide (Lasix), bumetanide (Bumex), and torsemide (Demadex).]

TOXICOLOGY

One case of anaphylactic reaction was reported following ingestion of *Bai Ji Li*.[7] [Note: Anaphylactic shock is the most severe type of allergic reaction. Unfortunately, it is very difficult, if not impossible, to predict when patients will have such serious reactions. Though there is one case of anaphylactic reaction reported, use of *Bai Ji Li* does not necessarily have a higher risk of allergy than other herbs.]

AUTHORS' COMMENTS

Bai Ji Li (Fructus Tribuli) is sometime confused with *Sha Yuan Ji Li*, the alternate name for *Sha Yuan Zi* (Semen Astragali Complanati). Although they both treat disorders of the eyes, they have very different functions.

- *Bai Ji Li* anchors Liver yang and relieves Liver qi stagnation, calming the Liver and dispelling wind-heat to brighten the eyes. It is used for red eyes with tears or pain.
- *Sha Yuan Zi* tonifies the Liver and Kidney (specifically Kidney yang), secures *jing* (essence) and improves vision by nourishing the Liver. It is used more for blurred vision or diminished visual acuity.

References

1. *Xian Dai Zhong Yao Yao Li Xue* (Contemporary Pharmacology of Chinese Herbs), 1997; 1115
2. *Chang Yong Zhong Yao Xian Dai Yan Jiu Yu Lin Chuan* (Recent Study & Clinical Application of Common Traditional Chinese Medicine), 1995; 510:511
3. Ibid.
4. *Xin Yi Xue* (New Medicine), 1976; 11:555
5. *He Bei Yi Yao* (*Hebei Medicine and Herbology*), 1981; 2:45
6. Chen, J. Recognition & prevention of Herb-drug interactions, *Medical Acupuncture*, Fall/Winter 1998/1999; volume 10/number 2; 9-13
7. *Chang Yong Zhong Yao Xian Dai Yan Jiu Yu Lin Chuan* (Recent Study & Clinical Application of Common Traditional Chinese Medicine), 1995; 510:511

Jue Ming Zi (Semen Cassiae)

决明子 决明子

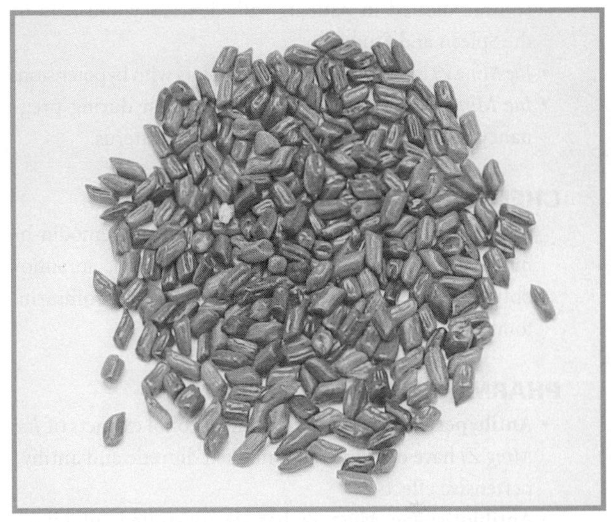

Pinyin Name: *Jue Ming Zi*
Literal Name: "seed of brightness"
Alternate Chinese Names: *Cao Jue Ming, Ma Ti Jue Ming*
Original Source: *Shen Nong Ben Cao Jing* (Divine Husbandman's Classic of the Materia Medica) in the second century
English Name: cassia seed
Botanical Name: *Cassia obtusifolia* L. (*Jue Ming*), *Cassia tora* L. (*Xiao Jue Ming*)
Pharmaceutical Name: Semen Cassiae
Properties: sweet, bitter, cool
Channels Entered: Liver, Large Intestine

CHINESE THERAPEUTIC ACTIONS

1. Clears Liver Heat and Benefits the Eyes

Liver heat or wind-heat in the Liver channel: *Jue Ming Zi* (Semen Cassiae) treats eye disorders such as redness, dryness, swelling and pain in the eyes, photophobia, cataracts and night blindness.

- Redness, swelling and pain of the eyes caused by Liver heat: use *Jue Ming Zi* with *Long Dan Cao* (Radix Gentianae), *Huang Qin* (Radix Scutellariae) and *Xia Ku Cao* (Spica Prunellae).
- Redness, swelling and pain of the eyes arising from wind-heat attacking the Liver channel: combine this herb with *Ju Hua* (Flos Chrysanthemi), *Man Jing Zi* (Fructus Viticis) and *Mu Zei* (Herba Equiseti Hiemalis).
- Cataract, optic atrophy, dryness and diminished vision caused by Liver and Kidney deficiencies: add *Jue Ming Zi* to *Sheng Di Huang* (Radix Rehmanniae), *Ju Hua* (Flos Chrysanthemi), *Shan Yao* (Rhizoma Dioscoreae), and *Xuan Shen* (Radix Scrophulariae).
- Night blindness and optic nerve degeneration: use *Jue Ming Zi* alone.

2. Calms the Liver and Anchors Liver Yang

Liver yang rising: Characteristic symptoms include headache, dizziness, vertigo, red face, red eyes, and irritability. Many patients with Liver yang rising also have hypertension. Bitter and cold, *Jue Ming Zi* clears Liver heat and calms Liver yang.

- Hypertension caused by rising Liver yang: use *Jue Ming Zi* with *Gou Teng* (Ramulus Uncariae cum Uncis), *Mu Li* (Concha Ostreae), and *Ju Hua* (Flos Chrysanthemi).

3. Clears Heat and Moistens Bowels

Constipation from dryness or heat: *Jue Ming Zi* treats dry stools and acute or chronic constipation arising from heat or dryness.

- Constipation: use it with *Hei Zhi Ma* (Semen Sesami Nigrum), *Sheng Di Huang* (Radix Rehmanniae) and *Dang Gui* (Radicis Angelicae Sinensis) to clear heat and lubricate the bowels.
- Mild constipation: use the herb individually as tea.

4. Cardiovascular Effect

Jue Ming Zi has excellent functions to reduce high cholesterol and treat atherosclerosis, used individually or in combination with other herbs.

- Cholesterol: use 30 grams of *Jue Ming Zi* with *Jiao Gu Lan* (Rhizoma seu Herba Gynostemmatis), *Da Huang* (Radix et Rhizoma Rhei), *Shan Zha* (Fructus Crataegi) and *Ze Xie* (Rhizoma Alismatis).
- Atherosclerosis: pair it with *Dan Shen* (Radix Salviae Miltiorrhizae).

DOSAGE

10 to 15 grams in decoction. Use 30 grams of *Jue Ming Zi* to lower cholesterol levels. *Jue Ming Zi* should be crushed prior to cooking in herbal decoction. The dosage range is 3 to 6 grams for use as powder.

The unprocessed herb is colder in nature than other forms, and has a stronger function to clear Liver fire and wind-heat attacking the Liver channel. It is usually used to treat acute eye disorders. Because of its cold nature, the unprocessed herb is sometimes associated with diarrhea. The dry-fried form is not as cold, and less likely to cause diarrhea. However, it is also less effective to clear Liver Heat.

CAUTIONS / CONTRAINDICATIONS

- Cold and sedating in nature, *Jue Ming Zi* is

Jue Ming Zi (Semen Cassiae)

contraindicated in patients with deficiency and cold of the Spleen and Stomach.

- *Jue Ming Zi* is contraindicated in patients with hypotension.
- *Jue Ming Zi* should be used with caution during pregnancy, as it stimulates contraction of the uterus.

CHEMICAL COMPOSITION

Chrysophanol, emodin, aloe-emodin, rhein, emodin-b-monoglucoside, emodinan, physcion, obtusin, aurantio-obtusin, torachrysone, rubrofusarin, nor-rubrofusarin, toratactone.[1]

PHARMACOLOGICAL EFFECTS

- **Antihypertensive:** Both water and alcohol extracts of *Jue Ming Zi* have demonstrated marked diuretic and antihypertensive effects.[2]
- **Antibiotic:** *Jue Ming Zi* has demonstrated inhibitory influence against *Staphylococcus aureus, Corynebacterium diphtheriae, E. coli,* and various species of bacillus and dermatophytes.[3]
- **Antihyperlipidemic:** *Jue Ming Zi* has been shown to lower blood cholesterol levels in both animal and human studies. In one study, administration of 10 grams of *Jue Ming Zi* per day lowered blood cholesterol levels in rabbits. In another study, incorporation of *Jue Ming Zi* as 7% of the diet in mice increased the blood HDL level.[4,5]
- **Purgative:** Oral administration of *Jue Ming Zi* in mice is associated with a purgative effect that peaks 3 to 5 hours after ingestion.[6]
- **Uterine stimulant:** Administration of *Jue Ming Zi* is associated with increased contraction of the uterus.[7]

CLINICAL STUDIES AND RESEARCH

- **Hyperlipidemia:** *Jue Ming Zi* in three separate dosage forms was used to treat 100 patients with high cholesterol levels. The first group received an herbal decoction (the decoction contains 50 grams of herb, and was taken in 2 equally-divided doses daily); the second group received herbal syrup (100 ml of the syrup contains 75 grams of herb, and 20 ml of syrup was given three times daily); and the third group received pills (each pill contains 3 grams of herb, 5 pills were given three times daily). The duration of treatment was six weeks, with evaluation taken at baseline and every 2 weeks until the completion of the study. The cholesterol levels of the subjects ranged between 210 and 484 mg/dL prior to treatment, and 110 and 208 mg/dL at the conclusion of the study. The mean decrease was 93.1 mg/dL. The patients demonstrated a progressive decline in cholesterol levels. Prior to the herbal treatment, all patients had cholesterol levels exceeding the normal level. The study reported that after 2 weeks, 86% were within normal ranges; after 4 weeks, 96%; and after 6 weeks, 98% were within normal levels.[8]
- **Hyperlipidemia:** According to one report, 48 patients were treated with 20 ml of *Jue Ming Zi* syrup (100 ml of the syrup contains 75 grams of herb) three times daily for 2 months. The study reported reduction in blood cholesterol in 95.8% of the patients, reduction in triglycerides in 86.7%, and reduction of β-lipoprotein in 89.5%.[9]
- **Vaginitis:** In one study, 22 patients were treated with *Jue Ming Zi* herbal solution used as a topical wash for one 15 to 20 minute application daily for 10 days, with good results.[10]

HERB-DRUG INTERACTION

- **Diuretics:** *Jue Ming Zi* has a diuretic effect. Though no instances of this potential interaction have been documented, concurrent use with diuretic drugs may lead to increased elimination of water and/or electrolytes.[11] [Note: Examples of diuretics include chlorothiazide, hydrochlorothiazide, furosemide (Lasix), bumetanide (Bumex), and torsemide (Demadex).]

TOXICOLOGY

The addition of *Jue Ming Zi* as 16 to 32% of the daily diet of rats for 8 days was associated with reduction of sperm count, reduction of red blood cells, and increased white blood cells and lymphocytes.[12]

AUTHORS' COMMENTS

Jue Ming Zi and *Shi Jue Ming* (Concha Haliotidis) both anchor rising Liver yang and treat dizziness, headache, vertigo, and redness, swelling and pain in the eyes. *Jue Ming Zi* is bitter and cold, and more effectively treats eye disorders caused by heat and wind in the Liver channel. It can also be used to resolve constipation. *Shi Jue Ming* is salty, sinking and stronger in anchoring rising Liver yang, and nourishes Liver yin.

References

1. *Xian Dai Zhong Yao Yao Li Xue* (Contemporary Pharmacology of Chinese Herbs), 1997; 1116-1117
2. *Zhong Yao Zhi* (Chinese Herbology Journal), 1984:352
3. *Zhi Wu Yao You Xiao Cheng Fen Shou Ce* (Manual of Plant Medicinals and Their Active Constituents), 1986; 41,212,384,829
4. *Zhong Yao Zhi* (Chinese Herbology Journal), 1984:352
5. *Zhong Cao Yao* (Chinese Herbal Medicine), 1991; 22(2):72
6. *Guo Wai Yi Xue Zhong Yi Zhong Yao Fen Ce* (Monograph of Chinese Herbology from Foreign Medicine), 1982; (6):48
7. *Zhong Cao Yao Yao Li Xue* (Herbology of Chinese Medicinals), 1983:113
8. *Xin Yi Yao Xue Za Zhi* (New Journal of Medicine and Herbology), 1974; 3:30
9. *Zhong Guo Yi Yuan Yao Xue Za Zhi* (Chinese Hospital Journal of Herbology), 1987, 9:395
10. *Jiang Su Yi Yao* (Jiangsu Journal of Medicine and Herbology), 1975; 6:45
11. Chen, J. Recognition & prevention of Herb-drug interactions, *Medical Acupuncture*, Fall/Winter 1998/1999; volume 10/number 2; 9-13
12. *Food Chem Toxicol*, 1990; 28(2):101

Gou Qi Gen (Radix Lycii)

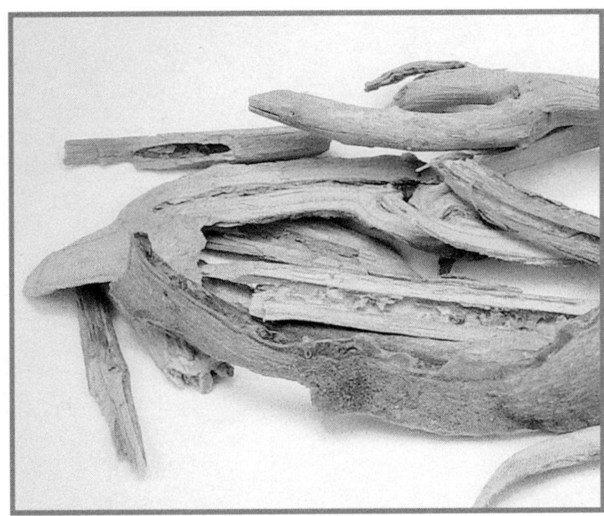

枸杞根

Pinyin Name: *Gou Qi Gen*
Alternate Chinese Names: *Qi Gen, Gou Qi Tou*
English Name: lycium root
Botanical Name: *Lycium chinense* Miller
Pharmaceutical Name: Radix Lycii
Properties: sweet, cold
Channels Entered: Liver

CHINESE THERAPEUTIC ACTIONS

Clears the Liver and Brightens the Eyes

Liver fire: *Gou Qi Gen* (Radix Lycii) treats Liver fire that manifests in redness, pain, excessive tearing, swelling of the eyes, hepatitis and tendonitis. It is also used for visual disorders associated with deficiency, that manifest in blurry or diminished vision.

- Conjunctivitis: use *Gou Qi Gen* with *Shu Wei Huang* (Herba Rostellulariae) and *Qian Li Guang* (Herba Senecionis Scandens).
- Blurred and diminished vision: combine it with white *Ju Hua* (Flos Chrysanthemi), *Shu Di Huang* (Radix Rehmanniae Preparata) and *Huang Jing* (Rhizoma Polygonati).
- Tendonitis: add it to *Shan Pu Tao* (Radix Vitis Amurensis) and *Shu Wei Huang* (Herba Rostellulariae).
- Hepatitis: pair *Gou Qi Gen* with *Huang Shui Qie* (Herba Solani).

DOSAGE

5 to 15 grams

CAUTIONS / CONTRAINDICATIONS

- Because of its cold thermal property, *Gou Qi Gen* should be used with caution in patients with Spleen deficiency.

Zhen Zhu (Margarita)

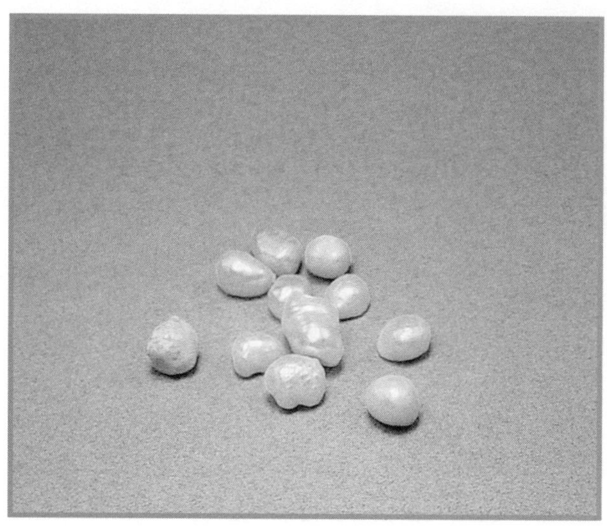

珍珠

Pinyin Name: *Zhen Zhu*
Literal Name: "precious ball"
Alternate Chinese Names: *Zhen Zhen Zhu, Lian Zhu*
Original Source: *Ri Hua Zi Ben Cao* (Materia Medica of Ri Hua-Zi) by Ri Hua-Zi in 713 A.D.
English Name: pearl
Zoological Name: *Pteria martensii* (Dunker) (*Zhen Zhu Bei*); *Hyriopsis cumingii* (Lea) (*San Jiao Fang Bang*); *Cristaria plicata* (Leach) (*Zhou Wen Guan Bang*); *Anodonta woodiana* (Lea) (*Bei Jiao Wu Chi Bang*)
Pharmaceutical Name: Margarita
Properties: sweet, salty, cold
Channels Entered: Heart, Liver

CHINESE THERAPEUTIC ACTIONS

1. Pacifies the Heart and Settles Tremors and Palpitations

***Shen* (spirit) disturbance:** *Zhen Zhu* (Margarita) treats both excess and deficient *shen* disturbances. **Excess** *shen* disturbance is characterized by Liver wind, with palpitations, seizures, tremors and childhood convulsions. **Deficient** *shen* disturbance is characterized by lack of nourishment to the Heart, with such symptoms as neurasthenia, being easily frightened, insomnia and palpitations.

- Excess *shen* disturbance: use *Zhen Zhu* with *Niu Huang* (Calculus Bovis), *Hu Po* (Succinum), *Dan Nan Xing* (Arisaema cum Bile) and *Tian Zhu Huang* (Concretio Silicea Bambusae).
- Deficient *shen* disturbance: combine it with *Fu Shen* (Poria Paradicis), *Suan Zao Ren* (Semen Zizyphi Spinosae) and *Wu Wei Zi* (Fructus Schisandrae Chinensis). Serve with honey.

2. Clears the Liver and Removes Superficial Visual Obstructions

Pterygium, blurred vision, painful eyes caused by Liver heat or Liver deficiency: *Zhen Zhu* is commonly used to treat eye disorders. It is usually used with other herbs topically as eye drops. It is rarely used internally for this function.

- Pterygium, eye pain: use *Zhen Zhu* with *Qing Xiang Zi* (Semen Celosiae), *Huang Qin* (Radix Scutellariae), *Ju Hua* (Flos Chrysanthemi), and *Shi Jue Ming* (Concha Haliotidis). Cook the herbs, and carefully direct the steam to the eyes as treatment.
- Red, painful eyes with superficial visual obstruction: pair this herb with *Bing Pian* (Borneolum Syntheticum) as an eye drop solution.

3. Promotes Healing and Helps Generate Flesh

Non-healing ulcers, sore throat with ulceration of the gums, eczema: *Zhen Zhu* treats toxic heat accumulation that is manifesting in ulcers or other dermatological disorders. It is usually used topically on non-healing ulcers to help generate flesh.

- Non-healing ulcers or macerated areas: combine *Zhen Zhu* with *Bing Pian* (Borneolum Syntheticum) and *Ru Xiang* (Gummi Olibanum) topically.
- Sores of the throat or ulcerated gums: use powdered *Zhen Zhu*, *Niu Huang* (Calculus Bovis) and *Qing Dai* (Indigo Naturalis) together, and apply topically.
- Burns and eczema: use *Zhen Zhu* alone as powder.

DOSAGE

0.3 to 1 gram. Generally used in powder or pill form. If used in decoction, crush *Zhen Zhu* into smaller pieces to facilitate the extraction of active constituents.

CHEMICAL COMPOSITION

Calcium carbonate (over 90%), magnesium, copper, iron, leucine, methionine, alanine, glycine, glutamic acid, aspartic acid, amino acids.[1]

PHARMACOLOGICAL EFFECTS

- **Smooth muscle relaxant:** Preparations of *Zhen Zhu* had an inhibitory effect on the smooth muscle of the intestines in rabbits.[2]

CLINICAL STUDIES AND RESEARCH

- **Stomatitis:** In one study, 319 patients with stomatitis from various causes were treated with a topical preparation with a rate of effectiveness of up to 92.79%. The preparation contained powdered *Zhen Zhu*, *Qing Dai*

Zhen Zhu (Margarita)

(Indigo Naturalis), *Bing Pian* (Borneolum Syntheticum), *Niu Huang* (Calculus Bovis), *Hua Shi* (Talcum), and other ingredients.[3]

AUTHORS' COMMENTS

Zhen Zhu (Margarita) and *Zhen Zhu Mu* (Concha Margaritaferae) both clear Liver fire, anchor rising yang, and pacify the Heart. *Zhen Zhu* more strongly sedates the Heart and calms the *shen* (spirit). *Zhen Zhu Mu* more effectively calms the Liver and brightens the eyes.

References

1. *Chang Yong Zhong Yao Cheng Fen Yu Yao Li Shou Ce* (A Handbook of the Composition and Pharmacology of Common Chinese Drugs), 1994; 1311
2. *Zhong Yao Da Ci Dien* (Dictionary of Chinese Herbs), 1977:1494
3. *Zhong Cheng Yao Yan Jiu* (Research of Chinese Patent Medicine), 1985; 1:21

Zhen Zhu Mu (Concha Margaritaferae)

珍珠母

Pinyin Name: *Zhen Zhu Mu*
Literal Name: "mother of pearl"
Original Source: *Tu Jing Ben Cao* (Illustrated Classic of the Materia Medica) by Su Song in 1061 A.D.
English Name: mother of pearl, nacre
Zoological Name: *Hyriopsis cumingii* (Lea) (*San Jiao Fang Bang*); *Cristaria plicata* (Leach) (*Zhou Wen Guan Bang*); *Pteria martensii* (Dunker) (*Ma Si Zhen Zhu Mu*)
Pharmaceutical Name: Concha Margaritaferae
Properties: salty, cold
Channels Entered: Heart, Liver

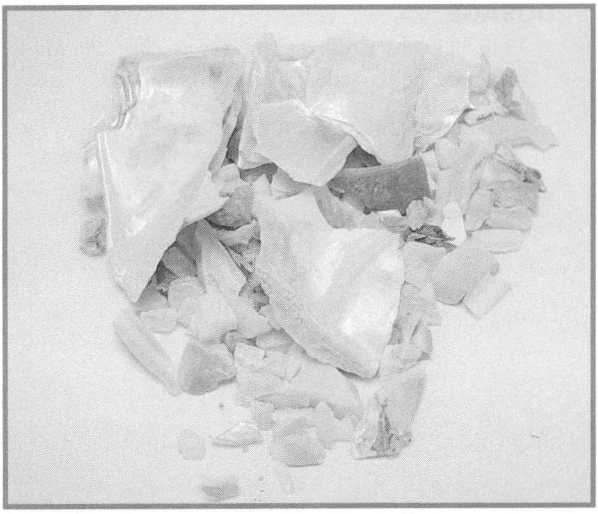

CHINESE THERAPEUTIC ACTIONS

1. Calms the Liver and Anchors Yang

Liver yang rising with Liver yin deficiency: *Zhen Zhu Mu* (Concha Margaritaferae) has a sinking nature and anchors rising Liver yang to treat symptoms such as dizziness, headache, tinnitus, irritability, frequent dreams, insomnia, palpitations and mania.

- Liver yang rising: use *Zhen Zhu Mu* with *Bai Shao* (Radix Paeoniae Alba), *Sheng Di Huang* (Radix Rehmanniae) and *Long Chi* (Dens Draconis).
- Neurasthenia: combine it with *Bai Shao* (Radix Paeoniae Alba), *Sheng Di Huang* (Radix Rehmanniae), *Bai Ji Li* (Fructus Tribuli), *Yuan Zhi* (Radix Polygalae), *Xiang Fu* (Rhizoma Cyperi), *Gou Teng* (Ramulus Uncariae cum Uncis) and *Dai Zhe Shi* (Haematitum).

2. Clears the Liver and Brightens Vision

Visual impairment due to Liver yin deficiency and Liver yang rising: Symptoms include dizziness, blurred vision, night blindness, photophobia, redness, swelling, burning and pain in the eyes.

- Dizziness, blurred vision, night blindness due to Liver deficiency: use *Zhen Zhu Mu* with *Cang Zhu* (Rhizoma Atractylodis), and pig or duck liver.
- Photophobia, redness, swelling and pain in the eyes: use it with *Ju Hua* (Flos Chrysanthemi), *Jue Ming Zi* (Semen Cassiae) and *Che Qian Zi* (Semen Plantaginis).

3. Pacifies Heart Fire

Secondary to Liver yang rising and phlegm misting the Pericardium, patients with Heart fire will show delirious speech, tremor, seizures or mania.

Zhen Zhu Mu (Concha Margaritaferae)

- Heart fire: combine *Zhen Zhu Mu* with *Yu Jin* (Radix Curcumae), *Huang Lian* (Rhizoma Coptidis), *Tian Zhu Huang* (Concretio Silicea Bambusae), *Dan Nan Xing* (Arisaema cum Bile), *Shi Chang Pu* (Rhizoma Acori), *Gou Teng* (Ramulus Uncariae cum Uncis) and *Quan Xie* (Scorpio).

4. Promotes Healing and Reduces Itching of the Skin

Eczema and itching can be treated with topical application of *Zhen Zhu Mu* alone, as powder.

5. Neutralizes Stomach Acid and Relieves Pain

Peptic ulcers with pain and acid regurgitation can be treated with *Zhen Zhu Mu*, which neutralizes stomach acid, stops acid regurgitation and relieves stomach pain.

DOSAGE

15 to 30 grams. Crush and pre-decoct *Zhen Zhu Mu* to maximize the extraction of active components.

CAUTIONS / CONTRAINDICATIONS

- *Zhen Zhu Mu* is contraindicated in cases of coldness and water accumulation in the Heart channel.

CHEMICAL COMPOSITION

$CaCO_3$, SiO_2, Al_2O_3, SO_2, K_2O, NaCl. The content of calcium is over 97%, among inorganic components.[1]

CLINICAL STUDIES AND RESEARCH

- **Immunologic:** Continuous administration of *Zhen Zhu Mu* powder at 1.5 to 3.0 grams per day for 2 months resulted in an improvement in memory, energy, concentration and cellular immunity in 146 geriatric patients.[2]

TOXICOLOGY

Zhen Zhu Mu is generally considered to be safe. The LD_{50} for oral ingestion is greater than 5000 mg/kg in rats.[3]

References

1. *Chang Yong Zhong Yao Cheng Fen Yu Yao Li Shou Ce* (A Handbook of the Composition and Pharmacology of Common Chinese Drugs), 1994; 1311-1312
2. *Lao Nian Xue Za Zhi* (Journal of Geriatrics), 1987; 7)1):50
3. *Hai Yang Yao Wu Za Zhi* (Journal of Herbs from the Sea), 1986; (1):16

Chapter 15 summary — Liver-Calming and Wind-Extinguishing Herbs

Name	Similarities	Differences
Ling Yang Jiao (Cornu Saigae Tataricae)	Calm Liver wind, clear Liver heat, relieve spasms	Strongly extinguishes Liver wind, brightens the eyes
Gou Teng (Ramulus Uncariae cum Uncis)		Calms Liver yang
Tian Ma (Rhizoma Gastrodiae)		Calms Liver wind, stops spasms, opens channels and collaterals
Quan Xie (Scorpio)	Calm Liver wind, stop tonic-clonic spasms and convulsions	Opens channels and collaterals to relieve pain, eliminates toxicity, disperses nodules, relieves twitching, treats tremor
Wu Gong (Scolopendra)		Opens channels and collaterals to relieve pain, eliminates toxicity and disperses nodules, treats tonic-clonic convulsions
Jiang Can (Bombyx Batryticatus)		Eliminates phlegm, dispels wind-heat
Di Long (Pheretima)		Clears heat, opens channels and collaterals, relieves wheezing, promotes urination
Shi Jue Ming (Concha Haliotidis)	Calm the Liver, sedate yang	Brightens the eyes
Mu Li (Concha Ostreae)		Softens hardness, reduces nodules, consolidates *jing* (essence)
Dai Zhe Shi (Haematitum)		Cools blood, stops bleeding, reverses rebellious Stomach qi
Bai Ji Li (Fructus Tribuli)		Disperses Liver qi stagnation, dispels wind to brighten the eyes and relieve itching
Jue Ming Zi (Semen Cassiae)		Brightens the eyes, relieves headache
Gou Qi Gen (Radix Lycii)		Clears the Liver and brightens the eyes
Zhen Zhu (Margarita)	Calm Liver yang, pacify the *shen* (spirit)	Generates tissue and heals skin when used externally
Zhen Zhu Mu (Concha Margaritaferae)		Clears Liver heat and brightens the eyes

General Characteristics of Liver-Calming and Wind-Extinguishing Herbs:

Taste: salty
Thermal property: cool, cold
Channels entered: Liver
Therapeutic actions: calm Liver wind, clear Liver heat, anchor Liver yang

These herbs address Liver wind, Liver heat and Liver yang disorders:

Liver wind is characterized by movement and by the mobile nature of the illness, with symptoms such as dizziness, vertigo, headache, seizures, convulsions, and stroke.

Liver yang rising is typified by internal heat surging upwards, with symptoms such as restlessness, irritability, anger, high blood pressure, and insomnia.

Liver fire is displayed by internal fire surging upwards, with symptoms such as flushed face, pain, redness, and swelling and pain of the eyes.

Ling Yang Jiao (Cornu Saigae Tataricae) is cold, with excellent functions to extinguish wind, and relieve spasms, in cases of endogenous wind secondary to excess heat. *Ling Yang Jiao* is one of the most important herbs for treating tremors, convulsions and seizures. In addition, it also sedates heat and eliminates toxins from the Liver. There is an old saying: "*Ling Yang Jiao* is a must when treating Liver disorders."

Chapter 15 summary

Gou Teng (Ramulus Uncariae cum Uncis) and ***Tian Ma*** (Rhizoma Gastrodiae) are often paired to treat the spasms and tremors of Liver wind.

Gou Teng more effectively clears wind secondary to heat in the Heart and Liver, and is best for childhood convulsions with high fever.

Tian Ma treats headache, dizziness and vertigo caused by excess or deficiency.

Quan Xie (Scorpio), ***Wu Gong*** (Scolopendra) and ***Jiang Can*** (Bombyx Batryticatus) are used clinically to strongly extinguish wind and relieve spasms.

Quan Xie and *Wu Gong* have essentially the same functions, with only minor differences. They are often used together to eliminate toxins, disperse stagnation to treat nodules, toxic swellings and masses. *Quan Xie* is more effective for twitching and tremors, while *Wu Gong* is more effective to relieve tonic-clonic convulsions. *Wu Gong* is warmer and drier than *Quan Xie*.

Jiang Can is the weakest of these three substances in extinguishing wind. However, it relieves pain and itching, dissolves phlegm and disperses stagnation.

Di Long (Pheretima), salty and cold, has descending and sedating characteristics. It relieves spasms, opens collaterals, relieves dyspnea, promotes urination and clears heat. *Di Long* stops tremor and spasms, treats hemiplegia, relieves cough due to Lung heat, and treats *re lin* (heat dysuria).

Shi Jue Ming (Concha Haliotidis) and ***Mu Li*** (Concha Ostreae) are important herbs to anchor the yang. They are most suitable in cases of underlying yin deficiency in which rising Liver yang manifests as dizziness, palpitations, vertigo and insomnia.

Shi Jue Ming clears the Liver and brightens the eyes to treat visual disorders.

Mu Li softens hardness, disperses stagnation and treat nodules and masses. Calcined *Mu Li* consolidates *jing* (essence) to treat spermatorrhea, leukorrhea and profuse sweating. It also neutralizes stomach acid to relieve gastric ulcer pains.

Dai Zhe Shi (Haematitum) anchors Liver yang, clears Liver fire, reverses rising Stomach qi to relieve nausea, vomiting and hiccups. It also cools the blood and stops bleeding.

Bai Ji Li (Fructus Tribuli) and ***Jue Ming Zi*** (Semen Cassiae) pacify the Liver, dispel wind and brighten the eyes.

Bai Ji Li more strongly disperses Liver qi stagnation.

Jue Ming Zi more effectively lubricates the intestines to treat constipation or dry stools.

Gou Qi Gen (Radix Lycii) clears the Liver to treat visual disorders.

Zhen Zhu (Margarita) and ***Zhen Zhu Mu*** (Concha Margaritaferae) clear Liver fire, anchor rising yang, and pacify the *shen* (spirit).

Zhen Zhu more strongly sedates the Heart and calms the *shen*. It is also used topically to promote healing and generation of tissue.

Zhen Zhu Mu more effectively calms the Liver and brightens the eyes. It is also used more frequently because it is more accessible and affordable than *Zhen Zhu*.

Chapter 15 summary

HERBS FROM OTHER FUNCTIONAL CATEGORIES WITH LIVER-CALMING AND WIND-EXTINGUISHING FUNCTIONS

Name	Functional Category
Bai Shao (Radix Paeoniae Alba)	Tonic Herbs (Chapter 17)
Bie Jia (Carapax Trionycis)	Tonic Herbs (Chapter 17)
Chan Tui (Periostracum Cicadae)	Exterior-Releasing Herbs (Chapter 1)
Ci Shi (Magnetitum)	*Shen*-Calming Herbs (Chapter 14)
Gui Ban (Plastrum Testudinis)	Tonic Herbs (Chapter 17)
Long Gu (Os Draconis)	*Shen*-Calming Herbs (Chapter 14)
Niu Huang (Calculus Bovis)	Heat-Clearing Herbs (Chapter 2)
Ju Hua (Flos Chrysanthemi)	Exterior-Releasing Herbs (Chapter 1)

Chapter 16

— Orifice-Opening Herbs

开窍药

Chapter 16 — Orifice-Opening Herbs

Chapter 16

开窍药 — Orifice-Opening Herbs

Definition: Herbs that are said to "open the orifices" act to dispel any pathogenic blockages in order to restore sensory function and induce consciousness.

Obstruction of the sensory orifices leads to altered consciousness. Acrid and aromatic in nature, herbs that open orifices disperse and dispel any obstructing substances, restore the five senses, and induce consciousness.

Orifice-opening herbs disperse and dispel obstructions, restore the five senses, and induce consciousness. These herbs ... relieve symptoms, but do not correct underlying causes of the symptoms.

Traditional Chinese medicine looks to the ***Heart*** in the presence of sensory or consciousness disorders, while allopathic medicine assesses the brain and central nervous system. Clinically speaking, loss of consciousness is a severe, acute symptom that is usually the result of circulatory or respiratory impairment. Therefore, herbs that open orifices also have a resuscitating function, acting in ways similar to cardiac stimulants. Clinical research has proven that some herbs in this category stimulate the central nervous system, excite respiratory and cardiac functions and increase blood pressure.

DIFFERENTIAL DIAGNOSIS AND TREATMENT

Loss of consciousness is a serious medical condition requiring immediate treatment. Possible causes of unconsciousness include ***febrile disorders***, ***heat trapped in the Pericardium***, and ***phlegm obstructing the sensory orifices***. Viewed from allopathic medicine perspectives, these disorders include seizures, epilepsy, and stroke.

When using herbs that open orifices in traditional Chinese medicine, the *Ba Gang Bian Zheng* (Eight Principle Differentiation) diagnostic approach must be incorporated. One must discern whether the loss of consciousness is caused by deficiency or excess, and by cold or heat, factors that provide critical information for effective treatment/resuscitation. Based on this differentiation, the practitioner then combines substances that open the orifices with appropriate herbs from other categories to address the particular patterns accompanying the primary disorder.

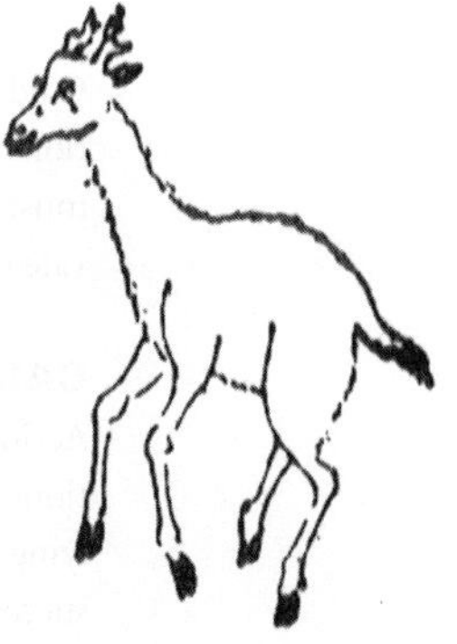

She Xiang (Moschus)
Ben Cao Gang Mu (Materia Medica), by Li Shi-Zhen, 1578 A.D.

1. Accurate differential diagnoses of *tuo zheng* (abandoned syndrome) and *bi zheng* (closed disorder) are of vital importance. The two are treated with radically different strategies, and selecting inappropriate treatment will delay or complicate recovery.

- ***Tuo zheng* (abandoned syndrome):** Unconsciousness due to ***deficiency*** is described as *tuo zheng* (abandoned syndrome), wherein the patient exhibits lax or 'open' symptomology with 'abandoned body functions:' open mouth, open hands, faint pulse, closed eyes, urinary incontinence, and perspiration. This condition should be treated with herbs that tonify qi and restore yang. Moxibustion below the umbilicus is also beneficial. Unconsciousness due to deficiency, or *tuo zheng*, should not be treated with herbs that open orifices, as this will further accentuate the weakness and deficiency the individual is already experiencing. (It may be helpful to think of the herbs that open orifices as being substances that open all of one's 'doors and windows': a person experiencing unconsciousness characterized by *tuo zheng* is already too 'wide open' and needs to have the orifices closed, or at least protected from further loss of vital qi or substances.)

Chapter 16 — Orifice-Opening Herbs

- ***Bi zheng* (closed disorder):** Unconsciousness due to ***excess*** is referred to as *bi zheng* (closed disorder), wherein the patient exhibits 'closed' symptomology with clenched jaws, closed mouth, tight fists and a forceful pulse. This condition is most appropriately treated with herbs that open the sensory orifices and restore consciousness. Resuscitating herbs are only applicable to *bi zheng* (closed disorder) or excess types. There are both warm and cold herbs in this category, used to treat *bi zheng* (closed disorder) arising from cold or heat, respectively. (Again, if one uses the analogy of doors and windows, a closed-type unconsciousness is one in which the individual is 'closed off' from receiving input, thus needing the assistance of herbs that open him or her up again to receive nourishment, oxygen, and sensory stimuli.)

Note: The pinyin names are exactly the same for 痹证 *bi zheng* (painful obstruction syndrome) and 闭证 *bi zheng* (closed disorder), though the Chinese characters are different. These two disorders have different symptomology, diagnoses, and treatments, and should not be incorrectly identified. Therefore, to avoid confusion, the term *bi zheng* (closed disorder) will be displayed with its translation throughout the entire text, without abbreviation.

2. In addition to differentiating between deficient and excess patterns of unconsciousness, one must also discern whether the disorder is cold or hot in nature.
   - ***Loss of consciousness due to cold*** is characterized by a blue or greenish facial complexion, a cold body, pale face, and slow pulse. Such conditions should be treated with warm herbs that open the orifices and restore consciousness. In allopathic terminology, unconsciousness due to cold is usually caused by cerebrovascular accidents and poisoning.
   - ***Loss of consciousness due to heat*** is characterized by a red face, warm body, yellow tongue coat, and rapid pulse. These conditions should be treated with cold herbs that open the orifices and restore consciousness. In the terminology of allopathic medicine, unconsciousness due to heat is often related to infectious diseases, meningitis, severe pneumonia, septicemia, heat stroke, liver disease, or toxic uremia.

Last, one must also consider any accompanying complications when treating these conditions. **Cold** conditions must be treated with herbs that dispel cold and warm the interior, **heat** conditions should be treated with herbs that clear heat and eliminate toxins, **seizures** and **convulsions** must be treated with herbs that calm Liver wind, and **pain** must be treated with herbs that activate qi and blood circulation.

CAUTIONS/CONTRAINDICATIONS

- Acrid and aromatic, herbs that open orifices consume qi and should be reserved for acute situations only. While they restore consciousness and relieve symptoms, they do not correct the underlying condition that causes the symptoms. Therefore, they must be combined with other herbs to successfully treat patients to the point of recovery and restored balance.
- The necessary dosage of orifice-opening herbs is usually low, and these substances should only be used for a short period of time, for symptomatic treatment *only*. These herbs are to be discontinued when the desired effect is achieved.

PROCESSING

All of the herbs in this category are acrid, travel in the organs and channels, and are able to disperse pathogenic elements (moving them outward from the body). Because the substances are aromatic, the preferred form of intake is either in pills or powder. They are seldom added to decoctions, as their effectiveness will be greatly compromised by cooking.

Chapter 16 — Orifice-Opening Herbs

PHARMACOLOGICAL EFFECTS

- **Effects on the central nervous system**: Some herbs in this category stimulate or inhibit the central nervous system (CNS), or exert *both* effects. *Bing Pian* (Borneolum Syntheticum) and *Zhang Nao* (Camphora) stimulate the CNS to increase heart rate, blood pressure, and respiration. The essential oil of *Shi Chang Pu* (Rhizoma Acori) is noted for its inhibitory effect on the central nervous system, which explains its use to treat seizures, epilepsy and convulsions. *She Xiang* (Moschus) has a regulating effect on the CNS, with a stimulating effect at low doses and an inhibiting effect when given in high doses.
- **Resuscitation**: Some orifice-opening herbs are used in formulations for emergency treatment of angina and myocardial infarction. These herbs have clearly demonstrated effectiveness in relieving pain, increasing resistance to hypoxia, and restoring normal blood perfusion to affected areas.

POTENTIAL HERB-DRUG INTERACTIONS

By the nature of disorders of sensory functioning, orifice-opening herbs are not used frequently or extensively. At the time of publication, there are no reported or documented interactions between these herbs and pharmaceuticals.

She Xiang (Moschus)

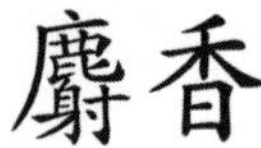

Pinyin Name: *She Xiang*
Alternate Chinese Names: *Dang Mei Zi, Yuan Cun Xiang*
Original Source: *Shen Nong Ben Cao Jing* (Divine Husbandman's Classic of the Materia Medica) in the second century
English Name: musk, navel gland secretions of the musk deer
Zoological Name: *Moschus berezovskii* Flerov (*Lin She*); *Moschus sifanicus* Przewalski (*Ma She*), *Moschus moschiferus* L. (*Yuan She*)
Pharmaceutical Name: Moschus
Properties: acrid, warm
Channels Entered: Heart, Liver, Spleen

CHINESE THERAPEUTIC ACTIONS

1. Opens Orifices, Awakes the *Shen* (Spirit) and Unblocks *Bi Zheng* (Closed Disorder)

***Bi zheng* (closed disorder):** *She Xiang* (Moschus) is one of the strongest substances in reviving the *shen* (spirit). It is the key, indispensable ingredient when treating diseases accompanied by impaired consciousness. Although it is warm, it treats both hot and cold types of *bi zheng* (closed disorder), when combined with other appropriate herbs.

***Bi zheng* (closed disorder) due to phlegm and heat:** *Bi zheng* (closed disorders) caused by phlegm and/or heat misting the Pericardium may present the following symptoms: impaired consciousness, unconsciousness, seizures, epilepsy, stroke, convulsions, stupor, fainting due to heat-stroke or extreme emotional stimulation, and tetanus.

- Impaired consciousness caused by heat and phlegm, stroke, convulsions, and/or heat stroke: use *She Xiang* with *Niu Huang* (Calculus Bovis), *Bing Pian* (Borneolum Syntheticum) and *Zhu Sha* (Cinnabaris). **Exemplar Formula:** *An Gong Niu Huang Wan* (Calm the Palace Pill with Cattle Gallstone).
- Infantile convulsions: combine it with *Niu Huang* (Calculus Bovis), *Tian Zhu Huang* (Concretio Silicea Bambusae) and *Zhu Sha* (Cinnabaris). **Exemplar Formula:** *Xiao Er Hui Chun Dan* (Return of Spring Special Pill (Pediatric)).
- Tremors and convulsions: use this substance with *Ling Yang Jiao* (Cornu Saigae Tataricae) and *Zhu Sha* (Cinnabaris).

***Bi zheng* (closed disorder) due to cold and phlegm:** Fainting from heatstroke, or extreme anger, that occurs at the end of summer and in the beginning of autumn, caused by infection, marked by fever, chest stuffiness, abdominal distention or vomiting and diarrhea.

- Impaired consciousness due to cold and phlegm: combine *She Xiang* with *Su He Xiang* (Styrax), *Tan Xiang* (Lignum Santali Albi) and *She Xiang* (Moschus). **Exemplar Formula:** *Su He Xiang Wan* (Liquid Styrax Pill).

2. Invigorates Blood Circulation, Opens Channels and Collaterals, Dissipates Clumps and Reduces Swelling

Carbuncles, sores, or hot swellings: *She Xiang* is usually applied topically when there is not yet an open lesion on the skin. This substance is aromatic and penetrating in nature and is most suitable to disperse stagnation in the *xue* (blood) level. It reduces swelling, invigorates blood, disperses stagnation and relieves pain. It is often combined with heat-clearing, toxin-eliminating and blood-invigorating herbs to relieve carbuncles and sores.

- Carbuncles, sores and hot swellings: use *She Xiang* with *Ru Xiang* (Gummi Olibanum) and *Mo Yao* (Myrrha).
- Sore throat: use it with *Niu Huang* (Calculus Bovis).
- Immobile palpable masses or organomegaly: use this substance alone, or with *Chi Shao* (Radix Paeoniae Rubrae), *San Leng* (Rhizoma Sparganii) and *E Zhu* (Rhizoma Curcumae).

Amenorrhea: *She Xiang* (Moschus) enters the *xue* (blood) level and strongly invigorates the blood to open the channels.

- Amenorrhea: use *She Xiang* with *Dan Shen* (Radix Salviae Miltiorrhizae), *Chi Shao* (Radix Paeoniae Rubrae), *Tao Ren* (Semen Persicae) and *Hong Hua* (Flos Carthami).

3. Relieves Pain

Traumatic injuries with blood stagnation: *She Xiang* is used frequently in the trauma departments of hospitals in China to relieve pain due to trauma, sprain, strain and bone fractures. This substance is used internally or topically to help the regeneration of tissues and bones, and to relieve pain and swelling. It also treats aches and pain of muscles and joints.

- Pain caused by traumatic injuries: use *She Xiang* with *Ru Xiang* (Gummi Olibanum), *Mo Yao* (Myrrha) and *Yan Hu Suo* (Rhizoma Corydalis). **Exemplar Formula:** *Qi Li San* (Seven-Thousandths of a Tael Powder).

She Xiang (Moschus)

- Angina pectoris, arteriosclerosis due to blood stagnation in the Heart: use this substance with *Mu Xiang* (Radix Aucklandiae) and *Tao Ren* (Semen Persicae).

4. Induces Labor in Stillbirth

Stillbirth: With its strong penetrating properties, *She Xiang* expels a dead fetus or a placenta that fails to descend. It is not used to induce labor in a viable pregnancy, as it is too strong and thus may hurt the fetus.

- Stillbirth: use *She Xiang* with *Rou Gui* (Cortex Cinnamomi).

She Xiang also treats paralysis of the intestines, infantile paralysis, or toxic snake bites.

DOSAGE

0.06 to 0.10 gram [60 to 100 mg] as powder or pills. The maximum dose of *She Xiang* is 1.0 (one) gram. This substance should not be decocted because of its strong aromatic property. Traditionally, it was mixed with water or vinegar prior to ingestion. Today, it is mostly used in the powder or pill forms, internally. It is also given sublingually for treatment of angina, with effects comparable to nitroglycerin.

CAUTIONS / CONTRAINDICATIONS

- Use of *She Xiang* is contraindicated in pregnancy. It has been proposed, though not confirmed, that topical treatment may cause miscarriage like internal use is known to do.
- Deficient patients, especially those with yin deficiency, should use *She Xiang* with caution, as it is strong and may easily damage the constitution.
- According to some classic texts, ingestion of garlic is contraindicated while taking *She Xiang*.

CHEMICAL COMPOSITION

Muscone, normuscone, muscopyridine, allantoin, androsterone, olein.[1,2]

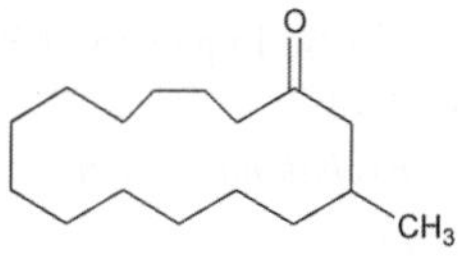

Muscone

PHARMACOLOGICAL EFFECTS

- **Effects on the central nervous system:** Small doses of *She Xiang* and muscone have a stimulating effect on the central nervous system, while large doses have an inhibiting effect. The effect of *She Xiang* to open the sensory orifices is associated with its function to reduce cerebral edema, increase blood perfusion to the brain, and increase resistance of the central nervous system to hypoxia.[3]
- **Cardiovascular:** The use of *She Xiang* is associated with a positive inotropic effect, a positive cardiotonic effect, and an increase in cardiac output in frog heart specimens. With intravenous injection, it significantly lowered blood pressure. *Muscone*, on the other hand, has demonstrated mixed effects on the cardiovascular system in various animal species.[4]
- **Antibiotic:** *Muscone* has an inhibitory effect against *Staphylococcus aureus* and *E. coli*.[5]
- **Uterine stimulant:** *She Xiang* and muscone both have a stimulating effect on the smooth muscles, leading to contraction of the uterus. Pregnant uteri are more strongly influenced by this than non-pregnant ones.[6]
- **Antineoplastic:** *She Xiang* and muscone have demonstrated preliminary effectiveness against ascites and carcinoma in mice.[7] In humans, it has been used to treat cancers of the esophagus, gastric glands, colon, and urinary bladder.[8]

CLINICAL STUDIES AND RESEARCH

- **Angina**: Sublingual administration of *She Xiang* has shown effectiveness in treating 367 patients with angina and coronary artery disease.[9] In another study of 287 patients, an herbal paste that incorporated *She Xiang* as the main ingredient showed marked effectiveness when placed on *Xinshu* (UB 15). The dressing was changed once every 24 hours.[10]
- **Hepatitis and cirrhosis**: Bilateral injection of 2 ml of 5% *She Xiang* (equivalent to 100mg) at *Zhangmen* (LR 13), alternating with *Qimen* (LR 14), one time per week for 4 weeks per course of treatment, showed satisfactory results in 32 patients with chronic hepatitis or early-stage liver cirrhosis.[11]
- **Low back pain:** According to one report, 21 patients with low back pain due to trauma were treated with satisfactory results using an injection of 2 to 4 ml of 0.2% *She Xiang* to *ah shi* points one time per week for 2 weeks.[12]
- **Vitiligo**: Subcutaneous injection of 0.4% *She Xiang* had 83.33% effectiveness in treating 78 patients with varying degrees of vitiligo. Injections were given twice a week, for 3 months per course of treatment, for a total of 2 to 3 courses of treatments.[13]
- **Cancer**: Injection of *She Xiang* has shown beneficial effects in treating 96 patients with various cancers, including esophagus, stomach, liver, colon, and rectal cancers. Beneficial results include increased appetite, reduced swelling, and improvement of other symptoms.[14]

TOXICOLOGY

Overdose of *She Xiang* in mice is associated with symptoms such as tremor, closed eyes, and respiratory depression. In one study, the LD_{50} of *She Xiang* via intraperitoneal

She Xiang (Moschus)

injection was 331.1 mg/kg. In another study, the LD_{50} of *She Xiang* via intravenous injection was 6 g/kg.[15,16,17]

AUTHORS' COMMENTS

She Xiang is considered the most potent of all aromatic substances, as it opens channels and collaterals to treat unconsciousness, carbuncles, immobile masses and amenorrhea. Its dispersing property treats pain in the chest or abdomen, or pain due to trauma or wind-damp obstruction. Because of its potent and broad dispersing effects, some classic texts state that *She Xiang* enters all twelve channels to treat stagnation.

She Xiang and *Su He Xiang* (Styrax) have similar effects in opening the orifices and awakening the *shen* (spirit).

- *She Xiang* is stronger in opening the orifices and is suitable for both cold and hot types of *bi zheng* (closed disorder). It invigorates the blood, dispels stagnation and stops pain.
- *Su He Xiang* is weaker than *She Xiang* and is primarily used for cold type *bi zheng* (closed disorder) caused by phlegm. It dispels dampness and treats pain and stifling sensations in the chest and abdomen.

References

1. *Xian Dai Zhong Yao Yao Li Xue* (Contemporary Pharmacology of Chinese Herbs), 1997; 1132-1133
2. *The Merck Index* 12th edition, Chapman & Hall/CRCnetBASE/Merck, 2000
3. *Zhong Yao Xue* (Chinese Herbology), 1998; 715:718
4. *Zhong Cheng Yao Yan Jiu* (Research of Chinese Patent Medicine), 1984; (7):1
5. *Zhong Yao Xue* (Chinese Herbology), 1998; 715:718
6. *Zhong Cheng Yao Yan Jiu* (Research of Chinese Patent Medicine), 1985; (3):5
7. *Ren Min Jun Yi* (Military Reserve Medicine), 1977, (7):54
8. *Zhong Yao Xue* (Chinese Herbology), 1998; 715:718
9. *Zhong Cheng Yao Yan Jiu* (Research of Chinese Patent Medicine), 1981; 9:13
10. *Zhong Xi Yi Jie He Za Zhi* (Journal of Integrated Chinese and Western Medicine), 1988; 7:409
11. *Tian Jing Zhong Yi* (Tianjing Chinese Medicine), 1987; 5:20
12. *Xin Zhong Yi* (New Chinese Medicine), 1985; 4:26
13. *Hu Nan Yi Xue Yuan Xue Bao* (Medical Journal of Hunan University of Medicine), 1980; 2:157
14. *Zhong Yi Yao Yan Jiu Can Kao* (Research and Discussion of Chinese Medicine and Herbology), 1975; 4:22
15. *Shang Hai Yao Wu Shi Yan* (Shanghai Research of Medicine), 1977
16. *Guo Wai Yi Xue Can Kao Zi Liao* (Foreign Reference of Medicine), 1974; (5):313
17. *Yao Xue Xue Bao* (Journal of Herbology), 1979; (11):685

Bing Pian (Borneolum Syntheticum)

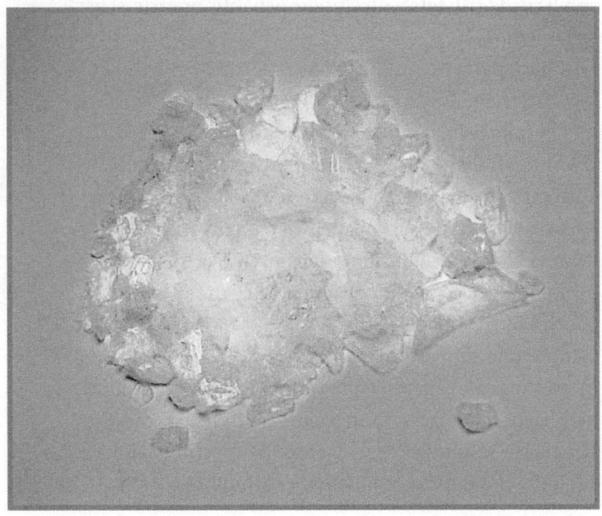

冰片

Pinyin Name: *Bing Pian*
Literal Name: "ice slice"
Alternate Chinese Names: *Nao Xiang, Mei Pian, Long Nao Xiang, Pian Nao, Mei Hua Niao, Mei Pian*
Original Source: *Xin Xiu Ben Cao* (Newly Revised Materia Medica) by Su Jing in 657-659 A.D.
English Name: borneol
Botanical Name: *Dryobalanops aromatica* Gaertn. f. (*Long Nao Xiang*)
Pharmaceutical Name: Borneolum Syntheticum
Properties: acrid, bitter, cool
Channels Entered: Heart, Spleen, Lung

Bing Pian (Borneolum Syntheticum)

CHINESE THERAPEUTIC ACTIONS

1. Opens the Orifices, Resuscitates and Revives the *Shen* (Spirit)

Fainting, unconsciousness, convulsions or childhood convulsions: *Bing Pian* (Borneolum Syntheticum) is commonly used to treat emergency cases of fainting and unconsciousness. Compared with *She Xiang* (Moschus), *Bing Pian* is milder but has similar effects.

- Convulsions due to heat: use *Bing Pian* with *Niu Huang* (Calculus Bovis), *Quan Xie* (Scorpio) and *She Xiang* (Moschus). **Exemplar Formula:** *An Gong Niu Huang Wan* (Calm the Palace Pill with Cattle Gallstone).
- Convulsions due to cold: use this substance with *Su He Xiang* (Styrax) and *She Xiang* (Moschus). **Exemplar Formula:** *Su He Xiang Wan* (Liquid Styrax Pill).

2. Clears Heat, Relieves Pain, Stops Itching

Toxic heat affecting the eyes, throat and skin: Common symptoms of toxic heat include sore throat, ulcers in the oral cavity, painful swollen gums, swelling, redness and pain in the eyes. This substance is not harmful to the skin or mucous membranes and thus can be applied topically to the throat and gums without adverse reactions. In addition to clearing heat and relieving pain, it also prevents decay and relieves itching. This is one of the best substances for topical use to reduce swelling, clear heat, eliminate toxins and help to regenerate flesh.

- Swollen and painful gums and throat, hoarse voice: mix *Bing Pian* with the powder of *Peng Sha* (Borax), *Yuan Ming Fen* (Matrii Sulfas Exsiccatus) and *Zhu Sha* (Cinnabaris), and apply topically.
- Thrush, white mouth or mycotic stomatitis: mix this substance with the powder of *Xiong Huang* (Realgar), *Peng Sha* (Borax) and *Gan Cao* (Radix Glycyrrhizae), and apply topically.
- Redness, swelling and painful eyes: use *Bing Pian* alone. This substance is often found in eye drops for relief of swelling.
- Ulceration with pain and swelling of the skin, ears or nose: apply it topically with the powder of *Niu Huang* (Calculus Bovis) and *Zhen Zhu* (Margarita).
- Toothache: apply this substance topically with *Zhu Sha* (Cinnabaris) powder.
- Suppuration with ulceration: combine it with *Chi Shi Zhi* (Halloysitum Rubrum), *Ru Xiang* (Gummi Olibanum), *Mo Yao* (Myrrha), *Qing Fen* (Calomelas), *Peng Sha* (Borax) and *Long Gu* (Os Draconis) to generate flesh.
- Redness, swelling and pain of the eyes, visual disturbance: use *Bing Pian* topically as a single remedy to clear heat and reduce swelling.

DOSAGE

0.15 to 0.30 gram in pill or powder form. *Bing Pian* is not used in decoctions.

CAUTIONS / CONTRAINDICATIONS

- Use of *Bing Pian* is contraindicated in pregnancy.
- Do not expose *Bing Pian* to fire or heat. Do <u>not</u> cook it in decoction.

CHEMICAL COMPOSITION

Borneol, isoborneol, camphor, humulene, β-elemene, caryophyllene, asiatic acid, erythrodid.[1,2]

H_3C CH_3 CH_3 H OH

Borneol

PHARMACOLOGICAL EFFECTS

- **Antibiotic**: *Bing Pian* has an inhibitory effect against *Staphylococcus aureus, Diplococcus pneumoniae, E. coli* and some dermatophytes.[3]
- **Effect on pregnancy**: Administration of *Bing Pian* during the second and third trimester induces labor in mice.[4]

CLINICAL STUDIES AND RESEARCH

- **Dizziness**: Topical application of *Bing Pian* on ear points was 97% effective in treating 77 patients with dizziness. The size of *Bing Pian* used was similar to a grain of rice. The points selected included *Shenmen*, Brain, Pituitary, Heart, and others. Two to three points were selected for each treatment, with seeds changed every three days. The total duration of treatment was 12 to 24 days.[5]
- **Dermatological use**: Topical application of *Bing Pian* and *Da Huang* (Radix et Rhizoma Rhei) at a 1:10 ratio was extremely effective in treating 230 patients with various abscesses and swellings. Herbal powder was applied to the affected area, with a dressing change every 2 to 3 days. Most patients reported complete recovery within three treatments.[6]
- **Otitis media**: In one study, 324 patients with acute or chronic suppurative otitis media were treated with topical application of an herbal formula, with complete recovery in 64.7% cases, and an overall rate of effectiveness of 93.4%. The treatment protocol was to apply the herbal powder sparingly to the affected area. The herbal formula contained *Bing Pian* 2.5g, *She Xiang* (Moschus) 0.5g, *Zhang Nao* (Camphora) 10g, *Long Gu* (Os Draconis) 15g, *Huang Lian* (Rhizoma Coptidis) 10g, and *Mu Li* (Concha Ostreae) 10g.[7]

Bing Pian (Borneolum Syntheticum)

- **Herpes zoster**: Topical application of *Bing Pian* was used to treat 30 patients with herpes zoster, with satisfactory results. The treatment protocol was to mix 10 to 30 grams of *Bing Pian* with rice water to make a 40% herbal paste, which was then placed on the affected area three to four times daily for 3 to 5 days.[8]

TOXICOLOGY

The LD_{50} for oral ingestion of *Bing Pian* is 2,269 to 2,879 mg/kg in mice.[9]

AUTHORS' COMMENTS

"*Bing Pian*" is available in both synthetic and natural forms. The synthetic form, *Bing Pian* (Borneolum Syntheticum), is the most commonly-used form, as it has similarly potent effects and is much less expensive than the natural form.

References

1. *Xian Dai Zhong Yao Yao Li Xue* (Contemporary Pharmacology of Chinese Herbs), 1997; 1141
2. *The Merck Index* 12th edition, Chapman & Hall/CRCnetBASE/Merck, 2000
3. *Zhong Yao Xue* (Chinese Herbology), 1998; 718:720
4. *Chang Yong Zhong Yao Xian Dai Yan Jiu Yu Lin Chuan* (Recent Study & Clinical Application of Common Traditional Chinese Medicine), 1995; 531:534
5. *He Nan Zhong Yi* (Henan Chinese Medicine), 1986; 4:14
6. *Zhong Xi Yi Jie He Za Zhi* (Journal of Integrated Chinese and Western Medicine), 1984; 5:272
7. *Zhong Yi Yao Xue Bao* (Report of Chinese Medicine and Herbology), 1986; 1:31
8. *Zhong Yao Xue* (Chinese Herbology), 1998; 718:720
9. *Chang Yong Zhong Yao Xian Dai Yan Jiu Yu Lin Chuan* (Recent Study & Clinical Application of Common Traditional Chinese Medicine), 1995; 531:534

Su He Xiang (Styrax)

蘇合香 苏合香

Pinyin Name: *Su He Xiang*
Literal Name: "revive and join fragrance"
Alternate Chinese Names: *Su He*
Original Source: *Ming Yi Za Zhu* (Miscellaneous Records of Famous Physicians) by Tao Hong-Jing in 500 A.D.
English Name: styrax, storesin
Botanical Name: *Liquidambar orientalis* Mill. (*Su He Xiang Shu*)
Pharmaceutical Name: Styrax
Properties: acrid, warm
Channels Entered: Heart, Spleen

CHINESE THERAPEUTIC ACTIONS

1. Opens Orifices and Disperses Turbidity

Stroke caused by phlegm, convulsions: *Su He Xiang* (Styrax) is aromatic and is best at warming channels, opening orifices, dispersing turbidity and relieving stagnation. It is effective for all stroke patients who experience sudden unconsciousness. It is most suitable for cold-type *bi zheng* (closed disorder).

- Sudden unconsciousness or cold-type *bi zheng* (closed disorder): use *Su He Xiang* with *She Xiang* (Moschus), *Bing Pian* (Borneolum Syntheticum) and *Zhu Sha* (Cinnabaris). **Exemplar Formula:** *Su He Xiang Wan* (Liquid Styrax Pill).

2. Relieves Pain

Chest and abdominal coldness and pain: *Su He Xiang* is excellent for chest or abdominal coldness and pain caused by qi, blood, cold or phlegm stagnation. The primary function of this substance is to dispel stagnation. *Su He Xiang* has been made into pills primarily for angina pectoris and coronary artery disorders.

- Chest and abdominal pain: use *Su He Xiang* with *Chen Xiang* (Lignum Aquilariae Resinatum), *Tan Xiang* (Lignum Santali Albi), *Xiang Fu* (Rhizoma Cyperi) and *Ding Xiang* (Flos Caryophylli).
- Angina: use this substance with *Bing Pian* (Borneolum Syntheticum), *Tan Xiang* (Lignum

Su He Xiang (Styrax)

Santali Albi), *Ru Xiang* (*Gummi* Olibanum) and *Qing Mu Xiang* (Radix Aristolochiae).

DOSAGE

0.3 to 1.0 gram in pill form. *Su He Xiang* is not suitable for decoction. For external use, it can be mixed with alcohol.

CAUTIONS / CONTRAINDICATIONS

- *Su He Xiang* is contraindicated in *bi zheng* (closed disorder) caused by heat or deficiency.

CHEMICAL COMPOSITION

Oleanonic acid, 3-epi-oleanonic acid.[1]

PHARMACOLOGICAL EFFECTS

- **Hematological**: *Su He Xiang* has antiplatelet action and prolongs clotting time.[2]
- **Cardiovascular**: *Su He Xiang* is commonly used to treat coronary artery disease. It benefits cardiac muscle by increasing blood perfusion, decreasing heart rate, decreasing oxygen consumption, and increasing muscle resistance to hypoxia.[3]
- **Others**: It has demonstrated mild antibiotic and anti-inflammatory effects.[4]

CLINICAL STUDIES AND RESEARCH

- **Coronary artery disease (CAD):** *Su He Xiang* has been incorporated into various herbal formulations for the treatment of CAD, with good success. In one study, 146 patients with CAD were treated with a 91.5% rate of effectiveness using an herbal formula containing *Su He Xiang*, *Bing Pian* (Borneolum Syntheticum), *Mu Xiang* (Radix Aucklandiae), *Zhu Sha* (Cinnabaris) and *Tan Xiang* (Lignum Santali Albi). In another study, 301 patients with CAD were treated with an 83.4% rate of effectiveness using an herbal formula containing *Su He Xiang* and *Bing Pian*.[5]
- **Biliary tract ascariasis:** One report states that 8 out of 9 patients with biliary tract ascariasis responded favorably to a preparation of *Su He Xiang* given two to three times daily with warm water.[6]

HERB-DRUG INTERACTION

- **Anticoagulant or antiplatelet drugs:** *Su He Xiang* has antiplatelet action, and should be used with caution in patients who take anticoagulant or antiplatelet medications. Though this potential interaction has not been documented, this substance may potentiate the effect of drugs such as warfarin.[7] [Note: Examples of anticoagulants include heparin, warfarin (Coumadin) and enoxaparin (Lovenox); and examples of antiplatelets include aspirin, dipyridamole (Persantine), and clopidogrel (Plavix).]

AUTHORS' COMMENTS

Su He Xiang and *She Xiang* (Moschus) are similar in their action to open the orifices and awaken the *shen* (spirit).

- *Su He Xiang* is weaker than *She Xiang*, and is primarily used for cold-type *bi zheng* (closed disorder), such as stroke or convulsion caused by phlegm. Furthermore, it dispels dampness and treats pain and stifling sensations in the chest and abdomen.
- *She Xiang* is stronger in opening the orifices and is suitable for both cold and hot-type *bi zheng* (closed disorders). It also invigorates the blood, dispels stagnation and stops pain.

References

1. *Xian Dai Zhong Yao Yao Li Xue* (Contemporary Pharmacology of Chinese Herbs), 1997; 1136-1137
2. *Zhong Cheng Yao* (Study of Chinese Patent Medicine), 1990; 12(9):31
3. *Yi Xue Xue Bao* (Report of Medicine), 1979; (11):655
4. *Zhong Yao Xue* (Chinese Herbology), 1998; 721:722
5. *Yi Xue Qing Kuang Jiao Liu* (Medical Information Exchange), 1977; 2:19
6. *Shan Xi Zhong Yi* (Shanxi Chinese Medicine), 1985; 7:322
7. Chen, J. Recognition & prevention of Herb-drug interactions, *Medical Acupuncture*, Fall/Winter 1998/1999; volume 10/number 2; 9-13

Shi Chang Pu (Rhizoma Acori)

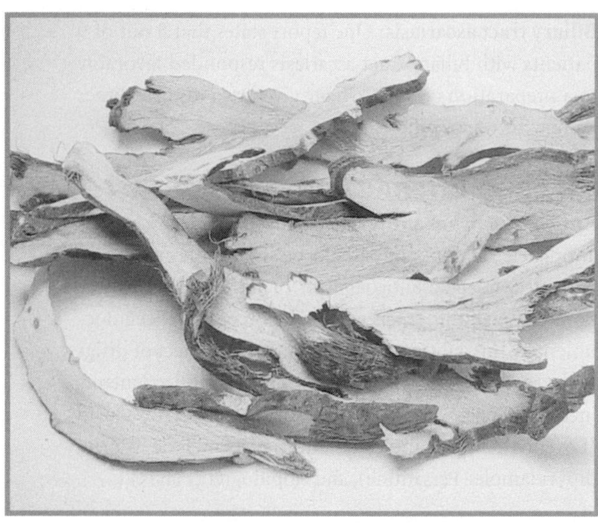

石菖蒲 石菖蒲

Pinyin Name: *Shi Chang Pu*

Alternate Chinese Names: *Chang Pu, Sui Chang Pu, Bai Chang*

Original Source: *Shen Nong Ben Cao Jing* (Divine Husbandman's Classic of the Materia Medica) in the second century

English Name: acorus, grass-leaf sweet-flag rhizome

Botanical Name: *Acorus tatarinowii* Schott; *Acorus gramineus* Soland.

Pharmaceutical Name: Rhizoma Acori

Properties: acrid, warm

Channels Entered: Heart, Stomach

CHINESE THERAPEUTIC ACTIONS

1. Opens Orifices, Vaporizes Turbid Phlegm

Obstruction caused by phlegm: *Shi Chang Pu* (Rhizoma Acori) is one of the best and the most potent substances at opening sensory orifices. It treats phlegm obstructing the sensory orifices causing coma, unconsciousness, manic behavior, delirium, high fever, seizures and epilepsy.

- High fever with coma or unconsciousness caused by hot phlegm: use it with *Yu Jin* (Radix Curcumae), *Lian Qiao* (Fructus Forsythiae), *Zhu Ye* (Herba Phyllostachys) and *Tian Zhu Huang* (Concretio Silicea Bambusae).
- Manic behavior with greasy tongue coat and slippery pulse: add it to *Yuan Zhi* (Radix Polygalae), *Dan Nan Xing* (Arisaema cum Bile), *Fu Shen* (Poria Paradicis) and *Sheng Tie Luo* (Frusta Ferri).
- Manic behavior with constipation: use this substance with *Da Huang* (Radix et Rhizoma Rhei), *Mang Xiao* (Natrii Sulfas), *Hou Po* (Cortex Magnoliae Officinalis) and *Zhi Shi* (Fructus Aurantii Immaturus).
- Epilepsy: use *Shi Chang Pu* alone, or with *Yu Jin* (Radix Curcumae), *Ming Fan* (Alumen) and *Zhu Sha* (Cinnabaris).

2. Opens Orifices, Pacifies *Shen* (Spirit)

Obstruction caused by phlegm: *Shi Chang Pu* effectively opens sensory orifices and pacifies *shen*, and improves sensory and cognitive functions. It treats forgetfulness, tinnitus, deafness, dizziness, and dulled sensorium.

- Forgetfulness or insomnia: combine *Shi Chang Pu* with *Ren Shen* (Radix Ginseng), *Fu Shen* (Poria Paradicis) or *Yuan Zhi* (Radix Polygalae).
- Tinnitus or deafness due to Kidney deficiency: pair this herb with *Ci Shi* (Magnetitum) or *Liu Wei Di Huang Wan* (Six-Ingredient Pill with Rehmannia).

3. Transforms Turbid Dampness, Harmonizes the Middle *Jiao*

Dampness accumulation in the middle *jiao*: Damp obstruction of the middle *jiao* results in impairment of the Spleen's transportation and transformation functions. Chief symptoms of this condition include chest and abdominal fullness, distention and pain, poor appetite, and a feeling of thick, copious saliva in the mouth.

- Dampness accumulation in the middle *jiao*: use *Shi Chang Pu* with *Huo Xiang* (Herba Agastache), *Cang Zhu* (Rhizoma Atractylodis), *Chen Pi* (Pericarpium Citri Reticulatae), *Fu Ling* (Poria) and *Hou Po* (Cortex Magnoliae Officinalis).
- Damp-heat diarrhea: use it with *Shi Lian Zi* (Herba Sinocrassulae Indicae), *Huang Lian* (Rhizoma Coptidis), *Chen Pi* (Pericarpium Citri Reticulatae) and *He Ye* (Folium Nelumbinis).
- Diarrhea with Spleen deficiency: add it to *Dang Shen* (Radix Codonopsis), and *Bai Zhu* (Rhizoma Atractylodis Macrocephalae).
- Diarrhea accompanied by exterior conditions: use this herb with *Shi Lian Zi* (Herba Sinocrassulae Indicae), *Ge Gen* (Radix Puerariae), *Huang Lian* (Rhizoma Coptidis) and *Huang Qin* (Radix Scutellariae).

4. Benefits the Throat

Hoarse voice: *Shi Chang Pu* benefits the throat to treat hoarse voice due to laryngitis or inflammation of the vocal cords.

- Hoarse voice and dry mouth: use *Shi Chang Pu* with *Pang Da Hai* (Semen Sterculiae Lychnophorae), *Gu Zhi Hua* (Semen Oroxyli), *Shi Hu* (Herba Dendrobii) and *Mai Men Dong* (Radix Ophiopogonis).

Shi Chang Pu (Rhizoma Acori)

5. Others

Shi Chang Pu treats eczema, carbuncles, boils and pain caused by trauma, or *bi zheng* (painful obstruction syndrome) characterized by wind-damp obstruction. *Shi Chang Pu* may be used internally or topically.

DOSAGE

5 to 10 grams for dried *Shi Chang Pu*, 10 to 20 grams for the fresh herb. *Shi Chang Pu* is often used in decoctions or pills. Grind it into powder or use as a decoction for an external wash, if applying this substance topically.

CAUTIONS / CONTRAINDICATIONS

- Use of *Shi Chang Pu* is not suitable for patients with spermatorrhea, sweating, or yin and blood deficiencies.

CHEMICAL COMPOSITION

α-asarone, β-asarone, caryophyllene, α-humulene, sekishone, asaronaldehyde.[1,2]

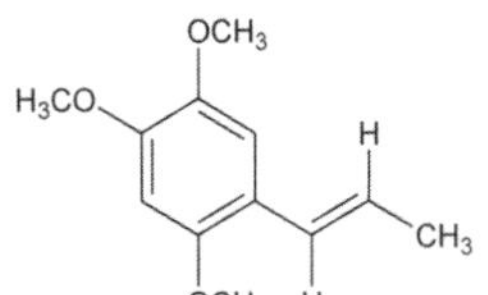

α-asarone 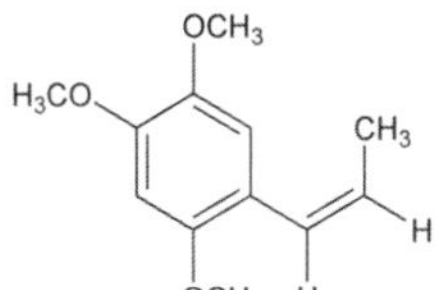 β-asarone

PHARMACOLOGICAL EFFECTS

- **CNS suppressant:** Hypnotic influence is observed with use of essential oil of *Shi Chang Pu*, antiseizure action is observed with the water extract, and sedative effects are observed with both.[3]
- **Effect on memory**: Administration of *Shi Chang Pu* is associated with an improvement in memory. In a laboratory study, 55 mice were divided into three groups, with group one receiving normal saline, group two receiving 0.1 g/kg of *Shi Chang Pu* and group three receiving 0.2 g/kg. The mice were then placed in a maze to test the time required to exit the maze and the number of mistakes committed. The same exercise was repeated daily for 6 days. At the end of the study, it was concluded that *Shi Chang Pu* has a dose-dependent effect in mice in reducing the time required and mistakes made to exit the maze.[4]
- **Gastrointestinal**: Decoction of *Shi Chang Pu* stimulates the secretion of gastric acid.[5]

CLINICAL STUDIES AND RESEARCH

- **Seizures and convulsions**: In one study, 50 mg of α-asarone given three times daily for 30 days per course of treatment was approximately 83.3% effective in controlling seizures and convulsions in 90 patients.[6]
- **Chronic obstructive pulmonary disease (COPD):** According to one report, 148 patients with COPD were treated with an 85.5% rate of effectiveness using 60 mg of α-asarone three times daily for 14 to 21 days.[7]
- **Mental retardation**: Use of an herbal treatment was associated with mild to moderate improvement in classroom performance in 30 children with low intelligence quotients (IQ). The herbal formula contained *Ren Shen* (Radix Ginseng), *Yuan Zhi* (Radix Polygalae), *Bu Gu Zhi* (Fructus Psoraleae), *Bai Dou Kou* (Fructus Amomi Rotundus), milk powder, cocoa, and sugar. Children were given 10 to 15 grams of the formula twice daily for 2 weeks per course of treatment, for a total of three months of treatment.[8]

HERB-DRUG INTERACTION

- **Ethanol:** In an *in vitro* study, a traditional Chinese medicinal preparation containing *Shi Chang Pu*, *Ren Shen* (Radix Ginseng), *Yuan Zhi* (Radix Polygalae), and *Fu Ling* (Poria) was found to reduce ethanol-induced impairment of memory registration. It also ameliorated scopolamine-induced memory registration deficit. These results suggest that this herbal preparation ameliorates the impairment effect of ethanol on learning and memory processes.[9]

TOXICOLOGY

The LD_{50} for water extract of *Shi Chang Pu* via intraperitoneal injection is 53 g/kg in mice. The LD_{50} for α-asarone via intraperitoneal injection is 338.5 mg/kg. Toxic effects include seizures, convulsion, slowed respiration rate, and death within 16 to 24 hours.[10]

SUPPLEMENT

- 九節菖蒲 / 九节菖蒲 *Jiu Jie Chang Pu* (Rhizoma Anemones Altaicae) is acrid and warm. The primary functions of *Jiu Jie Chang Pu* are to open sensory orifices, eliminate phlegm, and pacify the *shen* (spirit). It treats unconsciousness due to febrile diseases or phlegm obstruction, seizure, tinnitus, deafness, and chest and abdominal distention and pain. Compared to *Shi Chang Pu*, *Jiu Jie Chang Pu* does not contain essential oil, and is slightly toxic. Therefore, they should not be used interchangeably. The dosage for *Jiu Jie Chang Pu* is 3 to 5 grams.
- 水菖蒲 / 石菖蒲 *Shui Chang Pu* (Rhizoma Acori Calami) is acrid, bitter, warm, and enters the Heart, Spleen and Large Intestine. *Shui Chang Pu* dispels phlegm, opens sensory orifices, strengthens the Spleen, dissolves dampness, and kills parasites. *Shui Chang Pu* and *Shi Chang Pu* (Rhizoma Acori) are derived from the same genus and have similar functions, and are sometimes substituted for each other. Pharmacologically, *Shui Chang Pu* has an antibiotic effect against MRSA, and

Shi Chang Pu (Rhizoma Acori)

potentiates the antibiotic effect of chloramphenicol.[11] The dosage for *Shui Chang Pu* is 3 to 6 grams.

AUTHORS' COMMENTS

Shi Chang Pu and *Yuan Zhi* (Radix Polygalae) both improve memory and cognitive performance. *Shi Chang Pu* works by opening sensory orifices and improving alertness. *Yuan Zhi* works by calming the *shen* (spirit) and relieving hyperactivity and poor concentration.

According to Dr. Gan Zhu-Wang, *Shi Chang Pu* treats otitis media associated with frequent flying or changes of pressure within the ears.

References

1. *Xian Dai Zhong Yao Yao Li Xue* (Contemporary Pharmacology of Chinese Herbs), 1997; 1139
2. *The Merck Index* 12th edition, Chapman & Hall/CRCnetBASE/Merck, 2000
3. *Zhong Yao Xue* (Chinese Herbology), 1998; 722:725
4. *Zhong Cao Yao* (Chinese Herbal Medicine), 1992; 23(8):417
5. *Zhong Yao Xue* (Chinese Herbology), 1998; 722:725
6. *Yao Xue Tong Bao* (Report of Herbology), 1982; 9:50
7. *Xin Yao Yu Lin Chuang* (New Medicine and the Clinical Application), 1986; 4:210
8. *Zhong Cheng Yao Yan Jiu* (Research of Chinese Patent Medicine), 1982; 6:22
9. *Biological and Pharmaceutical Bulletin.* 17(11):1472-6, 1994 Nov.
10. *Zhong Yao Yao Li Yu Ying Yong* (Pharmacology and Applications of Chinese Herbs), 1983:292
11. Abascal K and Yarnell E, Herb and Drug Resistance – Clinical Implications of Research on Microbial Resistance to Antibiotics, *Alternative & Complementary Therapies*; vol 8, no 5, October 2002

Chapter 16 summary

— Orifice-Opening Herbs

Name	Similarities	Differences
She Xiang (Moschus)	Open the orifices	Invigorates blood circulation and disperses blood stagnation
Bing Pian (Borneolum Syntheticum)	and awaken	Clears heat and stops pain when used externally
Su He Xiang (Styrax)	the *shen* (spirit)	Warms the channels and disperses cold *bi zheng* (closed disorder)
Shi Chang Pu (Rhizoma Acori)		Dissolves dampness and harmonizes the middle *jiao*

General Characteristics of Orifice-Opening Herbs:

Taste: acrid
Thermal property: aromatic and warm
Channels entered: Heart
Therapeutic actions: open sensory orifices, awaken *shen* (spirit)

These herbs open the sensory orifices, awaken the *shen*, and restore normal sensory perceptions. They are taken internally or applied topically. Clinical applications include fire in the Heart or phlegm misting the Heart, manifesting in symptoms of tremor, spasms, stroke and convulsions.

She Xiang (Moschus), ***Bing Pian*** (Borneolum Syntheticum) and ***Su He Xiang*** (Styrax) are aromatic, extremely penetrating in nature, and treat a variety of disorders with excellent results, such as angina pectoris in coronary heart disease. In addition, they may be used to treat masses, accumulations, and *bi zheng* (closed disorder).

She Xiang (Moschus) and ***Bing Pian*** (Borneolum Syntheticum), are also used topically to treat toxic swellings, scrofulae, sores and furuncles. In addition, *She Xiang* treats traumatic injuries, amenorrhea, dysmenorrhea, difficult labor, eye disorders, sore throat and childhood convulsions.

Shi Chang Pu (Rhizoma Acori) treats mania, stupor and mental disorientation, forgetfulness and insomnia.

HERBS FROM OTHER FUNCTIONAL CATEGORIES WITH ORIFICE-OPENING FUNCTIONS

Name	Functional Category
Chan Su (Venenum Bufonis)	Substances for Topical Application (Chapter 20)
Niu Huang (Calculus Bovis)	Heat-Clearing Herbs (Chapter 2)
Xi Xin (Herba Asari)	Interior-Warming Herbs (Chapter 7)
Yuan Zhi (Radix Polygalae)	*Shen*-Calming Herbs (Chapter 14)
Zao Jiao (Fructus Gleditsiae)	Phlegm-Resolving and Coughing- and Wheezing-Relieving Herbs (Chapter 13)
Zhang Nao (Camphora)	Substances for Topical Application (Chapter 20)

Chapter 17

— Tonic Herbs

补虚药

Chapter 17 — Tonic Herbs

Section 1. Qi-Tonifying Herbs

Section 2. Yang-Tonifying Herbs

Section 3. Blood-Tonifying Herbs

Section 4. Yin-Tonifying Herbs

Chapter 17

— Tonic Herbs

Definition: To 'tonify' is to strengthen qi, tonify blood, nourish yin, and build yang. Tonic herbs improve functioning of internal organs, strengthen bodily constitution, boost immunity, and improve overall health.

Qi, yang, blood, and *yin* are fundamental elements in the body. Deficiencies of *qi* or *yang* represent a decline in physical function, while deficiencies of *blood* or *yin* represent shortages of bodily substance.

SUBCATEGORIES OF ACTION

1. ***Qi-tonifying herbs*** strengthen the ***Spleen*** and ***Lung*** to improve the functionality of these two organs. The ***Spleen*** is responsible for transportation of fluids and transformation of food, and Spleen qi deficiency is characterized by lethargy, lack of energy, weakness of the extremities, poor appetite, abdominal fullness and distention, diarrhea, weight loss, edema, organ prolapse (mostly stomach, uterus or rectum), and bleeding. The ***Lung*** is responsible for respiration, and Lung qi deficiency is characterized by shortness of breath, lack of desire to speak, wheezing and dyspnea following minimal physical activity, and perspiration.
2. ***Yang-tonifying herbs*** build ***Kidney yang***. Since Kidney yang is considered the source of yang for the entire body, tonifying Kidney yang will benefit patients with ***Spleen yang*** and ***Heart yang*** deficiencies. The Kidney is responsible for the reproductive and genitourinary systems. Kidney deficiency leads to disorders such as aversion to cold, lower back and knee weakness and pain, lower abdominal coldness and pain, infertility, premature ejaculation, impotence, leukorrhea with clear discharge, frequent nighttime urination, and urinary incontinence. Disorders characterized by yang deficiency may be effectively treated with Kidney yang tonic herbs.
3. ***Blood-tonifying herbs*** tonify blood. Blood deficiency has an impact on the ***Spleen***, ***Liver*** and ***Heart***, or it can also arise from weakness or failure of these organs. The Spleen *controls* blood, the Liver *stores* blood, and the Heart *controls blood vessels*. Inadequate supplies of blood adversely influence the ability of each organ to carry out its functions. Deficiency of blood is characterized by sallow facial appearance, pale lips and nails, excessive worries, palpitations, forgetfulness, insomnia, excessive dreaming, being easily frightened, weight loss, edema, diminished menses, light-colored menstrual flow, delayed menstruation, or amenorrhea.
4. ***Yin-tonifying herbs*** nourish yin and promote generation of body fluids. Yin deficiency occurs as a result of febrile disorders, chronic illnesses or injurious lifestyles, and is usually related to or adversely affects the ***Kidney*** and ***Liver***. Classic signs and symptoms of yin deficiency include emaciation, lower back and knee pain and soreness, muscle and bone weakness, decreased sperm production, dizziness, tinnitus, dry eyes, lightheadedness, and forgetfulness. Yin deficiency may be complicated by heat, due to the inability of yin to control yang. Yin-deficient heat is characterized by tidal fever, red cheeks, warm palms and soles, dry mouth and throat, spermatorrhea, night sweats, dry stools, red or cracked tongue, thin or absent tongue coating, and a thready, rapid pulse.

   In addition to the Liver and Kidney, yin deficiency also occurs in the ***Stomach*** and ***Lung***. Stomach yin deficiency is characterized by dry mouth, thirst, dry red tongue, dry heaves, and dry stools or constipation. Lung yin deficiency is characterized by dry cough, scanty or

Ren Shen (Radix Ginseng)
Ben Cao Gang Mu (Materia Medica), by Li Shi-Zhen, 1578 A.D.

Deficiencies of qi or yang represent a decline in physical function, while deficiencies of blood or yin represent shortages of bodily substance.

Chapter 17 — Tonic Herbs

no sputum, cough with scanty phlegm streaked with blood, dry mouth and tongue, and is recognized also by the chronic nature of the illness. Yin deficiency may occur in various organs with or without complications, and must be treated accordingly.

DIFFERENTIAL DIAGNOSIS AND TREATMENT

Tonic herbs build, strengthen, nourish or increase qi, blood, yin and yang. While deficiency in each of the substances may occur singly, it is far more common for deficiencies to appear in combinations.

Deficiencies may occur singly, but more commonly appear in combination.

- ***Deficiency of qi and yang***, each of which represent elements of body functionality, often occur together. Severe cases of qi deficiency may lead to yang deficiency, while yang deficiency is *always* accompanied by qi deficiency.
- ***Deficiency of qi and blood*** occur together frequently, as formation of one is dependant on the supply of the other. In other words, the production of qi requires an adequate supply of blood, and production of blood requires an adequate supply of qi. Therefore, qi and blood tonics are often used together.
- ***Deficiency of qi and yin*** often occur together, as febrile disorders or chronic illness greatly consume both elements. Herbs that nourish yin and promote generation of body fluids facilitate recovery of physical function and rehabilitation of qi. Therefore, qi and yin tonics have synergistic action in treating qi and yin deficiencies.
- ***Deficiency of yin and blood*** also occur together, as what affects yin will also affect blood, and vice-versa. When yin and blood deficiency occur together, tonics for both are used simultaneously.
- ***Deficiency of yin and yang*** may occur together, as the formation of one is dependant on the other. In other words, chronic yin deficiency will lead to yang deficiency, and chronic yang deficiency will lead to yin deficiency. Therefore, herbs that nourish yin and tonify yang are commonly used together.

Deficiency of qi, blood, yin and/or yang weakens the physical constitution, and increases the vulnerability of the body to additional imbalances. Thus, conditions arising from deficiency often include complications.

- Yang deficiency is often accompanied by ***cold***, and requires treatment to tonify yang and dispel cold.
- Yin deficiency is often accompanied by ***deficiency heat*** that requires treatment to nourish yin and clear deficiency heat.
- Qi deficiency is often accompanied by ***qi stagnation***, requiring treatment to tonify qi and invigorate qi circulation.
- Blood deficiency may lead to ***forgetfulness*** and ***insomnia***, and requires herbs to tonify blood and calm the *shen* (spirit).
- Qi deficiency may be complicated by the presence of an ***exterior syndrome***, which requires simultaneous treatment using herbs that tonify qi and release the exterior.

CAUTIONS/CONTRAINDICATIONS

- Qi-tonic herbs are sweet, sometimes cloying, and in the presence of weakness or other imbalance, they may create dampness and stagnation in the middle *jiao*.
- Yang-tonic herbs are warm and drying, and if indiscriminately prescribed, may damage yin and increase heat.
- Blood- and yin-tonic herbs are sometimes heavy or greasy, and thus may create dampness and interfere with normal digestive functions.

Note: Patients who are extremely deficient may not benefit immediately from administration of tonic herbs, as their body may be too weak to digest and absorb the nutrients involved. Astringent herbs or mild tonics should be used for a long period of time to ensure successful and complete recovery. Proper treatment in such situations requires patience and persistence, as aggressive tonic treatment may, in fact, delay recovery.

Chapter 17 — Tonic Herbs

PROCESSING

Tonic herbs require prolonged cooking to ensure complete extraction of active constituents. To improve patient compliance for long-term use, these herbs should be given in pill form or in herbal tincture.

PHARMACOLOGICAL EFFECTS

- **Immunologic:** Many tonic herbs enhance the immune system by increasing white blood cell and lymphocyte counts, and by enhancing both cellular and humoral immunity.

  Herbs that increase white blood cell counts in patients with chemotherapy-induced bone marrow suppression include *Dang Shen* (Radix Codonopsis), *Bai Zhu* (Rhizoma Atractylodis Macrocephalae), *Shu Di Huang* (Radix Rehmanniae Preparata), *Nu Zhen Zi* (Fructus Ligustri Lucidi), *Bai Shao* (Radix Paeoniae Alba) and *Gou Qi Zi* (Fructus Lycii).

  Herbs that effectively increase lymphocyte counts in cancer patients include *Yin Yang Huo* (Herba Epimedii), *He Shou Wu* (Radix Polygoni Multiflori), and *Sha Shen* (Radix Glehniae seu Adenophorae).

  Herbs that increase phagocytic activities of macrophages include *Ren Shen* (Radix Ginseng), *Dang Shen* (Radix Codonopsis), *Huang Qi* (Radix Astragali) and *Yin Yang Huo* (Herba Epimedii).

  Among herbs that increase the activities of T-lymphocytes and natural killer cells is *Dong Chong Xia Cao* (Cordyceps).

  Ren Shen (Radix Ginseng) increases IgM count. *Huang Qi* (Radix Astragali) increases IgE count.
- **Adaptogenic**: Tonic herbs influence various systems to enhance the body's ability to adapt to stressful situations. Mechanisms of adaptogenic effects are attributed to regulation of the cardiovascular, nervous, and respiratory systems.

  Increased resistance to radiation can be achieved with *Ren Shen* (Radix Ginseng) and *Ci Wu Jia* (Radix et Caulis Acanthopanacis Senticosi).

  Increased resistance to hypoxia can be accomplished with *Ren Shen* (Radix Ginseng), *Ci Wu Jia* (Radix et Caulis Acanthopanacis Senticosi), *Yu Zhu* (Rhizoma Polygonati Odorati), and *Shu Di Huang* (Radix Rehmanniae Preparata).

  Drug-induced liver damage can be minimized by use of *Ren Shen* (Radix Ginseng), *Wu Wei* Zi (Fructus Schisandrae Chinensis), *Shu Di Huang* (Radix Rehmanniae Preparata), *Dang Gui* (Radicis Angelicae Sinensis), *Gou Qi* Zi (Fructus Lycii) and *Huang Qi* (Radix Astragali).

  Mental and physical fatigue can be reversed with *Ren Shen* (Radix Ginseng), *Ci Wu Jia* (Radix et Caulis Acanthopanacis Senticosi) and *Wu Wei* Zi (Fructus Schisandrae Chinensis).
- **Endocrinological**: Some tonic herbs stimulate the endocrine system to increase secretion of endogenous hormones, including ACTH, thyroid hormone, adrenocortical hormones, male and female hormones and others.

  Herbs that regulate the adrenal cortex include *Ren Shen* (Radix Ginseng), *Ci Wu Jia* (Radix et Caulis Acanthopanacis Senticosi), *Wu Wei Zi* (Fructus Schisandrae Chinensis), and *Gan Cao* (Radix Glycyrrhizae).

  Herbs that stimulate the production of male hormones include *Lu Rong* (Cornu Cervi Pantotrichum), *Yin Yang Huo* (Herba Epimedii), and *Dong Chong Xia Cao* (Cordyceps).

  Herbs that stimulate the production of female hormones include *Bu Gu Zhi* (Fructus Psoraleae) and *She Chuang Zi* (Fructus Cnidii).
- **Metabolic**: Some substances lower plasma glucose and cholesterol levels, such as *Ren Shen* (Radix Ginseng), *Yu Zhu* (Rhizoma Polygonati Odorati), *Bai Zhu* (Rhizoma Atractylodis Macrocephalae), *Shu Di Huang* (Radix Rehmanniae Preparata), *Gou Qi Zi* (Fructus Lycii), *Huang Jing* (Rhizoma Polygonati) and *Yin Yang Huo* (Herba Epimedii). Herbs that lower plasma cholesterol levels include *Ren Shen*, *Nu Zhen Zi* (Fructus Ligustri Lucidi), *Dang Gui* (Radicis Angelicae Sinensis), *He Shou Wu* (Radix Polygoni Multiflori), *Gou Qi Zi*, *Huang Jing*, and *Yin Yang Huo*.
- **Cardiovascular**: Tonic herbs increase contractility of cardiac muscle, dilate blood vessels, decrease blood pressure, decrease oxygen requirement of cardiac muscles, treat arrhythmias, and increase blood perfusion to cardiac muscle.

~

Deficiency increases bodily vulnerability to additional imbalances.

~

Chapter 17 — Tonic Herbs

Herbs with cardiotonic properties include *Ren Shen* (Radix Ginseng), *Huang Qi* (Radix Astragali), *Ling Zhi* (Ganoderma), *Bai Shao* (Radix Paeoniae Alba), *Lu Rong* (Cornu Cervi Pantotrichum) and *Bu Gu Zhi* (Fructus Psoraleae).

Herbs with vasodilating effects include *Ren Shen* (Radix Ginseng), *Dang Shen* (Radix Codonopsis), *Huang Qi* (Radix Astragali), *Dang Gui* (Radicis Angelicae Sinensis), *Bai Shao* (Radix Paeoniae Alba), *Lu Rong* (Cornu Cervi Pantotrichum), *Yin Yang Huo* (Herba Epimedii), *Bu Gu Zhi* (Fructus Psoraleae) and *Mai Men Dong* (Radix Ophiopogonis).

- **Others**: Tonic herbs strengthen the body, improve physical and cognitive performance, improve sleep, improve appetite, and increase body weight.

With organ transplants or autoimmune disorders, enhancing the immune system may be undesirable.

POTENTIAL HERB-DRUG INTERACTIONS

- **Immunosuppressants**: Many tonic herbs serve to enhance the immune system. Though this is desirable in most cases, there are situations that warrant caution: in particular, patients who have received organ transplants or suffer from autoimmune disorders. In these cases, enhancing the immune system may interfere with immunosuppressants and increase the risk of organ rejection, or interfere with substances for regulation of immune function.
- **Hormones**: Herbs that stimulate the endocrine system promote the release of hormones, and should be used with caution in patients who are already receiving hormone supplementation with insulin, steroids, and sex hormones. Though the herbs and drugs all aim to treat the same disorder, concurrent use may potentiate the overall effect and cause undesirable reactions.
- **Cardiovascular agents**: Some tonic herbs act on the cardiovascular system. Herbs with cardiotonic influence may increase blood pressure, while herbs with vasodilating effects may lower blood pressure. Consequently, any concurrent use of these herbs with cardiotonic pharmaceuticals must be carefully chosen and monitored to prevent adverse interactions.
- **Dexamethasone**: It has been shown that dexamethasone-induced osteoporosis in male rats can be prevented and treated by using Kidney tonic herbs to regulate the endocrine system.[1]

References

1. Shen P. Chen D. Zhang G., Study on efficacy of Chinese Kidney-Tonifying Recipe in male rats with osteoporosis induced by dexamethasone and its mechanism. *Chung-Kuo Chung His I Chieh Ho Tsa Chih.* 18(5):290-2, 1998 May.

Section 1 — Qi-Tonifying Herbs

Ren Shen (Radix Ginseng)

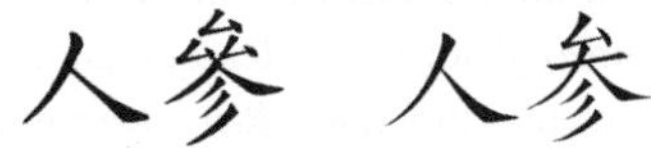

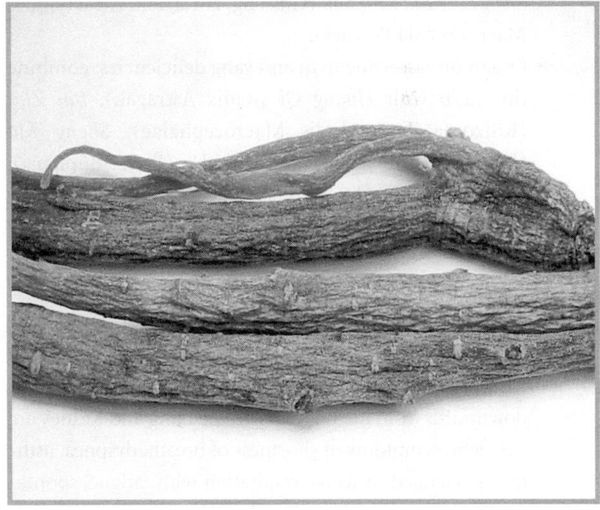

Pinyin Name: *Ren Shen*
Literal Name: "man's plant," "man root"
Alternate Chinese Names: *Gui Gai, Yi Shan Shen, Chao Xian Shen, Ren Xian*
Original Source: *Shen Nong Ben Cao Jing* (Divine Husbandman's Classic of the Materia Medica) in the second century
English Name: ginseng, ginseng root
Botanical Name: *Panax ginseng* C. A. Mey. (*Ren Shen*)
Pharmaceutical Name: Radix Ginseng
Properties: sweet, slightly bitter, slightly warm
Channels Entered: Lung, Spleen

CHINESE THERAPEUTIC ACTIONS

1. Greatly Tonifies *Yuan* (Source) *Qi*

Qi deficiency or depletion, fading pulse: *Yuan* (source) *qi* is the basis of all qi in the body. *Ren Shen* (Radix Ginseng) is the best herb to strengthen the body and restore vitality. It tonifies deficiency and restores the collapse of *yuan qi*, that may have become depleted after profuse perspiration, after excessive loss of fluids in severe vomiting or diarrhea, with excessive loss of blood, or due to other chronic illnesses. Clinical manifestations of such conditions include shallow respiration, shortness of breath, cold extremities, and feeble or barely palpable pulse. In those conditions, this herb can be used alone to greatly tonify and revitalize the body. Qi deficiency is often accompanied by yang deficiency, and qi collapse is often accompanied by yang collapse. As such, when treating cases of deficiency or collapse, interior-warming or yang-tonic herbs are usually added to *Ren Shen*.

- Collapse of *yuan* (source) *qi*: use *Ren Shen* as a single-herb remedy.
- Qi and yang deficiencies with profuse perspiration and cold extremities: use it with *Fu Zi* (Radix Aconiti Lateralis Praeparata). **Exemplar Formula**: *Shen Fu Tang* (Ginseng and Prepared Aconite Decoction).
- Qi and yin deficiencies: combine it with *Mai Men Dong* (Radix Ophiopogonis) and *Wu Wei Zi* (Fructus Schisandrae Chinensis). **Exemplar Formula:** *Sheng Mai San* (Generate the Pulse Powder).
- Qi and blood deficiencies: pair *Ren Shen* with *Shu Di Huang* (Radix Rehmanniae Preparata).

2. Tonifies the Spleen

Spleen qi deficiency: *Ren Shen* tonifies the Spleen and enhances its functions of transformation and transportation. With middle *jiao* deficiency, food cannot be transformed into energy, and thus, fatigue, lack of energy, nausea, vomiting, poor appetite, sallow complexion, low voice, listlessness, diarrhea, stomach and rectal prolapse and other conditions characterized by qi deficiency of the Spleen and Stomach will manifest.

Ren Shen (Radix Ginseng)

- Qi deficiency of the Spleen and Stomach: use *Ren Shen* with *Bai Zhu* (Rhizoma Atractylodis Macrocephalae).
- Qi deficiency of the Spleen and Stomach with dampness: use this herb with *Bai Zhu* (Rhizoma Atractylodis Macrocephalae), *Fu Ling* (Poria) and *Gan Cao* (Radix Glycyrrhizae). **Exemplar Formula:** *Si Jun Zi Tang* (Four-Gentlemen Decoction).
- Qi deficiency of the Spleen and Stomach with loose stools or diarrhea: add *Ren Shen* to *Bai Zhu* (Rhizoma Atractylodis Macrocephalae), *Fu Ling* (Poria), *Shan Yao* (Rhizoma Dioscoreae), *Bian Dou* (Semen Lablab Album), *Sha Ren* (Fructus Amomi) and *Chen Pi* (Pericarpium Citri Reticulatae). **Exemplar Formula:** *Shen Ling Bai Zhu San* (Ginseng, Poria, and Atractylodes Macrocephala Powder).
- Organ prolapse due to qi and yang deficiencies: combine this herb with *Huang Qi* (Radix Astragali), *Bai Zhu* (Rhizoma Atractylodis Macrocephalae), *Sheng Ma* (Rhizoma Cimicifugae) and *Chai Hu* (Radix Bupleuri). **Exemplar Formula:** *Bu Zhong Yi Qi Tang* (Tonify the Middle and Augment the Qi Decoction).

3. Tonifies the Lung

Lung deficiency: The Lung dominates the qi of the body and controls respiration. The Kidney dominates *yuan* (source) *qi*, consolidates *jing* (essence) and helps pull qi downwards from the Lung. When the Lung and Kidney are deficient, symptoms of shortness of breath, dyspnea, asthma, accelerated or feeble respiration with fatigue, spontaneous sweating and weak pulse, may appear. *Ren Shen* tonifies the Lung and enhances its respiratory effectiveness.

- Chronic cough due to Lung deficiency: use *Ren Shen* with *Kuan Dong Hua* (Flos Farfarae), *Zi Wan* (Radix Asteris), *Bai Bu* (Radix Stemonae) and *Wu Wei Zi* (Fructus Schisandrae Chinensis).
- Wheezing and shortness of breath due to Lung and Kidney deficiency: use this herb with *Ge Jie* (Gecko), *Hu Tao Ren* (Semen Juglandis) and *Wu Wei Zi* (Fructus Schisandrae Chinensis). **Exemplar Formula:** *Ren Shen Ge Jie San* (Ginseng and Gecko Powder).

4. Promotes Generation of Body Fluids and Relieves Thirst

***Xiao ke* (wasting and thirsting) syndrome, thirst from qi and yin deficiencies:** The production, distribution and elimination of body fluids require proper functioning of qi. Yin and qi deficiencies result in the thirst and related symptoms of *xiao ke* syndrome. *Ren Shen* tonifies qi, promotes generation of body fluids and relieves thirst. Should heat also be a factor contributing to thirst, additional symptoms may include heat sensations with thirst that cannot be quenched by water, excessive perspiration, and a big pulse that is revealed upon pressure to be weak.

- *Xiao ke* syndrome with thirst: combine *Ren Shen* with *Tian Hua Fen* (Radix Trichosanthis), *Mai Men Dong* (Radix Ophiopogonis) and *Zhi Mu* (Radix Anemarrhenae).
- Febrile disorders with heat damaging both qi and body fluids: use *Ren Shen* with *Shi Gao* (Gypsum Fibrosum), *Zhi Mu* (Radix Anemarrhenae), *Gan Cao* (Radix Glycyrrhizae), and *Geng Mi* (Semen Oryzae). **Exemplar Formula:** *Bai Hu Jia Ren Shen Tang* (White Tiger plus Ginseng Decoction).

5. Calms the *Shen* (Spirit), Improves Mental Function

Lack of qi and blood nourishment to the Heart *shen*: Abundant *yuan* (source) *qi* nourishes Heart qi, calms the *shen*, and improves mental functions. *Ren Shen* tonifies qi, calms the *shen*, and improves cognitive functions. It is commonly used alone to treat insomnia, disturbed sleep with excessive dreams, fright, confusion and forgetfulness caused by qi deficiency. When taken for a prolonged period of time, this herb treats neurasthenia involving symptoms of fatigue, headache and insomnia.

- Poor cognitive functions due to Heart and Spleen weakness with qi and blood deficiencies, with chief complaints of fatigue, excessive worrying and insomnia: use *Ren Shen* with *Huang Qi* (Radix Astragali), *Long Yan Rou* (Arillus Longan), and *Suan Zao Ren* (Semen Zizyphi Spinosae). **Exemplar Formula:** *Gui Pi Tang* (Restore the Spleen Decoction).
- Poor cognitive functions due to Heart and Kidney weakness with yin and blood deficiencies: combine this herb with *Sheng Di Huang* (Radix Rehmanniae), *Mai Men Dong* (Radix Ophiopogonis), *Dan Shen* (Radix Salviae Miltiorrhizae), and *Bai Zi Ren* (Semen Platycladi). **Exemplar Formula:** *Tian Wang Bu Xin Dan* (Emperor of Heaven's Special Pill to Tonify the Heart).
- Confusion and forgetfulness: add *Ren Shen* to *Shi Chang Pu* (Rhizoma Acori), *Yuan Zhi* (Radix Polygalae), *Fu Shen* (Poria Paradicis) and *Fu Ling* (Poria).

6. Tonifies Qi and Blood

Blood deficiency: *Ren Shen* tonifies qi and enhances the production of blood. It is commonly used to treat patients with sallow complexion revealing both qi and blood deficiencies.

- Qi and blood deficiencies: use *Ren Shen* with *Shu Di Huang* (Radix Rehmanniae Preparata), *Bai Shao* (Radix Paeoniae Alba), *Bai Zhu* (Rhizoma Atractylodis Macrocephalae), and *Fu Ling* (Poria). **Exemplar Formula:** *Ba Zhen Tang* (Eight-Treasure Decoction).

Ren Shen (Radix Ginseng)

7. Treats Impotence

This herb tonifies qi and yang and is commonly used with Kidney yang-tonic herbs to treat impotence. *Ren Shen* may be used singly as herbal tincture, or in combination with other herbs in an herbal formula.

- Impotence: use *Ren Shen* with *Lu Rong* (Cornu Cervi Pantotrichum), *Shu Di Huang* (Radix Rehmanniae Preparata), *Fu Zi* (Radix Aconiti Lateralis Praeparata), and *Bu Gu Zhi* (Fructus Psoraleae).

8. Tonifies Qi in Deficiency Patients with Exterior Conditions

Exterior disorder with interior deficiency: *Ren Shen* treats deficiency patients who have contracted external pathogenic factors. It boosts *wei* (defensive) *qi* to fight against external pathogenic factors.

- Exterior condition with interior deficiency: combine *Ren Shen* with *Qiang Huo* (Rhizoma et Radix Notopterygii), *Chai Hu* (Radix Bupleuri) and *Du Huo* (Radix Angelicae Pubescentis). **Exemplar Formula:** *Ren Shen Bai Du San* (Ginseng Powder to Overcome Pathogenic Influences).

DOSAGE

5 to 10 grams in decoction, 0.5 to 1.0 gram in powder. The dosage of *Ren Shen* may be increased to 15 to 30 grams to treat collapse of *yuan* (source) *qi*. The decoction should be taken in multiple small doses (instead of one large dose) when treating collapse. Due to the high cost of the herb, *Ren Shen* is usually decocted separately at relatively low temperatures to ensure complete extraction of active constituents.

CAUTIONS / CONTRAINDICATIONS

- Sweet and warm in nature, *Ren Shen* is contraindicated in cases of excess conditions, such as bleeding caused by heat in the blood, red eyes and dizziness due to Liver yang rising, wheezing and cough because of Lung heat, or phlegm accumulation, constipation, parasites, internal accumulation, heat or fire conditions.
- According to classic texts, *Ren Shen* is incompatible with *Li Lu* (Radix et Rhizoma Veratri), antagonized by *Zao Jiao* (Fructus Gleditsiae), and counteracted by *Wu Ling Zhi* (Excrementum Trogopteri seu Pteromi) and *Lai Fu Zi* (Semen Raphani Sativi).
- The effectiveness of *Ren Shen* may be reduced by concurrent consumption of turnips, daikon radishes, and tea.

OVERDOSAGE

Mild overdose of *Ren Shen* may lead to side effects such as dry mouth and lips, excitation, fidgeting, irritability, tremor, palpitations, blurred vision, headache, insomnia, increased body temperature, increased blood pressure, edema, decreased appetite, increased sexual desire, dizziness, itching, eczema, early morning diarrhea, bleeding, and fatigue. Such patients are advised to discontinue the herb and seek symptomatic treatment if necessary. Gross overdose may lead to such adverse reactions as nausea, vomiting, irritability, restlessness, urinary and bowel incontinence, fever, increased blood pressure, increased respiration, decreased sensitivity and reaction to light, decreased heart rate, cyanotic facial complexion, red face, seizures, convulsions, and delirium. Though the toxicity of this herb is mild, intake of large dosages may cause toxic side effects of pityriasis rosea, itching, headache, dizziness, sudden rise in temperature, or bleeding. Bleeding is characteristic of acute overdose of *Ren Shen*.[1]

Allergic reactions to *Ren Shen* are characterized by burning sensations of the extremities, itching, excitation, insomnia, dizziness, chest congestion and discomfort, nausea, vomiting, pale face, perspiration, cold extremities, low voice, a deep and thready pulse, and urinary and bowel incontinence.

TREATMENT OF OVERDOSAGE

An herbal decoction of 120 grams of *Gan Cao* (Radix Glycyrrhizae) treats general overdose of *Ren Shen*. Specific symptomatic treatments are also available. *Lai Fu Zi* (Semen Raphani Sativi) treats feelings of distention, dyspnea, or oppression associated with overdose of *Ren Shen*. *Tian Men Dong* (Radix Asparagi) and *Sheng Di Huang* (Radix Rehmanniae) treat increased heat in the body associated with overdose of *Ren Shen*. *Chen Pi* (Pericarpium Citri Reticulatae), *Sha Ren* (Fructus Amomi) and *Shan Zha* (Fructus Crataegi) treat bloating, which sometimes occurs with use of *Ren Shen*.[2]

Acute cases of overdose can be treated by emetic methods. Ingestion of 1.2 to 1.5 grams of *Li Lu* (Radix et Rhizoma Veratri) with warm water will usually induce vomiting of the ingested *Ren Shen* within a few minutes. Chronic cases of overdose can be relieved by ingestion of daikon radish. The treatment is to either ingest 500 to 1,000 grams of fresh daikon radish, or to cook 250 to 500 grams of dried daikon radish and administer via decoction.[3]

Severe cases of overdose characterized by epistaxis with bright red blood, red tongue and rapid pulse should be treated with herbs that clear heat, cool blood and stop bleeding. Herbal treatment includes 6 grams of powdered *Da Huang* (Radix et Rhizoma Rhei), 3 grams of *San Qi* (Radix Notoginseng), 3 grams of *Xi Jiao* (Cornu Rhinoceri), and 400 ml of juice squeezed from fresh daikon radish. [Note: *Shui Niu Jiao* (Cornu Bubali) is used as a substitute because of the protected status of *Xi Jiao* (Cornu Rhinoceri).]

Ren Shen (Radix Ginseng)

CHEMICAL COMPOSITION

Triterpene saponins, aglycone (20S)-protopanaxadiol (ginsenoside Ra0, Ra1, Ra2, Ra3, Rb1, Rb2, Rb3; notoginsenoside R4, Rs1, Rs2, Rs3, Rs4; malonylginsenoside Rb1, Rc, Rd), aglycone (20S)-protopanaxytriol (ginsenoside Re, Rf, Rg1, notoginsenoside R1), aglycone oleanolic acid (ginsenoside Ro, chikusetsusasaponin-V Rb1, Rb2, Rc, Rd, Re, Rg1), water-soluble polysaccharides (panaxane A to U), polyynes (falcarinol, falcarintriol).[4,5]

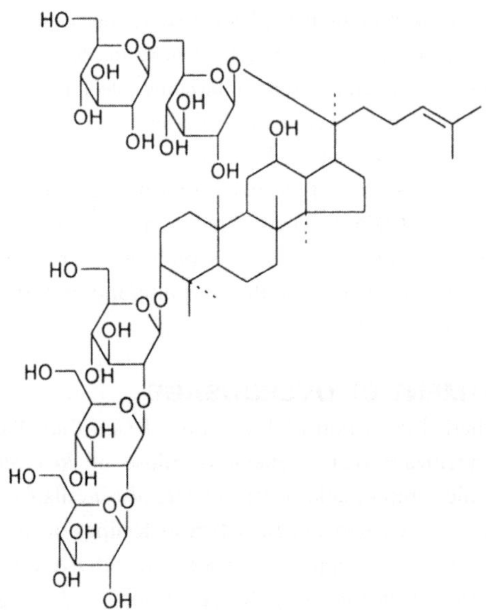

Ginsenoside Ra0

PHARMACOLOGICAL EFFECTS

- **Effects on the central nervous system**: Many laboratory and clinical studies have shown that administration of *Ren Shen* has a significant impact on the central nervous system. It has a stimulating effect in low doses, but an inhibiting effect in large doses. It was found that intraperitoneal injection at the dosage of 50 mg/kg for 5 days has a stimulating effect, as it increases the amounts of dopamine and norepinephrine in the brain stem. On the other hand, oral ingestion of a 40% *Ren Shen* solution has a sedative effect as it greatly decreases the physical activities of rats. Because of its dual functions of stimulation and inhibition, *Ren Shen* provides an adaptogenic effect for the body under various environmental stress.[6,7]
- **Cognitive**: Administration of *Ren Shen* has demonstrated a marked effect in improving memory and learning ability. Using the herbal extract at the dosage of 20 mg/kg/day (equivalent to 100 mg/kg/day of dried herb) for 3 days, there was a significant increase in cognitive capacity in rats as the time necessary to exit a maze was substantially reduced compared to the control group that did not receive any herbs. However, when the dosage of the herbal extract was increased to 100 mg/kg/day (equivalent to 500 mg/kg/day of dried herb), there was an opposite effect, with impairment of memory and learning capacity.[8]
- **Endocrinological**: Administration of *Ren Shen* has a marked influence on the endocrine system. In animal studies, it stimulates the pituitary gland to increase the secretion of ACTH, which in turn stimulates the adrenal glands and their activities. This finding was confirmed in subsequent studies in which *Ren Shen* did not increase activities of the adrenal glands in subjects whose pituitary glands had been surgically removed.[9] In another study, mice that were given *Ren Shen* had an increase in ACH and ACTH, and subsequently better physical performance. Mice that were given one dose of the herb had a 132% increase in swimming time, and mice that were given the herb for 7 days had a 179% increase. Interestingly, overdose of the herb had an opposite effect as it decreased swimming time.[10]
- **Immunostimulant**: *Ren Shen* has immune-enhancing effects. It increases the function of the reticuloendothelial system and increases the total count of IgM.[11]
- **Cardiovascular**: Administration of *Ren Shen* has a positive inotropic effect on the hearts of dogs, rabbits, cats and other animals. It increases the contractility of the heart, slightly increases blood pressure, and constricts blood vessels. It has shown beneficial effects in treatment of shock, arrhythmia and burns. At larger doses, however, it has an opposite effect as it causes an inhibitory influence on the cardiovascular system leading to decreased contractility of the heart, dilation of blood vessels, and a decreased heart rate.[12]
- **Hypoglycemic**: Administration of *Ren Shen* was effective in lowering blood glucose in dogs with hyperglycemia.[13]
- **Antihyperlipidemic**: The saponins in *Ren Shen* lower blood cholesterol levels and reduce the risk of atherosclerosis.[14]
- **Hepatoprotective:** *Ren Shen* has a protective effect in treating various liver disorders. The extract of the herb effectively lowered the elevated levels of liver enzymes in mice induced by acute or chronic consumption of ethanol.[15]
- **Reproductive**: *Ren Shen* has a stimulating effect on the pituitary gland to increase the secretion of gonadotropin. In young mice, it speeds up the development of the reproductive organs. In adult mice, it stimulates the production of sperm in males, and lengthens the estrus period in females. However, it has not demonstrated any direct effect on the sex hormones.[16]

CLINICAL STUDIES AND RESEARCH

- **Shock**: Ten patients in shock due to profuse bleeding were treated with a decoction of 30 grams of *Ren Shen*

Ren Shen (Radix Ginseng)

along with electro-acupuncture on *Baihui* (GV 20) with satisfactory results. All patients were treated in remote areas of China where hospitalization was not available.[17]

- **Cardiac ischemia**: Intravenous or intramuscular injection of an herbal preparation containing *Ren Shen, Mai Men Dong* (Radix Ophiopogonis) and *Wu Wei Zi* (Fructus Schisandrae Chinensis) was beneficial in treatment of cardiac ischemia and cardiogenic shock.[18]
- **Leukopenia**: *Ren Shen* demonstrated immune-enhancing effects in treatment of 52 cancer patients with leukopenia caused by chemotherapy. Administration of *Ren Shen* enabled the patients to complete the entire course of chemotherapy treatment.[19] According to another report, 38 patients with leukopenia were treated with 50 to 100 ml of a *Ren Shen* preparation given two to three times daily, with an 87% rate of effectiveness.[20]
- **Sexual dysfunction**: In one study, 27 patients with impotence were treated with 500 mg/day of *Ren Shen* extract with marked success. Out of 27 patients, 15 regained normal function, 9 had moderate improvement, and 3 showed no response. In another study, 24 patients with low sperm count were treated with a preparation of *Ren Shen* with an increase in sperm count noted in 70% of the patients, and an increase in sperm motility in 67% of the patients.[21]
- **Diabetes mellitus**: Administration of *Ren Shen* liquid extract at the dosage of 0.5 ml twice daily was beneficial for patients with diabetes mellitus. The average reduction of blood glucose was 40 to 50 mg/dL, and the therapeutic effect lasted for up to 2 weeks after discontinuation of herbal treatment. Patients with mild diabetes showed a marked reduction of blood glucose levels and an improvement in overall symptoms. Patients with moderate diabetes showed no significant change of blood glucose, but did show some improvement in signs and symptoms.[22]
- **Addison's disease**: In one study, 18 patients with Addison's disease were treated with a 20% ginseng preparation (made from leaves and branches) for an average of 121 days with good results. The initial dosage was 20 to 30 ml, taken three times daily, with a gradual increase to a daily dose of 150 to 300 ml. The study reported weight gain, increased blood pressure, increased grip strength, increased blood glucose levels, increased sodium content in the plasma, and increased levels of ACTH.[23]
- **Spleen deficiency**: Ten children diagnosed with Spleen deficiency according to traditional Chinese medicine were treated with decoction of *Ren Shen* twice daily for 7 to 14 days per course of treatment. Children under 3 years of age received 3 grams of *Ren Shen* cooked in 30 ml of water, and children over three years of age received 5 grams in 60 ml of water. After the herbal treatment, the children showed an increase in appetite, cessation of spontaneous perspiration, increase in body weight, and improvement in facial complexion.[24]
- **Hypertension and atherosclerosis**: Oral administration of 20 drops of a 20% *Ren Shen* preparation twice daily was beneficial in patients with hypertension, atherosclerosis, and chest pain. After herbal treatment, the patients reported overall symptomatic improvement, such as decreased chest pain, little or no headache, normal sleep, and relief of dyspnea. The improvement lasted for 6 to 9 months after discontinuation of the herbs.[25]
- **Hypercholesterolemia**: *Ren Shen* has a moderate effect in lowering blood cholesterol levels, but a significant effect in lowering triglycerides. Administration of *Ren Shen* in a group of elderly patients showed improvement in memory in 80%, improvement in sleep in 54%, relief of depression in 40%, and relief of headache in 75%.[26]
- **Coronary artery disease**: In one study, 31 patients with coronary artery disease were treated with intravenous infusion of *Ren Shen* once or twice daily with relief of pain in 93.54%, and improvement based on ECG evaluation in 76.66% of the patients. The *Ren Shen* injection was prepared by mixing 6 to 10 ml of herbal solution with 40 ml of D10W.[27]
- **Acute hepatitis**: Oral administration of *Ren Shen* was found to have beneficial effects in treatment of infectious hepatitis by reducing the duration of icteric jaundice and facilitating the recovery of liver functions.[28]

HERB-DRUG INTERACTION

- **Antidepressants:** It has been suggested, but not been documented, that induction of mania may occur in depressed patients who mix antidepressants and *Ren Shen.* In rare cases, the concurrent use of *Ren Shen* and phenelzine has led to manic-like symptoms.[29,30] [Note: Examples of similar antidepressants are as follows: monoamine oxidase inhibitors (MAOI) such as phenelzine (Nardil), tranylcypromine (Parnate), and isocarboxazid (Marplan).]
- **Ethanol:** In an *in vitro* study, an herbal preparation of *Ren Shen, Yuan Zhi* (Radix Polygalae), *Shi Chang Pu* (Rhizoma Acori) and *Fu Ling* (Poria) was found to reduce the ethanol-induced impairment of memory registration. It also ameliorated scopolamine-induced memory registration deficit. These results suggest that this herbal preparation ameliorates the impairment effect of ethanol on learning and memory processes.[31]
- **Antidiabetics:** The use of *Ren Shen* has been associated with reduction of fasting blood glucose levels. Therefore, it has been suggested that hypoglycemia may occur when *Ren Shen* is combined with drugs for treatment of diabetes mellitus.[32] [Note: Examples of antidiabetic drugs include insulin, tolbutamide (Orinase), glipizide (Glucotrol), and glyburide (DiaBeta/Micronase).]

Ren Shen (Radix Ginseng)

TOXICOLOGY

In animal toxicology studies, no significant side effects were reported in mice who received continuous oral ingestion of *Ren Shen* for one month at dosages of 100, 250 and 500 mg/kg. The LD_{50} for oral ingestion of the herb in mice is 5 g/kg. The LD_{50} for subcutaneous injection of the herbal extract in mice is 16.5 ml/kg.[33]

In human toxicology reports, oral ingestion of 100 ml of a 3% tincture may lead to mild discomfort. Oral ingestion of 200 ml of a 3% tincture may lead to rashes, itching, headaches, dizziness, increase in body temperature, and bleeding.[34]

SUPPLEMENT

- 人參葉 / 人参叶 *Ren Shen Ye* (Folium Ginseng), first cited in the *Ben Cao Cong Xin* (Thoroughly Revised Materia Medica) by Wu Yi-Luo in 1751, is derived from the leaf of the same plant as *Ren Shen*. *Ren Shen Ye* is bitter, slightly sweet and cold. It relieves summer-heat, generates body fluids and clears deficiency heat. Suitable conditions for use of *Ren Shen Ye* include thirst, febrile disorders with body fluid loss, Stomach yin deficiency, and toothache due to deficiency fire. Recommended dosage of *Ren Shen Ye* is 5 to 10 grams.

  According to the *Ben Cao Gang Mu* (Materia Medica) by Li Shi-Zhen in 1578, the leaf has no function and is extremely bitter and cold, and can damage qi and blood. However, according to *Ben Cao Shi Yi* (Omissions from the [Classic of the] Materia Medica) by Chen Cang-Qi in 741 A.D., the leaf can tonify the body, generate body fluids, clear summer-heat, clear deficiency heat, benefit the head and extremities and help patients regain sobriety after alcohol intake. Modern research has shown that the stem, leaves, flower and fruit of this plant all contain higher percentages of ginsenosides than the root. The stem has been shown to have similar functions to those of the root and ginsenoside has been used clinically to treat coronary heart disorders, high cholesterol, diabetes and tumors.
- 三七葉 / 三七叶 *San Qi Ye* (Folium Notoginseng) has tastes and actions similar to those of *Ren Shen Ye*, and is commonly used as a substitute.

AUTHORS' COMMENTS

According to Dr. Liu Zhi-Tong, in cases of difficult labor, *Ren Shen* greatly tonifies the *yuan* (source) qi, replenishes fluids, and dilates the cervix to facilitate delivery.

Wild-crafted *Ren Shen* has the strongest function and is reserved for the most severe cases of qi deficiency or collapse. Wild-crafted *Ren Shen* is generally not used because it is extremely expensive. Cultivated *Ren Shen* is also potent, and is the most common form of the herb sold commercially. In most cases, cultivated *Ren Shen* is very effective and affordable. The root of cultivated *Ren Shen* should be at least three years old before harvesting, to obtain therapeutic potency.

Different types of ginseng have slightly different functions:

- *Sheng Sai Shen*, sun-dried ginseng, is more suitable for qi and yin deficiencies.
- *Hong Shen*, red or steamed ginseng, is warmer and is mostly used for qi and yang deficiencies.
- The "tails" of *Ren Shen* are believed to have a weaker tonic effect.
- The "head" of *Ren Shen* is believed to have some effect to induce vomiting.

[Note: It has been found that the "head" and the "body" of *Ren Shen* have essentially the same constituents. Furthermore, in a study of 1500 volunteers who ingested various amounts of ginseng "head," there were no reports of nausea and vomiting. Therefore, it is now accepted that ginseng "head" does not cause nausea and vomiting.[35]]

References

1. *Zhong Yao Bu Liang Fan Ying Yu Zhi Liao* (Adverse Reactions and Treatment of Chinese Herbal Medicine), 1996; 218:220, 1996; 113:117
3. Ibid.
3. *Xin Yi Xue* (New Medicine), 6:619, 1958
4. *PDR for Herbal Medicine*, Medical Economics Company, 2000; 347
5. Yan X, Zhou J, Xie G, *Traditional Chinese Medicines Molecular Structures, Natural Sources and Applications*; Ashgate, 1999; 2598
6. *Zhong Yao Yao Li Yu Ying Yong* (Pharmacology and Applications of Chinese Herbs), 1983; 16
7. *Zhong Hua Yi Xue Za Zhi* (Chinese Journal of Medicine), 1985; 42(12):13
8. *Zhong Yao Ci Hai* (Encyclopedia of Chinese Herbs), 1994
9. *Bai Qiu En Yi Ke Da Xue Xue Bao* (Journal of Baiqiuen University of Medicine), 1980; 6(2):32
10. *Planta Med*, 1979; 30:43
11. *Zhong Yao Xue* (Chinese Herbology), 1998; 729:736
12. *CA*, 1992; 116:34223d
13. *Zhong Yao Xue* (Chinese Herbology), 1998; 729:736
14. Ibid.
15. *CA*, 1989; 111:148638v
16. *Zhong Cheng Yao* (Study of Chinese Patent Medicine), 1989; 11(9):30
17. *Zhong Yi Za Zhi* (Journal of Chinese Medicine), 1987; 4:13
18. *Zhong Cao Yao Tong Xun* (Journal of Chinese Herbal Medicine), 1972; 4:21
19. *Te Chan Ke Xue Shi Yan* (Research of Special Scientific Projects), 1984; 4:24
20. *Zhong Liu Yu Fang Yan Jiu* (Tumor Prevention and Research), 1987; 3:149
21. *Ji Lin Yi Xue* (Jilin Medicine), 1983; 5:54
22. Ibid.
23. Ibid.
24. *Chong Qing Yi Yao* (Chongching Medicine and Herbology), 1984; 6:41
25. *Ji Lin Yi Xue* (Jilin Medicine), 1983; 5:54
26. Ibid.
27. *An Hui Yi Xue* (Anhui Medicine), 1988; 3:51
28. *Ji Lin Yi Xue* (Jilin Medicine), 1983; 5:54

Ren Shen (Radix Ginseng)

29. *Lancet.* 355(9198):134-8, 2000 Jan 8
30. Brinker, Francis. *Herb Contraindications and Drug Interactions,* 1997; 51
31. *Biological and Pharmaceutical Bulletin.* 17(11):1472-6, 1994 Nov
32. *The IBIS Guide to Drug-Herb and Drug-Nutrient Interactions,* 1999
33. *Zhong Yao Yao Li Yu Ying Yong* (Pharmacology and Applications of Chinese Herbs), 1983: 16
34. *Chang Yong Zhong Yao Cheng Fen Yu Yao Li Shou Ce* (A Handbook of the Composition and Pharmacology of Common Chinese Drugs), 1994; 15:119
35. *Bei Jing Yi Xue* (Beijing Medicine), 1986; 1: 30

Xi Yang Shen (Radix Panacis Quinquefolii)

西洋參 西洋参

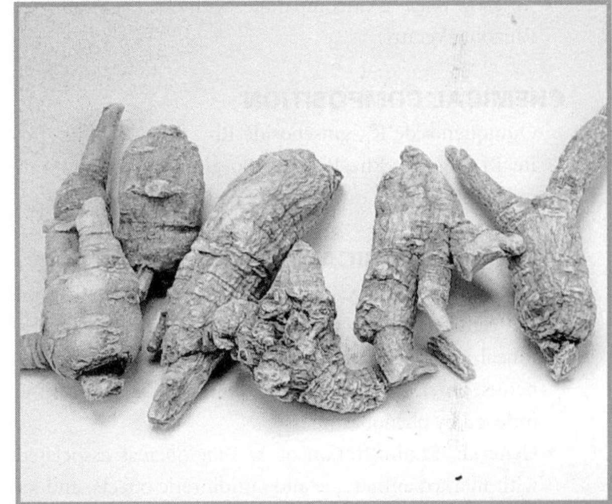

Pinyin Name: *Xi Yang Shen*
Literal Name: "western seas root," "western seas ginseng," "western ginseng"
Alternate Chinese Names: *Hua Qi Shen, Xi Shen, Yang Shen, Guan Dong Ren Shen*
Original Source: *Ben Cao Cong Xin* (Thoroughly Revised Materia Medica) by Wu Yi-Luo in 1751
English Name: American ginseng
Botanical Name: *Panax quinquefolium* (*Xi Yang Shen*)
Pharmaceutical Name: Radix Panacis Quinquefolii
Properties: sweet, bitter, cold
Channels Entered: Kidney, Heart, Lung

CHINESE THERAPEUTIC ACTIONS

1. Tonifies Qi and Nourishes Yin

Lung and Kidney yin deficiencies: *Xi Yang Shen* (Radix Panacis Quinquefolii) treats Lung and Kidney yin-deficient fire with cough, wheezing, scanty sputum that may or may not be streaked with blood, loss of voice, or hemoptysis. It is the best choice for tonifying and nourishing both the qi and yin of the Lung and Kidney.

- Qi and yin deficiencies due to chronic disorders: combine *Xi Yang Shen* with *Mai Men Dong* (Radix Ophiopogonis), *E Jiao* (Colla Corii Asini), *Zhi Mu* (Radix Anemarrhenae) and *Bei Mu* (Bulbus Fritillaria).

2. Clears Fire and Generates Body Fluids

Qi and body fluid deficiencies: Common symptoms include irritability, thirst and fatigue. *Xi Yang Shen* can sedate fire and generate body fluids at the same time. This herb has an excellent function in moistening the body to treat thirst, and dryness of the mouth and tongue. It is used both in cases where fire has damaged fluids, and in cases of yin-deficient heat.

- Yin and qi deficiencies: combine *Xi Yang Shen* with *Huang Qi* (Radix Astragali), *Shan Yao* (Rhizoma Dioscoreae) and *Tian Hua Fen* (Radix Trichosanthis).
- Yin deficiency with heat signs: combine this herb with *Sheng Di Huang* (Radix Rehmanniae), *Shi Hu* (Herba Dendrobii) and *Wu Wei Zi* (Fructus Schisandrae Chinensis).
- Diabetes: add it to *Shan Yao* (Rhizoma Dioscoreae), *Sheng Di Huang* (Radix Rehmanniae), *Shi Gao* (Gypsum Fibrosum) and *Zhi Mu* (Radix Anemarrhenae).
- Dryness of throat or mouth: incorporate this herb with *Tian Men Dong* (Radix Asparagi), *Mai Men Dong* (Radix Ophiopogonis), *Zhi Mu* (Radix Anemarrhenae), and *Yu Zhu* (Rhizoma Polygonati Odorati).
- Thirst: add it to *Huang Qi* (Radix Astragali), *Shan Yao* (Rhizoma Dioscoreae) and *Tian Hua Fen* (Radix Trichosanthis).

Xi Yang Shen (Radix Panacis Quinquefolii)

3. Sedates Heat in the Intestines and Stops Bleeding

Heat in the Intestines with hematochezia due to yin deficiency: combine *Xi Yang Shen* with *Long Yan Rou* (Arillus Longan).

DOSAGE

3 to 6 grams. Due to the high cost of *Xi Yang Shen*, it is often decocted separately from other herbs to ensure complete extraction.

CAUTIONS / CONTRAINDICATIONS

- Use of *Xi Yang Shen* is contraindicated in cases of excess fire with stagnation, or in Stomach damp-cold.
- *Xi Yang Shen* is incompatible with *Li Lu* (Radix et Rhizoma Veratri).

CHEMICAL COMPOSITION

Quinquenoside R_1, ginsenoside Rb_1, Rb $_2$, Rb_3, Rc, Rd, Re, Rf_2, Rg_1, R_0; Rh_1, Rg_3; pseudo-ginsenoside F_{11}, quinquefolans A, B, C; essential oils, rutin.[1]

PHARMACOLOGICAL EFFECTS

- **CNS suppressant:** *Xi Yang Shen* has a sedative effect on the central nervous system (CNS). In mice, intraperitoneal injection of this herb leads to decreased spontaneous physical activities and increased sleeping time induced by phenobarbitals.[2]
- **General:** Administration of *Xi Yang Shen* is associated with marked antifatigue and antidiuretic effects, and an increased resistance to hypoxia.[3]

CLINICAL STUDIES AND RESEARCH

- **Supportive therapy with radiation:** In one study, 20 patients with cancer of the nasal cavity were treated daily with decoction of 3 grams of *Xi Yang Shen* one time each day, starting two weeks prior to the chemotherapy and radiation therapies. The study reported a significant reduction of side effects related to chemotherapy and radiation, such as dry mouth, nausea and vomiting.[4]

TOXICOLOGY

One intraperitoneal injection daily of *Xi Yang Shen* at 450 mg/kg for 7 days showed no significant toxicity nor fatalities in laboratory animals.[5]

AUTHORS' COMMENTS

Xi Yang Shen and *Ren Shen* (Radix Ginseng) both tonify qi and generate body fluids.

- *Xi Yang Shen* is cool in nature and is stronger in nourishing the yin and sedating fire, while its qi-tonic action is weaker than that of *Ren Shen*. As such, *Xi Yang Shen* is best used for patients with both qi and yin deficiencies, as is often seen in Lung yin-deficient fire.
- *Ren Shen* is warm and stronger in tonifying qi and is used for patients experiencing deficiency and cold. *Ren Shen* is especially effective for severe conditions where there is exhaustion of qi, in which case the patients often show Spleen and Stomach deficiencies, Lung qi deficiency, qi and blood deficiencies or possible qi collapse.

References

1. *Xian Dai Zhong Yao Yao Li Xue* (Contemporary Pharmacology of Chinese Herbs), 1997; 1189-1190
2. *Chang Yong Zhong Yao Xian Dai Yan Jiu Yu Lin Chuan* (Recent Study & Clinical Application of Common Traditional Chinese Medicine), 1995; 549:551
3. *Zhong Yao Xue* (Chinese Herbology), 1998; 737:738
4. *Shang Hai Zhong Yi Yao Za Zhi* (Shanghai Journal of Chinese Medicine and Herbology), 1979; 4:29
5. *Chang Yong Zhong Yao Xian Dai Yan Jiu Yu Lin Chuan* (Recent Study & Clinical Application of Common Traditional Chinese Medicine), 1995; 549:551

Dang Shen (Radix Codonopsis)

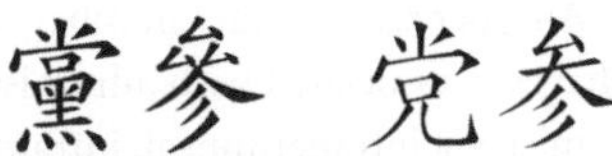

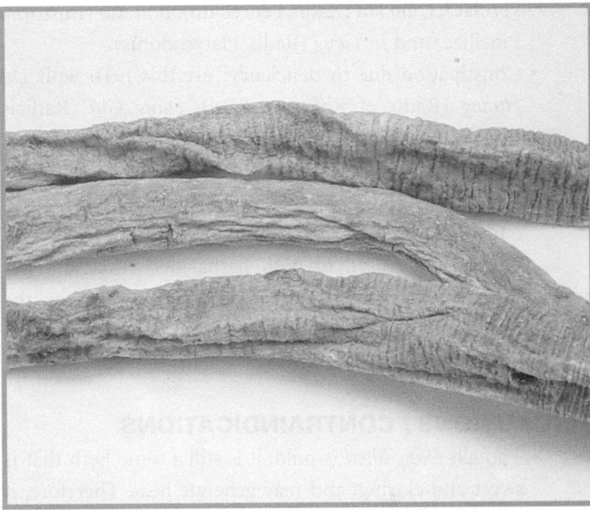

Pinyin Name: *Dang Shen*
Literal Name: "group root"
Alternate Chinese Names: *Tai Dang, Fang Dang, Shi Tou Shen, Lu Dang*
Original Source: *Ben Jing Feng Yuan* (Journey to the Origin of the Classic of Materia Medica) by Zhang Lu in 1670
English Name: codonopsis, pilose Asia bell root
Botanical Name: *Codonopsis pilosula* (Franch.) Nannf. (*Dang Shen*)
Pharmaceutical Name: Radix Codonopsis
Properties: sweet, neutral
Channels Entered: Spleen, Lung

CHINESE THERAPEUTIC ACTIONS

1. Tonifies Qi, Strengthens the Middle *Jiao*

***Zhong* (central) *qi* deficiency:** *Dang Shen* (Radix Codonopsis) tonifies the Spleen and Stomach to enhance their transportation and transformation functions. It is commonly used to treat qi deficiency characterized by fatigue, lack of appetite, weak extremities, and diarrhea.

- Qi deficiency: use *Dang Shen* with *Bai Zhu* (Rhizoma Atractylodis Macrocephalae).
- Indigestion, epigastric fullness and distention, and decreased food intake due to Spleen and Stomach deficiencies: use it with *Zhi Shi* (Fructus Aurantii Immaturus), *Shan Zha* (Fructus Crataegi), *Mai Ya* (Fructus Hordei Germinatus) and *Chen Pi* (Pericarpium Citri Reticulatae).
- Prolapse of organs due to qi and yang deficiencies: add *Dang Shen* to *Huang Qi* (Radix Astragali), *Sheng Ma* (Rhizoma Cimicifugae), *Zhi Ke* (Fructus Aurantii) and *Bai Zhu* (Rhizoma Atractylodis Macrocephalae).
- Constipation with qi deficiency: combine this herb with *Dang Gui* (Radicis Angelicae Sinensis), *Da Huang* (Radix et Rhizoma Rhei) and *Mang Xiao* (Natrii Sulfas).

2. Tonifies the Lung

Lung qi deficiency: *Dang Shen* tonifies the Lung to treat coughing, wheezing, shortness of breath, and low voice from Lung deficiency. In true Lung deficiency, all of the above symptoms worsen with exertion. This herb tonifies the Lung and is not drying in nature.

- Disorders characterized by Lung qi deficiency: incorporate *Dang Shen* with *Huang Qi* (Radix Astragali), *Wu Wei Zi* (Fructus Schisandrae Chinensis), *Zi Wan* (Radix Asteris), and *Sang Bai Pi* (Cortex Mori).

3. Nourishes Blood, Promotes Generation of Body Fluids

Deficiency of qi, body fluids, and blood: *Dang Shen* has an excellent effect to tonify qi, that in turn enhances the production of blood and body fluids. It is commonly used to treat cases of chronic illness characterized by qi and yin deficiencies, or qi and blood deficiencies.

- Qi and yin deficiencies: use *Dang Shen* with *Mai Men Dong* (Radix Ophiopogonis) and *Wu Wei Zi* (Fructus Schisandrae Chinensis).
- Blood deficiency: combine it with *Dang Gui* (Radicis Angelicae Sinensis), *Shu Di Huang* (Radix Rehmanniae Preparata) and *He Shou Wu* (Radix Polygoni Multiflori).
- Qi and blood deficiencies: use it with *Bai Zhu* (Rhizoma Atractylodis Macrocephalae), *Gan Cao* (Radix Glycyrrhizae), *Dang Gui* (Radicis Angelicae Sinensis) and *Bai Shao* (Radix Paeoniae Alba). **Exemplar Formula:** *Ba Zhen Tang* (Eight-Treasure Decoction).

4. Restores Constitution and Expels Pathogenic Factors

Excess accumulation of pathogenic factors with interior deficiency: *Dang Shen* is often used for patients with exterior conditions or interior excess meeting constitutional deficiency. This herb is mild, generates body fluids, and nourishes blood to help the body fight pathogenic factors. The most common clinical manifestations include common cold and constipation. Contraindicated for use alone in these conditions, *Dang Shen* should always be combined with appropriate herbs to expel the pathogenic factors.

- Wind-cold with aversion to cold, fever, headache, nasal obstruction, cough and sputum, in a constitutionally deficient patient: use this herb with *Zi Su Ye* (Folium

Dang Shen (Radix Codonopsis)

Perillae), *Qian Hu* (Radix Peucedani), *Ban Xia* (Rhizoma Pinelliae) and *Jie Geng* (Radix Platycodonis).

- Constipation due to deficiency: use this herb with *Da Huang* (Radix et Rhizoma Rhei), *Dang Gui* (Radicis Angelicae Sinensis) and *Mang Xiao* (Natrii Sulfas).

DOSAGE

6 to 10 grams, with a maximum of 30 grams. *Dang Shen* is commonly used in both herbal decoction and pill forms. Dry-fried, it more effectively strengthens the Spleen and stops diarrhea. Honey-baked, it more strongly tonifies the middle *jiao* and benefits the qi.

CAUTIONS / CONTRAINDICATIONS

- Though *Dang Shen* is mild, it is still a tonic herb that is sweet and cloying, and may generate heat. Therefore, it should be used with caution in cases of excess heat or fire.
- *Dang Shen* is incompatible with *Li Lu* (Radix et Rhizoma Veratri).
- It has been reported that dosages of *Dang Shen* above 63 grams may cause arrhythmia or discomfort in the left pectoral area. However, side effects subside when the herb is discontinued.[1]

CHEMICAL COMPOSITION

Alkaloids (codonopsine, codonopsinine), glycosides (inulin, fructose, syringin, glucopyranoside, fructofuranoside, tangshenoside I, II, III, IV), flavonoids (luteolin-7-glucoside, apigenin, apigenin-7-glucoside, luteolin, aynaroside, luteotin-7-rotinoside, luteotin-7-galactoside), triterpenoids (oleanolic acid, echino cystic acid, albigenic acid, taraxeryl acetate, taraxerol, friedelin), essential oils (palmitic acid, hexanoic acid, heptanoic acid, octanoic acid, nonanoic acid, dodecanoic acid, tetradecanoic acid, pentadecanoic acid, hexadecanoic acid, octadecoic acid, octadecadienoic acid), α-spinasterol, stimasterol, amino acids.[2]

PHARMACOLOGICAL EFFECTS

- **Adaptogenic:** *Dang Shen* has both stimulating and inhibiting effects on the central nervous system to help animals adapt to various stressful environments. According to studies, intraperitoneal injection of the herb greatly enhances resistance to hypoxia in mice.[3]
- **Gastrointestinal:** Administration of *Dang Shen* has marked preventative and treatment effects on peptic ulcers. Decoction of *Dang Shen* at various dosages ranging from 50 to 250 mg/kg increases gastric emptying time, decreases severity of ulceration, and increases the amount of prostaglandins in the stomach. Furthermore, administration of *Dang Shen* also showed a marked protective effect in relieving peptic ulcers induced by over-consumption of aspirin and non-steroidal-anti-inflammatory drugs.[4,5]
- **Immunostimulant:** An increase in the number and activities of macrophages is associated with administration of *Dang Shen* in mice via intraperitoneal, intramuscular or intravenous injections.[6]
- **Hematological:** Administration of water and alcohol extracts of *Dang Shen* is associated with an increase in red blood cells and hemoglobin, but a decrease in white blood cells and lymphocytes.[7]
- **Cardiovascular:** Intravenous injection of water and alcohol extracts of *Dang Shen* has a temporary effect to lower blood pressure in anesthetized rabbits and dogs. In anesthetized cats, intravenous injection of the herb increases cardiac output and blood perfusion to the brain, lower extremities, and internal organs.[8]

CLINICAL STUDIES AND RESEARCH

- **Uterine bleeding:** In one study, 37 patients with uterine bleeding were treated with decoction of *Dang Shen* at dosages of 30 to 60 grams twice daily for 5 days. Out of 37 patients, 5 made complete recovery, 14 showed marked improvement, 10 reported some improvement, and 8 showed no response.[9]
- **Hypotension:** Patients with hypotension were treated with an herbal preparation one time each day 15 days per course of treatment, for 1 to 2 courses total. Good results were reported in 28 out of 30 patients. The herbal preparation contained *Dang Shen* 15g, *Huang Jing* (Rhizoma Polygonati) 12g, *Rou Gui* (Cortex Cinnamomi) 10g, *Da Zao* (Fructus Jujubae) 10 pieces, and *Gan Cao* (Radix Glycyrrhizae) 6g.[10]

TOXICOLOGY

The LD_{50} for intraperitoneal injection of water extract of *Dang Shen* is 79.21 +/- 3.6 g/kg in mice. No fatalities or abnormal reactions were reported in mice following a bolus dose of 10 g/kg administered via oral ingestion.[11]

References

1. Jiang Ting Liang, *Research and Discussion of Chinese Medicine and Herbology,* 1976; 4:33
2. *Xian Dai Zhong Yao Yao Li Xue* (Contemporary Pharmacology of Chinese Herbs), 1997; 1166-1167
3. *Zhong Yao Tong Bao* (Journal of Chinese Herbology), 1986; 11(8):53
4. *Zhong Yao Yao Li Yu Lin Chuang* (Pharmacology and Clinical Applications of Chinese Herbs), 1990; 6(6):9
5. Ibid., 1991; 14(5):47
6. *Zhong Xi Yi Jie He Za Zhi* (Journal of Integrated Chinese and Western Medicine), 1985; 5(8):487
7. *Zhong Yao Xue* (Chinese Herbology), 1998; 739:741
8. Ibid.
9. *Zhe Jiang Zhong Yi Za Zhi* (Zhejiang Journal of Chinese Medicine), 1986; 5:207
10. *Guang Xi Zhong Yi Yao* (Guangxi Chinese Medicine and Herbology), 1985; 5:36
11. *Zhong Cao Yao* (Chinese Herbal Medicine), 1988; 19(8):21

Tai Zi Shen (Radix Pseudostellariae)

太子參 太子参

Pinyin Name: *Tai Zi Shen*
Literal Name: "prince root," "prince ginseng"
Alternate Chinese Names: *Hai Er Shen, Tong Shen*
Original Source: *Zhong Guo Yao Yong Zhi Wu Zi* (Chinese Journal of Medicinal Botanicals)
English Name: pseudostellaria, heterophylly false starwort root
Botanical Name: *Pseudostellaria heterophylla* (Miq.) Pax ex Pax et Hoffm. (*Hai Er Shen*)
Pharmaceutical Name: Radix Pseudostellariae
Properties: sweet, slightly bitter, neutral
Channels Entered: Lung, Spleen

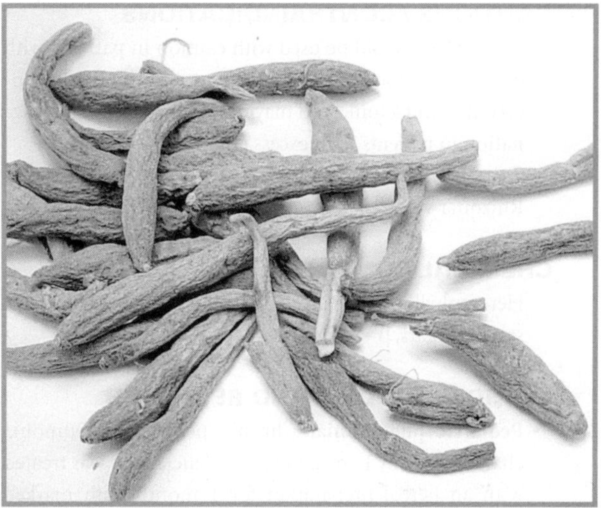

CHINESE THERAPEUTIC ACTIONS

1. Tonifies Qi

Spleen qi deficiency and Stomach yin deficiency: *Tai Zi Shen* (Radix Pseudostellariae) is a mild tonic especially useful in cases where patients are so deficient that they cannot fully benefit from strong tonics. It is also useful for patients recuperating from chronic illnesses. Clinical applications include fatigue, lack of energy, dry mouth, no appetite, and spontaneous perspiration. Compared to *Ren Shen* (Radix Ginseng), *Tai Zi Shen* has a similar, but weaker ability to tonify qi and promote generation of body fluids.

- Spleen and Stomach deficiencies: use *Tai Zi Shen* with *Shan Yao* (Rhizoma Dioscoreae) and *Bian Dou* (Semen Lablab Album).
- Poor appetite due to Spleen and Stomach deficiencies: combine it with *Bai Zhu* (Rhizoma Atractylodis Macrocephalae) and *Gu Ya* (Fructus Setariae Germinatus).
- Deficiencies of qi and yin accompanied by spontaneous perspiration: add this herb to *Mai Men Dong* (Radix Ophiopogonis), *Wu Wei Zi* (Fructus Schisandrae Chinensis), *Fu Xiao Mai* (Semen Tritici Aestivi Levis) and *Huang Qi* (Radix Astragali).

2. Tonifies the Lung

Lung deficiency: The Lung dominates respiration, prefers moisture, and dislikes dryness. It is most susceptible to the pathogenic factors of dryness and heat. *Tai Zi Shen* enters the Lung to tonify qi, promote generation of fluids and moisten dryness. It is commonly used to treat heat and dryness in the Lung that manifest in coughing with shortness of breath and scanty sputum.

- Dry cough due to heat drying the fluids in the Lung: use *Tai Zi Shen* with *Sha Shen* (Radix Glehniae seu Adenophorae), *Bai He* (Bulbus Lilii), *Mai Men Dong* (Radix Ophiopogonis), and *Bei Mu* (Bulbus Fritillaria).

3. Promotes Generation of Body Fluids and Treats Chronic Febrile Disorders

Qi and yin deficiencies with thirst, palpitations and insomnia: *Tai Zi Shen* is neutral to cool in thermal property. It tonifies the middle *jiao* and clears deficiency heat in patients with chronic febrile disorders that often lead to heat damaging the qi and drying yin. Clinical presentation of this condition is characterized by thirst, palpitations, insomnia, low-grade fever, thready pulse, and red tongue. *Tai Zi Shen* treats these conditions by promoting the generation of body fluids.

- Thirst due to qi and yin deficiencies with heat: add this herb to *Sheng Di Huang* (Radix Rehmanniae), *Zhi Mu* (Radix Anemarrhenae), *Mai Men Dong* (Radix Ophiopogonis), and *Zhu Ye* (Herba Phyllostachys).
- Insomnia and palpitations due to qi and yin deficiencies with heat: combine this herb with *Mai Men Dong* (Radix Ophiopogonis), *Wu Wei Zi* (Fructus Schisandrae Chinensis), *Suan Zao Ren* (Semen Zizyphi Spinosae) and *Bai Zi Ren* (Semen Platycladi).
- Persistent unremitting fever due to qi and yin deficiencies with heat, or summer heatstroke in children: add it to *Sha Shen* (Radix Glehniae seu Adenophorae), *Shi Hu* (Herba Dendrobii), *Bai Wei* (Radix Cynanchi Atrati), and *Qing Hao* (Herba Artemisiae Annuae).
- Acute or chronic hepatitis: incorporate *Tai Zi Shen* with *Wu Wei Zi* (Fructus Schisandrae Chinensis) and *Yu Mi Xu* (Stigma Maydis).

DOSAGE

10 to 30 grams in decoction.

Tai Zi Shen (Radix Pseudostellariae)

CAUTIONS / CONTRAINDICATIONS

- *Tai Zi Shen* should be used with caution in patients with excess conditions. Though it is neutral in thermal property, it is still a tonic and may create dampness and stagnation in patients with excess conditions.
- *Tai Zi Shen* is incompatible with *Li Lu* (Radix et Rhizoma Veratri).

CHEMICAL COMPOSITION

Heterophyllin A, B; glycerol l-monolinolate, saponins, starch, sugars, β-sitosterol.[1]

CLINICAL STUDIES AND RESEARCH

- **Pediatric pneumonia:** Chronic pediatric pneumonia characterized by Lung and Spleen deficiencies was treated with an herbal preparation for 1 month with marked improvement. The herbal preparation contained *Tai Zi Shen*, *Huang Qi* (Radix Astragali), *Mai Men Dong* (Radix Ophiopogonis), *Wu Wei Zi* (Fructus Schisandrae Chinensis), *Bai Zhu* (Rhizoma Atractylodis Macrocephalae), honey-processed *Zi Wan* (Radix Asteris) and honey-processed *Kuan Dong Hua* (Flos Farfarae).[2]
- **Hepatitis:** Long-term administration of *Tai Zi Shen* at 30 grams per dose is beneficial in patients with hepatitis or early liver cirrhosis accompanied by abnormal albumin and globulin levels.[3]

References

1. *Chang Yong Zhong Yao Cheng Fen Yu Yao Li Shou Ce* (A Handbook of the Composition and Pharmacology of Common Chinese Drugs), 1994; 553-554
2. *Zhong Yao Lin Zheng Ying Yong* (Clinical Applications of Chinese Herbs), 1980; :442
3. Ibid.

Dong Yang Shen (Radix Ginseng Japonica)

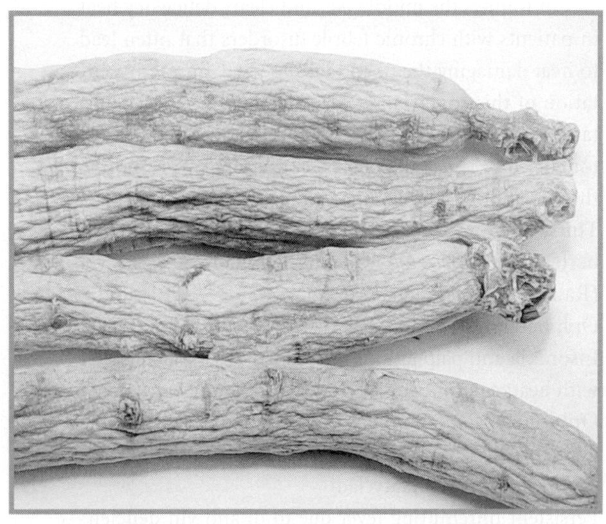

東洋參 东洋参

Pinyin Name: *Dong Yang Shen*
Literal Name: "eastern ginseng"
Alternate Chinese Names: *Yang Shen*
English Name: eastern ginseng, Japanese ginseng
Botanical Name: *Panax ginseng* C. A. Mey. (*Ren Shen*)
Pharmaceutical Name: Radix Ginseng Japonica
Properties: sweet, slightly bitter, cool
Channels Entered: Spleen, Lung

CHINESE THERAPEUTIC ACTIONS

1. Tonifies the Lung and Spleen, Nourishes the *Shen* (Spirit)

Spleen qi deficiency: *Dong Yang Shen* (Radix Ginseng Japonica) treats symptoms of fatigue, lassitude, poor appetite, loose stools, weak pulse, and a pale tongue with teeth marks.

- General Spleen qi deficiency: use *Dong Yang Shen* with *Bai Zhu* (Rhizoma Atractylodis Macrocephalae), *Fu Ling* (Poria), *Huang Qi* (Radix Astragali), and *Gan Cao* (Radix Glycyrrhizae).
- Loose stools: combine this herb with *Shan Yao* (Rhizoma Dioscoreae) and *Sha Ren* (Fructus Amomi).
- Poor appetite: use it with *Huo Xiang* (Herba Agastache) and *Mai Ya* (Fructus Hordei Germinatus).

Lung qi deficiency: Manifestations of this condition include feeble cough, shortened respiration, spontaneous

Dong Yang Shen (Radix Ginseng Japonica)

sweating, dyspnea and fatigue.

- Lung qi deficiency: add *Dong Yang Shen* to *Huang Qi* (Radix Astragali) and *Shan Yao* (Rhizoma Dioscoreae).
- Feeble cough: use it with *Wu Wei Zi* (Fructus Schisandrae Chinensis), *Zi Wan* (Radix Asteris) and *Kuan Dong Hua* (Flos Farfarae).
- Spontaneous sweating: combine this herb with *Fang Feng* (Radix Saposhnikoviae), *Huang Qi* (Radix Astragali) and *Bai Zhu* (Rhizoma Atractylodis Macrocephalae).

Lack of nourishment to the *shen* (spirit): Manifestations of this imbalance include excessive dreams or dream-disturbed sleep.

- *Shen* disturbance: combine *Dong Yang Shen* with *Yuan Zhi* (Radix Polygalae) and *Suan Zao Ren* (Semen Zizyphi Spinosae).

2. Regulates the Middle *Jiao* and Improves Appetite

Spleen and Stomach qi deficiencies: *Dong Yang Shen* can tonify and regulate the middle *jiao* to treat nausea, vomiting and poor appetite.

- Spleen and Stomach qi deficiencies: combine this herb with *Bai Zhu* (Rhizoma Atractylodis Macrocephalae), *Ban Xia* (Rhizoma Pinelliae) and *Sheng Jiang* (Rhizoma Zingiberis Recens).

DOSAGE

3 to 9 grams in decoction.

CAUTIONS / CONTRAINDICATIONS

- *Dong Yang Shen* is contraindicated in excess conditions, as the tonic nature of the herb may create dampness and stagnation.

AUTHORS' COMMENTS

Dong Yang Shen and *Ren Shen* (Radix Ginseng) are the same plant cultivated in different geographic climates. *Dong Yang Shen* is cultivated in Japan while *Ren Shen* is cultivated in Northern China and Korea. However, these two herbs do not have identical therapeutic effects because their growing environments are quite different. The characteristics of *Dong Yang Shen* are similar to those of *Xi Yang Shen* (Radix Panacis Quinquefolii). Both tonify but do not cause the dry heat seen in other warm and dry tonics. *Dong Yang Shen* tonifies and regulates the middle *jiao*. *Xi Yang Shen* is stronger in tonifying action than *Dong Yang Shen*.

Huang Qi (Radix Astragali)

黄耆 黄芪

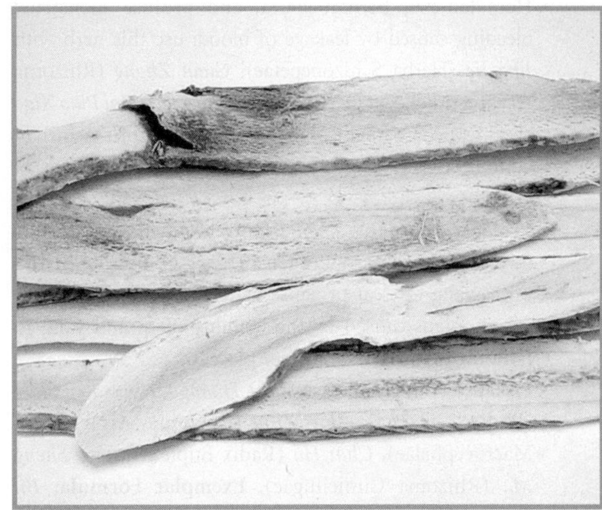

Pinyin Name: *Huang Qi*
Alternate Chinese Names: *Jin Huang Qi, Jian Qi, Kou Qi*
Original Source: *Shen Nong Ben Cao Jing* (Divine Husbandman's Classic of the Materia Medica) in the second century
English Name: astragalus, Mongolian milkvetch root, membranous milkvetch root
Botanical Name: *Astragalus membranaceus* Bge. var. *mongholicus* (Dge.) Hsiao (*Meng Gu Huang Qi*); *Astragalus membranaceus* (Fisch.) Bge. (*Mo Jiao Huang Qi*)
Pharmaceutical Name: Radix Astragali
Properties: sweet, slightly warm
Channels Entered: Spleen, Lung

Huang Qi (Radix Astragali)

CHINESE THERAPEUTIC ACTIONS

1. Tonifies Qi and Raises Yang

Spleen qi deficiency: *Huang Qi* (Radix Astragali) tonifies the Spleen to enhance its effectiveness in transformation and transportation. Clinical applications include pale or sallow facial appearance, fatigue, tired extremities, decreased food intake, diarrhea, and other conditions of Spleen deficiency.

- Fatigue and tired extremities due to Spleen deficiency: use *Huang Qi* individually, or combine it with *Dang Shen* (Radix Codonopsis) or *Ren Shen* (Radix Ginseng) for synergistic effect.
- Loose stools or diarrhea due to Spleen deficiency: add it to *Fu Ling* (Poria), *Shan Yao* (Rhizoma Dioscoreae), *Bian Dou* (Semen Lablab Album) and *Yi Yi Ren* (Semen Coicis).
- Spleen yang deficiency: use *Huang Qi* with yang tonics.

Inability of qi to control blood circulation: Proper flow and production of blood require an adequate supply of qi. In addition, Spleen qi controls the flow of blood and keeps it in the vessels. Deficiency of Spleen qi may lead to secondary blood deficiency and leakage of blood. Clinically, patients may exhibit fatigue, lethargy, shortness of breath, pale face, hematemesis, hematochezia, bruises, uterine bleeding, or other bleeding disorders. In short, patients with Spleen qi deficiency may bleed or bruise easily.

- Qi and blood deficiencies characterized by shortness of breath and pale face: combine *Huang Qi* with *Ren Shen* (Radix Ginseng), *Bai Zhu* (Rhizoma Atractylodis Macrocephalae), *Dang Gui* (Radicis Angelicae Sinensis) and *Suan Zao Ren* (Semen Zizyphi Spinosae). **Exemplar Formula:** *Gui Pi Tang* (Restore the Spleen Decoction).
- Hematemesis, hematochezia, and profuse menstrual bleeding caused by leakage of blood: use this herb with *Jing Jie* (Herba Schizonepetae), *Guan Zhong* (Rhizoma Dryopteridis), *San Qi* (Radix Notoginseng), *Hai Piao Xiao* (Endoconcha Sepiae) and *E Jiao* (Colla Corii Asini) in addition to *Gui Pi Tang* (Restore the Spleen Decoction).

Prolapse of organs: *Zhong* (central) *qi* deficiency results in prolapse of internal organs. *Huang Qi* tonifies qi and raises yang to treat prolapse of the stomach, rectum or other organs caused by the inability of qi and yang to hold the organs in the proper place.

- Prolapse of internal organs: use *Huang Qi* with *Ren Shen* (Radix Ginseng), *Bai Zhu* (Rhizoma Atractylodis Macrocephalae), *Chai Hu* (Radix Bupleuri), and *Sheng Ma* (Rhizoma Cimicifugae). **Exemplar Formula:** *Bu Zhong Yi Qi Tang* (Tonify the Middle and Augment the Qi Decoction). A large amount of *Zhi Ke* (Fructus Aurantii) may be added to enhance the overall effectiveness of the formula.

Lung and Spleen qi deficiencies: Clinical manifestations of compromised respiratory and digestive functions include cough, wheezing, shortness of breath, profuse white and watery sputum, pale face, low voice, fatigue, abdominal fullness and diarrhea. *Huang Qi* enters both Lung and Spleen channels to tonify qi. It is the herb of choice for treating qi deficiency of these organs.

- Lung and Spleen qi deficiencies: combine *Huang Qi* with *Dang Shen* (Radix Codonopsis), *Fu Ling* (Poria), *Zi Wan* (Radix Asteris), and *Chen Pi* (Pericarpium Citri Reticulatae).

Qi and blood deficiencies: This imbalance is characterized by sallow facial appearance, dizziness, vertigo, lack of energy, no desire to speak, spontaneous perspiration, palpitations and insomnia. Since qi is the leader of blood, tonification of qi enhances the production of blood.

- Qi and blood deficiencies: pair *Huang Qi* with *Dang Gui* (Radicis Angelicae Sinensis). **Exemplar Formula:** *Dang Gui Bu Xue Tang* (Tangkuei Decoction to Tonify the Blood).

Qi deficiency with deficiency heat symptoms: Spleen qi deficiency prohibits clear yang from disseminating throughout the body. If yang qi is trapped in the muscle level for a prolonged period of time, symptoms of irritability with low-grade fever or unremitting high fever with fatigue, spontaneous sweating and frequent contraction of exterior conditions will occur. *Huang Qi* treats this deficiency heat condition even though it is warm in nature. **Exemplar Formula:** *Bu Zhong Yi Qi Tang* (Tonify the Middle and Augment the Qi Decoction).

Cancer with qi deficiency caused by chemotherapy and radiation treatments: Patients with cancer often receive chemotherapy and radiation treatments that severely damage qi. Use of *Huang Qi* replenishes the qi and decreases the adverse side effects associated with such treatments.

- Qi deficiency due to chemotherapy and radiation: use *Huang Qi* with *Ling Zhi* (Ganoderma), *Nu Zhen Zi* (Fructus Ligustri Lucidi), *Dang Shen* (Radix Codonopsis), *Ren Shen* (Radix Ginseng), *Dong Chong Xia Cao* (Cordyceps) and *Shan Zhu Yu* (Fructus Corni).

Sudden qi collapse due to heavy blood loss: Qi and blood travel together in the vessels. When there is a sudden loss of blood, qi collapses as well. Symptoms include sudden facial pallor, profuse sweating, shortness of breath, and fading pulse. In severe cases, symptoms such as icy extremities, a sudden drop in blood pressure and body temperature, and sweating, may occur.

- Qi and blood collapse: use a large dose of *Huang Qi* (between 60 to 120 grams) with *Dang Gui* (Radicis

Huang Qi (Radix Astragali)

Angelicae Sinensis), *Ren Shen* (Radix Ginseng), *Fu Zi* (Radix Aconiti Lateralis Praeparata), *Mai Men Dong* (Radix Ophiopogonis), and *Wu Wei Zi* (Fructus Schisandrae Chinensis).

2. Tonifies *Wei* (Defensive) *Qi*, Consolidates the Exterior

Deficiency of the *wei* (defensive) *qi* with spontaneous sweating: Deficiency of the exterior leads to leakage of body fluids, resulting in spontaneous perspiration. This often leads to a compromised immune system and frequent contraction of exterior pathogenic infections.

- Spontaneous perspiration because of exterior deficiency: use *Huang Qi* with *Mu Li* (Concha Ostreae), *Ma Huang Gen* (Radix Ephedrae), and *Fu Xiao Mai* (Semen Tritici Aestivi Levis).
- Spontaneous perspiration with aversion to wind, weak pulse, and frequent contraction of bacterial and viral infections: use this herb with *Bai Zhu* (Rhizoma Atractylodis Macrocephalae) and *Fang Feng* (Radix Saposhnikoviae). **Exemplar Formula:** *Yu Ping Feng San* (Jade Windscreen Powder).
- Profuse perspiration and extreme fatigue due to yang deficiency: combine *Huang Qi* with *Fu Zi* (Radix Aconiti Lateralis Praeparata) and *Sheng Jiang* (Rhizoma Zingiberis Recens).
- Night sweating due to qi and yin deficiencies: use it with *Sheng Di Huang* (Radix Rehmanniae), *Mai Men Dong* (Radix Ophiopogonis), *Wu Wei Zi* (Fructus Schisandrae Chinensis), *Fu Xiao Mai* (Semen Tritici Aestivi Levis) and *Di Gu Pi* (Cortex Lycii).

3. Promotes the Discharge of Pus and Generates Flesh

Chronic non-healing ulcers and sores: *Huang Qi* treats chronic sores and ulcerations with underlying deficiencies of qi and blood. Use of *Huang Qi* facilitates the discharge of pus and abscess, and encourages healing through generation of new flesh.

- Chronic non-ulcerating sores with pus: combine *Huang Qi* with *Dang Gui* (Radicis Angelicae Sinensis), *Chuan Xiong* (Rhizoma Ligustici Chuanxiong), *Chuan Shan Jia* (Squama Manis), and *Zao Jiao Ci* (Spina Gleditsiae).
- Chronic sores with underlying deficiency: use this herb with *Ren Shen* (Radix Ginseng), *Dang Gui* (Radicis Angelicae Sinensis), *Chuan Xiong* (Rhizoma Ligustici Chuanxiong), *Bai Zhi* (Radix Angelicae Dahuricae) and *Fang Feng* (Radix Saposhnikoviae). **Exemplar Formula:** *Qian Jin Nei Tuo San* (Drain the Interior Powder Worthy of A Thousand Gold).
- Flat, chronic sores and non-healing ulcers: use it with *Dang Gui* (Radicis Angelicae Sinensis), *Shu Di Huang* (Radix Rehmanniae Preparata), *Ren Shen* (Radix Ginseng), *Bai Zhu* (Rhizoma Atractylodis Macrocephalae), and *Rou Gui* (Cortex Cinnamomi). **Exemplar Formula:** *Shi Quan Da Bu Tang* (All-Inclusive Great Tonifying Decoction).
- Qi deficiency lesions in children: add *Huang Qi* to *Ren Shen* (Radix Ginseng), *Rou Gui* (Cortex Cinnamomi), and *Zhi Gan Cao* (Radix Glycyrrhizae Preparata). **Exemplar Formula:** *Bao Yuan Tang* (Preserve the Basal Decoction).

4. Regulates Water Circulation, Reduces Edema

Edema due to qi deficiency: Spleen qi deficiency with an inability to carry out the transportation function results in retention of water in the body. *Huang Qi* tonifies qi and promotes normal circulation of water to treat conditions such as facial edema, superficial edema, sensations of heaviness in the body, spontaneous sweating and intolerance of wind. *Huang Qi* tonifies qi, and in turn facilitates the elimination of water. When used individually, the diuretic effect of *Huang Qi* is very mild and should be combined with diuretic herbs for stronger therapeutic results. However, this is the herb of choice when the patient presents deficiency along with water retention signs and symptoms. When using *Huang Qi* as a diuretic only, the recommended dosage is low, approximately 9 grams.

- Edema, heavy sensations of the body, spontaneous perspiration, and aversion to wind because of accumulation of water with an exterior wind condition: use *Huang Qi* with *Bai Zhu* (Rhizoma Atractylodis Macrocephalae), *Fen Fang Ji* (Radix Stephaniae Tetandrae), *Gan Cao* (Radix Glycyrrhizae) and *Sheng Jiang* (Rhizoma Zingiberis Recens). **Exemplar Formula:** *Fang Ji Huang Qi Tang* (Stephania and Astragalus Decoction).
- Superficial edema caused by yang deficiency: combine this herb with *Gui Zhi* (Ramulus Cinnamomi), *Fu Ling* (Poria) and *Fen Fang Ji* (Radix Stephaniae Tetandrae). **Exemplar Formula:** *Fang Ji Fu Ling Tang* (Stephania and Poria Decoction).
- Chronic nephritis with edema and proteinuria: use a high dose of *Huang Qi* (60 to 90 grams) with *Dang Shen* (Radix Codonopsis), *Shi Wei* (Folium Pyrrosiae), and *Shan Yao* (Rhizoma Dioscoreae) with *Fang Ji Huang Qi Tang* (Stephania and Astragalus Decoction) or *Fang Ji Fu Ling Tang* (Stephania and Poria Decoction).

5. Relieves Numbness and Pain

Numbness: Numbness of the muscles in this case is due to insufficient nourishment and circulation of qi and blood. *Huang Qi* has a strong effect to tonify qi, which, in turn, helps to generate blood and increase blood flow to the extremities. It tonifies and promotes normal circulation of qi to relieve skin and muscle numbness and pain.

Huang Qi (Radix Astragali)

- Skin and muscle numbness and pain caused by qi and blood deficiencies: use this herb with *Gui Zhi* (Ramulus Cinnamomi), *Bai Shao* (Radix Paeoniae Alba), *Sheng Jiang* (Rhizoma Zingiberis Recens) and *Da Zao* (Fructus Jujubae).
- Numbness and pain in the extremities due to deficiency at *ying* (nutritive) and *wei* (defense) levels and accumulation of wind and dampness: use *Huang Qi* with *Qiang Huo* (Rhizoma et Radix Notopterygii), *Fang Feng* (Radix Saposhnikoviae), *Jiang Huang* (Rhizoma Curcumae Longae), and *Dang Gui* (Radicis Angelicae Sinensis). **Exemplar Formula:** *Juan Bi Tang* (Remove Painful Obstruction Decoctions).

Stroke Sequelae: *Huang Qi* is commonly used to treat post-stroke complications, such as hemiplegia and deviation of the eyes and mouth, caused by qi deficiency and blood stagnation. It is important to note that *Huang Qi* is only suitable for post-stroke patients who are deficient in nature and the dosage used must be high. Use of *Huang Qi* is not recommended for those who are at risk of stroke due to Liver yang rising, such as in patients with hypertension.

- Post-stroke complications: use a high dose of *Huang Qi* with *Dang Gui Wei* (Extremitas Radicis Angelicae Sinensis), *Chuan Xiong* (Rhizoma Ligustici Chuanxiong), *Tao Ren* (Semen Persicae), *Hong Hua* (Flos Carthami) and *Di Long* (Pheretima). **Exemplar Formula:** *Bu Yang Huan Wu Tang* (Tonify the Yang to Restore Five Decoction).

6. Treats *Xiao Ke* (Wasting and Thirsting) Syndrome

***Xiao ke* syndrome:** *Huang Qi* tonifies qi, promotes generation of body fluids, and treats *xiao ke* syndrome accompanied by symptoms of thirst and fatigue.

- *Xiao ke* syndrome without interior heat: use *Huang Qi* with *Sheng Di Huang* (Radix Rehmanniae), *Shan Zhu Yu* (Fructus Corni), *Shan Yao* (Rhizoma Dioscoreae) and pig pancreas.
- *Xiao ke* syndrome with interior heat: combine this herb with *Zhi Mu* (Radix Anemarrhenae), *Ge Gen* (Radix Puerariae), *Tian Hua Fen* (Radix Trichosanthis) and *Shan Yao* (Rhizoma Dioscoreae).

DOSAGE

10 to 15 grams. The maximum dosage of *Huang Qi* is 120 grams. Unprocessed *Huang Qi* (fresh or dried) has qualities better suited to treat exterior disorders, as it tonifies *wei* (defensive) *qi*, stops perspiration, regulates circulation of water, reduces edema, and promotes generation of flesh. The honey-processed herb has an enhanced ability to treat imbalances of the interior, such as Spleen and Lung qi deficiencies and yang deficiency. It is also commonly used to treat chronic cases of fatigue, diarrhea, organ prolapse, and all cases of deficiency.

When preparing honey-fried *Huang Qi*, use 12.5 to 15 kg of honey with 50 kg of the dried herb. Mix and stir fry over low heat until the herb turns brown and is no longer sticky to the touch. [The amounts of honey and *Huang Qi* can be increased or decreased as long as they stay in the same proportion.]

CAUTIONS / CONTRAINDICATIONS

- Use of *Huang Qi* is contraindicated when pathogens are present at exterior levels of the body.
- It is contraindicated in cases characterized by an excess of qi, such as found in anger due to Liver qi stagnation.
- It is contraindicated in internal heat, excess fire, or deficiency and cold of the lower *jiao*.
- It is contraindicated with sores and lesions caused by heat in the blood.
- It is contraindicated in cases of stagnation.
- Pregnant women in the third trimester should use *Huang Qi* with caution. It has a diuretic effect and long-term use may decrease the quantity of amniotic fluid.[1]

CHEMICAL COMPOSITION

Acetylastragaloside I, astragaloside I-IV, isoastragaloside I-II, astramembrannin II, cycloastragenol, cyclosiversigenin, soyasaponin I, tragacantha, kumatakenin, fomononetin.[2,3]

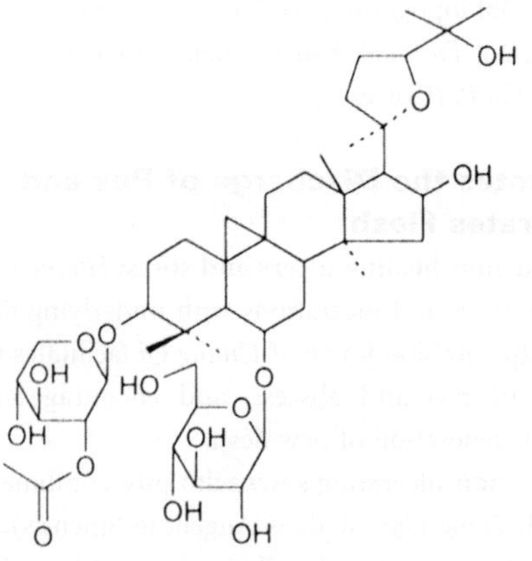

Astragaloside I

PHARMACOLOGICAL EFFECTS

- **Immunostimulant:** Subcutaneous injection of *Huang Qi* increases white blood cells and multinuclear leukocytes in mice. In addition, administration of *Huang Qi* is associated with an enhanced production of IgM in mice.[4,5]
- **Hematopoietic:** *Huang Qi* has been shown to increase the production and maturity of blood cells from the bone marrow.[6]

Huang Qi (Radix Astragali)

- **Metabolic:** Decoction of *Huang Qi* has been shown to increase the basal metabolic rate and cAMP in mice.[7]
- **Effect on cAMP and cGMP:** Decoction of *Huang Qi* is associated with increased cAMP but decreased cGMP in plasma, increased cAMP and cGMP in the spleen, and increased cGMP in the liver.[8]
- **Renal:** Oral use of *Huang Qi* powder decreases the amount of protein present in the urine of mice.[9]
- **Antihypertensive:** Intravenous injection of *Huang Qi* decreases blood pressure in anesthetized rabbits, dogs and cats. The mechanism of this effect is attributed to dilation of peripheral blood vessels.[10]
- **Hepatoprotective:** *Huang Qi* is commonly used to treat various types of chronic hepatitis. Furthermore, *Huang Qi* has significant hepatoprotective effects, especially against carbon tetrachloride.[11,12]
- **Antibiotic:** *Huang Qi* has been shown to inhibit the activity of *Bacillus dysenteriae, Bacillus anthracis,* β-hemolytic streptococcus, *Corynebacterium diphtheriae, Diplococcus pneumoniae,* and *Staphylococcus aureus.*[13]
- **Sedative and analgesic:** Intravenous injection of astragaloside has been shown to have mild sedative and analgesic effects in mice.[14]

CLINICAL STUDIES AND RESEARCH

- **Prevention of common colds and influenza:** In one study, 540 patients with past histories of frequent common colds and influenza were divided into two groups and received preventative treatment with *Huang Qi*. One group received 5 grams of *Huang Qi* in pills three times daily, and the other group received 15 grams of *Huang Qi* in decoction every other day. All patients had two courses of 10 days treatment, with 5 days of rest in between courses. The study reported that patients in both groups had similar results. Both had 2.7 times lower risk of infection, and a shortened duration of infection.[15]
- **Prevention of pulmonary tract infection:** An herbal tea of 15 grams of *Huang Qi* and 10 grams of *Da Zao* (Fructus Jujubae), given twice daily, demonstrated marked effectiveness in prevention of pulmonary tract infection in 160 patients with past histories of chronic bronchitis, bronchial asthma, and allergic rhinitis.[16]
- **Prevention of upper respiratory tract infection in children:** One report described that 2 ml of *Huang Qi* solution (equivalent to 2 grams of dried herb) given daily, showed 94% effectiveness in prevention of respiratory tract infection in 100 children.[17]
- **Rhinitis:** Local injection of a *Huang Qi* preparation every third day for 10 treatments showed a 93.26% rate of effectiveness in 47 patients with rhinitis.[18]
- **Prevention of asthma and cough:** A *Huang Qi* preparation was injected (equivalent to 1 gram of dried herb) into *Zusanli* (ST 36) bilaterally twice weekly for three months per course of treatment, for a total of 3 to 4 courses of treatment, with 2 weeks of rest between each course. Out of 41 patients, there was significant improvement in 85.4% and moderate improvement in 56.1%. Furthermore, most patients noticed an increase in appetite and energy, improvement in quality of sleep, and fewer episodes of infection.[19]
- **Peptic ulcer disease:** According to one report, patients with gastric ulcers, duodenal ulcers, or both, were treated with intramuscular injections of 2 ml of a *Huang Qi* preparation (equivalent to 2 grams of dried herb) twice daily. Many patients showed symptomatic improvement after 1 week. Most patients showed complete healing or moderate improvement after approximately one month.[20] According to another report, an herbal decoction containing *Huang Qi* 12g, *Bai Shao* (Radix Paeoniae Alba) 12g, *Gan Cao* (Radix Glycyrrhizae) 5g, *Gui Zhi* (Ramulus Cinnamomi) 10g, *Sheng Jiang* (Rhizoma Zingiberis Recens) 3g, *Da Zao* (Fructus Jujubae) 5 pieces, and *Yi Tang* (Saccharum Granorum) 30g, was given in two equally-divided doses twice daily for 25 to 53 days to treat patients with peptic ulcer disease. Out of 43 patients, 22 reported significant improvement, 17 reported moderate improvement, and 4 showed no improvement. The rate of effectiveness was 90.7%.[21]
- **Gastric prolapse:** Patients with gastric prolapse were treated with an herbal preparation of fresh *Huang Qi, Sheng Ma* (Rhizoma Cimicifugae), *Chai Hu* (Radix Bupleuri), and *Wu Wei Zi* (Fructus Schisandrae Chinensis). The treatment protocol was to inject the herbs (dosage equivalent to 1 gram of each herb) intramuscularly into *Zhongwan* (CV 12) and *Zusanli* (ST 36) every other day for 1 month. The rate of effectiveness was 84.9% among 42 patients who participated in the study.[22]
- **Rectal prolapse:** Daily administration of an herbal decoction containing 30 to 50 grams of fresh *Huang Qi*, 15 grams of *Dan Shen* (Radix Salviae Miltiorrhizae), 10 grams of *Shan Zha* (Fructus Crataegi), 3 grams of *Fang Feng* (Radix Saposhnikoviae), and 3 grams of *Sheng Ma* (Rhizoma Cimicifugae) showed marked effectiveness for treatment of rectal prolapse.[23]
- **Hepatitis:** In one study, 29 patients with chronic infectious hepatitis were treated with intramuscular injections of *Huang Qi* (equivalent to 4 grams of dried herb) for 1 to 3 months, with marked improvement.[24] Another report described 174 patients with positive HBsAg who were treated with an injection of a 100% *Huang Qi* preparation. The treatment protocol was to administer one injection every three days for a total of 2 months, alternating between two acupuncture points *Zusanli* (ST 36) and *Shenshu* (BL 23). Out of 174 patients, 131 (75.3%) became negative for HBsAg.[25]

Huang Qi (Radix Astragali)

- **Immune disorder:** According to one report, 14 patients with low white blood cell counts showed marked improvement with an herbal decoction of 30 grams of fresh *Huang Qi*, 15 grams of *Ren Shen* (Radix Ginseng), and 20 pieces of *Da Zao* (Fructus Jujubae).[26]
- **Reversal of immune suppression:** In an *in vivo* study, administration of *Huang Qi* was associated with reversal of cyclophosphamide-induced immune suppression.[27]
- **Leukopenia:** Administration of *Huang Qi* was associated with an obvious rise in white blood cell (WBC) counts in 115 patients with leukopenia.[28]
- **Immune restoration:** Administration of *Huang Qi* and *Nu Zhen Zi* (Fructus Ligustri Lucidi) was reported to act as a potent immune stimulant in 19 cancer patients.[29]
- **Nephritis:** Twenty patients with chronic nephritis were treated with 100g of *Huang Qi* in decoction, given in two equally-divided doses twice daily for 15 to 90 days. Out of 20 patients, 7 showed significant improvement, 9 showed marked improvement, and 4 showed no improvement. Most patients reported symptomatic improvement as well as a decrease of protein in the urine.[30]
- **Nephropathy:** *Huang Qi* in large doses has shown beneficial effects against nephropathy in mice and glomerulonephritis in rabbits. Furthermore, large doses of *Huang Qi* are commonly used to treat chronic nephritis in human clinical trials. It increases the volume of urine, and the excretion of chloride and ammonia.[31,32]
- **Glomerulonephritis:** In one study, 56 patients with chronic glomerulonephritis were treated with intramuscular injection of *Huang Qi* (equivalent to 3 grams of dried herb) for 1 month with marked reduction of protein in the urine (effective rate of 61.7%) and improved kidney function.[33]
- **Psoriasis:** Administration of *Huang Qi* (as powder, decoction, injection or topical cream) was used to treat patients with psoriasis with a 95.6% rate of effectiveness. Out of 204 patients, 42 reported marked improvement, 62 reported moderate improvement, 91 reported slight improvement, and 9 reported no improvement.[34]
- **Pulseless disease (Takayasu's disease):** In one study, 6 patients with this condition were treated with an herbal formula with significant improvement in 3 cases, moderate improvement in 2 cases, and slight improvement in 1 case. The herbal formula contained *Bu Yang Huan Wu Tang* (Tonify the Yang to Restore Five Decoction) with 60 grams of *Huang Qi* and additional blood-activating and blood stasis-removing herbs.[35]
- **Prostatic hypertrophy:** In one report, 52 patients with prostatic hypertrophy were treated with an herbal decoction taken on an empty stomach. The formula contained 100 grams of fresh *Huang Qi* and 30 grams of *Hua Shi* (Talcum) cooked in decoction, with 3 grams of *Hu Po* (Succinum) added prior to administration. At the conclusion of the study, 38 patients reported complete remission of symptoms, 13 reported improvement in flow rate and reduction in size of the prostate, and 1 reported no improvement.[36]

HERB-DRUG INTERACTION

- **Aminoglycosides**: In one study, a compound injection of *Huang Qi* and *Lu Han Cao* (Herba Pyrolae) in guinea pigs was found to be effective in preventing ototoxicity and nephrotoxicity associated with use of aminoglycosides.[37] [Note: Examples of aminoglycosides include gentamicin, tobramycin, amikacin.]
- It has been demonstrated that *Huang Qi* has an inhibitory influence on copper-induced oxidative stress. According to studies, the effect of *Huang Qi* is similar to that of mannitol and of superoxide dismutase as free radical scavengers.[38]

TOXICOLOGY

Huang Qi has very low toxicity. Oral ingestion of *Huang Qi* decoction (7.5 g/kg) cannot be determined in rats. The LD_{50} in mice for intraperitoneal injection is approximately 40 g/kg.[39]

AUTHORS' COMMENTS

According to Dr. Zhang Xiao-Ping, the combination of *Huang Qi* and *Shan Yao* (Rhizoma Dioscoreae) has excellent effects to lower plasma glucose levels to treat diabetes mellitus patients. These two herbs are especially effective in individuals with diabetes characterized by qi and yin deficiencies.

References

1. *Zhe Jiang Zhong Yi Za Zhi* (Zhejiang Journal of Chinese Medicine), 1987; 22(1): 36
2. *Xian Dai Zhong Yao Yao Li Xue* (Contemporary Pharmacology of Chinese Herbs), 1997; 1175-1176
3. Yan X, Zhou J, Xie G, *Traditional Chinese Medicines Molecular Structures, Natural Sources and Applications*; Ashgate, 1999; 509
4. *Shan Xi Yi Yao Za Zhi* (Shanxi Journal of Medicine and Herbology), 1974; 5-6:57
5. *Biol Pharm Bull*, 1977; 20(11)-1178-82
6. *Nan Jing Zhong Yi Xue Yuan Xue Bao* (Journal of Nanjing University of Traditional Chinese Medicine), 1989; 1:43
7. *Zhong Yao Yao Li Yu Lin Chuang* (Pharmacology and Clinical Applications of Chinese Herbs), 1985:193
8. *Zhong Cheng Yao Yan Jiu* (Research of Chinese Patent Medicine), 1984; 11:3
9. *Zhong Guo Sheng Li Ke Xue Hui, Di Er Ci Hui* (Chinese Convention on Biophysiology, 2nd Annual Convention), 1963:63
10. *Guo Wai Yi Xue Can Kao Za Zhi* (Foreign Journal of Medicine), 1977; 4:231
11. *Zhong Xi Yi Jie He Za Zhi* (Journal of Integrated Chinese and Western Medicine), 1990; 10(6):330
12. *Shang Hai Yi Yao Za Zhi* (Shanghai Journal of Medicine and Herbology), 1988:(4):4

Huang Qi (Radix Astragali)

13. *Zhong Yao Zhi* (Chinese Herbology Journal), 1949;(12):648
14. *Zhong Yao Tong Bao* (Journal of Chinese Herbology), 1986; 11(9):47
15. *Zhong Yi Za Zhi* (Journal of Chinese Medicine), 1980; 1:71
16. *Hu Nan Zhong Yi Xue Yuan Xue Bao* (Journal of Hunan University of Traditional Chinese Medicine), 1987; 4:13
17. *Jiang Su Zhong Yi* (Jiangsu Chinese Medicine), 1988; 9:32
18. *Nan Jing Yi Xue Yuan Xue Bao* (Journal of Nanjing University of Medicine), 1988; 3:246
19. *Zhong Hua Er Ke Za Zhi* (Chinese Journal of Pediatrics), 1978; 2:87
20. *Jiang Su Yi Yao* (Jiangsu Journal of Medicine and Herbology), 1977; 1:20
21. *Hu Nan Yi Yao Za Zhi* (Hunan Journal of Medicine and Herbology), 1977; 2:35
22. *Shan Xi Yi Yao Za Zhi* (Shanxi Journal of Medicine and Herbology), 1978; 2:31
23. *Shan Dong Zhong Yi Za Zhi* (Shandong Journal of Chinese Medicine), 1983; 2:43
24. *Zhe Jiang Zhong Yi Za Zhi* (Zhejiang Journal of Chinese Medicine), 1983; 3:103
25. *Ji Lin Zhong Yi Yao* (Jilin Chinese Medicine and Herbology), 1985; 5:24
26. *Yun Nan Zhong Yi Za Zhi* (Yunan Journal of Chinese Medicine), 1980; 2:28
27. *Journal of Clinical and Laboratory Immunology*, 1988 Mar. 25(3):125-9
28. *Zhong Guo Zhong Xi Yi Jie He Za Zhi* (Chinese Journal of Integrative Chinese and Western Medicine), 1995 Aug.; 15(8):462-4
29. *Cancer*, 1983 July; 52(1):70-3
30. *Hei Long Jiang Zhong Yi Yao* (Heilongjiang Chinese Medicine and Herbology), 1982; 1:39
31. *Zhong Hua Nei Ke Xue Za Zhi* (Journal of Chinese Internal Medicine), 1986; 25(4):222
32. *Jiang Su Yi Xue* (Jiangsu Medical Journal), 1989; 15(1):12
33. *Zhong Xi Yi Jie He Za Zhi* (Journal of Integrated Chinese and Western Medicine), 1987; 7:403
34. *Zhong Yi Za Zhi* (Journal of Chinese Medicine), 1982; 7:52
35. *Zhe Jiang Zhong Yi Za Zhi* (Zhejiang Journal of Chinese Medicine), 1981; 9:396
36. *Xin Zhong Yi* (New Chinese Medicine), 1987; 10:54
37. Xuan, W., Dong, M., and Dong, M. *Annals of Otology, Rhinology and Laryngology*, May 1995, vol. 104(5): 374-80
38. *Journal of Ethnopharmacology*. 68(1-3):331-3, 1999 Dec 15
39. *Yao Xue Xue Bao* (Journal of Herbology), 1965; 12(5):319

Jiao Gu Lan (Rhizoma seu Herba Gynostemmatis)

絞股藍 绞股蓝

Pinyin Name: *Jiao Gu Lan*

Alternate Chinese Names: *Qi Dan Ye, Xiao Ke Yao, Jin Si Hua Gua Long, Long Xu Teng, Pian Di Sheng Gen, Wu Ye Shen*

English Name: gynostemma

Botanical Name: *Gynostemma pentaphyllum* (Thunb.) Makino.

Pharmaceutical Name: Rhizoma seu Herba Gynostemmatis

Properties: slightly bitter, cold

Channels Entered: Lung, Heart

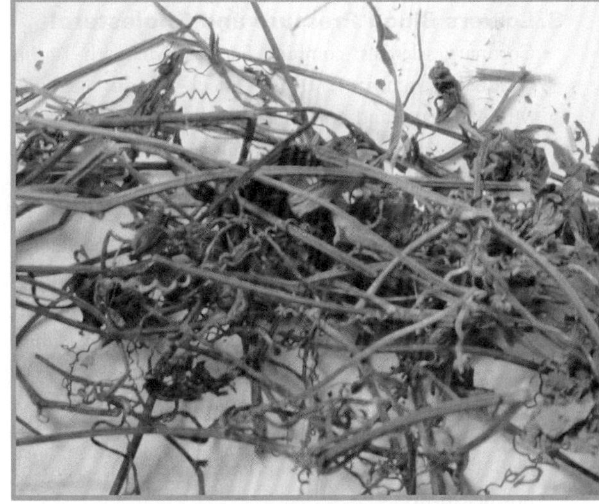

CHINESE THERAPEUTIC ACTIONS

1. Moistens Lung, Promotes Generation of Body Fluids, Dispels Phlegm

Jiao Gu Lan has a general effect to nourish and strengthen the body. It is commonly used to treat chronic disorders, such as asthma, migraines, neuralgia, impaired function of the respiratory and gastrointestinal tracts, and syndromes characterized by deficiency. Clinical manifestations may include vomiting or nausea with drooling of saliva, shortness of breath and chest congestion.

- Chronic bronchitis: use *Jiao Gu Lan* with *Fu Rong* (Radix Hibisci).

2. Clears Heat, Eliminates Toxins, Reduces Inflammation

Toxic heat accumulation: *Jiao Gu Lan* (Rhizoma seu

Jiao Gu Lan (Rhizoma seu Herba Gynostemmatis)

Herba Gynostemmatis) clears heat and eliminates toxins from the body to reduce swelling, inflammation and pain. Clinically, it treats gastric ulcers, duodenal ulcers, hyperlipidemia, nodules, cystitis, herpes zoster and other conditions characterized by dampness, heat and toxins. *Jiao Gu Lan* has also been used to treat various kinds of cancer and to help inhibit the spread of tumors.

- Gastric and duodenal ulcer: combine *Jiao Gu Lan* with *Bai Hua She She Cao* (Herba Oldenlandia), *Hai Piao Xiao* (Endoconcha Sepiae) and *Bei Mu* (Bulbus Fritillaria).
- Nodules: use this herb with *Bie Jia* (Carapax Trionycis), *Zhe Bei Mu* (Bulbus Fritillariae Thunbergii) or add it to *Zhen Ren Huo Ming Yin* (True Man Decoction to Revitalize Life).
- Tumors: add this herb to *Bai Hua She She Cao* (Herba Oldenlandia), *Ban Zhi Lian* (Herba Scutellariae Barbatae), *Ling Zhi* (Ganoderma), and *Dong Chong Xia Cao* (Cordyceps).
- Cystitis: use it with *Shui Ding Xiang* (Herba Ludwigiae Prostratae), and *Ding Shu Xiu* (Herba Elephantopus Scaber).
- Herpes zoster: add it to *Long Dan Cao* (Radix Gentianae) or *Long Dan Xie Gan Tang* (Gentiana Decoction to Drain the Liver). These herbs can be taken internally or applied topically.
- Liver spots: Mix *Jiao Gu Lan* powder with water, apply topically as paste.

3. Lowers Blood Pressure and Cholesterol

- Coronary sclerosis: combine *Jiao Gu Lan* with *Yu Jin* (Radix Curcumae), *Dan Shen* (Radix Salviae Miltiorrhizae), and *Shi Chang Pu* (Rhizoma Acori), or add it to *Xue Fu Zhu Yu Tang* (Drive Out Stasis in the Mansion of Blood Decoction).
- Hypertension: add it to *Hu Zhang* (Rhizoma Polygoni Cuspidati) and *Cha Chi Huang* (Herba Stellariae Aquaticae).
- Hyperlipidemia: use this herb with *Jue Ming Zi* (Semen Cassiae), *Shan Zha* (Fructus Crataegi), and *Da Huang* (Radix et Rhizoma Rhei).

DOSAGE

5 to 12 grams in decoction, and 0.75 to 1.0 gram in powder form.

CAUTIONS / CONTRAINDICATIONS

- *Jiao Gu Lan* may cause mild stomach discomfort when taken as tea on an empty stomach.
- Use of *Jiao Gu Lan* has been associated with potential side effects such as fatigue, lack of energy, dizziness, chest congestion, mild fever, perspiration, sore throat, rash, increased heartbeat, and increased respiration rate.[1]
- *Jiao Gu Lan* may caused drowsiness and sedation. Therefore, individuals who take this herb should exercise caution if driving or operating heavy machinery.

CHEMICAL COMPOSITION

Gynoside, ginsenoside, rutin, ombuoside.[2]

PHARMACOLOGICAL EFFECTS

- **Immunostimulant:** *Jiao Gu Lan* has been shown in animal studies to increase the weight of the spleen, the phagocytic activity of macrophages, and the number of T-lymphocytes and NK cells.[3,4,5,6]
- **Cardiovascular:** Decoction of *Jiao Gu Lan* (20 to 40%) has demonstrated positive inotropic and negative chronotropic effects in rabbits. In anesthetized cats, injection of *Jiao Gu Lan* at 50 mg/kg has a reliable anti-hypertensive effect for up to 30 minutes.[7,8]
- **Antihyperlipidemic:** Water extract of *Jiao Gu Lan* has demonstrated a marked effect to lower cholesterol and triglycerides in rats.[9]
- **Antineoplastic:** According to laboratory studies, preparations of *Jiao Gu Lan* have demonstrated an inhibiting influence on various kinds of cancer cells, including cancers of the stomach, abdomen, uterus, liver, mouth, esophagus, pancreas, brain, lung, kidney, tongue, breast, and skin. There is also an increase in life expectancy in mice that received the herb, in comparison to the placebo group.[10]
- **Antiaging:** Administration of *Jiao Gu Lan* is associated with prolonged life expectancy and delayed aging in animals. In one study, a group of old mice were divided into two groups. After 4 months, all mice in the control group died, while only 50% of the mice died in the herb group.[11]
- **Antiplatelet:** *Jiao Gu Lan* inhibits platelet aggregation and thrombus formation in mice.[12]
- **Endocrine:** Administration of *Jiao Gu Lan* is associated with an increase in plasma ACTH levels in rats.[13]
- **CNS suppressant:** Extract of *Jiao Gu Lan* has demonstrated sedative, hypnotic and analgesic effects that last up to 7 hours in mice. It prolonged sleeping time induced by barbiturates and reversed the effects of mescaline. Lastly, *Jiao Gu Lan* at 100 to 150 mg/kg has a significant analgesic effect in mice.[14,15,16]

CLINICAL STUDIES AND RESEARCH

- **Hypercholesterolemia:** In one clinical trial, 129 patients were divided into two groups with one receiving *Jiao Gu Lan* and the other receiving a placebo. After 1 month, the patients in the herb group showed a statistically significant reduction in both total cholesterol and triglyceride levels in comparison with the placebo group. Side effects

Jiao Gu Lan (Rhizoma seu Herba Gynostemmatis)

of *Jiao Gu Lan* included dizziness in 2 cases, poor appetite in 1 case, abdominal distention in 4 cases, weight loss in 42 patients, and weight gain in 28 patients.[17] In another study, the combination of *Jiao Gu Lan* and *Shan Zha* (Fructus Crataegi) reduced both triglyceride and cholesterol levels.[18]

- **Antiaging:** Administration of *Jiao Gu Lan* three times daily for 2 months was beneficial for 106 patients in reducing general signs and symptoms of aging, such as fatigue, lack of energy, aversion to cold, diarrhea, poor memory, decreased balance, insomnia and excessive dreams.[19]
- **Headache:** In one study, 50 patients with headaches due to various causes were treated with 30 to 50 grams of *Jiao Gu Lan* daily as tea with 79.6% rate of effectiveness.[20]
- **Chronic tracheitis:** A preparation of *Jiao Gu Lan* was used to treat patients with chronic tracheitis in one clinical study. Out of 86 patients, the study reported complete recovery in 12 patients, moderate improvement in 23 patients, some improvement in 45 patients, and no change in 6 patients.[21]
- **Chronic atrophic gastritis:** In one clinical study, 151 patients were treated with 10 grams of *Jiao Gu Lan* three times daily for 3 months. According to endoscopy, 28 patients showed significant improvement, 57 showed moderate improvement, 58 showed no change, and 8 showed deterioration in their condition. The overall effective rate was 56.26%. No significant side effects were reported.[22]

HERB-DRUG INTERACTION

- **Sedatives:** *Jiao Gu Lan* has sedative, hypnotic and analgesic effects. It potentiates the sedative effect of barbiturates and reverses the effect of mescaline.[23,24,25] [Note: Many categories of drugs induce sedation, such as antihistamines, narcotic analgesics, barbiturates, benzodiazepines and many others.]

TOXICOLOGY

No abnormalities were reported via blood panel, or in the liver, kidney, heart, and testes when *Jiao Gu Lan* was given to mice at 4 g/kg/day for 90 days. In acute toxicology studies, the LD_{50} for oral ingestion of extract is 48.94 g/kg, and the LD_{50} for intraperitoneal injection is 2,862 mg/kg.[26]

References

1. *Zhong Guo Zhong Yao Za Zhi* (People's Republic of China Journal of Chinese Herbology), 1989; 14(12):52
2. *Xian Dai Zhong Yao Yao Li Xue* (Contemporary Pharmacology of Chinese Herbs), 1997; 1227-1228
3. *Xin Zhong Yi* (New Chinese Medicine), 1988; 20(4):51
4. *Zhong Cao Yao* (Chinese Herbal Medicine), 1990; 21(7):25
5. *Shan Xi Zhong Yi* (Shanxi Chinese Medicine), 1991; 12(1):38
6. *Zhong Xi Yi Jie He Za Zhi* (Journal of Integrated Chinese and Western Medicine), 1990; 12(2):96
7. *Xin Zhong Yi* (New Chinese Medicine), 1988; 20(4):51
8. *Zhong Cao Yao* (Chinese Herbal Medicine), 1989; 20(4):2845
9. *Xian Dai Shi Yong Yao Xue* (Practical Applications of Modern Herbal Medicine), 1990; 7(1):42
10. *Zhong Yao Xian Dai Yan Jiu Yu Ying Yong* (Modern Study of Traditional Chinese Medicine), vol. IV, 3519:3556
11. *Zhong Cheng Yao* (Study of Chinese Patent Medicine), 1988; 10(3):25
12. *Zhong Guo Yao Li Xue Tong Bao* (Journal of Chinese Herbal Pharmacology), 1989; 5(4):213
13. *Chang Chun Zhong Yi Xue Yuan Xue Bao* (Journal of Changchun University of Chinese Medicine), 1994; 10(1):50-51
14. *Zhong Yao Xian Dai Yan Jiu Yu Ying Yong* (Modern Study of Traditional Chinese Medicine), vol. IV, 3519:3556
15. *JP*, 1981; 127316: 6-7
16. *JP*, 1983; 9941:74
17. *Hu Nan Yi Xue* (Hunan Medicine), 1991; 8(5):259
18. la Cour, B. et al. Traditional Chinese medicine in treatment of hyperlipidemia. *Journal of Ethnopharmacology.* 46(2):125-9, May 1996
19. *Hu Nan Yi Yao Za Zhi* (Hunan Journal of Medicine and Herbology), 1991; 7(2):56
20. *Zhong Guo Shi Yong Nei Ke Za Zhi* (Chinese Journal of Practical Internal Medicine), 1993; 13(12):725
21. *Hu Nan Zhong Yi Za Zhi* (Hunan Journal of Chinese Medicine), 1993; 9(4):11
22. *Zhong Xi Yi Jie He Za Zhi* (Journal of Integrated Chinese and Western Medicine), 1991; 11(12):713
23. *Zhong Yao Xian Dai Yan Jiu Yu Ying Yong* (Modern Study of Traditional Chinese Medicine), vol. IV, 3519:3556
24. *JP*, 1981; 127316: 6-7
25. *JP*, 1983; 9941:74
26. *Xin Zhong Yi* (New Chinese Medicine), 1988; 20(4):51

Bai Zhu (Rhizoma Atractylodis Macrocephalae)

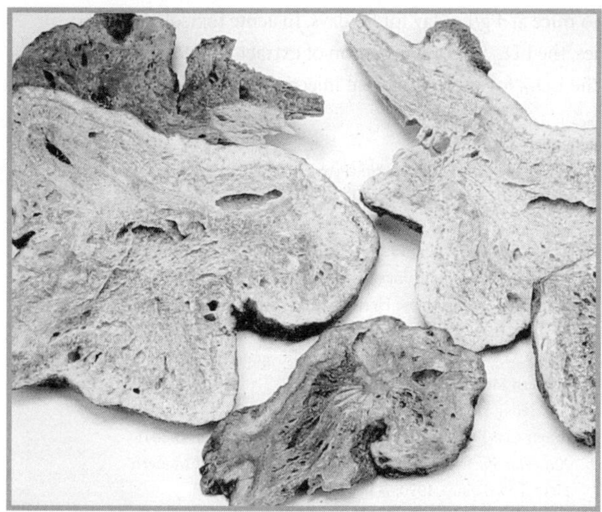

白朮

Pinyin Name: *Bai Zhu*
Literal Name: "white atractylodes"
Alternate Chinese Names: *Yu Zhu*
Original Source: *Shen Nong Ben Cao Jing* (Divine Husbandman's Classic of the Materia Medica) in the second century
English Name: white atractylodes, large-headed atractylodes rhizome
Botanical Name: *Atractylodes macrocephala* Koidz. (*Bai Zhu*)
Pharmaceutical Name: Rhizoma Atractylodis Macrocephalae
Properties: bitter, sweet, warm
Channels Entered: Spleen, Stomach

CHINESE THERAPEUTIC ACTIONS

1. Tonifies Qi, Strengthens Spleen

Spleen and Stomach qi deficiencies: *Bai Zhu* (Rhizoma Atractylodis Macrocephalae) tonifies the middle *jiao* to enhance transformation and transportation functions. Clinically, it treats disorders characterized by qi deficiency of the Spleen and Stomach, such as shortness of breath, fatigue, sallow facial appearance, decreased food intake, loose stools, and diarrhea.

- Qi deficiency of the Spleen and Stomach: combine *Bai Zhu* with *Ren Shen* (Radix Ginseng), *Fu Ling* (Poria) and *Gan Cao* (Radix Glycyrrhizae). **Exemplar Formula:** *Si Jun Zi Tang* (Four-Gentleman Decoction).
- Qi deficiency of the Spleen and Stomach, with food accumulation and qi stagnation: use this herb with *Ren Shen* (Radix Ginseng), *Fu Ling* (Poria), *Gan Cao* (Radix Glycyrrhizae) and *Zhi Shi* (Fructus Aurantii Immaturus).
- Deficiency and cold of the Spleen and Stomach: use it with *Gan Jiang* (Rhizoma Zingiberis), *Ren Shen* (Radix Ginseng) and *Zhi Gan Cao* (Radix Glycyrrhizae Preparata). **Exemplar Formula:** *Li Zhong Tang* (Regulate the Middle Decoction).

Spleen deficiency with accumulated dampness: Bitter and warm in nature, *Bai Zhu* has excellent functions to treat diarrhea by drying dampness and strengthening the Spleen.

- Diarrhea caused by summer-heat and dampness: use *Bai Zhu* with *Che Qian Zi* (Semen Plantaginis).
- Diarrhea due to deficiencies of the Spleen and Stomach, with accumulated dampness: use this herb with *Ren Shen* (Radix Ginseng), *Fu Ling* (Poria), *Yi Yi Ren* (Semen Coicis) and *Sha Ren* (Fructus Amomi). **Exemplar Formula:** *Shen Ling Bai Zhu San* (Ginseng, Poria, and Atractylodes Macrocephala Powder).
- Clear watery leukorrhea due to deficiency of the Spleen and accumulated dampness: add it to *Shan Yao* (Rhizoma Dioscoreae), *Cang Zhu* (Rhizoma Atractylodis) and *Che Qian Zi* (Semen Plantaginis). **Exemplar Formula:** *Wan Dai Tang* (End Discharge Decoction).

Blood deficiency: Blood deficiency may occur secondary to Spleen qi deficiency because the production of blood is dependent upon the availability of qi. *Bai Zhu* is used with other qi and blood tonics to tonify qi and enhance the production of blood.

- Blood deficiency: incorporate *Bai Zhu* with *Ren Shen* (Radix Ginseng), *Fu Ling* (Poria), *Dang Gui* (Radicis Angelicae Sinensis), *Bai Shao* (Radix Paeoniae Alba), *Chuan Xiong* (Rhizoma Ligustici Chuanxiong), *Shu Di Huang* (Radix Rehmanniae Preparata) and *Gan Cao* (Radix Glycyrrhizae). **Exemplar Formulas:** *Ren Shen Yang Ying Tang* (Ginseng Decoction to Nourish the Nutritive Qi) or *Ba Zhen Tang* (Eight-Treasure Decoction).

2. Dries Dampness, Eliminates Water Accumulation

Edema due to accumulation of water and dampness: Deficiency of the Spleen impairs its normal function to transform and transport water, leading to edema and other conditions of water accumulation. *Bai Zhu* is most suitable for edema with Spleen qi deficiency.

- Edema with Spleen deficiency: use *Bai Zhu* with *Fu Ling* (Poria), *Zhu Ling* (Polyporus), and *Ze Xie* (Rhizoma Alismatis). **Exemplar Formula:** *Si Ling San* (Four-Ingredient Powder with Poria).
- Edema with Spleen yang deficiency: add this herb to *Fu Ling* (Poria), *Zhu Ling* (Polyporus), *Ze Xie* (Rhizoma Alismatis) and *Gui Zhi* (Ramulus Cinnamomi). **Exemplar Formula:**

Bai Zhu (Rhizoma Atractylodis Macrocephalae)

Wu Ling San (Five-Ingredient Powder with Poria).

- Edema with Kidney yang deficiency: use this herb with *Fu Zi* (Radix Aconiti Lateralis Praeparata), *Fu Ling* (Poria), and *Sheng Jiang* (Rhizoma Zingiberis Recens). **Exemplar Formula:** *Zhen Wu Tang* (True Warrior Decoction).

Accumulation of phlegm: Deficiency of the Spleen impairs its normal function of transforming and transporting water, leading to accumulation of water, dampness and phlegm. Characteristic symptoms of this include dizziness, vertigo, palpitations and cough with clear sputum.

- Accumulation of phlegm: add *Bai Zhu* to *Gui Zhi* (Ramulus Cinnamomi), *Fu Ling* (Poria) and *Gan Cao* (Radix Glycyrrhizae). **Exemplar Formula:** *Ling Gui Zhu Gan Tang* (Poria, Cinnamon Twig, Atractylodes Macrocephala, and Licorice Decoction).
- Dizziness and vertigo due to accumulation of phlegm, with Liver wind: use this herb with *Ban Xia* (Rhizoma Pinelliae), *Tian Ma* (Rhizoma Gastrodiae), *Fu Ling* (Poria) and *Chen Pi* (Pericarpium Citri Reticulatae). **Exemplar Formula:** *Ban Xia Bai Zhu Tian Ma Tang* (Pinellia, Atractylodes Macrocephala, and Gastrodia Decoction).

3. Stops Spontaneous Perspiration

***Wei* (defensive) *qi* deficiency with spontaneous sweating:** *Bai Zhu* tonifies the Spleen, strengthens *wei qi*, and stops spontaneous perspiration. It may be used individually or in combination with other herbs. *Bai Zhu* is not generally used in patients with yin deficiency. However, if combined with appropriate herbs, it is effective for the treatment of night sweats caused by yin deficiency.

- Spontaneous perspiration: use *Bai Zhu* with *Huang Qi* (Radix Astragali), *Mu Li* (Concha Ostreae), *Ma Huang Gen* (Radix Ephedrae), and *Fu Xiao Mai* (Semen Tritici Aestivi Levis).
- Spontaneous perspiration and aversion to wind due to deficiency of *wei* (defensive) *qi*: add it to *Huang Qi* (Radix Astragali) and *Fang Feng* (Radix Saposhnikoviae). **Exemplar Formula:** *Yu Ping Feng San* (Jade Windscreen Powder).
- Night sweats arising from yin deficiency: combine it with *Shi Hu* (Herba Dendrobii), *Mu Li* (Concha Ostreae) and *Wu Wei Zi* (Fructus Schisandrae Chinensis).

4. Stabilizes Pregnancy

Restless fetus: Spleen qi deficiency in pregnant women can lead to malnutrition that causes restlessness in the fetus. *Bai Zhu* tonifies Spleen qi, then Spleen qi in turn nourishes the fetus and keeps it in place. *Bai Zhu* treats restless fetus and unstable pregnancy accompanied by Spleen qi deficiency.

- Unstable pregnancy with severe qi deficiency: use *Bai Zhu* with *Ren Shen* (Radix Ginseng), *Fu Ling* (Poria) and *Huang Qi* (Radix Astragali).
- Unstable pregnancy with qi deficiency and interior heat: use it with *Huang Qin* (Radix Scutellariae).
- Unstable pregnancy with Kidney deficiency: use this herb with *Sang Ji Sheng* (Herba Taxilli), *Du Zhong* (Cortex Eucommiae), *Xu Duan* (Radix Dipsaci) and *E Jiao* (Colla Corii Asini).
- Unstable pregnancy with qi stagnation: combine it with *Su Geng* (Caulis Perillae), *Sha Ren* (Fructus Amomi) and *Chen Pi* (Pericarpium Citri Reticulatae).
- Unstable pregnancy with blood deficiency: add *Bai Zhu* to *Shu Di Huang* (Radix Rehmanniae Preparata), *Dang Gui* (Radicis Angelicae Sinensis), and *Bai Shao* (Radix Paeoniae Alba).
- Unstable pregnancy with uterine bleeding: use this herb with *E Jiao* (Colla Corii Asini) and charred *Ai Ye* (Folium Artemisiae Argyi).
- Miscarriage with bleeding: combine *Bai Zhu* with *E Jiao* (Colla Corii Asini) and charred *Ai Ye* (Folium Artemisiae Argyi).

DOSAGE

5 to 15 grams in decoction. Unprocessed *Bai Zhu* more strongly dries dampness and eliminates water accumulation. The dry-fried herb is stronger to tonify qi, strengthen the Spleen, stop perspiration and stabilize pregnancy. The charred form is stronger to strengthen the Spleen and stop diarrhea. The fresh herb is also used to treat constipation, at larger dosages of 60 to 120 grams.

CAUTIONS / CONTRAINDICATIONS

- *Bai Zhu* is not recommended for sole use in cases of yin deficiency, yin deficiency with heat, and fluid deficiency. It must be combined with appropriate herbs to prevent accentuating deficiency.
- Use of *Bai Zhu* is contraindicated in cases of qi stagnation characterized by feelings of distention and oppression.

CHEMICAL COMPOSITION

Atractylol, atractylon, junipercamphor, atractylolide, hydroxyactyldide, sesquiterpenelon, β-eudesmol, hinesol, 8-β-ethoxyatractylenolide, palmitic acid, anhydroatractylolide, fructose, synanthrin.[1]

PHARMACOLOGICAL EFFECTS

- **Adaptogenic:** Decoction of *Bai Zhu*, given to mice is associated with an increase in body weight, and increased swimming performance.[2]
- **Immunostimulant:** Decoction of *Bai Zhu* increases the activity of the macrophages and reticuloendothelial

Bai Zhu (Rhizoma Atractylodis Macrocephalae)

system. It also increases the number of white blood cells, lymphocytes, and IgG.[3,4]

- **Gastrointestinal:** *Bai Zhu* has a dual effect on the gastrointestinal tract. At low doses between 5 to 15 grams, it treats diarrhea. At high doses between 60 and 120 grams, it treats constipation.[5]
- **Antiplatelet:** *Bai Zhu* has a marked effect to inhibit the aggregation of platelets. In a clinical study of healthy volunteers, administration of 5% *Bai Zhu* decoction three times daily for 4 days significantly prolonged the prothrombin time. This effect may last for up to 10 days after discontinuation.[6]
- **Diuretic:** *Bai Zhu* has a marked and prolonged diuretic effect when administered to rats, rabbits, dogs and other animals. The proposed mechanism of action is inhibition of sodium re-absorption leading to increased diuresis.[7]
- **Antidiabetic:** Administration of *Bai Zhu* is associated with a slight decrease of blood glucose in rabbits and rats.[8]
- **Antineoplastic:** Essential oil of *Bai Zhu* has demonstrated marked inhibitory action against esophageal cancer in *in vitro* studies.[9]

CLINICAL STUDIES AND RESEARCH

- **Diarrhea:** According to one report, 320 infants with diarrhea were treated with 3 to 4 grams of an herbal powder three times daily before meals with good results. Foods that are raw, cold, oily or greasy were removed from the diet during the treatment period. The herbal powder contained *Bai Zhu* 200g, *Shan Yao* (Rhizoma Dioscoreae) 200g, *Zao Shu Pi* (Cortex Zizyphi Jujubae) 150g, and *Che Qian Zi* (Semen Plantaginis) 150g, all dry-fried.[10]
- **Hepatic disorders:** Various hepatic disorders characterized by deficiency of the Spleen with accumulation of dampness were treated with herbal formulas based on *Bai Zhu* with good results. The dosage of *Bai Zhu* was 30 to 60 grams for ascites due to liver cirrhosis, 15 to 30 grams in infectious hepatitis, and 60 to 100 grams in liver cancer.[11]
- **Excessive salivation:** Infants with excessive salivation were treated with marked effectiveness using the juice of 10 grams of fresh *Bai Zhu* mixed with small amounts of water and sugar.[12]
- **Chronic back and leg pain:** In one study, 24 patients with chronic pain in the back and legs characterized by cold and dampness were treated with an herbal decoction twice daily for 2 to 3 days with satisfactory results. The herbal decoction contained 30 grams of *Bai Zhu*, 6 grams of *Chuan Shan Jia* (Squama Manis), and 100 ml of grain-based liquor.[13]
- **Meniere's disease:** Dizziness and vertigo due to Meniere's disease have been successfully treated using an herbal formula containing 30 grams each of dry-fried *Bai Zhu*, *Ze Xie* (Rhizoma Alismatis) and dry-fried *Yi Yi Ren* (Semen Coicis).[14]
- **Constipation:** In one study, 50 women with post-surgical constipation were treated with an herbal decoction one time daily for 1 to 4 days, with satisfactory results. The herbal decoction contained 60 grams of fresh *Bai Zhu*, 30 grams of *Sheng Di Huang* (Radix Rehmanniae) and 3 grams of *Sheng Ma* (Rhizoma Cimicifugae).[15] Another report stated that fresh *Bai Zhu* may be used as the main herb for treating mild to severe constipation with dosages between 30 and 150 grams. For modification, *Sheng Di Huang* (Radix Rehmanniae) may be added if there are dry stools; *Sheng Ma* (Rhizoma Cimicifugae) may be added to ascend the clear and descend the turbid substances; and *Rou Gui* (Cortex Cinnamomi), *Fu Zi* (Radix Aconiti Lateralis Praeparata), *Hou Po* (Cortex Magnoliae Officinalis) and *Gan Jiang* (Rhizoma Zingiberis) may be added if there are soft stools with difficulty in defecation, slippery and black/gray tongue coat, and thin, weak pulse.[16]

HERB-DRUG INTERACTION

- **Omeprazole:** It has been suggested that hinesol, one of the components of *Bai Zhu*, is a relatively specific inhibitor of H+, K+ -ATPase. Hinesol also enhanced the inhibitory effect of omeprazole on H+, K+ -ATPase, though the exact inhibitory sites are different.[17]
- **Anticoagulant or antiplatelet drugs:** *Bai Zhu* has antiplatelet effects, and should be used with caution in patients who take anticoagulant or antiplatelet medications. Though no instances of this potential interaction have been documented, this herb may potentiate the effect of drugs such as warfarin.[18] [Note: Examples of anticoagulants include heparin, warfarin (Coumadin) and enoxaparin (Lovenox); and examples of antiplatelets include aspirin, dipyridamole (Persantine), and clopidogrel (Plavix).]
- **Diuretics:** *Bai Zhu* has a diuretic effect. Though there is no actual report of instances of this potential interaction, concurrent use with diuretic drugs may lead to increased elimination of water and/or electrolytes.[19] [Note: Examples of diuretics include chlorothiazide, hydrochlorothiazide, furosemide (Lasix), bumetanide (Bumex), and torsemide (Demadex).]

TOXICOLOGY

The LD_{50} for decoction of *Bai Zhu* in mice via intraperitoneal injection is 13.3 g/kg. Following injection, most animals showed excitation followed by sedation.[20]

In another study, decoction of *Bai Zhu* at the dosage of 0.5 g/kg given one time daily for 14 days via oral ingestion showed a decrease in white blood cells, especially lymphocytes.[21]

Bai Zhu (Rhizoma Atractylodis Macrocephalae)

AUTHORS' COMMENTS

Historically, *Bai Zhu* (Rhizoma Atractylodis Macrocephalae) and *Cang Zhu* (Rhizoma Atractylodis) have been used interchangeably. In *Shen Nong Ben Cao Jing* (Divine Husbandman's Classic of the Materia Medica) in the second century, only "*Zhu*" was mentioned without stating whether it was *Cang Zhu* or *Bai Zhu*. They were used interchangeably until the Tang Dynasty. Starting from the Song dynasty, *Cang Zhu* and *Bai Zhu* began to be used separately. Though both belong to the Compositae family and both strengthen the Spleen to dispel dampness, *Bai Zhu* tonifies qi, stops perspiration, and stabilizes the fetus, while *Cang Zhu* more strongly dries dampness and induces perspiration to dispel external pathogenic factors. Today, *Bai Zhu* is used more with Spleen-deficient patients while *Cang Zhu* is used more for patients with dampness. But when both Spleen deficiency and dampness are prominent, both herbs can be combined.

Bai Zhu has an interesting ability to treat both diarrhea and constipation. Historically, it has been used within a normal dosage (5 to 15 grams) to strengthen the Spleen, improve digestive function, and treat diarrhea. More recently, it was found that a large dose (60 to 120 grams) of fresh *Bai Zhu* is also effective for treatment of constipation, presumably by strengthening the Spleen to push out the feces. *Bai Zhu* is used alone, or combined with *Sheng Di Huang* (Radix Rehmanniae) or *Sheng Ma* (Rhizoma Cimicifugae) for treatment of constipation.

There are four herbs that are commonly used to stabilize pregnancy:

- *Bai Zhu* (Rhizoma Atractylodis Macrocephalae) treats restless fetus from Spleen qi deficiency.
- *Sha Ren* (Fructus Amomi) regulates qi and calms restless fetus in the presence of qi stagnation and middle *jiao* deficiency.
- *Du Zhong* (Cortex Eucommiae) is most suitable to treat restless fetus caused by deficiency of the Kidney and Liver.
- *Huang Qin* (Radix Scutellariae) calms restless fetus caused by heat.

References

1. *Xian Dai Zhong Yao Yao Li Xue* (Contemporary Pharmacology of Chinese Herbs), 1997; 1180
2. *Xin Yi Yao Xue Za Zhi* (New Journal of Medicine and Herbology), 1974; 8:13
3. *Jun Shi Yi Xue Jian Xun* (Military Medicine Notes), 1977; 2:5
4. *Xin Yi Yao Xue Za Zhi* (New Journal of Medicine and Herbology), 1979; 6:60
5. *Chang Yong Zhong Yao Cheng Fen Yu Yao Li Shou Ce* (A Handbook of the Composition and Pharmacology of Common Chinese Drugs), 1994; 739:742
6. Ibid.
7. *Zhong Hua Yi Xue Za Zhi* (Chinese Journal of Medicine), 1961; 47(1):7
8. Ibid., 1958; 44(22):150
9. *Zhong Liu Yu Zhi Tong Xun* (Journal of Prevention and Treatment of Cancer), 1976; 2:40
10. *Shan Dong Zhong Yi Za Zhi* (Shandong Journal of Chinese Medicine), 1982; 2:107
11. *An Hui Zhong Yi Xue Yuan Xue Bao* (Journal of Anhui University School of Medicine), 1984; 2:25
12. *Liao Ning Zhong Yi Za Zhi* (Liaoning Journal of Chinese Medicine), 1986; 8:42
13. *Hu Bei Zhong Yi Za Zhi* (Hubei Journal of Chinese Medicine), 1982; 6:57
14. Ibid., 1983; 4:20
15. *Xin Yi Yao Xue Za Zhi* (New Journal of Medicine and Herbology), 1979; 6:27
16. Ibid., 1978; 4:9
17. *Biochem Pharmacol* 2000, April 1:59(7):881-6
18. Chen, J. Recognition & prevention of Herb-drug interactions, *Medical Acupuncture*, Fall/Winter 1998/1999; volume 10/number 2; 9-13
19. Ibid.
20. *Sheng Li Xue Bao* (Physiology News), 1961; 24(3,4):227
21. *Chang Yong Zhong Yao Cheng Fen Yu Yao Li Shou Ce* (A Handbook of the Composition and Pharmacology of Common Chinese Drugs), 1994; 739:742

Shan Yao (Rhizoma Dioscoreae)

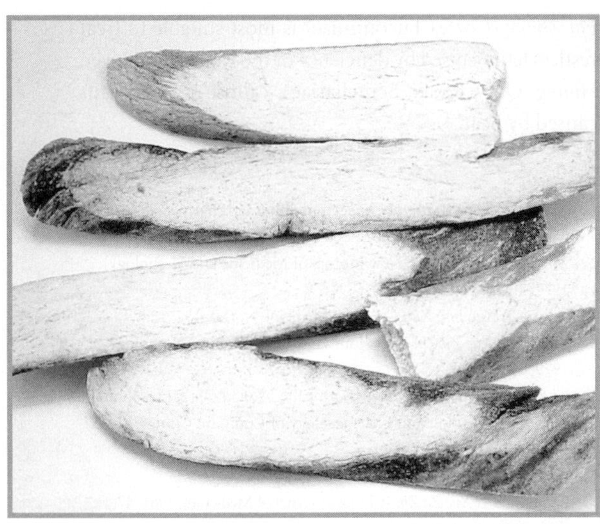

山藥 山药

Pinyin Name: *Shan Yao*
Literal Name: "mountain medicine"
Alternate Chinese Names: *Huai Shan Yao, Huai Shan*
English Name: dioscorea, common yam rhizome
Botanical Name: *Dioscorea opposita* Thunb. (*Shu Yu*)
Pharmaceutical Name: Rhizoma Dioscoreae
Properties: sweet, neutral
Channels Entered: Kidney, Lung, Spleen

CHINESE THERAPEUTIC ACTIONS

1. Tonifies Qi and Nourishes Spleen and Stomach Yin

Spleen and Stomach deficiencies: *Shan Yao* (Rhizoma Dioscoreae) enhances the transportation and transformation functions of the Spleen and Stomach to treat fatigue, lack of energy, decreased food intake, loose stools, diarrhea and other conditions characterized by deficiency of the middle *jiao*. *Shan Yao* is often used in an herbal formula for synergistic effect with the other herbs, but it may be used individually at a large dosage, in powder, if necessary. Sweet-tasting *Shan Yao* tonifies both the qi and the yin of the Spleen. It is also slightly astringent, as it has an effect to relieve diarrhea or loose stools.

- Decreased food intake and lack of energy due to Spleen deficiency: use *Shan Yao* with *Ren Shen* (Radix Ginseng) and *Bai Zhu* (Rhizoma Atractylodis Macrocephalae).
- Poor appetite, loose stools and diarrhea due to Spleen deficiency: use it with *Ren Shen* (Radix Ginseng), *Bai Zhu* (Rhizoma Atractylodis Macrocephalae), *Fu Ling* (Poria) and *Yi Yi Ren* (Semen Coicis). **Exemplar Formula:** *Shen Ling Bai Zhu San* (Ginseng, Poria, and Atractylodes Macrocephala Powder).
- Food stagnation due to deficiency of the Spleen and Stomach: combine this herb with *Yi Yi Ren* (Semen Coicis), *Shen Qu* (Massa Fermentata) and *Ji Nei Jin* (Endothelium Corneum Gigeriae Galli).
- Deficiency of the Spleen and Stomach with qi stagnation: add it to *Zhi Shi* (Fructus Aurantii Immaturus), *Chen Pi* (Pericarpium Citri Reticulatae), and *Sha Ren* (Fructus Amomi).
- Deficiency of the Spleen and Stomach with Stomach yin deficiency: use *Shan Yao* with *Mai Men Dong* (Radix Ophiopogonis), *Shi Hu* (Herba Dendrobii) and *Yu Zhu* (Rhizoma Polygonati Odorati).

Leukorrhea: Spleen deficiency causes accumulation of dampness and may lead to leukorrhea. Depending on the color and smell of the discharge, other herbs can be added accordingly.

- Red and white leukorrhea: combine *Shan Yao* with *Hai Piao Xiao* (Endoconcha Sepiae), *Long Gu* (Os Draconis), *Mu Li* (Concha Ostreae) and *Qian Cao* (Radix Rubiae). **Exemplar Formula:** *Qing Dai Tang* (Clear the Discharge Decoction).
- Yellow leukorrhea with foul odor, caused by deficiency of the Spleen and accumulation of damp-heat: use this herb with *Huang Bai* (Cortex Phellodendri), *Che Qian Zi* (Semen Plantaginis), *Zhi Shi* (Fructus Aurantii Immaturus) and *Bai Guo* (Semen Ginkgo). **Exemplar Formula:** *Yi Huang Tang* (Benefit the Yellow [Discharge] Decoction).
- Leukorrhea due to Spleen deficiency and Liver qi stagnation: use it with *Bai Zhu* (Rhizoma Atractylodis Macrocephalae), *Cang Zhu* (Rhizoma Atractylodis), *Ren Shen* (Radix Ginseng), *Chai Hu* (Radix Bupleuri) and *Bai Shao* (Radix Paeoniae Alba). **Exemplar Formula:** *Wan Dai Tang* (End Discharge Decoction).
- Leukorrhea due to Spleen and Kidney deficiencies: use *Shan Yao* with *Shan Zhu Yu* (Fructus Corni) and *Tu Si Zi* (Semen Cuscutae).

2. Tonifies Qi and Nourishes Lung Yin

Lung deficiency: The Lung dominates qi, prefers a moist environment, and dislikes dryness. Both Lung yin deficiency and qi deficiency can lead to coughing, wheezing, shallow breathing, with an absence of sputum or scanty, sticky, difficult-to-expectorate sputum. *Shan Yao* tonifies

Shan Yao (Rhizoma Dioscoreae)

both the qi and the yin of the Lung and is ideal for the conditions described above.

- Lung yin and fluid deficiencies: use *Shan Yao* with *Xuan Shen* (Radix Scrophulariae), *Ji Nei Jin* (Endothelium Corneum Gigeriae Galli) and *Niu Bang Zi* (Fructus Arctii).
- Lung yin and fluid deficiencies with heat: combine this herb with *Xuan Shen* (Radix Scrophulariae), *Ji Nei Jin* (Endothelium Corneum Gigeriae Galli), *Niu Bang Zi* (Fructus Arctii), and *Sheng Di Huang* (Radix Rehmanniae).
- Difficulty inhaling due to Kidney deficiency: use it with *Shu Di Huang* (Radix Rehmanniae Preparata), *Shan Zhu Yu* (Fructus Corni), *Ge Jie* (Gecko), and *Dong Chong Xia Cao* (Cordyceps).

3. Treats *Xiao Ke* (Wasting and Thirsting) Syndrome

***Xiao ke* syndrome:** This condition is characterized by yin deficiency and heat, or by qi and yin deficiencies. Unlike many other qi-tonic herbs that are drying in nature, *Shan Yao* is an excellent herb to tonify qi, nourish yin, and treat *xiao ke* syndrome. It may be used alone at a large dosage, or in combination with other herbs. This herb can be taken daily when made into porridge.

- *Xiao ke* syndrome: combine *Shan Yao* with *Huang Qi* (Radix Astragali), *Zhi Mu* (Radix Anemarrhenae), and *Ge Gen* (Radix Puerariae).
- *Xiao ke* syndrome with internal heat: use this herb with *Shi Gao* (Gypsum Fibrosum), *Zhi Mu* (Radix Anemarrhenae), *Mai Men Dong* (Radix Ophiopogonis) and *Tian Hua Fen* (Radix Trichosanthis).
- *Xiao ke* with more pronounced polyphagia and polydipsia: use it with *Shi Gao* (Gypsum Fibrosum), *Zhi Mu* (Radix Anemarrhenae), *Ge Gen* (Radix Puerariae), *Huang Jing* (Rhizoma Polygonati), *Tian Hua Fen* (Radix Trichosanthis) and *Sheng Di Huang* (Radix Rehmanniae).
- *Xiao ke* with more pronounced polyuria: add this herb to *Sheng Di Huang* (Radix Rehmanniae), *Shu Di Huang* (Radix Rehmanniae Preparata), *Shan Zhu Yu* (Fructus Corni), *Wu Wei Zi* (Fructus Schisandrae Chinensis), *Ze Xie* (Rhizoma Alismatis), *Mu Dan Pi* (Cortex Moutan) and *Lian Xu* (Stamen Nelumbinis).

4. Tonifies Kidney Yin

Nourishing in nature, *Shan Yao* tonifies Kidney yin to treat soreness and weakness of the knees and lower back, dizziness, light-headedness, tidal fever and night sweats. Astringent in nature, it consolidates the Kidney and treats leakage of fluids such as found in spermatorrhea, premature ejaculation, frequent urination and nocturnal enuresis. *Shan Yao* is relatively mild, and is often combined with other herbs for maximum effect.

- Kidney yin deficiency: add this herb to *Shu Di Huang* (Radix Rehmanniae Preparata), *Shan Zhu Yu* (Fructus Corni), *Mu Dan Pi* (Cortex Moutan), *Ze Xie* (Rhizoma Alismatis) and *Fu Ling* (Poria). **Exemplar Formula:** *Liu Wei Di Huang Wan* (Six-Ingredient Pill with Rehmannia).
- Spermatorrhea, premature ejaculation or nocturnal emissions due to Kidney deficiency: combine *Shan Yao* with *Qian Shi* (Semen Euryales) and *Lian Zi* (Semen Nelumbinis). **Exemplar Formula:** *Jin Suo Gu Jing Wan* (Metal Lock Pill to Stabilize the Essence).
- Frequent urination and nocturnal urination: use this herb with *Yi Zhi Ren* (Fructus Alpiniae Oxyphyllae) and *Wu Yao* (Radix Linderae). **Exemplar Formula:** *Suo Quan Wan* (Shut the Sluice Pill).

DOSAGE

10 to 30 grams, with a maximum of 250 grams, in decoction. *Shan Yao* is prescribed at 6 to 10 grams in powder form. It may be used internally or topically. The fresh herb is commonly used to tonify yin, while dried *Shan Yao* is more often used to strengthen the Spleen and Stomach. The dry-fried herb has a stronger function to tonify the Lung, Spleen and Stomach, and is commonly used to treat diarrhea and leukorrhea.

CAUTIONS / CONTRAINDICATIONS

- *Shan Yao* is contraindicated in cases of excess heat.
- *Shan Yao* should not be used as the sole herb in addressing cases of accumulated dampness.
- *Shan Yao* may sometimes cause abdominal fullness, distention or poor appetite. In cases of indigestion due to intake of this herb, add *Chen Pi* (Pericarpium Citri Reticulatae) to regulate qi and relieve these minor side effects.

CHEMICAL COMPOSITION

Choline, dopamine, batasine, abscisin, starch 16%, mannan, phytic acid.[1]

PHARMACOLOGICAL EFFECTS

- **Antidiabetic:** Administration of *Shan Yao* lowers blood glucose levels in mice. In one study, oral ingestion of the decoction at the dosage of 30 g/kg/day for 10 days lowered blood glucose levels in mice by approximately 10 to 30 mg/dL. In another study, oral ingestion of the decoction at the dosage of 30 g/kg effectively controlled the normally sharp increase of blood glucose following intraperitoneal injection of glucose at 2 g/kg.[2]
- **Gastrointestinal:** Decoction of *Shan Yao* stimulates the intestines and increases peristalsis in mice.[3]

CLINICAL STUDIES AND RESEARCH

- **Infantile diarrhea:** In one clinical study, 123 infants with diarrhea were divided into two groups: group one

Shan Yao (Rhizoma Dioscoreae)

received *Shan Yao* and group two received a placebo. The dosage of *Shan Yao* was as follows: 5 to 10 grams in children under one year old, 11 to 15 grams in children between one and two years old, and 16 to 20 grams in children between two to three years of age. The study concluded that improvement in the treatment group was significantly better than in the placebo group.[4] In another report, an herbal preparation given twice daily was effective in relieving infantile diarrhea within 3 days, as demonstrated in over 1,000 patients. The herbal formula was prepared by mixing 15 grams of *Shan Yao*, 10 grams of *Yi Yi Ren* (Semen Coicis) and one fresh chicken liver with a small portion of vinegar. The mixture was steamed until well-done before administration.[5]

- **Infantile indigestion:** Infants with indigestion were treated with an herbal decoction containing 10 grams of *Shan Yao* and 4 grams of *Che Qian Zi* (Semen Plantaginis) for approximately 6 months. Infants under 6 months of age received half the dosage, while infants over 2 years old received a 33% higher dosage. Infants with dehydration or other complications received slight modifications in herbal treatment, along with acupuncture. The study reported complete recovery in 96 out of 101 infants. [6]

HERB-DRUG INTERACTION

- **Antidiabetics:** It is prudent to use *Shan Yao* with caution when insulin, sulfonylureas, and other antidiabetic medications are present. Though no instances of this potential interaction have been documented, the combination of antidiabetic herbs and drugs may have a synergistic effect, leading to hypoglycemia.[7] [Note: Examples of antidiabetic drugs include insulin, tolbutamide (Orinase), glipizide (Glucotrol), and glyburide (DiaBeta/Micronase).]

AUTHORS' COMMENTS

According to Dr. Zhang Xiao-Ping, the combination of *Shan Yao* and *Huang Qi* (Radix Astragali) has excellent effects to lower plasma glucose levels to treat diabetes mellitus patients. These two herbs are especially effective in individuals with diabetes characterized by qi and yin deficiencies.

References

1. *Xian Dai Zhong Yao Yao Li Xue* (Contemporary Pharmacology of Chinese Herbs), 1997; 1204
2. *Zhong Guo Yao Ke Da Xue Xue Bao* (Journal of University of Chinese Herbology), 1991; 22(3):158
3. *Zhi Wu Zi Yuan Yu Huan Jing* (Source and Environment of Plants), 1992; 1(2):10
4. *Hu Nan Yi Yao Za Zhi* (Hunan Journal of Medicine and Herbology), 1982; 4:17
5. *Hu Bei Zhong Yi Za Zhi* (Hubei Journal of Chinese Medicine), 1985; 5:35
6. *Zhong Yi Za Zhi* (Journal of Chinese Medicine), 1984; 5:9
7. Chen, J. Recognition & prevention of Herb-drug interactions, *Medical Acupuncture*, Fall/Winter 1998/1999; volume 10/number 2; 9-13

Bian Dou (Semen Lablab Album)

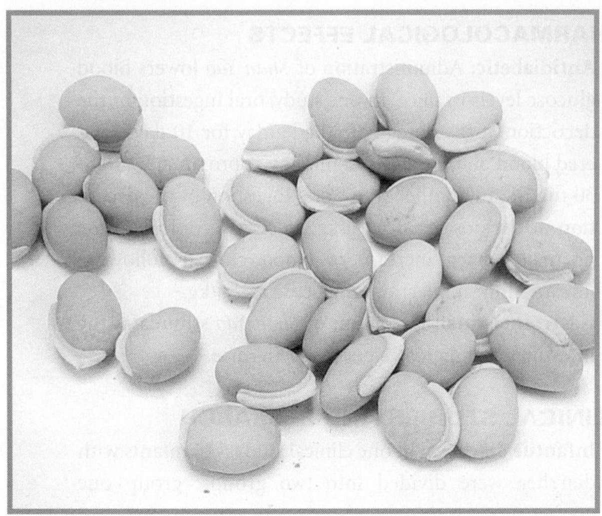

扁豆

Pinyin Name: *Bian Dou*
Literal Name: "flat bean"
Alternate Chinese Names: *Bai Bian Dou*
Original Source: *Ming Yi Za Zhu* (Miscellaneous Records of Famous Physicians) by Tao Hong-Jing in 500 A.D.
English Name: dolichos nut
Botanical Name: *Dolichos lablab* L. (*Bian Dou*)
Pharmaceutical Name: Semen Lablab Album
Properties: sweet, slightly warm
Channels Entered: Spleen, Stomach

Bian Dou (Semen Lablab Album)

CHINESE THERAPEUTIC ACTIONS

1. Strengthens Spleen

Spleen deficiency with dampness: Sweet and slightly warm, *Bian Dou* (Semen Lablab Album) enters and strengthens the Spleen and Stomach channels to treat disorders characterized by deficiency of the Spleen and Stomach with accumulated dampness. Moderate in its action, *Bian Dou* tonifies the Spleen without causing stagnation, and dissolves dampness without drying fluids. It is most suitable for weak, chronic or convalescing patients who cannot digest heavy tonics. It is usually the tonic herb of choice to use before administering stronger ones. Clinical applications include fatigue, lack of energy, decreased intake of food, loose stools, and diarrhea.

- Deficiency of the Spleen and Stomach with dampness: combine *Bian Dou* with *Ren Shen* (Radix Ginseng), *Bai Zhu* (Rhizoma Atractylodis Macrocephalae), *Fu Ling* (Poria) and *Yi Yi Ren* (Semen Coicis). **Exemplar Formula:** *Shen Ling Bai Zhu San* (Ginseng, Poria, and Atractylodes Macrocephala Powder).
- Slight deficiency of the Spleen and Stomach: use this herb with *Tai Zi Shen* (Radix Pseudostellariae), *Shan Yao* (Rhizoma Dioscoreae), and *Gu Ya* (Fructus Setariae Germinatus).

Gynecological disorders: *Bian Dou* strengthens the Spleen to stop excessive vaginal discharge.

- Vaginal discharge with fatigue: use this herb with *Bai Zhu* (Rhizoma Atractylodis Macrocephalae), *Qian Shi* (Semen Euryales) and *Hai Piao Xiao* (Endoconcha Sepiae).

2. Clears Summer-Heat and Dampness

Summer-heat and dampness: In Asia, summer is the season in which pathogenic dampness usually attacks the body, especially the middle *jiao*. *Bian Dou* is commonly used to treat nausea, vomiting and diarrhea associated with disharmony and stagnation of summer-heat and dampness in the middle *jiao*. The primary function of *Bian Dou* is to clear dampness, with the addition of other herbs needed help clear the summer-heat.

- Nausea and vomiting due to summer-heat and dampness: use *Bian Dou* with *Xiang Ru* (Herba Elsholtziae seu Moslae), *He Ye* (Folium Nelumbinis) and *Hou Po* (Cortex Magnoliae Officinalis). **Exemplar Formula:** *Xiang Ru Yin* (Elsholtzia Decoction).

3. Eliminates Toxins

Bian Dou is commonly used to treat food poisoning, alcohol intoxication, or ingestion of various types of toxins.

- Alcohol intoxication: use this herb with *Ge Hua* (Flos Puerariae), *Bai Dou Kou* (Fructus Amomi Rotundus) and *Sha Ren* (Fructus Amomi).
- Pufferfish poisoning: combine it with *Lu Gen* (Rhizoma Phragmitis), *Zi Su Ye* (Folium Perillae) and *Sheng Jiang* (Rhizoma Zingiberis Recens).
- Poultry poisoning: use *Bian Dou* individually.
- Arsenic poisoning: use this herb alone in powder form with water, or combine it with *Fang Feng* (Radix Saposhnikoviae), *Lu Dou* (Semen Phaseoli Radiati) and *Gan Cao* (Radix Glycyrrhizae).
- Calomel poisoning: use *Bian Dou* alone.

DOSAGE

10 to 30 grams in decoctions; 6 to 10 grams in powder. The maximum dosage of *Bian Dou* is 50 grams in decoction. The unprocessed herb is best to nourish the Stomach, dispel summer dampness and eliminate toxins. The dry-fried herb strengthens the Spleen and relieves diarrhea.

CAUTIONS / CONTRAINDICATIONS

- According to *Ben Cao Cong Xin* (Thoroughly Revised Materia Medica) by Wu Yi-Luo in 1751, dry-fried *Bian Dou* is the preferred form of this herb, as ingestion of an excessive amount of fresh *Bian Dou* (without cooking) is toxic. [Note: Fresh *Bian Dou* is considered toxic because it contains hemagglutinin A, the compound responsible for the adverse reactions. Heat-processed *Bian Dou* is not toxic, because hemagglutinin A is readily rendered inactive by heat.[1]]

CHEMICAL COMPOSITION

Protein 22.7%, lipids 1.8%, carbohydrates 57%, calcium 0.046%, phosphorus 0.052%, iron 1mg%, phytin 0.247%, stachyose, raffinose, L-pipecolic acid, hemagglutinin A, hemagglutinin B.[2]

TOXICOLOGY

Gross overdose of fresh *Bian Dou* (without cooking) is associated with growth inhibition and liver damage in mice.[3]

SUPPLEMENT

- 扁豆衣 *Bian Dou Yi* (Pericarpium Lablab Album), first cited in the Qing dynasty, is derived from the skin of the fruit of the same plant as *Bian Dou*. The taste, property and functions of *Bian Dou Yi* are the same as *Bian Dou*, but weaker. *Bian Dou Yi* does not clog the middle *jiao*. It is best for Spleen deficiency with dampness, or for summer-dampness nausea and vomiting, edema and leg *qi*. Recommended dosage of *Bian Dou Yi* is 5 to 10 grams in decoctions.
- 扁豆花 / 扁豆花 *Bian Dou Hua* (Flos Lablab Album), first cited in *Tu Jing Ben Cao* (Illustrated Classic of the Materia Medica) by Su Song in 1061, is the flower of this plant. It is harvested during July or August when the

Bian Dou (Semen Lablab Album)

flower has not fully blossomed. It is sweet and neutral, dispels summer-damp, and harmonizes the Stomach. It is mostly used to treat summer-damp with fever, diarrhea or dysentery. It can also be used to treat either red or white leukorrhea. The recommended dosage for *Bian Dou Yi* is 5 to 10 grams in decoction or in powder.

AUTHORS' COMMENTS

According to various sources, the thermal property of *Bian Dou* has been described as cool, neutral, and slightly warm. Presumably, the herb was described as cool because of its action to clear summer-heat and eliminate toxins. However, most texts now describe *Bian Dou* as a warm herb because its primary effect is to tonify the Spleen and strengthen the middle *jiao*.

Bian Dou can be white, black or dark red. *Bai Bian Dou*, literally "white flat bean," is generally used for medicinal purposes. *Hei Dou*, literally "black bean," is not used medicinally. *Hong Xue Dou*, literally "red blood bean," eliminates toxins from the Liver, reduces inflammation and treats superficial visual obstruction.

According to Dr. Zhu Shen-Yu, *Bian Dou* is one of the best herbs for the nausea and morning sickness associated with pregnancy. Other herbs that are beneficial include *Dao Dou* (Semen Canavaliae), *Sha Ren* (Fructus Amomi), *Huang Lian* (Rhizoma Coptidis), *Chen Pi* (Pericarpium Citri Reticulatae), *Zhu Ru* (Caulis Bambusae in Taenia) and *Bai Zhu* (Rhizoma Atractylodis Macrocephalae).

References

1. Osman HG, et al. Serological and chemical investigations on the glutinins of phaseolus montcalm. *J Chem*, 1963; 6(2):191.
2. *Xian Dai Zhong Yao Yao Li Xue* (Contemporary Pharmacology of Chinese Herbs), 1997; 1206-1207
3. Osman HG, et al. Serological and chemical investigations on the glutinins of phaseolus montcalm. *J Chem*, 1963; 6(2):191.

Ci Wu Jia (Radix et Caulis Acanthopanacis Senticosi)

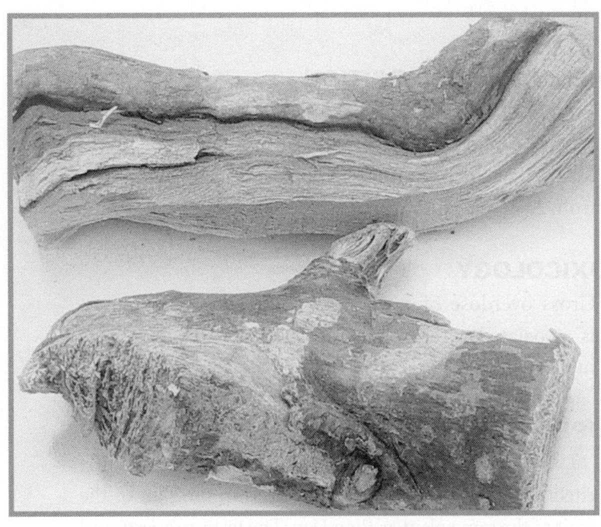

刺五加

Pinyin Name: *Ci Wu Jia*
Literal Name: "prickly acanthopanax"
Alternate Chinese Names: *Wu Jia Shen*
English Name: acanthopanax root, many-prickle acanthopanax root, eleuthero
Botanical Name: *Acanthopanax senticosus* (Rupr. et Maxim.) Harm. [also referred to as *Eleutherococcus senticosus* Rupr. et Maxim.) Harm.]
Pharmaceutical Name: Radix et Caulis Acanthopanacis Senticosi
Properties: acrid, slightly bitter, warm
Channels Entered: Spleen, Kidney, Heart

CHINESE THERAPEUTIC ACTIONS

1. Tonifies Qi, Strengthens the Spleen and Kidney

Spleen and Kidney yang deficiencies: *Ci Wu Jia* (Radix et Caulis Acanthopanacis Senticosi) commonly treats deficiency, characterized by fatigue, lack of energy, poor appetite, and soreness and pain of the lower back and knees. *Ci Wu Jia* is relatively mild and should be combined with other tonic herbs for maximum effectiveness.

- General fatigue, poor appetite: use *Ci Wu Jia* with *Ren Shen* (Radix Ginseng), *Bai Zhu* (Rhizoma Atractylodis Macrocephalae), *Fu Ling* (Poria) and *Gan Cao* (Radix Glycyrrhizae).
- Lower back and knee pain from Kidney yang deficiency: combine this herb with *Du Zhong* (Cortex Eucommiae), *Sang Ji Sheng* (Herba Taxilli) and other Kidney yang tonics.

Ci Wu Jia (Radix et Caulis Acanthopanacis Senticosi)

2. Calms the *Shen* (Spirit)

Disturbed sleep: *Ci Wu Jia* calms the *shen* to relieve insomnia or dream-disturbed sleep. Because of lack of nourishment to the *shen* of the Heart, patients may have excessive dreaming, and difficulty falling asleep or staying asleep. This herb should be combined with *shen*-calming herbs for maximum effectiveness.

- Disturbed sleep from deficiency: add *Ci Wu Jia* to *Long Yan Rou* (Arillus Longan), *Suan Zao Ren* (Semen Zizyphi Spinosae), and *Bai Zi Ren* (Semen Platycladi).

DOSAGE

9 to 27 grams in decoction.

CHEMICAL COMPOSITION

Eleutheroside A,B,C,D,E; daucosterin, siringine, ethyl-α-D-galactoside, isofraxidin glucoside, protoprimulagenin A, PES-A,B; chlorogenic acid, β-sitosterol, betulinic acid, amygdalin, isofraxidin.[1,2]

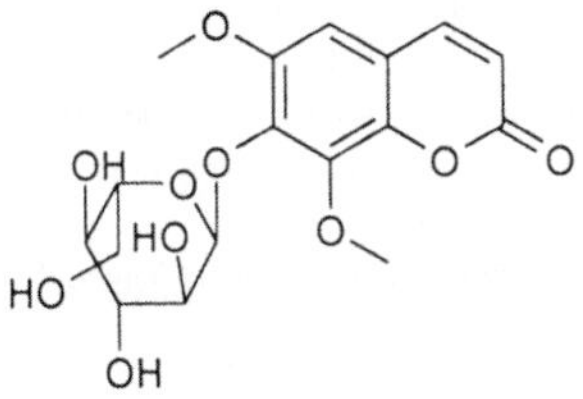

Eleutheroside B_1

PHARMACOLOGICAL EFFECTS

- **Sedative:** *Ci Wu Jia* is associated with a sedative effect on the central nervous system. Alcohol extract of the herb at 10 to 20 g/kg, given via intraperitoneal injection in mice, significantly reduced spontaneous activity and prolonged sleeping time induced by barbiturates.[3]
- **Cardiovascular:** In anesthetized cats and rabbits, intravenous injection of alcohol extract of *Ci Wu Jia* at 2 to 4 g/kg lowered blood pressure, but only for a short period of time. In other studies, administration of *Ci Wu Jia* is associated with increased blood perfusion to the brain and coronary arteries.[4,5]
- **Adaptogenic:** Administration of *Ci Wu Jia* is associated with marked adaptogenic effects in various stressful environments. In mice, administration of the herb prolonged swimming time by approximately 25%, improved resistance to cold temperatures by 42 to 72%, and provided protection against irradiation by minimizing damage to the bone marrow.[6,7]
- **Immunostimulant:** Administration of *Ci Wu Jia* is associated with an improvement of the immune system in both healthy and immune-suppressed subjects. Guinea pigs who received the herb once daily for 15 days showed an increase in phagocytic activity of the macrophages. In addition, other studies in mice indicated that *Ci Wu Jia* increased production of white blood cells and interferon.[8,9,10]
- **Metabolic:** Daily administration of *Ci Wu Jia* in rabbits for 30 days was associated with an increase in glucose levels in the blood and in glycogen levels in the liver and muscle tissues.[11]
- **Endocrinological:** Administration of *Ci Wu Jia* has a regulatory effect on the endocrine system, specifically the adrenal glands, thyroid and pancreas. It has been used to treat subjects with adrenocortical insufficiency, enlarged thyroid, and hyperglycemia, with good results.[12,13]

CLINICAL STUDIES AND RESEARCH

- **Coronary artery disease with hypercholesterolemia:** Administration of a *Ci Wu Jia* preparation three times daily for 1 to 3 months was 95.45% effective in treating 132 angina patients. The same preparation was also effective in lowering plasma cholesterol and triglyceride levels in 53 patients.[14]
- **Neurasthenia:** Oral administration of *Ci Wu Jia* was 90% effective in treating patients with neurasthenia, with symptoms such as fatigue, headache, insomnia, poor appetite, and increased body weight.[15]
- **Bone marrow suppression:** Administration of *Ci Wu Jia* was effective in increasing white blood cell counts in 84.2% of 43 cancer patients who had bone marrow suppression following chemotherapy and radiation treatments.[16]
- **Coronary artery disease:** Administration of a *Ci Wu Jia* preparation three times daily for 1 to 3 months was 95% effective for relief of angina, 88% effective for reducing plasma cholesterol levels, and 87% effective for reducing triglycerides.[17]
- **Hypercholesterolemia:** In a clinical study with 31 patients, administration of an herbal formula (3 parts *Ci Wu Jia* and 1 part *Xiang Ru* (Herba Elsholtziae seu Moslae)) at 30 ml/day for 10 days reduced β-lipoprotein by 32.6%, and increased HDL by 16.3%.[18]

HERB-DRUG INTERACTION

- **Digoxin:** An elevated serum digoxin level was documented in one patient taking both digoxin and *Ci Wu Jia*. When *Ci Wu Jia* was discontinued, the serum digoxin level returned to normal. When *Ci Wu Jia* was re-introduced, the serum digoxin level increased. The exact mechanism of this action is unclear. Proposed reasons included conversion of components in *Ci Wu Jia* to digoxin *in vivo*, interference with digoxin elimination, or false serum assay results.[19]
- **Barbiturates**: *Ci Wu Jia* increases the effect of hexobarbital, inhibiting its metabolic breakdown.[20]
- **Antibiotic**: *Ci Wu Jia* increases the efficacy of antibiotics, possibly increasing T-lymphocyte activity.[21]

Ci Wu Jia (Radix et Caulis Acanthopanacis Senticosi)

- **Adrenalin**: *Ci Wu Jia* stimulates the production of adrenalin by the adrenal glands.[22]

TOXICOLOGY

No adverse reactions were observed following oral administration of alcohol extract of *Ci Wu Jia* at 350 g/kg in mice. In a long-term toxicology study, oral administration of *Ci Wu Jia* in rabbits at 30 g/kg (100 times the normal adult dose in human) for 15 days did not cause any damage to the vital organs, including heart, liver, spleen, lungs and kidneys.[23,24]

AUTHORS' COMMENTS

Siberian ginseng is a common, but technically inaccurate, name of *Ci Wu Jia* (Radix et Caulis Acanthopanacis Senticosi). Siberian ginseng is not a species of Panax, although they belong in the same family, Araliaceae. The designation 'Siberian ginseng' was an attempt to give an expensive name to a relatively inexpensive herb. Eleuthero is now the common name of this herb. [Note: *Acanthopanax senticosus* is also referred to as *Eleutherococcus senticosus.*]

References

1. *Xian Dai Zhong Yao Yao Li Xue* (Contemporary Pharmacology of Chinese Herbs), 1997; 1222-1223
2. Yan X, Zhou J, Xie G, *Traditional Chinese Medicines Molecular Structures, Natural Sources and Applications*; Ashgate, 1999; 2063
3. *Zhong Yi Yao Xue Bao* (Report of Chinese Medicine and Herbology), 1985; (2):29
4. Ibid.
5. *Shan Xi Xin Yi Yao* (New Medicine and Herbology of Shanxi), 1982; 11(10):52
6. *Zhong Yi Yao Xue Bao* (Report of Chinese Medicine and Herbology), 1985; (2):29
7. *Hu Bei Yi Xue Yuan Xue Bao* (Journal of Hubei College of Medicine), 1989; 10(3):226
8. *Hei Long Jiang Zhong Yi Yao* (Heilongjiang Chinese Medicine and Herbology), 1981; (4):37
9. *Zhong Cao Yao* (Chinese Herbal Medicine), 1990j; 21(1):27
10. *CA*, 1972; 76:54331
11. *CA*, 1967; 66:51311
12. *CA*, 1964; 60:163896
13. *CA*, 1967; 68:19237
14. *Zhong Yi Yao Xin Xi* (Information on Chinese Medicine and Herbology), 1987; 4:36
15. *CA*, 1968; 69:104731
16. Ibid.
17. *Zhong Yi Yao Xin Xi* (Information on Chinese Medicine and Herbology), 1987; (4):36
18. *Zhong Xi Yi Jie He Za Zhi* (Journal of Integrated Chinese and Western Medicine), 1990; 10(3):155
19. *CMAJ*, 1996, Aug 1; 155(3):293-5
20. P.F.D'Arcy: *Adverse Reactions And Interactions With Herbal Medicine. Part 2 – Drug Interactions*. Adverse Drug React. Toxicol. Rev. 1993, 12(3) 147-162 Oxford University Press
21. Brinker, Francis. *Eclectic Dispensatory of Botanical Therapeutics*, vol II, 1995
22. Ibid.
23. *Int J Immunopharmacol*, 1991; 13(5):549
24. *Zhong Yao Xian Dai Yan Jiu Yu Ying Yong* (Modern Study of Traditional Chinese Medicine), 1994; 411

Gan Cao (Radix Glycyrrhizae)

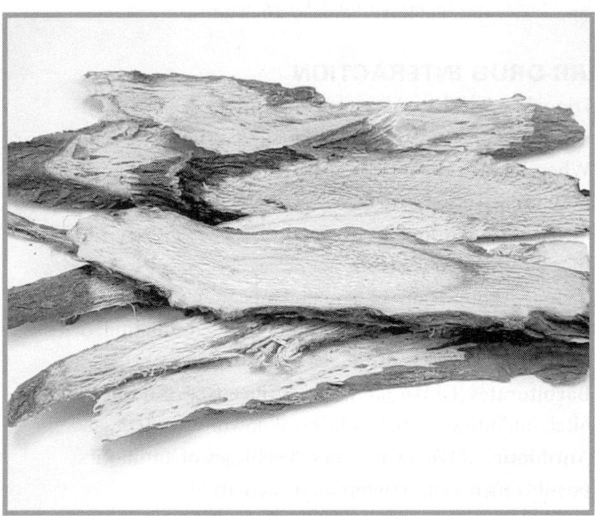

甘草 甘草

Pinyin Name: *Gan Cao*
Literal Name: "sweet herb," "sweet grass"
Alternate Chinese Names: *Guo Lao*
Original Source: *Shen Nong Ben Cao Jing* (Divine Husbandman's Classic of the Materia Medica) in the second century
English Name: licorice root (British spelling: liquorice)
Botanical Name: *Glycyrrhiza uralensis* Fisch. (*Gan Cao*); *Glycyrrhiza inflata* Bat. (*Zhang Guo Gan Cao*); *Glycyrrhiza qlabra* L. (*Guang Guo Gan Cao*)
Pharmaceutical Name: Radix Glycyrrhizae
Properties: sweet, neutral
Channels Entered: Spleen, Stomach, Lung and Heart

Gan Cao (Radix Glycyrrhizae)

CHINESE THERAPEUTIC ACTIONS

1. Tonifies Spleen, Benefits Qi

Spleen and Stomach deficiencies: *Gan Cao* (Radix Glycyrrhizae) tonifies the middle *jiao* to enhance the transformation and transportation functions of the Spleen and Stomach. Clinically, it treats disorders such as shortness of breath, fatigue, sallow facial appearance, decreased food intake, loose stools, and diarrhea. The honey-fried herb, *Zhi Gan Cao* (Radix Glycyrrhizae Preparata), is stronger than the unprocessed herb for tonification of qi.

- Deficiency of Spleen and Stomach qi: combine *Gan Cao* with *Ren Shen* (Radix Ginseng), *Bai Zhu* (Rhizoma Atractylodis Macrocephalae) and *Fu Ling* (Poria). **Exemplar Formula:** *Si Jun Zi Tang* (Four-Gentleman Decoction).

Palpitations, arrhythmia and intermittent pulse: These conditions may occur as a result of qi and blood deficiencies of the Heart. Clinically, *Gan Cao* treats patients with palpitations and irregular or intermittent pulse with deficiency and cold. Honey-fried *Gan Cao* is best used for this condition.

- Palpitations with irregular or intermittent pulse: use it with *Ren Shen* (Radix Ginseng), *Sheng Di Huang* (Radix Rehmanniae), *E Jiao* (Colla Corii Asini) and *Gui Zhi* (Ramulus Cinnamomi). **Exemplar Formula:** *Zhi Gan Cao Tang* (Honey-Fried Licorice Decoction).

***Zang zao* (dry organ) disorder:** This is a condition characterized by Heart deficiency and Liver qi stagnation with a wan appearance, disturbed sleep, and emotional instability. *Gan Cao* treats this condition by tonifying qi, nourishing the Heart and harmonizing the middle *jiao*.

- *Zang zao* disorder: use *Gan Cao* with *Da Zao* (Fructus Jujubae) and *Xiao Mai* (Fructus Tritici). **Exemplar Formula:** *Gan Mai Da Zao Tang* (Licorice, Wheat, and Jujube Decoction).
- *Zang zao* disorder with *shen* (spirit) disturbance: combine this herb with *Da Zao* (Fructus Jujubae), *Xiao Mai* (Fructus Tritici), *Long Gu* (Os Draconis), *Mu Li* (Concha Ostreae), *Suan Zao Ren* (Semen Zizyphi Spinosae) and *Bai Zi Ren* (Semen Platycladi).

2. Moistens the Lung, Stops Cough

Cough or dyspnea: *Gan Cao* moistens the Lung, nourishes qi, dispels phlegm and stops cough. Neutral in property and mild in action, it treats coughing and wheezing of various etiologies, including cold or heat, and deficiency or excess, with or without phlegm.

- *Wei* (atrophy) syndrome of the Lung with chronic cough: use *Gan Cao* alone.
- Cough and wheezing caused by wind-cold: use it with *Ma Huang* (Herba Ephedrae), *Xing Ren* (Semen Armeniacae Amarum) and *Sheng Jiang* (Rhizoma Zingiberis Recens). **Exemplar Formula:** *San Ao Tang* (Three-Unbinding Decoction).
- Cough and wheezing due to wind-heat: combine this herb with *Sang Ye* (Folium Mori), *Ju Hua* (Flos Chrysanthemi), *Jie Geng* (Radix Platycodonis) and *Xing Ren* (Semen Armeniacae Amarum). **Exemplar Formula:** *Sang Ju Yin* (Mulberry Leaf and Chrysanthemum Decoction).
- Cough and wheezing due to Lung heat: use this herb with *Shi Gao* (Gypsum Fibrosum), *Ma Huang* (Herba Ephedrae), and *Xing Ren* (Semen Armeniacae Amarum). **Exemplar Formula:** *Ma Xing Gan Shi Tang* (Ephedra, Apricot Kernel, Licorice, and Gypsum Decoction).
- Cough and wheezing due to Lung cold, with sputum: add it to *Gan Jiang* (Rhizoma Zingiberis), *Xi Xin* (Herba Asari), and *Wu Wei Zi* (Fructus Schisandrae Chinensis). **Exemplar Formula:** *Xiao Qing Long Tang* (Minor Bluegreen Dragon Decoction).
- Cough and wheezing because of dryness: use *Gan Cao* with *Bei Sha Shen* (Radix Glehniae), *Mai Men Dong* (Radix Ophiopogonis), *E Jiao* (Colla Corii Asini) and *Kuan Dong Hua* (Flos Farfarae).

3. Relieves Pain

Epigastric, abdominal, musculoskeletal and smooth muscle pain and cramps: The Spleen dominates muscles and the Liver controls tendons. Therefore, patients with Spleen deficiency and Liver excess often experience muscle cramps and pain, especially in epigastric and abdominal tissues. *Gan Cao* has excellent properties to relieve pain and cramps of smooth or skeletal muscles by tonifying the Spleen and replenishing qi.

- Pain and cramps of smooth or skeletal muscles: combine *Gan Cao* with *Bai Shao* (Radix Paeoniae Alba). **Exemplar Formula:** *Shao Yao Gan Cao Tang* (Peony and Licorice Decoction).
- Abdominal pain due to deficiency and cold of the middle *jiao*: use this herb with *Shan Yao* (Rhizoma Dioscoreae), *Yi Tang* (Saccharum Granorum), *Gui Zhi* (Ramulus Cinnamomi), *Sheng Jiang* (Rhizoma Zingiberis Recens) and *Da Zao* (Fructus Jujubae).
- Diarrhea, dysentery and abdominal pain caused by damp-heat: combine *Gan Cao* with *Bai Shao* (Radix Paeoniae Alba), *Huang Lian* (Rhizoma Coptidis), *Huang Qin* (Radix Scutellariae), *Da Huang* (Radix et Rhizoma Rhei) and *Bing Lang* (Semen Arecae). **Exemplar Formula:** *Shao Yao Tang* (Peony Decoction).
- Hypochondriac pain due to Liver qi stagnation: use this herb with *Bai Shao* (Radix Paeoniae Alba), *Chai Hu* (Radix Bupleuri), *Dang Gui* (Radicis Angelicae Sinensis)

Gan Cao (Radix Glycyrrhizae)

and *Bai Zhu* (Rhizoma Atractylodis Macrocephalae). **Exemplar Formula:** *Xiao Yao San* (Rambling Powder).

- Epigastric pain caused by stomach ulcer: add this herb to *Hai Piao Xiao* (Endoconcha Sepiae), *Wa Leng Zi* (Concha Arcae), *Chen Pi* (Pericarpium Citri Reticulatae) and honey.
- Leg cramps due to blood deficiency: use it with *Bai Shao* (Radix Paeoniae Alba), *Mu Gua* (Fructus Chaenomelis) and *Ji Xue Teng* (Caulis Spatholobi).

4. Clears Heat, Eliminates Toxins

Sores, swellings and carbuncles: The fresh or unprocessed form of *Gan Cao* is used to clear heat and eliminate toxins. It may be used internally or topically to treat various sores and ulcers characterized by heat and toxins.

- Uncomplicated sores or lesions: use *Gan Cao* alone, topically or internally.
- Erysipelas: use it alone as decoction and apply topically.
- Red lesions with eczema and itching: apply decoction of *Gan Cao* topically.
- Yang sores with redness, swelling and pain: use it with *Jin Yin Hua* (Flos Lonicerae), *Lian Qiao* (Fructus Forsythiae), *Zi Hua Di Ding* (Herba Violae) and *Pu Gong Ying* (Herba Taraxaci).
- Yin sores with dark-purplish appearance: add it to *Shu Di Huang* (Radix Rehmanniae Preparata), *Rou Gui* (Cortex Cinnamomi), *Lu Jiao Jiao* (Gelatinum Cornu Cervi) and *Bai Jie Zi* (Semen Sinapis). **Exemplar Formula:** *Yang He Tang* (Yang-Heartening Decoction).
- Burns: mix *Gan Cao* with honey for topical application. Frostbite: use it with an equal portion of *Yuan Hua* (Flos Genkwa) and apply topically as an herbal wash.

Sore throat: *Gan Cao* relieves soreness, swelling and pain in the throat, a condition characterized by the presence of heat and toxins. It may be used alone or in combination with other herbs. If heat is not severe and the throat is not extremely red, *Gan Cao* can be used alone.

- Sore throat: use it with *Jie Geng* (Radix Platycodonis). **Exemplar Formula:** *Jie Geng Tang* (Platycodon Decoction).
- Severe sore throat with redness, swelling, and pus: combine this herb with *Jie Geng* (Radix Platycodonis), *Shan Dou Gen* (Radix Sophorae Tonkinensis), *Xuan Shen* (Radix Scrophulariae), and *Niu Bang Zi* (Fructus Arctii).

5. Treats Poisoning

Poisoning: *Gan Cao* is useful as an antidote for various poisonings, including but not limited to food, herbs, herbicides, pesticides, drugs, and heavy metals.

- Food poisoning from beef: use *Gan Cao* alone as decoction.
- Drug poisoning: use *Gan Cao* with honey.
- Herbicide or pesticide poisoning: use 12 grams of *Gan Cao* and 15 grams of *Hua Shi* (Talcum) in herbal decoction, three times daily.
- Lead poisoning: use this herb with *Xing Ren* (Semen Armeniacae Amarum).
- Arsenic poisoning: use it with *Lu Dou* (Semen Phaseoli Radiati), *Hei Dou* (Semen Glycine Max) and *Jin Yin Hua* (Flos Lonicerae).

6. Harmonizes Other Herbs

Gan Cao harmonizes and moderates the harsh or adverse effects of other herbs, keeping them from damaging the middle *jiao*.

- It neutralizes the toxicity of *Fu Zi* (Radix Aconiti Lateralis Praeparata).
- *Gan Cao* controls the warm property of *Gan Jiang* (Rhizoma Zingiberis) to prevent damage to the yin.
- It prevents the cold properties of *Shi Gao* (Gypsum Fibrosum) and *Zhi Mu* (Radix Anemarrhenae) from damaging the Stomach.
- This herb reduces the initial drastic and potent purgative effects of *Da Huang* (Radix et Rhizoma Rhei) and *Mang Xiao* (Natrii Sulfas), and prolongs the overall duration of effect.
- It reduces the initial peak in effect of *Dang Shen* (Radix Codonopsis), *Bai Zhu* (Rhizoma Atractylodis Macrocephalae), *Shu Di Huang* (Radix Rehmanniae Preparata) and *Dang Gui* (Radicis Angelicae Sinensis) and prolongs the overall tonic effect.
- *Gan Cao* is used with both cold and hot herbs such as *Ban Xia* (Rhizoma Pinelliae), *Gan Jiang* (Rhizoma Zingiberis), *Huang Lian* (Rhizoma Coptidis) and *Huang Qin* (Radix Scutellariae), to harmonize the effect of the overall combination.

DOSAGE

3 to 10 grams, with a maximum of 15 to 30 grams. *Gan Cao* is used in herbal decoction, powder, pills or syrup. It is commonly used both internally and topically. The unprocessed herb more strongly purges fire, eliminates toxins, moistens the Lung, and stops cough; therefore, it is commonly used to treat throat soreness and pain, various infections with formation of pus and abscess, cough with hot phlegm, and food or drug poisoning. Honey-processed *Gan Cao* has a sweeter taste and warmer nature; therefore, it tonifies the Spleen, benefits qi, moistens the Lung, and stops cough. The honey-fried herb is stronger than the unprocessed herb for tonification of qi.

CAUTIONS / CONTRAINDICATIONS

- Sweet in nature, *Gan Cao* can create dampness and is, therefore, contraindicated in cases of nausea, vomiting,

Gan Cao (Radix Glycyrrhizae)

chest and abdominal fullness and distention due to accumulation of dampness.

- *Gan Cao* is incompatible with *Gan Sui* (Radix Euphorbiae Kansui), *Da Ji* (Radix Euphorbiae seu Knoxiae), *Yuan Hua* (Flos Genkwa), and *Hai Zao* (Sargassum).
- Large dosages or chronic usage of *Gan Cao* are contraindicated in cases of edema, kidney disorders, hypokalemia, hypertension, and congestive heart failure.

OVERDOSAGE

Overdose or chronic use of *Gan Cao* may cause edema, elevated blood pressure, weak extremities, numbness, sodium retention, potassium loss, dizziness, and headache.

TREATMENT OF OVERDOSAGE

Ze Xie (Rhizoma Alismatis) and *Fu Ling* (Poria) should be combined with *Gan Cao* to prevent sodium and water retention, especially if *Gan Cao* is to be used in a large dose or on a long-term basis. Reduction of sodium intake and supplementation of potassium are also recommended. Discontinue *Gan Cao* should the patient report edema, elevated blood pressure, or other adverse reactions.

CHEMICAL COMPOSITION

Triterpenoids (glycyrrhizin, glycyrrhizic acid, glycyrrhetinic acid, glycyrrhetic acid), flavonoids (liguiritin, isoliquiritin, liquiritigenin, uralenol-3-methylether, uralene).[1,2]

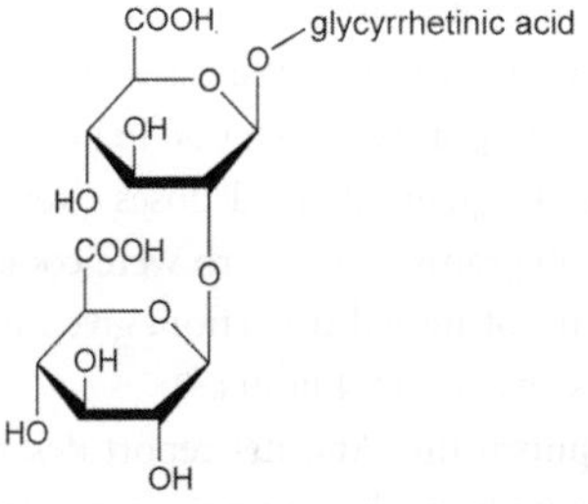

Glycyrrhizic Acid

PHARMACOLOGICAL EFFECTS

- **Mineralocorticoid:** Extract of *Gan Cao* or its compounds (glycyrrhizin and glycyrrhetinic acid) have all demonstrated mineralocorticoid effects, leading to increased re-absorption of sodium and water and excretion of potassium. Overdose or long-term ingestion may cause an increase in edema and blood pressure.[3]
- **Glucocorticoid:** Administration of glycyrrhizin and glycyrrhetinic acid clearly enhances the overall duration of effect of cortisone, as demonstrated by various laboratory studies. The proposed mechanisms of action vary among experts. Some believe that the enhanced cortisone effect is due to decreased metabolism by the liver, or increased plasma concentration caused by decreased protein binding.[4]
- **Anti-inflammatory:** Glycyrrhizin and glycyrrhetinic acid have demonstrated marked anti-inflammatory effects. Clinical applications include inflammation, edema, formation of granuloma, arthritis, and others. The proposed mechanism of anti-inflammatory action includes decreased permeability of the blood vessels, antihistamine functions, and decreased sensitivity to stimuli. The anti-inflammatory influence of glycyrrhizin and glycyrrhetinic acid is approximately 1/10th that of cortisone.[5]
- **Antiarrhythmic**: Extract of *Zhi Gan Cao* (Radix Glycyrrhizae Preparata) has shown marked effectiveness in treating arrhythmia induced by aconitine in rabbits.[6]
- **Immunologic:** Administration of *Gan Cao* may stimulate or inhibit the phagocytic activity of macrophages in mice. Under a stressful environment (cold, heat or hunger), the herb stimulates the immune system and increases phagocytic activities. In a normal environment, *Gan Cao* inhibits the immune system.[7]
- **Gastrointestinal:** Many components of *Gan Cao* have proven to prevent and treat peptic ulcers. The mechanisms of this action include inhibition of gastric acid secretion, binding and deactivation of gastric acid, and promotion of recovery from ulceration.[8]
- **Antispasmodic:** Both water and alcohol extracts of *Gan Cao* exert inhibitory influences on smooth muscle to stop spasms and cramps of the intestines and uterus. The antispasmodic effect is enhanced when *Bai Shao* (Radix Paeoniae Alba) is added.[9]
- **Antitoxin:** Glycyrrhizin, generally considered to be one of the main constituents of *Gan Cao,* has a marked detoxifying effect to treat poisoning, including but not limited to drug poisoning (chloral hydrate, urethane, cocaine, picrotoxin, caffeine, pilocarpine, nicotine, barbiturates, mercury and lead), food poisoning (tetrodotoxin, snake and mushrooms), and others (enterotoxin, herbicides and pesticides). On the other hand, *Gan Cao* is not effective in treating poisoning caused by atropine, morphine, and sulfonmethane. It may increase the toxicity of ephedrine. The exact mechanism of this action is unclear, but is thought to be related to its regulatory effect on the endocrine or hepatic systems. Oral ingestion of *Gan Cao* reduces the absorption of toxins via direct binding, an effect similar to that of activated charcoal. *Gan Cao* significantly reduces the toxicity of *Fu Zi* (Radix Aconiti Lateralis Praeparata) when the two herbs are decocted together.[10,11]
- **Hepatoprotective:** Studies in mice have shown that *Gan Cao* increases the amount of cytochrome p-450 in the liver, which is responsible for the protective effect of the herb on the liver against chemical or tetrachloride-induced liver damage and liver cancer.[12]

Gan Cao (Radix Glycyrrhizae)

- **Antitussive and expectorant:** Administration of *Gan Cao* is associated with marked antitussive and expectorant effects in guinea pigs. The antitussive effect is thought to be related to its effect on the central nervous system.[13]
- **Analgesic:** *Gan Cao* has an analgesic effect as demonstrated by studies in mice. The analgesic effect of *Gan Cao* is enhanced by concurrent use of *Bai Shao* (Radix Paeoniae Alba).[14]
- **Antibiotic:** *Gan Cao* inhibits the growth of *Staphylococcus aureus*, *Mycobacterium tuberculosis*, *E. coli*, amoebae and *Trichomonas vaginalis*.[15]
- **Antihyperlipidemic:** While glycyrrhizin has been shown to lower plasma cholesterol levels, *Gan Cao* has not demonstrated any preventative or treatment effect on atherosclerosis.[16]

CLINICAL STUDIES AND RESEARCH

- **Endocrine:** In one study, 8 out of 9 patients with declining pituitary function were treated successfully by 2 to 3 months of taking the following herbal combination: 15 to 30 grams of fresh *Gan Cao* and 6 grams of *Ren Shen* (Radix Ginseng). Modifications to the herbal formula were made if deemed necessary. For severe aversion to cold, 10 grams of *Fu Zi* (Radix Aconiti Lateralis Praeparata) were added. The duration of treatment was increased to 2 to 6 months. If elevated blood pressure and edema were noted, the dosage of *Gan Cao* was reduced by 50% and 10 grams each of *Fu Ling* (Poria), *Du Zhong* (Cortex Eucommiae) and *Wu Wei Zi* (Fructus Schisandrae Chinensis) were added.[17]
- **Addison's disease:** Extract of *Gan Cao* given three times daily for 25 to 40 days showed marked effectiveness in treating patients with Addison's disease. Patients with mild to moderate conditions required only 3 to 5 ml of the herb per dose. Patients with more severe conditions required up to 8 to 10 ml of the herb per dose, and supplements of adrenocortical steroids if necessary.[18]
- **Peptic ulcer:** One hundred patients with gastric or duodenal ulcers were treated with 15 ml of *Gan Cao* extract, four times daily for 6 weeks, with 90% rate of effectiveness.[19]
- **Tuberculosis:** In one study, 55 patients with pulmonary tuberculosis were treated with an herbal decoction three times daily for 30 to 90 days. There was significant improvement in 23 patients and some improvement in 32 patients. The main ingredient of the herbal formula was 18 grams of fresh *Gan Cao*, cooked to yield 150 ml of the decoction. Other herbs effective in treating tuberculosis were added based on the condition of each patient.[20]
- **Hepatitis:** Hepatitis B in 330 patients was treated with glycyrrhizin, with 77% effectiveness. The study reported that glycyrrhizin reduced the damage to and death of liver cells, reduced inflammatory reaction, promoted regeneration of liver cells, and decreased the risk of liver cirrhosis and necrosis.[21]
- **Arrhythmia:** An herbal decoction administered twice daily for 3 to 12 doses had satisfactory results in treating 23 patients with arrhythmia. The study reported that the patients had no subjective complaints and ECGs appeared normal. The herbal formula contained 30 grams each of *Gan Cao*, *Zhi Gan Cao* (Radix Glycyrrhizae Preparata), and *Ze Xie* (Rhizoma Alismatis).[22]
- **Back and leg pain:** According to one report, 27 patients with severe pain of the back and legs were treated by local injection of a *Gan Cao* solution, with complete relief of pain in 20 patients and moderate relief in 7 patients. Patients with acute conditions received injections every other day for 4 to 7 treatments; those with chronic conditions received injections every other day, for 8 to 14 treatments.[23]
- **Purpura:** Eight patients with purpura caused by thrombocytopenia were treated with decoction of *Gan Cao* (25 to 30 grams), three times daily, with significant improvement in 3 patients, moderate improvement in 4 patients and some improvement in 1 patient. The study reported that bleeding stopped for most patients within 3 to 4 days.[24]
- **Intestinal spasms:** In one study, 241 out of 254 patients (94.8%) with intestinal spasms showed significant improvement after receiving 10 to 15 ml of extract of *Gan Cao* three times daily for 3 to 6 days.[25]
- **Food poisoning:** Administration of a decoction of *Gan Cao* was used to treat 454 patients with various kinds of food poisoning, with satisfactory results in most cases. The treatment protocol for mild cases of food poisoning was to use 9 to 15 grams of *Gan Cao* in herbal decoction, given in 3 to 4 equally-divided doses over 2 hours. In severe cases, 30 grams of the herb were cooked in water to yield 300 ml of herbal decoction, given in 3 equally-divided doses, every 3 to 4 hours.[26]
- **Mushroom poisoning**: Another report describes 20 out of 22 patients with mushroom poisoning who had complete recovery, after being treated with an herbal decoction of *Gan Cao*. Two patients required hospitalization because immediate herbal treatment was not available. The herbal decoction was prepared by using 94 grams of *Gan Cao* cooked twice to yield 200 ml of final decoction. Patients were given 100 ml of the decoction immediately, followed by another 100 ml 30 minutes later.[27]
- **Profuse urination:** Two patients with profuse urination were treated with 5 grams of powdered *Gan Cao* four times daily with good results.[28]
- **Tonsillitis:** In one study, 34 out of 38 patients reported complete recovery from chronic tonsillitis after being treated with *Gan Cao* tea for 1 to 5 months. The treatment protocol was to soak 10 grams of the herb in hot water and drink throughout the day as tea. Patients were advised to

Gan Cao (Radix Glycyrrhizae)

avoid fish and spicy or sweet foods. Patients with mild conditions required 1 to 2 months of treatment, while those with severe conditions required 3 to 5 months.[29]

- **Phlebitis:** Three patients with phlebitis were treated with marked effectiveness using 15 ml of extract or 50 grams of *Gan Cao* in decoction three times daily, before meals. The study reported relief of pain, edema and other symptoms after herbal treatment.[30]
- **Acute mastitis:** According to one report, 27 patients with acute mastitis (without suppuration) were treated with satisfactory results using an herbal decoction containing 30 grams each of *Gan Cao* and *Chi Shao* (Radix Paeoniae Rubrae), given one time daily for 1 to 3 days.[31]
- **Frostbite:** Complete recovery from frostbite was reported in 58 out of 76 patients after being treated with an herbal solution applied topically three times daily. The herbal solution was prepared by cooking 10 grams each of *Gan Cao* and *Yuan Hua* (Flos Genkwa), to yield 2,000 ml of the herbal solution.[32]

HERB-DRUG INTERACTION

- **Corticosteroids:** It has been suggested that the use of *Gan Cao* may alter the therapeutic effects of systemic corticosteroids. Glycyrrhizin, one of the components of *Gan Cao*, is a strong inhibitor of 11 β-hydroxysteroid dehydrogenase and may prolong the biological half-life of the systemic corticosteroids.[33] [Note: Examples of corticosteroids include cortisone, prednisone (Orasone), dexamethasone (Decadron), hydrocortisone (Cortef), methylprednisolone (Medrol).]
- **Digoxin:** *Gan Cao* should be used with caution with cardiac glycosides, such as digoxin (Lanoxin), as potassium loss may increase the toxicity of the drug.[34]
- **Drug overdose:** *Gan Cao* speeds the metabolism of drugs such as chloral hydrate, urethane, cocaine, picrotoxin, caffeine, pilocarpine, nicotine, and barbiturates, and treats overdose of these agents.[35]

TOXICOLOGY

Administration of decoction of *Gan Cao* in mice at the dosage of 2 g/kg for 6 weeks resulted in no fatalities or signs of edema. In another study, an increase in body weight and decrease in function of the adrenal glands were associated with continuous administration of *Gan Cao* extract for 40 days in rabbits and guinea pigs.[36,37]

Glycyrrhetinic acid is associated with a reduction of thyroid function and a decrease in the basal metabolic rate in guinea pigs.[38]

The LD_{50} for water extract of *Gan Cao* in mice is 1.9432 +/- 0.467 g/kg via intravenous injection, 6.8466 g/kg via intraperitoneal injection, and 7.8192 g/kg via subcutaneous injection.[39]

SUPPLEMENT

- 炙甘草 / 炙甘草 *Zhi Gan Cao* (Radix Glycyrrhizae Preparata), sweet and warm, is the honey-processed form of *Gan Cao*. *Zhi Gan Cao* has a stronger effect than *Gan Cao* to tonify Spleen, benefit qi, moisten the Lung, and stop cough.

AUTHORS' COMMENTS

According to traditional texts, *Gan Cao* is incompatible with *Hai Zao* (Sargassum). However, throughout the history of Chinese medicine, there have been several formulas that incorporate both herbs, such as *Hai Zao Yu Hu Tang* (Sargassum Decoction for the Jade Flask). According to Jiang Te-Xie's article "*Hai Zao* is not incompatible with *Gan Cao*," 10 grams of *Gan Cao* with 15 grams of *Hai Zao* (when cooked in a decoction and administered to patients) did not present any adverse reactions.[40]

According to Dr. Zhang Xue-Wen, *Gan Cao*, *Lu Dou* (Semen Phaseoli Radiati), and *Bai Mao Gen* (Rhizoma Imperatae) are effective to treat food poisoning. *Gan Cao* and *Lu Dou* clear heat and toxins, and are commonly used to eliminate toxicity from herbs, drugs and food. *Bai Mao Gen* clears heat and promotes diuresis to quickly dispel toxins from the body, prevent internal bleeding, and protect the kidneys.

References

1. *Xian Dai Zhong Yao Yao Li Xue* (Contemporary Pharmacology of Chinese Herbs), 1997; 1183
2. *The Merck Index* 12th edition, Chapman & Hall/CRCnetBASE/Merck, 2000
3. *Zhong Yao Zhi* (Chinese Herbology Journal), 1993; 358
4. Ibid.
5. *Zhong Cao Yao* (Chinese Herbal Medicine), 1991; 22(10):452
6. *Jiang Su Zhong Yi Za Zhi* (Jiangsu Journal of Chinese Medicine), 1987; 8(10):688
7. *Zhong Yao Xue* (Chinese Herbology), 1998; 759:766
8. *Zhong Yao Zhi* (Chinese Herbology Journal), 1993; 358
9. Ibid.
10. *Zhong Yao Tong Bao* (Journal of Chinese Herbology), 1986; 11(10):55
11. Ibid.
12. Ibid.
13. *Zhong Yao Yao Li Yu Ying Yong* (Pharmacology and Applications of Chinese Herbs), 1983:264
14. *Zhong Yao Xue* (Chinese Herbology), 1998, 759:765
15. *Zhong Yao Zhi* (Chinese Herbology Journal), 1993; 358
16. *Zhong Yao Xue* (Chinese Herbology), 1998, 759:765
17. *Zhong Hua Yi Xue Za Zhi* (Chinese Journal of Medicine), 1975; 10:718
18. *Bai Qiu En Yi Ke Da Xue Xue Bao* (Journal of Baiqiuen University of Medicine), 1978; 4:54
19. *Zhong Hua Nei Ke Xue Za Zhi* (Journal of Chinese Internal Medicine), 1960; 3:226
20. *Jiang Xi Yi Yao* (Jiangxi Medicine and Herbology), 1965; 1:562
21. *Zhong Yao Tong Bao* (Journal of Chinese Herbology), 1987; 9:60
22. *Bei Jing Zhong Yi Xue Yuan Xue Bao* (Journal of Beijing University School of Medicine), 1983; 2:24

Gan Cao (Radix Glycyrrhizae)

23. *Zhe Jiang Zhong Yi Za Zhi* (Zhejiang Journal of Chinese Medicine), 1980; 2:60
24. *Zhong Hua Nei Ke Za Zhi* (Chinese Journal of Internal Medicine), 1981; 11:704
25. Ibid., 1960; 4:354
26. *Xin Zhong Yi* (New Chinese Medicine), 1985; 2:34
27. Ibid., 1978; 1:36
28. *Zhong Hua Nei Ke Za Zhi* (Chinese Journal of Internal Medicine), 1959; 12:1169
29. *Yun Nan Zhong Yi Xue Yuan Xue Bao* (Journal of Yunnan University School of Medicine), 1983; 1:20
30. *Zhong Hua Wai Ke Za Zhi* (Chinese Journal of External Medicine), 1959; 7:656
31. *Hu Nan Yi Yao Za Zhi* (Hunan Journal of Medicine and Herbology), 1976; 2:58
32. *Zhong Hua Wai Ke Za Zhi* (Chinese Journal of External Medicine), 1959; 10:1029
33. *Lancet* 2000 Jan 8; 355(9198):134-8
34. Wicht, M. *Herbal Drugs and Phytopharmaceuticals*, 1994
35. *Zhong Yao Tong Bao* (Journal of Chinese Herbology), 1986; 11(10):55
36. *Zhong Yao Zhi* (Chinese Herbology Journal), 1993; 358
37. *Zhong Yao Xue* (Chinese Herbology), 1998; 759:765
38. *Zhi Wu Yao You Xiao Cheng Fen Shou Ce* (Manual of Plant Medicinals and Their Active Constituents), 1986: 521; 522; 510; 672
39. *Zhong Cao Yao* (Chinese Herbal Medicine), 1991; 22(10):452
40. *Shan Dong Zhong Yi Za Zhi* (Shandong Journal of Chinese Medicine) (4): 7, 1984

Da Zao (Fructus Jujubae)

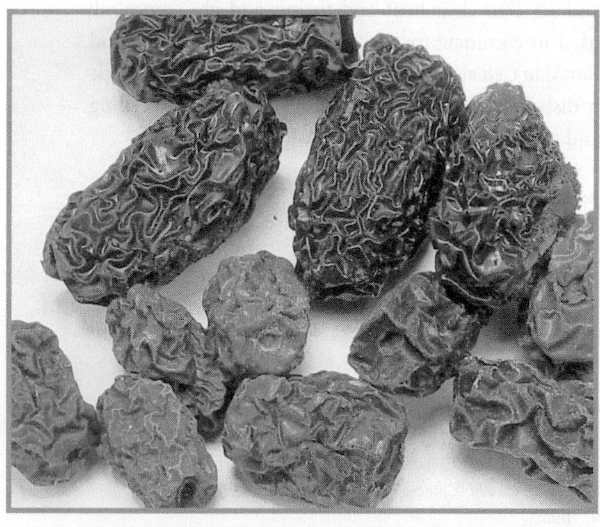

大棗 大枣

Pinyin Name: *Da Zao*
Literal Name: "big date"
Alternate Chinese Names: *Hong Da Zao, Hong Zao, Hei Da Zao, Hei Zao, Zao*
Original Source: *Shen Nong Ben Cao Jing* (Divine Husbandman's Classic of the Materia Medica) in the second century
English Name: jujube, date
Botanical Name: *Ziziphus jujuba* Mill. var. *inermis* (Bge.) Rehd. (*Zao*)
Pharmaceutical Name: Fructus Jujubae
Properties: sweet, warm
Channels Entered: Spleen, Stomach

CHINESE THERAPEUTIC ACTIONS

1. Tonifies the Spleen and Stomach, Benefits Qi

Middle *jiao* deficiency: *Da Zao* (Fructus Jujubae) tonifies the middle *jiao* to enhance the transformation and transportation functions of the Spleen and Stomach. Clinically, it treats disorders such as shortness of breath, fatigue, sallow facial appearance, decreased food intake, loose stools, and diarrhea. It may be used alone or in combination with other herbs. This herb is often made into porridge with rice and rock sugar. Because it is sweet, it is also made into cookies with digestive herbs for patients with weak digestive systems.

- Spleen and Stomach deficiencies: use *Da Zao* with *Ren Shen* (Radix Ginseng), *Bai Zhu* (Rhizoma Atractylodis Macrocephalae) and *Fu Ling* (Poria).
- Diarrhea and decreased food intake because of accumulation of dampness and cold in the Spleen and Stomach: use this herb with *Bai Zhu* (Rhizoma Atractylodis Macrocephalae), *Gan Jiang* (Rhizoma Zingiberis) and *Ji Nei Jin* (Endothelium Corneum Gigeriae Galli).

2. Tonifies Blood

Blood deficiency: *Da Zao* tonifies blood and treats disorders characterized by blood deficiency, such as yellow or sallow facial appearance, pale lips, weight loss, dizziness, blurred vision, pale nails, pale scanty menstrual discharge, and in severe cases, amenorrhea. *Da Zao* tonifies

Da Zao (Fructus Jujubae)

both qi and blood and is ideal as an adjunct herb to strengthen the body.

- Blood deficiency: use *Da Zao* as a single-herb remedy.
- Severe blood deficiency with irritability and insomnia: use this substance with *Shu Di Huang* (Radix Rehmanniae Preparata), *Dang Gui* (Radicis Angelicae Sinensis), *E Jiao* (Colla Corii Asini) and *Huang Qi* (Radix Astragali).

3. Calms the *Shen* (Spirit)

***Zang zao* (dry organ) disorder:** *Da Zao* calms the *shen* and treats irritability, disturbed sleep and emotional instability in *zang zao*, a condition characterized by Heart deficiency combined with Liver qi stagnation.

- *Zang zao* disorder: combine this herb with *Gan Cao* (Radix Glycyrrhizae) and *Xiao Mai* (Fructus Tritici). **Exemplar Formula:** *Gan Mai Da Zao Tang* (Licorice, Wheat, and Jujube Decoction).
- *Zang zao* disorder with *shen* disturbance: add this herb to *Gan Cao* (Radix Glycyrrhizae), *Xiao Mai* (Fructus Tritici), *Long Gu* (Os Draconis), *Mu Li* (Concha Ostreae), *Suan Zao Ren* (Semen Zizyphi Spinosae) and *Bai Zi Ren* (Semen Platycladi).

4. Harmonizes Other Herbs

Da Zao harmonizes the harsh and toxic effects of some other herbs and protects against damage to the internal organs.

- *Ting Li Zi* (Semen Descurainiae seu Lepidii): *Da Zao* is used with *Ting Li Zi* to prevent it from damaging Lung qi. The combination of these two herbs can be used to treat cough, wheezing and chest fullness caused by accumulation of phlegm in the chest.
- *Gan Sui* (Radix Euphorbiae Kansui), *Da Ji* (Radix Euphorbiae seu Knoxiae) and *Yuan Hua* (Flos Genkwa): *Da Zao* is used with these three herbs to prevent damage to Spleen and Stomach. The combination of these herbs treats ascites with severe accumulation of water and phlegm.
- *Sheng Jiang* (Rhizoma Zingiberis Recens): *Da Zao* is frequently combined with *Sheng Jiang* to treat exterior conditions. *Sheng Jiang* induces perspiration to release the exterior, while *Da Zao* promotes generation of body fluids to prevent the excessive loss of fluids that may occur with use of exterior-releasing herbs.

Lastly, spontaneous perspiration caused by deficiency can be treated by *Da Zao*, *Fu Xiao Mai* (Semen Tritici Aestivi Levis), *Wu Mei* (Fructus Mume) and *Sang Ye* (Folium Mori).

DOSAGE

3 to 12 fruits, or 10 to 30 grams. *Da Zao* should be cracked open when used in herbal decoction. Without breaking the fruit, only 1/7th of the active components can be extracted.[1]

CAUTIONS / CONTRAINDICATIONS

- Sweet in nature, *Da Zao* may create dampness, phlegm and heat. Therefore, it is contraindicated for use as a single remedy, or at a large dosage, in cases of excess dampness, excess heat, and hot phlegm.
- *Da Zao* is not recommended in cases of intestinal parasites.
- Excessive use of *Da Zao* may lead to tooth decay, due to the high sugar content of the herb.

CHEMICAL COMPOSITION

Betulinic acid, eanothic acid, oleanolic acid, crataegolic acid, alphitonic acid, zizyphus saponin I, II, III; jujuboside A, B; mashnic acid.[2,3,4]

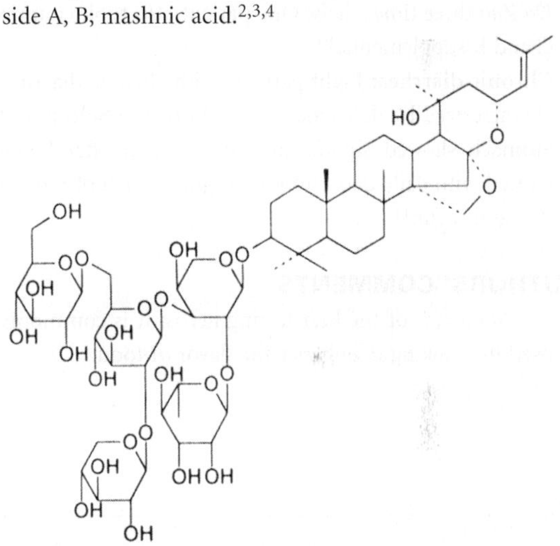

Jujuboside A

PHARMACOLOGICAL EFFECTS

- **Generalized:** In one study, 36 mice were divided equally into a treatment group and a placebo group. The treatment group received continuous administration of a 30% *Da Zao* decoction at the dosage of 0.3 ml/kg. After three weeks, the mice in the treatment group had a significant increase in body weight, muscle strength, and physical endurance when compared to the placebo group. The average weight gain was 3.0 grams in the treatment group, and 1.6 grams in placebo group. The duration of swimming time was 3 minutes and 50 seconds in treatment group, and 2 minutes and 30 seconds in placebo group.[5]
- **Antineoplastic:** Several components of *Da Zao* have demonstrated an inhibitory influence on cancer cells. Continuous administration of mashnic acid for 14 days was more effective than 5-Fluorouracil in inhibiting the growth of cancer cells.[6]
- **Sedative:** *Da Zao* has a sedative effect on the central

Da Zao (Fructus Jujubae)

nervous system. It lowers blood pressure and reduces spontaneous motor activities.[7]

- **Hepatoprotective:** *Da Zao* has a protective effect on the liver. In one study, rabbits that received injections of *Da Zao* recovered much faster from carbon tetrachloride-induced liver damage than the control group.[8]

CLINICAL STUDIES AND RESEARCH

- **Allergic purpura:** Decoction of 10 pieces of *Da Zao* given three times daily successfully treated 5 patients with allergic purpura who did not respond to vitamin C, K, diphenhydramine, or other pharmaceutical treatments.[9]
- **Allergic purpura with normal platelets:** Gradual improvement and eventual recovery from allergic purpura was reported in 6 patients who ingested 10 pieces of *Da Zao* three times daily. One patient also took vitamin C and K supplements.[10]
- **Chronic diarrhea:** Eight patients with chronic diarrhea characterized by deficiency and cold of the Spleen and Stomach showed significant improvement after being treated with daily decoction of 50 grams each of red *Da Zao* and sugar.[11]

AUTHORS' COMMENTS

Da Zao is one of the best-tasting herbs. It is commonly used for cooking to enhance the flavor of food.

Da Zao is available in black and red colors. The properties and applications of these two are essentially the same. *Hong Da Zao,* red jujube, is slightly stronger in tonifying qi. *Hei Da Zao,* black jujube, is slightly stronger in tonifying blood.

Da Zao and *Sheng Jiang* (Rhizoma Zingiberis Recens) are frequently paired. From a TCM perspective, this pair harmonizes the herbal formula and protects and/or tonifies the middle *jiao*. From the pharmacologic perspective, they promote digestive function and increase the absorption of herbs.

References

1. *Zhong Yao Tong Bao* (Journal of Chinese Herbology), 8 (3): 23-24, 1983
2. *Xian Dai Zhong Yao Yao Li Xue* (Contemporary Pharmacology of Chinese Herbs), 1997; 1207
3. *Chang Yong Zhong Yao Cheng Fen Yu Yao Li Shou Ce* (A Handbook of the Composition and Pharmacology of Common Chinese Drugs), 1994; 220
4. *Guo Wai Yi Xue Zhong Yi Zhong Yao Fen Ce* (Monograph of Chinese Herbology from Foreign Medicine), 1985; 7(4):48
5. Ibid.
6. Ibid.
7. Ibid.
8. *Guang Dong Zhong Yi* (Guangdong Chinese Medicine), 1962; 5:1
9. *Shang Hai Zhong Yi Yao Za Zhi* (Shanghai Journal of Chinese Medicine and Herbology), 1958; 11:29
10. Ibid., 1962; 4:22
11. *Xin Zhong Yi* (New Chinese Medicine), 1987; 6:56

Geng Mi (Semen Oryzae)

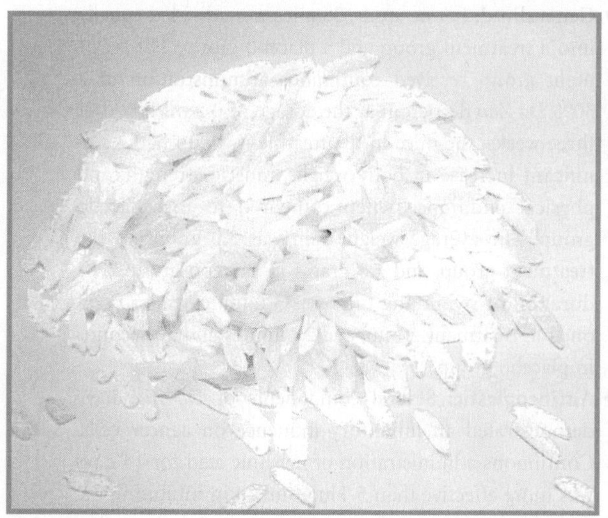

粳米

Pinyin Name: *Geng Mi*
Literal Name: "rice"
Alternate Chinese Names: *Da Mi*
English Name: rice
Botanical Name: *Oryza sativa* L. (*Dao*)
Pharmaceutical Name: Semen Oryzae
Properties: sweet, cool
Channels Entered: Spleen, Stomach

Geng Mi (Semen Oryzae)

CHINESE THERAPEUTIC ACTIONS

Tonifies the Lung, Spleen, and Intestines

Geng Mi (Semen Oryzae) tastes sweet, tonifies Lung qi, and strengthens the middle *jiao*. Clinically, it treats thirst, diarrhea, fatigue, and irritability. In addition, *Geng Mi* is sometimes used to strengthen the middle *jiao*, to prevent damage by cold and harsh herbs.

In addition, *Geng Mi* is often combined with *Shi Gao* (Gypsum Fibrosum) to prevent the cold property of the latter herb from damaging the middle *jiao*. **Exemplar Formula:** *Bai Hu Tang* (White Tiger Decoction).

DOSAGE

9 to 15 grams in decoction. This herb is commonly used as food.

Feng Mi (Mel)

蜂蜜

Pinyin Name: *Feng Mi*
Literal Name: "bee honey"
Alternate Chinese Names: *Bai Mi, Mi, Feng Tang*
Original Source: *Shen Nong Ben Cao Jing* (Divine Husbandman's Classic of the Materia Medica) in the second century
English Name: honey
Zoological Name: *Apis cerana* Fabricius; *Apis mellifera* L.
Pharmaceutical Name: Mel
Properties: sweet, neutral
Channels Entered: Spleen, Lung, Large Intestine

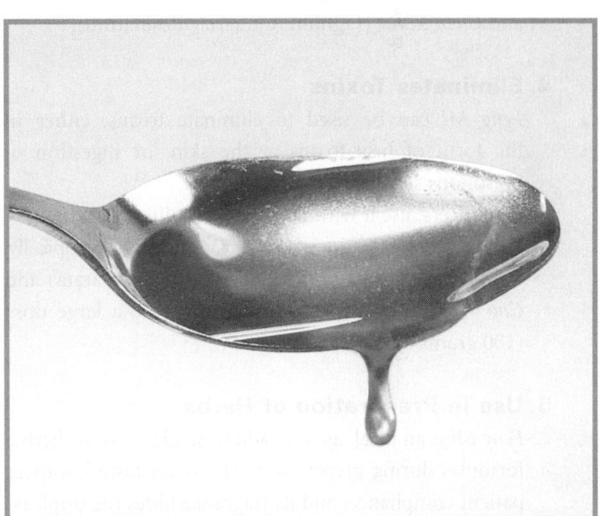

CHINESE THERAPEUTIC ACTIONS

1. Tonifies the Middle *Jiao*, Relieves Pain

Feng Mi (Mel) tonifies the Spleen and Stomach to relieve pain, increase energy, and improve appetite. It may be used individually or in combination in an herbal formula.

- Abdominal pain: use *Feng Mi* with *Bai Shao* (Radix Paeoniae Alba), *Gan Cao* (Radix Glycyrrhizae), *Gui Zhi* (Ramulus Cinnamomi) and *Gan Jiang* (Rhizoma Zingiberis).
- Hernial pain due to cold, with cold hands and feet: pair it with *Wu Tou* (Radix Aconiti).
- Deficiency of blood and body fluids: add this substance to *Sheng Di Huang* (Radix Rehmanniae), *Lu Jiao Jiao* (Gelatinum Cornu Cervi) and *Sheng Jiang* (Rhizoma Zingiberis Recens).
- Postpartum thirst and weakness: combine *Feng Mi* with *Sheng Di Huang* (Radix Rehmanniae), *Lu Jiao Jiao* (Gelatinum Cornu Cervi) and *Sheng Jiang* (Rhizoma Zingiberis Recens).

2. Moistens the Lung to Stop Cough

Feng Mi tonifies and moistens the Lung to treat chronic cases of Lung deficiency with cough.

- Chronic cough: use *Feng Mi* with juice of *Sheng Jiang* (Rhizoma Zingiberis Recens).
- Chronic cough: combine it with *Su Zi* (Fructus Perillae), the juice of *Sheng Jiang* (Rhizoma Zingiberis Recens), the juice of *Sheng Di Huang* (Radix Rehmanniae), and *Xing Ren* (Semen Armeniacae Amarum).
- Chronic cough with blood-streaked sputum: use this substance with *Ren Shen* (Radix Ginseng), *Sheng Di Huang* (Radix Rehmanniae) and *Fu Ling* (Poria).

3. Lubricates the Bowels to Relieve Constipation

Feng Mi lubricates the bowels to relieve constipation caused by dryness and lack of fluids. It may be used alone, as a suppository, or orally in combination with other herbs.

17 TONIC HERBS

Feng Mi (Mel)

- Constipation: use 30 to 60 grams of *Feng Mi* as a single remedy.
- Constipation with blood deficiency: use it with *Dang Gui* (Radicis Angelicae Sinensis), and *Hei Zhi Ma* (Semen Sesami Nigrum).
- Constipation with yin deficiency: add it to *Xuan Shen* (Radix Scrophulariae), *Zhi Mu* (Radix Anemarrhenae) and *Sheng Di Huang* (Radix Rehmanniae).
- Constipation with yang deficiency: combine this substance with *Suo Yang* (Herba Cynomorii) and *Rou Cong Rong* (Herba Cistanches).
- Constipation with interior heat: use it with *Jue Ming Zi* (Semen Cassiae), *Gua Lou Shi* (Fructus Trichosanthis), and *Da Huang* (Radix et Rhizoma Rhei).
- Constipation with qi stagnation: use *Feng Mi* with *Zhi Ke* (Fructus Aurantii), *Xing Ren* (Semen Armeniacae Amarum), and *Chen Xiang* (Lignum Aquilariae Resinatum).

4. Eliminates Toxins

Feng Mi can be used to eliminate toxins, either in the form of heat-toxins at the skin, or ingestion of poisonous substances.

- Oral ulcers: use it with *Da Qing Ye* (Folium Isatidis).
- Various sores and lesions: use *Feng Mi* individually topically.
- Poisoning by *Chuan Wu* (Radix Aconiti Preparata) and *Cao Wu* (Radix Aconiti Kusnezoffii): use a large dose (100 grams or more) of *Feng Mi*.

5. Use in Preparation of Herbs

Feng Mi is an ideal agent to add to single herbs or herbal formulas during preparation. The sweet taste improves patient compliance, and its fragrance hides the unpleasant smell of some herbs. Sticky in physical property, it combines well with powders to facilitate the process of making pills.

DOSAGE

15 to 30 grams orally. Use an adequate amount of *Feng Mi* for processing herbs, making pills, and for topical applications.

CAUTIONS / CONTRAINDICATIONS

- *Feng Mi* should be used with caution in cases of dampness, interior phlegm, or in patients with abdominal fullness and bloating.
- It should be used with caution in cases of loose stools or diarrhea.
- Allergic reaction is sometimes observed in children who ingest natural honey. Symptoms include urticaria and gastrointestinal disturbance.
- Ingestion of raw honey is not recommended for infants less than 12 months old because of infant botulism.

CHEMICAL COMPOSITION

Dextrose, fructose, sucrose, dextrin, malic and acetic acid.[1]

PHARMACOLOGICAL EFFECTS

- **Hepatoprotective:** Use of *Feng Mi* is associated with a hepatoprotective effect in rats treated with carbon tetrachloride.[2]
- **Antibiotic:** Raw *Feng Mi* has shown some antibiotic effects. However, most commercial products are devoid of such activity, possibly because the heat used during processing destroys these effects.[3]

CLINICAL STUDIES AND RESEARCH

- **Intestinal obstruction:** Patients with intestinal obstruction were treated with suppositories of *Feng Mi*. Out of 77 patients, 50 showed positive response within one dose. The suppositories were 3 to 6 cm long and were made by cooking *Feng Mi* until it turns solid.[4]
- **Overdose of *Wu Tou* (Radix Aconiti):** In one study, 11 cases of *Wu Tou* poisoning were treated with 50 to 100 grams of *Feng Mi*, taken with warm water. Most patients begin to show relief within 30 minutes, and all began to recover within 1 to 2 hours.[5]
- **Sinusitis and rhinitis:** Injection of a preparation containing 40% *Feng Mi* showed 94.6% effectiveness among 276 patients. The treatment protocol was to inject 2 to 4 ml of the preparation bilaterally into local areas surrounding the nose three times daily for 4 days per course of treatment. Patients with atrophic sinusitis or rhinitis were less responsive to the treatment.[6]
- **Burns:** Topical application of *Feng Mi* to the affected area four to five times daily showed marked effectiveness to relieve pain and facilitate recovery from the wounds.[7]

AUTHORS' COMMENTS

Feng Mi has two main functions when used to make herbal pills. It helps to bind the herbal powder together, and it acts as a reservoir to slowly release all the herbs into the gastrointestinal tract for extended absorption and therapeutic effect of the herbs. Use of *Feng Mi* in herbal pills improves patient compliance by reducing the frequency of dosing from three or four times daily to one or two doses daily.

References

1. *Zhong Yao Xue* (Chinese Herbology), 1998; 771-776
2. Ibid.
3. Ibid.
4. *Guang Zhou Yi Yao* (Guangzhou Medicine and Medicinals), 1984; 4:63
5. *He Bei Zhong Yi* (Hebei Chinese Medicine), 1986; 2:33
6. *He Bei Yi Yao* (Hebei Medicine and Herbology), 1981; 5:61
7. *Zhong Hua Wai Ke Za Zhi* (Chinese Journal of External Medicine), 1962; 2:110

Yi Tang (Saccharum Granorum)

飴糖 饴糖

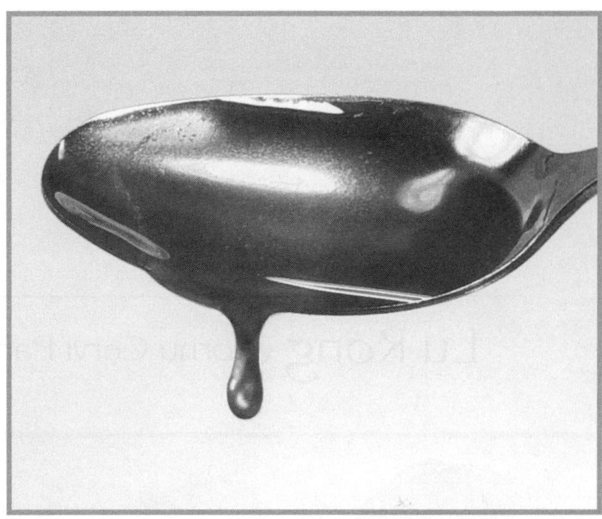

Pinyin Name: *Yi Tang*
Alternate Chinese Names: *Jiao Yi*
Original Source: *Ming Yi Za Zhu* (Miscellaneous Records of Famous Physicians) by Tao Hong-Jing in 500 A.D.
English Name: maltose, barley malt sugar
Pharmaceutical Name: Saccharum Granorum
Properties: sweet, warm
Channels Entered: Spleen, Stomach, Lung

CHINESE THERAPEUTIC ACTIONS

1. Tonifies the Spleen, Benefits Qi

Spleen and Stomach deficiencies: Sweet and warm, *Yi Tang* (Saccharum Granorum) treats fatigue, shortness of breath, and poor appetite caused by Spleen and Stomach deficiencies.

- Spleen and Stomach deficiencies: use *Yi Tang* with *Huang Qi* (Radix Astragali), *Dang Shen* (Radix Codonopsis), *Zhi Gan Cao* (Radix Glycyrrhizae Preparata), and *Da Zao* (Fructus Jujubae).

2. Relieves Pain

Abdominal pain: *Yi Tang* nourishes the middle *jiao* to treat abdominal pain caused by deficiency and cold. Such conditions are often characterized by pain that is alleviated by warmth and pressure, and by aversion to cold, and loose stools.

- Abdominal pain due to deficiency and cold: use *Yi Tang* with *Gui Zhi* (Ramulus Cinnamomi), *Sheng Jiang* (Rhizoma Zingiberis Recens), *Bai Shao* (Radix Paeoniae Alba), *Zhi Gan Cao* (Radix Glycyrrhizae Preparata) and *Da Zao* (Fructus Jujubae). **Exemplar Formula:** *Xiao Jian Zhong Tang* (Minor Construct the Middle Decoction).
- Abdominal pain from qi deficiency: use it with *Huang Qi* (Radix Astragali).
- Abdominal pain due to blood deficiency: combine this substance with *Dang Gui* (Radicis Angelicae Sinensis). **Exemplar Formula:** *Dang Gui Jian Zhong Tang* (Tangkuei Decoction to Construct the Middle).
- Chest and abdominal coldness and pain, cold limbs, nausea, and vomiting due to yang deficiency and cold stagnation: add *Yi Tang* to *Gan Jiang* (Rhizoma Zingiberis), *Hua Jiao* (Pericarpium Zanthoxyli), and *Ren Shen* (Radix Ginseng). **Exemplar Formula:** *Da Jian Zhong Tang* (Major Construct the Middle Decoction).

3. Moistens the Lung, Relieves Cough

Yi Tang treats cough caused by dryness in the Lung, or by qi deficiency, with or without sputum.

- Cough: use this substance with *Xing Ren* (Semen Armeniacae Amarum), *Bai Bu* (Radix Stemonae), and *Sha Shen* (Radix Glehniae seu Adenophorae).

4. Coats Foreign Objects

Yi Tang can be used to treat obstruction of the throat caused by fishbones or other objects. The patient should swallow small portions of the thick liquid slowly, so it can coat the obstructing substance and facilitate its passage.

DOSAGE

30 to 60 grams in decoction. *Yi Tang* is used in syrup or pill forms as well.

CAUTIONS / CONTRAINDICATIONS

- Use *Yi Tang* with caution in patients with middle *jiao* dampness, or those who are vomiting because of stagnation.
- Use of *Yi Tang* is contraindicated in patients with heat or phlegm.
- It is contraindicated in children with *gan ji* (infantile malnutrition) or cough caused by hot phlegm.

CHEMICAL COMPOSITION

Maltose, protein, lipid, vitamin B.[1]

AUTHORS' COMMENTS

Restless fetus and unstable pregnancy can be treated with the combination of *Yi Tang* and *Sha Ren* (Fructus Amomi).

References

1. *Zhong Yao Xue* (Chinese Herbology), 1998; 769-771

Section 2

— Yang-Tonifying Herbs

Lu Rong (Cornu Cervi Pantotrichum)

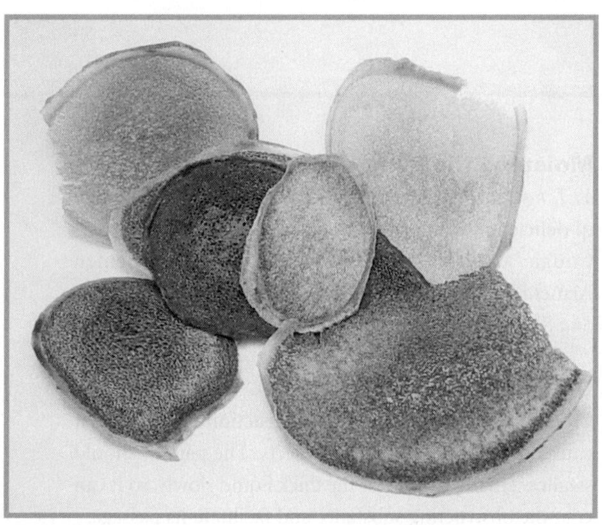

鹿茸 鹿茸

Pinyin Name: *Lu Rong*
Literal Name: "deer antler"
Original Source: *Shen Nong Ben Cao Jing* (Divine Husbandman's Classic of the Materia Medica) in the second century
English Name: deer antler, hairy deer horn, hairy antler
Zoological Name: *Cervus nippon* Temmiinck (*Mei Hua Lu*); *Cervus elaphus* L. (*Ma Lu*)
Pharmaceutical Name: Cornu Cervi Pantotrichum
Properties: sweet, salty, warm
Channels Entered: Kidney, Liver

CHINESE THERAPEUTIC ACTIONS

1. Tonifies Kidney Yang and Replenishes Kidney *Jing* (Essence)

Kidney yang deficiency with impotence: *Lu Rong* (Cornu Cervi Pantotrichum) treats Kidney yang and *jing* (essence) deficiencies with symptoms such as impotence, spermatorrhea, nocturnal emissions, soreness and weakness of the lower back and knees, weakness of sinews and joints, dizziness, lassitude and tinnitus.

- Impotence or spermatorrhea: combine *Lu Rong* with *Ren Shen* (Radix Ginseng), *Shu Di Huang* (Radix Rehmanniae Preparata), *Shan Yao* (Rhizoma Dioscoreae), *Gou Qi Zi* (Fructus Lycii), and *Yin Yang Huo* (Herba Epimedii). This formula may be taken as powder, or soaked in grain-based liquor to make medicinal tincture.

Infertility, leukorrhea: Insufficient Kidney fire results in deficiencies of the *ren* (conception) and *chong* (thoroughfare) channels. Clinical manifestations include clear, watery leukorrhea, constant uterine bleeding, or infertility in women. This substance warms Kidney yang and the uterus, regulates menstruation and helps to contract the uterus to stop bleeding.

- Infertility caused by deficiencies of Kidney yang and the *ren* (conception) and *chong* (thoroughfare) channels: use *Lu Rong* individually in powder.
- Uterine bleeding, clear vaginal discharge: combine it with *Shu Di Huang* (Radix Rehmanniae Preparata), *Rou Cong Rong* (Herba Cistanches), and *Hai Piao Xiao* (Endoconcha Sepiae).

2. Nourishes Blood, *Ren* (Conception) and *Chong* (Thoroughfare) Channels

Severe anemia due to blood and Kidney *jing* (essence) deficiencies: Blood and *jing* arise from the same source. In cases of severe blood deficiency or loss, *jing* will be lost as well. *Lu Rong* tonifies blood and nourishes *jing* to promote production of red blood cells and reticulocytes. Therefore, *Lu Rong* is best for thin and weak patients with severe blood and *jing* deficiencies.

- Severe anemia: combine *Lu Rong* with *Huang Qi* (Radix Astragali), *Dang Shen* (Radix Codonopsis), and *Dang Gui* (Radicis Angelicae Sinensis).

Lu Rong (Cornu Cervi Pantotrichum)

3. Strengthens Sinews and Bones

Weakness of sinews and bones: The Kidney stores *jing* (essence), which is vital to strong bones. The Liver stores blood and controls the sinews and tendons. When the Liver and Kidney are deficient, the bones, sinews and joints become weak. Deficiencies of Kidney yang and *jing* in children manifest in mental retardation, learning disabilities and delayed mental and physical growth. Deficiencies of Kidney yang and *jing* in elderly patients may lead to *wei* (atrophy) syndrome.

- Weakness of sinews and bones: use *Lu Rong* individually in powder form.
- Developmental delays in children: use *Lu Rong* individually in powder form.
- *Wei* (atrophy) syndrome: combine this substance with *Suo Yang* (Herba Cynomorii), *Niu Xi* (Radix Cyathulae seu Achyranthis), *Shu Di Huang* (Radix Rehmanniae Preparata), *Xu Duan* (Radix Dipsaci) and *Ji Xue Teng* (Caulis Spatholobi).

Delayed healing of broken or fractured bones: *Lu Rong* is often used in the trauma departments of hospitals in China to promote healing of bones.

- Delayed healing of broken or fractured bones: combine this substance with *Huang Qi* (Radix Astragali), *Wu Jia Pi* (Cortex Acanthopanacis), *Gu Sui Bu* (Rhizoma Drynariae), and *Yin Yang Huo* (Herba Epimedii).

4. Heals Chronic Yin Sores and Boils

Chronic yin sores and boils that are concave, discharging a clear fluid, slow-healing in nature, with dark, dull skin surrounding the lesion: apply *Lu Rong* powder topically.

DOSAGE

1 to 2 grams. Because *Lu Rong* is quite expensive, this substance is usually not decocted with other herbs. In powder form, it is taken with the decoction. *Lu Rong* can be used as powder or soaked in grain-based liquor to enhance its warming effect.

CAUTIONS / CONTRAINDICATIONS

- Use of *Lu Rong* is contraindicated in patients with yin-deficient heat, phlegm-heat in the Lung, Stomach fire, and excess or stagnant conditions caused by heat.
- It should not be used if the patient is bleeding because of yin-deficient fire.

OVERDOSAGE

Acute overdose of *Lu Rong* is characterized by tremor, dyspnea, tearing, gastrointestinal disturbances, and dermal redness and itching.[1]

CHEMICAL COMPOSITION

Pantocrine, lysophosphatidyl choline, ganglioside, putrescine, spermindine, spermine, PGE_1, PGE_2, PGF, condroitin sulfate, androgen, estradiol, oestrone, ceramide, lecithin, cephalin, cholesterol, lipids, ganglioside, sphingomyeline, calcium phosphate, calcium carbonate.[2]

PHARMACOLOGICAL EFFECTS

- **Cardiovascular:** As evaluated in various animal studies, the cardiovascular effect of *Lu Rong* varies according to dosage. At low doses, there is no significant change. At moderate doses, it displays positive chronotropic and inotropic effects, leading to increased cardiac output. At large doses, it has negative chronotropic and inotropic effects, leading to dilation of blood vessels and decreased blood pressure. Its clinical applications include treatment of arrhythmia and hypotension caused by profuse blood loss.[3]
- **Endocrine:** Plasma levels of testosterone were evaluated in mice who received oral administration of *Lu Rong* at the dosage of 100 to 200 mg/kg. Testosterone levels increased significantly in old and young mice, but no change was observed in normal adult mice.[4]
- **Gastrointestinal:** *Lu Rong* stimulates the production of PGE_2 and is commonly used for treatment of peptic ulcers.[5]
- **Effect on healing:** Pantocrine, one component of *Lu Rong*, has been shown to enhance healing of chronic wounds, ulcerations, and bone fractures.[6]
- **General strengthening:** Pantocrine, one component of *Lu Rong*, is a general tonic that has demonstrated marked effectiveness to increase work capacity, improve sleep, increase appetite, and decrease muscle fatigue. Long-term administration of *Lu Rong* is associated with an increase in body weight and red blood cell count.[7]

CLINICAL STUDIES AND RESEARCH

- **Hyperplasia of mammary glands:** An injectable preparation of *Lu Rong* showed 87.2% effectiveness in treating 86 women with hyperplasia of the mammary glands. The treatment protocol was to administer 2 ml via intramuscular injection, twice daily for 10 to 15 days prior to menstruation.[8]
- **Diarrhea:** Patients with diarrhea characterized by deficiency of Kidney yang were treated with one intramuscular injection of *Lu Rong* daily, or every other day, for a total of two doses. Out of 16 patients, 12 had complete recovery, 3 showed moderate improvement, and 1 showed no response.[9]
- **Impotence:** Intramuscular injection of *Lu Rong* given every other day and oral ingestion of herbs daily were used to treat 42 patients with impotence, with marked

Lu Rong (Cornu Cervi Pantotrichum)

effectiveness. The treatment protocol was to inject 0.5 ml of *Lu Rong* into the acupuncture points *Qihai* (CV 6), *Guanyuan* (CV 4), *Zhongji* (CV 3), *Qugu* (CV 2) and *Zusanli* (ST 36), and 1.0 ml into *Mingmen* (GV 4). The composition of the herbal formula varied depending on the presentation of each patient.[10]

- **Atrioventricular block:** In one study, 20 patients with atrioventricular block were treated with 2.0 ml intramuscular injection of *Lu Rong* for 25 to 30 days with an 85% effective rate.[11]

TOXICOLOGY

The LD_{50} of pantocrine in mice is 34.0 ml/kg via intravenous injection, 104 ml/kg via intraperitoneal injection, 114 ml/kg via subcutaneous injection, 97.8 ml/kg via intramuscular injection, and 117 ml/kg via oral ingestion.[12]

SUPPLEMENT

- 麋茸 / 麋茸 *Mi Rong* (Cornu Elaphuri Pantotrichum), first cited in the *Xin Xiu Ben Cao* (Newly Revised Materia Medica) by Su Jing in 657-659 A.D., is immature deer antler with hair. The taste, property, channels entered, functions, and contraindications are similar to those of *Lu Rong*.

AUTHORS' COMMENTS

According to the doctrine of similarity, it is believed that because animals are closer to human beings than plants or other substances, animal substances will be more beneficial than plants or minerals in tonifying the *jing* (essence) of the body.

According to *Ben Cao Gang Mu* (Materia Medica), deer are considered to be among the animals most helpful for tonifying yang and *jing* (essence). In addition to the horn and antler, many other deer parts tonify yang and replenish *jing*, such as deer blood, bone marrow, kidney and placenta.

References

1. *Yao Xue Xue Bao* (Journal of Herbology), 1991; 26(9):714
2. *Xian Dai Zhong Yao Yao Li Xue* (Contemporary Pharmacology of Chinese Herbs), 1997; 1232-1233
3. *Yi Xue Xue Bao* (Report of Medicine), 1991; 26(9):714
4. *Chem Pharm Bull*, 1988; 36:2587:2593
5. *Yao Xue Xue Bao* (Journal of Herbology), 1985; 20:321
6. Ibid., 1991; 26(9):714
7. *Zhong Yao Da Ci Dian* (Dictionary of Chinese Herbs), 1977:2232
8. *Shang Hai Zhong Yi Yao Za Zhi* (Shanghai Journal of Chinese Medicine and Herbology), 1980; 3:31
9. *Ji Lin Zhong Yi Yao* (Jilin Chinese Medicine and Herbology), 1985; 2:22
10. *Zhe Jiang Zhong Yi Za Zhi* (Zhejiang Journal of Chinese Medicine), 1983; 11:498
11. *Zhe Jiang Yi Xue* (Zhejiang Journal of Medicine), 1988; 1:22
12. *Yao Xue Xue Bao* (Journal of Herbology), 1991; 26(9):714

Lu Jiao (Cornu Cervi)

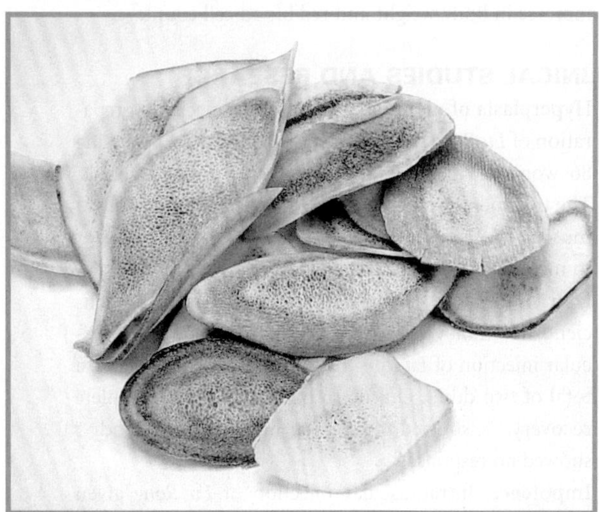

鹿角 鹿角

Pinyin Name: *Lu Jiao*
Literal Name: "deer horn"
Original Source: *Shen Nong Ben Cao Jing* (Divine Husbandman's Classic of the Materia Medica) in the second century
English Name: deer horn
Zoological Name: *Cervus nippon* Temmiinck (*Mei Hua Lu*); *Cervus elaphus* L. (*Ma Lu*)
Pharmaceutical Name: Cornu Cervi
Properties: salty, warm
Channels Entered: Kidney, Liver

Lu Jiao (Cornu Cervi)

CHINESE THERAPEUTIC ACTIONS

1. Tonifies Kidney Yang

Kidney yang deficiency: *Lu Jiao* (Cornu Cervi) is used as a less-expensive substitute for *Lu Rong* (Cornu Cervi Pantotrichum). However, *Lu Jiao* is much less potent than *Lu Rong*. *Lu Jiao* is applicable for patients who present with uterine bleeding, clear vaginal discharge, diarrhea and poor appetite caused by deficiencies of Spleen and Kidney yang and of the *ren* (conception) and *chong* (thoroughfare) channels.

- Back pain from yang deficiency: combine *Lu Jiao* with *Du Zhong* (Cortex Eucommiae), *Xu Duan* (Radix Dipsaci), *Bu Gu Zhi* (Fructus Psoraleae) and *Fu Zi* (Radix Aconiti Lateralis Praeparata).

2. Invigorates Blood Circulation and Disperses Blood Stasis

Lu Jiao treats low back and joint pain by tonifying the Kidney and regulating blood circulation.

- Pain in the back and joints: *Lu Jiao* can be taken individually, or with other herbs, to relieve pain.

3. Reduces Swelling

Lu Jiao treats toxic sores, breast abscesses and swellings caused by blood stagnation.

- Sores: apply *Lu Jiao* powder topically.

DOSAGE

5 to 10 grams. *Lu Jiao* can be cooked in decoctions, taken in powder internally, or applied topically.

CAUTIONS / CONTRAINDICATIONS

- *Lu Jiao* is contraindicated in patients with yin-deficient heat, phlegm-heat in the Lung, Stomach fire, or excess or stagnant conditions caused by heat. It should not be used if the patient is bleeding due to yin-deficient fire.

CHEMICAL COMPOSITION

Gelatin 25%, calcium phosphate 50-60%, calcium carbonate, amino acids.[1]

SUPPLEMENT

- 麋角 *Mi Jiao* (Cornu Elaphuri), first cited in *Ming Yi Za Zhu* (Miscellaneous Records of Famous Physicians) by Tao Hong-Jing in 500 A.D., is dried deer horn. Its taste, property, channels entered, and functions are similar to those of *Lu Jiao* (Cornu Cervi).

AUTHORS' COMMENTS

Lu Jiao is the horn of mature male deer. In comparison with *Lu Rong* (Cornu Cervi Pantotrichum), *Lu Jiao* more strongly reduces swelling and invigorates blood circulation, but has weaker action to tonify yang. *Lu Jiao* is less expensive, and is sometimes used as a substitute for *Lu Rong*.

References

1. *Chang Yong Zhong Yao Cheng Fen Yu Yao Li Shou Ce* (A Handbook of the Composition and Pharmacology of Common Chinese Drugs), 1994, 16151.

Lu Jiao Jiao (Gelatinum Cornu Cervi)

鹿角膠 鹿角胶

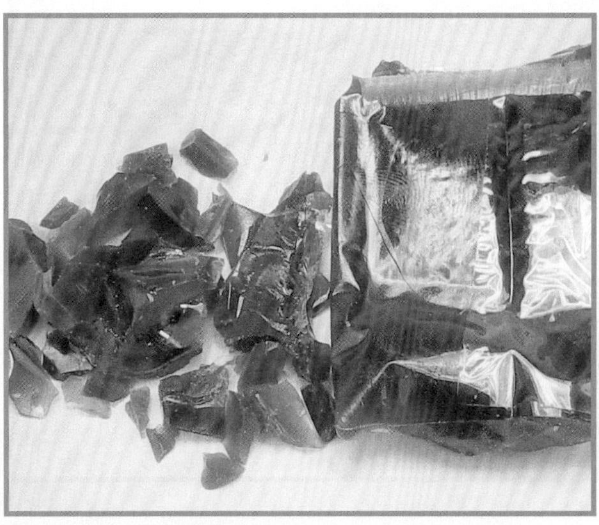

Pinyin Name: *Lu Jiao Jiao*
Literal Name: "deer horn gelatin"
Alternate Chinese Names: *Bai Jiao*
English Name: deer horn gelatin
Zoological Name: *Cervus nippon* Temmiinck (*Mei Hua Lu*); *Cervus elaphus* L. (*Ma Lu*)
Pharmaceutical Name: Gelatinum Cornu Cervi
Properties: sweet, salty, warm
Channels Entered: Liver, Kidney

Lu Jiao Jiao (Gelatinum Cornu Cervi)

CHINESE THERAPEUTIC ACTIONS

1. Tonifies the Liver and Kidney

Kidney yang and *jing* (essence) deficiencies: *Lu Jiao Jiao* (Gelatinum Cornu Cervi), though not as strong as *Lu Rong* (Cornu Cervi Pantotrichum) in tonifying the Kidney, is often used as a substitute because it is less expensive. It is best used when the patient has both Kidney yang deficiency and *jing* exhaustion. The applications include *wei* (atrophy) syndrome, weight loss, and various signs of bleeding such as abnormal uterine bleeding, epistaxis, urinary bleeding or hematemesis.

- Uterine bleeding, or clear, watery leukorrhea: combine *Lu Jiao Jiao* with *Pu Huang* (Pollen Typhae), and *Hai Piao Xiao* (Endoconcha Sepiae).
- Impotence: use this substance with *Du Zhong* (Cortex Eucommiae), *Rou Cong Rong* (Herba Cistanches) and *Yin Yang Huo* (Herba Epimedii).
- Malnutrition and delayed physical growth in children: use it with *Shu Di Huang* (Radix Rehmanniae Preparata), *Shan Zhu Yu* (Fructus Corni), *Shan Yao* (Rhizoma Dioscoreae) and *Fu Ling* (Poria).

2. Yin Sores

Lu Jiao Jiao can be used internally or topically to treat various types of sores and skin lesions.

- Yin sores: use *Lu Jiao Jiao* with *Ma Huang* (Herba Ephedrae), *Shu Di Huang* (Radix Rehmanniae Preparata), *Bai Jie Zi* (Semen Sinapis) and *Rou Gui* (Cortex Cinnamomi).
- Chronic yin sores and boils that are concave, discharging clear fluid and are slow-healing in nature: apply *Lu Jiao Jiao* powder topically.

DOSAGE

5 to 10 grams. Dissolve *Lu Jiao Jiao* in hot water, or in heated grain-based liquor. It can also be made into pills, powder or paste.

CAUTIONS / CONTRAINDICATIONS

- *Lu Jiao Jiao* is contraindicated in cases of yin-deficient fire.
- It is contraindicated in patients without exhaustion of *jing* (essence) and blood.
- It is also contraindicated in cases in which there is no deficiency of *ming men* (life gate) fire.

CHEMICAL COMPOSITION

See *Lu Jiao* (Cornu Cervi).

AUTHORS' COMMENTS

Lu Jiao Jiao is used mainly to warm the lower *jiao* (primarily the Kidney) to tonify the yin within the yang, generate *jing* (essence) and blood, and stop uterine bleeding. It has effects similar to, but weaker than those of *Lu Rong* (Cornu Cervi Pantotrichum).

Lu Jiao Shuang (Cornu Cervi Degelatinatum)

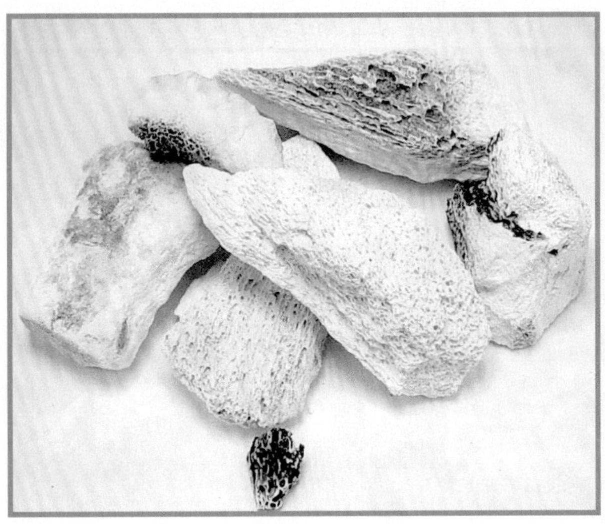

鹿角霜 鹿角霜

Pinyin Name: *Lu Jiao Shuang*
Literal Name: "deer horn fragments"
Original Source: *Ben Cao Pin Hui Jing Yao* (Essentials of Materia Medica) by Liu Wen-Tai in 1505
English Name: deer horn fragments
Zoological Name: *Cervus nippon* Temminck (*Mei Hua Lu*); *Cervus elaphus* L. (*Ma Lu*)
Pharmaceutical Name: Cornu Cervi Degelatinatum
Properties: sweet, salty, slightly warm
Channels Entered: Kidney, Liver, Heart, Pericardium

Lu Jiao Shuang (Cornu Cervi Degelatinatum)

CHINESE THERAPEUTIC ACTIONS

1. Tonifies Kidney Yang, Nourishes Blood in the *Ren* (Conception) and *Chong* (Thoroughfare) Channels

Spleen and Kidney yang deficiencies: *Lu Jiao Shuang* (Cornu Cervi Degelatinatum) is the sediment left after *Lu Jiao* (Cornu Cervi) is boiled and processed into *Lu Jiao Jiao* (Gelatinum Cornu Cervi). The yang-tonic function of this substance is weaker than that of *Lu Rong* (Cornu Cervi Pantotrichum), *Lu Jiao* and *Lu Jiao Jiao*. However, it is not cloying or greasy in nature, which makes it suitable for long-term use. It also has an astringent function that is best used for patients having diarrhea and poor appetite due to Spleen and Kidney yang deficiencies. Women with uterine bleeding and profuse, clear vaginal discharge due to Kidney yang deficiency may also use *Lu Jiao Shuang*.

2. Heals Ulcers and Stops Bleeding

- For slow-healing sores: apply *Lu Jiao Shuang* powder topically.
- Bleeding from knife cuts: use it topically.

DOSAGE

10 to 15 grams. The maximum dose of *Lu Jiao Shuang* is 25 to 30 grams.

CAUTIONS / CONTRAINDICATIONS

- Use of *Lu Jiao Shuang* is contraindicated in patients with yin-deficient heat, phlegm-heat in the Lung, Stomach fire, and excess or stagnant conditions caused by heat.
- It should not be used if the patient is bleeding because of yin-deficient fire.

CLINICAL STUDIES AND RESEARCH

- **Stones in the urinary tract:** In one study, 12 patients with stones were treated with satisfactory results, using an herbal formula containing 30 grams of *Lu Jiao Shuang* as the main ingredient.[1]

References

1. *Shang Hai Zhong Yi Yao Za Zhi* (Shanghai Journal of Chinese Medicine and Herbology), 1982; 10:3

17

TONIC HERBS

Dong Chong Xia Cao (Cordyceps)

冬蟲夏草
冬虫夏草

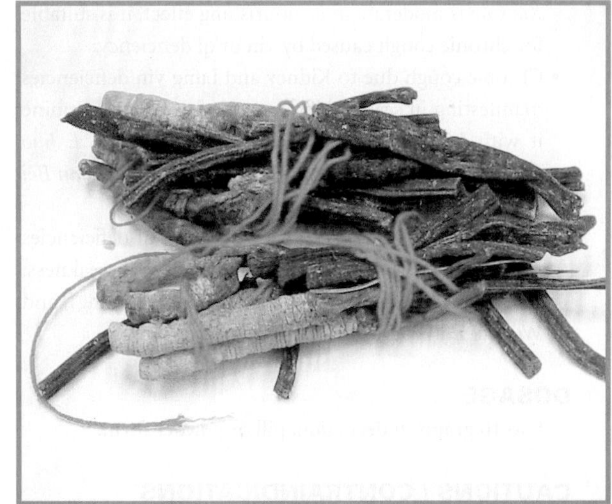

Pinyin Name: *Dong Chong Xia Cao*
Literal Name: "winter bug summer herb"
Alternate Chinese Names: *Chong Cao, Dong Chong Cao, Xia Cao Dong Chong*
Original Source: *Ben Cao Cong Xin* (Thoroughly Revised Materia Medica) by Wu Yi-Luo in 1751
English Name: cordyceps, Chinese caterpillar fungus
Botanical Name: *Cordyceps sinensis* (Berk.) Sacc. (*Dong Chong Xia Cao*); It is usually combined with the larval remains of *Hepialus varians* Staudinger.
Pharmaceutical Name: Cordyceps
Properties: sweet, warm
Channels Entered: Lung, Kidney

Dong Chong Xia Cao (Cordyceps)

CHINESE THERAPEUTIC ACTIONS

1. Tonifies Kidney Yang and Augments *Jing* (Essence)

Kidney yang and *jing* (essence) deficiencies: This condition is characterized by generalized soreness, lower back and knee weakness and pain, spermatorrhea, frequent urination, nocturnal emissions, impotence, premature ejaculation, tinnitus, forgetfulness, and poor memory. *Dong Chong Xia Cao* (Cordyceps) is also ideal for convalescing patients or those who are extremely weak, with spontaneous sweating.

- Bone and joint disorders: combine *Dong Chong Xia Cao* with *Du Zhong* (Cortex Eucommiae) and *Xu Duan* (Radix Dipsaci).
- Impotence: combine this substance with *Lu Rong* (Cornu Cervi Pantotrichum) and *Yin Yang Huo* (Herba Epimedii).
- Tinnitus: combine it with *Gou Qi Zi* (Fructus Lycii) and *Shan Zhu Yu* (Fructus Corni).
- Spontaneous sweating during recovery from chronic illness: use it with *Huang Qi* (Radix Astragali) to tonify the *wei* (defensive) *qi*. The herbs are cooked as soup with beef, lamb or duck.

2. Tonifies the Lung, Stops Bleeding and Dissolves Phlegm

Chronic respiratory disorders, cough: *Dong Chong Xia Cao* treats chronic respiratory disorders with Lung and Kidney deficiencies manifesting in consumptive cough with blood-streaked sputum. It helps to arrest cough, dispel sputum and stop bleeding. Because *Dong Chong Xia Cao* is moderate in its nourishing effect, it is suitable for chronic cough caused by yin or qi deficiency.

- Chronic cough due to Kidney and Lung yin deficiencies manifesting in scanty, blood-streaked sputum: combine it with *Mai Men Dong* (Radix Ophiopogonis), *E Jiao* (Colla Corii Asini), *Bai He* (Bulbus Lilii), and *Chuan Bei Mu* (Bulbus Fritillariae Cirrhosae).
- Chronic cough due to Kidney and Lung qi deficiencies resulting in manifesting of feeble cough and weakness: add it to *Ge Jie* (Gecko), *Ren Shen* (Radix Ginseng), and *Wu Wei Zi* (Fructus Schisandrae Chinensis).

DOSAGE

5 to 10 grams in decoction, pill or powder form.

CAUTIONS / CONTRAINDICATIONS

- Use *Dong Chong Xia Cao* with caution in exterior conditions.
- Side effects associated with the use of *Dong Chong Xia Cao* include headache, irritability, restlessness, edema and swelling of the face and extremities, epistaxis, decreased volume of urine, yellow, greasy tongue coat, and thready, rapid pulse.[1]

CHEMICAL COMPOSITION

Cordycepic acid 7 to 9%, cordycepin, 3-deoxyadenosine, amino acid approximately 25%.[2,3]

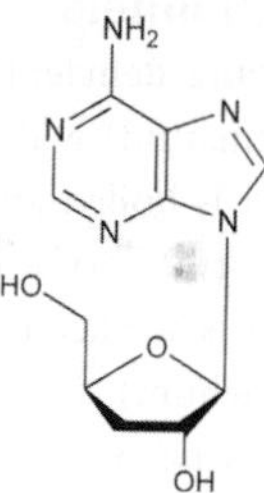

Cordycepin

PHARMACOLOGICAL EFFECTS

- **Adrenocortical:** *Dong Chong Xia Cao* has been shown to stimulate the secretion of adrenal gland hormones in mice.[4]
- **Immunostimulant:** *Dong Chong Xia Cao* has been shown to enhance the phagocytic activities of macrophages.[5]
- **Male reproductive:** Decoction of *Dong Chong Xia Cao* has been shown to increase sperm count and sperm motility in mice.[6]
- **Sedative and hypnotic:** Decoction of *Dong Chong Xia Cao* given to mice on a daily basis increases the duration and improves the quality of sleep.[7]
- **Cardiovascular:** Administration of *Dong Chong Xia Cao* is associated with a decrease in heart rate and blood pressure for over one hour. Furthermore, it decreases the oxygen requirement of the cardiac muscles in mice.[8]
- **Antiarrhythmic:** Administration of *Dong Chong Xia Cao* decreases the length and severity of aconite-induced cardiac arrhythmia in mice.[9]
- **Antihyperlipidemic:** Administration of *Dong Chong Xia Cao* lowers TG, TC, LDL and VLDL while increasing HDL in rats.[10]
- **Antibiotic:** *Dong Chong Xia Cao* has been shown to have antibiotic effect against *Staphylococcal* spp., *Streptococcal* spp., *Bacillus anthracis,* and some dermatophytes.[11]
- **Antineoplastic:** *Dong Chong Xia Cao* has demonstrated preliminary effectiveness against cancer cell activity in mice.[12]
- **Respiratory:** *Dong Chong Xia Cao* dilates and relaxes the bronchial muscles to relieve asthma. It, does not, however, have any antitussive or expectorant effects.[13]
- **Others:** Studies have demonstrated that *Dong Chong Xia Cao* increases colony-forming units (CFU) and platelets.[14,15]

CLINICAL STUDIES AND RESEARCH

- **Sexual dysfunction:** In one study, 197 patients with sexual disorders were treated with 1 gram of *Dong Chong Xia Cao* three times daily for 40 days. The rate of effectiveness

Dong Chong Xia Cao (Cordyceps)

was 64.15% in 159 patients who received cultivated *Dong Chong Xia Cao*, and 31.57% in 38 patients who received wild-crafted *Dong Chong Xia Cao*.[16]

- **Hyperlipidemia:** Administration of 1 gram of *Dong Chong Xia Cao* three times daily showed marked action to decrease LDL and TG and increase HDL in 273 patients with hyperlipidemia. Another study of 204 patients reported that *Dong Chong Xia Cao* decreases LDL but increases TG.[17,18]
- **Low platelet count:** Administration of *Dong Chong Xia Cao* is associated with an 83.3% success rate in raising platelet counts in 30 patients.[19]
- **Kidney impairment:** Compromised renal function in 117 patients was treated with 6 grams of *Dong Chong Xia Cao* three times daily, with good results.[20]
- **Tinnitus:** According to one report, 23 patients with tinnitus were treated with 6 grams of *Dong Chong Xia Cao* three times daily for up to 4 weeks, with good results.[21]
- **Arrhythmia:** An effective rate of 64.9% was reported in 57 patients with arrhythmia treated with 0.5 gram of *Dong Chong Xia Cao* three times daily for 2 weeks.[22]
- **Chronic tracheitis:** In one study, 656 patients with chronic tracheitis were treated with *Dong Chong Xia Cao* three times daily for 40 days, with good results.[23]
- **Allergic rhinitis:** Administration of 6 grams of *Dong Chong Xia Cao* three times daily for 4 weeks showed a 93% effective rate in treating 43 patients with allergic rhinitis.[24]
- **Cancer:** Malignant tumors in 30 patients were treated with 1.5 grams of *Dong Chong Xia Cao* three times daily for 2 months. The study reported improvement based on symptomatic assessment in 93% of patients.[25]

TOXICOLOGY

Dong Chong Xia Cao has an extremely low level of toxicity. Mice have been shown to tolerate up to 45 g/kg of *Dong Chong Xia Cao*, approximately 250 times the therapeutic dosage in humans. The LD_{50} in mice via intraperitoneal injection is 21.7 +/- 1.3 g/kg. Symptoms of overdose include generalized inhibition initially, followed by generalized excitation, spasms, convulsions, and respiratory depression.[26]

AUTHORS' COMMENTS

Dong Chong Xia Cao has been used recently to treat cancer, hyperlipidemia and hypertension. The cultivated herb is widely used today and the price is much lower, by comparison with the wild-crafted ones.

According to Dr. Cheng Jian-Hua, *Dong Chong Xia Cao*, *Mai Men Dong* (Radix Ophiopogonis), *Shi Hu* (Herba Dendrobii) and *Sheng Di Huang* (Radix Rehmanniae) served daily as a beverage is helpful in treating lung cancer.

References

1. *Zhong Yao Bu Liang Fan Ying Yu Zhi Liao* (Adverse Reactions and Treatment of Chinese Herbal Medicine), 1996; 218:220, 1996; 194:195
2. *Xian Dai Zhong Yao Yao Li Xue* (Contemporary Pharmacology of Chinese Herbs), 1997; 1250-1251
3. *The Merck Index* 12th edition, Chapman & Hall/CRCnetBASE/Merck, 2000
4. *Zhong Xi Yi Jie He Za Zhi* (Journal of Integrated Chinese and Western Medicine), 1990; 10(9):570
5. *Shang Hai Yi Yao Za Zhi* (Shanghai Journal of Medicine and Herbology), 1988; 1:48
6. *Zhong Yao Xue* (Chinese Herbology), 1998; 785:788
7. *Zhong Cao Yao* (Chinese Herbal Medicine), 1983; 14(5):32
8. Ibid., 1986; 17(5):17
9. Ibid., 1983; 14(5):32
10. *Zhong Yao Xue* (Chinese Herbology), 1998; 785:788
11. *Ren Min Wei Sheng Chu Ban She* (Journal of People's Public Health), 1983:358
12. *Zhong Yao Tong Bao* (Journal of Chinese Herbology), 1987; 12(2):53
13. *Fu Jian Yi Yao Za Zhi* (Fujian Journal of Medicine and Herbology), 1983; 5:311
14. *Hu Nan Yi Ke Da Xue Xue Bao* (Journal of Hunan University School of Medicine), 1989; 14(2):147
15. *Zhong Yao Tong Bao* (Journal of Chinese Herbology), 1987; 12(1):47
16. *Jiang Su Zhong Yi Yao* (Jiangsu Medicine and Herbology), 1985; 5:46
17. *Zhong Xi Yi Jie He Za Zhi* (Journal of Integrated Chinese and Western Medicine), 1985; 11:652
18. *Qing Hai Yi Yao Za Zhi* (Qinghai Journal of Medicine and Herbology), 1986; 3:22
19. *Hai Jun Yi Xue* (Navy Medicine), 1986; 2:10
20. *Shang Hai Zhong Yi Yao Za Zhi* (Shanghai Journal of Chinese Medicine and Herbology), 1986; 8:29
21. *Fu Jian Yi Yao Za Zhi* (Fujian Journal of Medicine and Herbology), 1985; 6:42
22. *Zhe Jiang Zhong Yi Xue Yuan Xue Bao* (Journal of Zhejiang University of Chinese Medicine), 1985; 6:28
23. *Zhong Cao Yao* (Chinese Herbal Medicine), 1987; 10:8
24. *Zhong Xi Yi Jie He Za Zhi* (Journal of Integrated Chinese and Western Medicine), 1987; 1:43
25. *Shang Hai Zhong Yi Yao Za Zhi* (Shanghai Journal of Chinese Medicine and Herbology), 1986; 10:25
26. *Zhong Yao Yao Li Yu Ying Yong* (Pharmacology and Applications of Chinese Herbs), 1983:358

Ge Jie (Gecko)

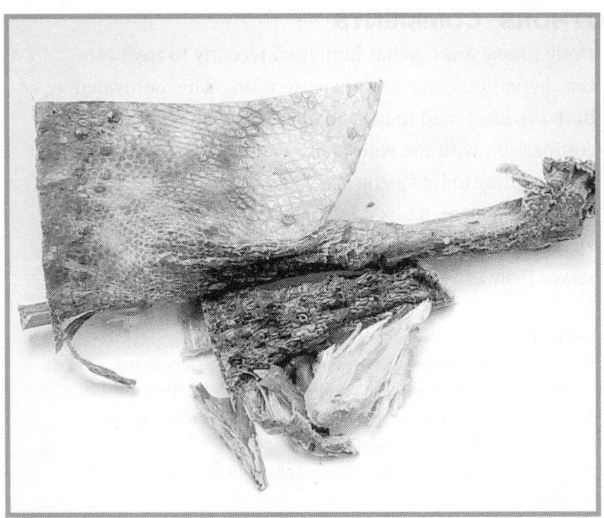

蛤蚧

Pinyin Name: *Ge Jie*
Alternate Chinese Names: *Xian Dan*
Original Source: *Shen Nong Ben Cao Jing* (Divine Husbandman's Classic of the Materia Medica) in the second century
English Name: gecko, tokay
Zoological Name: *Gekko gecko* L. (*Ge Jie*)
Pharmaceutical Name: Gecko
Properties: salty, neutral
Channels Entered: Lung, Kidney

CHINESE THERAPEUTIC ACTIONS

1. Tonifies Lung Qi and Relieves Cough and Dyspnea

Chronic cough, dyspnea and wheezing due to Lung and Kidney deficiencies: The Lung dominates qi and the Kidney is the root of qi. Chronic respiratory disorder is often characterized by both Lung and Kidney deficiencies. *Ge Jie* (Gecko) can be used to treat Lung and Kidney deficiencies with presentations of labored respiration, chronic coughing, consumptive cough with blood-streaked sputum, wheezing, low voice or inability to finish conversations (patient will need to pause to gasp for breath), shortened inhalation and prolonged exhalation, withered *shen* (spirit), spontaneous sweating, soreness, edema of the limbs, weakness of lower back and knees. The above symptoms will worsen with exertion.

- Chronic respiratory disorders with deficiency and cold signs: combine *Ge Jie* with *Ren Shen* (Radix Ginseng), *Bu Gu Zhi* (Fructus Psoraleae), *Hu Tao Ren* (Semen Juglandis). **Exemplar Formula:** *Ren Shen Ge Jie San* (Ginseng and Gecko Powder).
- Chronic respiratory disorders with yin-deficient signs of tidal fever, steaming bones sensations: combine this substance with *Xi Yang Shen* (Radix Panacis Quinquefolii), *Hu Huang Lian* (Rhizoma Picrorhizae), *Xuan Shen* (Radix Scrophulariae), and *Shu Di Huang* (Radix Rehmanniae Preparata).

2. Tonifies Kidney Yang, *Jing* (Essence) and Augments the Blood

Overindulgence in sexual activities injures the *jing* (essence) and blood. *Jing* deficiency eventually causes Kidney deficiency, and chronic blood deficiency results in Liver deficiency. Chronic deficiency of Kidney *jing* and Liver blood leads to lack of nourishment to the tendons and sinews, resulting in weakness and soreness especially of the lower back and knees.

- Impotence: combine *Ge Jie* with *Yin Yang Huo* (Herba Epimedii), *Lu Rong* (Cornu Cervi Pantotrichum) and *Shan Yao* (Rhizoma Dioscoreae). These four herbs can be soaked in grain-based liquor to make medicinal tincture.
- Weakness and soreness of bones and joints: combine this substance with *Du Zhong* (Cortex Eucommiae), *Xu Duan* (Radix Dipsaci) and *Du Huo* (Radix Angelicae Pubescentis).
- Daybreak (early morning) diarrhea: add *Ge Jie* to *Bu Gu Zhi* (Fructus Psoraleae), *Rou Dou Kou* (Semen Myristicae), and *Wu Wei Zi* (Fructus Schisandrae Chinensis).

DOSAGE

3 to 7 grams in decoctions, and 1 to 2 grams in powder form. *Ge Jie* is also used in tincture by soaking it in grain-based liquor. Liquor-fried (with grain-based liquor) *Ge Jie* has a stronger effect to tonify the Kidney. In addition, this processing facilitates the crushing and extraction of active components.

CAUTIONS / CONTRAINDICATIONS

Use of *Ge Jie* is contraindicated in cough caused by exterior conditions, or in cases of excess heat.

CHEMICAL COMPOSITION

Carnoside, carnitine, guanine, albumen, cholesterol, fatty acid, calcium, magnesium, iron, zinc, copper, sodium.[1]

PHARMACOLOGICAL EFFECTS

- **Reproductive:** In male mice, *Ge Jie* increased the weight of the testicles. In female mice, it prolonged estrus periods,

Ge Jie (Gecko)

increased the weight of the reproductive organs, and induced estrus in oophorectomized mice.[2]

- **Respiratory:** Alcohol extract of *Ge Jie* relaxes the bronchi and has marked antiasthmatic action. Water extract, on the other hand, has no significant effect.[3]
- **Immunostimulant:** Alcohol extract of the body and the tail of *Ge Jie* in mice increases the white blood cell count and phagocytic activities by the macrophages, and increases the weight of the spleen.[4]
- **Adrenocortical:** Administration of *Ge Jie* is associated with increased production of adrenocortical hormone.[5]

CLINICAL STUDIES AND RESEARCH

- **Male sexual disorder:** Patients with impotence and infertility were treated with an herbal formula containing *Ge Jie*, with satisfactory improvement within 3 treatments. The herbal formula was given with grain-based liquor two hours prior to sexual intercourse.[6]
- **Bronchitis:** In one study, 128 geriatric patients with chronic bronchitis were treated with an overall 85.9% rate of effectiveness using an herbal formula containing *Ge Jie* as the main ingredient.[7]

TOXICOLOGY

The LD_{50} in mice for oral ingestion is not available, as the dosage of 135 g/kg did not cause any fatalities. The LD_{50} in mice for water and alcohol extracts of *Ge Jie* via intraperitoneal injection is approximately 5.24 g/kg.[8]

AUTHORS' COMMENTS

The tail of *Ge Jie* has been proposed to be the most potent part. The validity of this concept, however, is currently under challenge. Studies have shown that both the tail and the body had similar active constituents and produced similar effects, when ethanol was used to extract the active components from both parts. As a result, most herbal pharmacies today will use both the body and the tail together.[9]

References

1. *Xian Dai Zhong Yao Yao Li Xue* (Contemporary Pharmacology of Chinese Herbs), 1997; 1266
2. *Zhong Yao Xue* (Chinese Herbology), 1998; 783:785
3. *Chang Yong Zhong Yao Cheng Fen Yu Yao Li Shou Ce* (A Handbook of the Composition and Pharmacology of Common Chinese Drugs), 1994, 1682:1685
4. *Zhong Cheng Yao Yan Jiu* (Research of Chinese Patent Medicine), 1991; 13(5):36
5. *Zhong Yao Xue* (Chinese Herbology), 1998; 783:785
6. *Xin Zhong Yi* (New Chinese Medicine), 1987; 2:3
7. *Zhong Yi Yao Yan Jiu* (Research of Chinese Medicine and Herbology), 1990,(2):36
8. *Zhong Cheng Yao Yan Jiu* (Research of Chinese Patent Medicine), 1991; 13(5):36
9. *Guang Xi Zhong Yi Yao* (Guangxi Chinese Medicine and Herbology), 1984; 5:48

Hu Tao Ren (Semen Juglandis)

胡桃仁 胡桃仁

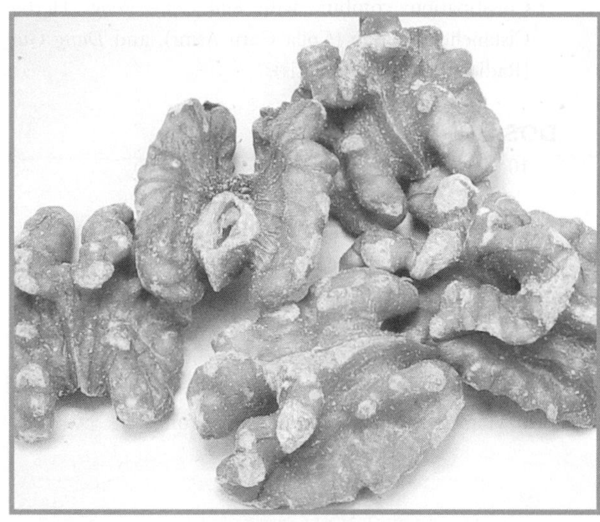

Pinyin Name: *Hu Tao Ren*
Literal Name: "barbarian peach pit"
Alternate Chinese Names: *He Tao Ren, He Tao, Qiang Tao, Hu Tao Rou*
Original Source: *Bei Ji Qian Jin Yao Fang* (Thousands of Golden Prescriptions for Emergencies)
English Name: walnut, English walnut, Persian walnut
Botanical Name: *Juglans regia* L. (*Hu Tao*)
Pharmaceutical Name: Semen Juglandis
Properties: sweet, warm
Channels Entered: Kidney, Lung, Large Intestine

Hu Tao Ren (Semen Juglandis)

CHINESE THERAPEUTIC ACTIONS

1. Tonifies the Kidney and Replenishes the *Jing* (Essence)

Kidney yang and *jing* (essence) deficiencies: Clinical manifestations of this condition include weakness of tendons and bones, back pain, prematurely gray hair, and blurry vision. *Hu Tao Ren* (Semen Juglandis) is sweet and rich in oil to nourish Kidney *jing*. This is also an important herb to strengthen the bones.

- Prematurely gray hair: combine this herb with *He Shou Wu* (Radix Polygoni Multiflori), *Nu Zhen Zi* (Fructus Ligustri Lucidi), and *Dang Gui* (Radicis Angelicae Sinensis).
- Blurry vision: use it with *Gou Qi Zi* (Fructus Lycii).
- Soreness and weakness of lower back and knees: add this herb to *Du Zhong* (Cortex Eucommiae) and *Xu Duan* (Radix Dipsaci).
- Arthritis: combine it with *Yin Yang Huo* (Herba Epimedii).

2. Warms the Lung and Arrests Wheezing

Cough and dyspnea due to cold and deficiency of the Lung: Kidney deficiency is characterized by an inability to grasp qi downwards, leading to difficulty in inhalation. When both the Lung and Kidney are deficient, there is a chronic, weak cough that worsens with exertion. *Hu Tao Ren* is most suitable for this type of chronic cough because it tonifies both Lung and Kidney.

- Chronic cough and dyspnea: serve *Hu Tao Ren* with honey.

3. Moistens the Intestines and Unblocks the Bowels

Constipation: Lack of either *jing* (essence) or blood or both leads to dry stools or constipation. *Hu Tao Ren* is rich in oil, which moistens the walls of the intestines and is most suitable for constipation that follows chronic illnesses with injured yin, or dry, difficult stools in the elderly.

- Constipation: combine with *Rou Cong Rong* (Herba Cistanches), *E Jiao* (Colla Corii Asini), and *Dang Gui* (Radicis Angelicae Sinensis).

DOSAGE

10 to 30 grams.

CAUTIONS / CONTRAINDICATIONS

- *Hu Tao Ren* should be used with caution in patients with yin-deficient fire, cough with yellow phlegm or loose stools.

CHEMICAL COMPOSITION

Linoleic acid, linolenic acid, oleic acid, carotene, vitamin B, vitamin E, calcium, phosphorus, iron.[1]

PHARMACOLOGICAL EFFECTS

- **Hematological:** Injection of *Hu Tao Ren* is associated with mild anticoagulant and thrombolytic effects in dogs.[2]
- **Anti-inflammatory:** Intravenous administration of a *Hu Tao Ren* preparation inhibited the inflammation process in mice with acute otitis media.[3]

CLINICAL STUDIES AND RESEARCH

- **Urinary stones:** *Hu Tao Ren* was shown to have a beneficial effect in treating stones in the urinary tract in two separate clinical studies.[4,5]
- **Dermatological disorders:** In one study, 170 patients with eczema or dermatitis were treated topically with a *Hu Tao Ren* preparation with a 76.2% rate of effectiveness. The topical paste was 30% *Hu Tao Ren* oil, and was prepared by stir-frying the herb to extract the oil.[6]

HERB-DRUG INTERACTION

- **Anticoagulant or antiplatelet drugs:** *Hu Tao Ren* has anticoagulant and thrombolytic effects, and should be used with caution in patients who take anticoagulant or antiplatelet medications. Though this potential interaction has not been documented, this herb may potentiate the effect of drugs such as warfarin.[7] [Note: Examples of anticoagulants include heparin, warfarin (Coumadin) and enoxaparin (Lovenox); and examples of antiplatelets include aspirin, dipyridamole (Persantine), and clopidogrel (Plavix).]

AUTHORS' COMMENTS

To arrest cough, use *Hu Tao Ren* with intact skin. To lubricate the intestines, peel and discard the skin.

References

1. *Xian Dai Zhong Yao Yao Li Xue* (Contemporary Pharmacology of Chinese Herbs), 1997; 1286
2. *Shang Hai Zhong Yi Yao Za Zhi* (Shanghai Journal of Chinese Medicine and Herbology), 1985(7):45
3. *Zhong Yao Tong Bao* (Journal of Chinese Herbology), 1986; 11(11):37
4. *Zhong Hua Wai Ke Za Zhi* (Chinese Journal of External Medicine), 1957; 8:681
5. *Shan Dong Yi Yao* (Shandong Medicine and Herbology), 1980; 9:55
6. *Xin Yi Yao Xue Za Zhi* (New Journal of Medicine and Herbology), 1973; 4:24
7. Chen, J. Recognition & prevention of Herb-drug interactions, *Medical Acupuncture*, Fall/Winter 1998/1999; volume 10/number 2; 9-13

Rou Cong Rong (Herba Cistanches)

肉蓯蓉 肉苁蓉

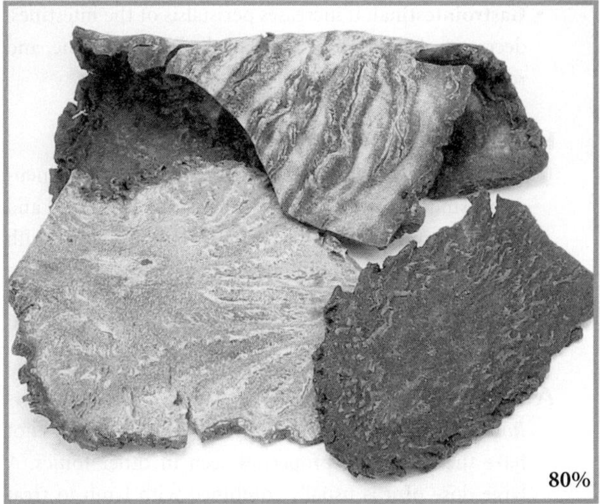
80%

Pinyin Name: *Rou Cong Rong*
Alternate Chinese Names: *Dan Da Yun, Da Yun, Cong Rong, Chang Yang*
Original Source: *Shen Nong Ben Cao Jing* (Divine Husbandman's Classic of the Materia Medica) in the second century
English Name: cistanche, desert-living cistanche
Botanical Name: *Cistanche salsa* (C.A. Mey.) G. Beck (*Rou Cong Rong*); *Cistanche deserticola* Y.C. Ma. (*Rou Cong Rong*)
Pharmaceutical Name: Herba Cistanches
Properties: sweet, salty, warm
Channels Entered: Kidney, Large Intestine

CHINESE THERAPEUTIC ACTIONS

1. Tonifies Kidney Yang, *Jing* (Essence) and Blood

Impotence, infertility: *Rou Cong Rong* (Herba Cistanches) treats impotence in men and infertility in women caused by Kidney yang deficiency with lack of *jing* (essence) and blood. *Rou Cong Rong* is a mild herb. Therefore, to achieve therapeutic effect, it is usually used in a formula, at a larger dose, and on a long-term basis.

- Impotence, infertility, spermatorrhea: use a large dose of *Rou Cong Rong* with *Lu Rong* (Cornu Cervi Pantotrichum), *Shan Yao* (Rhizoma Dioscoreae) and *Fu Ling* (Poria).
- Decreased sexual desire: combine this herb with *Yin Yang Huo* (Herba Epimedii).
- Forgetfulness, loss of hearing: use it with *Lu Rong* (Cornu Cervi Pantotrichum), *Shan Yao* (Rhizoma Dioscoreae) and *Fu Ling* (Poria).

Rou Cong Rong treats Kidney yang deficiency with such symptoms as lower back and knee soreness and pain, weakness in the joints and sinews, tinnitus, dizziness, forgetfulness, loss of hearing, clear vaginal discharge, amenorrhea or scanty menstrual flow.

- Soreness and weakness of joints: combine *Rou Cong Rong* with *Xu Duan* (Radix Dipsaci) and *Lu Rong* (Cornu Cervi Pantotrichum).

2. Moistens the Large Intestine and Facilitates the Passage of Stools

Constipation due to dryness: Chronic constipation may arise from a variety of causes, such as sudden loss of a large amount of blood, excessive perspiration, overuse of diuretic products, or simply as a result of chronic illnesses. Though *Rou Cong Rong* is warm, it is not drying. In fact, it moistens the Large Intestine and promotes bowel movement. It is best for constipation caused by yang deficiency with fluid deficiency and dryness.

- Constipation: combine it with *Huo Ma Ren* (Fructus Cannabis) and *Hei Zhi Ma* (Semen Sesami Nigrum).

DOSAGE

10 to 20 grams. The recommended dosage for *Rou Cong Rong* is relatively high, as small dosages usually do not show any immediate effect. *Rou Cong Rong* is usually fried with salt or steamed with grain-based liquor to direct the herb to the Kidney and enhance its effect to treat impotence, low back pain, and infertility.

CAUTIONS / CONTRAINDICATIONS

- *Rou Cong Rong* is contraindicated in patients with diarrhea or constipation from excess heat.
- Use of this herb is contraindicated in Kidney yin-deficient patients, or those who are easily aroused sexually but experience premature ejaculation.

CHEMICAL COMPOSITION

β-sitosterol, succinic acid, caffeic acid, amino acids, potassium, sodium, calcium, magnesium, iron, and zinc.[1]

PHARMACOLOGICAL EFFECTS

- **Immunostimulant:** Administration of water extract of *Rou Cong Rong* at the dosage of 50 to 100 mg/kg is associated with an increase in weight of the spleen, and increased phagocytic activities by the macrophages.[2]
- **Endocrine:** *Rou Cong Rong* has a stimulating effect on the endocrine system to increase secretion by the hypothalamus, pituitary gland, and reproductive organs.[3]

Rou Cong Rong (Herba Cistanches)

- **Gastrointestinal:** It increases peristalsis of the intestines, decreases absorption of water in the large intestine, and relieves constipation.[4]

HERB-DRUG INTERACTION

- **General:** *Rou Cong Rong* increases the activities of neurotransmitters, such as norepinephrine, dopamine and serotonin in the hypothalamus, and may interact with drugs such as sympathomimetics, monoamine oxidase inhibitors, selective serotonin reuptake inhibitors, and tricyclic antidepressants.[5]

AUTHORS' COMMENTS

Rou Cong Rong is a good Kidney yang tonic as it does not have the stagnating properties seen in other tonics. A large dose of it is usually combined with lamb to treat various signs of Kidney yang deficiency.

Rou Cong Rong has an effect similar to that of *Suo Yang* (Herba Cynomorii). *Rou Cong Rong* nourishes yang, *jing* (essence), and blood. *Suo Yang* similarly provides these functions, but more strongly as a yang tonic, less so as a *jing* and blood tonic. These herbs serve as a complementary team to treat the signs and symptoms associated with Kidney yang deficiency with *jing* depletion.

References

1. *Chang Yong Zhong Yao Cheng Fen Yu Yao Li Shou Ce* (A Handbook of the Composition and Pharmacology of Common Chinese Drugs), 1994; 858-859
2. *Zhong Xi Yi Jie He Za Zhi* (Journal of Integrated Chinese and Western Medicine), 1988; 8(12):736
3. *Zhong Yi Za Zhi* (Journal of Chinese Medicine), 1984; 7(7):63
4. *Chang Yong Zhong Yao Cheng Fen Yu Yao Li Shou Ce* (A Handbook of the Composition and Pharmacology of Common Chinese Drugs), 1994; 858:862
5. *Shang Hai Zhong Yi Xue Yuan Xue Bao* (Journal of Shanghai University of Chinese Medicine), 1987; 1(1):37

Suo Yang (Herba Cynomorii)

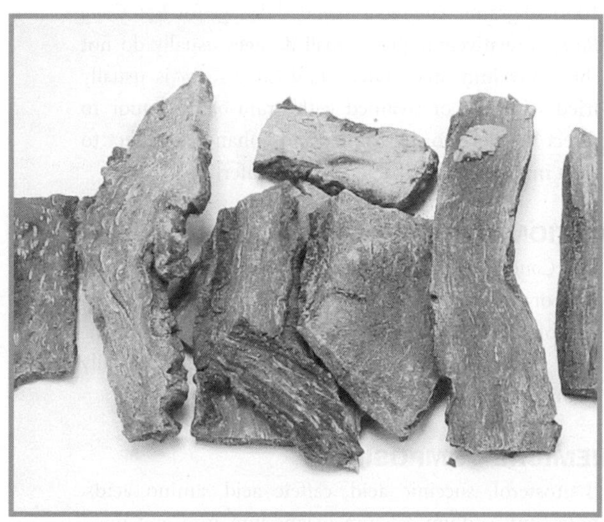

鎖陽 锁阳

Pinyin Name: *Suo Yang*
Literal Name: "lock yang," "yang locker"
Original Source: *Ben Cao Gang Mu Shi Yi* (Omissions from the Grand Materia Medica) by Zhao Xue-Min in 1765
English Name: cynomorium, songaria cynomorium
Botanical Name: *Cynomorium songaricum* Rupr. (*Suo Yang*)
Pharmaceutical Name: Herba Cynomorii
Properties: sweet, warm
Channels Entered: Liver, Kidney, Large Intestine

CHINESE THERAPEUTIC ACTIONS

1. Tonifies Kidney Yang

Impotence, infertility: Kidney *jing* (essence) deficiency, unable to support yang, causes impotence, amenorrhea and infertility. *Suo Yang* (Herba Cynomorii) nourishes Liver yin and warms Kidney yang. It more strongly assists yang and mildly nourishes *jing* and blood.

- Nocturnal emissions, impotence: use *Suo Yang* with *Rou Cong Rong* (Herba Cistanches), *Fu Ling* (Poria) and *Sang Piao Xiao* (Ootheca Mantidis) with honey.
- Soreness and weakness of the back and knees: combine it with *Shu Di Huang* (Radix Rehmanniae Preparata) and *Gui Ban* (Plastrum Testudinis). **Exemplar Formula:** *Hu Qian Wan* (Hidden Tiger Pill from the Analytic Collection).

Suo Yang (Herba Cynomorii)

2. Lubricates Intestines and Promotes Bowel Movement

Constipation due to dryness: Lack of nourishment to the intestines causes constipation or dry stools. *Suo Yang*, when used in large quantities over a prolonged period of time, moistens the intestines.

- Constipation: use *Suo Yang* with honey or with *Sang Shen Zi* (Fructus Mori).

DOSAGE

10 to 15 grams in decoction or pill form.

CAUTIONS / CONTRAINDICATIONS

- *Suo Yang* is contraindicated in patients with diarrhea caused by Spleen deficiency or constipation from excess heat.
- It is contraindicated in yin-deficient patients who are easily aroused sexually.

CHEMICAL COMPOSITION

Essential oils (ethylacetate, acetic acid, pyridine, n-hexanal, 2-furaldehyde, 2-furanacabinol, 2-heptanone, n-heptanal, 2,3,5-trimethyl-pyrazine, 2-ethyl-hexanol, tetramethyl-pyrazine, n-nonanol, methyl-n-nonanoate, ethyl-nonanoate, tetradecanoic acid, methyl hexadecanoate, methyl hexadecanoate, 2,6-diethyl-methyl-pyrarine, palmitic acid, 9-octadecenoic acid), β-sitosterol, ursolic acid, daucosterol, gallic acid, protocatechuic acid, catechin, and other inorganic components.[1,2]

PHARMACOLOGICAL EFFECTS

- **Gastrointestinal:** Oral administration of water extract of *Suo Yang* at 12.5 g/kg regulated bowel movement in mice. The initial onset of action is 20 minutes after ingestion.[3]
- **Immunostimulant:** Oral administration of alcohol extract of *Suo Yang* at 0.5 g/kg/day for 7 days increased the phagocytic activity of the macrophages in mice.[4]

References

1. *Xian Dai Zhong Yao Yao Li Xue* (Contemporary Pharmacology of Chinese Herbs), 1997; 1272
2. *Chang Yong Zhong Yao Cheng Fen Yu Yao Li Shou Ce* (A Handbook of the Composition and Pharmacology of Common Chinese Drugs), 1994; 1686-1691
3. *Zhong Yao Cai* (Study of Chinese Herbal Material), 1990; 13(10)36
4. *Zhong Guo Yi Yao Xue Bao* (Chinese Journal of Medicine and Herbology), 1989; 4(3):187

Ba Ji Tian (Radix Morindae Officinalis)

巴戟天

Pinyin Name: *Ba Ji Tian*
Alternate Chinese Names: *Ba Ji*
Original Source: *Shen Nong Ben Cao Jing* (Divine Husbandman's Classic of the Materia Medica) in the second century
English Name: morinda, medicinal Indian mulberry root
Botanical Name: *Morinda officinalis* How. (*Ba Ji Tian*)
Pharmaceutical Name: Radix Morindae Officinalis
Properties: acrid, sweet, slightly warm
Channels Entered: Kidney

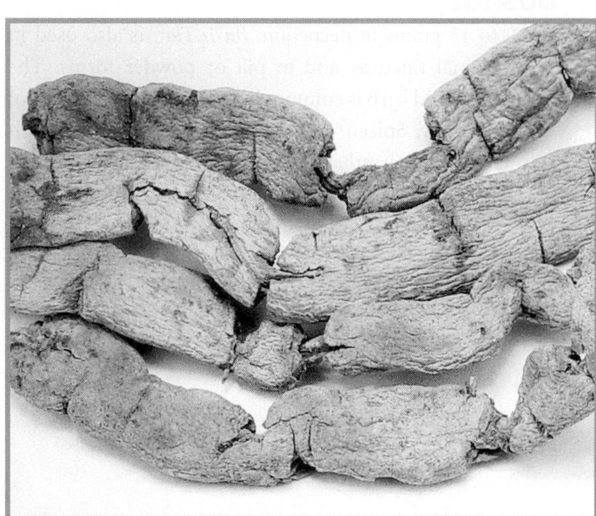

CHINESE THERAPEUTIC ACTIONS

1. Tonifies the Kidney and Assists the Yang

Impotence, infertility: In men, the chief manifestations of Kidney yang deficiency are impotence, spermatorrhea, premature ejaculation and urinary incontinence. In women, Kidney yang deficiency manifests in deficiency

Ba Ji Tian (Radix Morindae Officinalis)

and cold signs such as infertility, blood clots during menstruation, dull lower abdominal pain and coldness. *Ba Ji Tian* (Radix Morindae Officinalis) has a milder yang-tonic effect than other herbs in this category. However, it tonifies blood and *jing* (essence) at the same time.

- Urinary incontinence: combine *Ba Ji Tian* with *Yi Zhi Ren* (Fructus Alpiniae Oxyphyllae), *Sang Piao Xiao* (Ootheca Mantidis), *Tu Si Zi* (Semen Cuscutae), and salt water.
- Irregular menstruation, clear vaginal discharge and infertility: use this herb with *Rou Gui* (Cortex Cinnamomi), *Wu Zhu Yu* (Fructus Evodiae), *Gao Liang Jiang* (Rhizoma Alpiniae Officinarum), salt, and warm, grain-based liquor.
- Impotence: combine this herb with *Ren Shen* (Radix Ginseng), *Lu Rong* (Cornu Cervi Pantotrichum), *Shan Yao* (Rhizoma Dioscoreae) and *Yin Yang Huo* (Herba Epimedii).

2. Strengthens Sinews and Bones, Treats *Bi Zheng* (Painful Obstruction Syndrome)

***Bi zheng* caused by wind-cold-damp:** Bodily deficiency allows the pathogenic factors wind-cold-damp to invade the channels and collaterals of the body and obstruct the flow of qi and blood. Clinical manifestations include muscle spasms and cramps, joint pain, difficulty flexing the joints, back pain, and muscle atrophy.

- *Bi zheng*: combine *Ba Ji Tian* with *Niu Xi* (Radix Cyathulae seu Achyranthis), *Wu Jia Pi* (Cortex Acanthopanacis), and *Gui Xin* (Cortex Rasus Cinnamomi).

DOSAGE

10 to 15 grams in decoction. *Ba Ji Tian* is also used in medicinal tincture, and in pill or powder forms. The unprocessed herb is commonly used to warm the yang of the Kidney, Spleen and Stomach. Frying it with salt increases its warmth, but not its drying influence; thus, it more strongly tonifies the Kidney and strengthens the muscles and tendons. Long-term use of the salt-fried herb is also effective for treating premature ejaculation and incontinence caused by yang deficiency.

CAUTIONS / CONTRAINDICATIONS

- *Ba Ji Tian* should not be used as a single-herb remedy for patients with yin-deficient fire. It should be combined with yin, *jing* (essence) or blood tonics.
- This herb is contraindicated in patients with damp-heat.

CHEMICAL COMPOSITION

Morindin, monotropein, asperuloside tertraacetate, β-sitosterol, vitamin C.[1]

PHARMACOLOGICAL EFFECTS

- **General:** Administration of *Ba Ji Tian* is associated with an increase in body weight and an improvement in physical performance in mice, as measured by swimming endurance.[2]
- **Endocrine:** Administration of *Ba Ji Tian* is associated with an increase in the plasma levels of corticosteroids. The mechanism of this action is attributed to its stimulating effect on the pituitary gland and the adrenal cortex.[3]

TOXICOLOGY

No fatalities were reported in animal studies following oral ingestion of *Ba Ji Tian* decoction at the dosage of 250 g/kg.[4]

AUTHORS' COMMENTS

The yang-tonifying function of *Ba Ji Tian* is not as strong as that of *Yin Yang Huo* (Herba Epimedii) or *Lu Rong* (Cornu Cervi Pantotrichum). However, it also has a nourishing function to tonify *jing* (essence) and blood, which prevents other herbs from creating deficient fire in the body.

References

1. *Xian Dai Zhong Yao Yao Li Xue* (Contemporary Pharmacology of Chinese Herbs), 1997; 1255
2. *Zhong Xi Yi Jie He Za Zhi* (Journal of Integrated Chinese and Western Medicine), 1991; 11(7):415
3. *Guo Wai Yi Xue Zhong Yi Zhong Yao Fen Ce* (Monograph of Chinese Herbology from Foreign Medicine), 1990; 12(6):48
4. *Zhong Xi Yi Jie He Za Zhi* (Journal of Integrated Chinese and Western Medicine), 1991; 11(7):415

Yin Yang Huo (Herba Epimedii)

淫羊藿

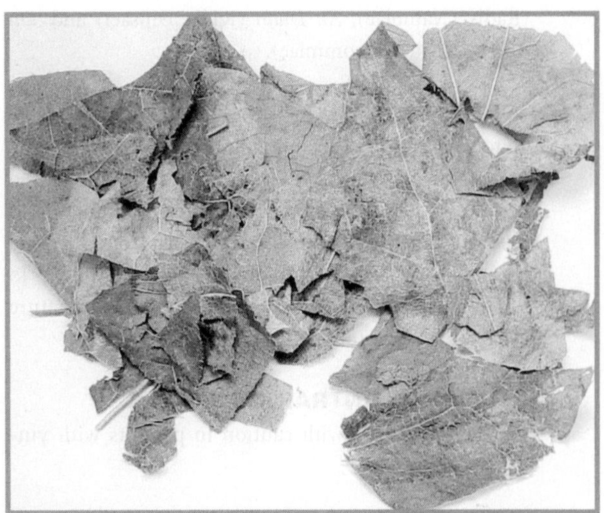

Pinyin Name: *Yin Yang Huo*
Literal Name: "horny goat herb," "horny goat weed"
Alternate Chinese Names: *Xian Ling Pi, San Zhi Jiu Ye Cao, Qi Zhang Cao, Qian Lian Jin*
Original Source: *Shen Nong Ben Cao Jing* (Divine Husbandman's Classic of the Materia Medica) in the second century
English Name: epimedium, short-horned epimedium, sagittate epimedium, pubescent epimedium, Korean epimedium
Botanical Name: *Epimedium grandiflorum* Morr. (*Yin Yang Huo*); *Epimedium sagittatum* (Sieb. et Zucc.) Maxim. (*Jian Ye Yin Yang Huo*); *Epimedium pubescens* Maxim. (*Rou Mao Yin Yang Huo*); *Epimedium brevicornum* Maxim. (*Xin Ye Yin Yang Huo*); *Epimedium koreanum* Nakai (*Chao Xian Yin Yang Huo*)
Pharmaceutical Name: Herba Epimedii
Properties: acrid, sweet, warm
Channels Entered: Kidney, Liver

CHINESE THERAPEUTIC ACTIONS

1. Tonifies the Kidney, Strengthens Yang and Increases Libido

Kidney yang deficiency: *Yin Yang Huo* (Herba Epimedii) primarily treats Kidney yang deficiency that manifests in sexual disorders such as impotence, lack of sexual desire, incomplete erection, premature ejaculation, spermatorrhea, low sperm count, soreness and weakness of the lower back and knees, and infertility. It also treats infertility in women arising from cold and deficiency of the Kidney. Patients with Kidney yang deficiency may also have Kidney yin or *jing* (essence) deficiencies. Therefore, it is advised that herbs that tonify *jing*, yin or blood be added to the overall formulation to achieve balance, as a pure Kidney yang-tonic formula may cause rising Kidney fire.

- Impotence: soak *Yin Yang Huo* in grain-based liquor for three days and drink the tincture.
- Kidney yang deficiency: combine this herb with *Shu Di Huang* (Radix Rehmanniae Preparata), *Gui Ban Jiao* (Gelatinum Plastrum Testudinis), and *Zi He Che* (Placenta Hominis).

2. Dispels Wind-Damp-Cold and Alleviates *Bi Zheng* (Painful Obstruction Syndrome)

Bi zheng: *Yin Yang Huo* treats *bi zheng* caused by wind-damp-cold attacking the channels and blocking the circulation of qi and yang to the extremities. Symptoms include pain and coldness of the limbs, numbness, and spasms and cramps of the tendons and muscles. If blood stagnation is prominent secondary to yang deficiency, severe cramps, convulsions, hemiplegia or facial paralysis may occur. Acrid, warm and dispersing in nature, *Yin Yang Huo* dispels wind-damp-cold from the channels and collaterals and promotes normal circulation of qi and blood to the extremities. This herb is also used for post-stroke patients in whom stiffness, numbness or paralysis indicate yang deficiency with stagnation in the channels.

- Wind-cold-damp *bi zheng*: combine *Yin Yang Huo* with *Qiang Huo* (Rhizoma et Radix Notopterygii), *Fang Feng* (Radix Saposhnikoviae), *Fu Zi* (Radix Aconiti Lateralis Praeparata), *Du Huo* (Radix Angelicae Pubescentis), and *Wu Jia Pi* (Cortex Acanthopanacis).
- Chronic numbness and pain of the extremities: soak the herb in grain-based liquor for at least four months, and drink a small amount of the tincture daily.
- Post-stroke hemiplegia: use it with *Du Huo* (Radix Angelicae Pubescentis), *Fang Feng* (Radix Saposhnikoviae), and *Wu Jia Pi* (Cortex Acanthopanacis).
- Myelanalosis or myelitis with weakness of lower extremities or lower-body paralysis, with urinary and bowel incontinence: add this herb to *Shu Di Huang* (Radix Rehmanniae Preparata), *Shan Zhu Yu* (Fructus Corni), *Shan Yao* (Rhizoma Dioscoreae), *Fu Ling* (Poria), *Fu Zi* (Radix Aconiti Lateralis Praeparata), *Rou Gui* (Cortex Cinnamomi), *Ba Ji Tian* (Radix Morindae Officinalis), *Rou Cong Rong* (Herba Cistanches), *Chuan Niu Xi*

17 TONIC HERBS

Yin Yang Huo (Herba Epimedii)

(Radix Cyathulae), *Xu Duan* (Radix Dipsaci) and *Du Zhong* (Cortex Eucommiae).

DOSAGE

10 to 15 grams in decoction. *Yin Yang Huo* is commonly used as herbal tincture, paste or pills. The unprocessed herb more strongly dispels wind and dampness and relieves *bi zheng* (painful obstruction syndrome). Frying the herb in oil (sesame or lamb oil) enhances its effect to tonify Kidney yang, and to treat impotence, premature ejaculation, and other sexual disorders.

CAUTIONS / CONTRAINDICATIONS

- Use *Yin Yang Huo* with caution in patients with yin-deficient fire.

CHEMICAL COMPOSITION

Icariine, des-o-methyicariine, β-anhydroicaritine, des-o-methy-β-anhydroicaritine, icarisid I, isoquercetin, icariin-3-o-d-rhamnoside, hyperin, sagittatosides A, B, C; epimedins A, B, C; wushanicariin.[1]

PHARMACOLOGICAL EFFECTS

- **Sexual and reproductive:** Administration of *Yin Yang Huo* increases sperm production, stimulates the sensory nerves, and increases sexual desire and activity. The leaves and root have the strongest therapeutic effect, followed by the fruit and stem. Other studies have shown *Yin Yang Huo* to increase the secretion of endogenous hormones, such as corticosterone, cortisol, and testosterone.[2,3]
- **Respiratory:** Preparation of *Yin Yang Huo* has shown marked antitussive, expectorant and antiasthmatic effects. The antitussive effect of the herb is attributed to its effect on the central nervous system.[4]
- **Antibiotic:** It has an inhibitory effect against *Staphylococcus albus, Staphylococcus aureus, Diplococcus pneumoniae,* and *Mycobacterium tuberculosis.*[5]
- **Cardiovascular:** Water and alcohol extracts of *Yin Yang Huo* have an antihypertensive effect, as demonstrated in rabbit, cat, rat and other animal studies. In rats with renal hypertension, *Yin Yang Huo* has an immediate antihypertensive effect, though the blood pressure rebounded upon discontinuation of the herb. The antihypertensive effect of *Yin Yang Huo* in cats was not reversed by injection of atropine.[6]
- **Antihyperlipidemic:** Rabbits with high plasma cholesterol levels were treated with 5 ml of decoction of *Yin Yang Huo* twice daily for 30 days. The study reported a decrease in cholesterol levels but an increase in triglyceride levels.[7]
- **Antidiabetic:** Extract of *Yin Yang Huo* given orally significantly lowered plasma glucose levels in rats, for up to 60 minutes.[8]
- **Anti-inflammatory:** A preparation of *Yin Yang Huo* injected subcutaneously decreased vascular permeability and decreased the extent of swelling and inflammation in rats.[9]

CLINICAL STUDIES AND RESEARCH

- **Coronary artery disease (CAD):** In one study, 130 patients with CAD were treated with 4 to 6 tablets of *Yin Yang Huo* (each tablet is equivalent to 2.7 grams of the dried herb) twice daily for 1 month, with marked symptomatic improvement.[10]
- **Neutropenia:** Administration of 15 grams of *Yin Yang Huo* given as tea for 30 to 45 days (three times daily for the first week, two times daily thereafter) has proven beneficial in treating patients with neutropenia. No other immune-enhancing agents or vitamins were given throughout the study. Out of 22 patients who enrolled in the study, 14 completed the study with 100% compliance. Of these 14 patients, 3 showed significant improvement, 4 showed marked improvement, 4 had some improvement, and 3 had no response. [11]
- **Chronic bronchitis:** In one study, 1,066 patients with chronic bronchitis were treated with pills of *Yin Yang Huo* with an overall effective rate of 74.6%. The rate of effectiveness was 86.8% for its antitussive function, 87.9% for its expectorant function, and 73.8% for its antiasthmatic function.[12]
- **Poliomyelitis:** Injection of *Yin Yang Huo* and *Sang Ji Sheng* (Herba Taxilli) was found to be effective in treating patients with acute onset and sequelae of poliomyelitis.[13]
- **Neurasthenia:** One report describes 228 patients with neurasthenia who were treated with three different preparations of *Yin Yang Huo*, with approximately 90% effectiveness in all three groups.[14]
- **Viral myocarditis:** Administration of 7 to 10 tablets of *Yin Yang Huo* (each tablet equivalent to 2.7 grams of the dried herb) given three times daily for 2 months showed beneficial effects in 36 patients with viral myocarditis.[15]

TOXICOLOGY

The LD_{50} for *Yin Yang Huo* extract in mice was 36 g/kg via intraperitoneal injection, and 56.8 g/kg via intravenous injection. Oral ingestion of *Yin Yang Huo* at the dosage of 450 g/kg for 3 days showed no abnormal effects. Symptoms of overdose included dilation of pupils, increased physical movement, mild spasms and cramps, and in severe cases, respiratory depression.[16,17]

AUTHORS' COMMENTS

Sexual disorders often involve both Kidney yin and yang deficiencies. When tonifying Kidney yang, one must also include yin-tonic herbs to balance the formula, thereby

Yin Yang Huo (Herba Epimedii)

avoiding the unwanted buildup of heat from the yang-tonic herbs. In addition, *Yin Yang Huo* is not recommended for long-term use as it may damage yin.

For impotence, *Yin Yang Huo* is often made into medicinal tincture by soaking it in a grain-based liquor with other herbs such as *Shan Zhu Yu* (Fructus Corni), *Xiao Mai* (Fructus Tritici), *Shu Di Huang* (Radix Rehmanniae Preparata), *Rou Cong Rong* (Herba Cistanches), *Gou Qi Zi* (Fructus Lycii), *Ba Ji Tian* (Radix Morindae Officinalis) and *Yang Qi Shi* (Actinolitum). It can also be prepared in pill form.

References

1. *Xian Dai Zhong Yao Yao Li Xue* (Contemporary Pharmacology of Chinese Herbs), 1997; 1238
2. *Zhong Yao Da Ci Dian* (Dictionary of Chinese Herbs), 1977:2251
3. *Zhong Xi Yi Jie He Za Zhi* (Journal of Integrated Chinese and Western Medicine), 1989; 9(12):737-8,710
4. *Zhong Yao Yao Li Yu Ying Yong* (Pharmacology and Applications of Chinese Herbs), 1983:1102
5. Ibid.
6. Ibid.
7. Ibid.
8. Ibid.
9. Ibid.
10. *Xin Yi Yao Xue Za Zhi* (New Journal of Medicine and Herbology), 1975; 12:26
11. *Zhong Xi Yi Jie He Za Zhi* (Journal of Integrated Chinese and Western Medicine), 1985; 12:719
12. *Hu Bei Wei Sheng* (Hubei Health), 1972; 7:15
13. *Zhong Cao Yao Tong Xun* (Journal of Chinese Herbal Medicine), 1972; 2:28
14. *Zhong Yi Za Zhi* (Journal of Chinese Medicine), 1982; 11:70
15. *Zhong Xi Yi Jie He Za Zhi* (Journal of Integrated Chinese and Western Medicine), 1984; 9:523
16. *Zhong Yao Da Ci Dian* (Dictionary of Chinese Herbs), 1977:2251
17. *Zhong Xi Yi Jie He Za Zhi* (Journal of Integrated Chinese and Western Medicine), 1985; 12:7191.

Xian Mao (Rhizoma Curculiginis)

仙茅 仙茅

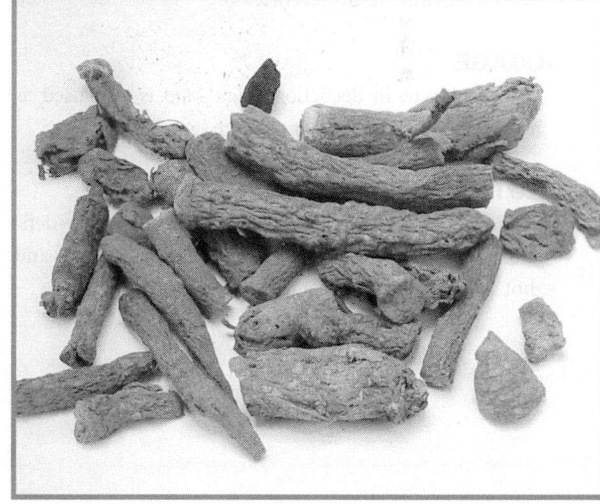

Pinyin Name: *Xian Mao*
Literal Name: "immortal grass"
Original Source: *Hai Yao Ben Cao* (Materia Medica of Herbs from [Across the] Seas) by Li Xun in 907-960 A.D.
English Name: curculigo, common curculigo rhizome
Botanical Name: *Curculigo orchioides* Gaertz. (*Xian Mao*)
Pharmaceutical Name: Rhizoma Curculiginis
Properties: acrid, hot
Channels Entered: Kidney
Safety Index: toxic

CHINESE THERAPEUTIC ACTIONS

1. Warms the Kidney and Fortifies Yang

Kidney yang deficiency: *Xian Mao* (Rhizoma Curculiginis) is one of the most potent Kidney yang-tonic herbs. It treats urinary incontinence, polyuria, impotence and spermatorrhea in men. In women, manifestations of Kidney yang deficiency are irregular menstruation and infertility.

- Impotence: combine *Xian Mao* with *Yin Yang Huo* (Herba Epimedii), and *Ba Ji Tian* (Radix Morindae Officinalis), in grain-based liquor.
- Polyuria, tinnitus or loss of hearing: combine this herb with *Jin Ying Zi* (Fructus Rosae Laevigatae).
- Spleen and Kidney yang deficiencies with epigastric fullness and pain, poor appetite, and vomiting of clear fluids: add *Xian Mao* to *Sha Ren* (Fructus Amomi), *Wu Zhu Yu* (Fructus Evodiae), *Mu Xiang* (Radix Aucklandiae), and *Gao Liang Jiang* (Rhizoma Alpiniae Officinarum).

17 TONIC HERBS

Xian Mao (Rhizoma Curculiginis)

- Urinary incontinence and frequent urination: use *Xian Mao* as a single herb.
- Irregular menstruation or hypertension during menopause: use it with *Yin Yang Huo* (Herba Epimedii), *Dang Gui* (Radicis Angelicae Sinensis) and *Zhi Mu* (Radix Anemarrhenae).
- Epigastric coldness with acid regurgitation and poor appetite: use this herb with *Sha Ren* (Fructus Amomi), *Wu Zhu Yu* (Fructus Evodiae), *Mu Xiang* (Radix Aucklandiae) and *Gao Liang Jiang* (Rhizoma Alpiniae Officinarum).

2. Dispels Cold and Damp, Treats *Bi Zheng* (Painful Obstruction Syndrome)

Bi zheng: Arthritis, pain, numbness and stiffness frequently occur as a result of constitutional deficiency of Kidney yang complicated by invasion of cold and damp obstructing the channels. *Xian Mao* strengthens the bones and dispels cold and damp from the channels to relieve pain.

- Feelings of weakness in the bones and sinews, and/or lower back and knee pain: combine *Xian Mao* with *Xu Duan* (Radix Dipsaci), *Du Zhong* (Cortex Eucommiae), *Yin Yang Huo* (Herba Epimedii), and *Wu Jia Pi* (Cortex Acanthopanacis). *Cao Wu* (Radix Aconiti Kusnezoffii) or *Chuan Wu* (Radix Aconiti Preparata) may be added to the formulation to dispel cold.

DOSAGE

3 to 10 grams in decoction. *Xian Mao* is also used as medicinal tincture, pills or powder.

CAUTIONS / CONTRAINDICATIONS

- *Xian Mao* is contraindicated in patients with yin-deficient fire or excess heat syndromes. *Xian Mao* is toxic and hot, and is not recommended for long-term use.
- Use of *Xian Mao* may be associated with side effects such as numbness or swelling of the tongue, which can be relieved by taking *Da Huang* (Radix et Rhizoma Rhei) or *Huang Qin* (Radix Scutellariae).

CHEMICAL COMPOSITION

Lycorine, yuccagenin, β-sitosterol, curculigoside, corchioside A, curculigoside B, curculigine A,B,C; orcinol glucoside.[1]

PHARMACOLOGICAL EFFECTS

- **Immunostimulant:** Administration of a 70% alcohol extract of *Xian Mao* once daily for 7 days increased the phagocytic activity of the macrophages in mice.[2]
- **CNS suppressant:** Intraperitoneal injection of alcohol extract of *Xian Mao* at 10 g/kg prolonged the sleeping time induced by phenobarbital at 40 mg/kg in mice.[3]
- **Reproductive:** *Xian Mao* stimulates the reproductive system to increase the weight of the ovaries and uterus in female mice,[4] and the weight of the testicles in male rats.[5]

TOXICOLOGY

Xian Mao has relatively low toxicity. No fatalities were observed with a loading dose of 150 g/kg via the oral route in mice.[6]

References

1. *Xian Dai Zhong Yao Yao Li Xue* (Contemporary Pharmacology of Chinese Herbs), 1997; 1256
2. *Zhong Guo Zhong Yao Za Zhi* (People's Republic of China Journal of Chinese Herbology), 1989; 14(10):42
3. Ibid.
4. *Zhong Yi Za Zhi* (Journal of Chinese Medicine), 1984; (7):63
5. *Zhong Guo Zhong Yao Za Zhi* (People's Republic of China Journal of Chinese Herbology), 1989; 14(10):42
6. Ibid.

Yang Qi Shi (Actinolitum)

陽起石 阳起石

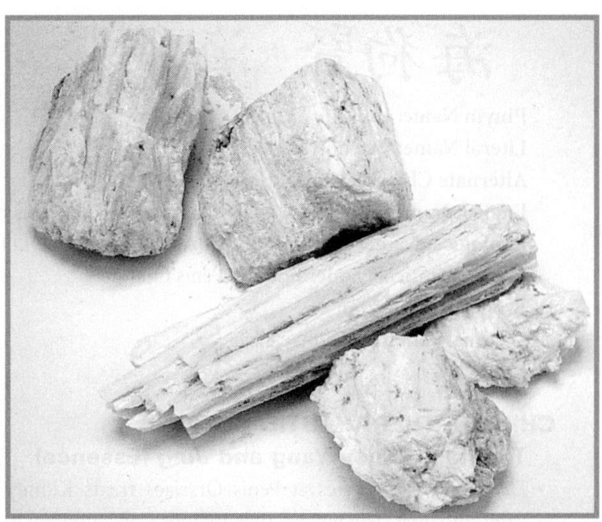

Pinyin Name: *Yang Qi Shi*
Literal Name: "yang rising stone"
Alternate Chinese Names: *Bai Shi, Shi Sheng, Tou Shan Shi*
Original Source: *Shen Nong Ben Cao Jing* (Divine Husbandman's Classic of the Materia Medica) in the second century
English Name: actinolite
Pharmaceutical Name: Actinolitum
Properties: salty, slightly warm
Channels Entered: Kidney

CHINESE THERAPEUTIC ACTIONS

Warms the Kidney and Fortifies Yang

Impotence, female infertility due to Kidney yang deficiency: *Yang Qi Shi* (Actinolitum) most often treats impotence caused by Kidney yang deficiency. Other symptoms include spermatorrhea, loose stools, soreness of the lower back and knees, premature ejaculation and coldness of the extremities. In women, Kidney yang deficiency manifests as infertility or lack of sexual desire.

- Kidney yang deficiency in men: combine *Yang Qi Shi* with *Lu Rong* (Cornu Cervi Pantotrichum) and *Tu Si Zi* (Semen Cuscutae).
- Infertility in women: add this substance to *Wu Zhu Yu* (Fructus Evodiae), *Gan Jiang* (Rhizoma Zingiberis), *Shu Di Huang* (Radix Rehmanniae Preparata) and *Huai Niu Xi* (Radix Achyranthis Bidentatae).

DOSAGE

3 to 6 grams in pill form. *Yang Qi Shi* should be calcined to facilitate the crushing and extraction of active constituents.

CAUTIONS / CONTRAINDICATIONS

- *Yang Qi Shi* is not suitable for long-term use.
- *Yang Qi Shi* is contraindicated for patients with yin-deficient heat.

CHEMICAL COMPOSITION

Actinolite.[1]

References

1. *Zhong Yao Xue* (Chinese Herbology), 1998; 814-815

Hai Gou Shen (Testes et Penis Otariae)

海狗腎 海狗肾

Pinyin Name: *Hai Gou Shen*
Literal Name: "sea dog kidneys"
Alternate Chinese Names: *Hai Gou Bian*
English Name: male seal sexual organs, testes and penis of an ursine seal
Zoological Name: *Callorhinus ursinus* L.; *Phoca vitulina* (L.)
Pharmaceutical Name: Testes et Penis Otariae
Properties: salty, hot
Channels Entered: Kidney, Liver

CHINESE THERAPEUTIC ACTIONS

Tonifies Kidney Yang and *Jing* (Essence)

Hai Gou Shen (Testes et Penis Otariae) treats Kidney yang and *jing* deficiencies that manifest as impotence, low sexual drive, intolerance to cold and cold extremities.

- Impotence: combine *Hai Gou Shen* with *Lu Rong* (Cornu Cervi Pantotrichum) and *Yin Yang Huo* (Herba Epimedii).
- Decreased sexual drive: use it with *Dong Chong Xia Cao* (Cordyceps).

DOSAGE

3 to 15 grams. Due to the unpleasant taste, *Hai Gou Shen* is usually taken as a powder.

CAUTIONS / CONTRAINDICATIONS

- Use of *Hai Gou Shen* is contraindicated for patients with yin-deficient fire.

AUTHORS' COMMENTS

The sex organs of deer and other animals are useful as replacements for the tonic functions served by seal testicles and penis.

Hai Shen (Strichopus Japonicus)

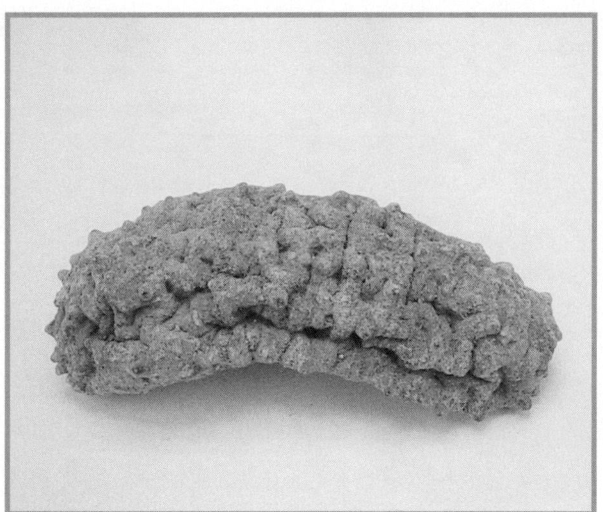

海參 海参

Pinyin Name: *Hai Shen*
Literal Name: "sea root"
English Name: sea cucumber, sea slug, trepang
Zoological Name: *Strichopus japonicus* Selenka
Pharmaceutical Name: Strichopus Japonicus
Properties: sweet, salty, warm
Channels Entered: Heart, Kidney

Hai Shen (Strichopus Japonicus)

CHINESE THERAPEUTIC ACTIONS

Tonifies Kidney Yang and *Jing* (Essence)

Hai Shen (Strichopus Japonicus) treats Kidney yang and *jing* deficiencies that manifest as impotence, nocturnal emissions and frequent urination.

DOSAGE

30 to 60 grams. *Hai Shen* is most commonly used as food.

CHEMICAL COMPOSITION

Acid mucopoly saccharide (SJAMO), holotoxin, holothurin, holothrin A, echinoside, stichoposides.[1]

References

1. *Xian Dai Zhong Yao Yao Li Xue* (Contemporary Pharmacology of Chinese Herbs), 1997; 1274

Hai Long (Syngnathus)

海龍 海龙

Pinyin Name: *Hai Long*
Literal Name: "sea dragon"
English Name: pipe fish
Zoological Name: *Syngnathus acus* L.; *Solenognathus hardwickii* (Gray); *Syngnathoides biaculeatus* (Bloch)
Pharmaceutical Name: Syngnathus
Properties: sweet, salty, slightly warm
Channels Entered: Kidney

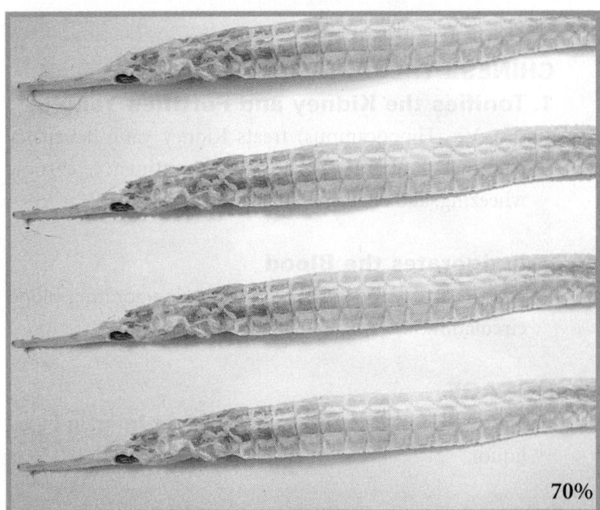

CHINESE THERAPEUTIC ACTIONS

1. Tonifies the Kidney and Fortifies Yang

Hai Long (Syngnathus) treats Kidney yang deficiency that manifests as impotence and debility, especially in the elderly.

2. Reduces Swelling and Dissipates Nodules

Hai Long treats scrofula by reducing the size and swelling of the nodules.

DOSAGE

3 to 9 grams in decoctions; 1.5 to 2.4 grams in pills or powder.

CHEMICAL COMPOSITION

Protein, cholesterol, palmitic acid, stearic acid, calcium, magnesium, sodium, phosphorus.[1]

References

1. *Xian Dai Zhong Yao Yao Li Xue* (Contemporary Pharmacology of Chinese Herbs), 1997; 1281

Hai Ma (Hippocampus)

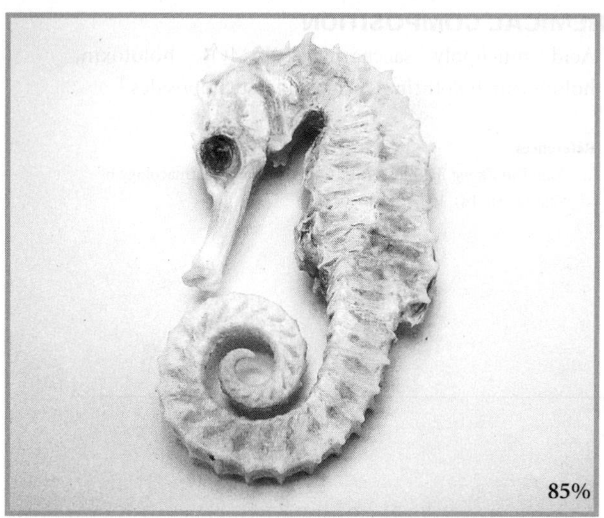
85%

海馬 海马

Pinyin Name: *Hai Ma*
Literal Name: "sea horse"
Alternate Chinese Names: *Shui Ma*
English Name: sea horse
Zoological Name: *Hippocampus kelloggi* Jordan et Snyder H. histrix Kaup; *Hippocampus trimacullatus* Leach
Pharmaceutical Name: Hippocampus
Properties: sweet, salty, warm
Channels Entered: Kidney, Liver

CHINESE THERAPEUTIC ACTIONS

1. Tonifies the Kidney and Fortifies Yang

Hai Ma (Hippocampus) treats Kidney yang deficiency patterns of impotence, urinary incontinence, chronic wheezing, and debility in the elderly.

2. Invigorates the Blood

Hai Ma treats abdominal masses by invigorating blood circulation.

DOSAGE

3 to 9 grams. *Hai Ma* is often steeped in grain-based liquor.

CAUTIONS / CONTRAINDICATIONS

- *Hai Ma* should be used with caution during pregnancy, and for patients with yin-deficient fire.

CHEMICAL COMPOSITION

Glutamic acid, glycine, arginine, sodium, potassium, magnesium calcium, iron.[1]

PHARMACOLOGICAL EFFECTS

- **Reproductive:** In female mice, administration of *Hai Ma* is associated with a prolonged estrus period and an increase in weight of the uterus and ovaries. In male mice, administration of *Hai Ma* is associated with an androgenic effect on the prostate gland and the testes. Compared to other herbs, *Hai Ma* is stronger than *Ge Jie* (Gecko), but weaker than *She Chuang Zi* (Fructus Cnidii) and *Yin Yang Huo* (Herba Epimedii) for exerting stimulating effects on the reproductive organs.[2]
- **Adaptogenic:** According to animal studies, administration of *Hai Ma* improves both mental and physical performance. It has been shown to increase swimming time in mice and to improve memory in other animals.[3]

CLINICAL STUDIES AND RESEARCH

- **Impotence:** In a clinical trial, 107 patients with impotence were treated with herbal tincture daily for 2 months, with an overall rate of effectiveness of 83.2%. The herbal tincture was prepared by soaking *Hai Ma*, *Ge Jie* (Gecko), *Lu Rong* (Cornu Cervi Pantotrichum), *Hai Shen* (Strichopus Japonicus), *Gou Qi Zi* (Fructus Lycii), *Yin Yang Huo* (Herba Epimedii) and *Wu Wei Zi* (Fructus Schisandrae Chinensis) in grain-based liquor for 7 days prior to consumption. The treatment protocol was to administer 35 grams of tincture daily, before bedtime.[4]

References

1. *Xian Dai Zhong Yao Yao Li Xue* (Contemporary Pharmacology of Chinese Herbs), 1997; 1280
2. *Zhong Yao Da Ci Dian* (Dictionary of Chinese Herbs), 1977; 1923
3. *Xian Dai Shi Yong Yao Xue* (Practical Applications of Modern Herbal Medicine), 1991; 8(3):1
4. *Ji Lin Zhong Yi Yao* (Jilin Chinese Medicine and Herbology), 1981; (1):17

Du Zhong (Cortex Eucommiae)

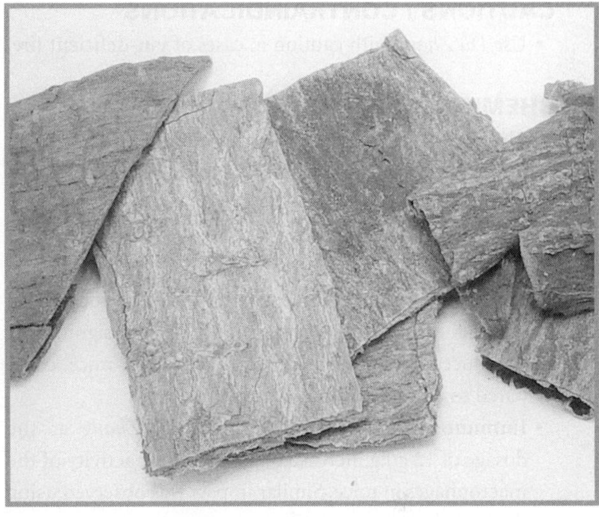

杜仲

Pinyin Name: *Du Zhong*
Alternate Chinese Names: *Bei Zhong, Si Mian Pi, Yu Zi Pi, Mu Mian*
Original Source: *Shen Nong Ben Cao Jing* (Divine Husbandman's Classic of the Materia Medica) in the second century
English Name: eucommia bark
Botanical Name: *Eucommia ulmoides* Oliv. (*Du Zhong*)
Pharmaceutical Name: Cortex Eucommiae
Properties: sweet, warm
Channels Entered: Kidney, Liver

CHINESE THERAPEUTIC ACTIONS

1. Tonifies the Liver and Kidney, Strengthens Bones and Sinews

Back pain due to Kidney deficiency: Deficient blood and *jing* (essence) of the Kidney and Liver often result in weakness and soreness of the lower back and knees. *Du Zhong* (Cortex Eucommiae) nourishes the Liver to benefit the tendons and sinews, and tonifies the Kidney to strengthen the bones. This herb can also be used for back pain and soreness during menstruation.

- Low back pain: fry *Du Zhong* with salt to guide it to the Kidney channel. Use it alone or soak it in grain-based liquor with *Gou Qi Zi* (Fructus Lycii).
- Cold legs and intolerance to cold: combine this herb with *Fu Zi* (Radix Aconiti Lateralis Praeparata), *Rou Gui* (Cortex Cinnamomi) and *Yin Yang Huo* (Herba Epimedii).
- Low back pain during or after menstruation: add this herb to *Sang Ji Sheng* (Herba Taxilli), *Dang Gui* (Radicis Angelicae Sinensis) and *Chuan Xiong* (Rhizoma Ligusticum Chuanxiong).
- Low back pain in the first three months of pregnancy, with a feeling of abdominal prolapse: use *Du Zhong* with *Sang Ji Sheng* (Herba Taxilli), *Xu Duan* (Radix Dipsaci), *Bai Zhu* (Rhizoma Atractylodis Macrocephalae), *Shu Di Huang* (Radix Rehmanniae Preparata), *Bai Shao* (Radix Paeoniae Alba), *Su Geng* (Caulis Perillae), and *Dang Gui* (Radicis Angelicae Sinensis).
- Fractured or broken bones: pair this herb and *Xu Duan* (Radix Dipsaci) to promote healing of the bones.

2. Calms the Fetus

Restless fetus, bleeding or miscarriage: Liver and Kidney deficiencies cause restless fetus, bleeding or miscarriage. *Du Zhong* tonifies these two organs to stabilize the fetus and prevent miscarriage.

- Unstable pregnancy with restless fetus and bleeding, previous history of miscarriage in the first trimester: combine *Du Zhong* with *Da Zao* (Fructus Jujubae), *Xu Duan* (Radix Dipsaci), and *Shan Yao* (Rhizoma Dioscoreae).
- Continuous bleeding after miscarriage: combine charred *Du Zhong* with charred *Xu Duan* (Radix Dipsaci), *Dang Gui* (Radicis Angelicae Sinensis), *Bai Shao* (Radix Paeoniae Alba), *E Jiao* (Colla Corii Asini) and *Ai Ye* (Folium Artemisiae Argyi).

3. Tonifies Kidney Yang

Du Zhong tonifies Kidney yang to treat reproductive and urinary disorders, such as impotence and incontinence.

- Impotence: incorporate *Du Zhong* with *Shan Zhu Yu* (Fructus Corni), *Xiao Hui Xiang* (Fructus Foeniculi) and *Che Qian Zi* (Semen Plantaginis).
- Urinary incontinence and dribbling of urine: use it with *Shan Zhu Yu* (Fructus Corni), *Xiao Hui Xiang* (Fructus Foeniculi), and *Che Qian Zi* (Semen Plantaginis).

4. Lowers Blood Pressure

Hypertension: *Du Zhong* has been used recently to treat hypertension with good success. It may be used alone, or in combination with *Huang Qin* (Radix Scutellariae) and *Xia Ku Cao* (Spica Prunellae) in decoction.

DOSAGE

10 to 15 grams in decoction or in pills. Dry-fried *Du Zhong* is more potent than the unprocessed form. Frying it with salt enhances its effect to tonify the Liver and Kidney by increasing the extraction of active components (by as much as 100%). Salt-fried *Du Zhong* is the preferred form to treat low back pain, spontaneous emission, and unstable pregnancy.

Du Zhong (Cortex Eucommiae)

CAUTIONS / CONTRAINDICATIONS

- Use *Du Zhong* with caution in cases of yin-deficient fire.

CHEMICAL COMPOSITION

Pinoresinol, gutta-percha, eucommioside I, eucommiol, ulmoprenol, eucommioside, alkaloids, proteins, amino acid, organic acid, vitamins, microelements.[1]

PHARMACOLOGICAL EFFECTS

- **Sedative:** *Du Zhong* has a sedative effect on the central nervous system. Administration of *Du Zhong* significantly reduced spontaneous physical activity in mice, compared to administration of normal saline.[2]
- **Immunostimulant:** Decoction of *Du Zhong* at the dosage of 12 g/kg increased the phagocytic activity of the macrophages in mice. Similar impact was observed using the bark, leaves, or twigs.[3]
- **Anti-inflammatory:** *Du Zhong* has demonstrated marked anti-inflammatory effects in rats. The mechanism of this effect is attributed to its stimulating effect on the endocrine system and consequent secretion of steroids from the adrenal cortex. The bark and leaves are stronger than the twigs for this action.[4]
- **Antihypertensive:** Administration of *Du Zhong* in various preparations significantly reduces blood pressure in anesthetized rabbits and dogs. Water extract was found to be stronger than alcohol extract. Dry-fried *Du Zhong* was determined to be more effective than the unprocessed herb. Tolerance was noted when *Du Zhong* was repeatedly injected intravenously within a short period of time. The mechanism of the action to reduce blood pressure was attributed to dilation of blood vessels.[5]
- **Uterine relaxant:** Administration of *Du Zhong* blocks stimulation and contraction of the uterus in a dose-dependant fashion. The water and alcohol extracts are comparable in potency. However, salt-fried *Du Zhong* is more effective than the unprocessed herb.[6]
- **Adaptogenic:** Administration of *Du Zhong* significantly prolonged swimming time in mice. The leaves, however, did not exhibit a statistically significant influence.[7]
- **Antibiotic:** Decoction of *Du Zhong* shows inhibitory influence on *Staphylococcus aureus*, *Bacillus dysenteriae*, *Pseudomonas aeruginosa*, *Bacillus anthracis*, *Diplococcus pneumoniae*, and β-hemolytic streptococcus.[8]

CLINICAL STUDIES AND RESEARCH

- **Hypertension:** In one study, 251 hypertensive patients were divided into two groups, with group one receiving *Du Zhong* and group two receiving *Du Zhong Ye* (Folium Eucommiae). The dosage of *Du Zhong Ye* was three times greater than *Du Zhong*. All other ingredients in the formula were the same. All patients received herbs three times daily for 30 days. Out of 104 patients who received *Du Zhong*, 44 showed significant improvement, 36 showed moderate improvement, and 24 showed no response (an overall rate of 76.9% effectiveness). Out of 147 patients that received *Du Zhong Ye*, 81 showed significant improvement, 44 showed moderate improvement, and 22 showed no response (an overall rate of 85% effectiveness).[9]
- **Sciatica:** Six patients with sciatica were successfully treated with an herbal formula one time each day for 7 to 10 doses. The treatment protocol was to cook 30 grams of *Du Zhong* with a pair of pig kidneys for half an hour, filter out the herbs and serve the soup and kidneys.[10]

TOXICOLOGY

No fatalities were reported in mice that received 500 g/kg of *Du Zhong* via intraperitoneal injection once daily for 6 days. Intraperitoneal injection of *Du Zhong* at 600 mg/kg led to decreased physical activity for 2 hours, with no long-term effect. The LD_{50} for intravenous injection of *Du Zhong* in mice is 574.1 g/kg.[11]

SUPPLEMENT

- 杜仲葉 / 杜仲叶 *Du Zhong Ye* (Folium Eucommiae) is derived from the leaves of the same plant as *Du Zhong*. Laboratory analysis has confirmed that *Du Zhong* and *Du Zhong Ye* have essentially the same constituents. Therefore, *Du Zhong Ye* is now used as an acceptable substitute for *Du Zhong*.

AUTHORS' COMMENTS

Du Zhong and *Xu Duan* (Radix Dipsaci) both tonify the Liver and Kidney, strengthen sinews and bones, calm restless fetus, stop uterine bleeding and treat weakness, soreness and pain in the lower back and knees. *Du Zhong* more strongly tonifies the Liver and Kidney, and thus is used more for low back pain, impotence, polyuria and dizziness. *Xu Duan* is less strengthening, but more effectively invigorates the flow of blood in the channels and collaterals. It is used for the pain of trauma, fractured or broken bones, *bi zheng* (painful obstruction syndrome), and sores.

Du Zhong and *Gou Ji* (Rhizoma Cibotii) both warm and tonify the Kidney and Liver to treat lower back and knee soreness and pain, impotence and polyuria. *Du Zhong* is warmer, and calms the fetus, while *Gou Ji* more effectively treats *bi zheng* (painful obstruction syndrome).

Warm and drying in nature, *Du Zhong* is sometimes combined with *Shu Di Huang* (Radix Rehmanniae Preparata) to reduce the stagnant, cloying side effects of *Shu Di Huang*.

Du Zhong has recently been successfully used to treat hypertension. The mechanism of its antihypertensive effect is attributed to dilation of the blood vessels. Dry-

Du Zhong (Cortex Eucommiae)

fried *Du Zhong* is the most potent for this function. Salt-fried *Du Zhong* should be avoided since salt may cause retention of water. If heat signs are prominent, *Huang Qin* (Radix Scutellariae) and *Xia Ku Cao* (Spica Prunellae) can be added.

There are four herbs that are commonly used to stabilize pregnancy:

- *Du Zhong* (Cortex Eucommiae) is most suitable to treat restless fetus caused by deficiency of the Kidney and Liver.
- *Sha Ren* (Fructus Amomi) regulates qi and calms restless fetus in the presence of qi stagnation and middle *jiao* deficiency.
- *Huang Qin* (Radix Scutellariae) calms restless fetus caused by heat.
- *Bai Zhu* (Rhizoma Atractylodis Macrocephalae) treats restless fetus from Spleen qi deficiency.

References

1. *Xian Dai Zhong Yao Yao Li Xue* (Contemporary Pharmacology of Chinese Herbs), 1995; 1259:1262
2. *Tong Ji Yi Ke Da Xue Xue Bao* (Journal of Tongji University of Medicine), 1989;(3):198
3. *Zhong Cao Yao* (Chinese Herbal Medicine), 1983; 14(8):27
4. Ibid., 1982; 13(6):24
5. *Zhong Yao Cai* (Study of Chinese Herbal Material), 1986; 6:33
6. Ibid.
7. *Tong Ji Yi Ke Da Xue Xue Bao* (Journal of Tongji University of Medicine), 1989;(3):198
8. *Zhong Yao Xue* (Chinese Herbology), 1998; 797:799
9. *Xin Yi Yao Xue Za Zhi* (New Journal of Medicine and Herbology), 1978; 10:30
10. *Zhong Yao Xue* (Chinese Herbology), 1998; 797:799
11. *Zhong Cao Yao* (Chinese Herbal Medicine), 1982; 13(6):24

Xu Duan (Radix Dipsaci)

續斷 续断

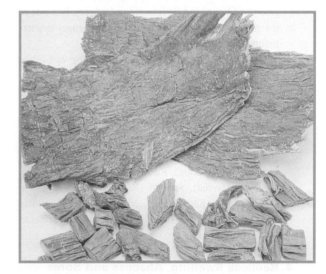

Pinyin Name: *Xu Duan*
Literal Name: "restore what is broken," "restore the broken," "reconnect broken parts"
Alternate Chinese Names: *Chuan Duan, Jie Gu Cao*
Original Source: *Shen Nong Ben Cao Jing* (Divine Husbandman's Classic of the Materia Medica) in the second century
English Name: dipsacus, Himalayan teasel root
Botanical Name: *Dipsacus asper* Wall. (*Chuan Xu Duan*)
Pharmaceutical Name: Radix Dipsaci
Properties: bitter, sweet, acrid, slightly warm
Channels Entered: Liver, Kidney

CHINESE THERAPEUTIC ACTIONS

1. Tonifies the Liver and Kidney

Liver and Kidney deficiencies: Liver and Kidney deficiencies are characterized by inability to nourish muscles and tendons, resulting in aches and pains in the lower extremities. Furthermore, deficiency of Kidney yang leads to compromised ability of the organ to contain body fluids, leading to symptoms such as polyuria and spermatorrhea. Clinically, *Xu Duan* (Radix Dipsaci) tonifies the Liver and Kidney to treat musculoskeletal and genitourinary disorders.

- Lower back and knee soreness and pain: combine *Xu Duan* with *Du Zhong* (Cortex Eucommiae), *Niu Xi* (Radix Cyathulae seu Achyranthis), *Gou Ji* (Rhizoma Cibotii), *Sheng Di Huang* (Radix Rehmanniae), *Shu Di Huang* (Radix Rehmanniae Preparata) and *Tu Si Zi* (Semen Cuscutae).
- Polyuria, spermatorrhea: use *Xu Duan* as a single-herb remedy.

17 TONIC HERBS

Xu Duan (Radix Dipsaci)

2. Calms the Fetus and Stops Uterine Bleeding

Restless fetus, habitual miscarriage, or uterine bleeding during pregnancy: These conditions often occur because of Liver and Kidney deficiencies and instability of the *ren* (conception) and *chong* (thoroughfare) channels.

- Uterine bleeding from Kidney deficiency: combine *Xu Duan* with *Tu Si Zi* (Semen Cuscutae), *E Jiao* (Colla Corii Asini), and *Sang Ji Sheng* (Herba Taxilli).
- Unstable pregnancy due to Kidney deficiency: use it with *Du Zhong* (Cortex Eucommiae).
- Restless fetus or habitual miscarriage in the first trimester, with uterine bleeding and severe low back pain: combine *Xu Duan* with *Du Zhong* (Cortex Eucommiae), *Da Zao* (Fructus Jujubae) and rice.

3. Invigorates Blood Circulation and Strengthens Tendons and Bones

Trauma, fractures, sprains and strains: Trauma causes fractured bones, damage to the tendons, and blood stagnation in the channels and collaterals, resulting in redness, swelling and pain. When blood stagnation is not resolved, swelling, pain and inflammation will not decrease. *Xu Duan* invigorates blood, strengthens tendons and bones, and alleviates pain. It promotes the growth of bones and flesh to aid in recovery. It is one of the most commonly used herbs in the trauma departments of hospitals in China.

- Traumatic injuries with severe pain, swelling, or broken bones: mix *Xu Duan*, *Gu Sui Bu* (Rhizoma Drynariae), *Dang Gui* (Radicis Angelicae Sinensis) and *Da Huang* (Radix et Rhizoma Rhei) powder with grain-based liquor and apply topically to the injury.
- Traumatic injuries: combine *Xu Duan* with *Dang Gui* (Radicis Angelicae Sinensis), *Chuan Xiong* (Rhizoma Ligustici Chuanxiong), *Ru Xiang* (Gummi Olibanum), *Mo Yao* (Myrrha), *San Qi* (Radix Notoginseng), *Du Zhong* (Cortex Eucommiae), *Niu Xi* (Radix Cyathulae seu Achyranthis), and *Gu Sui Bu* (Rhizoma Drynariae) to make a decoction.

4. Reduces Swelling, Abscess and Sores

Abscess and sores: *Xu Duan* dredges the channels and collaterals and reduces swelling and pain. It is often used with heat-clearing, toxins-eliminating herbs such as *Pu Gong Ying* (Herba Taraxaci) to treat toxic abscesses and sores.

- Breast abscesses: use this herb with *Pu Gong Ying* (Herba Taraxaci) and apply topically.

DOSAGE

10 to 20 grams in decoction. Use up to 30 grams of *Xu Duan* in severe cases. The dry-fried herb has a stronger function to stop uterine bleeding. *Xu Duan* is also used in powder or pill form.

CHEMICAL COMPOSITION

β-sitosterol, hederagenin, ursol aldehyde, ursolic acid.[1]

PHARMACOLOGICAL EFFECTS

- **Effect on nutritional deficiency:** *Xu Duan* has had beneficial effects on mice with vitamin E deficiency.[2]

TOXICOLOGY

Use of *Xu Duan* has been associated with 3 cases of severe skin allergy, characterized by redness, itching, and burning sensations.[3,4]

AUTHORS' COMMENTS

Xu Duan and *Du Zhong* (Cortex Eucommiae) both tonify the Liver and Kidney, strengthen sinews and bones, calm restless fetus, stop uterine bleeding and are used for weakness, soreness and pain in the lower back and knees. *Xu Duan* is milder in tonification but stronger in invigorating the flow of blood in the channels and collaterals. It alleviates pain of trauma, fractured or broken bones, *bi zheng* (painful obstruction syndrome), and sores. *Du Zhong* has a stronger Liver and Kidney tonifying function and thus is used more for low back pain, impotence, polyuria and dizziness.

References

1. *Xian Dai Zhong Yao Yao Li Xue* (Contemporary Pharmacology of Chinese Herbs), 1997; 1263
2. *Zhong Cao Yao Xue* (Study of Chinese Herbal Medicine), 1980:1089
3. *Si Chuan Zhong Yi* (Sichuan Chinese Medicine), 1984; 2(4):25
4. *Hei Long Jiang Zhong Yi Yao* (Heilongjiang Chinese Medicine and Herbology), 1989;(2):40

Gu Sui Bu (Rhizoma Drynariae)

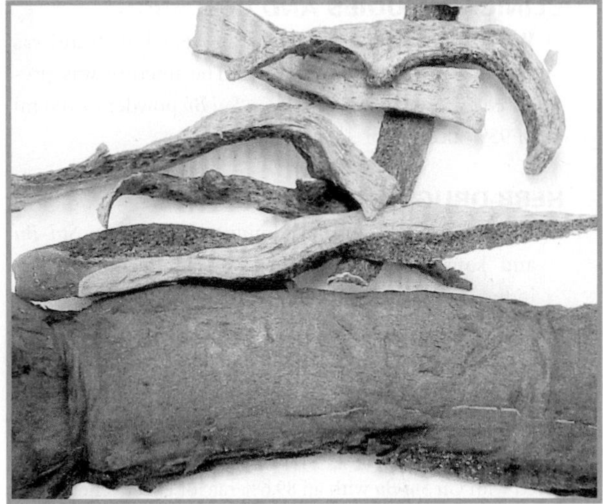

骨碎補 骨碎补

Pinyin Name: *Gu Sui Bu*
Literal Name: "mender of shattered bones," "bone fracture remedy"
Alternate Chinese Names: *Hou Jiang, Hu Sun Jiang, Kun Jiang, Shen Jiang, Mao Jiang*
Original Source: *Yao Xing Ben Cao* (Materia Medica of Medicinal Properties) by Zhen Quan in 600 A.D.
English Name: drynaria
Botanical Name: *Drynaria fortunei* (Kunze) J. Sm. (*Hu Jue*)
Pharmaceutical Name: Rhizoma Drynariae
Properties: bitter, warm
Channels Entered: Liver, Kidney

CHINESE THERAPEUTIC ACTIONS

1. Tonifies the Kidney and Strengthens the Bones

Kidney deficiency: *Gu Sui Bu* (Rhizoma Drynariae) treats Kidney deficiency symptoms such as loose teeth, soreness and weakness of the bones (especially of the back and knees), tinnitus or loss of hearing, frequent urination and diarrhea.

- Low back and knee pain: combine this herb with *Niu Xi* (Radix Cyathulae seu Achyranthis), *Bu Gu Zhi* (Fructus Psoraleae), and *Gui Xin* (Cortex Rasus Cinnamomi).
- Toothache, bleeding gums or loose teeth: use fresh *Gu Sui Bu* individually. It may be used in decoction, or the powder may be used to brush the teeth.
- Tinnitus, deafness, gradual loosening of teeth: use this herb with *Shu Di Huang* (Radix Rehmanniae Preparata), *Shan Zhu Yu* (Fructus Corni), *Fu Ling* (Poria), and *Ze Xie* (Rhizoma Alismatis).

2. Tonifies the Kidney and Benefits the Ears

The Kidney opens to the ears; thus, tonifying the Kidney directly benefits auditory functioning.

- Tinnitus or loss of hearing: combine *Gui Sui Bu* with *Shu Di Huang* (Radix Rehmanniae Preparata), *Shan Zhu Yu* (Fructus Corni), *Fu Ling* (Poria), and *Ze Xie* (Rhizoma Alismatis).

3. Promotes Mending of Bones and Relieves Pain

Trauma, fractures, sprains and strains: *Gu Sui Bu* dispels blood stasis, relieves swelling, and stops pain and bleeding. It is an essential herb when treating fractured or broken bones or other injuries such as traumatic contusions, sprains and ligament damage. It also promotes healing after surgery.

- Traumatic injuries with fractured bones, post-surgical recovery: add this herb to *Xu Duan*, *Zi Ran Tong* (Pyritum), *Gui Ban* (Plastrum Testudinis) and *Mo Yao* (Myrrha). Serve the decoction with warm liquor.

DOSAGE

10 to 20 grams in decoction. *Gui Sui Bu* must be cleaned thoroughly and dry-fried to facilitate extraction of active components. To relieve pain, fresh *Gu Sui Bu* is mixed with alcohol and applied topically.

CAUTIONS / CONTRAINDICATIONS

- Use of *Gui Sui Bu* is contraindicated in yin-deficient patients with heat, or in those who have no blood stagnation.

OVERDOSAGE

Acute adverse reaction has been reported following an overdose of *Gu Sui Bu* (250 grams in 2 days). Reactions included dry mouth, excessive speech, palpitations, fear, and chest oppression.[1]

CHEMICAL COMPOSITION

Naringin, naringenin, sugars.[2]

PHARMACOLOGICAL EFFECTS

- **Effect on calcium:** *Gu Sui Bu* increases bone absorption of calcium. It is commonly used to treat patients with bone fractures.[3]
- **Osteoarthritis:** Administration of *Gu Sui Bu* has demonstrated beneficial effects in 160 mice with osteoarthritis.[4]
- **Antihyperlipidemic:** It has preventative and therapeutic effects for high plasma cholesterol levels.[5]

Gu Sui Bu (Rhizoma Drynariae)

CLINICAL STUDIES AND RESEARCH

- **Warts:** Topical application of an herbal tincture was effective in treatment of warts. The tincture was prepared by soaking 9 grams of *Gu Sui Bu* powder in 100 ml of 95% alcohol for 3 days.[6]

HERB-DRUG INTERACTION

- **Kanamycin:** Concurrent administration of *Gu Sui Bu* and kanamycin has a preventative effect on drug-induced ototoxicity in mice. However, it did not reverse deafness once the damage had occurred.[7]
- **Streptomycin:** In one study, decoction of 30 grams of *Gu Sui Bu* was effective in treating 32 patients with tinnitus and numbness caused by streptomycin. In another study, 200 patients with adverse reactions to streptomycin were treated with *Gu Sui Bu* with an 89.6% rate of effectiveness.[8,9]

AUTHORS' COMMENTS

Gu Sui Bu and *Xu Duan* (Radix Dipsaci) both tonify the Liver and Kidney to strengthen tendons and bones, and invigorate blood circulation to treat traumatic injuries. They are an excellent pair to treat patients with bone fractures. They also prevent and treat osteoporosis by increasing bone mass density. *Gu Sui Bu* more strongly tonifies the Kidney to treat tinnitus, toothache, chronic diarrhea and loss of hearing. *Xu Duan* also treats restless fetus and stops bleeding.

References

1. *Zhe Jiang Zhong Yi Za Zhi* (Zhejiang Journal of Chinese Medicine), 1989; 24(12):546
2. *Xian Dai Zhong Yao Yao Li Xue* (Contemporary Pharmacology of Chinese Herbs), 1997; 1269
3. *Zhong Yao Xue* (Chinese Herbology), 1998; 802:803
4. *Zhong Yao Tong Bao* (Journal of Chinese Herbology), 1987; 12(10):41
5. *Zhong Yao Xue* (Chinese Herbology), 1998; 802:803
6. *Zhong Yi Za Zhi* (Journal of Chinese Medicine), 1964; 8:37
7. *Zhong Yao Xue* (Chinese Herbology), 1998; 802:803
8. *Zhong Yuan Yi Kan* (Resource Journal of Chinese Medicine), 1987; 2:33
9. *Antibiotic*, 1981; 4:52

Gou Ji (Rhizoma Cibotii)

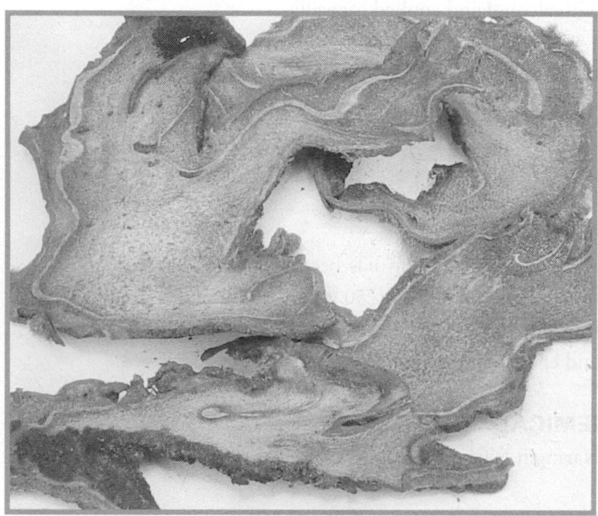

狗脊

Pinyin Name: *Gou Ji*
Literal Name: "dog's spine"
Alternate Chinese Names: *Jin Mao Gou Ji, Fu Jin, Gou Qing, Chi Jie*
Original Source: *Shen Nong Ben Cao Jing* (Divine Husbandman's Classic of the Materia Medica) in the second century
English Name: cibotium, east Asian tree fern rhizome, scythian lamb rhizome
Botanical Name: *Cibotium barometz* (L.) J. Sm. (*Jin Mao Gou Ji*)
Pharmaceutical Name: Rhizoma Cibotii
Properties: sweet, bitter, warm
Channels Entered: Liver, Kidney

CHINESE THERAPEUTIC ACTIONS

1. Tonifies the Liver and Kidney, Strengthens Bones and Sinews

Back pain and stiffness from Kidney deficiency: *Gou Ji* (Rhizoma Cibotii) treats chronic Liver and Kidney deficiencies complicated by invasion of cold, dampness and wind. Clinically, the chief complaint is back and knee pain and weakness, with stiffness and an inability to lie down flat without experiencing pain.

- Back pain: combine *Gou Ji* with *Du Zhong* (Cortex

Gou Ji (Rhizoma Cibotii)

Eucommiae), *Xu Duan* (Radix Dipsaci), and *Shu Di Huang* (Radix Rehmanniae Preparata).

2. Dispels Wind-Dampness and Relieves *Bi Zheng* (Painful Obstruction Syndrome)

***Bi zheng*:** *Gou Ji* relieves pain and stiffness caused by the invasion of pathogenic wind, damp and cold in individuals with deficient constitutions.

- Chronic low back pain with wind-cold-damp: combine *Gou Ji* with *Du Zhong* (Cortex Eucommiae), *Xu Duan* (Radix Dipsaci), *Hai Feng Teng* (Caulis Piperis Kadsurae), *Qin Jiao* (Radix Gentianae Macrophyllae), and *Du Huo* (Radix Angelicae Pubescentis).

3. Consolidates the *Jing* (Essence) and Prevents Leakage

Urinary incontinence, spermatorrhea, and profuse, clear vaginal discharge or hypermenorrhea: These leakage symptoms are associated with Kidney yang being unable to contain *jing*. *Gou Ji* has an astringent function to prevent leakage. It is a mild Kidney yang tonic and should always be used with other yang tonics.

- Urinary incontinence or continual dripping: combine *Gou Ji* with *Du Zhong* (Cortex Eucommiae), *Wu Jia Pi* (Cortex Acanthopanacis) and *Mu Gua* (Fructus Chaenomelis).
- Frequent urination: incorporate this herb with *Tu Si Zi* (Semen Cuscutae), *Wu Wei Zi* (Fructus Schisandrae Chinensis), and *Sang Piao Xiao* (Ootheca Mantidis).
- Profuse, clear vaginal discharge: add *Gou Ji* to *Bai Lian* (Radix Ampelopsis), *Ai Ye* (Folium Artemisiae Argyi), *Bai Zhu* (Rhizoma Atractylodis Macrocephalae), *Lu Rong* (Cornu Cervi Pantotrichum) and *Ji Guan Hua* (Flos Celosiae Cristatae). Serve with warm liquor.

DOSAGE

10 to 15 grams. Dry-frying *Gou Ji* will facilitate removal of its hair-like projections, and aid extraction of active components. The golden hair-like substance on *Gou Ji* can be used externally to stop bleeding.

CAUTIONS / CONTRAINDICATIONS

- *Gou Ji* is contraindicated in Kidney yin-deficient patients who show heat signs such as dysuria, scanty or dark yellow urine, or bitter and dry mouth.

CHEMICAL COMPOSITION

Onitin, starch, magnesium, calcium, potassium, aluminum.[1]

PHARMACOLOGICAL EFFECTS

- **Hemostatic:** The hair-like parts of *Gou Ji* have an effect to stop bleeding.[2]

CLINICAL STUDIES AND RESEARCH

- **Tooth extraction:** In one study, 213 patients with post tooth-extraction bleeding were treated topically with good results using an herbal preparation containing *Gou Ji*.[3]

AUTHORS' COMMENTS

Gou Ji has a weak function to tonify Kidney yang to remedy sexual dysfunction. But, the strength of this herb is in treating pain associated with Kidney deficiency or invasion of wind-damp.

References

1. *Xian Dai Zhong Yao Yao Li Xue* (Contemporary Pharmacology of Chinese Herbs), 1997; 1264
2. *Zhong Yao Xue* (Chinese Herbology), 1998; 801-802
3. *Zhong Xi Yi Jie He Za Zhi* (Journal of Integrated Chinese and Western Medicine), 1985; 8:483

Hu Lu Ba (Semen Trigonellae)

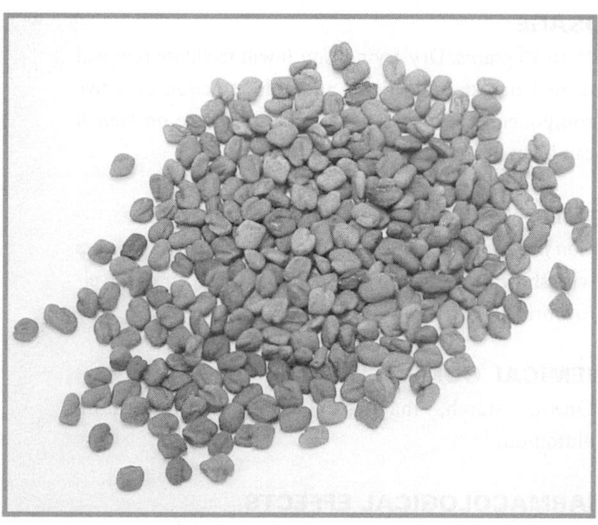

胡蘆巴 胡芦巴

Pinyin Name: *Hu Lu Ba*
Alternate Chinese Names: *Lu Ba Zi*
Original Source: *Jia You Ben Cao* (Materia Medica of the Jia You Era) by Zhang Yu-Xi and Su Song in 1057-1060
English Name: fenugreek seed, common fenugreek seed
Botanical Name: *Trigonella foenum-graecum* L. (*Hu Lu Ba*)
Pharmaceutical Name: Semen Trigonellae
Properties: bitter, warm
Channels Entered: Kidney, Liver

CHINESE THERAPEUTIC ACTIONS

1. Warms Kidney Yang

Abdominal coldness and pain, hernial pain: Deficient Kidney yang decreases in its ability to warm the middle *jiao*, and leads to subsequent Spleen yang deficiency allowing accumulation of cold, with pain and qi stagnation. *Hu Lu Ba* (Semen Trigonellae) treats Kidney and Spleen yang deficiencies with symptoms such as abdominal coldness, fullness and bloating or hypochondriac pain. Hernial pain and cold sensations of the scrotum are the result of lack of warmth in the Liver channel.

- Kidney yang deficiency with coldness, characterized by abdominal and hypochondriac fullness and pain: combine *Hu Lu Ba* with *Fu Zi* (Radix Aconiti Lateralis Praeparata) and *Wu Zhu Yu* (Fructus Evodiae).
- Severe hernial pain: add this herb to *Wu Zhu Yu* (Fructus Evodiae) and *Xiao Hui Xiang* (Fructus Foeniculi). Serve on an empty stomach with warm liquor.
- Gas in the intestines, colicky pain, feelings of genital prolapse: use it with *Wu Zhu Yu* (Fructus Evodiae), *Chuan Wu* (Radix Aconiti Preparata) and *Xiao Hui Xiang* (Fructus Foeniculi). Serve with grain-based liquor.

2. Dispels Damp-Cold and Relieves Pain

Leg *qi* due to damp-cold: Pain and cold sensations in the knees and feet are indications of cold-damp accumulation in the lower extremities, caused by Kidney yang deficiency and the inability to circulate qi and blood to the local area.

- Pain in the lower extremities: combine *Hu Lu Ba* with *Bu Gu Zhi* (Fructus Psoraleae) and *Mu Gua* (Fructus Chaenomelis).

DOSAGE

3 to 10 grams in decoction. *Hu Lu Ba* is also used in pill or powder form. Dry-frying the herb facilitates crushing and extraction of active constituents. Frying it with salt directs the function of the herb to the Kidney.

CAUTIONS / CONTRAINDICATIONS

- *Hu Lu Ba* is contraindicated in cases of yin-deficient fire or damp-heat.
- *Hu Lu Ba* should be used with caution during pregnancy, due to its emmenagogic effect.[1]

CHEMICAL COMPOSITION

Teigonelline, choline, diosgenin, yamogenin, tigogenin, neotigogenin, sitogenin, vitexin, saponaretin, vitexin-7-glucoside, orientin, isoorientin, vicenin I, vicenin, cholesterol, 4-hydroxyisoleucin, galactomannan, laueic acid, carpaine.[2]

PHARMACOLOGICAL EFFECTS

- **Antidiabetic:** Galactomannan lowers blood glucose levels.[3]

CLINICAL STUDIES AND RESEARCH

- **Diabetes mellitus:** Daily ingestion of 25 grams of *Hu Lu Ba* for 21 days has been found to decrease the quantity of glucose in blood and urine.[4]

TOXICOLOGY

Carpaine has a sedative effect on the central nervous system. Overdose in mice is associated with respiratory depression and cardiac arrest.[5]

AUTHORS' COMMENTS

Hu Lu Ba, *Fu Zi* (Radix Aconiti Lateralis Praeparata) and *Xian Mao* (Rhizoma Curculiginis) all warm Kidney yang and relieve pain. *Hu Lu Ba* is the mildest of the three.

Hu Lu Ba (Semen Trigonellae)

References
1. Brinker, Francis. *Herb Contraindications and Drug Interactions*, 1997; 47
2. *Xian Dai Zhong Yao Yao Li Xue* (Contemporary Pharmacology of Chinese Herbs), 1997; 1258
3. *CA*, 1984; 100:99862a
4. *Zhong Yao Xue* (Chinese Herbology), 1987; 812:813
5. *Zhi Wu Yao You Xiao Cheng Fen Shou Ce* (Manual of Plant Medicinals and Their Active Constituents), 1986:177

Bu Gu Zhi (Fructus Psoraleae)

補骨脂 补骨脂

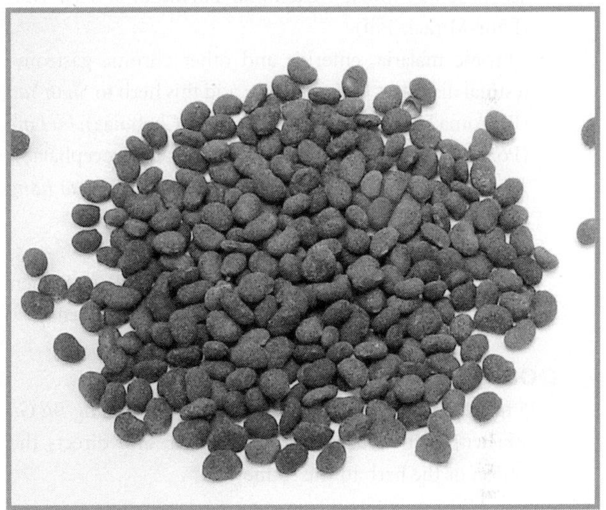

Pinyin Name: *Bu Gu Zhi*
Literal Name: "tonify the bone fat," "tonify bone resin"
Alternate Chinese Names: *Po Gu Zi*
Original Source: *Yao Xing Ben Cao* (Materia Medica of Medicinal Properties) by Zhen Quan in 600 A.D.
English Name: psoralea fruit
Botanical Name: *Psoralea corylifolia* L. (*Bu Gu Zhi*)
Pharmaceutical Name: Fructus Psoraleae
Properties: bitter, acrid, very warm
Channels Entered: Kidney, Spleen

CHINESE THERAPEUTIC ACTIONS

1. Tonifies the Kidney and Fortifies Yang, Consolidates *Jing* (Essence) and Retains Urine

Impotence, spermatorrhea, urinary incontinence, frequent urination: Deficiency of yang and *jing* allows wind and cold to invade the Kidney. Signs and symptoms of these deficiencies include spermatorrhea, impotence, premature ejaculation, cold and painful lower back, feelings of cold in the genital region (scrotum), feelings of prolapse, and decreased mobility in the back. *Bu Gu Zhi* (Fructus Psoraleae) is acrid, thus it disperses wind; and is warm, so it fortifies yang.

- Impotence due to over-indulgence in sexual activity, feelings of heaviness of the extremities, night sweats: combine *Bu Gu Zhi* with *Tu Si Zi* (Semen Cuscutae), *Hu Tao Ren* (Semen Juglandis), and *Chen Xiang* (Lignum Aquilariae Resinatum). This formula should be taken regularly with a small amount of salt water or warm liquor for 3 to 6 months.
- Nocturnal polyuria in the elderly: use this herb alone, served with rice porridge.
- Urinary incontinence and polyuria: combine it with *Sang Piao Xiao* (Ootheca Mantidis), *Tu Si Zi* (Semen Cuscutae), *Wu Yao* (Radix Linderae) and *Yi Zhi Ren* (Fructus Alpiniae Oxyphyllae).
- Chronic urinary incontinence in adolescents or adults: combine *Bu Gu Zhi* with *Sang Piao Xiao* (Ootheca Mantidis), *Fu Pen Zi* (Fructus Rubi), *Wu Yao* (Radix Linderae Strychnifolia), *Yi Zhi Ren* (Fructus Alpiniae Oxyphyllae), *Shu Di Huang* (Radix Rehmanniae Preparata), *Shan Zhu Yu* (Fructus Corni), *Ji Nei Jin* (Endothelium Corneum Gigeriae Galli), *Fu Ling* (Poria), calcined *Long Gu* (Os Draconis), calcined *Mu Li* (Concha Ostreae), and *Sang Ji Sheng* (Herba Taxilli).
- Low back pain: use *Bu Gu Zhi* alone as powder, and take it with warm liquor.
- Feeling of heaviness, coldness and extreme pain in the low back: combine this herb with *Du Zhong* (Cortex Eucommiae) and *Hu Tao Ren* (Semen Juglandis). Serve the decoction regularly with warm liquor.

Bu Gu Zhi (Fructus Psoraleae)

2. Warms the Spleen and Stops Diarrhea

Diarrhea from Spleen deficiency: In Spleen yang deficiency, normal transformation and transportation functions are compromised, leading to diarrhea, borborygmus, bloating, and poor appetite. *Bu Gu Zhi* is commonly used to treat chronic diarrhea caused by Spleen and Kidney yang deficiencies.

- Diarrhea from Spleen and Kidney yang deficiencies: use *Bu Gu Zhi* with *Rou Dou Kou* (Semen Myristicae).
- Diarrhea from Spleen and Kidney yang deficiencies with cold: combine it with *Rou Dou Kou* (Semen Myristicae), *Wu Wei Zi* (Fructus Schisandrae Chinensis), and *Wu Zhu Yu* (Fructus Evodiae). **Exemplar Formula:** *Si Shen Wan* (Four-Miracle Pill).
- Chronic malaria, enteritis and other chronic gastrointestinal disorders with diarrhea: add this herb to *Shan Yao* (Rhizoma Dioscoreae), *He Zi* (Fructus Chebulae), *Fu Ling* (Poria), *Bai Zhu* (Rhizoma Atractylodis Macrocephalae), *Fu Zi* (Radix Aconiti Lateralis Praeparata), and *Pao Jiang* (Rhizoma Zingiberis Preparatum).

Bu Gu Zhi, when combined with *Hu Tao Ren* (Semen Juglandis), treats asthma caused by Kidney deficiency.

DOSAGE

5 to 10 grams in decoction, pill or powder. Frying *Bu Gu Zhi* with salt reduces its drying effect, and directs the action of the herb to the Kidney.

CAUTIONS / CONTRAINDICATIONS

- *Bu Gu Zhi* is acrid, warm and drying; thus long-term use may lead to depletion of yin, characterized by side effects such as dry mouth, dry tongue, and sore throat.
- *Bu Gu Zhi* is contraindicated in cases involving yin-deficient heat, constipation, nocturnal emissions, hematuria, cystitis or urinary tract infection, red eyes, and a bitter taste in the mouth with a dry tongue.
- Use *Bu Gu Zhi* with caution during pregnancy.

CHEMICAL COMPOSITION

Psoralen, isopsoralen, coryfolin, corylifolinin, psoralidin, isopsoralidin, corylidin, 8-methoxypsoralen, isobavahin, bavachinin, bavachalcone, bavachromenn, bavachromanol, corylin, neobavaisofavane, corylinal, bakuchiol, psoraldehyde, isoneobavachalion, dihydrofuranochalcone bakuchalcone, chalcone bavachromanol, neobavachalcone, limonene, terpineol, stigmasterol, trilaurin, daidzin, coumstrol, angelicin.[1]

PHARMACOLOGICAL EFFECTS

- **Cardiovascular:** Administration of *Bu Gu Zhi* dilates the coronary artery and increases blood perfusion to the cardiac muscle in mice.[2]
- **Respiratory:** In a laboratory study, a preparation of *Bu Gu Zhi* was found to have marked antiasthmatic properties compared to a placebo.[3]
- **Antibiotic:** It has an inhibitory effect against *Staphylococcus aureus*, *Staphylococcus albus*, and others.[4]
- **Immunostimulant:** Administration of *Bu Gu Zhi* is associated with an increase in white blood cell counts in rats.[5]
- **Effects on smooth muscle:** According to animal studies, an extract of *Bu Gu Zhi* stimulated the smooth muscle of the intestines, but relaxed the smooth muscle of the uterus.[6]
- **Antineoplastic:** Preliminary studies have demonstrated that psoralen at the dosage of 250 μg/ml inhibits DNA synthesis of cancer cells in patients with sarcoma.[7]

CLINICAL STUDIES AND RESEARCH

- **Psoriasis:** In one study, 800 patients with psoriasis were treated with a 93% rate of effectiveness using intramuscular injection of alcohol extract of *Bu Gu Zhi* one time each day for 10 days. The same treatment was repeated if necessary, with 3 days of rest between 10-day courses.[8]
- **Neutropenia:** Three grams of *Bu Gu Zhi* powder given three times daily for 4 weeks per treatment period showed marked effectiveness in treating neutropenia. Out of 19 patients, 14 made complete recovery, 4 showed moderate improvement, and 1 experienced no response.[9]
- **Alopecia:** According to one report, 45 patients with alopecia were treated with 84.4% effectiveness using intramuscular injection of *Bu Gu Zhi* and UV ray therapy.[10]
- **White vulvar lesions:** Topical application of *Bu Gu Zhi* to the affected area every other day was effective in 50 out of 53 patients with white vulvar lesions. The herbal paste was prepared by mixing equal portions of *Bu Gu Zhi* and 95% alcohol for 1 week, followed by a gradual simmering until the liquid became a paste. 500 ml of solution generally yields 50 ml of paste.[11]
- **Uterine bleeding:** In one study, 326 patients with uterine bleeding from various causes were treated with over 90% effectiveness. The treatment protocol was to administer 1.5 grams each of *Bu Gu Zhi* and *Chi Shi Zhi* (Halloysitum Rubrum) three times daily for 3 days, or longer if necessary.[12]
- **Enuresis:** According to one report, bed-wetting in 6 children between 3 and 12 years of age was treated with complete success using dry-fried *Bu Gu Zhi* in powder daily, in one dose at bedtime. The dosage was 1.5 grams for children between 3 and 9 years of age, and 2.5 grams for children between 10 and 12 years of age.[13]

TOXICOLOGY

Injection of *Bu Gu Zhi* is occasionally associated with severe allergic reactions.[14]

Bu Gu Zhi (Fructus Psoraleae)

AUTHORS' COMMENTS

Bu Gu Zhi and *Yi Zhi Ren* (Fructus Alpiniae Oxyphyllae) tonify the Kidney and consolidate the *jing* (essence), treating impotence, spermatorrhea, urinary incontinence and diarrhea from Kidney yang deficiency. *Bu Gu Zhi* more strongly tonifies the Kidney in treating back pain and spermatorrhea. *Yi Zhi Ren* more effectively warms the middle *jiao* and treats reduced appetite and increased desire to sleep.

Asthma characterized by Lung and Kidney deficiencies can be treated effectively with *Bu Gu Zhi*, *Ge Jie* (Gecko) and *Dong Chong Xia Cao* (Cordyceps).

References

1. *Xian Dai Zhong Yao Yao Li Xue* (Contemporary Pharmacology of Chinese Herbs), 1997; 1244
2. *Zhong Cheng Yao Yan Jiu* (Research of Chinese Patent Medicine), 1987; (12):24
3. *Guang Dong Yi Xue* (Guangdong Medicine), 1984; 5(11):29
4. *Zhong Yao Xue* (Chinese Herbology), 1998; 804:806
5. *Zhong Cheng Yao Yan Jiu* (Research of Chinese Patent Medicine), 1987; (12):24
6. *Zhong Yao Xue* (Chinese Herbology), 1998; 804:806
7. *Shi Yong Kou Qiang Yi Xue Za Zhi* (Journal of Medical Stomatology), 1990; 11(9):427
8. *Zhong Yi Za Zhi* (Journal of Chinese Medicine), 1982; 9:31
9. *Xin Yi Xue* (New Medicine), 1975; 10:497
10. *Zhong Cao Yao Tong Xun* (Journal of Chinese Herbal Medicine), 1972; 1:41
11. *Xin Yi Xue* (New Medicine), 1977; 7:319
12. *Tian Jing Yi Yao* (Tianjing Medicine and Herbology), 1973; 1:36
13. *Xin Zhong Yi* (New Chinese Medicine), 1977; 7:319
14. *Zhong Hua Pi Fu Ke Xue Za Zhi* (Chinese Journal of Dermatology), 1983; (4):267

Yi Zhi Ren (Fructus Alpiniae Oxyphyllae)

益智仁

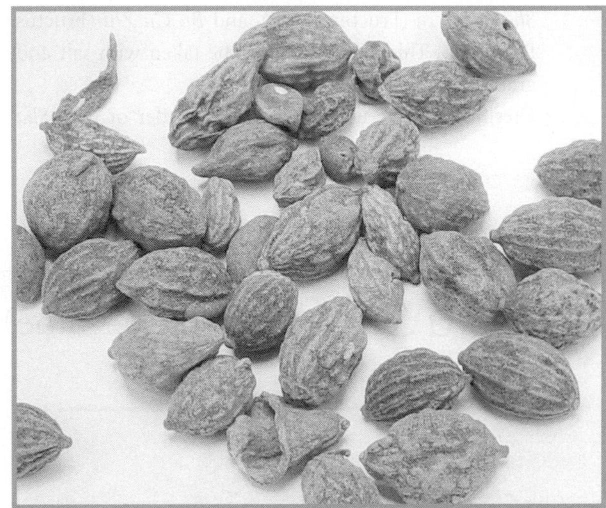

Pinyin Name: *Yi Zhi Ren*
Literal Name: "benefit the intelligence seed," "benefit intelligence nut"
Alternate Chinese Names: *Yi Zhi Zi*
Original Source: *Ben Cao Shi Yi* (Omissions from the [Classic of the] Materia Medica) by Chen Cang-Qi in 741 A.D.
English Name: alpinia fruit, sharp-leaf galangal fruit
Botanical Name: *Alpinia oxyphylla* Miq. (*Yi Zhi*)
Pharmaceutical Name: Fructus Alpiniae Oxyphyllae
Properties: acrid, warm
Channels Entered: Kidney, Spleen

CHINESE THERAPEUTIC ACTIONS

1. Warms the Spleen, Increases Appetite, Stops Excessive Salivation and Diarrhea

Diarrhea, epigastric and abdominal coldness and pain, excessive salivation: Deficiency and cold of the middle *jiao* manifest in symptoms of epigastric and abdominal coldness, fullness and pain, diarrhea, and profuse, clear salivation. Excessive salivation accompanies impairment of the Spleen's transportation function. *Yi Zhi Ren* (Fructus Alpiniae Oxyphyllae) stops salivation and diarrhea by warming the Spleen, restoring its transportation function and helping it distribute water evenly in the body. Abdominal pain and fullness are the result of Stomach qi not being able to descend properly because of stagnation. This herb increases appetite by warming the Spleen and Stomach and moving qi stagnation in the middle *jiao*.

- Diarrhea with abdominal distention: combine *Yi Zhi Ren* with *Sha Ren* (Fructus Amomi).
- Spleen qi and yang deficiencies: combine it with *Shan Yao*

Yi Zhi Ren (Fructus Alpiniae Oxyphyllae)

(Rhizoma Dioscoreae), *Bai Zhu* (Rhizoma Atractylodis Macrocephalae), and *Ren Shen* (Radix Ginseng).

- Profuse salivation, especially during the night: use this herb with *Cang Zhu* (Rhizoma Atractylodis), *Fu Ling* (Poria), *He Zi* (Fructus Chebulae), *Ban Xia* (Rhizoma Pinelliae) and *Chen Pi* (Pericarpium Citri Reticulatae).
- Vomiting of clear fluids: add this herb to *Ding Xiang* (Flos Caryophylli) and *Wu Zhu Yu* (Fructus Evodiae).
- Diarrhea with qi deficiency: use it with *Dang Shen* (Radix Codonopsis), *Bai Zhu* (Rhizoma Atractylodis Macrocephalae) and *Shan Yao* (Rhizoma Dioscoreae).

2. Warms the Kidney, Consolidates Fluids

Spermatorrhea, enuresis and uterine bleeding due to Kidney deficiency: *Yi Zhi Ren* treats Kidney yang deficiency with compromised ability to retain body fluids. Clinical manifestations include leakage of fluids from the body, such as frequent nocturnal urination, nocturnal emissions, frequent urinary urges, spermatorrhea or chronic uterine bleeding.

- Spermatorrhea or frequent nocturnal urinary urges: combine *Yi Zhi Ren* with *Wu Yao* (Radix Linderae), *Shan Yao* (Rhizoma Dioscoreae), *Sang Piao Xiao* (Ootheca Mantidis), *Wu Wei Zi* (Fructus Schisandrae Chinensis), *Shan Zhu Yu* (Fructus Corni), and *Bu Gu Zhi* (Fructus Psoraleae). This formula should be taken with salt and grain-based liquor.
- Uterine bleeding: use it alone as a powder or with *Sha Ren* (Fructus Amomi). This formula should be taken with salt and grain-based liquor.

DOSAGE

3 to 10 grams in decoction. *Yi Zhi Ren* is also used in pill or powder form. The unprocessed form has a strong drying effect, and is commonly used to treat excessive salivation, involuntary salivation, vomiting and diarrhea. Frying *Yi Zhi Ren* with salt directs its functions to the Kidney, thereby enhancing its effect to treat frequent urination, nocturnal urination, nocturnal emissions, premature ejaculation, and leukorrhea.

CAUTIONS / CONTRAINDICATIONS

- Use of *Yi Zhi Ren* is contraindicated in cases of yin-deficient fire, vomiting caused by qi stagnation or heat, urinary incontinence due to heat, and diarrhea from qi deficiency or heat.

CHEMICAL COMPOSITION

Yakuchinone A, nootkatol, cineole, zingberene, zingiberol.[1]

PHARMACOLOGICAL EFFECTS

Yi Zhi Ren has cardiotonic and antineoplastic effects.[2,3]

References

1. *Xian Dai Zhong Yao Yao Li Xue* (Contemporary Pharmacology of Chinese Herbs), 1997; 1265
2. *Planta Med*, 1984; 50(2):186
3. *Zhong Guo Zhong Yao Za Zhi* (People's Republic of China Journal of Chinese Herbology), 1990; 15(8):492

Tu Si Zi (Semen Cuscutae)

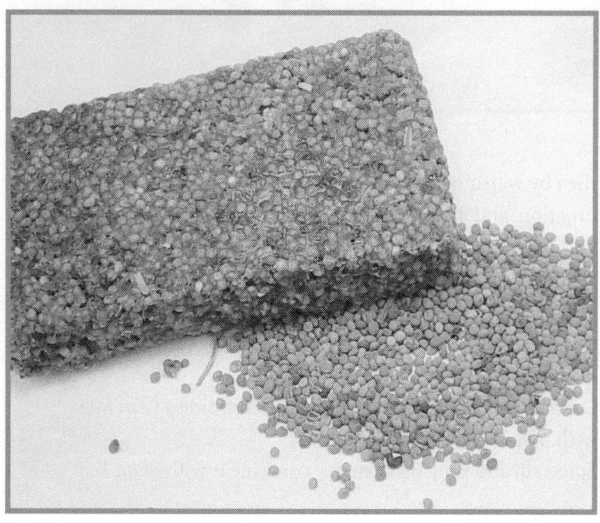

菟絲子 菟丝子

Pinyin Name: *Tu Si Zi*
Literal Name: "rabbit string seed," "hare silk seed"
Alternate Chinese Names: *Tu Si Bing, Jin Qian Cao Zi*
Original Source: *Shen Nong Ben Cao Jing* (Divine Husbandman's Classic of the Materia Medica) in the second century
English Name: cuscuta, dodder seed
Botanical Name: *Cuscuta chinensis* Lam. (*Tu Si Zi*); *Cuscuta japonica* Choisy (*Da Tu Si Zi*)
Pharmaceutical Name: Semen Cuscutae
Properties: acrid, sweet, neutral
Channels Entered: Liver, Kidney

Tu Si Zi (Semen Cuscutae)

CHINESE THERAPEUTIC ACTIONS

1. Tonifies Kidney Yin and Yang

Impotence, chronic uterine bleeding, leukorrhea: *Tu Si Zi* (Semen Cuscutae) treats prominent signs of Kidney yin and yang deficiencies such as impotence, back pain, urinary incontinence, spermatorrhea, uterine bleeding, and profuse, clear vaginal discharge. This herb is neutral and can be used alone at high dosages to treat the above-mentioned symptoms.

- Spermatorrhea, frequent dreams: use *Tu Si Zi* alone at high dosage, or combine it with *Wu Wei Zi* (Fructus Schisandrae Chinensis), *Lian Zi* (Semen Nelumbinis), *Yuan Zhi* (Radix Polygalae) and *Qian Shi* (Semen Euryales).
- Uterine bleeding, restless fetus, back pain with a feeling of prolapse: combine it with *Du Zhong* (Cortex Eucommiae), *Sang Ji Sheng* (Herba Taxilli), and *E Jiao* (Colla Corii Asini).
- Impotence: add this herb to *Bai Ji Li* (Fructus Tribuli), *Yin Yang Huo* (Herba Epimedii), *Gou Qi Zi* (Fructus Lycii) and *Ba Ji Tian* (Radix Morindae Officinalis).
- Heart qi deficiency from excessive worrying, with dribbling urination, white turbid urine and enuresis: use *Tu Si Zi* with *Fu Ling* (Poria) and *Lian Zi* (Semen Nelumbinis).

2. Consolidates Kidney *Jing* (Essence) and Reserves the Urine

Enuresis: Kidney qi deficiency results in the inability of the urinary bladder to hold urine. *Tu Si Zi* treats urinary disorders such as incontinence, terminal dripping, frequent urinary urges, polyuria, or turbid urine caused by qi and yang deficiencies.

- Urinary incontinence, frequent urinary urges, terminal dripping of turbid urine: combine *Tu Si Zi* with *Fu Ling* (Poria) and *Lian Zi* (Semen Nelumbinis).

3. Brightens the Eyes

Diminished vision: The Liver opens to the eyes. Lack of nourishment results in blurred vision, spots in front of the eyes, dryness of the eyes, and dizziness.

- Blurred vision: combine *Tu Si Zi* with *Shan Zhu Yu* (Fructus Corni), *Ju Hua* (Flos Chrysanthemi), and *Shu Di Huang* (Radix Rehmanniae Preparata).

4. Stops Diarrhea

Diarrhea and poor appetite are the results of Kidney yang deficiency and failure to warm Spleen yang. Unable to be transformed or transported, food, water and dampness accumulate in the intestines, and diarrhea occurs. *Tu Si Zi* warms the Spleen and Kidney to restore proper digestion and stop diarrhea.

- Diarrhea: combine *Tu Si Zi* with *Bu Gu Zhi* (Fructus Psoraleae), *Huang Qi* (Radix Astragali) and *Bai Zhu* (Rhizoma Atractylodis Macrocephalae).

5. Treats *Xiao Ke* (Wasting and Thirsting) Syndrome

Tu Si Zi is commonly used to treat *xiao ke* syndrome. The fresh juice of these seeds may be used as a single-herb remedy. Dried *Tu Si Zi* is commonly combined with other herbs in a formula.

DOSAGE

10 to 15 grams.

CAUTIONS / CONTRAINDICATIONS

- Though *Tu Si Zi* is neutral in thermal property, it tonifies Kidney yang more than it does Kidney yin. Therefore, it should be used with caution in cases of yin-deficient heat (especially those patients who are easily aroused sexually), or for patients with dryness, constipation or scanty, dark urine.

CHEMICAL COMPOSITION

Cholesterol, campesterol, β-sitosterol, stigmasterol, β-amyrin.[1]

PHARMACOLOGICAL EFFECTS

- **Hepatoprotective:** Administration of a 20% decoction of *Tu Si Zi* has a marked hepatoprotective effect in mice, especially against carbon tetrachloride.[2]
- **General strengthening:** Decoction of *Tu Si Zi* has been shown to increase resistance to hypoxia and increase swimming time in mice.[3]

CLINICAL STUDIES AND RESEARCH

- **Vitiligo:** Topical application of an herbal tincture two to three times daily provided good results in 8 out of 10 patients with vitiligo. The herbal tincture was prepared by soaking 25 grams of cuscuta seeds and twigs in 100 ml of 95% alcohol for 48 hours.[4]

References

1. *Xian Dai Zhong Yao Yao Li Xue* (Contemporary Pharmacology of Chinese Herbs), 1997; 1248
2. *Chang Yong Zhong Yao Cheng Fen Yu Yao Li Shou Ce* (A Handbook of the Composition and Pharmacology of Common Chinese Drugs), 1994; 1563:1564
3. Ibid.
4. *Xi An Yi Ke Da Xue Xue Bao* (Journal of Xian University School of Medicine), 1959; 6:88

Sha Yuan Zi (Semen Astragali Complanati)

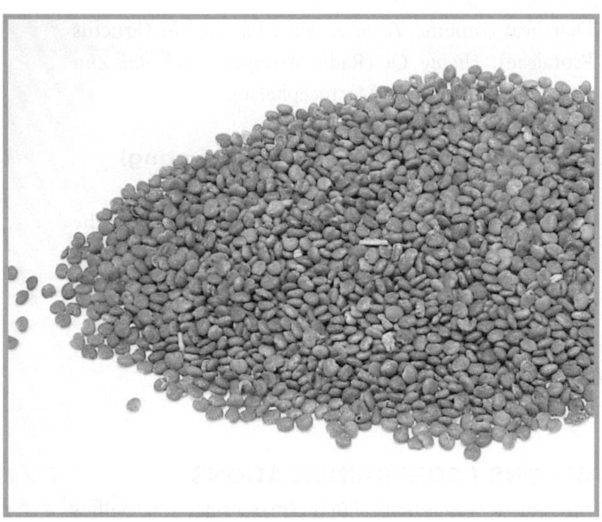

沙苑子 沙苑子

Pinyin Name: *Sha Yuan Zi*

Alternate Chinese Names: *Sha Yuan Ji Li, Tong Ji Li, Wai Sha Yuan, Tong Xi Li*

Original Source: *Tu Jing Ben Cao* (Illustrated Classic of the Materia Medica) by Su Song in 1061

English Name: astragalus seed, flat-stem milkvetch seed

Botanical Name: *Astragalus complanatus* R. Br. (*Sha Yuan Zi*)

Pharmaceutical Name: Semen Astragali Complanati

Properties: sweet, warm

Channels Entered: Kidney, Liver

CHINESE THERAPEUTIC ACTIONS

1. Tonifies the Kidney and Consolidates *Jing* (Essence)

Leakage of body fluids: Liver and Kidney deficiencies lead to leakage of *jing*. Symptoms of this problem include spermatorrhea, urinary incontinence, premature ejaculation, profuse clear vaginal discharge, and polyuria. *Sha Yuan Zi* (Semen Astragali Complanati) strengthens the Kidney and helps secure and prevent the loss of *jing*.

- General Kidney deficiency with leakage of *jing*: combine *Sha Yuan Zi* with *Lu Jiao Shuang* (Cornu Cervi Degelatinatum), *Qian Shi* (Semen Euryales) and *Shan Zhu Yu* (Fructus Corni).
- Impotence, spermatorrhea: combine this herb with *Shan Zhu Yu* (Fructus Corni), *Wu Wei Zi* (Fructus Schisandrae Chinensis), *Lian Xu* (Stamen Nelumbinis), *Long Gu* (Os Draconis), *Ba Ji Tian* (Radix Morindae Officinalis), and *Xian Mao* (Rhizoma Curculiginis).
- Polyuria or urinary incontinence: use *Sha Yuan Zi* with *Sang Piao Xiao* (Ootheca Mantidis), *Tu Si Zi* (Semen Cuscutae), *Fu Pen Zi* (Fructus Rubi), *Yi Zhi Ren* (Fructus Alpiniae Oxyphyllae) and *Bu Gu Zhi* (Fructus Psoraleae).

2. Nourishes the Liver and Brightens the Eyes

Visual disorders due to Liver and Kidney deficiencies: The Liver opens to the eyes: lack of nourishment to the Liver causes blurred vision, reduced visual acuity, and dizziness. *Sha Yuan Zi* is warm, yet not drying. It consolidates *jing* and nourishes Liver blood to benefit the eyes.

- Visual disturbances: combine this herb with *Gou Qi Zi* (Fructus Lycii), *Tu Si Zi* (Semen Cuscutae), *Bai Ji Li* (Fructus Tribuli), *Jue Ming Zi* (Semen Cassiae), and *Ju Hua* (Flos Chrysanthemi).

DOSAGE

10 to 20 grams in decoction. *Sha Yuan Zi* is also used in pill or powder form. The salt-fried herb has a dual effect to tonify yin and yang, and is commonly used to treat spermatorrhea, nocturnal emissions, and incontinence.

CAUTIONS / CONTRAINDICATIONS

- Use of *Sha Yuan Zi* is contraindicated in yin-deficient patients with heat signs, or those with hyperactive sex drive.

CHEMICAL COMPOSITION

Complanatuside, neocomplanoside, myricomplanoside, astragalin, kaempferide, myricetin, threonine, valine, methionine, leucine, isoleucine, phenylalanine.[1]

PHARMACOLOGICAL EFFECTS

- **Cardiovascular:** According to animal studies, injection of *Sha Yuan Zi* has been shown to decrease blood pressure, decrease heart rate, decrease peripheral vascular resistance and increase blood perfusion to the brain.[2]

TOXICOLOGY

The LD_{50} for intraperitoneal injection of *Sha Yuan Zi* is 37.75 g/kg in mice.[3]

AUTHORS' COMMENTS

Sha Yuan Ji Li, the alternate pinyin name for *Sha Yuan Zi*, is often confused with *Bai Ji Li* (Fructus Tribuli). Though they both treat disorders of the eyes, they have very different functions. *Sha Yuan Zi* tonifies the Liver and Kidney, secures *jing* and improves vision. It is used most often for blurred vision or diminished visual acuity. *Bai Ji Li* calms the Liver and dispels wind-heat to brighten the eyes. It treats red eyes with tears or pain.

Sha Yuan Zi (Semen Astragali Complanati)

Sha Yuan Zi and *Tu Si Zi* (Semen Cuscutae) both tonify the Kidney and benefit *jing*. *Sha Yuan Zi* warms Kidney yang, secures *jing* and is best used to treat impotence and spermatorrhea. *Tu Si Zi* is warm but not drying. It is best for infertility.

References

1. *Xian Dai Zhong Yao Yao Li Xue* (Contemporary Pharmacology of Chinese Herbs), 1997; 1270-1271
2. *Xi Bei Yi Yao Za Zhi* (Northwest Journal of Herbal Medicine), 1988, 3(2):17
3. *Shan Xi Yi Kan* (Shanxi Journal of Medicine), 1987; 16(5):61

Jiu Cai Zi (Semen Allii Tuberosi)

韭菜子 韭菜子

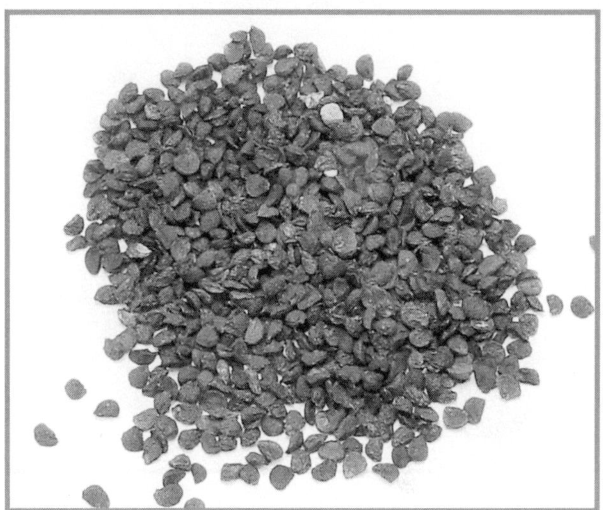

Pinyin Name: *Jiu Cai Zi*

Alternate Chinese Names: *Jiu Zi, Cao Zhong Ru, Qi Yang Cao*

Original Source: *Ming Yi Za Zhu* (Miscellaneous Records of Famous Physicians) by Tao Hong-Jing in 500 A.D.

English Name: allium seed, tuber onion seed

Botanical Name: *Allium tuberosum* Rottler (*Jiu Cai*)

Pharmaceutical Name: Semen Allii Tuberosi

Properties: acrid, sweet, warm

Channels Entered: Liver, Kidney

CHINESE THERAPEUTIC ACTIONS

1. Tonifies the Liver and Kidney, Fortifies Yang and Consolidates *Jing* (Essence)

Liver and Kidney deficiencies with yang deficiency: *Jiu Cai Zi* (Semen Allii Tuberosi) treats pain and coldness of the back and knees, impotence with spermatorrhea, clear leukorrhea, polyuria, infertility, and other conditions related to Liver and Kidney deficiencies.

- Kidney yang deficiency: use *Jiu Cai Zi* alone as powder and serve it with warm liquor or combine with *Tu Si Zi* (Semen Cuscutae) and *Lu Rong* (Cornu Cervi Pantotrichum).
- Profuse, clear vaginal discharge: combine this herb with *Long Gu* (Os Draconis) and *Hai Piao Xiao* (Endoconcha Sepiae).
- Polyuria: add it to *Bu Gu Zhi* (Fructus Psoraleae), *Yi Zhi Ren* (Fructus Alpiniae Oxyphyllae) and *Sang Piao Xiao* (Ootheca Mantidis).

2. Warms the Stomach and Treats Chronic Stomach Qi Reversal

Jiu Cai Zi treats vomiting and chronic stubborn hiccups caused by Stomach cold.

- Vomiting, hiccups: combine *Jiu Cai Zi* with *Wu Zhu Yu* (Fructus Evodiae) and *Gao Liang Jiang* (Rhizoma Alpiniae Officinarum).

DOSAGE

5 to 15 grams in decoction. *Jiu Cai Zi* is also used in pill or powder form.

CAUTIONS / CONTRAINDICATIONS

- *Jiu Cai Zi* is contraindicated in cases of yin-deficient fire.

CHEMICAL COMPOSITION

Alkaloids, saponin.[1]

CLINICAL STUDIES AND RESEARCH

- **Nausea:** In one study, 5 patients were treated with good results using 9 grams of *Jiu Cai Zi* powder twice daily. In another study, 33 out of 38 patients with nausea related to carcinoma showed good response after being treated with 1.5 to 3.0 grams of dry-fried *Jiu Cai Zi* powder one to three times daily.[2,3]

Jiu Cai Zi (Semen Allii Tuberosi)

References

1. *Chang Yong Zhong Yao Cheng Fen Yu Yao Li Shou Ce* (A Handbook of the Composition and Pharmacology of Common Chinese Drugs), 1994; 1415
2. *Xin Yi Yao Xue Za Zhi* (New Journal of Medicine and Herbology), 1975; 1:44
3. *Shang Hai Chi Jiao Yi Sheng Za Zhi* (Shanghai Journal of Barefoot Doctors), 1978; 5:53

Zi He Che (Placenta Hominis)

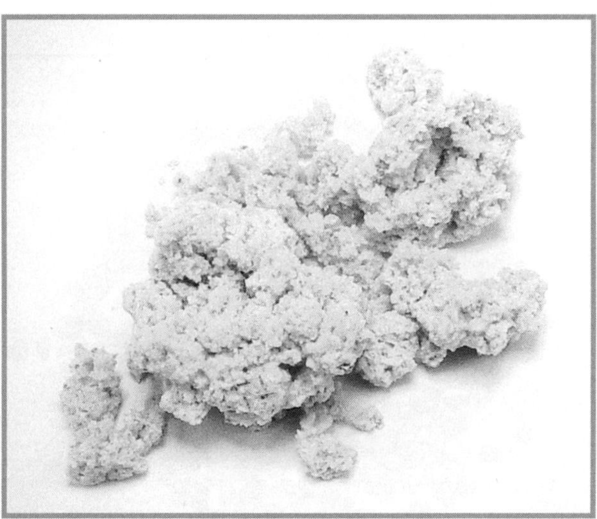

紫河車 紫河车

Pinyin Name: *Zi He Che*
Literal Name: "purple river vehicle"
Alternate Chinese Names: *Tai Pan, Ren Bao, Bai Yi, Hun Yuan Mu, Hun Tun Yi*
Original Source: *Ben Cao Shi Yi* (Omissions from the [Classic of the] Materia Medica) by Chen Cang-Qi in 741 A.D.
English Name: placenta, dried human placenta
Zoological Name: *Homo sapiens* (*Ren Bao*)
Pharmaceutical Name: Placenta Hominis
Properties: sweet, salty, warm
Channels Entered: Kidney, Lung, Liver

CHINESE THERAPEUTIC ACTIONS

1. Replenishes *Jing* (Essence)

Prenatal deficiency with insufficient *jing*: Kidney *jing* is derived from one's parents. When this is deficient, patients present with symptoms associated with Kidney yang, *jing* and blood deficiencies. Typical symptoms include immature development of the sexual organs, infertility in men and women, low sex drive, impotence, spermatorrhea, irregular menstruation, back and knees soreness and weakness, tinnitus, and dizziness. *Zi He Che* (Placenta Hominis) is the best choice to tonify *jing*, as it is the part of the body most directly involved with the development of a human being. It is the product of *jing* and blood from the father and the mother. It is therefore used to greatly tonify the blood at the *ying* (nutritive) level. Use of *Zi He Che* in women enhances the development of the reproductive organs such as the breast, vagina, uterus and ovaries. It can also be used to alleviate atrophy of the reproductive organs. Use of *Zi He Che* in men helps with the development of the genital organs, in addition to treating impotence, spermatorrhea, premature ejaculation, and infertility.

- *Jing* deficiency: combine *Zi He Che* with *Shu Di Huang* (Radix Rehmanniae Preparata), *Dong Chong Xia Cao* (Cordyceps), *Lu Jiao Jiao* (Gelatinum Cornu Cervi) and *Yin Yang Huo* (Herba Epimedii).

2. Nourishes Blood

Insufficient lactation: *Zi He Che* treats extremely weak postpartum women who have scanty or insufficient milk production caused by blood and *jing* (essence) deficiencies.

- Insufficient lactation due to blood deficiency: combine *Zi He Che* with *Dang Gui* (Radicis Angelicae Sinensis) and *Shu Di Huang* (Radix Rehmanniae Preparata).
- Insufficient lactation because of qi and blood deficiencies: combine this substance with *Huang Qi* (Radix Astragali), *Ren Shen* (Radix Ginseng), *Dang Gui* (Radicis Angelicae Sinensis) and *Shu Di Huang* (Radix Rehmanniae Preparata).

Qi and blood deficiencies: This substance is excellent for patients who are recovering from chronic illnesses. Other possible symptoms include fatigue, weight loss, shortness of breath, lack of desire to speak, sallow or dark and dull complexion.

Zi He Che (Placenta Hominis)

- Anemia: combine *Zi He Che* with *Dang Gui* (Radicis Angelicae Sinensis) and *Shu Di Huang* (Radix Rehmanniae Preparata).
- Qi and blood deficiencies: combine it with *Huang Qi* (Radix Astragali), *Ren Shen* (Radix Ginseng), *Dang Gui* (Radicis Angelicae Sinensis) and *Shu Di Huang* (Radix Rehmanniae Preparata).

3. Benefits Lung Qi

Chronic dyspnea and cough: The Lung dominates qi and the Kidney grasps it downward. When both organs are weakened by chronic coughing, the following symptoms will also be present: shortness of breath, interrupted respiration, and wheezing. *Zi He Che* is usually administered on a long-term basis to promote wellness and prevent recurrence of cough.

- Chronic respiratory disorders: combine *Zi He Che* with *Ge Jie* (Gecko).
- Chronic cough with yin-deficient heat, manifesting in scanty yellow sputum: use this substance with *Tian Men Dong* (Radix Asparagi), *Gui Ban* (Plastrum Testudinis) and *Huang Bai* (Cortex Phellodendri).

DOSAGE

1.5 to 3 grams as powder two to three times daily. The dosage of *Zi He Che* may be doubled in severe cases.

CAUTIONS / CONTRAINDICATIONS

- *Zi He Che* should not be used alone for yin-deficient patients with heat signs.

CHEMICAL COMPOSITION

The composition of *Zi He Che* is extremely complex. The main components include protein, amino acids, enzymes and hormones (human chorionic gonadotropin, prolactin, oxytocin, thyroid-stimulating hormone, and sex hormones).[1,2]

PHARMACOLOGICAL EFFECTS

- **Immunostimulant:** Oral administration of *Zi He Che* at 6.6 g/kg in mice once daily for 7 days is associated with increased immunity and elevated IgM count.[3]

CLINICAL STUDIES AND RESEARCH

- **Chronic tracheitis:** In one study, 609 patients with chronic tracheitis were treated with intramuscular injections of *Zi He Che* every day or every other day, with an overall rate of effectiveness of 82.37 to 87.6%.[4]
- **Bronchial asthma:** Two patients with bronchial asthma were treated with marked success using 2 to 4 grams of *Zi He Che* three times daily after meals.[5]
- **Lung cancer:** According to one report, 31 out of 33 patients showed improvement after daily treatment with an herbal decoction containing *Zi He Che*, *Gua Lou Shi* (Fructus Trichosanthis), *Chen Pi* (Pericarpium Citri Reticulatae), *Yi Yi Ren* (Semen Coicis), *E Zhu* (Rhizoma Curcumae), *Xia Ku Cao* (Spica Prunellae), *Shan Dou Gen* (Radix Sophorae Tonkinensis) and *Bai Guo* (Semen Ginkgo).[6]

TOXICOLOGY

Subcutaneous injection in mice of *Zi He Che* at normal therapeutic doses for 3 to 6 months showed no abnormality in functions or development. At high doses, however, it causes tremor, constriction of pores, and swelling at the site of injection. At 300 times the therapeutic dose, there is an abnormal effect on the liver, kidneys, and spleen.[7]

SUPPLEMENT

- 臍帶 / 脐带 *Qi Dai* (Corda Umbilicalis Hominis), first cited in *Ben Cao Shi Yi* (Omissions from the [Classic of the] Materia Medica) by Chen Cang-Qi in 741 A.D., is the umbilical cord. It treats wheezing and night sweats caused by Kidney yang and *jing* (essence) deficiencies. *Qi Dai* is often decocted with *Jin Yin Hua* (Flos Lonicerae), and *Gan Cao* (Radix Glycyrrhizae) in grain-based liquor.

AUTHORS' COMMENTS

Human placenta is generally not used, for many reasons. Instead, placentae from pigs and cattle are used as substitutes.

References

1. *Xian Dai Zhong Yao Yao Li Xue* (Contemporary Pharmacology of Chinese Herbs), 1997; 1268
2. *Xian Dai Ben Cao Gang Mu* (Contemporary Materia Medica), 2000; 2802
3. *Shan Xi Yi Yao Za Zhi* (Shanxi Journal of Medicine and Herbology), 1988; 17(9):53
4. *Hu Nan Yi Yao Za Zhi* (Hunan Journal of Medicine and Herbology), 1979; 2:8
5. *Ji Lin Yi Sheng* (Jilin Doctor), 1960; (11):4
6. *He Bei Zhong Yi* (Hebei Chinese Medicine), 1991; 13(5):19
7. *Chang Yong Zhong Yao Xian Dai Yan Jiu Yu Lin Chuan* (Recent Study & Clinical Application of Common Traditional Chinese Medicine), 1995; 616:618

Section 3 — Blood-Tonifying Herbs

Dang Gui (Radicis Angelicae Sinensis)

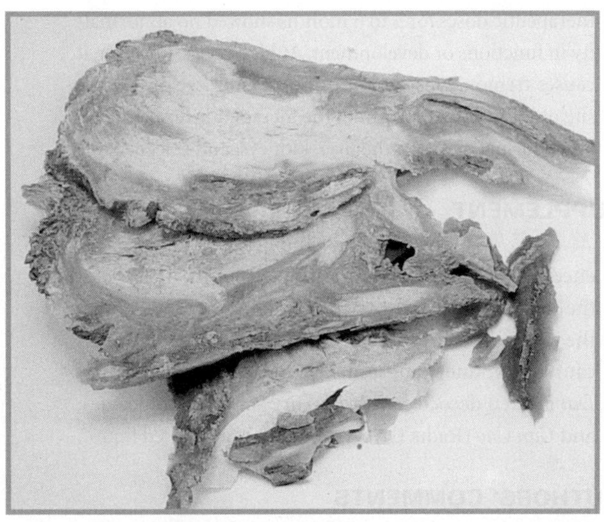

當歸 当归

Pinyin Name: *Dang Gui*
Literal Name: "state of return," "ought to return"
Alternate Chinese Names: *Xi Gui, Gan Gui, Quan Dang Gui, Qin Dang Gui, Yun Dang Gui, Chuan Dang Gui*
Original Source: *Shen Nong Ben Cao Jing* (Divine Husbandman's Classic of the Materia Medica) in the second century
English Name: tangkuei, angelica root, dong quai, Chinese angelica
Botanical Name: *Angelica sinensis* (Oliv.) Diels (*Dang Gui*)
Pharmaceutical Name: Radicis Angelicae Sinensis
Properties: sweet, acrid, warm
Channels Entered: Heart, Liver, Spleen

CHINESE THERAPEUTIC ACTIONS

1. Tonifies Blood

Heart and Liver blood deficiencies: Symptoms of Heart and Liver blood deficiencies include anemia, pale complexion, brittle nails, dry hair, dizziness, blurred vision, and palpitations. *Dang Gui* (Radicis Angelicae Sinensis), warm in nature, is most suitable for cold-type blood-deficient patients. It also treats abdominal pain related to blood deficiency and coldness.

- Blood deficiency: combine *Dang Gui* with *Shu Di Huang* (Radix Rehmanniae Preparata), *Bai Shao* (Radix Paeoniae Alba), and *Chuan Xiong* (Rhizoma Ligustici Chuanxiong) to enhance the blood-tonifying effect. **Exemplar Formula:** *Si Wu Tang* (Four-Substance Decoction). This formula tonifies blood, regulates the menstrual cycle and is used for various patterns of blood deficiency.
- Blood and qi deficiencies: pair it with *Huang Qi* (Radix Astragali). **Exemplar Formula:** *Dang Gui Bu Xue Tang* (Tangkuei Decoction to Tonify the Blood). This formula is commonly used as a tonic for postpartum fatigue and weakness.
- Spleen and Heart deficiencies characterized by insomnia with excessive dreaming and worry, fatigue, palpitations, forgetfulness and difficulty falling asleep: combine *Dang Gui* with *Ren Shen* (Radix Ginseng), *Bai Zhu* (Rhizoma Atractylodis Macrocephalae), *Long Yan Rou* (Arillus Longan), *Suan Zao Ren* (Semen Zizyphi Spinosae), and similar tonics. **Exemplar Formula:** *Gui Pi Tang* (Restore the Spleen Decoction).
- Blood deficiency with deficiency-heat symptoms, hot flashes, irritability, flushed cheeks: use it with *Mu Dan Pi* (Cortex Moutan), *Sheng Di Huang* (Radix Rehmanniae), *Chi Shao* (Radix Paeoniae Rubrae), and *Huang Qin* (Radix Scutellariae).
- Epigastric and abdominal pain and coldness due to blood deficiency and Spleen and Stomach deficiencies: use *Dang Gui* with *Sheng Jiang* (Rhizoma Zingiberis Recens), *Gui Zhi* (Ramulus Cinnamomi), *Bai Shao* (Radix Paeoniae Alba) and *Yi Tang* (Saccharum Granorum). *Dang Gui* is commonly cooked with lamb to make soup.

Dang Gui (Radicis Angelicae Sinensis)

2. Invigorates Blood Circulation and Relieves Pain

Menstrual disorders: Blood deficiency, blood stagnation or qi stagnation all result in menstrual disorders such as irregular menstrual cycle, dysmenorrhea, amenorrhea and other gynecological disorders. Because of the warm property of *Dang Gui* and its action to nourish the blood and invigorate circulation, it is most suitable for treatment of cold types of menstrual disorders with blood and qi stagnation.

- Amenorrhea due to blood deficiency and stagnation: combine *Dang Gui* with *Hong Hua* (Flos Carthami), *Tao Ren* (Semen Persicae), *Chuan Xiong* (Rhizoma Ligustici Chuanxiong), and *Chi Shao* (Radix Paeoniae Rubrae). **Exemplar Formulas:** *Tao Hong Si Wu Tang* (Four-Substance Decoction with Safflower and Peach Pit) and *Shao Fu Zhu Yu Tang* (Drive Out Blood Stasis in the Lower Abdomen Decoction).
- Amenorrhea or irregular menstruation because of cold and deficiency: combine it with *Wu Zhu Yu* (Fructus Evodiae), *Gui Zhi* (Ramulus Cinnamomi), *Ren Shen* (Radix Ginseng), and *Chuan Xiong* (Rhizoma Ligustici Chuanxiong). **Exemplar Formula:** *Wen Jing Tang* (Warm the Menses Decoction).
- Dysmenorrhea due to cold and deficiency: use this herb with *Wu Ling Zhi* (Excrementum Trogopteri seu Pteromi), *Pu Huang* (Pollen Typhae) and *Yan Hu Suo* (Rhizoma Corydalis). **Exemplar Formula:** *Shi Xiao San* (Sudden Smile Powder).
- Pre-menstrual syndrome, irregular menstruation caused by Liver qi stagnation: add it to *Chai Hu* (Radix Bupleuri), *Bai Shao* (Radix Paeoniae Alba), *Bai Zhu* (Rhizoma Atractylodis Macrocephalae), and *Fu Ling* (Poria). **Exemplar Formula:** *Xiao Yao San* (Rambling Powder).
- Early menstruation, bloating during menstruation, irritability from heat and qi stagnation: add *Dang Gui* to *Mu Dan Pi* (Cortex Moutan), *Zhi Zi* (Fructus Gardeniae), *Chai Hu* (Radix Bupleuri) and *Bai Shao* (Radix Paeoniae Alba). **Exemplar Formula:** *Jia Wei Xiao Yao San* (Augmented Rambling Powder).
- General menstrual disorders with fatigue and weakness due to qi and blood deficiencies: combine this herb with *Ren Shen* (Radix Ginseng), *Bai Zhu* (Rhizoma Atractylodis Macrocephalae), *Shu Di Huang* (Radix Rehmanniae Preparata) and *Bai Shao* (Radix Paeoniae Alba). **Exemplar Formula:** *Ba Zhen Tang* (Eight-Treasure Decoction).
- Menopausal symptoms due to yin deficiency with heat: use *Dang Gui* with *Xian Mao* (Rhizoma Curculiginis), *Yin Yang Huo* (Herba Epimedii), *Zhi Mu* (Radix Anemarrhenae), *Huang Bai* (Cortex Phellodendri), and *Ba Ji Tian* (Radix Morindae Officinalis). **Exemplar Formula:** *Er Xian Tang* (Two-Immortal Decoction).

Gestational and postpartum disorders: *Dang Gui* enters the *xue* (blood) level. It functions to tonify yet does not have the stagnant side effects seen in other tonic herbs. It is also frequently used to treat disorders caused by cold, blood deficiency and blood stagnation before or after deliveries.

- Abdominal pain during pregnancy: combine *Dang Gui* with *Chuan Xiong* (Rhizoma Ligusticum Chuanxiong).
- Pain and diarrhea during pregnancy: use it with *Bai Shao* (Radix Paeoniae Alba), *Fu Ling* (Poria), *Bai Zhu* (Rhizoma Atractylodis Macrocephalae), and *Ze Xie* (Rhizoma Alismatis).
- Restless fetus, lower back soreness, abdominal pain and breech presentation of the fetus: incorporate it with *Chuan Xiong* (Rhizoma Ligustici Chuanxiong), *Jing Jie* (Herba Schizonepetae), *Tu Si Zi* (Semen Cuscutae), *Ai Ye* (Folium Artemisiae Argyi), and *Hou Po* (Cortex Magnoliae Officinalis). **Exemplar Formula:** *Bao Chan Wu You Fang* (Preserve Pregnancy and Care Free Decoction).
- Postpartum spontaneous sweating, fever, shortness of breath, and back and leg pain accompanied by an inability to turn from side to side: combine this herb with *Huang Qi* (Radix Astragali), *Bai Shao* (Radix Paeoniae Alba), and *Sheng Jiang* (Rhizoma Zingiberis Recens).
- Postpartum bleeding, lower abdominal coldness and pain caused by blood deficiency with cold: use it with *Chuan Xiong* (Rhizoma Ligustici Chuanxiong), *Tao Ren* (Semen Persicae), *Pao Jiang* (Rhizoma Zingiberis Preparatum), and *Gan Cao* (Radix Glycyrrhizae). **Exemplar Formula:** *Sheng Hua Tang* (Generation and Transformation Decoction).
- Insufficient milk due to blood and qi deficiencies: add this herb to *Ren Shen* (Radix Ginseng), *Huang Qi* (Radix Astragali), *Mai Men Dong* (Radix Ophiopogonis), *Chuan Mu Tong* (Caulis Clematidis Armandii), peanuts and pig's feet.
- Postpartum *bi zheng* (painful obstruction syndrome): combine *Dang Gui* with *Qiang Huo* (Rhizoma et Radix Notopterygii), *Chuan Xiong* (Rhizoma Ligustici Chuanxiong), and *Qin Jiao* (Radix Gentianae Macrophyllae).

Traumatic Injuries: *Dang Gui*, acrid in taste, activates blood circulation and disperses blood stagnation. If blood stagnation is dispersed, swelling will automatically subside. *Dang Gui* is commonly used in trauma departments in hospitals in China, along with blood-activating herbs, to treat the following symptoms: bruises, fractured or broken bones, swelling, and injuries of the tendons.

- Traumatic injuries of the thoracic cavity: combine *Dang Gui* with *Chai Hu* (Radix Bupleuri), *Chuan Shan Jia* (Squama Manis), *Da Huang* (Radix et Rhizoma Rhei), and *Hong Hua* (Flos Carthami). **Exemplar Formulas:**

Dang Gui (Radicis Angelicae Sinensis)

Xue Fu Zhu Yu Tang (Drive Out Stasis in the Mansion of Blood Decoction) or *Fu Yuan Huo Xue Tang* (Revive Health by Invigorating the Blood Decoction).

- Bruises, swelling and redness from traumatic injuries: add this herb to *Su Mu* (Lignum Sappan), *Ru Xiang* (Gummi Olibanum), *Mo Yao* (Myrrha), and *Di Bie Chong* (Eupolyphaga).
- Broken or fractured bones: use it with *Ru Xiang* (Gummi Olibanum), *Mo Yao* (Myrrha), *Zi Ran Tong* (Pyritum), and *Gu Sui Bu* (Rhizoma Drynariae).

***Bi zheng* (painful obstruction syndrome) with numbness and pain:** Besides tonifying blood and invigorating circulation, *Dang Gui* stops pain and disperses coldness. By dispersing stagnation and promoting nourishment in the channels and tendons, *Dang Gui* treats numbness and pain in the limbs and extremities. It is used for pain caused by blood deficiency, blood deficiency complicated by coldness and wind, or qi and blood deficiencies.

- Numbness due to blood deficiency: combine *Dang Gui* with *Huang Qi* (Radix Astragali), *Chi Shao* (Radix Paeoniae Rubrae), *Shu Di Huang* (Radix Rehmanniae Preparata), and *Chuan Xiong* (Rhizoma Ligustici Chuanxiong).
- Coldness of the extremities, back, and/or buttocks due to blood and yang deficiencies: add this herb to *Gui Zhi* (Ramulus Cinnamomi), *Bai Shao* (Radix Paeoniae Alba), *Xi Xin* (Herba Asari), and *Chuan Mu Tong* (Caulis Clematidis Armandii). **Exemplar Formula:** *Dang Gui Si Ni Tang* (Tangkuei Decoction for Frigid Extremities).
- *Bi zheng* (painful obstruction syndrome), painful joints, and/or numbness due to *ying* (nutritive) and *wei* (defensive) deficiencies: combine this herb with *Huang Qi* (Radix Astragali), *Jiang Huang* (Rhizoma Curcumae Longae), *Chi Shao* (Radix Paeoniae Rubrae), and *Fang Feng* (Radix Saposhnikoviae). **Exemplar Formula:** *Juan Bi Tang* (Remove Painful Obstruction Decoction).
- Soreness and weakness of lower back and knees due to qi, blood, Liver and Kidney deficiencies: use it with *Du Huo* (Radix Angelicae Pubescentis), *Sang Ji Sheng* (Herba Taxilli), *Qin Jiao* (Radix Gentianae Macrophyllae), and *Sheng Di Huang* (Radix Rehmanniae). **Exemplar Formula:** *Du Huo Ji Sheng Tang* (Angelica Pubescens and Taxillus Decoction).

Sores and abscesses: Applied topically, *Dang Gui* reduces swelling, expels pus, generates flesh and relieves pain. Because it is warm and nourishing in nature, it is most suitable when taken internally for slow healing sores from qi and blood deficiencies.

- Slow-healing sores due to qi and blood deficiencies: *Dang Gui* is used alone topically, or combined with *Huang Qi* (Radix Astragali), *Jin Yin Hua* (Flos Lonicerae), *Gan Cao* (Radix Glycyrrhizae), *Bai Zhi* (Radix Angelicae Dahuricae), and red *Da Zao* (Fructus Jujubae) for internal use.
- Toxic ulcers with pus: add this herb to *Huang Qi* (Radix Astragali), *Chuan Shan Jia* (Squama Manis), *Chuan Xiong* (Rhizoma Ligustici Chuanxiong), and *Zao Jiao Ci* (Spina Gleditsiae), to drain pus.
- Redness, swelling and burning toxic sores: combine *Dang Gui* with *Jin Yin Hua* (Flos Lonicerae), *Chi Shao* (Radix Paeoniae Rubrae), *Zhe Bei Mu* (Bulbus Fritillariae Thunbergii), *Tian Hua Fen* (Radix Trichosanthis), and *Chuan Shan Jia* (Squama Manis). **Exemplar Formula:** *Zhen Ren Huo Ming Yin* (True Man Decoction to Revitalize Life).
- Ulcerated sores with redness, swelling and pain: use *Dang Gui* with a large dose of *Jin Yin Hua* (Flos Lonicerae), *Gan Cao* (Radix Glycyrrhizae), and *Xuan Shen* (Radix Scrophulariae). **Exemplar Formula:** *Si Miao Yong An Tang* (Four-Valiant Decoction for Well-Being).
- Chronic non-healing ulcerated sores caused by qi and blood deficiencies: use *Dang Gui* with *Huang Qi* (Radix Astragali), *Rou Gui* (Cortex Cinnamomi), *Shu Di Huang* (Radix Rehmanniae Preparata) and *Ren Shen* (Radix Ginseng). **Exemplar Formula:** *Shi Quan Da Bu Tang* (All-Inclusive Great Tonifying Decoction).

3. Moistens Intestines and Unblocks the Bowels

Constipation due to blood deficiency: When the bowels are not properly nourished by blood, constipation or dry stools result. Usually the elderly, or those who have chronic constipation, or are postpartum women, or are in late or recovery stages of chronic disorders suffer this type of constipation. *Dang Gui* nourishes the blood and moistens the intestines to promote bowel movement.

- Constipation due to blood deficiency: combine *Dang Gui* with *He Shou Wu* (Radix Polygoni Multiflori), *Huo Ma Ren* (Fructus Cannabis), *Tao Ren* (Semen Persicae), *Rou Cong Rong* (Herba Cistanches), *Sheng Di Huang* (Radix Rehmanniae), *Shu Di Huang* (Radix Rehmanniae Preparata), and *Da Huang* (Radix et Rhizoma Rhei). **Exemplar Formula:** *Ji Chuan Jian* (Benefit the River [Flow] Decoction).

4. Stops Cough and Treats Dyspnea

Cough and dyspnea: *Dang Gui* is often used with herbs that transform phlegm and stop cough.

- Cough, dyspnea, shortness of breath, and profuse sputum: combine this herb with *Su Zi* (Fructus Perillae), *Ban Xia* (Rhizoma Pinelliae), *Hou Po* (Cortex Magnoliae Officinalis), and *Qian Hu* (Radix Peucedani). **Exemplar Formula:** *Su Zi Jiang Qi Tang* (Perilla Fruit Decoction for Directing Qi Downward).

Dang Gui (Radicis Angelicae Sinensis)

- Coughing during the night, dyspnea, profuse, salty-tasting sputum caused by Kidney and Lung yin deficiencies: combine *Dang Gui* with a large dose of *Chen Pi* (Pericarpium Citri Reticulatae), *Ban Xia* (Rhizoma Pinelliae), *Fu Ling* (Poria), and *Gan Cao* (Radix Glycyrrhizae).

DOSAGE

5 to 15 grams. *Dang Gui* is used in decoctions, herbal tincture, plasters, pills, or powder. Unprocessed *Dang Gui* is commonly used to tonify the blood, regulate menstruation, and lubricate the bowels. *Dang Gui* dry-fried with grain-based liquor more strongly moves the blood, and is commonly used to treat menstrual pain, traumatic bruises and pain, *bi zheng* (painful obstruction syndrome), and cases of blood stagnation. Dry-frying increases its warmth, which makes it an ideal agent to tonify the blood without causing diarrhea. The charred herb stops bleeding.

CAUTIONS / CONTRAINDICATIONS

- Use *Dang Gui* with caution for patients with abdominal distention, Spleen deficiency, or those with loose stools or diarrhea.
- *Dang Gui* is contraindicated in excess conditions, or for patients with yin-deficient heat signs.

CHEMICAL COMPOSITION

Essential oils 0.2 to 0.4% (ligustilide, n-butylidene phthalide, n-butylphthalide, n-valero-phenone-O-carboxylic acid); ferulic acid, scopletin.[1,2]

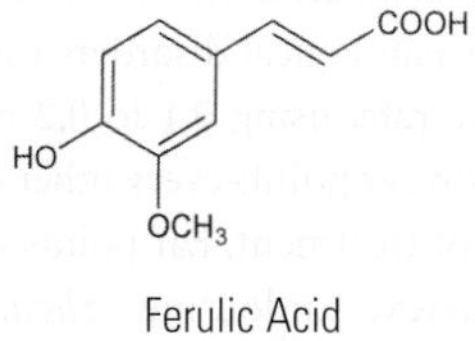

COOH
HO
OCH_3

Ferulic Acid

PHARMACOLOGICAL EFFECTS

- **Effects on the uterus:** Administration of *Dang Gui* is associated with both stimulating and inhibiting effects on the smooth muscle of the uterus. Laboratory studies have shown that water and alcohol extracts tend to stimulate the uterus, while the essential oil inhibits it.[3] Furthermore, clinical studies have shown that when the uterus is in a state of relaxation, *Dang Gui* can induce contraction. Conversely, if the uterus is in a contracted state, then *Dang Gui* promotes relaxation. This dual action is credited for the therapeutic effect of relieving spasms and stopping pain.[4]
- **Cardiovascular:** In one laboratory study using frog specimens, intravenous injection of *Dang Gui* was associated initially with an inhibitory influence on the heart, followed by a negative chronotropic effect and positive inotropic effect. It improves overall blood circulation by decreasing the whole blood specific viscosity, or improving the hemorrheological changes in "blood stagnation." It also has an antiarrhythmic effect, especially against arrhythmia induced by epinephrine, cardiac glycosides, aconitine, and barium chloride. Administration of *Dang Gui* is associated with reduction of plasma cholesterol and triglyceride levels, and a decreased risk of atherosclerosis, as demonstrated in laboratory studies.[5,6,7,8]
- **Antiplatelet:** Administration of *Dang Gui* in rats is associated with a marked antiplatelet effect, similar to that of aspirin.[9] Other studies have demonstrated that *Dang Gui* also inhibits thrombus formation.[10]
- **Immunostimulant:** Administration of *Dang Gui* is associated with an increase in phagocytic activity by the macrophages.[11]
- **Respiratory:** *Dang Gui* has demonstrated a beneficial effect in treating wheezing and dyspnea caused by bronchospasm.[12]
- **Hepatoprotective:** *Dang Gui* promotes the generation of hepatocytes and has demonstrated a marked hepatoprotective effect.[13]
- **Antibiotic:** It shows inhibitory activity against *Salmonella typhi*, *E. coli*, *Corynebacterium diphtheriae*, *Vibrio cholerae*, α-hemolytic streptococcus and β-hemolytic streptococcus.[14]
- **Analgesic and anti-inflammatory:** Extract of *Dang Gui* has analgesic and anti-inflammatory effects similar to those of acetylsalicylic acid. It decreases vascular permeability to reduce inflammation.[15] Its anti-inflammatory effect is approximately 1.1 times stronger than acetylsalicylic acid, and its analgesic effect is approximately 1.7 times stronger than acetylsalicylic acid.[16,17]

CLINICAL STUDIES AND RESEARCH

- **Cough and wheezing:** In one clinical study, essential oil of *Dang Gui* given three times daily for 7 days was found to be 90.2% effective in treating 51 patients with coughing and wheezing. Most patients began to respond to the herbal treatment within 2 to 3 hours, with maximum effect shown at 8 to 24 hours.[18]
- **Low back and leg pain:** An herbal injection containing *Dang Gui* and *Chuan Xiong* (Rhizoma Ligustici Chuanxiong) was found to be 97% effective in relieving pain when administered to the affected area once daily or every other day for 10 days.[19]
- **Arrhythmia:** According to one report, 100 patients with arrhythmia were treated with two *Dang Gui* preparations, with 83.3% rate of effectiveness. The first preparation was intravenous infusion of 60 to 120 ml of 25 to 50% *Dang Gui* preparation once daily for 15 days. The

17 TONIC HERBS

Dang Gui (Radicis Angelicae Sinensis)

second preparation was 20 ml of 150% *Dang Gui* syrup given three times daily for 15 days.[20]

- **Stroke:** Patients with ischemic stroke were treated with intravenous infusion of *Dang Gui* one time daily for 15 to 30 doses per course of treatment. Of 40 patients, the study reported complete recovery in 12 patients, marked improvement in 13 patients, slight improvement in 11 patients, and no response in 4 patients.[21]
- **Migraine:** A preparation of *Dang Gui* demonstrated an 82.9% rate of effectiveness in 35 patients with migraine headache.[22]
- **Nephritis:** In one study, 33 patients with acute nephritis were treated with one injection of a 20% *Dang Gui* solution to acupuncture points daily, with good results. No restrictions were made in regards to intake of water and salt. Acupuncture points selected include *Shenshu* (BL 23), *Zhongji* (CV 3), *Shuiquan* (KI 5), and *ah shi* points. Out of 33 patients, 11 also received drug treatment.[23]
- **Pain:** Local injection of a 5% *Dang Gui* solution was found to have satisfactory effects to relieve post-surgical pain in patients who had chest operation. Out of 105 patients, 84 had excellent response, 16 had good response, and 5 had poor response.[24]
- **Upper gastrointestinal bleeding:** In a clinical study, patients with upper gastrointestinal bleeding were treated with 4.5 grams of powdered *Dang Gui* three times daily with marked effectiveness. Out of 40 patients, the study reported remarkable improvement in 30 patients, moderate improvement in 4 patients, and no response in 6 patients.[25]
- **Liver disease:** One intramuscular injection of *Dang Gui* (equivalent to 4 grams of the dried herb) daily for 2 months stimulated symptomatic improvement in 17 patients with chronic hepatitis and 10 patients with liver cirrhosis.[26]
- **Enuresis:** According to one report, 87 patients who had enuresis for more than 2 years were treated with daily injection of 5% *Dang Gui* solution to acupuncture points for 1 week with a 90% rate of effectiveness. The treatment protocol was to inject 0.5 to 1.0 ml of *Dang Gui* solution into each point one time daily. Three to four acupuncture points were selected for each treatment. Points selected included *Shenshu* (BL 23), *Dachangshu* (BL 25), *Pangguangshu* (BL 28), *Guanyuan* (CV 4), *Zhongji* (CV 3), *Sanyinjiao* (SP 6), and *Yiniao* (Extra).[27]
- **Menstrual pain**: Essential oil of *Dang Gui* given three times daily for 15 to 20 days was 76.79% effective in relieving menstrual pain in 112 patients.[28]
- **Uterine prolapse:** In a clinical study, 67 patients with uterine prolapse were treated with injections of *Dang Gui*, with complete recovery in 27 patients, moderate improvement in 34 patients, and no response in 6 patient. The overall rate of effectiveness was 90%. The treatment protocol was to inject 2 ml of a 50% *Dang Gui* solution daily into the acupuncture points *Sanyinjiao* (SP 6) and *Zusanli* (ST 36), alternating sides with each treatment.[29]
- **Insomnia:** Injection of 2 ml of a 5% *Dang Gui* solution bilaterally into *Anmian* points one time daily or every other day for 10 treatments was found to be 88% effective in treating insomnia in 50 patients.[30]
- **Thromboangiitis obliterans:** In one study, 52 patients were treated with an injection of a 5% *Dang Gui* solution daily, 6 days per week for a total of 4 weeks, with an 88.5% rate of effectiveness. Effectiveness was defined as relief of pain, improvement of blood circulation, increase of peripheral body temperature, and enhancement of recovery.[31]
- **Herpes zoster:** One report describes 54 patients with herpes zoster who all recovered within 6 to 7 days after being treated with 0.5 to 1.0 gram of *Dang Gui* powder every 4 to 6 hours.[32]
- **Alopecia areata:** Oral administration of 9 grams of an herbal formula three times daily after meals showed satisfactory results in 40 patients with alopecia areata. The herbal formula was prepared by mixing 500 grams each of *Dang Gui* and *Bai Zi Ren* (Semen Platycladi) with honey to make pills.[33]
- **Psoriasis:** In a clinical study, 100 patients with psoriasis were treated with a combination injection, with complete recovery in 80 patients, moderate improvement in 15 patients, and slight improvement in 5 patients. The treatment protocol consisted of daily injection of 2% *Dang Gui* solution and 2% novocaine.[34]
- **Dermatological disorders:** In one study, 353 patients with various dermatological disorders were treated with a 90.7% effective rate, using 0.1 to 0.2 ml injectable of 0.5% *Dang Gui* on ear points every other day for 10 to 20 days per course of treatment. Ear points selected included Adrenal Cortex, Endocrine, *Shenmen*, Pituitary Gland, and Lung.[35]
- **Deafness:** Patients with acute-onset deafness were treated with intravenous infusion of 20 ml of 200% *Dang Gui* solution in 20 ml of D5W. The treatment protocol was to administer daily injections for 5 days per course of treatment, for a total of 4 to 5 courses. Out of 105 patients, the study reported complete recovery in 21 patients, marked improvement in 29 patients, moderate improvement in 29 patients, and no effect in 26 patients. The overall rate of effective was 75%.[36]
- **Anal fissure:** According to one study, the combination injection of *Dang Gui* and 1% lidocaine to the affected area in 114 patients had an rate of effectiveness of 96.5%.[37]
- **Chronic hypertrophic rhinitis:** According to one report, 43 patients were treated with a 90.7% rate of effectiveness using injection of herbs. The treatment protocol was to

Dang Gui (Radicis Angelicae Sinensis)

inject to the affected area 0.5 ml of a 5% *Dang Gui* solution and 0.3 ml of a 0.1% *Hong Hua* (Flos Carthami) solution.[38]

- **Chronic pharyngitis:** In one clinical study of 130 patients, injection of a *Dang Gui* preparation one time daily for 10 days provided satisfactory results. The treatment protocol was to inject the herb into *ah shi* points around T3 and T4.[39]
- **Fibrous cavernositis of the penis:** Two patients recovered completely after treatment by one injection of 2 ml of a 10% *Dang Gui* and 1 ml of 2% novocaine into the affected area each week for 5 to 10 weeks.[40]

HERB-DRUG INTERACTION

- **Anticoagulant or antiplatelet drugs:** It has been suggested that concurrent use of *Dang Gui* and warfarin may potentiate the effect of warfarin. In one *in vitro* study, it was discovered that while *Dang Gui* treatment did not affect prothrombin time on its own, it significantly lowered prothrombin time values when given concurrently with warfarin.[41,42,43] [Note: Examples of anticoagulants include heparin, warfarin (Coumadin) and enoxaparin (Lovenox); and examples of antiplatelets include aspirin, dipyridamole (Persantine), and clopidogrel (Plavix).]
- **Scopolamine and cycloheximide**: Administration of *Dang Gui* extract at 1 g/kg was found to be effective in treating scopolamine- and cycloheximide-induced amnesia in rats.[44]
- **Acetaminophen**: It has been shown that *Dang Gui* treats acetaminophen-induced liver damage, presumably because *Dang Gui* promotes the generation of hepatocytes.[45,46]

TOXICOLOGY

Dang Gui has very low toxicity. The LD_{50} of *Dang Gui* in mice is 100 g/kg via injection. Overdose is characterized by fatigue, drowsiness, itching, stomach discomfort, and abdominal pain. Long-term ingestion at the dosage of 6 g/kg showed no abnormality in physical activities, food intake, body weight, urine examination, or hematological examination. There was a slight increase in cytochrome P-450.[47,48]

SUPPLEMENT

In traditional texts, different segments of *Dang Gui* are said to have slightly different actions:

- 當歸頭 / 当归头 *Dang Gui Tou* (Caput Radicis Angelicae Sinensis), the head of the root, is said to be the most tonifying part. It has hemostatic effects as well as an ascending nature that directs the flow of blood upwards.
- 當歸身 / 当归身 *Dang Gui Shen* (Corpus Radicis Angelicae Sinensis), the body, has stronger blood nourishing than blood-invigorating properties.
- 當歸尾 / 当归尾 *Dang Gui Wei* (Extremitas Radicis Angelicae Sinensis), the tail, is most effective in invigorating blood and directing the flow outwards, to the channels and collaterals of the extremities.

AUTHORS' COMMENTS

Traditional Chinese medicine considers *Dang Gui* to be a blood tonic, and it is thus commonly used to treat pregnant women who have blood deficiency. In fact, several classic formulas specifically use *Dang Gui* to tonify blood and stabilize pregnancy, such as *Bao Chan Wu You Fang* (Preserve Pregnancy and Care Free Decoction) from *Zeng Bu Nei Jing Shi Yi* (Supplement to the Formulas Omitted from the Inner Classic). However, when caring for pregnant women, one should always exercise caution and use medicinal substances only when the benefits outweigh the risks.

Dang Gui and *Bai Shao* (Radix Paeoniae Alba) are both blood tonics. *Dang Gui* is warm and dispersing, and more suitable for blood-deficient patients with yang deficiency and coldness. *Bai Shao* is cool and stable, and is used for blood and yin-deficient patients with heat.

According to Dr. Richard Tan, the use of *Dang Gui* (Radicis Angelicae Sinensis) and *Huang Qi* (Radix Astragali), such as in *Dang Gui Bu Xue Tang* (Tangkuei Decoction to Tonify the Blood), can be used to raise WBC and RBC counts in patients receiving chemotherapy or radiation treatments.

References

1. *Xian Dai Zhong Yao Yao Li Xue* (Contemporary Pharmacology of Chinese Herbs), 1997; 1290-1291
2. *The Merck Index* 12th edition, Chapman & Hall/CRCnetBASE/Merck, 2000.
3. *Zhong Hua Yi Xue Za Zhi* (Chinese Journal of Medicine), 1954; 40(9):670
4. *Zhong Yao Xue* (Chinese Herbology), 1998; 815:823
5. *Jiang Su Zhong Yi* (Jiangsu Chinese Medicine), 1965; (3):22
6. Xue, JX. et al. Effects of the combination of astragalus membranaceus (Fisch.) Bge. (AM), angelica sinensis (Oliv.) Diels (TAS), cyperus rotundus L. (CR), ligusticum chuanxiong Hort (LC) and paeonia veitchii lynch (PV) on the hemorrheological changes in "blood stagnating" rats. *Chung Kuo Chung Yao Tsa Chih*; 19(2):108-10, 128. Feb 1994
7. *Lan Zhou Yi Xue Yuan Xue Bao* (Journal of Lanzhou University of Medicine), 1989; 15(3):125
8. *Zhong Cao Yao Tong Xun* (Journal of Chinese Herbal Medicine), 1976; (3):30
9. *Yao Xue Xue Bao* (Journal of Herbology), 1980; 15(6):321
10. *Zhong Guo Yao Li Xue Tong Bao* (Journal of Chinese Herbal Pharmacology), 1981; 2(1):35
11. *Zhong Hua Yi Xue Za Zhi* (Chinese Journal of Medicine), 1978; 17(8):87
12. *Zhong Cao Yao* (Chinese Herbal Medicine), 1983; 14(8):45
13. *Chong Qing Yi Yao* (Chongching Medicine and Herbology), 1989; 18(4):39

Dang Gui (Radicis Angelicae Sinensis)

14. *Huo Xue Hua Yu Yan Jiu* (Research on Blood-Activating and Stasis-Eliminating Herbs), 1981:335
15. *Xin Yi Yao Xue Za Zhi* (New Journal of Medicine and Herbology), 1975; (6):34
16. *Yao Xue Za Zhi* (Journal of Medicinals), 1971; (91):1098
17. Ibid.
18. *Tian Jing Zhong Yi* (Tianjing Chinese Medicine), 1986; 1:4
19. *Xin Zhong Yi* (New Chinese Medicine), 1980; 2:34
20. *Zhong Yi Za Zhi* (Journal of Chinese Medicine), 1981; 7:54
21. *Shen Jing Jing Shen Ji Bing Za Zhi* (Journal of Psychiatric Disorders), 1981; 4:222
22. *Bei Jing Yi Xue* (Beijing Medicine), 1988; 2:95
23. *Xin Yi Xue* (New Medicine), 1976; 6:294
24. *Xin Yi Yao Xue Za Zhi* (New Journal of Medicine and Herbology), 1976; 12:26
25. *Liao Ning Zhong Yi Za Zhi* (Liaoning Journal of Chinese Medicine), 1982; 6:40
26. *Zhong Yi Yao Xin Xi* (Information on Chinese Medicine and Herbology), 1985; 3:18
27. *Chi Jiao Yi Sheng Za Zhi* (Journal of Barefoot Doctors), 1977; 4:21
28. *Lan Zhou Yi Xue Yuan Xue Bao* (Journal of Lanzhou University of Medicine), 1988; 1:36
29. *Yao Xue Tong Bao* (Report of Herbology), 1979; 7:310
30. *Zhong Xi Yi Jie He Za Zhi* (Journal of Integrated Chinese and Western Medicine), 1983; 5:319
31. *Xin Yi Yao Xue Za Zhi* (New Journal of Medicine and Herbology), 1977; 11:35
32. *Zhong Hua Yi Xue Za Zhi* (Chinese Journal of Medicine), 1961; 5:317
33. *Shan Xi Zhong Yi* (Shanxi Chinese Medicine), 1987; 9:419
34. *Zhong Yi Yao Xue Bao* (Report of Chinese Medicine and Herbology), 1981; 4:34
35. *Shan Xi Yi Yao Za Zhi* (Shanxi Journal of Medicine and Herbology), 1975; 5:69
36. *Zhong Xi Yi Jie He Za Zhi* (Journal of Integrated Chinese and Western Medicine), 1986; 9:536
37. *Tian Jing Zhong Yi* (Tianjing Chinese Medicine), 1986; 4:10
38. *Hu Bei Zhong Yi Za Zhi* (Hubei Journal of Chinese Medicine), 1986; 5:49
39. *Liao Ning Zhong Yi Za Zhi* (Liaoning Journal of Chinese Medicine), 1986; 4:36
40. *Bei Jing Yi Xue* (Beijing Medicine), 1980; 1:47
41. Chan-K. Lo-AC, Yeung-JH, and Woo-KS. *Journal of Pharmacy and Pharmacology*, (1995, May) vol. 47(5):402-6
42. *Pharmacotherapy* 1999, July; 19(7):870-876
43. *European Journal of Drug Metabolism and Pharmacokinetics*. 20(1):55-60, 1995
44. Hsieh MT et al., Radix Angelica Sinensis extracts ameliorate scopolamine- and cycloheximide-induced amnesia, but not p-chloroamphetamine-induced amnesia in rats. *American Journal of Chinese Medicine*. 28(2):263-72, 2000
45. *Zhong Guo Yao Li Tong Xun* (Journal of Chinese Herbal Studies), 1992; 9(1):52
46. *Chong Qing Yi Yao* (Chongching Medicine and Herbology), 1989; 18(4):39
47. *Zhong Cao Yao* (Chinese Herbal Medicine), 1981; 12(7):33
48. *Guo Wai Yi Yao Zhi Wu Yao Fen Ce* (Monograph of Foreign Botanical Medicine), 1993; 8(3):116

Shu Di Huang (Radix Rehmanniae Preparata)

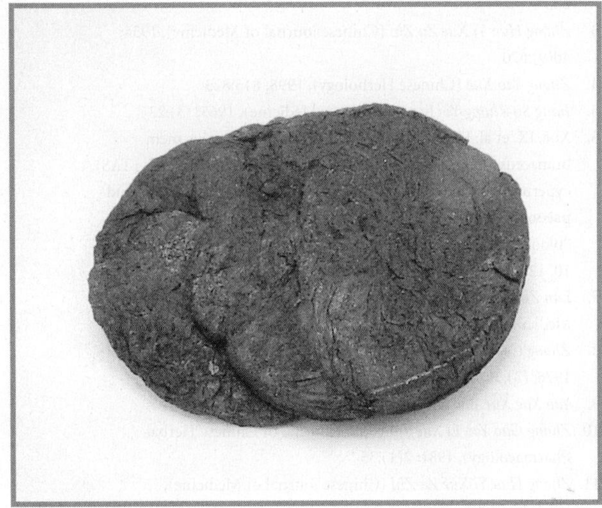

熟地黄

Pinyin Name: *Shu Di Huang*

Literal Name: "cooked earth's yellowness," "cooked earth yellow"

Alternate Chinese Names: *Shu Di, Da Di Huang*

Original Source: *Bei Ji Qian Jin Yao Fang* (Thousands of Golden Prescriptions for Emergencies)

English Name: cooked rehmannia, prepared rhizome of adhesive rehmannia

Botanical Name: *Rehmannia glutinosa* Libosch (*Di Huang*)

Pharmaceutical Name: Radix Rehmanniae Preparata

Properties: sweet, slightly warm

Channels Entered: Liver, Kidney

Shu Di Huang (Radix Rehmanniae Preparata)

CHINESE THERAPEUTIC ACTIONS

1. Nourishes Blood

Blood deficiency: *Shu Di Huang* (Radix Rehmanniae Preparata) treats blood deficiency and the consequent lack of nourishment to the Liver and Heart. Proper circulation of blood is dependent on the volume of blood being circulated. In anemic or blood-deficient patients, there is insufficient blood to nourish the organs. Typical signs include sallow or pale complexion, dizziness, palpitations, and insomnia. *Shu Di Huang* strongly nourishes and tonifies the blood.

- Anemia: combine *Shu Di Huang* with *Dang Gui* (Radicis Angelicae Sinensis), *Bai Shao* (Radix Paeoniae Alba), and *Chuan Xiong* (Rhizoma Ligustici Chuanxiong). **Exemplar Formula:** *Si Wu Tang* (Four-Substance Decoction).
- Anemia with fatigue and weakness: use this herb with *Ren Shen* (Radix Ginseng), *Bai Zhu* (Rhizoma Atractylodis Macrocephalae), *Fu Ling* (Poria), *Dang Gui* (Radicis Angelicae Sinensis), and *Bai Shao* (Radix Paeoniae Alba). **Exemplar Formula:** *Ba Zhen Tang* (Eight-Treasure Decoction).

Menstrual disorders: Blood belongs to the yin element and is the foundation of women's health. Irregular menstruation is often caused by blood stagnation or blood deficiency. Because the rich nature of *Shu Di Huang* may cause stagnation, it should only be used for patients with irregular menstruation arising from blood deficiency, and not for those with blood stagnation.

- Irregular menstruation: combine this herb with *Dang Gui* (Radicis Angelicae Sinensis), *Chuan Xiong* (Rhizoma Ligustici Chuanxiong), *Yi Mu Cao* (Herba Leonuri), and *Bai Shao* (Radix Paeoniae Alba).
- Hypermenorrhea because of blood deficiency: use charred *Shu Di Huang* with *Bai Shao* (Radix Paeoniae Alba), *Dang Gui* (Radicis Angelicae Sinensis), *Shan Zhu Yu* (Fructus Corni) and charred *Jing Jie* (Herba Schizonepetae).
- Chronic uterine bleeding resulting in yin and blood deficiencies: use it with charred *Jing Jie* (Herba Schizonepetae), *Hai Piao Xiao* (Endoconcha Sepiae), *E Jiao* (Colla Corii Asini), and charred *Ai Ye* (Folium Artemisiae Argyi).
- Infertility due to *ren* (conception) and *chong* (thoroughfare) channel deficiencies with blood deficiency and heat: use this herb with *Huang Lian* (Rhizoma Coptidis) and *Dang Gui* (Radicis Angelicae Sinensis).

Gestational and postpartum disorders: *Shu Di Huang* treats restless fetus, habitual miscarriage, and postpartum complications. *Shu Di Huang* is used as the main herb in formulas that treat lower abdominal pain, edema, nausea, and vomiting caused by deficiency from sudden loss of blood in postpartum women.

- Restless fetus or habitual miscarriage: combine it with *Ren Shen* (Radix Ginseng), *Bai Zhu* (Rhizoma Atractylodis Macrocephalae), *Dang Gui* (Radicis Angelicae Sinensis), *Xu Duan* (Radix Dipsaci), and *Sha Ren* (Fructus Amomi). **Exemplar Formula:** *Tai Shan Pan Shi San* (Powder that Gives the Stability of Mount Tai).

2. Tonifies Liver and Kidney Yin

Liver and Kidney yin deficiencies: Clinical presentations include soreness and weakness of the lower back and knees, dizziness, vertigo, tinnitus, diminished hearing, tidal fever, night sweats, nocturnal emissions, a thready, rapid pulse, and a dry, cracked tongue with scanty or no coating. *Shu Di Huang* nourishes the yin and blood of the Liver and Kidney. It is often combined with yang-tonic herbs to fortify Kidney yang as well.

- Liver and Kidney yin deficiencies: combine *Shu Di Huang* with *Shan Yao* (Rhizoma Dioscoreae), *Shan Zhu Yu* (Fructus Corni), *Mu Dan Pi* (Cortex Moutan), *Fu Ling* (Poria), and *Ze Xie* (Rhizoma Alismatis). **Exemplar Formula:** *Liu Wei Di Huang Wan* (Six-Ingredient Pill with Rehmannia).
- Kidney yin-deficient fire: use it with *Zhi Mu* (Radix Anemarrhenae), *Huang Bai* (Cortex Phellodendri), *Gui Ban* (Plastrum Testudinis) and the bone marrow of pigs. **Exemplar Formula:** *Da Bu Yin Wan* (Great Tonify the Yin Pill).
- Weakness and soreness of the knees because of Kidney yin-deficient fire: add *Shu Di Huang* to *Gui Ban* (Plastrum Testudinis), *Suo Yang* (Herba Cynomorii), and *Zhi Mu* (Radix Anemarrhenae). **Exemplar Formula:** *Hu Qian Wan* (Hidden Tiger Pill from the Analytic Collection).
- Kidney yin and yang deficiencies: combine this herb with *Gou Qi Zi* (Fructus Lycii), *Shan Yao* (Rhizoma Dioscoreae), *Shan Zhu Yu* (Fructus Corni), *Fu Zi* (Radix Aconiti Lateralis Praeparata), and *Rou Gui* (Cortex Cinnamomi). **Exemplar Formula:** *You Gui Wan* (Restore the Right [Kidney] Pill).

***Xiao ke* (wasting and thirsting) syndrome:** *Shu Di Huang* strongly tonifies yin for treatment of *xiao ke*, and is especially effective for polyuria.

- *Xiao ke* syndrome with predominant polyuria: combine this herb with *Shan Yao* (Rhizoma Dioscoreae), *Shan Zhu Yu* (Fructus Corni), and *Ze Xie* (Rhizoma Alismatis).
- *Xiao ke* syndrome with qi deficiency: add it to with *Ren Shen* (Radix Ginseng), *Huang Qi* (Radix Astragali), and *Xi Yang Shen* (Radix Panacis Quinquefolii).
- *Xiao ke* syndrome with yin-deficient fire: use *Shu Di Huang* with *Shi Gao* (Gypsum Fibrosum), *Zhi Mu* (Radix Anemarrhenae), *Di Gu Pi* (Cortex Lycii) and *Tian Hua Fen* (Radix Trichosanthis).

Shu Di Huang (Radix Rehmanniae Preparata)

3. Replenishes *Jing* (Essence) and Fills the Marrow

Developmental delay and premature aging: *Jing* and blood are derived from the same source. *Shu Di Huang* tonifies blood and nourishes *jing*. Deficiencies of *jing* and blood cause both physical and mental developmental delays in children. The manifestations of these deficiencies in adults include prematurely gray hair, forgetfulness, dizziness, blurry vision, impotence, tinnitus, and other signs of early aging.

- Developmental delay in children and premature aging: combine *Shu Di Huang* with *He Shou Wu* (Radix Polygoni Multiflori), *Gou Qi Zi* (Fructus Lycii), *Lu Jiao Jiao* (Gelatinum Cornu Cervi), *Gui Ban Jiao* (Gelatinum Plastrum Testudinis), and *Tu Si Zi* (Semen Cuscutae).

4. Arrests Cough and Wheezing

Respiratory disorders: This type of deficient cough, wheezing, and asthma is associated with Kidney deficiency with inability to grasp the qi downwards. The prolonged, labored inhalation process results in accelerated respiration and shortness of breath.

- Cough, wheezing, and sputum due to Kidney deficiency: combine *Shu Di Huang* with *Ban Xia* (Rhizoma Pinelliae), *Chen Pi* (Pericarpium Citri Reticulatae), *Fu Ling* (Poria), *Gan Cao* (Radix Glycyrrhizae) and *Dang Gui* (Radicis Angelicae Sinensis).
- Cough, shortness of breath, accelerated respiration: incorporate this herb with *Wu Wei Zi* (Fructus Schisandrae Chinensis), *Shan Yao* (Rhizoma Dioscoreae), *Fu Ling* (Poria), and *Shan Zhu Yu* (Fructus Corni).

DOSAGE

10 to 30 grams in decoction. *Shu Di Huang* is also used in pill, powder and paste forms. *Shu Di Huang* is prepared by steaming the herb with water or grain-based liquor, followed by slicing and drying. Traditionally, charred *Shu Di Huang* is used to stop bleeding.

CAUTIONS / CONTRAINDICATIONS

- Use *Shu Di Huang* with caution in patients with Spleen and Stomach deficiencies. Because the stagnating and cloying nature of *Shu Di Huang* may impair digestion, it is contraindicated in excess conditions with dampness, phlegm or qi stagnation.

CHEMICAL COMPOSITION

Catalpol, 6-o-acetylcatalpol, aucubin, melittoside, rehmanniosides A,B,C,D; rehmaglutins A,B,C,D; glutinoside, rehmannans A,B,C; stachyose, D-mannitol.[1]

PHARMACOLOGICAL EFFECTS

See *Sheng Di Huang* (Radix Rehmanniae).

CLINICAL STUDIES AND RESEARCH

- **Hypertension:** According to one report, 62 patients with cardiovascular disorders were treated with 30 to 50 grams of *Shu Di Huang* daily for 2 weeks. There was a reduction of blood pressure, total cholesterol levels, and triglycerides. There was also an improvement in cerebral blood flow and in ECG results.[2]
- **Myelitis:** In one clinical study on retrogressive myelitis in 1,000 patients, administration of an herbal formula two to three times daily for 1 to 2 months provided significant improvement in 803 patients, moderate improvement in 141 patients, and no response in 56 patients. The herbal formula contained *Shu Di Huang*, *Rou Cong Rong* (Herba Cistanches), *Lu Han Cao* (Herba Pyrolae), *Gu Sui Bu* (Rhizoma Drynariae), *Yin Yang Huo* (Herba Epimedii), *Ji Xue Teng* (Caulis Spatholobi), and *Lai Fu Zi* (Semen Raphani).[3]
- **Electric ophthalmitis:** One study reported that placing a 2 mm slice of *Shu Di Huang* on the eye showed good therapeutic effect in treating patients with electric ophthalmitis.[4]

AUTHORS' COMMENTS

Shu Di Huang is frequently used with *Dang Gui* (Radicis Angelicae Sinensis) and *Chuan Xiong* (Rhizoma Ligustici Chuanxiong). The combination of these three herbs has a maximum tonifying effect, with minimal side effects, as the stagnating tendencies of the tonics are offset by the blood-invigorating activities.

Sha Ren (Fructus Amomi) or *Chen Pi* (Pericarpium Citri Reticulatae) is commonly used with *Shu Di Huang* to offset its stagnating nature. In addition, the concurrent use of *Sha Ren* or *Chen Pi* will protect the Spleen and Stomach and promote digestion.

See *Sang Shen Zi* (Fructus Mori) for comparison of these two herbs.

There are three types of *Di Huang* (Rehmanniae): *Xian Di Huang* (Radix Rehmanniae Recens), *Sheng Di Huang* (Radix Rehmanniae), and *Shu Di Huang* (Radix Rehmanniae Preparata). All three nourish yin and generate body fluids to treat yin and blood deficiencies. Despite similarities between the three, there are also differences.

- *Xian Di Huang* is the fresh root. It is bitter, sweet and very cold. In comparison with the others, *Xian Di Huang* has a weaker function to nourish yin, but a stronger function to clear heat, cool blood, relieve thirst and dispel irritability. Also, it is less stagnating in nature, and thus is used mostly for patients with heat in the blood and yin deficiency.
- *Sheng Di Huang* is the dried, unprocessed root. It is

Shu Di Huang (Radix Rehmanniae Preparata)

weaker than *Xian Di Huang* for clearing heat and cooling the blood. It is mostly used to address heat in the blood that is injuring body fluids, *jing* (essence) or blood.

- *Shu Di Huang* is the processed root (processed by steaming with water or grain-based liquor). It has the strongest tonifying action of the three, and is most suitable for use to alleviate *jing* (essence), blood, and yin deficiencies.

References

1. *Chang Yong Zhong Yao Cheng Fen Yu Yao Li Shou Ce* (A Handbook of the Composition and Pharmacology of Common Chinese Drugs), 1994; 792-793
2. Ibid.
3. *Liao Ning Zhong Yi Za Zhi* (Liaoning Journal of Chinese Medicine), 1982; 3:40
4. *Xin Zhong Yi* (New Chinese Medicine), 1979; 5:41

He Shou Wu (Radix Polygoni Multiflori)

何首烏 何首乌

Pinyin Name: *He Shou Wu*
Literal Name: "black haired Mr. He," "Mr. He's black hair"
Alternate Chinese Names: *Shou Wu, Sheng Shou Wu, Zhi Shou Wu*
Original Source: *Ri Hua Zi Ben Cao* (Materia Medica of Ri Hua-Zi) by Ri Hua-Zi in 713 A.D.
English Name: polygonum, fo-ti root, fleece flower root, multiflower knotweed tuber
Botanical Name: *Polygonum multiflorum* Thunb. (*He Shou Wu*)
Pharmaceutical Name: Radix Polygoni Multiflori
Properties: sweet, bitter, astringent, slightly warm
Channels Entered: Kidney, Liver

CHINESE THERAPEUTIC ACTIONS

1. Replenishes *Jing* (Essence) and Nourishes the Blood of the Liver and Kidney

Blood and *jing* deficiencies: *He Shou Wu* (Radix Polygoni Multiflori) treats blood and *jing* deficiencies that manifest as dizziness, blurred vision, gray hair, soreness and weakness of the lower back and knees, and spermatorrhea. It tonifies the *jing* and blood of the Liver and Kidney. This herb is one of the best tonics, as it is warm yet not drying, tonifying yet not stagnating like other tonics. Processed *He Shou Wu* is most effective for this function.

- Prematurely gray hair: combine *He Shou Wu* with *Da Zao* (Fructus Jujubae), *Gou Qi Zi* (Fructus Lycii), *Tu Si Zi* (Semen Cuscutae), *Dang Gui* (Radicis Angelicae Sinensis), *Huai Niu Xi* (Radix Achyranthis Bidentatae), *Nu Zhen Zi* (Fructus Ligustri Lucidi), *Han Lian Cao* (Herba Ecliptae) and *Hei Zhi Ma* (Semen Sesami Nigrum). **Exemplar Formula:** *Qi Bao Mei Ran Wan* (Seven-Treasure Special Pill for Beautiful Whiskers).
- Early signs of aging as described above: combine this herb with *Sang Shen Zi* (Fructus Mori), *Hei Zhi Ma* (Semen Sesami Nigrum), *Shu Di Huang* (Radix Rehmanniae Preparata), and *Du Zhong* (Cortex Eucommiae).
- Nocturnal emissions, spermatorrhea, vaginal discharge: add it to *Shan Zhu Yu* (Fructus Corni), *Shan Yao* (Rhizoma Dioscoreae), *Qian Shi* (Semen Euryales), *Wu Wei Zi* (Fructus Schisandrae Chinensis), *Long Gu* (Os Draconis), *Mu Li* (Concha Ostreae) and *Yuan Zhi* (Radix Polygalae).
- Anemia: use it with *Dang Gui* (Radicis Angelicae Sinensis), *Bai Shao* (Radix Paeoniae Alba), *Chuan Xiong* (Rhizoma Ligustici Chuanxiong), and *Shu Di Huang* (Radix Rehmanniae Preparata).
- Dizziness, blurred vision, tinnitus, numbness of limbs, soreness and weakness of the lower back and knees: use *He Shou Wu* with *Xi Xian Cao* (Herba Siegesbeckiae), *Sang Shen Zi* (Fructus Mori), *Hei Zhi Ma* (Semen Sesami Nigrum), *Shu Di Huang* (Radix Rehmanniae Preparata) and *Du Zhong* (Cortex Eucommiae).

He Shou Wu (Radix Polygoni Multiflori)

Menstrual disorders: The Liver stores blood and is essential in regulating periods. Deficient Liver blood usually results in symptoms of irregular menstruation and abnormal uterine bleeding. Dry-fried *He Shou Wu* is preferred for this particular application.

- Menstrual disorders: combine dry-fried *He Shou Wu* with *Dang Gui* (Radicis Angelicae Sinensis), *Bai Shao* (Radix Paeoniae Alba), *Chuan Xiong* (Rhizoma Ligustici Chuanxiong), and *Shu Di Huang* (Radix Rehmanniae Preparata).

2. Eliminates Toxins

Toxic sores: Unprocessed *He Shou Wu* is cold, and effectively clears heat and eliminates toxins. It treats abscesses, scrofula, goiter and neck lumps, chronic, non-healing sores with pus and ulceration, that damage yin and blood.

- Scrofula, goiter and neck lumps: use unprocessed *He Shou Wu* with *Ku Shen Gen* (Radix Sophorae Flavescentis), *Fang Feng* (Radix Saposhnikoviae), *Bo He* (Herba Menthae), and alcohol.
- Abscesses and swellings of various parts of the body: combine this herb with *Fang Feng* (Radix Saposhnikoviae), *Jing Jie* (Herba Schizonepetae), *Jin Yin Hua* (Flos Lonicerae) and *Ku Shen Gen* (Radix Sophorae Flavescentis).
- Swellings and nodules caused by fire toxins and yin and blood deficiencies: combine it with *Xia Ku Cao* (Spica Prunellae), *Chuan Xiong* (Rhizoma Ligustici Chuanxiong), *Dang Gui* (Radicis Angelicae Sinensis), *Bai Zhi* (Radix Angelicae Dahuricae) and *Chuan Mu Tong* (Caulis Clematidis Armandii). It can also be used alone topically to eliminate toxins and relieve swelling.

3. Treats Malarial Disorders

Unprocessed *He Shou Wu* acts to tonify and eliminates toxins at the same time. It can be used to treat malaria characterized by yin and blood deficiencies that involves more heat than cold.

- Malarial disorders: combine 25 to 30 grams of *He Shou Wu* with 3 grams of *Gan Cao* (Radix Glycyrrhizae).
- Malarial disorders with more fever than chills (due to yin and blood deficiencies): combine this herb with *Bie Jia* (Carapax Trionycis) and *Zhu Sha* (Cinnabaris).
- Malarial disorders with more qi deficiency: add it to *Qing Hao* (Herba Artemisiae Annuae) and *Chang Shan* (Radix Dichroae).

4. Moistens the Intestines and Unblocks the Bowels

Constipation because of intestinal dryness: Regular bowel movements are dependent on proper nourishment of the intestines. When body fluids and blood are deficient, constipation or dry stools may occur. This condition is usually present in anemic patients, postpartum women, the elderly, or in patients who have just recovered from a chronic illness. Unprocessed *He Shou Wu* is preferred for this application.

- Constipation or dry stools: *He Shou Wu* is used alone, or combined with *Dang Gui* (Radicis Angelicae Sinensis), *Huo Ma Ren* (Fructus Cannabis), and *Hei Zhi Ma* (Semen Sesami Nigrum) to lubricate the bowels.

5. Lowers Cholesterol, Treats Cardiovascular Disorders

He Shou Wu has been used recently to lower cholesterol, treat atherosclerosis and prevent cholesterol from remaining in the liver. For this application, use equal portions of unprocessed and dry-fried *He Shou Wu.*

- Angina, coronary heart disorder, hypertension, or epigastric pain: combine both processed and unprocessed forms of *He Shou Wu* with *Dan Shen* (Radix Salviae Miltiorrhizae).

DOSAGE

10 to 30 grams in herbal decoction. *He Shou Wu* is used in the form of pills, decoction, grain-based liquor, powder or paste. External use can be either in the form of powder or herbal soaks. The unprocessed herb is bitter, and has a strong action to eliminate heat, disperse nodules, and induce bowel movement. Diarrhea or loose stools is one of the main side effects when the unprocessed herb is consumed. To minimize this effect, *He Shou Wu* is processed by steaming it with the juice of black beans and then drying it under the sun. Processing the herb with black beans eliminates the side effect of diarrhea, and potentiates the therapeutic effect to strengthen the Liver and Kidney, benefit blood and *jing* (essence), and enhance its action to benefit hair.

CAUTIONS / CONTRAINDICATIONS

- *He Shou Wu* should neither be decocted nor stored in metal containers. It should not be combined with *Ci Shi* (Magnetitum), *Dai Zhe Shi* (Haematitum), *Yu Yu Liang* (Limonitum) or *Sheng Tie Luo* (Frusta Ferri).
- *He Shou Wu* should be used with caution in patients with Spleen deficiency, loose stools, or diarrhea. It is not suitable for patients with dampness or phlegm.

CHEMICAL COMPOSITION

Chrysophanol, emodin, sennoside, physcion, questin, citrosein, questinol, 2-acetylemodin, chein, chrysophanol anthrone, rhapontin, tricin, calcium, iron, zinc, copper.[1]

PHARMACOLOGICAL EFFECTS

- **Cardiovascular:** Injection of a 20% *He Shou Wu* preparation has a marked effect to reduce the heart

He Shou Wu (Radix Polygoni Multiflori)

rate in frog specimens. This effect is milder than meperidine hydrochloride.[2]

- **Antihyperlipidemic:** Administration of *He Shou Wu* is associated with an increase in HDL and a decrease in triglycerides and cholesterol, as demonstrated in various laboratory studies.[3]
- **Antiaging:** Administration of *He Shou Wu* retards the aging process and increases the life expectancy of subjects in many laboratory studies.[4]
- **Immunostimulant:** Administration of *He Shou Wu* is associated with an increase in T-lymphocytes and white blood cells, and increased activity of the macrophages in mice.[5]
- **Gastrointestinal:** *He Shou Wu* increases intestinal peristalsis, moistens the bowel, and promotes bowel movement.[6]
- **Endocrine:** Administration of *He Shou Wu* is associated with an increase in hormonal secretion by the adrenal and thyroid glands.[7]

CLINICAL STUDIES AND RESEARCH

- **Hypercholesterolemia:** In one study, 178 patients with hypercholesterolemia were treated with *He Shou Wu* extract (dosage equivalent to 4 to 5 grams of dried herb) three times daily for 2 to 12 weeks (up to 14 months in rare cases) and showed marked improvement in 38.2% and moderate improvement in 23.6% of the patients. The average reduction of cholesterol was 39 mg/dL.[8]
- **Whooping cough:** An herbal decoction containing 6 to 12 grams of *He Shou Wu*, and 1.5 to 3 grams of *Gan Cao* (Radix Glycyrrhizae) was taken in 4 to 6 equally-divided doses daily to treat whooping cough. Small portions of *He Zi* (Fructus Chebulae) or *Ying Su Ke* (Pericarpium Papaveris) were added if necessary to stop diarrhea. Out of 35 patients, 19 recovered completely, 8 had significant improvement, 4 showed moderate improvement, and 4 had no response.[9]
- **Insomnia:** According to one report, 141 patients with insomnia were treated with both intramuscular injection and oral ingestion of *He Shou Wu* for 20 to 30 days with marked improvement in 53.9% and moderate improvement in 44.7% of the patients. The overall rate of effectiveness was 98.6%.[10]
- **Schizophrenia:** In one study, the combination of herbal decoction and prescription drugs was used to treat 95 patients with schizophrenia. The herbal decoction was given twice daily, and contained 94 grams of fresh *He Shou Wu*, 94 grams of fresh *Ye Jiao Teng* (Caulis Polygoni Multiflori), and 2 to 6 pieces of *Da Zao* (Fructus Jujubae). Promethazine and chlorpromazine were also given to the patients as needed. Out of 95 patients, 8 recovered completely, 47 improved significantly, 11 showed moderate improvement, and 29 showed no improvement. The overall rate of effectiveness was 58%.[11]
- **Prematurely gray hair:** In one clinical study, an herbal formula was 88.98% effective in treating 36 patients with prematurely gray hair. The herbal formula was prepared by soaking 30 grams of processed *He Shou Wu*, 30 grams of *Shu Di Huang* (Radix Rehmanniae Preparata) and 15 grams of *Dang Gui* (Radicis Angelicae Sinensis) in 1,000 ml of rice wine for 10 to 15 days prior to ingestion. Patients were advised to take 15 to 30 ml of the tincture daily.[12]
- **Malaria:** Seventeen children with malaria were treated with satisfactory results using an herbal decoction containing 18 to 25 grams of *He Shou Wu* and 1.5 to 3 grams of *Gan Cao* (Radix Glycyrrhizae). The herbs were cooked for 2 hours, and the decoction was taken in three equally-divided doses three times daily, before meals.[13]

TOXICOLOGY

No fatalities were reported when *He Shou Wu* was given in mice at dosages up to 1,000 g/kg. The LD_{50} for *He Shou Wu* in mice via intraperitoneal injection is 169.4 g/kg.[14]

AUTHORS' COMMENTS

According to Dr. Tsai Wen-Qi, use of *He Shou Wu*, such as in *Qi Bao Mei Ran Wan* (Seven-Treasure Special Pill for Beautiful Whiskers), promotes hair growth and increases sperm count and mobility.

References

1. *Xian Dai Zhong Yao Yao Li Xue* (Contemporary Pharmacology of Chinese Herbs), 1997; 1306
2. *Zhong Yao Yao Li Yu Ying Yong* (Pharmacology and Applications of Chinese Herbs), 1983: 533
3. *Zhong Cao Yao* (Chinese Herbal Medicine), 1991; 22(3):117
4. *Zhong Yao Yao Li Yu Lin Chuang* (Pharmacology and Clinical Applications of Chinese Herbs), 1989; 5(3):19
5. Ibid., 5(1):24
6. *Chang Yong Zhong Yao De Ying Yong* (Application of Commonly-Used Chinese Herbs), 1983:117-118
7. *Zhong Yao Yao Li Yu Lin Chuang* (Pharmacology and Clinical Applications of Chinese Herbs), 1989; 5(3):19
8. *Yi Yao Gong Ye* (Pharmaceutical Industry), 1974; 6:1
9. *Jiang Su Zhong Yi* (Jiangsu Chinese Medicine), 1965; 3:10
10. *Zhong Cao Yao Tong Xun* (Journal of Chinese Herbal Medicine), 1974; 5:38
11. *Yi Xue Yan Jiu Tong Xun* (Report of Medical Studies), 1976; 4:30
12. *Shan Dong Zhong Yi Za Zhi* (Shandong Journal of Chinese Medicine), 1983; 4:41
13. *Guang Dong Yi Xue* (Guangdong Medicine), 1964; 4:31
14. *Zhong Cheng Yao Yan Jiu* (Research of Chinese Patent Medicine), 1982; (1):21

Bai Shao (Radix Paeoniae Alba)

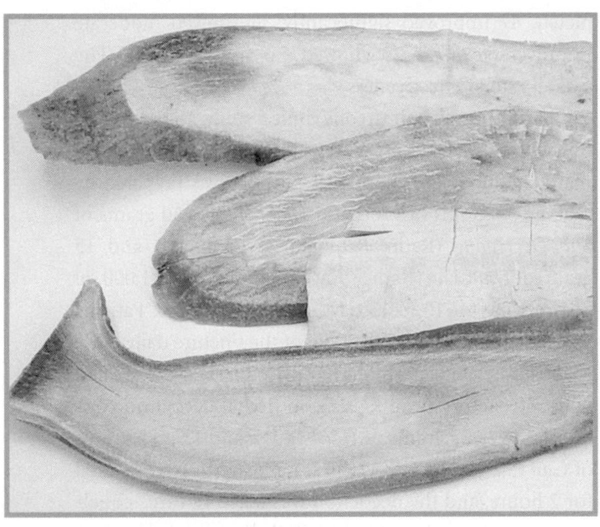

白芍 白芍

Pinyin Name: *Bai Shao*
Literal Name: "white peony"
Alternate Chinese Names: *Bai Shao Yao, Shao Yao, Hao Bai Shao, Jin Shao Yao*
Original Source: *Shen Nong Ben Cao Jing* (Divine Husbandman's Classic of the Materia Medica) in the second century
English Name: white peony root
Botanical Name: *Paeonia lactiflora* Pall. (*Shao Yao*)
Pharmaceutical Name: Radix Paeoniae Alba
Properties: bitter, sour, cool
Channels Entered: Liver, Spleen

CHINESE THERAPEUTIC ACTIONS

1. Nourishes Blood and Preserves Yin

Liver blood deficiency: The chief manifestations of Liver blood deficiency include: dull and pale complexion, dizziness, tinnitus, and brittle, pale nails. *Bai Shao* (Radix Paeoniae Alba), cool in thermal property, nourishes the blood and yin and is best for blood-deficient patients with heat signs.

- Blood deficiency or anemia: combine *Bai Shao* with *Shu Di Huang* (Radix Rehmanniae Preparata), *Dang Gui* (Radicis Angelicae Sinensis), *He Shou Wu* (Radix Polygoni Multiflori), *E Jiao* (Colla Corii Asini), and *Lu Jiao Jiao* (Gelatinum Cornu Cervi).

Obstetric/gynecological disorders, irregular menstruation, gestational and postpartum disorders: Chronic deficiency of Liver blood results in deficiencies of the *ren* (conception) and *chong* (thoroughfare) channels. The symptoms may include: irregular menstruation, dysmenorrhea, uterine bleeding, and gestational and postpartum disorders. *Bai Shao* nourishes blood, softens the Liver and is an important herb to regulate menstruation and alleviate pain. It is best for patients with blood-deficient heat or Liver yang rising with underlying yin or blood deficiencies.

- Menstrual disorders with blood stagnation signs such as dysmenorrhea and clots, delayed onset or amenorrhea: combine *Bai Shao* with *Wu Ling Zhi* (Excrementum Trogopteri seu Pteromi), *Pu Huang* (Pollen Typhae), *Gan Cao* (Radix Glycyrrhizae), *Yan Hu Suo* (Rhizoma Corydalis), *Tao Ren* (Semen Persicae), and *Hong Hua* (Flos Carthami).
- Menstrual disorders with cold signs such as cold extremities, dark purple clots, pain aggravated by cold, delayed menstruation: use baked *Bai Shao* with *Pao Jiang* (Rhizoma Zingiberis Preparatum), *Rou Gui* (Cortex Cinnamomi), and *Ai Ye* (Folium Artemisiae Argyi).
- Menstrual disorders with heat signs such as profuse flow of fresh, red blood, heat sensations, or early menstruation: combine *Bai Shao* with *Huang Qin* (Radix Scutellariae), *Huang Lian* (Rhizoma Coptidis), and *Mu Dan Pi* (Cortex Moutan).
- Menstrual disorders with Liver qi stagnation, pre-menstrual syndrome, bloating, irritability, distended breasts: add this herb to *Chai Hu* (Radix Bupleuri), *Xiang Fu* (Rhizoma Cyperi), *Su Geng* (Caulis Perillae), and *Qing Pi* (Pericarpium Citri Reticulatae Viride).
- Menstrual disorders with qi deficiency signs such as fatigue, weakness, pale and scanty menstruation: combine *Bai Shao* with *Dang Shen* (Radix Codonopsis), *Huang Qi* (Radix Astragali), *Ren Shen* (Radix Ginseng), and *Bai Zhu* (Rhizoma Atractylodis Macrocephalae).
- Lower back pain or restless fetus due to Kidney deficiency: add it to *Du Zhong* (Cortex Eucommiae), *Xu Duan* (Radix Dipsaci), *Sang Ji Sheng* (Herba Taxilli), and *Tu Si Zi* (Semen Cuscutae).
- Abnormal uterine bleeding: combine this herb with *E Jiao* (Colla Corii Asini), *Han Lian Cao* (Herba Ecliptae), *Xian He Cao* (Herba Agrimoniae), and *Hai Piao Xiao* (Endoconcha Sepiae) to stop bleeding.

Weak constitution, with spontaneous or night sweating: Night sweating is indicative of yin deficiency and spontaneous sweating is suggestive of qi deficiency. Night sweating by definition is perspiration that takes place during sleep but stops upon awakening. Night sweating does not necessarily have to happen during the night but any perspiration during sleep would qualify as night sweating, which occurs as yang retreats to the interior

Bai Shao (Radix Paeoniae Alba)

during sleep and pushes out body fluids. Spontaneous sweating occurs while one is awake, regardless of day or night, with or without exertion, as it is the result of weakness of the *wei* (defense) *qi* with inability to control the opening and closing of the pores. *Bai Shao* may be used to stop both night and spontaneous sweating by nourishing the *ying* (nutritive) level and preserving yin.

- Night sweating: combine *Bai Shao* with *Wu Wei Zi* (Fructus Schisandrae Chinensis), *Fu Xiao Mai* (Semen Tritici Aestivi Levis), *Bai Zi Ren* (Semen Platycladi), and *Mu Li* (Concha Ostreae).
- Spontaneous sweating: use it with *Gui Zhi* (Ramulus Cinnamomi), *Sheng Jiang* (Rhizoma Zingiberis Recens), *Da Zao* (Fructus Jujubae), *Long Gu* (Os Draconis), and *Mu Li* (Concha Ostreae) to help consolidate the *ying* (nutritive) and *wei* (defensive) levels to prevent leakage of sweat. **Exemplar Formula:** *Gui Zhi Jia Long Mu Tang* (Cinnamon Twig Decoction plus Dragon Bone and Oyster Shell).
- Wind-cold with deficiency and perspiration: combine it with *Gui Zhi* (Ramulus Cinnamomi), *Sheng Jiang* (Rhizoma Zingiberis Recens), and *Da Zao* (Fructus Jujubae). **Exemplar Formula:** *Gui Zhi Tang* (Cinnamon Twig Decoction).
- Excessive perspiration caused by misuse of diaphoretic herbs to treat wind-cold syndrome: incorporate *Bai Shao* with *Gui Zhi* (Ramulus Cinnamomi), *Fu Zi* (Radix Aconiti Lateralis Praeparata), *Sheng Jiang* (Rhizoma Zingiberis Recens), and *Da Zao* (Fructus Jujubae).

Liver wind rising with yin and blood deficiencies: Liver yin and blood deficiencies often occur when there has been long-standing retention of pathogenic heat from a warm-febrile disease, or are caused by the misuse of heat-clearing, purgative or diaphoretic herbs. Symptoms include muscle spasms, twitches, tremors, alternating flexion and extension of the extremities, tonic-clonic spasms or convulsions in severe cases.

- Muscle spasms: combine *Bai Shao* with *Sheng Di Huang* (Radix Rehmanniae), *E Jiao* (Colla Corii Asini), *Mu Li* (Concha Ostreae), *Bie Jia* (Carapax Trionycis), *Gui Ban* (Plastrum Testudinis), *Mai Men Dong* (Radix Ophiopogonis) and egg yolks. **Exemplar Formula:** *Da Ding Feng Zhu* (Major Arrest Wind Pearl).

***Bi zheng* (painful obstruction syndrome):** *Bi zheng* due to blood deficiency often causes symptoms such as numbness (especially in the extremities), tightness of the tendons, and impaired agility.

- *Bi zheng*: incorporate *Bai Shao* with *Huang Qi* (Radix Astragali), *Gui Zhi* (Ramulus Cinnamomi), *Sheng Jiang* (Rhizoma Zingiberis Recens), and *Da Zao* (Fructus Jujubae).
- Bone spurs: combine it with *Mu Gua* (Fructus Chaenomelis), *Ji Xue Teng* (Caulis Spatholobi), *Wei Ling Xian* (Radix Clematidis), *Gan Cao* (Radix Glycyrrhizae) and *Po Bu Zi Ye* (Folium Cordia Dichotoma).

2. Nourishes the Liver to Calm Liver Yang and Liver Wind

Liver yang rising: Symptoms of Liver yang rising because of deficient Liver yin and blood include: dizziness, tinnitus, flushed face, red eyes, irritability, bad temper, headache, vertigo, and poor balance (feeling of heaviness on top and lightness at the feet). In severe cases, convulsions, delirium, and loss of consciousness may occur. *Bai Shao* nourishes blood, preserves yin and softens the Liver. It is cool in nature, which helps to disperse heat. The Liver governs the sinews: excess accumulation of heat in the body injures the fluids and deprives the tendons and sinews of nourishment.

- Liver yang rising: combine *Bai Shao* with *Sheng Di Huang* (Radix Rehmanniae), *Huai Niu Xi* (Radix Achyranthis Bidentatae), *Dai Zhe Shi* (Haematitum), and *Mu Li* (Concha Ostreae) to nourish the yin and calm the yang. **Exemplar Formula:** *Jian Ling Tang* (Construct Roof Tiles Decoction).
- Liver yang rising with Liver wind: Treat these symptoms by combining *Bai Shao* with *Ju Hua* (Flos Chrysanthemi), *Sang Ye* (Folium Mori), *Sheng Di Huang* (Radix Rehmanniae), *Mu Li* (Concha Ostreae), *Shi Jue Ming* (Concha Haliotidis), and *Tian Ma* (Rhizoma Gastrodiae).

3. Softens the Liver and Relieves Pain

Pain and spasms: *Bai Shao* is often used for pain in the muscles, tendons and sinews caused by lack of nourishment. *Bai Shao* softens the liver and also relieves epigastric, intercostal, hypochondriac and abdominal pain, and spasms and cramps of the smooth muscles and tendons.

- Epigastric, hypochondriac or flank pain and spasms: combine *Bai Shao* with *Gan Cao* (Radix Glycyrrhizae) to relieve smooth muscle spasms. **Exemplar Formula:** *Shao Yao Gan Cao Tang* (Peony and Licorice Decoction).
- Severe epigastric or abdominal pain or cramps caused by the Liver overacting on the deficient, cold, middle *jiao:* add this herb to *Gui Zhi* (Ramulus Cinnamomi), *Yi Tang* (Saccharum Granorum), *Da Zao* (Fructus Jujubae), *Gan Cao* (Radix Glycyrrhizae), and *Sheng Jiang* (Rhizoma Zingiberis Recens) to warm the middle *jiao* and disperse cold. **Exemplar Formula:** *Xiao Jian Zhong Tang* (Minor Construct the Middle Decoction).
- Numbness, spasms, and pain in the limbs from blood deficiency: combine this herb with *Gan Cao* (Radix Glycyrrhizae).

Bai Shao (Radix Paeoniae Alba)

- *Bi zheng* (painful obstruction syndrome) due to coldness and blood deficiency: incorporate it with *Mu Gua* (Fructus Chaenomelis), *Gui Zhi* (Ramulus Cinnamomi), *Ji Xue Teng* (Caulis Spatholobi), *Dang Gui Wei* (Extremitas Radicis Angelicae Sinensis), and *Shen Jin Cao* (Herba Lycopodii).
- Chronic *bi zheng* (painful obstruction syndrome) due to wind, cold and dampness with blood deficiency: combine *Bai Shao* with *Du Huo* (Radix Angelicae Pubescentis), *Qin Jiao* (Radix Gentianae Macrophyllae), *Ren Shen* (Radix Ginseng), *Dang Gui* (Radicis Angelicae Sinensis), and *Gan Cao* (Radix Glycyrrhizae). **Exemplar Formula:** *San Bi Tang* (Three-Painful Obstruction Decoction).

Breast distention, pre-menstrual syndrome: Breast distention and symptoms of pre-menstrual syndrome such as mood swings, irritability, restlessness, and bad temper are associated with Liver qi stagnation with underlying Liver blood and yin deficiencies.

- Pre-menstrual syndrome: combine *Bai Shao* with *Chai Hu* (Radix Bupleuri), *Dang Gui* (Radicis Angelicae Sinensis), *Bai Zhu* (Rhizoma Atractylodis Macrocephalae), and *Gan Cao* (Radix Glycyrrhizae) to relieve Liver qi stagnation, nourish the blood and stop pain. **Exemplar Formula:** *Xiao Yao San* (Rambling Powder).

Diarrhea, borborygmus with abdominal pain: The Liver overacting on the Spleen creates stagnant qi with symptoms of borborygmus, and abdominal pain that is relieved by diarrhea.

- Diarrhea, borborygmus and abdominal pain: combine dry-fried *Bai Shao* with dry-fried *Bai Zhu* (Rhizoma Atractylodis Macrocephalae), *Chen Pi* (Pericarpium Citri Reticulatae) and *Fang Feng* (Radix Saposhnikoviae). **Exemplar Formula:** *Tong Xie Yao Fang* (Important Formula for Painful Diarrhea).

Dysenteric disorders with rectal tenesmus: Dysenteric disorders due to damp-heat accumulation in the lower *jiao* can result in burning diarrhea with rectal tenesmus and burning sensations in the anus.

- Dysenteric disorders with rectal tenesmus: incorporate *Bai Shao* with *Huang Qin* (Radix Scutellariae), *Huang Lian* (Rhizoma Coptidis), *Da Huang* (Radix et Rhizoma Rhei), *Ge Gen* (Radix Puerariae), *Bai Tou Weng* (Radix Pulsatillae), *Mu Xiang* (Radix Aucklandiae), and *Gan Cao* (Radix Glycyrrhizae). **Exemplar Formula:** *Shao Yao Tang* (Peony Decoction).

DOSAGE

5 to 10 grams in decoction. In severe cases, up to 30 grams of *Bai Shao* can be used. This herb is also used in pill or powder forms. The fresh or unprocessed herb has a stronger function to preserve yin and calm the Liver, and is commonly used to treat headaches, dizziness, tinnitus, and other conditions in which Liver yang is rising. The dry-fried form is warmer, and more effective to tonify blood and preserve yin. Dried-fried *Bai Shao* is best for abdominal pain, diarrhea, and borborygmus. Frying *Bai Shao* with grain-based liquor converts its cool property to neutral and improves its blood-invigorating effect, and is best for spasms, cramps, hypochondriac and abdominal pain from qi and blood stagnation.

CAUTIONS / CONTRAINDICATIONS

- *Bai Shao* is incompatible with *Li Lu* (Radix et Rhizoma Veratri).
- *Bai Shao* is contraindicated in cases of middle *jiao* yang deficiency with cold.
- Because of its astringent nature, *Bai Shao* is contraindicated in patients with eczema or rashes from exterior wind attack with incomplete expression.
- Use of *Bai Shao* is contraindicated in postpartum patients with blood stagnation, or for those who are still bleeding.
- Use of *Bai Shao* may be associated with drowsiness and sedation. Therefore, individuals who take this herb should exercise caution if driving or operating heavy machinery.

CHEMICAL COMPOSITION

Paeoniflorin, albiflorin, oxypaeoniflorin, benzoylpaeoniflorin, paeonin, hydroxypaeoniflorin.[1]

PHARMACOLOGICAL EFFECTS

- **CNS suppressant:** Subcutaneous injection of *Bai Shao* has demonstrated marked sedative and suppressant effects on the central nervous system (CNS) in mice. It prolonged the sleeping time induced by barbiturates, and has a protective effect against seizures induced by cardiazol.[2]
- **Gastrointestinal:** *Bai Shao* has an inhibitory influence on the smooth muscles of the intestines and the uterus. In addition, it inhibits the secretion of gastric acid to treat peptic ulcers in mice.[3]
- **Antibiotic:** Decoction of *Bai Shao* has been shown to have inhibitory action against *Bacillus dysenteriae, E. coli, Salmonella typhi, Pseudomonas aeruginosa, Staphylococcus aureus*, β-hemolytic streptococcus, *Diplococcus pneumoniae*, and some dermatophytes.[4]
- **Antipyretic and anti-inflammatory:** Paeoniflorin has demonstrated marked antipyretic and anti-inflammatory effects.[5]
- **Antiplatelet:** Paeoniflorin has a mild influence to inhibit emboli formation through delayed aggregation of platelets.[6]
- **Cardiovascular:** *Bai Shao* has demonstrated a marked

Bai Shao (Radix Paeoniae Alba)

action to relax blood vessels, dilate peripheral blood vessels, and cause a slight decrease in blood pressure.[7]

CLINICAL STUDIES AND RESEARCH

- **Intestinal spasm:** In one study, 85 patients with intestinal cramps and spasms were treated with one dose of an herbal decoction daily. Most patients reported complete remission of spasms and cramps without recurrence. The formula contained *Bai Shao* 30g, *Gui Zhi* (Ramulus Cinnamomi) 15g, *Gan Cao* (Radix Glycyrrhizae) 15g, and *Mu Gua* (Fructus Chaenomelis) 10g.[8]
- **Pain:** Intramuscular injection of 4 ml of an herbal preparation (equivalent to 4 grams of *Bai Shao* and 1 gram of *Gan Cao* (Radix Glycyrrhizae)) showed marked analgesic effect within 30 minutes without significant side effects. The analgesic action was 84.67% effective (105 out of 124 subjects) in patients with deficiency-type pain, and 50.98% effective (26 out of 51 subjects) in patients with excess-type pain.[9]
- **Trigeminal neuralgia:** The combination of *Bai Shao* and *Gan Cao* (Radix Glycyrrhizae) was effective in relieving pain in 30 out of 42 patients.[10]
- **Muscle spasms and twitching in the facial region:** The combination of *Bai Shao* and *Gan Cao* (Radix Glycyrrhizae) was effective in reducing the frequency and severity of muscle spasms and twitching in 11 out of 11 patients.[11]
- **Pain in the lower back and legs:** The combination of *Bai Shao* and *Gan Cao* (Radix Glycyrrhizae) was effective in relieving pain. Out of 33 elderly patients, 12 reported significant improvement, 16 reported moderate improvement, 4 reported slight improvement and 1 reported no improvement.[12]
- **Myotonia:** An herbal decoction was given orally one time daily for 50 days for treatment of myotonia. Out of 10 patients with congenital myotonia, 1 showed marked improvement, 4 showed moderate improvement, and 5 showed slight improvement. Out of 10 patients with atrophic myotonia, 2 showed marked improvement, 4 showed moderate improvement, and 4 showed slight improvement. The formula contained *Bai Shao* 40g, *Gan Cao* (Radix Glycyrrhizae) 25g, *Mu Gua* (Fructus Chaenomelis) 25g, *Niu Xi* (Radix Cyathulae seu Achyranthis) 25g, *Chan Tui* (Periostracum Cicadae) 12g, *Jiang Can* (Bombyx Batryticatus) 12g, and *Yi Yi Ren* (Semen Coicis) 30g.[13]
- **Habitual constipation:** According to one report, over 60 patients with chronic habitual constipation were treated with Chinese herbs, with great success. The basic herbal treatment consisted of 24 to 40 grams of fresh *Bai Shao* and 10 to 15 grams of fresh *Gan Cao* (Radix Glycyrrhizae) taken as herbal decoction twice daily. The herbal formula was modified specifically according to the following conditions: 24 to 32 grams of fresh *Bai Zhu* (Rhizoma Atractylodis Macrocephalae) were added for qi deficiency; 10 to 15 grams of *Fu Zi* (Radix Aconiti Lateralis Praeparata) were added for excess cold and stagnation; 9 to 15 grams of *E Jiao* (Colla Corii Asini) were added for yin deficiency and blood dryness; 9 to 15 grams of *Dang Gui* (Radicis Angelicae Sinensis) were added for blood deficiency with coldness; 10 grams of *Mai Ya* (Fructus Hordei Germinatus) were added for qi stagnation; 20 to 30 grams of *Dai Zhe Shi* (Haematitum) were added and *Gan Cao* (Radix Glycyrrhizae) removed for hypertension with Liver yang excess; *Ban Xia* (Rhizoma Pinelliae) and *Chen Pi* (Pericarpium Citri Reticulatae) were added and *Gan Cao* (Radix Glycyrrhizae) removed for hypertension with excessive dampness accumulation. Most patients reported normal bowel movements within 2 to 4 doses without rebound constipation. Severe constipation required up to one week of continuous herbal therapy.[14]
- **Peptic ulcer:** In one study, patients with peptic ulcers were treated with Chinese herbs with marked success. Out of 120 patients, 83 reported marked improvement, 33 reported moderate improvement, and 4 reported no response. Patients with peptic ulcers caused by qi and blood stagnation were most responsive to the treatment. The treatment included *Bai Shao* 15 to 20g and *Zhi Gan Cao* (Radix Glycyrrhizae Preparata) 12 to 15g as the core combination. The herbal formula was modified specifically according to the following conditions: *Dang Shen* (Radix Codonopsis) 12g, *Huang Qi* (Radix Astragali) 12g, *Fu Ling* (Poria) 20g, and *Gan Jiang* (Rhizoma Zingiberis) 10g for deficiency and cold of the Spleen and Stomach; *Sha Shen* (Radix Glehniae seu Adenophorae) 10g, *Mai Men Dong* (Radix Ophiopogonis) 12g, *Dang Gui* (Radicis Angelicae Sinensis) 12g, and *Sheng Di Huang* (Radix Rehmanniae) 15g for Stomach yin deficiency; *Ru Xiang* (Gummi Olibanum) 10g, *Mo Yao* (Myrrha) 10g, *Dan Shen* (Radix Salviae Miltiorrhizae) 15g, and *Chuan Xiong* (Rhizoma Ligusticum Chuanxiong) 15g for qi and blood stagnation; and *Chai Hu* (Radix Bupleuri) 10g, *Bai Zhu* (Rhizoma Atractylodis Macrocephalae) 10g, *Chen Pi* (Pericarpium Citri Reticulatae) 10g, and *Fu Ling* (Poria) 20g for Liver and Stomach disharmony.[15]
- **Hyperosteogeny:** In one study, patients with hyperosteogeny were treated with an herbal decoction once daily with good success. Out of 160 patients, 109 showed marked improvement, 42 showed moderate improvement, and 9 showed slight improvement. The herbal formula contained *Bai Shao* 30 to 60g, *Mu Gua* (Fructus Chaenomelis) 12g, *Ji Xue Teng* (Caulis Spatholobi) 15g, *Wei Ling Xian* (Radix Clematidis) 15g, *Gan Cao* (Radix Glycyrrhizae) 12g, and others if necessary.[16]

Bai Shao (Radix Paeoniae Alba)

- **Whooping cough:** According to one report, 33 patients with whooping cough were treated with an herbal decoction with marked success. The core combination consisted of 15 grams of *Bai Shao* and 5 grams of *Gan Cao* (Radix Glycyrrhizae). *Bai Bu* (Radix Stemonae) and *Bai He* (Bulbus Lilii) were added to suppress cough; *Di Long* (Pheretima), *Ting Li Zi* (Semen Descurainiae seu Lepidii) and *Wu Gong* (Scolopendra) were added to relieve wheezing and resolve phlegm production. No antibiotic drugs were given throughout the treatment.[17]
- **Asthma:** Patients with acute wheezing and dyspnea were treated with an herbal decoction of 20 grams of *Bai Shao* and 10 grams of *Gan Cao* (Radix Glycyrrhizae) powder, mixed with 100 to 150 ml of water, and cooked for only 3 to 5 minutes. Out of 35 patients, 8 showed significant response to the herbs, 23 showed marked response, and 4 showed no change. With regard to initial onset of action, 26 patients noticed marked improvement within 30 to 60 minutes, and 4 noticed marked improvement within 1 to 2 hours.[18]
- **Restless leg syndrome:** Oral administration of an herbal decoction (15 grams of *Bai Shao* and 15 grams of *Gan Cao* (Radix Glycyrrhizae)) was given twice daily to treat restless leg syndrome. The therapy showed a 100% rate of effectiveness in 54 patients. However, 6 patients experienced recurrence after the cessation of herbal treatment.[19]
- **Diabetes mellitus:** According to one journal, 180 patients with diabetes mellitus were given an herbal formula three times daily. The formula contained 40 grams of *Bai Shao* and 8 grams of *Gan Cao* (Radix Glycyrrhizae). The herbal therapy lowered blood glucose levels in 73.9% of patients (54 with marked effects, 67 with moderate effects, 12 with slight response, and 47 with no response).[20]

HERB-DRUG INTERACTION

- **Anticoagulant or antiplatelet drugs:** *Bai Shao* has been shown to have a mild inhibitory effect on platelet aggregation and prevention of emboli formation. Therefore, it should be taken with caution by patients who are taking anticoagulant or antiplatelet drugs.[21] [Note: Examples of anticoagulants include heparin, warfarin (Coumadin) and enoxaparin (Lovenox); and examples of antiplatelets include aspirin, dipyridamole (Persantine), and clopidogrel (Plavix).]
- **Antidiabetics:** It is prudent to use *Bai Shao* with caution with insulin, sulfonylureas, and other antidiabetic medications as the combination may have synergistic effects, leading to hypoglycemia.[22] [Note: Examples of antidiabetic drugs include insulin, tolbutamide (Orinase), glipizide (Glucotrol), and glyburide (DiaBeta/Micronase).]
- **Sedatives:** *Bai Shao* has sedative and analgesic effects on the central nervous system. It prolonged the sleeping time induced by barbiturates, and has a protective effect against seizures induced by cardiazol.[23] [Note: Many categories of drugs induce sedation, such as antihistamines, narcotic analgesics, barbiturates, benzodiazepines and many others.]

TOXICOLOGY

The LD_{50} for paeoniflorin in mice is 3,530 mg/kg via intravenous injection and 9,530 mg/kg via intraperitoneal injection.

AUTHORS' COMMENTS

Bai Shao is often combined with *Gui Zhi* (Ramulus Cinnamomi) to relieve exterior conditions in deficient patients. *Bai Shao* and *Gui Zhi* together harmonize the *ying* (nutritive) and the *wei* (defensive) levels to promote diaphoresis and at the same time prevent leakage of sweat and nourish fluids.

According to Dr. Zhang Liang-Lin, *Bai Shao* and *Wu Yao* (Radix Linderae) are an excellent pair to treat the lower abdominal bloating and pain associated with dysmenorrhea.

Please refer to *Chi Shao* (Radix Paeoniae Rubrae) for comparison of *Bai Shao* and *Chi Shao*.

References

1. *Xian Dai Zhong Yao Yao Li Xue* (Contemporary Pharmacology of Chinese Herbs), 1997; 1313
2. *Zhong Yao Tong Bao* (Journal of Chinese Herbology), 1985; 10(6):43
3. *Zhong Yao Zhi* (Chinese Herbology Journal), 1993:183
4. *Xin Zhong Yi* (New Chinese Medicine), 1989; 21(3):51
5. *Zhong Yao Zhi* (Chinese Herbology Journal), 1993:183
6. *Zhong Yao Xue* (Chinese Herbology), 1998; 831:836
7. *Zhong Guo Yao Li Xue Tong Bao* (Journal of Chinese Herbal Pharmacology), 1986; 2(5):26
8. *Zhong Yi Za Zhi* (Journal of Chinese Medicine), 1985; 6:50
9. *Shang Hai Zhong Yi Yao Za Zhi* (Shanghai Journal of Chinese Medicine and Herbology), 1983; 4:14
10. *Zhong Yi Za Zhi* (Journal of Chinese Medicine), 1983; 11:9
11. *Hu Nan Zhong Yi* (Hunan Journal of Traditional Chinese Medicine), 1989; 2:7
12. *Yun Nan Zhong Yi* (Yunnan Journal of Traditional Chinese Medicine), 1990; 4:15
13. *Zhong Xi Yi Jie He Za Zhi* (Journal of Integrated Chinese and Western Medicine), 1984; 8:497
14. *Zhong Yi Za Zhi* (Journal of Chinese Medicine), 1983; 8:79
15. *Shan Dong Zhong Yi Za Zhi* (Shandong Journal of Chinese Medicine), 1984; 2:22
16. *Xin Zhong Yi* (New Chinese Medicine), 1980; 1:18
17. *Hu Nan Zhong Yi Za Zhi* (Hunan Journal of Chinese Medicine), 1988; 1:48
18. *Zhong Yi Za Zhi* (Journal of Chinese Medicine), 1987; 9:66
19. *He Bei Zhong Yi* (Hebei Chinese Medicine), 1984,3:29
20. *Zhong Xi Yi Jie He Za Zhi* (Journal of Integrated Chinese and Western Medicine), 1986; 10:593
21. Chen, J. Recognition & prevention of herb-drug interactions, *Medical Acupuncture*, Fall/Winter 1998/1999; volume 10/number 2; 9-13
22. Ibid.
23. *Zhong Yao Tong Bao* (Journal of Chinese Herbology), 1985; 10(6):43

E Jiao (Colla Corii Asini)

阿膠 阿胶

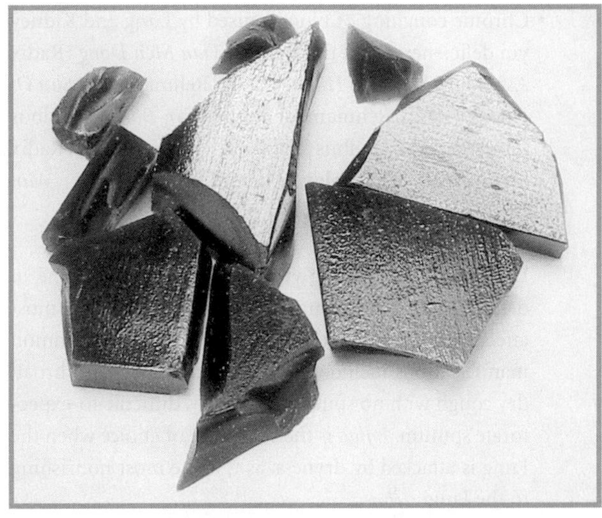

Pinyin Name: *E Jiao*
Literal Name: "gelatin"
Alternate Chinese Names: *Lu Pi Jiao, Pen Fu Jiao, Bo Zhi Jiao, Yang Jiao, E Jiao Zhu*
Original Source: *Shen Nong Ben Cao Jing* (Divine Husbandman's Classic of the Materia Medica) in the second century
English Name: ass-hide glue, donkey-hide gelatin, gelatin
Zoological Name: *Equus asinus* L. (*Lu*)
Pharmaceutical Name: Colla Corii Asini
Properties: sweet, neutral
Channels Entered: Lung, Liver, Kidney

CHINESE THERAPEUTIC ACTIONS

1. Tonifies Blood and Stops Bleeding

Blood deficiency of the Liver and Heart: Clinical manifestations include pale or sallow complexion, dizziness, and palpitations. *E Jiao* (Colla Corii Asini) tonifies blood and treats various menstrual disorders such as irregularity, dysmenorrhea, and gestational and postpartum disorders.

- Anemia: combine *E Jiao* with *Dang Gui* (Radicis Angelicae Sinensis), *Bai Shao* (Radix Paeoniae Alba), and *Shu Di Huang* (Radix Rehmanniae Preparata).
- Anemia with qi deficiency: combine this substance with *Huang Qi* (Radix Astragali), *Dang Gui* (Radicis Angelicae Sinensis), *Shu Di Huang* (Radix Rehmanniae Preparata) and *Dang Shen* (Radix Codonopsis).

Bleeding: *E Jiao* is neutral, sweet and sticky in nature. It stops bleeding caused by yin deficiency in various parts of the body (hematemesis, epistaxis, bleeding gums, hematochezia, hematuria and uterine bleeding). The charred form is preferred, for it has a stronger hemostatic function. *E Jiao* can be used alone or with other hemostatic herbs.

- Bleeding during pregnancy: use dry-fried *E Jiao* as powder.
- Profuse hematemesis or bleeding from the ears: combine this substance with *Pu Huang* (Pollen Typhae) and *Sheng Di Huang* (Radix Rehmanniae) juice.
- Bleeding associated with Spleen qi and yang deficiencies, such as hematemesis, epistaxis, hematochezia and uterine bleeding: combine *E Jiao* with *Shu Di Huang* (Radix Rehmanniae Preparata), *Bai Zhu* (Rhizoma Atractylodis Macrocephalae), and *Fu Zi* (Radix Aconiti Lateralis Praeparata).
- Hypermenorrhea, uterine bleeding, bleeding during pregnancy, or bleeding from miscarriage: add this substance to *Ai Ye* (Folium Artemisiae Argyi), *Shu Di Huang* (Radix Rehmanniae Preparata), *Bai Shao* (Radix Paeoniae Alba), and *Gan Cao* (Radix Glycyrrhizae).
- Hematochezia or bleeding hemorrhoids: use it with *Huang Qin* (Radix Scutellariae), *Ku Shen Gen* (Radix Sophorae Flavescentis), charred *Huai Hua* (Flos Sophorae), charred *Di Yu* (Radix Sanguisorbae), and *Fang Feng* (Radix Saposhnikoviae).
- Hemoptysis: combine it with *Mai Men Dong* (Radix Ophiopogonis), *Bai He* (Bulbus Lilii), *Bai Ji* (Rhizoma Bletillae), *Sha Shen* (Radix Glehniae seu Adenophorae), charred *Zhi Zi* (Fructus Gardeniae), and *Ou Jie* (Nodus Nelumbinis Rhizomatis).

2. Nourishes Yin and Moistens the Lung

Lung yin deficiency: The Lung is among the most tender organs in the body, and is very susceptible to damage, especially from dryness. Dryness usually results from chronic respiratory disorders, and manifests in symptoms such as cough, dyspnea, and shortness of breath upon exertion. *E Jiao* is sweet, neutral and moistening in nature, and is effective in nourishing Lung yin. However, in order to avoid producing phlegm, *E Jiao* should be used with phlegm-eliminating herbs so that both the root of yin deficiency and the symptoms are treated.

- Loud, labored and accelerated respiration caused by Lung yin deficiency with fire: combine *E Jiao* with *Niu Bang Zi* (Fructus Arctii), *Xing Ren* (Semen Armeniacae Amarum), and *Gan Cao* (Radix Glycyrrhizae).
- Chronic cough, asthma and spontaneous sweating caused by Lung qi and yin deficiencies: combine this substance with *Wu Wei Zi* (Fructus Schisandrae Chinensis), *Ren Shen* (Radix Ginseng), *Kuan Dong Hua* (Flos Farfarae), and *Bei Mu* (Bulbus Fritillaria).

E Jiao (Colla Corii Asini)

- Chronic coughing of blood caused by Lung and Kidney yin deficiencies: add this herb to *Tian Men Dong* (Radix Asparagi), *Sheng Di Huang* (Radix Rehmanniae), *Shu Di Huang* (Radix Rehmanniae Preparata), *Bai He* (Bulbus Lilii), *Bei Mu* (Bulbus Fritillaria), and *Bai Bu* (Radix Stemonae). **Exemplar Formula:** *Yue Hua Wan* (Moonlight Pill).

Dryness injuring Lung yin: The Lung, the first line of defense against environmental factors, is the organ most affected by the pathogenic factor dryness. Common manifestations include: dryness of the nose and throat, dry cough with no sputum, or scanty, difficult-to-expectorate sputum. *E Jiao* is the substance of choice when the Lung is attacked by dryness, as it is the most nourishing to the Lung.

- Symptoms of dryness injuring Lung yin: combine *E Jiao* with *Sang Ye* (Folium Mori), *Shi Gao* (Gypsum Fibrosum), *Mai Men Dong* (Radix Ophiopogonis), *Pi Pa Ye* (Folium Eriobotryae), and *Xing Ren* (Semen Armeniacae Amarum). **Exemplar Formula:** *Qing Zao Jiu Fei Tang* (Eliminate Dryness and Rescue the Lungs Decoction).

Late-stage chronic illnesses with deficiency heat signs: Chronic illness often consumes yin and body fluids, leading to yin-deficient heat with low grade fever and steaming bones sensations.

- Low-grade fever, steaming bones sensations: combine *E Jiao* with *Sheng Di Huang* (Radix Rehmanniae), *Bie Jia* (Carapax Trionycis), *Gui Ban* (Plastrum Testudinis), *Qin Jiao* (Radix Gentianae Macrophyllae), *Yin Chai Hu* (Radix Stellariae), and *Qing Hao* (Herba Artemisiae Annuae).

3. Moistens the Intestines and Unblocks the Bowels:

Regular bowel movement is dependent on proper nourishment of the intestines. When body fluids and blood are deficient, constipation or dry stools may occur. This condition usually is present in anemic, postpartum, or elderly patients, or in those recovering from a chronic illness.

- Constipation or dry stools: combine this herb with honey, *Cong Bai* (Bulbus Allii Fistulosi) and *Zhi Ke* (Fructus Aurantii).

4. Others

- Water retention manifesting in dysuria with edema: use *E Jiao* with *Zhu Ling* (Polyporus), *Hua Shi* (Talcum), *Ze Xie* (Rhizoma Alismatis) and *Fu Ling* (Poria) to tonify yin and clear heat. **Exemplar Formula:** *Zhu Ling Tang* (Polyporus Decoction).
- For diarrhea during pregnancy with abdominal pain: use it with *Huang Lian* (Rhizoma Coptidis), *Shi Liu Pi* (Pericarpium Granati) and *Dang Gui* (Radicis Angelicae Sinensis).

DOSAGE

5 to 10 grams. Dissolve *E Jiao* in warm decoction, hot water or heated grain-based liquor, and take orally. It is also used in powder or pill form. *E Jiao* is sometimes dry-fried with other herbs to reduce its odor and minimize stickiness.

CAUTIONS / CONTRAINDICATIONS

- Because *E Jiao* is sticky, it is contraindicated in patients with Spleen and Stomach deficiencies that manifest as loose stools, diarrhea, or poor appetite.
- *E Jiao* should not be used for patients with phlegm or damp accumulation.

CHEMICAL COMPOSITION

Collagen, amino acids (lysine, arginine, histadine, glycine, cysteine), sodium, potassium, calcium, magnesium, aluminum, and zinc.[1]

PHARMACOLOGICAL EFFECTS

- **Hematological:** A group of dogs with post-hemorrhage anemia were divided into three groups: those that received a placebo, those that received iron, and those that received *E Jiao*. Increase in red blood cell count and hemoglobin was most prominent in the *E Jiao* group, followed by the iron group, and lastly, the placebo group.[2]
- **Cardiovascular:** Intravenous infusion of 5 to 6% *E Jiao* was beneficial in treating cats with post-hemorrhage shock.[3]
- **Effect on calcium metabolism:** Daily ingestion of 30 grams of *E Jiao* in dogs increased the absorption and utilization of calcium carbonate. Plasma levels of calcium also increased.[4]

CLINICAL STUDIES AND RESEARCH

- **Pulmonary tuberculosis:** In one clinical trial, patients with hemoptysis caused by pulmonary tuberculosis were treated with 20 to 30 grams of *E Jiao* powder two to three times daily, with warm water. Those with profuse hemoptysis were also treated with pharmaceutical drugs to stop bleeding. In addition to herbal treatment, all patients received antibiotics to treat the tuberculosis. Out of 56 patients, the study reported marked improvement in 37 patients, moderate improvement in 15 patients, and no improvement in 4 patients. The overall rate of effectiveness in relieving hemoptysis was 92.7%.[5]
- **Chronic ulceration of the legs:** It was reported in one study that 24 patients with chronic ulceration of the legs recovered completely after topical treatment with *E Jiao* cream for 20 days. The cream was prepared by mixing 30 grams of *E Jiao* in 70 ml of water and cooked until the

E Jiao (Colla Corii Asini)

preparation turned into paste. The daily treatment protocol was to first cleanse the affected area, apply the cream, then cover the area with gauze. The procedure was repeated daily until complete recovery was achieved.[6]

- **Leukopenia and anemia:** An herbal formula containing *E Jiao*, *Ren Shen* (Radix Ginseng), *Shu Di Huang* (Radix Rehmanniae Preparata), *Dang Shen* (Radix Codonopsis), *Shan Zha* (Fructus Crataegi) and others was 79.33% effective in raising white blood cell counts, and 67.8% effective in treating anemia caused by lack of iron.[7]
- **Unstable pregnancy:** A formula containing 12 grams of *E Jiao*, 2 eggs, and 30 grams of sugar showed 83.3% effectiveness in 36 patients with restless fetus or unstable pregnancies.[8]

AUTHORS' COMMENTS

The use of *E Jiao* started approximately in the Tang dynasty. At that time, gelatin from many animals was used, including cattle, pigs, horses, donkeys and camels. Gelatin derived from cattle has weaker tonic functions but stronger blood-invigorating and toxin-eliminating effects. Gelatin derived from pigs has similar blood-tonic and hemostatic functions. From a clinical perspective, these gelatin substances treat anemia, primary thrombocytopenia, dysfunctional uterine bleeding and aplastic anemia.

To enhance the hemostatic properties, *E Jiao* should be processed with *Pu Huang* (Pollen Typhae). To enhance the nourishing function to the Lung, process *E Jiao* with *Hai Ge Fen* (Concha Meretricis seu Cyclinae).

References

1. *Xian Dai Zhong Yao Yao Li Xue* (Contemporary Pharmacology of Chinese Herbs), 1997; 1320
2. *Zhong Cheng Yao Yan Jiu* (Research of Chinese Patent Medicine), 1981; (5):31
3. *Chang Yong Zhong Yao Cheng Fen Yu Yao Li Shou Ce* (A Handbook of the Composition and Pharmacology of Common Chinese Drugs), 1994, 1124:1131
4. *Chin J Physiol*, 1935; 9(4):383
5. *Liao Ning Zhong Yi Za Zhi* (Liaoning Journal of Chinese Medicine), 1987; 9:39
6. *Zhong Xi Yi Jie He Za Zhi* (Journal of Integrated Chinese and Western Medicine), 1987; 4:241
7. *Shan Dong Yi Yao Gong Ye* (Shandong Pharmaceutical Industry), 1986; 3:21
8. *Shan Xi Zhong Yi* (Shanxi Chinese Medicine), 1987; 2:35

Long Yan Rou (Arillus Longan)

龍眼肉 龙眼肉

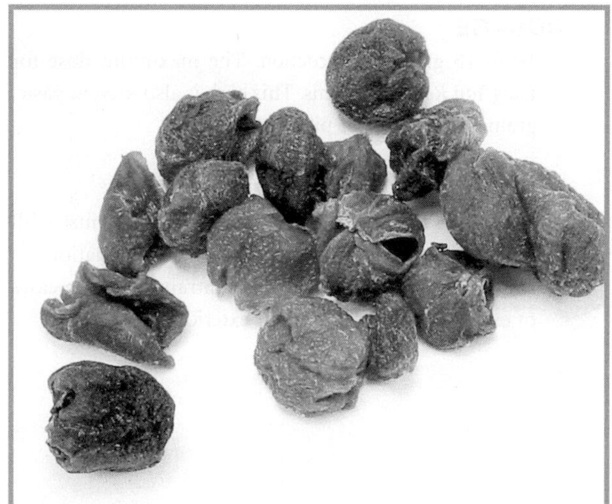

Pinyin Name: *Long Yan Rou*
Literal Name: "dragon eye flesh"
Alternate Chinese Names: *Gui Yuan Rou, Gui Yuan, Yi Zhi*
Original Source: *Shen Nong Ben Cao Jing* (Divine Husbandman's Classic of the Materia Medica) in the second century
English Name: longan fruit, dried longan pulp
Botanical Name: *Euphoria longan [Dimocarpus longan]* (Lour.) Steud. (*Long Yan*)
Pharmaceutical Name: Arillus Longan
Properties: sweet, warm
Channels Entered: Heart, Spleen

CHINESE THERAPEUTIC ACTIONS

1. Tonifies Heart and Spleen

Spleen and Heart deficiencies: The Heart governs the blood vessels and the *shen* (spirit). The Spleen transforms food into *gu* (food) *qi*. Excessive worrying or pensiveness damages the Heart and Spleen and causes palpitations,

Long Yan Rou (Arillus Longan)

insomnia, difficulty falling and staying asleep, forgetfulness, withered *shen* (spirit), and fatigue. *Long Yan Rou* (Arillus Longan) is sweet, warm and not stagnating in nature. It enters and nourishes the Heart and Spleen, and can be used alone or with other tonic herbs.

- Spleen and Heart deficiencies with the symptoms listed above: use *Long Yan Rou* alone, or with *Ren Shen* (Radix Ginseng), *Huang Qi* (Radix Astragali), *Dang Gui* (Radicis Angelicae Sinensis), and *Suan Zao Ren* (Semen Zizyphi Spinosae). **Exemplar Formula:** *Gui Pi Tang* (Restore the Spleen Decoction).
- Diarrhea from Spleen deficiency: combine this herb with *Sheng Jiang* (Rhizoma Zingiberis Recens), *Bai Zhu* (Rhizoma Atractylodis Macrocephalae), *Shan Yao* (Rhizoma Dioscoreae), and *Yi Yi Ren* (Semen Coicis).

2. Benefits Qi and Blood

Qi and blood deficiencies: This condition is commonly seen in the chronically ill and the elderly. Typical symptoms associated with qi and blood deficiencies include fatigue, weakness, shortness of breath, spontaneous sweating, and a pale or sallow complexion.

- Qi and blood deficiencies: combine *Long Yan Rou* with *Huang Qi* (Radix Astragali), and *Ren Shen* (Radix Ginseng), or *Xi Yang Shen* (Radix Panacis Quinquefolii).
- Edema in postpartum women: use it with *Sheng Jiang* (Rhizoma Zingiberis Recens) and *Da Zao* (Fructus Jujubae).
- Qi and blood deficiencies with cold due to yang deficiency: soak this herb in grain-based liquor and drink daily.

DOSAGE

10 to 15 grams in decoction. The maximum dose for *Long Yan Rou* is 30 grams. This herb is also used in paste, grain-based liquor or pill forms.

CAUTIONS / CONTRAINDICATIONS

- *Long Yan Rou* is contraindicated for patients with phlegm-fire and middle *jiao* dampness or stagnation.
- *Long Yan Rou* is warm and thus contraindicated in cases of excess or deficiency heat, or exterior conditions.

CHEMICAL COMPOSITION

Vitamin A, B_1, B_2, C; adenine, choline, glucose, sucrose.[1]

PHARMACOLOGICAL EFFECTS

- **Antibiotic:** The water extract of *Long Yan Rou* (1:2) exerts inhibitory influences against some pathogenic fungi.[2]

SUPPLEMENT

- 龍眼花 / 龙眼花 *Long Yan Hua* (Flos Longan) is derived from the flower of the same plant as *Long Yan Rou*. *Long Yan Hua* is bland, sour, astringent, cold, and enters the Liver and Kidney channels. Clinically, it consolidates Kidney *jing* (essence) and restrains vaginal discharge. For Kidney dysfunction with proteinuria, *Long Yan Hua* is used with *Xian Feng Cao* (Herba Bidentis) and *Ding Shu Xiu* (Herba Elephantopus Scaber). For white vaginal discharge, it is combined with *Ji Guan Hua* (Flos Celosiae Cristatae), *Fu Ling* (Poria), *Chen Pi* (Pericarpium Citri Reticulatae), *Ban Xia* (Rhizoma Pinelliae) and *Gan Cao* (Radix Glycyrrhizae). For foul-smelling yellow vaginal discharge, *Long Yan Hua* is added to *Long Dan Cao* (Radix Gentianae), *Qu Mai* (Herba Dianthi), *Bian Xu* (Herba Polygoni Avicularis), *Huang Bai* (Cortex Phellodendri) and *Ku Shen Gen* (Radix Sophorae Flavescentis). For diabetes mellitus, it is used with *Bi Zi Cao* (Herba Pogonantheri Criniti). The dosage for *Long Yan Hua* is 6 to 15 grams in decoction.

AUTHORS' COMMENTS

Long Yan Rou soaked in grain-based liquor is used to treat patients suffering from deficiency and cold who have insomnia or difficulty sleeping. A small portion is taken before sleep.

Long Yan Rou, *Sang Shen Zi* (Fructus Mori) and *Gou Qi Zi* (Fructus Lycii) are tonics that can be safely taken over a long period of time without creating an imbalance in the body.

References

1. *Xian Dai Zhong Yao Yao Li Xue* (Contemporary Pharmacology of Chinese Herbs), 1997; 1335
2. *Zhong Yao Xue* (Chinese Herbology), 1998; 840:841

Section 4

— Yin-Tonifying Herbs

Bei Sha Shen (Radix Glehniae)

北沙参 北沙参

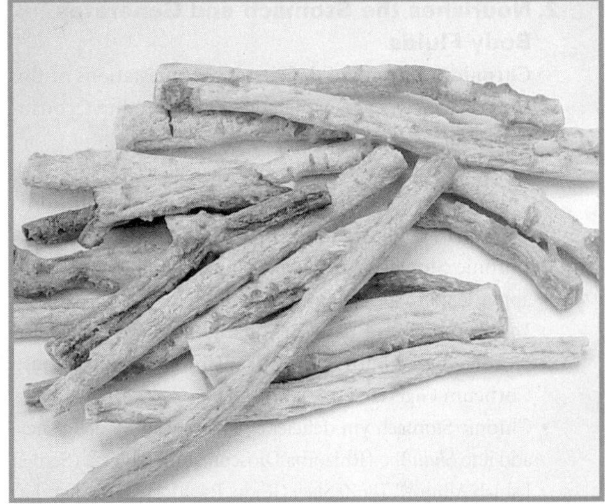

Pinyin Name: *Bei Sha Shen*
Literal Name: "sand root from the north"
Alternate Chinese Names: *Yin Tiao Shen, Lai Yang Sha Shen, Liao Sha Shen*
Original Source: *Ben Cao Hui Yan* (Treasury of Words on the Materia Medica) by Ni Zhu-Mo in 1624
English Name: glehnia, coastal glehnia root
Botanical Name: *Glehnia littoralis* F. Schmidt ex Miq. (*Shan Hu Cai*)
Pharmaceutical Name: Radix Glehniae
Properties: sweet, cool
Channels Entered: Lung, Stomach

CHINESE THERAPEUTIC ACTIONS

1. Nourishes Yin, Clears the Lung

Lung dryness: *Bei Sha Shen* (Radix Glehniae) treats Lung yin deficiency with fire, that manifests as dry mouth, dry throat, dryness of the nasal cavity, voice loss, sore throat, dry cough with no sputum, or scanty, difficult-to-expectorate sputum. In some cases, blood-streaked sputum may be present. *Bei Sha Shen* moistens the Lung and treats dry cough with heat signs. It is often used for chronic respiratory disorders such as tuberculosis or chronic bronchitis.

- Dry cough: combine *Bei Sha Shen* with *Mai Men Dong* (Radix Ophiopogonis), *Tian Hua Fen* (Radix Trichosanthis), *Yu Zhu* (Rhizoma Polygonati Odorati) and *Sang Ye* (Folium Mori).
- Dry cough with fire: use it with *Shi Gao* (Gypsum Fibrosum), *Zhi Mu* (Radix Anemarrhenae), *Zhe Bei Mu* (Bulbus Fritillariae Thunbergii), *Sang Bai Pi* (Cortex Mori), *Di Gu Pi* (Cortex Lycii), *Qian Hu* (Radix Peucedani), *Gua Lou Shi* (Fructus Trichosanthis) and *Tian Men Dong* (Radix Asparagi).
- Dry cough with scanty, yellow, difficult-to-expectorate sputum: combine this herb with *Mai Men Dong* (Radix Ophiopogonis), *Zhi Mu* (Radix Anemarrhenae), *Chuan Bei Mu* (Bulbus Fritillariae Cirrhosae), *Bie Jia* (Carapax Trionycis) and *Di Gu Pi* (Cortex Lycii).
- Dry cough with blood or blood-streaked sputum: add it to *E Jiao* (Colla Corii Asini), *Bai Ji* (Rhizoma Bletillae) and *Bai Mao Gen* (Rhizoma Imperatae).
- Wind-heat with aversion to cold: use this herb with *Sang Ye* (Folium Mori), *Dan Dou Chi* (Semen Sojae Praeparatum), *Xing Ren* (Semen Armeniacae Amarum) and *Zhe Bei Mu* (Bulbus Fritillariae Thunbergii).

Cough due to Lung heat: *Bei Sha Shen* clears Lung heat and alleviates cough. It nourishes yin and treats cough with sticky, scanty, yellow sputum.

- Lung heat with cough and yellow sputum: use this herb with *Sang Bai Pi* (Cortex Mori), *Di Gu Pi* (Cortex Lycii), *Qian Hu* (Radix Peucedani) and *Gua Lou Shi* (Fructus Trichosanthis).

Lung yin deficiency with dryness: Chief manifestations of this imbalance include dry cough with or without scanty, difficult-to-expectorate sputum. In some cases,

17 TONIC HERBS

Bei Sha Shen (Radix Glehniae)

hemoptysis or blood-streaked sputum may also be present. *Bei Sha Shen* strongly nourishes Lung yin and is best to treat yin deficiency with rising fire.

- Lung yin deficiency with dryness and rising deficient fire causing dry cough, scanty or absence of sputum: use *Bei Sha Shen* with *Mai Men Dong* (Radix Ophiopogonis), *Zhi Mu* (Radix Anemarrhenae), *Chuan Bei Mu* (Bulbus Fritillariae Cirrhosae), *Bie Jia* (Carapax Trionycis) and *Di Gu Pi* (Cortex Lycii).
- Cough with blood or blood-streaked sputum: combine it with *E Jiao* (Colla Corii Asini), *Bai Ji* (Rhizoma Bletillae) and *Bai Mao Gen* (Rhizoma Imperatae).

2. Nourishes the Stomach and Generates Body Fluids

Chronic Stomach yin deficiency: Manifestations of this chronic deficiency may include dry throat, thirst, constipation and a dry, red tongue.

- Chronic Stomach yin deficiency: use *Bei Sha Shen* with *Mai Men Dong* (Radix Ophiopogonis), *Yu Zhu* (Rhizoma Polygonati Odorati) and *Shi Hu* (Herba Dendrobii).
- Chronic Stomach yin deficiency accompanied by poor appetite or food stagnation: combine this herb with *Gu Ya* (Fructus Setariae Germinatus), *Mai Ya* (Fructus Hordei Germinatus) and *Ji Nei Jin* (Endothelium Corneum Gigeriae Galli).
- Chronic Stomach yin deficiency with Spleen qi deficiency: add it to *Shan Yao* (Rhizoma Dioscoreae), *Bian Dou* (Semen Lablab Album), *Tai Zi Shen* (Radix Pseudostellariae) and *Xi Yang Shen* (Radix Panacis Quinquefolii).

3. Tonifies Liver and Kidney Yin

Bei Sha Shen treats Liver and Kidney yin deficiencies, characterized by dryness or blood and qi stagnation causing hypochondriac pain, acid reflux, dry mouth and throat, and red tongue.

- Liver and Kidney yin deficiencies with symptoms listed above: use it with *Mai Men Dong* (Radix Ophiopogonis), *Sheng Di Huang* (Radix Rehmanniae), *Gou Qi Zi* (Fructus Lycii), and *Chuan Lian Zi* (Fructus Toosendan).

Exemplar Formula: *Yi Guan Jian* (Linking Decoction).

DOSAGE

10 to 15 grams for the dried herb, 20 to 30 grams for the fresh herb, in decoction. *Bei Sha Shen* is also used in pill, powder or paste forms.

CAUTIONS / CONTRAINDICATIONS

- Use of *Bei Sha Shen* is contraindicated for cough caused by wind-cold, cold-damp, or cases of deficiency and cold of the Spleen and Stomach.
- *Bei Sha Shen* antagonizes *Fen Fang Ji* (Radix Stephaniae Tetandrae).
- *Bei Sha Shen* is incompatible with *Li Lu* (Radix et Rhizoma Veratri).

CHEMICAL COMPOSITION

Phellopterin, bergapten, psoralen, xanthotoxin, marmesin, bergaptin, imperatorin, isoimperatorin, cnidilin.[1,2]

PHARMACOLOGICAL EFFECTS

- **Effect on temperature regulation:** Alcohol extract of *Bei Sha Shen* has been shown to lower body temperature in rabbits with a normal temperature, or with a fever induced by typhoid vaccination.[3]
- **Cardiovascular:** Water extract of *Bei Sha Shen* has a cardiotonic effect on frog heart specimens. At high doses, however, it may inhibit cardiac contraction. In anesthetized rabbits, intravenous injection raises blood pressure and increases respiration.[4]

SUPPLEMENT

- 沙參 / 沙参 *Sha Shen* (Radix Glehniae seu Adenophorae) is the generic name that refers to both *Bei Sha Shen* (Radix Glehniae) and *Nan Sha Shen* (Radix Adenophorae). Many classic texts did not distinguish between these two herbs, as they have similar functions, and have historically been used interchangeably.

AUTHORS' COMMENTS

Bei Sha Shen (Radix Glehniae) and *Nan Sha Shen* (Radix Adenophorae) are sweet and cool, moisten Lung yin, nourish the Stomach and generate body fluids. *Bei Sha Shen*, stronger in nourishing the yin and clearing heat, is often used for post febrile disorders when the injury to yin manifests as thirst, dry throat and a dry, scarlet tongue. *Nan Sha Shen* nourishes yin, dispels phlegm, and is more suitable for dryness and heat that have damaged Lung yin, manifesting in symptoms of dry cough, scanty sputum that may be blood-streaked or hemoptysis, with thirst and dryness.

When treating cough, *Bei Sha Shen* is heavier in texture and suitable only for dry cough due to Lung yin deficiency; *Nan Sha Shen* is lighter in texture and is more suitable for dry cough caused by Lung yin deficiency or wind-heat.

References

1. *Chang Yong Zhong Yao Cheng Fen Yu Yao Li Shou Ce* (A Handbook of the Composition and Pharmacology of Common Chinese Drugs), 1994; 708-709
2. *Xian Dai Zhong Yao Yao Li Xue* (Contemporary Pharmacology of Chinese Herbs), 1997; 1342
3. *Yi Xue Zhong Yang Za Zhi* (Central Journal of Medicine), 1961; 164:154
4. *Chang Yong Zhong Yao Cheng Fen Yu Yao Li Shou Ce* (A Handbook of the Composition and Pharmacology of Common Chinese Drugs), 1994, 708:709

Nan Sha Shen (Radix Adenophorae)

南沙参 南沙参

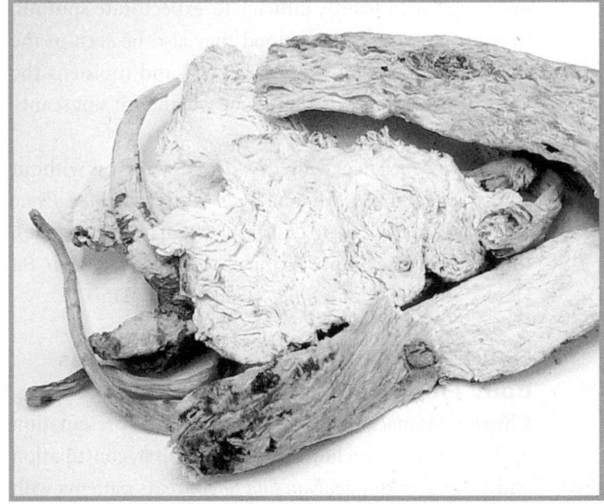

Pinyin Name: *Nan Sha Shen*
Literal Name: "sand root from the south"
Original Source: *Shen Nong Ben Cao Jing* (Divine Husbandman's Classic of the Materia Medica) in the second century
English Name: adenophora, four-leaf lady-bell root, upright lady-bell root
Botanical Name: *Adenophora tetraphylla* (Thunb.) Fisch. (*Lun Ye Sha Shen*); *Adenophora stricta* Miq. (*Sha Shen*); *Adenophora hunanensis* Nannf. (*Xing Ye Sha Shen*)
Pharmaceutical Name: Radix Adenophorae
Properties: sweet, slightly bitter, cool
Channels Entered: Lung, Stomach

CHINESE THERAPEUTIC ACTIONS

1. Nourishes Yin, Clears the Lung and Dispels Phlegm

Lung dryness: *Nan Sha Shen* (Radix Adenophorae) treats pathogenic dryness attacking the Lung that results in injury of Lung yin, with symptoms of dry mouth, dry throat, dryness of the nasal cavity, voice loss, sore throat, dry cough with no sputum, or scanty, difficult-to-expectorate sputum. In some cases, blood-streaked sputum may be present. *Nan Sha Shen* moistens the Lung and treats dry cough accompanied by heat signs. It can be used for both chronic Lung yin-deficient coughs or cough caused by attack of external pathogenic dryness.

- Initial exterior stage of warm febrile disorders with dryness, characterized by acute dry cough with yellow sputum, fever and aversion to cold: combine *Nan Sha Shen* with *Sang Ye* (Folium Mori), *Dan Dou Chi* (Semen Sojae Praeparatum), *Zhe Bei Mu* (Bulbus Fritillariae Thunbergii) and *Xing Ren* (Semen Armeniacae Amarum). **Exemplar Formula:** *Sang Xing Tang* (Mulberry Leaf and Apricot Kernel Decoction).
- Dry heat damaging Lung and Stomach yin, characterized by dry cough with dry throat, thirst or scanty sputum: use this herb with *Mai Men Dong* (Radix Ophiopogonis), *Yu Zhu* (Rhizoma Polygonati Odorati), *Tian Hua Fen* (Radix Trichosanthis) and *Sang Ye* (Folium Mori). **Exemplar Formula:** *Sha Shen Mai Dong Tang* (Glehnia and Ophiopogonis Decoction).
- Dry cough with blood-streaked sputum caused by dryness and heat turning into fire: add *Nan Sha Shen* to *Tian Men Dong* (Radix Asparagi), *Zhi Mu* (Radix Anemarrhenae), *Zhe Bei Mu* (Bulbus Fritillariae Thunbergii), *Di Gu Pi* (Cortex Lycii) and *Zi Zhu* (Folium Callicarpae).
- Dry cough with difficult-to-expectorate sputum: combine this herb with *Sang Bai Pi* (Cortex Mori), *Di Gu Pi* (Cortex Lycii), *Zhe Bei Mu* (Bulbus Fritillariae Thunbergii), *Gua Lou Shi* (Fructus Trichosanthis), *Shi Gao* (Gypsum Fibrosum) and *Huang Qin* (Radix Scutellariae).
- Chronic dry cough with no sputum: use *Nan Sha Shen*, *Tian Men Dong* (Radix Asparagi), *Sheng Di Huang* (Radix Rehmanniae), *Chuan Bei Mu* (Bulbus Fritillariae Cirrhosae), *Bai Bu* (Radix Stemonae) and *E Jiao* (Colla Corii Asini). **Exemplar Formula:** *Yue Hua Wan* (Moonlight Pill).
- Tuberculosis or other chronic respiratory disorders with dry cough, scanty or blood-streaked sputum, tidal fever, flushed cheeks, night sweats, *wu xin re* (five-center heat), and weight loss: combine this herb with *Sheng Di Huang* (Radix Rehmanniae), *Xuan Shen* (Radix Scrophulariae), *Bie Jia* (Carapax Trionycis), *Qin Jiao* (Radix Gentianae Macrophyllae), *Di Gu Pi* (Cortex Lycii), *Yin Chai Hu* (Radix Stellariae), *Chuan Bei Mu* (Bulbus Fritillariae Cirrhosae), *Bai Bu* (Radix Stemonae) and *Bai Ji* (Rhizoma Bletillae).

Cough due to Lung heat: Heat invading the Lung produces symptoms of cough or dyspnea with sticky yellow sputum. *Nan Sha Shen* clears and moistens the Lung without causing dampness. It also dispels phlegm, which makes it the ideal herb to treat Lung heat with yellow and difficult-to-expectorate sputum.

- Lung heat with cough and yellow phlegm: use *Nan Sha Shen* with *Sang Bai Pi* (Cortex Mori), *Di Gu Pi* (Cortex Lycii), *Zhe Bei Mu* (Bulbus Fritillariae Thunbergii), *Gua Lou Shi* (Fructus Trichosanthis), *Shi Gao* (Gypsum Fibrosum) and *Huang Qin* (Radix Scutellariae).

Yin-deficient cough: In chronic respiratory disorders involving Lung yin deficiency, the chief manifestation is

Nan Sha Shen (Radix Adenophorae)

dry cough with scanty, difficult-to-expectorate sputum. In some cases, streaks of blood may also be seen in the sputum. *Nan Sha Shen* nourishes yin and moistens the Lung. It treats Lung yin deficiency whether or not scanty sputum is present.

- Lung yin deficiency with dry cough with or without scanty sputum: use *Nan Sha Shen* with *Tian Men Dong* (Radix Asparagi), *Sheng Di Huang* (Radix Rehmanniae), *Chuan Bei Mu* (Bulbus Fritillariae Cirrhosae), *Bai Bu* (Radix Stemonae) and *E Jiao* (Colla Corii Asini).

2. Nourishes the Stomach and Generates Body Fluids

Chronic Stomach yin deficiency: Clinical presentation of this imbalance includes dry throat, thirst, constipation and a dry, red tongue. *Nan Sha Shen* treats patients with Stomach yin deficiency and a peeled tongue coating from late-stage febrile disorders or chronic illnesses.

- Stomach yin deficiency with the symptoms described above: combine *Nan Sha Shen* with *Yu Zhu* (Rhizoma Polygonati Odorati), *Mai Men Dong* (Radix Ophiopogonis), *Sheng Di Huang* (Radix Rehmanniae), *Shi Hu* (Herba Dendrobii), *Tian Hua Fen* (Radix Trichosanthis) and *Bai Shao* (Radix Paeoniae Alba).
- Stomach yin deficiency with poor appetite: add this herb to *Mai Ya* (Fructus Hordei Germinatus), *Mu Gua* (Fructus Chaenomelis) and *Ji Nei Jin* (Endothelium Corneum Gigeriae Galli).

DOSAGE

10 to 15 grams of the dried herb, 15 to 60 grams of the fresh herb, in decoction. *Nan Sha Shen* is also used in pill or powder forms. The fresh herb more effectively clears Lung heat and generates fluids, thus is usually used in treatment of Lung heat with injured yin.

CAUTIONS / CONTRAINDICATIONS

- *Nan Sha Shen* is contraindicated in cough caused by wind-cold.
- *Nan Sha Shen* antagonizes *Fen Fang Ji* (Radix Stephaniae Tetandrae).
- *Nan Sha Shen* is incompatible with *Li Lu* (Radix et Rhizoma Veratri).

CHEMICAL COMPOSITION

Taraxerone, β-sitosterol, shashenoside I, II, III; syringinoside, linoleic acid, ikshusterol, sessili folic 3-o-isovalerate, camphene, eucalyptol, camphor, azulene, bornyl acetate, daucosterol.[1,2]

PHARMACOLOGICAL EFFECTS

- **Antitussive:** Decoction of *Nan Sha Shen* has an antitussive effect in rabbits that lasts approximately 4 hours.[3]
- **Cardiovascular:** Administration of a 1% solution of *Nan Sha Shen* demonstrated a cardiotonic effect that lasted approximately 5 minutes on the heart of frog specimens.[4]
- **Antibiotic:** *Nan Sha Shen* has an antifungal effect against various pathogenic fungus and dermatophytes.[5]

AUTHORS' COMMENTS

Nan Sha Shen is a light, moistening tonic that does not create stagnation in the body or induce production of phlegm. For that reason, it is often used for chronic respiratory disorders involving Lung yin deficiency. Fresh *Nan Sha Shen* more strongly clears heat and generates body fluids. It is more often used for excess heat damaging the body fluids, and less frequently for deficient patients with injured yin.

An herbal pharmacy will generally supply *Bei Sha Shen* (Radix Glehniae) when "*Sha Shen*" is written on the prescription. Doctors must specify "*Nan*" if *Nan Sha Shen* (Radix Adenophorae) is to be prescribed. Please refer to *Bei Sha Shen* for comparison of these two herbs.

In folk medicine, large doses of *Nan Sha Shen* and *Xing Ren Ye* (Folium Pruni Armeniacae) cooked with eggs, treat toothache caused by yin-deficient fire. Some other records have shown that this pair, combined with pork, can treat postpartum milk insufficiency.

References

1. *Xian Dai Zhong Yao Yao Li Xue* (Contemporary Pharmacology of Chinese Herbs), 1997; 1363
2. *Chang Yong Zhong Yao Cheng Fen Yu Yao Li Shou Ce* (A Handbook of the Composition and Pharmacology of Common Chinese Drugs), 1994; 1352-1353
3. *Zhong Hua Yi Xue Za Zhi* (Chinese Journal of Medicine), 1956; 42(10):959
4. *Chang Yong Zhong Yao Cheng Fen Yu Yao Li Shou Ce* (A Handbook of the Composition and Pharmacology of Common Chinese Drugs), 1994; 1352:1353
5. *Zhong Hua Pi Fu Ke Xue Za Zhi* (Chinese Journal of Dermatology), 1957; 5(4):286

Mai Men Dong (Radix Ophiopogonis)

麥門冬 麦门冬

Pinyin Name: *Mai Men Dong*
Literal Name: "lush winter wheat"
Alternate Chinese Names: *Mai Dong, Cun Dong, Da Mai Dong*
Original Source: *Shen Nong Ben Cao Jing* (Divine Husbandman's Classic of the Materia Medica) in the second century
English Name: ophiopogon
Botanical Name: *Ophiopogon japonicus* Ker-Gawl (*Men Dong*)
Pharmaceutical Name: Radix Ophiopogonis
Properties: sweet, slightly bitter, cool
Channels Entered: Spleen, Stomach, Heart

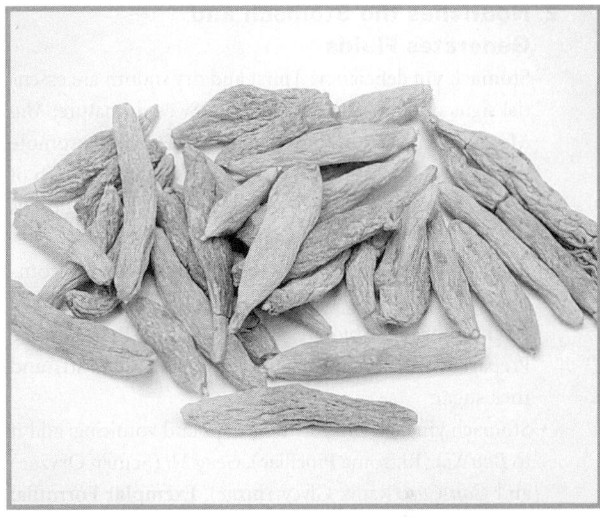

CHINESE THERAPEUTIC ACTIONS

1. Nourishes Yin and Moistens the Lung

Pathogenic dryness attacking the Lung: Injured Lung yin as a result of dryness attacking the Lung may result in symptoms of dry mouth, dry throat, dry cough with no sputum, or scanty, difficult-to-expectorate sputum. In some cases, hemoptysis or blood-streaked sputum may be present. *Mai Men Dong* (Radix Ophiopogonis) moistens the Lung and at the same time sedates Lung heat, and is best used for febrile disorders involving dryness or fire such as bronchitis, tuberculosis and pertussis.

- Heat and dryness in the Lung characterized by dyspnea, dry cough, chest fullness and pain: combine *Mai Men Dong* with *Sang Ye* (Folium Mori), *Shi Gao* (Gypsum Fibrosum), *Pi Pa Ye* (Folium Eriobotryae) and *E Jiao* (Colla Corii Asini). **Exemplar Formula:** *Qing Zao Jiu Fei Tang* (Eliminate Dryness and Rescue the Lungs Decoction).
- Fire and dryness in the Lung characterized by coughing with blood, and/or thick, yellow, difficult-to-expectorate sputum, and chest pain: incorporate this herb with *Tian Men Dong* (Radix Asparagi), *Zhi Mu* (Radix Anemarrhenae), *Bei Mu* (Bulbus Fritillaria), *Gua Lou Shi* (Fructus Trichosanthis), *Huang Qin* (Radix Scutellariae), *Zhi Zi* (Fructus Gardeniae), *Bai Ji* (Rhizoma Bletillae), *Han Lian Cao* (Herba Ecliptae) and *Bai Mao Gen* (Rhizoma Imperatae).

Chronic dry cough from Lung yin deficiency: Chronic febrile disorders consume a tremendous amount of yin and lead to chronic coughing with blood-streaked sputum. Deficiency heat signs of low-grade fever, flushed cheeks and irritability may also be present. *Mai Men Dong*, too mild to be used alone in this case, is usually combined with other yin tonics to achieve maximum effectiveness.

- Sore throat with epistaxis, hematemesis or blood-streaked sputum: combine this herb with *Sheng Di Huang* (Radix Rehmanniae), *Xuan Shen* (Radix Scrophulariae), *Bei Mu* (Bulbus Fritillaria) and *Mu Dan Pi* (Cortex Moutan). **Exemplar Formula:** *Yang Yin Qing Fei Tang* (Nourish the Yin and Clear the Lungs Decoction).
- Loss of voice, dry throat, thirst: combine *Mai Men Dong* with *Xuan Shen* (Radix Scrophulariae), *Sheng Di Huang* (Radix Rehmanniae), *Jie Geng* (Radix Platycodonis), *Gan Cao* (Radix Glycyrrhizae), *Shan Dou Gen* (Radix Sophorae Tonkinensis), and *Zhi Mu* (Radix Anemarrhenae).
- Lung and Kidney yin deficiencies with excessive hemoptysis: use this herb with *Bai Ji* (Rhizoma Bletillae), *Bai Mao Gen* (Rhizoma Imperatae) and *Han Lian Cao* (Herba Ecliptae).

Yin-deficient heat: In patients with chronic yin deficiency, the condition may be complicated by the presence of excess heat in the body. Clinical manifestations include soreness and swelling of the throat, hematemesis or epistaxis. *Mai Men Dong* and herbs that clear excess heat must be used simultaneously.

- Soreness and swelling of the throat due to yin deficiency and excess heat: combine this herb with *Sheng Di Huang* (Radix Rehmanniae), *Xuan Shen* (Radix Scrophulariae), *Bei Mu* (Bulbus Fritillaria) and *Mu Dan Pi (Cortex Moutan)* . **Exemplar Formula:** *Yang Yin Qing Fei Tang* (Nourish the Yin and Clear the Lungs Decoction).
- Diphtheria with sore throat: combine it with *Sheng Di Huang* (Radix Rehmanniae), *Xuan Shen* (Radix Scrophulariae), *Bei Mu* (Bulbus Fritillaria), and *Mu Dan Pi* (Cortex Moutan).
- Hematemesis or epistaxis due to yin deficiency and excess heat: use it with *Sheng Di Huang* (Radix Rehmanniae).

Mai Men Dong (Radix Ophiopogonis)

2. Nourishes the Stomach and Generates Fluids

Stomach yin deficiency: Thirst and dry mouth are essential signs of Stomach yin deficiency. Sweet in nature, *Mai Men Dong* enters the Stomach to nourish yin and promote the generation of fluids. It is often considered the herb of choice to tonify Stomach yin, because its tonic effect is much less stagnating than that of other tonic herbs.

- Stomach yin deficiency with thirst and dry mouth: combine *Mai Men Dong* with *Sha Shen* (Radix Glehniae seu Adenophorae), *Shu Di Huang* (Radix Rehmanniae Preparata), *Yu Zhu* (Rhizoma Polygonati Odorati) and rock sugar.
- Stomach yin deficiency with hiccups and vomiting: add it to *Ban Xia* (Rhizoma Pinelliae), *Geng Mi* (Semen Oryzae) and *Gan Cao* (Radix Glycyrrhizae). **Exemplar Formula:** *Mai Men Dong Tang* (Ophiopogonis Decoction).
- Qi and yin deficiencies with fatigue, shortness of breath, thirst and dry mouth: combine this herb with *Ren Shen* (Radix Ginseng) and *Wu Wei Zi* (Fructus Schisandrae Chinensis). **Exemplar Formula:** *Sheng Mai San* (Generate the Pulse Powder).

***Xiao ke* (wasting and thirsting) syndrome:** This condition frequently occurs as a result of chronic febrile disorders damaging yin in the body. *Mai Men Dong* enters the Spleen and Stomach and is commonly used to treat *xiao ke* syndrome of the upper and middle *jiaos,* characterized by dry mouth, thirst, polydipsia and polyphagia.

- *Xiao ke* syndrome with extreme thirst: combine *Mai Men Dong* with *Xi Yang Shen* (Radix Panacis Quinquefolii), *Shan Yao* (Rhizoma Dioscoreae), *Tian Hua Fen* (Radix Trichosanthis), *Shi Gao* (Gypsum Fibrosum), *Zhi Mu* (Radix Anemarrhenae), and *Wu Mei* (Fructus Mume).
- *Xiao ke* syndrome with heat and thirst: use this herb with *Huang Lian* (Rhizoma Coptidis), the juices of *Xian Di Huang* (Radix Rehmanniae Recens) and fresh *Tian Hua Fen* (Radix Trichosanthis), and milk.

3. Clears the Heart and Eliminates Irritability

Irritability and insomnia: With deficiencies of yin and blood, heat rises upwards and disturbs the *shen* (spirit) of the Heart. Clinical manifestations of this condition include insomnia, restlessness and irritability. Sweet and cold in nature, *Mai Men Dong* enters the Heart to clear heat and nourish yin and blood to relieve irritability.

- Yin and blood deficiencies of the Heart with heat, characterized by insomnia, palpitations, irritability, night fever, or restless sleep: combine *Mai Men Dong* with *Huang Lian* (Rhizoma Coptidis), *E Jiao* (Colla Corii Asini), *Bei Mu* (Bulbus Fritillaria), *Sheng Di Huang* (Radix Rehmanniae), *Xuan Shen* (Radix Scrophulariae), *Dan Shen* (Radix Salviae Miltiorrhizae), *Zhen Zhu Mu* (Concha Margaritaferae) and *Yuan Zhi* (Radix Polygalae).
- Heat in the *ying* (nutritive) stage characterized by nocturnal fever, irritability and insomnia: use this herb with *Sheng Di Huang* (Radix Rehmanniae), *Dan Shen* (Radix Salviae Miltiorrhizae) and *Jin Yin Hua* (Flos Lonicerae). **Exemplar Formula:** *Qing Ying Tang* (Clear the Nutrition Level Decoction).
- Qi and blood deficiencies caused by chronic febrile disorder, with irritability and insomnia: combine this herb with *Zhu Ye* (Herba Phyllostachys), *Shi Gao* (Gypsum Fibrosum), *Ren Shen* (Radix Ginseng) and *Ban Xia* (Rhizoma Pinelliae). **Exemplar Formula:** *Zhu Ye Shi Gao Tang* (Lophatherum and Gypsum Decoction).
- Yin and blood deficiencies characterized by restlessness, irritability, insomnia, palpitations, fatigue, red tongue and little tongue coat: use *Mai Men Dong* with *Sheng Di Huang* (Radix Rehmanniae), *Dan Shen* (Radix Salviae Miltiorrhizae), *Yuan Zhi* (Radix Polygalae) and *Suan Zao Ren* (Semen Zizyphi Spinosae). **Exemplar Formula:** *Tian Wang Bu Xin Dan* (Emperor of Heaven's Special Pill to Tonify the Heart).
- Disharmony of the Kidney and Heart characterized by insomnia, forgetfulness, night sweats, and palpitations: combine this herb with *Bai Zi Ren* (Semen Platycladi), *Gou Qi Zi* (Fructus Lycii), *Fu Shen* (Poria Paradicis) and *Shi Chang Pu* (Rhizoma Acori).

4. Moistens the Intestines

Intestinal dryness, constipation: Deficiencies of yin and fluids leading to dryness is a major cause of constipation. *Mai Men Dong* nourishes yin, lubricates the intestines and promotes bowel movement.

- Constipation: combine it with *Xuan Shen* (Radix Scrophulariae), and *Shu Di Huang* (Radix Rehmanniae Preparata).
- Post-febrile disease with constipation: use this herb with *Huo Ma Ren* (Fructus Cannabis), *Sheng Di Huang* (Radix Rehmanniae), *Xuan Shen* (Radix Scrophulariae), *Gua Lou Ren* (Semen Trichosanthis) and *Zhi Shi* (Fructus Aurantii Immaturus).

DOSAGE

10 to 15 grams in decoction. *Mai Men Dong* should be crushed to increase surface area and facilitate the extraction of active constituents. It is also used in paste, pill or powder form.

CAUTIONS / CONTRAINDICATIONS

- Use of *Mai Men Dong* is contraindicated in patients with coughing caused by wind-cold or damp-phlegm accumulation.

Mai Men Dong (Radix Ophiopogonis)

- It is also contraindicated for patients experiencing diarrhea from cold and deficiency of the middle *jiao*.
- Use of this herb may be associated with drowsiness and sedation. Therefore, individuals who take this herb should exercise caution if driving or operating heavy machinery.

CHEMICAL COMPOSITION

Ophiopogonin A,B,C,D; ruscogenin, β-sitosterol, stigmasterol, β-sitosterol-β-glucoside, ophioside, kaempferol-3-galactoglucoside.[1]

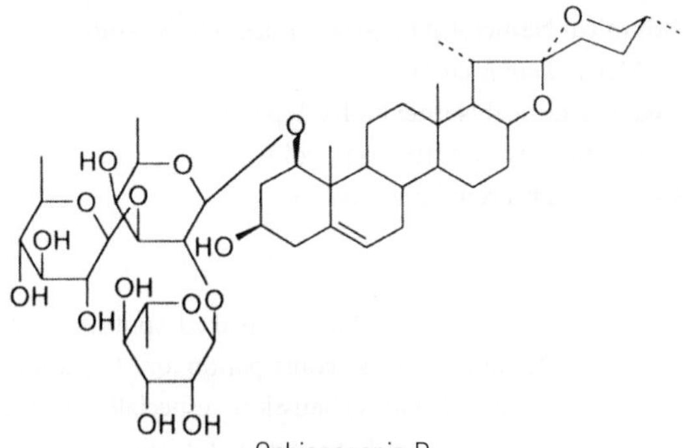

Ophiopogonin D

PHARMACOLOGICAL EFFECTS

- **Antiarrhythmic:** Intravenous injection of *Mai Men Dong* is effective in treating drug-induced arrhythmia in rats. However, the duration of its antiarrhythmic effect is relatively short, as arrhythmia tends to recur.[2]
- **Cardiovascular:** Ophiopogonin has a positive inotropic effect and increases cardiac output in frog heart specimens. At a large dosage, however, it decreases cardiac contractility and cardiac output.[3]
- **Antibiotic:** *Mai Men Dong* has an inhibiting influence on *Staphylococcus albus*, *Bacillus subtilis*, *E. coli* and *Salmonella typhi*.[4]

CLINICAL STUDIES AND RESEARCH

- **Coronary artery disorder:** In one clinical study, 101 patients with coronary artery disorders were divided into three groups and treated with oral, intramuscular injection, or intravenous injection of *Mai Men Dong*. Oral treatment consisted of 10 ml of decoction given three times daily (equivalent to 45 grams of dried herb per day) for 3 to 18 months; intramuscular injection consisted of 4 ml of injection per day given via one or two equally-divided injections (equivalent to 8 grams of dried herb per day) for 2 to 4 months; and intravenous injection consisted of 40 ml of injection per day (equivalent to 40 grams of dried herb per day) for one week. The rate of effectiveness was 74% for 50 patients who received oral treatment, 83.7% for 31 patients who received intramuscular treatment, and 80% in the 20 patients who received intravenous treatment.[5]
- **Use in elderly patients:** According to one report, 100 geriatric patients treated with *Mai Men Dong* daily for four months noticed a significant improvement in their overall health. There was a marked reduction of dizziness, blurred vision, tinnitus, back pain, fatigue, abdominal distention and palpitations. Furthermore, those with hypertension showed a reduction of both systolic and diastolic blood pressures. Those with pre-existing chronic gastritis experienced diarrhea, which stopped following discontinuation of the herb. No significant abnormalities were noted through heart, liver, kidney and blood examinations.[6]

TOXICOLOGY

Mice and rats that were fed large dosages of *Mai Men Dong* over a period of 90 days showed no abnormalities in liver, kidney and blood examinations.[7]

AUTHORS' COMMENTS

Some classic texts have stated that the center part of *Mai Men Dong* must be removed before cooking. However, it has been shown that the center is only approximately 3% of the herb and contains essentially the same basic chemical components as the rest of the herb. Furthermore, some herbalists have tried taking *Mai Men Dong* (15 to 30 grams) themselves with the center part intact, for five to ten days, and did not experience any adverse side effects. Therefore, it is now generally accepted that removal of the center part is not necessary.

Mai Men Dong, *Chuan Mu Tong* (Caulis Clematidis Armandii), *Huang Lian* (Rhizoma Coptidis), and *Tian Zhu Huang* (Concretio Silicea Bambusae) all clear the Heart and eliminate irritability.

- *Mai Men Dong* is a tonic used for deficient Heart yin with heat that manifests as irritability and insomnia.
- *Chuan Mu Tong* is a diuretic that clears damp-heat to relieve irritability with oral ulcers and yellow urine.
- *Huang Lian* is used for febrile disease with excess fire in the Heart disturbing *shen* (spirit), thus manifesting in irritability and insomnia.
- *Tian Zhu Huang* dissolves hot phlegm and is best for irritability with spasms and convulsions.

References

1. *Xian Dai Zhong Yao Yao Li Xue* (Contemporary Pharmacology of Chinese Herbs), 1997; 1337
2. *Zhong Cao Yao* (Chinese Herbal Medicine), 1982; 13(9); 27-32
3. *Hua Xi Yao Xue Za Zhi* (Huaxi Herbal Journal), 1991; 6(1):13
4. *Zhong Yao Xue* (Chinese Herbology), 1998; 845:848
5. *Xin Yi Yao Xue Za Zhi* (New Journal of Medicine and Herbology), 1977; 5:39
6. *Zhong Guo Zhong Yao Za Zhi* (People's Republic of China Journal of Chinese Herbology), 1992; 17(1):21
7. *Zhong Guo Zhong Yao Za Zhi* (People's Republic of China Journal of Chinese Herbology), 1992; 17(1):21

17 TONIC HERBS

Tian Men Dong (Radix Asparagi)

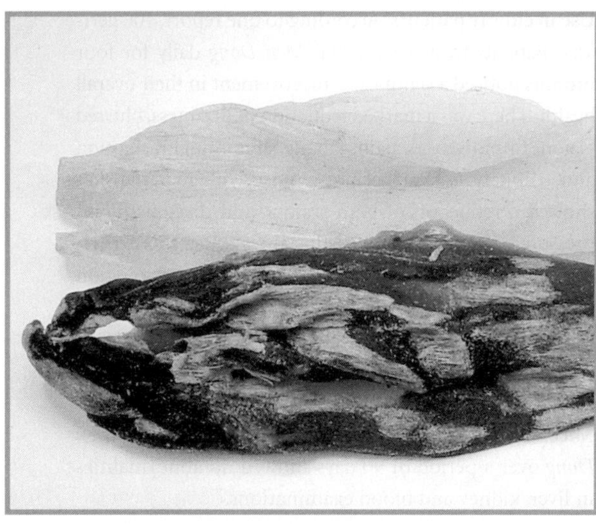

天門冬 天门冬

Pinyin Name: *Tian Men Dong*
Literal Name: "lush winter aerial plant"
Alternate Chinese Names: *Tian Dong, Ming Tian Dong, Wan Sui Teng*
Original Source: *Shen Nong Ben Cao Jing* (Divine Husbandman's Classic of the Materia Medica) in the second century
English Name: asparagus tuber
Botanical Name: *Asparagus cochinchinensis* (Lour.) Merr. (*Tian Men Dong*)
Pharmaceutical Name: Radix Asparagi
Properties: sweet, bitter, very cold
Channels Entered: Lung, Kidney

CHINESE THERAPEUTIC ACTIONS

1. Clears Lung Heat, Sedates Fire

In addition to moistening dryness, *Tian Men Dong* (Radix Asparagi) is very cold and is best used to clear Lung heat and sedate fire characterized by fever, aversion to wind and cold, chest pain and blood-streaked sputum or hemoptysis. *Tian Men Dong* treats cases in which pathogenic dryness has attacked the Lung and is causing symptoms of non-productive dry cough or dry cough with scanty, sticky sputum that may or may not be blood-streaked and difficult to expectorate.

- Wind-heat attack with dryness: combine *Tian Men Dong* with *Sang Ye* (Folium Mori), *Dan Dou Chi* (Semen Sojae Praeparatum), *Nan Sha Shen* (Radix Adenophorae) and *Xing Ren* (Semen Armeniacae Amarum).
- Mild dry cough: use this herb individually.
- Moderate dry cough: pair it with *Mai Men Dong* (Radix Ophiopogonis).
- Chronic dry cough with blood: combine it with *Zhi Mu* (Radix Anemarrhenae), *Bei Mu* (Bulbus Fritillaria), *E Jiao* (Colla Corii Asini), *Ce Bai Ye* (Cacumen Platycladi) and *Gua Lou Shi* (Fructus Trichosanthis).
- Chronic cough due to Lung heat, with scanty, yellow, difficult-to-expectorate sputum: combine this herb with *Di Gu Pi* (Cortex Lycii), *Sang Bai Pi* (Cortex Mori), *Shi Gao* (Gypsum Fibrosum), *Gua Lou Shi* (Fructus Trichosanthis), and *Zhe Bei Mu* (Bulbus Fritillariae Thunbergii).

2. Nourishes the Yin and Moistens Dryness

Chronic febrile disorders injuring the yin: Chronic febrile diseases consume a tremendous amount of the body's yin. With gradual recovery, the heat slowly dissipates, but yin deficiency may become more prominent. Clinically, patients may experience muscle wasting, thirst, consumptive cough with blood-streaked sputum, low-grade or afternoon fevers, constipation or dry stools. These are signs of yin exhaustion, especially of the Kidney. Western medical diagnoses for such illnesses include tuberculosis, diabetes mellitus, and cancer.

- Aftermath of febrile disorders with heat and dryness symptoms: pair *Tian Men Dong* with *Mai Men Dong* (Radix Ophiopogonis).
- Yin and qi deficiencies: combine this herb with *Xi Yang Shen* (Radix Panacis Quinquefolii) and *Shu Di Huang* (Radix Rehmanniae Preparata).
- Steaming bones sensations, flushed cheeks, night sweats: add it to *Qin Jiao* (Radix Gentianae Macrophyllae), *Bai Wei* (Radix Cynanchi Atrati), *Bie Jia* (Carapax Trionycis), *Di Gu Pi* (Cortex Lycii), *Yin Chai Hu* (Radix Stellariae), *Sheng Di Huang* (Radix Rehmanniae), *Gui Ban* (Plastrum Testudinis), *Huang Bai* (Cortex Phellodendri) and *Zhi Mu* (Radix Anemarrhenae).
- *Xiao ke* (wasting and thirsting) syndrome in the upper *jiao* with polydipsia: combine this herb with *Mai Men Dong* (Radix Ophiopogonis), *Tian Hua Fen* (Radix Trichosanthis), *Zhi Mu* (Radix Anemarrhenae), and *Huang Qin* (Radix Scutellariae).
- *Xiao ke* (wasting and thirsting) syndrome in the middle *jiao* with polyphagia: incorporate *Tian Men Dong* with *Shi Gao* (Gypsum Fibrosum), *Zhi Mu* (Radix Anemarrhenae) and *Sheng Di Huang* (Radix Rehmanniae).
- *Xiao ke* (wasting and thirsting) syndrome in the lower *jiao* with polyuria: combine it with *Zhi Mu* (Radix Anemarrhenae), *Huang Bai* (Cortex Phellodendri), *Shu Di Huang* (Radix Rehmanniae Preparata), *Wu Wei Zi* (Fructus Schisandrae Chinensis), *Shan Zhu Yu* (Fructus Corni) and *Lian Xu* (Stamen Nelumbinis).

Tian Men Dong (Radix Asparagi)

- Chronic respiratory disorders such as tuberculosis or cancer: combine this herb with *Mai Men Dong* (Radix Ophiopogonis), *Bai Bu* (Radix Stemonae), *Sheng Di Huang* (Radix Rehmanniae), *Shi Hu* (Herba Dendrobii) and *E Jiao* (Colla Corii Asini).

Moistens the intestines: *Tian Men Dong* is very cold and moistening and is best used to treat constipation caused by dryness and heat accumulation.

- Constipation due to yin deficiency and heat: combine this herb with *Xuan Shen* (Radix Scrophulariae), *Mai Men Dong* (Radix Ophiopogonis), *Sheng Di Huang* (Radix Rehmanniae) and *Zhi Mu* (Radix Anemarrhenae).
- Constipation from blood deficiency with heat: add it to *Dang Gui* (Radicis Angelicae Sinensis), a large dose of *Bai Shao* (Radix Paeoniae Alba), *He Shou Wu* (Radix Polygoni Multiflori) and honey.

Sore throat: The Kidney channel travels through the throat to reach the tongue. Kidney yin deficiency with rising fire will cause throat swelling and pain.

- Sore throat due to deficient fire: combine *Tian Men Dong* with *Shu Di Huang* (Radix Rehmanniae Preparata), *Xuan Shen* (Radix Scrophulariae), *Mai Men Dong* (Radix Ophiopogonis) and *Shi Hu* (Herba Dendrobii).
- Sore throat due to Lung heat: add this herb to *Ban Lan Gen* (Radix Isatidis), *Shan Dou Gen* (Radix Sophorae Tonkinensis), *Jie Geng* (Radix Platycodonis) and *Gan Cao* (Radix Glycyrrhizae).

DOSAGE

6 to 15 grams in decoction. *Tian Men Dong* is also used in paste, powder and pill forms.

CAUTIONS / CONTRAINDICATIONS

- Use of *Tian Men Dong* is contraindicated when there is diarrhea due to deficiency and cold of the middle *jiao*, or cough due to wind-cold.

CHEMICAL COMPOSITION

Asparagine, β-sitosterol, 5-methoxy-methylfurfural, smilagenin, neo-ketose.[1]

PHARMACOLOGICAL EFFECTS

- **Antibiotic:** Decoction of *Tian Men Dong* has an inhibitory effect against *Bacillus anthracis*, α-hemolytic streptococcus, β-hemolytic streptococcus, *Diplococcus pneumoniae*, *Staphylococcus aureus*, *Corynebacterium diphtheriae*, and *Bacillus subtilis*.[2]
- **Antineoplastic:** Alcohol extract of *Tian Men Dong* has demonstrated an inhibitory effect against sarcoma in mice.[3]

CLINICAL STUDIES AND RESEARCH

- **Breast tumor:** In one clinical study, 42 patients with lobular hypertrophy of the mammary glands were treated with an overall 83% rate of effectiveness using oral, intramuscular, or intravenous injection of *Tian Men Dong*. In another study, 72 patients with mammary cancer showed marked improvement using the same treatment protocols. For oral administration, the protocol was to weigh out 63 grams of the herb, remove the outer layer of the root, add a small quantity of grain-based liquor, steam the preparation for 30-60 minutes, and ingest the herbs in three equally-divided doses daily. Detailed guidelines for intramuscular or intravenous injection were not available at the time of publication.[4]
- **Malignant lymphoma:** According to one report, 41 patients were treated with an overall 87.9% rate of effectiveness using an integrative approach of both Chinese and western medicine. Out of 41 patients, 23 received herbal treatment only and 18 received the combination of herbal and chemotherapy treatment. The study reported an 82.5% rate of effectiveness for the herbal treatment. The herbal treatment consisted of intravenous injection of *Tian Men Dong* and intramuscular injection of *Bai Hua She She Cao* (Herba Oldenlandia) twice daily for 3 to 6 months. The injectables contained dosage equivalent in decoction to 10 to 40 grams (with a maximum of 120 grams) for *Tian Men Dong*, and 8 grams for *Bai Hua She She Cao*. Those who could not tolerate injection were converted to oral ingestion of herbs three times daily.[5]

AUTHORS' COMMENTS

Some texts state that ingestion of *Tian Men Dong* with meat increases the production of milk for nursing mothers.

Recently, *Tian Men Dong* and *Bai Hua She She Cao* (Herba Oldenlandia) have been used together to treat fibrocystic breast disorders, and cancers of the breast and the lymphatic system.

Tian Men Dong and *Mai Men Dong* (Radix Ophiopogonis) clear heat, nourish yin and moisten dryness. They can be used for patients with Lung yin deficiency with dry cough, scanty sputum, coughing of blood, and constipation. However, *Tian Men Dong* is very cold and is usually used with other herbs that clear deficient heat to treat Kidney yin-deficient fire with low-grade fever, night sweating and nocturnal emissions. *Mai Men Dong* treats Heart yin deficiency with fire caused by heat in the *ying* (nutritive) level manifesting in irritability, insomnia and palpitations.

Tian Men Dong (Radix Asparagi)

References

1. *Xian Dai Zhong Yao Yao Li Xue* (Contemporary Pharmacology of Chinese Herbs), 1997; 1369
2. *Jiang Su Yi Yao* (Jiangsu Journal of Medicine and Herbology), 1976; (4):33
3. *Yao Li Shi Yan Fang Fa Xue* (Research Methodology of Herbal Medicine), 1982; 363
4. *Jiang Su Yi Yao* (Jiangsu Journal of Medicine and Herbology), 1976; 4:33
5. *Xin Yi Xue* (New Medicine), 1975; 4:193

Shi Hu (Herba Dendrobii)

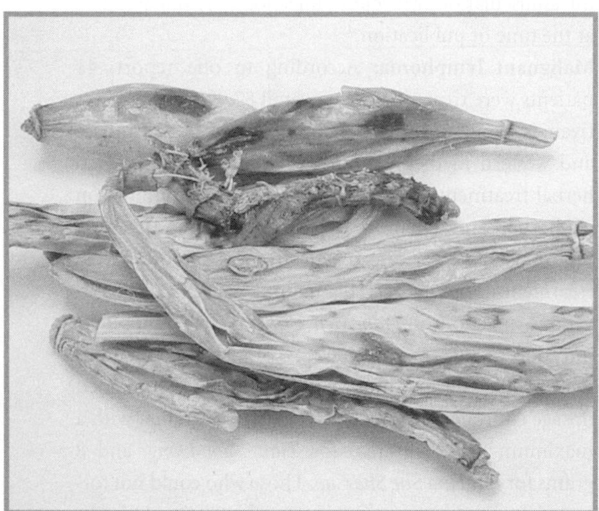

石斛 石斛

Pinyin Name: *Shi Hu*
Literal Name: "stone bushel," "bushel of stone"
Alternate Chinese Names: *Jin Chai Shi Hu, Tie Pi Shi Hu, Huo Shan Shi Hu, Er Huan Shi Hu, Jin Shi Hu, Huang Cao, Jin Si Hu, Jin Shu Hu, Xiao Huan Chai*
Original Source: *Shen Nong Ben Cao Jing* (Divine Husbandman's Classic of the Materia Medica) in the second century
English Name: dendrobium, dendrobium stem
Botanical Name: *Dendrobium loddigesii* Rolfe. (*Huan Cao Shi Hu*); *Dendrobium fimbriatum* Hook. var. *oculatum* Hook. (*Ma Bian Shi Hu*); *Dendrobium chrysanthum* Wall. (*Huang Cao Shi Hu*); *Dendrobium candidum* Wall. ex Lindl. (*Tie Pi Shi Hu*); *Dendrobium nobile* Lindl. (*Jin Cha Shi Hu*)
Pharmaceutical Name: Herba Dendrobii
Properties: sweet, cool
Channels Entered: Kidney, Stomach

CHINESE THERAPEUTIC ACTIONS

1. Nourishes the Stomach and Generates Body Fluids

Febrile disorders with injured yin: Thirst, dry mouth and throat, irritability, and perspiration are symptoms of febrile disease injuring body fluids. *Shi Hu* (Herba Dendrobii), especially the fresh form, is most suitable to clear heat and generate body fluids. Because this herb is relatively mild in function, it is commonly combined with other herbs that nourish yin, clear heat, and promote generation of body fluids.

- For severe heat with extreme thirst and irritability, dry tongue with a black coating: combine *Shi Hu* with *Tian Hua Fen* (Radix Trichosanthis), *Sheng Di Huang* (Radix Rehmanniae), *Mai Men Dong* (Radix Ophiopogonis) and *Lian Qiao* (Fructus Forsythiae).
- Post-febrile disorder with qi and yin deficiencies characterized by fatigue, no desire to speak, dry lips, and in severe cases, incoherence: use this herb with *Ren Shen* (Radix Ginseng) or *Xi Yang Shen* (Radix Panacis Quinquefolii), *Mai Men Dong* (Radix Ophiopogonis), *Mu Gua* (Fructus Chaenomelis), and *Lian Zi* (Semen Nelumbinis).
- *Xiao ke* (wasting and thirsting) syndrome: combine it with *Shi Gao* (Gypsum Fibrosum), *Tian Hua Fen* (Radix Trichosanthis) and *Shan Yao* (Rhizoma Dioscoreae).

Stomach yin deficiency: Dry mouth and throat, dry red tongue, thirst, dry heaves, dull epigastric pain and constipation are indications of Stomach yin deficiency. Sweet and cool, *Shi Hu* enters the Stomach to nourish yin and clear heat.

- Mild cases of Stomach yin deficiency: drink *Shi Hu* as tea daily.
- Moderate cases of Stomach yin deficiency: combine this

Shi Hu (Herba Dendrobii)

herb with *Sha Shen* (Radix Glehniae seu Adenophorae), *Mai Men Dong* (Radix Ophiopogonis), *Yu Zhu* (Rhizoma Polygonati Odorati), *Mu Gua* (Fructus Chaenomelis), *Gu Ya* (Fructus Setariae Germinatus) and *Shan Zha* (Fructus Crataegi).

2. Nourishes Yin and Clears Heat

Yin deficiency with heat: Yin deficiency with interior heat is characterized by unremitting low-grade fever. This condition is treated by herbs that nourish yin and eliminate deficiency heat.

- Unremitting low-grade fever: combine *Shi Hu* with *Sheng Di Huang* (Radix Rehmanniae), *Mai Men Dong* (Radix Ophiopogonis), *Bai Wei* (Radix Cynanchi Atrati) and *Qing Hao* (Herba Artemisiae Annuae).
- Chronic dry cough with low-grade fever, night sweats, and dry mouth: add this herb to *Sheng Di Huang* (Radix Rehmanniae), *Mai Men Dong* (Radix Ophiopogonis), *Bai He* (Bulbus Lilii), *Qin Jiao* (Radix Gentianae Macrophyllae), *Yin Chai Hu* (Radix Stellariae) and *Di Gu Pi* (Cortex Lycii).

3. Brightens the Eyes and Strengthens the Back, Tendons and Bones

Blurred vision and dizziness due to yin deficiency: The Liver opens to the eyes, and the presence of Liver yin is directly dependent on the availability of Kidney yin. Kidney yin deficiency leads to Liver yin deficiency, which eventually results in malnourishment of the eyes and compromised visual function. This might show up as diminished visual acuity, blurred vision, dizziness, platycoria or spots in front of the eyes. Sweet and cold in nature, *Shi Hu* is most suitable to treat conditions characterized by yin deficiency with rising deficiency heat.

- Blurred vision, dilated pupils, and dizziness caused by yin deficiency with heat: combine *Shi Hu* with *Gou Qi Zi* (Fructus Lycii), *Shu Di Huang* (Radix Rehmanniae Preparata), *Tian Men Dong* (Radix Asparagi), *Ju Hua* (Flos Chrysanthemi), *Sha Yuan Zi* (Semen Astragali Complanati), and *Jue Ming Zi* (Semen Cassiae). **Exemplar Formula:** *Shi Hu Ye Guang Wan* (Dendrobium Pill for Night Vision).
- Spots in front of the eyes: add this herb to *Cang Zhu* (Rhizoma Atractylodis) and *Yin Yang Huo* (Herba Epimedii).

Pain, soreness and weakness of the back and knees: The Kidney resides in the lower back, stores *jing* (essence) and dominates the bones; lack of nourishment to the Kidney creates a dull, sore, aching pain. *Shi Hu* nourishes Kidney yin and strengthens the back.

- Soreness, weakness and pain in the back and knees: combine *Shi Hu* with *Shu Di Huang* (Radix Rehmanniae Preparata), *Huai Niu Xi* (Radix Achyranthis Bidentatae), *Sang Ji Sheng* (Herba Taxilli) and *Fu Pen Zi* (Fructus Rubi).
- Numbness of extremities or *wei* (atrophy) syndrome: incorporate this herb with *Huai Niu Xi* (Radix Achyranthis Bidentatae), *Huang Bai* (Cortex Phellodendri), *Xu Duan* (Radix Dipsaci), *Shu Di Huang* (Radix Rehmanniae Preparata), *Shan Yao* (Rhizoma Dioscoreae), *Qin Jiao* (Radix Gentianae Macrophyllae) and *Mu Gua* (Fructus Chaenomelis).

DOSAGE

6 to 15 grams of the dried herb, 15 to 30 grams of the fresh herb, in decoction. *Shi Hu* is also used in pill, paste or powder forms. Pre-cook this herb when making a decoction. Fresh *Shi Hu* strongly clears heat and promotes generation of body fluids to treat febrile diseases involving damaged body fluids, thirst, and red tongue. Dried *Shi Hu* moderately clears heat and promotes generation of body fluids in cases of mild-to-moderate severity. Use both forms to treat febrile disorders with injured yin.

CAUTIONS / CONTRAINDICATIONS

- Use of *Shi Hu* is contraindicated in excess febrile disorders, damp and phlegm accumulation, and the exterior stage of a disease.
- *Shi Hu* is not suitable for use during the early stages of warm-febrile disorders.

CHEMICAL COMPOSITION

Dendrobine, nobilonine, dendramine, dendroxine, dendrine, and 6-hydroxydendroxine.[1]

PHARMACOLOGICAL EFFECTS

- **Gastrointestinal:** Administration of a diluted solution of *Shi Hu* is associated with an increase in gastric acid secretion and intestinal peristalsis. A concentrated solution, however, inhibits intestinal peristalsis.[2]
- **Antipyretic and analgesic:** Dendrobine has antipyretic and analgesic effects, similar to but slightly weaker than phenacetin.[3]

CLINICAL STUDIES AND RESEARCH

- **Atrophic gastritis:** In one clinical study, 156 patients with atrophic gastritis were treated with herbal formulas with complete recovery in 87 patients, improvement in 66 patients, and no response in 3 patients. The standard herbal formula contained *Shi Hu*, *Mai Men Dong* (Radix Ophiopogonis), *Sheng Di Huang* (Radix Rehmanniae), *Yu Zhu* (Rhizoma Polygonati Odorati), *Tian Hua Fen* (Radix Trichosanthis), *Wu Mei* (Fructus Mume), *Shan Zha*

Shi Hu (Herba Dendrobii)

(Fructus Crataegi), *Bai Shao* (Radix Paeoniae Alba), *Gan Cao* (Radix Glycyrrhizae) and *San Qi* (Radix Notoginseng). *Shi Gao* (Gypsum Fibrosum) and *Pu Gong Ying* (Herba Taraxaci) were added if excess Stomach heat was present. *Zhi Shi* (Fructus Aurantii Immaturus) and *Hou Po* (Cortex Magnoliae Officinalis) were added if there was epigastric distention due to qi stagnation. *Pu Huang* (Pollen Typhae) and *Wu Ling Zhi* (Excrementum Trogopteri seu Pteromi) were added if there was stabbing pain in the epigastrium. *Huo Ma Ren* (Fructus Cannabis) and *Yu Li Ren* (Semen Pruni) were added if there were dry stools or constipation. The herbal formula was administered as a decoction twice daily for three months.[4]

TOXICOLOGY

Shi Hu is very safe. However, seizures have been associated with gross overdose.[5]

AUTHORS' COMMENTS

Shi Hu and *Yu Zhu* (Rhizoma Polygonati Odorati) both tonify yin, generate body fluids and nourish Stomach yin. Common manifestations of these deficiencies include dry cough, irritability and constipation. *Shi Hu* more strongly generates body fluids and relieves thirst. It also nourishes Kidney yin to dispel deficiency fire. Milder and lighter, *Yu Zhu* does not create stagnation like other tonics. It is also used for yin-deficient patients who have wind-heat manifesting in dry cough, sore throat and thirst.

Shi Hu and *Tian Hua Fen* (Radix Trichosanthis) both generate body fluids and alleviate thirst. *Shi Hu* more strongly nourishes Kidney yin and brightens the eyes. *Tian Hua Fen* more effectively sedates fire and nourishes Stomach yin.

References

1. *Zhong Cao Yao Cheng Fen Hua Xue* (Composition and Chemistry of Chinese Herbs), 1977:814
2. *Zhong Yao Xue* (Chinese Herbology), 1998; 851:852
3. *J Am Chem Soc*, 1977; 99(3):1612
4. *Shan Xi Zhong Yi* (Shanxi Chinese Medicine), 1990; 11(8):344
5. *Chang Yong Zhong Yao Xian Dai Yan Jiu Yu Lin Chuan* (Recent Study & Clinical Application of Common Traditional Chinese Medicine), 1995; 649:651

Yu Zhu (Rhizoma Polygonati Odorati)

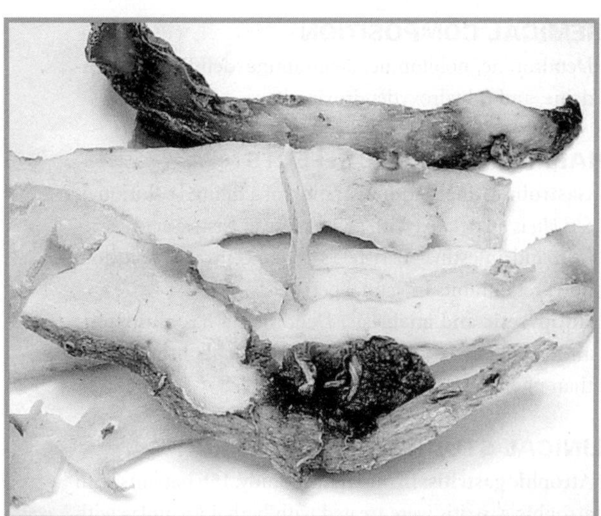

玉竹

Pinyin Name: *Yu Zhu*
Literal Name: "jade bamboo"
Alternate Chinese Names: *Wei Rui, Ming Yu Zhu, Shan Wei Shen, Di Jie*
Original Source: *Shen Nong Ben Cao Jing* (Divine Husbandman's Classic of the Materia Medica) in the second century
English Name: polygonatum rhizome, fragrant Solomon's seal rhizome
Botanical Name: *Polygonatum odoratum* (Mill.) Druce (*Yu Zhu*)
Pharmaceutical Name: Rhizoma Polygonati Odorati
Properties: sweet, neutral
Channels Entered: Lung, Stomach

CHINESE THERAPEUTIC ACTIONS

1. Nourishes Yin and Moistens the Lung

Dryness attacking the Lung: Pathogenic dryness often attacks the Lung during autumn. With dryness injuring Lung yin, patients may have a non-productive dry cough, or dry cough with scanty and sticky sputum, and dry mouth and throat. *Yu Zhu* (Rhizoma Polygonati Odorati) has abundant juice that helps to moisten both

Yu Zhu (Rhizoma Polygonati Odorati)

the Lung and Stomach. This herb tonifies without stagnating, which makes it ideal for treating yin deficiency accompanied by heat.

- Dry cough: combine *Yu Zhu* with *Nan Sha Shen* (Radix Adenophorae), *Bei Sha Shen* (Radix Glehniae), *Shi Hu* (Herba Dendrobii), *Mai Men Dong* (Radix Ophiopogonis), *Sang Ye* (Folium Mori), and *Tian Hua Fen* (Radix Trichosanthis). **Exemplar Formula:** *Sha Shen Mai Dong Tang* (Glehnia and Ophiopogonis Decoction).
- Lung dryness and cold: use it with *Sang Ye* (Folium Mori), *Xing Ren* (Semen Armeniacae Amarum), *Qian Hu* (Radix Peucedani) and *Jie Geng* (Radix Platycodonis).

Consumptive cough: Chronic respiratory disorders often lead to consumption of Lung yin, a condition characterized by feeble, dry cough, with scanty, difficult-to-expectorate sputum. Sweet in nature, *Yu Zhu* enters the Lung to nourish yin. It does not, however, sedate deficiency fire or dispel phlegm. Therefore, it must be combined with herbs that accomplish those functions.

- Chronic cough with relatively more deficiency heat: combine *Yu Zhu* with *Sheng Di Huang* (Radix Rehmanniae), *Zhi Mu* (Radix Anemarrhenae), and *Di Gu Pi* (Cortex Lycii).
- Chronic cough with relatively more yin deficiency: use this herb with *Bei Mu* (Bulbus Fritillaria), and *Bai Bu* (Radix Stemonae).

2. Generates Body Fluids and Nourishes the Stomach

Stomach yin deficiency: This condition may result from a febrile disorder or heat in the interior. Clinical manifestations include hunger but no desire to eat, dull epigastric pain, stomach discomfort, and dry mouth and tongue. Sweet in nature, *Yu Zhu* enters the Stomach to nourish yin and promote generation of fluids. It is most suitable for treating late-stage febrile disorders with yin deficiency or disharmony between organs because of heat injuring the body fluids.

- Stomach yin deficiency: combine *Yu Zhu* with *Sha Shen* (Radix Glehniae seu Adenophorae), *Shi Hu* (Herba Dendrobii), *Mai Men Dong* (Radix Ophiopogonis), *Mai Ya* (Fructus Hordei Germinatus) and rock sugar.

Yin deficiency with exterior wind-heat invasion: This chronic yin deficiency is complicated by recent exposure to exterior pathogens. Clinical manifestations include aversion to wind, fever, dry cough, scanty sputum, dizziness, irritability, and dry mouth. Such conditions must be treated with herbs that concurrently tonify yin and eliminate exterior wind-heat. Moderate in action and non-stagnating in nature, *Yu Zhu* nourishes yin and is less likely than other yin tonics to retain exterior pathogenic factors in the body.

- Yin deficiency with exterior wind-heat: combine *Yu Zhu* with *Bo He* (Herba Menthae), *Bai Wei* (Radix Cynanchi Atrati), *Dan Dou Chi* (Semen Sojae Praeparatum) and *Jie Geng* (Radix Platycodonis).

***Xiao ke* (wasting and thirsting) syndrome**: Lastly, *Yu Zhu* treats *xiao ke* syndrome characterized by yin deficiency of the Lung, Stomach and Kidney. *Yu Zhu* nourishes yin and promotes generation of body fluids.

- *Xiao ke* syndrome: combine *Yu Zhu* with *Tian Hua Fen* (Radix Trichosanthis), fresh *Ge Gen* (Radix Puerariae), fresh *Shan Yao* (Rhizoma Dioscoreae) and fresh *Shu Di Huang* (Radix Rehmanniae Preparata).
- *Xiao ke* in the upper *jiao* with polydipsia: use this herb with *Mai Men Dong* (Radix Ophiopogonis), *Zhi Mu* (Radix Anemarrhenae), *Huang Qin* (Radix Scutellariae) and *Tian Hua Fen* (Radix Trichosanthis).
- *Xiao ke* in the middle *jiao* with polyphagia: add it to *Shi Gao* (Gypsum Fibrosum), *Zhi Mu* (Radix Anemarrhenae) and *Sheng Di Huang* (Radix Rehmanniae).
- *Xiao ke* in the lower *jiao* with polyuria: combine it with *Zhi Mu* (Radix Anemarrhenae), *Huang Bai* (Cortex Phellodendri), *Shu Di Huang* (Radix Rehmanniae Preparata), *Wu Wei Zi* (Fructus Schisandrae Chinensis) and *Shan Zhu Yu* (Fructus Corni).

DOSAGE

10 to 15 grams in decoction. *Yu Zhu* is also used in paste, pill or powder forms. Fresh *Yu Zhu* more effectively treats yin-deficient heat. The dried herb is better to remedy mild yin-deficient heat.

CAUTIONS / CONTRAINDICATIONS

- *Yu Zhu* is not recommended in cases of Spleen deficiency, accumulation of dampness, phlegm stagnation or qi stagnation.

CHEMICAL COMPOSITION

Convallamarin, convallarin, polygonatiin, polygonotin, quercitol, vitamin A, starch.[1]

PHARMACOLOGICAL EFFECTS

- **Cardiovascular:** Administration of *Yu Zhu* is associated with dilation of blood vessels and reduction of blood pressure in laboratory animals. In frog heart specimens, a small dose of *Yu Zhu* has a positive inotropic effect while a large dose has a negative inotropic effect. No significant change in heart rate was observed.[2]
- **Effects on smooth muscle:** A 20% decoction of *Yu Zhu* has a mild stimulating effect on the uterus in mice. It also

Yu Zhu (Rhizoma Polygonati Odorati)

has an initial stimulating, followed by inhibiting, effect on the smooth muscle of the intestines in mice.[3]

- **Antidiabetic:** Oral administration of *Yu Zhu* inhibits hyperglycemia associated with epinephrine and glucose intake.[4]

CLINICAL STUDIES AND RESEARCH

- **Congestive heart failure:** According to one report, congestive heart failure in 5 patients was stabilized in 5 to 10 days by daily treatment with 15 grams of *Yu Zhu* decoction.[5]

TOXICOLOGY

No fatalities in mice were reported following oral ingestion of *Yu Zhu* decoction at the dosage of 10 g/kg for one week. The LD_{50} for 100% *Yu Zhu* solution was 112.5 g/kg.[6]

AUTHORS' COMMENTS

Yu Zhu and *Huang Jing* (Rhizoma Polygonati) both nourish the Lung and Stomach. *Yu Zhu* more strongly tonifies Stomach yin with symptoms of dry mouth and thirst, while *Huang Jing* more effectively tonifies Kidney yin with symptoms of dizziness, and soreness and weakness of the lower back and knees.

See *Shi Hu* (Herba Dendrobii) for comparison of these two herbs.

References

1. *Xian Dai Zhong Yao Yao Li Xue* (Contemporary Pharmacology of Chinese Herbs), 1997; 1358
2. *Jin Yi Ke Ji* (Jinyi Science and Technology), 1979; (9):5
3. *Qing Dao Yi Xue Yuan Xue Bao* (Journal of Qingdao Institution of Medicine), 1959; (2):11
4. *Yi Xue Zhong Yang Za Zhi* (Central Journal of Medicine), 1972; 280:718
5. *Ke Ji Tong Xun* (Journal of Science and Technology), 1972; (1):26
6. *Ha Er Bing Yi Ke Da Xue* (Haerbing University of Medicine), 1959:14

Huang Jing (Rhizoma Polygonati)

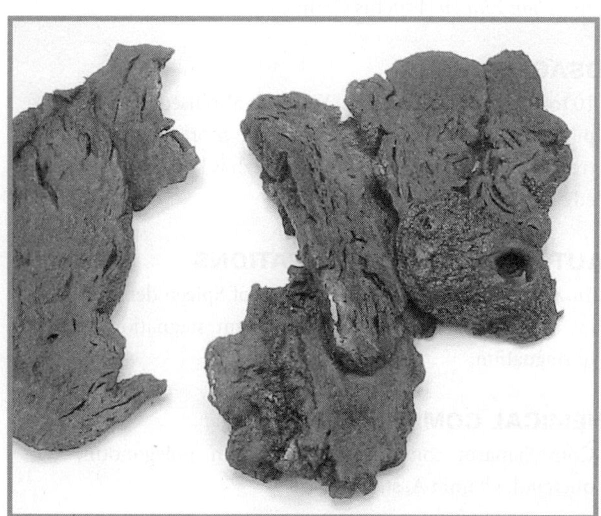

黄精

Pinyin Name: *Huang Jing*
Literal Name: "yellow essence," "yellow pure substance"
Alternate Chinese Names: *Mi Pu*
Original Source: *Ming Yi Za Zhu* (Miscellaneous Records of Famous Physicians) by Tao Hong-Jing in 500 A.D.
English Name: polygonatum root, king Solomon's seal rhizome, Siberian Solomon's seal rhizome, many-flower Solomon's seal rhizome
Botanical Name: *Polygonatum kingianum* Coll et hemsl. (*Dian Huang Jing*); *Polygonatum sibiricum* Red. (*Huang Jing*); *Polygonatum cyrtonema* Hua. (*Nang Si Huang Jing*)
Pharmaceutical Name: Rhizoma Polygonati
Properties: sweet, neutral
Channels Entered: Spleen, Lung, Kidney

CHINESE THERAPEUTIC ACTIONS

1. Nourishes Yin, Moistens the Lung

Chronic yin-deficient cough: Sweet and neutral, *Huang Jing* (Rhizoma Polygonati) nourishes yin, moistens the Lung, and tonifies qi. It is commonly used to treat coughing caused by yin deficiency or yin-deficient heat, characterized by a dry, non-productive cough. If heat dries fluids and damages the Lung, streaks of blood may be present with coughing, or in the sputum. Patients with deficiency heat may have flushed cheeks and irritability.

Huang Jing (Rhizoma Polygonati)

Chronic coughing consumes Lung qi causing shortness of breath and fatigue. *Huang Jing* is the ideal herb to treat yin-deficient cough, nourish the Lung and also benefit qi. *Huang Jing* may be used alone or in combination with other herbs.

- Chronic cough associated with yin deficiency: use *Huang Jing* with *Sha Shen* (Radix Glehniae seu Adenophorae), *Zhi Mu* (Radix Anemarrhenae), *Bei Mu* (Bulbus Fritillaria) and *Bai Bu* (Radix Stemonae).
- Coughing with streaks of blood: use this herb with *E Jiao* (Colla Corii Asini), *Bai Ji* (Rhizoma Bletillae), and *Han Lian Cao* (Herba Ecliptae).

Cough due to dryness: *Huang Jing* is commonly used to treat cough by nourishing yin and moistening dryness. Dryness in the Lung consumes body fluids and leads to dry nose, itchy throat, dry non-productive coughing, or coughing with sticky, difficult-to-expectorate sputum that may be streaked with blood. Dryness may be accompanied by heat or cold factors, and must be addressed accordingly. *Huang Jing* is neutral and thus suitable for use for coughing caused by either cold or heat.

- Cough due to cold and dryness: use *Huang Jing* with *Zi Su Ye* (Folium Perillae), *Xing Ren* (Semen Armeniacae Amarum), *Zi Wan* (Radix Asteris), and *Kuan Dong Hua* (Flos Farfarae).
- Cough from heat and dryness: combine this herb with *Sang Ye* (Folium Mori), *Xing Ren* (Semen Armeniacae Amarum), *Zhe Bei Mu* (Bulbus Fritillariae Thunbergii), and *Nan Sha Shen* (Radix Adenophorae).

2. Tonifies Kidney *Jing* (Essence)

Huang Jing enters the Kidney to tonify *jing*, promote generation of marrow and improve cognitive functions. It is commonly used to treat Kidney deficiency characterized by symptoms such as soreness of the back, weakness of the knees, dizziness, vertigo, prematurely gray hair, and blurred vision. It may be used individually with pork, beef or chicken as soup or in combination with other herbs in powder, pills or decoction.

- Kidney *jing* deficiency: use *Huang Jing* with small portions of *Gan Jiang* (Rhizoma Zingiberis) and *Rou Gui* (Cortex Cinnamomi) to potentiate the tonic function.
- Kidney *jing* and Liver yin deficiencies: combine it with *Gou Qi Zi* (Fructus Lycii).
- Kidney *jing* and blood deficiencies: add *Dang Gui* (Radicis Angelicae Sinensis).

3. Relieves *Xiao Ke* (Wasting and Thirsting) Syndrome

***Xiao ke* syndrome:** This syndrome is characterized by yin-deficient heat with symptoms such as polyuria, polyphagia, and polydipsia. Other symptoms include emaciation, irritability and fatigue. *Huang Jing* enters and nourishes the Lung, Spleen and Kidney, the organs commonly affected by this syndrome. Therefore, it may be used to treat upper, middle, and lower *xiao ke* syndromes. *Huang Jing* may be used with other herbs, or individually in large doses. Due to the neutral thermal property of *Huang Jing* and the fact that this herb tonifies both qi and yin, it is ideal for treatment of chronic *xiao ke* syndrome with yin and qi deficiencies.

- *Xiao ke* with relatively more heat: use *Huang Jing* with *Tian Hua Fen* (Radix Trichosanthis), *Shi Gao* (Gypsum Fibrosum), *Zhi Mu* (Radix Anemarrhenae) and *Huang Lian* (Rhizoma Coptidis).
- *Xiao ke* with severe yin deficiency: combine it with *Sheng Di Huang* (Radix Rehmanniae), *Shu Di Huang* (Radix Rehmanniae Preparata), *Tian Men Dong* (Radix Asparagi) and *Shi Hu* (Herba Dendrobii).
- *Xiao ke* with deficiencies of yin and yang: use this herb with *Shu Di Huang* (Radix Rehmanniae Preparata), *Shan Yao* (Rhizoma Dioscoreae), *Shan Zhu Yu* (Fructus Corni), *Rou Gui* (Cortex Cinnamomi) and *Fu Zi* (Radix Aconiti Lateralis Praeparata).
- *Xiao ke* with deficiencies of qi and yin: combine it with *Huang Qi* (Radix Astragali), *Shan Yao* (Rhizoma Dioscoreae), *Xi Yang Shen* (Radix Panacis Quinquefolii), and *Tai Zi Shen* (Radix Pseudostellariae).

4. Tonifies the Spleen and Benefits Qi

Spleen and Stomach deficiencies: *Huang Jing* tonifies Spleen qi and yin to relieve symptoms such as fatigue, poor appetite, weak pulse, dry mouth, poor appetite, and a red tongue with no coating. In these cases, *Huang Jing* is commonly used with other herbs, as its Spleen-tonic function is rather mild.

- Spleen and Stomach qi deficiencies: use *Huang Jing* with *Dang Shen* (Radix Codonopsis), *Fu Ling* (Poria), *Bai Zhu* (Rhizoma Atractylodis Macrocephalae) and *Yi Yi Ren* (Semen Coicis).
- Spleen and Stomach yin deficiencies: combine it with *Sha Shen* (Radix Glehniae seu Adenophorae), *Mai Men Dong* (Radix Ophiopogonis), *Yu Zhu* (Rhizoma Polygonati Odorati) and *Gu Ya* (Fructus Setariae Germinatus).
- Spleen and Stomach qi and yin deficiencies: use it with *Dang Shen* (Radix Codonopsis), *Mai Men Dong* (Radix Ophiopogonis), *Wu Wei Zi* (Fructus Schisandrae Chinensis) and *Shan Yao* (Rhizoma Dioscoreae).

DOSAGE

10 to 15 grams for dried *Huang Jing*, 30 to 60 grams for the fresh herb, in decoction. *Huang Jing* is commonly used in decoction, pills, or powder forms. For topical

Huang Jing (Rhizoma Polygonati)

application, this herb is generally processed first by cooking with water or soaking in alcohol or vinegar. For oral use, *Huang Jing* is often processed by steaming with water or grain-based liquor, as the unprocessed herb may be slightly irritating to the throat.

CAUTIONS / CONTRAINDICATIONS

- Sticky and greasy in nature, *Huang Jing* may create dampness and stagnation.
- Because of the potential for stagnation, this herb is not recommended for use in cases of dampness with Spleen deficiency, cough with profuse sputum, diarrhea due to cold, or fullness and distention caused by qi stagnation.

CHEMICAL COMPOSITION

Azetidine-2-carboxylic acid, aspartic acid, homoserine, diaminobutyric acid, digitalis glycoside, vitexin xyloside.[1]

PHARMACOLOGICAL EFFECTS

- **Antibiotic:** Extract of *Huang Jing* has demonstrated inhibitory action against *Staphylococcus aureus*, acid-fast bacilli, and some dermatophytes.[2]
- **Antidiabetic:** Administration of *Huang Jing* extract is associated with an initial elevation followed by a reduction of plasma glucose levels in rabbits. Extract of *Huang Jing* is especially effective in reducing plasma glucose levels raised by adrenaline.[3]
- **Adaptogenic:** Intraperitoneal injection of *Huang Jing* prolonged the swimming time of mice.[4]
- **Cardiovascular:** *Huang Jing* is associated with an increase in heart rate, reduction in blood pressure, and dilation of the coronary arteries.[5,6,7]
- **Antihyperlipidemic:** Administration of *Huang Jing* extract for 30 days showed a marked reduction in triglycerides and cholesterol levels in rats.[8]

CLINICAL STUDIES AND RESEARCH

- **Hypotension:** Ten hypotensive patients were treated with an herbal decoction with good immediate results, but less than satisfactory long-term effects. The herbal formula contained 30 grams of *Huang Jing*, 30 grams of *Dang Shen* (Radix Codonopsis), and 10 grams of *Zhi Gan Cao* (Radix Glycyrrhizae Preparata).[9]
- **Hypercholesterolemia:** High plasma cholesterol levels in 86 patients showed an average reduction of 38.2 mg/dL after two months of taking an herbal formula containing *Huang Jing*, *He Shou Wu* (Radix Polygoni Multiflori) and *Sang Ji Sheng* (Herba Taxilli).[10]
- **Near-sightedness:** An herbal formula containing *Huang Jing* and *Hei Dou* (Semen Glycine Max) was 59.75% effective in improving the vision of 41 patients with near-sightedness.[11]
- **Pulmonary tuberculosis:** In one study, 19 patients with pulmonary tuberculosis were treated with *Huang Jing* four times daily for 2 months, with satisfactory results. The study reported negative findings in the sputum, normal range of ESR, improvement in symptoms, and weight gain.[12]
- **Fungal infection:** Topical application of a *Huang Jing* tincture was effective in treating 55 out of 67 patients with fungal infections. The tincture was prepared by soaking 100 grams of the herb in 250 ml of 75% alcohol for 15 days. The tincture is then mixed with 150 ml of rice vinegar before application.[13]
- **Deafness:** Patients with deafness caused by poisoning were treated with intramuscular injection of *Huang Jing*, vitamin B1, and vitamin A three times daily. Out of 100 patients, 9 had complete recovery, 22 showed some improvement, 3 showed slight improvement, and the rest showed no response.[14]

AUTHORS' COMMENTS

Huang Jing and *Yu Zhu* (Rhizoma Polygonati Odorati) both nourish the Lung and Stomach. *Huang Jing* is stronger in tonifying Kidney yin with symptoms of dizziness, and soreness and weakness of the lower back and knees. *Yu Zhu* is stronger in tonifying Stomach yin with symptoms of dry mouth and thirst.

References

1. *Xian Dai Zhong Yao Yao Li Xue* (Contemporary Pharmacology of Chinese Herbs), 1997; 1353
2. *Gui Zhou Yao Xun* (Guizhou Journal of Herbology), 1988; 1:3
3. *Ri Ben Yao Wu Xue Za Zhi* (Japan Journal of Pharmacology), 1927; 6(4):466
4. *Zhong Yao Yao Li Du Li Yu Lin Chuang* (Pharmacology, Toxicology and Clinical Applications of Chinese Herbs), 1990; 6(3):28
5. *Zhong Yao Yao Li Yu Ying Yong* (Pharmacology and Applications of Chinese Herbs), 1983:998
6. *Zhong Guo Yi Yao Ke Xue Yuan Lun Wen Zhai Yao* (Abstract from Chinese University of Medicine and Science), 1956; II:70
7. *Si Chuan Zhong Cao Yao Tong Xun* (Sichuan Journal of Chinese Herbology), 1974; (2):20
8. *Jiang Su Zhong Yi* (Jiangsu Chinese Medicine), 1988; (7):41
9. *Hu Bei Zhong Yi Za Zhi* (Hubei Journal of Chinese Medicine), 1981; 12:31
10. *Xin Yi Xue* (New Medicine), 1977; 45:211
11. Ibid., 1981; 6:40
12. *Zhe Jiang Yi Xue* (Zhejiang Journal of Medicine), 1960; 4:43
13. *Shan Dong Zhong Yi Za Zhi* (Shandong Journal of Chinese Medicine), 1986; 5:47
14. *Zhong Xi Yi Jie He Za Zhi* (Journal of Integrated Chinese and Western Medicine), 1982; 1:19

Bai He (Bulbus Lilii)

百合

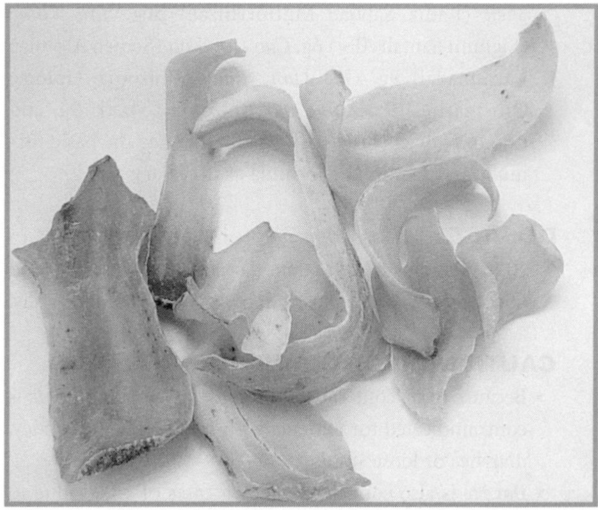

Pinyin Name: *Bai He*
Literal Name: "hundred meetings"
Alternate Chinese Names: *Bai Hua Bai He*
Original Source: *Shen Nong Ben Cao Jing* (Divine Husbandman's Classic of the Materia Medica) in the second century
English Name: lily, lily bulb
Botanical Name: *Lilium brownii* F. E. Brown. (*Bai He*); *Lilium alancifolium* Thunb. (*Juan He*); *Lilium pumilum* DC. (*Xi Ye Bai He*)
Pharmaceutical Name: Bulbus Lilii
Properties: sweet, cool
Channels Entered: Lung, Heart

CHINESE THERAPEUTIC ACTIONS

1. Moistens the Lung and Arrests Cough

Consumptive cough due to Lung deficiency: Chronic coughing causes qi deficiency and loss of moisture in the Lung. The chief manifestations of Lung yin deficiency include: chronic, consumptive, dry cough, shortness of breath, and difficult-to-expectorate white or yellow scanty, sticky sputum that may contain streaks of blood. Besides moistening the Lung, *Bai He* (Bulbus Lilii) treats Lung yin deficiency with heat signs such as tidal fever, night sweats, the absence of sputum, and hemoptysis. Clinical applications include: chronic respiratory disorders such as tuberculosis, bronchiectasis, asthma, and lung abscesses.

- Dry cough: combine *Bai He* with *Kuan Dong Hua* (Flos Farfarae), *Sheng Di Huang* (Radix Rehmanniae), *Mai Men Dong* (Radix Ophiopogonis), *Sha Shen* (Radix Glehniae seu Adenophorae) and pear skins.
- Dry cough with blood-streaked sputum: add this herb to *Sheng Di Huang* (Radix Rehmanniae), *Xuan Shen* (Radix Scrophulariae), *Chuan Bei Mu* (Bulbus Fritillariae Cirrhosae), and *Mai Men Dong* (Radix Ophiopogonis).
Exemplar Formula: *Bai He Gu Jin Tang* (Lily Bulb Decoction to Preserve the Metal).
- Bronchiectasis, hemoptysis: use this herb with *Bai Ji* (Rhizoma Bletillae), *Bai Bu* (Radix Stemonae) and the powder of *Hai Ge Fen* (Concha Meretricis seu Cyclinae), with honey, to make pills.
- Lung abscess: use *Bai He* alone. Drink the decoction and eat the herb.
- Non-ulcerating sores: crush fresh *Bai He* and apply it topically as a paste.

2. Clears the Heart and Calms the *Shen* (Spirit)

Restless *shen*: The Heart governs the blood vessels and houses the *shen*. Lung yin deficiency directly affects its neighbor, the Heart. Possible symptoms may include inability to concentrate, disorientation in speech and action, sensory impairment, a bitter taste in the mouth, dark yellow urine, and a thready, rapid pulse. *Bai He*, sweet and cool, nourishes Lung yin and clears Heart fire. It tonifies deficiency and at the same time calms the *shen*.

- Palpitations, insomnia, restlessness, dark urine, and inability to concentrate, due to the aftermath of febrile disease: combine *Bai He* with *Zhi Mu* (Radix Anemarrhenae), and *Sheng Di Huang* (Radix Rehmanniae).
- Difficulty falling and staying asleep: use it with *Suan Zao Ren* (Semen Zizyphi Spinosae).
- Irritability and thirst due to perspiration, resulting from misuse of diaphoretic herbs: add this herb to *Zhi Mu* (Radix Anemarrhenae).
- Dark urine or dysuria: use *Bai He* with *Hua Shi* (Talcum).
- Vomiting or hiccups: use it with *Dai Zhe Shi* (Haematitum).

3. Nourishes Stomach Yin and Harmonizes the Middle *Jiao*

Bai He has recently been found to be effective in harmonizing the middle *jiao* and easing the dull pain associated with Stomach yin deficiency. It is often used in late-stage stomach disorders such as atrophic gastritis, ulcers and stomach cancer.

- Atrophic gastritis due to Stomach yin deficiency: use *Bai He* with *Bai Shao* (Radix Paeoniae Alba), *Shan Yao* (Rhizoma Dioscoreae) and *Huang Qi* (Radix Astragali).
- Chronic stomach pain from unknown causes: use *Bai He* (Bulbus Lilii) 30g, *Wu Yao* (Radix Linderae) 9g, *Dan*

Bai He (Bulbus Lilii)

Shen (Radix Salviae Miltiorrhizae) 30g, *Tan Xiang* (Lignum Santali Albi) 6g, *Cao Dou Kou* (Semen Alpiniae Katsumadai) 9g, *Gao Liang Jiang* (Rhizoma Alpiniae Officinarum) 9g, *Xiang Fu* (Rhizoma Cyperi) 9g, and *Chuan Lian Zi* (Fructus Toosendan) 6g as the basic formula, and modify the formula as necessary.

DOSAGE

10 to 30 grams in decoction. *Bai He* is often used as food in congees or soups. The fresh herb may be used topically.

CAUTIONS / CONTRAINDICATIONS

- Because of its cold and moistening properties, *Bai He* is contraindicated for patients with middle *jiao* deficiency, diarrhea or loose stools.
- *Bai He* is also contraindicated in cases of cough due to wind-cold or phlegm.
- Use of *Bai He* may be associated with drowsiness and sedation. Therefore, individuals who take this herb should exercise caution if driving or operating heavy machinery.

OVERDOSAGE

Gross overdose of *Bai He* is associated with adverse reactions such as nausea, vomiting, decreased appetite, diarrhea and constipation. Rare instances of hair loss and changes in ECG have also been reported. Injection of this herb has been associated with necrosis of local tissues.[1]

CHEMICAL COMPOSITION

Colchicine, starch, protein, lipids, sugars, organ acids, calcium, magnesium, iron, aluminum, iron, potassium, zinc.[2]

PHARMACOLOGICAL EFFECTS

- **Respiratory:** Administration of *Bai He* is associated with marked antitussive and expectorant effects in mice.[3]
- **Adaptogenic:** Administration of *Bai He* in mice is associated with an increase resistance to hypoxia and increased swimming time.[4]

CLINICAL STUDIES AND RESEARCH

- **Atrophic gastritis:** In one study, 56 patients with atrophic gastritis were treated with herbal medicine for three months with marked effectiveness in 22 cases, moderate results in 28 cases and no response in 6 cases. The overall rate of effectiveness was 89.3%. The herbal decoction contained *Bai He* 30g, *Wu Yao* (Radix Linderae Strychnifolia) 9g, *Bai Shao* (Radix Paeoniae Alba) 15g, *Hong Hua* (Flos Carthami) 15g, *Shan Yao* (Rhizoma Dioscoreae) 20g, *Huang Qi* (Radix Astragali) 20g, *Chen Pi* (Pericarpium Citri Reticulatae) 10g, *Gan Cao* (Radix Glycyrrhizae) 5g, *Huang Lian* (Rhizoma Coptidis) 3g, and others, depending on the condition of each patient.[5]
- **Sores:** Topical application of *Bai He* powder provides effective treatment for sores. According to one report, good results were observed following topical application of the herb powder, with the affected area covered with gauze, and the dressing changed once every 2 to 3 days in summer and every 5 to 8 days in winter.[6]
- **Bleeding:** According to one report, 100 patients with post-surgical nasal bleeding were treated topically with *Bai He* cream, with good results. The cream was prepared by mixing 15 grams of *Bai He* powder with distilled water, then stirring the solution while gradually heating it to 60° C, to obtain a paste-like cream. The cream was then cooled and sterilized prior to topical application. The treatment protocol was to apply a small amount of the cream into the nasal cavity to stop bleeding. The cream generally begin to dissolve after 3 hours, and completely disappeared after 14 hours. No allergic or adverse reactions were reported.[7]

HERB-DRUG INTERACTION

- **Sedatives:** Oral ingestion of *Bai He* prolonged sleeping time induced by barbiturates.[8] [Note: Many categories of drugs induce sedation, such as antihistamines, narcotic analgesics, barbiturates, benzodiazepines and many others.]

AUTHORS' COMMENTS

Because of its pleasant taste and neutral property, *Bai He* is often used as food and cooked with porridge to nourish Lung yin.

References

1. *Zhong Yao Yao Li Du Li Yu Lin Chuang* (Pharmacology, Toxicology and Clinical Applications of Chinese Herbs), 1992; 376
2. *Xian Dai Zhong Yao Yao Li Xue* (Contemporary Pharmacology of Chinese Herbs), 1997; 1361
3. *Zhong Yao Cai* (Study of Chinese Herbal Material), 1990; 13(6):31
4. Ibid.
5. *Liao Ning Zhong Yi Za Zhi* (Liaoning Journal of Chinese Medicine), 1988; 4:18
6. *Zhong Cheng Yao Yan Jiu* (Research of Chinese Patent Medicine), 1985; 1:45
7. *Zhong Hua Er Bi Hou Ke Za Zhi* (Chinese Journal of ENT), 1954; 1:20
8. *Zhong Yao Cai* (Study of Chinese Herbal Material), 1990; 13(6):31

Gou Qi Zi (Fructus Lycii)

枸杞子

Pinyin Name: *Gou Qi Zi*
Literal Name: "thorny stalk seed," "aspen-willow fruit"
Alternate Chinese Names: *Di Gu Zi, Gan Qi, Qi Zi, Xue Qi, Ku Qi, Gou Ji, Tian Jing Zi, Tu Gou Qi*
Original Source: *Ming Yi Za Zhu* (Miscellaneous Records of Famous Physicians) by Tao Hong-Jing in 500 A.D.
English Name: lycium fruit, matrimony vine fruit, barbary wolfberry
Botanical Name: *Lycium barbarum* L. (*Ning Xia Gou Qi*); *Lycium chinense* Mill. (*Gou Qi*)
Pharmaceutical Name: Fructus Lycii
Properties: sweet, neutral
Channels Entered: Liver, Kidney, Lung

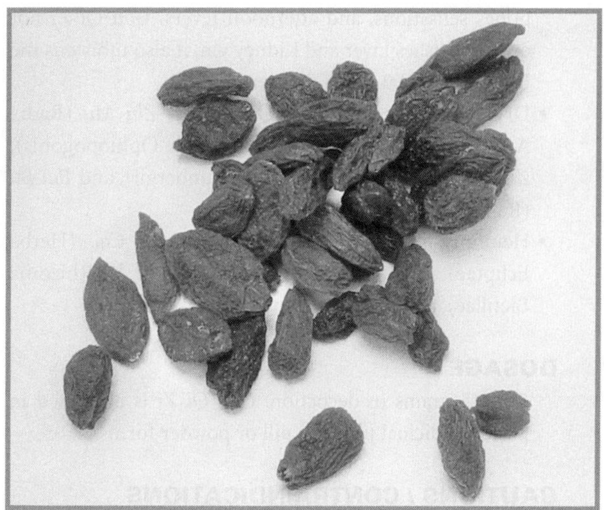

CHINESE THERAPEUTIC ACTIONS

1. Tonifies Liver and Kidney Yin, Brightens the Eyes

Liver and Kidney yin deficiencies: The Liver opens to the eyes: insufficient yin of the Liver and Kidney may lead to dizziness, blurry vision, nocturnal emissions, infertility, soreness and weakness of the lower back and knees, prematurely gray hair, *xiao ke* (wasting and thirsting) syndrome, night sweats, thirst, and diminished visual acuity. *Gou Qi Zi* (Fructus Lycii) is neutral and has a light, moistening yet non-stagnating, nature that effectively nourishes different parts of the body without the side effect of creating stagnation. It is excellent for deficient patients who need mild tonics for a prolonged period of time. *Gou Qi Zi* is the herb of choice for treating visual disorders caused by Liver and Kidney yin deficiencies.

- Blurry vision: use *Gou Qi Zi* alone, soaked in grain-based liquor.
- Dizziness, diminished visual acuity, dryness or tearing with exposure to wind: combine this herb with *Ju Hua* (Flos Chrysanthemi) and *Liu Wei Di Huang Wan* (Six-Ingredient Pill with Rehmannia). **Exemplar Formula:** *Qi Ju Di Huang Wan* (Lycium Fruit, Chrysanthemum, and Rehmannia Pill).
- Soreness and weakness of the lower back and knees: add *Gou Qi Zi* to *Gu Sui Bu* (Rhizoma Drynariae), *Du Zhong* (Cortex Eucommiae), *Xu Duan* (Radix Dipsaci), and *Sang Ji Sheng* (Herba Taxilli).
- Nocturnal emissions, night sweating, blurry vision, tinnitus: combine this herb with *Shu Di Huang* (Radix Rehmanniae Preparata), *Shan Yao* (Rhizoma Dioscoreae), *Shan Zhu Yu* (Fructus Corni), and *Gui Ban Jiao* (Gelatinum Plastrum Testudinis). **Exemplar Formula:** *Zuo Gui Wan* (Restore the Left [Kidney] Pill).
- Impotence and nocturnal emissions from Kidney yin and yang deficiencies: incorporate this herb with *Shu Di Huang* (Radix Rehmanniae Preparata), *Shan Zhu Yu* (Fructus Corni), *Rou Gui* (Cortex Cinnamomi), and *Fu Zi* (Radix Aconiti Lateralis Praeparata). **Exemplar Formula:** *You Gui Wan* (Restore the Right [Kidney] Pill).
- *Xiao ke* (wasting and thirsting) syndrome: combine *Gou Qi Zi* with *Tian Men Dong* (Radix Asparagi), *Mai Men Dong* (Radix Ophiopogonis), *Shan Yao* (Rhizoma Dioscoreae), *Yu Zhu* (Rhizoma Polygonati Odorati), *Sheng Di Huang* (Radix Rehmanniae), *Zhi Mu* (Radix Anemarrhenae), and *Shi Gao* (Gypsum Fibrosum).
- Sallow appearance, prematurely gray hair, insomnia, and frequent dreams: use *Gou Qi Zi* with *Long Yan Rou* (Arillus Longan) and *He Shou Wu* (Radix Polygoni Multiflori).
- Prematurely gray hair, loose teeth: combine this herb with *He Shou Wu* (Radix Polygoni Multiflori), *Dang Gui* (Radicis Angelicae Sinensis), *Huai Niu Xi* (Radix Achyranthis Bidentatae), and *Tu Si Zi* (Semen Cuscutae).
- Steaming bones sensations: combine it with *Di Gu Pi* (Cortex Lycii).
- Emaciation, spermatorrhea, impotence, dizziness, and blurred vision: add it to *Ren Shen* (Radix Ginseng), *Lu Jiao* (Cornu Cervi), and *Gui Ban* (Plastrum Testudinis). **Exemplar Formula:** *Gui Lu Er Xian Jiao* (Tortoise Shell and Deer Antler Syrup).

2. Moistens Lung Yin

Chronic respiratory disorders with Lung yin deficiency: Symptoms include dry cough, without sputum or with scanty sputum that is difficult to expectorate, possibly coughing with blood or blood streaks, steaming

Gou Qi Zi (Fructus Lycii)

bones sensations, and afternoon fevers. *Gou Qi Zi* not only nourishes Liver and Kidney yin, it also moistens the Lung to treat Lung yin deficiency.

- Dry cough: combine *Gou Qi Zi* with *Zhi Mu* (Radix Anemarrhenae), *Mai Men Dong* (Radix Ophiopogonis), *Zhe Bei Mu* (Bulbus Fritillariae Thunbergii), and *Bai Bu* (Radix Stemonae).
- Hemoptysis: combine it with *Han Lian Cao* (Herba Ecliptae), *E Jiao* (Colla Corii Asini), *Bai Ji* (Rhizoma Bletillae), and *Zi Zhu* (Folium Callicarpae).

DOSAGE

5 to 15 grams in decoction. *Gou Qi Zi* is also used in paste, medicinal tincture, pill or powder forms.

CAUTIONS / CONTRAINDICATIONS

- Though *Gou Qi Zi* is not stagnating in nature, it should still be used with caution for patients who have diarrhea from Spleen and Stomach deficiencies.
- Use of *Gou Qi Zi* is contraindicated for patients with excess or exterior conditions.
- *Gou Qi Zi* should be used with caution during pregnancy, as it stimulates contraction of the uterus.

CHEMICAL COMPOSITION

Betaine, solavetivone, zeaxanthin, physalien, β-sitosterol, linoleic acid, sodium, calcium, potassium, magnesium, copper, zinc, iron.[1]

PHARMACOLOGICAL EFFECTS

- **Immunostimulant:** Administration of *Gou Qi Zi* is associated with an increase in non-specific immunity. It increases phagocytic activity of the macrophages and the total number of T cells.[2]
- **Hematological:** Decoction of *Gou Qi Zi* has been shown to increase the production of red blood cells and white blood cells in mice.[3]
- **Cardiovascular:** Intravenous injection of water extract of *Gou Qi Zi* at 20 mg/kg lowers blood pressure in rabbits. This cardiovascular effect may be reversed by injection of atropine.[4]
- **Uterine stimulant:** Decoction of *Gou Qi Zi* has a stimulating effect on the uterus in rabbits.[5]
- **Antineoplastic:** *Gou Qi Zi* enhances the immune system and suppresses the growth of cancer cells in mice.[6]

CLINICAL STUDIES AND RESEARCH

- **Male infertility:** In one clinical study, men with a low sperm count and poor sperm motility were treated with 15 grams of fresh *Gou Qi Zi* taken as food each night for 1 month per course of treatment. The patients were advised to avoid sexual activity during the treatment. Out of 42 patients, 23 patients showed normal sperm count and motility after 1 month, 10 patients had similar results after 2 months, and 9 showed no change. In follow-up visits two years after the initial treatment, the 33 who had normal sperm counts and motility had successfully conceived children.[7]
- **Chronic atrophic gastritis:** Patients with chronic atrophic gastritis were treated with 10 grams of *Gou Qi Zi* twice daily [20 grams per day] on an empty stomach for 2 months per course of treatment. All other herbal or drug treatments were discontinued during the treatment with *Gou Qi Zi*. Out of 20 patients, the study reported marked improvement in 15 patients and moderate improvement in 5 patients, after 2 to 4 months of treatment.[8]

TOXICOLOGY

The LD_{50} for intraperitoneal injection of water extract of *Gou Qi Zi* is 83.2 g/kg in mice.[9]

SUPPLEMENT

- 枸杞葉 / 枸杞叶 *Gou Qi Ye* (Folium Lycii), the leaf, is sometimes used as a substitute for *Gou Qi Zi*.

AUTHORS' COMMENTS

Gou Qi Zi is used with a large dose of *Bai Mao Gen* (Rhizoma Imperatae) to treat chronic hepatic disorders with bleeding gums.

When applied topically, a large dose of *Gou Qi Zi* powder mixed with vaseline or olive oil treats burns, redness and swelling.

Gou Qi Zi and *Ju Hua* (Flos Chrysanthemi) both brighten the eyes. *Gou Qi Zi* focuses on nourishing the Liver and Kidney to brighten the eyes. It is used for deficiency types of eye disorders with dryness and soreness. *Ju Hua* disperses wind, clears heat and brightens the eyes by calming rising Liver yang. It is used for excess types of eye disorders with redness, swelling and pain. The two herbs are often used together for patients with Liver yin deficiency and rising Liver yang.

References

1. *Xian Dai Zhong Yao Yao Li Xue* (Contemporary Pharmacology of Chinese Herbs), 1997; 1343
2. *Zhong Cao Yao* (Chinese Herbal Medicine), 19(7):25
3. *Zhong Yao Xue* (Chinese Herbology), 1998; 860:862
4. *Zhong Yao Zhi* (Chinese Herbology Journal), 1984:484
5. *Zhong Yao Xue* (Chinese Herbology), 1998; 860:862
6. *Zhong Guo Yao Li Xue Yu Du Li Xue Za Zhi* (Journal of Herbology and Toxicology), 1985; 2(2):127
7. *Xin Zhong Yi* (New Chinese Medicine), 1988; 2:20
8. *Zhong Yi Za Zhi* (Journal of Chinese Medicine), 1987; 2:92
9. *Zhong Yao Zhi* (Chinese Herbology Journal), 1984:484

Sang Shen Zi (Fructus Mori)

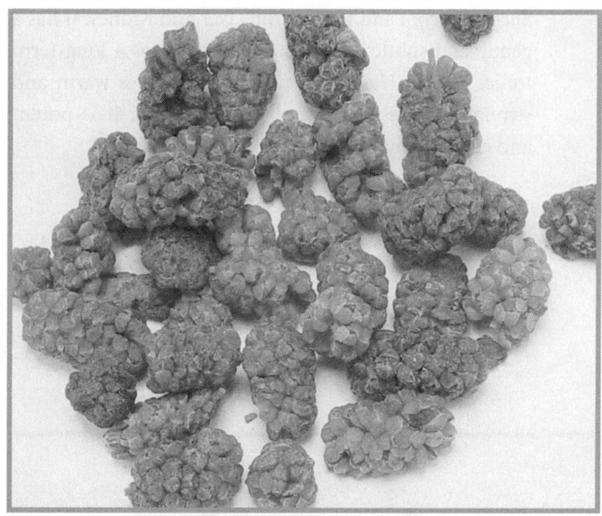

桑椹子

Pinyin Name: *Sang Shen Zi*
Literal Name: "mori seed"
Alternate Chinese Names: *Sang Shen*
Original Source: *Xin Xiu Ben Cao* (Newly Revised Materia Medica) by Su Jing in 657-659 A.D.
English Name: mulberry fruit
Botanical Name: *Morus alba* L. (*Sang*)
Pharmaceutical Name: Fructus Mori
Properties: sweet, cold
Channels Entered: Heart, Liver, Kidney

CHINESE THERAPEUTIC ACTIONS

1. Tonifies Yin and Nourishes Blood

Yin and blood deficiencies of the Liver and Kidney: This condition is characterized by symptoms such as dizziness, vertigo, blurry vision, prematurely gray hair, soreness and weakness of the lower back and knees, tinnitus, and insomnia. *Sang Shen Zi* (Fructus Mori) is a sweet fruit with light tonic properties that make it suitable for long-term use. The decoction, powdered or fresh form of this fruit is often mixed with honey.

- Yin and blood deficiencies of the Liver and Kidney: combine *Sang Shen Zi* with honey.
- Prematurely gray hair: use this herb with *He Shou Wu* (Radix Polygoni Multiflori), *Han Lian Cao* (Herba Ecliptae), *Nu Zhen Zi* (Fructus Ligustri Lucidi), and *Sheng Di Huang* (Radix Rehmanniae).
- Amenorrhea caused by anemia: add it to *Ji Xue Teng* (Caulis Spatholobi) and *Hong Hua* (Flos Carthami), and cook with grain-based liquor and water.

2. Generates Body Fluids

Thirst and body fluid deficiency: *Sang Shen Zi* generates body fluids, replenishes yin, and tonifies blood.

- Thirst, with heat sensations: combine *Sang Shen Zi* with *Sheng Di Huang* (Radix Rehmanniae), *Shi Hu* (Herba Dendrobii), *Mai Men Dong* (Radix Ophiopogonis), *Yu Zhu* (Rhizoma Polygonati Odorati), and *Sha Shen* (Radix Glehniae seu Adenophorae).
- Thirst and hot flashes: add this herb to *Shi Gao* (Gypsum Fibrosum), *Zhi Mu* (Radix Anemarrhenae), *Tian Men Dong* (Radix Asparagi), and *Tian Hua Fen* (Radix Trichosanthis).
- Thirst and fatigue from qi deficiency: use it with *Xi Yang Shen* (Radix Panacis Quinquefolii), *Tai Zi Shen* (Radix Pseudostellariae), and *Huang Qi* (Radix Astragali).

3. Lubricates the Intestines

Constipation caused by dryness: Lack of nourishment to the bowels leads to dry stools or constipation. *Sang Shen Zi* nourishes yin and blood to lubricate the Large Intestine and promote bowel movement. It can be used alone for mild cases of constipation.

- Constipation or dry stools: use *Sang Shen Zi* alone, cooked in a large quantity of water and served with honey.
- Chronic constipation: combine it with *He Shou Wu* (Radix Polygoni Multiflori), *Rou Cong Rong* (Herba Cistanches), *Hei Zhi Ma* (Semen Sesami Nigrum) and *Huo Ma Ren* (Fructus Cannabis).
- Constipation and dry stools with abdominal bloating: use it with *Zhi Ke* (Fructus Aurantii).

DOSAGE

10 to 15 grams in decoction. *Sang Shen Zi* is also used in paste, grain-based liquor, pill or powder forms.

CAUTIONS / CONTRAINDICATIONS

- Use *Sang Shen Zi* with caution in Spleen- and Stomach-deficient patients who have diarrhea or loose stools.

CHEMICAL COMPOSITION

Rutin, carotene, vitamin A, B_1, B_2, C; protein, sugars, anthocyanidinglucoside, lipids, cyanidin.

AUTHORS' COMMENTS

Sang Shen Zi and *Gou Qi Zi* (Fructus Lycii) are mild tonics that can be taken over a long period of time to enhance general health and promote longevity.

Sang Shen Zi and *Shu Di Huang* (Radix Rehmanniae Preparata) are both excellent yin and blood tonics. *Sang*

17 TONIC HERBS

Sang Shen Zi (Fructus Mori)

Shen Zi is cool and tonifies the Liver and Kidney. It has a gentle and subtle effect, and works well as a long-term tonic. *Shu Di Huang*, on the other hand, is warm and strongly nourishes yin and tonifies blood. It is potent and exerts immediate effects.

References

1. *Xian Dai Zhong Yao Yao Li Xue* (Contemporary Pharmacology of Chinese Herbs), 1997; 1364

Han Lian Cao (Herba Ecliptae)

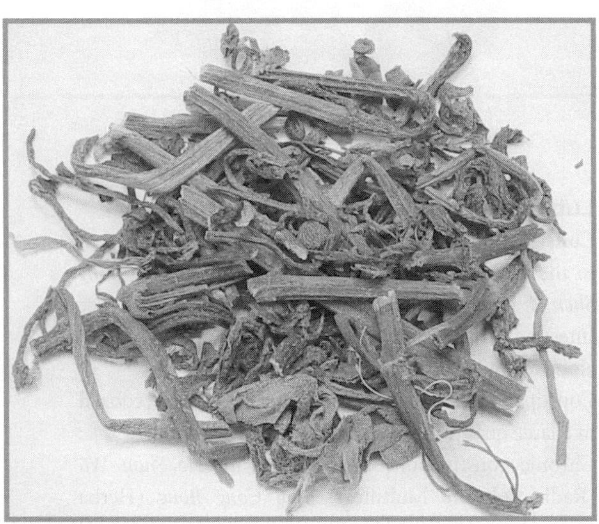

旱蓮草 旱莲草

Pinyin Name: *Han Lian Cao*
Alternate Chinese Names: *Mo Han Lian, Li Chang*
English Name: eclipta
Botanical Name: *Eclipta prostrata* L.
Pharmaceutical Name: Herba Ecliptae
Properties: sweet, sour, cold
Channels Entered: Liver, Kidney

CHINESE THERAPEUTIC ACTIONS

1. Nourishes Yin and Tonifies the Kidney

Liver and Kidney yin deficiencies: The Liver stores blood and opens to the eyes. The Kidney dominates the bones and generates *jing* (essence) and marrow. Signs of Liver and Kidney yin deficiencies include dizziness, vertigo, blurred vision, prematurely gray hair, and soreness and weakness of the lower back and knees. Because *Han Lian Cao* (Herba Ecliptae) is sour and cold, it is excellent to treat yin-deficient heat.

- Yin deficiency of the Liver and Kidney: pair *Han Lian Cao* with *Nu Zhen Zi* (Fructus Ligustri Lucidi). **Exemplar Formula:** *Er Zhi Wan* (Two-Ultimate Pill).
- Prematurely gray hair: combine this herb with *He Shou Wu* (Radix Polygoni Multiflori), *Sang Shen Zi* (Fructus Mori) and *Nu Zhen Zi* (Fructus Ligustri Lucidi).

2. Cools the Blood and Stops Bleeding

Bleeding caused by heat in the vessels: Excess heat in the vessels pushes blood out, creating symptoms of vomiting, hemoptysis, epistaxis, uterine bleeding, hematuria, hematochezia, subcutaneous bleeding or purpura. *Han Lian Cao* is an essential herb that enters the Liver channel to cool the blood and stop bleeding. The fresh herb is usually used for this function as it is stronger in cooling the blood than the dried form.

- General bleeding: combine *Han Lian Cao* with *Sheng Di Huang* (Radix Rehmanniae), *Bai Mao Gen* (Rhizoma Imperatae), *E Jiao* (Colla Corii Asini), *Ce Bai Ye* (Cacumen Platycladi) and *Pu Huang* (Pollen Typhae).
- Hematuria: incorporate this herb with *Sheng Di Huang* (Radix Rehmanniae), *Xuan Shen* (Radix Scrophulariae), *Bai Mao Gen* (Rhizoma Imperatae), charred *Huang Bai* (Cortex Phellodendri), *Da Ji* (Herba seu Radix Cirsii Japonici), *Xiao Ji* (Herba Cirisii), *Qu Mai* (Herba Dianthi) and *Ze Xie* (Rhizoma Alismatis).
- Hematemesis: use it with *Shi Gao* (Gypsum Fibrosum), *Zhi Mu* (Radix Anemarrhenae), *Huang Qin* (Radix Scutellariae), *Bai Ji* (Rhizoma Bletillae) and charred *Ou Jie* (Nodus Nelumbinis Rhizomatis).
- Hematochezia: combine this herb with *Di Yu* (Radix Sanguisorbae), charred *Huai Hua* (Flos Sophorae),

Han Lian Cao (Herba Ecliptae)

Huang Bai (Cortex Phellodendri) and *Fang Feng* (Radix Saposhnikoviae).

- External bleeding due to trauma: mash fresh *Han Lian Cao* into a paste or use the powdered form and apply topically to stop bleeding.

DOSAGE

10 to 30 grams in decoction. *Han Lian Cao* is also used in paste, juice, pill or powder forms. The fresh herb has a stronger function to clear heat and cool the blood than the dried herb.

CAUTIONS / CONTRAINDICATIONS

- Use *Han Lian Cao* with caution for Spleen and Kidney deficiencies, and patients experiencing cold and diarrhea.
- Use it with caution for Spleen qi-deficient patients who have food stagnation.

CHEMICAL COMPOSITION

Wedololactone, demethyl wedelolactone, α-terthienyl, α-terthienylmethanol, α-formyl-α-terthienyl, ecliptine.[1]

PHARMACOLOGICAL EFFECTS

- **Hemostatic:** In dogs with external bleeding, good hemostatic results were achieved following topical application of *Han Lian Cao* powder or powdered extract, with slight pressure, on the wound.[2]
- **Antibiotic:** This herb has inhibitory action on *Staphylococcus aureus* and *Bacillus dysenteriae*.[3]

CLINICAL STUDIES AND RESEARCH

- **Dysentery:** An herbal decoction containing *Han Lian Cao* and sugar has shown remarkable effectiveness for treatment of dysentery. Response was observed following the first dose, with complete recovery within 3 to 4 doses in most cases. The herbal formula contained 125 grams of *Han Lian Cao* and 31 grams of sugar. White (refined) sugar was used for patients with bloody dysentery, and brown sugar was used for patients with white mucus dysentery.[4]
- **Coronary artery disease (CAD):** In one study, 30 patients with CAD were treated with 96.7% effectiveness using a water extract of *Han Lian Cao*. The treatment protocol was to administer 15 grams of the extract (equivalent to 30 grams of dried herb) twice daily for one month per course of treatment. Marked improvement was noted in most patients after 2 to 4 months of herbal therapy. The effectiveness was attributed to the function of the herb to dilate the coronary artery, increase blood perfusion to the cardiac muscle, and increase resistance to hypoxia.[5]
- **Bleeding:** Two patients with profuse bleeding experienced complete recovery following treatment with *Han Lian Cao*. The diagnosis according to traditional Chinese medicine was excessive heat in the interior with yin deficiency, leading to reckless movement of the blood. The treatment protocol was to administer 2,000 ml of juice from fresh *Han Lian Cao*. A decoction of other herbs was also used as supportive treatment.[6]

SUPPLEMENT

- 紅旱連 / 红旱连 *Hong Han Lian* (Herba Hypericum Ascyron) is sometimes used as a substitute for *Han Lian Cao*. *Hong Han Lian* is stronger in cooling the blood, invigorating blood circulation, and healing sores and ulcers. *Han Lian Cao* is more effective in tonifying the Kidney yin and stops bleeding.

AUTHORS' COMMENTS

The juice of *Han Lian Cao* treats diphtheria and dysentery when ingested orally, and treats headaches when applied topically to the nasal cavity.

Han Lian Cao and *Nu Zhen Zi* (Fructus Ligustri Lucidi) both tonify Liver and Kidney yin and treat symptoms of dizziness, tinnitus, vertigo, premature graying of hair, and soreness and weakness of the lower back and knees. *Han Lian Cao* is stronger in cooling the blood to stop various kinds of bleeding. *Nu Zhen Zi* treats hot flashes and steaming bones sensations arising from deficiency heat.

According to Dr. Zhang You-Fen, the following tincture promotes hair growth. Steam 20 grams of *Han Lian Cao* for 20 minutes. Allow it to cool, then soak the steamed herb in 75% alcohol for three days. Apply the tincture generously to bald areas. After it dries, use a plum blossom needle to tap the area for 5 minutes. Repeat daily.

References

1. *Xian Dai Zhong Yao Yao Li Xue* (Contemporary Pharmacology of Chinese Herbs), 1997; 1366-1367
2. *Yi Yao Za Zhi* (Journal of Medicine and Herbology), 1981, 101(6):501
3. *Xin Hua Ben Cao Gang Mu* (New Chinese Materia Medica), 1990:415
4. *Zhong Yi Za Zhi* (Journal of Chinese Medicine), 1965; 5:29
5. *Tian Jing Yi Yao* (Tianjing Medicine and Herbology), 1986; 8:490
6. *Zhe Jiang Zhong Yi Za Zhi* (Zhejiang Journal of Chinese Medicine), 1988; 2:55

Nu Zhen Zi (Fructus Ligustri Lucidi)

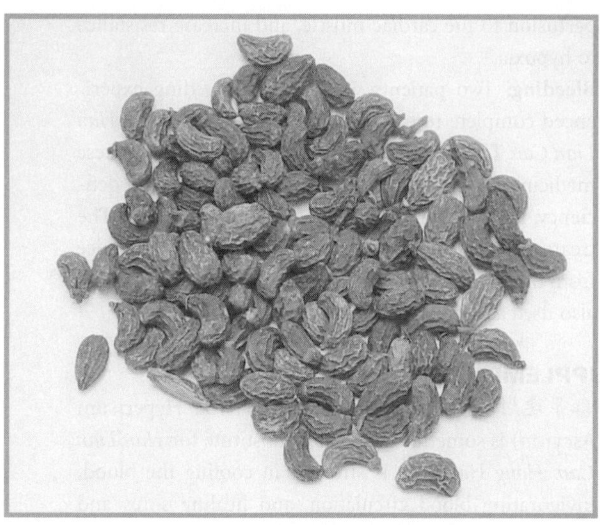

女貞子 女贞子

Pinyin Name: *Nu Zhen Zi*
Literal Name: "female chastity seed"
Alternate Chinese Names: *Nu Zhen, Dong Qing Zi, Nu Zhen Shi*
Original Source: *Shen Nong Ben Cao Jing* (Divine Husbandman's Classic of the Materia Medica) in the second century
English Name: ligustrum, glossy privet fruit
Botanical Name: *Ligustrum lucidum* Ait. (*Nu Zhen*)
Pharmaceutical Name: Fructus Ligustri Lucidi
Properties: sweet, bitter, cool
Channels Entered: Liver, Kidney

CHINESE THERAPEUTIC ACTIONS

1. Tonifies the Liver and Kidney

Liver and Kidney yin and *jing* (essence) deficiencies: Manifestations include dizziness, tinnitus, vertigo, prematurely gray hair, and soreness and weakness of the lower back and knees. *Nu Zhen Zi* (Fructus Ligustri Lucidi) is a light tonic that is not stagnating in nature, and is suitable for use over a long period of time. It is best for yin deficiency with heat.

- Prematurely gray hair: combine *Nu Zhen Zi* with *Han Lian Cao* (Herba Ecliptae), *He Shou Wu* (Radix Polygoni Multiflori), *Sang Shen Zi* (Fructus Mori), and *Hei Zhi Ma* (Semen Sesami Nigrum).
- Dizziness, tinnitus, loose teeth, and soreness and weakness of the lower back and knees: add this herb to *Sang Shen Zi* (Fructus Mori), *Shu Di Huang* (Radix Rehmanniae Preparata), *Du Zhong* (Cortex Eucommiae), *Shan Yao* (Rhizoma Dioscoreae), and *Han Lian Cao* (Herba Ecliptae).
- Constipation: combine this herb with *Huo Ma Ren* (Fructus Cannabis) and *Yu Li Ren* (Semen Pruni).

Yin-deficient heat, menopause: *Nu Zhen Zi* nourishes yin and dispels deficiency heat to treat symptoms of irritability, tidal fever, hot flashes, thirst, night sweats, mood swings, steaming bones sensations and other symptoms and signs of Liver and Kidney yin and *jing* deficiencies.

- Irritability and mood swings: combine *Nu Zhen Zi* with *Han Lian Cao* (Herba Ecliptae), *Yin Chai Hu* (Radix Stellariae), *He Huan Hua* (Flos Albiziae), *Long Gu* (Os Draconis) and *Mu Li* (Concha Ostreae).
- Hot flashes and steaming bones sensations: add it to *Di Gu Pi* (Cortex Lycii), *Mu Dan Pi* (Cortex Moutan), *Qing Hao* (Herba Artemisiae Annuae), *Bai Wei* (Radix Cynanchi Atrati) and *Hu Huang Lian* (Rhizoma Picrorhizae).
- Thirst: combine this herb with *Mai Men Dong* (Radix Ophiopogonis), *Sheng Di Huang* (Radix Rehmanniae), and *Zhi Mu* (Radix Anemarrhenae).
- Night sweats: incorporate *Nu Zhen Zi* with *Fu Xiao Mai* (Semen Tritici Aestivi Levis) and *Wu Wei Zi* (Fructus Schisandrae Chinensis).

2. Clears Heat and Brightens the Eyes

Eye disorders: The Liver opens to the eyes and lack of nourishment from the Liver results in diminished vision, blurred vision, and dry eyes. Rising Liver yang also causes redness and pain in the eyes. *Nu Zhen Zi* can be used in both excess and deficient types of eye disorders.

- Red and painful eyes due to Liver yang rising: combine *Nu Zhen Zi* with *Jue Ming Zi* (Semen Cassiae), *Xia Ku Cao* (Spica Prunellae) and *Qing Xiang Zi* (Semen Celosiae).
- Blurred vision from deficiency: use it with *Gou Qi Zi* (Fructus Lycii), *Shu Di Huang* (Radix Rehmanniae Preparata), *Tu Si Zi* (Semen Cuscutae), *Fu Pen Zi* (Fructus Rubi) and *Chu Shi Zi* (Fructus Broussonetiae).

DOSAGE

10 to 15 grams in decoction. *Nu Zhen Zi* is also used as paste or pills. The unprocessed herb has a stronger effect to nourish yin and moisten dryness, and is commonly used to treat dizziness, vertigo and constipation. The steamed herb (with grain-based liquor) has a stronger effect to tonify the Liver and Kidney, and is commonly used to treat dizziness, vertigo, tinnitus, blurred vision, and prematurely gray hair.

CAUTIONS / CONTRAINDICATIONS

- Use of *Nu Zhen Zi* is contraindicated for patients who

Nu Zhen Zi (Fructus Ligustri Lucidi)

have yang deficiency, or deficiency and cold of the Spleen and Stomach, characterized by diarrhea.

CHEMICAL COMPOSITION

Oleanolic acid, nuzhenide, ligustroside, olenropein, betulin, lupeol, salidroside, ursolic acid, palmitic acid, ursolic acid, rutin, quercetin.[1,2]

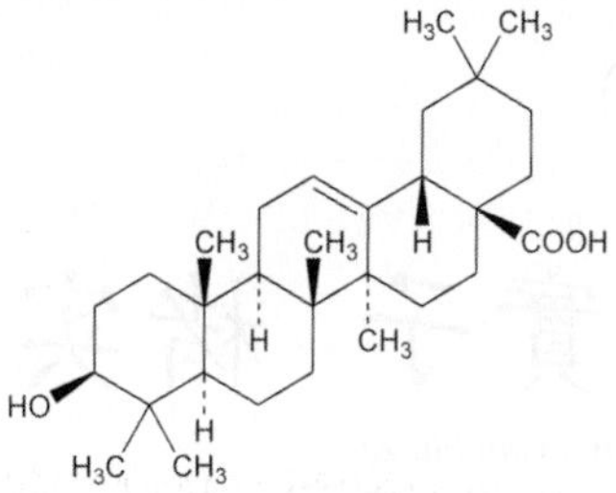

Oleanolic Acid

PHARMACOLOGICAL EFFECTS

- **Immunostimulant:** Administration of *Nu Zhen Zi* is associated with an increase in white blood cells. It is also effective in reversing neutropenia induced by chemotherapy treatment.[3]
- **Antidiabetic:** Decoction of *Nu Zhen Zi* is associated with a marked reduction of plasma glucose levels. It also counters the sharp rise of plasma glucose levels associated with epinephrine and ingestion of glucose. It is commonly used for prevention and treatment of diabetes mellitus.[4]
- **Antihyperlipidemic:** Administration of *Nu Zhen Zi* powder in rabbits at the dosage of 20 grams per day for 46 days showed a significant reduction of plasma cholesterol and triglyceride levels.[5]
- **Hematological:** Administration of *Nu Zhen Zi* stimulates the production of blood in mice.[6]
- **Anti-inflammatory:** Administration of *Nu Zhen Zi* at dosages of 12.5 to 25.0 g/kg in mice is associated with a reduction in swelling, inflammation and permeability of the blood vessels.[7]
- **Hepatoprotective:** Oleanolic acid has been shown to lower elevated liver enzyme levels and prevent liver damage caused by carbon tetrachloride.[8]
- **Antibiotic:** *Nu Zhen Zi* has an inhibitory effect against *Staphylococcus aureus*, *Bacillus dysenteriae*, *Salmonella typhi*, *Pseudomonas aeruginosa*, and *E. coli*.[9]

CLINICAL STUDIES AND RESEARCH

- **Chronic hepatitis:** In one study, 222 patients with chronic hepatitis were treated with an herbal preparation with an overall rate of effectiveness of 69.8%. The herbal treatment contained oleanolic acid isolated from *Nu Zhen Zi* and *Qing Ye Dan* (Herba Swertiae Mileensis).[10]
- **Neutropenia:** Intramuscular injection of 100% *Nu Zhen Zi* is commonly used as the supportive treatment in patients with neutropenia due to chemotherapy and radiation treatments. [11]
- **Hypercholesterolemia:** According to one report, 30 patients with high cholesterol were treated with a preparation of *Nu Zhen Zi* (equivalent to 5.3 grams of dried herb per day) for one month. Reduction of total cholesterol and β-lipoprotein levels was reported in 70.6% of patients.[12]

HERB-DRUG INTERACTION

- **Antidiabetics:** Herbs that lower plasma glucose levels, such as *Nu Zhen Zi,* should be used with caution with insulin, sulfonylureas, and other antidiabetic medications, as the combination may have a synergistic effect, leading to hypoglycemia.[13] [Note: Examples of antidiabetic drugs include insulin, tolbutamide (Orinase), glipizide (Glucotrol), and glyburide (DiaBeta/Micronase).]

TOXICOLOGY

Nu Zhen Zi is very safe. No side effects or adverse reactions were observed following one-time ingestion of 75 grams of the herb by rabbits.[14]

AUTHORS' COMMENTS

Nu Zhen Zi also treats tuberculosis of the lung or lymph nodes in patients with signs of yin deficiency and tidal fever.

Nu Zhen Zi and *Gou Qi Zi* (Fructus Lycii) are both mild tonics for the Liver and Kidney. *Nu Zhen Zi* nourishes only yin. *Gou Qi Zi* tonifies both yin and qi.

Nu Zhen Zi and *Han Lian Cao* (Herba Ecliptae) both tonify Liver and Kidney yin and treat common symptoms of dizziness, tinnitus, vertigo, premature graying of hair, and soreness and weakness of the lower back and knees. *Nu Zhen Zi* also treats hot flashes and steaming bones sensations from deficiency heat. *Han Lian Cao* more strongly cools the blood to stop various kinds of bleeding.

References

1. *Xian Dai Zhong Yao Yao Li Xue* (Contemporary Pharmacology of Chinese Herbs), 1997; 1374
2. *The Merck Index* 12th edition, Chapman & Hall/CRCnetBASE/Merck, 2000
3. *Zhong Cheng Yao Yan Jiu* (Research of Chinese Patent Medicine), 1982; (1):42
4. *Zhong Guo Zhong Yao Za Zhi* (People's Republic of China Journal of Chinese Herbology), 1992; 17(7):429
5. *Jin Zhou Yi Xue Yuan Xue Bao* (Journal of Jinzhou University of Medicine), 1983; 4(1):40
6. *Zhong Yao Tong Bao* (Journal of Chinese Herbology), 1983; 8(6):35
7. *Zhong Guo Zhong Yao Za Zhi* (People's Republic of China Journal of Chinese Herbology), 1989; 14(7):47
8. Ibid., 1992; 17(9):531
9. *Zhong Yao Xue* (Chinese Herbology), 1998; 865:867
10. *Zhong Cao Yao* (Chinese Herbal Medicine), 1980; 10:443

Nu Zhen Zi (Fructus Ligustri Lucidi)

11. *Zhong Yao Yao Li Yu Ying Yong* (Pharmacology and Applications of Chinese Herbs), 1983
12. *Liao Ning Zhong Yi Za Zhi* (Liaoning Journal of Chinese Medicine), 1981; 6:36
13. Chen, J. Recognition & prevention of herb-drug interactions, *Medical Acupuncture*, Fall/Winter 1998/1999; volume 10/number 2; 9-13
14. *Zhong Yao Yao Li Yu Ying Yong* (Pharmacology and Applications of Chinese Herbs), 1983:130

Chu Shi Zi (Fructus Broussonetiae)

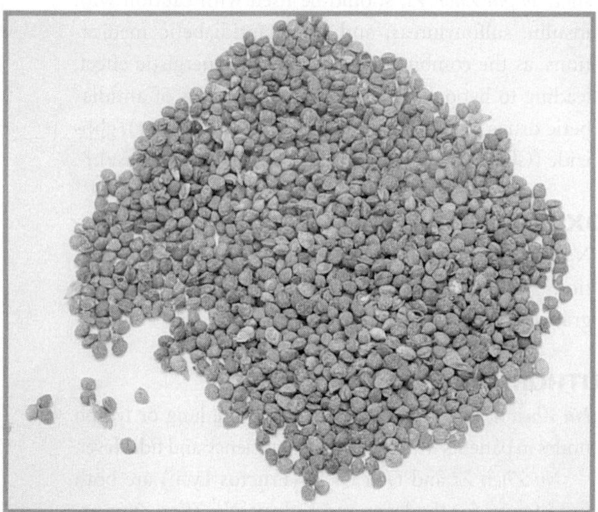

楮實子 楮实子

Pinyin Name: *Chu Shi Zi*
Original Source: *Shen Nong Ben Cao Jing* (Divine Husbandman's Classic of the Materia Medica) in the second century
English Name: broussonetia, paper mulberry fruit
Botanical Name: *Broussonetia papyrifera* (L.) Vent.
Pharmaceutical Name: Fructus Broussonetiae
Properties: sweet, cold
Channels Entered: Kidney, Liver

CHINESE THERAPEUTIC ACTIONS

Tonifies the Kidney and Liver

Chu Shi Zi (Fructus Broussonetiae) tonifies the Kidney and Liver to treat disorders such as weakness and deficiency, dizziness, blurred vision, and edema. It may be used internally or topically.

DOSAGE

6 to 15 grams.

Gui Ban (Plastrum Testudinis)

龜板 龟板

Pinyin Name: *Gui Ban*
Literal Name: "tortoise shell"
Alternate Chinese Names: *Gui Jia, Bai Gui Ban, Zhi Kan Ban, Yuan Wu Ban*
Original Source: *Shen Nong Ben Cao Jing* (Divine Husbandman's Classic of the Materia Medica) in the second century
English Name: testudinis shell (ventral side), tortoise plastron
Zoological Name: *Chinemys reevesii* (Gray) (*Wu Gui*)
Pharmaceutical Name: Plastrum Testudinis
Properties: salty, sweet, cold
Channels Entered: Liver, Kidney, Heart

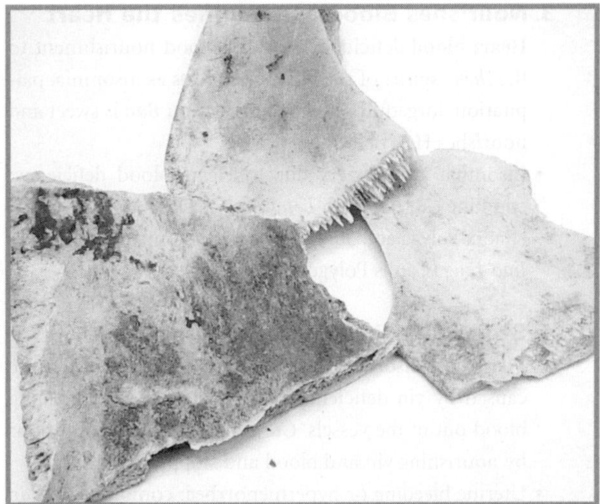

CHINESE THERAPEUTIC ACTIONS

1. Nourishes Yin and Anchors Yang

Liver yin deficiency with rising fire: Dizziness, vertigo, headache, flushed face, red eyes, irritability, and short temper are manifestations of Liver and Kidney yin deficiencies with an inability to control the rising yang. *Gui Ban* (Plastrum Testudinis), cold and heavy in nature, has a sinking tendency that helps anchor yang and nourish yin.

- Liver yang rising: combine *Gui Ban* with *Bai Shao* (Radix Paeoniae Alba), *Huai Niu Xi* (Radix Achyranthis Bidentatae), *Dai Zhe Shi* (Haematitum), *Long Gu* (Os Draconis) and *Shi Jue Ming* (Concha Haliotidis). **Exemplar Formula:** *Zhen Gan Xi Feng Tang* (Sedate the Liver and Extinguish Wind Decoction).
- Red and painful eyes: use it with *Jue Ming Zi* (Semen Cassiae), *Ju Hua* (Flos Chrysanthemi), *Shi Jue Ming* (Concha Haliotidis) and *Xia Ku Cao* (Spica Prunellae).
- Steaming bones sensations, tidal fevers, night sweats, nocturnal emissions: combine this substance with *Shu Di Huang* (Radix Rehmanniae Preparata), *Zhi Mu* (Radix Anemarrhenae), *Mu Dan Pi* (Cortex Moutan) and *Di Gu Pi* (Cortex Lycii).

Liver yin deficiency with Liver wind: The Liver governs the tendons; lack of blood and yin nourishment of the Liver causes stiffness. Prolonged yin deficiency due to febrile disease results in internal movement of Liver wind. Manifestations of these combined pathologies include tremors, dizziness, tinnitus, headache, flushed face, red eyes, short temper, afternoon fever, irritability during the night, convulsions, and in severe cases, stroke and paralysis.

- Liver wind: combine *Gui Ban* with a high dose of *Bai Shao* (Radix Paeoniae Alba), *Gou Teng* (Ramulus Uncariae cum Uncis), *E Jiao* (Colla Corii Asini), *Bie Jia* (Carapax Trionycis) and *Mu Li* (Concha Ostreae).

Yin-deficient heat: *Gui Ban* strongly nourishes yin and dispels deficiency heat. It treats rising deficiency fire that manifests as steaming bones sensations, tidal fevers, night sweats, nocturnal emissions and irritability.

- Yin-deficient heat: use *Gui Ban* with *Shu Di Huang* (Radix Rehmanniae Preparata), *Zhi Mu* (Radix Anemarrhenae) and *Huang Bai* (Cortex Phellodendri).

2. Tonifies the Kidney and Strengthens Bones

Kidney yin and *jing* (essence) deficiencies with weak bones: Kidney *jing*, stored in the marrow, is essential to the health and development of bones. *Jing* deficiency manifests as weakness and soreness of the back and knees, weakness in the legs, retarded skeletal development in children or failure of the fontanelle to close. *Gui Ban* fortifies the bones and strengthens tendons.

- Weakness and soreness of the back and knees: combine this substance with *Shu Di Huang* (Radix Rehmanniae Preparata), *Huai Niu Xi* (Radix Achyranthis Bidentatae), *Shan Yao* (Rhizoma Dioscoreae), *Shan Zhu Yu* (Fructus Corni), *Xu Duan* (Radix Dipsaci), *Du Zhong* (Cortex Eucommiae), *Zhi Mu* (Radix Anemarrhenae) and *Bai Shao* (Radix Paeoniae Alba).
- Kidney yin and yang deficiencies with weak bones, spermatorrhea or nocturnal emissions, weight loss, and blurred vision: add *Gui Ban* to *Lu Rong* (Cornu Cervi Pantotrichum), *Gou Qi Zi* (Fructus Lycii) and *Ren Shen* (Radix Ginseng). **Exemplar Formula:** *Gui Lu Er Xian Jiao* (Tortoise Shell and Deer Antler Syrup).

Guí Ban (Plastrum Testudinis)

3. Nourishes Blood and Tonifies the Heart

Heart blood deficiency: Lack of blood nourishment to the *shen* (spirit) of the Heart manifests as insomnia, palpitation, forgetfulness, and anxiety. *Gui Ban* is sweet and nourishes Heart blood.

- Insomnia and anxiety due to Heart blood deficiency: combine *Gui Ban* with *Long Gu* (Os Draconis), *Yuan Zhi* (Radix Polygalae), *Shi Chang Pu* (Rhizoma Acori) and *Ye Jiao Teng* (Caulis Polygoni Multiflori).

4. Stops Bleeding

Menstrual disorders: Irregular uterine bleeding may be caused by yin deficiency, with deficiency heat pushing blood out of the vessels. *Gui Ban* treats such conditions by nourishing yin and blood and stopping bleeding.

- Uterine bleeding or hypermenorrhea: combine *Gui Ban* with *Sheng Di Huang* (Radix Rehmanniae), *Xuan Shen* (Radix Scrophulariae), *E Jiao* (Colla Corii Asini), *Huang Qin* (Radix Scutellariae), *Bai Shao* (Radix Paeoniae Alba), *Huang Bai* (Cortex Phellodendri), *Bai Mao Gen* (Rhizoma Imperatae), charred *Ce Bai Ye* (Cacumen Platycladi) and *Qian Cao* (Radix Rubiae).

5. Promotes Healing of Sores

Non-healing sores and ulcerations: Calcined *Gui Ban* powder is used topically to treat non-healing sores and ulcerations.

DOSAGE

10 to 30 grams in decoction. *Gui Ban* is also used in paste, pill or powder form. It should be crushed to increase surface area and pre-decocted to facilitate extraction. The unprocessed form is used for nourishing yin and dispelling deficiency heat. The vinegar-processed form dissipates nodules and softens masses.

CAUTIONS / CONTRAINDICATIONS

- Use of *Gui Ban* is contraindicated during pregnancy and for patients with diarrhea, deficiency-related cold, or damp-cold.

CHEMICAL COMPOSITION

Collagen, protein, lipids, amino acids, calcium, phosphorus.[1]

PHARMACOLOGICAL EFFECTS

- **Hepatic:** Preliminary reports have indicated that *Gui Ban* is beneficial for treatment of sarcoma and liver cirrhosis with ascites.[2]

CLINICAL STUDIES AND RESEARCH

- **Scrofula:** An ointment containing *Gui Ban* powder and petroleum jelly has been shown to be beneficial in treatment of scrofula. With daily application, recovery is generally reported within 6 to 7 treatments.[3]
- **Burns:** In one study, 53 patients with burns were treated by topical application of an herbal preparation, with marked success. The herbal formula was prepared by mixing equal portions of fine powder of charred *Gui Ban* and charred *Di Yu* (Radix Sanguisorbae) with sesame oil, to make a paste. The treatment protocol was to clean the wound first, then apply the herbal paste to the affected area, twice daily until recovery.[4]

SUPPLEMENT

- 龜板膠 / 龟板胶 *Gui Ban Jiao* (Gelatinum Plastrum Testudinis), first cited in *Ben Cao Zheng* (Rectification of the Materia Medica), is the gelatin made from turtle shells. Compared to *Gui Ban*, it has similar properties but a richer function to tonify yin and stop bleeding. The usual dosage for *Gui Ban Jiao* is 3 to 10 grams. It is usually dissolved with the decoction prior to ingestion, rather than cooked in the decoction.

AUTHORS' COMMENTS

Gui Ban and *Bie Jia* (Carapax Trionycis) both nourish Liver yin and anchor yang. Please refer to *Bie Jia* for comparative functions.

Originally, only the ventral part (yin side) of the shell was used as a yin tonic. Currently, both the ventral and dorsal sides are used. Research has shown the active components to be the same for both the dorsal and ventral sides. Also, it was found that the dorsal shell has twice as much gelatin as the ventral part.

References

1. *Xian Dai Zhong Yao Yao Li Xue* (Contemporary Pharmacology of Chinese Herbs), 1997; 1370
2. *Chang Yong Zhong Yao Xian Dai Yan Jiu Yu Lin Chuan* (Recent Study & Clinical Application of Common Traditional Chinese Medicine), 1995, 660:661
3. *Zhong Ji Yi Kan* (Medium Medical Journal), 1960; (5):34
4. *Chi Jiao Yi Sheng Za Zhi* (Journal of Barefoot Doctors), 1974; (4):44

Bie Jia (Carapax Trionycis)

鱉甲 鳖甲

Pinyin Name: *Bie Jia*
Literal Name: "turtle shell"
Original Source: *Shen Nong Ben Cao Jing* (Divine Husbandman's Classic of the Materia Medica) in the second century
English Name: tortoise shell (dorsal side), turtle shell
Zoological Name: *Trionyx sinensis* Wiegmann (*Bie*)
Pharmaceutical Name: Carapax Trionycis
Properties: salty, cold
Channels Entered: Liver

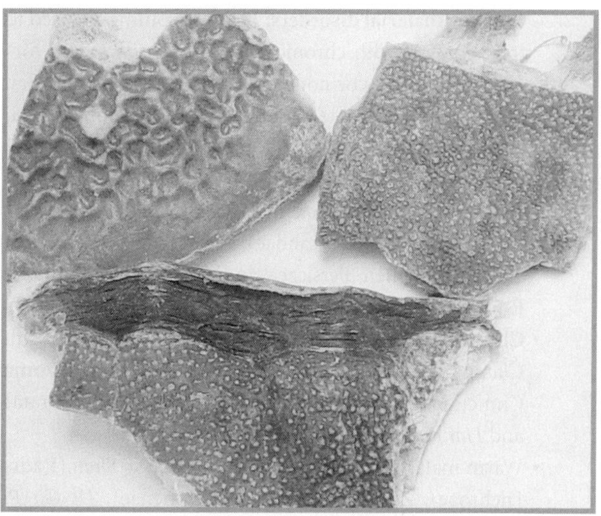

CHINESE THERAPEUTIC ACTIONS

1. Nourishes Yin and Anchors Yang

Yin-deficiency with Liver wind: The Liver governs the tendons and stores blood. Liver yin deficiency can cause tendons to be stiff. Prolonged Liver yin deficiency not only causes yang to rise, but also creates internal movement of Liver wind, which then manifests in tremors, dizziness, tinnitus, headaches, flushed face, red eyes, short temper, muscle spasms, convulsions, and in severe cases, stroke and paralysis. *Bie Jia* (Carapax Trionycis) nourishes yin, anchors yang and is best to address late-stage febrile disease in which both yin and blood are injured.

- Liver wind: combine *Bie Jia* with a high dose of *Bai Shao* (Radix Paeoniae Alba), *Sheng Di Huang* (Radix Rehmanniae), *E Jiao* (Colla Corii Asini), and *Mai Men Dong* (Radix Ophiopogonis). **Exemplar Formula:** *Da Ding Feng Zhu* (Major Arrest Wind Pearl).

Yin-deficient heat: *Bie Jia* treats post-febrile deficiency heat symptoms such as unremitting low-grade fever, afternoon fevers, steaming bones sensations, thirst and night sweats. This substance simultaneously nourishes yin and dispels deficiency heat.

- Yin-deficient heat with feelings of heat during the night and cold during the day, low-grade fever in the absence of perspiration, red tongue, scanty coating and a thready, rapid pulse: combine *Bie Jia* with *Qing Hao* (Herba Artemisiae Annuae), *Mu Dan Pi* (Cortex Moutan), *Sheng Di Huang* (Radix Rehmanniae), and *Zhi Mu* (Radix Anemarrhenae). **Exemplar Formula:** *Qing Hao Bie Jia Tang* (Artemisia Annua and Soft-shelled Turtle Shell Decoction).
- Steaming bones sensations, nighttime fever and night sweats, weight loss, cough and fatigue: combine this substance with *Qin Jiao* (Radix Gentianae Macrophyllae), *Di Gu Pi* (Cortex Lycii), *Chai Hu* (Radix Bupleuri) and *Zhi Mu* (Radix Anemarrhenae). **Exemplar Formula:** *Qin Jiao Bie Jia San* (Gentiana Macrophylla and Soft-shelled Turtle Shell Powder).
- Severe steaming bones sensations: add it to *Di Gu Pi* (Cortex Lycii), *Yin Chai Hu* (Radix Stellariae), *Qing Hao* (Herba Artemisiae Annuae) and *Hu Huang Lian* (Rhizoma Picrorhizae). **Exemplar Formula:** *Qing Gu San* (Cool the Bones Powder).
- Tuberculosis with chronic consumptive dry cough, blood-streaked sputum: combine *Bie Jia* with *Yin Chai Hu* (Radix Stellariae), *Qin Jiao* (Radix Gentianae Macrophyllae), *Qing Hao* (Herba Artemisiae Annuae), *Di Gu Pi* (Cortex Lycii), *Zhi Mu* (Radix Anemarrhenae), *Dang Gui* (Radicis Angelicae Sinensis), *Wu Mei* (Fructus Mume), *Bai Shao* (Radix Paeoniae Alba), *Sheng Di Huang* (Radix Rehmanniae) and *Xuan Shen* (Radix Scrophulariae).

2. Softens Hardness and Dissipates Nodules

Amenorrhea: *Bie Jia* softens hardness and dissipates nodules to treat amenorrhea and masses in the lower *jiao* characterized by blood stagnation. It may also treat amenorrhea caused by yin and blood deficiencies failing to nourish the *ren* (conception) and *chong* (thoroughfare) channels. *Bie Jia* should be combined with other blood-invigorating herbs to enhance overall effectiveness. The vinegar-processed form is often used for this function.

- Amenorrhea or masses from blood stagnation: combine this substance with *Da Huang* (Radix et Rhizoma Rhei), *Tao Ren* (Semen Persicae), *Hong Hua* (Flos Carthami), *Dang Gui Wei* (Extremitas Radicis Angelicae Sinensis), *Chi Shao* (Radix Paeoniae Rubrae), *San Leng* (Rhizoma Sparganii), *E Zhu* (Rhizoma Curcumae), *Gui Zhi* (Ramulus Cinnamomi) and *Chuan Shan Jia* (Squama Manis).

Bie Jia (Carapax Trionycis)

Chronic malarial disorders: *Bie Jia* is commonly used to treat patients with chronic malarial disorders with formation of masses or nodules. *Bie Jia* functions to soften hardness and dissipate nodules. When used alone, *Bie Jia* is relatively weak, thus, it is usually combined with other herbs to amplify its effects.

- Abdominal masses from malaria: use *Bie Jia* with *She Gan* (Rhizoma Belamcandae), *Meng Chong* (Tabanus), *Tao Ren* (Semen Persicae) and *Da Huang* (Radix et Rhizoma Rhei).
- Chronic malarial disorders: combine this substance with *Chang Shan* (Radix Dichroae), *Sheng Ma* (Rhizoma Cimicifugae), *Fu Zi* (Radix Aconiti Lateralis Praeparata) and *Hai Piao Xiao* (Endoconcha Sepiae).
- Warm malarial disorders: use it with *Chang Shan* (Radix Dichroae), *Zhi Mu* (Radix Anemarrhenae), *Di Gu Pi* (Cortex Lycii), *Zhu Ye* (Herba Phyllostachys) and *Shi Gao* (Gypsum Fibrosum).

Organomegaly: *Bie Jia* treats enlargement of internal organs, such as the liver, spleen and thyroid.

- Hepatomegaly or splenomegaly: combine this substance with *Dan Shen* (Radix Salviae Miltiorrhizae), *Hu Zhang* (Rhizoma Polygoni Cuspidati), *Yu Jin* (Radix Curcumae), *Xuan Shen* (Radix Scrophulariae) and *Bai Shao* (Radix Paeoniae Alba).
- Goiter: use *Bie Jia* with *Xuan Shen* (Radix Scrophulariae), *Zhi Mu* (Radix Anemarrhenae), *Zhi Zi* (Fructus Gardeniae), *Xia Ku Cao* (Spica Prunellae), *Chuan Niu Xi* (Radix Cyathulae) and *Mu Li* (Concha Ostreae).
- Intestinal abscesses and abdominal pain: use the calcined form of *Bie Jia* powder.

DOSAGE

10 to 30 grams in decoction. *Bie Jia* is also used in paste, pill or powder forms. It should be crushed to increase surface area, and pre-decocted to facilitate extraction. The calcined powder form of this substance is used externally. The unprocessed form is used for nourishing yin and dispelling deficiency heat. The vinegar-processed form dissipates nodules and softens masses.

CAUTIONS / CONTRAINDICATIONS

- *Bie Jia* is contraindicated during pregnancy, as it has dissipating and dispersing functions.
- It is also contraindicated for Spleen-deficient patients with loose stools or diarrhea, and for patients who have not completely recovered from an exterior disorder.
- Use of *Bie Jia* is associated with occasional cases of allergic response.[1]

CHEMICAL COMPOSITION

Gelatin, collagen, colloid, keratin, iodine, vitamin D.[2]

PHARMACOLOGICAL EFFECTS

- **Effect on the connective tissue:** *Bie Jia* has been shown to inhibit proliferation of connective tissue, and dissolve masses and nodules.[3]
- **Hematological:** It increases plasma protein and treats anemia caused by liver disorders.[4]

CLINICAL STUDIES AND RESEARCH

- **Costal chondritis:** In one study, 48 patients with costal chondritis were divided into two groups: 30 patients treated with Chinese herbs and 18 treated with drugs. The majority of the patients were young adults, slightly more were female than male, and the affected area was generally from the second to the fourth rib. The study reported a 96.67% rate of effectiveness for the herbal group and 55.56% rate of effectiveness for the drug group. The herbal formula contained *Bie Jia*, *Gui Ban* (Plastrum Testudinis), *Chuan Shan Jia* (Squama Manis), *San Leng* (Rhizoma Sparganii), *Zhi Ke* (Fructus Aurantii), *Ding Xiang* (Flos Caryophylli), and *Gan Cao* (Radix Glycyrrhizae). The details of the drug treatment were not available at the time of publication.[5]

SUPPLEMENT

- 鱉甲膠 / 鳖甲胶 *Bie Jia Jiao* (Gelatinum Carapax Trionycis) is the gelatin made from processing *Bie Jia*. It is similar to *Bie Jia*, but *Bie Jia Jiao* is stronger in nourishing yin and is usually used to treat deficiency heat symptoms, including bleeding. Dissolve *Bie Jia Jiao* in decoction prior to ingesting, or take it separately with hot water or warm liquor. It is contraindicated during pregnancy, in cases of Spleen deficiency with loose stools or diarrhea, and for patients who have not completely recovered from an exterior disorder. The usual dosage of *Bie Jia Jiao* is 3 to 10 grams.

AUTHORS' COMMENTS

Bie Jia and *Gui Ban* (Plastrum Testudinis) both nourish Liver yin and anchor yang. Common applicable symptoms include steaming bones sensations, night sweats, nocturnal emissions, tremors, or convulsions. *Bie Jia* softens nodules and breaks stagnation. It is best used for organomegaly or palpable masses in the abdomen. *Gui Ban* strengthens bones to treat weakness of sinews and bones, soreness and pain in the back and knees, and failure of the fontanelle to close. It also calms the *shen* (spirit) and treats palpitations and insomnia.

Bie Jia (Carapax Trionycis)

References

1. *Zhong Yao Tong Bao* (Journal of Chinese Herbology), 1987; 12(6):57
2. *Xian Dai Zhong Yao Yao Li Xue* (Contemporary Pharmacology of Chinese Herbs), 1997; 1373
3. *Zhong Cao Yao Xue* (Study of Chinese Herbal Medicine), 1980:1445
4. Ibid.
5. *Zhong Xi Yi Jie He Za Zhi* (Journal of Integrated Chinese and Western Medicine), 1989; 9(3):179

Hei Zhi Ma (Semen Sesami Nigrum)

黑芝麻

Pinyin Name: *Hei Zhi Ma*
Literal Name: "black sesame seed"
Alternate Chinese Names: *Hu Ma Ren, Zi Ma, Ju Sheng Zi*
Original Source: *Shen Nong Ben Cao Jing* (Divine Husbandman's Classic of the Materia Medica) in the second century
English Name: sesame seed
Botanical Name: *Sesamum indicum* L. (*Zhi Ma*)
Pharmaceutical Name: Semen Sesami Nigrum
Properties: sweet, neutral
Channels Entered: Liver, Kidney

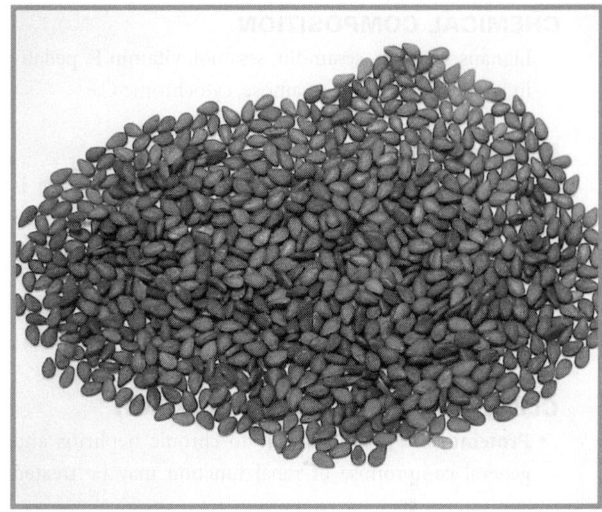

CHINESE THERAPEUTIC ACTIONS

1. Tonifies *Jing* (Essence) and Blood

***Jing* and blood deficiencies:** Liver blood and Kidney *jing* deficiencies cause premature graying, dizziness and blurred vision. *Hei Zhi Ma* (Semen Sesami Nigrum) is mild, and thus not likely to cause stagnation or damage to the Spleen and Stomach. It is suitable for long-term use either by itself or with other herbs. This herb is often served as food with honey or dates, made into congee or used on pancakes.

- Premature gray hair: combine *Hei Zhi Ma* with *He Shou Wu* (Radix Polygoni Multiflori), *Sang Shen Zi* (Fructus Mori), *Han Lian Cao* (Herba Ecliptae) and *Nu Zhen Zi* (Fructus Ligustri Lucidi).
- Blurred vision: add this herb to *Gou Qi Zi* (Fructus Lycii), *Bai Ji Li* (Fructus Tribuli), *Ju Hua* (Flos Chrysanthemi), *Shu Di Huang* (Radix Rehmanniae Preparata) and *Sang Ye* (Folium Mori), with honey.
- Dizziness and tinnitus: incorporate it with *Dang Gui* (Radicis Angelicae Sinensis), *Shu Di Huang* (Radix Rehmanniae Preparata), *Huang Jing* (Rhizoma Polygonati), *E Jiao* (Colla Corii Asini) and *Nu Zhen Zi* (Fructus Ligustri Lucidi).
- Insufficient milk in nursing women because of blood deficiency: combine these seeds with *Huang Qi* (Radix Astragali), *Dang Gui* (Radicis Angelicae Sinensis), *Dang Shen* (Radix Codonopsis), *Chuan Shan Jia* (Squama Manis) and *Wang Bu Liu Xing* (Semen Vaccariae).

2. Moistens Dryness and Lubricates the Intestines

Constipation or dry stools: *Hei Zhi Ma* is rich in oil and lubricates the intestines to treat constipation from lack of blood and body fluids.

- Constipation: combine *Hei Zhi Ma* with *Dang Gui* (Radicis Angelicae Sinensis), *Huo Ma Ren* (Fructus Cannabis), *Bai Zi Ren* (Semen Platycladi) and *Rou Cong Rong* (Herba Cistanches).

DOSAGE

10 to 30 grams in decoction. *Hei Zhi Ma* is also used in the form of pills or powders. It is applied topically as a

Hei Zhi Ma (Semen Sesami Nigrum)

wash, paste or powder. The dry-fried herb is most suitable for internal use.

CAUTIONS / CONTRAINDICATIONS

- Use *Hei Zhi Ma* with caution for patients who have diarrhea.
- Use it with caution for toothache from rising fire.

OVERDOSAGE

Overdose of *Hei Zhi Ma* may cause loose stools and diarrhea.[1]

CHEMICAL COMPOSITION

Lignans, sesamin, sesamdin, sesamol, vitamin E, pedaliin, protein, planteose, sesamose, cytochrome C.[2]

PHARMACOLOGICAL EFFECTS

- **Metabolic:** Administration of *Hei Zhi Ma* in mice is associated with reduction of plasma glucose levels and increased glycogen storage in the liver and muscle tissues. At very large doses, it reduces glycogen storage.[3]
- **Gastrointestinal:** The lipid content of *Hei Zhi Ma* helps to moisten the bowel and relieve constipation.[4]

CLINICAL STUDIES AND RESEARCH

- **Proteinuria:** Proteinuria due to chronic nephritis and general compromise of renal function may be treated effectively within one course of treatment using an herbal formula containing 500 grams each of *Hei Zhi Ma*, *Hu Tao Ren* (Semen Juglandis) and *Da Zao* (Fructus Jujubae). The treatment protocol is to ingest 20 grams of herbal powder with 7 pieces of *Da Zao* three times daily.[5]

AUTHORS' COMMENTS

Hei Zhi Ma treats sores and insect bites when crushed and applied topically. Sesame oil applied topically also treats acute burns.

Hei Zhi Ma is also known as *Hu Ma Ren*, an alternate name. *Hu Ma Ren* (Semen Sesami Nigrum) and *Huo Ma Ren* (Fructus Cannabis) have similar pinyin names, but different functions. *Hu Ma Ren* tonifies the Liver and Kidney, nourishing blood and *jing* (essence) to moisten dryness. *Huo Ma Ren* generates body fluids and treats constipation.

Another seed that should not be confused with or used interchangeably with *Hei Zhi Ma* is the triangularly-shaped *Chong Wei Zi* (Semen Leonuri), which is sweet and cold, and invigorates blood circulation, dispels stagnation, cools the Liver and brightens vision.

References

1. *CA*, 1987; 106:192768h
2. *Xian Dai Zhong Yao Yao Li Xue* (Contemporary Pharmacology of Chinese Herbs), 1997; 1380
3. *Zhong Yao Da Ci Dian* (Dictionary of Chinese Herbs), 1977:2388
4. *Zhong Yao Xue* (Chinese Herbology), 1998; 873:874
5. *He Bei Zhong Yi* (Hebei Chinese Medicine), 1985; 6:21

Bai Mu Er (Fructificatio Tremellae Fuciformis)

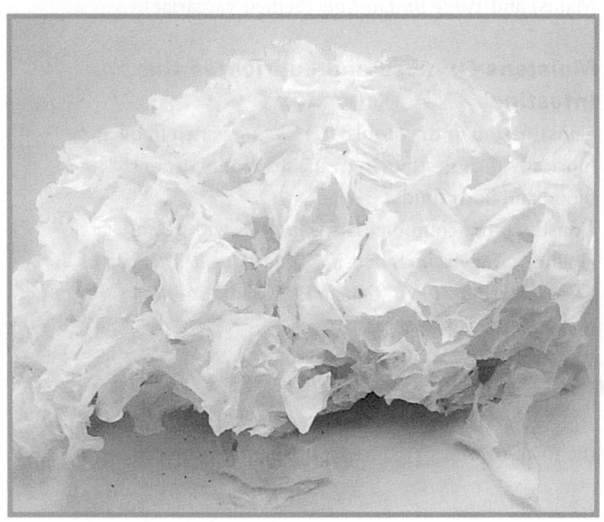

白木耳

Pinyin Name: *Bai Mu Er*
Literal Name: "white wood ear"
Alternate Chinese Names: *Mu Er, Yin Er*
English Name: wood ear, fruiting body of tremella
Botanical Name: *Tremella fuciformis* Berk.
Pharmaceutical Name: Fructificatio Tremellae Fuciformis
Properties: sweet, bland, neutral
Channels Entered: Lung, Stomach

Bai Mu Er (Fructificatio Tremellae Fuciformis)

CHINESE THERAPEUTIC ACTIONS

1. Nourishes Stomach Yin and Generates Body Fluids

Yin deficiency with heat: *Bai Mu Er* (Fructificatio Tremellae Fuciformis) treats yin-deficient heat with emaciation and *wu xin re* (five-center heat).

- *Wu xin re* (five-center heat): combine *Bai Mu Er* with *Di Gu Pi* (Cortex Lycii), *Mu Dan Pi* (Cortex Moutan) and *Yin Chai Hu* (Radix Stellariae).

2. Nourishes Lung Yin and Moistens Dryness

Lung yin deficiency: *Bai Mu Er* treats consumptive dry cough that is non-productive, or is accompanied by scanty, blood-streaked and difficult-to-expectorate sputum.

DOSAGE

3 to 9 grams.

CHEMICAL COMPOSITION

Tremella polysaccharide.[1]

AUTHORS' COMMENTS

Because of its pleasant taste, *Bai Mu Er* is often eaten as a dessert, cooked with *Lian Zi* (Semen Nelumbinis) and rock sugar in water.

References

1. *Xian Dai Zhong Yao Yao Li Xue* (Contemporary Pharmacology of Chinese Herbs), 1997; 1381

Zhi Ju Zi (Fructus Hoveniae)

枳椇子

Pinyin Name: *Zhi Ju Zi*
Alternate Chinese Names: *Ji Ju Zi, Zhi Ju Zi, Mu Shan Hu, Guai Zao Zi, Ji Zua Zi*
English Name: hovenia, trifoliate orange root bark
Botanical Name: *Hovenia dulcis* Thunb.
Pharmaceutical Name: Fructus Hoveniae
Properties: sweet, neutral
Channels Entered: Stomach

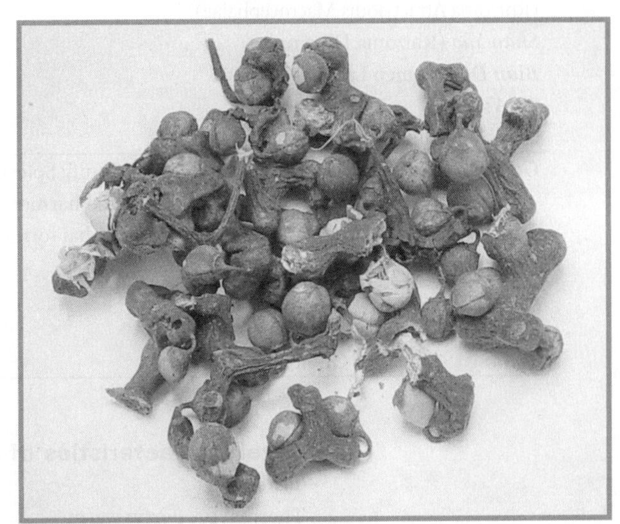

CHINESE THERAPEUTIC ACTIONS

1. Generates Body Fluids

Zhi Ju Zi (Fructus Hoveniae) generates body fluids, and alleviates thirst in cases of febrile disorders or diabetes mellitus.

- Febrile disorders with thirst: use *Zhi Ju Zi* with *Shi Hu* (Herba Dendrobii), *Mai Men Dong* (Radix Ophiopogonis), *Shi Gao* (Gypsum Fibrosum) and *Zhi Mu* (Radix Anemarrhenae).
- Diabetes with thirst: combine this herb with *Shi Gao* (Gypsum Fibrosum), *Zhi Mu* (Radix Anemarrhenae) and *Geng Mi* (Semen Oryzae).

2. Resolves Alcohol Toxicity

- Hangover or alcohol poisoning: use *Zhi Ju Zi* with *Ge Hua* (Flos Puerariae).

DOSAGE

3 to 9 grams.

CHEMICAL COMPOSITION

Sugar, K_2O, potassium, magnesium.

Chapter 17 summary — Tonic Herbs

SECTION 1: QI-TONIFYING HERBS

Name	Similarities	Differences
Ren Shen (Radix Ginseng)	Tonify Spleen and Lung qi	Greatly tonifies *yuan* (source) *qi*, rescues collapse, generates fluids
Xi Yang Shen (Radix Panacis Quinquefolii)		Same as *Ren Shen* but cold in property and stronger in nourishing body fluids
Dang Shen (Radix Codonopsis)		Same as *Ren Shen* but weaker
Tai Zi Shen (Radix Pseudostellariae)		Same as *Ren Shen* but weaker, more suitable for weak patients who cannot take high doses of tonics
Dong Yang Shen (Radix Ginseng Japonica)		Harmonizes middle *jiao*, improves appetite
Huang Qi (Radix Astragali)		Ascends yang qi, consolidates *wei* (defensive) *qi*, dispels water, promotes healing of sores and carbuncles
Jiao Gu Lan (Rhizoma seu Herba Gynostemmatis)	Tonify Lung and Heart	Clears heat, eliminates toxins
Bai Zhu (Rhizoma Atractylodis Macrocephalae)	Tonify Spleen	Dries dampness, dispels water, stops perspiration, stabilizes fetus
Shan Yao (Rhizoma Dioscoreae)		Nourishes yin, benefits Lung and Kidney
Bian Dou (Semen Lablab Album)		Dispels dampness
Ci Wu Jia (Radix et Caulis Acanthopanacis Senticosi)		Tonifies Spleen and Kidney, calms *shen* (spirit)
Gan Cao (Radix Glycyrrhizae)	Tonify Spleen and harmonize herbal formulas	Tonifies Heart qi, moistens the Lung, sedates fire, detoxifies
Da Zao (Fructus Jujubae)		Tonifies blood
Geng Mi (Semen Oryzae)		Strengthens the Spleen and Stomach
Feng Mi (Mel)		Moistens the Lung and intestines, clears heat and eliminates toxins
Yi Tang (Saccharum Granorum)		Reduces pain, relieves cough

General Characteristics of Qi-Tonifying Herbs:

Taste: sweet
Thermal property: warm
Channels entered: Spleen, Lung
Therapeutic actions: tonify Spleen and Lung qi

These herbs tonify Spleen and Lung qi to treat fatigue, lethargy, weak voice, cough or dyspnea, minimal body movement, poor appetite, vomiting, diarrhea or spontaneous sweating.

Ren Shen (Radix Ginseng), ***Xi Yang Shen*** (Radix Panacis Quinquefolii), ***Dang Shen*** (Radix Codonopsis), ***Tai Zi Shen*** (Radix Pseudostellariae), and ***Dong Yang Shen*** (Radix Ginseng Japonica) all tonify Spleen and Lung qi.

Ren Shen is the essential herb to tonify qi and treat qi collapse. It greatly tonifies *yuan* (source) *qi*, and the Spleen and Lung, generates body fluids, relieves thirst and improves cognition. It is most suitable for qi deficiency, qi collapse, deficiency of the Lung and Spleen, thirst, and lack of nourishment to the *shen* (spirit).

Chapter 17 summary

Xi Yang Shen is cold, tonifies qi, nourishes yin, clears fire and generates body fluids. Although *Xi Yang Shen* and *Ren Shen* are both referred to as "ginseng," they differ greatly in therapeutic properties and functions.

Dang Shen, sweet and neutral, is less potent than *Ren Shen*. *Dang Shen* tonifies the middle *jiao*, benefits qi, generates body fluids, and nourishes blood. It is most suitable for patients with qi deficiency of the Lung and Spleen, body fluid loss or blood deficiency. *Dang Shen* is frequently used as an effective and affordable substitute for *Ren Shen*.

Tai Zi Shen, sweet and neutral, and shares similar functions to *Xi Yang Shen* to tonify qi and generate body fluids. *Tai Zi Shen* is mild, and best for qi and body fluid deficiencies with few or no signs of heat.

Dong Yang Shen (cultivated in Japan) is the same plant as *Ren Shen* (grows in northern China and Korea). They have essentially the same functions. *Dong Yang Shen* is described as slightly less potent to tonify qi, but more effective to regulate the middle *jiao*.

Huang Qi (Radix Astragali), sweet and warm, causes yang qi to ascend and is one of the most important herbs when treating chronic deficiency. It tonifies the middle *jiao*, raises yang qi to treat prolapse, tonifies the Lung to strengthen the *wei* (defensive) *qi* and stop spontaneous sweating, promotes healing of sores and carbuncles by generating flesh, and dispels water to relieve edema. *Huang Qi* generates blood and tonifies qi simultaneously, therefore making it ideal for treating *xiao ke* (wasting and thirsting) syndrome, numbness from blood deficiency or post-stroke symptoms.

Jiao Gu Lan (Rhizoma seu Herba Gynostemmatis), though technically not in the "ginseng family," contains ginsenoside and has qi-tonic action. It strengthens the Lung and promotes generation of fluids. It also clears heat, eliminates toxins, and reduces inflammation to treat infection.

Bai Zhu (Rhizoma Atractylodis Macrocephalae), ***Shan Yao*** (Rhizoma Dioscoreae) and ***Bian Dou*** (Semen Lablab Album) all strengthen the Spleen and stop diarrhea.

Bai Zhu most strongly tonifies qi of the middle *jiao*, dries dampness, dispels water, relieves perspiration, and stabilizes the fetus. *Bai Zhu* is best for Spleen qi deficiency with accumulated dampness manifesting as edema and phlegm accumulation, and for spontaneous sweating and restless fetus due to qi deficiency.

Shan Yao tonifies qi, nourishes yin, and benefits the Lung and Kidney. Though mild in potency, it exerts an astringent effect to treat chronic or feeble cough, spermatorrhea, and *xiao ke* (wasting and thirsting) syndrome.

Bian Dou is a less potent qi tonic than the other two. However, it is not stagnating in nature and is an excellent mild tonic for convalescing patients who cannot take heavy tonics. It dissolves summer-damp and clears summer-heat with irritability and thirst.

Ci Wu Jia (Radix et Caulis Acanthopanacis Senticosi), sometimes used as a low-cost substitute for *Ren Shen* (Radix Ginseng), does not have the same effects but adequately tonifies the Spleen and Kidney and calms the *shen* (spirit).

Gan Cao (Radix Glycyrrhizae) and ***Da Zao*** (Fructus Jujubae) tonify the Spleen and are frequently used to harmonize herbal formulas.

Gan Cao tonifies the Spleen, benefits qi, moistens the Lung, relieves cough, clears heat, eliminates toxins, and relieves pain. It has a wide range of functions to treat a variety of disorders. It is also used in many formulas to harmonize other herbs and alleviate unwanted side effects.

Da Zao tonifies the middle *jiao*, benefits qi, and nourishes blood to tranquilize the *shen* (spirit).

Geng Mi (Semen Oryzae) tonifies the Spleen and Stomach and treats digestive disorders. It prevents cold or harsh herbs from damaging the middle *jiao*.

Chapter 17 summary

Feng Mi (Mel) moistens dryness of the Lung, relieves cough, tonifies the middle *jiao*, lubricates the intestines and relieves pain. It treats abdominal pain resulting from deficiency, Lung deficiency with feeble dry cough, and constipation or dry stools. It clears toxins to treat sores, carbuncles, abscesses, burns and eye disorders.

Yi Tang (Saccharum Granorum) tonifies the Spleen, benefits qi and moistens the Lung to relieve cough.

SECTION 2: YANG-TONIFYING HERBS

Name	Similarities	Differences
Lu Rong (Cornu Cervi Pantotrichum)	Tonify Kidney yang	Most strongly tonifies Kidney yang, replenishes *jing* (essence) and blood, strengthens bones and tendons
Lu Jiao (Cornu Cervi)		Strongly tonifies Kidney yang, invigorates blood circulation and disperses blood stasis
Lu Jiao Jiao (Gelatinum Cornu Cervi)		Moderately tonifies Kidney yang and *jing* (essence)
Lu Jiao Shuang (Cornu Cervi Degelatinatum)		Mildly tonifies Spleen and Kidney yang
Dong Chong Xia Cao (Cordyceps)	Tonify Lung and Kidney to stop cough and wheezing	Tonifies Kidney yang and nourishes Lung yin
Ge Jie (Gecko)		Stops wheezing
Hu Tao Ren (Semen Juglandis)		Strengthens the back, moistens bowels, relieves constipation
Rou Cong Rong (Herba Cistanches)	Tonify Kidney yang to treat reproductive disorders	Moistens the bowel, relieves constipation, replenishes *jing* (essence) and blood
Suo Yang (Herba Cynomorii)		Moistens the bowel, relieves constipation
Ba Ji Tian (Radix Morindae Officinalis)		Dispels wind-cold-damp
Yin Yang Huo (Herba Epimedii)		Dispels wind-cold-damp, increases libido, not for long-term use
Xian Mao (Rhizoma Curculiginis)		Dispels wind-cold-damp, not for long-term use
Yang Qi Shi (Actinolitum)		Treats impotence and infertility, not for long-term use
Hai Gou Shen (Testes et Penis Otariae)	Tonify Kidney yang	Tonifies Kidney yang and *jing* (essence)
Hai Shen (Strichopus Japonicus)		Tonifies Kidney yang and *jing* (essence)
Hai Long (Syngnathus)		Tonifies Kidney yang
Hai Ma (Hippocampus)		Tonifies Kidney yang, invigorates blood circulation
Du Zhong (Cortex Eucommiae)	Tonify Liver and Kidney to strengthen bones and tendons	Stabilizes pregnancy, relieves Liver yang rising
Xu Duan (Radix Dipsaci)		Stabilizes pregnancy, connects bones and tendons
Gu Sui Bu (Rhizoma Drynariae)		Connects bones and tendons
Gou Ji (Rhizoma Cibotii)		Dispels wind and dampness, restrains leakage of body fluids
Hu Lu Ba (Semen Trigonellae)		Warms Kidney yang, treats hernia due to cold, dispels wind, cold, or damp
Bu Gu Zhi (Fructus Psoraleae)	Warm Spleen and Kidney yang to treat diarrhea	Warms Kidney yang
Yi Zhi Ren (Fructus Alpiniae Oxyphyllae)		Warms Spleen, retains body fluids
Tu Si Zi (Semen Cuscutae)	Tonify Kidney and Liver, consolidate *jing* (essence)	Retains *jing* (essence), benefits the eyes, stops diarrhea
Sha Yuan Zi (Semen Astragali Complanati)		Retains *jing*, benefits the eyes
Jiu Cai Zi (Semen Allii Tuberosi)		Strengthens yang and consolidates yin
Zi He Che (Placenta Hominis)		Replenishes *jing* and blood, treats degenerative disorders, benefits Lung qi

Chapter 17 summary

General Characteristics of Yang-Tonifying Herbs:

Taste: sweet
Thermal property: warm
Channels entered: Kidney, Spleen, Heart
Therapeutic actions: tonify Kidney, Spleen and Heart yang

Yang-tonic herbs fortify yang and are most suitable for intolerance to cold, cold extremities, soreness and weakness of the lower back and knees, diarrhea, polyuria, enuresis, frequent urinary urges (especially during the night), impotence, infertility and lack of libido in both men and women.

Lu Rong (Cornu Cervi Pantotrichum), ***Lu Jiao*** (Cornu Cervi), ***Lu Jiao Jiao*** (Gelatinum Cornu Cervi), and ***Lu Jiao Shuang*** (Cornu Cervi Degelatinatum) are Kidney yang tonics derived from deer.

Lu Rong tonifies Kidney yang, benefits *jing* (essence) and blood, strengthens tendons and bones, and is extremely effective to replenish the bodily constitution.

Lu Jiao is a similar but weaker substitute for *Lu Rong*. It invigorates blood circulation and reduces swelling to treat sores, swellings, and pain in the low back, or pain affecting bones and tendons.

Lu Jiao Jiao moderately tonifies the Liver and Kidney and benefits *jing* and blood. It treats Kidney yang, *jing* and blood deficiencies in patients who are thin or have bleeding due to deficiency and cold.

Lu Jiao Shuang mildly tonifies Kidney yang. One advantage is that it will not cause indigestion, abdominal fullness, or distention in Kidney yang deficient patients with weak digestive functions. It also has an astringent effect to stop bleeding.

Dong Chong Xia Cao (Cordyceps), ***Ge Jie*** (Gecko) and ***Hu Tao Ren*** (Semen Juglandis) tonify the Lung and Kidney to treat respiratory disorders.

Dong Chong Xia Cao effectively tonifies the Lung and Kidney to treat chronic cough, wheezing and dyspnea with bloody sputum. It is also effective for patients with impotence or spontaneous sweating due to extreme deficiency.

Ge Jie tonifies Lung qi, fortifies Kidney yang, benefits *jing* (essence) and blood, and treats chronic cough, dyspnea and wheezing. This substance also treats impotence due to Kidney yang deficiency.

Hu Tao Ren tonifies the Kidney, benefits *jing* (essence), and warms the Lung to relieve coughing due to Lung qi and Kidney yang deficiencies. It also moistens the intestines and treats constipation due to dryness in the intestines.

Rou Cong Rong (Herba Cistanches) and ***Suo Yang*** (Herba Cynomorii) tonify Kidney yang to enhance sexual and reproductive functions.

Rou Cong Rong more effectively tonifies *jing* (essence) and blood.

Suo Yang more strongly tonifies Kidney yang to treat impotence and infertility. Because *Suo Yang* is a warmer herb, it is also more likely to cause side effects such as dryness or thirst.

Ba Ji Tian (Radix Morindae Officinalis), ***Yin Yang Huo*** (Herba Epimedii) and ***Xian Mao*** (Rhizoma Curculiginis) all tonify the Kidney and fortify yang to treat infertility and impotence. In addition, they dispel wind-dampness to relieve *bi zheng* (painful obstruction syndromes).

Acrid and slightly warm, *Ba Ji Tian* tonifies *jing* (essence) and blood, and treats irregular menstruation caused by deficiency and cold.

Acrid, sweet and warm, *Yin Yang Huo* more strongly tonifies the Kidney. It may be used alone or in combination with other herbs.

Acrid, hot and toxic, *Xian Mao* most strongly tonifies the Kidney and disperses coldness and dampness. In comparison with the herbs above, *Xian Mao* is drier and hotter and must be used with caution, as overdose can injure the yin.

Chapter 17 summary

Yang Qi Shi (Actinolitum) warms and strengthens Kidney yang to treat impotence.

Hai Gou Shen (Testes et Penis Otariae), ***Hai Shen*** (Strichopus Japonicus), ***Hai Long*** (Syngnathus) and ***Hai Ma*** (Hippocampus) are four substances from the ocean that tonify yang.

Hai Gou Shen and *Hai Shen* tonify Kidney yang and *jing* (essence).

Hai Long tonifies Kidney yang, reduces swelling, and dissipates nodules.

Hai Ma tonifies Kidney yang and invigorates blood circulation.

Du Zhong (Cortex Eucommiae), ***Xu Duan*** (Radix Dipsaci), ***Gu Sui Bu*** (Rhizoma Drynariae) and ***Gou Ji*** (Rhizoma Cibotii) all tonify the Liver and Kidney and strengthen tendons and bones, treating weakness and soreness of the back, legs and tendons. They are often used together for synergistic effect.

Du Zhong is the strongest yang tonic of the four. It also calms the fetus and lowers blood pressure.

Xu Duan moderately tonifies yang and stabilizes the fetus. Its strength is to invigorate blood circulation and reconnect tendons and bones. Because of its effect to invigorate blood circulation, it has an excellent ability to tonify without causing stagnation.

Gu Sui Bu tonifies the Kidney, strengthens the bones, relieves pain, and facilitates reconnection of the bones and tendons.

Gou Ji dispels wind-dampness and strongly relieves pain in and around the spine, such as found in *bi zheng* (painful obstruction syndrome) with pain and difficulty bending. *Gou Ji* consolidates Kidney qi to treat urinary incontinence and profuse vaginal discharge.

Hu Lu Ba (Semen Trigonellae), bitter and warm, warms Kidney yang, dispels cold and dampness, and dispels cold attacking the Liver channel.

Bu Gu Zhi (Fructus Psoraleae) and ***Yi Zhi Ren*** (Fructus Alpiniae Oxyphyllae) warm and tonify Spleen and Kidney yang, consolidate *jing* (essence) and retain urine.

Bu Gu Zhi is hot and has a very strong yang-tonic function to strengthen the Kidney, fortify yang, and warm the Spleen to stop diarrhea. Clinical manifestations include impotence, spermatorrhea, enuresis, cough, dyspnea and chronic diarrhea. Soaking this herb in alcohol and applying it topically can treat vitiligo.

Yi Zhi Ren is warm and has a weaker function than *Bu Gu Zhi* to fortify the yang. It tonifies the Spleen to disperse cold and relieve excess saliva or drooling, and warms the Kidney to consolidate *jing* (essence) and retain urine. Clinical applications include abdominal coldness and pain, vomiting, diarrhea, poor appetite, excess salivation and spermatorrhea.

Tu Si Zi (Semen Cuscutae) and ***Sha Yuan Zi*** (Semen Astragali Complanati) tonify the Kidney and Liver, fortify yang, brighten the eyes, consolidate *jing* (essence) and retain urine. Clinical applications include back pain, spermatorrhea, enuresis, diminished vision, dizziness and profuse vaginal discharge from Kidney yang deficiency.

Tu Si Zi, acrid and neutral, tonifies Kidney yin and yang. It is not drying or stagnating, which makes it easy to digest and absorb. It tonifies the Spleen to relieve diarrhea, stabilize the fetus and aid in *xiao ke* (wasting and thirsting) syndrome.

Sha Yuan Zi, sweet, warm and not drying, strongly consolidates fluids.

Jiu Cai Zi (Semen Allii Tuberosi) is warm, tonifies the Liver and Kidney, warms the back and knees, consolidates *jing* (essence) and fortifies yang.

Zi He Che (Placenta Hominis) is considered by some to be the most essential, irreplaceable herb to tonify Kidney *jing* (essence). It is said to have great effectiveness for treating reproductive disorders, promoting normal development of organs, nourishing blood and benefiting Lung qi.

Chapter 17 summary

SECTION 3: BLOOD-TONIFYING HERBS

Name	Similarities	Differences
Dang Gui (Radicis Angelicae Sinensis)	Tonify blood	Invigorates blood circulation, regulates menstruation, relieves pain, lubricates the intestines
Shu Di Huang (Radix Rehmanniae Preparata)		Tonifies Kidney and Liver yin
He Shou Wu (Radix Polygoni Multiflori)		Tonifies Kidney and Liver yin, nourishes *jing* (essence), grows hair, lubricates the intestines, eliminates toxins
Bai Shao (Radix Paeoniae Alba)		Softens the Liver, relieves smooth and skeletal muscle pain and spasms
E Jiao (Colla Corii Asini)		Stops bleeding, nourishes yin, moistens dryness
Long Yan Rou (Arillus Longan)		Tranquilizes the *shen* (spirit)

General Characteristics of Blood-Tonifying Herbs:

Taste: sweet
Thermal property: warm
Channels entered: Spleen, Liver, Heart
Therapeutic actions: tonify blood, nourish yin

Blood-tonic herbs tonify blood and nourish yin to treat pale lips, face and nails, dizziness, tinnitus, palpitations, insomnia, irregular menstruation and anemia.

Dang Gui (Radicis Angelicae Sinensis) is warm, and an excellent herb to tonify blood, invigorate blood circulation, and relieve pain, for any patient with blood deficiency or blood stagnation. Symptoms include irregular menstruation, amenorrhea, dysmenorrhea, gestational and postpartum disorders, sores, abscesses, trauma-related pain, *bi zheng* (painful obstruction syndrome) and various problems of blood deficiency and blood stagnation. *Dang Gui* also lubricates the intestines, for constipation or dry stools caused by blood deficiency.

Shu Di Huang (Radix Rehmanniae Preparata), sweet and slightly warm, nourishes both blood and yin. It is the essential herb in replenishing *jing* (essence) and marrow, and treats Liver blood deficiency and Kidney yin and *jing* deficiencies. Heavy and stagnating in nature, *Shu Di Huang* should be combined with *Sha Ren* (Fructus Amomi) or other digestive herbs.

He Shou Wu (Radix Polygoni Multiflori) is similar to *Shu Di Huang* (Radix Rehmanniae Preparata) in its tonic effect, but slightly milder, with the advantage of not creating stagnations while gently stabilizing and binding.

Prepared *He Shou Wu* tonifies blood, yin, and *jing* (essence).

Unprepared *He Shou Wu* eliminates heat, disperses nodules, and induces bowel movement.

Bai Shao (Radix Paeoniae Alba), cool in thermal property, nourishes blood, astringes yin, sedates rising Liver yang, softens the Liver and relieves pain. Clinical applications include Liver blood deficiency, irregular menstruation, obstetric/gynecologic disorders, deficiency with perspiration, yin deficiency with Liver wind, Liver yang rising and pain associated with lack of nourishment to the Liver.

Dang Gui is more suitable for blood-deficient patients with coldness or blood stagnation.

Bai Shao is more useful for blood deficiency with heat or Liver yang rising, or Liver qi stagnation.

E Jiao (Colla Corii Asini), neutral and sweet, effectively tonifies blood, stops bleeding, nourishes yin and moistens the Lung. It treats blood deficiency and Lung yin deficiency with dry, feeble cough (possibly with blood). *E Jiao* is sticky and not suitable for patients with weak stomachs.

Chapter 17 summary

Long Yan Rou (Arillus Longan) tonifies the blood and calms the *shen* (spirit). It has an excellent effect to tonify qi and blood without creating stagnation such as indigestion, fullness or bloating.

SECTION 4: YIN-TONIFYING HERBS

Name	Similarities	Differences
Bei Sha Shen (Radix Glehniae)	Tonify Lung yin, and promote generation of body fluids	Nourishes Stomach yin
Nan Sha Shen (Radix Adenophorae)		Nourishes Stomach yin, dissolves phlegm
Mai Men Dong (Radix Ophiopogonis)		Nourishes Heart and Spleen yin, relieves constipation
Tian Men Dong (Radix Asparagi)		Nourishes Kidney yin, clears Lung heat and fire
Shi Hu (Herba Dendrobii)		Nourishes Stomach yin, benefits eyes
Yu Zhu (Rhizoma Polygonati Odorati)		Nourishes Lung and Stomach yin
Huang Jing (Rhizoma Polygonati)		Tonifies the Spleen
Bai He (Bulbus Lilii)		Nourishes Stomach yin, clears the Heart and calms *shen* (spirit)
Gou Qi Zi (Fructus Lycii)	Tonify Liver and Kidney yin	Nourishes the Liver, benefits the eyes
Sang Shen Zi (Fructus Mori)		Tonifies Lung yin, promotes generation of body fluids, tonifies blood
Han Lian Cao (Herba Ecliptae)		Tonifies yin, cools blood and stops bleeding
Nu Zhen Zi (Fructus Ligustri Lucidi)		Clears heat, brightens eyes, and increases white blood cell counts
Chu Shi Zi (Fructus Broussonetiae)		Treats dizziness and blurred vision
Gui Ban (Plastrum Testudinis)	Nourish yin and anchor yang	Nourishes Kidney yin to strengthen bones, stops bleeding
Bie Jia (Carapax Trionycis)		Clears deficiency heat, softens hardness and nodules
Hei Zhi Ma (Semen Sesami Nigrum)	Tonify *jing* (essence) and blood	Relieves constipation
Bai Mu Er (Fructificatio Tremellae Fuciformis)	Nourish Stomach yin	Nourishes Lung and Stomach yin
Zhi Ju Zi (Fructus Hoveniae)		Relieves alcohol poisoning

General Characteristics of Yin-Tonifying Herbs:

Taste: sweet
Thermal property: neutral, cool
Channels entered: Kidney, Liver, Stomach, Lung
Therapeutic actions: tonify yin, promote generation of body fluid, anchor yang

Yin-tonic herbs nourish yin, generate body fluids and moisten dryness, treating yin deficiency involving emaciation, dry mouth, dry throat, tidal fever, night sweats, chronic cough with sticky, scanty, difficult-to-expectorate sputum, nocturnal emissions, dry stools or constipation.

Bei Sha Shen (Radix Glehniae) and ***Nan Sha Shen*** (Radix Adenophorae), cool in thermal property, nourish yin, clear and benefit the Lung and generate body fluids, in all types of Lung and Stomach yin deficiency involving heat or injury of body fluids.

Bei Sha Shen, from northern China, more strongly nourishes yin.
Nan Sha Shen, from southern China, more effectively eliminates phlegm.

Mai Men Dong (Radix Ophiopogonis) and ***Tian Men Dong*** (Radix Asparagi) nourish yin, clear the Lung, moisten dryness and generate body fluids for injured yin involving thirst, chronic dry cough, dry stools or constipation.

Chapter 17 summary

Mai Men Dong, cool in thermal property, clears the Heart, reduces irritability and nourishes Stomach yin. It is milder in potency, but less stagnating than *Tian Men Dong*.

Tian Men Dong, stronger in nourishing yin, moistens dryness to clear heat and generate body fluids, treats Kidney yin deficiency and eliminates breast nodules.

Shi Hu (Herba Dendrobii), cool in thermal property, nourishes Stomach yin, generates body fluids, and dispels heat. It also brightens the eyes, strengthens the back and knees, and treats deteriorating vision caused by Liver and Kidney deficiencies.

Yu Zhu (Rhizoma Polygonati Odorati), neutral, mild and moistening, nourishes Lung yin, generates body fluids and nourishes the Stomach, treating Lung and Stomach yin deficiencies, cough due to dryness and heat, and thirst with a dry tongue coat. Mild in potency and gradual in its delivery of therapeutic effects, *Yu Zhu* is less stagnating than other yin tonics and less likely to cause side effects.

Huang Jing (Rhizoma Polygonati), neutral, sweet and rich in fluids, markedly nourishes Lung yin and benefits Spleen qi, for yin deficiency with chronic dry cough, *xiao ke* (wasting and thirsting) syndrome, and Spleen and Stomach deficiency. It replenishes *jing* (essence), generates marrow and is used for various signs and symptoms of Kidney *jing* deficiency.

Bai He (Bulbus Lilii) moistens the Lung to relieve coughing from Lung heat, or chronic coughing with blood. It clears the Heart and calm the *shen* (spirit) to treat irritability, palpitations, insomnia and excessive dreaming.

Gou Qi Zi (Fructus Lycii), sweet and neutral, nourishes the Liver and Kidney, brightens the eyes, and treats dizziness and blurred vision due to Kidney and Liver yin deficiencies. It also nourishes the Lung to treat yin-deficient cough. Mild and non-stagnating in its tonic effect, *Gou Qi Zi* used on a long-term basis will not cause stagnation and dampness in the middle *jiao*.

Sang Shen Zi (Fructus Mori), sweet, cold and moistening, nourishes yin, tonifies blood, generates body fluids, and lubricates the intestines, treating all yin-deficient conditions of damaged body fluids and intestinal dryness. Pleasant tasting and mild, it is suitable for long-term use, but is contraindicated in yang deficiency cold, or dampness arising from Spleen and Stomach deficiency, or food stagnation.

Han Lian Cao (Herba Ecliptae) and ***Nu Zhen Zi*** (Fructus Ligustri Lucidi) nourish Liver and Kidney yin to treat dizziness, vertigo, soreness and weakness of the lower back and knees, and prematurely gray hair.

Han Lian Cao is cold, clears heat, stops bleeding, and treats various bleeding disorders caused by yin deficiency with heat in the blood.

Nu Zhen Zi is cool, tonifies without creating stagnation, brightens the eyes to treat diminished or blurry vision from Liver and Kidney yin deficiencies, and clears yin-deficient heat.

Chu Shi Zi (Fructus Broussonetiae) mildly tonifies the Liver and Kidney.

Gui Ban (Plastrum Testudinis) and ***Bie Jia*** (Carapax Trionycis) nourish yin, anchor yang, and clear deficiency heat, treating steaming bones sensations of yin deficiency, Liver wind rising from yin deficiency, and Liver yang rising.

Gui Ban more strongly nourishes the yin. It also tonifies the Kidney, strengthens the bones, nourishes blood, tonifies the Heart, softens hardness, dispels blood stagnation and stops bleeding.

Bie Jia more effectively clears heat, softens hardness and disperses stagnation.

Chapter 17 summary

Hei Zhi Ma (Semen Sesami Nigrum), sweet, neutral and rich in oil, tonifies *jing* (essence) and blood, lubricates the intestines and treats blood deficiency with dryness in the intestines.

Bai Mu Er (Fructificatio Tremellae Fuciformis) and ***Zhi Ju Zi*** (Fructus Hoveniae) nourish Stomach yin.

Bai Mu Er nourishes both Lung and Stomach, promotes generation of fluids, and moistens dryness.

Zhi Ju Zi nourishes Stomach yin and treats alcohol poisoning and hangover.

HERBS FROM OTHER FUNCTIONAL CATEGORIES WITH TONIC FUNCTIONS

Name	Functional Category
Bai Zi Ren (Semen Platycladi)	*Shen*-Calming Herbs (Chapter 14)
Fu Ling (Poria)	Water-Regulating and Damp-Resolving Herbs (Chapter 6)
Fu Pen Zi (Fructus Rubi)	Astringent Herbs (Chapter 18)
Fu Zi (Radix Aconiti Lateralis Praeparata)	Interior-Warming Herbs (Chapter 7)
Lian Zi (Semen Nelumbinis)	Astringent Herbs (Chapter 18)
Niu Xi (Radix Cyathulae seu Achyranthis)	Blood-Invigorating and Stasis-Removing Herbs (Chapter 12)
Rou Gui (Cortex Cinnamomi)	Interior-Warming Herbs (Chapter 7)
Sang Ji Sheng (Herba Taxilli)	Wind-Damp Dispelling Herbs (Chapter 4)
Shan Zhu Yu (Fructus Corni)	Astringent Herbs (Chapter 18)
Sheng Di Huang (Radix Rehmanniae)	Heat-Clearing Herbs (Chapter 2)
Suan Zao Ren (Semen Zizyphi Spinosae)	*Shen*-Calming Herbs (Chapter 14)
Wu Wei Zi (Fructus Schisandrae Chinensis)	Astringent Herbs (Chapter 18)
Xiao Mai (Fructus Tritici)	*Shen*-Calming Herbs (Chapter 14)
Xuan Shen (Radix Scrophulariae)	Heat-Clearing Herbs (Chapter 2)
Yi Yi Ren (Semen Coicis)	Water-Regulating and Damp-Resolving Herbs (Chapter 6)

Chapter 18

— Astringent Herbs

收澀药

Chapter 18 — Astringent Herbs

Chapter 18

收澀葯 — Astringent Herbs

Definition: Astringent herbs bind, retain, restrain, and prevent the loss of precious body fluids and substances.

Qi, blood, *jing* (essence) and *jin ye* (body fluids) are bodily substances essential to health maintenance. In the normal course of life, these four substances are continually produced, and consumed. Maintenance of health requires the level of production to be equal to, or greater than, that of consumption. When consumption exceeds production, organ function is compromised, leading to deterioration of overall health. This imbalance must be treated as early as possible to restore normal balance. If not, the condition will continue to deteriorate, leading to deep deficiency. While tonic herbs are often beneficial in the initial stages of deficiency, they are not as useful in chronic situations, as the patient is often too weak to metabolize tonics and will be unable to benefit fully from the tonic substances. In such cases, astringent herbs are prescribed to prevent further loss of these four vital substances.

Sour in taste, astringent herbs enter the ***Heart***, ***Lung***, ***Liver***, ***Kidney***, and ***Large Intestine*** to bind, retain and prevent the loss of valuable body fluids and other substances. They are often prescribed for patients who have chronic illnesses with profound deficiency and inability to hold fluids within the body, leading to leakage. Clinical indications for use of astringent herbs include profuse menstruation, perspiration, diarrhea, coughing, spermatorrhea, nocturnal emissions, frequent urination, and bleeding.

DIFFERENTIAL DIAGNOSIS AND TREATMENT

It is important to keep in mind that while astringent herbs prevent the loss of bodily substances, they do not intrinsically restore normal balance. Therefore, while astringents can be used in patients with chronic illnesses, they should not be used on a long-term basis. Clinically, they should first be used for a short period of time to stop further losses in chronic illnesses. When the condition stabilizes, differential diagnosis must be made again and appropriate herbs be prescribed. That is, once stable, patients with spontaneous perspiration due to qi deficiency should be treated with qi tonics; patients with loose stools and diarrhea due to Spleen and Stomach deficiencies must be treated with Spleen and Stomach tonics; and patients with frequent urination and incontinence associated with Kidney deficiency must be treated with Kidney tonics. In short, for adequate treatment, use astringent herbs to ease the urgency of the condition, then use tonics to treat the underlying causes of the disease.

Wu Bei Zi (Galla Chinensis)
Ben Cao Gang Mu (Materia Medica),
by Li Shi-Zhen, 1578 A.D.

CAUTIONS/CONTRAINDICATIONS

As astringent herbs function to bind and restrain, the use of such herbs will keep any pathogenic factors within the body. Therefore, astringent herbs should not be used in conditions characterized by the presence of pathogenic factors inside the body, such as perspiration due to febrile disorders, food stagnation with diarrhea, profuse menstrual bleeding due to heat in the blood, or frequent urination due to heat in the lower *jiao*.

Chapter 18 — Astringent Herbs

Astringent herbs should not be used when pathogenic factors are in the body, as these herbs may keep the pathogens inside the body.

PHARMACOLOGICAL EFFECTS

- **Hemostatic**: Many astringent herbs stop bleeding, such as *Wu Bei Zi* (Galla Chinensis), *Shi Liu Pi* (Pericarpium Granati), *He Zi* (Fructus Chebulae), and *Chi Shi Zhi* (Halloysitum Rubrum).
- **Antidiarrheal**: Many herbs stop diarrhea, through various mechanisms of action. *Chi Shi Zhi* (Halloysitum Rubrum) has an absorbent effect, binding to various endototoxins and irritants to relieve diarrhea. *Rou Dou Kou* (Semen Myristicae) has a regulating influence on intestinal peristalsis, and at large doses, inhibits intestinal motility and relieves diarrhea. *Ying Su Ke* (Pericarpium Papaveris) slows intestinal motility and reduces the fluid in the intestines to relieve diarrhea.
- **Antibiotic**: Many astringent herbs have antibacterial and antiviral effects. Herbs with antibacterial actions include *Wu Bei Zi* (Galla Chinensis), *Wu Mei* (Fructus Mume), *Jin Ying Zi* (Fructus Rosae Laevigatae), *Shi Liu Pi* (Pericarpium Granati), *Fu Pen Zi* (Fructus Rubi) and *He Zi* (Fructus Chebulae). Herbs with antiviral properties include *Wu Bei Zi* (Galla Chinensis), *Jin Ying Zi* (Fructus Rosae Laevigatae), and *Shi Liu Pi* (Pericarpium Granati).
- **Immunostimulant**: Some herbs stimulate the immune system, such as *Shan Zhu Yu* (Fructus Corni) and *Jin Ying Zi* (Fructus Rosae Laevigatae).

POTENTIAL HERB-DRUG INTERACTIONS

- **Absorption**: *Yu Yu Liang* (Limonitum) and *Chi Shi Zhi* (Halloysitum Rubrum) have strong binding effects, and are commonly used to treat diarrhea and accidental ingestion of toxins and/or poisons. However, because of their strong binding effect, they should not be ingested at the same time as pharmaceuticals, as their binding will inherently decrease absorption of the drugs. Administer these herbs separately from drugs, with a gap of at least two to three hours between them.

Wu Wei Zi (Fructus Schisandrae Chinensis)

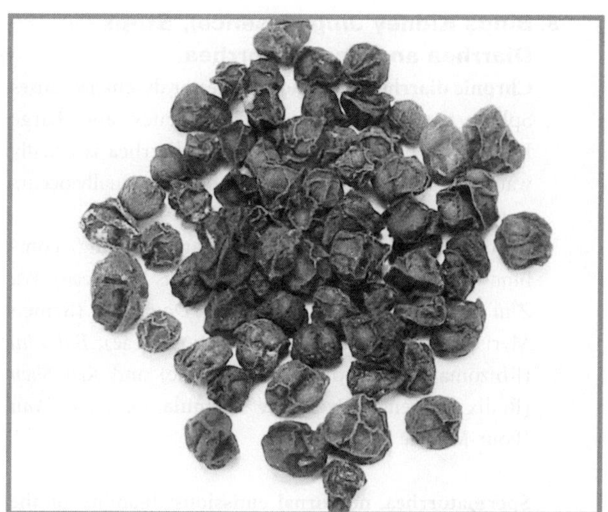

五味子

Pinyin Name: *Wu Wei Zi*
Literal Name: "five-flavored seed"
Alternate Chinese Names: *Bei Wu Wei, Wu Mei Zi, Bei Wu Wei Zi*
Original Source: *Shen Nong Ben Cao Jing* (Divine Husbandman's Classic of the Materia Medica) in the second century
English Name: schisandra, Chinese magnolia vine fruit, orange magnolia vine fruit
Botanical Name: *Schisandra chinensis* Baill. (*Bei Wu Wei Zi*); *Schisandra sphenanthera Rehd.* et Wils. (*Nan Wu Wei Zi*)
Pharmaceutical Name: Fructus Schisandrae Chinensis
Properties: sour, warm
Channels Entered: Kidney, Lung, Heart

CHINESE THERAPEUTIC ACTIONS

1. Contains the Leakage of Lung Qi, Arrests Cough, Nourishes the Kidney

Chronic cough, dyspnea or asthma: Chronic dry cough may cause yin and qi deficiencies of the Lung and Kidney. Manifestations include dry cough, loss of voice, shortness of breath, labored respiration, fatigue, weakness, and a lusterless complexion. *Wu Wei Zi* (Fructus Schisandrae Chinensis) enters the Lung to stop leakage of Lung qi and enters the Kidney to nourish the Kidney and help it grasp qi.

- Chronic consumptive cough: combine *Wu Wei Zi* with *Bai He* (Bulbus Lilii), *Sheng Di Huang* (Radix Rehmanniae), *Shan Zhu Yu* (Fructus Corni), *Zi Wan* (Radix Asteris), and *Pi Pa Ye* (Folium Eriobotryae).
- Asthma: combine it with *Ren Shen* (Radix Ginseng) and *Ge Jie* (Gecko).
- Cough due to wind-cold: a small quantity of *Wu Wei Zi* is used with *Ma Huang* (Herba Ephedrae) and *Xi Xin* (Herba Asari). **Exemplar Formula:** *Xiao Qing Long Tang* (Minor Bluegreen Dragon Decoction).

2. Generates Body Fluids, Inhibits Sweating

Spontaneous sweating: When Lung qi and *wei* (defensive) *qi* are unable to control the pores, body fluids leak out and spontaneous sweating occurs at any time of the day.

- Spontaneous sweating: combine *Wu Wei Zi* with *Huang Qi* (Radix Astragali), *Fu Xiao Mai* (Semen Tritici Aestivi Levis), *Ma Huang Gen* (Radix Ephedrae) and *Suan Zao Ren* (Semen Zizyphi Spinosae).
- Spontaneous and night sweating with qi deficiency: add this herb to *Ren Shen* (Radix Ginseng) and *Mai Men Dong* (Radix Ophiopogonis) **Exemplar Formula:** *Sheng Mai San* (Generate the Pulse Powder).

Night sweating: Yang qi rises to circulate in the *wei* (defensive) and *qi* (energy) levels during the day, and returns to the *ying* (nutritive) and *xue* (blood) levels at night. If deficient yin or *jing* cannot keep the yang in check, yang will push yin or *jing* outwards (in the form of sweating) when yang returns to the *ying* and *xue* levels at night. In other words, night sweats represent loss of body fluids paradoxically caused by yin or *jing* deficiency.

- Night sweats: combine *Wu Wei Zi* with *Mai Men Dong* (Radix Ophiopogonis), *Sheng Di Huang* (Radix Rehmanniae), *Xuan Shen* (Radix Scrophulariae), *Shan Zhu Yu* (Fructus Corni), *Long Gu* (Os Draconis), *Mu Li* (Concha Ostreae), *Huang Bai* (Cortex Phellodendri) and *Wu Mei* (Fructus Mume).

Thirst: Excessive loss of body fluids causes thirst, as do Liver and Kidney yin deficiencies. *Wu Wei Zi* can be used effectively with yin tonics to retain body fluids. *Wu Wei Zi* is commonly used in *xiao ke* (wasting and thirsting) syndrome when the patient has extreme thirst.

- Thirst: combine *Wu Wei Zi* with *Mai Men Dong* (Radix Ophiopogonis), *Shi Hu* (Herba Dendrobii), *Sheng Di Huang* (Radix Rehmanniae), *Xuan Shen* (Radix Scrophulariae) and *Wu Mei* (Fructus Mume).
- Thirst in *xiao ke* disorders: add this herb to *Shu Di Huang* (Radix Rehmanniae Preparata), *Shan Yao* (Rhizoma Dioscoreae), *Tian Hua Fen* (Radix Trichosanthis), *Shi Gao* (Gypsum Fibrosum) and *Zhi Mu* (Radix Anemarrhenae).

Wu Wei Zi (Fructus Schisandrae Chinensis)

3. Binds Kidney *Jing* (Essence), Stops Diarrhea and Spermatorrhea

Chronic diarrhea: Chronic diarrhea or dysentery causes Spleen yang deficiency, *jing* deficiency and Large Intestine qi deficiency. This type of diarrhea is usually watery, may contain undigested food, and usually occurs in the early morning.

- Chronic diarrhea (especially in the early morning): combine *Wu Wei Zi* with *Bu Gu Zhi* (Fructus Psoraleae), *Wu Zhu Yu* (Fructus Evodiae), *Rou Dou Kou* (Semen Myristicae), *Shan Yao* (Rhizoma Dioscoreae), *Bai Zhu* (Rhizoma Atractylodis Macrocephalae) and *Ren Shen* (Radix Ginseng). **Exemplar Formula:** *Si Shen Wan* (Four-Miracle Pill).

Spermatorrhea, nocturnal emissions: Inability of the Kidney to retain *jing* (essence) because of deficiency.

- Spermatorrhea: combine *Wu Wei Zi* with *Sang Piao Xiao* (Ootheca Mantidis), *Jin Ying Zi* (Fructus Rosae Laevigatae) and *Shan Zhu Yu* (Fructus Corni).
- Nocturnal emissions: add this herb to *Long Gu* (Os Draconis), *Mu Li* (Concha Ostreae), *Sheng Di Huang* (Radix Rehmanniae), *Shan Zhu Yu* (Fructus Corni), *Jin Ying Zi* (Fructus Rosae Laevigatae), and *Mu Dan Pi* (Cortex Moutan).

Polyuria or urinary incontinence: This type of excessive urination is caused by inability of Kidney qi to retain urine. It is usually light in color and is not accompanied by burning pain.

- Polyuria: combine *Wu Wei Zi* with *Wu Yao* (Radix Linderae Strychnifolia), *Yi Zhi Ren* (Fructus Alpiniae Oxyphyllae), *Shan Zhu Yu* (Fructus Corni), *Shan Yao* (Rhizoma Dioscoreae) and *Dang Shen* (Radix Codonopsis).
- Enuresis or urinary incontinence: add this herb to *Sang Piao Xiao* (Ootheca Mantidis), *Shu Di Huang* (Radix Rehmanniae Preparata), *Shan Zhu Yu* (Fructus Corni), *Shan Yao* (Rhizoma Dioscoreae), *Yi Zhi Ren* (Fructus Alpiniae Oxyphyllae), *Fu Pen Zi* (Fructus Rubi), *Ji Nei Jin* (Endothelium Corneum Gigeriae Galli) and *Xu Duan* (Radix Dipsaci).

4. Tranquilizes the Heart, Calms the *Shen* (Spirit)

Yin and blood deficiencies: Common symptoms of inability of blood to nourish *shen* include: palpitations, anxiety, insomnia and dream-disturbed sleep. *Wu Wei Zi* is often combined with tonic herbs to nourish the Heart and calm the *shen*.

- Insomnia caused by Heart and Kidney yin and blood deficiencies: combine *Wu Wei Zi* with *Bai Zi Ren* (Semen Platycladi), *Yuan Zhi* (Radix Polygalae), *Fu Shen* (Poria Paradicis), *Long Chi* (Dens Draconis), *Zhen Zhu Mu* (Concha Margaritaferae), *Long Yan Rou* (Arillus Longan) and *Dang Shen* (Radix Codonopsis). **Exemplar Formula:** *Tian Wang Bu Xin Dan* (Emperor of Heaven's Special Pill to Tonify the Heart).

DOSAGE

2 to 6 grams in decoction, 1 to 3 grams in powder.

- Unprocessed *Wu Wei Zi* more strongly promotes generation of body fluids and stops perspiration. It is commonly used to treat spontaneous perspiration, night perspiration, and thirst due to loss of body fluids.
- Steaming with vinegar increases the sour taste and enhances the astringent function of this herb. It treats cough, wheezing, spermatorrhea, and chronic diarrhea.
- Steaming *Wu Wei Zi* with grain-based liquor increases the effect of tonifying the Kidney and consolidating *jing* (essence). This preparation treats spermatorrhea and nocturnal emissions.

CAUTIONS / CONTRAINDICATIONS

- Use of *Wu Wei Zi* is contraindicated in excess conditions such as heat, damp-phlegm, Liver fire, wind-heat or rashes that have not cleared.
- It is also contraindicated in the initial stages of common colds, cough, rashes or any exterior condition, as *Wu Wei Zi* may trap pathogenic factors inside the body.
- Two rare incidences of adverse reactions associated with *Wu Wei Zi* have been reported. In case one, following the ingestion of an herbal decoction including *Wu Wei Zi*, the patient reported palpitations, shortness of breath, chest congestion, increased heart rate and pre-ventricular contraction.[1] In case two, the patient reported respiratory suppression following the ingestion of an herbal decoction including *Wu Wei Zi*.[2]

CHEMICAL COMPOSITION

Deoxyschisandrin, kadsuranin, schisanhenol, schisanhenol acetate, gomisin, schisandrin, isoschisandrin, schisandrol, angeloylgomisin, tiggoylgomisin, benzoylgomisin, rubschisandrin, epigomisin, schisantherin, andeloylgomisin, tigloylgomisin, binankadsurin, angeloylbinankadsurin, isobutyroylibinankadsurin, benzoylbinankadsurin, rubschisantherin.[3]

PHARMACOLOGICAL EFFECTS

- **CNS stimulant:** *Wu Wei Zi* stimulates the central nervous system. It increases mental alertness, improves work efficiency, and quickens reflexes.[4]
- **Hepatoprotective:** Administration of *Wu Wei Zi* is associated with marked hepatoprotective effect against various types of drugs and/or chemical-induced toxicity.[5] In

Wu Wei Zi (Fructus Schisandrae Chinensis)

one study, a preparation of *Wu Wei Zi* significantly lowered liver enzymes in mice with elevated SGPT levels caused by intraperitoneal injection of 0.1% carbon tetrachloride. In a follow-up study with rats, mice and rabbits, administration of schisandrol (dosages equivalent to 2.5 and 10.0 g/kg of dried herb) demonstrated marked preventative and treatment effects for carbon tetrachloride-induced liver damage. The mechanisms of hepatoprotective function of *Wu Wei Zi* are attributed to alteration of liver cell-membrane permeability to prevent the entry of toxic substances, and increased blood flow to the liver and increased regeneration of liver cells.[6,7]

- **Gastrointestinal:** Deoxyschizandrin inhibits secretion of gastric acid in rats, and has shown beneficial effects in treatment of gastric ulcers. The effective dose of deoxyschizandrin is 50 to 100 mg/kg.[8]
- **Cardiovascular:** *Wu Wei Zi* appears to have a regulating effect on the cardiovascular system. While it may decrease blood pressure in normal subjects, it may increase blood pressure in those with weakened constitutions. Laboratory studies indicate *Wu Wei Zi* has vasodilating and cardiotonic effects.[9]
- **Respiratory:** Both water and alcohol extracts of *Wu Wei Zi* stimulate the lungs to increase the rate and depth of respiration. They have also been shown to reverse respiratory depression associated with morphine.[10]
- **Reproductive:** Administration of *Wu Wei Zi* powder at a dosage of 1 g/kg for 30 days in mice is associated with a stimulating effect on reproductive organs. The study reported an increase in weight of the testicles in males and an increase in ovulation in females.[11]
- **Immunostimulant:** Administration of *Wu Wei Zi* is associated with stimulation of non-specific immunity.[12]
- **Antibiotic:** Alcohol extract of *Wu Wei Zi* has an inhibitory effect *in vitro* against *Staphylococcus aureus, Bacillus anthracis, Salmonella typhi, Bacillus dysenteriae, Diplococcus pneumoniae, Vibrio cholerae,* and *Pseudomonas aeruginosa.*[13]

CLINICAL STUDIES AND RESEARCH

- **Dysentery:** Children with dysentery were successfully treated with various *Wu Wei Zi* preparations, including 0.25 to 0.5 gram of dried herb, 30 to 40 drops of tincture, or 0.5 gram of extract.[14]
- **Meniere's Syndrome:** In one study, 20 patients were given 4 to 5 doses of an herbal formula with marked effectiveness. The herbal formula contained *Wu Wei Zi, Suan Zao Ren* (Semen Zizyphi Spinosae), *Dang Gui* (Radicis Angelicae Sinensis), *Long Yan Rou* (Arillus Longan) and other herbs.[15]
- **Hepatitis:** An herbal formula was used with a 97% rate of effectiveness (33 out of 34 patients) in treatment of chronic hepatitis. The herbal formula contained *Wu Wei Zi, Ling Zhi* (Ganoderma), *Dan Shen* (Radix Salviae Miltiorrhizae) and *Chai Hu* (Radix Bupleuri). Patients were advised to take the herbs 30 minutes after meals for 30 days per course of treatment, for a total of three courses.[16]
- **Asthma:** Patients with severe asthma were treated with an herbal formula for 7 months to 2 years, with good results. Out of 50 patients, the study reported complete recovery in 1 case, stability in 47 cases, and no response in 2 cases. The herbal formula contained 30 to 50 grams of *Wu Wei Zi*, 9 to 12 grams of *Di Long* (Pheretima), and 30 to 80 grams of *Yu Xing Cao* (Herba Houttuyniae). Patients were advised to first soak the herbs in water for 2 to 4 hours, then cook the herbs for 15 to 20 minutes, and take the decoction twice daily, at 4 and 8 pm.[17]
- **Prolonged labor:** According to one report, 72 out of 80 women experiencing prolonged labor were treated with good results using 20 to 25 drops of 70% *Wu Wei Zi* tincture every hour for 3 hours. The mechanism of action is attributed to the uterine stimulant effect of the herb.[18]

TOXICOLOGY

In one study, 70 mice were given a 15 g/kg bolus dose of *Wu Wei Zi*. Observation over the next 72 hours showed no change in appetite, no abnormal behavior, and no fatalities. However, the LD_{50} for oral ingestion of essential oil of *Wu Wei Zi* is 8.75 +/- 2.41 g/kg in mice.[19]

HERB-DRUG INTERACTION

- **Cycloheximide**: *Wu Wei Zi* has been found to significantly counteract cycloheximide-induced amnesia in rats. The beneficial effect of the herb is amplified by treatment with serotonergic receptor antagonists, but reduced by serotonergic receptor agonists as well as GABA(A)and cholinergic receptor antagonists.[20]

AUTHORS' COMMENTS

Wu Wei Zi and *Wu Bei Zi* (Galla Chinensis) both stop sweating, diarrhea and spermatorrhea. *Wu Wei Zi* tonifies the Kidney and generates body fluids, nourishes the Heart and calms the *shen* (spirit), while *Wu Bei Zi* cools deficiency heat and stops bleeding.

References

1. *He Bei Zhong Yi* (Hebei Chinese Medicine), 1991; (4):21
2. *Hei Long Jiang Zhong Yi Yao* (Heilongjiang Chinese Medicine and Herbology), 1987; (5):469
3. *Xian Dai Zhong Yao Yao Li Xue* (Contemporary Pharmacology of Chinese Herbs), 1997; 1388-1390
4. *Zhong Yao Xue* (Chinese Herbology), 1998; 878:881
5. *Zhong Hua Yi Xue Za Zhi* (Chinese Journal of Medicine), 1974; (5):275
6. Nagai, H. et al. *Planta Medica.* 55(1):13-17. 1989
7. Takeda, S. et al. *Nippon Yakurigaku Zasshi.* 88(4):321-30. 1986

Wu Wei Zi (Fructus Schisandrae Chinensis)

8. *Ri Ben Yao Li Xue Za Zhi* (Japanese Journal of Herbology), 1986; 87(3):209
9. *Zhong Yao Xue* (Chinese Herbology), 1998; 878:890
10. *Zhong Yao Yao Li Yu Ying Yong* (Pharmacology and Applications of Chinese Herbs), 1983, 1983: 177
11. *Shang Hai Zhong Yi Yao Za Zhi* (Shanghai Journal of Chinese Medicine and Herbology), 1989; 2:43
12. *Zhong Yao Xue* (Chinese Herbology), 1998; 878:881
13. Ibid.
14. *Tian Jing Yi Xue Za Zhi* (Journal of Tianjing Medicine and Herbology), 1965; 4:338
15. *Zhong Hua Er Bi Hou Ke Za Zhi* (Chinese Journal of ENT), 1960; 1:25
16. *Shan Xi Zhong Yi* (Shanxi Chinese Medicine), 1988; 3:106
17. *Zhong Yi Za Zhi* (Journal of Chinese Medicine), 1988; 9:47
18. *Zhong Yao Xue* (Chinese Herbology), 1998; 878:881
19. *Bei Jing Yi Ke Da Xue Xue Bao* (Journal of Beijing University of Medicine), 1988, 20(10):457
20. Hsieh MT. Wu CR. Wang WH. Lin LW., The ameliorating effect of the water layer of Fructus Schisandrae on cycloheximide-induced amnesia in rats: interaction with drugs acting at neurotransmitter receptors. *Pharmacological Research*. 43(1):17-22, 2001 Jan

Wu Mei (Fructus Mume)

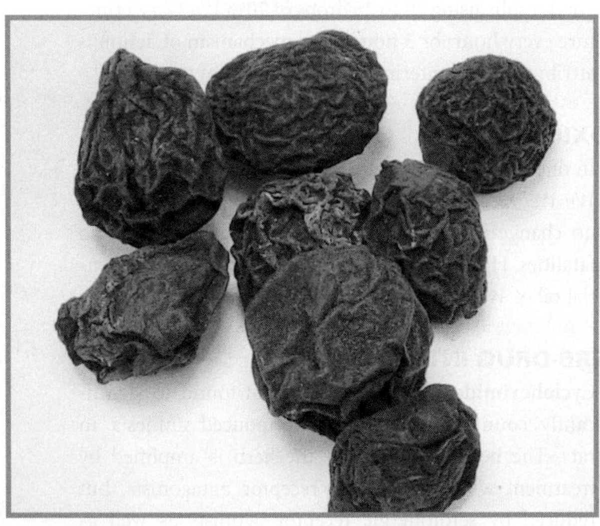

烏梅 乌梅

Pinyin Name: *Wu Mei*
Literal Name: "dark plum"
Alternate Chinese Names: *Suan Mei, Mei Shi, Xun Mei, Chun Mei, Mei Zi, Mei*
Original Source: *Shen Nong Ben Cao Jing* (Divine Husbandman's Classic of the Materia Medica) in the second century
English Name: mume, smoked plum, dark plum
Botanical Name: *Prunus mume* (Sieb.) Sieb. et Zucc. (*Mei Shu*)
Pharmaceutical Name: Fructus Mume
Properties: sour, neutral
Channels Entered: Liver, Spleen, Lung , Large Intestine

CHINESE THERAPEUTIC ACTIONS

1. Inhibits Leakage of Lung Qi and Stops Leakage of Sweat

Lung qi deficiency: *Wu Mei* (Fructus Mume) treats chronic respiratory diseases typified by a dry, feeble cough and a voice low in volume.

- Chronic cough: use *Wu Mei* with *Wu Wei Zi* (Fructus Schisandrae Chinensis), *Bai He* (Bulbus Lilii), *Zi Wan* (Radix Asteris), *Xing Ren* (Semen Armeniacae Amarum), *E Jiao* (Colla Corii Asini) and *Ban Xia* (Rhizoma Pinelliae).

2. Binds the Intestines

Diarrhea or dysentery: *Wu Mei* treats chronic diarrhea or unremitting dysentery from qi deficiency.

- Chronic diarrhea or dysentery: use charred *Wu Mei* alone, or in combination with *He Zi* (Fructus Chebulae), *Ying Su Ke* (Pericarpium Papaveris) and *Rou Dou Kou* (Semen Myristicae).

Rectal prolapse: This generally occurs as result of chronic diarrhea causing Spleen qi depletion.

- Rectal prolapse: combine *Wu Mei* with *Huang Qi* (Radix Astragali), *Dang Shen* (Radix Codonopsis), *Sheng Ma* (Rhizoma Cimicifugae), *Chai Hu* (Radix Bupleuri) and *Bai Zhu* (Rhizoma Atractylodis Macrocephalae).

Dysentery: *Wu Mei* is combined with heat-clearing and dampness-drying herbs to treat both the symptoms and the causes of dysentery.

- Dysentery with burning sensations caused by damp-heat: use with *Huang Lian* (Rhizoma Coptidis).

Wu Mei (Fructus Mume)

3. Generates Body Fluids

Thirst: *Wu Mei* relieves thirst and generates body fluids. It treats patients with chronic yin-deficient heat manifesting in thirst, weight loss, and irritability.

- Thirst in diabetes, diabetes insipidus and hyperthyroidism: combine this herb with *Xi Yang Shen* (Radix Panacis Quinquefolii), *Mai Men Dong* (Radix Ophiopogonis), *Tian Hua Fen* (Radix Trichosanthis), *Sheng Di Huang* (Radix Rehmanniae), *Shi Gao* (Gypsum Fibrosum), *Shan Yao* (Rhizoma Dioscoreae) or *Ge Gen* (Radix Puerariae).
- Thirst and summer-heat: *Wu Mei* is often taken with sugar as a beverage during the summer, to generate fluids.

4. Expels Parasites

Abdominal pain and vomiting due to parasites: *Wu Mei* not only relieves pain associated with parasites, but also the sour taste calms and weakens the parasites and facilitates their expulsion, when combined with other purgative and antiparasitic herbs. This herb has recently been used to effectively treat ascariasis of the biliary tract.

- Roundworms and hookworms: use *Wu Mei* with *Xi Xin* (Herba Asari), *Fu Zi* (Radix Aconiti Lateralis Praeparata), *Huang Lian* (Rhizoma Coptidis), *Shi Jun Zi* (Fructus Quisqualis), and *Hua Jiao* (Pericarpium Zanthoxyli). **Exemplar Formula:** *Wu Mei Wan* (Mume Pill).

5. Stops Uterine Bleeding

Charred *Wu Mei* treats chronic uterine bleeding resulting from deficiency.

6. Treats Corns and Warts

- **Corns and warts:** Soak 30 grams of *Wu Mei* in salt water for 24 hours. Pit the fruit and add vinegar, to make a paste. Apply the paste to affected areas and remove it in 2 or 3 days. This topical application is also used to treat ulcers and sores.

DOSAGE

10 to 30 grams in decoction, with a maximum of 30 grams. Unprocessed *Wu Mei* is often used to inhibit the leakage of Lung qi, bind the intestines to stop diarrhea, promote the generation of fluids, and kill parasites. The charred herb stops bleeding and diarrhea.

CAUTIONS / CONTRAINDICATIONS

- Because *Wu Mei* has a restraining effect, it is not suitable for sole use to treat acute diarrhea, or diarrhea caused by food poisoning or infections. It should be combined with other herbs to address the root of the condition.
- *Wu Mei* is contraindicated for patients having excess heat or stagnation.

CHEMICAL COMPOSITION

Organic acids, oleanolic acid, sitosterol.[1]

PHARMACOLOGICAL EFFECTS

- **Antibiotic:** *Wu Mei* has demonstrated an inhibitory effect against *Staphylococcus aureus*, *Salmonella typhi*, *Bacillus subtilis*, *Bacillus dysenteriae*, *E. coli*, *Mycobacterium tuberculosis* and some dermatophytes.[2]
- **Skeletal muscle relaxant:** Administration of a 100% decoction of *Wu Mei* is associated with an inhibitory effect on the intestines of rabbits.[3]
- **Antiparasitic:** According to laboratory studies, there is a moderate reduction of movement in roundworms when placed in a 5% *Wu Mei* solution, and significant reduction of movement when placed in a 30% solution.[4]
- **Antiaging:** *Wu Mei* has an antiaging effect. [5]

CLINICAL STUDIES AND RESEARCH

- **Internal hemorrhoids:** Injection of a *Wu Mei* solution to the affected area showed effectiveness in treating 110 patients with internal hemorrhoids. Most patients received 5 to 20 ml (a maximum of 30 ml) of solution per injection, with each ml of injection containing 0.4 gram of dried herb.[6]
- **Viral hepatitis:** According to one report, 66 of 74 patients showed significant improvement following an herbal treatment, with decreased liver enzyme levels, relief of jaundice, and symptomatic improvement. The treatment protocol was to cook 40 to 50 grams of *Wu Mei* in 500 ml of water to yield 250 ml of decoction, taken in two equally-divided doses daily. Patients were also advised to take vitamins B and C.[7]
- **Bacterial dysentery:** Patients with bacterial dysentery were effectively treated using 5 grams of *Wu Mei* powder (0.1 g/kg in children) every 6 hours.[8]
- **Chronic cholecystitis:** Patients with cholecystitis were treated with good results using an herbal decoction containing Wu *Mei* 5g, *Jiang Huang* (Rhizoma Curcumae Longae) 9g, *Yin Chen Hao* (Herba Artemisiae Scopariae) 15g, *Zhi Zi* (Fructus Gardeniae) 10g, *Da Huang* (Radix et Rhizoma Rhei) 9g, *Ji Nei Jin* (Endothelium Corneum Gigeriae Galli) 9g, *Fo Shou* (Fructus Citri Sarcodactylis) 9g, *Zhi Shi* (Fructus Aurantii Immaturus) 9g, *Hua Shi* (Talcum) 30g, and *Gan Cao* (Radix Glycyrrhizae) 3g.[9]
- **Infantile diarrhea:** In one study, 65 out of 67 infants (98.5%) with diarrhea showed complete recovery following an herbal treatment. Infants under one year of age were given 1 gram of *Wu Mei* and 0.25 gram of soda, and those over one year of age were given 1.5 gram of *Wu Mei* and 0.25 grams of soda. The herbs were given three times daily, for 3 days per treatment course.[10]

Wu Mei (Fructus Mume)

- **Biliary ascariasis:** Patients with biliary ascariasis were treated with a *Wu Mei* vinegar solution with remarkable results. Out of 50 participants, the study reported pain relief within half an hour in 30 patients, and complete recovery in 48 patients within 2 days. The herbal solution was prepared by mixing 500 grams of *Wu Mei* in 1,000 ml of vinegar for 24 hours. Patients were given 10 to 20 ml of the vinegar solution three times daily.[11]
- **Treatment of hookworm:** Following an herbal treatment that lasted between 5 and 23 days, 14 of 20 patients recovered from hookworm infestation. The treatment protocol was to cook 15 to 30 grams of *Wu Mei* in 500 ml of water, to yield 120 ml of decoction. The decoction was taken twice daily on an empty stomach, before breakfast and lunch.[12]

AUTHORS' COMMENTS

Records have shown that when treating parasites, herbs that are usually used are sour, bitter, acrid and warm. The sour taste softens the worms, the bitter purges them, the acrid weakens the worms and the heat calms them. *Wu Mei Wan* (Mume Pill) is the representative formula of this principle, as it contains all four tastes and properties.

References

1. *Xian Dai Zhong Yao Yao Li Xue* (Contemporary Pharmacology of Chinese Herbs), 1997; 747
2. *Zhong Yi Za Zhi* (Journal of Chinese Medicine), 1984:262
3. Ibid.
4. *Chang Yong Zhong Yao Xian Dai Yan Jiu Yu Lin Chuan* (Recent Study & Clinical Application of Common Traditional Chinese Medicine), 1995, 669:672
5. Ibid.
6. *Jiang Su Zhong Yi Za Zhi* (Jiangsu Journal of Chinese Medicine), 1980; 5:29
7. *Zhong Xi Yi Jie He Za Zhi* (Journal of Integrated Chinese and Western Medicine), 1986; 11:694
8. *Liao Ning Zhong Yi Za Zhi* (Liaoning Journal of Chinese Medicine), 1979; (4):15
9. *Shang Hai Zhong Yi Yao Za Zhi* (Shanghai Journal of Chinese Medicine and Herbology), 1981; (12):27
10. *Zhong Xi Yi Jie He Za Zhi* (Journal of Integrated Chinese and Western Medicine), 1988; 6:566
11. *Fu Jian Zhong Yi Yao* (Fujian Chinese Medicine and Herbology), 1982; (2):54
12. *Zhong Yi Za Zhi* (Journal of Chinese Medicine), 1959; (3):153

Wu Bei Zi (Galla Chinensis)

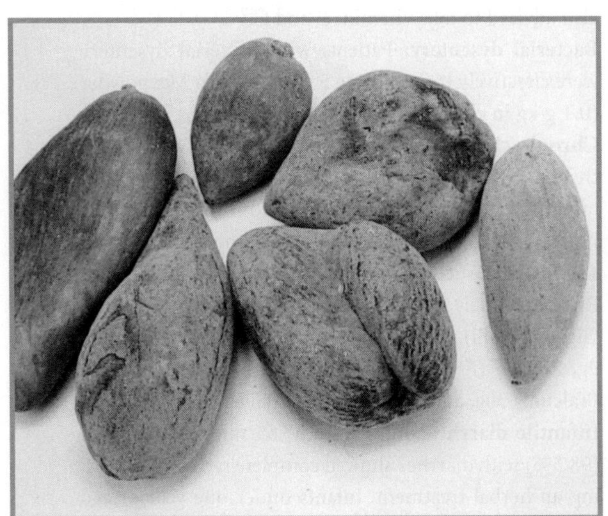

五倍子

Pinyin Name: *Wu Bei Zi*
Literal Name: "five multiples seed"
Alternate Chinese Names: *Wen Ge, Bai Chong Chang*
Original Source: *Ben Cao Shi Yi* (Omissions from the [Classic of the] Materia Medica) by Chen Cang-Qi in 741 A.D.
English Name: nut galls, Chinese nut galls
Botanical Name: *Rhus chinensis* Mill. (*Yan Fu Mu*); *Rhus potaninii* Maxim. (*Qing Fu Yang*); *Rhus punjabensis* Stew. var. *sinica* (Diels) Rehd. et Wils. (*Hong Fu Yang*); *Melaphis chinensis* (Bell) Baker (*Wu Bei Zi Ya*)
Pharmaceutical Name: Galla Chinensis
Properties: salty, sour, cold
Channels Entered: Lung, Large Intestine, Kidney

Wu Bei Zi (Galla Chinensis)

CHINESE THERAPEUTIC ACTIONS

1. Contains Leakage of Lung Qi to Arrest Cough, Cools Deficiency Fire

Chronic cough due to Lung deficiency: Sour, astringent and cold, *Wu Bei Zi* (Galla Chinensis) enters the Lung to contain leakage of Lung qi and clear deficiency fire. It is commonly used to treat chronic cough with blood or blood-streaked sputum due to yin deficiency and deficiency heat of the Lung. It cools deficiency fire to prevent further loss of Lung yin, and arrests cough to prevent leakage of Lung qi.

- Chronic cough: use *Wu Bei Zi* with *Wu Wei Zi* (Fructus Schisandrae Chinensis), *Tian Men Dong* (Radix Asparagi) and *Xuan Shen* (Radix Scrophulariae).

2. Binds the Intestines

Chronic diarrhea, dysentery or rectal prolapse: *Wu Bei Zi* binds the intestines to treat chronic diarrhea, chronic dysentery and rectal prolapse. It may be used individually or in combination with other herbs.

- Chronic diarrhea, dysentery during the summer: fry *Wu Bei Zi* with vinegar and grind it into powder. Serve with rice soup.
- Rectal prolapse: use it with *Ming Fan* (Alumen) as an external wash or soak.
- Postpartum uterine prolapse: use this herb alone as powder.

3. Consolidates Kidney *Jing* (Essence)

Leakage of *jing*: *Wu Bei Zi* treats Kidney deficiency with leakage of *jing*. Symptoms of this deficiency include spermatorrhea, enuresis, white or turbid urine, nocturnal emissions, night fevers, irritability and a dull, dark complexion.

- Leakage of *jing*: use this herb with *Long Gu* (Os Draconis) and *Fu Ling* (Poria). Add a small portion of salt to the decoction and take it on an empty stomach.

4. Stops Sweating

Spontaneous or night sweating: *Wu Bei Zi* effectively treats both spontaneous and night sweating. Mix this herb with water to make a paste and apply it topically to the umbilicus.

5. Stops Bleeding

Various bleeding disorders: *Wu Bei Zi* has an astringent function to treat various bleeding disorders, such as uterine bleeding, hematochezia, bleeding gums, hematuria, and epistaxis. It may be used individually or in combination with other herbs, via oral or topical administration.

- Uterine bleeding, bleeding due to miscarriage: use *Wu Bei Zi* with *Ming Fan* (Alumen), *He Zi* (Fructus Chebulae) and *Hai Piao Xiao* (Endoconcha Sepiae).
- Hematochezia, hematuria: use it alone as powder.
- Epistaxis, gum bleeding: use this herb as powder and apply it topically.

6. Eliminates Toxins and Reduces Swelling

Wu Bei Zi helps to heal sores as it eliminates toxins and reduces swelling. It is used topically on various carbuncles, sores, swellings, and oozing or ulcerated lesions.

- Non-healing sores, ulcerations and carbuncles with oozing fluids: apply *Wu Bei Zi* topically as powder or as a wash.

DOSAGE

1.5 to 6 grams.

CAUTIONS / CONTRAINDICATIONS

- *Wu Bei Zi* should be used with caution in cases of excess, heat, accumulation, or stagnation.

CHEMICAL COMPOSITION

Gallotannin, gallotannic acid, gallic acid.[1]

PHARMACOLOGICAL EFFECTS

- **Antibiotic:** *Wu Bei Zi* has an *in vitro* inhibitory effect against *Staphylococcus aureus, Diplococcus pneumoniae, Salmonella typhi*, and *Pseudomonas aeruginosa*.[2]

CLINICAL STUDIES AND RESEARCH

- **Gastrointestinal bleeding:** In one clinical study, 33 patients with upper gastrointestinal bleeding were treated with an herbal formula with marked effectiveness. The treatment protocol was to cook 6 grams of *Wu Bei Zi* in water to yield 100 ml of decoction, which was taken in three equally-divided doses daily. Those with severe blood loss received blood infusions. Those with hematemesis were instructed not to ingest food orally. Following one week of treatment, 29 out of 33 (91%) patients tested negative for blood in the stool. Three more patients were negative after 9 to 11 days. One patient with stomach cancer did not respond to the herbal treatment.[3]
- **Spermatorrhea:** According to one report, 35 patients with spermatorrhea were treated by topical application of herbs, with marked improvement in 9 patients, moderate improvement in 19, and no improvement in 7. The herbal paste was prepared by mixing powdered *Wu Bei Zi* with normal saline solution. The herbal paste was applied bilaterally to *Siman* (Extra) points, covered with gauze, and re-applied every three days. *Siman* (Extra) is located 2 *cun* below and 0.5 *cun* lateral to the umbilicus.[4]
- **Scars from burns:** A topical herbal preparation showed good therapeutic benefit in treatment of patients with scars from burns. The herbal preparation contained 100 grams of *Wu Bei Zi* in powder, 1 *Wu Gong* (Scolopendra),

Wu Bei Zi (Galla Chinensis)

and 18 grams of honey, mixed with 250 ml of black vinegar to make a paste. The compound was applied topically to the wound, and changed every 3 to 5 days.[5]

- **Thrush:** In one study, 20 patients with thrush or myocotic stomatitis due to monilia candida recovered completely after being treated twice daily by topical application of an herbal powder containing 20 grams of *Wu Bei Zi* and 3 grams of *Bing Pian* (Borneolum Syntheticum).[6]

HERB-DRUG INTERACTION

- **Absorption:** *Wu Bei Zi* has a strong binding affinity, and when it physically binds to another substance, the result is a large, insoluble complex that cannot be absorbed. Therefore, it is recommended that the ingestion of drugs and this herb be separated by at least 2 hours to avoid interference with proper absorption.[7]

TOXICOLOGY

Decoction of *Wu Bei Zi* at the dosage of 20 g/kg showed no abnormalities in mice. However, subcutaneous injection at 20 g/kg produced necrosis of local tissue and some fatalities in mice within 24 hours.[8]

AUTHORS' COMMENTS

Please refer to *Wu Wei Zi* (Fructus Schisandrae Chinensis) for a comparison of *Wu Bei Zi* and *Wu Wei Zi.*

Historically, *Wu Bei Zi* has been used as a generic antidote to treat the accidental ingestion of poisonous substances. It has a strong binding affinity, and when it physically binds to another substance, the result is a large, insoluble complex that cannot be absorbed. The poisonous substance is then eliminated from the body via the stool with minimal systemic absorption.

References

1. *Xian Dai Zhong Yao Yao Li Xue* (Contemporary Pharmacology of Chinese Herbs), 1997; 848
2. *Zhong Yao Da Ci Dian* (Dictionary of Chinese Herbs), 1975; 391
3. *Zhe Jiang Zhong Yi Xue Yuan Xue Bao* (Journal of Zhejiang University of Chinese Medicine), 1987; 6:20
4. *Xin Jiang Zhong Yi Yao* (Xinjiang Chinese Medicine and Herbology), 1986; 4:4
5. *Xin Zhong Yi* (New Chinese Medicine), 1986; 12:8
6. *He Bei Zhong Yi* (Hebei Chinese Medicine), 1987; 6:48
7. Chen, J. *The Herbal Safety Course,* National Alliance Conference, 2002
8. *Zhong Yao Da Ci Dian* (Dictionary of Chinese Herbs), 1975; 391

He Zi (Fructus Chebulae)

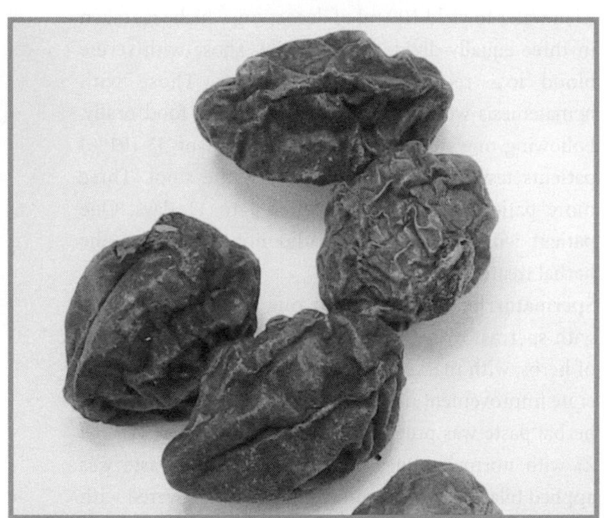

訶子 诃子

Pinyin Name: *He Zi*
Alternate Chinese Names: *He Li Le, He Li*
Original Source: *Yao Xing Ben Cao* (Materia Medica of Medicinal Properties) by Zhen Quan in 600 A.D.
English Name: chebule, medicine terminalia fruit
Botanical Name: *Terminalia chebula* Retz. (*He Zi*); *Terminalia chebula* Retz. var. *tomentella* Kurt. (*Rong Mao He Zi*)
Pharmaceutical Name: Fructus Chebulae
Properties: bitter, astringent, neutral
Channels Entered: Lung, Large Intestine

He Zi (Fructus Chebulae) most effectively treats Lung deficiency in which rebellious, deficient qi manifests as chronic coughing, dyspnea and loss of voice. Clinical applications of this herb include chronic dyspnea, coughing,

CHINESE THERAPEUTIC ACTIONS

1. Restrains the Lung, Directs Lung Qi Downwards, Benefits the Throat

Cough and dyspnea from Lung deficiency, loss of voice:

He Zi (Fructus Chebulae)

loss of voice, shortness of breath due to chronic respiratory disorders, chronic pharyngitis and laryngitis.

- Lung qi deficiency with chronic cough, dyspnea and asthma: use *He Zi* with *Ge Jie* (Gecko), *Wu Wei Zi* (Fructus Schisandrae Chinensis) and *Ren Shen* (Radix Ginseng).
- Chronic cough: use this herb with *Bai He* (Bulbus Lilii), *Wu Mei* (Fructus Mume), *Wu Wei Zi* (Fructus Schisandrae Chinensis), *Mai Men Dong* (Radix Ophiopogonis) and *Ma Dou Ling* (Fructus Aristolochiae).
- Chronic laryngitis and pharyngitis with loss of voice: combine it with *Wu Mei* (Fructus Mume), *She Gan* (Rhizoma Belamcandae), *Chan Tui* (Periostracum Cicadae), and *Xuan Fu Hua* (Flos Inulae).
- Chronic cough leading to loss of voice: drink a decoction of *He Zi* daily.

2. Binds the Intestines and Stops Diarrhea

He Zi treats chronic diarrhea from deficiency and cold, or from heat, depending on what other herbs are combined in the formula. After processing, *He Zi* has a warm property. Used alone, it is best for chronic diarrhea or dysentery resulting from deficiency and cold.

- Chronic diarrhea caused by deficiency and cold: combine it with *Rou Dou Kou* (Semen Myristicae), *Qian Shi* (Semen Euryales), *Mu Xiang* (Radix Aucklandiae), *Wu Zhu Yu* (Fructus Evodiae), *Bu Gu Zhi* (Fructus Psoraleae) and *Bai Zhu* (Rhizoma Atractylodis Macrocephalae).
- Chronic dysentery: use *He Zi* with *Chi Shi Zhi* (Halloysitum Rubrum), *Wu Mei* (Fructus Mume) and *Si Shen Wan* (Four-Miracle Pill).
- Chronic diarrhea caused by damp-heat: add it to *Huang Lian* (Rhizoma Coptidis), *Mu Xiang* (Radix Aucklandiae) and *Gan Cao* (Radix Glycyrrhizae).
- Bloody diarrhea: combine it with *Fang Feng* (Radix Saposhnikoviae), charred *Huai Hua* (Flos Sophorae), charred *Di Yu* (Radix Sanguisorbae), charred *Huang Bai* (Cortex Phellodendri) and *Bai Zhu* (Rhizoma Atractylodis Macrocephalae).

DOSAGE

3 to 10 grams. The unprocessed form clears the Lung and benefits the voice. Roasted *He Zi* stops diarrhea.

CAUTIONS / CONTRAINDICATIONS

- *He Zi* should not be used alone when treating exterior conditions or internal accumulations of damp-heat. Before using this herb, one must be certain there are no lingering pathogenic factors in the Lung or the intestines.

CHEMICAL COMPOSITION

Chebulinic acid, chebulagic acid, corilagin, terchebin, glucogallin, ellagic acid, gallic acid, chebulin, sennoside A, terchebulin, punicalagin, terflavin A, shikimic acid, dehydroshikimic acid, quinic acid, arabinose, fructose, glucose, sucrose, rhamnose, amino acids, tannase, polyphenol oxidase, peroxydase, ascorbic acid oxidase, β-sitosterol, daucosterol, triacontanoic acid, palmitic acid.[1]

PHARMACOLOGICAL EFFECTS

- **Antibiotic:** Decoction of *He Zi* has an inhibiting influence on *Pseudomonas aeruginosa*, *Corynebacterium diphtheriae*, *Staphylococcus aureus*, *E. coli*, *Diplococcus pneumoniae*, β-hemolytic streptococcus and *Bacillus proteus*.[2]
- **Antispasmodic:** Chebulin may relieve spasms and cramps of the smooth muscles with an effect similar to papaverine.[3]
- **Gastrointestinal:** *He Zi* has a complicated effect on the gastrointestinal tract that includes initial purgative and subsequent astringent effects. The initial purgative effect is attributed to sennoside A, which is a mild to moderate purgative. The subsequent astringent effect is attributed to the high content of tannin, that stops diarrhea.[4]

CLINICAL STUDIES AND RESEARCH

- **Infantile diarrhea:** In one study, 227 of 230 infants were successfully treated with an herbal formulation containing *He Zi* 5-10 g, *Fang Feng* (Radix Saposhnikoviae) 5-10g, *Chen Pi* (Pericarpium Citri Reticulatae) 5-10g, *Mai Ya* (Fructus Hordei Germinatus) 5-10g, *Ge Gen* (Radix Puerariae) 5-20g, and *Shan Zha* (Fructus Crataegi) 5-20g. For excessive damp-heat, *Huang Qin* (Radix Scutellariae) 5-10g and *Qin Pi* (Cortex Fraxini) 5-10g were added. For Spleen deficiency, *Wu Yao* (Radix Linderae Strychnifolia) 5-10g and *Ying Su Ke* (Pericarpium Papaveris) 3-5g were added.[5]
- **Bacterial dysentery:** According to one report, 23 out of 25 patients reported complete recovery from bacterial dysentery within 3 days following treatment with *He Zi* preparations. The treatment protocol included both oral and rectal administration of *He Zi*. For oral treatment, enteric-coated *He Zi* tablets were given 2 hours before meals, three to four times daily. For rectal treatment, 10 to 40 ml of 20% *He Zi* solution was given as enema twice daily.[6]
- **Lobar pneumonia:** An herbal decoction containing 15 grams of *He Zi*, 15 grams of *Gua Lou Shi* (Fructus Trichosanthis) and 9 grams of *Bai Bu* (Radix Stemonae) was used to treat 20 patients with lobar pneumonia, with good results. Most patients reported reduction in fever within 1 to 3 days, gradual decline of white blood cell count to normal within 3 to 6 days, and complete recovery within 6 to 11 days. No adverse reactions were reported.[7]

TOXICOLOGY

The LD_{50} for chebulin in mice is 550 mg/kg.[8]

He Zi (Fructus Chebulae)

AUTHORS' COMMENTS

He Zi and *Rou Dou Kou* (Semen Myristicae) both treat chronic diarrhea. *He Zi* focuses on the upper *jiao*, and treats wheezing and chronic cough with loss of voice from Lung qi deficiency. *Rou Dou Kou* focuses on the middle *jiao*, and treats abdominal fullness and pain, poor appetite and nausea caused by cold, Spleen deficiency and qi stagnation.

According to Dr. Lu Zhi-Zheng, *He Zi* and *Wu Mei* (Fructus Mume), used for colitis patients with diarrhea, bind the intestines and prevent prolapse.

References

1. *Chang Yong Zhong Yao Cheng Fen Yu Yao Li Shou Ce* (A Handbook of the Composition and Pharmacology of Common Chinese Drugs), 1994; 1110-1111
2. *Zhi Wu Yao You Xiao Cheng Fen Shou Ce* (Manual of Plant Medicinals and Their Active Constituents), 1986: 952
3. *Zhong Yao Zhi* (Chinese Herbology Journal), 1984; 428
4. *Zhi Wu Yao You Xiao Cheng Fen Shou Ce* (Manual of Plant Medicinals and Their Active Constituents), 1986: 952
5. *Ji Lin Zhong Yi Yao* (Jilin Chinese Medicine and Herbology), 1983; 1:25
6. *Zhong Hua Nei Ke Za Zhi* (Chinese Journal of Internal Medicine), 1960; (4):361
7. *Wu Han Xin Yi Yao* (Wuhan New Medicine and Herbology), 1971; (1):25
8. *Zhi Wu Yao You Xiao Cheng Fen Shou Ce* (Manual of Plant Medicinals and Their Active Constituents), 1986: 952

Yíng Sù Ké (Pericarpium Papaveris)

罌粟殼 罂粟壳

Pinyin Name: *Ying Su Ke*
Alternate Chinese Names: *Mi Ke, Yu Mi Ke*
Original Source: *Yi Xue Qi Yuan* (Origins of the Medicine) by Zhang Yuan-Su in Yuan Dynasty
English Name: opium shells, opium husks
Botanical Name: *Papaver somniferum* L. (*Ying Su*)
Pharmaceutical Name: Pericarpium Papaveris
Properties: sour, astringent, neutral
Channels Entered: Kidney, Large Intestine, Lung
Safety Index: toxic

CHINESE THERAPEUTIC ACTIONS

1. Contains the Lung

Chronic cough because of Lung qi deficiency: *Ying Su Ke* (Pericarpium Papaveris) restrains the leakage of Lung qi to treat chronic cough.

- Cough: use *Ying Su Ke* individually for symptomatic treatment of coughing.
- Chronic cough: use this herb with *Bai Zhu* (Rhizoma Atractylodis Macrocephalae), *Shan Yao* (Rhizoma Dioscoreae), and *Gan Cao* (Radix Glycyrrhizae).

2. Binds the Large Intestine

Chronic diarrhea with pain: *Ying Su Ke* restrains leakage of fluids from the Large Intestine to stop diarrhea.

- Diarrhea: use it with *He Zi* (Fructus Chebulae) and *Rou Dou Kou* (Semen Myristicae).
- Diarrhea with Spleen deficiency: combine this herb with *Ren Shen* (Radix Ginseng), *Bai Zhu* (Rhizoma Atractylodis Macrocephalae) and *Fu Ling* (Poria).

3. Relieves Pain

Pain in the chest, abdomen, tendons and bones: *Ying Su Ke* has a strong pain-relieving function. It is commonly used for acute pain, including stomach and abdominal pain, cancer-related pain, and pain from external injuries, among others. It may be used individually or in combination with other herbs.

DOSAGE

10 to 30 grams in decoction. Honey-processed *Ying Su Ke* is stronger in antitussive function. The vinegar-processed herb is more effective in antidiarrheal and pain-relieving actions.

Ying Su Ke (Pericarpium Papaveris)

CAUTIONS / CONTRAINDICATIONS

- Early stages of cough, diarrhea or dysentery should not be treated with *Ying Su Ke* alone.
- Use of *Ying Su Ke*, or its constituents, is habit-forming. Avoid long-term use.

OVERDOSAGE

Symptoms of overdose associated with *Ying Su Ke* include headache, dizziness, nausea, vomiting, constipation, difficulty urinating, perspiration, and biliary colic. Respiratory depression is the single most dangerous side effect and is the limiting factor restricting high doses of all opioids. In overdose, respiration may be suppressed to 2 to 4 breaths per minute. Acute overdose is generally detected by drowsiness, miosis, and respiratory depression. Use of opioids is strongly discouraged in newborns, young children, and patients with hypothyroid or pre-existing respiratory conditions. Furthermore, long-term use of opioids should be avoided whenever possible due to risks of developing tolerance and addiction. Because of the high abuse potential of a substance like this, use of the herb and its components is highly regulated in most countries.[1]

CHEMICAL COMPOSITION

Morphine, codeine, thebaine, narcotine, papaverine, narcotoline, sedoheptulose, D-mannoheptulose, myoinositol, erythritol.[2,3]

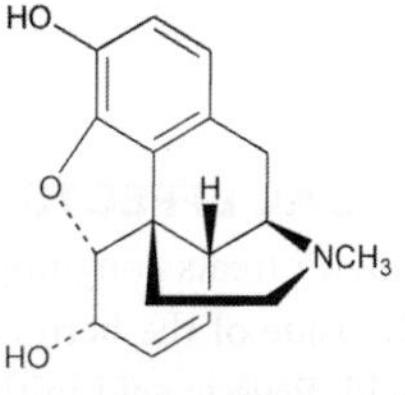

Morphine

PHARMACOLOGICAL EFFECTS

- **Analgesic:** Morphine, one of the components of *Ying Su Ke,* is one of the strongest analgesic substances to relieve all types of pain – visceral, somatic and cutaneous. In fact, it is the standard by which all other analgesic medications are measured for dosing and conversion. Morphine relieves pain by raising the threshold of pain perception and reducing discomfort. In other words, a patient on morphine may still be aware of the presence of pain but will not be distressed by it.[4]
- **Antitussive:** Both morphine and codeine have marked antitussive functions. However, morphine is not an ideal antitussive agent because of its side effects and adverse reactions, such as the developing of tolerance, constipation, and respiratory depression.[5]
- **Respiratory:** Respiratory depression and respiratory failure are the major complications of use of morphine and opioid medications. In fact, patients may begin to experience respiratory difficulties prior to achieving analgesia. Respiratory depression occurs because the medications cause a decreased sensitivity of the respiratory center to carbon dioxide.[6]
- **CNS suppressant:** Administration of *Ying Su Ke* is associated with sedation and drowsiness. It is not an effective hypnotic agent, as the sleep is shallow and the subject may be easily awakened.[7]
- **Gastrointestinal:** Morphine and codeine may both cause constipation by delaying gastric emptying time, decreasing the propulsive peristaltic movement of the intestines and reducing the secretion of digestive fluids. Furthermore, they may cause nausea and vomiting by stimulating the chemoreceptor zone.[8]
- **Others:** In addition to the pharmacological effects listed above, opioids may also cause paradoxical excitation, changes in the endocrine system, alteration of body temperature, release of histamine, and allergic reactions.

CLINICAL STUDIES AND RESEARCH

- **Chronic gastroenteritis:** Patients with chronic gastroenteritis were treated with an herbal formula containing 10 grams of *Ying Su Ke*, 30 grams of *Jin Yin Hua* (Flos Lonicerae), and 30 grams of *Shan Yao* (Rhizoma Dioscoreae). The formula was given as decoction, twice daily.[9]

HERB-DRUG INTERACTION

- **Depressant effect**: Phenothiazines, monoamine oxidase inhibitors, and tricyclic antidepressants may exaggerate and prolong the depressant effect of *Ying Su Ke.* [10]

TOXICOLOGY

For *Ying Su Ke*, the LD_{50} via oral ingestion is approximately 1.8 to 2.2 g/kg in mice, rabbits, cats, and dogs. For its components, the LD_{50} for morphine in mice is 531 mg/kg via subcutaneous injection and 500 mg/kg via intraperitoneal injection; the LD_{50} for codeine in mice is 300 mg/kg via subcutaneous injection; and the LD_{50} for papaverine in mice via oral ingestion is 2500 mg/kg.[11]

AUTHORS' COMMENTS

The first documentation of opium use is found in the writings of the Greek Theophratus in the third century, B.C. Since then, it has been used medicinally, but also abused, by many cultures all around the world. In 1806, Serturner successfully isolated morphine from opium. This is considered to be a major breakthrough in the history of allopathic medicine, as most analgesics prescribed today are originally from components of opium or their derivatives.

Ying Su Ke (Pericarpium Papaveris)

For patients in severe pain, *Yan Hu Suo* (Rhizoma Corydalis) may be used as a substitute, as *Ying Su Ke* may not be available in many countries.

References

1. *Zhong Yao Da Ci Dian* (Dictionary of Chinese Herbs), 1977; 2650
2. *Chang Yong Zhong Yao Cheng Fen Yu Yao Li Shou Ce* (A Handbook of the Composition and Pharmacology of Common Chinese Drugs), 1994
3. *The Merck Index* 12th edition, Chapman & Hall/CRCnetBASE/Merck, 2000
4. Kalant H, and Roschlau W, *Principles of Medical Pharmacology*, 6th edition, Oxford University Press, 1998; 262:277
5. *Zhong Cao Yao Xue* (Study of Chinese Herbal Medicine), 1976; 355
6. Ibid.
7. Ibid.
8. *Zhong Yao Da Ci Dian* (Dictionary of Chinese Herbs), 1977; 2650
9. *Si Chuan Zhong Yi* (Sichuan Chinese Medicine), 1985; 3(2):18
10. Gilman A, Rall T, et al., *Goodman and Gilman's The Pharmacological Basis of Therapeutics*, 8th edition, Pergamon Press, 1990;99
11. *Chang Yong Zhong Yao Cheng Fen Yu Yao Li Shou Ce* (A Handbook of the Composition and Pharmacology of Common Chinese Drugs), 1994

Ye Ying Pi (Pericarpium Prunus Pseudocerasus)

野樱皮 野櫻皮

Pinyin Name: *Ye Ying Pi*
Literal Name: "wild cherry bark"
English Name: wild black cherry bark
Botanical Name: *Prunus serotina*
Pharmaceutical Name: Pericarpium Prunus
Properties: sour, bitter, cool
Channels Entered: Lung

CHINESE THERAPEUTIC ACTIONS

Relieves Cough

Ye Ying Pi (Pericarpium Prunus Pseudocerasus) redirects inappropriately rising Lung qi and relieves cough. As an antitussive agent, this herb may be used individually or in combination with other herbs.

- Cough: combine *Ye Ying Pi* with *Xing Ren* (Semen Armeniacae Amarum) and *Ma Huang* (Herba Ephedrae).

DOSAGE

3 to 5 grams.

CHEMICAL COMPOSITION

Cyanogenic glycosides, coumarins, volatile oil, tannins, resins.

PHARMACOLOGICAL EFFECTS

- **Antitussive:** *Ye Ying Pi* treats coughing. After ingestion, the cyanogenic glycoside of the herb is converted in the body to prussic acid. Prussic acid initially increases respiratory functioning of the lung, followed by sedation of the sensory nerve that provokes cough.

TOXICOLOGY

Prussic acid is slightly toxic. However, use of the herb is safe, as the content of cyanogenic glycoside and the degree to which it is converted to prussic acid are relatively low (0.07 to 0.16%).

Chi Shi Zhi (Halloysitum Rubrum)

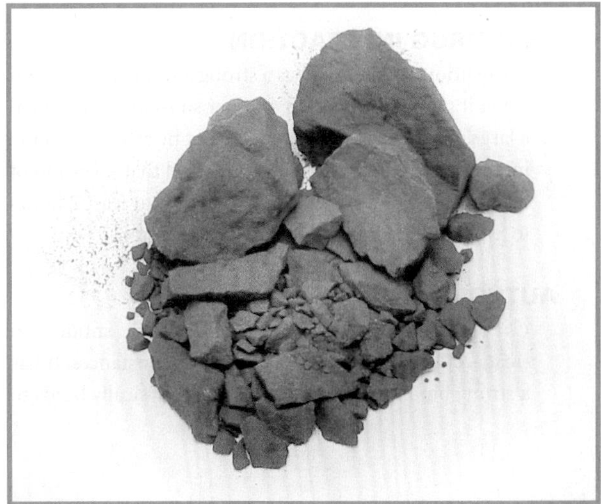

赤石脂

Pinyin Name: *Chi Shi Zhi*
Literal Name: "crimson stone resin"
Alternate Chinese Names: *Hong Gao Ling, Chi Shi Tu*
Original Source: *Shen Nong Ben Cao Jing* (Divine Husbandman's Classic of the Materia Medica) in the second century
English Name: halloysite, red halloysite
Pharmaceutical Name: Halloysitum Rubrum
Properties: sweet, sour, astringent, warm
Channels Entered: Stomach, Large Intestine

CHINESE THERAPEUTIC ACTIONS

1. Binds the Intestines and Stops Diarrhea

Chronic unremitting diarrhea or dysentery, rectal prolapse: Large Intestine qi deficiency occurs when diarrhea persists for a long time. When Spleen qi also becomes deficient, organ prolapse, especially of the rectum, occurs. In addition to diarrhea, the patient will feel fatigue, weak limbs, dull abdominal pain, and a preference for pressure and warmth. *Chi Shi Zhi* (Halloysitum Rubrum) stops chronic diarrhea in ulcerative colitis, chronic enteritis, dysentery and intestinal tuberculosis.

- Chronic diarrhea and/or rectal prolapse: combine *Chi Shi Zhi* with *Yu Yu Liang* (Limonitum).
- Dysentery with pus and bleeding from deficiency and cold: use it with *Gan Jiang* (Rhizoma Zingiberis) and *Geng Mi* (Semen Oryzae).

2. Stops Bleeding

Uterine bleeding and leukorrhea: Profuse uterine bleeding or spotting between periods is the result of Liver and Kidney deficiencies with an inability to nourish the *ren* (conception) and *chong* (thoroughfare) channels.

- Uterine bleeding: use *Chi Shi Zhi* with *Hai Piao Xiao* (Endoconcha Sepiae), charred *Ai Ye* (Folium Artemisiae Argyi), *E Jiao* (Colla Corii Asini), *Bai Shao* (Radix Paeoniae Alba) and *Huang Qi* (Radix Astragali).
- Blood in vaginal discharge: use this mineral with *Qian Shi* (Semen Euryales), *Lu Jiao Shuang* (Cornu Cervi Degelatinatum) and *She Chuang Zi* (Fructus Cnidii).

3. Promotes Healing of Sores and Ulcers

- **Chronic non-healing ulcers, weeping damp sores or bleeding:** use *Chi Shi Zhi* as powder with *Ru Xiang* (Gummi Olibanum), and *Xue Jie* (Sanguis Draconis). Apply topically.

DOSAGE

10 to 20 grams. The maximum dose for *Chi Shi Zhi* is 30 grams. Use it as powder externally.

CAUTIONS / CONTRAINDICATIONS

- *Chi Shi Zhi* is contraindicated for patients with damp-heat and stagnation.
- It is also contraindicated in hot diarrhea or early stages of dysenteric disorders.
- *Chi Shi Zhi* should be prescribed with caution for pregnant patients.

CHEMICAL COMPOSITION

Aluminum silicate, $Al_4(Si_4O_{10})(OH)_{8+}4H_2O$.[1]

PHARMACOLOGICAL EFFECTS

- **Binding:** *Chi Shi Zhi* contains a large amount of aluminum silicate. Following oral ingestion of *Chi Shi Zhi*, the aluminum silicate binds to, and subsequently eliminates, various substances present in the gastrointestinal tract, including, but not limited to, phosphorus, mercury, and bacterial endotoxins.[2]
- **Hemostatic:** Administration of *Chi Shi Zhi* may decrease bleeding time in rabbits.[3]

CLINICAL STUDIES AND RESEARCH

- **Prolapsed rectum:** One report describes 14 patients with rectal prolapse who were effectively treated using an herbal decoction containing *Chi Shi Zhi* 15g, *Yu Yu Liang* (Limonitum) 15g, *Tu Si Zi* (Semen Cuscutae) 9g, *Bai Zhu* (Rhizoma Atractylodis Macrocephalae) 9g, *Bu Gu Zhi* (Fructus Psoraleae) 6g, *Zhi Gan Cao* (Radix Glycyrrhizae Preparata) 4.5g, *Sheng Ma* (Rhizoma Cimicifugae) 4.5g, *Pao Jiang* (Rhizoma Zingiberis Preparatum) 4.5g, and others, depending on the condition of the individual patient.[4]

Chi Shi Zhi (Halloysitum Rubrum)

HERB-DRUG INTERACTION

- **Absorption:** *Chi Shi Zhi* has a strong binding affinity, and when it physically binds to another substance, they form a large, insoluble complex that cannot be absorbed in the intestines. Therefore, it is recommended that ingestion of drugs and this substance be separated by at least 2 hours to avoid interference with proper absorption.[5]

AUTHORS' COMMENTS

Chi Shi Zhi is historically used as a generic antidote to treat accidental ingestion of poisonous substances. It has a strong binding affinity, and when it physically binds to another substance, the result is a large, insoluble complex that cannot be absorbed through the gastrointestinal tract. The poisonous substance is then eliminated from the body via the stool with minimal systemic absorption.

References

1. *Zhong Yao Xue* (Chinese Herbology), 1998; 892-893
2. *Chang Yong Zhong Yao Xian Dai Yan Jiu Yu Lin Chuan* (Recent Study & Clinical Application of Common Traditional Chinese Medicine), 1995, 679:680
3. *Zhong Yao Xue* (Chinese Herbology), 1998; 892:893
4. *Zhe Jiang Zhong Yi Za Zhi* (Zhejiang Journal of Chinese Medicine), 1966; 9(2):22
5. Chen, J. *The Herbal Safety Course*, National Alliance Conference, 2002

Yu Yu Liang (Limonitum)

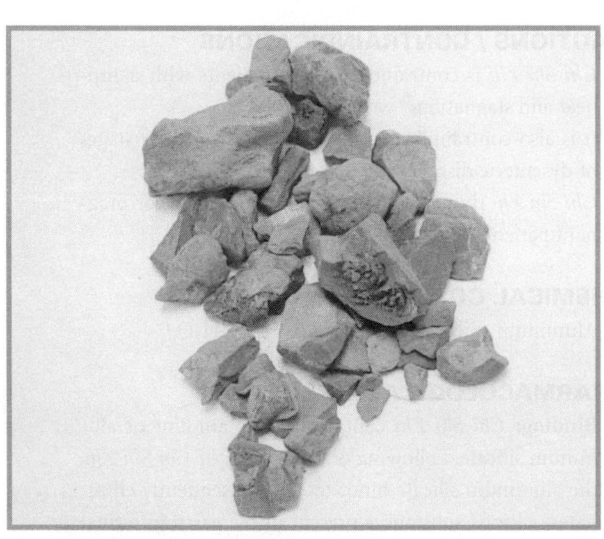

禹餘糧 禹馀粮

Pinyin Name: *Yu Yu Liang*
Literal Name: "surplus grain"
Alternate Chinese Names: *Yu Liang Shi, Yu Lang Shi, Tai Yi Yu Liang*
Original Source: *Shen Nong Ben Cao Jing* (Divine Husbandman's Classic of the Materia Medica) in the second century
English Name: limonite
Pharmaceutical Name: Limonitum
Properties: sweet, astringent, neutral
Channels Entered: Large Intestine, Stomach

CHINESE THERAPEUTIC ACTIONS

1. Binds the Intestines, Stops Diarrhea

Chronic diarrhea and dysentery: Sweet and astringent, *Yu Yu Liang* (Limonitum) binds the intestines to stop chronic diarrhea arising from qi deficiency of the Large Intestine and its inability to retain fluids. Its astringent effect in treatment of diarrhea is similar to that of *Chi Shi Zhi* (Halloysitum Rubrum).

- Diarrhea caused by deficiency of the middle *jiao*: use *Yu Yu Liang* with *Gui Zhi* (Ramulus Cinnamomi), *Gan Jiang* (Rhizoma Zingiberis) and *Bai Zhu* (Rhizoma Atractylodis Macrocephalae).

2. Restrains Leakage of Body Fluids, Stops Bleeding

Uterine bleeding, leukorrhea: *Yu Yu Liang* restrains the leakage of body fluids to stop bleeding and profuse leukorrhea.

- Profuse menstrual bleeding: use *Yu Yu Liang* with *Chi Shi Zhi* (Halloysitum Rubrum), charred *Guan Zhong* (Rhizoma Dryopteridis), and charred *Lian Fang* (Receptaculum Nelumbinis).
- Profuse leukorrhea and feeling of dampness and cold in the genital region caused by yang deficiency: combine it with *Hua Jiao* (Pericarpium Zanthoxyli) and *She Chuang Zi* (Fructus Cnidii).

Yu Yu Liang (Limonitum)

DOSAGE

10 to 20 grams.

CAUTIONS / CONTRAINDICATIONS

- *Yu Yu Liang* is contraindicated in cases of excess, to avoid retention of any pathogenic factors.

CHEMICAL COMPOSITION

Aluminum, magnesium, potassium, sodium, FeO_3.[1]

HERB-DRUG INTERACTION

- **Absorption:** *Yu Yu Liang* has a strong binding affinity, and when it physically binds to another substance, the result is a large, insoluble complex that cannot be absorbed through the intestines. Therefore, it is recommended that the ingestion of drugs and this herb be separated by at least 2 hours to avoid interference with proper absorption.[2]

AUTHORS' COMMENTS

Yu Yu Liang has historically been used as a generic antidote to treat accidental ingestion of poisonous substances. It has a strong binding affinity, and when it physically binds to another substance, the result is a large, insoluble complex that cannot be absorbed in the gastrointestinal system. The poisonous substance is then eliminated from the body via the stool with minimal systemic absorption.

References

1. *Chang Yong Zhong Yao Cheng Fen Yu Yao Li Shou Ce* (A Handbook of the Composition and Pharmacology of Common Chinese Drugs), 1994; 680-681
2. Chen, J. *The Herbal Safety Course*, National Alliance Conference, 2002

Rou Dou Kou (Semen Myristicae)

肉豆蔻 肉豆蔻

Pinyin Name: *Rou Dou Kou*
Literal Name: "fleshy cardamon"
Alternate Chinese Names: *Rou Guo, Yu Guo*
Original Source: *Yao Xing Ben Cao* (Materia Medica of Medicinal Properties) by Zhen Quan in 600 A.D.
English Name: myristica, nutmeg
Botanical Name: *Myristica fragrans* Houtt. (*Rou Dou Kou Shu*)
Pharmaceutical Name: Semen Myristicae
Properties: acrid, warm
Channels Entered: Large Intestine, Spleen, Stomach

CHINESE THERAPEUTIC ACTIONS

1. Binds the Intestines and Stops Diarrhea

Spleen yang deficiency: *Rou Dou Kou* (Semen Myristicae) treats chronic diarrhea caused by Spleen yang deficiency, with rectal prolapse, abdominal fullness and distention, vomiting and poor appetite. In severe cases where Kidney yang is also deficient, early morning diarrhea, also known as "5 a.m. diarrhea," will occur.

- Spleen yang deficiency: combine *Rou Dou Kou* with *Bai Zhu* (Rhizoma Atractylodis Macrocephalae), *Dang Shen* (Radix Codonopsis), *Fu Ling* (Poria), *Mu Xiang* (Radix Aucklandiae), *Qian Shi* (Semen Euryales) and *Sha Ren* (Fructus Amomi).
- Early morning diarrhea (5 a.m. diarrhea) with cold abdomen: add it to *Wu Zhu Yu* (Fructus Evodiae), *Wu Wei Zi* (Fructus Schisandrae Chinensis) and *Bu Gu Zhi* (Fructus Psoraleae). **Exemplar Formula:** *Si Shen Wan* (Four-Miracle Pill).

18 ASTRINGENT HERBS

Rou Dou Kou (Semen Myristicae)

- Chronic enteritis or dysentery with diarrhea: incorporate this herb with *Wu Zhu Yu* (Fructus Evodiae), *Wu Wei Zi* (Fructus Schisandrae Chinensis), *Bu Gu Zhi* (Fructus Psoraleae), *Dang Shen* (Radix Codonopsis), *Bai Zhu* (Rhizoma Atractylodis Macrocephalae), *Fu Ling* (Poria), *He Zi* (Fructus Chebulae), *Shan Yao* (Rhizoma Dioscoreae), *Shan Zhu Yu* (Fructus Corni), *Rou Gui* (Cortex Cinnamomi), *Fu Zi* (Radix Aconiti Lateralis Praeparata), *Gan Jiang* (Rhizoma Zingiberis) and *Wu Yao* (Radix Linderae). Modify as needed.

2. Warms the Middle *Jiao,* Regulates Qi and Stops Pain

Epigastric and abdominal coldness, pain, distention and fullness: Spleen yang deficiency with qi stagnation causes epigastric and abdominal bloating, fullness and distention, poor appetite, indigestion, and a feeling of cold in the abdomen.

- Chronic diarrhea with bloating and fullness: add *Rou Dou Kou* to *Mu Xiang* (Radix Aucklandiae) and *Xiang Fu* (Rhizoma Cyperi).
- Chronic diarrhea with feelings of abdominal cold: use this herb with *Fu Zi* (Radix Aconiti Lateralis Praeparata) and *Gao Liang Jiang* (Rhizoma Alpiniae Officinarum).
- Chronic diarrhea with abdominal pain: combine it with *Ying Su Ke* (Pericarpium Papaveris) and *Bai Shao* (Radix Paeoniae Alba).
- Chronic diarrhea with poor appetite and weakness: use *Rou Dou Kou* with *Dang Shen* (Radix Codonopsis), *Huang Qi* (Radix Astragali), *Bai Zhu* (Rhizoma Atractylodis Macrocephalae) and *Fu Ling* (Poria).

DOSAGE

3 to 10 grams in decoctions; 1.5 to 3 grams as powder. *Rou Dou Kou* is almost always used in its roasted form for the functions described above, and is best for warming the middle *jiao* and stopping diarrhea. The fresh or unprocessed form is contraindicated in patients with deficiency and cold of the middle *jiao*, as it contains essential oil that stimulates the intestines and causes diarrhea.

CAUTIONS / CONTRAINDICATIONS

- Use of *Rou Dou Kou* is contraindicated for patients who have excess or heat conditions (e.g., diarrhea or dysentery caused by heat).

OVERDOSAGE

Dizziness, incoherent speech or stupor, and hypersomnia have been reported following ingestion of 7.5 grams or more of *Rou Dou Kou* powder. Use of myristicin has been associated with hallucination in humans.[1]

CHEMICAL COMPOSITION

Pinene, sabinene, camphene, myristicin, eugenol, safrol, elemicin, α-thujene, carene, dipentene, geraniol, dehydrodisoeugenol, terpinene, myristin, olein, diarylpropanoids.[2,3]

H_2C … OCH_3

Myristicin

PHARMACOLOGICAL EFFECTS

- **Sedative and hypnotic:** The essential oil of *Rou Dou Kou* has demonstrated an inhibitory effect on the central nervous system. Following intravenous injection at the dosage of 50 mg/kg in rabbits, there is a significant inhibition of perception of pain and olfactory stimulation. It also prolonged sleeping time induced by pentobarbital.[4]
- **Antibiotic:** *Rou Dou Kou* has an inhibitory effect on *Staphylococcus aureus, Diplococcus pneumoniae,* and *Bacillus subtilis.*[5]
- **Anesthetic:** The essential oil of *Rou Dou Kou* has shown anesthetic functions in mice, rabbit, cat and dog studies.[6]

CLINICAL STUDIES AND RESEARCH

- **Ulcerative colitis:** Ulcerative colitis in 62 patients was treated with an herbal decoction with complete recovery in 44 patients, moderate improvement in 16, and no response in 2. The herbal decoction contained *Rou Dou Kou, Bai Zhu* (Rhizoma Atractylodis Macrocephalae), *He Zi* (Fructus Chebulae), *Ren Shen* (Radix Ginseng), *Mu Xiang* (Radix Aucklandiae), *Dang Gui* (Radicis Angelicae Sinensis), *Rou Gui* (Cortex Cinnamomi), *Zhi Gan Cao* (Radix Glycyrrhizae Preparata), *Bai Shao* (Radix Paeoniae Alba), and *Ying Su Ke* (Pericarpium Papaveris). *Fu Ling* (Poria) and *Yi Yi Ren* (Semen Coicis) were added for dampness; *Huang Qi* (Radix Astragali) and *Sheng Ma* (Rhizoma Cimicifugae) were added for qi deficiency; *Fu Zi* (Radix Aconiti Lateralis Praeparata) and *Pao Jiang* (Rhizoma Zingiberis Preparatum) were added for excess cold; *Huang Lian* (Rhizoma Coptidis) and *Da Huang* (Radix et Rhizoma Rhei) were added for excess heat; *Shan Zha* (Fructus Crataegi) and *Bing Lang* (Semen Arecae) were added for food stagnation; *Yan Hu Suo* (Rhizoma Corydalis) and a large dosage of *Bai Shao* (Radix Paeoniae Alba) were added for excess pain; and charred *Di Yu* (Radix Sanguisorbae) and *San Qi* (Radix Notoginseng) were added for rectal bleeding.[7]
- **Infantile diarrhea:** According to one report, 285 infants were treated effectively using an herbal formula containing *Shan Yao* (Rhizoma Dioscoreae), *Ma Chi Xian*

Rou Dou Kou (Semen Myristicae)

(Herba Portulacae), *Cang Zhu* (Rhizoma Atractylodis), *Che Qian Zi* (Semen Plantaginis), *Rou Dou Kou* (Semen Myristicae), *Gan Cao* (Radix Glycyrrhizae), *Da Huang* (Radix et Rhizoma Rhei), and *Ding Xiang* (Flos Caryophylli). The herbs were given in powder form four times daily.[8]

TOXICOLOGY

The LD_{50} for myristicin in cats is 0.5 to 1.0 ml/kg. Subcutaneous injection of myristicin at the dosage of 0.12 ml may lead to hepatic disorders. Ingestion of *Rou Dou Kou* powder in cats at the dosage of 1.8 g/kg may induce drowsiness, and possibly fatality within 24 hours.[9]

SUPPLEMENT

- 肉豆根 *Rou Dou Gen* (Radix Myristicae) is derived from the root of the same plant as *Rou Dou Kou*. It is acrid, bitter and cold. Its functions and indications include regulating the menses to treat irregular menstruation, promoting urination to treat dysuria, and clearing heat to reduce pain and inflammation of the eyes and ears. The dosage for *Rou Dou Gen* is 10 to 15 grams.

AUTHORS' COMMENTS

Rou Dou Kou and *He Zi* (Fructus Chebulae) both treat chronic diarrhea. *Rou Dou Kou* focuses on the middle *jiao* and treats abdominal fullness and pain, poor appetite and nausea due to cold, Spleen deficiency and qi stagnation. *He Zi* focuses on the upper *jiao* and treats wheezing and chronic cough with loss of voice from Lung qi deficiency.

Rou Dou Kou and *Bai Dou Kou* (Fructus Amomi Rotundus) both warm the middle *jiao* and regulate qi. They are both suitable for deficiency and cold of the Spleen and Stomach with qi stagnation causing symptoms such as epigastric and abdominal fullness and pain, diarrhea, and vomiting. *Rou Dou Kou* is also an astringent and stops chronic diarrhea (especially early morning diarrhea caused by Spleen and Kidney yang deficiencies). *Bai Dou Kou* regulates qi and relieves nausea and vomiting. It more commonly is used to dry dampness of the middle *jiao* and relieve abdominal fullness and poor appetite.

Rou Dou Kou (Semen Myristicae), *Bai Dou Kou* (Fructus Amomi Rotundus), and *Cao Dou Kou* (Semen Alpiniae Katsumadai) have similar pinyin names, but different functions. They should not be abbreviated as "*Dou Kou*," to avoid error and confusion.

- *Rou Dou Kou* binds the intestines and stops diarrhea.
- *Bai Dou Kou* regulates qi, dissolves dampness, and strengthens the Stomach.
- *Cao Dou Kou* warms the middle *jiao* and dries dampness.

References

1. *Zhong Yao Xue* (Chinese Herbology), 1998; 891:892
2. *Xian Dai Zhong Yao Yao Li Xue* (Contemporary Pharmacology of Chinese Herbs), 1997; 1401
3. *The Merck Index* 12th edition, Chapman & Hall/CRCnetBASE/Merck, 2000
4. *Zhi Wu Yao You Xiao Cheng Fen Shou Ce* (Manual of Plant Medicinals and Their Active Constituents), 1986: 722
5. *J of Nat Prod*, 1991; 54(3):856
6. *Zhong Cao Yao Tong Xun* (Journal of Chinese Herbal Medicine), 1978; (9):7
7. *Shan Dong Yi Yao* (Shandong Medicine and Herbology), 1990; 30(9):29
8. *Si Chuan Zhong Yi* (Sichuan Chinese Medicine), 1990; 8(6):27
9. *Chang Yong Zhong Yao Cheng Fen Yu Yao Li Shou Ce* (A Handbook of the Composition and Pharmacology of Common Chinese Drugs), 1994; 855:858

Shi Liu Pi (Pericarpium Granati)

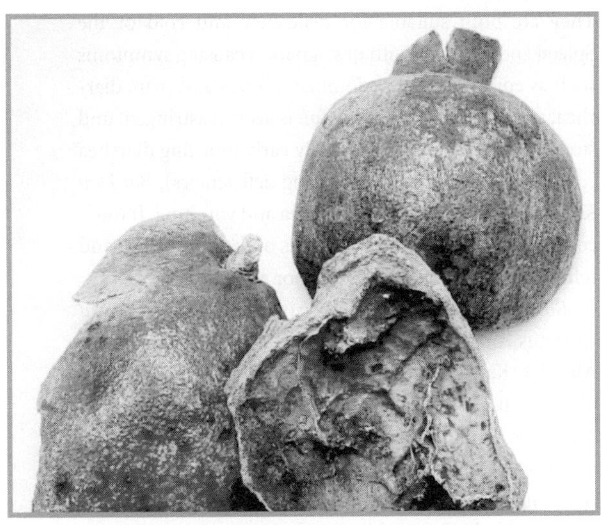

石榴皮

Pinyin Name: *Shi Liu Pi*
Alternate Chinese Names: *Shi Liu Ke, Suan Liu Pi, Suan Shi Liu Pi*
Original Source: *Ming Yi Za Zhu* (Miscellaneous Records of Famous Physicians) by Tao Hong-Jing in 500 A.D.
English Name: granatum rind
Botanical Name: *Punica granatum* L. (*Shi Liu*)
Pharmaceutical Name: Pericarpium Granati
Properties: sour, astringent, warm
Channels Entered: Stomach, Large Intestine

CHINESE THERAPEUTIC ACTIONS

1. Binds the Intestines and Stops Diarrhea

Chronic diarrhea, dysentery, and rectal prolapse: Sour and astringent, *Shi Liu Pi* (Pericarpium Granati) enters the Large Intestine to bind and stop chronic watery diarrhea. It is commonly used to treat chronic diarrhea, dysentery, and rectal prolapse caused by either Spleen yang deficiency or damp-heat accumulation. *Shi Liu Pi* may be used individually or in combination with other herbs.

- Chronic diarrhea due to Spleen yang deficiency: combine *Shi Liu Pi* with *Bai Zhu* (Rhizoma Atractylodis Macrocephalae), *Dang Shen* (Radix Codonopsis) and *Fu Ling* (Poria).
- Chronic damp-heat dysentery: use this herb with *Huang Lian* (Rhizoma Coptidis) and *Huang Bai* (Cortex Phellodendri).
- Rectal prolapse: use it with *Ming Fan* (Alumen), and *Jin Ying Zi* (Fructus Rosae Laevigatae) as an external soak. In addition, apply *Wu Bei Zi* (Galla Chinensis) powder topically to the affected area.

2. Kills Parasites

Shi Liu Pi kills intestinal parasites and relieves pain.

- Tapeworms and roundworms with abdominal pain: use this herb with *Bing Lang* (Semen Arecae).
- Amoebic dysentery: use alone as decoction three times daily, for six days.

3. Stops Bleeding

Shi Liu Pi is used in powder form externally to stop bleeding caused by trauma. Internally, it is used in decoction to treat uterine bleeding and leukorrhea.

- Bleeding due to traumatic injuries: apply it topically as a powder.
- Uterine bleeding: combine this herb with charred *Di Yu* (Radix Sanguisorbae), charred *Jing Jie* (Herba Schizonepetae), *Da Ji* (Herba seu Radix Cirsii Japonici) and *Xiao Ji* (Herba Cirisii).

Shi Liu Pi is also used topically to treat psoriasis.

DOSAGE

3 to 10 grams in decoction. Use *Shi Liu Pi* externally as powder or as a wash.

CAUTIONS / CONTRAINDICATIONS

- *Shi Liu Pi* is contraindicated in the acute or beginning stages of diarrhea or dysentery. When using this herb to kill parasites, dietary fats and oils should be avoided, as they may interfere with absorption of the herb.

CHEMICAL COMPOSITION

Pelletierine, methyl-pelletierine, pseudo-pelletierine, dl-isopelletierine, methyl-dl-isopelletierine, isoquercitrin, inulin, mannitol, tannin, mallic acid, punicine, calcium oxalate.[1]

PHARMACOLOGICAL EFFECTS

- **Antibiotic:** Decoction of *Shi Liu Pi* has an inhibitory effect against *Corynebacterium diphtheriae, Staphylococcus aureus, Bacillus dysenteriae*, and various pathogenic fungi and dermatophytes.[2]
- **Antiparasitic:** Decoction of *Shi Liu Pi* has demonstrated a marked antiparasitic effect against tapeworms.[3]

CLINICAL STUDIES AND RESEARCH

- **Burns:** In one study, 45 patients with first- and second-degree burns showed remarkable improvement and

Shi Liu Pi (Pericarpium Granati)

complete recovery after topical treatment with *Shi Liu Pi* solution. The treatment protocol was to cook 500 grams of the herb in water to yield 250 ml of solution. The herb residue was filtered out and the solution applied to the burned area topically.[4]

TOXICOLOGY

The alkaloids of *Shi Liu Pi*, approximately 25 times more toxic than the fresh herb, are responsible for most adverse reactions, such as dizziness, weakness, visual disturbances, tinnitus, tremor, nausea, vomiting, abdominal pain, and diarrhea. The side effects are relieved by discontinuation of the herb. In animal toxicology studies, respiratory suppression has been reported following gross overdose.[5]

AUTHORS' COMMENTS

According to Dr. Gan Zhu-Wang, *Shi Liu Pi*, *He Zi* (Fructus Chebulae) and *Yi Zhi Ren* (Fructus Alpiniae Oxyphyllae) added to a base formula, treat incessant nasal discharge.

References

1. *Xian Dai Zhong Yao Yao Li Xue* (Contemporary Pharmacology of Chinese Herbs), 1997; 755
2. *Zhong Cao Yao Xue* (Study of Chinese Herbal Medicine), 1976; 694
3. *Chang Yong Zhong Yao Xian Dai Yan Jiu Yu Lin Chuan* (Recent Study & Clinical Application of Common Traditional Chinese Medicine), 1995; 675:676
4. *Ji Lin Zhong Yi Yao* (Jilin Chinese Medicine and Herbology), 1983; 4:29
5. *Chang Yong Zhong Yao Xian Dai Yan Jiu Yu Lin Chuan* (Recent Study & Clinical Application of Common Traditional Chinese Medicine), 1995; 675:676

Chun Gen Pi (Cortex Ailanthi)

椿根皮 樗根皮

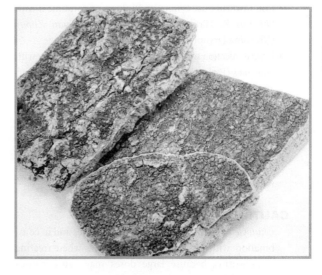

Pinyin Name: *Chun Gen Pi*
Alternate Chinese Names: *Chou Chun Pi, Chu Pi, Chu Bai Pi*
Original Source: *Yao Xing Ben Cao* (Materia Medica of Medicinal Properties) by Zhen Quan in 600 A.D.
English Name: ailanthus bark
Botanical Name: *Ailanthus altissima* (Mill.) Swingle (*Chou Chun*)
Pharmaceutical Name: Cortex Ailanthi
Properties: bitter, astringent, cold
Channels Entered: Large Intestine, Stomach, Liver

CHINESE THERAPEUTIC ACTIONS

1. Clears Heat, Dries Dampness and Binds the Intestines

Dysentery or diarrhea: Bitter and cold, *Chun Gen Pi* (Cortex Ailanthi) enters the Large Intestine to clear heat and dry dampness. Because it is astringent, this herb also binds the intestines. It commonly treats chronic diarrhea or dysentery accompanying damp-heat accumulation in the Large Intestine. Use of *Chun Gen Pi* is most effective when diarrhea or dysentery is accompanied by blood or pus. It may be used individually or in combination, as decoction or enema.

- Chronic dysentery or diarrhea with pus and blood: use *Chun Gen Pi* alone as an enema, or use it with *Huang Lian* (Rhizoma Coptidis), *Huang Bai* (Cortex Phellodendri) and *Huang Qin* (Radix Scutellariae).
- Chronic diarrhea with deficiency and cold signs: combine this herb with *Bu Gu Zhi* (Fructus Psoraleae), *Wu Zhu Yu* (Fructus Evodiae), and *Rou Dou Kou* (Semen Myristicae).
- Toxic heat dysentery: add it to *Huang Lian* (Rhizoma Coptidis), *Huang Bai* (Cortex Phellodendri) and *Huang Qin* (Radix Scutellariae).

Chun Gen Pi (Cortex Ailanthi)

2. Stops Bleeding

Uterine bleeding, red or white leukorrhea: Astringent in nature, *Chun Gen Pi* treats various causes of bleeding, including uterine bleeding from yin deficiency, and vaginal discharge or bleeding caused by damp-heat accumulation.

- Uterine bleeding: combine it with *Gui Ban* (Plastrum Testudinis), *Bai Shao* (Radix Paeoniae Alba), *Xiang Fu* (Rhizoma Cyperi) and *Huang Qin* (Radix Scutellariae).
- Vaginal bleeding due to damp-heat with red and white vaginal discharge: add it to *Huang Bai* (Cortex Phellodendri), *Zhi Zi* (Fructus Gardeniae), *Qian Shi* (Semen Euryales) and *Lian Zi* (Semen Nelumbinis).
- Postpartum rectal prolapse: use this herb with *Hua Jiao* (Pericarpium Zanthoxyli) as a wash.

3. Kills Parasites

Roundworms, fungus: *Chun Gen Pi* effectively treats intestinal parasites and fungus. It may be used individually or in combination with other herbs. However, individual use of *Chun Gen Pi* often requires a large dosage that may cause side effects such as nausea and vomiting. In order to keep the dosage at a useful level without side effects, other antiparasitic herbs should be added.

- Roundworms: use *Chun Gen Pi* alone, or combine it with *Shi Jun Zi* (Fructus Quisqualis) and *Guan Zhong* (Rhizoma Dryopteridis).
- Fungal infection with itching: use this herb externally with *Hua Jiao* (Pericarpium Zanthoxyli), *Ming Fan* (Alumen) and *Li Lu* (Radix et Rhizoma Veratri) as an external wash.

DOSAGE

3 to 5 grams for internal use. Externally, *Chun Gen Pi* is used in the form of a wash or ointment. The charred form more strongly functions to bind the intestines and relieve diarrhea.

CAUTIONS / CONTRAINDICATIONS

Chun Gen Pi is often used in smaller dosages and in combination with other antiparasitic herbs when treating roundworms, because large doses may cause nausea and vomiting.

CHEMICAL COMPOSITION

Quassin, ailanthone.[1,2]

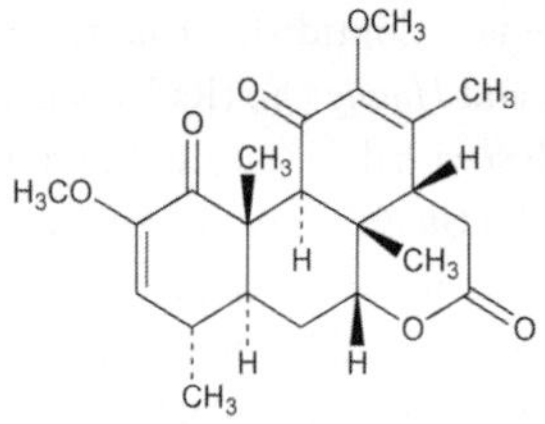

Quassin

PHARMACOLOGICAL EFFECTS

- **Antineoplastic:** Quassin and ailanthone have demonstrated preliminary antineoplastic effects against nose and throat cancers.[3]

CLINICAL STUDIES AND RESEARCH

- **Hematochezia:** In one study, an herbal decoction effectively helped all of 46 patients with blood in the stool due to various causes. The herbal formula used 120 grams of *Chun Gen Pi* as the main ingredient, and the decoction was administered three times daily.[4]

SUPPLEMENT

- 椿根 / 桩根 *Chun Gen* (Radix Ailanthi) is the entire root used as the medicinal part of the plant, while *Chun Gen Pi* is the bark. *Chun Gen* is bitter and astringent, and enters the Stomach channel. It functions to dry dampness from the middle *jiao*, bind the intestines to relieve diarrhea, clear heat to reduce swelling and inflammation, and release the exterior to promote eruption of measles. Clinically, it treats chronic diarrhea, chronic dysentery, hematochezia, profuse menstrual discharge, and cancers of the rectum and cervix. It is contraindicated in cases of deficiency and cold of the Spleen and Stomach. The dosage for *Chun Gen* is 3 to 5 grams.

AUTHORS' COMMENTS

Chun Gen Pi and *Shi Liu Pi* (Pericarpium Granati) bind the intestines, stop diarrhea and kill parasites. Both herbs are used internally and externally.

- *Chun Gen Pi* is cold, and treats chronic damp-heat diarrhea, possibly including blood or mucus in the stools. Externally, *Chun Gen Pi* is used as a wash or paste to treat dermatological disorders.
- *Shi Liu Pi* is warm, and treats chronic diarrhea with rectal prolapse caused by Spleen qi or yang deficiency. It is also used externally as a soak or powder.

References

1. *Zhong Yao Xue* (Chinese Herbology), 1998; 888
2. *The Merck Index* 12th edition, Chapman & Hall/CRCnetBASE/Merck, 2000.
3. *Zhi Wu Yao You Xiao Cheng Fen Shou Ce* (Manual of Plant Medicinals and Their Active Constituents), 1986: 26:875
4. *An Hui Zhong Yi Xue Yuan Xue Bao* (Journal of Anhui University School of Medicine); 1985; 2:62

Shan Zhu Yu (Fructus Corni)

山茱萸 山茱萸

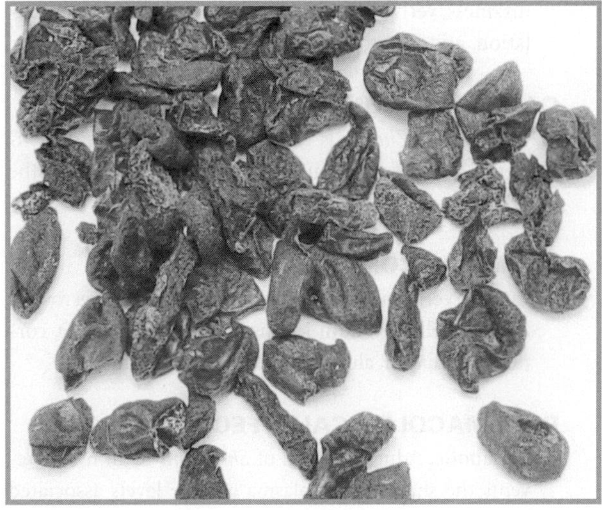

Pinyin Name: *Shan Zhu Yu*
Literal Name: "sour mountain herb," "wild date"
Alternate Chinese Names: *Zao Rou, Shan Yu Rou, Zao Pi*
Original Source: *Shen Nong Ben Cao Jing* (Divine Husbandman's Classic of the Materia Medica) in the second century
English Name: cornus, medicinal cornel fruit, asiatic cornelian cherry fruit, Japanese cornel dogwood fruit
Botanical Name: *Cornus officinalis* Sieb. et Zucc. (*Shan Zhu Yu*)
Pharmaceutical Name: Fructus Corni
Properties: sour, slightly warm
Channels Entered: Kidney, Liver

CHINESE THERAPEUTIC ACTIONS

1. Tonifies the Liver and Kidney

Liver and Kidney deficiencies: Lack of nourishment of Liver blood and Kidney *jing* (essence) leads to symptoms such as dizziness, vertigo, light-headedness, soreness and weakness of the lower back and knees, impotence and spermatorrhea. *Shan Zhu Yu* (Fructus Corni) tonifies Liver blood, Kidney *jing* and yang.

- Liver and Kidney yin deficiencies: combine *Shan Zhu Yu* with *Shu Di Huang* (Radix Rehmanniae Preparata), *Shan Yao* (Rhizoma Dioscoreae), *Mu Dan Pi* (Cortex Moutan), *Ze Xie* (Rhizoma Alismatis) and *Fu Ling* (Poria). **Exemplar Formula:** *Liu Wei Di Huang Wan* (Six-Ingredient Pill with Rehmannia).
- Tinnitus, blurred vision from Kidney yin deficiency: add it to *Shu Di Huang* (Radix Rehmanniae Preparata), *Shan Yao* (Rhizoma Dioscoreae), *Gui Ban Jiao* (Gelatinum Plastrum Testudinis), *Lu Jiao Jiao* (Gelatinum Cornu Cervi) and *Gou Qi Zi* (Fructus Lycii).
- Impotence and spermatorrhea because of Kidney yang deficiency: combine this herb with *Bu Gu Zhi* (Fructus Psoraleae), *Suo Yang* (Herba Cynomorii), *Jin Ying Zi* (Fructus Rosae Laevigatae) and *Yin Yang Huo* (Herba Epimedii).
- Back pain: use it with *Xu Duan* (Radix Dipsaci) and *Du Zhong* (Cortex Eucommiae).

2. Retains *Jing* (Essence) and Body Fluids

Excessive perspiration arising from deficiency: When there is a deficiency in *zheng* (upright) *qi*, perspiration occurs, as there is insufficient qi to close the pores. Also as seen in shock, devastated yang or collapse, qi becomes unable to control the pores, and excessive sweating and coldness occur.

- Excessive sweating: combine *Shan Zhu Yu* with *Wu Wei Zi* (Fructus Schisandrae Chinensis), *Mai Men Dong* (Radix Ophiopogonis), *Huang Qi* (Radix Astragali), *Long Gu* (Os Draconis) and *Mu Li* (Concha Ostreae).
- Shock, drastic drop in blood pressure, and excessive perspiration: incorporate this herb with *Ren Shen* (Radix Ginseng) and *Fu Zi* (Radix Aconiti Lateralis Praeparata).

Uterine bleeding

- Excessive uterine bleeding: combine *Shan Zhu Yu* with charred *Huang Bai* (Cortex Phellodendri), *E Jiao* (Colla Corii Asini) and charred *Ai Ye* (Folium Artemisiae Argyi).

Urinary incontinence or polyuria: Kidney yang deficiency is often a cause of an inability to retain urine.

- Frequent urination, polyuria (light in color with no dysuria): combine *Shan Zhu Yu* with *Sang Piao Xiao* (Ootheca Mantidis), *Yi Zhi Ren* (Fructus Alpiniae Oxyphyllae), *Fu Pen Zi* (Fructus Rubi), *Wu Yao* (Radix Linderae Strychnifolia), *Shu Di Huang* (Radix Rehmanniae Preparata), *Shan Yao* (Rhizoma Dioscoreae) and *Wu Wei Zi* (Fructus Schisandrae Chinensis).
- Terminal dripping following urination: use this herb with *Fu Pen Zi* (Fructus Rubi), *Tu Si Zi* (Semen Cuscutae), *Jin Ying Zi* (Fructus Rosae Laevigatae) and *Sha Yuan Zi* (Semen Astragali Complanati).

DOSAGE

6 to 12 grams. In severe cases, use up to 30 grams of *Shan Zhu Yu*. The unprocessed herb has a stronger binding function to treat spontaneous or night perspiration. The steamed form (with grain-based liquor) has a warmer and stronger tonic effect for the Liver and Kidney, and is commonly used to treat low back pain,

18 ASTRINGENT HERBS

Shan Zhu Yu (Fructus Corni)

dizziness, vertigo, tinnitus, impotence, premature ejaculation, and incontinence.

CAUTIONS / CONTRAINDICATIONS

- Use of *Shan Zhu Yu* is contraindicated in cases of deficient Kidney fire, or in dysuria caused by heat in the lower *jiao*.

CHEMICAL COMPOSITION

Cornin, verbenalin, ursolic acid, morroniside, sweroside, loganin, tellmagrandin I, II; isoterchebin, gemin D, cornusin A, B; iron, aluminum, and magnesium.[1]

PHARMACOLOGICAL EFFECTS

- **Metabolic:** Administration of *Shan Zhu Yu* in mice prevents the sharp rise in plasma glucose levels associated with epinephrine or ingestion of a large dose of glucose. With long-term ingestion, there is an increase in glycogen storage in the liver but no significant change to the triglyceride or total cholesterol levels.[2]
- **Anti-inflammatory:** In one laboratory study with mice, 5 g/kg of *Shan Zhu Yu* demonstrated an anti-inflammatory effect similar to 50 mg/kg of aspirin, and both treatments significantly reduced swelling.[3]
- **Antibiotic:** *Shan Zhu Yu* has an inhibitory effect against *Staphylococcus aureus, Salmonella typhi, Bacillus dysenteriae* and some pathogenic fungi.[4]
- **Diuretic:** In anesthetized dogs, extract of *Shan Zhu Yu* induces diuresis and lowers blood pressure.[5]

HERB-DRUG INTERACTION

- **Diuretics:** *Shan Zhu Yu* has a diuretic effect. Though no instances of this potential interaction have been documented, concurrent use with diuretic drugs may lead to increased elimination of water and/or electrolytes.[6] [Note: Examples of diuretics include chlorothiazide, hydrochlorothiazide, furosemide (Lasix), bumetanide (Bumex), and torsemide (Demadex).]

TOXICOLOGY

Shan Zhu Yu has very low toxicity.[7]

References

1. *Chang Yong Zhong Yao Cheng Fen Yu Yao Li Shou Ce* (A Handbook of the Composition and Pharmacology of Common Chinese Drugs), 1994; 368-369
2. *Zhong Yao Yao Li Yu Lin Chuang* (Pharmacology and Clinical Applications of Chinese Herbs), 1989; 5(1):36
3. *Chang Yong Zhong Yao Cheng Fen Yu Yao Li Shou Ce* (A Handbook of the Composition and Pharmacology of Common Chinese Drugs), 1994, 368:376
4. *CA*, 1953; 47:12652g
5. *Chang Yong Zhong Yao Cheng Fen Yu Yao Li Shou Ce* (A Handbook of the Composition and Pharmacology of Common Chinese Drugs), 1994, 368:376
6. Chen, J. Recognition & prevention of herb-drug interactions, *Medical Acupuncture*, Fall/Winter 1998/1999; volume 10/number 2; 9-13
7. *Zhong Yao Tong Bao* (Journal of Chinese Herbology), 1987; 12:(11):38

Jin Ying Zi (Fructus Rosae Laevigatae)

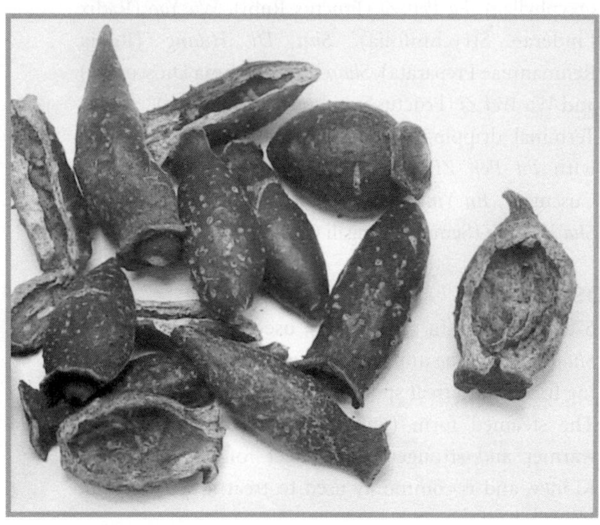

金櫻子 金樱子

Pinyin Name: *Jin Ying Zi*

Literal Name: "golden cherry fruit," "golden-tassel seed," "golden-cherry seed"

Original Source: *Shu Ben Cao* (Materia Medica of Sichuan) by Han Bao-Sheng in 935-960 A.D.

English Name: rosa laevigata, golden tassel seed, cherokee rose fruit

Botanical Name: *Rosa laevigata* Michx.

Pharmaceutical Name: Fructus Rosae Laevigatae

Properties: sour, astringent, neutral

Channels Entered: Kidney, Urinary Bladder, Large Intestine

Jin Ying Zi (Fructus Rosae Laevigatae)

CHINESE THERAPEUTIC ACTIONS

1. Consolidates *Jing* (Essence) and Restrains Urine

Spermatorrhea, polyuria, profuse vaginal discharge: *Jin Ying Zi* (Fructus Rosae Laevigatae) treats various disorders characterized by leakage of body fluids from the lower *jiao*, such as frequent urination, urinary incontinence, spermatorrhea, profuse vaginal discharge, and other urinary disorders caused by Kidney deficiency. *Jin Ying Zi* may be used individually or in combination with other herbs.

- Urinary disorders: combine this herb with *Qian Shi* (Semen Euryales).
- Spermatorrhea or nocturnal emissions: use *Jin Ying Zi* alone.

2. Binds the Intestines and Stops Diarrhea

Chronic diarrhea: *Jin Ying Zi* treats chronic diarrhea or dysentery resulting from Spleen qi deficiency. It effectively helps prolapse of the rectum or uterus, or profuse uterine bleeding. It may be used individually or in combination with other herbs.

- Chronic diarrhea: combine *Jin Ying Zi* with *Bai Zhu* (Rhizoma Atractylodis Macrocephalae), *Dang Shen* (Radix Codonopsis), *Shan Yao* (Rhizoma Dioscoreae) and *Fu Ling* (Poria).

DOSAGE

6 to 18 grams in decoction.

CAUTIONS / CONTRAINDICATIONS

- *Jin Ying Zi* is contraindicated in cases of excess fire or exterior disorders.
- Potential side effects of *Jin Ying Zi* include constipation, abdominal pain, abdominal fullness and cough.[1]

CHEMICAL COMPOSITION

Saponins, limonene, citric acid, mallic acid, fructose, sucrose, tannin, resin, vitamin C.[2]

PHARMACOLOGICAL EFFECTS

- **Antihyperlipidemic:** In rabbits with artificially-induced atherosclerosis, daily administration of *Jin Ying Zi* for 2 to 3 weeks significantly reduced total cholesterol and β-lipoprotein, compared to the placebo group. A decrease in fat content in the heart and the liver was also observed.[3]
- **Antibiotic:** Decoction of *Jin Ying Zi* has an inhibitory effect against various influenza viruses. A 25% solution has a limiting influence on *Staphylococcus aureus*, *E. coli*, and *Pseudomonas aeruginosa*.[4]

CLINICAL STUDIES AND RESEARCH

- **Prolapsed uterus:** In one clinical study, 203 patients experiencing uterine prolapse were treated with a 76% rate of effectiveness using an herbal decoction. The decoction was prepared by soaking 3,000 grams of *Jin Ying Zi* in water for 24 hours, then cooking it slowly in water to yield 3,000 ml in the final decoction. Patients were instructed to take 60 ml of the decoction with warm water twice daily for 3 days, followed by 3 days of rest, and conclude with 3 more days of treatment. Out of 203 patients, the study reported complete recovery in 16 patients and improvement in 138 patients.[5]
- **Infantile diarrhea:** According to one report, 20 infants with diarrhea were treated with a decoction of *Jin Ying Zi* with complete recovery in 13 cases, improvement in 6 cases, and no response in 1 case. The herbal decoction was prepared by cooking 3,000 grams of the herb in 3,000 ml of water, to yield 1,500 ml of the final decoction. Patients were given the decoction three times daily on an empty stomach. The dosage was 10 ml for infants under 1 year of age, 15 ml for infants between 1 and 2 years of age, and 20 ml for those over 2 years of age.[6]

TOXICOLOGY

Subcutaneous injection of *Jin Ying Zi* in developing mice at the dosage of 500 to 1,100 mg/kg showed a decreased rate of weight gain, an increase in white blood cell counts, and a decrease in red blood cell counts. No abnormalities were observed in liver enzymes and blood examination, nor were abnormalities noted in biopsy of heart, liver, kidney, spleen, intestines, and adrenal cortex tissues.[7]

AUTHORS' COMMENTS

Jin Ying Zi and *He Zi* (Fructus Chebulae) are both astringents. *Jin Ying Zi* more strongly consolidates the *jing* (essence) whereas *He Zi* more effectively binds the intestines to stop diarrhea.

Jin Ying Zi and *Fu Pen Zi* (Fructus Rubi) both treat spermatorrhea and premature ejaculation. However, *Jin Ying Zi* also treats diarrhea and dysentery. *Fu Pen Zi* treats urinary incontinence and enuresis.

References

1. *Chang Yong Zhong Yao Xian Dai Yan Jiu Yu Lin Chuan* (Recent Study & Clinical Application of Common Traditional Chinese Medicine), 1995; 489:690
2. *Zhong Yao Xue* (Chinese Herbology), 1998; 900-901
3. *Chang Yong Zhong Yao Xian Dai Yan Jiu Yu Lin Chuan* (Recent Study & Clinical Application of Common Traditional Chinese Medicine), 1995; 489:690
4. Ibid.
5. *Zhe Jiang Zhong Yi Za Zhi* (Zhejiang Journal of Chinese Medicine), 1960; (3):126
6. *Zhong Yi Za Zhi* (Journal of Chinese Medicine), 1985; 26(6):71
7. *Chang Yong Zhong Yao Xian Dai Yan Jiu Yu Lin Chuan* (Recent Study & Clinical Application of Common Traditional Chinese Medicine), 1995; 489:690

Sang Piao Xiao (Ootheca Mantidis)

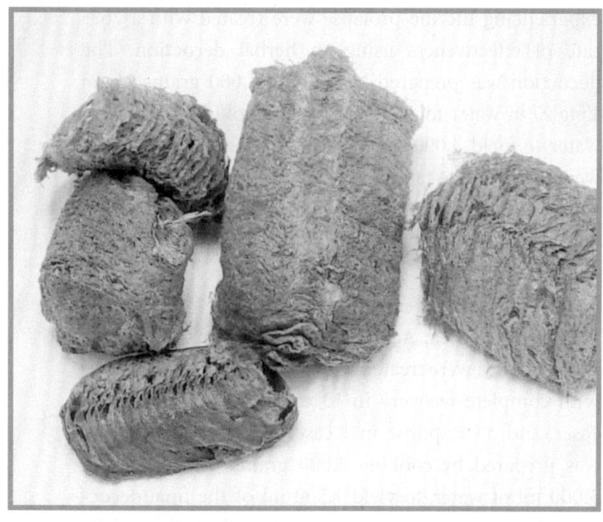

桑螵蛸

Pinyin Name: *Sang Piao Xiao*
Original Source: *Shen Nong Ben Cao Jing* (Divine Husbandman's Classic of the Materia Medica) in the second century
English Name: mantis, mantis egg case
Zoological Name: *Mantis religiosa* L. (*Bao Chi Tang Lang*); *Paratenodera sinensis* Saussure (*Da Dao Lang*); *Statilia maculata* Thunb. (*Xiao Dao Lang*); *Hierodula patellifera* Serville (*Ju Fu Tang Lang*)
Pharmaceutical Name: Ootheca Mantidis
Properties: sweet, salty, neutral
Channels Entered: Liver, Kidney

CHINESE THERAPEUTIC ACTIONS

Tonifies Kidney Yang, Consolidates *Jing* (Essence) and Restrains Urine

Spermatorrhea, frequent urination, profuse vaginal discharge: *Sang Piao Xiao* (Ootheca Mantidis) treats Kidney yang deficiency manifesting as an inability to hold the *jing* in place. Symptoms of this deficiency include spermatorrhea, polyuria, frequent urination, profuse white vaginal discharge, dribbling urine, nocturnal emissions, frequent urination in pregnant women and enuresis in children. *Sang Piao Xiao* in powder form also treats insufficient urination or urinary blockage. *Sang Piao Xiao* exerts a dual effect to regulate the urinary bladder to retain urine, and to promote urination.

- Spermatorrhea and nocturnal emissions due to Heart and Kidney deficiencies: combine it with *Long Gu* (Os Draconis), *Gui Ban* (Plastrum Testudinis), *Fu Shen* (Poria Paradicis) and *Yuan Zhi* (Radix Polygalae). **Exemplar Formula:** *Sang Piao Xiao San* (Mantis Egg-Case Powder).
- Enuresis from Kidney yang deficiency: decoct *Sang Piao Xiao* 12g, *Yi Zhi Ren* (Fructus Alpiniae Oxyphyllae) 9g, *Wu Yao* (Radix Linderae) 12g, *Fu Pen Zi* (Fructus Rubi) 12g, *Xu Duan* (Radix Dipsaci) 15g, *Yin Yang Huo* (Herba Epimedii) 12g, *Rou Gui* (Cortex Cinnamomi) 4g, *Fu Zi* (Radix Aconiti Lateralis Praeparata) 6g, *Suo Yang* (Herba Cynomorii) 12g, *Ji Nei Jin* (Endothelium Corneum Gigeriae Galli) 12g, *Shu Di Huang* (Radix Rehmanniae Preparata) 24g, and *Sang Ji Sheng* (Herba Taxilli) 30g.
- Frequent urination during pregnancy: use this herb alone as powder.
- Dysuria: use this herb alone as powder and serve with rice soup.
- Frequent urination and spermatorrhea caused by Kidney deficiency: use it with *Ren Shen* (Radix Ginseng), *Suan Zao Ren* (Semen Zizyphi Spinosae), *Lian Zi* (Semen Nelumbinis), *Shi Chang Pu* (Rhizoma Acori) and *Yuan Zhi* (Radix Polygalae).

Profuse vaginal discharge, impotence: *Sang Piao Xiao* tonifies Kidney yang and retains essence. Because it is neutral, it is often used with Kidney yang tonics.

- Profuse vaginal discharge or impotence caused by Kidney yang deficiency: add this herb to *Bu Gu Zhi* (Fructus Psoraleae), *Tu Si Zi* (Semen Cuscutae), *Sha Yuan Zi* (Semen Astragali Complanati), *She Chuang Zi* (Fructus Cnidii) and *Lu Jiao Shuang* (Cornu Cervi Degelatinatum).

DOSAGE

3 to 10 grams. Use of unprocessed *Sang Piao Xiao* is sometimes associated with diarrhea. The steamed form is warmer than the unprocessed one, and less likely to cause diarrhea.

CAUTIONS / CONTRAINDICATIONS

- Use of *Sang Piao Xiao* is contraindicated in patients with yin-deficient fire or cystitis with heat accumulation in the urinary bladder.

CHEMICAL COMPOSITION

Protein, amino acids, iron, calcium.[1]

CLINICAL STUDIES AND RESEARCH

- **Enuresis:** According to one report, 11 patients with bed-wetting were treated one time per day with an herbal decoction containing *Sang Piao Xiao* and *Yi Zhi Ren* (Fructus Alpiniae Oxyphyllae), with marked improvement. The dosage was 47 grams of each herb for adults, and 31 grams of each herb for children between 5 and 12

Sang Piao Xiao (Ootheca Mantidis)

years of age.[2] In another study, 45 out of 50 patients experiencing bed-wetting showed complete recovery after treatment with an herbal decoction of *Sang Piao Xiao*, calcined *Mu Li* (Concha Ostreae), *Jiu Cai Zi* (Semen Allii Tuberosi) and other herbs.[3]

AUTHORS' COMMENTS

Sang Piao Xiao, Yi Zhi Ren (Fructus Alpiniae Oxyphyllae), *Fu Pen Zi* (Fructus Rubi), and *Wu Yao* (Radix Linderae) all cause appropriate retention of urine.

- *Sang Piao Xiao* consolidates *jing* (essence).
- *Yi Zhi Ren* more strongly tonifies the Spleen and Kidney.
- *Fu Pen Zi* more effectively tonifies the Liver and Kidney.
- *Wu Yao* warms the Kidney and Urinary Bladder to regulate the qi, and treat frequent urination.

References

1. *Chang Yong Zhong Yao Cheng Fen Yu Yao Li Shou Ce* (A Handbook of the Composition and Pharmacology of Common Chinese Drugs), 1994; 1559-1560
2. *Zhong Yi Za Zhi* (Journal of Chinese Medicine), 1965; 11:30
3. *Xin Yi Xue* (New Medicine), 1974; 3:139

Fu Pen Zi (Fructus Rubi)

覆盆子

Pinyin Name: *Fu Pen Zi*
Literal Name: "overturned bowl fruit"
Alternate Chinese Names: *Fu Pen*
Original Source: *Ming Yi Za Zhu* (Miscellaneous Records of Famous Physicians) by Tao Hong-Jing in 500 A.D.
English Name: rubus, palm-leaf raspberry fruit
Botanical Name: *Rubus chingii* Hu. (*Fu Peng Zi*)
Pharmaceutical Name: Fructus Rubi
Properties: sweet, sour, slightly warm
Channels Entered: Kidney, Liver

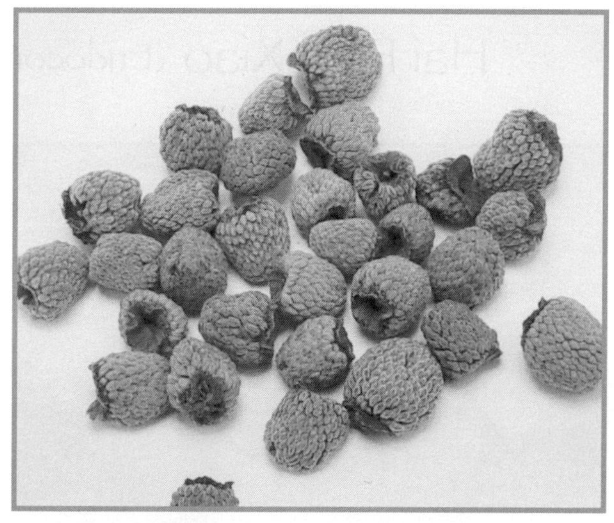

18 ASTRINGENT HERBS

CHINESE THERAPEUTIC ACTIONS

1. Tonifies the Kidney, Consolidates *Jing* (Essence) and Retains Urine

Spermatorrhea and polyuria due to Kidney deficiency: *Fu Pen Zi* (Fructus Rubi) treats Kidney deficiency with signs and symptoms such as spermatorrhea, premature ejaculation, nocturnal emissions and urinary frequency or enuresis. It may be used individually or in combination with other herbs.

- Spermatorrhea, nocturnal emissions, premature ejaculation, impotence: use *Fu Pen Zi* alone as powder, or with *Sha Yuan Zi* (Semen Astragali Complanati), *Shan Zhu Yu* (Fructus Corni) and *Qian Shi* (Semen Euryales).
- Urinary frequency or enuresis: combine this herb with *Sang Piao Xiao* (Ootheca Mantidis), *Yi Zhi Ren* (Fructus Alpiniae Oxyphyllae) and *Jin Ying Zi* (Fructus Rosae Laevigatae).
- Diabetes insipidus with polyuria: add it to *Sang Piao Xiao* (Ootheca Mantidis), *Wu Wei Zi* (Fructus Schisandrae Chinensis), *Shan Zhu Yu* (Fructus Corni), *Wu Yao* (Radix Linderae) and *Yi Zhi Ren* (Fructus Alpiniae Oxyphyllae).

2. Tonifies the Liver and Improves Vision

Impaired vision: *Fu Pen Zi* tonifies the Liver and Kidney, nourishes blood and *jing* (essence) to treat deterioration of visual acuity characterized by blurry vision, dizziness and diminished vision.

Fu Pen Zi (Fructus Rubi)

- Impaired vision: use this herb with *Gou Qi Zi* (Fructus Lycii), *Che Qian Zi* (Semen Plantaginis), *Tu Si Zi* (Semen Cuscutae), *Wu Wei Zi* (Fructus Schisandrae Chinensis), *Sha Yuan Zi* (Semen Astragali Complanati), and *Ye Ming Sha* (Excrementum Vespertilionis Murini).

DOSAGE

3 to 10 grams.

CAUTIONS / CONTRAINDICATIONS

- Use of *Fu Pen Zi* is not suitable for patients who have burning dysuria caused by damp-heat accumulation in the lower *jiao*.
- *Fu Pen Zi* should also be used with caution for Kidney yin deficient patients with heat.

CHEMICAL COMPOSITION

Rubusoside, fupenzic acid, ellagic acid, β-sitosterol.[1]

PHARMACOLOGICAL EFFECTS

- **Antibiotic:** Decoction of *Fu Pen Zi* has an inhibitory effect on *Staphylococcus aureus* and *Vibrio cholerae*.[2]
- **Hormonal:** *Fu Pen Zi* exerts estrogen-like activity on the vaginal mucosa of rats and rabbits.[3]

References

1. *Chang Yong Zhong Yao Cheng Fen Yu Yao Li Shou Ce* (A Handbook of the Composition and Pharmacology of Common Chinese Drugs), 1994; 1843
2. *Zhong Cao Yao Xue* (Study of Chinese Herbal Medicine), 425
3. *Chang Yong Zhong Yao Xian Dai Yan Jiu Yu Lin Chuan* (Recent Study & Clinical Application of Common Traditional Chinese Medicine), 1995; 691:692

Hai Piao Xiao (Endoconcha Sepiae)

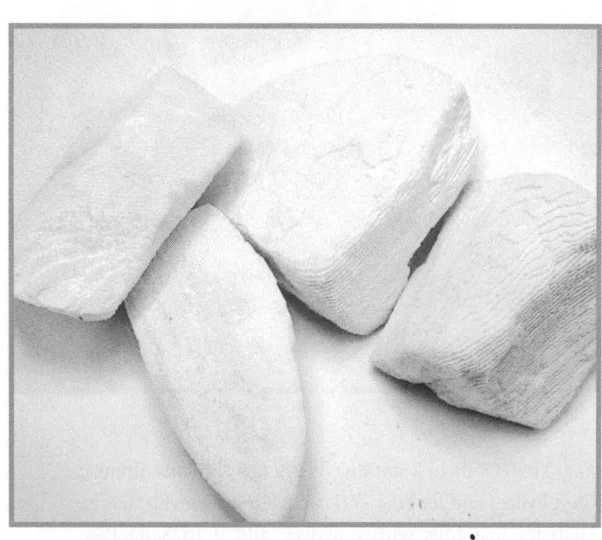

海螵蛸

Pinyin Name: *Hai Piao Xiao*
Alternate Chinese Names: *Wu Zei Gu*
Original Source: *Shen Nong Ben Cao Jing* (Divine Husbandman's Classic of the Materia Medica) in the second century
English Name: cuttlebone, cuttlefish bone
Zoological Name: *Sepiella maindroni* de Rochebrune. (*Wu Zhen Wu Ce*); *Sepia esculenta* Hoyle. (*Jin Wu Ce*)
Pharmaceutical Name: Endoconcha Sepiae
Properties: salty, astringent, slightly warm
Channels Entered: Liver, Kidney

CHINESE THERAPEUTIC ACTIONS

1. Stops Bleeding

Hai Piao Xiao (Endoconcha Sepiae) most effectively treats bleeding from the lungs, stomach and uterus caused by qi deficiency with inability of Spleen to keep the blood circulating within the vessels. It is also used for trauma-related bleeding when applied topically. It may be used individually or in combination, internally or topically.

- Hematemesis: use *Hai Piao Xiao* with *Bai Ji* (Rhizoma Bletillae) and *Chuan Bei Mu* (Bulbus Fritillariae Cirrhosae).
- Bleeding from the lungs or stomach: combine this substance with *Bai Ji* (Rhizoma Bletillae), *Zhe Bei Mu* (Bulbus Fritillariae Thunbergii), *Da Huang* (Radix et Rhizoma Rhei) and *Gan Cao* (Radix Glycyrrhizae).
- Uterine bleeding: add it to calcined *Long Gu* (Os Draconis), calcined *Mu Li* (Concha Ostreae), *Shan Zhu Yu* (Fructus Corni), *Huang Qi* (Radix Astragali), *Wu Wei Zi* (Fructus Schisandrae Chinensis), *Tu Si Zi* (Semen Cuscutae), *Qian Cao* (Radix Rubiae) and *Wu Bei Zi* (Galla Chinensis).

Hai Piao Xiao (Endoconcha Sepiae)

- External bleeding due to trauma: apply this substance topically with *San Qi* (Radix Notoginseng).
- Bleeding due to tooth extraction or nasal surgery: use *Hai Piao Xiao* powder topically to stop bleeding.

2. Consolidates *Jing* (Essence) and Stops Leukorrhea

Spermatorrhea and leukorrhea: *Hai Piao Xiao* treats leakage of Kidney *jing* caused by Kidney qi deficiency and inability to hold the *jing*.

- Spermatorrhea: use *Hai Piao Xiao* with *Shan Zhu Yu* (Fructus Corni), *Sha Yuan Zi* (Semen Astragali Complanati) and *Tu Si Zi* (Semen Cuscutae).
- Profuse red, white or clear vaginal discharge: use it with *Shan Yao* (Rhizoma Dioscoreae), *Long Gu* (Os Draconis) and *Mu Li* (Concha Ostreae).

3. Neutralizes Stomach Acid and Relieves Pain

Stomach pain with acid regurgitation: Burning stomach or epigastric pain, acid regurgitation, and distasteful belching are typical signs of patients suffering from gastritis, or gastric or duodenal ulcers. *Hai Piao Xiao* may be used individually or in combination with other herbs to neutralize acid to relieve pain.

- Stomach pain with acid regurgitation: use *Hai Piao Xiao* with *Zhe Bei Mu* (Bulbus Fritillariae Thunbergii).
- Stomach pain with bleeding: combine it with *Bai Ji* (Rhizoma Bletillae) and *Zhe Bei Mu* (Bulbus Fritillariae Thunbergii).
- Bitter taste in the mouth: add it to *Huang Lian* (Rhizoma Coptidis) and *Wu Zhu Yu* (Fructus Evodiae). **Exemplar Formula:** *Zuo Jin Wan* (Left Metal Pill).
- Stomach pain due to stress: combine *Hai Piao Xiao* with *Xiao Yao San* (Rambling Powder).

4. Resolves Dampness and Promotes Healing

Chronic non-healing sores, ulcers or damp rashes: When applied topically, *Hai Piao Xiao* reduces secretions, generates growth of new skin and promotes healing.

- Eczema and dermatitis: use this substance with *Huang Bai* (Cortex Phellodendri), *Qing Dai* (Indigo Naturalis) and *Bing Pian* (Borneolum Syntheticum). Use as powder and apply topically.

DOSAGE

6 to 12 grams in decoction, 1.5 to 3 grams as powder.

CAUTIONS / CONTRAINDICATIONS

- *Hai Piao Xiao* should be used with caution in yin-deficient patients with heat or exterior conditions.

CHEMICAL COMPOSITION

Calcium carbonate, sodium chloride, calcium phosphate, magnesium chloride, chitin.[1]

PHARMACOLOGICAL EFFECTS

- **Gastrointestinal:** With a high content of calcium carbonate, *Hai Piao Xiao* is an effective antacid to neutralize gastric acid.[2]
- **Effect on healing of bone fractures:** Administration of *Hai Piao Xiao* was associated with shortened recovery time in rabbits with bone fractures.[3]

CLINICAL STUDIES AND RESEARCH

- **Ulceration of the skin:** Patients with skin ulcers were treated by topical application of *Hai Piao Xiao* powder, with excellent results. Out of 100 patients, the study reported complete recovery in 83 patients and moderate improvement in 11 patients, within 3 to 5 treatments. The treatment protocol was to sprinkle powdered *Hai Piao Xiao* onto the affected area, cover it with gauze, and change the dressing every 2 to 3 days.[4]
- **Upper gastrointestinal bleeding:** Equal portions of *Hai Piao Xiao* and *Da Huang* (Radix et Rhizoma Rhei) were ground into powder and placed into capsules with a net weight of 500 mg per capsule. The treatment protocol was to administer 4 to 6 capsules every 4 to 6 hours, with warm water. The treatment was effective in treating upper gastrointestinal bleeding in 49 out of 50 patients. The time required for hemostasis was 12 to 72 hours.[5]
- **Peptic ulcer:** In one study, 58 out of 62 patients with gastric or duodenal ulcers showed significant improvement when treated with 2 to 5 grams of an herbal formula, three times daily. The herbal formula contained 85% *Hai Piao Xiao* and 15% *Zhe Bei Mu* (Bulbus Fritillariae Thunbergii). In another study, an herbal formula containing 10 parts *Hai Piao Xiao* and 1 part *Ban Xia* (Rhizoma Pinelliae), given in doses of 2 to 5 grams per dose, three times daily before meals, showed marked effectiveness in treating peptic ulcers.[6,7]

AUTHORS' COMMENTS

Hai Piao Xiao has been found to be an excellent source of calcium and collagen. High in calcium carbonate, it works well as an antacid, and exerts immediate effect.

Use of *Hai Piao Xiao* is sometimes associated with constipation. Adding a small amount of *Da Huang* (Radix et Rhizoma Rhei) alleviates this side effect.

References

1. *Xian Dai Zhong Yao Yao Li Xue* (Contemporary Pharmacology of Chinese Herbs), 1997; 859
2. *Zhong Yao Xue* (Chinese Herbology), 1998; 903:904

18 ASTRINGENT HERBS

Hai Piao Xiao (Endoconcha Sepiae)

3. *Fu Jian Zhong Yi Yao* (Fujian Chinese Medicine and Herbology), 1988; 19(3):49
4. *Zhong Xi Yi Jie He Za Zhi* (Journal of Integrated Chinese and Western Medicine), 1987; 11:697
5. Ibid., 1986; (11):665
6. *Zhong Hua Nei Ke Za Zhi* (Chinese Journal of Internal Medicine), 1959; 7(11):8
7. *Zhong Yao Tong Bao* (Journal of Chinese Herbology), 1958; 4(6):194

Qian Shi (Semen Euryales)

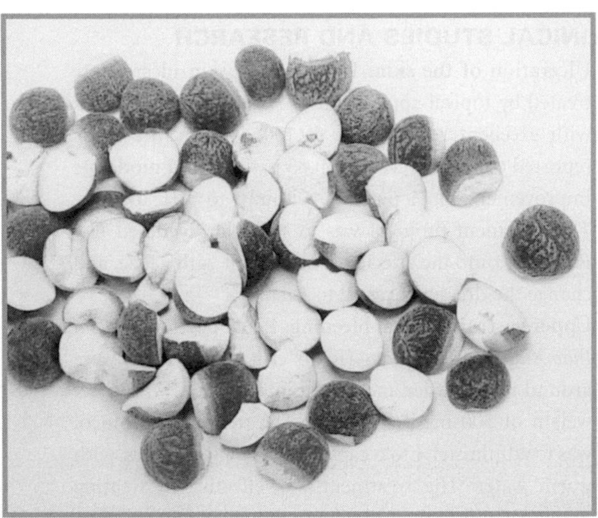

芡實 芡实

Pinyin Name: *Qian Shi*
Literal Name: "gorgon fruit"
Alternate Chinese Names: *Ji Tou Shi, Ji Tou, Yan Tou, Ji Tou Mi*
English Name: euryale, euryale seed
Botanical Name: *Euryale ferox* Salisb.
Pharmaceutical Name: Semen Euryales
Properties: sweet, astringent, neutral
Channels Entered: Kidney, Spleen

CHINESE THERAPEUTIC ACTIONS

1. Tonifies the Spleen and Dispels Dampness

Chronic diarrhea: *Qian Shi* (Semen Euryales) commonly treats chronic diarrhea caused by Spleen deficiency. Deficiency compromises the Spleen function of absorbing water into the body, and subsequently leads to flooding of water into the intestines, and thus to diarrhea. *Qian Shi* relieves diarrhea by tonifying the Spleen and drying intestinal dampness.

- Chronic diarrhea caused by Spleen deficiency: use *Qian Shi* with *Bai Zhu* (Rhizoma Atractylodis Macrocephalae), *Dang Shen* (Radix Codonopsis) and *Fu Ling* (Poria).

2. Tonifies the Kidney and Consolidates *Jing* (Essence)

Spermatorrhea, enuresis, profuse vaginal discharge: Loss of Kidney *jing* is due in part to deficient Kidney qi that has become unable to hold in the *jing*. Clinically, *Qian Shi* treats symptoms such as spermatorrhea, profuse vaginal discharge, and urinary incontinence.

- Spermatorrhea: combine *Qian Shi* with *Jin Ying Zi* (Fructus Rosae Laevigatae).
- Urinary incontinence: add this herb to *Jin Ying Zi* (Fructus Rosae Laevigatae) and *Sang Piao Xiao* (Ootheca Mantidis).
- Profuse clear vaginal discharge: use it with *Jin Ying Zi* (Fructus Rosae Laevigatae) and *Shan Yao* (Rhizoma Dioscoreae).
- Profuse yellow foul-smelling vaginal discharge due to damp-heat accumulation: incorporate *Qian Shi* with *Huang Bai* (Cortex Phellodendri), *Ku Shen Gen* (Radix Sophorae Flavescentis) and *Che Qian Zi* (Semen Plantaginis).

DOSAGE

10 to 15 grams. The maximum dose of *Qian Shi* is 30 grams. Dry-fried, the herb functions better to tonify the Spleen to stop diarrhea, and warm the Kidney to prevent the loss of *jing* (essence).

CHEMICAL COMPOSITION

Starch, protein, lipid, carbohydrates, fiber, thiamine, riboflavine, nicotinic acid, carotene, tryptophan, cysteine, cystine, amylose, amylopectin.[1]

Qian Shi (Semen Euryales)

CLINICAL STUDIES AND RESEARCH

- **Proteinuria:** In one study, 73 patients with proteinuria due to glomerulonephritis were treated with an 89.1% rate of effectiveness. The treatment protocol was daily administration of an herbal formula as porridge for 10 days per course of treatment, for 2 to 4 courses total, with 2 days of intermission between each course. The herbal formula contained 30 grams of *Qian Shi*, 10 pieces of *Bai Guo* (Semen Ginkgo), and 30 grams of sticky rice.[2]

AUTHORS' COMMENTS

According to Dr. Zhu Lang-Chun, *Qian Shi*, *Jin Ying Zi* (Fructus Rosae Laevigatae), and *Yi Zhi Ren* (Fructus Alpiniae Oxyphyllae) have synergistic action to treat proteinuria.

References

1. *Chang Yong Zhong Yao Cheng Fen Yu Yao Li Shou Ce* (A Handbook of the Composition and Pharmacology of Common Chinese Drugs), 1994; 988
2. *Zhong Yi Za Zhi* (Journal of Chinese Medicine), 1985; 9:47

Lian Zi (Semen Nelumbinis)

蓮子 莲子

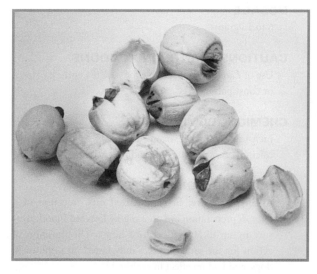

Pinyin Name: *Lian Zi*
Literal Name: "lotus seed"
Alternate Chinese Names: *Lian Zi Rou, Ou Shi, Lian Rou, Lian Shi, Lian Ren*
Original Source: *Shen Nong Ben Cao Jing* (Divine Husbandman's Classic of the Materia Medica) in the second century
English Name: lotus seed
Botanical Name: *Nelumbo nucifera* Gaertn. (*Lian*)
Pharmaceutical Name: Semen Nelumbinis
Properties: sweet, astringent, neutral
Channels Entered: Heart, Kidney, Spleen

CHINESE THERAPEUTIC ACTIONS

1. Tonifies the Spleen and Stops Diarrhea

Chronic diarrhea: *Lian Zi* (Semen Nelumbinis) commonly treats chronic diarrhea caused by Spleen deficiency and inability to transport and transform water. In this instance, water accumulates in the Large Intestine, resulting in diarrhea. Other symptoms associated with Spleen deficiency include poor appetite, weight loss, sallow complexion, poor digestion and generalized weakness. *Lian Zi* treats the root cause and the symptom of diarrhea from Spleen deficiency by tonifying the organ and stopping leakage of body fluids.

- Chronic diarrhea: use *Lian Zi* with *Ren Shen* (Radix Ginseng), *Bai Zhu* (Rhizoma Atractylodis Macrocephalae) and *Shan Yao* (Rhizoma Dioscoreae). **Exemplar Formula:** *Shen Ling Bai Zhu San* (Ginseng, Poria, and Atractylodes Macrocephala Powder).

2. Tonifies the Kidney and Consolidates *Jing* (Essence)

Spermatorrhea, leukorrhea due to Kidney deficiency: *Lian Zi* treats Kidney deficiency characterized by premature ejaculation, spermatorrhea, or profuse, clear or white vaginal discharge. Not only does it tonify the Spleen and Kidney, it also has astringent action to stop leakage of body fluids.

- Premature ejaculation, spermatorrhea: use *Lian Zi* with *Sha Yuan Zi* (Semen Astragali Complanati), *Tu Si Zi* (Semen Cuscutae), *Lian Xu* (Stamen Nelumbinis) and *Lu Rong* (Cornu Cervi Pantotrichum).

Lian Zi (Semen Nelumbinis)

- Vaginal discharge: combine it with *Bai Guo* (Semen Ginkgo), *Qian Shi* (Semen Euryales), *Ji Guan Hua* (Flos Celosiae Cristatae) and *Jin Ying Zi* (Fructus Rosae Laevigatae).

3. Nourishes the Heart and Calms the *Shen* (Spirit)

Irritability, palpitations, insomnia: When there is a lack of nourishment of yin or blood to the *shen* of the Heart, symptoms of irritability, anxiety, dream-disturbed sleep or insomnia may occur.

- Irritability, anxiety, dream-disturbed sleep or insomnia: combine *Lian Zi* with *Mai Men Dong* (Radix Ophiopogonis), *Bai Zi Ren* (Semen Platycladi), *Fu Shen* (Poria Paradicis), *Yuan Zhi* (Radix Polygalae), *Zhen Zhu Mu* (Concha Margaritaferae) and *Suan Zao Ren* (Semen Zizyphi Spinosae).

DOSAGE

6 to 15 grams.

CAUTIONS / CONTRAINDICATIONS

- Use of *Lian Zi* is not suitable for patients with dry stools or constipation.

CHEMICAL COMPOSITION

Liensinine, raffinose, oxoushisunine, N-norarmepavine, calcium, phosphorus, iron, sodium, zinc, magnesium.[1,2]

PHARMACOLOGICAL EFFECTS

- **Antihypertensive:** In anesthetized cats, injection of a *Lian Zi* preparation at 1 to 2 mg/kg lowered blood pressure by up to 50% for 2 to 3 hours. The duration of action for the same product only lasted 30 minutes in dogs, and had no effect in rabbits.[3,4]

SUPPLEMENT

The lotus and its various parts are among the most versatile herbs in Chinese herbal medicine. Every part of the plant has separate and distinct properties. Overall, eight different parts of the lotus plant are used medicinally. A brief summary of all the parts is listed below for comparative purposes. [Note: Additional information on these herbs can be found in the individual monographs. *He Di* (Calyx Nelumbinis) and *He Geng* (Caulis Nelumbinis) are not frequently used, and do not have further description elsewhere.]

- 蓮子 / 莲子 *Lian Zi* (Semen Nelumbinis), sweet, astringent and neutral, tonifies the Spleen and Kidney to stop diarrhea, spermatorrhea, uterine bleeding and vaginal discharge. It also nourishes the Heart and calms the *shen* (spirit).
- 蓮子蕊 / 莲子蕊 *Lian Zi Xin* (Plumula Nelumbinis), bitter and cold, clears heat. It treats irritability, delirium and other heat signs associated with febrile disorders.
- 蓮鬚 / 莲须 *Lian Xu* (Stamen Nelumbinis), astringent and neutral, clears heat, consolidates *jing* (essence) and stops bleeding. It is often used to treat nocturnal emissions, spermatorrhea, frequent urination, enuresis, uterine bleeding, and hematemesis.
- 荷葉 / 荷叶 *He Ye* (Folium Nelumbinis), astringent, bitter and neutral, clears summer-heat, ascends clear yang, stops bleeding, and is used for disorders associated with heat stroke. It also treats diarrhea or bleeding from Spleen deficiency.
- 荷蒂 / 荷蒂 *He Di* (Calyx Nelumbinis), bitter and sweet, clears summer-heat, harmonizes the middle *jiao*, calms restless fetus and treats diarrhea or dysentery accompanied by blood and mucus.
- 荷梗 / 荷梗 *He Geng* (Caulis Nelumbinis), bitter and neutral, regulates chest qi and most effectively addresses feelings of chest congestion caused by dampness in the summer.
- 蓮房 / 莲房 *Lian Fang* (Receptaculum Nelumbinis), bitter, astringent and warm, enters the *xue* (blood) level and disperses blood stagnation, stops bleeding and treats uterine bleeding, or blood in the stool or urine. It also treats hemorrhoids, rectal prolapse and eczema.
- 藕節 / 藕节 *Ou Jie* (Nodus Nelumbinis Rhizomatis), sweet, astringent and neutral, disperses blood stagnation.

References

1. *Zhong Yao Xue* (Chinese Herbology), 1998; 897
2. *Xian Dai Ben Cao Gang Mu* (Contemporary Materia Medica), 2000; 2115
3. *Zhong Yao Xue* (Chinese Herbology), 1998; 897
4. *Chang Yong Zhong Yao Xian Dai Yan Jiu Yu Lin Chuan* (Recent Study & Clinical Application of Common Traditional Chinese Medicine), 1995; 685:686

Lian Zi Xin (Plumula Nelumbinis)

蓮子蕊 莲子蕊

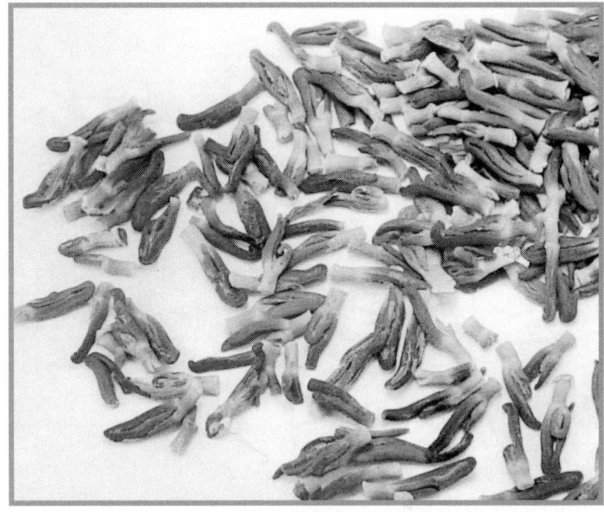

Pinyin Name: *Lian Zi Xin*
Literal Name: "lotus seed heart"
Alternate Chinese Names: *Lian Yi*
English Name: lotus embryo, lotus plumule
Botanical Name: *Nelumbo nucifera* Gaertn. (*Lian*)
Pharmaceutical Name: Plumula Nelumbinis
Properties: bitter, cold
Channels Entered: Heart, Pericardium

CHINESE THERAPEUTIC ACTIONS

1. Clears the Heart and Relieves Irritability

Bitter and cold, *Lian Zi Xin* (Plumula Nelumbinis) clears heat from the Heart and Pericardium. Mild cases of heat affecting the Heart are characterized by irritability. Severe cases of heat attacking the Heart and covering the Pericardium are characterized by irritability, fever and delirium.

- Irritability due to heat affecting the Heart: use *Lian Zi Xin* with *Dan Zhu Ye* (Herba Lophatheri), *Deng Xin Cao* (Medulla Junci) and *Zhi Zi* (Fructus Gardeniae).
- Irritability, fever, and delirium due to heat attacking the Heart and Pericardium: combine this herb with *Xuan Shen* (Radix Scrophulariae), *Mai Men Dong* (Radix Ophiopogonis) and *Zhu Ye* (Herba Phyllostachys).

2. Clears Heat from the Blood and Stops Bleeding

Lian Zi Xin clears heat, cools blood, and stops bleeding. It treats various bleeding disorders, such as hematemesis, epistaxis, and excessive menstrual bleeding, that are caused by heat in the blood.

- Bleeding due to heat in the blood: use with *Sheng Di Huang* (Radix Rehmanniae) and *Bai Mao Gen* (Rhizoma Imperatae) to cool blood and stop bleeding.

3. Treats Spermatorrhea due to Kidney Deficiency

Lian Zi Xin has an astringent action and treats spermatorrhea caused by Kidney deficiency.

- Spermatorrhea: use this herb with *Sang Piao Xiao* (Ootheca Mantidis), *Sha Yuan Zi* (Semen Astragali Complanati) and *Jin Ying Zi* (Fructus Rosae Laevigatae).

DOSAGE

1.5 to 3 grams. The maximum dosage for *Lian Zi Xin* is 10 grams.

CAUTIONS / CONTRAINDICATIONS

- *Lian Zi Xin* is contraindicated in patients with abdominal masses and constipation.

CHEMICAL COMPOSITION

Liensinine, isoliensinine, alkaloids.[1]

PHARMACOLOGICAL EFFECTS

- **Antihypertensive:** Liensinine lowers blood pressure by dilating peripheral blood vessels. It has a short duration of action.[2]

AUTHORS' COMMENTS

Eight parts of the lotus plant are used as medicines. Please refer to *Lian Zi* (Semen Nelumbinis) for complete description of the substances and their uses.

References

1. *Xian Dai Zhong Yao Yao Li Xue* (Contemporary Pharmacology of Chinese Herbs), 1997; 298
2. *Zhong Yao Xue* (Chinese Herbology), 1998; 897

Lian Xu (Stamen Nelumbinis)

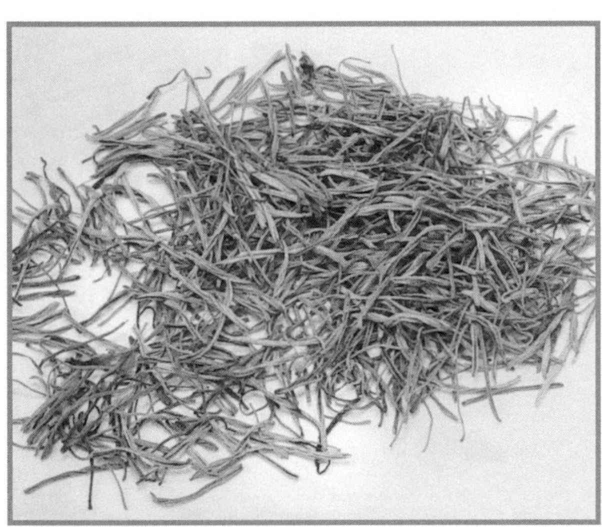

蓮鬚 莲须

Pinyin Name: *Lian Xu*
Alternate Chinese Names: *Jin Ying Cao*
Original Source: *Ben Cao Pin Hui Jing Yao* (Essentials of Materia Medica) by Liu Wen-Tai in 1505
English Name: lotus stamen
Botanical Name: *Nelumbo nucifera* Gaertn. (*Lian*)
Pharmaceutical Name: Stamen Nelumbinis
Properties: sweet, astringent, neutral
Channels Entered: Heart, Kidney

CHINESE THERAPEUTIC ACTIONS

1. Consolidates the Kidney

Lian Xu (Stamen Nelumbinis) restrains the leakage of body fluids allowed by Kidney deficiency. Clinically, it treats spermatorrhea, nocturnal emissions, and frequent urination.

- Spermatorrhea or nocturnal emissions: use with *Sha Yuan Zi* (Semen Astragali Complanati), *Qian Shi* (Semen Euryales), *Long Gu* (Os Draconis) and *Mu Li* (Concha Ostreae). **Exemplar Formula:** *Jin Suo Gu Jing Wan* (Metal Lock Pill to Stabilize the Essence).

2. Clears the Heart

Lian Xu clears the Heart and stops excessive dreaming at night.

3. Stops Bleeding

Lian Xu also treats bleeding disorders such as epistaxis, hematemesis, and profuse uterine bleeding.

DOSAGE

1.5 to 5.0 grams.

AUTHORS' COMMENTS

Eight parts of the lotus plant are used as medicines. Please refer to *Lian Zi* (Semen Nelumbinis) for complete description of the substances and their uses.

Fu Xiao Mai (Semen Tritici Aestivi Levis)

浮小麥 浮小麦

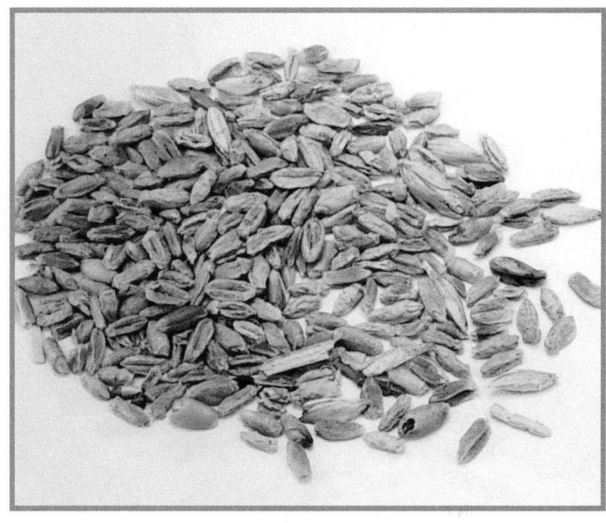

Pinyin Name: *Fu Xiao Mai*
Literal Name: "floating little wheat"
Alternate Chinese Names: *Fu Sui Mai, Fu Mai*
Original Source: *Ben Cao Meng Quan* (Hidden Aspects of the Materia Medica) by Chen Jia-Mo in 1565
English Name: wheat levis, light wheat, shriveled wheat
Botanical Name: *Triticum aestivum* L. (*Xiao Mai*)
Pharmaceutical Name: Semen Tritici Aestivi Levis
Properties: sweet, cool
Channels Entered: Heart

CHINESE THERAPEUTIC ACTIONS

Benefits Qi, Clears Heat and Stops Sweating

Spontaneous sweating: Sweet in taste, *Fu Xiao Mai* (Semen Tritici Aestivi Levis) tonifies Spleen and Lung qi, increases the ability of *wei* (defensive) *qi* to control the opening and closing of the skin pores, and stops spontaneous sweating. It is cool in thermal property to benefit Heart yin and dispel the heat that is causing the perspiration.

- Spontaneous sweating due to qi deficiency: combine *Fu Xiao Mai* with *Huang Qi* (Radix Astragali), *Ma Huang Gen* (Radix Ephedrae), *Wu Wei Zi* (Fructus Schisandrae Chinensis) and *Mu Li* (Concha Ostreae). **Exemplar Formula:** *Mu Li San* (Oyster Shell Powder).

Night sweating: *Fu Xiao Mai* clears yin-deficient heat and stops night sweating. Other symptoms of yin-deficient heat include low-grade fever, steaming bones sensations and feelings of warmth in the palms and soles.

- Night sweating due to yin-deficient heat: use this herb with *Sheng Di Huang* (Radix Rehmanniae), *Mai Men Dong* (Radix Ophiopogonis), *Di Gu Pi* (Cortex Lycii), and *Xuan Shen* (Radix Scrophulariae).

Steaming bones sensations: This type of sensation occurs when there is depletion of yin and qi. This herb tonifies qi, nurtures the body and treats steaming bones sensations and heat sensations caused by yin deficiency.

- Steaming bones sensations: combine *Fu Xiao Mai* with *Sheng Di Huang* (Radix Rehmanniae), *Mai Men Dong* (Radix Ophiopogonis), *Di Gu Pi* (Cortex Lycii) and *Xuan Shen* (Radix Scrophulariae).

DOSAGE

15 to 30 grams. *Fu Xiao Mai* is used in decoction or as powder.

CHEMICAL COMPOSITION

Starch, proteins, carbohydrates, lipids, fiber, enzymes, vitamins.[1]

AUTHORS' COMMENTS

Fu Xiao Mai (Semen Tritici Aestivi Levis) and *Xiao Mai* (Fructus Tritici) are derived from the same plant, but have different characteristics and functions. When *Fu Xiao Mai* and *Xiao Mai* are both placed in water, *Fu Xiao Mai* floats and *Xiao Mai* sinks. *Fu Xiao Mai* has astringent functions to stop sweating, while *Xiao Mai* can nourish the Heart and calm *shen* (spirit).

References

1. *Xian Dai Ben Cao Gang Mu* (Contemporary Materia Medica), 2000; 200

Ma Huang Gen (Radix Ephedrae)

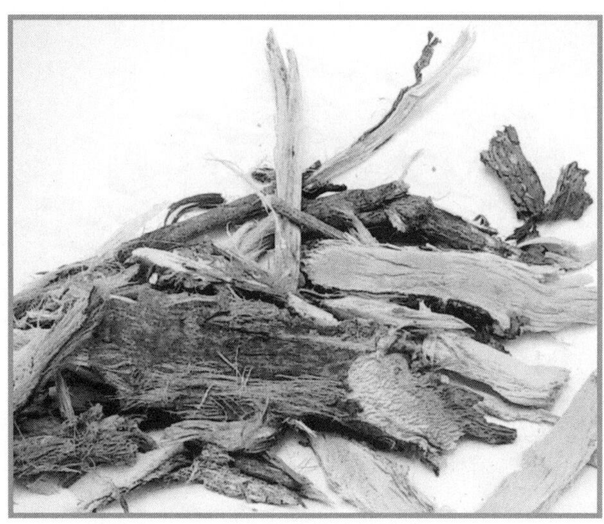

麻黄根

Pinyin Name: *Ma Huang Gen*
Literal Name: "hemp yellow root," "ephedra root"
Original Source: *Ming Yi Za Zhu* (Miscellaneous Records of Famous Physicians) by Tao Hong-Jing in 500 A.D.
English Name: ephedra root
Botanical Name: *Ephedra sinica* Stapf. (*Cao Ma Huang*); *Ephedra equisetina* Bge. (*Mu Zei Ma Huang*); *Ephedra intermedia* Schrenk et Mey. (*Zhong Ma Huang*)
Pharmaceutical Name: Radix Ephedrae
Properties: sweet, neutral
Channels Entered: Lung

CHINESE THERAPEUTIC ACTIONS

Stops Perspiration

Ma Huang Gen (Radix Ephedrae) is an excellent herb to treat both spontaneous and night sweating caused by qi or yin deficiencies. However, *Ma Huang Gen* only treats the symptom of sweating, and does not address the cause.

- Spontaneous sweating: combine *Ma Huang Gen* with *Huang Qi* (Radix Astragali) and *Fu Xiao Mai* (Semen Tritici Aestivi Levis).
- Night sweating or postpartum sweating: use this herb with *Mu Li* (Concha Ostreae), *Wu Wei Zi* (Fructus Schisandrae Chinensis), *Sheng Di Huang* (Radix Rehmanniae), *Shan Zhu Yu* (Fructus Corni), and *Long Gu* (Os Draconis).

DOSAGE

3 to 10 grams. *Ma Huang Gen* is also used as powder.

CAUTIONS / CONTRAINDICATIONS

- Use of *Ma Huang Gen* is contraindicated in exterior conditions, as the astringent function of *Ma Huang Gen* may keep the pathogenic factor trapped inside the body.

CHEMICAL COMPOSITION

Maokonine, tyrosine betaine, ephedradines A, B, C, D; mahuannins A, B, C, D; ephedrannin.[1]

PHARMACOLOGICAL EFFECTS

- **Cardiovascular:** In animal studies, maokonine increases blood pressure, ephedradine A decreases blood pressure, and extract of *Ma Huang Gen* decreases contractility of the heart.[2]
- **Smooth muscle stimulant:** *Ma Huang Gen* has a stimulating effect on the smooth muscles of the intestines and the uterus.[3]

AUTHORS' COMMENTS

Derived from different parts of the same plant, *Ma Huang* (Herba Ephedrae) and *Ma Huang Gen* (Radix Ephedrae) have completely different and opposite functions. *Ma Huang* is a diaphoretic and strongly induces perspiration. Use of *Ma Huang* is contraindicated in individuals with perspiration due to qi or yin deficiency. On the other hand, *Ma Huang Gen* stops spontaneous or night sweating. Use of *Ma Huang Gen* is contraindicated in patients who have exterior wind-heat or wind-cold conditions.

References

1. *Chang Yong Zhong Yao Cheng Fen Yu Yao Li Shou Ce* (A Handbook of the Composition and Pharmacology of Common Chinese Drugs), 1994; 1630
2. *Zhong Cheng Yao Yan Jiu* (Research of Chinese Patent Medicine), 1985; (10):20
3. *Zhong Yao Xue* (Chinese Herbology), 1998; 886:887

Chapter 18 summary

— Astringent Herbs

Name	Similarities	Differences
Wu Wei Zi (Fructus Schisandrae Chinensis)	Constrict the Lung to arrest coughing, bind the intestines to stop diarrhea	Stops loss of body fluids (sweating, diarrhea, sperm, urine), promotes generation of body fluids
Wu Mei (Fructus Mume)		Promotes generation of body fluids, kills parasites
Wu Bei Zi (Galla Chinensis)		Stops sweating and loss of sperm and urine
He Zi (Fructus Chebulae)		Benefits voice
Ying Su Ke (Pericarpium Papaveris)		Relieves pain
Ye Ying Pi (Pericarpium Prunus Pseudocerasus)		Relieves cough
Chi Shi Zhi (Halloysitum Rubrum)	Bind the intestines, stop diarrhea	Strongly binds the intestines, stops vaginal and uterine bleeding
Yu Yu Liang (Limonitum)		Stops uterine bleeding and leukorrhea
Rou Dou Kou (Semen Myristicae)		Warms the middle *jiao*, regulates qi circulation
Shi Liu Pi (Pericarpium Granati)		Stops bleeding, kills parasites, more effective for Spleen yang deficiency
Chun Gen Pi (Cortex Ailanthi)		Stops bleeding, kills parasites
Shan Zhu Yu (Fructus Corni)	Restrain leakage of fluids from the lower *jiao*	Tonifies Liver and Kidney yin
Jin Ying Zi (Fructus Rosae Laevigatae)		Binds the intestines, treats rectal and uterine prolapse
Sang Piao Xiao (Ootheca Mantidis)		Tonifies Kidney yang
Fu Pen Zi (Fructus Rubi)		Tonifies Kidney, improves vision
Hai Piao Xiao (Endoconcha Sepiae)		Stops bleeding, treats gastrointestinal disorders
Qian Shi (Semen Euryales)		Tonifies Spleen to stop diarrhea
Lian Zi (Semen Nelumbinis)		Tonifies Spleen to stop diarrhea, nourishes the Heart
Lian Zi Xin (Plumula Nelumbinis)		Clears the Heart, relieves irritability, clears heat from the blood, stops bleeding
Lian Xu (Stamen Nelumbinis)		Clears the Heart, stops bleeding
Fu Xiao Mai (Semen Tritici Aestivi Levis)	Stop sweating	Stops spontaneous and night perspiration
Ma Huang Gen (Radix Ephedrae)		Stops spontaneous and night perspiration

General Characteristics of Astringent Herbs:

Taste: sour, astringent
Thermal property: varies
Channels entered: Heart, Lung, Liver, Kidney, Large Intestine
Therapeutic actions: restrain the loss of qi and body fluids

Astringent herbs consolidate and minimize the loss of substances from the body. They are used mainly for deficiency patients with leakage of fluids seen as spontaneous sweating, night sweating, chronic diarrhea, chronic dysentery, rectal prolapse, spermatorrhea, premature ejaculation, enuresis, frequent urination, leukorrhea, uterine bleeding and chronic cough due to deficiency. Leakage of fluids occurs when deficiency causes the body to become unable to retain fluids within itself. Though astringent herbs restrain and prevent leakage, most of them do not have tonic functions to treat the root of the problem. Thus they are mainly used to treat the symptoms, not causes, of the disease. Therefore, most of the herbs in this category are combined with tonic herbs to achieve maximum results. In cases involving dampness, excess heat, or exterior pathogens, the strong restraining action of astringent herbs would be contraindicated.

Chapter 18 summary

Wu Wei Zi (Fructus Schisandrae Chinensis), ***Wu Mei*** (Fructus Mume), ***Wu Bei Zi*** (Galla Chinensis), ***He Zi*** (Fructus Chebulae), ***Ying Su Ke*** (Pericarpium Papaveris) and ***Ye Ying Pi*** (Pericarpium Prunus Pseudocerasus) all restrain the Lung to stop coughing, and bind the intestines to stop diarrhea. Clinical applications include chronic Lung deficiency cough, chronic diarrhea or dysentery.

Wu Wei Zi functions to stabilize and bind, nourish and moisten the Lung and Kidney. Clinically, it treats disorders of the Lung and Kidney, such as chronic cough, thirst with dry mouth, spontaneous sweating, night sweating, spermatorrhea, diarrhea, enuresis, polyuria, chronic diarrhea, and conditions characterized by deficiency of these two organs.

Wu Mei generates body fluids to relieve thirst, improve appetite and promote digestion. It is mostly used in patients with body fluid deficiency manifesting in thirst, poor appetite and decreased dietary intake. With its sour taste, *Wu Mei* also calms and expels parasites and relieves pain associated with an infestation. Finally, when this herb is used topically, it treats corns, warts, ulcers and sores.

Wu Bei Zi is sour, and has the strongest effect of this group to stabilize and bind. Cold in thermal property, it clears heat and purges fire. *Wu Bei Zi* is commonly used to treat deficiency of the Lung with heat, chronic cough with phlegm and streaks of blood, chronic diarrhea, rectal prolapse, or continuous dysentery. It is also used for profuse sweating, hematochezia, spermatorrhea, nocturnal emissions, profuse uterine bleeding, and nocturnal urination. When used topically, it treats various sores, carbuncles, furuncles, and skin lesions.

He Zi is sour, astringent, bitter and descending in nature. It clears the Lung and benefits the throat and vocal cords. It is most suitable for chronic cough with voice loss due to Lung deficiency. More specifically, the roasted form binds the intestines to stop diarrhea, while the unprocessed form restrains the Lung, redirects rebellious Lung qi downward and relieves coughing.

Ying Su Ke has a marked ability to stabilize and bind, and treats chronic chough from Lung deficiency, chronic diarrhea or dysentery. It has excellent analgesic functions and treats pain in the chest, abdomen, tendons and bones.

Ye Ying Pi is primarily used to relieve cough.

Chi Shi Zhi (Halloysitum Rubrum), ***Yu Yu Liang*** (Limonitum), ***Rou Dou Kou*** (Semen Myristicae), ***Shi Liu Pi*** (Pericarpium Granati), and ***Chun Gen Pi*** (Cortex Ailanthi) bind the intestines to stop chronic diarrhea and dysentery.

Chi Shi Zhi is sour, sweet and warm, with an effect to stabilize, bind and tonify. It is commonly used to tonify and regulate the middle *jiao* to treat chronic diarrhea, rectal prolapse, hematochezia, uterine bleeding or profuse leukorrhea caused by qi deficiency. *Chi Shi Zhi* also promotes generation of flesh, and therefore can also be used externally to treat non-healing ulcers.

Yu Yu Liang functions similarly to *Chi Shi Zhi* to bind the intestines, stop diarrhea and stop uterine bleeding and leukorrhea. They are often used together clinically for stronger synergistic effect. The main difference between the two herbs is that *Chi Shi Zhi* is warm, tonifies qi and regulates the middle *jiao*, while *Yu Yu Liang* is neutral and more effectively stops bleeding and leukorrhea.

Rou Dou Kou, acrid, aromatic and warm, acts as an astringent in the intestines to stop diarrhea, and regulates the middle *jiao* to awaken the Spleen and improve appetite. Clinical applications include bloating, abdominal pain, rectal prolapse, chronic diarrhea, and conditions characterized by deficiency and cold of the Spleen and Stomach.

Shi Liu Pi is astringent and warm to bind the intestines and stop diarrhea. It also stops bleeding in cases of uterine bleeding and bleeding from trauma. In addition, *Shi Liu Pi* kills parasites, particularly roundworms and pinworms.

Chun Gen Pi binds the intestines and clears damp-heat. It is effective for treating both diarrhea and dysentery. In addition, it stops uterine and vaginal bleeding.

Shan Zhu Yu (Fructus Corni), ***Jin Ying Zi*** (Fructus Rosae Laevigatae), ***Sang Piao Xiao*** (Ootheca Mantidis), ***Fu Pen Zi*** (Fructus Rubi), ***Hai Piao Xiao*** (Endoconcha Sepiae), and ***Qian Shi*** (Semen

Chapter 18 summary

Euryales) consolidate the Kidney, and retain *jing* (essence) and urine. They treat spermatorrhea, premature ejaculation and enuresis, dripping or polyuria from Kidney deficiency.

Shan Zhu Yu is sour and slightly warm. It tonifies the Liver and Kidney, and replenishes blood, *jing* and yang. Clinical applications include sweating, profuse menstrual discharge, spermatorrhea, polyuria, and uterine bleeding.

Jin Ying Zi is sour, with marked stabilizing and binding effects. It is most often used to retain urine and stop diarrhea.

Sang Piao Xiao is sweet, salty and neutral, with an effect to stabilize, bind and tonify. It treats spermatorrhea, leukorrhea, impotence, enuresis, polyuria, and other disorders of Kidney yang deficiency.

Fu Pen Zi is sweet, sour and slightly warm but not drying. It is best used to tonify the Kidney, consolidate *jing* and retain urine. Clinical applications include impotence, premature ejaculation, enuresis and frequent urination associated with Kidney yang deficiency. It can also be used to treat diminished or weakened vision due to *jing* and blood deficiencies.

Hai Piao Xiao stops bleeding and leukorrhea, neutralizes acid and helps the healing of weeping wounds or sores. It treats uterine bleeding, hematemesis, bleeding ulcers, and acid regurgitation with stomach pain.

Qian Shi is sweet, astringent and neutral. It tonifies the Spleen to relieve diarrhea, and consolidates the Kidney to stop spermatorrhea and leukorrhea.

Lian Zi (Semen Nelumbinis), ***Lian Zi Xin*** (Plumula Nelumbinis) and ***Lian Xu*** (Stamen Nelumbinis) are three astringent herbs from the same plant.

Lian Zi is sweet, astringent and neutral. It tonifies the Kidney to consolidates *jing* (essence), tonifies the Spleen to stop diarrhea, and nourishes the Heart to calm the *shen* (spirit). Clinical applications include insomnia, fear and fright, spermatorrhea, leukorrhea and chronic diarrhea from Spleen deficiency.

Lian Zi Xin clears heat from the Heart to relieve irritability, and cools blood to stop bleeding.

Lian Xu has similar, but weaker, effects to those of *Lian Zi Xin.*

Ma Huang Gen (Radix Ephedrae) and ***Fu Xiao Mai*** (Semen Tritici Aestivi Levis) both stop night or spontaneous perspiration.

Ma Huang Gen is mostly used to stop excessive perspiration due to weakness of *wei* (defensive) *qi.*

Fu Xiao Mai is sweet and cool, and stops spontaneous or night sweating. In addition, it clears deficiency heat in chronic cases and treats steaming bones sensations caused by yin deficiency. It also tonifies qi and benefits the Heart.

HERBS FROM OTHER FUNCTIONAL CATEGORIES WITH ASTRINGENT FUNCTIONS

Name	Functional Category
Bai Ji (Rhizoma Bletillae)	Stop-Bleeding Herbs (Chapter 11)
Da Huang (Radix et Rhizoma Rhei), charred	Downward Draining Herbs (Chapter 3)
Er Cha (Catechu)	Substances for Topical Application (Chapter 20)
Long Gu (Os Draconis)	*Shen*-Calming Herbs (Chapter 14)
Ming Fan (Alumen)	Substances for Topical Application (Chapter 20)
Mu Li (Concha Ostreae)	Liver-Calming and Wind-Extinguishing Herbs (Chapter 15)
Xian He Cao (Herba Agrimoniae)	Stop-Bleeding Herbs (Chapter 11)
Xue Jie (Sanguis Draconis)	Substances for Topical Application (Chapter 20)
Zi Zhu (Folium Callicarpae)	Stop-Bleeding Herbs (Chapter 11)

Chapter 19

— Emetic Herbs

湧吐药

Chapter 19 — Emetic Herbs

Chapter 19

湧吐药 — Emetic Herbs

Definition: Emetic herbs provoke vomiting, causing the stomach to eject its contents, such as stagnant food, excess mucus, or toxins.

Vomiting is a treatment strategy reserved for cases of accidental poisoning, food stagnation, and phlegm obstruction. The function of emetic herbs is to remove, or assist the body in rejecting, pathogenic and/or obstructing elements, which allows the body to return to self-regulation when freed from the pathogens.

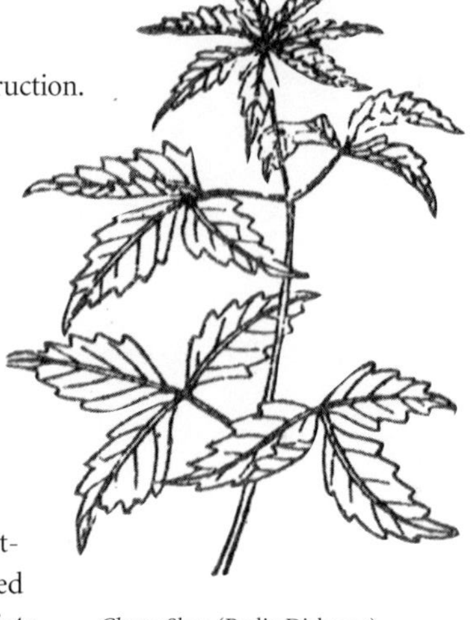

Chang Shan (Radix Dichroae)
Ben Cao Gang Mu (Materia Medica), by Li Shi-Zhen, 1578 A.D.

DIFFERENTIAL DIAGNOSIS AND TREATMENT

Emetic herbs are used for accidental poisoning, food stagnation, and phlegm obstruction.

- **Accidental poisonings** show different symptoms and signs depending on the substance ingested. Use of emetic herbs is justified within a short period of time following ingestion of a poisonous substance, while the injurious matter is still in the stomach and can be ejected by vomiting.
- **Food stagnation** is characterized by obstruction of the epigastrium by undigested food, that leads to fullness, distention and pain.
- **Phlegm obstruction** is identified by the presence of altered consciousness, mania, and/or seizures.

CAUTIONS/CONTRAINDICATIONS

> **Extremely toxic, irritating, and potent, emetic herbs must be used with extreme caution, according to appropriate guidelines, and only when necessary.**

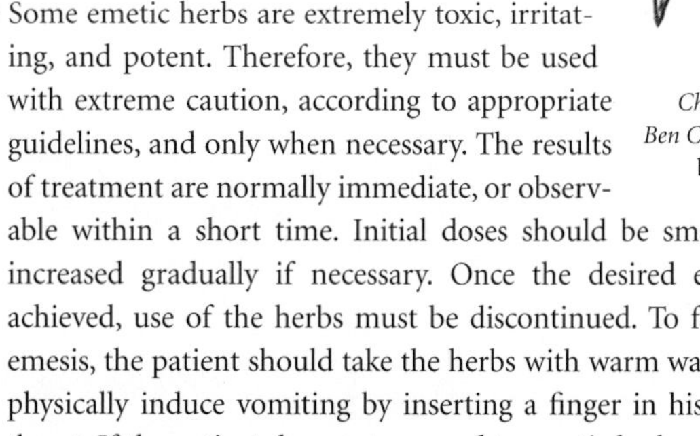

- Some emetic herbs are extremely toxic, irritating, and potent. Therefore, they must be used with extreme caution, according to appropriate guidelines, and only when necessary. The results of treatment are normally immediate, or observable within a short time. Initial doses should be small, and increased gradually if necessary. Once the desired effect is achieved, use of the herbs must be discontinued. To facilitate emesis, the patient should take the herbs with warm water, and physically induce vomiting by inserting a finger in his or her throat. If the patient does not respond to emetic herbs, or relief is not evident, he or she must immediately seek emergency medical treatment.
- Emetic herbs injure the ***Spleen*** and ***Stomach***, consuming ***qi*** and ***yin***. Therefore, even when indicated, they must be used with extreme caution, especially in patients who are very young or very old, those who are pregnant, postpartum, anemic, hypertensive, or suffer from heart disease or peptic ulcers.
- Following emesis, patients must be instructed not to resume eating solid foods immediately: the Spleen and Stomach energy may still be disordered, weak or vulnerable. Easily-digestible juices or liquid foods should be given until the patient is recovered sufficiently to re-introduce small amounts of readily-assimilable foods.
- Emetic substances should not be used to provoke vomiting if corrosive substances were ingested; this would only cause additional damage to the upper gastrointestinal tract when the corrosive elements are ejected as vomitus. Select other methods to neutralize or remove the toxic substances.

Chapter 19 — Emetic Herbs

PHARMACOLOGICAL EFFECTS

- **Emetic:** These herbs induce vomiting via direct stimulation of the gastrointestinal tract or the central nervous system.

POTENTIAL HERB-DRUG INTERACTIONS

- **Absorption:** Emetic herbs induce vomiting, and should not be given concurrently with other herbs or drugs. If taken together, the emetic effect of the herbs would cause ejection of other substances before they could be absorbed or implemented by the body.

Gua Di (Pedicellus Cucumeris)

瓜蒂 瓜蒂

Pinyin Name: *Gua Di*
Literal Name: "melon stalk"
Alternate Chinese Names: *Gua Ding, Ku Ding Xiang*
Original Source: *Shen Nong Ben Cao Jing* (Divine Husbandman's Classic of the Materia Medica) in the second century
English Name: melon pedicle
Botanical Name: *Cucumis melo* L. (*Tian Gua*)
Pharmaceutical Name: Pedicellus Cucumeris
Properties: bitter, cold
Channels Entered: Stomach
Safety Index: toxic

CHINESE THERAPEUTIC ACTIONS

1. Induces Vomiting

Hot phlegm accumulation: *Gua Di* (Pedicellus Cucumeris) induces vomiting to eliminate accumulation of hot phlegm, a condition characterized by seizures, epilepsy, sore throat, wheezing, dyspnea, irritability, restlessness, and insomnia.

- Hot phlegm: use *Gua Di* with *Chi Xiao Dou* (Semen Phaseoli), and *Xiang Fu* (Rhizoma Cyperi).

Food retention: *Gua Di* induces vomiting to eliminate retention of food, a condition characterized by fullness and pain in the chest and epigastrium, nausea, and vomiting.

- Retention of food: use this herb individually.

2. Dispels Damp-Heat

Headache and jaundice: The powder of *Gua Di* can be blown into the nostrils to treat headache and jaundice caused by damp-heat. After intranasal administration, there will be yellow nasal discharge dripping from the nose, an indication of damp-heat being successfully eliminated from the body. Herbs should be discontinued once yellow fluids have dripped from the nose.

DOSAGE

2.5 to 5.0 grams in decoction, and 0.3 to 1.0 gram in powder form. The antiemetic effect of *Gua Di* may be enhanced with ingestion of rock sugar immediately following the herb.

CAUTIONS / CONTRAINDICATIONS

- Use of *Gua Di* is contraindicated in cases of deficiency, bleeding, or patients who do not have an excess condition.

OVERDOSAGE

Symptoms associated with overdose of *Gua Di* usually occur within 30 minutes after ingestion. Clinical presentation includes dizziness, lightheadedness, upper abdominal discomfort, burning sensations and pain in the stomach, nausea, vomiting, vomitus of food and bile, severe diarrhea, restlessness, thirst, cold extremities, and hypotension. Laboratory analysis may show elevated white blood cell counts, decreased platelet counts, and the presence of protein in the urine.

TREATMENT OF OVERDOSAGE

Adverse reactions characterized by nausea and vomiting can be treated with 5 ml juice of *Sheng Jiang* (Rhizoma Zingiberis Recens). An herbal decoction of 10 grams of *Ban Xia* (Rhizoma Pinelliae) and 6 grams of *Gan Cao* (Radix Glycyrrhizae) is also effective. Ingestion of 0.1 to 0.15 gram of *She Xiang* (Moschus) has also been used with good success to relieve continuous nausea and vomiting.

CHEMICAL COMPOSITION

Cucurbitacin B, cucurbitacin E, cucurbitacin D, isocucurbitacin B, cucurbitacin, β-2-O-β-D-pyranoglucoside.[1,2]

PHARMACOLOGICAL EFFECTS

- **Emetic:** Administration of *Gua Di* is associated with an emetic effect due to its stimulation of the central nervous system and the gastrointestinal tract.[3]
- **Hepatoprotective:** Preparations of *Gua Di* have been shown to have a hepatoprotective effective by minimizing damage to and enhancing the recovery of the liver.[4]

CLINICAL STUDIES AND RESEARCH

- **Hepatitis:** Administration of *Gua Di* via intranasal or oral routes have proven effective in treatment of acute and chronic hepatitis. In 103 cases of acute hepatitis, the treatment protocol was to soak 5 grams of *Gua Di* in 100 ml of water for 10 days, taking the solution in two equally-divided doses after meals. In 18 cases of chronic hepatitis without jaundice, *Gua Di* powder was administered into the nostrils.[5]

Gua Di (Pedicellus Cucumeris)

- **Liver cancer:** According to one report, 169 patients with liver cancer were treated with a preparation of *Gua Di* three times daily after meals, for three months per course of treatment. The study reported that there was marked improvement, such as relief of pain, decreased tumor size, and increased strength in the patients. No significant side effects were noted.[6]

TOXICOLOGY

The LD_{50} of a *Gua Di* preparation is 1.1 g/kg in laboratory studies. Autopsy showed various degrees of bleeding in internal organs.[7]

References

1. *Xian Dai Ben Cao Gang Mu* (Contemporary Materia Medica), 2000; 871
2. *Zhong Yao Xue* (Chinese Herbology), 1998; 908-909
3. Ibid., 908-910
4. Ibid., 908-910
5. *Xin Yi Yao Xue Za Zhi* (New Journal of Medicine and Herbology), 1976; 9:42
6. *Zhong Cao Yao* (Chinese Herbal Medicine), 1987; 18(10):21
7. *Zhong Yao Xue* (Chinese Herbology), 1998; 908:910

Chang Shan (Radix Dichroae)

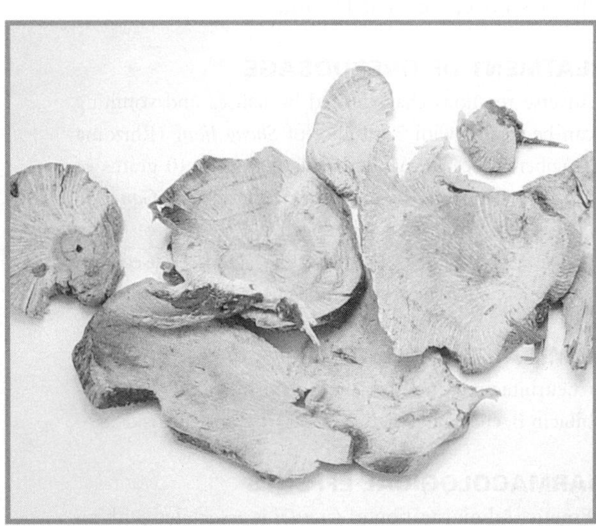

常山

Pinyin Name: *Chang Shan*
Literal Name: "eternal mountain," "constant mountain"
Alternate Chinese Names: *Heng Shan, Ji Gu Chang Shan*
Original Source: *Shen Nong Ben Cao Jing* (Divine Husbandman's Classic of the Materia Medica) in the second century
English Name: dichroa root, anti-febrile dichroa root
Botanical Name: *Dichroa febrifuga* Lour. (*Huang Chang Shan*)
Pharmaceutical Name: Radix Dichroae
Properties: acrid, bitter, cold
Channels Entered: Lung, Heart, Liver
Safety Index: toxic

CHINESE THERAPEUTIC ACTIONS

1. Expels Phlegm by Inducing Vomiting

Phlegm obstructing the chest and diaphragm prevents the proper flow of qi, manifesting as chest and epigastric fullness, distention and pain. *Chang Shan* (Radix Dichroae) strongly disperses stagnation, and enters the Heart and Lung channels to expand the chest by inducing vomiting. It may be used individually or in combination with other herbs.

- Phlegm obstruction in the chest: use *Chang Shan* with *Gan Cao* (Radix Glycyrrhizae) and honey.

2. Treats Malaria

Chang Shan is commonly used to treat various malarial disorders characterized by alternation of fever and chills.

- Malaria: soak *Chang Shan* in grain-based liquor and serve daily until symptoms subside. *Bing Lang* (Semen Arecae) is usually given concurrently to relieve vomiting.

DOSAGE

5 to 10 grams. The fresh herb is commonly used to induce vomiting. *Chang Shan* processed with grain-based liquor is commonly used to treat malaria.

CAUTIONS / CONTRAINDICATIONS

- *Chang Shan* has a strong emetic function and may injure qi. It should be prescribed with caution for those who are weak or experiencing deficiencies.

Chang Shan (Radix Dichroae)

CHEMICAL COMPOSITION

α-dichroine, β-dichroine, γ-dichroine, isofrifugine, febrifugine, dichroidine, 4-quinazolone, umbelliferone.[1]

PHARMACOLOGICAL EFFECTS

- **Antimalarial:** *Chang Shan* has demonstrated potent antimalarial action in various studies. In comparison with quinine, γ-dichroine is 150 times more potent, β-dichroine is 100 times more potent, and α-dichroine is equally as potent. The leaves are approximately five times more potent than the roots for treating malaria. Both water and alcohol extracts of *Chang Shan* are effective against *P. gallinaceum, P. lophurae, P. relictum,* and *P. cynomolgi*.[2]
- **Antiamebic:** β-dichroine has an inhibitory action *in vitro* against amoebae, with an effect 100% stronger than emetine hydrochloride. The minimum inhibitory concentration (MIC) for β-dichroine via oral ingestion is 1.0 mg/kg.[3]
- **Antipyretic:** Oral ingestion of *Chang Shan* decoction at 2 g/kg was effective in reducing body temperature in rabbits with artificially-induced fevers.[4] Comparatively, the antipyretic effect of *Chang Shan* is stronger than *Chai Hu* (Radix Bupleuri) and is similar to that of aspirin.[5]
- **Cardiovascular:** It has been proposed that α-, β-, and γ-dichroine all lower the blood pressure through inhibition of the cardiovascular system and dilation of the blood vessels. There is a positive correlation between dosage, therapeutic effect, and duration of action.[6]
- **Emetic:** α-, β-, and γ-dichroine have all demonstrated emetic effects in dogs, cats and pigeons. The effective dose in dogs and cats is 0.04 and 0.15 mg/kg, respectively.[7]

CLINICAL STUDIES AND RESEARCH

- **Malaria:** According to one report, 5,984 carriers of malaria were treated with two injections of *Chang Shan* with good results. All carriers were 10 years of age or under. The two injections were given 25 days apart.[8]
- **Arrhythmia:** In one clinical study, 35 patients with pre-ventricular contractions were treated with an herbal decoction twice daily for 30 days with significant improvement in 12 patients and moderate improvement in 16 patients. The herbal formula contained 10 grams each of *Chang Shan, Bai Zi Ren* (Semen Platycladi), and *Zhi Gan Cao* (Radix Glycyrrhizae Preparata), and 30 grams each of *Ku Shen Gen* (Radix Sophorae Flavescentis), *Dan Shen* (Radix Salviae Miltiorrhizae) and *Dang Shen* (Radix Codonopsis). All other herbal or pharmaceutical medicines were discontinued during the study.[9]

TOXICOLOGY

The LD_{50} for mice via oral ingestion is 570 mg/kg for α-dichroine, 6.57 mg/kg for β-dichroine, 6.45 mg/kg for γ-dichroine, and 7.79 mg/kg for total alkaloids.[10] Following oral administration, the most common adverse reactions in mice were vomiting, diarrhea, and blood in the stool.[11]

SUPPLEMENT

- 蜀漆 *Shu Qi* (Folium Dichroae), first cited in *Shen Nong Ben Cao Jing* (Divine Husbandman's Classic of the Materia Medica) in the second century, is the soft branches and leaves of the same plant as *Chang Shan*. *Chang Shan* and *Shu Qi* have similar tastes, channels, functions, indications and cautions. The only difference is that *Shu Qi* is more effective for treatment of malaria. The dosage for *Shu Qi* is 3 to 6 grams.

AUTHORS' COMMENTS

According to Dr. Zhang Xiao-Ping, pre-ventricular contraction (PVC) can be treated successfully with *Chang Shan, Ku Shen Gen* (Radix Sophorae Flavescentis), *Ban Xia* (Rhizoma Pinelliae) and *Zhi Gan Cao* (Radix Glycyrrhizae Preparata).

References

1. *Xian Dai Zhong Yao Yao Li Xue* (Contemporary Pharmacology of Chinese Herbs), 1997; 764
2. *Zhong Yao Yao Li Yu Ying Yong* (Pharmacology and Applications of Chinese Herbs), 1983, 1983: 1024
3. *Wu Han Yi Xue Yuan Xue Bao* (Journal of Wuhan University School of Medicine), 1958; 1:11
4. *Zhong Hua Yi Xue Za Zhi* (Chinese Journal of Medicine), 1956; 42(10):964
5. Ibid., 1954; 40(11):873
6. *Sheng Li Xue Bao* (Physiology News), 1956; 20(1):30
7. Ibid., 1961; 24(3,4):180
8. *Yun Nan Yi Xue Za Zhi* (Yunan Journal of Medicine), 1961; 3:8
9. *Fu Jian Zhong Yi Yao* (Fujian Chinese Medicine and Herbology), 1983; 6:26
10. *Zhong Yao Yao Li Yu Ying Yong* (Pharmacology and Applications of Chinese Herbs), 1983, 1983: 1024
11. *Zhong Yao Yao Li Du Li Yu Lin Chuang* (Pharmacology, Toxicology and Clinical Applications of Chinese Herbs), 1992:135

Li Lu (Radix et Rhizoma Veratri)

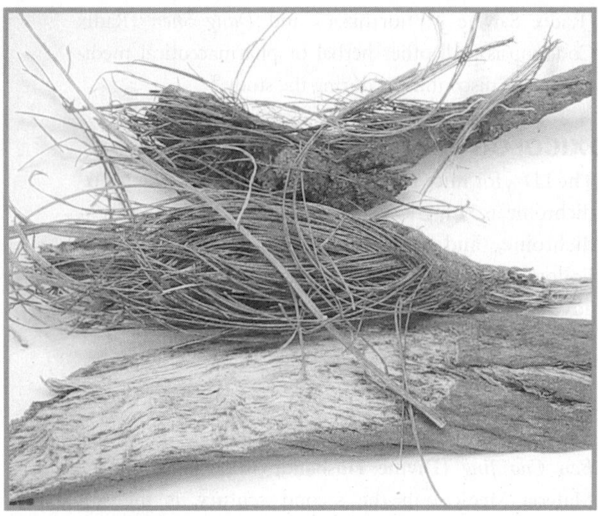

黎蘆 黎芦

Pinyin Name: *Li Lu*
Literal Name: "lack false hellebore," "vanity grass"
Alternate Chinese Names: *Shan Cong, Lu Cong*
Original Source: *Shen Nong Ben Cao Jing* (Divine Husbandman's Classic of the Materia Medica) in the second century
English Name: veratrum root and rhizome, false-hellebore rhizome and root
Botanical Name: *Veratrum nigrum* L. (*Hei Li Lu*)
Pharmaceutical Name: Radix et Rhizoma Veratri
Properties: acrid, bitter, cold
Channels Entered: Lung, Liver, Stomach
Safety Index: toxic

CHINESE THERAPEUTIC ACTIONS

1. Induces Vomiting

Profuse accumulation of phlegm, ingestion of a toxic substance: *Li Lu* (Radix et Rhizoma Veratri) induces vomiting to eliminate phlegm, poisons, and toxic substances in the stomach.

- Ingestion of a toxic substance: use *Li Lu* alone in powder form.

Li Lu also treats wind-stroke, epilepsy, seizures, and painful obstruction of the throat.

- Phlegm obstruction: use this herb with *Yu Jin* (Radix Curcumae) or *Tian Nan Xing* (Rhizoma Arisaematis).

2. Kills Parasites and Relieves Itching

Li Lu is effective against scabies, ringworm, lice, and fungus. Mix it with oil and apply topically. *Li Lu* is also used to kill mosquitoes, flies, maggots and larvae.

DOSAGE

0.3 to 0.9 gram in powder or pill form. *Li Lu* may be used internally with extreme caution. It is applied topically when mixed with oil.

CAUTIONS / CONTRAINDICATIONS

- Oral ingestion of *Li Lu* should be used with extreme caution, because of the potential side effects.
- *Li Lu* is contraindicated in cases of deficiency, blood loss, and pregnancy.
- *Li Lu* is incompatible with *Xi Xin* (Herba Asari), *Bai Shao* (Radix Paeoniae Alba), *Ren Shen* (Radix Ginseng), *Dang Shen* (Radix Codonopsis), *Sha Shen* (Radix Glehniae seu Adenophorae), and *Ku Shen Gen* (Radix Sophorae Flavescentis).

OVERDOSAGE

In a toxicology study in healthy volunteers, it was noted that 70 mg of *Li Lu* induced reactions such as numbness of the mouth, difficulty swallowing, diarrhea, and chest oppression. Other adverse reactions associated with *Li Lu* include nausea, vomiting, irregular heartbeat, hypotension, and respiratory depression.[1]

TREATMENT OF OVERDOSAGE

Continuous vomiting following overdose of *Li Lu* can be alleviated with a decoction of 3 grams of *Rou Gui* (Cortex Cinnamomi) or 5 ml of juice from *Sheng Jiang* (Rhizoma Zingiberis Recens).

In cases of systemic toxicity characterized by visual disturbance (yellow tint seen visually), an antidote formula should be used with such herbs as *Long Yan Rou* (Arillus Longan) 30g, *Gou Qi Zi* (Fructus Lycii) 15g, *Huang Qi* (Radix Astragali) 45g, *Yin Chen Hao* (Herba Artemisiae Scopariae) 20g, *Che Qian Zi* (Semen Plantaginis) 15g, and *Fu Pen Zi* (Fructus Rubi) 15g.

Another formula that has been used successfully for general detoxification includes *Jin Yin Hua* (Flos Lonicerae), *Gan Cao* (Radix Glycyrrhizae), *Hei Dou* (Semen Glycine Max), *Lu Dou* (Semen Phaseoli Radiati), *Chi Xiao Dou* (Semen Phaseoli) and honey.[2]

CHEMICAL COMPOSITION

Veratric acid, verazine, veramarine, protoveratrine A, germidine, veratroyl-zygadenine, rubijervine, isorubijervine, pseudojervine, jervine, veramine, verussurinine.[3,4,5]

Li Lu (Radix et Rhizoma Veratri)

COOH, OCH_3, OCH_3

Veratric Acid

AUTHORS' COMMENTS

It is important to note that vomiting is both a desired effect and a side effect, depending on the context. When *Li Lu* is used to treat ingestion of a poisonous substance, vomiting is the desired effect. However, excessive or prolonged vomiting can cause dehydration and depletion of body fluids. Therefore, it is extremely important that this herb not be used unless the benefits outweigh the risks.

References

1. *Zhong Yao Xue* (Chinese Herbology), 1998; 912:914
2. *Lin Chuang Shou Ce You Du Zhong Yao Shi Yong* (Clinical Handbook on Applications of Toxic Chinese Herbs), 1992; 71-72
3. *Xian Dai Ben Cao Gang Mu* (Contemporary Materia Medica), 2000; 3208
4. *Zhong Yao Xue* (Chinese Herbology), 1998; 912-914
5. *The Merck Index* 12th edition, Chapman & Hall/CRCnetBASE/Merck, 2000

Chapter 19 summary — Emetic Herbs

Name	Similarities	Differences
Gua Di (Pedicellus Cucumeris)	Induce vomiting	Treats jaundice and migraine headaches
Chang Shan (Radix Dichroae)		Treats malaria and arrhythmia
Li Lu (Radix et Rhizoma Veratri)		Kills parasites and relieves itching when used topically

General Characteristics of Emetic Herbs:

Taste: acrid, bitter
Thermal property: cold
Channels entered: Stomach
Therapeutic actions: induce vomiting
Safety index: toxic

Emetic herbs are quite potent and are used only in cases of excess, in particular to induce vomiting to treat ingestion of toxic substances, food stagnation, and phlegm accumulation in the chest or throat. Because these are toxic substances of varying degrees, inappropriate or careless treatment will injure the middle *jiao*, body fluids and qi. Thus, low dosages are employed, and gradually increased to achieve the desired effect. Emetic treatment should be discontinued immediately when the symptoms of excess are relieved.

Gua Di (Pedicellus Cucumeris), ***Chang Shan*** (Radix Dichroae) and ***Li Lu*** (Radix et Rhizoma Veratri) induce vomiting to treat food and phlegm accumulation, and ingestion of toxic substances. All three herbs are toxic, and must be used with extreme caution.

HERBS FROM OTHER FUNCTIONAL CATEGORIES WITH EMETIC FUNCTIONS

Name	Functional Category
Ming Fan (Alumen)	Substances for Topical Application (Chapter 20)
Zao Jiao (Fructus Gleditsiae)	Phlegm-Resolving and Coughing- and Wheezing-Relieving Herbs (Chapter 13)
Yuan Zhi (Radix Polygalae)	*Shen*-Calming Herbs (Chapter 14)

Chapter 20

— Substances for Topical Application

外用药

Chapter 20 — Substances for Topical Application

Chapter 20

外用藥 — Substances for Topical Application

Definition: Herbs for topical application function to eliminate toxins, kill parasites, reduce swelling, relieve pain, treat ulcerations, drain pus and abscesses, promote generation of flesh, relieve itching, and stop bleeding.

Substances for topical application are generally reserved for external uses, to treat disorders affecting the external parts of the body. When necessary, these substances may be used to treat internal disorders, either by topical application or internal ingestion.

Topical herbs have a broad range of properties that allow for versatile application to a wide variety of imbalances. They help to resolve conditions affecting the skin and superficial layers, restoring the health and integrity of the skin, and/or penetrating beyond the surface to remove pathogens and restore internal balance.

- For ***external*** disorders, herbs are absorbed by skin, membranes, and local tissue in the affected area. External application is most effective for rashes, itching, eczema, carbuncles, furuncles, scabies, arthritis, burns, insect and animal bites, traumatic injuries, and other skin and soft tissue disorders. Herbs are also used topically to treat various ear, nose and throat disorders.
- For ***internal*** disorders, topically-applied herbs are absorbed through the skin into the blood and distributed throughout the body. Diseases that may be treated with topical application of herbs include asthma, malaria, jaundice, edema, and numerous pediatric and gynecological disorders.

Some substances in this chapter are no longer in use but are important to include here for academic and informational purposes. Their historical uses serve to provide reminders and possible templates for future refinements and research.

Dosage forms and routes of administration vary depending on both the medicinal substances and the diseases treated. Common dosage forms include creams, ointments, herbal pastes and plasters, powder, pills, pellets, capsules, tablets, solutions, and decoctions.

These substances are delivered to the affected area via various routes of administration, such as topical application (creams, ointments, pastes, plasters and powder), oral ingestion (pills, pellets, capsules, and tablets), local instillation (ear drops, eye drops), and others (solution as mouth gargle, decoction as herbal wash, steam for inhalation, etc). In short, there is a wide selection of dosage forms and routes of administration available to treat various external and internal disorders.

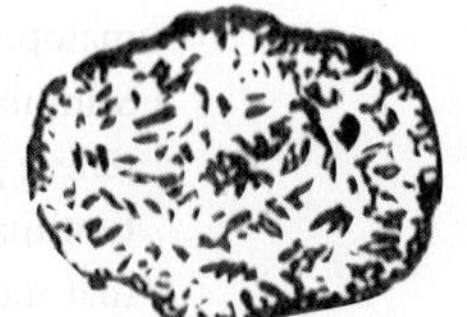

Mi Tuo Seng (Lithargyum)
Ben Cao Gang Mu (Materia Medica), by Li Shi-Zhen, 1578 A.D.

SUBCATEGORIES OF ACTION

Substances for topical application are derived from a wide variety of plant, animal and mineral sources. Though they are not divided into subcategories, they do have distinct characteristics. Some are cold, others are hot. Some potent herbs take immediate action, while milder ones exert sustained action. Some are toxic and should be reserved for topical use only. There are herbs that eliminate heat and toxins to treat sores and ulceration, and others that eliminate wind to relieve itching. Some drain pus and abscesses, while others directly promote healing of wounds.

Chapter 20 — Substances for Topical Application

DIFFERENTIAL DIAGNOSIS AND TREATMENT

As is true in internal medicine, differential diagnosis is essential for successful treatment with topical substances. One must clearly determine whether a disease is deficient or excess, cold or hot, primarily affecting the interior or exterior, and whether or not toxins are present. Optimal treatment requires precise identification of disease patterns and proper application of the appropriate herbal remedy. When necessary, to achieve maximum effectiveness, herbs from other functional categories are added.

Examples of dosage forms and applications to address two major distinguishing factors:

- ***Wet*** disorders, such as ulcerations with pus and abscesses, are treated with ***powdered*** herbs, to dry the affected area.
- ***Dry*** disorders, such as rashes and itching, are treated with herbal ***pastes*** to moisten the skin and facilitate recovery.

Arthritis and ***soft tissue injuries*** are treated with herbal ***plasters*** for continuous, sustained therapeutic effects.

~

Toxic herbs for external application should not be used internally, nor for prolonged periods of time, or at large dosages.

~

CAUTIONS/CONTRAINDICATIONS

- Many herbs for external application are toxic, and thus should not be used internally, nor for prolonged periods of time, or at large dosages.
- Toxic substances should not be applied over a large surface area or near sensory orifices, as there is an increased chance of local irritation or excessive systemic absorption. If adverse reactions are observed, immediate and appropriate treatment should be applied.
- Herbs should be used with caution if applied over a large surface area with damaged or broken skin, such as in cases of severe burns, because of the risk of overdose via topical absorption.

PROCESSING

Many substances in this chapter must be processed appropriately to insure safety for either external or internal uses, particularly to alleviate toxicity.

PHARMACOLOGICAL EFFECTS

A general rule of thumb to follow when using herbs topically is that herbs that are used orally can be use topically, but herbs that are used topically may or may not be used orally. Many herbs that are used orally (discussed in chapters 1 to 19) can also be used topically, and are listed below as examples. The pharmacological effects of substances for topical application are as follows:

- **Antibiotic:** Many substances for topical application kill bacteria, viruses, fungi, parasites, and dermatophytes.
- **Stimulant:** The action of stimulant topicals serves to reduce inflammation and swelling, and to relieve pain, such as *Bo He* (Herba Menthae) and *Zhang Nao* (Camphora). However, the stimulation may also cause irritation with redness, flushing and formation of blisters. Stimulant herbs that may be more irritating to the skin include *Ba Dou* (Fructus Crotonis), *Ya Dan Zi* (Fructus Bruceae) and *Ban Mao* (Mylabris).
- **Hemostatic:** Specific topical substances stop bleeding, including *Er Cha* (Catechu), *Wu Bei Zi* (Galla Chinensis), *Hu Zhang* (Rhizoma Polygoni Cuspidati), and *Di Yu* (Radix Sanguisorbae).
- **Astringent:** Binding and restraining topicals facilitate healing, minimize discharge and promote regeneration of tissues. Examples include *Er Cha* (Catechu), *Wu Bei Zi* (Galla Chinensis) and *Ming Fan* (Alumen).
- **Analgesic and anesthetic:** Pain-relieving topical herbs include *Wu Tou* (Radix Aconiti), *Ban Xia* (Rhizoma Pinelliae), *Tian Nan Xing* (Rhizoma Arisaematis), *Xi Xin* (Herba Asari) and *Bai Fu Zi* (Rhizoma Typhonii).
- **Moistening:** Some herbs, like *Hei Zhi Ma* (Semen Sesami Nigrum), are oil soluble. When applied topically, they form a protective barrier, moisten the skin and prevent dryness. Others, such as *Hua Shi* (Talcum), reduce swelling and inflammation when applied topically, by drawing water out of the affected area to the outside of the body.

Chapter 20 — Substances for Topical Application

POTENTIAL HERB-DRUG INTERACTIONS

There are no known or documented interactions between topical herbs and pharmaceutical medicines at the time of publication.

Note: Although many of the substances listed in this chapter can influence internal conditions, many are too toxic for internal use, thus are used via external application or not at all. Some are no longer in use but are important to include here for academic and informational purposes. The historical uses of these substances in traditional Chinese medicine serve to provide reminders and possible templates for future refinements and research.

Liu Huang (Sulfur)

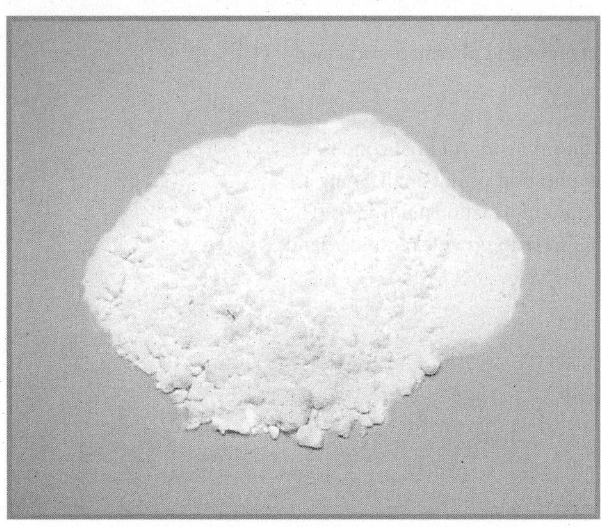

硫黄

Pinyin Name: *Liu Huang*
Literal Name: "Sulfur yellow"
Alternate Chinese Names: *Shi Liu Huang*
Original Source: *Shen Nong Ben Cao Jing* (Divine Husbandman's Classic of the Materia Medica) in the second century
English Name: sulfur
Pharmaceutical Name: Sulfur
Properties: sour, warm
Channels Entered: Kidney, Large Intestine
Safety Index: toxic

CHINESE THERAPEUTIC ACTIONS

1. Relieves Toxicity, Kills Parasites and Stops Itching

Dermatological disorders: Topical application of *Liu Huang* (Sulfur) acts to kill parasites and relieve itching. Clinical applications include eczema, scabies, ringworm, yin sores, damp sores, ulcers and carbuncles. *Liu Huang* may be used alone topically with sesame oil, or in combination with other herbs.

- Scabies, herpetic lesions, sores and fungal infections: use *Liu Huang* individually, topically.
- Scabies: combine this substance with *Xiong Huang* (Realgar) and lard.
- Rash on the scrotum: use it with *Qing Dai* (Indigo Naturalis).
- Diaper rash: combine it with *Xiong Huang* (Realgar), *Han Shui Shi* (Mirabilite), and *Zhang Nao* (Camphora).

2. Tonifies the Yang of the *Ming Men* (Life Gate)

Kidney yang deficiency or collapse: *Liu Huang* is taken internally to treat soreness, weakness and coldness of the lower limbs, enuresis, impotence, decreased libido, asthma and constipation.

- Impotence, weak and cold lower limbs: use *Liu Huang* with *Shu Di Huang* (Radix Rehmanniae Preparata), *Ba Ji Tian* (Radix Morindae Officinalis), *Yin Yang Huo* (Herba Epimedii), *Rou Gui* (Cortex Cinnamomi), *Fu Zi* (Radix Aconiti Lateralis Praeparata) and *Ren Shen* (Radix Ginseng).
- Asthma caused by Kidney yang deficiency and cold: use this substance with *Fu Zi* (Radix Aconiti Lateralis Praeparata), *Chen Xiang* (Lignum Aquilariae Resinatum) and *Rou Gui* (Cortex Cinnamomi).

Constipation from deficiency and cold: *Liu Huang* revitalizes the intestines and promotes bowel movement.

- Constipation from cold and deficiency: use it with *Ban Xia* (Rhizoma Pinelliae) and *Sheng Jiang* (Rhizoma Zingiberis Recens).

DOSAGE

1 to 3 grams for internal use in pills or powder. *Liu Huang* is most often used topically as a powder, paste or ointment.

CAUTIONS / CONTRAINDICATIONS

- *Liu Huang* is toxic, and contraindicated in pregnancy and in cases of yin deficiency with heat signs.
- Large dosages and long-term use of *Liu Huang* should be avoided.

OVERDOSAGE

Adverse reaction to *Liu Huang* may occur as quickly as within a few minutes following exposure to the substance. The toxic dose for humans is 10 to 20 grams per dose, with warning signs such as poor appetite, decrease in spontaneous activities, abdominal distention, and difficulty breathing.

Mild overdose of *Liu Huang* is characterized by increased sensitivity to light, tearing, runny nose, burning sensations of the nose and throat, and visual disturbances.

Moderate overdose is characterized by headache, dizziness, lethargy, nausea, vomiting, dyspnea, cyanotic face, hepatomegaly, jaundice, impaired liver function and visual disturbances.

Severe overdose is characterized by headache, palpitations, delirium, anxiety, restlessness, convulsions, unconsciousness, and if untreated, respiratory depression and death.[1]

Liu Huang (Sulfur)

TREATMENT OF OVERDOSAGE

Treatment of overdose includes the following methods:

- An herbal decoction of 30 grams of *Hei Dou* (Semen Glycine Max) and 15 grams of *Gan Cao* (Radix Glycyrrhizae).
- Administration of 15 grams of *Lu Dou* (Semen Phaseoli Radiati), taken as powder with warm water.
- Administration of 30 grams of *Wu Mei* (Fructus Mume) and 15 grams of sugar with water.
- An herbal solution with 250 grams of *Lu Dou* (Semen Phaseoli Radiati) and 60 grams of *Gan Cao* (Radix Glycyrrhizae) taken as solution.[2]

CHEMICAL COMPOSITION

Sulfur. Other impurities may be present.[3]

PHARMACOLOGICAL EFFECTS

- **Gastrointestinal:** Oral administration of *Liu Huang* may stimulate the gastrointestinal tract, increase intestinal peristalsis, and promote bowel movement.[4]
- **Respiratory:** Oral administration of *Liu Huang* is associated with a marked antitussive effect in mice.[5]

TOXICOLOGY

The LD_{50} for oral administration of *Liu Huang* is 20 g/kg in mice.[6]

AUTHORS' COMMENTS

Arsenic is sometimes present in *Liu Huang* as an impurity. Processing *Liu Huang* with heat is considered to be a standard process to minimize toxicity and prevent arsenic poisoning.[7]

References

1. *Zhong Yao Bu Liang Fan Ying Yu Zhi Liao* (Adverse Reactions and Treatment of Chinese Herbal Medicine), 1996; 218:220, 1996; 270:272
2. Ibid.
3. *Xian Dai Zhong Yao Yao Li Xue* (Contemporary Pharmacology of Chinese Herbs), 1997; 1405
4. *Zhong Yao Da Ci Dian* (Dictionary of Chinese Herbs), 1986; 616
5. *Zhong Yao Yao Li Xue* (Study of Chinese Herbology), 1985; 312
6. *Zhong Yao Xue* (Chinese Herbology), 1998; 908
7. Ibid.

Xiong Huang (Realgar)

雄黄

Pinyin Name: *Xiong Huang*
Literal Name: "male yellow"
Alternate Chinese Names: *Ming Xiong Huang, Xiong Jing, Yao Huang*
Original Source: *Shen Nong Ben Cao Jing* (Divine Husbandman's Classic of the Materia Medica) in the second century
English Name: realgar
Pharmaceutical Name: Realgar
Properties: acrid, bitter, warm
Channels Entered: Heart, Liver, Kidney
Safety Index: toxic

CHINESE THERAPEUTIC ACTIONS

1. Eliminates Toxins, Dries Dampness

Sores and ulcers: *Xiong Huang* (Realgar) is used to treat lesions characterized by swelling, abscess, and ulceration. It may be used internally or topically, individually or in combination with other herbs.

- Sores with redness, swelling, itching and pain: mix *Xiong Huang* with *Ming Fan* (Alumen) and apply the powder topically.
- Abscess and hard suppurative lesions: use this mineral with *She Xiang* (Moschus), *Ru Xiang* (Gummi Olibanum) and *Mo Yao* (Myrrha).
- Toxic sores and swellings: drain the pus, then apply the powder topically.

Fungal infection: Topical application of *Xiong Huang* effectively treats fungal infections.

- Fungal infection: mix it with *Huang Lian* (Rhizoma Coptidis) and apply topically.

Xiong Huang (Realgar)

Insect or animal bites: *Xiong Huang* is used to treat insect and animal bites. Mild cases are treated by topical application only, while severe cases are treated both internally and topically.

- Insect and snake bites: use it with *Wu Ling Zhi* (Excrementum Trogopteri seu Pteromi) and grain-based liquor. The powder may be applied topically or taken internally.
- Rabies: combine this mineral with *Xi Xin* (Herba Asari), *Bi Ba* (Fructus Piperis Longi), and *She Xiang* (Moschus), in grain-based liquor.

Syphilitic chancres:

- Syphilitic chancres: mix *Xiong Huang* with *Xing Ren* (Semen Armeniacae Amarum), *Qing Fen* (Calomelas), and *Zhu Dan* (Fel Porcus) and apply topically.

2. Kills Parasites

Oral ingestion of *Xiong Huang* is effective in killing various parasites. It also treats abdominal pain caused by parasitic accumulation.

- Intestinal parasites with abdominal pain: use this substance with processed *Ba Dou* (Fructus Crotonis), *Ku Lian Pi* (Cortex Meliae), *Bing Lang* (Semen Arecae), and *Gan Qi* (Resina Toxicodendri).
- Cerebral cysticercosis: combine *Xiong Huang* with *Gan Qi* (Resina Toxicodendri), *Chuan Shan Jia* (Squama Manis), and *Lei Wan* (Omphalia).

3. Eliminates Phlegm, Treats Malaria and Settles Wind

Xiong Huang eliminates phlegm to treat disorders such as asthma, malaria, seizures and tetanus. It is commonly used internally within an herbal formula for synergistic action.

- Asthma: use it individually, three times daily, with warm water.
- Malaria: combine it with *Shan Ci Gu* (Pseudobulbus Cremastrae), *Zhu Sha* (Cinnabaris), and *Qian Jin Zi* (Semen Euphorbiae).
- Seizures, epilepsy and convulsions: use it with *Zhu Sha* (Cinnabaris).
- Tetanus: use *Xiong Huang* with *Fang Feng* (Radix Saposhnikoviae) and *Cao Wu* (Radix Aconiti Kusnezoffii), with warm grain-based liquor.

Xiong Huang has recently been used to treat cancer. It is usually combined with other herbs internally or applied externally, and used primarily for skin and cervical cancers.

DOSAGE

0.15 to 0.30 gram for internal use as pills.

CAUTIONS / CONTRAINDICATIONS

- *Xiong Huang* is contraindicated in cases of yin deficiency, blood deficiency, or pregnancy.
- *Xiong Huang* is toxic. Therefore, it is not suitable for long-term use or application over a large surface area.
- *Xiong Huang* should not be used in decoction or mixed with hot water. Exposure to heat produces As_2S_2, which is extremely toxic.

OVERDOSAGE

Acute overdose is characterized by severe vomiting and diarrhea. Chronic overdose is characterized by lack of appetite, fatigue, slow reactions, hair loss, blurred vision, dizziness, restlessness, irritability, numbness of the extremities, and leg pain.[1]

TREATMENT OF OVERDOSAGE

Mild cases of overdose may be treated with an herbal decoction containing *Gan Cao* (Radix Glycyrrhizae) and *Lu Dou* (Semen Phaseoli Radiati). Patients with severe overdose must be admitted to the hospital immediately.[2]

CHEMICAL COMPOSITION

Arsenic sulfide (AsS or As_2S_2).[3]

PHARMACOLOGICAL EFFECTS

- **Antibiotic:** *Xiong Huang* has an inhibitory effect against various pathogenic bacteria and dermatophytes.[4]

CLINICAL STUDIES AND RESEARCH

- **Malaria:** Chronic malaria in 29 patients was treated successfully using an herbal formula containing 0.3 gram of *Xiong Huang* and 2 grams of *Liu Yi San* (Six-to-One Powder). The powder was divided into two doses, with one taken 2 hours before the outbreak, and the other 4 to 6 hours later.[5]
- **Pinworm:** In one clinical study, 240 patients with pinworm infestations were treated with an herbal formula, with complete recovery in 203 patients. The herbal formula contained *Xiong Huang* 6g, *Shi Jun Zi* (Fructus Quisqualis) 6g, *Gan Cao* (Radix Glycyrrhizae) 3g, *Xing Ren* (Semen Armeniacae Amarum) 3g, *Yu Jin* (Radix Curcumae) 3g, and *Ba Dou* (Fructus Crotonis) 2g. All herbs were ground into fine powder, mixed with honey, and made into 48 pills. The treatment protocol was to administer 2 pills to infants between 6 months and 1 year of age; 4 pills to infants between 1 and 2 years of age; and 6 pills to children between 2 and 3 years of age. The patients were instructed to take one dose of herbs daily in the morning, on an empty stomach.[6]
- **Dysentery:** Ten patients with dysentery and discharge of mucus were treated with an herbal formula with good

Xiong Huang (Realgar)

results. The herbal formula contained *Xiong Huang*, *Da Huang* (Radix et Rhizoma Rhei), and *Huang Bai* (Cortex Phellodendri), in equal proportions. The patients were given 1.5 grams of the herbal formula in powder form, three times daily for 10 days.[7]

- **Pulmonary tuberculosis:** In one study, 6 of 9 patients with pulmonary tuberculosis responded well to treatment with a formula containing equal amounts of *Xiong Huang* and *Liu Huang* (Sulfur). The substances were ground into powder, mixed with bovine bile, and made into pills. The patients were instructed to take 0.3 gram of the pills, three times daily.[8]

References

1. *Zhong Yao Du Li Xue* (Toxicology of Chinese Herbs), 1989; 193:194
2. Ibid.
3. *Xian Dai Zhong Yao Yao Li Xue* (Contemporary Pharmacology of Chinese Herbs), 1997; 1406
4. *Zhong Yao Xue* (Chinese Herbology), 1998; 919:922
5. *Zhong Cheng Yao Yan Jiu* (Research of Chinese Patent Medicine), 1982; 7:46
6. *He Bei Zhong Yi* (Hebei Chinese Medicine), 1988; 5:17
7. *Zhong Yao Xue* (Chinese Herbology), 1998; 919:922
8. Ibid.

Qing Fen (Calomelas)

輕粉 轻粉

Pinyin Name: *Qing Fen*
Literal Name: "light powder"
Alternate Chinese Names: *Xiao Fen, Ni Fen*
Original Source: *Ben Cao Shi Yi* (Omissions from the [Classic of the] Materia Medica) by Chen Cang-Qi in 741 A.D.
English Name: calomel
Pharmaceutical Name: Calomelas
Properties: acrid, cold
Channels Entered: Liver, Kidney
Safety Index: toxic

CHINESE THERAPEUTIC ACTIONS

1. Eliminates Toxins

Ulceration, syphilis, dermatological disorders, rosacea, pimples: *Qing Fen* (Calomelas) is used to treat dermatological disorders characterized by toxins, such as ulcerations of the skin and flesh, discharge of pus, and infection. It dispels heat, eliminates toxins, and relieves itching. *Qing Fen* is dry, strong and extremely toxic. It is mostly used in powder form externally, for dermatological disorders caused by heat and toxicity.

- Ulcerations of the skin and flesh: combine *Qing Fen* with *Huang Bai* (Cortex Phellodendri), and calcined *Shi Gao* (Gypsum Fibrosum). All herbs are ground into fine powder, mixed with water or sesame oil, and applied topically.
- Skin sores: use it with *Huang Lian* (Rhizoma Coptidis) and *Zhu Dan* (Fel Porcus), topically.
- Rosacea and pimples: mix this mineral with *Da Huang* (Radix et Rhizoma Rhei), *Liu Huang* (Sulfur) powder, sesame oil, petroleum jelly, honey and cold water. Apply topically.
- Chancre: ingest *Qing Fen* with *Hu Tao Ren* (Semen Juglandis), *Huai Hua* (Flos Sophorae), *Da Zao* (Fructus Jujubae). This method is no longer recommended because of the toxicity of *Qing Fen*.

2. Kills Parasites

Topical application of *Qing Fen* effectively treats skin parasites and inhibits the growth of dermatophytes. Clinically, it treats scabies, fungal infection of the skin, and relieves itching.

- Scabies: use *Qing Fen* with *Xiong Huang* (Realgar) and *Da Feng Zi* (Semen Hydnocarpi) as powder, topically.
- General fungal infections: combine it with *Liu Huang* (Sulfur) and *Qian Dan* (Minium) topically.
- Fungal infection with severe itching: use this substance with *Lang Du* (Radix Euphorbiae Fischerianae), *Xi Xin*

Qing Fen (Calomelas)

(Herba Asari), and *Shui Yin* (Hydrargyum). The herbs are ground into fine powder, mixed with beeswax, and applied topically.

3. Promotes Normal Urination and Bowel Movement

Oral ingestion of *Qing Fen* unblocks the bladder and the bowels. It treats edema, urinary retention and constipation. It can be used with cathartic herbs to dispel internal stagnation.

- Mild edema with difficulties in urination and bowel movement: use *Qing Fen* individually.
- Moderate edema with difficulties in urination and bowel movement: add it to *Da Ji* (Radix Euphorbiae seu Knoxiae), *Yuan Hua* (Flos Genkwa) and *Qian Niu Zi* (Semen Pharbitidis).
- Severe edema with difficulties with urination and bowel movement: combine it with *Da Ji* (Radix Euphorbiae seu Knoxiae), *Yuan Hua* (Flos Genkwa), *Qian Niu Zi* (Semen Pharbitidis), *Qing Pi* (Pericarpium Citri Reticulatae Viride) and *Bing Lang* (Semen Arecae).
- Constipation: use it with *Da Zao* (Fructus Jujubae).

DOSAGE

Qing Fen is ground into fine powder for topical use. For oral use, the dosage is 0.06 to 0.15 gram [60 to 150 mg] and it should not be taken more than twice daily. Use of *Qing Fen* in decoction is contraindicated, as cooking increases its toxicity.

CAUTIONS / CONTRAINDICATIONS

- *Qing Fen* is extremely toxic, and if used internally must be prescribed with extreme caution. It is contraindicated during pregnancy and for those with deficient constitutions.
- *Qing Fen* may be used for edema associated with cardiovascular disorders. However, it is contraindicated in cases of edema or ascites caused by kidney or liver disease.
- *Qing Fen* should be used with caution for patients with hypersensitive skin, as instances of contact dermatitis have been reported.
- Because heat increases the toxicity of *Qing Fen*, this mineral must be handled with caution. When making a topical preparation, *Qing Fen* should be added at the very end, after the water or beeswax has cooled to room temperature. Mixing *Qing Fen* in a hot medium increases the risk of contact dermatitis.

OVERDOSAGE

Overdose of *Qing Fen* is characterized by erosive gastritis, a metallic taste in the mouth, redness and swelling of the oral cavity, thirst, nausea, vomiting, hematemesis, hematuria, decreased urinary volume, difficulty breathing, and in severe cases, necrosis of kidney tissue.

TREATMENT OF OVERDOSAGE

Overdose may be treated by ingestion of milk or egg whites to decrease absorption of the substance. It may also be treated by use of an herbal decoction of *Jin Yin Hua* (Flos Lonicerae), *Lu Dou* (Semen Phaseoli Radiati), *Gan Cao* (Radix Glycyrrhizae) and *Tu Fu Ling* (Rhizoma Smilacis Glabrae).

CHEMICAL COMPOSITION

Mercurous chloride (Hg_2Cl_2) 99.6%.[1]

PHARMACOLOGICAL EFFECTS

- **Antibiotic:** *Qing Fen* has an inhibitory effect *in vitro* against various pathogenic bacteria and fungi.[2]
- **Gastrointestinal:** After oral ingestion, *Qing Fen* binds with bile in the intestines to become bivalent mercury ions. These ions interfere with the normal breakdown and digestion of food in the intestines, leading to increased elimination of electrolytes, water, and bile. Therefore, patients ingesting this substance commonly report diarrhea and green discoloration of the stool.[3]
- **Urinary:** Systemic absorption of bivalent mercury ions interferes with re-absorption of water in the kidney, leading to increased urination and diuresis.[4]

CLINICAL STUDIES AND RESEARCH

- **Body odor:** In one report, 100 patients with body odor were treated with topical application of *Qing Fen* and *Hua Shi* (Talcum) to the underarm, with satisfactory results.[5]

TOXICOLOGY

The LD_{50} for *Qing Fen* is 410 mg/kg in mice and 1,740 mg/kg in rats.[6]

References

1. *Zhong Yao Xue* (Chinese Herbology), 1998; 925-927
2. *Chang Yong Zhong Yao Xian Dai Yan Jiu Yu Lin Chuan* (Recent Study & Clinical Application of Common Traditional Chinese Medicine), 1995; 699:701
3. *Zhong Yao Xue* (Chinese Herbology), 1998; 925:928
4. Ibid.
5. *Zhong Cheng Yao Yan Jiu* (Research of Chinese Patent Medicine), 1982; 7:45
6. *Zhong Yao Xue* (Chinese Herbology), 1998; 925:928

Qian Dan (Minium)

鉛丹 铅丹

Pinyin Name: *Qian Dan*
Literal Name: "lead elixir," "lead pills"
Alternate Chinese Names: *Guang Dan, Huang Dan, Dong Dan*
Original Source: *Shen Nong Ben Cao Jing* (Divine Husbandman's Classic of the Materia Medica) in the second century
English Name: minium
Pharmaceutical Name: Minium
Properties: bitter, cool
Channels Entered: Heart, Liver
Safety Index: toxic

CHINESE THERAPEUTIC ACTIONS

1. External Use

External application of *Qian Dan* (Minium) functions to eliminate toxins, dispel dampness, promote the generation of flesh and facilitate recovery of sores and ulcerations. Its clinical applications include treatment of sores, ulcerations, abscesses, eczema, body odor, and similar damp surface problems. *Qian Dan* is to be used topically for all the indications listed below:

- Sores with or without pus: mix 30 grams each of *Qian Dan* and *E Jiao* (Colla Corii Asini) and cook in water until these substances become liquid.
- Chronic ulceration with necrosis of local tissue: use this mineral with calcined *Shi Gao* (Gypsum Fibrosum), *Qing Fen* (Calomelas) and *Bing Pian* (Borneolum Syntheticum).
- Chronic non-healing ulcerations with pus and abscess: combine it with calcined *Shi Gao* (Gypsum Fibrosum), *Qing Fen* (Calomelas), *Long Gu* (Os Draconis), *Ru Xiang* (Gummi Olibanum) and *Mo Yao* (Myrrha).
- Body odor: use it with *Qing Fen* (Calomelas), *Huang Bai* (Cortex Phellodendri), *Huang Lian* (Rhizoma Coptidis) and *She Xiang* (Moschus).
- General itching and pain: add it to *Qing Fen* (Calomelas) and *Chuan Shan Jia* (Squama Manis).

2. Internal Use

Internal ingestion of *Qian Dan* effectively dispels phlegm to treat seizures and convulsions. Traditional formulas sometimes use *Qian Dan* to treat seizures, convulsions, epilepsy and delirium. However, internal ingestion should be avoided if possible, because of the toxicity of this substance.

- Seizure or epilepsy: *Qian Dan* has been used historically with *Chai Hu Jia Long Mu Tang* (Bupleurum plus Dragon Bone and Oyster Shell Decoction).

Internal ingestion of *Qian Dan* has been used historically to eliminate toxins and kill parasites. It may be used individually or in combination with other herbs.

- Malaria: this substance was used with *Chang Shan* (Radix Dichroae), *Qing Hao* (Herba Artemisiae Annuae) and *Da Suan* (Bulbus Alli Sativi).

DOSAGE

0.3 to 0.6 gram for internal use. *Qian Dan* may be used as pills or powder.

CAUTIONS / CONTRAINDICATIONS

- Cold and toxic, *Qian Dan* is contraindicated in pregnant women, or in cases of nausea and vomiting characterized by cold in the body.
- *Qian Dan* is toxic when absorbed systemically. Therefore, long-term use or application over a large surface area of the body can be dangerous.
- Internal use of *Qian Dan* is frequently associated with toxicity. Therefore, it must be used only with extreme caution.
- Due to the toxicity of this substance, oral ingestion of *Qian Dan* is rarely recommended.

OVERDOSAGE

Oral ingestion of *Qian Dan* is toxic to the gastrointestinal tract, central nervous system, hematological, and cardiovascular systems of the body. Acute overdose of *Qian Dan* is characterized by dryness of the mouth and throat, thirst, burning sensations and pain in the upper esophagus, a metallic taste in the mouth, salivation, nausea, vomiting, severe abdominal pain, constipation or diarrhea, black tarry stools, and in severe cases, shock. Chronic overdose of *Qian Dan* is characterized by a lack of diagnostic symptoms in early stages, followed by neuritis, abdominal pain, anemia, disturbances of the central nervous system, joint pain, muscle spasms and cramps, muscle paralysis, dark-purplish discoloration of the gums, poor appetite, abdominal distention and pain, slight relief of pain by pressure, palpitations, shortness of breath, fatigue, enlargement of the liver, proteinuria and

Qian Dan (Minium)

irregular menstruation. Acute poisoning may occur following a bolus dose of 15 grams of *Qian Dan*, and chronic poisoning has been reported following daily ingestion of 2 mg of this mineral.[1]

TREATMENT OF OVERDOSAGE

Overdose of *Qian Dan* may be treated by one or more of the following methods:

- An herbal decoction with *Hai Zao* (Sargassum) and *Kun Bu* (Thallus Laminariae seu Eckloniae).
- An herbal decoction of *Jin Qian Cao* (Herba Lysimachiae), *Ju Hua* (Flos Chrysanthemi) and *Gan Cao* (Radix Glycyrrhizae).
- Ingestion of egg whites, milk, soy milk, or *Lu Dou* (Semen Phaseoli Radiati).[2]

CHEMICAL COMPOSITION

Lead oxide red (Pb_3O_4).[3]

References

1. *Xian Dai Zhong Yao Yao Li Xue* (Contemporary Pharmacology of Chinese Herbs), 1997; 1425
2. Ibid.
3. Ibid.

Mi Tuo Seng (Lithargyum)

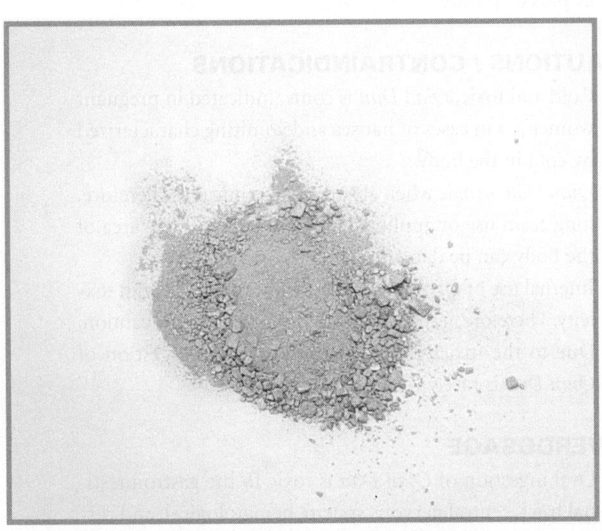

密陀僧

Pinyin Name: *Mi Tuo Seng*
Literal Name: "elusive reclusive monk"
Alternate Chinese Names: *Mo Duo Seng, Yin Chi, Jin Lu Di*
Original Source: *Lei Gong Pao Zhi Lun* (Grandfather Lei's Discussions of Herb Preparation) by Lei Xiao in 470 A.D.
English Name: litharge
Pharmaceutical Name: Lithargyum
Properties: salty, acrid, neutral
Channels Entered: Liver, Spleen
Safety Index: toxic

CHINESE THERAPEUTIC ACTIONS

1. Eliminates Toxins

Mi Tuo Seng (Lithargyrum) eliminates toxins and treats various dermatological conditions when used topically. It is often made into an ointment or paste for chronic ulcers and sores with suppuration. Clinical applications include scabies, ringworm, damp rashes, abscesses, suppurative inflammations, ulcerations, sores and other dermatological conditions. *Mi Tuo Seng* is to be used topically for all indications listed below:

- Chronic non-healing bedsores and ulceration: use *Mi Tuo Seng* with *Xiong Huang* (Realgar) and *Liu Huang* (Sulfur).
- Fungal infection: use this mineral individually.
- General dermatological disorders: grind 30 grams of *Mi Tuo Seng* and 3 grams of *Qing Fen* (Calomelas) into fine powder, mix with petroleum jelly, and apply to the affected area.
- Body odor or excessive perspiration: use it with *Qing Fen* (Calomelas), *Ming Fan* (Alumen) and *Bing Pian* (Borneolum Syntheticum) and apply to the affected area.

2. Kills Parasites

Mi Tuo Seng has only moderate strength in treating parasitic infections, and must be combined with other herbs for maximum effectiveness. Clinical applications include tinea versicolor, vitiligo, scabies and rosacea.

Mi Tuo Seng (Lithargyum)

DOSAGE

Mi Tuo Seng is primarily used topically. The maximum dose for oral ingestion is 0.3 to 1.0 gram daily.

CAUTIONS / CONTRAINDICATIONS

- Oral ingestion of *Mi Tuo Seng* is commonly associated with toxicity and overdose. Therefore, long-term use or large doses are strongly discouraged.

CHEMICAL COMPOSITION

Lead oxide (PbO).[1]

PHARMACOLOGICAL EFFECTS

- **Antibiotic:** *Mi Tuo Seng* has a mild inhibiting influence on some pathogenic fungi at 2% and 4% concentrations.[2]

CLINICAL STUDIES AND RESEARCH

- **Eczema:** In one study, 48 out of 50 patients showed complete recovery after treatment with an herbal formula containing 10 grams of *Mi Tuo Seng*, 5 grams of *Huang Bai* (Cortex Phellodendri), and 2.5 grams of *Bing Pian* (Borneolum Syntheticum). The herbs were ground into fine powder, mixed with an oil-based carrier, and applied topically.[3]
- **Tinea versicolor:** Treatment of 40 patients with tinea versicolor resulted in complete recovery within 1 or 2 treatments using topical application of *Mi Tuo Seng* and *Liu Huang* (Sulfur). The ingredients were ground into fine powder, mixed with 76% rubbing alcohol to make a paste, and applied topically to the affected area.[4]

References

1. *Zhong Yao Xue* (Chinese Herbology), 1998; 934-936
2. Ibid., 934:935
3. *Zhong Hua Pi Fu Ke Xue Za Zhi* (Chinese Journal of Dermatology), 1966; 1:44
4. *Fu Jian Yi Yao Za Zhi* (Fujian Journal of Medicine and Herbology), 1980; 5:48

Ming Fan (Alumen)

明礬 明矾

Pinyin Name: *Ming Fan*
Alternate Chinese Names: *Bai Fan*
Original Source: *Shen Nong Ben Cao Jing* (Divine Husbandman's Classic of the Materia Medica) in the second century
English Name: alum
Pharmaceutical Name: Alumen
Properties: sour, cold
Channels Entered: Lung, Liver, Spleen, Stomach, Large Intestine
Safety Index: toxic

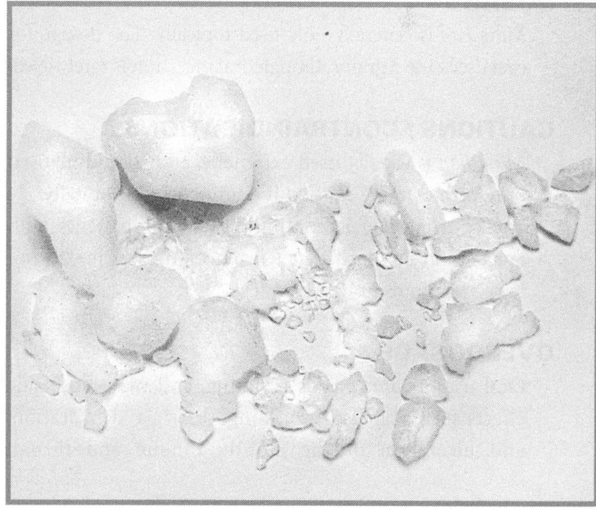

CHINESE THERAPEUTIC ACTIONS

1. Eliminates Toxins, Kills Parasites, Dries Dampness and Stops Itching

Dermatological disorders: *Ming Fan* (Alumen) treats scabies, ringworm, rashes, oral sores, eczema, vaginal discharge, genital itching and itching lesions. *Ming Fan* also eliminates toxins to treat lung and breast abscesses, hemorrhoids, and other disorders due to toxic swellings.

- Vaginal discharge, genital itching, eczema: combine *Ming Fan* with *She Chuang Zi* (Fructus Cnidii) as an external soak or wash.
- Swelling without pus or suppuration: crush this mineral with *Cong Bai* (Bulbus Allii Fistulosi), and ingest with grain-based alcohol.

Ming Fan (Alumen)

2. Stops Bleeding, Relieves Diarrhea

Bleeding and diarrhea: *Ming Fan* has an astringent effect that stops the loss of body fluids, and stops bleeding and diarrhea. Clinical applications include hemoptysis, epistaxis, gastrointestinal bleeding, bleeding from traumatic injuries, diarrhea and dysentery.

- Epistaxis, hemoptysis, upper gastrointestinal bleeding: use *Ming Fan* with *Er Cha* (Catechu) internally or apply topically.
- Chronic diarrhea or dysentery: combine this substance with *He Zi* (Fructus Chebulae), *Liu Huang* (Sulfur), *Bai Tou Weng* (Radix Pulsatillae) and *Huang Lian* (Rhizoma Coptidis).

3. Clears Heat and Expels Phlegm

Wind-phlegm disorder: Irritability, mania, epilepsy, and vomiting of phlegm are common presentations of this condition.

- Wind-phlegm disorders: use *Ming Fan* with *Yu Jin* (Radix Curcumae), *Bo He* (Herba Menthae) and *Zao Jiao* (Fructus Gleditsiae).

4. Clears Damp-Heat

Jaundice: *Ming Fan* treats jaundice caused by damp-heat.

- Jaundice: use it with *Yin Chen Hao* (Herba Artemisiae Scopariae).

DOSAGE

Ming Fan is generally only used topically. The dosage for oral use is 1 to 3 grams, though oral ingestion is rarely used.

CAUTIONS / CONTRAINDICATIONS

- *Ming Fan* is usually used externally, and should be used only with extreme caution if administered internally.
- Use of *Ming Fan* is contraindicated for patients with Spleen and Stomach deficiencies, or those who do not have symptoms of damp-heat.

OVERDOSAGE

Oral use of *Ming Fan* is irritating, and may cause side effects such as nausea, vomiting, diarrhea, dehydration, and ulceration of the mouth, tongue and throat. Overdose may cause vomiting, diarrhea and shock. Therefore, *Ming Fan* is almost always used topically.[1]

CHEMICAL COMPOSITION

$KAl_2(SO_4)_2(OH)_6$.[2]

PHARMACOLOGICAL EFFECTS

- **Antibiotic:** *Ming Fan* has an inhibitory effect *in vitro* against *Bacillus proteus*, *Pseudomonas aeruginosa*, *Staphylococcus aureus*, and *Candida albicans*. It has an inhibitory effect on various gram-positive and gram-negative bacteria, including but not limited to *Staphylococcus aureus*, *Bacillus proteus*, *E. coli*, *Pseudomonas aeruginosa*, *Bacillus anthracis*, *Bacillus dysenteriae*, *Salmonella typhi*, β-hemolytic streptococcus, *Diplococcus* and *Streptococcus pneumoniae*.[3,4]

CLINICAL STUDIES AND RESEARCH

- **Infectious parotitis:** According to one report, 16 patients with parotitis were treated topically with a formulation, and reported complete recovery within three days. The paste was prepared by mixing *Ming Fan*, *Xiong Huang* (Realgar) and *Bing Pian* (Borneolum Syntheticum) with rubbing alcohol.[5]

TOXICOLOGY

Intramuscular injection of an 8% *Ming Fan* solution in rabbits and dogs caused severe irritation and necrosis of the local tissues. Oral administration of *Ming Fan* solution is associated with severe burning sensations, nausea, vomiting, diarrhea, and dehydration.[6]

References

1. *Zhong Yao Da Ci Dian* (Dictionary of Chinese Herbs), 1986; 680
2. *Xian Dai Zhong Yao Yao Li Xue* (Contemporary Pharmacology of Chinese Herbs), 1997; 1416
3. Ibid., 1416-1417
4. *Chang Yong Zhong Yao Xian Dai Yan Jiu Yu Lin Chuan* (Recent Study & Clinical Application of Common Traditional Chinese Medicine), 1995; 705:707
5. *Wu Han Yi Xue Za Zhi* (Wuhan Journal of Medicine), 1965; (3):24
6. *Chang Yong Zhong Yao Xian Dai Yan Jiu Yu Lin Chuan* (Recent Study & Clinical Application of Common Traditional Chinese Medicine), 1995; 705:707

Da Suan (Bulbus Alli Sativi)

大蒜 大蒜

Pinyin Name: *Da Suan*
Original Source: *Ming Yi Za Zhu* (Miscellaneous Records of Famous Physicians) by Tao Hong-Jing in 500 A.D.
English Name: garlic bulb, garlic
Botanical Name: *Allium sativum* L. (*Da Suan*)
Pharmaceutical Name: Bulbus Alli Sativi
Properties: acrid, warm
Channels Entered: Spleen, Stomach, Lung

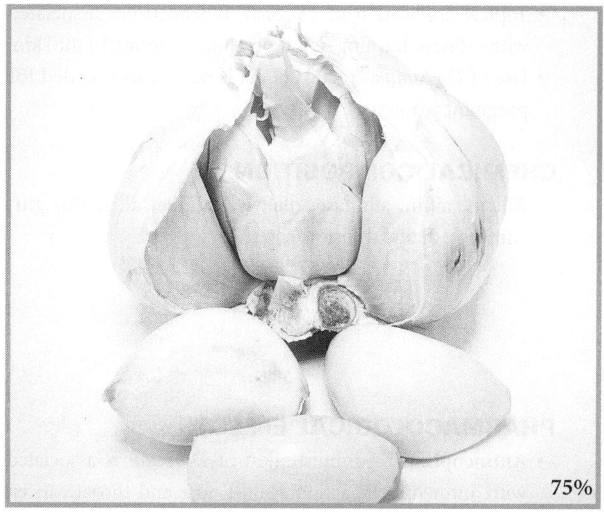
75%

CHINESE THERAPEUTIC ACTIONS

1. Reduces Swelling, Relieves Toxicity

Dermatological disorders: *Da Suan* (Bulbus Alli Sativi) effectively addresses various disorders characterized by swelling and toxins. It is commonly used both internally and topically, individually or in combination with other herbs. Clinical applications include sores, swellings, carbuncles, tuberculosis, whooping cough, dysentery, diarrhea, and influenza.

- Rashes, itching and swelling of the skin: grind *Da Suan* with sesame oil and mix with salt into a paste, apply topically.
- Whooping cough: crush 30 grams of *Da Suan* into paste and soak it (in twice as much water as garlic) for 12 hours. Filter out the solution and mix it with a small portion of sugar. The final preparation is given three times daily for 10 to 15 days per course of treatment.
- Diarrhea or dysentery: use the fresh herb or its decoction one time each day for 6 days. It can also be used as an enema.
- Prevention of viral infection: take 5 to 10 grams of *Da Suan* with meals daily, or use a 10% *Da Suan* solution as nasal drops.
- Tuberculosis: use 30 grams each of *Da Suan*, *Geng Mi* (Semen Oryzae) with 3 grams of *Bai Ji* (Rhizoma Bletillae). The formula is prepared by removing and discarding the skin of *Da Suan* and cooking the herb in boiling water for 1 to 1.5 minutes. *Da Suan* is then removed, and *Geng Mi* added and cooked until the decoction becomes porridge. Add the already-cooked *Da Suan* back to the porridge with 3 grams of *Bai Ji* before ingestion. Take twice daily (morning and night) for 3 months.

2. Kills Parasites

It effectively prevents and treats intestinal parasitic infestations such as hookworm and pinworm.

- Intestinal parasitic infestation: use *Da Suan* with *Bing Lang* (Semen Arecae), *Ku Lian Pi* (Cortex Meliae), and *He Shi* (Fructus Carpesii).
- Prevention of hookworm: apply it topically to the extremities prior to entering agricultural fields.
- Pinworms: mix this herb with vegetable oil and apply topically around the anus.
- Vaginitis due to amoebae or trichomonas: apply *Da Suan* paste topically.
- Influenza, encephalitis, and other infectious diseases: Apply 10% *Da Suan* juice into the nostrils and take 5 to 10 grams of *Da Suan* with every meal.

3. Relieves Food Poisoning

Decoction of *Da Suan* is beneficial in treating fish and crab poisoning. It is generally combined with *Zi Su Ye* (Folium Perillae) and *Sheng Jiang* (Rhizoma Zingiberis Recens) to treat various types of food poisoning. *Da Suan* also helps to neutralize toxins and relieve pain caused by centipede bites.

DOSAGE

3 to 5 pieces. *Da Suan* is commonly used both internally and topically. It may be used as fresh herb, decoction, food supplement, or syrup. The juice may be used as a rectal enema. To enhance the effect of moxa, *Da Suan* is cut into thin slices and placed on the skin at the desired points before moxa is applied.

CAUTIONS / CONTRAINDICATIONS

- Acrid and warm, *Da Suan* is contraindicated in cases of yin-deficient heat.
- *Da Suan* is contraindicated in cases of excess heat affecting the eyes, throat, mouth, tongue and gums.

Da Suan (Bulbus Alli Sativi)

- Topical application of *Da Suan* is sometimes associated with redness, burning sensations, and blistering of the skin.
- Use of *Da Suan* as rectal enema is not recommended for pregnant women.

CHEMICAL COMPOSITION

Allicin, alliin, alliinase, diallyl disulfide, allistatin, glucominol, diallyl thiosulfonate.[1,2]

$H_2C{=}CH{-}CH_2{-}S({=}O){-}S{-}CH_2{-}CH{=}CH_2$

Allicin

PHARMACOLOGICAL EFFECTS

- **Antineoplastic:** Administration of *Da Suan* is associated with antineoplastic action against nose and throat cancer, leukemia, stomach cancer, liver cancer with ascites, and lymphatic cancer. Allicin and allitridin are two of the active components responsible for the antineoplastic effect.[3,4,5,6,7]
- **Cardiovascular:** Administration of *Da Suan* is associated with reduction of blood pressure, blood cholesterol levels, and atherosclerosis. In dogs, daily administration of *Da Suan* for 7 to 10 days lowered blood pressure by as much as 50 mmHg.[8] *Da Suan* also demonstrated marked effectiveness to lower plasma cholesterol and triglyceride levels in rabbits and decreased the risk of atherosclerosis.[9]
- **Antibiotic:** *Da Suan* has an antiviral effect against cytomegalovirus, and an antibiotic effect against *Candida albicans, Mycobacterium tuberculosis, Bacillus dysenteriae, Salmonella typhi, Vibrio cholerae,* and *Bacillus paratyphosus.*[10]
- **Hepatoprotective:** *Da Suan* has a protective effect against carbon tetrachloride-induced liver damage in rats.[11]
- **Antidiabetic:** Oral administration of *Da Suan* in mice is associated with a 17.9 to 26.2% drop in plasma glucose levels, two hours after the initial dose.[12]

CLINICAL STUDIES AND RESEARCH

- **Pneumonomoniliasis:** Two patients with pneumonomoniliasis resistant to antibiotics were treated with 20 ml of 10% *Da Suan* solution administered via oral inhalation, with good results.[13]
- **Hypercholesterolemia:** Oral administration of a *Da Suan* preparation (equivalent to 50 grams per day of the herb) was given to 274 patients for 30 days. The study reported an increase in HDL and a decrease in LDL.[14]
- **Nephritis:** Acute nephritis in 21 patients was treated with *Da Suan* and *Xi Gua* (Fructus Citrulli), with complete recovery in 14 patients, moderate improvement in 5 patients, and no response in 2 patients. The treatment protocol was to insert 250 grams of *Da Suan* through a small hole into watermelon and shave off the outer skin. The *Da Suan*-injected *Xi Gua* is to be steamed and ingested within one day; and the outer skin is to be cooked and ingested as tea.[15]
- **Alopecia areata:** Topical application of *Da Suan* and oral ingestion of *Shi Quan Da Bu Tang* (All-Inclusive Great Tonifying Decoction) were effective for 856 patients with alopecia areata. The duration of treatment was between 17 and 46 days.[16]

HERB-DRUG INTERACTION

- **Antidiabetics:** Herbs that lower the plasma glucose levels, such as *Da Suan,* should be used cautiously with insulin, sulfonylureas, and other antidiabetic medications as the combination may have a synergistic effect, leading to hypoglycemia.[17] [Note: Examples of antidiabetic drugs include insulin, tolbutamide (Orinase), glipizide (Glucotrol), and glyburide (DiaBeta/Micronase).]
- **Antibiotic:** Fresh *Da Suan* and its constituent allicin reduced the minimum inhibitory concentration (MIC) of vancomycin for vancomycin-resistant enterococci.[18]

TOXICOLOGY

The LD_{50} for oral ingestion of allicin in rats is 265 mg/kg, and the LD_{50} for intravenous injection of essential oil of *Da Suan* in mice is 134 mg/kg.[19]

AUTHORS' COMMENTS

Da Suan is commonly taken as food. According to various contemporary studies, this herb is good for the cardiovascular system and also has certain cancer-fighting attributes. It can be taken daily to promote health, but excessive use is sometimes associated with eye deterioration.

Breath odor from ingesting *Da Suan* may be neutralized by chewing a small portion of tea leaves or a small slice of *Dang Gui* (Radicis Angelicae Sinensis).

References

1. *Xian Dai Zhong Yao Yao Li Xue* (Contemporary Pharmacology of Chinese Herbs), 1997; 757
2. *The Merck Index* 12th edition, Chapman & Hall/CRCnetBASE/Merck, 2000.
3. *Shi Yong Zhong Liu Xue Za Zhi* (Practical Journal of Cancer), 1990; 4:25
4. *Zhong Hua Zhong Liu Za Zhi* (Chinese Journal of Cancer), 1985; 7(2)103
5. *Zhong Cheng Yao Yan Jiu* (Research of Chinese Patent Medicine), 1987; 10:26
6. *Chang Yong Zhong Yao Cheng Fen Yu Yao Li Shou Ce* (A Handbook of the Composition and Pharmacology of Common Chinese Drugs), 1994; 328:351
7. *Zhong Yao Xue* (Chinese Herbology), 1998; 956:959
8. *Qing Dao Yi Xue Yuan Xue Bao* (Journal of Qingdao Institution of Medicine), 1957; 1:14
9. *Chang Yong Zhong Yao Cheng Fen Yu Yao Li Shou Ce* (A Handbook of the Composition and Pharmacology of Common Chinese Drugs), 1994; 328:351

Da Suan (Bulbus Alli Sativi)

10. *Zhong Ji Yi Kan* (Medium Medical Journal), 1981; 8:7
11. *Planta Medica*, 1986; 3:163
12. *Shang Hai Zhong Yi Yao Za Zhi* (Shanghai Journal of Chinese Medicine and Herbology), 1989; 5:45
13. *Zhong Xi Yi Jie He Za Zhi* (Journal of Integrated Chinese and Western Medicine), 1986; 12:760
14. *Zhong Yi Za Zhi* (Journal of Chinese Medicine), 1985; 2:42
15. *Zhong Xi Yi Jie He Za Zhi* (Journal of Integrated Chinese and Western Medicine), 1983; 4:228
16. *Ji Lin Yi Xue* (Jilin Medicine), 1985; 5:24
17. Chen, J. Recognition & prevention of herb-drug interactions, *Medical Acupuncture*, Fall/Winter 1998/1999; volume 10/number 2; 9-13
18. Abascal K and Yarnell E, Herb and Drug Resistance – Clinical Implications of Research on Microbial Resistance to Antibiotics, *Alternative & Complementary Therapies*; vol 8, no 5, October 2002
19. *Chang Yong Zhong Yao Cheng Fen Yu Yao Li Shou Ce* (A Handbook of the Composition and Pharmacology of Common Chinese Drugs), 1994; 328:351

Ban Mao (Mylabris)

斑蝥

Pinyin Name: *Ban Mao*
Alternate Chinese Names: *Hua Ban Mao*
Original Source: *Shen Nong Ben Cao Jing* (Divine Husbandman's Classic of the Materia Medica) in the second century
English Name: mylabris, blister beetle, large blister beetle, lesser blister beetle, telini fly
Zoological Name: *Mylabris phalerata* Pall. (*Da Ban Mao*); *Mylabris cichorii* L. (*Huang Hei Xiao Ban Mao*)
Pharmaceutical Name: Mylabris
Properties: acrid, cold
Channels Entered: Large Intestine, Small Intestine, Liver, Kidney
Safety Index: toxic

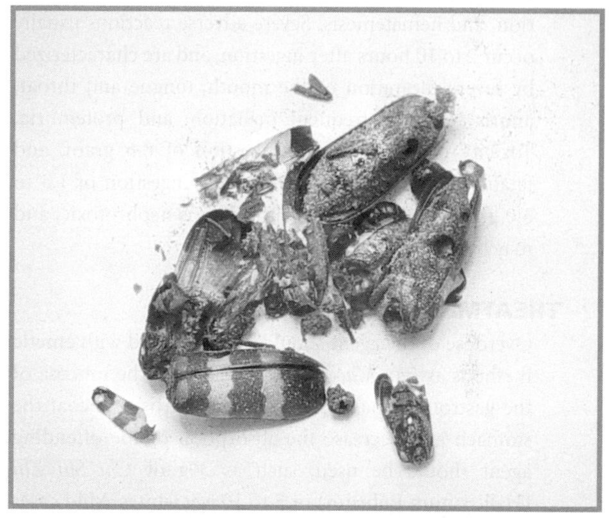

CHINESE THERAPEUTIC ACTIONS

1. Attacks Toxins and Dispels Sores

According to the doctrine of similarity, the toxic effect of *Ban Mao* (Mylabris) attacks toxins. Clinical applications include sores, carbuncles, furuncles, scrofula, psoriasis, toxic nodules and other conditions characterized by heat and toxins.

- Sores, carbuncles and furuncles: mix *Ban Mao* with garlic and apply topically. Other substances that can be used for the same purpose include *Xiong Huang* (Realgar), *Pi Shi* (Arsenolite) and *Peng Sha* (Borax).
- Psoriasis or fungal infection: mix it with *Gan Sui* (Radix Euphorbiae Kansui) and vinegar and apply several times daily.
- Scrofula: combine it with *Bo He* (Herba Menthae) and egg whites and take it internally.

2. Breaks Blood Stagnation to Disperse Nodules and Open Blood Circulation

Ban Mao treats palpable masses or nodules. It may also treat amenorrhea from blood stagnation.

- Liver or gastrointestinal cancer and tumors: use *Ban Mao* orally.
- Amenorrhea from blood stagnation: combine it with *Tao Ren* (Semen Persicae) and *Da Huang* (Radix et Rhizoma Rhei).

Ban Mao also helps to treat facial paralysis, *bi zheng* (painful obstruction syndrome), alopecia areata, and verruca wart.

DOSAGE

0.03 to 0.06 gram [30 to 60 mg] for oral use. The unprocessed form of *Ban Mao* is toxic and has a distinct

Ban Mao (Mylabris)

odor. Therefore, it must be dry-fried to reduce the toxicity and odor.

CAUTIONS / CONTRAINDICATIONS

- *Ban Mao* has a very strong stimulating and irritating effect on the skin and mucous membranes. Topical use may cause redness, burning sensations, irritation and death of the local tissues. Do not apply over a large surface area or over a long period of time.
- Use of *Ban Mao* is contraindicated in cases of general deficiency or in pregnancy.

OVERDOSAGE

Ban Mao is very toxic, even at small doses. Initial adverse reactions usually occur 10 minutes to 2 hours after ingestion, and are characterized by nausea, vomiting, salivation, and hematemesis. Severe adverse reactions usually occur 2 to 10 hours after ingestion, and are characterized by severe ulceration of the mouth, tongue and throat, anuria, oliguria, frequent urination, and proteinuria. Toxicity occurs following ingestion of 0.6 gram, and fatality has been reported following ingestion of 1.3 to 3.0 grams of *Ban Mao*. Cantharidin is nephrotoxic, and may be fatal at 30mg.[1]

TREATMENT OF OVERDOSAGE

Overdose of the agent should not be treated with emetic methods as *Ban Mao* is very irritating to the mucosa of the gastrointestinal system. Instead, herbs that coat the stomach and decrease the absorption of the offending agent should be used, such as 30g of *Chi Shi Zhi* (Halloysitum Rubrum) or 5 to 10 egg whites. Mild cases of overdose may be treated by an herbal decoction containing 30 grams of *Lu Dou* (Semen Phaseoli Radiati), 10 grams of *Gan Cao* (Radix Glycyrrhizae), and 3 grams of *Huang Lian* (Rhizoma Coptidis). An herbal decoction with 60 grams of *Lu Cha* (Folium Camellia Sinensis) can also be used to clear heat, promote urination and facilitate elimination of the toxin. Another effective formula includes 30 grams of *Gan Cao* (Radix Glycyrrhizae) and 15 grams of *Da Qing Ye* (Folium Isatidis). Adverse reaction associated with topical application of *Ban Mao* can be alleviated with topical application of *Huang Lian* (Rhizoma Coptidis) or *Bing Pian* (Borneolum Syntheticum). Lastly, patients with overdose of *Ban Mao* should avoid eating lipophilic foods, such as fat, meat and milk, as they will increase the absorption of the agent and increase toxicity.[2]

CHEMICAL COMPOSITION

Cantharidin, 1 to 1.2%.[3,4]

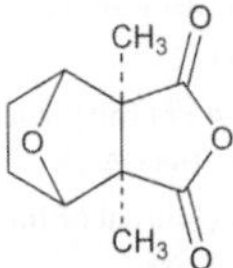

Cantharidin

PHARMACOLOGICAL EFFECTS

- **Immunologic:** It has been noted that a small dosage of cantharidin may increase white blood cell count and enhance immunity in some patients, while a large dosage may suppress the immune system.[5]
- **Antineoplastic:** Cantharidin has demonstrated an inhibitory effect on cancer cells in cases of hepatic carcinoma and sarcoma in mice.[6]

CLINICAL STUDIES AND RESEARCH

- **Liver cancer:** According to one report, 300 patients with liver cancer were treated with cantharidin and chemotherapy or radiation. The protocol for cantharidin was 0.25 to 0.5 mg three times daily. In addition to cantharidin, patients were encouraged to drink green tea on a daily basis. The study reported an overall rate of effectiveness of 65%, based on symptomatic evaluation and the size of the liver tumor.[7] In another study, 2 to 6 pills of a preparation (each pill contained 0.25 mg of cantharidin, *Bai Ji* (Rhizoma Bletillae), aluminum hydroxide, and others) were given to 800 patients with liver cancer three times daily, with 45 to 60% showing positive results. There were reduction of symptoms, decrease in tumor size, and 12.7% of the patients remained alive after 1 year.[8]
- **Facial paralysis:** Topical application of *Ban Mao* and *Ba Dou* (Fructus Crotonis) on acupuncture points was effective in treating patients with facial paralysis. Points selected were *Xiaguan* (ST 7), *Taiyang* (Extra), *Sibai* (ST 2), *Yingxiang* (LI 20), and others. Out of 38 cases, 30 reported complete recovery, 4 showed marked improvement, 2 showed mild improvement, and 2 showed no response.[9]

References

1. *Zhong Yao Du Li Xue* (Toxicology of Chinese Herbs), 1989; 174-176
2. Ibid.
3. *Xian Dai Zhong Yao Yao Li Xue* (Contemporary Pharmacology of Chinese Herbs), 1997; 1408
4. *The Merck Index* 12th edition, Chapman & Hall/CRCnetBASE/Merck, 2000.
5. *Yao Xue Tong Bao* (Report of Herbology), 1987; 22(9): 517
6. *Zhong Yao Yao Li Yu Ying Yong* (Pharmacology and Applications of Chinese Herbs), 1983, 1983; 1113
7. *Zhong Hua Yi Xue Za Zhi* (Chinese Journal of Medicine), 1975; 7:503
8. *Yao Xue Tong Bao* (Report of Herbology), 1980; 3:23
9. *Zhong Guo Kang Fu Yi Xue Za Zhi* (Chinese Journal of Rehabilitation), 1987; 3:130

Chan Su (Venenum Bufonis)

蟾酥

Pinyin Name: *Chan Su*
Original Source: *Yao Xing Ben Cao* (Materia Medica of Medicinal Properties) by Zhen Quan in 600 A.D.
English Name: toad venum, cake of toad skin secretion, dried venom of toads, toad-cake
Zoological Name: *Bufo bufo gargarizans* Cantor (*Zhong Hua Da Chan Su*); *Bufo bufo melanostictus* Schneider (*Hei Kuang Chan Su*)
Pharmaceutical Name: Venenum Bufonis
Properties: acrid, sweet, warm
Channels Entered: Heart
Safety Index: toxic

CHINESE THERAPEUTIC ACTIONS

1. Relieves Toxicity, Reduces Swelling

Chan Su (Venenum Bufonis), used topically or internally, treats various disorders characterized by heat, toxins and swelling. Clinical application of *Chan Su* includes sores, carbuncles, ulcers, sore throat, cancer, nodules and scrofula.

- Dermatological disorders characterized by heat and toxins: use *Chan Su* with *Xiong Huang* (Realgar), *She Xiang* (Moschus) and *Zhu Sha* (Cinnabaris).
- Extreme soreness and pain in the throat, scarlet fever, tonsillitis: combine it with *Niu Huang* (Calculus Bovis), *Xiong Huang* (Realgar), *She Xiang* (Moschus), and *Bing Pian* (Borneolum Syntheticum).
- Intestinal cancer: use this substance with *Bai Hua She She Cao* (Herba Oldenlandia), and *Ban Zhi Lian* (Herba Scutellariae Barbatae).
- Scrofula: add it to *Han Shui Shi* (Mirabilite) and *Ba Dou* (Fructus Crotonis).
- Liver cancer: combine it with *Long Kui* (Herba Solanum Nigrum), *Xia Ku Cao* (Spica Prunellae) and *Hu Zhang* (Rhizoma Polygoni Cuspidati).

2. Relieves Pain

Chan Su has a very strong analgesic effect. It is especially effective for toothache, regardless of the cause. It may be used as a topical anesthetic for minor surgery.

- Toothache: mix together *Chan Su* 30%, *Xiong Huang* (Realgar) 30%, *Gan Cao* (Radix Glycyrrhizae) 20% and *Peng Sha* (Borax) 20%. Grind the herbs into a fine powder and apply a small amount topically on the affected tooth.
- Local anesthetic for minor surgeries of the five sensory organs: mix *Chan Su* together with unprocessed *Chuan Wu* (Radix Aconiti Preparata), unprocessed *Cao Wu* (Radix Aconiti Kusnezoffii), unprocessed *Tian Nan Xing* (Rhizoma Arisaematis), unprocessed *Ban Xia* (Rhizoma Pinelliae) and warm grain-based liquor. Apply the herbs topically and begin surgery when anesthesia has been achieved. [Note: The combination of the unprocessed herbs listed above must be used topically only. Do not use these unprocessed herbs internally, as there is a high risk of toxicity.]

3. Opens the Orifices and Awakens the *Shen* (Spirit)

Chan Su treats patients with nausea, vomiting, and diarrhea in extreme cases of turbid summerheat. *Chan Su* may be used like smelling salts to awaken the patient in cases of loss of consciousness.

- Nausea, vomiting, and diarrhea in extreme cases of turbid summerheat: use *Chan Su* with *Cang Zhu* (Rhizoma Atractylodis), *She Xiang* (Moschus), *Ding Xiang* (Flos Caryophylli) and *Xiong Huang* (Realgar), and blow the powder into the patient's nostrils.

DOSAGE

0.015 to 0.030 gram [15 to 30 mg] for oral use. Because of the drastic and toxic effects of *Chan Su*, it must be used only at a small dose for a short period of time. It is also used externally as a powder or a paste. Frying it with grain-based liquor will facilitate the crushing and extraction of the active components.

CAUTIONS / CONTRAINDICATIONS

- *Chan Su* is toxic. It must be used with extreme caution, following precise instructions, when given via oral ingestion.
- It is contraindicated during pregnancy, as it induces contraction of the uterus.

OVERDOSAGE

Adverse reaction to *Chan Su* is directly associated with overdose, and may occur within 0.5 to 2 hours after ingestion. Overdose is characterized by interference with the gastrointestinal system (severe and recurrent nausea, vomiting, abdominal pain, diarrhea, and possibly dehydration), cardiovascular system (chest congestion, palpitations, bradycardia, arrhythmia, a thin, thready pulse,

Chan Su (Venenum Bufonis)

cold extremities, hypotension and shock), and nervous system (dizziness, headache, numbness of the mouth and lips, numbness of the extremities, lethargy, perspiration, delayed response to stimulus, absence of patellar reflex, and possibly seizures and convulsions).[1]

TREATMENT OF OVERDOSAGE

Early stage overdose can be treated via emetic methods followed by ingestion of egg whites. Ingestion of a large amount of water or concentrated tea is also beneficial. If available, 120 grams of fresh *Lu Gen* (Rhizoma Phragmitis) can be ground into juice and given to the patient. A purgative method using 15 grams of *Da Huang* (Radix et Rhizoma Rhei) can also be employed to eliminate the offending agent from the digestive tract.

Mild systemic reaction can be treated by ingestion of *Sheng Jiang* (Rhizoma Zingiberis Recens) or *Gan Cao* (Radix Glycyrrhizae). Adverse reactions characterized by repeated nausea and vomiting, abdominal pain and diarrhea and slow pulse can be treated with *Huo Xiang Zheng Qi San* (Agastache Powder to Rectify the Qi).

Direct physical contact of *Chan Su* with the eyes can cause extreme redness, swelling and pain. Such reactions can be alleviated by use of a saline wash or by rinsing with the juice of *Zi Cao Gen* (Radix Lithospermi).

Atropine has been used successfully to treat overdose of *Chan Su*, while epinephrine is ineffective.[1,2]

CHEMICAL COMPOSITION

Bufotoxins, bufogenins, cinobufalin, cinobufotalin, cinobufagin, cinobufatalin, telocinobufagin, gamabufotalin, gamabufogenin, resibufogenin, bufotalin, bufotanine, bufalin, bufotalinin, bufotalidin, bufotenine, bufotenidine.[3,4]

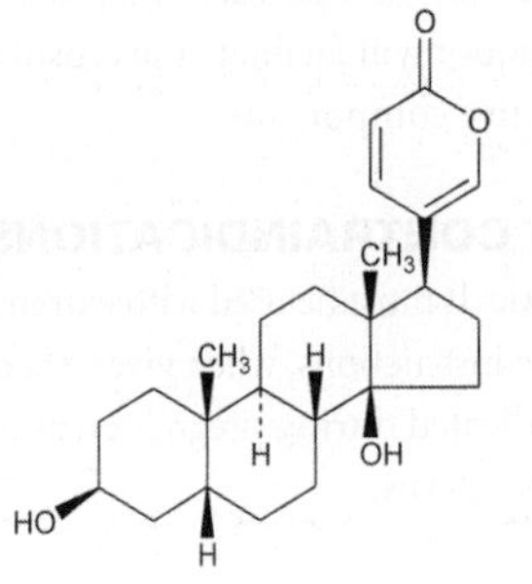

Bufalin

PHARMACOLOGICAL EFFECTS

- **Cardiotonic:** According to laboratory studies in anesthetized cats, dogs, rabbits and frogs, a small amount of *Chan Su* has been associated with marked inotropic effect while a larger dose is associated with an anesthetic effect. The cardiotonic effect is similar to that of digitalis, but is weaker, and has only a short active duration.[5]
- **Respiratory:** Cinobufalin, cinobufotalin, and numerous constituents of *Chan Su* have all demonstrated a stimulatory effect on the respiratory tract by increasing the respiration rate in anesthetized animals.[6] It was also noted that the stimulatory effect may counter the respiratory depression induced by morphine.[7]
- **Antineoplastic:** Administration of *Chan Su* is associated with an inhibitory effect on cancer cells in mice with liver cancer. The life expectancy of these mice is increased when they are treated with *Chan Su*.[8]

TOXICOLOGY

The LD_{50} for *Chan Su* in mice is 41.0 mg/kg via intravenous injection, 96.6 mg/kg via subcutaneous injection, and 26.81 mg/kg via intraperitoneal injection.[9]

AUTHORS' COMMENTS

Many research studies demonstrate successful use of *Chan Su* in treatment of various types of cancer, such as leukemia, lung, liver, and breast cancers.

References

1. *Zhong Yao Xue* (Chinese Herbology), 1998; 962:966
2. *Zhong Yao Du Li Xue* (Toxicology of Chinese Herbs), 1989; 181-184
3. *Xian Dai Zhong Yao Yao Li Xue* (Contemporary Pharmacology of Chinese Herbs), 1997; 1412
4. *The Merck Index* 12th edition, Chapman & Hall/CRCnetBASE/Merck, 2000.
5. *Zhong Guo Yi Yuan Yao Xue Za Zhi* (Chinese Hospital Journal of Herbology), 1991; 302
6. *Zhong Yao Yao Li Yu Ying Yong* (Pharmacology and Applications of Chinese Herbs), 1983, 1983; 1258
7. *Zhong Yao Yao Li Yu Du Li Za Zhi* (Journal of Pharmacology and Toxicology of Chinese Herbs), 1990; (1):71
8. *Zhong Yao Yao Li Yu Ying Yong* (Pharmacology and Applications of Chinese Herbs), 1983, 1983; 1258
9. *Zhong Yao Xue* (Chinese Herbology), 1998; 962:966

Ma Qian Zi (Semen Strychni)

馬錢子 马钱子

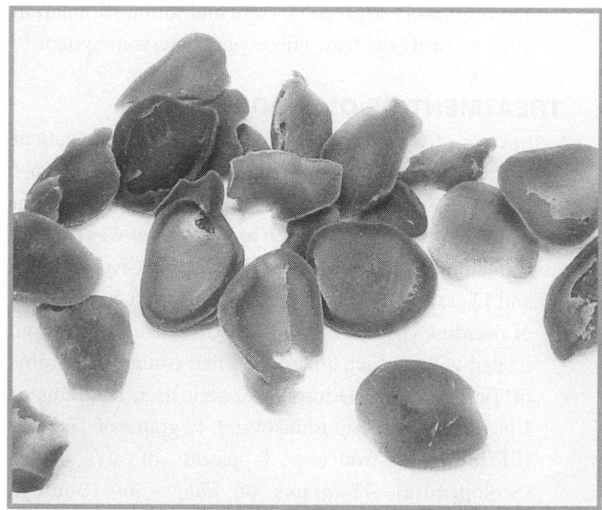

Pinyin Name: *Ma Qian Zi*
Literal Name: "horse money seed"
Alternate Chinese Names: *Ma Qian*
Original Source: *Ben Cao Gang Mu* (Materia Medica) by Li Shi-Zhen in 1578
English Name: nux vomica
Botanical Name: *Strychnos pierriana* A.W. Hill (*Yun Nan Ma Qian*); *Strychnos nux-vomica* L. (*Ma Qian*)
Pharmaceutical Name: Semen Strychni
Properties: bitter, cold
Channels Entered: Liver, Spleen
Safety Index: extremely toxic

CHINESE THERAPEUTIC ACTIONS

1. Reduces Swelling, Disperses Nodules

Abscesses, sores, carbuncles: Bitter and draining, *Ma Qian Zi* (Semen Strychni) eliminates toxins to reduce swelling and pain. It is commonly used externally to treat various dermatological disorders, such as abscesses, sores, and ulcerations. It is generally used via topical application, individually or in combination with other herbs.

- Soreness and inflammation of the throat: deep fry *Ma Qian Zi* in sesame oil, grind it into powder, and apply topically to the throat.
- Female genital lesions or ulcerations: soak *Ma Qian Zi* in water for several days, remove the skin, sun dry it, deep-fry in sesame oil, grind it into powder, and apply it topically.
- Sores with or without pus and abscesses: use this herb with *Chuan Shan Jia* (Squama Manis) and *Ru Xiang* (Gummi Olibanum).

2. Unblocks Channels and Collaterals and Relieves Pain

Various musculoskeletal disorders characterized by stagnation and pain: Clinical applications include muscle spasms and cramps, numbness, paralysis, and arthritic pain.

- Muscle aches and pains: use equal quantities of *Ma Qian Zi*, *Ma Huang* (Herba Ephedrae), *Ru Xiang* (Gummi Olibanum) and *Mo Yao* (Myrrha) and take with grain-based liquor every 3 hours as needed to relieve pain. The same combination can be used topically to reduce swelling and relieve pain.
- Chronic and severe *bi zheng* (painful obstruction syndrome) due to wind and dampness: use it with *Ma Huang* (Herba Ephedrae), *Ru Xiang* (Gummi Olibanum), *Quan Xie* (Scorpio), *Cang Zhu* (Rhizoma Atractylodis) and *Niu Xi* (Radix Cyathulae seu Achyranthis).
- Numbness and paralysis of the extremities: combine this herb with *Gan Cao* (Radix Glycyrrhizae).
- Facial paralysis, myasthenia gravis, atrophy and numbness of the extremities: add *Ma Qian Zi* to *Ren Shen* (Radix Ginseng), *Dang Gui* (Radicis Angelicae Sinensis), *Ru Xiang* (Gummi Olibanum) and *Chuan Shan Jia* (Squama Manis).

DOSAGE

0.3 to 0.6 gram for internal use. The unprocessed form is extremely toxic, and is contraindicated for internal use. *Ma Qian Zi* must be dry-fried to reduce toxicity and facilitate extraction of active components. The dry-fried herb is administered internally either in pills or powder. For external use, the powdered herb can either be sprayed onto the throat or applied topically with vinegar.

CAUTIONS / CONTRAINDICATIONS

- Use of unprocessed *Ma Qian Zi* orally is contraindicated.
- *Ma Qian Zi* is contraindicated in pregnancy, and in cases involving general deficiency.
- Long-term use of *Ma Qian Zi* or large dosages should be avoided because of toxicity.
- For internal use, *Ma Qian Zi* must be processed first by dry-frying or deep-frying in sesame oil to reduce toxicity.
- Topical application of *Ma Qian Zi* will lead to systemic absorption. Therefore, it should be used with extreme caution when applied over a large surface area or over mucous membranes.

OVERDOSAGE

Overdose of *Ma Qian Zi* is characterized by dry mouth, dizziness, numbness of the extremities, headache, palpitations, tonic-clonic convulsions, difficulty swallowing,

Ma Qian Zi (Semen Strychni)

and respiratory depression. Light and sound stimulation often intensify the toxic effects on the nervous system.[1]

TREATMENT OF OVERDOSAGE

In cases of overdose and overdose reactions, the patient should first be placed in a dark and quiet room to avoid light and sound stimulation. Mild cases of overdose can be relieved by decoction of 6 grams of *Rou Gui* (Cortex Cinnamomi), 60 grams of *Gan Cao* (Radix Glycyrrhizae), and 12 grams of *Wu Bei Zi* (Galla Chinensis). Severe cases of overdose characterized by muscle convulsions can be treated with an herbal decoction that contains 12 grams of *Tian Nan Xing* (Rhizoma Arisaematis), 12 grams of *Fang Feng* (Radix Saposhnikoviae), 12 grams of *Tian Ma* (Rhizoma Gastrodiae), 3 pieces of *Wu Gong* (Scolopendra), 15 grams of *Jiang Can* (Bombyx Batryticatus), 6 grams of *Quan Xie* (Scorpio), and 10 grams of *Gan Cao* (Radix Glycyrrhizae).[2]

CHEMICAL COMPOSITION

Strychnine, brucine, isobrucine, α-colubrine, β-colubrine, pseudostrychnine, strychnine N-oxide, brucine N-oxide, novacine, icajine, vomicine, protostrychnine, 15-hydroxystrychnine, loganin, chlorogenic acid.[3,4]

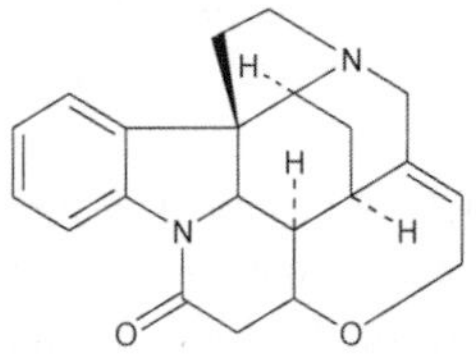

Strychnine

PHARMACOLOGICAL EFFECTS

- **CNS stimulant:** Strychnine has a strong stimulating effect on the central nervous system. The effect is characterized by an increase in spinal reflexes and sensory centers of the cerebral cortex.[5]
- **Respiratory:** Oral administration of isobrucine at 50 mg/kg has demonstrated marked antitussive and expectorant, and mild antiasthmatic effects. The expectorant effect was similar to that of ammonium chloride.[6]
- **Gastrointestinal:** *Ma Qian Zi* has a stimulating effect on the gastrointestinal system to increase secretion of gastric acid and improve appetite. It has no effect on the smooth muscle of the intestines.[7]

CLINICAL STUDIES AND RESEARCH

- **Myasthenia gravis:** In one study, 8 patients with myasthenia gravis were treated with *Ma Qian Zi*, with complete recovery in 4 patients, improvement in 1 patient, and no response from 3 patients. The treatment protocol was to initiate treatment with 0.2 gram of the herb in a capsule three times daily after meals, with warm water. The dosage was increased gradually by adding one more capsule every 2 to 4 days, until a maximum of 7 capsules per day was reached. Patients who experienced muscle spasms and twitching during the dosage titration period required reduction of dosage or discontinuation of herbs. Other herbs were given for supportive treatment if deemed necessary.[8]
- **Facial paralysis:** According to one report, 52 patients within 6 to 21 days of onset of facial paralysis were treated with 100% effectiveness within 1 or 2 treatments. The treatment protocol was to soak the herb in water for 24 hours, cut the herb into 0.1 cm slices, and apply it topically to the affected area. The old herb slice was removed and a new one applied every 7 days.[9]
- **Wind-cold-damp *bi zheng* (painful obstruction syndrome):** Chronic *bi zheng* refractory to other therapies in 16 patients was treated with an herbal formula with great success within 1 or 2 doses. The treatment protocol was to grind 30 grams of processed *Ma Qian Zi*, and 60 grams of *Xue Jie* (Sanguis Draconis) into powder and administer 1.5 grams twice daily. *Ma Qian Zi* is deep fried until it is golden yellow in color.[10]

TOXICOLOGY

The LD_{50} for oral administration of strychnine and isobrucine in mice is 3.27 and 233 mg/kg, respectively. The LD_{50} for intravenous administration of isobrucine in dogs is 8 mg/kg. In humans, oral ingestion of strychnine may cause poisoning at 5 to 10 mg, and fatality at 30 mg.[11]

References

1. *Zhong Yao Xue* (Chinese Herbology), 1998; 966:969
2. *Zhong Yao Du Li Xue* (Toxicology of Chinese Herbs), 48-51; 1989
3. *Xian Dai Zhong Yao Yao Li Xue* (Contemporary Pharmacology of Chinese Herbs), 1997; 430
4. *The Merck Index* 12th edition, Chapman & Hall/CRCnetBASE/Merck, 2000.
5. *Zhong Yao Xue* (Chinese Herbology), 1998; 966:969
6. *Zhong Yao Yao Li Yu Ying Yong* (Pharmacology and Applications of Chinese Herbs), 1983, 1983; 137
7. *Pharmacology*, 1962; 92
8. *Zhe Jiang Zhong Yi Za Zhi* (Zhejiang Journal of Chinese Medicine), 1986; 1:27
9. *Zhong Ji Yi Kan* (Medium Medical Journal), 1989; 1:45
10. *Shan Dong Zhong Yi Za Zhi* (Shandong Journal of Chinese Medicine), 1986; 1:49
11. *Zhong Yao Yao Li Yu Ying Yong* (Pharmacology and Applications of Chinese Herbs), 1983, 1983; 137

She Chuang Zi (Fructus Cnidii)

蛇床子

Pinyin Name: *She Chuang Zi*
Literal Name: "snake's bed seeds"
Alternate Chinese Names: *She Chuang Shi*
Original Source: *Shen Nong Ben Cao Jing* (Divine Husbandman's Classic of the Materia Medica) in the second century
English Name: cnidium fruit, common cnidium fruit
Botanical Name: *Cnidium monnieri* (L.) Cusson (*She Chuan*)
Pharmaceutical Name: Fructus Cnidii
Properties: acrid, bitter, warm
Channels Entered: Kidney

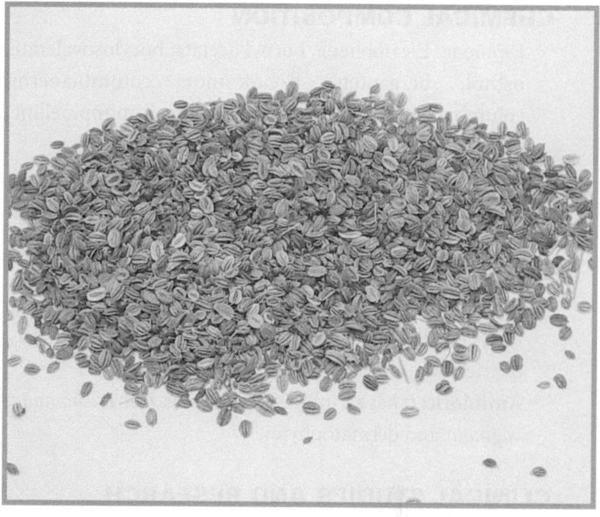

CHINESE THERAPEUTIC ACTIONS

1. Dries Dampness, Kills Parasites and Stops Itching

Clinical manifestations include damp accumulation in the lower body manifesting in weeping, itching skin lesions, especially around the genital area and the toes. Other skin disorders include eczema (of the scrotum, genital area, feet and anus), trichomoniasis, genital itching or vaginal discharge in females due to vaginitis, hemorrhoids, scabies and ringworm. *She Chuang Zi* (Fructus Cnidii) is warm, and most effective against dermatological disorders caused by wind and cold. When treating lesions due to heat or dampness, heat-clearing and dampness-drying herbs should be added. This herb can be used both internally and externally. *She Chuang Zi* dries dampness and effectively dispels wind to relieve itching.

- Genital itching: use *She Chuang Zi* with *Hua Jiao* (Pericarpium Zanthoxyli), *Bai Bu* (Radix Stemonae), *Ming Fan* (Alumen) and *Ku Shen Gen* (Radix Sophorae Flavescentis) as an external wash. Soak the affected area for 10 to 15 minutes one time each day. Take it with *Long Dan Xie Gan Tang* (Gentiana Decoction to Drain the Liver) internally.
- Swollen, painful scrotum: use powdered *She Chuang Zi* mixed with egg yolk, applied topically.
- Hemorrhoid pain: use it alone as an external wash or soak.
- Scabies: use it alone as powder topically.
- Weeping skin lesions: use this herb with *Ming Fan* (Alumen), *Liu Huang* (Sulfur) and *Xiong Huang* (Realgar).
- Itching lesions in patches: mix powdered *She Chuang Zi* with sesame oil and apply topically.

2. Disperses Cold and Dispels Wind

Turbid white vaginal discharge: This condition is usually caused by deficiencies of the Spleen, Kidney, *ren* (conception) and *chong* (thoroughfare) channels.

- Vaginal discharge: use powdered *She Chuang Zi* as vaginal suppository. It may be combined with *Ming Fan* (Alumen). Take it with *Sha Yuan Zi* (Semen Astragali Complanati), *Shan Zhu Yu* (Fructus Corni) and *Hai Piao Xiao* (Endoconcha Sepiae) and *Lu Rong* (Cornu Cervi Pantotrichum) for internal use.

Lower back: *She Chuang Zi* is effective to treat low back pain caused by wind-damp-cold and Kidney yang deficiency.

- Low back pain: use *She Chuang Zi* with *Sang Ji Sheng* (Herba Taxilli), *Du Zhong* (Cortex Eucommiae), *Gou Ji* (Rhizoma Cibotii) and *Du Huo* (Radix Angelicae Pubescentis).

3. Warms the Kidney and Strengthens Yang

Impotence and infertility: *She Chuang Zi* effectively treats impotence and infertility in men and women due to Kidney yang deficiency.

- Impotence or infertility: combine it with *Yin Yang Huo* (Herba Epimedii), *Tu Si Zi* (Semen Cuscutae), *Wu Wei Zi* (Fructus Schisandrae Chinensis) and *Du Zhong* (Cortex Eucommiae). Serve it with alcohol and honey.

DOSAGE

15 to 30 grams when *She Chuang Zi* is used as an external wash or soak, mixed with water or oil. For oral use, incorporate 3 to 9 grams in decoctions, pill or powder.

CAUTIONS / CONTRAINDICATIONS

- Use of *She Chuang Zi* is contraindicated in Kidney yin deficiency with heat signs, in excess heat or in damp-heat in the lower *jiao*.

She Chuang Zi (Fructus Cnidii)

CHEMICAL COMPOSITION

L-pinene, L-camphene, bornyl acetate, borylosovalerate, osthol, bergapten, β-eudesmol, columbianetin, columbianadin, archangelicin, edultin, isopimpinelline, o-isovalerylcolumbianetin, anthotoxol.[1]

PHARMACOLOGICAL EFFECTS

- **Endocrinologic:** Subcutaneous injection of alcohol extract of *She Chuang Zi* daily for 32 days in mice lengthened the latent period and shortened the estrus period in mice. Furthermore, it increased the weight of the uterus, ovaries, and testicles in mice.[2]
- **Antibiotic:** It has an inhibitory effect against *Trichomonas vaginalis* and dermatophytes.[3]

CLINICAL STUDIES AND RESEARCH

- **Trichomonal vaginitis:** Patients with trichomonal vaginitis were treated with vaginal wash and vaginal suppository of *She Chuang Zi* with great success. The treatment protocol was to use 500 ml of a 10% solution as a vaginal wash first, followed by insertion of two vaginal suppositories (0.5 gram each). Each course of treatment lasted 5 to 7 days, with a total treatment period of 2 months.[4]
- **Acute eczema or dermatitis:** In one study, 280 patients with acute eczema and 100 patients with acute dermatitis were successfully treated with topical application of an herbal solution. The herbal solution was prepared by cooking 60 grams of *She Chuang Zi* alone, or the combination containing 15 grams each of *She Chuang Zi*, *Fang Feng* (Radix Saposhnikoviae), *Jing Jie* (Herba Schizonepetae) and *Dang Shen* (Radix Codonopsis).[5]
- **Itching:** Intramuscular injection of *She Chuang Zi* and *Cang Er Cao* (Herba Xanthii) twice daily for 10 to 15 days per course of treatment was 83.6% effective in treating 607 patients with severe itching of the skin.[6]
- **Fungal infection:** Topical application of an herbal preparation was used effectively to treat 28 patients with fungal skin infections. The herbal preparation was made by mixing 500 grams of *She Chuang Zi*, 250 grams of *Qing Dai* (Indigo Naturalis), 50 grams of fish liver oil, and petroleum jelly. The herbal preparation was applied topically two to four times daily for 2 months.[7]

References

1. *Xian Dai Zhong Yao Yao Li Xue* (Contemporary Pharmacology of Chinese Herbs), 1997; 1282
2. *Zhong Yao Da Ci Dian* (Dictionary of Chinese Herbs), 1977; 2121
3. *Zhong Yao Xue* (Chinese Herbology), 1998; 969:972
4. *Zhong Yi Za Zhi* (Journal of Chinese Medicine), 1956; 5:250
5. *Wu Han Xin Yi Yao* (Wuhan New Medicine and Herbology), 1972; 1:36
6. *Lin Chuang Pi Fu Ke Za Zhi* (Journal of Clinical Dermatology), 1983; 1:15
7. *Zhong Guo Yi Yuan Yao Xue Za Zhi* (Chinese Hospital Journal of Herbology), 1988; 8:379

Lu Feng Fang (Nidus Vespae)

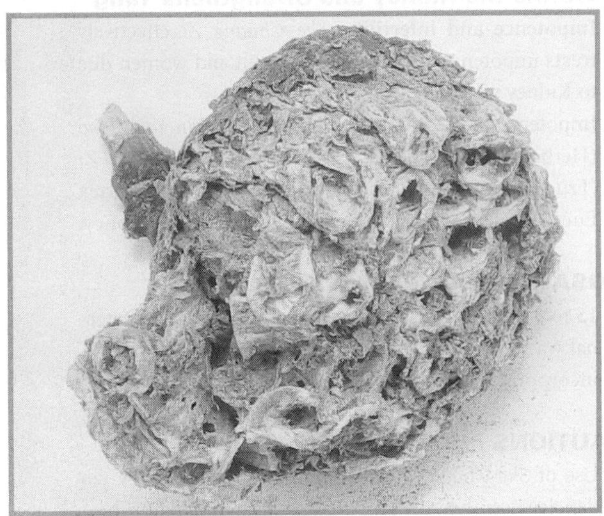

露蜂房

Pinyin Name: *Lu Feng Fang*
Alternate Chinese Names: *Feng Fang*
Original Source: *Shen Nong Ben Cao Jing* (Divine Husbandman's Classic of the Materia Medica) in the second century
English Name: hornet nest
Zoological Name: *Polistes olivaceous* (De Geer) (*Guo Ma Feng*); *Polistes japonicus* Saussure (*Ri Ben Chang Jiao Hu Feng*); *Parapolybia varia* Fabricius (*Yi Fu Hu Feng*)
Pharmaceutical Name: Nidus Vespae
Properties: sweet, neutral
Channels Entered: Stomach, Lung
Safety Index: toxic

Lu Feng Fang (Nidus Vespae)

CHINESE THERAPEUTIC ACTIONS

1. Relieves Toxicity, Dispels Wind, Stops Pain

Toxicity, sores and carbuncles, mastitis: *Lu Feng Fang* (Nidus Vespae) is toxic and treats toxic disorders, such as sores, mastitis, and carbuncles that have either recently developed or have existed for a long time.

- Sores and carbuncles: mix *Lu Feng Fang* with *Tian Nan Xing* (Rhizoma Arisaematis), *Ming Fan* (Alumen), unprocessed *Cao Wu* (Radix Aconiti Kusnezoffii), *Chi Xiao Dou* (Semen Phaseoli) and vinegar, and apply it topically.
- Mastitis: use 6 grams of dry-fried *Lu Feng Fang* in decoction.
- Soft or ulcerated sores: deep fry 21 pieces of *Ba Dou* (Fructus Crotonis) in sesame oil and use the oil to mix with powdered *Lu Feng Fang*. Apply topically.
- Ulceration with pus: combine it with *Wu Gong* (Scolopendra) and *Xiong Huang* (Realgar).

Urticaria, recent or chronic rash with or without itching, rubella, scabies:

- Wind rash with extreme itching: use the dry-fried *Lu Feng Fang* with *Chan Tui* (Periostracum Cicadae) as powder and serve it with grain-based liquor.

Sore throat, toothache, swollen and painful tongue: *Lu Feng Fang* enters the Stomach channel and treats pain in the digestive tract.

- Swollen, painful throat in children: grind dry-fried *Lu Feng Fang* with *Jiang Can* (Bombyx Batryticatus) into fine powder. Serve 1.5 grams with decoction of *Ru Xiang* (Gummi Olibanum).
- Tooth pain radiating to the side of the face, swollen gums (possibly manifesting as feeling like worms moving, or tingling in the teeth): use *Lu Feng Fang* with *Xi Xin* (Herba Asari) and *Ru Xiang* (Gummi Olibanum) as a gargle. Also, 3 grams of *Lu Feng Fang* and 3 grams of *Ming Fan* (Alumen) can be mixed and used as gargle.
- Swollen and painful tongue in children: mix powder of *Lu Feng Fang* with grain-based liquor and apply topically.

Cancer, tumors, palpable masses, scrofulae:

- Scrofula or recalcitrant purulent scrofula: apply *Lu Feng Fang* topically with *Huang Qi* (Radix Astragali), *She Tui* (Periostracum Serpentis) and *Xuan Shen* (Radix Scrophulariae) as a paste.
- Breast tumors, mastitis, fibrocystic breast disorders, abscesses or necrosing nodules in the breast with pain: use it with *Ku Lian Pi* (Cortex Meliae), and *Qing Pi* (Pericarpium Citri Reticulatae Viride). Take 10 grams and serve one dose with grain-based liquor every two days.
- Nasopharyngeal carcinoma, laryngocarcinoma, lymphatic metastasis: combine this substance with *Quan Xie* (Scorpio) and *Jiang Can* (Bombyx Batryticatus).

***Bi zheng* (painful obstruction syndrome):** Clinical applications of *Lu Feng Fang* include rheumatoid arthritis, reduced mobility of joints, and swollen or deformed joints.

- Rheumatoid arthritis: apply *Lu Feng Fang* topically with *Da Suan* (Bulbus Alli Sativi).
- Arthritis, osteomyelitis: mix it with *Quan Xie* (Scorpio), *Wu Gong* (Scolopendra) and *Di Bie Chong* (Eupolyphaga) to make powder. Serve three grams twice daily.

2. Kills Parasites

Ringworms and pinworms: *Lu Feng Fang* is effective against ringworms and pinworms. Despite traditional use of this substance in expelling parasites, it is rarely used clinically because it is toxic. Antiparasitic herbs are usually used instead.

DOSAGE

2.5 to 4.5 grams in decoctions. *Lu Feng Fang* is also used at 1 to 2 grams per serving in powder or pill form, taken twice daily. This substance can be used as powder or as a wash, externally.

CAUTIONS / CONTRAINDICATIONS

- Use of *Lu Feng Fang* is contraindicated in qi- and blood-deficient patients, or individuals with suppurated sores.

CHEMICAL COMPOSITION

Beeswax, resin, calcium, iron, protein.[1]

PHARMACOLOGICAL EFFECTS

- **Hematological:** Alcohol, ether and acetone extracts of *Lu Feng Fang* all shorten coagulation time, with acetone extract being the strongest.[2]
- **Antiparasitic:** Essential oil of *Lu Feng Fang* has a strong effect to kill tapeworms and earthworms.[3]
- **Antineoplastic:** It has an inhibitory effect *in vitro* on liver and stomach cancer cells.[4]

CLINICAL STUDIES AND RESEARCH

- **Acute mastitis:** Four patients with acute mastitis were treated with *Lu Feng Fang* with surprisingly good results. *Lu Feng Fang* was prepared by dry-frying it until it was a light yellow color. The patients were given 1 to 2 grams of the powder every 6 hours with 30 ml of grain-based liquor. In a follow-up study to confirm effectiveness, the same treatment protocol was applied to 26 women with acute mastitis. The study reported complete recovery in 23 patients, significant improvement in 1 patient, and no response in 2 patients. The overall rate of effectiveness was 92.3%.[5]
- **Suppurative infection:** According to one report, 30 grams of *Lu Feng Fang* were cooked at boiling temperature

Lu Feng Fang (Nidus Vespae)

in 1,000 ml of water for 15 minutes to yield an herbal solution for topical application. The herbal solution was used as a wash or soak one to two times daily to treat various suppurated dermatological infections, with good results.[7]

- **Toothache:** In one clinical study, a small amount of *Lu Feng Fang* was placed in alcohol and burned until it turned into ashes. The ashes were applied topically to the affected area and pain relief was achieved in most patients within 4 to 5 minutes. Out of 58 patients, the study reported significant results in 21 patients, moderate effects in 33 patients, and no response in 4 patients.[8]
- **Chronic sinusitis:** Extract of *Lu Feng Fang* was used to treat 158 patients with chronic sinusitis with an 85% effective rate.[9]

References

1. *Xian Dai Zhong Yao Yao Li Xue* (Contemporary Pharmacology of Chinese Herbs), 1997; 1424
2. *Zhong Yao Xue* (Chinese Herbology), 1998; 972:975
3. Ibid.
4. Ibid.
5. *Zhong Yi Za Zhi* (Journal of Chinese Medicine), 1959; 5:40
6. *Journal of Chinese Medicine*, 1963; 11:407
7. *Zhong Yao Xue* (Chinese Herbology), 1998; 972:975
8. *Xin Zhong Yi* (New Chinese Medicine), 1982; 12:51
9. *Zhong Cao Yao Tong Xun* (Journal of Chinese Herbal Medicine), 1979; 10:22

Xue Jie (Sanguis Draconis)

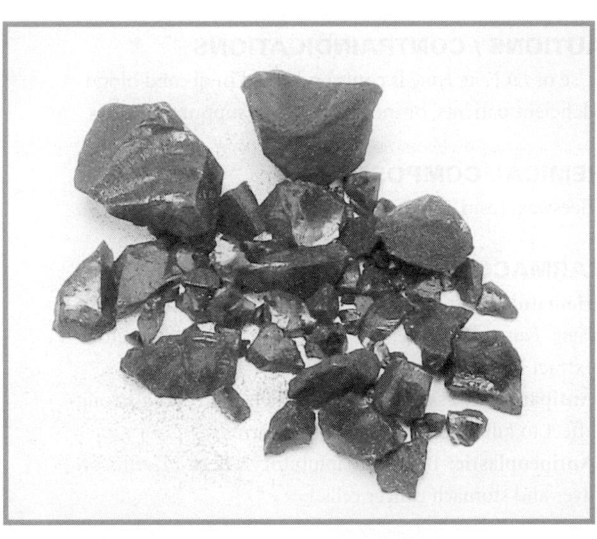

血竭

Pinyin Name: *Xue Jie*
Literal Name: "exhausted blood"
Alternate Chinese Names: *Qi Lin Xue*
Original Source: *Lei Gong Pao Zhi Lun* (Grandfather Lei's Discussions of Herb Preparation) by Lei Xiao in 470 A.D.
English Name: dragon's blood, resinous discharge
Botanical Name: *Daemonorops draco* Bl. (*Qi Lin Jie*)
Pharmaceutical Name: Sanguis Draconis
Properties: sweet, salty, neutral
Channels Entered: Heart, Liver

CHINESE THERAPEUTIC ACTIONS

1. External Use: Stops Bleeding, Promotes Generation of Flesh, Contains Ulceration

Bleeding from traumatic injuries, non-healing ulcers, hemorrhoids with swelling and pain: Topical use of *Xue Jie* (Sanguis Draconis) treats both acute and chronic skin conditions. It stops bleeding in acute conditions, and promotes the healing of wounds in chronic conditions by facilitating the generation of flesh and prevents the spread of ulcerations. It can be used alone topically or combined with other herbs for maximum effectiveness.

- Bleeding due to external injury: use *Xue Jie* with *Er Cha* (Catechu), *Ru Xiang* (Gummi Olibanum) and *Mo Yao* (Myrrha) topically. **Exemplar Formula:** *Qi Li San* (Seven-Thousandths of a Tael Powder).
- Open sores with discharge of pus: combine it with *Da Huang* (Radix et Rhizoma Rhei) and *Da Zao* (Fructus Jujubae) topically.

2. Internal Use: Activates Blood Circulation, Removes Blood Stasis, Relieves Pain

Blood stagnation with swelling and pain, amenorrhea, dysmenorrhea: Internal use of *Xue Jie* treats both acute and chronic disorders characterized by blood stasis, swelling and pain. *Xue Jie* activates blood and treats various pain or blood stagnation disorders in acute or

Xue Jie (Sanguis Draconis)

chronic cases. Clinical applications include amenorrhea, menstrual pain, and external or traumatic injuries.

- Amenorrhea and menstrual pain with abdominal masses caused by blood stasis: use *Xue Jie* with *Mo Yao* (Myrrha), *Hua Shi* (Talcum), and *Mu Dan Pi* (Cortex Moutan).
- External or traumatic injuries with excruciating pain: combine this substance with *Dang Gui* (Radicis Angelicae Sinensis), *Mo Yao* (Myrrha), *Chi Shao* (Radix Paeoniae Rubrae), *Bai Zhi* (Radix Angelicae Dahuricae) and *Gui Xin* (Cortex Rasus Cinnamomi) as powder. Serve this combination with grain-based liquor.
- Postpartum chest congestion and dyspnea: add *Xue Jie* to *Mo Yao* (Myrrha), *Hua Shi* (Talcum) and *Mu Dan Pi* (Cortex Moutan), combine with vinegar and serve with grain-based liquor and urine from a child.

DOSAGE

1.0 to 1.5 grams as herbal powder or pills internally. *Xue Jie* is used topically as powder, paste or plaster.

CAUTIONS / CONTRAINDICATIONS

- Use of *Xue Jie* is contraindicated during pregnancy or in the absence of blood stasis.

CHEMICAL COMPOSITION

Dracorubin, dracorhodin, nordracorhodin, nordracorubin, dracoresene, pimaric acid, sandaracopimaric acid.[1]

PHARMACOLOGICAL EFFECTS

- **Antibiotic:** *Xue Jie* has inhibitory action against various species of pathogenic fungi and dermatophytes.[2]

CLINICAL STUDIES AND RESEARCH

- **Arthritis:** Patients with chronic arthritis characterized by wind-damp were treated with an herbal formula twice daily for 45 days. The herbal formula was prepared by mixing 120 grams of *Xue Jie* powder and 30 grams of *Ma Qian Zi* (Semen Strychni) powder. The herbal powder was divided into 80 portions with each portion considered to be one dose. Out of 150 patients, the study reported marked effectiveness in 126 patients, moderate effects in 15 patients, and no effect in 9 patients.[3]
- **Upper gastrointestinal bleeding:** In one study, 270 patients with upper gastrointestinal bleeding were treated with one gram of *Xue Jie* four times daily with warm water. After the bleeding stopped, the dosage was decreased to one gram twice daily for 2 days. The study reported a 95.8% overall rate of effectiveness.[4]

References

1. *Xian Dai Zhong Yao Yao Li Xue* (Contemporary Pharmacology of Chinese Herbs), 1997; 930
2. *Zhong Yao Xue* (Chinese Herbology), 1998; 987:988
3. *Shan Xi Zhong Yi* (Shanxi Chinese Medicine), 1985; 6(4):162
4. *Zhe Jiang Zhong Yi Za Zhi* (Zhejiang Journal of Chinese Medicine), 1984; 7:303

Zhang Nao (Camphora)

樟腦 樟脑

Pinyin Name: *Zhang Nao*
Alternate Chinese Names: *Chao Nao, Nao Zi*
Original Source: *Ben Cao Pin Hui Jing Yao* (Essentials of Materia Medica) by Liu Wen-Tai in 1505
English Name: camphor
Botanical Name: *Cinnamomum camphora* (L.) Presl (*Mu Zhang*)
Pharmaceutical Name: Camphora
Properties: acrid, hot
Channels Entered: Heart, Spleen
Safety Index: toxic

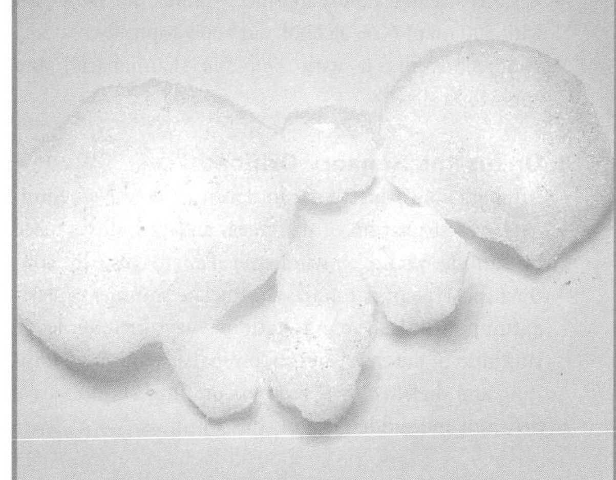

Zhang Nao (Camphora)

CHINESE THERAPEUTIC ACTIONS

1. Dispels Dampness, Kills Parasites

Zhang Nao (Camphora), commonly used topically, treats various dermatological disorders such as scabies, ringworms, sores, and fungal infections. It is mostly used in herbal formulas, as the antiparasitic effect is rather weak when used alone. *Zhang Nao* can also be used to treat burns.

- Itching: use it with *Liu Huang* (Sulfur) and *Qing Fen* (Calomelas) topically.
- Scabies, or sores and furuncles with pus: combine *Zhang Nao* with *Liu Huang* (Sulfur) and *Ming Fan* (Alumen) topically.
- Fungal infection: use this substance with *Tian Nan Xing* (Rhizoma Arisaematis), *Mu Bie Zi* (Semen Momordicae), *Ban Mao* (Mylabris), and *Chan Su* (Venenum Bufonis). Mix with rubbing alcohol.
- Itching eruptions, swelling and ulceration due to wind and heat in the blood: add it to *Huang Lian* (Rhizoma Coptidis), *Bai Zhi* (Radix Angelicae Dahuricae), *Hua Jiao* (Pericarpium Zanthoxyli) and *Qing Fen* (Calomelas). Mix with vegetable oil.
- Dry sores on the feet: mix it with sesame oil, *Ming Fan* (Alumen) and *Qing Fen* (Calomelas) and apply topically.
- Wet sores on the feet: mix *Zhang Nao* with *Ming Fan* (Alumen) and *Qing Fen* (Calomelas) and apply as powder.
- Burns: apply *Zhang Nao* with sesame oil. If there are blisters, apply the powder only, omitting the sesame oil.
- Fungal infection of the feet: mix 3 grams of *Zhang Nao* and 2 pieces of tofu and apply topically.

2. Disperses Cold and Relieves Pain

Toothache, pain of traumatic injuries: Acrid and warm, *Zhang Nao* has a strong dispersing effect to dispel cold and relieve pain.

- Frostbite: cook 10 grams of *Zhang Nao* and 30 grams of lard for 10 minutes to make a gel. Apply topically.
- Various swellings and pain: mix 9 grams of *Zhang Nao* with 500 ml of 60% alcohol and apply topically.
- Toothache: mix it with *Zhu Sha* (Cinnabaris) and apply topically.

3. Opens the Sensory Orifices

Aromatic and penetrating in nature, *Zhang Nao* eliminates the stagnation of dampness and turbidity caused by summer-damp or wind-cold. Patients usually contract this type of dampness during late summer or early autumn. Clinical manifestations may include fever, stuffiness of the chest, and abdominal distention or vomiting and diarrhea. It is used via oral ingestion to treat delirium and sudden loss of consciousness.

DOSAGE

0.1 to 0.2 gram for oral use, either in powder or tincture form. *Zhang Nao* is also used topically. Do not process *Zhang Nao* with heat, as heat will make this substance less effective.

CAUTIONS / CONTRAINDICATIONS

- Topical application of *Zhang Nao* over a large surface area may cause irritation and pain.
- Acrid, warm and drying, *Zhang Nao* is contraindicated in cases of excess heat, or when there is deficiency of qi or yin.
- *Zhang Nao* is contraindicated during pregnancy.

OVERDOSAGE

Zhang Nao is toxic when used internally. Overdose may occur after ingestion of 0.5 to 1.0 gram of the herb, and is characterized by dizziness, headache, feelings of warmth throughout the body, excitation and delirium. Dosage over 2 grams may cause severe muscle spasms and convulsions. Dosages over 7 to 15 grams may cause fatality.[1]

TREATMENT OF OVERDOSAGE

Overdose can be diagnosed by smelling the patient's breath, which will have a strong and characteristic odor of camphor. Acute overdose (within 2 to 3 hours) should be treated with emetic methods, followed by ingestion of 5 to 7 egg whites. An herbal decoction used with good success includes such herbs as *Shan Zhu Yu* (Fructus Corni) 15g, *Hu Zhang* (Rhizoma Polygoni Cuspidati) 10g, *Nu Zhen Zi* (Fructus Ligustri Lucidi) 15g, *Han Lian Cao* (Herba Ecliptae) 15g, *Dan Shen* (Radix Salviae Miltiorrhizae) 20g, *Long Yan Rou* (Arillus Longan) 30g, and *He Ye* (Folium Nelumbinis) 10g.[2]

When treating overdosage of *Zhang Nao*, antidotes containing opium or its derivatives are contraindicated as they have an inhibiting effect on respiration. Oil, milk, and alcohol are also contraindicated, as they promote the breakdown of the remaining *Zhang Nao* in the digestive tract.

CHEMICAL COMPOSITION

d-camphora.[3]

PHARMACOLOGICAL EFFECTS

- **CNS stimulant:** Subcutaneous injection of *Zhang Nao* has a marked stimulating effect on the central nervous system and the respiratory system.[4]
- **Cardiovascular**: *Zhang Nao* has a mixed effect on cardiac muscle. In a healthy person, a normal dosage of *Zhang Nao* exerts little or no effect while a large dosage has an inhibitory effect on the heart. In persons with heart failure, *Zhang Nao* has a stimulating effect.[5]
- **Gastrointestinal:** A small dosage of *Zhang Nao* has a

Zhang Nao (Camphora)

mild stimulatory effect on the stomach while a large dosage may cause nausea and vomiting.[6]

CLINICAL STUDIES AND RESEARCH

- **Rash and itching of the anus:** The following treatment protocol was recommended in one report: mix 2 grams of *Zhang Nao*, 2 grams of *Ming Fan* (Alumen), and 20 grams of *Mang Xiao* (Natrii Sulfas) in 600 ml of hot water. Sit in the solution twice daily.[7]

References

1. *Zhong Yao Xue* (Chinese Herbology), 1998; 989:991
2. *Zhong Yao Du Li Xue* (Toxicology of Chinese Herbs), 1989; 161-162
3. *Xian Dai Zhong Yao Yao Li Xue* (Contemporary Pharmacology of Chinese Herbs), 1997; 1138
4. *Zhong Yao Xue* (Chinese Herbology), 1998; 989:991
5. Ibid.
6. Ibid.
7. Ibid.

Da Feng Zi (Semen Hydnocarpi)

大風子 大风子

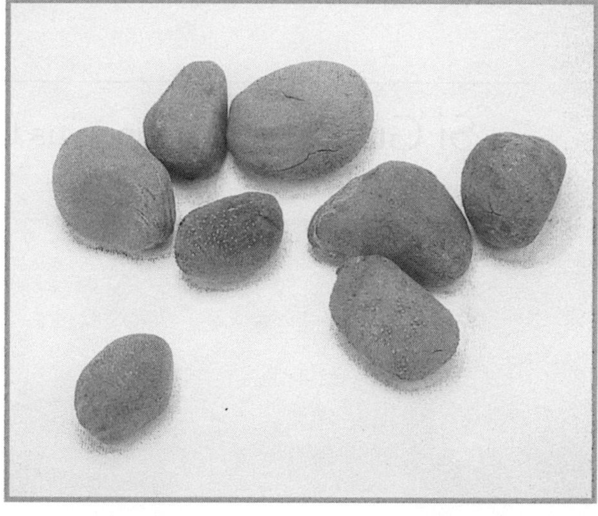

Pinyin Name: *Da Feng Zi*
Literal Name: "big wind seed," "big maple seeds"
Original Source: *Ben Cao Pin Hui Jing Yao* (Essentials of Materia Medica) by Liu Wen-Tai in 1505
English Name: hydnocarpus, chaulmoogra seed
Botanical Name: *Hydnocarpus anthelmintica* Pier. (*Tai Guo Da Feng Zi*); *Hydnocarpus hainanensis* (Merr.) Sleum (*Hai Nan Da Feng Zi*)
Pharmaceutical Name: Semen Hydnocarpi
Properties: acrid, hot
Channels Entered: Liver, Spleen, Kidney
Safety Index: extremely toxic

CHINESE THERAPEUTIC ACTIONS

Dispels Wind, Dries Dampness, Eliminates Toxins and Kills Parasites

Leprosy, syphilis, sarcoptidosis, scabies, tinea, rashes and itching: *Da Feng Zi* (Semen Hydnocarpi) is acrid, hot, drying, strong and toxic. It kills parasites and is commonly used for leprosy. This herb also treats rosacea, pimples and skin cracks. It is seldom used alone and is usually used with other herbs either internally or externally. When *Da Feng Zi* is properly processed, it can be used internally. Today however, due to its toxicity, it is rarely used internally.

- Leprosy: use *Da Feng Zi* with *Ku Shen Gen* (Radix Sophorae Flavescentis), *Fang Feng* (Radix Saposhnikoviae), *Chan Tui* (Periostracum Cicadae) and *Quan Xie* (Scorpio). Serve with tea.
- Ulcers associated with leprosy: use the powder of this herb with *Qing Fen* (Calomelas) and mix with sesame oil to apply topically.
- For oozing ulcers: use the powder of this herb with *Qing Fen* (Calomelas) and apply topically.
- Syphilitic sores: use 6 grams of *Da Feng Zi* with 3 grams of *Qing Fen* (Calomelas) and apply topically.
- Sarcoptidosis, rashes, itching, pus and sores: mix it with *Ming Fan* (Alumen), and *Qing Fen* (Calomelas) in sesame oil and apply topically.
- Itching of various dermatological disorders: mix *Da Feng Zi* with *Liu Huang* (Sulfur), *Xiong Huang* (Realgar), *Ming Fan* (Alumen) and apply topically.

DOSAGE

The calcined form or powder of *Da Feng Zi* is used externally as a paste or powder. For internal use, administer

Da Feng Zi (Semen Hydnocarpi)

0.3 to 1 gram of the appropriately-processed substance in pill form.

CAUTIONS / CONTRAINDICATIONS

- *Da Feng Zi* is highly toxic and should only be used topically.
- Use with extreme caution if taken internally. *Da Feng Zi* is contraindicated for long-term use or in high dosages.

OVERDOSAGE

Overdose of *Da Feng Zi* may cause hemolytic anemia, proteinuria, nephritis, headache, chest pain, fever, insomnia, and fatty liver.[1]

TREATMENT OF OVERDOSAGE

Treat early-stage overdose with emetic or purgative methods. Ingestion of activated charcoal is also beneficial to reduce absorption of the offending agent. One herbal formula has been used with success in treatment of *Da Feng Zi* overdose. The ingredients are *Lu Dou* (Semen Phaseoli Radiati) 60g, *Hei Dou* (Semen Glycine Max) 30g, *Chi Xiao Dou* (Semen Phaseoli) 30g, *Bai Mao Gen* (Rhizoma Imperatae) 30g, *Che Qian Zi* (Semen Plantaginis) 30g and *Gan Cao* (Radix Glycyrrhizae) 9g.[2]

CHEMICAL COMPOSITION

Chaulmoogric acid, hydnocarpic acid.[3]

References

1. *Yao Li Xue* (Pharmacology), 1965; 319
2. Ibid.
3. *Xian Dai Zhong Yao Yao Li Xue* (Contemporary Pharmacology of Chinese Herbs), 1997; 1428

Si Gua Luo (Retinervus Luffae Fructus)

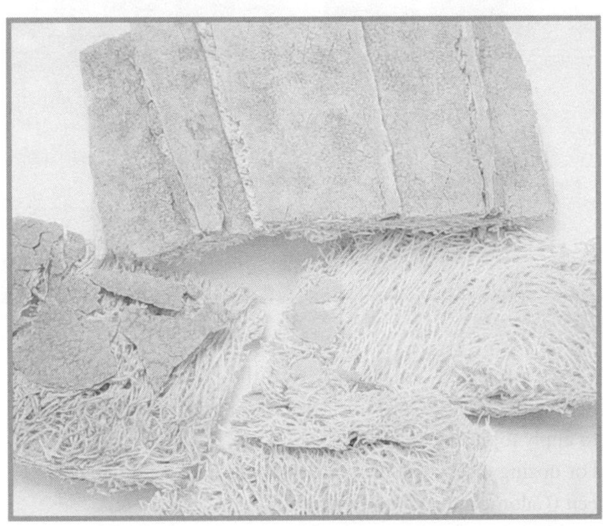

絲瓜絡 丝瓜络

Pinyin Name: *Si Gua Luo*
Literal Name: "net of string melon"
Original Source: *Ben Cao Meng Quan* (Hidden Aspects of the Materia Medica) by Chen Jia-Mo in 1565
English Name: luffa fiber, luffa vegetable sponge, towel-gourd vegetable sponge
Botanical Name: *Luffa cylindrica* (L.) Roem. (*Si Gua*)
Pharmaceutical Name: Retinervus Luffae Fructus
Properties: sweet, neutral
Channels Entered: Lung, Stomach, Liver

CHINESE THERAPEUTIC ACTIONS

1. Eliminates Toxins, Dissolves Phlegm

Toxic swellings, sores, abscesses and lesions: *Si Gua Luo* (Retinervus Luffae Fructus) treats accumulation of toxins and phlegm by clearing heat and reducing swelling. *Si Gua Luo* is generally used in calcined form, alone or with grain-based liquor.

- Breast abscess: use calcined *Si Gua Luo* with *Jin Yin Hua* (Flos Lonicerae), *Lian Qiao* (Fructus Forsythiae), *Pu Gong Ying* (Herba Taraxaci), and *Zi Hua Di Ding* (Herba Violae). *Si Gua Luo* is also mixed with sesame oil and applied topically.

2. Opens Peripheral Channels and Collaterals, and Dispels Wind

***Bi zheng* (painful obstruction syndrome), stiffness, tightness of the tendons:** *Si Gua Luo* dispels wind and dampness from peripheral channels and collaterals to relieve pain, cramps and spasms. It also relieves chest and hypochondriac pain by eliminating stagnation of

Si Gua Luo (Retinervus Luffae Fructus)

phlegm, qi, or blood. Because this herb is neutral to cool in property, it is more suitable for *bi zheng* caused by heat.

- *Bi zheng*: use *Si Gua Luo* with *Sang Zhi* (Ramulus Mori), *Luo Shi Teng* (Caulis Trachelospermi), *Qin Jiao* (Radix Gentianae Macrophyllae) and *Hai Feng Teng* (Caulis Piperis Kadsurae).
- Pain of qi and blood stagnation: use it with *Gua Lou Pi* (Pericarpium Trichosanthis), *Zhi Ke* (Fructus Aurantii), *Yu Jin* (Radix Curcumae), *Chai Hu* (Radix Bupleuri) and *Chuan Xiong* (Rhizoma Ligustici Chuanxiong).
- Pain arising from phlegm stagnation: add this herb to *Gua Lou Shi* (Fructus Trichosanthis), *Xie Bai* (Bulbus Allii Macrostemonis), *Ban Xia* (Rhizoma Pinelliae), *Bei Mu* (Bulbus Fritillaria) and *Qing Pi* (Pericarpium Citri Reticulatae Viride).

3. Opens Peripheral Channels and Collaterals in the Breast

Breast distention, breast tenderness, insufficient milk or obstruction: *Si Gua Luo* promotes lactation, treats lactation problems, and relieves breast distention and pain. Depending on the imbalance, appropriate herbs from other categories should be added, as *Si Gua Luo* is too mild to be used by itself.

- To promote lactation: use it with *Chuan Shan Jia* (Squama Manis), *Wang Bu Liu Xing* (Semen Vaccariae), and *Lu Lu Tong* (Fructus Liquidambaris).
- Lack of breast milk secretion because of qi deficiency: combine this herb with *Dang Shen* (Radix Codonopsis) and *Huang Qi* (Radix Astragali).
- Lack of breast milk secretion caused by blood deficiency: add it to *Shu Di Huang* (Radix Rehmanniae Preparata) and *Dang Gui* (Radicis Angelicae Sinensis).
- Breast distention and pain due to Liver qi stagnation: use it with *Chai Hu* (Radix Bupleuri) and *Xiang Fu* (Rhizoma Cyperi).
- Swelling and burning sensations of the breast: incorporate it with *Pu Gong Ying* (Herba Taraxaci), *Jin Yin Hua* (Flos Lonicerae), and *Tian Men Dong* (Radix Asparagi).

4. Dissolves Phlegm

Cough with profuse phlegm and chest pain: *Si Gua Luo* treats cough and chest congestion and pain caused by phlegm obstruction in the chest. This function is rather mild, thus the herb must be used with other herbs to clear heat and eliminate phlegm.

- Cough with sputum arising from Lung heat: combine *Si Gua Luo* with *Gua Lou Shi* (Fructus Trichosanthis), *Sang Bai Pi* (Cortex Mori), *Bei Mu* (Bulbus Fritillaria) and *Qian Hu* (Radix Peucedani).
- Cough with sputum accompanying an exterior condition: add it to *Niu Bang Zi* (Fructus Arctii), *Sang Ye* (Folium Mori), *Qian Hu* (Radix Peucedani) and *Xing Ren* (Semen Armeniacae Amarum).
- Cough due to cold: use it with *Xing Ren* (Semen Armeniacae Amarum), *Kuan Dong Hua* (Flos Farfarae), *Zi Wan* (Radix Asteris) and *Bai Bu* (Radix Stemonae).

5. Stops Bleeding

Charred *Si Gua Luo* stops bleeding, such as hematochezia or profuse menstrual bleeding.

DOSAGE

For internal use, 10 to 15 grams in decoction or as powder. *Si Gua Luo* is commonly used internally and topically in calcined form.

CHEMICAL COMPOSITION

Xylan, mannan, galactan.[1]

PHARMACOLOGICAL EFFECTS

- **Hepatoprotective:** Administration of *Si Gua Luo* in rats had a protective effect against liver damage induced by carbon tetrachloride.[2]
- **Others:** *Si Gua Luo* has been shown to have mild cardiotonic and diuretic effects.[3]

TOXICOLOGY

Oral administration of *Si Gua Luo* in animals at 100 times the therapeutic dose for humans, for 10 days, showed no significant changes to the brain, heart, liver, kidney and other internal organs. The herb is considered very safe, with little or no toxicity.[4]

References

1. *Xian Dai Zhong Yao Yao Li Xue* (Contemporary Pharmacology of Chinese Herbs), 1997; 442
2. *Zhong Yao Yao Li Du Li Yu Lin Chuang* (Pharmacology, Toxicology and Clinical Applications of Chinese Herbs), 1992:58
3. Ibid.
4. Ibid.

Er Cha (Catechu)

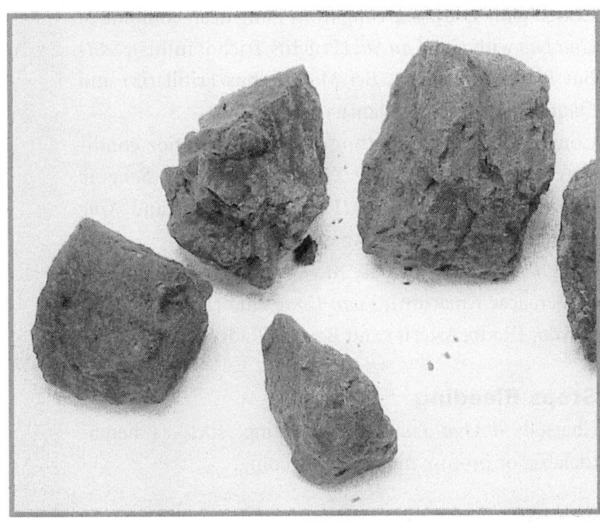

兒茶 儿茶

Pinyin Name: *Er Cha*
Literal Name: "child's tea"
Alternate Chinese Names: *Wu Die Ni, Hai Er Cha*
Original Source: *Yin Shan Zheng Yao* (Correct Guide to Eating and Drinking)
English Name: catechu, black catechu
Botanical Name: *Acacia catechu* (L.) Willd. (*Er Cha*); *Uncaria gambier* Roxb. (*Er Cha Gou Teng*)
Pharmaceutical Name: Catechu
Properties: bitter, astringent, cool
Channels Entered: Lung

CHINESE THERAPEUTIC ACTIONS

1. Drains Dampness and Absorbs Seepage

Oozing sores, non-healing ulcerations, canker sores caused by dampness: Clinical manifestations include sores that are filled with purulent fluid, chronic non-healing sores, and ulcers or sores of the oral cavity. *Er Cha* (Catechu) is used alone or with other herbs for maximum effectiveness.

- Non-healing sores, weeping lesions: mix *Er Cha* with *Ru Xiang* (Gummi Olibanum), *Mo Yao* (Myrrha), *Bing Pian* (Borneolum Syntheticum), *Xue Jie* (Sanguis Draconis) and *Long Gu* (Os Draconis). Apply topically as powder.
- Ulcers with necrosis of tissue: apply this herb topically as powder with *Qing Fen* (Calomelas) and *Xue Jie* (Sanguis Draconis).
- Oral ulcers and sores: apply it topically as powder with *Peng Sha* (Borax).
- Genital sores: apply *Er Cha* powder topically with *Hu Huang Lian* (Rhizoma Picrorhizae).
- Hemorrhoids: apply this herb topically with *She Xiang* (Moschus).

2. Generates Flesh and Stops Bleeding

Bleeding: *Er Cha*, applied topically as powder or served internally as decoction, stops bleeding, especially if bleeding is caused by heat. Clinical applications include gastrointestinal bleeding, bleeding gums, epistaxis, hematochezia, hemorrhage caused by trauma, or abnormal uterine bleeding.

- Traumatic hemorrhage: apply *Er Cha* powder topically with calcined *Long Gu* (Os Draconis), *Xue Jie* (Sanguis Draconis) and *Bai Ji* (Rhizoma Bletillae).
- Other kinds of bleeding: use it with *San Qi* (Radix Notoginseng) and *Hai Piao Xiao* (Endoconcha Sepiae) internally or externally.
- Burns: apply this herb topically with *Bing Pian* (Borneolum Syntheticum) and *Ge Jie* (Gecko).

3. Clears Heat and Dispels Phlegm

Lung heat with phlegm: *Er Cha* treats cough with yellow phlegm.

- Cough with yellow phlegm: use it with *Ma Huang* (Herba Ephedrae), *Xing Ren* (Semen Armeniacae Amarum), *Shi Gao* (Gypsum Fibrosum), and *Gan Cao* (Radix Glycyrrhizae).

4. Generates Fluids and Stops Diarrhea

Summer-heat: *Er Cha* treats thirst, diarrhea, and dysenteric disorders caused by summer-heat.

- Thirst: combine *Er Cha* with *He Ye* (Folium Nelumbinis), *Gan Cao* (Radix Glycyrrhizae), *Hua Shi* (Talcum), and *Qing Hao* (Herba Artemisiae Annuae).
- Diarrhea and dysenteric disorders with rectal tenesmus or burning sensations: use this herb with *Ge Gen* (Radix Puerariae), *Huang Lian* (Rhizoma Coptidis), *Huang Qin* (Radix Scutellariae) and *Huang Bai* (Cortex Phellodendri).

5. Relieves Food Stagnation in Children and Promotes Digestion

- Indigestion or food stagnation in children: use *Er Cha* with *Ji Nei Jin* (Endothelium Corneum Gigeriae Galli). Serve the powder with water.

DOSAGE

1 to 3 grams in decoction, 0.1 to 0.9 gram in pills or powders. When used topically, *Er Cha* is generally ground into powder and mixed with other herbs to make a paste.

Er Cha (Catechu)

CHEMICAL COMPOSITION

Catechim, catechu-tannic acid, dl-catechin, dl-epicatechin, phlobatannin, fesetin, quercetin, quercetagenin, kaempferol, dihydrokaempferol, taxifolin, isorhamnetin, protocatechu tannins, pyrogallic tannins.[1]

PHARMACOLOGICAL EFFECTS

- **Antibiotic:** Water extract of *Er Cha* has an inhibitory effect *in vitro* on *Staphylococcus aureus, Pseudomonas aeruginosa, Corynebacterium diphtheriae, Bacillus proteus, Bacillus dysenteriae,* and *Salmonella typhi.*[2]
- **Hepatoprotective:** According to one report, catechim has marked hepatoprotective effects. Catechim effectively reduced the elevated level of SGPT artificially induced by carbon tetrachloride in 27 rats.[3]

CLINICAL STUDIES AND RESEARCH

- **Burns:** Topical application of a formula with *Er Cha* and *Bing Pian* (Borneolum Syntheticum) as main ingredients effectively relieved pain and promoted healing in burn patients.[4]
- **Ulceration:** Ten patients with ulcerations of the skin and tissue of the lower extremities were treated with *Er Cha, Huang Lian* (Rhizoma Coptidis), *Huang Bai* (Cortex Phellodendri) and others, with complete recovery occurring within 5 to 15 days.[5]
- **Peptic ulcer disease:** In a clinical study, patients with gastric and duodenal ulcers were divided into three groups, with group one receiving *Er Cha* and *Da Huang* (Radix et Rhizoma Rhei) in powder, group two receiving *Er Cha* and *San Qi* (Radix Notoginseng), and group three receiving drug treatment (aminocaproic acid, Adrenosem salicylate, and vitamin K). Out of 34 patients in each group, the rate of effectiveness was 88.24% in group one (16 patients with significant and 14 patients with moderate improvement), 85.29% for group two (9 patients with significant and 20 patients with moderate improvement), and 58.82% for group three (7 patients with significant and 13 patients with moderate improvement).[6]
- **Diarrhea:** In one study, 110 patients with diarrhea were treated by oral ingestion of *Er Cha*, with satisfactory results. The dosage was 6 to 9 g/day for adults, and 150 to 250 mg/kg/day for children, given in three to four equally-divided doses with warm water.[7]
- **Galacturia:** According to one report, 60 grams each of *Er Cha, Ming Fan* (Alumen) and *Shen Qu* (Massa Fermentata) were ground into fine powder and encapsulated for treatment of galacturia. Patients were instructed to take 15 capsules (0.3 gram per capsule, 4.5 grams of herbs per dose) twice daily for 10 days per course of treatment. The authors reported that doctors who have used this treatment in clinical practice for over 10 years reported satisfactory results.[8]

TOXICOLOGY

The LD_{50} for catechim in mice is 1.37 g/kg.[9]

References

1. *Xian Dai Zhong Yao Yao Li Xue* (Contemporary Pharmacology of Chinese Herbs), 1997; 1420
2. *Zhong Cao Yao Xue* (Study of Chinese Herbal Medicine), 1976; 431
3. *Zhong Guo Yi Xue Ke Xue Xue Bao* (Journal of Chinese Medical Science University), 1990; 12(5):379
4. *He Bei Zhong Yi* (Hebei Chinese Medicine), 1984; 3:11
5. *Si Chuan Zhong Yi* (Sichuan Chinese Medicine), 1987; 5:29
6. *Zhong Xi Yi Jie He Za Zhi* (Journal of Integrated Chinese and Western Medicine), 1984; 4(4):226
7. *Liao Ning Zhong Yi Za Zhi* (Liaoning Journal of Chinese Medicine), 1980; 5:48
8. *Shan Dong Zhong Yi Za Zhi* (Shandong Journal of Chinese Medicine), 1987; 6:43
9. *Xian Dai Shi Yong Yao Xue* (Practical Applications of Modern Herbal Medicine), 1987; 4(3): 17

Wa Leng Zi (Concha Arcae)

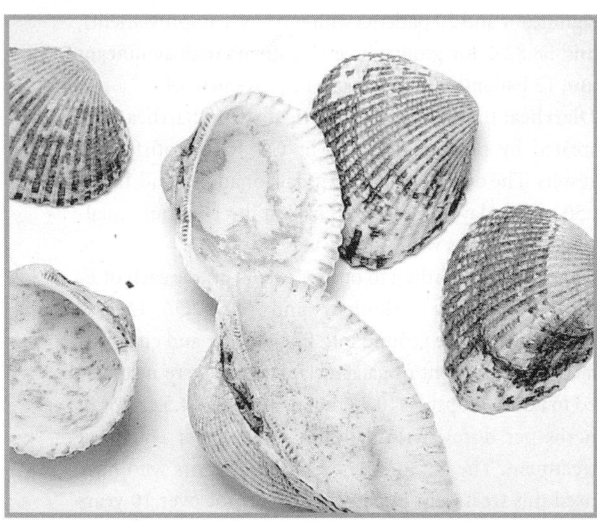

瓦楞子

Pinyin Name: *Wa Leng Zi*
Original Source: *Ben Cao Shi Yi* (Omissions from the [Classic of the] Materia Medica) by Chen Cang-Qi in 741 A.D.
English Name: ark shell
Zoological Name: *Arca subcrenata* Lischke (*Mao Han*); *Arca granosa* Linnaeus (*Ni Han*); *Arca inflata* Reeve (*Gui Han*)
Pharmaceutical Name: Concha Arcae
Properties: salty, neutral
Channels Entered: Liver, Stomach, Lung

CHINESE THERAPEUTIC ACTIONS

1. Dissolves Phlegm, Resolves Stagnation, Softens Hardness, Disperses Nodules

Mobile or immobile masses characterized by accumulation of qi, blood or phlegm: Clinical applications of *Wa Leng Zi* (Concha Arcae) include scrofula, goiter, abdominal masses, hepatomegaly and splenomegaly. It also treats chronic stubborn phlegm found in chronic coughing. The action of *Wa Leng Zi* is mild when it is used alone. Therefore, it is usually combined with other herbs for maximum effectiveness. *Wa Leng Zi* is also effective in treatment of goiter caused by Liver qi stagnation and improper food intake.

- Scrofula from phlegm and fire: use *Wa Leng Zi* with *Bei Mu* (Bulbus Fritillaria), *Xia Ku Cao* (Spica Prunellae), and *Lian Qiao* (Fructus Forsythiae).
- Goiter caused by accumulation of blood and phlegm: combine it with *Hai Zao* (Sargassum), *Kun Bu* (Thallus Laminariae seu Eckloniae), and *Hai Dai* (Thallus Laminariae).
- Immobile or mobile masses characterized by accumulations of qi, blood or phlegm: use this herb with *E Zhu* (Rhizoma Curcumae), *San Leng* (Rhizoma Sparganii), *Bie Jia* (Carapax Trionycis) and *Dan Shen* (Radix Salviae Miltiorrhizae). These herbs are also used for hepatomegaly, splenomegaly and tumors of the gastrointestinal tract.
- Chronic cough and phlegm: add this herb to *Bei Mu* (Bulbus Fritillaria), *Zi Wan* (Radix Asteris), *Kuan Dong Hua* (Flos Farfarae) and *Fu Hai Shi* (Pumice).

2. Controls Stomach Acid, Relieves Pain

Stomach pain with acid regurgitation: Vinegar-processed *Wa Leng Zi* has marked effectiveness to stop secretion of gastric acid and relieve pain. It treats acid reflux, and gastric and duodenal ulcers.

- Acid reflux: use this substance with *Hai Piao Xiao* (Endoconcha Sepiae) and *Chen Pi* (Pericarpium Citri Reticulatae).
- Gastric and duodenal ulcers: combine it with other herbs based on differential diagnosis.

3. Regulates Qi and Blood Circulation, Relieves Pain

Wa Leng Zi treats menstrual pain caused by stagnation of qi and blood.

- Menstrual pain: use it with *Xiang Fu* (Rhizoma Cyperi), *Tao Ren* (Semen Persicae), *Mu Dan Pi* (Cortex Moutan) and *Dang Gui* (Radicis Angelicae Sinensis).

DOSAGE

10 to 30 grams in herbal decoction, 1 to 3 grams in powder or pills. *Wa Leng Zi* should be cooked for an extended period of time to ensure maximum extraction of active components. Fresh *Wa Leng Zi* more strongly disperses nodules and softens hardness. Vinegar-treated *Wa Leng Zi* more effectively stops the secretion of gastric acid and relieves pain.

CHEMICAL COMPOSITION

Calcium carbonate, magnesium, iron, sodium phosphate.[1]

CLINICAL STUDIES AND RESEARCH

- **Peptic ulcer:** Stomach or duodenal ulcer patients were treated with an herbal formula with significant improvement. The herbal formula contained (in powder form) 5 parts calcined *Wa Leng Zi* and 1 part *Gan Cao* (Radix Glycyrrhizae). Patients received 10 grams of the powder three times daily, before meals. Patients with rhythmic

Wa Leng Zi (Concha Arcae)

cycles of pain were given 20 grams of the powder 20 minutes before the next onset of pain. The duration of treatment ranged between 20 and 56 days. Of 124 patients, 59 experienced complete recovery, 48 reported improvement, and 17 had no response. The overall rate of effectiveness was 89.12%.[2]

References

1. *Xian Dai Zhong Yao Yao Li Xue* (Contemporary Pharmacology of Chinese Herbs), 1997
2. *Liao Ning Yi Yao* (Liaoning Medicine and Herbology), 1971; 3:25

Peng Sha (Borax)

硼砂

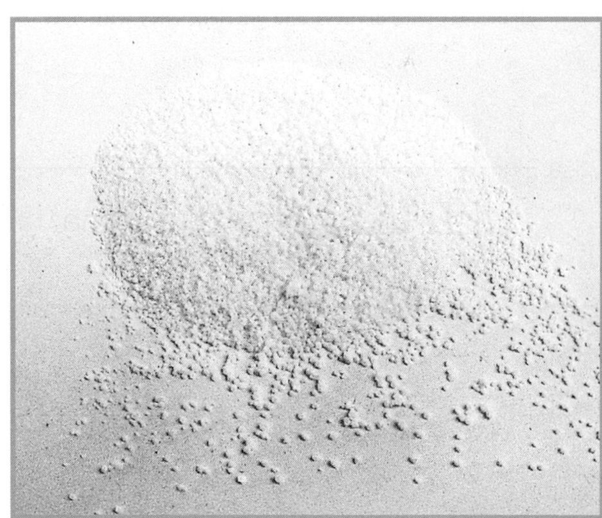

Pinyin Name: *Peng Sha*
Alternate Chinese Names: *Yue Shi, Pen Sha*
Original Source: *Ri Hua Zi Ben Cao* (Materia Medica of Ri Hua-Zi) by Ri Hua-Zi in 713 A.D.
English Name: borax
Pharmaceutical Name: Borax
Properties: sweet, salty, cool
Channels Entered: Lung, Stomach

CHINESE THERAPEUTIC ACTIONS

1. Clears Heat, Eliminates Toxins, and Reduces Swelling

Sore and swollen throat, oral ulcers, redness and swelling of the eyes, conjunctivitis: Sweet, salty and cool, *Peng Sha* (Borax) treats disorders characterized by the presence of heat and toxins. Clinical presentations include thrush, stomatitis, throat disorders with difficulty speaking and swallowing, locked jaw, aphasia, cyanosis, throat infection, tonsillitis, and sensations of having a heavy tongue.

- Ulceration of the mouth or sore throat: combine *Peng Sha* with *Mang Xiao* (Natrii Sulfas), *Bing Pian* (Borneolum Syntheticum), *Zhen Zhu* (Margarita) and *Zhu Sha* (Cinnabaris). Grind all ingredients into fine powder and apply topically.
- General disorders of the oral cavity: combine this substance with *Er Cha* (Catechu) and *Zhen Zhu* (Margarita).
- General disorders of the oral cavity characterized by heat and toxins: use it with *Qing Dai* (Indigo Naturalis) and *Huang Lian* (Rhizoma Coptidis).
- Skin sores and ulcerations: use unprocessed *Peng Sha* to clear heat and eliminate toxins, use calcined *Peng Sha* to drain pus and enhance recovery.
- Eye redness, swelling and pain: boil *Peng Sha* in water, let it cool and use the liquid as eyewash. Or apply powdered *Peng Sha* with *Bing Pian* (Borneolum Syntheticum) and powder of *Yuan Ming Fen* (Natrii Sulfas Praeparata) to the corner of the eyes three times daily.
- Bleeding lesions: use *Peng Sha* with charred *Pu Huang* (Pollen Typhae).

2. Clears Heat in the Lung, Dissolves Phlegm

Cough caused by hot phlegm: Oral ingestion of *Peng Sha* clears heat, dissolves phlegm, and eliminates toxins. It treats cough, sore throat or hoarse voice caused by phlegm and heat attacking the Lung.

- Chronic cough with sore throat, yellow, sticky, difficult-to-expectorate sputum: use *Peng Sha* with *Nan Sha Shen* (Radix Adenophorae), *Bei Mu* (Bulbus Fritillaria), *Gua*

Peng Sha (Borax)

Lou Shi (Fructus Trichosanthis), *Sang Bai Pi* (Cortex Mori) and *Huang Qin* (Radix Scutellariae).

DOSAGE

1.5 to 3.0 grams in pill or powder form for oral ingestion. *Peng Sha* is also used topically as fine powder or as topical wash. The unprocessed form more strongly clears heat and eliminates toxins, while the calcined form more effectively reduces swelling and eliminates dampness to treat oral ulcers.

CAUTIONS / CONTRAINDICATIONS

- *Peng Sha* should be administered with caution for oral use.
- *Peng Sha* should be used with caution in cases of yin deficiency with dryness, and yin deficiency with heat.

CHEMICAL COMPOSITION

Sodium tetraborate.[1]

PHARMACOLOGICAL EFFECTS

- **Antibiotic:** *Peng Sha* has an inhibitory effect against *E. coli*, *Pseudomonas aeruginosa*, *Bacillus anthracis*, *Bacillus dysenteriae*, *Salmonella typhi*, *Bacillus proteus*, *Staphylococcus aureus*, *Corynebacterium diphtheriae*, *Diplococcus meningitidis*, β-hemolytic streptococcus, and some pathogenic fungi.[2]

References

1. *Xian Dai Zhong Yao Yao Li Xue* (Contemporary Pharmacology of Chinese Herbs), 1997; 1418
2. *Zhong Yao Xue* (Chinese Herbology), 1998; 937:940

Lu Gan Shi (Galamina)

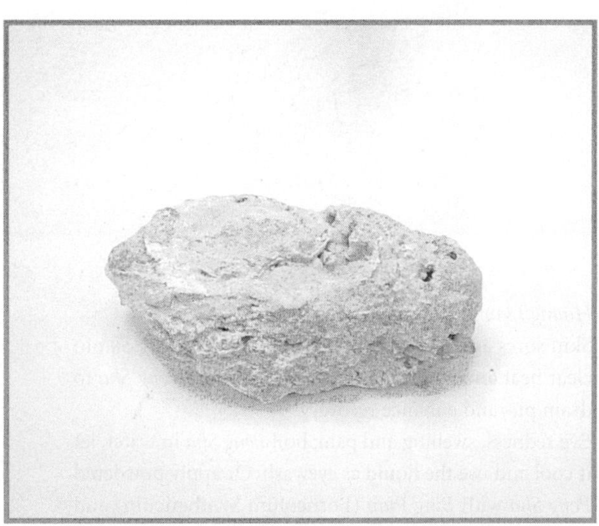

爐甘石 炉甘石

Pinyin Name: *Lu Gan Shi*
Literal Name: "stove sweet stone"
Alternate Chinese Names: *Gan Shi*, *Bai Gan Shi*
Original Source: *Wai Dan Ben Cao* (Materia Medica For External Elixirs)
English Name: galamina
Pharmaceutical Name: Galamina
Properties: sweet, neutral
Channels Entered: Liver, Stomach

CHINESE THERAPEUTIC ACTIONS

1. Eliminates Toxins and Brightens the Eyes

Lu Gan Shi (Galamina), commonly used topically, treats various eye disorders, such as redness, swelling and pain, excessive tearing, increased sensitivity to light, and pterygium.

- Eye redness and swelling: combine *Lu Gan Shi* with *Yuan Ming Fen* (Matrii Sulfas Exsiccatus).
- Excessive tearing: use it with *Hai Piao Xiao* (Endoconcha Sepiae).
- General eye problems: add *Zhu Sha* (Cinnabaris), *Peng Sha* (Borax) and *She Xiang* (Moschus) to *Lu Gan Shi.*

2. Dries Dampness, Generates Flesh, and Relieves Itching

Lu Gan Shi eliminates dampness and toxins from the skin to treat a variety of dermatological disorders. It is usually used topically, in combination with other herbs, for dermatological disorders with or without open sores.

- Diaper rash: mix 30 grams of calcined *Lu Gan Shi* and 3

Lu Gan Shi (Galamina)

grams of *Qing Fen* (Calomelas) and apply the combination topically to the affected area.

- Chronic ulceration: use this substance with calcined *Long Gu* (Os Draconis) and calcined *Shi Gao* (Gypsum Fibrosum) topically.
- Dermatitis: mix it with glycerin and apply topically.
- Eczema in the genital area: apply the powder topically.
- Genital ulcers: mix it with *Er Cha* (Catechu) and sesame oil, and apply topically.

DOSAGE

For ophthalmic application, *Lu Gan Shi* must be processed using the method called *shui fei* (refining with water). Do not use it internally.

CAUTIONS / CONTRAINDICATIONS

- Do not use *Lu Gan Shi* internally.

CHEMICAL COMPOSITION

Zinc carbonate, calcium oxide, magnesium oxide, ferric oxide, manganese oxide, copper, and lead.[1]

CLINICAL STUDIES AND RESEARCH

- **Chapped nipples:** Topical application of a formula to chapped nipples, two to three times daily, has shown satisfactory results in numerous patients. The formulation was prepared by mixing 10 grams each of *Lu Gan Shi*, *Hua Rui Shi* (Ophicalcitum), *Han Shui Shi* (Mirabilite), and a small amount of *Bing Pian* (Borneolum Syntheticum), in an oil base.[2]

References

1. *Xian Dai Zhong Yao Yao Li Xue* (Contemporary Pharmacology of Chinese Herbs), 1997; 1416
2. *Xin Zhong Yi* (New Chinese Medicine), 1974; 6:53

Mu Bie Zi (Semen Momordicae)

木鱉子 木鼈子

Pinyin Name: *Mu Bie Zi*
Literal Name: "wooden turtle seeds"
Original Source: *Ri Hua Zi Ben Cao* (Materia Medica of Ri Hua-Zi) by Ri Hua-Zi in 713 A.D.
English Name: momordica seeds, cochinchina momordica seed
Botanical Name: *Momordica cochinchinensis* (Lour.) Spreng. (*Mu Bie Zi*)
Pharmaceutical Name: Semen Momordicae
Properties: bitter, slightly sweet, warm
Channels Entered: Large Intestine, Liver, Stomach
Safety Index: toxic

CHINESE THERAPEUTIC ACTIONS

Reduces Swelling, Disperses Nodules, and Eliminates Toxins

Mu Bie Zi (Semen Momordicae) treats sores, ulcerations, abscesses, nodules, cysts, hemorrhoid, scrofulae and disorders characterized by the presence of heat and toxins. It may be used internally or topically.

- Throat soreness, swelling and pain: combine *Mu Bie Zi* with *Shan Dou Gen* (Radix Sophorae Tonkinensis).
- Abscess: use it with *Huang Qin* (Radix Scutellariae) and *Huang Bai* (Cortex Phellodendri).

DOSAGE

0.5 to 1.0 gram in pills.

CAUTIONS / CONTRAINDICATIONS

- *Mu Bie Zi* is contraindicated in pregnancy, or in individuals with weak constitutions.

Mu Bie Zi (Semen Momordicae)

CHEMICAL COMPOSITION

Momordin, gypsogenin, momordic acid, d-eleostearic acid.[1]

TOXICOLOGY

The LD_{50} for *Mu Bie Zi* in mice is 32.35 mg/kg via intravenous injection, and 37.34 mg/kg via intraperitoneal injection.[2]

References

1. *Chang Yong Zhong Yao Cheng Fen Yu Yao Li Shou Ce* (A Handbook of the Composition and Pharmacology of Common Chinese Drugs), 1994; 514
2. *Zhong Yao Da Ci Dian* (Dictionary of Chinese Herbs), 1975: 369

Wu Ming Yi (Pyrolusitum)

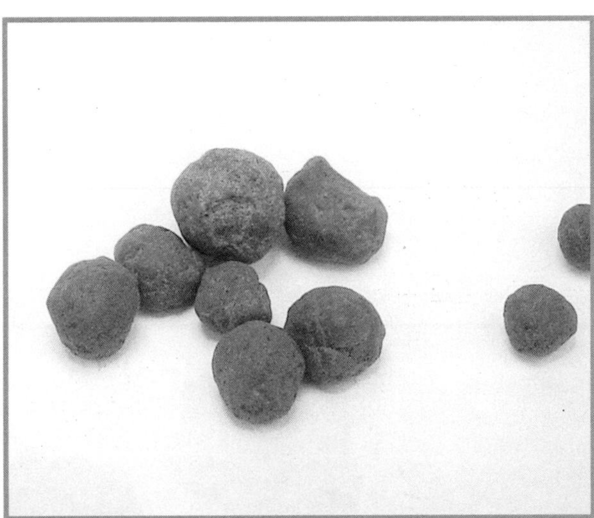

無名異 无名异

Pinyin Name: *Wu Ming Yi*
Original Source: *Shen Nong Ben Cao Jing* (Divine Husbandman's Classic of the Materia Medica) in the second century
English Name: pyrolusite
Pharmaceutical Name: Pyrolusitum
Properties: sweet, neutral
Channels Entered: Liver, Kidney

CHINESE THERAPEUTIC ACTIONS

Reduces Swelling and Pain, Stops Bleeding, Promotes Generation of Flesh

Wu Ming Yi (Pyrolusitum) is commonly used to address various traumatic and external injuries. Clinical applications include trauma, broken bones, wounds, bruises, bleeding, swelling, inflammation, and infection.

- Trauma with pain and inflammation: apply *Wu Ming Yi* topically.
- Bone fracture: use it with *Ru Xiang* (Gummi Olibanum) and *Mo Yao* (Myrrha).

DOSAGE

6 to 15 grams.

CHEMICAL COMPOSITION

MnO_2

Chapter 20 summary

SUBSTANCES FOR TOPICAL APPLICATION

Although many of the substances listed in this chapter can influence internal conditions, many are too toxic for internal use, thus are used via external application or not at all. Some are no longer in use but are important to include here for academic and informational purposes. The historical uses of these substances in traditional Chinese medicine serve to provide reminders and possible templates for future refinements and research.

The columns below are marked to indicate qualities or uses appropriate to each herb:

Tox (toxicity) – presence of toxicity

Drm (dermatology) – dermatological application to treat itching, eczema, parasites or fungus

Trm (trauma) – trauma or external injuries, such as sores, ulcers, abscesses, damage to flesh, bruises, or similar wounds

Name	Tox	Drm	Trm	Unique Functions
Liu Huang (Sulfur)	X	X		Ext: treats itching, kills parasites and fungi Int: tonifies Kidney yang, promotes bowel movement
Xiong Huang (Realgar)	X	X		Ext: kills fungi, treats insect and snake bites Int: dispels phlegm, treats seizures and malaria
Qing Fen (Calomelas)	X	X		Ext: treats ulcers, sores and syphilis Int: dispels water, promotes bowel movement
Qian Dan (Minium)	X		X	Ext: promotes generation of flesh, treats ulcers Int: dispels phlegm, treats seizure
Mi Tuo Seng (Lithargyrum)	X	X	X	Ext: treats oozing, non-healing sores Int: too toxic for internal use
Ming Fan (Alumen)		X	X	Ext: treats various itching skin disorders Int: stops bleeding, dispels phlegm
Da Suan (Bulbus Alli Sativi)		X		Ext: reduces swelling, eliminates toxins, kills parasites. Int: treats respiratory disorders, prevents infectious disease
Ban Mao (Mylabris)	X	X		Ext: eliminates heat toxins Int: breaks blood stagnation, disperses stagnation
Chan Su (Venenum Bufonis)	X	X	X	Ext: eliminates toxins, reduces swelling, relieves pain Int: opens orifices, eliminates toxins, relieves pain
Ma Qian Zi (Semen Strychni)	X	X	X	Ext: reduces swelling, disperses stagnation, opens channels and relieves pain Int: relieves muscle numbness and paralysis
She Chuang Zi (Fructus Cnidii)		X	X	Ext: relieves itching, kills parasites, dispels wind-cold Int: tonifies Kidney yang
Lu Feng Fang (Nidus Vespae)	X	X	X	Ext: eliminates toxins, dispels wind, kills parasites, relieves pain Int: disperses nodules to treat cancer, tumors, palpable masses, and scrofula
Xue Jie (Sanguis Draconis)			X	Ext: generates production of blood and flesh, heals sores and wounds Int: invigorates blood circulation, eliminates blood stasis
Zhang Nao (Camphora)	X	X	X	Ext: dries dampness, kills parasites, relieves pain Int: opens sensory orifices, relieves pain
Da Feng Zi (Semen Hydnocarpi)	X	X		Ext: dispels wind, dries dampness, eliminates toxins, kills parasites Int: avoid internal use
Si Gua Luo (Retinervus Luffae Fructus)		X	X	Ext: eliminates toxins, dispels phlegm, dispels wind, opens channels and collaterals Int: alleviates pain, relieves cough and chest pain
Er Cha (Catechu)			X	Ext: dries dampness, treats ulcers, generates flesh, stops bleeding Int: clears heat, relieves cough, generates body fluids, stops diarrhea.
Wa Leng Zi (Concha Arcae)				Ext: dispels phlegm, dissolves bruises, softens hardness, disperses nodules Int: neutralizes gastric acid, relieves stomach pain
Peng Sha (Borax)	X		X	Ext: breaks blood stagnation, disperses nodules, softens hardness Int: treats sores, ulcers, swollen throat
Lu Gan Shi (Galamina)		X	X	Ext: eliminates toxins, dries dampness, generates flesh, relieves itching Int: not used internally
Mu Bie Zi (Semen Momordicae)	X	X	X	Ext: reduces swelling, disperses nodules, eliminates toxins Int: treats sores and ulcers
Wu Ming Yi (Pyrolusitum)		X	X	Ext: reduces swelling and pain, stops bleeding, promotes generation of flesh Int: trauma

Chapter 20 summary

In TCM hospitals in China, substances for topical application are used in surgery, trauma, dermatology, and in eye, ear, nose and throat departments. They are also used for internal medicine, obstetric/gynecologic and pediatric disorders. Most of the herbs in this category are toxic and should be used carefully, within appropriate guidelines.

Liu Huang (Sulfur) is most effective against furuncles and scabies. When taken internally, it strengthens Kidney yang to treat impotence.

Xiong Huang (Realgar) contains arsenic, and is used externally to treat sores and carbuncles, and insect and snake bites. When taken internally, it can dispel phlegm, treat malaria and settle wind to treat fright.

Qing Fen (Calomelas) contains mercury, and is used externally to eliminate toxins and kill parasites.

Qian Dan (Minium) contains lead, and is used externally to treat ulcers and promote the generation of flesh. When taken internally, it dispels phlegm and treats seizures.

Mi Tuo Seng (Lithargyum) contains lead, and is used externally to generate flesh, treat sores, ulcers and wounds with oozing fluids. It also treats eczema. It is rarely used internally because of toxicity.

Ming Fan (Alumen) clears toxins, kills parasites, dries dampness, relieves itching, and stops bleeding. Used externally, it treats sores, carbuncles, eczema, scabies, fungal infections and itching. Used internally, it stops diarrhea and bleeding, clears heat, and dispels phlegm. Clinical applications of *Ming Fan* include hematemesis, epistaxis, epilepsy, mania and jaundice.

Da Suan (Bulbus Alli Sativi) reduces swelling, eliminates toxins and kills parasites. It can be used externally to treat swellings and sores, and relieve itching due to fungal infection. When used internally, it can treat chronic Lung disorders such as tuberculosis, and whooping cough. It can also be used to treat dysentery and prevent infectious disorders.

Ban Mao (Mylabris) eliminates heat and toxins when used externally, and invigorates blood circulation when used internally.

Chan Su (Venenum Bufonis) eliminates toxins, reduces swelling, relieves pain, and opens the sensory orifices to disperse stagnation. External and internal uses treat swelling, sores, scrofula, pain of masses, and abdominal pain with vomiting and diarrhea.

Ma Qian Zi (Semen Strychni) reduces swelling, disperses stagnation, opens channels and collaterals, relieves pain to treat swellings and sores, and treats pain, stiffness and paralysis caused by traumatic injuries.

She Chuang Zi (Fructus Cnidii) dries dampness, kills parasites, disperses cold and wind, and tonifies Kidney yang. Used externally, it treats various itching skin disorders. Used internally, it treats leukorrhea, back pain, or impotence due to cold and dampness.

Lu Feng Fang (Nidus Vespae) dispels wind, kills parasites, relieves pain and eliminates toxins. It treats toxic sores, carbuncles, masses and swellings, sore throat, toothache and itching skin disorders.

Chapter 20 summary

Xue Jie (Sanguis Draconis), when used externally, generates flesh, heals sores and wounds, and treats non-healing sores and wounds or bleeding due to traumatic injuries. *Xue Jie*, when taken internally, invigorates blood, disperses stagnation and relieves pain. Clinical applications of *Xue Jie* include blood stagnation, swelling, pain, amenorrhea and dysmenorrhea.

Zhang Nao (Camphora) is aromatic, dry and toxic. Used externally, it dispels dampness, kills parasites and relieves pain. It treats scabies, ringworms, fungal infections and toothache. Taken internally, it opens the orifices, and warms the body to relieve pain.

Da Feng Zi (Semen Hydnocarpi), extremely toxic, dispels wind, dries dampness, eliminates toxins, kills parasites and treats leprosy and syphilis. Taken internally, it treats leukorrhea, dysentery, hematochezia and bleeding.

Si Gua Luo (Retinervus Luffae Fructus) eliminates toxins, dissolves phlegm, dispels wind, opens channels and collaterals, and treats sores and swellings. Taken internally, it treats *bi zheng* (painful obstruction syndrome), cough with chest pain, or obstruction of breast milk. *Si Gua Luo* is relatively mild, and should be used at a high dosage for maximum results.

Er Cha (Catechu) dries dampness and treats wet sores and lesions. It is excellent to generate flesh and stop bleeding in treatment of non-healing ulcers, wet lesions, oral ulcers and various bleeding disorders. Taken internally, *Er Cha* clears heat, dispels phlegm, stops diarrhea, generates body fluids, arrests cough from Lung heat, and relieves diarrhea and thirst during summertime.

Unprocessed ***Wa Leng Zi*** (Concha Arcae) dispels phlegm, disperses stagnation and softens hardness for treatment of scrofula, goiter, and chronic cough with scanty, sticky, difficult-to-expectorate sputum. Processed *Wa Leng Zi* is often taken internally to treat stomach pain with acid reflux.

Peng Sha (Borax) is not toxic and is used externally to clear heat, eliminates toxins, reduce swelling and prevent decay. It can be used to treat swollen and painful throats, oral ulcers, and swelling and pain in the eyes. When taken internally, it clears the Lung, dissolves phlegm and treats cough with phlegm due to heat in the Lung.

Lu Gan Shi (Galamina) eliminates toxins, dries dampness, generates flesh, and relieves itching, primarily for skin and eye disorders.

Mu Bie Zi (Semen Momordicae) reduces swelling, disperses nodules, eliminates toxins, and treats sores and abscesses.

Wu Ming Yi (Pyrolusitum) reduces swelling and pain, stops bleeding, and promotes generation of flesh in traumatic and external injuries.

SUBSTANCES FOR TOPICAL USE FROM OTHER FUNCTIONAL CATEGORIES

Many substances used primarily for internal treatment also have topical uses. Please consult individual herb monographs for details.

Part III — Additional Resources

索引

Appendix 1 — Cross-reference Based on Traditional Chinese Medicine Diagnosis

The listing of any herb under a diagnosis does not insure that that substance can be unquestioningly prescribed for the named symptom or syndrome. Selection and combination of herbs must be based on careful differential diagnosis, guided by informed understanding and training in Chinese Herbal Medicine.

1. Abdominal pain

Qi stagnation

Chen Xiang (Lignum Aquilariae Resinatum)
Chuan Lian Zi (Fructus Toosendan)
Fo Shou (Fructus Citri Sarcodactylis)
Hou Po (Cortex Magnoliae Officinalis)
Mu Xiang (Radix Aucklandiae)
Qing Mu Xiang (Radix Aristolochiae)
Qing Pi (Pericarpium Citri Reticulatae Viride)
Rou Dou Kou (Semen Myristicae)
Sha Ren (Fructus Amomi)
Tan Xiang (Lignum Santali Albi)
Wu Yao (Radix Linderae)
Xiang Fu (Rhizoma Cyperi)
Yi Zhi Ren (Fructus Alpiniae Oxyphyllae)
Zhi Shi (Fructus Aurantii Immaturus)

Blood stagnation

Bai Jiang Cao (Herba cum Radice Patriniae)
E Zhu (Rhizoma Curcumae)
Gui Zhi (Ramulus Cinnamomi)
Hong Hua (Flos Carthami)
Liu Ji Nu (Herba Artemisiae Anomalae)
San Leng (Rhizoma Sparganii)
Shan Zha (Fructus Crataegi)
Su Mu (Lignum Sappan)
Tao Ren (Semen Persicae)
Wu Ling Zhi (Excrementum Trogopteri seu Pteromi)
Yan Hu Suo (Rhizoma Corydalis)
Yi Mu Cao (Herba Leonuri)

Food stagnation

Mai Ya (Fructus Hordei Germinatus)
Shan Zha (Fructus Crataegi)
Shen Qu (Massa Fermentata)

Blood deficiency

Dang Gui (Radicis Angelicae Sinensis)
Shu Di Huang (Radix Rehmanniae Preparata)

Deficiency and cold

Ai Ye (Folium Artemisiae Argyi)
Yi Tang (Saccharum Granorum)

Intestinal abscess

Bai Jiang Cao (Herba cum Radice Patriniae)
Chi Shao (Radix Paeoniae Rubrae)
Da Huang (Radix et Rhizoma Rhei)
Hong Teng (Caulis Sargentodoxae)
Mu Dan Pi (Cortex Moutan)
Tao Ren (Semen Persicae)

2. Anxiety

Heart fire

Zhu Sha (Cinnabaris)

Liver yang rising

Ci Shi (Magnetitum)
Long Gu (Os Draconis)
Mu Li (Concha Ostreae)
Zhen Zhu (Margarita)

Phlegm stagnation

Yuan Zhi (Radix Polygalae)
Zhu Li (Succus Bambusae)

Heat
Ling Yang Jiao (Cornu Saigae Tataricae)

Yin deficiency
Bai He (Bulbus Lilii)
Mai Men Dong (Radix Ophiopogonis)
Tian Men Dong (Radix Asparagi)

Blood deficiency
Bai Zi Ren (Semen Platycladi)
E Jiao (Colla Corii Asini)
Gui Ban (Plastrum Testudinis)
He Huan Pi (Cortex Albiziae)
Lian Zi (Semen Nelumbinis)
Long Yan Rou (Arillus Longan)
Sang Shen Zi (Fructus Mori)
Suan Zao Ren (Semen Zizyphi Spinosae)
Ye Jiao Teng (Caulis Polygoni Multiflori)

Qi and blood deficiency
Ren Shen (Radix Ginseng)
Sha Shen (Radix Glehniae seu Adenophorae)
Xi Yang Shen (Radix Panacis Quinquefolii)

Qi and yin deficiency
Wu Wei Zi (Fructus Schisandrae Chinensis)

3. *Ben tun* (running piglet)
Li Zhi He (Semen Litchi)

4. *Bi zheng* (closed disorder)
She Xiang (Moschus)
Su He Xiang (Styrax)
Zao Jiao (Fructus Gleditsiae)
Zhu Li (Succus Bambusae)

5. *Bi zheng* (painful obstruction syndrome)

***Xing bi* (mobile painful obstruction)**
Bai Hua She (Bungarus Parvus)
Chuan Xiong (Rhizoma Ligustici Chuanxiong)
Fang Feng (Radix Saposhnikoviae)
Gao Ben (Rhizoma Ligustici)
Hai Feng Teng (Caulis Piperis Kadsurae)
Lu Feng Fang (Nidus Vespae)
Luo Shi Teng (Caulis Trachelospermi)
Ma Qian Zi (Semen Strychni)
Man Jing Zi (Fructus Viticis)
Qian Nian Jian (Rhizoma Homalomenae)
Qiang Huo (Rhizoma et Radix Notopterygii)
Qin Jiao (Radix Gentianae Macrophyllae)
Quan Xie (Scorpio)
She Tui (Periostracum Serpentis)
Si Gua Luo (Retinervus Luffae Fructus)
Tian Ma (Rhizoma Gastrodiae)
Wu Gong (Scolopendra)
Wu Shao She (Zaocys)
Xu Chang Qing (Radix Cynanchi Paniculati)
Xun Gu Feng (Herba Aristolochiae Mollissimae)

***Tong bi* (extremely painful obstruction)**
Cao Wu (Radix Aconiti Kusnezoffii)
Chuan Wu (Radix Aconiti Preparata)
Fu Zi (Radix Aconiti Lateralis Praeparata)
Gao Ben (Rhizoma Ligustici)
Gui Zhi (Ramulus Cinnamomi)
Hu Lu Ba (Semen Trigonellae)
Ma Huang (Herba Ephedrae)
Rou Gui (Cortex Cinnamomi)
Xi Xin (Herba Asari)
Xian Mao (Rhizoma Curculiginis)
Yin Yang Huo (Herba Epimedii)

***Zhuo bi* (fixed painful obstruction)**
Bi Xie (Rhizoma Dioscoreae Hypoglaucae)
Can Sha (Excrementum Bombycis Mori)
Cang Er Zi (Fructus Xanthii)
Cang Zhu (Rhizoma Atractylodis)
Du Huo (Radix Angelicae Pubescentis)
Mu Gua (Fructus Chaenomelis)
Qiang Huo (Rhizoma et Radix Notopterygii)
Shi Chang Pu (Rhizoma Acori)
Song Jie (Lignum Pini Nodi)
Yi Yi Ren (Semen Coicis)

***Shi re bi* (damp-heat painful obstruction)**
Chou Wu Tong (Folium Clerodendri Trichotomi)
Chuan Mu Tong (Caulis Clematidis Armandii)
Di Long (Pheretima)
Fen Fang Ji (Radix Stephaniae Tetandrae)
Hai Tong Pi (Cortex Erythrinae)
Huang Bai (Cortex Phellodendri)
Luo Shi Teng (Caulis Trachelospermi)
Qin Jiao (Radix Gentianae Macrophyllae)
Xi Xian Cao (Herba Siegesbeckiae)

***Re bi* (heat painful obstruction)**
Bai Xian Pi (Cortex Dictamni)
Hong Teng (Caulis Sargentodoxae)
Ren Dong Teng (Caulis Lonicerae)
Sang Zhi (Ramulus Mori)

6. Bleeding

Cold in the blood
Ai Ye (Folium Artemisiae Argyi)
Fu Long Gan (Terra Flava Usta)

Heat in the blood
Bai Mao Gen (Rhizoma Imperatae)
Ce Bai Ye (Cacumen Platycladi)
Da Huang (Radix et Rhizoma Rhei)
Da Ji (Herba seu Radix Cirsii Japonici)
Dai Zhe Shi (Haematitum)
Di Gu Pi (Cortex Lycii)
Di Yu (Radix Sanguisorbae)
Guan Zhong (Rhizoma Dryopteridis)
Huai Hua (Flos Sophorae)
Huai Jiao (Fructus Sophorae)
Huang Qin (Radix Scutellariae)
Ma Bo (Lasiosphaera seu Calvatia)
Mu Zei (Herba Equiseti Hiemalis)
Niu Xi (Radix Cyathulae seu Achyranthis)
Qian Cao (Radix Rubiae)
Sang Ye (Folium Mori)
Shi Wei (Folium Pyrrosiae)
Xi Yang Shen (Radix Panacis Quinquefolii)
Xiao Ji (Herba Cirisii)
Yu Jin (Radix Curcumae)
Zhi Zi (Fructus Gardeniae)

Blood stagnation
Hua Rui Shi (Ophicalcitum)
San Qi (Radix Notoginseng)

Others
Bai Ji (Rhizoma Bletillae)
Hai Piao Xiao (Endoconcha Sepiae)
Ou Jie (Nodus Nelumbinis Rhizomatis)
Pu Huang (Pollen Typhae)
Xian He Cao (Herba Agrimoniae)
Zi Zhu (Folium Callicarpae)
Zong Lu Pi (Fibra Stipulae Trachycarpi)

7. Breast abscess
Bai Zhi (Radix Angelicae Dahuricae)

Ban Xia (Rhizoma Pinelliae)
Chuan Bei Mu (Bulbus Fritillariae Cirrhosae)
Gua Lou Ren (Semen Trichosanthis)
Lou Lu (Radix Rhapontici)
Mang Xiao (Natrii Sulfas)
Ming Fan (Alumen)
Pu Gong Ying (Herba Taraxaci)
Si Gua Luo (Retinervus Luffae Fructus)
Tian Hua Fen (Radix Trichosanthis)
Wang Bu Liu Xing (Semen Vaccariae)

8. Burns

Bai Wei (Radix Cynanchi Atrati)
Ce Bai Ye (Cacumen Platycladi)
Da Huang (Radix et Rhizoma Rhei)
Di Yu (Radix Sanguisorbae)
Han Shui Shi (Mirabilite)
Hu Zhang (Rhizoma Polygoni Cuspidati)
Huang Bai (Cortex Phellodendri)
Shi Gao (Gypsum Fibrosum)
Zi Zhu (Folium Callicarpae)

9. Cancer

Stomach
Bai Hua She She Cao (Herba Oldenlandia)
Long Kui (Herba Solanum Nigrum)
Peng Sha (Borax)

Lung
Bai Hua She She Cao (Herba Oldenlandia)
Ban Zhi Lian (Herba Scutellariae Barbatae)

Liver
Ban Mao (Mylabris)
Ban Zhi Lian (Herba Scutellariae Barbatae)
Ma Qian Zi (Semen Strychni)

Throat
Shan Dou Gen (Radix Sophorae Tonkinensis)
Tian Kui Zi (Radix Semiaquilegiae)

Urinary bladder
Tian Kui Zi (Radix Semiaquilegiae)

Rectal
Er Cha (Catechu)
Huang Jing (Rhizoma Polygonati)
Peng Sha (Borax)

Lymphatic
Tian Kui Zi (Radix Semiaquilegiae)

Breast
Lu Feng Fang (Nidus Vespae)
Shan Ci Gu (Pseudobulbus Cremastrae)
Tian Kui Zi (Radix Semiaquilegiae)

Cervical
E Zhu (Rhizoma Curcumae)
Long Kui (Herba Solanum Nigrum)

10. Carbuncles and furuncles

Yang type
Bai Hua She She Cao (Herba Oldenlandia)
Bai Ji (Rhizoma Bletillae)
Bai Jiang Cao (Herba cum Radice Patriniae)
Bai Wei (Radix Cynanchi Atrati)
Bai Xian Pi (Cortex Dictamni)
Bai Zhi (Radix Angelicae Dahuricae)
Ban Mao (Mylabris)
Ban Xia (Rhizoma Pinelliae)
Bei Mu (Bulbus Fritillaria)
Chi Shao (Radix Paeoniae Rubrae)
Chi Xiao Dou (Semen Phaseoli)
Chuan Shan Jia (Squama Manis)
Chuan Xin Lian (Herba Andrographis)
Chuan Xiong (Rhizoma Ligustici Chuanxiong)
Cong Bai (Bulbus Allii Fistulosi)
Da Huang (Radix et Rhizoma Rhei)
Da Ji (Radix Euphorbiae seu Knoxiae)
Dan Shen (Radix Salviae Miltiorrhizae)
Gan Cao (Radix Glycyrrhizae)
Gan Sui (Radix Euphorbiae Kansui)
He Huan Pi (Cortex Albiziae)
He Shou Wu (Radix Polygoni Multiflori)
Hu Zhang (Rhizoma Polygoni Cuspidati)
Huang Bai (Cortex Phellodendri)
Huang Lian (Rhizoma Coptidis)
Huang Qin (Radix Scutellariae)
Huang Yao Zi (Herba Dioscoreae Bulbiferae)
Jiang Can (Bombyx Batryticatus)
Jin Qian Cao (Herba Lysimachiae)
Jin Yin Hua (Flos Lonicerae)
Jing Jie (Herba Schizonepetae)
Lian Qiao (Fructus Forsythiae)
Lou Lu (Radix Rhapontici)
Lu Dou (Semen Phaseoli Radiati)
Ma Chi Xian (Herba Portulacae)
Mang Xiao (Natrii Sulfas)
Ming Fan (Alumen)
Mu Dan Pi (Cortex Moutan)
Niu Bang Zi (Fructus Arctii)
Niu Huang (Calculus Bovis)
Pu Gong Ying (Herba Taraxaci)
Qian Niu Zi (Semen Pharbitidis)
Qing Dai (Indigo Naturalis)
Quan Xie (Scorpio)
Ru Xiang (Gummi Olibanum)
Shan Ci Gu (Pseudobulbus Cremastrae)
Shan Dou Gen (Radix Sophorae Tonkinensis)
Sheng Ma (Rhizoma Cimicifugae)
Si Gua Luo (Retinervus Luffae Fructus)
Tian Hua Fen (Radix Trichosanthis)
Tu Fu Ling (Rhizoma Smilacis Glabrae)
Wu Gong (Scolopendra)
Xi Xian Cao (Herba Siegesbeckiae)
Xia Ku Cao (Spica Prunellae)
Xiao Ji (Herba Cirisii)
Xiong Huang (Realgar)
Xu Duan (Radix Dipsaci)
Xuan Shen (Radix Scrophulariae)
Yi Mu Cao (Herba Leonuri)
Yu Xing Cao (Herba Houttuyniae)
Yuan Zhi (Radix Polygalae)
Zao Jiao (Fructus Gleditsiae)
Zao Jiao Ci (Spina Gleditsiae)
Ze Lan (Herba Lycopi)
Zhu Dan (Fel Porcus)
Zhu Sha (Cinnabaris)
Zi Hua Di Ding (Herba Violae)
Zi Zhu (Folium Callicarpae)

Yin type
Bai Ji (Rhizoma Bletillae)
Bai Jie Zi (Semen Sinapis)
Ban Mao (Mylabris)
Ban Xia (Rhizoma Pinelliae)
Chuan Shan Jia (Squama Manis)
Dang Gui (Radicis Angelicae Sinensis)
Dang Shen (Radix Codonopsis)
E Jiao (Colla Corii Asini)
Er Cha (Catechu)
Hai Piao Xiao (Endoconcha Sepiae)
Huang Qi (Radix Astragali)
Long Gu (Os Draconis)
Lu Lu Tong (Fructus Liquidambaris)
Ma Huang (Herba Ephedrae)
Ma Qian Zi (Semen Strychni)
Ming Fan (Alumen)
Mo Yao (Myrrha)
Qian Dan (Minium)
Qing Fen (Calomelas)
Ren Shen (Radix Ginseng)
Rou Gui (Cortex Cinnamomi)
Ru Xiang (Gummi Olibanum)

Shi Gao (Gypsum Fibrosum)
Shu Di Huang (Radix Rehmanniae Preparata)
Xue Jie (Sanguis Draconis)
Zao Jiao Ci (Spina Gleditsiae)
Zhen Zhu (Margarita)

11. *Chang feng* (intestinal wind)

Ding Shu Xiu (Herba Elephantopus Scaber)
Fang Feng (Radix Saposhnikoviae)
Guan Ye Lian Qiao (Herba Hypericum)
Pao Zai Cao (Herba Physalis Angulatae)
Zong Lu Pi (Fibra Stipulae Trachycarpi)

12. Chest pain

Qi deficiency
Dang Shen (Radix Codonopsis)
Huang Qi (Radix Astragali)
Ren Shen (Radix Ginseng)
Tai Zi Shen (Radix Pseudostellariae)
Wu Wei Zi (Fructus Schisandrae Chinensis)
Xi Yang Shen (Radix Panacis Quinquefolii)

Qi stagnation
Chen Xiang (Lignum Aquilariae Resinatum)
Qing Mu Xiang (Radix Aristolochiae)
Tan Xiang (Lignum Santali Albi)
Wu Yao (Radix Linderae)
Zhi Ke (Fructus Aurantii)
Zhi Shi (Fructus Aurantii Immaturus)

Blood stagnation
Bai Jiang Cao (Herba cum Radice Patriniae)
Chuan Xiong (Rhizoma Ligustici Chuanxiong)
Dan Shen (Radix Salviae Miltiorrhizae)
Hong Hua (Flos Carthami)
Jiang Huang (Rhizoma Curcumae Longae)
Jiang Xiang (Lignum Dalbergiae Odoriferae)
Mao Dong Qing (Radix Ilicis Pubescentis)
Shan Zha (Fructus Crataegi)
Wu Ling Zhi (Excrementum Trogopteri seu Pteromi)
Yan Hu Suo (Rhizoma Corydalis)
Yu Jin (Radix Curcumae)

Phlegm stagnation
Bai Jie Zi (Semen Sinapis)
Ban Xia (Rhizoma Pinelliae)
Chen Pi (Pericarpium Citri Reticulatae)
Gua Lou Shi (Fructus Trichosanthis)
Gui Zhi (Ramulus Cinnamomi)
Hou Po (Cortex Magnoliae Officinalis)
Xie Bai (Bulbus Allii Macrostemonis)
Zhi Shi (Fructus Aurantii Immaturus)

Yang deficiency
Fu Zi (Radix Aconiti Lateralis Praeparata)
Gui Zhi (Ramulus Cinnamomi)
Xie Bai (Bulbus Allii Macrostemonis)
Yin Yang Huo (Herba Epimedii)

13. Constipation

Excess heat
Da Huang (Radix et Rhizoma Rhei)
Fan Xie Ye (Folium Sennae)
Hou Po (Cortex Magnoliae Officinalis)
Hu Zhang (Rhizoma Polygoni Cuspidati)
Jue Ming Zi (Semen Cassiae)
Lu Hui (Aloe)
Mang Xiao (Natrii Sulfas)
Zhi Shi (Fructus Aurantii Immaturus)
Zhu Dan (Fel Porcus)

Heat and dryness
Dang Gui (Radicis Angelicae Sinensis)
Dong Kui Zi (Semen Malvae)
Feng Mi (Mel)
Gua Lou Ren (Semen Trichosanthis)
He Shou Wu (Radix Polygoni Multiflori)
Hei Zhi Ma (Semen Sesami Nigrum)
Hu Tao Ren (Semen Juglandis)
Huo Ma Ren (Fructus Cannabis)
Jue Ming Zi (Semen Cassiae)
Rou Cong Rong (Herba Cistanches)
Sang Shen Zi (Fructus Mori)
Sheng Di Huang (Radix Rehmanniae)
Su Zi (Fructus Perillae)
Suo Yang (Herba Cynomorii)
Tao Ren (Semen Persicae)
Tian Men Dong (Radix Asparagi)
Xing Ren (Semen Armeniacae Amarum)
Yu Li Ren (Semen Pruni)

Qi stagnation
Bing Lang (Semen Arecae)
Chen Xiang (Lignum Aquilariae Resinatum)
Zhi Ke (Fructus Aurantii)

Deficiency
Bai Zhu (Rhizoma Atractylodis Macrocephalae)
Bai Zi Ren (Semen Platycladi)
Feng Mi (Mel)
Hei Zhi Ma (Semen Sesami Nigrum)

Cold
Ba Dou (Fructus Crotonis)
Hei Zhi Ma (Semen Sesami Nigrum)
Liu Huang (Sulfur)
Rou Cong Rong (Herba Cistanches)

Collapse of *zhong* (central) *qi*
Chai Hu (Radix Bupleuri)
Ge Gen (Radix Puerariae)
Gui Zhi (Ramulus Cinnamomi)
Huang Qi (Radix Astragali)
Ren Shen (Radix Ginseng)
Sheng Ma (Rhizoma Cimicifugae)
Zhi Ke (Fructus Aurantii)
Zhi Shi (Fructus Aurantii Immaturus)

14. Convulsions

Excess heat
Long Dan Cao (Radix Gentianae)
Niu Huang (Calculus Bovis)
Qing Dai (Indigo Naturalis)

Febrile disorders
Ling Yang Jiao (Cornu Saigae Tataricae)
Niu Huang (Calculus Bovis)
She Xiang (Moschus)

Heat and phlegm
Jiang Can (Bombyx Batryticatus)
Niu Huang (Calculus Bovis)

Liver yang rising
Gui Ban (Plastrum Testudinis)
Hu Po (Succinum)
Long Gu (Os Draconis)
Zhen Zhu (Margarita)

Wind and phlegm
Bai Fu Zi (Rhizoma Typhonii)
Bai Hua She (Bungarus Parvus)
Gan Sui (Radix Euphorbiae Kansui)
Hu Po (Succinum)
Li Lu (Radix et Rhizoma Veratri)
Meng Shi (Lapis Micae seu Chloriti)
Ming Fan (Alumen)
Quan Xie (Scorpio)
Tian Nan Xing (Rhizoma Arisaematis)
Tian Zhu Huang (Concretio Silicea Bambusae)

Wu Gong (Scolopendra)
Wu Shao She (Zaocys)
Xiong Huang (Realgar)
Zao Jiao (Fructus Gleditsiae)
Zhu Li (Succus Bambusae)

15. Cough

Wind-cold
Bai Qian (Rhizoma Cynanchi Stauntonii)
Ma Huang (Herba Ephedrae)
Sheng Jiang (Rhizoma Zingiberis Recens)
Xing Ren (Semen Armeniacae Amarum)
Zi Su Ye (Folium Perillae)

Wind-heat
Jie Geng (Radix Platycodonis)
Ju Hua (Flos Chrysanthemi)
Lu Gen (Rhizoma Phragmitis)
Niu Bang Zi (Fructus Arctii)
Qian Hu (Radix Peucedani)
Sang Ye (Folium Mori)

Dry-heat
Bai Bu (Radix Stemonae)
Chuan Bei Mu (Bulbus Fritillariae Cirrhosae)
Fei Zi (Semen Torreyae)
Gan Cao (Radix Glycyrrhizae)
Kuan Dong Hua (Flos Farfarae)
Sang Ye (Folium Mori)
Zhi Mu (Radix Anemarrhenae)
Zi Wan (Radix Asteris)

Cold phlegm
Bai Jie Zi (Semen Sinapis)
Bai Qian (Rhizoma Cynanchi Stauntonii)
Gan Jiang (Rhizoma Zingiberis)
Lai Fu Zi (Semen Raphani)
Tian Nan Xing (Rhizoma Arisaematis)
Xuan Fu Hua (Flos Inulae)
Yuan Hua (Flos Genkwa)

Damp phlegm
Ban Xia (Rhizoma Pinelliae)
Chen Pi (Pericarpium Citri Reticulatae)
Lai Fu Zi (Semen Raphani)
Su Zi (Fructus Perillae)
Tian Nan Xing (Rhizoma Arisaematis)
Xiang Yuan (Fructus Citri)
Yuan Hua (Flos Genkwa)

Hot phlegm
Ce Bai Ye (Cacumen Platycladi)
Che Qian Zi (Semen Plantaginis)
Chuan Bei Mu (Bulbus Fritillariae Cirrhosae)
Chuan Xin Lian (Herba Andrographis)
Dan Nan Xing (Arisaema cum Bile)
Di Gu Pi (Cortex Lycii)
Gua Lou Shi (Fructus Trichosanthis)
Hai Ge Fen (Concha Meretricis seu Cyclinae)
Hu Zhang (Rhizoma Polygoni Cuspidati)
Ma Dou Ling (Fructus Aristolochiae)
Meng Shi (Lapis Micae seu Chloriti)
Pang Da Hai (Semen Sterculiae Lychnophorae)
Peng Sha (Borax)
Qian Hu (Radix Peucedani)
Qing Dai (Indigo Naturalis)
Sang Bai Pi (Cortex Mori)
Shan Dou Gen (Radix Sophorae Tonkinensis)
She Gan (Rhizoma Belamcandae)
Shi Wei (Folium Pyrrosiae)
Tian Zhu Huang (Concretio Silicea Bambusae)
Zhe Bei Mu (Bulbus Fritillariae Thunbergii)
Zhi Mu (Radix Anemarrhenae)
Zhu Dan (Fel Porcus)
Zhu Li (Succus Bambusae)
Zhu Ru (Caulis Bambusae in Taenia)

Qi deficiency
Dang Shen (Radix Codonopsis)
Feng Mi (Mel)
Ge Jie (Gecko)
He Zi (Fructus Chebulae)
Hu Tao Ren (Semen Juglandis)
Huang Qi (Radix Astragali)
Ren Shen (Radix Ginseng)
Shan Yao (Rhizoma Dioscoreae)
Tai Zi Shen (Radix Pseudostellariae)
Wu Bei Zi (Galla Chinensis)
Wu Mei (Fructus Mume)
Wu Wei Zi (Fructus Schisandrae Chinensis)
Xi Yang Shen (Radix Panacis Quinquefolii)
Yi Tang (Saccharum Granorum)
Ying Su Ke (Pericarpium Papaveris Somniferi)

Yin deficiency
Bai Bu (Radix Stemonae)
Bai He (Bulbus Lilii)
Chuan Bei Mu (Bulbus Fritillariae Cirrhosae)
E Jiao (Colla Corii Asini)
Gou Qi Zi (Fructus Lycii)
Huang Jing (Rhizoma Polygonati)
Mai Men Dong (Radix Ophiopogonis)
Sha Shen (Radix Glehniae seu Adenophorae)
Tian Men Dong (Radix Asparagi)
Yu Zhu (Rhizoma Polygonati Odorati)
Zhi Mu (Radix Anemarrhenae)

Lung heat
Bai Mao Gen (Rhizoma Imperatae)
Che Qian Zi (Semen Plantaginis)
Chuan Xin Lian (Herba Andrographis)
Di Gu Pi (Cortex Lycii)
Er Cha (Catechu)
Hu Zhang (Rhizoma Polygoni Cuspidati)
Huang Qin (Radix Scutellariae)
Lu Gen (Rhizoma Phragmitis)
Ma Bo (Lasiosphaera seu Calvatia)
Ma Dou Ling (Fructus Aristolochiae)
Shi Gao (Gypsum Fibrosum)
Shi Wei (Folium Pyrrosiae)
Tian Hua Fen (Radix Trichosanthis)
Xia Ku Cao (Spica Prunellae)
Yu Xing Cao (Herba Houttuyniae)
Zhi Mu (Radix Anemarrhenae)
Zhu Dan (Fel Porcus)
Zhu Ru (Caulis Bambusae in Taenia)

16. Diarrhea

Qi stagnation
Bing Lang (Semen Arecae)
Xiang Fu (Rhizoma Cyperi)

Damp-cold
Cao Dou Kou (Semen Alpiniae Katsumadai)
Cao Guo (Fructus Tsaoko)
Sha Ren (Fructus Amomi)

Accumulation of water and dampness
Fu Ling (Poria)
Ze Xie (Rhizoma Alismatis)

Accumulation of summer-heat and dampness
Che Qian Zi (Semen Plantaginis)
Hua Shi (Talcum)

Spleen deficiency
Ai Ye (Folium Artemisiae Argyi)
Bai Zhu (Rhizoma Atractylodis Macrocephalae)
Bian Dou (Semen Lablab Album)
Fu Ling (Poria)
Gan Cao (Radix Glycyrrhizae)
Ge Gen (Radix Puerariae)
Lian Zi (Semen Nelumbinis)
Qian Shi (Semen Euryales)
Shan Yao (Rhizoma Dioscoreae)
Sheng Ma (Rhizoma Cimicifugae)
Tu Si Zi (Semen Cuscutae)
Xian He Cao (Herba Agrimoniae)
Yi Yi Ren (Semen Coicis)

Kidney deficiency
Bu Gu Zhi (Fructus Psoraleae)
Wu Wei Zi (Fructus Schisandrae Chinensis)
Wu Zhu Yu (Fructus Evodiae)
Yi Zhi Ren (Fructus Alpiniae Oxyphyllae)

Spleen and Kidney deficiencies
Chi Shi Zhi (Halloysitum Rubrum)
Chun Gen Pi (Cortex Ailanthi)
He Zi (Fructus Chebulae)
Jin Ying Zi (Fructus Rosae Laevigatae)
Rou Dou Kou (Semen Myristicae)
Shi Liu Pi (Pericarpium Granati)
Wu Bei Zi (Galla Chinensis)
Wu Mei (Fructus Mume)
Wu Wei Zi (Fructus Schisandrae Chinensis)
Ying Su Ke (Pericarpium Papaveris Somniferi)
Yu Yu Liang (Limonitum)

17. Dizziness

Liver yang rising
Bai Ji Li (Fructus Tribuli)
Bai Shao (Radix Paeoniae Alba)
Ci Shi (Magnetitum)
Dai Zhe Shi (Haematitum)
Du Zhong (Cortex Eucommiae)
Gou Teng (Ramulus Uncariae cum Uncis)
Gui Ban (Plastrum Testudinis)
Ju Hua (Flos Chrysanthemi)
Jue Ming Zi (Semen Cassiae)
Ling Yang Jiao (Cornu Saigae Tataricae)
Long Gu (Os Draconis)
Lu Dou Yi (Pericarpium Phaseoli Radiati)
Mu Li (Concha Ostreae)
Qing Xiang Zi (Semen Celosiae)
Shi Jue Ming (Concha Haliotidis)
Tian Ma (Rhizoma Gastrodiae)
Xia Ku Cao (Spica Prunellae)
Zhen Zhu Mu (Concha Margaritafẽrae)

Liver fire rising
Gou Teng (Ramulus Uncariae cum Uncis)
Hua Jiao (Pericarpium Zanthoxyli)
Huai Hua (Flos Sophorae)
Ju Hua (Flos Chrysanthemi)
Ling Yang Jiao (Cornu Saigae Tataricae)
Long Dan Cao (Radix Gentianae)
Lu Hui (Aloe)
Qing Xiang Zi (Semen Celosiae)
Xia Ku Cao (Spica Prunellae)

Liver wind rising
Gou Teng (Ramulus Uncariae cum Uncis)
Ju Hua (Flos Chrysanthemi)
Ling Yang Jiao (Cornu Saigae Tataricae)
Tian Ma (Rhizoma Gastrodiae)

Blood deficiency
Bai Shao (Radix Paeoniae Alba)
Dang Gui (Radicis Angelicae Sinensis)
E Jiao (Colla Corii Asini)
He Shou Wu (Radix Polygoni Multiflori)
Long Yan Rou (Arillus Longan)
Lu Dou Yi (Pericarpium Phaseoli Radiati)
Sang Shen Zi (Fructus Mori)
Shu Di Huang (Radix Rehmanniae Preparata)
Zi He Che (Placenta Hominis)

Qi deficiency
Dang Shen (Radix Codonopsis)
Huang Qi (Radix Astragali)
Ren Shen (Radix Ginseng)
Tai Zi Shen (Radix Pseudostellariae)
Xi Yang Shen (Radix Panacis Quinquefolii)

Yin deficiency
Gou Qi Zi (Fructus Lycii)
He Shou Wu (Radix Polygoni Multiflori)
Hei Zhi Ma (Semen Sesami Nigrum)
Huang Jing (Rhizoma Polygonati)
Nu Zhen Zi (Fructus Ligustri Lucidi)
Sang Shen Zi (Fructus Mori)
Shan Yao (Rhizoma Dioscoreae)
Shan Zhu Yu (Fructus Corni)
Shu Di Huang (Radix Rehmanniae Preparata)
Zi He Che (Placenta Hominis)

Yang deficiency
Lu Lu Tong (Fructus Liquidambaris)
Sha Yuan Zi (Semen Astragali Complanati)
Shan Zhu Yu (Fructus Corni)
Tu Si Zi (Semen Cuscutae)
Zi He Che (Placenta Hominis)

Phlegm stagnation
Bai Zhu (Rhizoma Atractylodis Macrocephalae)
Ban Xia (Rhizoma Pinelliae)
Fu Ling (Poria)
Tian Nan Xing (Rhizoma Arisaematis)
Ze Xie (Rhizoma Alismatis)
Zhu Ru (Caulis Bambusae in Taenia)

18. Dysentery

Damp-heat
Bai Tou Weng (Radix Pulsatillae)
Chuan Xin Lian (Herba Andrographis)
Da Huang (Radix et Rhizoma Rhei)
Huang Bai (Cortex Phellodendri)
Huang Lian (Rhizoma Coptidis)
Huang Qin (Radix Scutellariae)
Jin Yin Hua (Flos Lonicerae)
Ku Shen Gen (Radix Sophorae Flavescentis)
Ma Chi Xian (Herba Portulacae)
Qin Pi (Cortex Fraxini)
Xian He Cao (Herba Agrimoniae)
Ya Dan Zi (Fructus Bruceae)

Damp-cold
Cang Zhu (Rhizoma Atractylodis)
Hou Po (Cortex Magnoliae Officinalis)
Mu Xiang (Radix Aucklandiae)
Pao Jiang (Rhizoma Zingiberis Preparatum)
Rou Gui (Cortex Cinnamomi)

Fulminant dysentery
Bai Tou Weng (Radix Pulsatillae)
Chi Shao (Radix Paeoniae Rubrae)
Huang Bai (Cortex Phellodendri)
Huang Lian (Rhizoma Coptidis)
Jin Yin Hua (Flos Lonicerae)
Qin Pi (Cortex Fraxini)
Ya Dan Zi (Fructus Bruceae)
Zhu Dan (Fel Porcus)

Recurrent dysentery
Bai Tou Weng (Radix Pulsatillae)
Huang Lian (Rhizoma Coptidis)

Ku Shen Gen (Radix Sophorae Flavescentis)
Ya Dan Zi (Fructus Bruceae)

Fasting dysentery
Shi Chang Pu (Rhizoma Acori)
Shi Lian Zi (Herba Sinocrassulae Indicae)

19. Edema

Edema with exterior syndrome
Fu Ping (Herba Spirodelae)
Gui Zhi (Ramulus Cinnamomi)
Ma Huang (Herba Ephedrae)
Xiang Ru (Herba Elsholtziae seu Moslae)

Edema (General)
Da Fu Pi (Pericarpium Arecae)
Sang Bai Pi (Cortex Mori)
Sheng Jiang Pi (Pericarpium Zingiberis Recens)
Wu Jia Pi (Cortex Acanthopanacis)

Yang deficiency
Fu Zi (Radix Aconiti Lateralis Praeparata)
Gui Zhi (Ramulus Cinnamomi)
Rou Gui (Cortex Cinnamomi)

Spleen deficiency
Bai Zhu (Rhizoma Atractylodis Macrocephalae)
Fu Ling (Poria)
Yi Yi Ren (Semen Coicis)

Damp-cold
Fu Zi (Radix Aconiti Lateralis Praeparata)
Gui Zhi (Ramulus Cinnamomi)
Wu Jia Pi (Cortex Acanthopanacis)

Accumulation of water
Chi Xiao Dou (Semen Phaseoli)
Sang Bai Pi (Cortex Mori)
Shi Wei (Folium Pyrrosiae)
Ting Li Zi (Semen Descurainiae seu Lepidii)
Wu Jia Pi (Cortex Acanthopanacis)
Yi Mu Cao (Herba Leonuri)
Ze Lan (Herba Lycopi)
Ze Xie (Rhizoma Alismatis)

Damp-heat
Ba Dou (Fructus Crotonis)
Bai Mao Gen (Rhizoma Imperatae)
Ban Bian Lian (Herba Lobeliae Chinensis)
Che Qian Zi (Semen Plantaginis)
Da Ji (Radix Euphorbiae seu Knoxiae)
Dong Gua Pi (Exocarpium Benincasae)
Dong Kui Zi (Semen Malvae)
Fen Fang Ji (Radix Stephaniae Tetandrae)
Gan Sui (Radix Euphorbiae Kansui)
Hai Zao (Sargassum)
Kun Bu (Thallus Laminariae seu Eckloniae)
Qian Niu Zi (Semen Pharbitidis)
Shi Wei (Folium Pyrrosiae)
Ting Li Zi (Semen Descurainiae seu Lepidii)
Yuan Hua (Flos Genkwa)

20. Eye disorders

Wind-heat
Bai Ji Li (Fructus Tribuli)
Bo He (Herba Menthae)
Chan Tui (Periostracum Cicadae)
Chi Shao (Radix Paeoniae Rubrae)
Gu Jing Cao (Flos Eriocauli)
Jiang Can (Bombyx Batryticatus)
Ju Hua (Flos Chrysanthemi)
Jue Ming Zi (Semen Cassiae)
Man Jing Zi (Fructus Viticis)
Mu Zei (Herba Equiseti Hiemalis)
Sang Ye (Folium Mori)

Liver heat
Che Qian Cao (Herba Plantaginis)
Chi Shao (Radix Paeoniae Rubrae)
Chong Wei Zi (Semen Leonuri)
Da Huang (Radix et Rhizoma Rhei)
Jiang Can (Bombyx Batryticatus)
Ju Hua (Flos Chrysanthemi)
Jue Ming Zi (Semen Cassiae)
Ling Yang Jiao (Cornu Saigae Tataricae)
Mang Xiao (Natrii Sulfas)
Mi Meng Hua (Flos Buddlejae)
Qing Pi (Pericarpium Citri Reticulatae Viride)
Qing Xiang Zi (Semen Celosiae)
Sang Ye (Folium Mori)
Shi Jue Ming (Concha Haliotidis)
Xia Ku Cao (Spica Prunellae)
Zhen Zhu Mu (Concha Margaritaferae)
Zi Hua Di Ding (Herba Violae)

Dizziness due to Liver deficiency
Gou Qi Zi (Fructus Lycii)
Hei Zhi Ma (Semen Sesami Nigrum)
Nu Zhen Zi (Fructus Ligustri Lucidi)
Sang Shen Zi (Fructus Mori)
Sha Yuan Zi (Semen Astragali Complanati)
Shi Hu (Herba Dendrobii)
Tu Si Zi (Semen Cuscutae)

21. Fever

Yin deficiency heat
Bai Wei (Radix Cynanchi Atrati)
Bie Jia (Carapax Trionycis)
Di Gu Pi (Cortex Lycii)
Hu Huang Lian (Rhizoma Picrorhizae)
Huang Lian (Rhizoma Coptidis)
Mu Dan Pi (Cortex Moutan)
Qin Jiao (Radix Gentianae Macrophyllae)
Qing Hao (Herba Artemisiae Annuae)
Yin Chai Hu (Radix Stellariae)
Zhi Mu (Radix Anemarrhenae)

Qi deficiency with heat
Gan Cao (Radix Glycyrrhizae)
Huang Qi (Radix Astragali)
Ren Shen (Radix Ginseng)

Liver qi stagnation and Liver heat
Bo He (Herba Menthae)
Chai Hu (Radix Bupleuri)
Long Dan Cao (Radix Gentianae)
Mu Dan Pi (Cortex Moutan)
Zhi Zi (Fructus Gardeniae)

Blood stagnation with heat
Chi Shao (Radix Paeoniae Rubrae)
Dan Shen (Radix Salviae Miltiorrhizae)
Mu Dan Pi (Cortex Moutan)
Niu Xi (Radix Cyathulae seu Achyranthis)
Pu Huang (Pollen Typhae)
Wu Ling Zhi (Excrementum Trogopteri seu Pteromi)
Yi Mu Cao (Herba Leonuri)

22. Fungal infection

Ba Dou (Fructus Crotonis)
Ban Mao (Mylabris)
Chuan Lian Zi (Fructus Toosendan)
Ci Shi (Magnetitum)
Da Feng Zi (Semen Hydnocarpi)
Da Suan (Bulbus Alli Sativi)
Hai Tong Pi (Cortex Erythrinae)
Ku Lian Zi (Fructus Meliae)
Lu Hui (Aloe)
Qing Fen (Calomelas)
She Chuang Zi (Fructus Cnidii)
Wu Yi (Fructus Ulmi Praeparatus)

Xiong Huang (Realgar)
Xu Chang Qing (Radix Cynanchi Paniculati)
Yuan Hua (Flos Genkwa)
Zhang Nao (Camphora)

23. *Gan ji* (infantile malnutrition)

Di Gu Pi (Cortex Lycii)
Hu Huang Lian (Rhizoma Picrorhizae)
Ji Nei Jin (Endothelium Corneum Gigeriae Galli)
Shi Jun Zi (Fructus Quisqualis)
Yi Tang (Saccharum Granorum)
Yin Chai Hu (Radix Stellariae)

24. Headache

Wind-cold
Bai Zhi (Radix Angelicae Dahuricae)
Cang Er Zi (Fructus Xanthii)
Chuan Xiong (Rhizoma Ligustici Chuanxiong)
Du Huo (Radix Angelicae Pubescentis)
Fang Feng (Radix Saposhnikoviae)
Gao Ben (Rhizoma Ligustici)
Gui Zhi (Ramulus Cinnamomi)
Jing Jie (Herba Schizonepetae)
Ma Huang (Herba Ephedrae)
Qiang Huo (Rhizoma et Radix Notopterygii)
Xi Xin (Herba Asari)
Xiang Ru (Herba Elsholtziae seu Moslae)
Xin Yi Hua (Flos Magnoliae)
Zi Su Ye (Folium Perillae)

Wind-heat
Bo He (Herba Menthae)
Chan Tui (Periostracum Cicadae)
Dan Dou Chi (Semen Sojae Praeparatum)
Jiang Can (Bombyx Batryticatus)
Jin Yin Hua (Flos Lonicerae)
Jing Jie (Herba Schizonepetae)
Ju Hua (Flos Chrysanthemi)
Lian Qiao (Fructus Forsythiae)
Mu Zei (Herba Equiseti Hiemalis)
Niu Bang Zi (Fructus Arctii)
Sang Ye (Folium Mori)

Wind-dampness
Bai Zhi (Radix Angelicae Dahuricae)
Cang Er Zi (Fructus Xanthii)
Chuan Xiong (Rhizoma Ligustici Chuanxiong)
Du Huo (Radix Angelicae Pubescentis)
Fang Feng (Radix Saposhnikoviae)
Gao Ben (Rhizoma Ligustici)
Qiang Huo (Rhizoma et Radix Notopterygii)

Liver yang rising
Bai Ji Li (Fructus Tribuli)
Ci Shi (Magnetitum)
Dai Zhe Shi (Haematitum)
Gou Teng (Ramulus Uncariae cum Uncis)
Huai Hua (Flos Sophorae)
Huai Jiao (Fructus Sophorae)
Ju Hua (Flos Chrysanthemi)
Ling Yang Jiao (Cornu Saigae Tataricae)
Long Gu (Os Draconis)
Mu Li (Concha Ostreae)
Shi Jue Ming (Concha Haliotidis)
Tian Ma (Rhizoma Gastrodiae)
Zhen Zhu Mu (Concha Margaritaferae)

Qi deficiency
Chai Hu (Radix Bupleuri)
Dang Shen (Radix Codonopsis)
Ge Gen (Radix Puerariae)
Huang Qi (Radix Astragali)
Ren Shen (Radix Ginseng)
Sheng Ma (Rhizoma Cimicifugae)
Tai Zi Shen (Radix Pseudostellariae)
Xi Yang Shen (Radix Panacis Quinquefolii)

Kidney deficiency
Gou Qi Zi (Fructus Lycii)
He Shou Wu (Radix Polygoni Multiflori)
Shan Zhu Yu (Fructus Corni)
Shu Di Huang (Radix Rehmanniae Preparata)

Blood deficiency
Bai Shao (Radix Paeoniae Alba)
Dang Gui (Radicis Angelicae Sinensis)
Gou Qi Zi (Fructus Lycii)
He Shou Wu (Radix Polygoni Multiflori)
Lu Dou Yi (Pericarpium Phaseoli Radiati)
Sang Shen Zi (Fructus Mori)
Shu Di Huang (Radix Rehmanniae Preparata)

Blood stagnation
Chuan Niu Xi (Radix Cyathulae)
Chuan Xiong (Rhizoma Ligustici Chuanxiong)

Phlegm stagnation
Bai Fu Zi (Rhizoma Typhonii)
Bai Zhu (Rhizoma Atractylodis Macrocephalae)
Ban Xia (Rhizoma Pinelliae)

Stubborn headache
Bai Fu Zi (Rhizoma Typhonii)
Quan Xie (Scorpio)
Wu Gong (Scolopendra)
Xi Xin (Herba Asari)

Channel guiding herbs
Taiyang channels: *Qiang Huo* (Rhizoma et Radix Notopterygii)
Shaoyang channels: *Chai Hu* (Radix Bupleuri)
Yangming channels: *Bai Zhi* (Radix Angelicae Dahuricae)
Taiyin channels: *Cang Zhu* (Rhizoma Atractylodis)
Shaoyin channels: *Xi Xin* (Herba Asari)
Jueyin channels: *Wu Zhu Yu* (Fructus Evodiae)

25. Hepatitis

Ai Ye (Folium Artemisiae Argyi)
Bai Shao (Radix Paeoniae Alba)
Bai Tou Weng (Radix Pulsatillae)
Ban Lan Gen (Radix Isatidis)
Ban Mao (Mylabris)
Chai Hu (Radix Bupleuri)
Che Qian Cao (Herba Plantaginis)
Chi Shao (Radix Paeoniae Rubrae)
Chui Pen Cao (Herba Sedi)
Da Ji (Radix Euphorbiae seu Knoxiae)
Da Qing Ye (Folium Isatidis)
Dan Shen (Radix Salviae Miltiorrhizae)
Dang Gui (Radicis Angelicae Sinensis)
Dong Chong Xia Cao (Cordyceps)
Fo Shou (Fructus Citri Sarcodactylis)
Gou Qi Zi (Fructus Lycii)
Guan Zhong (Rhizoma Dryopteridis)
Hai Jin Sha (Herba Lygodii)
Hu Zhang (Rhizoma Polygoni Cuspidati)
Huang Jing (Rhizoma Polygonati)
Huang Qi (Radix Astragali)
Huang Qin (Radix Scutellariae)
Huo Xiang (Herba Agastache)
Jiao Gu Lan (Rhizoma seu Herba Gynostemmatis)
Ling Zhi (Ganoderma)
Lu Cha (Folium Camellia Sinensis)
Lu Hui (Aloe)
Ma Bian Cao (Herba Verbenae)
Ma Dou Ling (Fructus Aristolochiae)
Ming Fan (Alumen)

Mu Gua (Fructus Chaenomelis)
Mu Zei (Herba Equiseti Hiemalis)
Nu Zhen Zi (Fructus Ligustri Lucidi)
Qin Jiao (Radix Gentianae Macrophyllae)
Ren Dong Teng (Caulis Lonicerae)
Shan Dou Gen (Radix Sophorae Tonkinensis)
Shan Yao (Rhizoma Dioscoreae)
Shan Zha (Fructus Crataegi)
Shang Lu (Radix Phytolaccae)
She Xiang (Moschus)
Shui Niu Jiao (Cornu Bubali)
Wu Gong (Scolopendra)
Wu Long Cha (Folium Camellia Sinensis Fermentata)
Wu Mei (Fructus Mume)
Wu Wei Zi (Fructus Schisandrae Chinensis)
Xia Ku Cao (Spica Prunellae)
Xiao Ji (Herba Cirisii)
Yi Yi Ren (Semen Coicis)
Yin Chen Hao (Herba Artemisiae Scopariae)
Zhu Dan (Fel Porcus)

26. Hernial pain

Chuan Lian Zi (Fructus Toosendan)
Li Zhi He (Semen Litchi)
Qing Pi (Pericarpium Citri Reticulatae Viride)
Wu Yao (Radix Linderae)
Wu Zhu Yu (Fructus Evodiae)
Xiao Hui Xiang (Fructus Foeniculi)

27. Hiccups

Bi Cheng Qie (Fructus Litseae)
Chen Xiang (Lignum Aquilariae Resinatum)
Dai Zhe Shi (Haematitum)
Dao Dou (Semen Canavaliae)
Ding Xiang (Flos Caryophylli)
Shi Di (Calyx Kaki)
Xuan Fu Hua (Flos Inulae)

28. Hypochondriac pain

Qi stagnation

Ba Yue Zha (Fructus Akebiae)
Bo He (Herba Menthae)
Chai Hu (Radix Bupleuri)
Chuan Lian Zi (Fructus Toosendan)
Fo Shou (Fructus Citri Sarcodactylis)
Li Zhi He (Semen Litchi)
Qing Mu Xiang (Radix Aristolochiae)
Qing Pi (Pericarpium Citri Reticulatae Viride)
Wu Yao (Radix Linderae)
Xiang Fu (Rhizoma Cyperi)
Zhi Ke (Fructus Aurantii)

Blood stagnation

Chuan Xiong (Rhizoma Ligustici Chuanxiong)
Jiang Xiang (Lignum Dalbergiae Odoriferae)
Pu Huang (Pollen Typhae)
Yan Hu Suo (Rhizoma Corydalis)
Yu Jin (Radix Curcumae)

Alternation of cold and heat

Chai Hu (Radix Bupleuri)
Huang Qin (Radix Scutellariae)
Yu Jin (Radix Curcumae)

Hypochondriac fullness and pain

Chai Hu (Radix Bupleuri)
Qing Pi (Pericarpium Citri Reticulatae Viride)
Xiang Fu (Rhizoma Cyperi)
Zhi Ke (Fructus Aurantii)

Stabbing pain in the hypochondrium

Chuan Xiong (Rhizoma Ligustici Chuanxiong)
Dan Shen (Radix Salviae Miltiorrhizae)
Hong Hua (Flos Carthami)
Yan Hu Suo (Rhizoma Corydalis)

Hardness and pain of the hypochondrium

Bie Jia (Carapax Trionycis)
Chuan Shan Jia (Squama Manis)
Gui Ban (Plastrum Testudinis)
Mu Li (Concha Ostreae)

With prolonged edema

Ting Li Zi (Semen Descurainiae seu Lepidii)

With liver abscess

Bai Shao (Radix Paeoniae Alba)
Chuan Lian Zi (Fructus Toosendan)
He Huan Pi (Cortex Albiziae)
Mu Dan Pi (Cortex Moutan)

29. Indigestion

Ban Xia (Rhizoma Pinelliae)
Cang Zhu (Rhizoma Atractylodis)
Da Huang (Radix et Rhizoma Rhei)
Ji Nei Jin (Endothelium Corneum Gigeriae Galli)
Lu Cha (Folium Camellia Sinensis)
Mai Ya (Fructus Hordei Germinatus)
Rou Dou Kou (Semen Myristicae)
Shan Zha (Fructus Crataegi)
Wu Long Cha (Folium Camellia Sinensis Fermentata)
Wu Zhu Yu (Fructus Evodiae)
Zhu Dan (Fel Porcus)

30. Insomnia

Bai He (Bulbus Lilii)
Bai Jiang Cao (Herba cum Radice Patriniae)
Bai Shao (Radix Paeoniae Alba)
Chan Tui (Periostracum Cicadae)
Hou Po (Cortex Magnoliae Officinalis)
Jiao Gu Lan (Rhizoma seu Herba Gynostemmatis)
Long Dan Cao (Radix Gentianae)
Mai Men Dong (Radix Ophiopogonis)
Qin Jiao (Radix Gentianae Macrophyllae)
Suan Zao Ren (Semen Zizyphi Spinosae)
Tian Ma (Rhizoma Gastrodiae)
Tian Nan Xing (Rhizoma Arisaematis)
Wu Jia Pi (Cortex Acanthopanacis)
Xie Cao (Radix et Rhizoma Valerianae)
Zhi Zi (Fructus Gardeniae)

31. Intestinal abscess

Bai Hua She She Cao (Herba Oldenlandia)
Bai Jiang Cao (Herba cum Radice Patriniae)
Dong Gua Zi (Semen Benincasae)
Gua Lou Ren (Semen Trichosanthis)
Gua Lou Shi (Fructus Trichosanthis)
Hong Hua (Flos Carthami)
Hong Teng (Caulis Sargentodoxae)
Jin Yin Hua (Flos Lonicerae)
Ma Chi Xian (Herba Portulacae)
Mo Yao (Myrrha)
Mu Dan Pi (Cortex Moutan)
Ru Xiang (Gummi Olibanum)
Tao Ren (Semen Persicae)
Yi Yi Ren (Semen Coicis)
Zi Hua Di Ding (Herba Violae)

32. Jaundice

Damp-heat

Bai Mao Gen (Rhizoma Imperatae)
Bai Xian Pi (Cortex Dictamni)
Chi Xiao Dou (Semen Phaseoli)
Da Huang (Radix et Rhizoma Rhei)
Hu Zhang (Rhizoma Polygoni Cuspidati)

Huang Bai (Cortex Phellodendri)
Huang Lian (Rhizoma Coptidis)
Huang Qin (Radix Scutellariae)
Jin Qian Cao (Herba Lysimachiae)
Ku Shen Gen (Radix Sophorae Flavescentis)
Long Dan Cao (Radix Gentianae)
Pu Gong Ying (Herba Taraxaci)
Qin Jiao (Radix Gentianae Macrophyllae)
Shan Dou Gen (Radix Sophorae Tonkinensis)
Yin Chen Hao (Herba Artemisiae Scopariae)
Yu Jin (Radix Curcumae)
Zhi Zi (Fructus Gardeniae)
Zhu Dan (Fel Porcus)

Damp-cold
Bai Zhu (Rhizoma Atractylodis Macrocephalae)
Fu Ling (Poria)
Fu Zi (Radix Aconiti Lateralis Praeparata)
Gan Jiang (Rhizoma Zingiberis)
Rou Gui (Cortex Cinnamomi)
Yin Chen Hao (Herba Artemisiae Scopariae)

33. Lactation difficulties
Bai Ji Li (Fructus Tribuli)
Chuan Mu Tong (Caulis Clematidis Armandii)
Chuan Shan Jia (Squama Manis)
Dong Kui Zi (Semen Malvae)
Lou Lu (Radix Rhapontici)
Lu Lu Tong (Fructus Liquidambaris)
Si Gua Luo (Retinervus Luffae Fructus)
Tong Cao (Medulla Tetrapanacis)
Wang Bu Liu Xing (Semen Vaccariae)

34. Leg *qi*
Bing Lang (Semen Arecae)
Ding Shu Xiu (Herba Elephantopus Scaber)
Gan Song (Radix seu Rhizoma Nardostachys)
Hu Lu Ba (Semen Trigonellae)
Ma Bian Cao (Herba Verbenae)
Qing Feng Teng (Caulis Sinomenii)

35. Leukorrhea
Damp-heat
Huang Bai (Cortex Phellodendri)
Huang Lian (Rhizoma Coptidis)
Ku Shen Gen (Radix Sophorae Flavescentis)
Ze Xie (Rhizoma Alismatis)

Deficiency and cold
Ai Ye (Folium Artemisiae Argyi)
Gou Ji (Rhizoma Cibotii)
Lu Lu Tong (Fructus Liquidambaris)
Yin Guo Ye (Folium Ginkgo)

Damp-cold
Ai Ye (Folium Artemisiae Argyi)
Bai Zhi (Radix Angelicae Dahuricae)
Bai Zhu (Rhizoma Atractylodis Macrocephalae)
Cang Zhu (Rhizoma Atractylodis)
Hai Piao Xiao (Endoconcha Sepiae)

Kidney deficiency
Hai Piao Xiao (Endoconcha Sepiae)
Jin Ying Zi (Fructus Rosae Laevigatae)
Lian Zi (Semen Nelumbinis)
Long Gu (Os Draconis)
Mu Li (Concha Ostreae)
Qian Shi (Semen Euryales)
Sang Piao Xiao (Ootheca Mantidis)
Sha Yuan Zi (Semen Astragali Complanati)
Tu Si Zi (Semen Cuscutae)

Genital swelling and itching
Bai Bu (Radix Stemonae)
Bai Xian Pi (Cortex Dictamni)
Bian Xu (Herba Polygoni Avicularis)
Cang Zhu (Rhizoma Atractylodis)
Di Fu Zi (Fructus Kochiae)
Hua Jiao (Pericarpium Zanthoxyli)
Huang Bai (Cortex Phellodendri)
Ku Shen Gen (Radix Sophorae Flavescentis)
Long Dan Cao (Radix Gentianae)
She Chuang Zi (Fructus Cnidii)
Xian He Cao (Herba Agrimoniae)

36. Lightheadedness
Febrile disorders
Bing Pian (Borneolum Syntheticum)
She Xiang (Moschus)
Su He Xiang (Styrax)

Accumulation of dampness
Shi Chang Pu (Rhizoma Acori)
Yuan Zhi (Radix Polygalae)

37. *Lin zheng* (dysuria syndrome)
***Re lin* (heat dysuria)**
Bai Hua She (Bungarus Parvus)
Bai Mao Gen (Rhizoma Imperatae)
Bai Wei (Radix Cynanchi Atrati)
Bian Xu (Herba Polygoni Avicularis)
Che Qian Zi (Semen Plantaginis)
Chi Shao (Radix Paeoniae Rubrae)
Chuan Mu Tong (Caulis Clematidis Armandii)
Chuan Xin Lian (Herba Andrographis)
Da Huang (Radix et Rhizoma Rhei)
Deng Xin Cao (Medulla Junci)
Di Fu Zi (Fructus Kochiae)
Di Long (Pheretima)
Dong Kui Zi (Semen Malvae)
Hai Jin Sha (Herba Lygodii)
Hu Po (Succinum)
Hu Zhang (Rhizoma Polygoni Cuspidati)
Hua Shi (Talcum)
Huang Bai (Cortex Phellodendri)
Huang Qin (Radix Scutellariae)
Jin Qian Cao (Herba Lysimachiae)
Ku Shen Gen (Radix Sophorae Flavescentis)
Lu Gen (Rhizoma Phragmitis)
Pu Gong Ying (Herba Taraxaci)
Qu Mai (Herba Dianthi)
Shi Wei (Folium Pyrrosiae)
Tong Cao (Medulla Tetrapanacis)
Tu Fu Ling (Rhizoma Smilacis Glabrae)
Yu Xing Cao (Herba Houttuyniae)
Ze Xie (Rhizoma Alismatis)
Zhi Zi (Fructus Gardeniae)
Zhu Ye (Herba Phyllostachys)

***Xue lin* (bloody dysuria)**
Bai Mao Gen (Rhizoma Imperatae)
Bai Wei (Radix Cynanchi Atrati)
Chi Shao (Radix Paeoniae Rubrae)
Da Ji (Herba seu Radix Cirsii Japonici)
Hai Jin Sha (Herba Lygodii)
Hu Po (Succinum)
Niu Xi (Radix Cyathulae seu Achyranthis)
Pu Huang (Pollen Typhae)
Sheng Di Huang (Radix Rehmanniae)
Shi Wei (Folium Pyrrosiae)
Xiao Ji (Herba Cirisii)

***Shi lin* (stone dysuria)**
Hai Jin Sha (Herba Lygodii)
Hu Po (Succinum)
Ji Nei Jin (Endothelium Corneum Gigeriae Galli)
Jin Qian Cao (Herba Lysimachiae)
Shi Wei (Folium Pyrrosiae)

Gao lin (cloudy dysuria)
Bi Xie (Rhizoma Dioscoreae Hypoglaucae)
Hai Jin Sha (Herba Lygodii)
Shi Chang Pu (Rhizoma Acori)

***Lin zheng* (dysuria syndrome) due to yin deficiency**
Huang Bai (Cortex Phellodendri)
Sheng Di Huang (Radix Rehmanniae)
Zhi Mu (Radix Anemarrhenae)

38. Loss of voice

Wind-cold
Gan Cao (Radix Glycyrrhizae)
Ma Huang (Herba Ephedrae)
Xing Ren (Semen Armeniacae Amarum)

Wind-heat
Chan Tui (Periostracum Cicadae)
Pang Da Hai (Semen Sterculiae Lychnophorae)

Lung yin deficiency
He Zi (Fructus Chebulae)
Mai Men Dong (Radix Ophiopogonis)
Sha Shen (Radix Glehniae seu Adenophorae)

39. Low back pain

Kidney deficiency
Bu Gu Zhi (Fructus Psoraleae)
Dong Chong Xia Cao (Cordyceps)
Du Zhong (Cortex Eucommiae)
Gou Ji (Rhizoma Cibotii)
Gu Sui Bu (Rhizoma Drynariae)
Hu Tao Ren (Semen Juglandis)
Sang Ji Sheng (Herba Taxilli)
Sha Yuan Zi (Semen Astragali Complanati)
Tu Si Zi (Semen Cuscutae)
Xu Duan (Radix Dipsaci)

40. Lung abscess

Bai Jiang Cao (Herba cum Radice Patriniae)
Chuan Xin Lian (Herba Andrographis)
Dong Gua Zi (Semen Benincasae)
Jie Geng (Radix Platycodonis)
Jin Yin Hua (Flos Lonicerae)
Lu Gen (Rhizoma Phragmitis)
Pu Gong Ying (Herba Taraxaci)
Xia Ku Cao (Spica Prunellae)
Yi Yi Ren (Semen Coicis)
Yu Xing Cao (Herba Houttuyniae)

41. Maculae and papules

Heat in the blood
Chi Shao (Radix Paeoniae Rubrae)
Da Qing Ye (Folium Isatidis)
Mu Dan Pi (Cortex Moutan)
Qing Dai (Indigo Naturalis)
Sheng Di Huang (Radix Rehmanniae)
Xuan Shen (Radix Scrophulariae)
Zhang Hong Hua (Flos Crocus Sativus)
Zi Cao Gen (Radix Lithospermi)

Measles
Bo He (Herba Menthae)
Chan Tui (Periostracum Cicadae)
Fu Ping (Herba Spirodelae)
Ge Gen (Radix Puerariae)
Jing Jie (Herba Schizonepetae)
Niu Bang Zi (Fructus Arctii)
Sheng Ma (Rhizoma Cimicifugae)
Xiang Ru (Herba Elsholtziae seu Moslae)
Zi Cao Gen (Radix Lithospermi)

Urticaria
Bai Ji Li (Fructus Tribuli)
Bai Zhi (Radix Angelicae Dahuricae)
Chan Tui (Periostracum Cicadae)
Di Fu Zi (Fructus Kochiae)
Fang Feng (Radix Saposhnikoviae)
Jing Jie (Herba Schizonepetae)
Ku Shen Gen (Radix Sophorae Flavescentis)
She Chuang Zi (Fructus Cnidii)

Eczema
Bai Xian Pi (Cortex Dictamni)
Can Sha (Excrementum Bombycis Mori)
Chuan Xin Lian (Herba Andrographis)
Di Yu (Radix Sanguisorbae)
Hai Piao Xiao (Endoconcha Sepiae)
Hai Tong Pi (Cortex Erythrinae)
Huang Qin (Radix Scutellariae)
Huo Xiang (Herba Agastache)
Liu Huang (Sulfur)
Long Gu (Os Draconis)
Ming Fan (Alumen)
She Chuang Zi (Fructus Cnidii)
Tong Cao (Medulla Tetrapanacis)
Xu Chang Qing (Radix Cynanchi Paniculati)
Zhen Zhu Mu (Concha Margaritaferae)

42. Malaria

Bing Lang (Semen Arecae)
Cao Guo (Fructus Tsaoko)
Chai Hu (Radix Bupleuri)
Chang Shan (Radix Dichroae)
He Shou Wu (Radix Polygoni Multiflori)
Huang Qin (Radix Scutellariae)
Ma Bian Cao (Herba Verbenae)
Qian Dan (Minium)
Qing Hao (Herba Artemisiae Annuae)
Xian He Cao (Herba Agrimoniae)
Xiong Huang (Realgar)
Ya Dan Zi (Fructus Bruceae)
Zhu Sha (Cinnabaris)

43. Menstrual pain

Qi stagnation
Bo He (Herba Menthae)
Chai Hu (Radix Bupleuri)
Chuan Lian Zi (Fructus Toosendan)
Li Zhi He (Semen Litchi)
Wu Yao (Radix Linderae)
Xiang Fu (Rhizoma Cyperi)
Yu Jin (Radix Curcumae)

Blood stagnation
Bai Hua She (Bungarus Parvus)
Chi Shao (Radix Paeoniae Rubrae)
Chuan Shan Jia (Squama Manis)
Chuan Xiong (Rhizoma Ligustici Chuanxiong)
Dan Shen (Radix Salviae Miltiorrhizae)
Dang Gui (Radicis Angelicae Sinensis)
E Zhu (Rhizoma Curcumae)
Gui Zhi (Ramulus Cinnamomi)
Hong Hua (Flos Carthami)
Hong Teng (Caulis Sargentodoxae)
Hu Po (Succinum)
Hu Zhang (Rhizoma Polygoni Cuspidati)
Ji Xue Teng (Caulis Spatholobi)
Jiang Huang (Rhizoma Curcumae Longae)
Liu Ji Nu (Herba Artemisiae Anomalae)
Mo Yao (Myrrha)
Mu Dan Pi (Cortex Moutan)
Niu Xi (Radix Cyathulae seu Achyranthis)
Pu Huang (Pollen Typhae)
Qian Cao (Radix Rubiae)
Qu Mai (Herba Dianthi)
Ru Xiang (Gummi Olibanum)
San Leng (Rhizoma Sparganii)
Shan Zha (Fructus Crataegi)
She Xiang (Moschus)
Shui Zhi (Hirudo)
Su Mu (Lignum Sappan)
Tao Ren (Semen Persicae)
Wang Bu Liu Xing (Semen Vaccariae)

Wu Ling Zhi (Excrementum Trogopteri seu Pteromi)
Xue Jie (Sanguis Draconis)
Yan Hu Suo (Rhizoma Corydalis)
Yi Mu Cao (Herba Leonuri)
Yu Jin (Radix Curcumae)
Ze Lan (Herba Lycopi)

Damp-cold
Ai Ye (Folium Artemisiae Argyi)
Gui Zhi (Ramulus Cinnamomi)
Pao Jiang (Rhizoma Zingiberis Preparatum)
Rou Gui (Cortex Cinnamomi)
Wu Yao (Radix Linderae)
Wu Zhu Yu (Fructus Evodiae)

Qi deficiency
Dang Shen (Radix Codonopsis)
Huang Qi (Radix Astragali)
Ren Shen (Radix Ginseng)

Blood deficiency
Bai Shao (Radix Paeoniae Alba)
Dang Gui (Radicis Angelicae Sinensis)
Ji Xue Teng (Caulis Spatholobi)
Shu Di Huang (Radix Rehmanniae Preparata)

44. Nausea and vomiting

Wind-cold
Huo Xiang (Herba Agastache)
Pei Lan (Herba Eupatorii)
Sheng Jiang (Rhizoma Zingiberis Recens)
Xiang Ru (Herba Elsholtziae seu Moslae)
Zi Su Ye (Folium Perillae)

Stomach cold
Bai Dou Kou (Fructus Amomi Rotundus)
Ban Xia (Rhizoma Pinelliae)
Bi Cheng Qie (Fructus Litseae)
Cao Guo (Fructus Tsaoko)
Chen Xiang (Lignum Aquilariae Resinatum)
Dao Dou (Semen Canavaliae)
Ding Xiang (Flos Caryophylli)
Gan Jiang (Rhizoma Zingiberis)
Gao Liang Jiang (Rhizoma Alpiniae Officinarum)
Hu Jiao (Fructus Piper)
Hua Jiao (Pericarpium Zanthoxyli)
Sha Ren (Fructus Amomi)
Sheng Jiang (Rhizoma Zingiberis Recens)
Tan Xiang (Lignum Santali Albi)
Wu Zhu Yu (Fructus Evodiae)
Xiao Hui Xiang (Fructus Foeniculi)

Stomach heat
Bai Mao Gen (Rhizoma Imperatae)
Huang Lian (Rhizoma Coptidis)
Lu Gen (Rhizoma Phragmitis)
Pi Pa Ye (Folium Eriobotryae)
Zhu Ru (Caulis Bambusae in Taenia)

Qi stagnation
Bai Dou Kou (Fructus Amomi Rotundus)
Cao Dou Kou (Semen Alpiniae Katsumadai)
Chen Pi (Pericarpium Citri Reticulatae)
Chen Xiang (Lignum Aquilariae Resinatum)
Dao Dou (Semen Canavaliae)
Fo Shou (Fructus Citri Sarcodactylis)
Mu Xiang (Radix Aucklandiae)
Sha Ren (Fructus Amomi)
Shi Di (Calyx Kaki)
Tan Xiang (Lignum Santali Albi)
Wu Zhu Yu (Fructus Evodiae)
Xiang Yuan (Fructus Citri)
Xuan Fu Hua (Flos Inulae)
Zi Su Ye (Folium Perillae)

Overindulgence in food
Ji Nei Jin (Endothelium Corneum Gigeriae Galli)
Lai Fu Zi (Semen Raphani)
Mai Ya (Fructus Hordei Germinatus)
Shan Zha (Fructus Crataegi)
Shen Qu (Massa Fermentata)

Phlegm stagnation
Ban Xia (Rhizoma Pinelliae)
Chen Pi (Pericarpium Citri Reticulatae)
Fu Ling (Poria)
Sheng Jiang (Rhizoma Zingiberis Recens)
Xuan Fu Hua (Flos Inulae)

Damp-heat
Huang Lian (Rhizoma Coptidis)
Huang Qin (Radix Scutellariae)
Long Dan Cao (Radix Gentianae)

Nausea
Ban Xia (Rhizoma Pinelliae)
Chen Xiang (Lignum Aquilariae Resinatum)
Ding Xiang (Flos Caryophylli)

45. Nodules

Bai Fu Zi (Rhizoma Typhonii)
Ban Mao (Mylabris)
Bei Mu (Bulbus Fritillaria)
Chuan Shan Jia (Squama Manis)
Da Ji (Radix Euphorbiae seu Knoxiae)
Hai Ge Fen (Concha Meretricis seu Cyclinae)
Hai Zao (Sargassum)
Huang Yao Zi (Herba Dioscoreae Bulbiferae)
Jiang Can (Bombyx Batryticatus)
Kun Bu (Thallus Laminariae seu Eckloniae)
Lian Qiao (Fructus Forsythiae)
Lu Feng Fang (Nidus Vespae)
Mu Li (Concha Ostreae)
Quan Xie (Scorpio)
She Xiang (Moschus)
Wa Leng Zi (Concha Arcae)
Wu Gong (Scolopendra)
Xia Ku Cao (Spica Prunellae)
Xiong Huang (Realgar)
Xuan Shen (Radix Scrophulariae)

46. Pain

Bai Jie Zi (Semen Sinapis)
Bai Zhi (Radix Angelicae Dahuricae)
Ban Xia (Rhizoma Pinelliae)
Bi Ba (Fructus Piperis Longi)
Bi Cheng Qie (Fructus Litseae)
Bian Xu (Herba Polygoni Avicularis)
Bing Lang (Semen Arecae)
Chuan Xiong (Rhizoma Ligustici Chuanxiong)
Dang Gui (Radicis Angelicae Sinensis)
Di Fu Zi (Fructus Kochiae)
Di Yu (Radix Sanguisorbae)
Ding Xiang (Flos Caryophylli)
Fang Feng (Radix Saposhnikoviae)
Gan Jiang (Rhizoma Zingiberis)
Gao Ben (Rhizoma Ligustici)
Ge Gen (Radix Puerariae)
Hai Shen (Strichopus Japonicus)
Han Lian Cao (Herba Ecliptae)
Hong Hua (Flos Carthami)
Huang Jing (Rhizoma Polygonati)
Ku Lian Pi (Cortex Meliae)
Lian Zi Xin (Plumula Nelumbinis)
Ma Ti Jin (Herba Dichondrae Repentis)
Qin Jiao (Radix Gentianae Macrophyllae)
Qing Mu Xiang (Radix Aristolochiae)
San Qi (Radix Notoginseng)
Shan Zha (Fructus Crataegi)
Sheng Jiang (Rhizoma Zingiberis Recens)

Sheng Ma (Rhizoma Cimicifugae)
Su He Xiang (Styrax)
Su Mu (Lignum Sappan)
Suan Zao Ren (Semen Zizyphi Spinosae)
Tian Nan Xing (Rhizoma Arisaematis)
Tian Zhu Huang (Concretio Silicea Bambusae)
Wei Ling Xian (Radix Clematidis)
Wu Mei (Fructus Mume)
Xi Xin (Herba Asari)
Xiang Fu (Rhizoma Cyperi)
Xu Chang Qing (Radix Cynanchi Paniculati)
Xun Gu Feng (Herba Aristolochiae Mollissimae)
Yan Hu Suo (Rhizoma Corydalis)
Yi Yi Ren (Semen Coicis)
Ze Lan (Herba Lycopi)
Zhu Sha (Cinnabaris)

47. Parasitic infestation

Roundworms
Bing Lang (Semen Arecae)
Chuan Lian Zi (Fructus Toosendan)
Fei Zi (Semen Torreyae)
He Shi (Fructus Carpesii)
Hua Jiao (Pericarpium Zanthoxyli)
Lei Wan (Omphalia)
Lu Hui (Aloe)
Nan Gua Zi (Semen Cucurbitae Moschatae)
Qian Niu Zi (Semen Pharbitidis)
Shi Jun Zi (Fructus Quisqualis)
Wu Mei (Fructus Mume)
Wu Yi (Fructus Ulmi Praeparatus)
Xiong Huang (Realgar)

Hookworms
Bing Lang (Semen Arecae)
Fei Zi (Semen Torreyae)
Guan Zhong (Rhizoma Dryopteridis)
Ku Lian Pi (Cortex Meliae)
Lei Wan (Omphalia)

Pinworms
Bai Bu (Radix Stemonae)
Bing Lang (Semen Arecae)
Fei Zi (Semen Torreyae)
Guan Zhong (Rhizoma Dryopteridis)
Ku Lian Pi (Cortex Meliae)

Tapeworms
Bing Lang (Semen Arecae)
Fei Zi (Semen Torreyae)
Guan Zhong (Rhizoma Dryopteridis)
Lei Wan (Omphalia)
Nan Gua Zi (Semen Cucurbitae Moschatae)

48. Perspiration

Spontaneous perspiration due to disharmony of *wei* (defensive) and *ying* (nutritive) levels
Bai Shao (Radix Paeoniae Alba)
Gui Zhi (Ramulus Cinnamomi)

Spontaneous perspiration due to Lung qi deficiency
Huang Qi (Radix Astragali)
Wu Wei Zi (Fructus Schisandrae Chinensis)

Night sweating due to deficiency of Heart blood
Fu Xiao Mai (Semen Tritici Aestivi Levis)
Suan Zao Ren (Semen Zizyphi Spinosae)
Wu Wei Zi (Fructus Schisandrae Chinensis)

Night sweating due to deficiency heat
Di Gu Pi (Cortex Lycii)
Ma Huang Gen (Radix Ephedrae)
Shan Zhu Yu (Fructus Corni)
Wu Mei (Fructus Mume)
Zhi Mu (Radix Anemarrhenae)

Perspiration due to shock
Bai Zhu (Rhizoma Atractylodis Macrocephalae)
Fu Zi (Radix Aconiti Lateralis Praeparata)
Huang Qi (Radix Astragali)
Long Gu (Os Draconis)
Mu Li (Concha Ostreae)
Ren Shen (Radix Ginseng)
Wu Wei Zi (Fructus Schisandrae Chinensis)

Perspiration with yellow discoloration
Yin Chen Hao (Herba Artemisiae Scopariae)
Zhi Zi (Fructus Gardeniae)

49. Plum pit syndrome

Ban Xia (Rhizoma Pinelliae)
Fu Ling (Poria)
Hou Po (Cortex Magnoliae Officinalis)
Sheng Jiang (Rhizoma Zingiberis Recens)
Zi Su Ye (Folium Perillae)

50. Poisoning

Mercury
Tu Fu Ling (Rhizoma Smilacis Glabrae)

Arsenic
Fang Feng (Radix Saposhnikoviae)
Gan Cao (Radix Glycyrrhizae)
Lu Dou (Semen Phaseoli Radiati)

Fish and crab
Lu Gen (Rhizoma Phragmitis)
Sheng Jiang (Rhizoma Zingiberis Recens)
Zi Su Ye (Folium Perillae)

Aconite
Lu Dou (Semen Phaseoli Radiati)
Sheng Jiang (Rhizoma Zingiberis Recens)

***Chan Su* (Venenum Bufonis)**
Zi Cao Gen (Radix Lithospermi)

***Bai Guo* (Semen Ginkgo)**
Gan Cao (Radix Glycyrrhizae)

***Xing Ren* (Semen Armeniacae Amarum)**
Gan Cao (Radix Glycyrrhizae)
Lu Dou (Semen Phaseoli Radiati)

***Ban Xia* (Rhizoma Pinelliae) and *Tian Nan Xing* (Rhizoma Arisaematis)**
Gan Cao (Radix Glycyrrhizae)
Lu Dou (Semen Phaseoli Radiati)
Sheng Jiang (Rhizoma Zingiberis Recens)

General poisoning
Gan Cao (Radix Glycyrrhizae)
Lu Dou (Semen Phaseoli Radiati)

Streptomycin
Gu Sui Bu (Rhizoma Drynariae)

51. Rectal prolapse

Chai Hu (Radix Bupleuri)
Ge Gen (Radix Puerariae)
Huang Qi (Radix Astragali)
Jie Geng (Radix Platycodonis)
Sheng Ma (Rhizoma Cimicifugae)

Wu Bei Zi (Galla Chinensis)
Zhi Ke (Fructus Aurantii)
Zhi Shi (Fructus Aurantii Immaturus)

52. Restless fetus

Bai Shao (Radix Paeoniae Alba)
Bai Zhu (Rhizoma Atractylodis Macrocephalae)
Dang Gui (Radicis Angelicae Sinensis)
Du Zhong (Cortex Eucommiae)
E Jiao (Colla Corii Asini)
Gu Sui Bu (Rhizoma Drynariae)
Huang Qin (Radix Scutellariae)
Sang Ji Sheng (Herba Taxilli)
Sha Ren (Fructus Amomi)
Shu Di Huang (Radix Rehmanniae Preparata)
Tu Si Zi (Semen Cuscutae)
Xu Duan (Radix Dipsaci)
Yi Tang (Saccharum Granorum)
Zi Su Ye (Folium Perillae)
Zong Lu Pi (Fibra Stipulae Trachycarpi)

53. Seizures

Chai Hu (Radix Bupleuri)
Gan Song (Radix seu Rhizoma Nardostachys)
Gui Zhi (Ramulus Cinnamomi)
Hai Shen (Strichopus Japonicus)
Hu Jiao (Fructus Piper)
Jiang Can (Bombyx Batryticatus)
Peng Sha (Borax)
Quan Xie (Scorpio)
Shi Chang Pu (Rhizoma Acori)
Tian Ma (Rhizoma Gastrodiae)
Tian Nan Xing (Rhizoma Arisaematis)
Wu Mei (Fructus Mume)

54. Snake and insect bites

Bai Fu Zi (Rhizoma Typhonii)
Bai Hua She She Cao (Herba Oldenlandia)
Ban Bian Lian (Herba Lobeliae Chinensis)
Ban Zhi Lian (Herba Scutellariae Barbatae)
Chuan Xin Lian (Herba Andrographis)
Hu Zhang (Rhizoma Polygoni Cuspidati)
Huang Yao Zi (Herba Dioscoreae Bulbiferae)
Jin Qian Cao (Herba Lysimachiae)
Ma Chi Xian (Herba Portulacae)
Qing Mu Xiang (Radix Aristolochiae)
Wu Ling Zhi (Excrementum Trogopteri seu Pteromi)
Xiong Huang (Realgar)
Xu Chang Qing (Radix Cynanchi Paniculati)
Zi Hua Di Ding (Herba Violae)

55. Sore throat

Wind-heat
Bo He (Herba Menthae)
Jiang Can (Bombyx Batryticatus)
Niu Bang Zi (Fructus Arctii)
Sang Ye (Folium Mori)
Sheng Ma (Rhizoma Cimicifugae)

Deficiency heat
Huang Bai (Cortex Phellodendri)
Sheng Di Huang (Radix Rehmanniae)
Xuan Shen (Radix Scrophulariae)
Zhi Mu (Radix Anemarrhenae)

Excess heat
Gan Cao (Radix Glycyrrhizae)
Jie Geng (Radix Platycodonis)
Jing Jie (Herba Schizonepetae)
Lian Qiao (Fructus Forsythiae)
Ma Bo (Lasiosphaera seu Calvatia)
Niu Bang Zi (Fructus Arctii)
Shan Dou Gen (Radix Sophorae Tonkinensis)
She Gan (Rhizoma Belamcandae)

Heat-toxins
Bai Hua She She Cao (Herba Oldenlandia)
Ban Lan Gen (Radix Isatidis)
Chuan Xin Lian (Herba Andrographis)
Da Huang (Radix et Rhizoma Rhei)
Da Qing Ye (Folium Isatidis)
Deng Xin Cao (Medulla Junci)
Han Shui Shi (Mirabilite)
Jin Yin Hua (Flos Lonicerae)
Lian Qiao (Fructus Forsythiae)
Mang Xiao (Natrii Sulfas)
Niu Huang (Calculus Bovis)
Xia Ku Cao (Spica Prunellae)
Zhu Dan (Fel Porcus)
Zhu Sha (Cinnabaris)

With ulceration
Bing Pian (Borneolum Syntheticum)
Chan Su (Venenum Bufonis)
Ma Bo (Lasiosphaera seu Calvatia)

56. Spermatorrhea

Ba Ji Tian (Radix Morindae Officinalis)
Bai Guo (Semen Ginkgo)
Bu Gu Zhi (Fructus Psoraleae)
Dong Chong Xia Cao (Cordyceps)
Fu Pen Zi (Fructus Rubi)
Gou Ji (Rhizoma Cibotii)
Hai Piao Xiao (Endoconcha Sepiae)
He Shou Wu (Radix Polygoni Multiflori)
Jiu Cai Zi (Semen Allii Tuberosi)
Lian Xu (Stamen Nelumbinis)
Lian Zi Xin (Plumula Nelumbinis)
Long Gu (Os Draconis)
Lu Rong (Cornu Cervi Pantotrichum)
Mu Li (Concha Ostreae)
Qian Shi (Semen Euryales)
Rou Cong Rong (Herba Cistanches)
Sha Yuan Zi (Semen Astragali Complanati)
Shan Yao (Rhizoma Dioscoreae)
Shan Zhu Yu (Fructus Corni)
Tu Si Zi (Semen Cuscutae)
Wu Bei Zi (Galla Chinensis)
Wu Wei Zi (Fructus Schisandrae Chinensis)
Xian Mao (Rhizoma Curculiginis)
Xu Duan (Radix Dipsaci)
Yi Zhi Ren (Fructus Alpiniae Oxyphyllae)
Yin Yang Huo (Herba Epimedii)
Yuan Zhi (Radix Polygalae)

57. Stomach pain

Deficiency
Bai Zhu (Rhizoma Atractylodis Macrocephalae)
Dang Shen (Radix Codonopsis)
Gan Cao (Radix Glycyrrhizae)
Huang Qi (Radix Astragali)
Shan Yao (Rhizoma Dioscoreae)
Yi Tang (Saccharum Granorum)

Qi stagnation
Ba Yue Zha (Fructus Akebiae)
Chen Pi (Pericarpium Citri Reticulatae)
Chuan Lian Zi (Fructus Toosendan)
Fo Shou (Fructus Citri Sarcodactylis)
Gan Song (Radix seu Rhizoma Nardostachys)
Li Zhi He (Semen Litchi)
Mu Xiang (Radix Aucklandiae)
Qing Mu Xiang (Radix Aristolochiae)
Sha Ren (Fructus Amomi)
Tan Xiang (Lignum Santali Albi)
Wu Yao (Radix Linderae)
Xiang Fu (Rhizoma Cyperi)
Xiang Yuan (Fructus Citri)
Zhi Ke (Fructus Aurantii)

Cold
Bai Dou Kou (Fructus Amomi Rotundus)
Bi Cheng Qie (Fructus Litseae)
Cao Guo (Fructus Tsaoko)
Fu Zi (Radix Aconiti Lateralis Praeparata)
Gan Jiang (Rhizoma Zingiberis)
Gan Song (Radix seu Rhizoma Nardostachys)
Gao Liang Jiang (Rhizoma Alpiniae Officinarum)
Hua Jiao (Pericarpium Zanthoxyli)
Rou Gui (Cortex Cinnamomi)
Sha Ren (Fructus Amomi)
Sheng Jiang (Rhizoma Zingiberis Recens)
Tan Xiang (Lignum Santali Albi)
Wu Zhu Yu (Fructus Evodiae)

Heat
Chuan Lian Zi (Fructus Toosendan)
Da Huang (Radix et Rhizoma Rhei)
Huang Lian (Rhizoma Coptidis)
Shi Gao (Gypsum Fibrosum)
Zhi Zi (Fructus Gardeniae)
Zhu Ru (Caulis Bambusae in Taenia)

Stagnation
Chuan Lian Zi (Fructus Toosendan)
E Zhu (Rhizoma Curcumae)
Mo Yao (Myrrha)
Pu Huang (Pollen Typhae)
Ru Xiang (Gummi Olibanum)
San Leng (Rhizoma Sparganii)
Wu Ling Zhi (Excrementum Trogopteri seu Pteromi)
Yan Hu Suo (Rhizoma Corydalis)

Pain with food intake
Gu Ya (Fructus Setariae Germinatus)
Ji Nei Jin (Endothelium Corneum Gigeriae Galli)
Liu Ji Nu (Herba Artemisiae Anomalae)
Mai Ya (Fructus Hordei Germinatus)
Qing Pi (Pericarpium Citri Reticulatae Viride)
Shan Zha (Fructus Crataegi)
Shen Qu (Massa Fermentata)

Parasitic infestation
Bing Lang (Semen Arecae)
Ku Lian Pi (Cortex Meliae)
Qian Niu Zi (Semen Pharbitidis)
Shi Jun Zi (Fructus Quisqualis)
Wu Mei (Fructus Mume)

58. Syphilis and leprosy

Syphilis
Da Feng Zi (Semen Hydnocarpi)
Ku Shen Gen (Radix Sophorae Flavescentis)
Tu Fu Ling (Rhizoma Smilacis Glabrae)

Leprosy
Da Feng Zi (Semen Hydnocarpi)
Ku Shen Gen (Radix Sophorae Flavescentis)
She Tui (Periostracum Serpentis)
Zao Jiao (Fructus Gleditsiae)
Zao Jiao Ci (Spina Gleditsiae)

59. Thirst

Wind-heat
Ge Gen (Radix Puerariae)
Lu Gen (Rhizoma Phragmitis)

Stomach heat
Shi Gao (Gypsum Fibrosum)
Zhi Mu (Radix Anemarrhenae)

Intestinal heat
Da Huang (Radix et Rhizoma Rhei)
Mang Xiao (Natrii Sulfas)

Heat-toxins
Sheng Di Huang (Radix Rehmanniae)
Xuan Shen (Radix Scrophulariae)

Damaged yin
Shi Hu (Herba Dendrobii)
Tian Hua Fen (Radix Trichosanthis)
Yu Zhu (Rhizoma Polygonati Odorati)

Water accumulation
Ban Xia (Rhizoma Pinelliae)
Fu Ling (Poria)

With bitter taste in the mouth
Long Dan Cao (Radix Gentianae)
Yin Chen Hao (Herba Artemisiae Scopariae)

With sweet taste in the mouth
Fu Ling (Poria)
Pei Lan (Herba Eupatorii)

60. Toothache

Stomach fire
Bai Zhi (Radix Angelicae Dahuricae)
Da Huang (Radix et Rhizoma Rhei)
Huang Lian (Rhizoma Coptidis)
Sheng Ma (Rhizoma Cimicifugae)
Shi Gao (Gypsum Fibrosum)
Zhu Ye (Herba Phyllostachys)

Kidney deficiency
Gu Sui Bu (Rhizoma Drynariae)
Niu Xi (Radix Cyathulae seu Achyranthis)
Xi Xin (Herba Asari)

Wind-cold
Bai Zhi (Radix Angelicae Dahuricae)
Gao Ben (Rhizoma Ligustici)
Xi Xin (Herba Asari)

Cold stagnation
Bi Ba (Fructus Piperis Longi)

Wind
Xu Chang Qing (Radix Cynanchi Paniculati)
Xun Gu Feng (Herba Aristolochiae Mollissimae)

61. Traumatic injuries

Chi Shao (Radix Paeoniae Rubrae)
Chuan Xiong (Rhizoma Ligustici Chuanxiong)
Da Huang (Radix et Rhizoma Rhei)
Dang Gui (Radicis Angelicae Sinensis)
Hai Feng Teng (Caulis Piperis Kadsurae)
He Huan Pi (Cortex Albiziae)
Hong Hua (Flos Carthami)
Hong Teng (Caulis Sargentodoxae)
Hu Zhang (Rhizoma Polygoni Cuspidati)
Jiang Xiang (Lignum Dalbergiae Odoriferae)
Liu Ji Nu (Herba Artemisiae Anomalae)
Ma Qian Zi (Semen Strychni)
Meng Chong (Tabanus)
Mo Yao (Myrrha)
Mu Dan Pi (Cortex Moutan)
Niu Xi (Radix Cyathulae seu Achyranthis)
Ru Xiang (Gummi Olibanum)
San Qi (Radix Notoginseng)
She Xiang (Moschus)
Shui Zhi (Hirudo)
Song Jie (Lignum Pini Nodi)
Su Mu (Lignum Sappan)
Tao Ren (Semen Persicae)
Xu Chang Qing (Radix Cynanchi Paniculati)
Xu Duan (Radix Dipsaci)
Xue Jie (Sanguis Draconis)

Xun Gu Feng (Herba Aristolochiae Mollissimae)
Ze Lan (Herba Lycopi)
Zhang Nao (Camphora)
Zi Ran Tong (Pyritum)

62. Unstable pregnancy

Qi deficiency
Bai Zhu (Rhizoma Atractylodis Macrocephalae)
Huang Qi (Radix Astragali)
Ren Shen (Radix Ginseng)

Blood deficiency
Bai Shao (Radix Paeoniae Alba)
Dang Gui (Radicis Angelicae Sinensis)
E Jiao (Colla Corii Asini)
Shu Di Huang (Radix Rehmanniae Preparata)

Kidney deficiency
Du Zhong (Cortex Eucommiae)
Sang Ji Sheng (Herba Taxilli)
Tu Si Zi (Semen Cuscutae)
Xu Duan (Radix Dipsaci)

Heat in the blood
Huang Qin (Radix Scutellariae)

Qi stagnation
Sha Ren (Fructus Amomi)
Su Geng (Caulis Perillae)

63. Wheezing and dyspnea

Cold
Bai Jie Zi (Semen Sinapis)
Ci Shi (Magnetitum)
Gan Jiang (Rhizoma Zingiberis)
Lai Fu Zi (Semen Raphani)
Ma Huang (Herba Ephedrae)
Su Zi (Fructus Perillae)
Xi Xin (Herba Asari)
Xing Ren (Semen Armeniacae Amarum)

Heat
Bai Guo (Semen Ginkgo)
Hai Ge Fen (Concha Meretricis seu Cyclinae)
Huang Qin (Radix Scutellariae)
Ma Dou Ling (Fructus Aristolochiae)
Pi Pa Ye (Folium Eriobotryae)
Qian Hu (Radix Peucedani)
Sang Bai Pi (Cortex Mori)
Shi Wei (Folium Pyrrosiae)
Ting Li Zi (Semen Descurainiae seu Lepidii)

Phlegm
Hou Po (Cortex Magnoliae Officinalis)
Xiong Huang (Realgar)
Yin Guo Ye (Folium Ginkgo)

Lung deficiency
Dang Shen (Radix Codonopsis)
Mai Men Dong (Radix Ophiopogonis)
Ren Shen (Radix Ginseng)
Shan Yao (Rhizoma Dioscoreae)
Wu Wei Zi (Fructus Schisandrae Chinensis)

Kidney yang deficiency
Bu Gu Zhi (Fructus Psoraleae)
Fu Zi (Radix Aconiti Lateralis Praeparata)
Ge Jie (Gecko)

Lung and Kidney deficiencies
Ci Shi (Magnetitum)
Dong Chong Xia Cao (Cordyceps)
Ge Jie (Gecko)
Hu Tao Ren (Semen Juglandis)
Zi He Che (Placenta Hominis)

64. *Wu xin re* (five-center heat)

Bai Bu (Radix Stemonae)
Bai Mu Er (Fructificatio Tremellae Fuciformis)
Bai Wei (Radix Cynanchi Atrati)
Huang Lian (Rhizoma Coptidis)
Nan Sha Shen (Radix Adenophorae)
Qing Hao (Herba Artemisiae Annuae)
Sheng Di Huang (Radix Rehmanniae)
Yin Chai Hu (Radix Stellariae)
Zhi Mu (Radix Anemarrhenae)

65. *Xiao ke* (wasting and thirsting) syndrome

Upper *jiao*
Mai Men Dong (Radix Ophiopogonis)
Ren Shen (Radix Ginseng)
Tian Hua Fen (Radix Trichosanthis)
Wu Wei Zi (Fructus Schisandrae Chinensis)

Middle *jiao*
Ge Gen (Radix Puerariae)
Huang Jing (Rhizoma Polygonati)
Shi Hu (Herba Dendrobii)
Tian Hua Fen (Radix Trichosanthis)

Lower *jiao*
Shan Zhu Yu (Fructus Corni)
Shu Di Huang (Radix Rehmanniae Preparata)
Wu Wei Zi (Fructus Schisandrae Chinensis)
Zhi Mu (Radix Anemarrhenae)

66. *Zang zao* (dry organ) disorder

Da Zao (Fructus Jujubae)
Gan Cao (Radix Glycyrrhizae)
Xiao Mai (Fructus Tritici)

Appendix 2 — Cross-reference Based on Western Medical Diagnosis

The listing of any herb under a diagnosis does not insure that that substance can be unquestioningly prescribed for the named symptom or syndrome. Selection and combination of herbs must be based on careful differential diagnosis, guided by informed understanding and training in Chinese Herbal Medicine.

1. Acid reflux

Bei Sha Shen (Radix Glehniae)
Ding Xiang (Flos Caryophylli)
Hai Ge Fen (Concha Cyclinae)
Hai Piao Xiao (Endoconcha Sepiae)
Huang Lian (Rhizoma Coptidis)
Mu Li (Concha Ostreae)
Wa Leng Zi (Concha Arcae)
Wu Zhu Yu (Fructus Evodiae)
Zhe Bei Mu (Bulbus Fritillariae Thunbergii)

2. Allergies

Chan Tui (Periostracum Cicadae)
Fang Feng (Radix Saposhnikoviae)
Zi Su Ye (Folium Perillae)

3. Amoebae

Bai Tou Weng (Radix Pulsatillae)
Bi Cheng Qie (Fructus Litseae)
Lu Cha (Folium Camellia Sinensis)

Wu Long Cha (Folium Camellia Sinensis Fermentata)
Ya Dan Zi (Fructus Bruceae)

4. Anemia
Dang Shen (Radix Codonopsis)
E Jiao (Colla Corii Asini)
Hai Shen (Strichopus Japonicus)
Lu Lu Tong (Fructus Liquidambaris)
Ma Qian Zi (Semen Strychni)
Ren Shen (Radix Ginseng)
Sang Shen Zi (Fructus Mori)

5. Angina
Chen Xiang (Lignum Aquilariae Resinatum)
Chuan Xiong (Rhizoma Ligusticum Chuanxiong)
Dan Shen (Radix Salviae Miltiorrhizae)
Ge Gen (Radix Puerariae)
Gua Lou Shi (Fructus Trichosanthis)
Gui Zhi (Ramulus Cinnamomi)
Hong Hua (Flos Carthami)
San Qi (Radix Notoginseng)
Shan Zha (Fructus Crataegi)
She Xiang (Moschus)
Su He Xiang (Styrax)
Tan Xiang (Lignum Santali Albi)
Xie Bai (Bulbus Allii Macrostemonis)
Yan Hu Suo (Rhizoma Corydalis)
Zhi Shi (Fructus Aurantii Immaturus)

6. Appendicitis
Ba Dou (Fructus Crotonis)
Gua Lou Shi (Fructus Trichosanthis)
Shi Liu Pi (Pericarpium Granati)
Yi Yi Ren (Semen Coicis)

7. Arrhythmia
Bai Jie Zi (Semen Sinapis)
Chang Shan (Radix Dichroae)
Dang Gui (Radicis Angelicae Sinensis)
Dong Chong Xia Cao (Cordyceps)
Fu Zi (Radix Aconiti Lateralis Praeparata)
Gan Song (Radix seu Rhizoma Nardostachys)
Ge Gen (Radix Puerariae)
Gua Lou Shi (Fructus Trichosanthis)
Huang Lian (Rhizoma Coptidis)
Ku Shen Gen (Radix Sophorae Flavescentis)
Ling Zhi (Ganoderma)
Qiang Huo (Rhizoma et Radix Notopterygii)
Sang Ji Sheng (Herba Taxilli)
Shan Dou Gen (Radix Sophorae Tonkinensis)

8. Arthritis
Ba Ji Tian (Radix Morindae Officinalis)
Cao Wu (Radix Aconiti Kusnezoffii)
Chai Hu (Radix Bupleuri)
Chou Wu Tong (Folium Clerodendri Trichotomi)
Chuan Wu (Radix Aconiti Preparata)
Du Huo (Radix Angelicae Pubescentis)
Du Zhong (Cortex Eucommiae)
Fang Feng (Radix Saposhnikoviae)
Gan Jiang (Rhizoma Zingiberis)
Gou Ji (Rhizoma Cibotii)
Gui Zhi (Ramulus Cinnamomi)
Hai Ma (Hippocampus)
Lao Guan Cao (Herba Erodii seu Geranii)
Lei Gong Teng (Radix Tripterygii Wilfordii)
Ma Huang (Herba Ephedrae)
Mu Gua (Fructus Chaenomelis)
Qin Jiao (Radix Gentianae Macrophyllae)
Qing Feng Teng (Caulis Sinomenii)
Sang Zhi (Ramulus Mori)
Sheng Jiang (Rhizoma Zingiberis Recens)
Shui Niu Jiao (Cornu Bubali)
Wei Ling Xian (Radix Clematidis)
Wu Jia Pi (Cortex Acanthopanacis)
Wu Yao (Radix Linderae)
Xi Xian Cao (Herba Siegesbeckiae)
Xu Chang Qing (Radix Cynanchi Paniculati)
Xun Gu Feng (Herba Aristolochiae Mollissimae)
Zao Xiu (Rhizoma Paridis)

9. Ascites
Ba Dou (Fructus Crotonis)
Ban Bian Lian (Herba Lobeliae Chinensis)
Ban Zhi Lian (Herba Scutellariae Barbatae)
Bing Lang (Semen Arecae)
Chi Xiao Dou (Semen Phaseoli)
Da Ji (Radix Euphorbiae seu Knoxiae)
Da Suan (Bulbus Alli Sativi)
Gan Sui (Radix Euphorbiae Kansui)
Ma Bian Cao (Herba Verbenae)
Qian Niu Zi (Semen Pharbitidis)
Qing Fen (Calomelas)
Shang Lu (Radix Phytolaccae)
She Xiang (Moschus)
Yuan Hua (Flos Genkwa)
Ze Qi (Herba Euphorbiae Helioscopiae)

10. Asthma
Bai Jie Zi (Semen Sinapis)
Chen Xiang (Lignum Aquilariae Resinatum)
E Jiao (Colla Corii Asini)
Fo Shou (Fructus Citri Sarcodactylis)
Ge Jie (Gecko)
Gui Zhi (Ramulus Cinnamomi)
Hai Piao Xiao (Endoconcha Sepiae)
Jie Geng (Radix Platycodonis)
Jing Jie (Herba Schizonepetae)
Ku Shen Gen (Radix Sophorae Flavescentis)
Ma Huang (Herba Ephedrae)
Mu Xiang (Radix Aucklandiae)
Qian Niu Zi (Semen Pharbitidis)
Rou Gui (Cortex Cinnamomi)
Shan Dou Gen (Radix Sophorae Tonkinensis)
She Chuang Zi (Fructus Cnidii)
She Gan (Rhizoma Belamcandae)
Shi Chang Pu (Rhizoma Acori)
Shi Wei (Folium Pyrrosiae)
Wei Ling Xian (Radix Clematidis)
Xie Bai (Bulbus Allii Macrostemonis)
Xiong Huang (Realgar)
Zao Xiu (Rhizoma Paridis)

11. Atherosclerosis
Chen Pi (Pericarpium Citri Reticulatae)
Chi Shao (Radix Paeoniae Rubrae)
Chuan Shan Long (Rhizoma Dioscoreae Nipponicae)
Da Suan (Bulbus Alli Sativi)
Dang Gui (Radicis Angelicae Sinensis)
Gu Sui Bu (Rhizoma Drynariae)
Gui Ban (Plastrum Testudinis)
He Shou Wu (Radix Polygoni Multiflori)
Jiao Gu Lan (Rhizoma seu Herba Gynostemmatis)
Jin Ying Zi (Fructus Rosae Laevigatae)
Jue Ming Zi (Semen Cassiae)
Kun Bu (Thallus Laminariae seu Eckloniae)
Mu Dan Pi (Cortex Moutan)
Pu Huang (Pollen Typhae)
Ren Shen (Radix Ginseng)
San Qi (Radix Notoginseng)
Shan Zha (Fructus Crataegi)
Xie Bai (Bulbus Allii Macrostemonis)
Xu Chang Qing (Radix Cynanchi Paniculati)

12. Bleeding disorders

Ai Ye (Folium Artemisiae Argyi)
Bai Guo (Semen Ginkgo)
Bai He (Bulbus Lilii)
Bai Ji (Rhizoma Bletillae)
Bai Mao Gen (Rhizoma Imperatae)
Can Sha (Excrementum Bombycis Mori)
Che Qian Zi (Semen Plantaginis)
Chen Pi (Pericarpium Citri Reticulatae)
Da Huang (Radix et Rhizoma Rhei)
Da Ji (Herba seu Radix Cirsii Japonici)
Dang Gui (Radicis Angelicae Sinensis)
Di Gu Pi (Cortex Lycii)
Di Jin Cao (Herba Euphorbiae Humifusae)
Di Yu (Radix Sanguisorbae)
Fan Xie Ye (Folium Sennae)
Fu Long Gan (Terra Flava Usta)
Gu Sui Bu (Rhizoma Drynariae)
Guan Zhong (Rhizoma Dryopteridis)
Hai Piao Xiao (Endoconcha Sepiae)
Han Lian Cao (Herba Ecliptae)
Hu Zhang (Rhizoma Polygoni Cuspidati)
Hua Rui Shi (Ophicalcitum)
Huai Hua (Flos Sophorae)
Ji Guan Hua (Flos Celosiae Cristatae)
Lian Fang (Receptaculum Nelumbinis)
Long Gu (Os Draconis)
Lu Hui (Aloe)
Ma Huang (Herba Ephedrae)
Ou Jie (Nodus Nelumbinis Rhizomatis)
San Qi (Radix Notoginseng)
Su Zi (Fructus Perillae)
Wu Bei Zi (Galla Chinensis)
Wu Zhu Yu (Fructus Evodiae)
Xian He Cao (Herba Agrimoniae)
Xiao Ji (Herba Cirisii)
Xue Jie (Sanguis Draconis)
Xue Yu Tan (Crinis Carbonisatus)
Yi Mu Cao (Herba Leonuri)
Yu Xing Cao (Herba Houttuyniae)
Zhi Zi (Fructus Gardeniae)
Zi Zhu (Folium Callicarpae)
Zong Lu Pi (Fibra Stipulae Trachycarpi)

13. Blood flukes

Ba Dou (Fructus Crotonis)
Bing Lang (Semen Arecae)
Gan Jiang (Rhizoma Zingiberis)
Hai Zao (Sargassum)
He Cao Ya (Gemma Agrimoniae)
Jin Qian Cao (Herba Lysimachiae)
Ku Lian Pi (Cortex Meliae)
Ma Bian Cao (Herba Verbenae)
Nan Gua Zi (Semen Cucurbitae Moschatae)
Qing Hao (Herba Artemisiae Annuae)
Qu Mai (Herba Dianthi)
Wa Leng Zi (Concha Arcae)
Wu Mei (Fructus Mume)
Xian He Cao (Herba Agrimoniae)
Xiong Huang (Realgar)
Ya Dan Zi (Fructus Bruceae)

14. Bone fracture

Gu Sui Bu (Rhizoma Drynariae)
Ju Ye San Qi (Herba seu Radix Gynura Segetum)
Ma Ti Jin (Herba Dichondrae Repentis)

15. Bronchiectasis

Bai He (Bulbus Lilii)
Bai Ji (Rhizoma Bletillae)
San Qi (Radix Notoginseng)

16. Bronchitis

Ai Ye (Folium Artemisiae Argyi)
Bai Bu (Radix Stemonae)
Bai He (Bulbus Lilii)
Bai Jie Zi (Semen Sinapis)
Bai Mao Gen (Rhizoma Imperatae)
Bi Cheng Qie (Fructus Litseae)
Bu Gu Zhi (Fructus Psoraleae)
Cang Zhu (Rhizoma Atractylodis)
Che Qian Cao (Herba Plantaginis)
Chuan Bei Mu (Bulbus Fritillariae Cirrhosae)
Di Long (Pheretima)
E Jiao (Colla Corii Asini)
Fang Feng (Radix Saposhnikoviae)
Fo Shou (Fructus Citri Sarcodactylis)
Gua Di (Pedicellus Cucumeris)
He Shi (Fructus Carpesii)
Huang Jing (Rhizoma Polygonati)
Jie Geng (Radix Platycodonis)
Kuan Dong Hua (Flos Farfarae)
Ling Zhi (Ganoderma)
Liu Huang (Sulfur)
Ma Dou Ling (Fructus Aristolochiae)
Ma Huang (Herba Ephedrae)
Man Jing Zi (Fructus Viticis)
Nan Sha Shen (Radix Adenophorae)
Nu Zhen Zi (Fructus Ligustri Lucidi)
Pi Pa Ye (Folium Eriobotryae)
Qin Pi (Cortex Fraxini)
Qing Hao (Herba Artemisiae Annuae)
Ren Dong Teng (Caulis Lonicerae)
Sang Bai Pi (Cortex Mori)
She Chuang Zi (Fructus Cnidii)
She Gan (Rhizoma Belamcandae)
Tu Si Zi (Semen Cuscutae)
Wu Mei (Fructus Mume)
Xiong Huang (Realgar)
Xuan Fu Hua (Flos Inulae)
Yin Guo Ye (Folium Ginkgo)
Yin Yang Huo (Herba Epimedii)
Yuan Zhi (Radix Polygalae)
Ze Qi (Herba Euphorbiae Helioscopiae)
Zhu Dan (Fel Porcus)
Zi He Che (Placenta Hominis)
Zi Wan (Radix Asteris)

17. Burns

Bai Ji (Rhizoma Bletillae)
Bai Zhi (Radix Angelicae Dahuricae)
Di Yu (Radix Sanguisorbae)
Er Cha (Catechu)
Hu Zhang (Rhizoma Polygoni Cuspidati)
Huang Bai (Cortex Phellodendri)
Huang Lian (Rhizoma Coptidis)
Xue Yu Tan (Crinis Carbonisatus)
Zi Cao Gen (Radix Lithospermi)
Zi Zhu (Folium Callicarpae)

18. Cancer

Ba Dou (Fructus Crotonis)
Bai Tou Weng (Radix Pulsatillae)
Bai Zhu (Rhizoma Atractylodis Macrocephalae)
Ban Mao (Mylabris)
Bie Jia (Carapax Trionycis)
Chan Su (Venenum Bufonis)
Chuan Wu (Radix Aconiti Preparata)
Chuan Xin Lian (Herba Andrographis)
E Zhu (Rhizoma Curcumae)
Guan Zhong (Rhizoma Dryopteridis)
Gui Zhi (Ramulus Cinnamomi)
Huang Yao Zi (Herba Dioscoreae Bulbiferae)
Jiang Huang (Rhizoma Curcumae Longae)
Jiao Gu Lan (Rhizoma seu Herba Gynostemmatis)
Nu Zhen Zi (Fructus Ligustri Lucidi)
Qing Mu Xiang (Radix Aristolochiae)
San Qi (Radix Notoginseng)
Sang Bai Pi (Cortex Mori)
Shan Dou Gen (Radix Sophorae Tonkinensis)
She Xiang (Moschus)
Shen Qu (Massa Fermentata)
Su Mu (Lignum Sappan)
Tian Hua Fen (Radix Trichosanthis)
Tian Men Dong (Radix Asparagi)
Tian Nan Xing (Rhizoma Arisaematis)

Wei Ling Xian (Radix Clematidis)
Wu Mei (Fructus Mume)
Xian He Cao (Herba Agrimoniae)
Xuan Shen (Radix Scrophulariae)
Ya Dan Zi (Fructus Bruceae)
Yi Yi Ren (Semen Coicis)
Zhu Ling (Polyporus)
Zong Lu Pi (Fibra Stipulae Trachycarpi)

19. Carbuncles, furuncles and sores

Ba Dou (Fructus Crotonis)
Bai He (Bulbus Lilii)
Bai Tou Weng (Radix Pulsatillae)
Di Jin Cao (Herba Euphorbiae Humifusae)
Hai Piao Xiao (Endoconcha Sepiae)
Hai Zao (Sargassum)
Kun Bu (Thallus Laminariae seu Eckloniae)
Ma Bian Cao (Herba Verbenae)
Pi Pa Ye (Folium Eriobotryae)
Shui Zhi (Hirudo)
Wu Bei Zi (Galla Chinensis)

20. Cardiac ischemia

Bi Ba (Fructus Piperis Longi)
Bi Cheng Qie (Fructus Litseae)
Bing Pian (Borneolum Syntheticum)
Chuan Xiong (Rhizoma Ligustici Chuanxiong)
Ci Wu Jia (Radix et Caulis Acanthopanacis Senticosi)
Dang Gui (Radicis Angelicae Sinensis)
Dang Shen (Radix Codonopsis)
Fen Fang Ji (Radix Stephaniae Tetandrae)
Gan Song (Radix seu Rhizoma Nardostachys)
Ge Gen (Radix Puerariae)
Gou Ji (Rhizoma Cibotii)
Gua Lou Shi (Fructus Trichosanthis)
He Shou Wu (Radix Polygoni Multiflori)
Hong Hua (Flos Carthami)
Huang Jing (Rhizoma Polygonati)
Jiang Huang (Rhizoma Curcumae Longae)
Jiao Gu Lan (Rhizoma seu Herba Gynostemmatis)
Ku Shen Gen (Radix Sophorae Flavescentis)
Mai Men Dong (Radix Ophiopogonis)
Mao Dong Qing (Radix Ilicis Pubescentis)
Mu Dan Pi (Cortex Moutan)
Qiang Huo (Rhizoma et Radix Notopterygii)
Ren Shen (Radix Ginseng)
Rou Gui (Cortex Cinnamomi)
San Qi (Radix Notoginseng)
Yan Hu Suo (Rhizoma Corydalis)
Ye Ju Hua (Flos Chrysanthemi Indici)
Yi Mu Cao (Herba Leonuri)
Yin Yang Huo (Herba Epimedii)

21. Cholecystitis

Ba Dou (Fructus Crotonis)
Bai Tou Weng (Radix Pulsatillae)
Chai Hu (Radix Bupleuri)
Jin Qian Cao (Herba Lysimachiae)
Mang Xiao (Natrii Sulfas)
Wei Ling Xian (Radix Clematidis)
Wu Mei (Fructus Mume)
Yin Chen Hao (Herba Artemisiae Scopariae)
Zao Xiu (Rhizoma Paridis)

22. Chronic obstructive pulmonary disease (COPD)

E Zhu (Rhizoma Curcumae)
Fen Fang Ji (Radix Stephaniae Tetandrae)
Ma Bian Cao (Herba Verbenae)

23. Clotting disorders

Bi Cheng Qie (Fructus Litseae)
Ci Wu Jia (Radix et Caulis Acanthopanacis Senticosi)
Dang Gui (Radicis Angelicae Sinensis)
Di Long (Pheretima)
Ge Gen (Radix Puerariae)
Hai Feng Teng (Caulis Piperis Kadsurae)
Hai Shen (Strichopus Japonicus)
Hong Hua (Flos Carthami)
Mao Dong Qing (Radix Ilicis Pubescentis)
Shui Zhi (Hirudo)
Xuan Shen (Radix Scrophulariae)

24. Common colds and influenza

Bi Ba (Fructus Piperis Longi)
Bo He (Herba Menthae)
Cang Zhu (Rhizoma Atractylodis)
Cong Bai (Bulbus Allii Fistulosi)
Fang Feng (Radix Saposhnikoviae)
Guan Zhong (Rhizoma Dryopteridis)
Gui Zhi (Ramulus Cinnamomi)
Huo Xiang (Herba Agastache)
Jin Yin Hua (Flos Lonicerae)
Jing Jie (Herba Schizonepetae)
Ma Bian Cao (Herba Verbenae)
Ma Huang (Herba Ephedrae)
Niu Bang Zi (Fructus Arctii)
Sang Ye (Folium Mori)
Sheng Jiang (Rhizoma Zingiberis Recens)
Xiang Ru (Herba Elsholtziae seu Moslae)
Xin Yi Hua (Flos Magnoliae)
Yin Chen Hao (Herba Artemisiae Scopariae)

25. Conjunctivitis

Bai Tou Weng (Radix Pulsatillae)
Bo He (Herba Menthae)
Chai Hu (Radix Bupleuri)
Chan Tui (Periostracum Cicadae)
Da Qing Ye (Folium Isatidis)
Fang Feng (Radix Saposhnikoviae)
Lao Guan Cao (Herba Erodii seu Geranii)
Qiang Huo (Rhizoma et Radix Notopterygii)
Wu Mei (Fructus Mume)
Zi Cao Gen (Radix Lithospermi)

26. Constipation

Bai Zhu (Rhizoma Atractylodis Macrocephalae)
Da Huang (Radix et Rhizoma Rhei)
Fan Xie Ye (Folium Sennae)
Fei Zi (Semen Torreyae)
Gua Lou Shi (Fructus Trichosanthis)
Hei Zhi Ma (Semen Sesami Nigrum)
Lai Fu Zi (Semen Raphani)
Luo Han Guo (Fructus Momordicae)
Mang Xiao (Natrii Sulfas)
Sang Shen Zi (Fructus Mori)
Zhi Shi (Fructus Aurantii Immaturus)

27. Coronary artery disease

Bai Ji Li (Fructus Tribuli)
Bai Jie Zi (Semen Sinapis)
Ban Xia (Rhizoma Pinelliae)
Bi Cheng Qie (Fructus Litseae)
Bing Pian (Borneolum Syntheticum)
Chi Shao (Radix Paeoniae Rubrae)
Chuan Shan Long (Rhizoma Dioscoreae Nipponicae)
Chuan Xiong (Rhizoma Ligustici Chuanxiong)
Ci Wu Jia (Radix et Caulis Acanthopanacis Senticosi)
Dan Shen (Radix Salviae Miltiorrhizae)
Dang Shen (Radix Codonopsis)
Fen Fang Ji (Radix Stephaniae Tetandrae)
Gao Liang Jiang (Rhizoma Alpiniae Officinarum)

Ge Gen (Radix Puerariae)
Gua Lou Shi (Fructus Trichosanthis)
Gui Zhi (Ramulus Cinnamomi)
Hai Feng Teng (Caulis Piperis Kadsurae)
Han Lian Cao (Herba Ecliptae)
Hong Hua (Flos Carthami)
Huang Jing (Rhizoma Polygonati)
Jiang Huang (Rhizoma Curcumae Longae)
Ju Hua (Flos Chrysanthemi)
Ling Zhi (Ganoderma)
Lu Cha (Folium Camellia Sinensis)
Mai Men Dong (Radix Ophiopogonis)
Nan Sha Shen (Radix Adenophorae)
Ren Shen (Radix Ginseng)
San Qi (Radix Notoginseng)
Sang Ji Sheng (Herba Taxilli)
Shan Zha (Fructus Crataegi)
She Xiang (Moschus)
Shui Zhi (Hirudo)
Su He Xiang (Styrax)
Tian Nan Xing (Rhizoma Arisaematis)
Tian Zhu Huang (Concretio Silicea Bambusae)
Wu Bei Zi (Galla Chinensis)
Wu Long Cha (Folium Camellia Sinensis Fermentata)
Xi Xian Cao (Herba Siegesbeckiae)
Ye Ju Hua (Flos Chrysanthemi Indici)
Yi Mu Cao (Herba Leonuri)
Yin Guo Ye (Folium Ginkgo)
Yin Yang Huo (Herba Epimedii)
Yuan Zhi (Radix Polygalae)

28. Coughing and wheezing

Bai He (Bulbus Lilii)
Ge Jie (Gecko)
Gu Zhi Hua (Semen Oroxyli)
Liu Huang (Sulfur)
Luo Han Guo (Fructus Momordicae)
Tian Nan Xing (Rhizoma Arisaematis)
Ting Li Zi (Semen Descurainiae seu Lepidii)
Wang Bu Liu Xing (Semen Vaccariae)
Xian He Cao (Herba Agrimoniae)
Zhe Bei Mu (Bulbus Fritillariae Thunbergii)
Zhu Li (Succus Bambusae)

29. Dementia

Shi Chang Pu (Rhizoma Acori)
Yin Guo Ye (Folium Ginkgo)

30. Dermatological disorders

Bai Ji (Rhizoma Bletillae)
Bai Zhi (Radix Angelicae Dahuricae)
Ban Mao (Mylabris)
Ban Xia (Rhizoma Pinelliae)
Bing Lang (Semen Arecae)
Bu Gu Zhi (Fructus Psoraleae)
Cang Zhu (Rhizoma Atractylodis)
Chi Xiao Dou (Semen Phaseoli)
Da Suan (Bulbus Alli Sativi)
Da Zao (Fructus Jujubae)
Dang Gui (Radicis Angelicae Sinensis)
Dang Shen (Radix Codonopsis)
Di Fu Zi (Fructus Kochiae)
Di Yu (Radix Sanguisorbae)
Ding Xiang (Flos Caryophylli)
Fang Feng (Radix Saposhnikoviae)
Ge Gen (Radix Puerariae)
Gou Qi Zi (Fructus Lycii)
Hai Shen (Strichopus Japonicus)
Huai Hua (Flos Sophorae)
Huang Bai (Cortex Phellodendri)
Huo Xiang (Herba Agastache)
Jin Yin Hua (Flos Lonicerae)
Ku Lian Pi (Cortex Meliae)
Lei Gong Teng (Radix Tripterygii Wilfordii)
Liu Huang (Sulfur)
Long Dan Cao (Radix Gentianae)
Mu Zei (Herba Equiseti Hiemalis)
Qian Dan (Minium)
San Qi (Radix Notoginseng)
She Chuang Zi (Fructus Cnidii)
Sheng Ma (Rhizoma Cimicifugae)
Shi Liu Pi (Pericarpium Granati)
Wei Ling Xian (Radix Clematidis)
Wu Bei Zi (Galla Chinensis)
Wu Mei (Fructus Mume)
Xu Chang Qing (Radix Cynanchi Paniculati)
Ya Dan Zi (Fructus Bruceae)
Yin Chen Hao (Herba Artemisiae Scopariae)
Zhu Ling (Polyporus)
Zi Su Ye (Folium Perillae)

31. Diabetes mellitus

Di Gu Pi (Cortex Lycii)
Hei Zhi Ma (Semen Sesami Nigrum)
Huang Jing (Rhizoma Polygonati)
Huang Lian (Rhizoma Coptidis)
Jiang Can (Bombyx Batryticatus)
Kun Bu (Thallus Laminariae seu Eckloniae)
Li Zhi He (Semen Litchi)
Mai Ya (Fructus Hordei Germinatus)
Nu Zhen Zi (Fructus Ligustri Lucidi)
Ren Shen (Radix Ginseng)
Shan Yao (Rhizoma Dioscoreae)
Wu Bei Zi (Galla Chinensis)
Wu Mei (Fructus Mume)
Yu Mi Xu (Stigma Maydis)
Ze Xie (Rhizoma Alismatis)

32. Diarrhea

Che Qian Zi (Semen Plantaginis)
Da Suan (Bulbus Alli Sativi)
Fu Ling (Poria)
Fu Long Gan (Terra Flava Usta)
Ge Gen (Radix Puerariae)
Huo Xiang (Herba Agastache)
Lian Fang (Receptaculum Nelumbinis)
Ma Huang (Herba Ephedrae)
Shan Yao (Rhizoma Dioscoreae)
Sheng Jiang (Rhizoma Zingiberis Recens)
Shi Liu Pi (Pericarpium Granati)
Shu Di Huang (Radix Rehmanniae Preparata)
Wu Bei Zi (Galla Chinensis)
Wu Mei (Fructus Mume)
Wu Zhu Yu (Fructus Evodiae)
Xiang Ru (Herba Elsholtziae seu Moslae)
Ze Xie (Rhizoma Alismatis)
Zhu Ling (Polyporus)

33. Diphtheria

Ba Dou (Fructus Crotonis)
Ma Bian Cao (Herba Verbenae)
Zhu Dan (Fel Porcus)

34. Dysentery

Ba Dou (Fructus Crotonis)
Bai Tou Weng (Radix Pulsatillae)
Bi Cheng Qie (Fructus Litseae)
Bing Lang (Semen Arecae)
Che Qian Cao (Herba Plantaginis)
Chuan Xin Lian (Herba Andrographis)
Di Yu (Radix Sanguisorbae)
Gan Jiang (Rhizoma Zingiberis)
Hai Piao Xiao (Endoconcha Sepiae)
Huang Lian (Rhizoma Coptidis)
Huang Qin (Radix Scutellariae)
Ji Guan Hua (Flos Celosiae Cristatae)
Jin Yin Hua (Flos Lonicerae)
Lu Cha (Folium Camellia Sinensis)
Ma Bian Cao (Herba Verbenae)
Mu Gua (Fructus Chaenomelis)
Nu Zhen Zi (Fructus Ligustri Lucidi)
Qin Pi (Cortex Fraxini)
Ren Dong Teng (Caulis Lonicerae)
Rou Gui (Cortex Cinnamomi)
Shan Dou Gen (Radix Sophorae Tonkinensis)

Shan Zha (Fructus Crataegi)
Sheng Jiang (Rhizoma Zingiberis Recens)
Sheng Ma (Rhizoma Cimicifugae)
Shi Liu Pi (Pericarpium Granati)
Shi Wei (Folium Pyrrosiae)
Wu Bei Zi (Galla Chinensis)
Wu Long Cha (Folium Camellia Sinensis Fermentata)
Wu Mei (Fructus Mume)
Wu Wei Zi (Fructus Schisandrae Chinensis)
Xia Ku Cao (Spica Prunellae)
Xian He Cao (Herba Agrimoniae)
Xiang Ru (Herba Elsholtziae seu Moslae)
Xiao Ji (Herba Cirisii)
Ya Dan Zi (Fructus Bruceae)
Ze Qi (Herba Euphorbiae Helioscopiae)
Zong Lu Pi (Fibra Stipulae Trachycarpi)

35. Edema
Bai Zhu (Rhizoma Atractylodis Macrocephalae)
Ban Bian Lian (Herba Lobeliae Chinensis)
Che Qian Zi (Semen Plantaginis)
Chi Xiao Dou (Semen Phaseoli)
Da Fu Pi (Pericarpium Arecae)
Dong Gua Pi (Exocarpium Benincasae)
Dong Kui Zi (Semen Malvae)
Fen Fang Ji (Radix Stephaniae Tetandrae)
Fu Ling (Poria)
Fu Ping (Herba Spirodelae)
Gan Sui (Radix Euphorbiae Kansui)
Gui Zhi (Ramulus Cinnamomi)
Ma Huang (Herba Ephedrae)
Sang Bai Pi (Cortex Mori)
Sheng Jiang Pi (Pericarpium Zingiberis Recens)
Shi Wei (Folium Pyrrosiae)
Ting Li Zi (Semen Descurainiae seu Lepidii)
Wu Jia Pi (Cortex Acanthopanacis)
Xiang Ru (Herba Elsholtziae seu Moslae)
Yi Mu Cao (Herba Leonuri)
Yi Yi Ren (Semen Coicis)
Yuan Hua (Flos Genkwa)
Ze Lan (Herba Lycopi)
Ze Xie (Rhizoma Alismatis)

36. Encephalitis
Da Qing Ye (Folium Isatidis)
Da Suan (Bulbus Alli Sativi)
Di Long (Pheretima)
Qin Jiao (Radix Gentianae Macrophyllae)
Shan Dou Gen (Radix Sophorae Tonkinensis)
Shi Chang Pu (Rhizoma Acori)

37. Enteritis
Ba Dou (Fructus Crotonis)
Bai Zhi (Radix Angelicae Dahuricae)
Bing Lang (Semen Arecae)
Chuan Xin Lian (Herba Andrographis)
Da Huang (Radix et Rhizoma Rhei)
Er Cha (Catechu)
Hai Piao Xiao (Endoconcha Sepiae)
Ku Shen Gen (Radix Sophorae Flavescentis)
Lao Guan Cao (Herba Erodii seu Geranii)
Lu Han Cao (Herba Pyrolae)
Ma Bian Cao (Herba Verbenae)
Qin Jiao (Radix Gentianae Macrophyllae)
Ren Dong Teng (Caulis Lonicerae)
Shan Zha (Fructus Crataegi)
Wu Bei Zi (Galla Chinensis)
Wu Mei (Fructus Mume)
Xian He Cao (Herba Agrimoniae)
Ya Dan Zi (Fructus Bruceae)
Zao Xiu (Rhizoma Paridis)
Zhu Dan (Fel Porcus)

38. Facial paralysis
Ba Dou (Fructus Crotonis)
Bai Jie Zi (Semen Sinapis)
Ban Mao (Mylabris)
Cao Wu (Radix Aconiti Kusnezoffii)
E Bu Shi Cao (Herba Centipedae)
Fang Feng (Radix Saposhnikoviae)
Ma Qian Zi (Semen Strychni)
Niu Bang Zi (Fructus Arctii)
Quan Xie (Scorpio)
Zhang Nao (Camphora)

39. Fever
Bie Jia (Carapax Trionycis)
Chai Hu (Radix Bupleuri)
Fu Long Gan (Terra Flava Usta)
Ge Gen (Radix Puerariae)
Han Lian Cao (Herba Ecliptae)
Ling Yang Jiao (Cornu Saigae Tataricae)
Niu Huang (Calculus Bovis)
Qing Hao (Herba Artemisiae Annuae)
Shi Gao (Gypsum Fibrosum)

40. Frostbite
Bai Ji (Rhizoma Bletillae)
Gui Zhi (Ramulus Cinnamomi)
Sang Ji Sheng (Herba Taxilli)
Zhang Nao (Camphora)

41. Gastritis
Bai He (Bulbus Lilii)
Bing Lang (Semen Arecae)
Da Huang (Radix et Rhizoma Rhei)
Da Suan (Bulbus Alli Sativi)
Er Cha (Catechu)
Fo Shou (Fructus Citri Sarcodactylis)
Huang Lian (Rhizoma Coptidis)
Lu Cha (Folium Camellia Sinensis)
Ma Bian Cao (Herba Verbenae)
Wu Long Cha (Folium Camellia Sinensis Fermentata)
Wu Mei (Fructus Mume)

42. Gout
Ding Shu Xiu (Herba Elephantopus Scaber)
Pu Yin (Radix Wikstroemia Indica)
Wan Dian Jin (Radix Ilicis Asprellae)

43. Headache
Bai Zhi (Radix Angelicae Dahuricae)
Bo He (Herba Menthae)
Chai Hu (Radix Bupleuri)
Chuan Xiong (Rhizoma Ligustici Chuanxiong)
Dang Gui (Radicis Angelicae Sinensis)
Du Huo (Radix Angelicae Pubescentis)
Fang Feng (Radix Saposhnikoviae)
Gao Ben (Rhizoma Ligustici)
Ge Gen (Radix Puerariae)
Gou Teng (Ramulus Uncariae cum Uncis)
Gui Zhi (Ramulus Cinnamomi)
He Shou Wu (Radix Polygoni Multiflori)
Jing Jie (Herba Schizonepetae)
Ju Hua (Flos Chrysanthemi)
Qiang Huo (Rhizoma et Radix Notopterygii)
Tian Ma (Rhizoma Gastrodiae)
Wu Zhu Yu (Fructus Evodiae)
Xi Xin (Herba Asari)

44. Heart failure
Chan Su (Venenum Bufonis)
Fu Zi (Radix Aconiti Lateralis Praeparata)
Ting Li Zi (Semen Descurainiae seu Lepidii)
Yu Zhu (Rhizoma Polygonati Odorati)
Zhi Shi (Fructus Aurantii Immaturus)

45. Hemorrhoids

Bai Guo (Semen Ginkgo)
Bai Ji (Rhizoma Bletillae)
Chi Xiao Dou (Semen Phaseoli)
Huai Hua (Flos Sophorae)
Lian Fang (Receptaculum Nelumbinis)
Ming Fan (Alumen)
Wang Bu Liu Xing (Semen Vaccariae)
Wu Bei Zi (Galla Chinensis)
Xian He Cao (Herba Agrimoniae)
Ya Dan Zi (Fructus Bruceae)
Zi Zhu (Folium Callicarpae)

46. Hepatitis

Ai Ye (Folium Artemisiae Argyi)
Bai Shao (Radix Paeoniae Alba)
Bai Tou Weng (Radix Pulsatillae)
Ban Lan Gen (Radix Isatidis)
Ban Mao (Mylabris)
Chai Hu (Radix Bupleuri)
Che Qian Cao (Herba Plantaginis)
Chi Shao (Radix Paeoniae Rubrae)
Chui Pen Cao (Herba Sedi)
Da Ji (Radix Euphorbiae seu Knoxiae)
Da Qing Ye (Folium Isatidis)
Dan Shen (Radix Salviae Miltiorrhizae)
Dang Gui (Radicis Angelicae Sinensis)
Dong Chong Xia Cao (Cordyceps)
Fo Shou (Fructus Citri Sarcodactylis)
Gou Qi Zi (Fructus Lycii)
Guan Zhong (Rhizoma Dryopteridis)
Hai Jin Sha (Herba Lygodii)
Hu Zhang (Rhizoma Polygoni Cuspidati)
Huang Jing (Rhizoma Polygonati)
Huang Qi (Radix Astragali)
Huang Qin (Radix Scutellariae)
Huo Xiang (Herba Agastache)
Jiao Gu Lan (Rhizoma seu Herba Gynostemmatis)
Ling Zhi (Ganoderma)
Lu Cha (Folium Camellia Sinensis)
Lu Hui (Aloe)
Ma Bian Cao (Herba Verbenae)
Ma Dou Ling (Fructus Aristolochiae)
Ming Fan (Alumen)
Mu Gua (Fructus Chaenomelis)
Mu Zei (Herba Equiseti Hiemalis)
Nu Zhen Zi (Fructus Ligustri Lucidi)
Qin Jiao (Radix Gentianae Macrophyllae)
Ren Dong Teng (Caulis Lonicerae)
Shan Dou Gen (Radix Sophorae Tonkinensis)
Shan Yao (Rhizoma Dioscoreae)
Shan Zha (Fructus Crataegi)
Shang Lu (Radix Phytolaccae)
She Xiang (Moschus)
Shui Niu Jiao (Cornu Bubali)
Wu Gong (Scolopendra)
Wu Long Cha (Folium Camellia Sinensis Fermentata)
Wu Mei (Fructus Mume)
Wu Wei Zi (Fructus Schisandrae Chinensis)
Xia Ku Cao (Spica Prunellae)
Xiao Ji (Herba Cirisii)
Yi Yi Ren (Semen Coicis)
Yin Chen Hao (Herba Artemisiae Scopariae)
Zhu Dan (Fel Porcus)

47. Hepatomegaly

Bie Jia (Carapax Trionycis)
Dan Shen (Radix Salviae Miltiorrhizae)
Hong Hua (Flos Carthami)
Ku Lian Pi (Cortex Meliae)
Kun Bu (Thallus Laminariae seu Eckloniae)
Liu Ji Nu (Herba Artemisiae Anomalae)
Mu Li (Concha Ostreae)
San Leng (Rhizoma Sparganii Stoloniferi)
She Gan (Rhizoma Belamcandae)
Xia Ku Cao (Spica Prunellae)
Xing Ren (Semen Armeniacae Amarum)

48. Hyperlipidemia

Chai Hu (Radix Bupleuri)
Ci Wu Jia (Radix et Caulis Acanthopanacis Senticosi)
Cong Bai (Bulbus Allii Fistulosi)
Da Huang (Radix et Rhizoma Rhei)
Da Suan (Bulbus Alli Sativi)
Dang Gui (Radicis Angelicae Sinensis)
E Zhu (Rhizoma Curcumae)
Ge Gen (Radix Puerariae)
He Shou Wu (Radix Polygoni Multiflori)
Hu Zhang (Rhizoma Polygoni Cuspidati)
Huang Jing (Rhizoma Polygonati)
Jiang Huang (Rhizoma Curcumae Longae)
Jiao Gu Lan (Rhizoma seu Herba Gynostemmatis)
Jue Ming Zi (Semen Cassiae)
Kun Bu (Thallus Laminariae seu Eckloniae)
Lu Cha (Folium Camellia Sinensis)
Nu Zhen Zi (Fructus Ligustri Lucidi)
Ren Shen (Radix Ginseng)
San Qi (Radix Notoginseng)
Shan Zha (Fructus Crataegi)
Shui Zhi (Hirudo)
Tian Ma (Rhizoma Gastrodiae)
Tian Nan Xing (Rhizoma Arisaematis)
Wu Long Cha (Folium Camellia Sinensis Fermentata)
Xiang Ru (Herba Elsholtziae seu Moslae)
Xie Bai (Bulbus Allii Macrostemonis)
Xu Chang Qing (Radix Cynanchi Paniculati)
Ye Ju Hua (Flos Chrysanthemi Indici)
Yin Guo Ye (Folium Ginkgo)
Yu Zhu (Rhizoma Polygonati Odorati)
Ze Xie (Rhizoma Alismatis)

49. Hyperosteogeny

Bai Shao (Radix Paeoniae Alba)
Cao Wu (Radix Aconiti Kusnezoffii)
Chuan Wu (Radix Aconiti Preparata)
Du Huo (Radix Angelicae Pubescentis)
Gui Zhi (Ramulus Cinnamomi)
Lei Gong Teng (Radix Tripterygii Wilfordii)
Ma Qian Zi (Semen Strychni)
She Xiang (Moschus)
Wei Ling Xian (Radix Clematidis)
Xu Duan (Radix Dipsaci)

50. Hypertension

Bo He (Herba Menthae)
Che Qian Zi (Semen Plantaginis)
Chou Wu Tong (Folium Clerodendri Trichotomi)
Da Ji (Herba seu Radix Cirsii Japonici)
Di Gu Pi (Cortex Lycii)
Di Long (Pheretima)
Du Zhong (Cortex Eucommiae)
Fen Fang Ji (Radix Stephaniae Tetandrae)
Gou Teng (Ramulus Uncariae cum Uncis)
Huai Hua (Flos Sophorae)
Huang Lian (Rhizoma Coptidis)
Ju Hua (Flos Chrysanthemi)
Jue Ming Zi (Semen Cassiae)
Lai Fu Zi (Semen Raphani)
Ling Zhi (Ganoderma)
Liu Huang (Sulfur)
Lu Cha (Folium Camellia Sinensis)
Mu Zei (Herba Equiseti Hiemalis)
Qing Mu Xiang (Radix Aristolochiae)
Sang Shen Zi (Fructus Mori)
Shan Zha (Fructus Crataegi)
Shui Zhi (Hirudo)

Wang Bu Liu Xing (Semen Vaccariae)
Wu Long Cha (Folium Camellia Sinensis Fermentata)
Wu Mei (Fructus Mume)
Wu Zhu Yu (Fructus Evodiae)
Xi Xian Cao (Herba Siegesbeckiae)
Xia Ku Cao (Spica Prunellae)
Xia Tian Wu (Rhizoma Corydalis Decumbentis)
Xuan Shen (Radix Scrophulariae)
Ye Ju Hua (Flos Chrysanthemi Indici)
Yin Yang Huo (Herba Epimedii)
Ze Xie (Rhizoma Alismatis)
Zong Lu Pi (Fibra Stipulae Trachycarpi)

51. Hyperthyroidism
Hai Zao (Sargassum)
Huang Yao Zi (Herba Dioscoreae Bulbiferae)
Kun Bu (Thallus Laminariae seu Eckloniae)
Mu Li (Concha Ostreae)
Shi Gao (Gypsum Fibrosum)
Tian Hua Fen (Radix Trichosanthis)
Zhi Mu (Radix Anemarrhenae)

52. Hypothyroidism
Fu Zi (Radix Aconiti Lateralis Praeparata)
Hai Zao (Sargassum)
Kun Bu (Thallus Laminariae seu Eckloniae)
Rou Gui (Cortex Cinnamomi)

53. Hypoxia
Bai He (Bulbus Lilii)
Bai Shao (Radix Paeoniae Alba)
Bi Ba (Fructus Piperis Longi)
Bie Jia (Carapax Trionycis)
Ci Wu Jia (Radix et Caulis Acanthopanacis Senticosi)
Dan Shen (Radix Salviae Miltiorrhizae)
Dang Gui (Radicis Angelicae Sinensis)
Ding Xiang (Flos Caryophylli)
E Jiao (Colla Corii Asini)
Gan Jiang (Rhizoma Zingiberis)
Gan Song (Radix seu Rhizoma Nardostachys)
Ge Gen (Radix Puerariae)
Gua Lou Shi (Fructus Trichosanthis)
Gui Ban (Plastrum Testudinis)
Hai Feng Teng (Caulis Piperis Kadsurae)
Hai Long (Syngnathus)
Han Lian Cao (Herba Ecliptae)
Ling Zhi (Ganoderma)
Mai Men Dong (Radix Ophiopogonis)
Nu Zhen Zi (Fructus Ligustri Lucidi)
Ren Shen (Radix Ginseng)
Suan Zao Ren (Semen Zizyphi Spinosae)
Tian Ma (Rhizoma Gastrodiae)
Xi Yang Shen (Radix Panacis Quinquefolii)

54. Impotence
Ba Ji Tian (Radix Morindae Officinalis)
Bu Gu Zhi (Fructus Psoraleae)
Dong Chong Xia Cao (Cordyceps)
Du Zhong (*Cortex* Eucommiae)
Fu Zi (Radix Aconiti Lateralis Praeparata)
Ge Jie (Gecko)
Gou Qi Zi (Fructus Lycii)
Hai Ma (Hippocampus)
Jiu Cai Zi (Semen Allii Tuberosi)
Lu Rong (Cornu Cervi Pantotrichum)
Ren Shen (Radix Ginseng)
Rou Cong Rong (Herba Cistanches)
Rou Gui (Cortex Cinnamomi)
Sha Yuan Zi (Semen Astragali Complanati)
She Chuang Zi (Fructus Cnidii)
Shu Di Huang (Radix Rehmanniae Preparata)
Suo Yang (Herba Cynomorii)
Tu Si Zi (Semen Cuscutae)
Xian Mao (Rhizoma Curculiginis)
Xu Duan (Radix Dipsaci)
Yin Yang Huo (Herba Epimedii)
Zi He Che (Placenta Hominis)

55. Indigestion
Ban Xia (Rhizoma Pinelliae)
Cang Zhu (Rhizoma Atractylodis)
Da Huang (Radix et Rhizoma Rhei)
Ji Nei Jin (Endothelium Corneum Gigeriae Galli)
Lu Cha (Folium Camellia Sinensis)
Mai Ya (Fructus Hordei Germinatus)
Rou Dou Kou (Semen Myristicae)
Shan Zha (Fructus Crataegi)
Wu Long Cha (Folium Camellia Sinensis Fermentata)
Wu Zhu Yu (Fructus Evodiae)
Zhu Dan (Fel Porcus)

56. Infantile paralysis
Dang Gui (Radicis Angelicae Sinensis)
Xia Tian Wu (Rhizoma Corydalis Decumbentis)
Yin Yang Huo (Herba Epimedii)

57. Infantile stomatitis
Ba Dou (Fructus Crotonis)
Ban Lan Gen (Radix Isatidis)
Wu Zhu Yu (Fructus Evodiae)
Ye Ju Hua (Flos Chrysanthemi Indici)

58. Infection
Bing Pian (Borneolum Syntheticum)
Chi Shao (Radix Paeoniae Rubrae)
Chi Xiao Dou (Semen Phaseoli)
E Bu Shi Cao (Herba Centipedae)
Huang Bai (Cortex Phellodendri)
Huang Lian (Rhizoma Coptidis)
Huang Qin (Radix Scutellariae)
Lian Qiao (Fructus Forsythiae)
Ma Qian Zi (Semen Strychni)
Mao Dong Qing (Radix Ilicis Pubescentis)
Pu Gong Ying (Herba Taraxaci)
Qing Mu Xiang (Radix Aristolochiae)
She Tui (Periostracum Serpentis)
Xiao Ji (Herba Cirisii)
Xun Gu Feng (Herba Aristolochiae Mollissimae)
Ye Ju Hua (Flos Chrysanthemi Indici)
Ze Qi (Herba Euphorbiae Helioscopiae)

59. Infection (upper respiratory tract)
Ban Lan Gen (Radix Isatidis)
Chang Shan (Radix Dichroae)
Chuan Xin Lian (Herba Andrographis)
Da Qing Ye (Folium Isatidis)
Huang Qin (Radix Scutellariae)
Jin Yin Hua (Flos Lonicerae)
Jing Jie (Herba Schizonepetae)
Lian Qiao (Fructus Forsythiae)
Ma Huang (Herba Ephedrae)
Man Jing Zi (Fructus Viticis)
Niu Huang (Calculus Bovis)
Pu Gong Ying (Herba Taraxaci)
Sang Ye (Folium Mori)
Sang Zhi (Ramulus Mori)
Shi Gao (Gypsum Fibrosum)
Xi Xin (Herba Asari)
Ye Ju Hua (Flos Chrysanthemi Indici)
Yu Xing Cao (Herba Houttuyniae)
Zi Su Ye (Folium Perillae)

60. Infection (urinary tract)
Bai Tou Weng (Radix Pulsatillae)
Che Qian Cao (Herba Plantaginis)
Che Qian Zi (Semen Plantaginis)
Chuan Mu Tong (Caulis Clematidis Armandii)
Di Yu (Radix Sanguisorbae)
Guang Jin Qian Cao (Herba Desmodii Styracifolii)

Hai Jin Sha (Herba Lygodii)
Ma Bian Cao (Herba Verbenae)
Nan Gua Zi (Semen Cucurbitae Moschatae)
Qu Mai (Herba Dianthi)
Yu Mi Xu (Stigma Maydis)
Ze Xie (Rhizoma Alismatis)
Zhi Mu (Radix Anemarrhenae)
Zhu Ling (Polyporus)

61. Infertility

Bie Jia (Carapax Trionycis)
E Jiao (Colla Corii Asini)
Gui Ban (Plastrum Testudinis)
Huang Jing (Rhizoma Polygonati)
She Chuang Zi (Fructus Cnidii)
Tu Si Zi (Semen Cuscutae)
Xu Duan (Radix Dipsaci)
Zi He Che (Placenta Hominis)

62. Inflammation of the female reproductive system

Bai Jie Zi (Semen Sinapis)
Bai Tou Weng (Radix Pulsatillae)
Hu Zhang (Rhizoma Polygoni Cuspidati)
Hua Jiao (Pericarpium Zanthoxyli)
Huang Bai (Cortex Phellodendri)
Huang Qi (Radix Astragali)
Jue Ming Zi (Semen Cassiae)
Long Dan Cao (Radix Gentianae)
Ma Bian Cao (Herba Verbenae)
Peng Sha (Borax)
Shan Dou Gen (Radix Sophorae Tonkinensis)
She Chuang Zi (Fructus Cnidii)
Shi Liu Pi (Pericarpium Granati)
Wu Bei Zi (Galla Chinensis)
Ya Dan Zi (Fructus Bruceae)
Ye Ju Hua (Flos Chrysanthemi Indici)
Yu Xing Cao (Herba Houttuyniae)
Yuan Zhi (Radix Polygalae)
Zhu Dan (Fel Porcus)
Zi Cao Gen (Radix Lithospermi)

63. Inflammation of the male reproductive system

Che Qian Cao (Herba Plantaginis)
Che Qian Zi (Semen Plantaginis)
Chi Xiao Dou (Semen Phaseoli)
Chuan Bei Mu (Bulbus Fritillariae Cirrhosae)
Chuan Mu Tong (Caulis Clematidis Armandii)
Dang Gui (Radicis Angelicae Sinensis)
Guan Mu Tong (Caulis Aristolochiae Manshuriensis)
Guan Zhong (Rhizoma Dryopteridis)
Huang Bai (Cortex Phellodendri)
Long Dan Cao (Radix Gentianae)
Pu Gong Ying (Herba Taraxaci)
Qu Mai (Herba Dianthi)
Tu Si Zi (Semen Cuscutae)
Wei Ling Xian (Radix Clematidis)
Wu Mei (Fructus Mume)
Xuan Shen (Radix Scrophulariae)
Ye Ju Hua (Flos Chrysanthemi Indici)
Yu Xing Cao (Herba Houttuyniae)
Ze Xie (Rhizoma Alismatis)
Zhi Mu (Radix Anemarrhenae)

64. Intestinal obstruction

Ba Dou (Fructus Crotonis)
Ding Xiang (Flos Caryophylli)
Fan Xie Ye (Folium Sennae)
Gan Jiang (Rhizoma Zingiberis)
Hua Jiao (Pericarpium Zanthoxyli)
Wu Mei (Fructus Mume)
Zhu Dan (Fel Porcus)

65. Jaundice

Bai Mao Gen (Rhizoma Imperatae)
Bai Xian Pi (Cortex Dictamni)
Bai Zhu (Rhizoma Atractylodis Macrocephalae)
Chi Xiao Dou (Semen Phaseoli)
Da Huang (Radix et Rhizoma Rhei)
Fu Ling (Poria)
Fu Zi (Radix Aconiti Lateralis Praeparata)
Gan Jiang (Rhizoma Zingiberis)
Hu Zhang (Rhizoma Polygoni Cuspidati)
Huang Bai (Cortex Phellodendri)
Huang Lian (Rhizoma Coptidis)
Huang Qin (Radix Scutellariae)
Jin Qian Cao (Herba Lysimachiae)
Ku Shen Gen (Radix Sophorae Flavescentis)
Long Dan Cao (Radix Gentianae)
Pu Gong Ying (Herba Taraxaci)
Qin Jiao (Radix Gentianae Macrophyllae)
Rou Gui (Cortex Cinnamomi)
Shan Dou Gen (Radix Sophorae Tonkinensis)
Yin Chen Hao (Herba Artemisiae Scopariae)
Yu Jin (Radix Curcumae)
Zhi Zi (Fructus Gardeniae)
Zhu Dan (Fel Porcus)

66. Leprosy

Cang Er Zi (Fructus Xanthii)
Da Feng Zi (Semen Hydnocarpi)
Mao Dong Qing (Radix Ilicis Pubescentis)
Xia Tian Wu (Rhizoma Corydalis Decumbentis)

67. Leptospirosis

Jin Yin Hua (Flos Lonicerae)
Shan Dou Gen (Radix Sophorae Tonkinensis)
Xian He Cao (Herba Agrimoniae)

68. Leukopenia

Bu Gu Zhi (Fructus Psoraleae)
Can Sha (Excrementum Bombycis Mori)
Chan Su (Venenum Bufonis)
Ci Wu Jia (Radix et Caulis Acanthopanacis Senticosi)
Huang Jing (Rhizoma Polygonati)
Ling Zhi (Ganoderma)
Lu Lu Tong (Fructus Liquidambaris)
Nu Zhen Zi (Fructus Ligustri Lucidi)
Rou Gui (Cortex Cinnamomi)
Shan Dou Gen (Radix Sophorae Tonkinensis)
Yin Yang Huo (Herba Epimedii)

69. Liver cirrhosis

Ban Bian Lian (Herba Lobeliae Chinensis)
Ban Zhi Lian (Herba Scutellariae Barbatae)
Chai Hu (Radix Bupleuri)
Dan Shen (Radix Salviae Miltiorrhizae)
Gui Ban (Plastrum Testudinis)
Ling Zhi (Ganoderma)
She Xiang (Moschus)
Tai Zi Shen (Radix Pseudostellariae)
Tao Ren (Semen Persicae)

70. Liver diseases

Bai Zhi (Radix Angelicae Dahuricae)
Bie Jia (Carapax Trionycis)
Gan Sui (Radix Euphorbiae Kansui)
Gou Qi Zi (Fructus Lycii)
Hua Shi (Talcum)
Jin Qian Cao (Herba Lysimachiae)
Ma Dou Ling (Fructus Aristolochiae)
San Qi (Radix Notoginseng)
Shan Yao (Rhizoma Dioscoreae)
Shen Qu (Massa Fermentata)
Shui Zhi (Hirudo)
Wu Mei (Fructus Mume)

Zhi Zi (Fructus Gardeniae)

71. Malaria

Ai Ye (Folium Artemisiae Argyi)
Ba Dou (Fructus Crotonis)
Chang Shan (Radix Dichroae)
Chou Wu Tong (Folium Clerodendri Trichotomi)
Di Gu Pi (Cortex Lycii)
E Bu Shi Cao (Herba Centipedae)
Hai Piao Xiao (Endoconcha Sepiae)
Ma Bian Cao (Herba Verbenae)
Qing Hao (Herba Artemisiae Annuae)
Xian He Cao (Herba Agrimoniae)
Xiong Huang (Realgar)
Xu Chang Qing (Radix Cynanchi Paniculati)
Xun Gu Feng (Herba Aristolochiae Mollissimae)
Ya Dan Zi (Fructus Bruceae)
Ze Qi (Herba Euphorbiae Helioscopiae)

72. Mastitis

Bai Jie Zi (Semen Sinapis)
Bi Ba (Fructus Piperis Longi)
Bo He (Herba Menthae)
Chuan Lian Zi (Fructus Toosendan)
Cong Bai (Bulbus Allii Fistulosi)
Da Suan (Bulbus Alli Sativi)
Di Fu Zi (Fructus Kochiae)
Ding Xiang (Flos Caryophylli)
Gua Lou Shi (Fructus Trichosanthis)
Hai Zao (Sargassum)
Huai Hua (Flos Sophorae)
Jin Qian Cao (Herba Lysimachiae)
Ju He (Semen Citri Rubrum)
Lao Guan Cao (Herba Erodii seu Geranii)
Ma Huang (Herba Ephedrae)
Pu Gong Ying (Herba Taraxaci)
Shang Lu (Radix Phytolaccae)
Shen Qu (Massa Fermentata)
Si Gua Luo (Retinervus Luffae Fructus)
Tian Nan Xing (Rhizoma Arisaematis)
Xia Tian Wu (Rhizoma Corydalis Decumbentis)

73. Myelitis

Ba Dou (Fructus Crotonis)
Huang Lian (Rhizoma Coptidis)
Kuan Dong Hua (Flos Farfarae)

74. Myocardial infarction

Dan Shen (Radix Salviae Miltiorrhizae)
Gui Zhi (Ramulus Cinnamomi)
Sang Ji Sheng (Herba Taxilli)
Tian Ma (Rhizoma Gastrodiae)
Yan Hu Suo (Rhizoma Corydalis)

75. Myocarditis

Nan Sha Shen (Radix Adenophorae)
Yin Yang Huo (Herba Epimedii)
Yuan Zhi (Radix Polygalae)

76. Nausea and vomiting

Ban Xia (Rhizoma Pinelliae)
Fu Ling (Poria)
Fu Long Gan (Terra Flava Usta)
Gao Liang Jiang (Rhizoma Alpiniae Officinarum)
Pi Pa Ye (Folium Eriobotryae)
Sheng Jiang (Rhizoma Zingiberis Recens)
Su Zi (Fructus Perillae)
Wu Zhu Yu (Fructus Evodiae)
Xuan Fu Hua (Flos Inulae)
Zhu Ru (Caulis Bambusae in Taenia)

77. Nephritis

Bai Mao Gen (Rhizoma Imperatae)
Bei Sha Shen (Radix Glehniae)
Che Qian Cao (Herba Plantaginis)
Che Qian Zi (Semen Plantaginis)
Chi Xiao Dou (Semen Phaseoli)
Chuan Mu Tong (Caulis Clematidis Armandii)
Da Suan (Bulbus Alli Sativi)
Dang Shen (Radix Codonopsis)
Di Fu Zi (Fructus Kochiae)
Fu Ling (Poria)
Fu Ping (Herba Spirodelae)
Gui Ban (Plastrum Testudinis)
Huang Bai (Cortex Phellodendri)
Huang Qi (Radix Astragali)
Huang Lian (Rhizoma Coptidis)
Huo Xiang (Herba Agastache)
Lei Gong Teng (Radix Tripterygii Wilfordii)
Lu Han Cao (Herba Pyrolae)
Ma Huang (Herba Ephedrae)
Pi Pa Ye (Folium Eriobotryae)
San Qi (Radix Notoginseng)
Shan Zha (Fructus Crataegi)
Shan Zhu Yu (Fructus Corni)
Shang Lu (Radix Phytolaccae)
Shi Wei (Folium Pyrrosiae)
Shui Zhi (Hirudo)
Xiao Ji (Herba Cirisii)
Yi Mu Cao (Herba Leonuri)
Yi Yi Ren (Semen Coicis)
Yu Mi Xu (Stigma Maydis)
Ze Qi (Herba Euphorbiae Helioscopiae)
Zhu Ling (Polyporus)

78. Nephrotic syndrome

Dong Chong Xia Cao (Cordyceps)
Mang Xiao (Natrii Sulfas)
Shui Zhi (Hirudo)

79. Neuralgia

Bai Shao (Radix Paeoniae Alba)
Bai Zhi (Radix Angelicae Dahuricae)
Cao Wu (Radix Aconiti Kusnezoffii)
Chuan Wu (Radix Aconiti Preparata)
Du Huo (Radix Angelicae Pubescentis)
Fen Fang Ji (Radix Stephaniae Tetandrae)
Gui Zhi (Ramulus Cinnamomi)
Long Dan Cao (Radix Gentianae)
Ma Qian Zi (Semen Strychni)
Quan Xie (Scorpio)
Tian Ma (Rhizoma Gastrodiae)
Wu Mei (Fructus Mume)
Xia Tian Wu (Rhizoma Corydalis Decumbentis)
Xun Gu Feng (Herba Aristolochiae Mollissimae)
Yi Yi Ren (Semen Coicis)
Zao Xiu (Rhizoma Paridis)

80. Neurodermatitis

Bai Bu (Radix Stemonae)
Bai Tou Weng (Radix Pulsatillae)
Chi Shao (Radix Paeoniae Rubrae)
Gao Ben (Rhizoma Ligustici)
Qing Hao (Herba Artemisiae Annuae)
Sheng Di Huang (Radix Rehmanniae)
Shu Di Huang (Radix Rehmanniae Preparata)
Tian Nan Xing (Rhizoma Arisaematis)
Zi Cao Gen (Radix Lithospermi)

81. Neurosis

Ba Dou (Fructus Crotonis)
Bai He (Bulbus Lilii)
Chai Hu (Radix Bupleuri)
Ci Wu Jia (Radix et Caulis Acanthopanacis Senticosi)
Dang Shen (Radix Codonopsis)
Gou Teng (Ramulus Uncariae cum Uncis)
Gui Ban (Plastrum Testudinis)
He Huan Hua (Flos Albiziae)
He Huan Pi (Cortex Albiziae)
He Shou Wu (Radix Polygoni Multiflori)
Hou Po (Cortex Magnoliae Officinalis)
Huang Jing (Rhizoma Polygonati)
Ling Zhi (Ganoderma)

Lu Cha (Folium Camellia Sinensis)
Lu Lu Tong (Fructus Liquidambaris)
Ren Shen (Radix Ginseng)
Shan Yao (Rhizoma Dioscoreae)
Suan Zao Ren (Semen Zizyphi Spinosae)
Tian Ma (Rhizoma Gastrodiae)
Wang Bu Liu Xing (Semen Vaccariae)
Wu Long Cha (Folium Camellia Sinensis Fermentata)
Wu Mei (Fructus Mume)
Wu Wei Zi (Fructus Schisandrae Chinensis)
Xi Yang Shen (Radix Panacis Quinquefolii)
Xie Cao (Radix et Rhizoma Valerianae)
Xu Chang Qing (Radix Cynanchi Paniculati)
Yan Hu Suo (Rhizoma Corydalis)
Ye Jiao Teng (Caulis Polygoni Multiflori)
Yin Yang Huo (Herba Epimedii)
Yuan Zhi (Radix Polygalae)

82. Obesity

He Ye (Folium Nelumbinis)
Lu Cha (Folium Camellia Sinensis)
Zao Jiao (Fructus Gleditsiae)

83. Osteoporosis

Gou Ji (Rhizoma Cibotii)
Gu Sui Bu (Rhizoma Drynariae)
Gui Ban (Plastrum Testudinis)
Lu Rong (Cornu Cervi Pantotrichum)
Xu Duan (Radix Dipsaci)

84. Otitis media

Bing Pian (Borneolum Syntheticum)
Gan Cao (Radix Glycyrrhizae)
Huang Bai (Cortex Phellodendri)
Long Dan Cao (Radix Gentianae)
Ming Fan (Alumen)
She Tui (Periostracum Serpentis)
Xu Chang Qing (Radix Cynanchi Paniculati)
Yu Xing Cao (Herba Houttuyniae)
Ze Xie (Rhizoma Alismatis)
Zhu Dan (Fel Porcus)

85. Pain

Bai Jie Zi (Semen Sinapis)
Bai Zhi (Radix Angelicae Dahuricae)
Ban Xia (Rhizoma Pinelliae)
Bi Ba (Fructus Piperis Longi)
Bi Cheng Qie (Fructus Litseae)
Bian Xu (Herba Polygoni Avicularis)
Bing Lang (Semen Arecae)
Chuan Xiong (Rhizoma Ligustici Chuanxiong)
Dang Gui (Radicis Angelicae Sinensis)
Di Fu Zi (Fructus Kochiae)
Di Yu (Radix Sanguisorbae)
Ding Xiang (Flos Caryophylli)
Fang Feng (Radix Saposhnikoviae)
Gan Jiang (Rhizoma Zingiberis)
Gao Ben (Rhizoma Ligustici)
Ge Gen (Radix Puerariae)
Hai Shen (Strichopus Japonicus)
Han Lian Cao (Herba Ecliptae)
Hong Hua (Flos Carthami)
Huang Jing (Rhizoma Polygonati)
Ku Lian Pi (Cortex Meliae)
Lian Zi Xin (Plumula Nelumbinis)
Ma Ti Jin (Herba Dichondrae Repentis)
Qin Jiao (Radix Gentianae Macrophyllae)
Qing Mu Xiang (Radix Aristolochiae)
San Qi (Radix Notoginseng)
Shan Zha (Fructus Crataegi)
Sheng Jiang (Rhizoma Zingiberis Recens)
Sheng Ma (Rhizoma Cimicifugae)
Su He Xiang (Styrax)
Su Mu (Lignum Sappan)
Suan Zao Ren (Semen Zizyphi Spinosae)
Tian Nan Xing (Rhizoma Arisaematis)
Tian Zhu Huang (Concretio Silicea Bambusae)
Wei Ling Xian (Radix Clematidis)
Wu Mei (Fructus Mume)
Xi Xin (Herba Asari)
Xiang Fu (Rhizoma Cyperi)
Xu Chang Qing (Radix Cynanchi Paniculati)
Xun Gu Feng (Herba Aristolochiae Mollissimae)
Yan Hu Suo (Rhizoma Corydalis)
Yi Yi Ren (Semen Coicis)
Ze Lan (Herba Lycopi)
Zhu Sha (Cinnabaris)

86. Pancreatitis

Bai Shao (Radix Paeoniae Alba)
Chai Hu (Radix Bupleuri)

87. Paralysis

Da Suan (Bulbus Alli Sativi)
Fang Feng (Radix Saposhnikoviae)
He Shou Wu (Radix Polygoni Multiflori)

88. Parasitic infestation (intestinal)

Ai Ye (Folium Artemisiae Argyi)
Bai Bu (Radix Stemonae)
Bing Lang (Semen Arecae)
Chang Shan (Radix Dichroae)
Chuan Lian Zi (Fructus Toosendan)
Cong Bai (Bulbus Allii Fistulosi)
Fei Zi (Semen Torreyae)
Guan Zhong (Rhizoma Dryopteridis)
He Shi (Fructus Carpesii)
Ku Lian Pi (Cortex Meliae)
Lei Wan (Omphalia)
Ma Bian Cao (Herba Verbenae)
Nan Gua Zi (Semen Cucurbitae Moschatae)
Pi Pa Ye (Folium Eriobotryae)
Shi Jun Zi (Fructus Quisqualis)
Wei Ling Xian (Radix Clematidis)
Wu Mei (Fructus Mume)
Xun Gu Feng (Herba Aristolochiae Mollissimae)

89. Parotitis

Bai Jie Zi (Semen Sinapis)
Bian Xu (Herba Polygoni Avicularis)
Cang Zhu (Rhizoma Atractylodis)
Chi Xiao Dou (Semen Phaseoli)
Di Long (Pheretima)
Jiang Can (Bombyx Batryticatus)
Pu Gong Ying (Herba Taraxaci)
She Tui (Periostracum Serpentis)
Tian Nan Xing (Rhizoma Arisaematis)
Wei Ling Xian (Radix Clematidis)
Xiong Huang (Realgar)
Ze Qi (Herba Euphorbiae Helioscopiae)

90. Parotitis and tonsillitis

Ban Lan Gen (Radix Isatidis)
Ban Mao (Mylabris)
Bo He (Herba Menthae)
Che Qian Cao (Herba Plantaginis)
Dang Gui (Radicis Angelicae Sinensis)
Hai Zao (Sargassum)
Jie Geng (Radix Platycodonis)
Ju Hua (Flos Chrysanthemi)
Niu Bang Zi (Fructus Arctii)
Niu Huang (Calculus Bovis)
Pang Da Hai (Semen Sterculiae Lychnophorae)
Pu Gong Ying (Herba Taraxaci)
Shan Dou Gen (Radix Sophorae Tonkinensis)
Wei Ling Xian (Radix Clematidis)
Xuan Shen (Radix Scrophulariae)
Xue Yu Tan (Crinis Carbonisatus)
Yu Xing Cao (Herba Houttuyniae)
Ze Qi (Herba Euphorbiae Helioscopiae)
Zhu Sha (Cinnabaris)

91. Peptic ulcer
Bai Ji (Rhizoma Bletillae)
Gan Jiang (Rhizoma Zingiberis)
Huang Qi (Radix Astragali)
Ming Fan (Alumen)
Tian Nan Xing (Rhizoma Arisaematis)
Wa Leng Zi (Concha Arcae)
Wu Bei Zi (Galla Chinensis)
Wu Mei (Fructus Mume)
Yan Hu Suo (Rhizoma Corydalis)

92. Phlebitis
Dang Gui (Radicis Angelicae Sinensis)
Ma Qian Zi (Semen Strychni)
Mao Dong Qing (Radix Ilicis Pubescentis)
Shui Zhi (Hirudo)

93. Pneumonia
Bing Lang (Semen Arecae)
Da Suan (Bulbus Alli Sativi)
He Shi (Fructus Carpesii)
Hu Zhang (Rhizoma Polygoni Cuspidati)
Jin Yin Hua (Flos Lonicerae)
Lu Han Cao (Herba Pyrolae)
Ma Dou Ling (Fructus Aristolochiae)
Ma Huang (Herba Ephedrae)
She Gan (Rhizoma Belamcandae)
Sheng Ma (Rhizoma Cimicifugae)

94. Poisoning
Can Sha (Excrementum Bombycis Mori)
Ge Gen (Radix Puerariae)
Huang Qin (Radix Scutellariae)
Xian He Cao (Herba Agrimoniae)

95. Psoriasis
Bai Hua She (Bungarus Parvus)
Bai Zhi (Radix Angelicae Dahuricae)
Du Huo (Radix Angelicae Pubescentis)
Hu Zhang (Rhizoma Polygoni Cuspidati)
Qing Dai (Indigo Naturalis)
Shang Lu (Radix Phytolaccae)
Tu Fu Ling (Rhizoma Smilacis Glabrae)
Wu Shao She (Zaocys)
Zhu Ling (Polyporus)

96. Purpura due to lack of platelets
Bie Jia (Carapax Trionycis)
Bu Gu Zhi (Fructus Psoraleae)
Di Yu (Radix Sanguisorbae)
Dong Chong Xia Cao (Cordyceps)
Hei Zhi Ma (Semen Sesami Nigrum)
Ling Zhi (Ganoderma)
Mu Dan Pi (Cortex Moutan)
Qiang Huo (Rhizoma et Radix Notopterygii)
Shang Lu (Radix Phytolaccae)
Shui Niu Jiao (Cornu Bubali)
Suo Yang (Herba Cynomorii)
Zhi Zi (Fructus Gardeniae)

97. Rhinitis
Bai Zhi (Radix Angelicae Dahuricae)
Ban Mao (Mylabris)
Cang Er Zi (Fructus Xanthii)
E Bu Shi Cao (Herba Centipedae)
Fang Feng (Radix Saposhnikoviae)
Gan Cao (Radix Glycyrrhizae)
Hei Zhi Ma (Semen Sesami Nigrum)
Jie Geng (Radix Platycodonis)
Jin Yin Hua (Flos Lonicerae)
Mao Dong Qing (Radix Ilicis Pubescentis)
Xin Yi Hua (Flos Magnoliae)
Yu Xing Cao (Herba Houttuyniae)
Zi Zhu (Folium Callicarpae)

98. Roundworm infestation
Ba Dou (Fructus Crotonis)
Bing Lang (Semen Arecae)
Da Huang (Radix et Rhizoma Rhei)
Fei Zi (Semen Torreyae)
Guan Zhong (Rhizoma Dryopteridis)
He Shi (Fructus Carpesii)
Hua Jiao (Pericarpium Zanthoxyli)
Jin Qian Cao (Herba Lysimachiae)
Ku Lian Pi (Cortex Meliae)
Lei Wan (Omphalia)
Nan Gua Zi (Semen Cucurbitae Moschatae)
Shi Jun Zi (Fructus Quisqualis)
Shi Liu Pi (Pericarpium Granati)
Su He Xiang (Styrax)
Su Zi (Fructus Perillae)
Wu Mei (Fructus Mume)
Yin Chen Hao (Herba Artemisiae Scopariae)

99. Schizophrenia
Fu Ling (Poria)
Shui Niu Jiao (Cornu Bubali)
Wu Mei (Fructus Mume)

100. Seizures
Chai Hu (Radix Bupleuri)
Gan Song (Radix seu Rhizoma Nardostachys)
Gui Zhi (Ramulus Cinnamomi)
Hai Shen (Strichopus Japonicus)
Hu Jiao (Fructus Piper)
Jiang Can (Bombyx Batryticatus)
Peng Sha (Borax)
Quan Xie (Scorpio)
Shi Chang Pu (Rhizoma Acori)
Tian Ma (Rhizoma Gastrodiae)
Tian Nan Xing (Rhizoma Arisaematis)
Wu Mei (Fructus Mume)

101. Sexual dysfunction
Che Qian Zi (Semen Plantaginis)
Dang Gui (Radicis Angelicae Sinensis)
Dong Chong Xia Cao (Cordyceps)
Ge Jie (Gecko)
Guan Mu Tong (Caulis Aristolochiae Manshuriensis)
Hai Ma (Hippocampus)
Hai Shen (Strichopus Japonicus)
Long Gu (Os Draconis)
Ren Shen (Radix Ginseng)
Xian Mao (Rhizoma Curculiginis)
Yin Yang Huo (Herba Epimedii)
Ze Xie (Rhizoma Alismatis)

102. Shingles
Dang Gui (Radicis Angelicae Sinensis)
Jiang Huang (Rhizoma Curcumae Longae)
Si Gua Luo (Retinervus Luffae Fructus)
Wang Bu Liu Xing (Semen Vaccariae)
Xiong Huang (Realgar)
Zao Xiu (Rhizoma Paridis)

103. Shock
Chen Pi (Pericarpium Citri Reticulatae)
Mu Gua (Fructus Chaenomelis)
Qing Pi (Pericarpium Citri Reticulatae Viride)
Zhi Shi (Fructus Aurantii Immaturus)

104. Snake and insect bites
Bai Ji (Rhizoma Bletillae)
Hai Ma (Hippocampus)
Jing Tian San Qi (Herba seu Radix Sedum Aizoom)
Wei Ling Xian (Radix Clematidis)
Xu Chang Qing (Radix Cynanchi Paniculati)

105. Stomatitis and esophagitis
Ai Ye (Folium Artemisiae Argyi)
Chan Su (Venenum Bufonis)
Chuan Wu (Radix Aconiti Preparata)

Er Cha (Catechu)
Hou Po (Cortex Magnoliae Officinalis)
Jiang Huang (Rhizoma Curcumae Longae)
Jie Geng (Radix Platycodonis)
Jin Yin Hua (Flos Lonicerae)
Ma Bian Cao (Herba Verbenae)
Pang Da Hai (Semen Sterculiae Lychnophorae)
Qin Jiao (Radix Gentianae Macrophyllae)
Sheng Ma (Rhizoma Cimicifugae)
Shi Gao (Gypsum Fibrosum)
Yi Yi Ren (Semen Coicis)
Ze Qi (Herba Euphorbiae Helioscopiae)

106. Stone formation

Chen Pi (Pericarpium Citri Reticulatae)
Chi Xiao Dou (Semen Phaseoli)
Chuan Mu Tong (Caulis Clematidis Armandii)
Di Fu Zi (Fructus Kochiae)
Gua Lou Shi (Fructus Trichosanthis)
Guan Mu Tong (Caulis Aristolochiae Manshuriensis)
Guang Jin Qian Cao (Herba Desmodii Styracifolii)
Hai Jin Sha (Herba Lygodii)
Hua Shi (Talcum)
Jin Qian Cao (Herba Lysimachiae)
Shi Wei (Folium Pyrrosiae)
Su He Xiang (Styrax)
Wei Ling Xian (Radix Clematidis)
Yin Chen Hao (Herba Artemisiae Scopariae)
Yu Mi Xu (Stigma Maydis)

107. Stroke

Cao Wu (Radix Aconiti Kusnezoffii)
Chuan Wu (Radix Aconiti Preparata)
Dan Shen (Radix Salviae Miltiorrhizae)
Dang Gui (Radicis Angelicae Sinensis)
Fu Ling (Poria)
Hong Hua (Flos Carthami)
Huang Jing (Rhizoma Polygonati)
Kun Bu (Thallus Laminariae seu Eckloniae)
Mao Dong Qing (Radix Ilicis Pubescentis)
She Xiang (Moschus)
Shi Chang Pu (Rhizoma Acori)
Shui Zhi (Hirudo)
Tian Nan Xing (Rhizoma Arisaematis)
Xia Tian Wu (Rhizoma Corydalis Decumbentis)
Zhu Li (Succus Bambusae)

108. Tapeworm infestation

Bai Jie Zi (Semen Sinapis)
Ban Xia (Rhizoma Pinelliae)
Bing Lang (Semen Arecae)
Chuan Lian Zi (Fructus Toosendan)
Fei Zi (Semen Torreyae)
Hua Jiao (Pericarpium Zanthoxyli)
Lei Wan (Omphalia)
Nan Gua Zi (Semen Cucurbitae Moschatae)
Shi Liu Pi (Pericarpium Granati)
Xian He Cao (Herba Agrimoniae)

109. Tetanus

Chan Tui (Periostracum Cicadae)
Tian Nan Xing (Rhizoma Arisaematis)
Wu Mei (Fructus Mume)

110. Trauma

Ju Ye San Qi (Herba seu Radix Gynura Segetum)
San Qi (Radix Notoginseng)
She Xiang (Moschus)
Su Mu (Lignum Sappan)
Xu Chang Qing (Radix Cynanchi Paniculati)
Ze Lan (Herba Lycopi)
Zhi Zi (Fructus Gardeniae)

111. Trichomoniasis

Bai Bu (Radix Stemonae)
Bu Gu Zhi (Fructus Psoraleae)
Ku Lian Pi (Cortex Meliae)
Ku Shen Gen (Radix Sophorae Flavescentis)
Lei Wan (Omphalia)
She Chuang Zi (Fructus Cnidii)
Shi Jun Zi (Fructus Quisqualis)
Xian He Cao (Herba Agrimoniae)
Yuan Zhi (Radix Polygalae)

112. Tuberculosis

Ai Ye (Folium Artemisiae Argyi)
Bai Bu (Radix Stemonae)
Bai Guo (Semen Ginkgo)
Bai Ji (Rhizoma Bletillae)
Bai Jie Zi (Semen Sinapis)
Bai Tou Weng (Radix Pulsatillae)
Bie Jia (Carapax Trionycis)
Chan Su (Venenum Bufonis)
Da Ji (Radix Euphorbiae seu Knoxiae)
Da Suan (Bulbus Alli Sativi)
Di Yu (Radix Sanguisorbae)
Gan Cao (Radix Glycyrrhizae)
Gui Ban (Plastrum Testudinis)
Hai Zao (Sargassum)
Hua Rui Shi (Ophicalcitum)
Hua Shi (Talcum)
Huang Jing (Rhizoma Polygonati)
Ma Dou Ling (Fructus Aristolochiae)
Shan Yao (Rhizoma Dioscoreae)
She Tui (Periostracum Serpentis)
Wu Gong (Scolopendra)
Ze Qi (Herba Euphorbiae Helioscopiae)

113. Ulcer

Bai He (Bulbus Lilii)
Bai Zhi (Radix Angelicae Dahuricae)
Chui Pen Cao (Herba Sedi)
Dang Shen (Radix Codonopsis)
Gan Cao (Radix Glycyrrhizae)
Hai Ma (Hippocampus)
Hai Piao Xiao (Endoconcha Sepiae)
Hai Zao (Sargassum)
Huang Lian (Rhizoma Coptidis)
Mao Dong Qing (Radix Ilicis Pubescentis)
Mu Xiang (Radix Aucklandiae)
Pu Gong Ying (Herba Taraxaci)
Shan Yao (Rhizoma Dioscoreae)
Sheng Jiang (Rhizoma Zingiberis Recens)
Sheng Ma (Rhizoma Cimicifugae)
Wu Bei Zi (Galla Chinensis)
Wu Gong (Scolopendra)
Xuan Shen (Radix Scrophulariae)
Xue Yu Tan (Crinis Carbonisatus)
Ze Qi (Herba Euphorbiae Helioscopiae)
Zhu Dan (Fel Porcus)
Zi Cao Gen (Radix Lithospermi)

114. Vertigo

Bai Ji Li (Fructus Tribuli)
Bai Zhu (Rhizoma Atractylodis Macrocephalae)
Ban Xia (Rhizoma Pinelliae)
Gou Teng (Ramulus Uncariae cum Uncis)
Ju Hua (Flos Chrysanthemi)
Jue Ming Zi (Semen Cassiae)
Ling Yang Jiao (Cornu Saigae Tataricae)
Long Gu (Os Draconis)
Man Jing Zi (Fructus Viticis)
Shi Jue Ming (Concha Haliotidis)
Suan Zao Ren (Semen Zizyphi Spinosae)

Tian Ma (Rhizoma Gastrodiae)
Tian Nan Xing (Rhizoma Arisaematis)
Ze Xie (Rhizoma Alismatis)

115. Whooping cough

Bai Bu (Radix Stemonae)
Bai Ji (Rhizoma Bletillae)
Bo He (Herba Menthae)
Chuan Bei Mu (Bulbus Fritillariae Cirrhosae)
Da Suan (Bulbus Alli Sativi)
E Bu Shi Cao (Herba Centipedae)
Ma Huang (Herba Ephedrae)
Nan Gua Zi (Semen Cucurbitae Moschatae)
Pi Pa Ye (Folium Eriobotryae)
Sang Ye (Folium Mori)
Zhu Dan (Fel Porcus)
Zi Wan (Radix Asteris)

Appendix 3 — Cross-reference Based on Pharmacological Effects

The listing of any herb under a diagnosis does not insure that that substance can be unquestioningly prescribed for the named symptom or syndrome. Selection and combination of herbs must be based on careful differential diagnosis, guided by informed understanding and training in Chinese Herbal Medicine.

1. Adaptogenic
2. Analgesic
3. Anesthetic
4. Anesthetic (local)
5. Antacid
6. Antiaging
7. Antiallergic
8. Antiamebic
9. Antiarrhythmic
10. Antiasthmatic
11. Antibacterial
12. Anticoagulant
13. Anticonvulsant
14. Antidermatophyte
15. Antidiabetic
16. Antidiarrheal
17. Antiemetic
18. Antifatigue
19. Antifertility
20. Antifungal
21. Antihistamine
22. Antihyperlipidemic
23. Antihypertensive
24. Anti-inflammatory
25. Antimalarial
26. Antimutagenic
27. Antineoplastic
28. Antioxidant
29. Antiparasitic
30. Antiparasitic (intestinal)
31. Antiplatelet
32. Antipyretic
33. Antiseizure, antiepileptic
34. Antitrichomonal
35. Antitussive
36. Antiulcer
37. Antiviral
38. Anxiolytic
39. Bronchodilator
40. Cardiotonic
41. Cholagogic
42. CNS stimulant
43. CNS suppressant
44. Cognitive
45. Detox (eliminate toxins)
46. Dissolve/expel stones
47. Diuretic
48. Emetic
49. Endocrine (adrenal)
50. Expectorant
51. External wounds (facilitates healing)
52. Hematopoietic (red blood cells)
53. Hematopoietic (white blood cells)
54. Hemostatic
55. Hepatoprotective
56. Hormone-like (estrogen and testosterone)
57. Hyperglycemic
58. Hypertensive
59. Hypotensive
60. Immunostimulant
61. Immunosuppressive
62. Laxative
63. Metabolic
64. Radiation (protective effect)
65. Sedative and hypnotic
66. Smooth muscle relaxant
67. Smooth muscle stimulant
68. Thrombolytic
69. Uterine stimulant
70. Vasoconstrictor (peripheral)
71. Vasodilator (coronary artery)
72. Vasodilator (peripheral)

1. Adaptogenic

Dang Shen (Radix Codonopsis)
Ren Shen (Radix Ginseng)
Wu Jia Pi (Cortex Acanthopanacis)
Xian Mao (Rhizoma Curculiginis)

2. Analgesic

Bai Bu (Radix Stemonae)
Bai Shao (Radix Paeoniae Alba)
Bai Tou Weng (Radix Pulsatillae)
Bai Zhi (Radix Angelicae Dahuricae)
Bei Dou Gen (Rhizoma Menispermi)
Bei Sha Shen (Radix Glehniae)
Bi Cheng Qie (Fructus Litseae)
Bing Pian (Borneolum Syntheticum)
Cao Wu (Radix Aconiti Kusnezoffii)
Chai Hu (Radix Bupleuri)
Chan Su (Venenum Bufonis)
Chan Tui (Periostracum Cicadae)
Chi Shao (Radix Paeoniae Rubrae)
Chou Wu Tong (Folium Clerodendri Trichotomi)
Chuan Wu (Radix Aconiti Preparata)
Dang Gui (Radicis Angelicae Sinensis)
Dang Shen (Radix Codonopsis)
Ding Xiang (Flos Caryophylli)
Du Huo (Radix Angelicae Pubescentis)
Du Zhong (Cortex Eucommiae)
Fang Feng (Radix Saposhnikoviae)
Fang Feng (Radix Saposhnikoviae)
Fen Fang Ji (Radix Stephaniae Tetandrae)
Fu Zi (Radix Aconiti Lateralis Praeparata)
Gan Jiang (Rhizoma Zingiberis)
Gao Ben (Rhizoma Ligustici)
Gao Liang Jiang (Rhizoma Alpiniae Officinarum)
Gui Zhi (Ramulus Cinnamomi)
Hai Shen (Strichopus Japonicus)
Hong Hua (Flos Carthami)
Hua Jiao (Pericarpium Zanthoxyli)
Hua Jiao (Pericarpium Zanthoxyli)
Jiao Gu Lan (Rhizoma seu Herba Gynostemmatis)
Jin Qian Cao (Herba Lysimachiae)
Jing Jie (Herba Schizonepetae)
Ju Ye San Qi (Herba seu Radix Gynura Segetum)
Ling Zhi (Ganoderma)
Man Jing Zi (Fructus Viticis)
Mu Dan Pi (Cortex Moutan)
Mu Zei (Herba Equiseti Hiemalis)
Niu Xi (Radix Cyathulae seu Achyranthis)
Qiang Huo (Rhizoma et Radix Notopterygii)
Qin Pi (Cortex Fraxini)
Qing Feng Teng (Caulis Sinomenii)
Quan Xie (Scorpio)
Rou Gui (Cortex Cinnamomi)
San Qi (Radix Notoginseng)
Sang Bai Pi (Cortex Mori)
She Xiang (Moschus).
Sheng Jiang (Rhizoma Zingiberis Recens)
Sheng Ma (Rhizoma Cimicifugae)

Suan Zao Ren (Semen Zizyphi Spinosae)
Tian Ma (Rhizoma Gastrodiae)
Tian Zhu Huang (Concretio Silicea Bambusae)
Wei Ling Xian (Radix Clematidis)
Wu Zhu Yu (Fructus Evodiae)
Xi Xin (Herba Asari)
Xiang Fu (Rhizoma Cyperi)
Xiao Hui Xiang (Fructus Foeniculi)
Xu Chang Qing (Radix Cynanchi Paniculati)
Xun Gu Feng (Herba Aristolochiae Mollissimae)
Yan Hu Suo (Rhizoma Corydalis)
Ying Su Ke (Pericarpium Papaveris)
Zao Xiu (Rhizoma Paridis)

3. Anesthetic
Chan Su (Venenum Bufonis)
Chuan Wu (Radix Aconiti Preparata)
Da Suan (Bulbus Alli Sativi)

4. Anesthetic (local)
Cao Wu (Radix Aconiti Kusnezoffii)
Chan Su (Venenum Bufonis)
Chuan Wu (Radix Aconiti Preparata)
Fo Shou (Fructus Citri Sarcodactylis)
Hua Jiao (Pericarpium Zanthoxyli)
She Chuang Zi (Fructus Cnidii)
Xi Xin (Herba Asari)
Xiang Fu (Rhizoma Cyperi)
Xin Yi Hua (Flos Magnoliae)

5. Antacid
Hai Ge Fen (Concha Cyclinae)
Hai Piao Xiao (Endoconcha Sepiae)
Mu Li (Concha Ostreae)

6. Antiaging
Bai Ji Li (Fructus Tribuli)
Dong Chong Xia Cao (Cordyceps)
Ge Jie (Gecko)
Hai Ma (Hippocampus)
He Shou Wu (Radix Polygoni Multiflori)
Jiao Gu Lan (Rhizoma seu Herba Gynostemmatis)
Ju Hua (Flos Chrysanthemi)
Lu Cha (Folium Camellia Sinensis)
Ren Shen (Radix Ginseng)
San Qi (Radix Notoginseng)
Shan Yao (Rhizoma Dioscoreae)
Sheng Di Huang (Radix Rehmanniae)
Shu Di Huang (Radix Rehmanniae Preparata)
Tu Si Zi (Semen Cuscutae)
Wu Long Cha (Folium Camellia Sinensis Fermentata)
Wu Mei (Fructus Mume)
Yin Yang Huo (Herba Epimedii)

7. Antiallergic
Bai He (Bulbus Lilii)
Bi Cheng Qie (Fructus Litseae)
Chan Tui (Periostracum Cicadae)
Chen Xiang (Lignum Aquilariae Resinatum)
Da Zao (Fructus Jujubae)
Di Long (Pheretima)
E Bu Shi Cao (Herba Centipedae)
Fang Feng (Radix Saposhnikoviae)
Fen Fang Ji (Radix Stephaniae Tetandrae)
Jing Jie (Herba Schizonepetae)
Lian Qiao (Fructus Forsythiae)
Ling Zhi (Ganoderma)
Ma Huang (Herba Ephedrae)
Qiang Huo (Rhizoma et Radix Notopterygii)
Qin Jiao (Radix Gentianae Macrophyllae)
Qin Pi (Cortex Fraxini)
She Xiang (Moschus)
Tao Ren (Semen Persicae)
Wu Mei (Fructus Mume)
Wu Yao (Radix Linderae)
Xi Xin (Herba Asari)
Xin Yi Hua (Flos Magnoliae)
Xu Chang Qing (Radix Cynanchi Paniculati)
Yu Xing Cao (Herba Houttuyniae)
Zhi Shi (Fructus Aurantii Immaturus)
Zhu Dan (Fel Porcus)

8. Antiamebic
Ba Dou (Fructus Crotonis)
Bai Tou Weng (Radix Pulsatillae)
Chang Shan (Radix Dichroae)
Da Suan (Bulbus Alli Sativi)
Ya Dan Zi (Fructus Bruceae)

9. Antiarrhythmic
Bi Ba (Fructus Piperis Longi)
Bi Cheng Qie (Fructus Litseae)
Di Long (Pheretima)
Du Huo (Radix Angelicae Pubescentis)
Fen Fang Ji (Radix Stephaniae Tetandrae)
Fu Zi (Radix Aconiti Lateralis Praeparata)
Gan Cao (Radix Glycyrrhizae)
Gan Song (Radix seu Rhizoma Nardostachys)
Ge Gen (Radix Puerariae)
Gou Teng (Ramulus Uncariae cum Uncis)
Gua Lou Shi (Fructus Trichosanthis)
He Shou Wu (Radix Polygoni Multiflori)
Huang Bai (Cortex Phellodendri)
Huang Lian (Rhizoma Coptidis)
Ku Shen Gen (Radix Sophorae Flavescentis)
Ling Zhi (Ganoderma)
Mai Men Dong (Radix Ophiopogonis)
Mu Dan Pi (Cortex Moutan)
Qiang Huo (Rhizoma et Radix Notopterygii)
San Qi (Radix Notoginseng)
Shan Dou Gen (Radix Sophorae Tonkinensis)
She Chuang Zi (Fructus Cnidii)
Shi Di (Calyx Kaki)
Xi Yang Shen (Radix Panacis Quinquefolii)
Xie Cao (Radix et Rhizoma Valerianae)
Yin Yang Huo (Herba Epimedii)

10. Antiasthmatic
Ai Ye (Folium Artemisiae Argyi)
Bai Bu (Radix Stemonae)
Bai He (Bulbus Lilii)
Bi Cheng Qie (Fructus Litseae)
Chan Su (Venenum Bufonis)
Che Qian Zi (Semen Plantaginis)
Chen Pi (Pericarpium Citri Reticulatae)
Dang Gui (Radicis Angelicae Sinensis)
Di Long (Pheretima)
E Bu Shi Cao (Herba Centipedae)
Fo Shou (Fructus Citri Sarcodactylis)
Gao Ben (Rhizoma Ligustici)
Ge Jie (Gecko)
Gou Teng (Ramulus Uncariae cum Uncis)
Hu Zhang (Rhizoma Polygoni Cuspidati)
Jing Jie (Herba Schizonepetae)
Kuan Dong Hua (Flos Farfarae)
Kun Bu (Thallus Laminariae seu Eckloniae)
Lao Guan Cao (Herba Erodii seu Geranii)
Ling Zhi (Ganoderma)
Ma Dou Ling (Fructus Aristolochiae)
Ma Huang (Herba Ephedrae)
Ma Qian Zi (Semen Strychni)
Pi Pa Ye (Folium Eriobotryae)
Qin Pi (Cortex Fraxini)
Qing Pi (Pericarpium Citri Reticulatae Viride)
Ren Dong Teng (Caulis Lonicerae)

Shan Dou Gen (Radix Sophorae Tonkinensis)
Shang Lu (Radix Phytolaccae)
She Chuang Zi (Fructus Cnidii)
Shi Chang Pu (Rhizoma Acori)
Si Gua Luo (Retinervus Luffae Fructus)
Xiao Hui Xiang (Fructus Foeniculi)
Xing Ren (Semen Armeniacae Amarum)
Xuan Fu Hua (Flos Inulae)
Ye Jiao Teng (Caulis Polygoni Multiflori)
Zhu Dan (Fel Porcus)
Zi Su Ye (Folium Perillae)

11. Antibacterial

Ai Ye (Folium Artemisiae Argyi)
Bai Bu (Radix Stemonae)
Bai Guo (Semen Ginkgo)
Bai Ji (Rhizoma Bletillae)
Bai Jie Zi (Semen Sinapis)
Bai Mao Gen (Rhizoma Imperatae)
Bai Shao (Radix Paeoniae Alba)
Bai Tou Weng (Radix Pulsatillae)
Bai Xian Pi (Cortex Dictamni)
Bai Zhi (Radix Angelicae Dahuricae)
Bai Zhu (Rhizoma Atractylodis Macrocephalae)
Ban Lan Gen (Radix Isatidis)
Bi Ba (Fructus Piperis Longi)
Bi Cheng Qie (Fructus Litseae)
Bian Dou (Semen Lablab Album)
Bian Xu (Herba Polygoni Avicularis)
Bing Pian (Borneolum Syntheticum)
Bo He (Herba Menthae)
Bu Gu Zhi (Fructus Psoraleae)
Can Sha (Excrementum Bombycis Mori)
Cang Er Zi (Fructus Xanthii)
Chai Hu (Radix Bupleuri)
Chi Shao (Radix Paeoniae Rubrae)
Chi Xiao Dou (Semen Phaseoli)
Chuan Bei Mu (Bulbus Fritillariae Cirrhosae)
Chuan Lian Zi (Fructus Toosendan)
Chuan Xin Lian (Herba Andrographis)
Cong Bai (Bulbus Allii Fistulosi)
Da Feng Zi (Semen Hydnocarpi)
Da Huang (Radix et Rhizoma Rhei)
Da Ji (Radix Euphorbiae seu Knoxiae)
Da Qing Ye (Folium Isatidis)
Da Suan (Bulbus Alli Sativi)
Dan Shen (Radix Salviae Miltiorrhizae)
Dang Gui (Radicis Angelicae Sinensis)
Dang Shen (Radix Codonopsis)
Di Fu Zi (Fructus Kochiae)
Di Gu Pi (Cortex Lycii)
Di Jin Cao (Herba Euphorbiae Humifusae)
Di Yu (Radix Sanguisorbae)
Ding Xiang (Flos Caryophylli)
E Zhu (Rhizoma Curcumae)
Er Cha (Catechu)
Fan Xie Ye (Folium Sennae)
Fang Feng (Radix Saposhnikoviae)
Fen Fang Ji (Radix Stephaniae Tetandrae)
Fu Ling (Poria)
Gan Jiang (Rhizoma Zingiberis)
Gan Song (Radix seu Rhizoma Nardostachys)
Gao Ben (Rhizoma Ligustici)
Gao Liang Jiang (Rhizoma Alpiniae Officinarum)
Gu Sui Bu (Rhizoma Drynariae)
Guan Mu Tong (Caulis Aristolochiae Manshuriensis)
Guan Zhong (Rhizoma Dryopteridis)
Gui Zhi (Ramulus Cinnamomi)
Hai Jin Sha (Herba Lygodii)
Hai Zao (Sargassum)
Han Lian Cao (Herba Ecliptae)
He Huan Pi (Cortex Albiziae)
He Shi (Fructus Carpesii)
Hong Dou Kou (Fructus Alphiniae Galangae)
Hu Zhang (Rhizoma Polygoni Cuspidati)
Hua Jiao (Pericarpium Zanthoxyli)
Hua Shi (Talcum)
Huai Hua (Flos Sophorae)
Huang Bai (Cortex Phellodendri)
Huang Qin (Radix Scutellariae)
Huang Yao Zi (Herba Dioscoreae Bulbiferae)
Ji Guan Hua (Flos Celosiae Cristatae)
Jiang Huang (Rhizoma Curcumae Longae)
Jin Qian Cao (Herba Lysimachiae)
Jin Yin Hua (Flos Lonicerae)
Jing Jie (Herba Schizonepetae)
Jing Tian San Qi (Herba seu Radix Sedum Aizoom)
Ju Hua (Flos Chrysanthemi)
Jue Ming Zi (Semen Cassiae)
Ku Shen Gen (Radix Sophorae Flavescentis)
Lao Guan Cao (Herba Erodii seu Geranii)
Lian Fang (Receptaculum Nelumbinis)
Lian Qian Cao (Herba Glechomae)
Lian Qiao (Fructus Forsythiae)
Ling Zhi (Ganoderma)
Liu Huang (Sulfur)
Long Dan Cao (Radix Gentianae)
Long Yan Rou (Arillus Longan)
Lu Cha (Folium Camellia Sinensis)
Lu Han Cao (Herba Pyrolae)
Lu Hui (Aloe)
Ma Bian Cao (Herba Verbenae)
Ma Dou Ling (Fructus Aristolochiae)
Ma Huang (Herba Ephedrae)
Ma Qian Zi (Semen Strychni)
Ma Ti Jin (Herba Dichondrae Repentis)
Man Jing Zi (Fructus Viticis)
Mao Dong Qing (Radix Ilicis Pubescentis)
Ming Fan (Alumen)
Mu Dan Pi (Cortex Moutan)
Mu Gua (Fructus Chaenomelis)
Mu Xiang (Radix Aucklandiae)
Mu Zei (Herba Equiseti Hiemalis)
Niu Bang Zi (Fructus Arctii)
Peng Sha (Borax)
Pi Pa Ye (Folium Eriobotryae)
Pu Gong Ying (Herba Taraxaci)
Qian Dan (Minium)
Qin Jiao (Radix Gentianae Macrophyllae)
Qin Pi (Cortex Fraxini)
Qing Hao (Herba Artemisiae Annuae)
Qing Mu Xiang (Radix Aristolochiae)
Qu Mai (Herba Dianthi)
Ren Dong Teng (Caulis Lonicerae)
Rou Dou Kou (Semen Myristicae)
Rou Gui (Cortex Cinnamomi)
Sang Ji Sheng (Herba Taxilli)
Sang Ye (Folium Mori)
Shan Dou Gen (Radix Sophorae Tonkinensis)
Shan Zha (Fructus Crataegi)
She Gan (Rhizoma Belamcandae)
Sheng Jiang (Rhizoma Zingiberis Recens)
Sheng Ma (Rhizoma Cimicifugae)
Shi Liu Pi (Pericarpium Granati)
Shi Wei (Folium Pyrrosiae)
Si Gua Luo (Retinervus Luffae Fructus)
Su He Xiang (Styrax)
Su Mu (Lignum Sappan)
Su Zi (Fructus Perillae)
Tian Hua Fen (Radix Trichosanthis)
Tian Men Dong (Radix Asparagi)
Tu Si Zi (Semen Cuscutae)
Wei Ling Xian (Radix Clematidis)
Wu Bei Zi (Galla Chinensis)
Wu Gong (Scolopendra)
Wu Long Cha (Folium Camellia Sinensis Fermentata)
Wu Mei (Fructus Mume)

Wu Wei Zi (Fructus Schisandrae Chinensis)
Wu Yao (Radix Linderae)
Wu Yi (Fructus Ulmi Praeparatus)
Wu Zhu Yu (Fructus Evodiae)
Xi Xin (Herba Asari)
Xia Ku Cao (Spica Prunellae)
Xiang Fu (Rhizoma Cyperi)
Xiang Ru (Herba Elsholtziae seu Moslae)
Xiao Hui Xiang (Fructus Foeniculi)
Xiao Ji (Herba Cirisii)
Xie Bai (Bulbus Allii Macrostemonis)
Xin Yi Hua (Flos Magnoliae)
Xing Ren (Semen Armeniacae Amarum)
Xiong Huang (Realgar)
Xu Chang Qing (Radix Cynanchi Paniculati)
Xu Duan (Radix Dipsaci)
Xuan Fu Hua (Flos Inulae)
Xuan Shen (Radix Scrophulariae)
Xue Jie (Sanguis Draconis)
Xue Yu Tan (Crinis Carbonisatus)
Xun Gu Feng (Herba Aristolochiae Mollissimae)
Ye Jiao Teng (Caulis Polygoni Multiflori)
Ye Ju Hua (Flos Chrysanthemi Indici)
Yin Chen Hao (Herba Artemisiae Scopariae)
Yin Yang Huo (Herba Epimedii)
Yu Xing Cao (Herba Houttuyniae)
Yuan Zhi (Radix Polygalae)
Ze Qi (Herba Euphorbiae Helioscopiae)
Zhi Mu (Radix Anemarrhenae)
Zhu Dan (Fel Porcus)
Zhu Ling (Polyporus)
Zhu Ru (Caulis Bambusae in Taenia)
Zi Cao Gen (Radix Lithospermi)
Zi Su Ye (Folium Perillae)
Zi Wan (Radix Asteris)
Zi Zhu (Folium Callicarpae)

12. Anticoagulant

Bi Cheng Qie (Fructus Litseae)
Bian Dou (Semen Lablab Album)
Chi Shao (Radix Paeoniae Rubrae)
Chuan Xiong (Rhizoma Ligustici Chuanxiong)
Da Fu Pi (Pericarpium Arecae)
Dan Shen (Radix Salviae Miltiorrhizae)
Dang Gui (Radicis Angelicae Sinensis)
Dang Shen (Radix Codonopsis)
Di Long (Pheretima)
Ding Xiang (Flos Caryophylli)
Du Huo (Radix Angelicae Pubescentis)
E Zhu (Rhizoma Curcumae)
Fu Zi (Radix Aconiti Lateralis Praeparata)
Gan Jiang (Rhizoma Zingiberis)
Gao Liang Jiang (Rhizoma Alpiniae Officinarum)
Gou Teng (Ramulus Uncariae cum Uncis)
Gui Zhi (Ramulus Cinnamomi)
Hai Zao (Sargassum)
Hong Hua (Flos Carthami)
Hua Jiao (Pericarpium Zanthoxyli)
Kun Bu (Thallus Laminariae seu Eckloniae)
Ling Zhi (Ganoderma)
Lu Cha (Folium Camellia Sinensis)
Ma Huang (Herba Ephedrae)
Man Jing Zi (Fructus Viticis)
Mao Dong Qing (Radix Ilicis Pubescentis)
Mu Dan Pi (Cortex Moutan)
Mu Xiang (Radix Aucklandiae)
Mu Zei (Herba Equiseti Hiemalis)
Nan Sha Shen (Radix Adenophorae)
Sheng Ma (Rhizoma Cimicifugae)
Shui Zhi (Hirudo)
Su He Xiang (Styrax)
Tao Ren (Semen Persicae)
Tian Zhu Huang (Concretio Silicea Bambusae)
Wu Gong (Scolopendra)
Wu Long Cha (Folium Camellia Sinensis Fermentata)
Wu Yao (Radix Linderae)
Xi Xian Cao (Herba Siegesbeckiae)
Xiao Hui Xiang (Fructus Foeniculi)
Xue Jie (Sanguis Draconis)
Yi Mu Cao (Herba Leonuri)

13. Anticonvulsant

Gou Teng (Ramulus Uncariae cum Uncis)
Niu Huang (Calculus Bovis)
Tian Ma (Rhizoma Gastrodiae)
Tian Nan Xing (Rhizoma Arisaematis)

14. Antidermatophyte

Bai Xian Pi (Cortex Dictamni)
Bai Zhi (Radix Angelicae Dahuricae)
Ban Mao (Mylabris)
Bing Lang (Semen Arecae)
Cong Bai (Bulbus Allii Fistulosi)
Da Huang (Radix et Rhizoma Rhei)
Da Suan (Bulbus Alli Sativi)
Hai Shen (Strichopus Japonicus)
Hu Huang Lian (Rhizoma Picrorhizae)
Huang Bai (Cortex Phellodendri)
Huang Lian (Rhizoma Coptidis)
Huo Xiang (Herba Agastache)
Ju Hua (Flos Chrysanthemi)
Ku Lian Pi (Cortex Meliae)
Ku Shen Gen (Radix Sophorae Flavescentis)
Nan Sha Shen (Radix Adenophorae)
Qing Hao (Herba Artemisiae Annuae)
San Qi (Radix Notoginseng)
Sheng Ma (Rhizoma Cimicifugae)
Shi Jun Zi (Fructus Quisqualis)
Wu Bei Zi (Galla Chinensis)
Wu Mei (Fructus Mume)
Xie Cao (Radix et Rhizoma Valerianae)
Xuan Shen (Radix Scrophulariae)
Zhang Nao (Camphora)
Zhi Zi (Fructus Gardeniae)
Zi Su Ye (Folium Perillae)

15. Antidiabetic

Bai Zhu (Rhizoma Atractylodis Macrocephalae)
Cang Er Zi (Fructus Xanthii)
Cang Zhu (Rhizoma Atractylodis)
Chuan Wu (Radix Aconiti Preparata)
Da Suan (Bulbus Alli Sativi)
Di Gu Pi (Cortex Lycii)
Gan Cao (Radix Glycyrrhizae)
Ge Gen (Radix Puerariae)
Ge Jie (Gecko)
Gou Qi Zi (Fructus Lycii)
Hu Zhang (Rhizoma Polygoni Cuspidati)
Huang Jing (Rhizoma Polygonati)
Huang Lian (Rhizoma Coptidis)
Li Zhi He (Semen Litchi)
Ling Zhi (Ganoderma)
Mai Ya (Fructus Hordei Germinatus)
Niu Bang Zi (Fructus Arctii)
Ren Shen (Radix Ginseng)
Sang Ye (Folium Mori)
Shan Yao (Rhizoma Dioscoreae)
Xia Ku Cao (Spica Prunellae)
Xing Ren (Semen Armeniacae Amarum)
Yi Yi Ren (Semen Coicis)
Yin Yang Huo (Herba Epimedii)
Yu Zhu (Rhizoma Polygonati Odorati)
Ze Xie (Rhizoma Alismatis)
Zhi Mu (Radix Anemarrhenae)
Zi Cao Gen (Radix Lithospermi)

16. Antidiarrheal

Ai Ye (Folium Artemisiae Argyi)
Bai Zhu (Rhizoma Atractylodis Macrocephalae)

Bian Dou (Semen Lablab Album)
Bing Lang (Semen Arecae)
Bu Gu Zhi (Fructus Psoraleae)
Cao Dou Kou (Semen Alpiniae Katsumadai)
Cao Guo (Fructus Tsaoko)
Che Qian Zi (Semen Plantaginis)
Chi Shi Zhi (Halloysitum Rubrum)
Chun Gen Pi (Cortex Ailanthi)
Fu Ling (Poria)
Gan Cao (Radix Glycyrrhizae)
Ge Gen (Radix Puerariae)
He Zi (Fructus Chebulae)
Hua Shi (Talcum)
Jin Ying Zi (Fructus Rosae Laevigatae)
Lian Zi (Semen Nelumbinis)
Qian Shi (Semen Euryales)
Rou Dou Kou (Semen Myristicae)
Sha Ren (Fructus Amomi)
Shan Yao (Rhizoma Dioscoreae)
Sheng Ma (Rhizoma Cimicifugae)
Shi Liu Pi (Pericarpium Granati)
Tu Si Zi (Semen Cuscutae)
Wu Bei Zi (Galla Chinensis)
Wu Mei (Fructus Mume)
Wu Wei Zi (Fructus Schisandrae Chinensis)
Wu Zhu Yu (Fructus Evodiae)
Xian He Cao (Herba Agrimoniae)
Xiang Fu (Rhizoma Cyperi)
Yi Yi Ren (Semen Coicis)
Yi Zhi Ren (Fructus Alpiniae Oxyphyllae)
Ying Su Ke (Pericarpium Papaveris)
Yu Yu Liang (Limonitum)
Ze Xie (Rhizoma Alismatis)

17. Antiemetic

Ban Xia (Rhizoma Pinelliae)
Fu Long Gan (Terra Flava Usta)
Gan Jiang (Rhizoma Zingiberis)
Huo Xiang (Herba Agastache)
Lian Qiao (Fructus Forsythiae)
Sheng Jiang (Rhizoma Zingiberis Recens)

18. Antifatigue

Bie Jia (Carapax Trionycis)
Ci Wu Jia (Radix et Caulis Acanthopanacis Senticosi)
E Jiao (Colla Corii Asini)
Ma Huang (Herba Ephedrae)
Ren Shen (Radix Ginseng)
Wu Mei (Fructus Mume)
Xi Yang Shen (Radix Panacis Quinquefolii)

19. Antifertility

Ban Xia (Rhizoma Pinelliae)
Bing Pian (Borneolum Syntheticum)
Chuan Xin Lian (Herba Andrographis)
Di Long (Pheretima)
E Zhu (Rhizoma Curcumae)
Gan Sui (Radix Euphorbiae Kansui)
Guan Zhong (Rhizoma Dryopteridis)
He Huan Pi (Cortex Albiziae)
Jin Yin Hua (Flos Lonicerae)
Lei Gong Teng (Radix Tripterygii Wilfordii)
Lu Cha (Folium Camellia Sinensis)
Lu Han Cao (Herba Pyrolae)
Ma Dou Ling (Fructus Aristolochiae)
Mu Dan Pi (Cortex Moutan)
Niu Xi (Radix Cyathulae seu Achyranthis)
She Xiang (Moschus).
Shui Zhi (Hirudo)
Wang Bu Liu Xing (Semen Vaccariae)
Wei Ling Xian (Radix Clematidis)
Wu Bei Zi (Galla Chinensis)
Wu Long Cha (Folium Camellia Sinensis Fermentata)
Xi Xian Cao (Herba Siegesbeckiae)
Xiong Huang (Realgar)
Xun Gu Feng (Herba Aristolochiae Mollissimae)
Zong Lu Zi (Fructus Trachycarpi)

20. Antifungal

Ba Dou (Fructus Crotonis)
Ban Mao (Mylabris)
Chuan Lian Zi (Fructus Toosendan)
Ci Shi (Magnetitum)
Da Feng Zi (Semen Hydnocarpi)
Da Suan (Bulbus Alli Sativi)
Hai Tong Pi (Cortex Erythrinae)
Ku Lian Zi (Fructus Meliae)
Lu Hui (Aloe)
Qing Fen (Calomelas)
She Chuang Zi (Fructus Cnidii)
Wu Yi (Fructus Ulmi Praeparatus)
Xiong Huang (Realgar)
Xu Chang Qing (Radix Cynanchi Paniculati)
Yuan Hua (Flos Genkwa)
Zhang Nao (Camphora)

21. Antihistamine

Chan Tui (Periostracum Cicadae)
Chen Pi (Pericarpium Citri Reticulatae)
Fang Feng (Radix Saposhnikoviae)

22. Antihyperlipidemic

Bi Ba (Fructus Piperis Longi)
Da Suan (Bulbus Alli Sativi)
Dan Shen (Radix Salviae Miltiorrhizae)
Dang Gui (Radicis Angelicae Sinensis)
Di Gu Pi (Cortex Lycii)
Du Zhong (Cortex Eucommiae)
Ge Gen (Radix Puerariae)
Gou Qi Zi (Fructus Lycii)
Gui Ban (Plastrum Testudinis)
Hai Zao (Sargassum)
He Shou Wu (Radix Polygoni Multiflori)
Hong Hua (Flos Carthami)
Hei Zhi Ma (Semen Sesami Nigrum)
Hu Zhang (Rhizoma Polygoni Cuspidati)
Huai Hua (Flos Sophorae)
Huang Jing (Rhizoma Polygonati)
Huang Lian (Rhizoma Coptidis)
Huang Qin (Radix Scutellariae)
Huo Ma Ren (Fructus Cannabis)
Jiang Huang (Rhizoma Curcumae Longae)
Jiao Gu Lan (Rhizoma seu Herba Gynostemmatis)
Jin Yin Hua (Flos Lonicerae)
Jue Ming Zi (Semen Cassiae)
Kun Bu (Thallus Laminariae seu Eckloniae)
Lu Cha (Folium Camellia Sinensis)
Nu Zhen Zi (Fructus Ligustri Lucidi)
Ren Dong Teng (Caulis Lonicerae)
Sha Yuan Zi (Semen Astragali Complanati)
Shan Dou Gen (Radix Sophorae Tonkinensis)
Shan Zha (Fructus Crataegi)
Sheng Ma (Rhizoma Cimicifugae)
Shui Niu Jiao (Cornu Bubali)
Shui Zhi (Hirudo)
Suan Zao Ren (Semen Zizyphi Spinosae)
Wu Long Cha (Folium Camellia Sinensis Fermentata)
Xi Yang Shen (Radix Panacis Quinquefolii)
Xu Chang Qing (Radix Cynanchi Paniculati)
Ye Jiao Teng (Caulis Polygoni Multiflori)
Yin Guo Ye (Folium Ginkgo)
Yin Yang Huo (Herba Epimedii)
Yu Zhu (Rhizoma Polygonati Odorati)
Ze Xie (Rhizoma Alismatis)
Zi Su Ye (Folium Perillae)

23. Antihypertensive

Bo He (Herba Menthae)
Che Qian Zi (Semen Plantaginis)
Chou Wu Tong (Folium Clerodendri Trichotomi)
Da Ji (Herba seu Radix Cirsii Japonici)
Di Gu Pi (Cortex Lycii)
Di Long (Pheretima)
Du Zhong (Cortex Eucommiae)
Fen Fang Ji (Radix Stephaniae Tetandrae)
Gou Teng (Ramulus Uncariae cum Uncis)
Huai Hua (Flos Sophorae)
Huang Lian (Rhizoma Coptidis)
Ju Hua (Flos Chrysanthemi)
Jue Ming Zi (Semen Cassiae)
Lai Fu Zi (Semen Raphani)
Ling Zhi (Ganoderma)
Liu Huang (Sulfur)
Lu Cha (Folium Camellia Sinensis)
Mu Zei (Herba Equiseti Hiemalis)
Qing Mu Xiang (Radix Aristolochiae)
Sang Shen Zi (Fructus Mori)
Shan Zha (Fructus Crataegi)
Shui Zhi (Hirudo)
Wang Bu Liu Xing (Semen Vaccariae)
Wu Long Cha (Folium Camellia Sinensis Fermentata)
Wu Mei (Fructus Mume)
Wu Zhu Yu (Fructus Evodiae)
Xi Xian Cao (Herba Siegesbeckiae)
Xia Ku Cao (Spica Prunellae)
Xia Tian Wu (Rhizoma Corydalis Decumbentis)
Xuan Shen (Radix Scrophulariae)
Ye Ju Hua (Flos Chrysanthemi Indici)
Yin Yang Huo (Herba Epimedii)
Ze Xie (Rhizoma Alismatis)
Zong Lu Pi (Fibra Stipulae Trachycarpi)

24. Anti-inflammatory

Ba Ji Tian (Radix Morindae Officinalis)
Bai Shao (Radix Paeoniae Alba)
Bai Zhi (Radix Angelicae Dahuricae)
Bing Pian (Borneolum Syntheticum)
Cang Er Zi (Fructus Xanthii)
Cao Wu (Radix Aconiti Kusnezoffii)
Chai Hu (Radix Bupleuri)
Chan Su (Venenum Bufonis)
Chi Shao (Radix Paeoniae Rubrae)
Chou Wu Tong (Folium Clerodendri Trichotomi)
Chuan Wu (Radix Aconiti Preparata)
Chuan Xin Lian (Herba Andrographis)
Da Huang (Radix et Rhizoma Rhei)
Da Qing Ye (Folium Isatidis)
Dan Shen (Radix Salviae Miltiorrhizae)
Dang Gui (Radicis Angelicae Sinensis)
Dang Shen (Radix Codonopsis)
Di Yu (Radix Sanguisorbae)
Du Huo (Radix Angelicae Pubescentis)
Du Zhong (Cortex Eucommiae)
Fang Feng (Radix Saposhnikoviae)
Fang Feng (Radix Saposhnikoviae)
Fen Fang Ji (Radix Stephaniae Tetandrae)
Fu Zi (Radix Aconiti Lateralis Praeparata)
Gan Jiang (Rhizoma Zingiberis)
Gao Ben (Rhizoma Ligustici)
Ge Jie (Gecko)
Gu Sui Bu (Rhizoma Drynariae)
Guang Jin Qian Cao (Herba Desmodii Styracifolii)
Hai Ge Fen (Concha Meretricis seu Cyclinae)
Hong Hua (Flos Carthami)
Hei Zhi Ma (Semen Sesami Nigrum)
Hu Zhang (Rhizoma Polygoni Cuspidati)
Huai Hua (Flos Sophorae)
Huang Lian (Rhizoma Coptidis)
Huang Qi (Radix Astragali)
Huang Qin (Radix Scutellariae)
Jiang Huang (Rhizoma Curcumae Longae)
Jie Geng (Radix Platycodonis)
Jin Qian Cao (Herba Lysimachiae)
Jin Yin Hua (Flos Lonicerae)
Jing Jie (Herba Schizonepetae)
Ju Ye San Qi (Herba seu Radix Gynura Segetum)
Ku Shen Gen (Radix Sophorae Flavescentis)
Kuan Dong Hua (Flos Farfarae)
Lai Fu Zi (Semen Raphani)
Lei Gong Teng (Radix Tripterygii Wilfordii)
Lei Wan (Omphalia)
Lian Qiao (Fructus Forsythiae)
Liu Huang (Sulfur)
Lu Hui (Aloes)
Lu Lu Tong (Fructus Liquidambaris)
Ma Bian Cao (Herba Verbenae)
Ma Dou Ling (Fructus Aristolochiae)
Ma Huang (Herba Ephedrae)
Man Jing Zi (Fructus Viticis)
Mao Dong Qing (Radix Ilicis Pubescentis)
Mu Dan Pi (Cortex Moutan)
Niu Huang (Calculus Bovis)
Nu Zhen Zi (Fructus Ligustri Lucidi)
Pi Pa Ye (Folium Eriobotryae)
Qiang Huo (Rhizoma et Radix Notopterygii)
Qin Jiao (Radix Gentianae Macrophyllae)
Qin Pi (Cortex Fraxini)
Qing Feng Teng (Caulis Sinomenii)
Ren Dong Teng (Caulis Lonicerae)
San Qi (Radix Notoginseng)
Sha Yuan Zi (Semen Astragali Complanati)
Shan Dou Gen (Radix Sophorae Tonkinensis)
Shang Lu (Radix Phytolaccae)
She Gan (Rhizoma Belamcandae)
She Tui (Periostracum Serpentis)
She Xiang (Moschus).
Sheng Jiang (Rhizoma Zingiberis Recens)
Sheng Ma (Rhizoma Cimicifugae)
Su Mu (Lignum Sappan)
Tao Ren (Semen Persicae)
Tian Ma (Rhizoma Gastrodiae)
Wu Jia Pi (Cortex Acanthopanacis)
Xi Xian Cao (Herba Siegesbeckiae)
Xi Xin (Herba Asari)
Xia Ku Cao (Spica Prunellae)
Xian Mao (Rhizoma Curculiginis)
Xiang Fu (Rhizoma Cyperi)
Xiao Ji (Herba Cirisii)
Xu Chang Qing (Radix Cynanchi Paniculati)
Xue Jie (Sanguis Draconis)
Xue Yu Tan (Crinis Carbonisatus)
Xun Gu Feng (Herba Aristolochiae Mollissimae)
Ye Ju Hua (Flos Chrysanthemi Indici)
Yin Yang Huo (Herba Epimedii)
Yu Xing Cao (Herba Houttuyniae)
Ze Xie (Rhizoma Alismatis)
Zhi Zi (Fructus Gardeniae)
Zi Cao Gen (Radix Lithospermi)

25. Antimalarial

Chang Shan (Radix Dichroae)
He Cao Ya (Gemma Agrimoniae)
Ma Bian Cao (Herba Verbenae)
Qing Hao (Herba Artemisiae Annuae)
Wei Ling Xian (Radix Clematidis)
Ya Dan Zi (Fructus Bruceae)

26. Antimutagenic

Chai Hu (Radix Bupleuri)
Da Zao (Fructus Jujubae)
E Bu Shi Cao (Herba Centipedae)

Jiang Huang (Rhizoma Curcumae Longae)
Lao Guan Cao (Herba Erodii seu Geranii)
Lu Cha (Folium Camellia Sinensis)
Niu Bang Zi (Fructus Arctii)
She Chuang Zi (Fructus Cnidii)
Sheng Jiang (Rhizoma Zingiberis Recens)
Wu Long Cha (Folium Camellia Sinensis Fermentata)
Xi Yang Shen (Radix Panacis Quinquefolii)
Xing Ren (Semen Armeniacae Amarum)
Zhu Ling (Polyporus)

27. Antineoplastic

Bai Xian Pi (Cortex Dictamni)
Bai Zhu (Rhizoma Atractylodis Macrocephalae)
Ban Mao (Mylabris)
Bi Ba (Fructus Piperis Longi)
Bie Jia (Carapax Trionycis)
Bu Gu Zhi (Fructus Psoraleae)
Can Sha (Excrementum Bombycis Mori)
Cao Wu (Radix Aconiti Kusnezoffii)
Chai Hu (Radix Bupleuri)
Chan Su (Venenum Bufonis)
Chan Tui (Periostracum Cicadae)
Chang Shan (Radix Dichroae)
Chi Shao (Radix Paeoniae Rubrae)
Chuan Wu (Radix Aconiti Preparata)
Chuan Xin Lian (Herba Andrographis)
Ci Wu Jia (Radix et Caulis Acanthopanacis Senticosi)
Cong Bai (Bulbus Allii Fistulosi)
Da Huang (Radix et Rhizoma Rhei)
Da Suan (Bulbus Alli Sativi)
Da Zao (Fructus Jujubae)
Dang Gui (Radicis Angelicae Sinensis)
Dang Shen (Radix Codonopsis)
Dao Dou (Semen Canavaliae)
Deng Xin Cao (Medulla Junci)
Di Long (Pheretima)
Di Yu (Radix Sanguisorbae)
Dong Chong Xia Cao (Cordyceps)
Du Huo (Radix Angelicae Pubescentis)
E Zhu (Rhizoma Curcumae)
Er Cha (Catechu)
Fen Fang Ji (Radix Stephaniae Tetandrae)
Fu Ling (Poria)
Gan Cao (Radix Glycyrrhizae)
Gan Sui (Radix Euphorbiae Kansui)
Gua Lou Shi (Fructus Trichosanthis)
Guan Zhong (Rhizoma Dryopteridis)
Gui Ban (Plastrum Testudinis)
Hai Ge Fen (Concha Meretricis seu Cyclinae)
Hai Long (Syngnathus)
Hai Shen (Strichopus Japonicus)
Hong Dou Kou (Fructus Alphiniae Galangae)
Hu Zhang (Rhizoma Polygoni Cuspidati)
Jiang Can (Bombyx Batryticatus)
Jiang Huang (Rhizoma Curcumae Longae)
Jiao Gu Lan (Rhizoma seu Herba Gynostemmatis)
Ju Ye San Qi (Herba seu Radix Gynura Segetum)
Ku Shen Gen (Radix Sophorae Flavescentis)
Kun Bu (Thallus Laminariae seu Eckloniae)
Lao Guan Cao (Herba Erodii seu Geranii)
Lei Gong Teng (Radix Tripterygii Wilfordii)
Ling Zhi (Ganoderma)
Long Yan Rou (Arillus Longan)
Lu Cha (Folium Camellia Sinensis)
Lu Hui (Aloe)
Lu Lu Tong (Fructus Liquidambaris)
Ma Qian Zi (Semen Strychni)
Mu Gua (Fructus Chaenomelis)
Niu Bang Zi (Fructus Arctii)
Nu Zhen Zi (Fructus Ligustri Lucidi)
Pi Pa Ye (Folium Eriobotryae)
Ren Shen (Radix Ginseng)
San Qi (Radix Notoginseng)
Shan Dou Gen (Radix Sophorae Tonkinensis)
Su Mu (Lignum Sappan)
Tao Ren (Semen Persicae)
Tian Hua Fen (Radix Trichosanthis)
Tian Men Dong (Radix Asparagi)
Tian Nan Xing (Rhizoma Arisaematis)
Tu Si Zi (Semen Cuscutae)
Wu Long Cha (Folium Camellia Sinensis Fermentata)
Xian He Cao (Herba Agrimoniae)
Xiao Hui Xiang (Fructus Foeniculi)
Xie Cao (Radix et Rhizoma Valerianae)
Xing Ren (Semen Armeniacae Amarum)
Xun Gu Feng (Herba Aristolochiae Mollissimae)
Ya Dan Zi (Fructus Bruceae)
Ye Jiao Teng (Caulis Polygoni Multiflori)
Yi Yi Ren (Semen Coicis)
Yi Zhi Ren (Fructus Alpiniae Oxyphyllae)
Yu Xing Cao (Herba Houttuyniae)
Yuan Zhi (Radix Polygalae)
Zhu Ling (Polyporus)
Zi Cao Gen (Radix Lithospermi)
Zi Wan (Radix Asteris)
Zong Lu Pi (Fibra Stipulae Trachycarpi)

28. Antioxidant

Chai Hu (Radix Bupleuri)
Chen Pi (Pericarpium Citri Reticulatae)
Da Suan (Bulbus Alli Sativi)
Da Zao (Fructus Jujubae)
Dang Gui (Radicis Angelicae Sinensis)
Gan Cao (Radix Glycyrrhizae)
Hu Zhang (Rhizoma Polygoni Cuspidati)
Huai Hua (Flos Sophorae)
Huang Jing (Rhizoma Polygonati)
Lao Guan Cao (Herba Erodii seu Geranii)
Lu Cha (Folium Camellia Sinensis)
Lu Lu Tong (Fructus Liquidambaris)
Nu Zhen Zi (Fructus Ligustri Lucidi)
Ren Shen (Radix Ginseng)
Shan Zha (Fructus Crataegi)
Su Zi (Fructus Perillae)
Wu Bei Zi (Galla Chinensis)
Wu Long Cha (Folium Camellia Sinensis Fermentata)
Wu Wei Zi (Fructus Schisandrae Chinensis)
Xi Yang Shen (Radix Panacis Quinquefolii)
Xu Chang Qing (Radix Cynanchi Paniculati)

29. Antiparasitic

Bu Gu Zhi (Fructus Psoraleae)
Hu Jiao (Fructus Piper)
Liu Huang (Sulfur)
Wu Yi (Fructus Ulmi Praeparatus)

30. Antiparasitic (intestinal)

Bing Lang (Semen Arecae)
Chuan Lian Zi (Fructus Toosendan)
Ding Xiang (Flos Caryophylli)
Fei Zi (Semen Torreyae)
Guan Zhong (Rhizoma Dryopteridis)
He Huan Pi (Cortex Albiziae)
He Shi (Fructus Carpesii)
Hu Lu Ba (Semen Trigonellae)
Hua Jiao (Pericarpium Zanthoxyli)

Ku Lian Pi (Cortex Meliae)
Lei Wan (Omphalia)
Nan Gua Zi (Semen Cucurbitae Moschatae)
Qian Dan (Minium)
Sheng Jiang (Rhizoma Zingiberis Recens)
Shi Jun Zi (Fructus Quisqualis)
Shi Liu Pi (Pericarpium Granati)
Wu Mei (Fructus Mume)
Xian He Cao (Herba Agrimoniae)
Ya Dan Zi (Fructus Bruceae)
Yin Chen Hao (Herba Artemisiae Scopariae)

31. Antiplatelet

Ai Ye (Folium Artemisiae Argyi)
Ban Lan Gen (Radix Isatidis)
Chi Shao (Radix Paeoniae Rubrae)
Chuan Xin Lian (Herba Andrographis)
Da Suan (Bulbus Alli Sativi)
Dang Gui (Radicis Angelicae Sinensis)
Dang Shen (Radix Codonopsis)
Ding Xiang (Flos Caryophylli)
Du Huo (Radix Angelicae Pubescentis)
Fang Feng (Radix Saposhnikoviae)
Fen Fang Ji (Radix Stephaniae Tetandrae)
Gan Jiang (Rhizoma Zingiberis)
Gao Liang Jiang (Rhizoma Alpiniae Officinarum)
Ge Gen (Radix Puerariae)
Gou Teng (Ramulus Uncariae cum Uncis)
Gua Lou Shi (Fructus Trichosanthis)
Gui Zhi (Ramulus Cinnamomi)
Hu Zhang (Rhizoma Polygoni Cuspidati)
Huang Lian (Rhizoma Coptidis)
Jiang Huang (Rhizoma Curcumae Longae)
Jiao Gu Lan (Rhizoma seu Herba Gynostemmatis)
Ling Zhi (Ganoderma)
Lu Cha (Folium Camellia Sinensis)
Niu Huang (Calculus Bovis)
Ren Shen (Radix Ginseng)
Rou Gui (Cortex Cinnamomi)
Sang Ji Sheng (Herba Taxilli)
Sheng Jiang (Rhizoma Zingiberis Recens)
Su He Xiang (Styrax)
Suan Zao Ren (Semen Zizyphi Spinosae)
Wu Long Cha (Folium Camellia Sinensis Fermentata)
Xia Tian Wu (Rhizoma Corydalis Decumbentis)
Xie Bai (Bulbus Allii Macrostemonis)
Xin Yi Hua (Flos Magnoliae)
Xue Jie (Sanguis Draconis)
Ye Ju Hua (Flos Chrysanthemi Indici)
Zhi Mu (Radix Anemarrhenae)

32. Antipyretic

Bai Zhi (Radix Angelicae Dahuricae)
Bei Sha Shen (Radix Glehniae)
Chai Hu (Radix Bupleuri)
Chan Tui (Periostracum Cicadae)
Chang Shan (Radix Dichroae)
Chi Shao (Radix Paeoniae Rubrae)
Chuan Xin Lian (Herba Andrographis)
Da Qing Ye (Folium Isatidis)
Di Gu Pi (Cortex Lycii)
Di Long (Pheretima)
Fang Feng (Radix Saposhnikoviae)
Fu Ping (Herba Spirodelae)
Gan Jiang (Rhizoma Zingiberis)
Gao Ben (Rhizoma Ligustici).
Ge Gen (Radix Puerariae)
Gui Zhi (Ramulus Cinnamomi)
Gui Zhi (Ramulus Cinnamomi)
Jin Yin Hua (Flos Lonicerae)
Jing Jie (Herba Schizonepetae)
Ku Shen Gen (Radix Sophorae Flavescentis)
Lian Qiao (Fructus Forsythiae)
Ling Yang Jiao (Cornu Saigae Tataricae)
Ma Huang (Herba Ephedrae)
Mu Dan Pi (Cortex Moutan)
Niu Huang (Calculus Bovis)
Qiang Huo (Rhizoma et Radix Notopterygii)
Qing Hao (Herba Artemisiae Annuae)
Sang Bai Pi (Cortex Mori)
Shan Dou Gen (Radix Sophorae Tonkinensis)
She Gan (Rhizoma Belamcandae)
Sheng Jiang (Rhizoma Zingiberis Recens)
Sheng Ma (Rhizoma Cimicifugae)
Shi Gao (Gypsum Fibrosum)
Suan Zao Ren (Semen Zizyphi Spinosae)
Xi Xin (Herba Asari)
Xiang Fu (Rhizoma Cyperi)
Xu Chang Qing (Radix Cynanchi Paniculati)
Ye Ju Hua (Flos Chrysanthemi Indici)
Yin Chen Hao (Herba Artemisiae Scopariae)
Ze Qi (Herba Euphorbiae Helioscopiae)
Zhi Mu (Radix Anemarrhenae)
Zi Cao Gen (Radix Lithospermi)
Zi Su Ye (Folium Perillae)

33. Antiseizure, antiepileptic

Chan Tui (Periostracum Cicadae)
Chi Shao (Radix Paeoniae Rubrae)
Dang Shen (Radix Codonopsis)
Di Long (Pheretima)
Ding Xiang (Flos Caryophylli)
Gou Teng (Ramulus Uncariae cum Uncis)
Gui Zhi (Ramulus Cinnamomi)
Hu Jiao (Fructus Piper)
Jiang Can (Bombyx Batryticatus)
Ju Ye San Qi (Herba seu Radix Gynura Segetum)
Ling Yang Jiao (Cornu Saigae Tataricae)
Ling Zhi (Ganoderma)
Long Chi (Dens Draconis)
Long Gu (Os Draconis)
Mu Dan Pi (Cortex Moutan)
Niu Huang (Calculus Bovis)
Peng Sha (Borax)
Qin Pi (Cortex Fraxini)
Quan Xie (Scorpio)
Sang Bai Pi (Cortex Mori)
Sheng Jiang (Rhizoma Zingiberis Recens)
Sheng Ma (Rhizoma Cimicifugae)
Shi Chang Pu (Rhizoma Acori)
Suan Zao Ren (Semen Zizyphi Spinosae)
Tian Ma (Rhizoma Gastrodiae)
Tian Nan Xing (Rhizoma Arisaematis)
Wu Gong (Scolopendra)
Xi Yang Shen (Radix Panacis Quinquefolii)
Xian Mao (Rhizoma Curculiginis)
Xie Cao (Radix et Rhizoma Valerianae)
Zao Xiu (Rhizoma Paridis)
Zhu Sha (Cinnabaris)

34. Antitrichomonal

Bai Tou Weng (Radix Pulsatillae)
Bai Xian Pi (Cortex Dictamni)
Bi Cheng Qie (Fructus Litseae)
Da Suan (Bulbus Alli Sativi)
He Cao Ya (Gemma Agrimoniae)
Ku Shen Gen (Radix Sophorae Flavescentis)
Lei Wan (Omphalia)
Ming Fan (Alumen)

35. Antitussive

Ai Ye (Folium Artemisiae Argyi)

Bai Bu (Radix Stemonae)
Bai He (Bulbus Lilii)
Ban Xia (Rhizoma Pinelliae)
Bi Cheng Qie (Fructus Litseae)
Chai Hu (Radix Bupleuri)
Chan Su (Venenum Bufonis)
Che Qian Cao (Herba Plantaginis)
Chuan Bei Mu (Bulbus Fritillariae Cirrhosae)
Da Zao (Fructus Jujubae)
E Bu Shi Cao (Herba Centipedae)
Gan Cao (Radix Glycyrrhizae)
Hu Zhang (Rhizoma Polygoni Cuspidati)
Jie Geng (Radix Platycodonis)
Kuan Dong Hua (Flos Farfarae)
Kun Bu (Thallus Laminariae seu Eckloniae)
Lao Guan Cao (Herba Erodii seu Geranii)
Ma Bian Cao (Herba Verbenae)
Ma Dou Ling (Fructus Aristolochiae)
Ma Qian Zi (Semen Strychni)
Pi Pa Ye (Folium Eriobotryae)
Qin Pi (Cortex Fraxini)
Qing Feng Teng (Caulis Sinomenii)
Ren Dong Teng (Caulis Lonicerae)
Sang Bai Pi (Cortex Mori)
Shi Chang Pu (Rhizoma Acori)
Shi Wei (Folium Pyrrosiae)
Si Gua Luo (Retinervus Luffae Fructus)
Tao Ren (Semen Persicae)
Xing Ren (Semen Armeniacae Amarum)
Xuan Fu Hua (Flos Inulae)
Zhe Bei Mu (Bulbus Fritillariae Thunbergii)
Zhu Dan (Fel Porcus)
Zhu Li (Succus Bambusae)
Zi Su Ye (Folium Perillae)
Zi Wan (Radix Asteris)

36. Antiulcer

Bai Ji (Rhizoma Bletillae)
Bai Zhu (Rhizoma Atractylodis Macrocephalae)
Bi Ba (Fructus Piperis Longi)
Bi Cheng Qie (Fructus Litseae)
Cang Zhu (Rhizoma Atractylodis)
Chai Hu (Radix Bupleuri)
Da Huang (Radix et Rhizoma Rhei)
Ding Xiang (Flos Caryophylli)
Gan Cao (Radix Glycyrrhizae)
Gan Jiang (Rhizoma Zingiberis)
Gua Lou Shi (Fructus Trichosanthis)
Hai Piao Xiao (Endoconcha Sepiae)
Hou Po (Cortex Magnoliae Officinalis)
Hua Jiao (Pericarpium Zanthoxyli)
Huai Hua (Flos Sophorae)
Huang Bai (Cortex Phellodendri)
Jiao Gu Lan (Rhizoma seu Herba Gynostemmatis)
Ku Shen Gen (Radix Sophorae Flavescentis)
Lian Qian Cao (Herba Glechomae)
Lu Lu Tong (Fructus Liquidambaris)
Mu Xiang (Radix Aucklandiae)
Pu Gong Ying (Herba Taraxaci)
Ren Shen (Radix Ginseng)
Rou Gui (Cortex Cinnamomi)
Shan Dou Gen (Radix Sophorae Tonkinensis)
She Xiang (Moschus)
Sheng Jiang (Rhizoma Zingiberis Recens)
Wu Jia Pi (Cortex Acanthopanacis)
Wu Wei Zi (Fructus Schisandrae Chinensis)
Wu Zhu Yu (Fructus Evodiae)
Xiao Hui Xiang (Fructus Foeniculi)
Ya Dan Zi (Fructus Bruceae)
Yan Hu Suo (Rhizoma Corydalis)

37. Antiviral

Bai Bu (Radix Stemonae)
Ban Lan Gen (Radix Isatidis)
Ban Mao (Mylabris)
Bi Ba (Fructus Piperis Longi)
Bi Cheng Qie (Fructus Litseae)
Bing Lang (Semen Arecae)
Bo He (Herba Menthae)
Can Sha (Excrementum Bombycis Mori)
Chai Hu (Radix Bupleuri)
Chang Shan (Radix Dichroae)
Chen Pi (Pericarpium Citri Reticulatae)
Da Huang (Radix et Rhizoma Rhei)
Da Qing Ye (Folium Isatidis)
Da Suan (Bulbus Alli Sativi)
Gan Cao (Radix Glycyrrhizae)
Guan Zhong (Rhizoma Dryopteridis)
Gui Zhi (Ramulus Cinnamomi)
Hai Shen (Strichopus Japonicus)
Hua Ju Hong (Exocarpium Citri Grandis)
Huang Lian (Rhizoma Coptidis)
Huang Yao Zi (Herba Dioscoreae Bulbiferae)
Jiang Huang (Rhizoma Curcumae Longae)
Jin Yin Hua (Flos Lonicerae)
Lao Guan Cao (Herba Erodii seu Geranii)
Lian Qiao (Fructus Forsythiae)
Ma Huang (Herba Ephedrae)
Man Jing Zi (Fructus Viticis)
Qing Hao (Herba Artemisiae Annuae)
San Qi (Radix Notoginseng)
Sang Ji Sheng (Herba Taxilli)
Shi Liu Pi (Pericarpium Granati)
Wu Bei Zi (Galla Chinensis)
Wu Zhu Yu (Fructus Evodiae)
Xi Yang Shen (Radix Panacis Quinquefolii)
Xiang Ru (Herba Elsholtziae seu Moslae)
Ye Ju Hua (Flos Chrysanthemi Indici)
Yin Chen Hao (Herba Artemisiae Scopariae)
Yin Yang Huo (Herba Epimedii)
Zi Cao Gen (Radix Lithospermi)

38. Anxiolytic

Ba Ji Tian (Radix Morindae Officinalis)
Dong Chong Xia Cao (Cordyceps)
Gou Qi Zi (Fructus Lycii)
Hua Jiao (Pericarpium Zanthoxyli)
Huang Qi (Radix Astragali)
Long Yan Rou (Arillus Longan)
Lu Lu Tong (Fructus Liquidambaris)
Ren Shen (Radix Ginseng)
San Qi (Radix Notoginseng)
Wu Wei Zi (Fructus Schisandrae Chinensis)
Xi Yang Shen (Radix Panacis Quinquefolii)

39. Bronchodilator

Bai Guo (Semen Ginkgo)
Di Long (Pheretima)
Jing Jie (Herba Schizonepetae)
Ma Huang (Herba Ephedrae)
Xi Xin (Herba Asari)
Zi Su Ye (Folium Perillae)

40. Cardiotonic

Chan Su (Venenum Bufonis)
Chuan Shan Long (Rhizoma Dioscoreae Nipponicae)
Chuan Wu (Radix Aconiti Preparata)
Chuan Xiong (Rhizoma Ligustici Chuanxiong)
Du Zhong (Cortex Eucommiae)
Fang Feng (Radix Saposhnikoviae)
Fo Shou (Fructus Citri Sarcodactylis)
Fu Zi (Radix Aconiti Lateralis Praeparata)
He Shou Wu (Radix Polygoni Multiflori)
Huang Jing (Rhizoma Polygonati)

Huang Qi (Radix Astragali)
Ling Yang Jiao (Cornu Saigae Tataricae)
Ling Zhi (Ganoderma)
Ma Huang (Herba Ephedrae)
Mai Men Dong (Radix Ophiopogonis)
Nan Sha Shen (Radix Adenophorae)
Niu Huang (Calculus Bovis)
Qing Pi (Pericarpium Citri Reticulatae Viride)
Ren Shen (Radix Ginseng)
Shan Zha (Fructus Crataegi)
She Xiang (Moschus)
Sheng Jiang (Rhizoma Zingiberis Recens)
Suan Zao Ren (Semen Zizyphi Spinosae)
Ting Li Zi (Semen Descurainiae seu Lepidii)
Wu Gong (Scolopendra)
Xi Xin (Herba Asari)
Xiang Fu (Rhizoma Cyperi)
Yin Yang Huo (Herba Epimedii)
Yu Zhu (Rhizoma Polygonati Odorati)
Zhang Nao (Camphora)
Zhi Ke (Fructus Aurantii)
Zhi Shi (Fructus Aurantii Immaturus)

41. Cholagogic

Ai Ye (Folium Artemisiae Argyi)
Bi Cheng Qie (Fructus Litseae)
Bian Xu (Herba Polygoni Avicularis)
Bo He (Herba Menthae)
Da Huang (Radix et Rhizoma Rhei)
Ding Xiang (Flos Caryophylli)
E Zhu (Rhizoma Curcumae)
Gan Jiang (Rhizoma Zingiberis)
Hai Jin Sha (Herba Lygodii)
Hu Huang Lian (Rhizoma Picrorhizae)
Jiang Huang (Rhizoma Curcumae Longae)
Jin Qian Cao (Herba Lysimachiae)
Jin Yin Hua (Flos Lonicerae)
Long Dan Cao (Radix Gentianae)
Niu Huang (Calculus Bovis)
Pu Gong Ying (Herba Taraxaci)
Sheng Jiang (Rhizoma Zingiberis Recens)
Wei Ling Xian (Radix Clematidis)
Xiao Hui Xiang (Fructus Foeniculi)
Yin Chen Hao (Herba Artemisiae Scopariae)
Zhi Zi (Fructus Gardeniae)

42. CNS stimulant

Ma Huang (Herba Ephedrae)
Ma Qian Zi (Semen Strychni)
She Xiang (Moschus).
Wu Wei Zi (Fructus Schisandrae Chinensis)
Xia Tian Wu (Rhizoma Corydalis Decumbentis)
Xin Yi Hua (Flos Magnoliae)
Zhang Nao (Camphora)

43. CNS suppressant

Cang Zhu (Rhizoma Atractylodis)
Chuan Lian Zi (Fructus Toosendan)
Dan Shen (Radix Salviae Miltiorrhizae)
Fo Shou (Fructus Citri Sarcodactylis)
Fu Zi (Radix Aconiti Lateralis Praeparata)
Hou Po (Cortex Magnoliae Officinalis)
Hu Lu Ba (Semen Trigonellae)
Huang Lian (Rhizoma Coptidis)
Qin Jiao (Radix Gentianae Macrophyllae)
Rou Dou Kou (Semen Myristicae)
San Qi (Radix Notoginseng)
Shan Dou Gen (Radix Sophorae Tonkinensis)
Su Mu (Lignum Sappan)
Xiao Hui Xiang (Fructus Foeniculi)
Zi Su Ye (Folium Perillae)

44. Cognitive

Dang Shen (Radix Codonopsis)
Ling Zhi (Ganoderma)
Lu Lu Tong (Fructus Liquidambaris)
Ren Shen (Radix Ginseng)
Shi Chang Pu (Rhizoma Acori)

45. Detox (eliminate toxins)

Ban Xia (Rhizoma Pinelliae)
Bian Dou (Semen Lablab Album)
E Zhu (Rhizoma Curcumae)
Gan Cao (Radix Glycyrrhizae)
Ge Gen (Radix Puerariae)
Huang Qi (Radix Astragali)
Jin Yin Hua (Flos Lonicerae)
Lai Fu Zi (Semen Raphani)
Wu Bei Zi (Galla Chinensis)
Wu Wei Zi (Fructus Schisandrae Chinensis)

46. Dissolve/expel stones

Chen Pi (Pericarpium Citri Reticulatae)
Hai Jin Sha (Herba Lygodii)
Jin Qian Cao (Herba Lysimachiae)
Shi Wei (Folium Pyrrosiae)

47. Diuretic

Bai Mao Gen (Rhizoma Imperatae)
Bai Zhu (Rhizoma Atractylodis Macrocephalae)
Bian Xu (Herba Polygoni Avicularis)
Che Qian Cao (Herba Plantaginis)
Che Qian Zi (Semen Plantaginis)
Chuan Mu Tong (Caulis Clematidis Armandii)
Di Fu Zi (Fructus Kochiae)
Du Zhong (Cortex Eucommiae)
Fang Feng (Radix Saposhnikoviae)
Fu Ling (Poria)
Fu Ping (Herba Spirodelae)
Guan Mu Tong (Caulis Aristolochiae Manshuriensis)
Hai Jin Sha (Herba Lygodii)
Huang Qi (Radix Astragali)
Jin Qian Cao (Herba Lysimachiae)
Lian Qian Cao (Herba Glechomae)
Ma Huang (Herba Ephedrae)
Ma Ti Jin (Herba Dichondrae Repentis)
Mu Dan Pi (Cortex Moutan)
Qu Mai (Herba Dianthi)
Sang Bai Pi (Cortex Mori)
Sang Ji Sheng (Herba Taxilli)
Shi Hu (Herba Dendrobii)
Ting Li Zi (Semen Descurainiae seu Lepidii)
Wu Zhu Yu (Fructus Evodiae)
Ze Xie (Rhizoma Alismatis)
Zhu Ling (Polyporus)

48. Emetic

Chang Shan (Radix Dichroae)
Li Lu (Radix et Rhizoma Veratri)
Qing Mu Xiang (Radix Aristolochiae)

49. Endocrine (adrenal)

Chai Hu (Radix Bupleuri)
Chuan Xin Lian (Herba Andrographis)
Gan Cao (Radix Glycyrrhizae)
He Shou Wu (Radix Polygoni Multiflori)
Ren Shen (Radix Ginseng)
Sheng Di Huang (Radix Rehmanniae)
Shu Di Huang (Radix Rehmanniae Preparata)

50. Expectorant

Ai Ye (Folium Artemisiae Argyi)
Bai Bu (Radix Stemonae)
Bai Jie Zi (Semen Sinapis)
Ban Xia (Rhizoma Pinelliae)
Bi Cheng Qie (Fructus Litseae)
Bo He (Herba Menthae)
Chan Su (Venenum Bufonis)
Che Qian Cao (Herba Plantaginis)
Chen Pi (Pericarpium Citri Reticulatae)

Chuan Bei Mu (Bulbus Fritillariae Cirrhosae)
Da Zao (Fructus Jujubae)
Fo Shou (Fructus Citri Sarcodactylis)
Gan Cao (Radix Glycyrrhizae)
Gua Lou Shi (Fructus Trichosanthis)
Hua Rui Shi (Ophicalcitum)
Jie Geng (Radix Platycodonis),
Jing Jie (Herba Schizonepetae)
Kuan Dong Hua (Flos Farfarae)
Lao Guan Cao (Herba Erodii seu Geranii)
Ling Zhi (Ganoderma)
Liu Huang (Sulfur)
Ma Dou Ling (Fructus Aristolochiae)
Ma Qian Zi (Semen Strychni)
Pi Pa Ye (Folium Eriobotryae)
Qin Pi (Cortex Fraxini)
Qing Pi (Pericarpium Citri Reticulatae Viride)
Ren Dong Teng (Caulis Lonicerae)
Shang Lu (Radix Phytolaccae)
Shi Wei (Folium Pyrrosiae)
Si Gua Luo (Retinervus Luffae Fructus)
Tian Nan Xing (Rhizoma Arisaematis)
Xiao Hui Xiang (Fructus Foeniculi)
Yuan Zhi (Radix Polygalae)
Ze Qi (Herba Euphorbiae Helioscopiae)
Zhu Dan (Fel Porcus)
Zhu Li (Succus Bambusae)
Zi Su Ye (Folium Perillae)
Zi Wan (Radix Asteris)

51. External wounds (facilitates healing)

Di Yu (Radix Sanguisorbae)
Gu Sui Bu (Rhizoma Drynariae)
Lu Hui (Aloe)
Lu Lu Tong (Fructus Liquidambaris)
Shan Yao (Rhizoma Dioscoreae)

52. Hematopoietic (red blood cells)

Can Sha (Excrementum Bombycis Mori)
Dang Gui (Radicis Angelicae Sinensis)
Dang Shen (Radix Codonopsis)
E Jiao (Colla Corii Asini)
He Shou Wu (Radix Polygoni Multiflori)
Ma Huang (Herba Ephedrae)
Niu Huang (Calculus Bovis)
Sang Shen Zi (Fructus Mori)

53. Hematopoietic (white blood cells)

Bai He (Bulbus Lilii)
Ban Mao (Mylabris)
Bu Gu Zhi (Fructus Psoraleae)
Chan Su (Venenum Bufonis).
Di Yu (Radix Sanguisorbae)
Hu Zhang (Rhizoma Polygoni Cuspidati)
Nu Zhen Zi (Fructus Ligustri Lucidi)
Rou Gui (Cortex Cinnamomi)
Sang Shen Zi (Fructus Mori)

54. Hemostatic

Ai Ye (Folium Artemisiae Argyi)
Bai Ji (Rhizoma Bletillae)
Bai Mao Gen (Rhizoma Imperatae)
Da Huang (Radix et Rhizoma Rhei)
Da Ji (Herba seu Radix Cirsii Japonici)
Di Jin Cao (Herba Euphorbiae Humifusae)
Fang Feng (Radix Saposhnikoviae)
Fu Long Gan (Terra Flava Usta)
Guan Zhong (Rhizoma Dryopteridis)
Han Lian Cao (Herba Ecliptae)
Hu Zhang (Rhizoma Polygoni Cuspidati)
Hua Rui Shi (Ophicalcitum)
Huai Hua (Flos Sophorae)
Jin Yin Hua (Flos Lonicerae)
Jing Tian San Qi (Herba seu Radix Sedum Aizoom)
Ju Ye San Qi (Herba seu Radix Gynura Segetum)
Lian Fang (Receptaculum Nelumbinis)
Long Chi (Dens Draconis)
Long Gu (Os Draconis)
Ma Bian Cao (Herba Verbenae)
Ou Jie (Nodus Nelumbinis Rhizomatis)
San Qi (Radix Notoginseng)
Shi Liu Pi (Pericarpium Granati)
Su Mu (Lignum Sappan)
Xi Yang Shen (Radix Panacis Quinquefolii)
Xian He Cao (Herba Agrimoniae)
Xiao Ji (Herba Cirisii)
Xue Yu Tan (Crinis Carbonisatus)
Yin Yang Huo (Herba Epimedii)
Zi Cao Gen (Radix Lithospermi)
Zi Zhu (Folium Callicarpae)
Zong Lu Zi (Fructus Trachycarpi)

55. Hepatoprotective

Bai Shao (Radix Paeoniae Alba)
Bai Zhu (Rhizoma Atractylodis Macrocephalae)
Bie Jia (Carapax Trionycis)
Chai Hu (Radix Bupleuri)
Chuan Xin Lian (Herba Andrographis)
Chui Pen Cao (Herba Sedi)
Da Huang (Radix et Rhizoma Rhei)
Da Suan (Bulbus Alli Sativi)
Dang Gui (Radicis Angelicae Sinensis)
Dang Shen (Radix Codonopsis)
Er Cha (Catechu)
Fu Ling (Poria)
Gan Cao (Radix Glycyrrhizae)
Gou Qi Zi (Fructus Lycii)
Han Lian Cao (Herba Ecliptae)
He Shou Wu (Radix Polygoni Multiflori)
Hu Zhang (Rhizoma Polygoni Cuspidati)
Hua Jiao (Pericarpium Zanthoxyli)
Jiang Huang (Rhizoma Curcumae Longae)
Jin Yin Hua (Flos Lonicerae)
Lao Guan Cao (Herba Erodii seu Geranii)
Lian Qiao (Fructus Forsythiae)
Ling Zhi (Ganoderma)
Long Dan Cao (Radix Gentianae)
Lu Hui (Aloe)
Mu Gua (Fructus Chaenomelis)
Nu Zhen Zi (Fructus Ligustri Lucidi)
Pu Gong Ying (Herba Taraxaci)
Qing Hao (Herba Artemisiae Annuae)
San Qi (Radix Notoginseng)
Sha Yuan Zi (Semen Astragali Complanati)
Shan Dou Gen (Radix Sophorae Tonkinensis)
Sheng Jiang (Rhizoma Zingiberis Recens)
Sheng Ma (Rhizoma Cimicifugae)
Wu Wei Zi (Fructus Schisandrae Chinensis)
Wu Zhu Yu (Fructus Evodiae)
Xiao Ji (Herba Cirisii)
Xie Cao (Radix et Rhizoma Valerianae)
Yin Chen Hao (Herba Artemisiae Scopariae)
Ze Xie (Rhizoma Alismatis)
Zhi Zi (Fructus Gardeniae)
Zhu Ling (Polyporus)

56. Hormone-like (estrogen and testosterone)

Ba Ji Tian (Radix Morindae Officinalis)
Bai Ji Li (Fructus Tribuli)
Ban Mao (Mylabris)
Bu Gu Zhi (Fructus Psoraleae)
Ge Jie (Gecko)
Guan Zhong (Rhizoma Dryopteridis)
Gui Ban (Plastrum Testudinis)
Hai Ma (Hippocampus)
Lu Lu Tong (Fructus Liquidambaris)
She Chuang Zi (Fructus Cnidii)

She Xiang (Moschus)
Suo Yang (Herba Cynomorii)
Tu Si Zi (Semen Cuscutae)
Wu Jia Pi (Cortex Acanthopanacis)
Xian Mao (Rhizoma Curculiginis)
Xiang Fu (Rhizoma Cyperi)
Xiao Hui Xiang (Fructus Foeniculi)
Yin Yang Huo (Herba Epimedii)

57. Hyperglycemic

Chai Hu (Radix Bupleuri)
Dang Shen (Radix Codonopsis)
Qin Jiao (Radix Gentianae Macrophyllae)
Xuan Shen (Radix Scrophulariae)
Zi Su Ye (Folium Perillae)

58. Hypertensive

Chan Su (Venenum Bufonis)
Chen Pi (Pericarpium Citri Reticulatae)
Kuan Dong Hua (Flos Farfarae)
Ma Huang (Herba Ephedrae)
Qing Pi (Pericarpium Citri Reticulatae Viride)
Ze Xie (Rhizoma Alismatis)
Zhi Ke (Fructus Aurantii)
Zhi Shi (Fructus Aurantii Immaturus)

59. Hypotensive

Bai Guo (Semen Ginkgo)
Bai Ji Li (Fructus Tribuli)
Bi Ba (Fructus Piperis Longi)
Bi Cheng Qie (Fructus Litseae)
Chang Shan (Radix Dichroae)
Che Qian Zi (Semen Plantaginis)
Chen Xiang (Lignum Aquilariae Resinatum)
Chi Shao (Radix Paeoniae Rubrae)
Chou Wu Tong (Folium Clerodendri Trichotomi)
Chuan Bei Mu (Bulbus Fritillariae Cirrhosae)
Chuan Wu (Radix Aconiti Preparata)
Ci Wu Jia (Radix et Caulis Acanthopanacis Senticosi)
Da Ji (Herba seu Radix Cirsii Japonici)
Di Gu Pi (Cortex Lycii)
Di Long (Pheretima)
Di Yu (Radix Sanguisorbae)
Er Cha (Catechu)
Fo Shou (Fructus Citri Sarcodactylis)
Gan Song (Radix seu Rhizoma Nardostachys)
Gao Ben (Rhizoma Ligustici)
Ge Gen (Radix Puerariae)
Gou Teng (Ramulus Uncariae cum Uncis)
Hu Jiao (Fructus Piper)
Hu Zhang (Rhizoma Polygoni Cuspidati)
Huai Hua (Flos Sophorae)
Huang Bai (Cortex Phellodendri)
Huang Lian (Rhizoma Coptidis)
Huang Qin (Radix Scutellariae)
Huo Ma Ren (Fructus Cannabis)
Jing Tian San Qi (Herba seu Radix Sedum Aizoom)
Jue Ming Zi (Semen Cassiae)
Ku Lian Pi (Cortex Meliae)
Kun Bu (Thallus Laminariae seu Eckloniae)
Lai Fu Zi (Semen Raphani)
Lian Zi Xin (Plumula Nelumbinis)
Ling Yang Jiao (Cornu Saigae Tataricae)
Ling Zhi (Ganoderma)
Lu Lu Tong (Fructus Liquidambaris)
Man Jing Zi (Fructus Viticis)
Mu Dan Pi (Cortex Moutan)
Mu Zei (Herba Equiseti Hiemalis)
Niu Bang Zi (Fructus Arctii)
Niu Huang (Calculus Bovis)
Pang Da Hai (Semen Sterculiae Lychnophorae)
Qing Feng Teng (Caulis Sinomenii)
Qing Hao (Herba Artemisiae Annuae)
Qing Mu Xiang (Radix Aristolochiae)
Ren Dong Teng (Caulis Lonicerae)
Ren Shen (Radix Ginseng)
San Qi (Radix Notoginseng)
Sang Bai Pi (Cortex Mori)
Sang Ji Sheng (Herba Taxilli)
Sha Yuan Zi (Semen Astragali Complanati)
Shan Dou Gen (Radix Sophorae Tonkinensis)
Shan Zha (Fructus Crataegi)
Sheng Jiang (Rhizoma Zingiberis Recens)
Shui Niu Jiao (Cornu Bubali)
Suan Zao Ren (Semen Zizyphi Spinosae)
Tian Ma (Rhizoma Gastrodiae)
Tu Si Zi (Semen Cuscutae)
Wu Zhu Yu (Fructus Evodiae)
Xi Xian Cao (Herba Siegesbeckiae)
Xia Ku Cao (Spica Prunellae)
Xiang Fu (Rhizoma Cyperi)
Xie Cao (Radix et Rhizoma Valerianae)
Xin Yi Hua (Flos Magnoliae)
Xu Chang Qing (Radix Cynanchi Paniculati)
Xuan Shen (Radix Scrophulariae)
Ye Ju Hua (Flos Chrysanthemi Indici)
Yin Yang Huo (Herba Epimedii)
Yu Zhu (Rhizoma Polygonati Odorati)
Yuan Zhi (Radix Polygalae)

60. Immunostimulant

Ba Ji Tian (Radix Morindae Officinalis)
Bai Shao (Radix Paeoniae Alba)
Ban Lan Gen (Radix Isatidis)
Bian Dou (Semen Lablab Album)
Bie Jia (Carapax Trionycis)
Chan Su (Venenum Bufonis)
Ci Wu Jia (Radix et Caulis Acanthopanacis Senticosi)
Da Suan (Bulbus Alli Sativi)
Dang Gui (Radicis Angelicae Sinensis)
Dang Shen (Radix Codonopsis)
Dong Chong Xia Cao (Cordyceps)
Du Zhong (Cortex Eucommiae)
E Jiao (Colla Corii Asini)
Fang Feng (Radix Saposhnikoviae)
Fu Ling (Poria)
Fu Zi (Radix Aconiti Lateralis Praeparata)
Gan Cao (Radix Glycyrrhizae)
Ge Jie (Gecko)
Gou Qi Zi (Fructus Lycii)
Gui Ban (Plastrum Testudinis)
Hai Ge Fen (Concha Meretricis seu Cyclinae)
Hai Shen (Strichopus Japonicus)
He Shou Wu (Radix Polygoni Multiflori)
Huang Jing (Rhizoma Polygonati)
Huang Lian (Rhizoma Coptidis)
Huang Qi (Radix Astragali)
Jiao Gu Lan (Rhizoma seu Herba Gynostemmatis)
Jin Yin Hua (Flos Lonicerae)
Ling Zhi (Ganoderma)
Long Dan Cao (Radix Gentianae)
Long Yan Rou (Arillus Longan)
Lu Han Cao (Herba Pyrolae)
Mai Men Dong (Radix Ophiopogonis)
Nu Zhen Zi (Fructus Ligustri Lucidi)
Pu Gong Ying (Herba Taraxaci)
Qing Mu Xiang (Radix Aristolochiae)
Ren Shen (Radix Ginseng)
San Qi (Radix Notoginseng)
Sang Shen Zi (Fructus Mori)
Sha Yuan Zi (Semen Astragali Complanati)
Shan Yao (Rhizoma Dioscoreae)
Shan Zha (Fructus Crataegi)
She Xiang (Moschus)
Shi Gao (Gypsum Fibrosum)
Suan Zao Ren (Semen Zizyphi Spinosae)

Suo Yang (Herba Cynomorii)
Tian Ma (Rhizoma Gastrodiae)
Tu Si Zi (Semen Cuscutae)
Wu Mei (Fructus Mume)
Xian Mao (Rhizoma Curculiginis)
Xiang Ru (Herba Elsholtziae seu Moslae)
Yin Yang Huo (Herba Epimedii)
Yu Xing Cao (Herba Houttuyniae)
Zhu Ling (Polyporus)
Zi He Che (Placenta Hominis)

61. Immunosuppressive

Bei Sha Shen (Radix Glehniae)
Chai Hu (Radix Bupleuri)
Chan Tui (Periostracum Cicadae)
Chuan Shan Long (Rhizoma Dioscoreae Nipponicae)
Chuan Wu (Radix Aconiti Preparata)
Chuan Xin Lian (Herba Andrographis)
Gan Sui (Radix Euphorbiae Kansui)
Hong Hua (Flos Carthami)
Huang Qin (Radix Scutellariae)
Ku Shen Gen (Radix Sophorae Flavescentis)
Lei Gong Teng (Radix Tripterygii Wilfordii)
Shan Dou Gen (Radix Sophorae Tonkinensis)
She Chuang Zi (Fructus Cnidii)
Shu Di Huang (Radix Rehmanniae Preparata)
Tian Hua Fen (Radix Trichosanthis)
Tian Men Dong (Radix Asparagi)
Wu Jia Pi (Cortex Acanthopanacis)
Wu Wei Zi (Fructus Schisandrae Chinensis)
Xia Ku Cao (Spica Prunellae)
Ze Xie (Rhizoma Alismatis)

62. Laxative

Da Huang (Radix et Rhizoma Rhei)
Fan Xie Ye (Folium Sennae)
Gan Sui (Radix Euphorbiae Kansui)
Gua Lou Ren (Semen Trichosanthis)
He Shou Wu (Radix Polygoni Multiflori)
Huo Ma Ren (Fructus Cannabis)
Liu Huang (Sulfur)
Lu Hui (Aloe)
Mang Xiao (Natrii Sulfas)
Pang Da Hai (Semen Sterculiae Lychnophorae)
Qian Niu Zi (Semen Pharbitidis)
Tao Ren (Semen Persicae)

63. Metabolic

Bai Zhu (Rhizoma Atractylodis Macrocephalae)
Ci Wu Jia (Radix et Caulis Acanthopanacis Senticosi)
Gou Qi Zi (Fructus Lycii)
Gui Ban (Plastrum Testudinis)
Huang Qi (Radix Astragali)
Long Yan Rou (Arillus Longan)
Lu Lu Tong (Fructus Liquidambaris)
Niu Xi (Radix Cyathulae seu Achyranthis)
Ren Shen (Radix Ginseng)
San Qi (Radix Notoginseng)
Wu Jia Pi (Cortex Acanthopanacis)
Wu Wei Zi (Fructus Schisandrae Chinensis)
Xi Yang Shen (Radix Panacis Quinquefolii)

64. Radiation (protective effect)

Can Sha (Excrementum Bombycis Mori)
Chai Hu (Radix Bupleuri)
Chan Su (Venenum Bufonis)
Chuan Xiong (Rhizoma Ligustici Chuanxiong)
Dang Gui (Radicis Angelicae Sinensis)
E Jiao (Colla Corii Asini)
Hai Piao Xiao (Endoconcha Sepiae)
Hai Shen (Strichopus Japonicus)
Huai Hua (Flos Sophorae)
Kun Bu (Thallus Laminariae seu Eckloniae)
Ling Zhi (Ganoderma)
Lu Cha (Folium Camellia Sinensis)
Ren Shen (Radix Ginseng)
Rou Gui (Cortex Cinnamomi)
San Qi (Radix Notoginseng)
Wu Long Cha (Folium Camellia Sinensis Fermentata)
Wu Mei (Fructus Mume)
Zhu Ling (Polyporus)

65. Sedative and hypnotic

Ai Ye (Folium Artemisiae Argyi)
Bai He (Bulbus Lilii)
Bai Shao (Radix Paeoniae Alba)
Bai Tou Weng (Radix Pulsatillae)
Chi Shao (Radix Paeoniae Rubrae)
Di Long (Pheretima)
Dong Chong Xia Cao (Cordyceps)
Du Zhong (Cortex Eucommiae)
Fang Feng (Radix Saposhnikoviae)
Gan Song (Radix seu Rhizoma Nardostachys)
Gui Ban (Plastrum Testudinis)
He Huan Hua (Flos Albiziae)
Hong Hua (Flos Carthami)
Long Chi (Dens Draconis)
Long Gu (Os Draconis)
Mu Dan Pi (Cortex Moutan)
Mu Zei (Herba Equiseti Hiemalis)
Niu Huang (Calculus Bovis)
Sheng Jiang (Rhizoma Zingiberis Recens)
Sheng Ma (Rhizoma Cimicifugae)
Shi Chang Pu (Rhizoma Acori)
Tian Ma (Rhizoma Gastrodiae)
Tian Nan Xing (Rhizoma Arisaematis)
Wu Wei Zi (Fructus Schisandrae Chinensis)
Xian Mao (Rhizoma Curculiginis)
Xiao Ji (Herba Cirisii)
Yan Hu Suo (Rhizoma Corydalis)
Yu Mi Xu (Stigma Maydis)
Yuan Zhi (Radix Polygalae)
Zao Xiu (Rhizoma Paridis)
Zhu Sha (Cinnabaris)

66. Smooth muscle relaxant

Bai Zhi (Radix Angelicae Dahuricae)
Bi Ba (Fructus Piperis Longi)
Bo He (Herba Menthae)
Chan Su (Venenum Bufonis).
Chen Pi (Pericarpium Citri Reticulatae)
Chen Xiang (Lignum Aquilariae Resinatum)
Chi Shao (Radix Paeoniae Rubrae)
Chuan Bei Mu (Bulbus Fritillariae Cirrhosae)
Ding Xiang (Flos Caryophylli)
Fo Shou (Fructus Citri Sarcodactylis)
Gan Jiang (Rhizoma Zingiberis)
Gan Song (Radix seu Rhizoma Nardostachys)
Gao Ben (Rhizoma Ligustici)
Ge Gen (Radix Puerariae)
Hai Shen (Strichopus Japonicus)
Huai Hua (Flos Sophorae)
Huang Yao Zi (Herba Dioscoreae Bulbiferae)
Huo Xiang (Herba Agastache)
Kuan Dong Hua (Flos Farfarae)
Ling Zhi (Ganoderma)
Ma Huang (Herba Ephedrae)
Mu Xiang (Radix Aucklandiae)
Niu Huang (Calculus Bovis)
Qing Pi (Pericarpium Citri Reticulatae Viride)
Ren Dong Teng (Caulis Lonicerae)

Shan Dou Gen (Radix Sophorae Tonkinensis)
Shan Yao (Rhizoma Dioscoreae)
She Chuang Zi (Fructus Cnidii)
Sheng Ma (Rhizoma Cimicifugae)
Wei Ling Xian (Radix Clematidis)
Wu Mei (Fructus Mume)
Xi Xin (Herba Asari)
Xiang Ru (Herba Elsholtziae seu Moslae)
Yin Guo Ye (Folium Ginkgo)
Zao Xiu (Rhizoma Paridis)
Zhi Ke (Fructus Aurantii)

67. Smooth muscle stimulant
Ba Dou (Fructus Crotonis)
Chuan Lian Zi (Fructus Toosendan)
Ji Nei Jin (Endothelium Corneum Gigeriae Galli)
Ku Lian Pi (Cortex Meliae)
Lai Fu Zi (Semen Raphani)
Luo Han Guo (Fructus Momordicae)
Qian Niu Zi (Semen Pharbitidis)
Qu Mai (Herba Dianthi)
Sang Bai Pi (Cortex Mori)
Shan Yao (Rhizoma Dioscoreae)
Suo Yang (Herba Cynomorii)
Xiao Hui Xiang (Fructus Foeniculi)
Xiao Ji (Herba Cirisii)
Ya Dan Zi (Fructus Bruceae)
Zhi Zi (Fructus Gardeniae)
Zi Su Ye (Folium Perillae)

68. Thrombolytic
Qu Mai (Herba Dianthi)
Yuan Zhi (Radix Polygalae)

69. Uterine stimulant
Bo He (Herba Menthae)
Chang Shan (Radix Dichroae)
Di Long (Pheretima)
Du Zhong (Cortex Eucommiae)
Fei Zi (Semen Torreyae)
Gui Ban (Plastrum Testudinis)
Hai Long (Syngnathus)
Hong Hua (Flos Carthami)
Niu Xi (Radix Cyathulae seu Achyranthis)
Qu Mai (Herba Dianthi)
Tao Ren (Semen Persicae)
Wu Wei Zi (Fructus Schisandrae Chinensis)
Xu Duan (Radix Dipsaci)
Yi Mu Cao (Herba Leonuri)
Yuan Zhi (Radix Polygalae)

70. Vasoconstrictor (peripheral)
Ma Huang (Herba Ephedrae)
Yi Zhi Ren (Fructus Alpiniae Oxyphyllae)

71. Vasodilator (coronary artery)
Bai Ji Li (Fructus Tribuli)
Bu Gu Zhi (Fructus Psoraleae)
Chi Shao (Radix Paeoniae Rubrae)
Chuan Xiong (Rhizoma Ligustici Chuanxiong)
Dan Shen (Radix Salviae Miltiorrhizae)
Fu Zi (Radix Aconiti Lateralis Praeparata)
Hai Feng Teng (Caulis Piperis Kadsurae)
He Shou Wu (Radix Polygoni Multiflori)
Hong Hua (Flos Carthami)
Huang Jing (Rhizoma Polygonati)
Jing Tian San Qi (Herba seu Radix Sedum Aizoom)
Ju Hua (Flos Chrysanthemi)
Ling Zhi (Ganoderma)
Lu Han Cao (Herba Pyrolae)
San Qi (Radix Notoginseng)
Sang Ji Sheng (Herba Taxilli)
Shan Zha (Fructus Crataegi)
She Xiang (Moschus).
Shi Chang Pu (Rhizoma Acori)
Shui Zhi (Hirudo)
Su He Xiang (Styrax)
Wu Wei Zi (Fructus Schisandrae Chinensis)
Xie Cao (Radix et Rhizoma Valerianae)
Xuan Shen (Radix Scrophulariae)
Yan Hu Suo (Rhizoma Corydalis)
Yi Mu Cao (Herba Leonuri)
Yin Yang Huo (Herba Epimedii)
Zhi Shi (Fructus Aurantii Immaturus)

72. Vasodilator (peripheral)
Bai Shao (Radix Paeoniae Alba)
Chuan Wu (Radix Aconiti Preparata)
Chuan Xiong (Rhizoma Ligustici Chuanxiong)
Ci Wu Jia (Radix et Caulis Acanthopanacis Senticosi)
Dang Gui (Radicis Angelicae Sinensis)
Du Zhong (Cortex Eucommiae)
Ge Gen (Radix Puerariae)
Gua Lou Shi (Fructus Trichosanthis)
Gui Zhi (Ramulus Cinnamomi)
Hai Feng Teng (Caulis Piperis Kadsurae)
Mu Zei (Herba Equiseti Hiemalis)
Ren Shen (Radix Ginseng)
Sang Ji Sheng (Herba Taxilli)
Tao Ren (Semen Persicae)
Xie Cao (Radix et Rhizoma Valerianae).
Xin Yi Hua (Flos Magnoliae)
Yin Guo Ye (Folium Ginkgo)

Appendix 4 — Cross-reference of Single Herb Names

Pinyin Names	Pharmaceutical Names	Chinese Names
Ai Ye	Folium Artemisiae Argyi	艾叶
Ba Dou	Fructus Crotonis	巴豆
Ba Ji Tian	Radix Morindae Officinalis	巴戟天
Ba Yue Zha	Fructus Akebiae	八月札
Bai Bu	Radix Stemonae	百部
Bai Dou Kou	Fructus Amomi Rotundus	白豆蔻
Bai Dou Kou Ke	Pericarpium Amomi Rotundus	白豆蔻壳
Bai Fu Ling	Poria Alba	白茯苓
Bai Fu Zi	Rhizoma Typhonii	白附子
Bai Guo	Semen Ginkgo	白果
Bai He	Bulbus Lilii	百合
Bai Hua She	Bungarus Parvus	白花蛇
Bai Hua She She Cao	Herba Oldenlandia	白花蛇舌草
Bai Ji	Rhizoma Bletillae	白及
Bai Ji Li	Fructus Tribuli	白蒺藜
Bai Jiang Cao	Herba cum Radice Patriniae	败酱草
Bai Jie Zi	Semen Sinapis	白芥子
Bai Lian	Radix Ampelopsis	白蔹
Bai Long Chuan Hua Tou	Radix Clerodendron Paniculatum	白龙船花头
Bai Mao Gen	Rhizoma Imperatae	白茅根
Bai Mao Hua	Flos Imperatae	白茅花
Bai Mu Er	Fructificatio Tremellae Fuciformis	白木耳
Bai Mu Tong	Caulis Akebia Trifoliata Australis	白木通
Bai Qian	Rhizoma Cynanchi Stauntonii	白前
Bai Shao	Radix Paeoniae Alba	白芍
Bai Tou Weng	Radix Pulsatillae	白头翁
Bai Tou Weng Jing	Caulis Pulsatillae	白头翁茎
Bai Tou Weng Ye	Folium Pulsatillae	白头翁叶
Bai Wei	Radix Cynanchi Atrati	白薇
Bai Xian Pi	Cortex Dictamni	白鲜皮
Bai Zhi	Radix Angelicae Dahuricae	白芷
Bai Zhu	Rhizoma Atractylodis Macrocephalae	白术
Bai Zi Ren	Semen Platycladi	柏子仁
Ban Bian Lian	Herba Lobeliae Chinensis	半边莲
Ban Lan Gen	Radix Isatidis	板蓝根
Ban Mao	Mylabris	斑蝥
Ban Xia	Rhizoma Pinelliae	半夏
Ban Zhi Lian	Herba Scutellariae Barbatae	半枝莲
Bei Chai Hu	Radix Bupleurum Chinensis	北柴胡
Bei Dou Gen	Rhizoma Menispermi	北豆根
Bei Mu	Bulbus Fritillaria	贝母
Bei Sha Shen	Radix Glehniae	北沙参
Bei Ting Li Zi	Semen Lepidii	北葶苈子
Bei Wu Jia Pi	Cortex Periploca Sepium Radicis	北五加皮
Bi Ba	Fructus Piperis Longi	荜茇
Bi Cheng Qie	Fructus Litseae	荜澄茄
Bi Xie	Rhizoma Dioscoreae Hypoglaucae	萆薢
Bi Zi Cao	Herba Pogonantheri Criniti	笔仔草
Bian Dou	Semen Lablab Album	扁豆
Bian Dou Hua	Flos Lablab Album	扁豆花
Bian Dou Yi	Pericarpium Lablab Album	扁豆衣
Bian Xu	Herba Polygoni Avicularis	萹蓄

Pinyin Names	Pharmaceutical Names	Chinese Names
Bie Jia	Carapax Trionycis	鳖甲
Bie Jia Jiao	Gelatinum Carapax Trionycis	鳖甲胶
Bing Lang	Semen Arecae	槟榔
Bing Pian	Borneolum Syntheticum	冰片
Bo He	Herba Menthae	薄荷
Bu Gu Zhi	Fructus Psoraleae	补骨脂
Can Sha	Excrementum Bombycis Mori	蚕砂
Cang Er Cao	Herba Xanthii	苍耳草
Cang Er Gen	Radix Xanthii	苍耳根
Cang Er Zi	Fructus Xanthii	苍耳子
Cang Zhu	Rhizoma Atractylodis	苍术
Cao Dou Kou	Semen Alpiniae Katsumadai	草豆蔻
Cao Guo	Fructus Tsaoko	草果
Cao Wu	Radix Aconiti Kusnezoffii	草乌
Ce Bai Ye	Cacumen Platycladi	侧柏叶
Cha Chi Huang	Herba Stellariae Aquaticae	茶匙癀
Chai Hu	Radix Bupleuri	柴胡
Chan Su	Venenum Bufonis	蟾酥
Chan Tui	Periostracum Cicadae	蝉蜕
Chang Shan	Radix Dichroae	常山
Che Qian Cao	Herba Plantaginis	车前草
Che Qian Zi	Semen Plantaginis	车前子
Chen Pi	Pericarpium Citri Reticulatae	陈皮
Chen Xiang	Lignum Aquilariae Resinatum	沉香
Chi Fu Ling	Poria Rubrae	赤茯苓
Chi Shao	Radix Paeoniae Rubrae	赤芍
Chi Shi Zhi	Halloysitum Rubrum	赤石脂
Chi Xiao Dou	Semen Phaseoli	赤小豆
Chong Wei Zi	Semen Leonuri	茺蔚子
Chou Wu Tong	Folium Clerodendri Trichotomi	臭梧桐
Chu Shi Zi	Fructus Broussonetiae	楮实子
Chuan Bei Mu	Bulbus Fritillariae Cirrhosae	川贝母
Chuan Lian Zi	Fructus Toosendan	川楝子
Chuan Mu Tong	Caulis Clematidis Armandii	川木通
Chuan Niu Xi	Radix Cyathulae	川牛膝
Chuan Shan Jia	Squama Manis	穿山甲
Chuan Shan Long	Rhizoma Dioscoreae Nipponicae	穿山龙
Chuan Wu	Radix Aconiti Preparata	川乌
Chuan Xin Lian	Herba Andrographis	穿心莲
Chuan Xiong	Rhizoma Ligusticum Chuanxiong	川芎
Chui Pen Cao	Herba Sedi	垂盆草
Chun Gen	Radix Ailanthi	椿根
Chun Gen Pi	Cortex Ailanthi	椿根皮
Ci Shi	Magnetitum	磁石
Ci Wu Jia	Radix et Caulis Acanthopanacis Senticosi	刺五加
Cong Bai	Bulbus Allii Fistulosi	葱白
Da Ding Huang	Caulis Euonymi	大疔癀
Da Dou Huang Juan	Semen Glycines Germinatum	大豆黄卷
Da Feng Zi	Semen Hydnocarpi	大风子
Da Fu Pi	Pericarpium Arecae	大腹皮
Da Huang	Radix et Rhizoma Rhei	大黄
Da Hui Xiang	Fructus Anisi Stellati	大茴香
Da Ji	Herba seu Radix Cirsii Japonici	大蓟
Da Ji	Radix Euphorbiae seu Knoxiae	大戟

Pinyin Names	Pharmaceutical Names	Chinese Names
Da Ji Gen	Radix Cirsii Japonici	大蓟根
Da Ji Ye	Folium Cirsii Japonici	大蓟叶
Da Qing Ye	Folium Isatidis	大青叶
Da Suan	Bulbus Alli Sativi	大蒜
Da Xiao Ji		大小蓟
Da Ye Ma Dou Ling	Caulis Aristolochiae Kaempferi	大叶马兜铃
Da Zao	Fructus Jujubae	大枣
Dai Zhe Shi	Haematitum	代赭石
Dan Dou Chi	Semen Sojae Praeparatum	淡豆鼓
Dan Nan Xing	Arisaema cum Bile	胆南星
Dan Shen	Radix Salviae Miltiorrhizae	丹参
Dan Zhu Ye	Herba Lophatheri	淡竹叶
Dang Gui	Radicis Angelicae Sinensis	当归
Dang Gui Shen	Corpus Radicis Angelicae Sinensis	当归身
Dang Gui Tou	Caput Radicis Angelicae Sinensis	当归头
Dang Gui Wei	Extremitas Radicis Angelicae Sinensis	当归尾
Dang Shen	Radix Codonopsis	党参
Dao Di Wu Gong	Rhizoma Heliminthostachytis	倒地蜈蚣
Dao Diao Jin Zhong	Melothria Maderospatana	倒吊金钟
Dao Dou	Semen Canavaliae	刀豆
Deng Xin Cao	Medulla Junci	灯心草
Di Bie Chong	Eupolyphaga	地鳖虫
Di Fu Zi	Fructus Kochiae	地肤子
Di Gu Pi	Cortex Lycii	地骨皮
Di Long	Pheretima	地龙
Di Yu	Radix Sanguisorbae	地榆
Ding Jing Cao	Herba Linderniae	定经草
Ding Shu Xiu	Herba Elephantopus Scaber	丁竖杇
Ding Xiang	Flos Caryophylli	丁香
Ding Xiang Pi	Cortex Caryophylli	丁香皮
Dong Chong Xia Cao	Cordyceps	冬虫夏草
Dong Gua Pi	Exocarpium Benincasae	冬瓜皮
Dong Gua Zi	Semen Benincasae	冬瓜子
Dong Kui Zi	Semen Malvae	冬葵子
Dong Ling Cao	Herba Rabdosiae	冬凌草
Dong Qing Ye	Folium Ilexis	冬青叶
Dong Yang Shen	Radix Ginseng Japonica	东洋参
Du Huo	Radix Angelicae Pubescentis	独活
Du Zhong	Cortex Eucommiae	杜仲
Du Zhong Ye	Folium Eucommiae	杜仲叶
Duan Shi Gao	Gypsum Fibrosum Preparata	煅石膏
E Bu Shi Cao	Herba Centipedae	鹅不食草
E Jiao	Colla Corii Asini	阿胶
E Zhu	Rhizoma Curcumae	莪术
Er Cha	Catechu	儿茶
Fan Xie Ye	Folium Sennae	番泻叶
Fang Feng	Radix Saposhnikoviae	防风
Fang Jie Shi	Calcitum	方解石
Fei Zi	Semen Torreyae	榧子
Fen Fang Ji	Radix Stephaniae Tetandrae	粉防己
Feng Mi	Mel	蜂蜜
Feng Wei Cao	Herba Pteris	凤尾草
Fo Shou	Fructus Citri Sarcodactylis	佛手
Fo Shou Hua	Flos Citri Sarcodactylis	佛手花

Pinyin Names	Pharmaceutical Names	Chinese Names
Fu Hai Shi	Pumice	浮海石
Fu Ling	Poria	茯苓
Fu Ling Pi	Cortex Poria	茯苓皮
Fu Long Gan	Terra Flava Usta	伏龙肝
Fu Pen Zi	Fructus Rubi	覆盆子
Fu Ping	Herba Spirodelae	浮萍
Fu Rong	Radix Hibisci	芙蓉
Fu Rong Ye	Folium Hibisci	芙蓉草
Fu Shen	Poria Pararadicis	茯神
Fu Xiao Mai	Semen Tritici Aestivi Levis	浮小麦
Fu Zi	Radix Aconiti Lateralis Praeparata	附子
Gan Cao	Radix Glycyrrhizae	甘草
Gan Jiang	Rhizoma Zingiberis	乾姜
Gan Qi	Resina Toxicodendri	干漆
Gan Song	Radix seu Rhizoma Nardostachys	甘松
Gan Sui	Radix Euphorbiae Kansui	甘遂
Gao Ben	Rhizoma Ligustici	藁本
Gao Liang Jiang	Rhizoma Alpiniae Officinarum	高良姜
Ge Gen	Radix Puerariae	葛根
Ge Hua	Flos Puerariae	葛花
Ge Jie	Gecko	蛤蚧
Geng Mi	Semen Oryzae	粳米
Geng Tong Cao	Ramulus Aeschynomene Indica	梗通草
Gou Gu	Os Canitis	狗骨
Gou Ji	Rhizoma Cibotii	狗脊
Gou Qi Gen	Radix Lycii	枸杞根
Gou Qi Ye	Folium Lycii	枸杞叶
Gou Qi Zi	Fructus Lycii	枸杞子
Gou Teng	Ramulus Uncariae cum Uncis	钩藤
Gu Jing Cao	Flos Eriocauli	谷精草
Gu Sui Bu	Rhizoma Drynariae	骨碎补
Gu Ya	Fructus Setariae Germinatus	谷芽
Gu Zhi Hua	Semen Oroxyli	故纸花
Gua Di	Pedicellus Cucumeris	瓜蒂
Gua Lou Pi	Pericarpium Trichosanthis	瓜蒌皮
Gua Lou Ren	Semen Trichosanthis	瓜蒌仁
Gua Lou Shi	Fructus Trichosanthis	瓜蒌实
Guan Bai Fu	Rhizoma Aconitum Coreanum	关白附
Guan Mu Tong	Caulis Aristolochiae Manshuriensis	关木通
Guan Ye Lian Qiao	Herba Hypericum	贯叶连翘
Guan Zhong	Rhizoma Dryopteridis	贯众
Guang Fang Ji	Radix Aristolochiae Fangchi	广防己
Guang Huo Xiang	Herba Pogostemonis	广藿香
Guang Jin Qian Cao	Herba Desmodii Styracifolii	广金钱草
Gui Ban	Plastrum Testudinis	龟板
Gui Ban Jiao	Gelatinum Plastrum Testudinis	龟板胶
Gui Xin	Cortex Rasus Cinnamomi	桂心
Gui Zhi	Ramulus Cinnamomi	桂枝
Hai Dai	Thallus Laminariae	海带
Hai Feng Teng	Caulis Piperis Kadsurae	海风藤
Hai Fu Rong	Herba Limonium Wrightii	海芙蓉
Hai Ge Fen	Concha Meretricis seu Cyclinae	海蛤粉
Hai Gou Shen	Testes et Penis Otariae	海狗肾
Hai Jin Sha	Herba Lygodii	海金砂

Pinyin Names	Pharmaceutical Names	Chinese Names
Hai Long	Syngnathus	海龙
Hai Ma	Hippocampus	海马
Hai Piao Xiao	Endoconcha Sepiae	海螵蛸
Hai Shen	Strichopus Japonicus	海参
Hai Tong Pi	Cortex Erythrinae	海桐皮
Hai Zao	Sargassum	海藻
Han Lian Cao	Herba Ecliptae	旱莲草
Han Shui Shi	Mirabilite	寒水石
He Cao Ya	Gemma Agrimoniae	鹤草芽
He Di	Calyx Nelumbinis	荷蒂
He Geng	Caulis Nelumbinis	荷梗
He Huan Hua	Flos Albiziae	合欢花
He Huan Pi	Cortex Albiziae	合欢皮
He Shi	Fructus Carpesii	鹤虱
He Shou Wu	Radix Polygoni Multiflori	何首乌
He Tao Qiu Pi	Cortex Juglandis	核桃楸皮
He Ye	Folium Nelumbinis	荷叶
He Zi	Fructus Chebulae	诃子
Hei Dou	Semen Glycine Max	黑豆
Hei Zhi Ma	Semen Sesami Nigrum	黑芝麻
Hong Da Ji	Radix Knoxiae	红大戟
Hong Dou Kou	Fructus Alphiniae Galangae	红豆蔻
Hong Gu She	Radix Kadsura Japonicae	红骨蛇
Hong Han Lian	Herba Hypericum Ascyron	红旱连
Hong Hua	Flos Carthami	红花
Hong Qu	Monascus	红曲
Hong Shi Gao	Gypsum Rubrae	红石膏
Hong Teng	Caulis Sargentodoxae	红藤
Hou Po	Cortex Magnoliae Officinalis	厚朴
Hou Po Hua	Flos Magnoliae Officinalis	厚朴花
Hu Gu	Os Tigris	虎骨
Hu Huang Lian	Rhizoma Picrorhizae	胡黄连
Hu Jiao	Fructus Piper	胡椒
Hu Lu Ba	Semen Trigonellae	胡芦巴
Hu Po	Succinum	琥珀
Hu Tao Ren	Semen Juglandis	胡桃仁
Hu Yao Huang	Herba Leucas Mollissimae	虎咬癀
Hu Zhang	Rhizoma Polygoni Cuspidati	虎杖
Hua Jiao	Pericarpium Zanthoxyli	花椒
Hua Ju Hong	Exocarpium Citri Grandis	化橘红
Hua Rui Shi	Ophicalcitum	花蕊石
Hua Shi	Talcum	滑石
Hua Shi Cao	Herba Orthosiphon Aristatus	化石草
Huai Hua	Flos Sophorae	槐花
Huai Jiao	Fructus Sophorae	槐角
Huai Niu Xi	Radix Achyranthis Bidentatae	淮牛膝
Huai Tong Ma Dou Ling	Caulis Aristolochiae Moupinensis	淮通马兜铃
Huang Bai	Cortex Phellodendri	黄柏
Huang Jin Gui	Caulis Vanieriae	黄金桂
Huang Jing	Rhizoma Polygonati	黄精
Huang Lian	Rhizoma Coptidis	黄连
Huang Niu Jiao	Cornus Bovis	黄牛角
Huang Qi	Radix Astragali	黄芪
Huang Qin	Radix Scutellariae	黄芩

Pinyin Names	Pharmaceutical Names	Chinese Names
Huang Shui Qie	Herba Solani	黄水茄
Huang Teng	Caulis Fibraurea	黄藤
Huang Yang Jiao	Cornu Procapra Gutturosa	黄羊角
Huang Yao Zi	Herba Dioscoreae Bulbiferae	黄药子
Huo Ma Ren	Fructus Cannabis	火麻仁
Huo Xiang	Herba Agastache	藿香
Ji Gu Cao	Herba Abri	鸡骨草
Ji Guan Hua	Flos Celosiae Cristatae	鸡冠花
Ji Nei Jin	Endothelium Corneum Gigeriae Galli	鸡内金
Ji Xiang Teng	Caulis Paederiae	鸡香藤
Ji Xue Cao	Herba Centellae	积雪草
Ji Xue Teng	Caulis Spatholobi	鸡血藤
Jian Shen Qu	Massa Fermentata Praeparata	建神曲
Jiang Can	Bombyx Batryticatus	僵蚕
Jiang Huang	Rhizoma Curcumae Longae	姜黄
Jiang Xiang	Lignum Dalbergiae Odoriferae	降香
Jiao Gu Lan	Rhizoma seu Herba Gynostemmatis	绞股蓝
Jiao Mu	Semen Zanthoxyli Bungeani	椒目
Jie Geng	Radix Platycodonis	桔梗
Jin Bu Huan	Herba Lycopodii Serrati	金不换
Jin Fei Cao	Herba Inulae	金沸草
Jin Guo Lan	Radix Tinosporae	金果榄
Jin Qian Cao	Herba Lysimachiae	金钱草
Jin Yin Hua	Flos Lonicerae	金银花
Jin Ying Zi	Fructus Rosae Laevigatae	金樱子
Jing Da Ji	Radix Euphorbiae Pekinensis	京大戟
Jing Jie	Herba Schizonepetae	荆芥
Jing Sui	Flos Schizonepetae	荆穗
Jing Tian San Qi	Herba seu Radix Sedum Aizoom	景天三七
Jiu Cai Zi	Semen Allii Tuberosi	韭菜子
Jiu Ceng Ta	Herba Ocimi Basilici	九层塔
Jiu Jie Chang Pu	Rhizoma Anemones Altaicae	九节菖蒲
Ju He	Semen Citri Rubrum	橘核
Ju Hong	Exocarpium Citri Rubrum	橘红
Ju Hua	Flos Chrysanthemi	菊花
Ju Luo	Fibra Citri Rubrum	橘络
Ju Ye	Folium Citri Rubrum	橘叶
Ju Ye San Qi	Herba seu Radix Gynura Segetum	菊叶三七
Jue Ming Zi	Semen Cassiae	决明子
Ku Lian Pi	Cortex Meliae	苦楝皮
Ku Lian Zi	Fructus Meliae	苦楝子
Ku Shen Gen	Radix Sophorae Flavescentis	苦参根
Kuan Dong Hua	Flos Farfarae	款冬花
Kun Bu	Thallus Laminariae seu Eckloniae	昆布
Lai Fu Zi	Semen Raphani	莱菔子
Lang Du	Radix Euphorbiae Fischerianae	狼毒
Lao Guan Cao	Herba Erodii seu Geranii	老鹳草
Lei Gong Teng	Radix Tripterygii Wilfordii	雷公藤
Lei Wan	Omphalia	雷丸
Li Lu	Radix et Rhizoma Veratri	藜芦
Li Zhi He	Semen Litchi	荔枝核
Lian Fang	Receptaculum Nelumbinis	莲房
Lian Qian Cao	Herba Glechomae	连钱草
Lian Qiao	Fructus Forsythiae	连翘

Pinyin Names	Pharmaceutical Names	Chinese Names
Lian Xu	Stamen Nelumbinis	莲须
Lian Zi	Semen Nelumbinis	莲子
Lian Zi Xin	Plumula Nelumbinis	莲子心
Ling Yang Jiao	Cornu Saigae Tataricae	羚羊角
Ling Yin Chen	Herba Siphonostegia Chinensis	铃茵陈
Ling Zhi	Ganoderma	灵芝
Liu Huang	Sulfur	硫黄
Liu Ji Nu	Herba Artemisiae Anomalae	刘寄奴
Liu Ye	Folium Salicis Babylonicae	柳叶
Liu Zhi Huang	Herba Solidaginis	柳枝癀
Long Chi	Dens Draconis	龙齿
Long Dan Cao	Radix Gentianae	龙胆草
Long Gu	Os Draconis	龙骨
Long Kui	Herba Solanum Nigrum	龙葵
Long Yan Hua	Flos Longan	龙眼花
Long Yan Rou	Arillus Longan	龙眼肉
Lou Lu	Radix Rhapontici	漏芦
Lu Cha	Folium Camellia Sinensis	绿茶
Lu Dou	Semen Phaseoli Radiati	绿豆
Lu Dou Yi	Pericarpium Phaseoli Radiati	绿豆衣
Lu Feng Fang	Nidus Vespae	露蜂房
Lu Gan Shi	Galamina	炉甘石
Lu Gen	Rhizoma Phragmitis	芦根
Lu Han Cao	Herba Pyrolae	鹿含草
Lu Hui	Aloe	芦荟
Lu Jiao	Cornu Cervi	鹿角
Lu Jiao Jiao	Gelatinum Cornu Cervi	鹿角胶
Lu Jiao Shuang	Cornu Cervi Degelatinatum	鹿角霜
Lu Lu Tong	Fructus Liquidambaris	路路通
Lu Rong	Cornu Cervi Pantotrichum	鹿茸
Luo Han Guo	Fructus Momordicae	罗汉果
Luo Han Guo Ye	Folium Momordicae	罗汉果叶
Luo Shi Teng	Caulis Trachelospermi	络石藤
Ma An Teng	Herba Ipomoea Pes-caprae	马鞍藤
Ma Bian Cao	Herba Verbenae	马鞭草
Ma Bo	Lasiosphaera seu Calvatia	马勃
Ma Chi Xian	Herba Portulacae	马齿苋
Ma Dou Ling	Fructus Aristolochiae	马兜铃
Ma Huang	Herba Ephedrae	麻黄
Ma Huang Gen	Radix Ephedrae	麻黄根
Ma Qian Zi	Semen Strychni	马钱子
Ma Ti Jin	Herba Dichondrae Repentis	马蹄金
Mai Men Dong	Radix Ophiopogonis	麦门冬
Mai Ya	Fructus Hordei Germinatus	麦芽
Man Jing Zi	Fructus Viticis	蔓荆子
Mang Cao	Fructus Illicium Lanceolatum	莽草
Mang Xiao	Natrii Sulfas	芒硝
Mao Dong Qing	Radix Ilicis Pubescentis	毛冬青
Mao Zi Dun Tou	Herba Abutilon Indicum	帽仔盾头
Meng Chong	Tabanus	虻虫
Meng Shi	Lapis Micae seu Chloriti	礞石
Mi Jiao	Cornu Elaphuri	麋角
Mi Meng Hua	Flos Buddlejae	密蒙花
Mi Rong	Cornu Elaphuri Pantotrichum	麋茸

Pinyin Names	Pharmaceutical Names	Chinese Names
Mi Tuo Seng	Lithargyum	密陀僧
Ming Fan	Alumen	明矾
Mo Gu Xiao	Caulis Hyptis Capitatae	冇骨消
Mo Yao	Myrrha	没药
Mu Bie Zi	Semen Momordicae	木鳖子
Mu Dan Pi	Cortex Moutan	牡丹皮
Mu Dan Ye	Folium Moutan	牡丹叶
Mu Ding Xiang	Fructus Caryophylli	母丁香
Mu Fang Ji	Radix Cocculi Trilobi	木防己
Mu Gua	Fructus Chaenomelis	木瓜
Mu Li	Concha Ostreae	牡蛎
Mu Xiang	Radix Aucklandiae	木香
Mu Zei	Herba Equiseti Hiemalis	木贼
Nan Chai Hu	Radix Bupleurum Scorzonerifolfium	南柴胡
Nan Gua Zi	Semen Cucurbitae Moschatae	南瓜子
Nan Sha Shen	Radix Adenophorae	南沙参
Nan Ting Li Zi	Semen Descurainiae	南葶苈子
Niao Bu Su	Ramus Kalopanax Pictus	鸟不宿
Niu Bang Gen	Radix Arctii	牛蒡根
Niu Bang Zi	Fructus Arctii	牛蒡子
Niu Dan	Fel Bovis	牛胆
Niu Huang	Calculus Bovis	牛黄
Niu Xi	Radix Cyathulae seu Achyranthis	牛膝
Nu Zhen Zi	Fructus Ligustri Lucidi	女贞子
Ou Jie	Nodus Nelumbinis Rhizomatis	藕节
Pang Da Hai	Semen Sterculiae Lychnophorae	胖大海
Pao Jiang	Rhizoma Zingiberis Preparatum	炮姜
Pao Zai Cao	Herba Physalis Angulatae	炮仔草
Pei Lan	Herba Eupatorii	佩兰
Peng Sha	Borax	硼砂
Pi Pa Ye	Folium Eriobotryae	枇杷叶
Po Bu Zi Ye	Folium Cordia Dichotoma	破布子叶
Po Xiao	Sal Glauberis	朴硝
Pu Gong Ying	Herba Taraxaci	蒲公英
Pu Huang	Pollen Typhae	蒲黄
Pu Yin	Radix Wikstroemia Indica	埔银
Qi Dai	Corda Umbilicalis Hominis	脐带
Qi She	Agkistrodon	蕲蛇
Qi Ye Lian	Radix Schefflerae	七叶莲
Qian Cao	Radix Rubiae	茜草
Qian Dan	Minium	铅丹
Qian Hu	Radix Peucedani	前胡
Qian Li Guang	Herba Senecionis Scandens	千里光
Qian Nian Jian	Rhizoma Homalomenae	千年健
Qian Niu Zi	Semen Pharbitidis	牵牛子
Qian Shi	Semen Euryales	芡实
Qiang Huo	Rhizoma et Radix Notopterygii	羌活
Qin Jiao	Radix Gentianae Macrophyllae	秦艽
Qin Pi	Cortex Fraxini	秦皮
Qing Dai	Indigo Naturalis	青黛
Qing Fen	Calomelas	轻粉
Qing Feng Teng	Caulis Sinomenii	青风藤
Qing Guo Gen	Radix Canarium Album	青果根
Qing Hao	Herba Artemisiae Annuae	青蒿

Pinyin Names	Pharmaceutical Names	Chinese Names
Qing Ma Zi	Semen Abutili	苘麻子
Qing Mu Xiang	Radix Aristolochiae	青木香
Qing Niu Jiao Fen	Cornus Bovis	青牛角粉
Qing Pi	Pericarpium Citri Reticulatae Viride	青皮
Qing Xiang Zi	Semen Celosiae	青葙子
Qu Mai	Herba Dianthi	瞿麦
Quan Xie	Scorpio	全蝎
Ren Dong Teng	Caulis Lonicerae	忍冬藤
Ren Gong Niu Huang	Calculus Bovis Syntheticum	人工牛黄
Ren Shen	Radix Ginseng	人参
Ren Shen Ye	Folium Ginseng	人参叶
Ren Zhong Bai	Urinae Hominis Sedimen	人中白
Rou Cong Rong	Herba Cistanches	肉苁蓉
Rou Dou Gen	Radix Myristicae	肉豆根
Rou Dou Kou	Semen Myristicae	肉豆蔻
Rou Gui	Cortex Cinnamomi	肉桂
Ru Xiang	Gummi Olibanum	乳香
Rui Ren	Semen Prinsepiae	蕤仁
San Leng	Rhizoma Sparganii	三棱
San Qi	Radix Notoginseng	三七
San Qi Ye	Folium Notoginseng	三七叶
San Ye Mu Tong	Caulis Trifoliata	三叶木通
Sang Bai Pi	Cortex Mori	桑白皮
Sang Ji Sheng	Herba Taxilli	桑寄生
Sang Piao Xiao	Ootheca Mantidis	桑螵蛸
Sang Shen Zi	Fructus Mori	桑椹子
Sang Ye	Folium Mori	桑叶
Sang Zhi	Ramulus Mori	桑枝
Sha Ren	Fructus Amomi	砂仁
Sha Ren Ke	Pericarpium Amomi	砂仁壳
Sha Shen	Radix Glehniae seu Adenophorae	沙参
Sha Yuan Zi	Semen Astragali Complanati	沙苑子
Shan Ci Gu	Pseudobulbus Cremastrae	山慈姑
Shan Dou Gen	Radix Sophorae Tonkinensis	山豆根
Shan Ma Ti	Radix Rauvolfiae Hainanensis	山马蹄
Shan Pu Tao	Radix Vitis Amurensis	山葡萄
Shan Yang Jiao	Cornu Naemorhedis	山羊角
Shan Yao	Rhizoma Dioscoreae	山药
Shan Zha	Fructus Crataegi	山楂
Shan Zhu Yu	Fructus Corni	山茱萸
Shang Lu	Radix Phytolaccae	商陆
She Chuang Zi	Fructus Cnidii	蛇床子
She Gan	Rhizoma Belamcandae	射干
She Tui	Periostracum Serpentis	蛇蜕
She Xiang	Moschus	麝香
Shen Jin Cao	Herba Lycopodii	伸筋草
Shen Qu	Massa Fermentata	神曲
Sheng Di Huang	Radix Rehmanniae	生地黄
Sheng Jiang	Rhizoma Zingiberis Recens	生姜
Sheng Jiang Pi	Pericarpium Zingiberis Recens	生姜皮
Sheng Ma	Rhizoma Cimicifugae	升麻
Sheng Tie Luo	Frusta Ferri	生铁落
Shi Chang Pu	Rhizoma Acori	石菖蒲
Shi Di	Calyx Kaki	柿蒂

Pinyin Names	Pharmaceutical Names	Chinese Names
Shi Gao	Gypsum Fibrosum	石膏
Shi Hu	Herba Dendrobii	石斛
Shi Jue Ming	Concha Haliotidis	石决明
Shi Jun Zi	Fructus Quisqualis	使君子
Shi Lian Zi	Herba Sinocrassulae Indicae	石莲子
Shi Liu Pi	Pericarpium Granati	石榴皮
Shi Luo	Fructus Anethum Graveolens	莳萝
Shi Nan Teng	Ramulus Piper	石南藤
Shi Wei	Folium Pyrrosiae	石韦
Shu Di Huang	Radix Rehmanniae Preparata	熟地黄
Shu Hua Sha Shen	Radix Adenophorae Remotiflora	疏花沙参
Shu Qi	Folium Dichroae	蜀漆
Shu Wei Huang	Herba Rostellulariae	鼠尾癀
Shuang Liu Huang	Herba Vernoniae Patulae	双柳黄
Shui Chang Pu	Rhizoma Acori Calami	水菖蒲
Shui Ding Xiang	Herba Ludwigiae Prostratae	水丁香
Shui Niu Jiao	Cornu Bubali	水牛角
Shui Zhi	Hirudo	水蛭
Si Chuan Da Jin Qian Cao	Herba Lysimachia Christinae	四川大金钱
Si Gua Luo	Retinervus Luffae Fructus	丝瓜络
Song Guo	Fructus Pini	松果
Song Jie	Lignum Pini Nodi	松节
Song Ye	Folium Pini	松叶
Su Geng	Caulis Perillae	苏梗
Su He Xiang	Styrax	苏合香
Su Mu	Lignum Sappan	苏木
Su Zi	Fructus Perillae	苏子
Suan Zao Ren	Semen Zizyphi Spinosae	酸枣仁
Suo Luo Zi	Semen Aesculi	娑罗子
Suo Yang	Herba Cynomorii	锁阳
Tai Zi Shen	Radix Pseudostellariae	太子参
Tan Xiang	Lignum Santali Albi	檀香
Tao Ren	Semen Persicae	桃仁
Tian Hua Fen	Radix Trichosanthis	天花粉
Tian Kui Zi	Radix Semiaquilegiae	天葵子
Tian Ma	Rhizoma Gastrodiae	天麻
Tian Men Dong	Radix Asparagi	天门冬
Tian Nan Xing	Rhizoma Arisaematis	天南星
Tian Xian Teng	Herba Aristolochiae	天仙藤
Tian Zhu Huang	Concretio Silicea Bambusae	天竺黄
Ting Li Zi	Semen Descurainiae seu Lepidii	葶苈子
Tong Cao	Medulla Tetrapanacis	通草
Tou Gu Cao	Caulis Impatientis	透骨草
Tu Bei Mu	Bulbus Bolbostemma Paniculatum	土贝母
Tu Fu Ling	Rhizoma Smilacis Glabrae	土茯苓
Tu Niu Xi	Radix Achyranthes Longifolia	土牛膝
Tu Rou Gui	Cortex Cinnamomum Burmannium	土肉桂
Tu Si Zi	Semen Cuscutae	菟丝子
Tu Xi Xin	Herba Asari Forbgesii	土细辛
Wa Leng Zi	Concha Arcae	瓦楞子
Wan Dian Jin	Radix Ilicis Asprellae	万点金
Wan Nian Song	Herba Selaginellae	万年松
Wang Bu Liu Xing	Semen Vaccariae	王不留行
Wei Ling Xian	Radix Clematidis	威灵仙

Pinyin Names	Pharmaceutical Names	Chinese Names
Wu Bei Zi	Galla Chinensis	五倍子
Wu Gong	Scolopendra	蜈蚣
Wu Jia Pi	Cortex Acanthopanacis	五加皮
Wu Ling Zhi	Excrementum Trogopteri seu Pteromi	五灵脂
Wu Long Cha	Folium Camellia Sinensis Fermentata	乌龙茶
Wu Mei	Fructus Mume	乌梅
Wu Ming Yi	Pyrolusitum	无名异
Wu Shao She	Zaocys	乌蛸蛇
Wu Teng	Ramulus Linderae	乌藤
Wu Tian	Radix et Folium Viticis Quinatae	乌甜
Wu Tou	Radix Aconiti	乌头
Wu Wei Zi	Fructus Schisandrae Chinensis	五味子
Wu Yao	Radix Linderae	乌药
Wu Ye Mu Tong	Caulis Quinata	五叶木通
Wu Yi	Fructus Ulmi Praeparatus	芜荑
Wu Zhu Yu	Fructus Evodiae	吴茱萸
Xi Gua	Frucutus Citrulli	西瓜
Xi Gua Cui Pi	Exocarpium Citrulli	西瓜翠皮
Xi Gua Pi	Pericarpium Citrulli	西瓜皮
Xi Jiao	Cornu Rhinoceri	犀角
Xi Xian Cao	Herba Siegesbeckiae	豨莶草
Xi Xin	Herba Asari	细辛
Xi Yang Shen	Radix Panacis Quinquefolii	西洋参
Xia Ku Cao	Spica Prunellae	夏枯草
Xia Ku Hua	Flos Prunellae	夏枯花
Xia Tian Wu	Rhizoma Corydalis Decumbentis	夏天无
Xian Di Huang	Radix Rehmanniae Recens	鲜地黄
Xian Feng Cao	Herba Bidentis	咸丰草
Xian He Cao	Herba Agrimoniae	仙鹤草
Xian Mao	Rhizoma Curculiginis	仙茅
Xiang Fu	Rhizoma Cyperi	香附
Xiang Ru	Herba Elsholtziae seu Moslae	香薷
Xiang Si Cao	Herba Eupatorii Formosani	相思草
Xiang Si Zi	Semen Abrus Precatoris	相思子
Xiang Yuan	Fructus Citri	香橼
Xiao Hui Xiang	Fructus Foeniculi	小茴香
Xiao Ji	Herba Cirisii	小蓟
Xiao Jin Ying	Fructus Rosae Cymosae	小金樱
Xiao Mai	Fructus Tritici	小麦
Xie Bai	Bulbus Allii Macrostemonis	薤白
Xie Cao	Radix et Rhizoma Valerianae	缬草
Xin Yi Hua	Flos Magnoliae	辛夷花
Xing Ren	Semen Armeniacae Amarum	杏仁
Xing Ren Shu Pi	Cortex Pruni Armeniacae	杏仁树皮
Xiong Dan	Fel Ursi	熊胆
Xiong Huang	Realgar	雄黄
Xu Chang Qing	Radix Cynanchi Paniculati	徐长卿
Xu Duan	Radix Dipsaci	续断
Xuan Fu Hua	Flos Inulae	旋覆花
Xuan Shen	Radix Scrophulariae	玄参
Xue Jie	Sanguis Draconis	血竭
Xue Yu Tan	Crinis Carbonisatus	血余炭
Xun Gu Feng	Herba Aristolochiae Mollissimae	寻骨风
Ya Dan Zi	Fructus Bruceae	鸦胆子

Pinyin Names	Pharmaceutical Names	Chinese Names
Ya She Huang	Herba Lippiae	鸭舌癀
Yan Hu Suo	Rhizoma Corydalis	延胡索
Yang Qi Shi	Actinolitum	阳起石
Ye Jiao Teng	Caulis Polygoni Multiflori	夜交藤
Ye Ju Hua	Flos Chrysanthemi Indici	野菊花
Ye Ming Sha	Excrementum Vespertilionis Murini	夜明砂
Ye Ying Pi	Pericarpium Prunus Pseudocerasus	野樱皮
Yi Mu Cao	Herba Leonuri	益母草
Yi Tang	Saccharum Granorum	饴糖
Yi Tiao Gen	Radix Moghaniae	一条根
Yi Wu Gen	Radix Elaeagni	宜梧根
Yi Yi Gen	Radix Coicis	薏苡根
Yi Yi Ren	Semen Coicis	薏苡仁
Yi Zhi Ren	Fructus Alpiniae Oxyphyllae	益智仁
Yi Zhi Xiang	Herba Vernoniae Cinereae	一枝香
Yin Chai Hu	Radix Stellariae	银柴胡
Yin Chen Hao	Herba Artemisiae Scopariae	茵陈蒿
Yin Guo Ye	Folium Ginkgo	银果叶
Yin Yang Huo	Herba Epimedii	淫羊藿
Ying Su Ke	Pericarpium Papaveris	罂粟壳
Yu Bai Fu	Rhizoma Typhonium Giganteum	禹白附
Yu Jin	Radix Curcumae	郁金
Yu Li Ren	Semen Pruni	郁李仁
Yu Mi Xu	Stigma Maydis	玉米须
Yu Xing Cao	Herba Houttuyniae	鱼腥草
Yu Yu Liang	Limonitum	禹余粮
Yu Zhu	Rhizoma Polygonati Odorati	玉竹
Yuan Hua	Flos Genkwa	芫花
Yuan Ming Fen	Matrii Sulfas Exsiccatus	元明粉
Yuan Zhi	Radix Polygalae	远志
Zao Jiao	Fructus Gleditsiae	皂角
Zao Jiao Ci	Spina Gleditsiae	皂角刺
Zao Xiu	Rhizoma Paridis	蚤休
Ze Lan	Herba Lycopi	泽兰
Ze Qi	Herba Euphorbiae Helioscopiae	泽漆
Ze Xie	Rhizoma Alismatis	泽泻
Zhang Hong Hua	Flos Crocus Sativus	藏红花
Zhang Nao	Camphora	樟脑
Zhe Bei Mu	Bulbus Fritillariae Thunbergii	浙贝母
Zhen Zhu	Margarita	珍珠
Zhen Zhu Mu	Concha Margaritaferae	珍珠母
Zhi Gan Cao	Radix Glycyrrhizae Preparata	炙甘草
Zhi Ju Zi	Fructus Hoveniae	枳椇子
Zhi Ke	Fructus Aurantii	枳壳
Zhi Mu	Radix Anemarrhenae	知母
Zhi Shi	Fructus Aurantii Immaturus	枳实
Zhi Zi	Fructus Gardeniae	栀子
Zhi Zi Pi	Pericarpium Gardeniae	栀子皮
Zhi Zi Ren	Semen Gardeniae	栀子仁
Zhong Ru Shi	Stalactitum	钟乳石
Zhu Dan	Fel Porcus	猪胆
Zhu Fan Hua Tou	Rhizoma Mirabilidis	煮饭花头
Zhu Gu	Os Porcus	猪骨
Zhu Li	Succus Bambusae	竹沥

Pinyin Names	Pharmaceutical Names	Chinese Names
Zhu Ling	Polyporus	猪苓
Zhu Ru	Caulis Bambusae in Taenia	竹茹
Zhu Sha	Cinnabaris	朱砂
Zhu Ye	Herba Phyllostachys	竹叶
Zhu Zi Cao	Herba Euphorbiae Thymifoliae	珠仔草
Zi Bei Tian Kui	Herba Semiaquilegiae	紫背天葵
Zi Cao Gen	Radix Lithospermi	紫草根
Zi He Che	Placenta Hominis	紫河车
Zi Hua Di Ding	Herba Violae	紫花地丁
Zi Ran Tong	Pyritum	自然铜
Zi Shi Ying	Fluoritum	紫石英
Zi Su Ye	Folium Perillae	紫苏叶
Zi Wan	Radix Asteris	紫菀
Zi Zhu	Folium Callicarpae	紫珠
Zong Lu Pi	Fibra Stipulae Trachycarpi	棕榈皮
Zong Lu Zi	Fructus Trachycarpi	棕榈子
Zou Ma Tai	Rhizoma Ardisiae	走马胎

Appendix 5 — Cross-reference of Herbal Formula Names

Pinyin Names	Translational Names	Chinese Names
Ai Fu Nuan Gong Wan	Mugwort and Prepared Aconite Pill for Warming the Womb	艾附暖宫丸
An Gong Niu Huang Wan	Calm the Palace Pill with Cattle Gallstone	安宫牛黄丸
An Zhong San	Calm the Middle Powder	安中散
Ba Wei Dai Xia Fang	Eight-Ingredient Formula for Leukorrhea	八味带下方
Ba Wei Di Huang Wan	Eight-Ingredient Pill with Rehmannia	八味地黄丸
Ba Zhen Tang	Eight-Treasure Decoction	八珍汤
Ba Zheng San	Eight-Herb Powder for Rectification	八正散
Bai He Gu Jin Tang	Lily Bulb Decoction to Preserve the Metal	百合固金汤
Bai Hu Jia Cang Zhu Tang	White Tiger plus Atractylodes Decoction	白虎加苍术汤
Bai Hu Jia Gui Zhi Tang	White Tiger plus Cinnamon Twig Decoction	白虎加桂枝汤
Bai Hu Jia Ren Shen Tang	White Tiger plus Ginseng Decoction	白虎加人参汤
Bai Hu Tang	White Tiger Decoction	白虎汤
Bai Tong Tang	White Penetrating Decoction	白通汤
Bai Tou Weng Jia Gan Cao E Jiao Tang	Pulsatilla Decoction plus Licorice and Ass-Hide Gelatin	白头翁加甘草阿胶汤
Bai Tou Weng Tang	Pulsatilla Decoction	白头翁汤
Ban Xia Bai Zhu Tian Ma Tang	Pinellia, Atractylodes Macrocephala, and Gastrodia Decoction	半夏白术天麻汤
Ban Xia Hou Po Tang	Pinellia and Magnolia Bark Decoction	半夏厚朴汤
Ban Xia Xie Xin Tang	Pinellia Decoction to Drain the Epigastrium	半夏泻心汤
Bao Chan Wu You Fang	Preserve Pregnancy and Care-Free Decoction	保产无忧方
Bao He Wan	Preserve Harmony Pill from the Precious Mirror	保和丸
Bao Yuan Tang	Preserve the Basal Decoction	保元汤
Bei Mu Gua Lou San	Fritillaria and Trichosanthes Fruit Powder	贝母瓜蒌散
Bei Xie Fen Qing Yin	Dioscorea Hypoglauca Decoction to Separate the Clear	萆薢分清饮
Bi Yu San	Jasper Powder	碧玉散
Bu Dai Wan	Cloth Sack Pill	布袋丸
Bu Fei E Jiao San	Tonify the Lung Decoction with Ass-Hide Gelatin	补肺阿胶散
Bu Fei Tang	Tonify the Lung Decoction	补肺汤
Bu Huan Jin Zheng Qi San	Rectify the Qi Powder Worth More than Gold	不换金正气散
Bu Yang Huan Wu Tang	Tonify the Yang to Restore Five Decoction	补阳还五汤
Bu Zhong Yi Qi Tang	Tonify the Middle and Augment the Qi Decoction	补中益气汤
Can Shi Tang	Silkworm Droppings Decoction	蚕矢汤
Cang Er San	Xanthium Powder	苍耳散
Cang Lin San	Old Rice Granary Powder	仓廪散
Chai Ge Jie Ji Tang	Bupleurum and Kudzu Decoction to Release the Muscle Layer	柴葛解肌汤
Chai Hu Gui Zhi Gan Jiang Tang	Bupleurum, Cinnamon Twig, and Ginger Decoction	柴胡桂枝乾姜汤
Chai Hu Gui Zhi Tang	Bupleurum and Cinnamon Twig Decoction	柴胡桂枝汤
Chai Hu Jia Long Mu Tang	Bupleurum plus Dragon Bone and Oyster Shell Decoction	柴胡加龙牡汤
Chai Hu Qing Gan Tang	Bupleurum Decoction to Clear the Liver	柴胡清肝汤
Chai Hu Shu Gan Tang	Bupleurum Powder to Spread the Liver	柴胡疏肝汤
Chai Hu Xian Xiong Tang	Bupleurum Decoction for Sinking into the Chest	柴胡陷胸汤
Chai Hu Zhi Jie Tang	Bupleurum, Bitter Orange, and Platycodon Decoction	柴胡枳桔汤
Chai Ling Tang	Bupleurum and Poria Decoction	柴苓汤
Chai Ping Tang	Bupleurum and Calm the Stomach Decoction	柴平汤
Chai Xian Tang	Bupleurum Decoction to Raise the Sunken	柴陷汤
Cheng Qi Yang Ying Tang	Order the Qi and Nourish the Nutritive Qi Decoction	承气养营汤
Cheng Shi Chai Ge Jie Ji Tang	Cheng's Bupleurum and Kudzu Decoction to Release the Muscle Layer	程氏柴葛解肌汤
Chi Shi Zhi Yu Liang Shi Tang	Halloysitum and Limonite Decoction	赤石脂禹余粮汤
Chuan Xiong Cha Tiao San	Ligusticum Chuanxiong Powder to be Taken with Green Tea	川芎茶调散
Ci Zhu Wan	Magnetite and Cinnabar Pills	磁朱丸
Cong Bai Qi Wei Yin	Scallion Decoction with Seven Ingredients	葱白七味饮

Pinyin Names	Translational Names	Chinese Names
Cong Chi Jie Geng Tang	Scallion, Prepared Soybean, and Platycodon Decoction	葱豉桔梗汤
Cong Chi Tang	Scallion and Prepared Soybean Decoction	葱豉汤
Da An Wan	Great Tranquility Pill	大安丸
Da Bu Yin Wan	Great Tonify the Yin Pill	大补阴丸
Da Chai Hu Tang	Major Bupleurum Decoction	大柴胡汤
Da Cheng Qi Tang	Major Order the Qi Decoction	大承气汤
Da Ding Feng Zhu	Major Arrest Wind Pearl	大定风珠
Da Fang Feng Tang	Major Saposhnikovia Decoction	大防风汤
Da Huang Fu Zi Tang	Rhubarb and Prepared Aconite Decoction	大黄附子汤
Da Huang Mu Dan Tang	Rhubarb and Moutan Decoction	大黄牡丹汤
Da Jian Zhong Tang	Major Construct the Middle Decoction	大建中汤
Da Qiang Huo Tang	Major Notopterygium Decoction	大羌活汤
Da Qin Jiao Tang	Major Gentiana Macrophylla Decoction	大秦艽汤
Da Qing Long Tang	Major Bluegreen Dragon Decoction	大青龙汤
Da Xian Xiong Tang	Major Sinking into the Chest Decoction	大陷胸汤
Da Xian Xiong Wan	Major Sinking into the Chest Pill	大陷胸丸
Dang Gui Bu Xue Tang	Tangkuei Decoction to Tonify the Blood	当归补血汤
Dang Gui Jian Zhong Tang	Tangkuei Decoction to Construct the Middle	当归建中汤
Dang Gui Liu Huang Tang	Tangkuei and Six-Yellow Decoction	当归六黄汤
Dang Gui Long Hui Wan	Tangkuei, Gentiana and Aloe Pills	当归龙荟丸
Dang Gui Nian Tong Tang	Tangkuei Decoction to Lift the Pain	当归拈痛汤
Dang Gui San	Tangkuei Powder	当归散
Dang Gui Shao Yao San	Tangkuei and Peony Powder	当归芍药散
Dang Gui Si Ni Jia Wu Zhu Yu Sheng Jiang Tang	Tangkuei Decoction for Frigid Extremities plus Evodia and Fresh Ginger	当归四逆加吴茱萸生姜汤
Dang Gui Si Ni Tang	Tangkuei Decoction for Frigid Extremities	当归四逆汤
Dang Gui Yin Zi	Tangkuei Decoction	当归饮子
Dao Chi San	Guide Out the Red Powder	导赤散
Dao Qi Tang	Conduct the Qi Decoction	导气汤
Dao Shui Fu Ling Tang	Poria Decoction to Drain Water	导水茯苓汤
Dao Tan Tang	Guide Out Phlegm Decoction	导痰汤
Di Huang Yin Zi	Rehmannia Decoction	地黄饮子
Di Tan Tang	Scour Phlegm Decoction	涤痰汤
Ding Chuan Tang	Arrest Wheezing Decoction	定喘汤
Ding Xian Wan	Arrest Seizures Pill	定痫丸
Ding Xiang Shi Di Tang	Clove and Persimmon Calyx Decoction	丁香柿蒂汤
Du Huo Ji Sheng Tang	Angelica Pubescens and Taxillus Decoction	独活寄生汤
Du Qi Wan	Capital Qi Pill	都气丸
Dun Sou San	Long-Bout Cough Powder	顿嗽散
E Jiao Ji Zi Huang Tang	Ass-Hide Gelatin and Egg Yolk Decoction	阿胶鸡子黄汤
Er Chen Tang	Two-Cured Decoction	二陈汤
Er Long Zuo Ci Wan	Pill for Deafness that Is Kind to the Left [Kidney]	耳聋左慈丸
Er Miao San	Two-Marvel Powder	二妙散
Er Xian Tang	Two-Immortal Decoction	二仙汤
Er Zhi Wan	Two-Ultimate Pill	二至丸
Er Zhu Tang	Two-Atractylodes Decoction	二术汤
Fang Feng Tong Sheng San	Saposhnikovia Powder that Sagely Unblocks	防风通圣散
Fang Ji Fu Ling Tang	Stephania and Poria Decoction	防己茯苓汤
Fang Ji Huang Qi Tang	Stephania and Astragalus Decoction	防己黄芪汤
Fen Xiao Tang	Separate and Reduce Decoction	分消汤
Fu Fang Da Cheng Qi Tang	Revised Major Order the Qi Decoction	复方大承气汤
Fu Ling Wan	Poria Pill	茯苓丸
Fu Ling Yin	Poria Decoction	茯苓饮
Fu Tu Dan	Poria and Cuscuta Special Pill	茯菟丹

Pinyin Names	Translational Names	Chinese Names
Fu Yuan Huo Xue Tang	Revive Health by Invigorating the Blood Decoction	复元活血汤
Fu Zi Li Zhong Wan	Prepared Aconite Pill to Regulate the Middle	附子理中丸
Fu Zi Tang	Prepared Aconite Decoction	附子汤
Gan Cao Gan Jiang Fu Ling Bai Zhu Tang	Licorice, Ginger, Poria and Atractylodes Macrocephala Decoction	甘草干姜茯苓白术汤
Gan Cao Xie Xin Tang	Licorice Decoction to Drain the Epigastrium	甘草泻心汤
Gan Jiang Ren Shen Ban Xia Wan	Ginger, Ginseng, and Pinellia Pills	干姜人参半夏丸
Gan Lu Xiao Du Dan	Sweet Dew Special Pill to Eliminate Toxin	甘露消毒丹
Gan Lu Yin	Sweet Dew Decoction	甘露饮
Gan Mai Da Zao Tang	Licorice, Wheat, and Jujube Decoction	甘麦大枣汤
Ge Gen Huang Qin Huang Lian Tang	Kudzu, Coptis, and Scutellaria Decoction	葛根黄芩黄连汤
Ge Gen Tang	Kudzu Decoction	葛根汤
Ge Hua Jie Cheng San	Pueraria Flower Powder for Detoxification and Awakening	葛花解酲散
Ge Xia Zhu Yu Tang	Drive Out Blood Stasis Below the Diaphragm Decoction	膈下逐瘀汤
Gou Teng San	Uncaria Powder	钩藤散
Gou Teng Yin	Uncaria Decoction	钩藤饮
Gu Chong Tang	Stabilize Gushing Decoction	固冲汤
Gu Jing Wan	Stabilize the Menses Pill	固经丸
Gua Di San	Melon Pedicle Powder	瓜蒂散
Gua Lou Xie Bai Bai Jiu Tang	Trichosanthes Fruit, Chinese Chive, and Wine Decoction	瓜蒌薤白白酒汤
Gua Lou Xie Bai Ban Xia Tang	Trichosanthes Fruit, Chinese Chive, and Pinellia Decoction	瓜蒌薤白半夏汤
Gua Lou Zhi Shi Tang	Trichosanthes Fruit and Immature Bitter Orange Decoction	瓜蒌枳实汤
Guan Xin Su He Wan	Coronary Styrax Pills	冠心苏合丸
Gui Ling Gan Lu Yin	Cinnamon and Poria Sweet Dew Decoction	桂苓甘露饮
Gui Lu Er Xian Jiao	Tortoise Shell and Deer Antler Syrup	龟鹿二仙胶
Gui Pi Tang	Restore the Spleen Decoction	归脾汤
Gui Qi Jian Zhong Tang	Tangkuei and Astragalus Decoction to Construct the Middle	归芪建中汤
Gui Zhi Fu Ling Wan	Cinnamon Twig and Poria Pills	桂枝茯苓丸
Gui Zhi Jia Ge Gen Tang	Cinnamon Twig Decoction plus Kudzu	桂枝加葛根汤
Gui Zhi Jia Hou Po Xing Zi Tang	Cinnamon Twig Decoction plus Magnolia Bark and Apricot Kernel	桂枝加厚朴杏子汤
Gui Zhi Jia Long Mu Tang	Cinnamon Twig Decoction plus Dragon Bone and Oyster Shell	桂枝加龙牡汤
Gui Zhi Jia Shao Yao Tang	Cinnamon Twig Decoction plus Peony	桂枝加芍药汤
Gui Zhi Ma Huang Ge Ban Tang	Combined Cinnamon Twig and Ephedra Decoction	桂枝麻黄各半汤
Gui Zhi Ren Shen Tang	Cinnamon Twig and Ginseng Decoction	桂枝人参汤
Gui Zhi Shao Yao Zhi Mu Tang	Cinnamon Twig, Peony, and Anemarrhena Decoction	桂枝芍药知母汤
Gui Zhi Tang	Cinnamon Twig Decoction	桂枝汤
Gun Tan Wan	Vaporize Phlegm Pill	滚痰丸
Guo Qi Yin	Delayed Menstruation Decoction	过期饮
Hai Zao Yu Hu Tang	Sargassum Decoction for the Jade Flask	海藻玉壶汤
Hao Qin Qing Dan Tang	Artemisia Annua and Scutellaria Decoction to Clear the Gallbladder	蒿芩清胆汤
Hei Xiao Yao San	Black Rambling Powder	黑逍遥散
Hou Po Qi Wu Tang	Seven-Substance Decoction with Magnolia Bark	厚朴七物汤
Hou Po Wen Zhong Tang	Magnolia Bark Decoction for Warming the Middle	厚朴温中汤
Hu Qian Wan	Hidden Tiger Pill from the Analytic Collection	虎潜丸
Hua Chong Wan	Dissolve Parasites Pills	化虫丸
Hua Gai San	Canopy Powder	华盖散
Huai Hua San	Sophora Japonica Flower Powder	槐花散
Huai Jiao Wan	Sophora Japonica Fruit Pills	槐角丸
Huan Shao Dan	Return to Youth Pills	还少丹
Huang Lian Jie Du Tang	Coptis Decoction to Relieve Toxicity	黄连解毒汤
Huang Lian Shang Qing Wan	Coptis Pills to Clear the Upper	黄连上清丸
Huang Lian Tang	Coptis Decoction	黄连汤

Pinyin Names	Translational Names	Chinese Names
Huang Long Tang	Yellow Dragon Decoction	黄龙汤
Huang Qi Jian Zhong Tang	Astragalus Decoction to Construct the Middle	黄芪建中汤
Huang Qi Wu Wu Tang	Astragalus Five Decoction	黄芪五物汤
Huang Qin Hua Shi Tang	Scutellaria and Talcum Decoction	黄芩滑石汤
Huang Qin Tang	Scutellaria Decoction	黄芩汤
Huang Tu Tang	Yellow Earth Decoction	黄土汤
Hui Yang Jiu Ji Tang	Restore and Revive the Yang Decoction	回阳救急汤
Huo Luo Xiao Ling Dan	Fantastically Effective Pill to Invigorate the Collaterals	活络效灵丹
Huo Po Xia Ling Tang	Agastache, Magnolia Bark, Pinellia and Poria Decoction	藿朴夏苓汤
Huo Ren Cong Chi Tang	Scallion and Prepared Soybean Decoction from the Book to Safeguard Life	活人葱豉汤
Huo Xiang Zheng Qi San	Agastache Powder to Rectify the Qi	藿香正气散
Ji Chuan Jian	Benefit the River [Flow] Decoction	济川煎
Ji Ming San	Powder to Take at Cock's Crow	鸡鸣散
Ji Sheng Shen Qi Wan	Kidney Qi Pill from Formulas that Aid the Living	济生肾气丸
Ji Su San	Peppermint Powder	鸡苏散
Jia Jian Fu Mai Tang	Modified Restore the Pulse Decoction	加减复脉汤
Jia Jian Wei Rui Tang	Modified Polygonatum Odoratum Decoction	加减葳蕤汤
Jia Wei Ba Zheng San	Modified Eight Herb Powder for Rectification	加味八正散
Jia Wei Ping Wei San	Modified Calm the Stomach Powder	加味平胃散
Jia Wei Shen Qi Wan	Modified Kidney Qi Pill	加味肾气丸
Jia Wei Xiang Su San	Augmented Cyperus and Perilla Leaf Powder	加味香苏散
Jia Wei Xiao Yao San	Augmented Rambling Powder	加味逍遥散
Jian Ling Tang	Construct Roof Tiles Decoction	建瓴汤
Jian Pi Wan	Strengthen the Spleen Pills	健脾丸
Jiao Ai Tang	Ass-Hide Gelatin and Mugwort Decoction	胶艾汤
Jie Geng Tang	Platycodon Decoction	桔梗汤
Jin Fei Cao San	Inula Powder	金沸草散
Jin Gui Shen Qi Wan	Kidney Qi Pill from the Golden Cabinet	金匮肾气丸
Jin Jian Fei Er Wan	Golden Pill to Construct a Fat Child	金鉴肥儿丸
Jin Ling Zi San	Melia Toosendan Powder	金铃子散
Jin Suo Gu Jing Wan	Metal Lock Pill to Stabilize the Essence	金锁固精丸
Jing Fang Bai Du San	Schizonepeta and Saposhnikovia Powder to Overcome Pathogenic Influences	荆防败毒散
Jing Jie Lian Qiao Tang	Schizonepeta and Forsythia Decoction	荆芥连翘汤
Jiu Wei Bing Lang Jia Wu Fu Tang	Areca Nine Decoction plus Evodia and Poria	九味槟榔加吴茯汤
Jiu Wei Qiang Huo Tang	Nine-Herb Decoction with Notopterygium	九味羌活汤
Jiu Xian San	Nine-Immortal Powder	九仙散
Ju Ban Zhi Zhu Wan	Tangerine Peel, Pinellia, Immature Bitter Orange and Atractylodes Macrocephala Pill	橘半枳术丸
Ju He Wan	Tangerine Seed Pill	橘核丸
Ju Hua Cha Tiao San	Chrysanthemum Powder to be Taken with Green Tea	菊花茶调散
Ju Pi Zhu Ru Tang	Tangerine Peel and Bamboo Shaving Decoction	橘皮竹茹汤
Ju Yuan Jian	Lift the Source Decoction	举元煎
Juan Bi Tang	Remove Painful Obstruction Decoction	蠲痹汤
Ke Xue Fang	Coughing of Blood Formula	咳血方
Kong Xian Dan	Control Mucus Special Pill	控涎丹
Li Zhong An Hui Tang	Regulate the Middle and Calm Roundworm Decoction	理中安蛔汤
Li Zhong Hua Tan Wan	Regulate the Middle and Transform Phlegm Pills	理中化痰丸
Li Zhong Tang	Regulate the Middle Decoction	理中汤
Li Zhong Wan	Regulate the Middle Pills	理中丸
Lian Mei An Hui Tang	Picrorhiza and Mume Decoction to Calm Roundworm	连梅安蛔汤
Lian Po Yin	Coptis and Magnolia Bark Decoction	连朴饮
Lian Qiao Bai Du San	Forsythia Powder to Overcome Pathogenic Influences	连翘败毒散

Pinyin Names	Translational Names	Chinese Names
Liang Fu Wan	Galangal and Cyperus Pill	良附丸
Liang Ge San	Cool the Diaphragm Powder	凉膈散
Ling Gan Jiang Wei Xin Xia Ren Tang	Poria, Licorice, Ginger, Schisandra, Asarum, Pinellia and Apricot Seed Decoction	苓甘姜味辛夏仁汤
Ling Gan Wu Wei Jiang Xin Tang	Poria, Licorice, Schisandra, Ginger, and Asarum Decoction	苓甘五味姜辛汤
Ling Gui Zhu Gan Tang	Poria, Cinnamon Twig, Atractylodes Macrocephala, and Licorice Decoction	苓桂术甘汤
Ling Jiao Gou Teng Tang	Antelope Horn and Uncaria Decoction	羚角钩藤汤
Liu He Tang	Harmonize the Six Decoction	六和汤
Liu Jun Zi Tang	Six-Gentlemen Decoction	六君子汤
Liu Wei Di Huang Wan	Six-Ingredient Pill with Rehmannia	六味地黄丸
Liu Wei Gu Jing Wan	Rehmannia Six and Lotus Stamen Pills	六味固精丸
Liu Yi San	Six-to-One Powder	六一散
Long Dan Xie Gan Tang	Gentiana Decoction to Drain the Liver	龙胆泻肝汤
Ma Huang Fu Zi Gan Cao Tang	Ephedra, Prepared Aconite, and Licorice Decoction	麻黄附子甘草汤
Ma Huang Fu Zi Xi Xin Tang	Ephedra, Asarum, and Prepared Aconite Decoction	麻黄附子细辛汤
Ma Huang Jia Zhu Tang	Ephedra Decoction plus Atractylodes	麻黄加术汤
Ma Huang Tang	Ephedra Decoction	麻黄汤
Ma Xing Gan Shi Tang	Ephedra, Apricot Kernel, Licorice, and Gypsum Decoction	麻杏甘石汤
Ma Xing Yi Gan Tang	Ephedra, Apricot Kernel, Coicis, and Licorice Decoction	麻杏薏甘汤
Ma Zi Ren Wan	Hemp Seed Pill	麻子仁丸
Mai Men Dong Tang	Ophiopogonis Decoction	麦门冬汤
Mai Wei Di Huang Wan	Ophiopogonis, Schisandra and Rehmannia Pills	麦味地黄丸
Ming Mu Di Huang Wan	Improve Vision Pill with Rehmannia	明目地黄丸
Mu Fang Ji Tang	Cocculus Decoction	木防己汤
Mu Li San	Oyster Shell Powder	牡蛎散
Mu Xiang Bing Lang Wan	Aucklandia and Betel Nut Pills	木香槟榔丸
Nei Bu Huang Qi Tang	Tonify the Interior Decoction with Astragalus	内补黄芪汤
Ning Sou Wan	Quiet the Cough Pills	宁嗽丸
Niu Bang Jie Ji Tang	Arctium Decoction to Release the Muscle Layer	牛蒡解肌汤
Niu Huang Qing Xin Dan	Cattle Gallstone Pill to Clear the Heart	牛黄清心丸
Nu Ke Bai Zi Ren Wan	Platycladus Seed Pills for Females	女科柏子仁丸
Nuan Gan Jian	Warm the Liver Decoction	暖肝煎
Pai Nong San	Drain the Pus Powder	排脓散
Ping Wei San	Calm the Stomach Powder	平胃散
Pu Ji Xiao Du Yin	Universal Benefit Decoction to Eliminate Toxin	普济消毒饮
Qi Bao Mei Ran Wan	Seven-Treasure Special Pill for Beautiful Whiskers	七宝美髯丸
Qi Ju Di Huang Wan	Lycium Fruit, Chrysanthemum, and Rehmannia Pills	杞菊地黄丸
Qi Li San	Seven-Thousandths of a Tael Powder	七厘散
Qi Pi Wan	Guide the Spleen Pills	启脾丸
Qi Wei Bai Zhu San	Seven-Ingredient Powder with Atractylodes Macrocephala	七味白术散
Qian Jin Nei Tuo San	Drain-the-Interior Powder Worthy of a Thousand Gold	千金内托散
Qian Zheng San	Lead to Symmetry Powder	牵正散
Qiang Huo Sheng Shi Tang	Notopterygium Decoction to Overcome Dampness	羌活胜湿汤
Qin Jiao Bie Jia San	Gentiana Macrophylla and Soft-shelled Turtle Shell Powder	秦艽鳖甲散
Qing Bi Tang	Clear the Nose Decoction	清鼻汤
Qing Dai Tang	Clear Discharge Decoction	清带汤
Qing Fei Tang	Clear the Lung Decoction	清肺汤
Qing Fei Yin	Clear the Lung Drink	清肺饮
Qing Gu San	Cool the Bones Powder	清骨散
Qing Hao Bie Jia Tang	Artemisia Annua and Soft-shelled Turtle Shell Decoction	青蒿鳖甲汤
Qing Liang Yin	Clearing and Cooling Decoction	清凉饮
Qing Luo Yin	Clear the Collaterals Decoction	清络饮
Qing Qi Hua Tan Wan	Clear the Qi and Transform Phlegm Pill	清气化痰丸

Pinyin Names	Translational Names	Chinese Names
Qing Shang Fang Feng Tang	Clear the Upper and Guard the Wind Decoction	清上防风汤
Qing Shu Yi Qi Tang	Clear Summerheat and Augment the Qi Decoction	清暑益气汤
Qing Wei San	Clear the Stomach Powder	清胃散
Qing Wen Bai Du Yin	Clear Epidemics and Overcome Toxin Decoction	清瘟败毒饮
Qing Xin Li Ge Tang	Clear the Epigastrium and Benefit the Diaphragm Decoction	清心利膈汤
Qing Xin Lian Zi Yin	Lotus Seed Decoction to Clear the Heart	清心莲子饮
Qing Ying Tang	Clear the Nutrition Level Decoction	清营汤
Qing Zao Jiu Fei Tang	Eliminate Dryness and Rescue the Lung Decoction	清燥救肺汤
Qiong Yu Gao	Beautiful Jade Paste	琼玉膏
Qu Mai Zhi Zhu Wan	Medicated Leaven, Barley Sprout, Immature Bitter Orange, and Atractylodes Macrocephala Pill	曲糵枳术丸
Ren Shen Bai Du San	Ginseng Powder to Overcome Pathogenic Influences	人参败毒散
Ren Shen Dang Shao San	Ginseng, Tangkuei and Poria Powder	人参当芍散
Ren Shen Ge Jie San	Ginseng and Gecko Powder	人参蛤蚧散
Ren Shen Hu Tao Tang	Ginseng and Walnut Decoction	人参胡桃汤
Ren Shen Xie Fei Tang	Ginseng Decoction to Sedate the Lung	人参泻肺汤
Ren Shen Yang Ying Tang	Ginseng Decoction to Nourish the Nutritive Qi	人参养荣汤
Run Chang Wan	Moisten the Intestines Pill	润肠丸
San Ao Tang	Three-Unbinding Decoction	三拗汤
San Bi Tang	Three-Painful Obstruction Decoction	三痹汤
San Ceng Hui Xiang Wan	Fennel Seed Pill with Three Levels	三层茴香丸
San Huang Shi Gao Tang	Three-Yellow and Gypsum Decoction	三黄石膏汤
San Huang Xie Xin Tang	Three-Yellow Decoction to Sedate the Epigastrium	三黄泻心汤
San Miao San	Three-Marvel Powder	三妙散
San Miao Wan	Three-Marvel Pill	三妙丸
San Ren Tang	Three-Nut Decoction	三仁汤
San Sheng San	Three-Sage Powder	三圣散
San Wu Bei Ji Wan	Three-Substance Pill for Emergencies	三物备急丸
San Wu Xiang Ru Yin	Elsholtzia Three Decoction	三物香薷饮
San Zhong Kui Jian Tang	Disperse the Swelling and Break the Hardness Decoction	散肿溃坚汤
San Zi Yang Qin Tang	Three-Seed Decoction to Nourish One's Parents	三子养亲汤
Sang Ju Yin	Mulberry Leaf and Chrysanthemum Decoction	桑菊饮
Sang Ma Wan	Mulberry Leaf and Sesame Seed Pills	桑麻丸
Sang Piao Xiao San	Mantis Egg-Case Powder	桑螵蛸散
Sang Xing Tang	Mulberry Leaf and Apricot Kernel Decoction	桑杏汤
Sha Shen Mai Dong Tang	Glehnia and Ophiopogonis Decoction	沙参麦冬汤
Shang Zhong Xia Tong Yong Tong Feng Wan	Upper, Middle and Lower General Use Pills for Wind-Pain	上中下通用痛风丸
Shao Fu Zhu Yu Tang	Drive Out Blood Stasis in the Lower Abdomen Decoction	少腹逐瘀汤
Shao Yao Gan Cao Tang	Peony and Licorice Decoction	芍药甘草汤
Shao Yao Tang	Peony Decoction	芍药汤
She Gan Ma Huang Tang	Belamcanda and Ephedra Decoction	射干麻黄汤
Shen Fu Tang	Ginseng and Prepared Aconite Decoction	参附汤
Shen Ling Bai Zhu San	Ginseng, Poria, and Atractylodes Macrocephala Powder	参苓白术散
Shen Mi Tang	Mysterious Decoction	神秘汤
Shen Su Yin	Ginseng and Perilla Leaf Decoction	参苏饮
Shen Tong Zhu Yu Tang	Drive Out Blood Stasis from a Painful Body Decoction	身痛逐瘀汤
Shen Zhuo Tang	Kidney Fixity Decoction	肾著汤
Sheng Hua Tang	Generation and Transformation Decoction	生化汤
Sheng Jiang Xie Xin Tang	Fresh Ginger Decoction to Drain the Epigastrium	生姜泻心汤
Sheng Ma Ge Gen Tang	Cimicifuga and Kudzu Decoction	升麻葛根汤
Sheng Mai San	Generate the Pulse Powder	生脉散
Sheng Xian Tang	Raise the Sinking Decoction	升陷汤
Sheng Yang San Huo Tang	Raise the Yang and Disperse the Fire Decoction	升阳散火汤
Sheng Yu Tang	Sage-like Healing Decoction	圣愈汤

Pinyin Names	Translational Names	Chinese Names
Shi Bu Wan	Ten-Tonic Pills	十补丸
Shi Di Tang	Persimmon Calyx Decoction	柿蒂汤
Shi Gao Tang	Gypsum Decoction	石膏汤
Shi Hu Ye Guang Wan	Dendrobium Pill for Night Vision	石斛夜光丸
Shi Hui San	Ten Partially-charred Substances Powder	十灰散
Shi Liu Wei Liu Qi Yin	Sixteen-Ingredient Decoction to Flow Qi	十六味流气饮
Shi Pi San	Bolster the Spleen Powder	实脾散
Shi Quan Da Bu Tang	All-Inclusive Great Tonifying Decoction	十全大补汤
Shi Shen Tang	Ten-Immortal Decoction	十神汤
Shi Wei Bai Du Tang	Ten-Ingredient Decoction to Defeat Toxin	十味败毒汤
Shi Wei Wen Dan Tang	Ten-Ingredient Decoction to Warm the Gallbladder	十味温胆汤
Shi Wei Xiang Ru Yin	Ten-Ingredient Decoction with Elsholtzia	十味香薷饮
Shi Xiao San	Sudden Smile Powder	失笑散
Shi Zao Tang	Ten-Jujube Decoction	十枣汤
Shou Nian San	Pinch Powder	手拈散
Shu Gan Tang	Spread the Liver Decoction	疏肝汤
Shu Jin Li An San	Relax the Tendons and Instill Peace Powder	疏筋立安散
Shu Jing Huo Xue Tang	Relax the Channels and Invigorate the Blood Decoction	疏经活血汤
Shuang Jie Tong Sheng San	Double Relieve Powder that Sagely Unblocks	双解通圣散
Shui Lu Er Xian Dan	Water and Earth Immortals Special Pill	水陆二仙丹
Si Jun Zi Tang	Four-Gentlemen Decoction	四君子汤
Si Ling San	Four-Ingredient Powder with Poria	四苓散
Si Miao San	Four-Marvel Powder	四妙散
Si Miao Wan	Four-Marvel Pill	四妙丸
Si Miao Yong An Tang	Four-Valiant Decoction for Well-being	四妙勇安汤
Si Mo Tang	Four Milled-Herbs Decoction	四磨汤
Si Ni Jia Ren Shen Tang	Frigid Extremities Decoction plus Ginseng	四逆加人参汤
Si Ni San	Frigid Extremities Powder	四逆散
Si Ni Tang	Frigid Extremities Decoction	四逆汤
Si Shen Wan	Four-Miracle Pill	四神丸
Si Sheng Wan	Four-Fresh Pill	四生丸
Si Wu Tang	Four-Substance Decoction	四物汤
Si Wu Xiao Feng Yin	Eliminate Wind Decoction with the Four Substances	四物消风饮
Su He Xiang Wan	Liquid Styrax Pill	苏合香丸
Su Zao Yin Zi	Spread and Unblock Decoction	疏凿饮子
Su Zi Jiang Qi Tang	Perilla Fruit Decoction for Directing Qi Downward	苏子降气汤
Suan Zao Ren Tang	Sour Jujube Decoction	酸枣仁汤
Suo Quan Wan	Shut the Sluice Pill	缩泉丸
Tai Shan Pan Shi San	Powder that Gives the Stability of Mount Tai	泰山磐石散
Tao Hong Si Wu Tang	Four-Substance Decoction with Safflower and Peach Pit	桃红四物汤
Tao Hua Tang	Peach Blossom Decoction	桃花汤
Tao Ren Cheng Qi Tang	Peach Pit Decoction to Order the Qi	桃仁承气汤
Tian Ma Gou Teng Yin	Gastrodia and Uncaria Decoction	天麻钩藤饮
Tian Tai Wu Yao San	Top-Quality Lindera Powder	天台乌药散
Tian Wang Bu Xin Dan	Emperor of Heaven's Special Pill to Tonify the Heart	天王补心丹
Tiao Wei Cheng Qi Tang	Regulate the Stomach and Order the Qi Decoction	调胃承气汤
Ting Li Da Zao Xie Fei Tang	Descurainia and Jujube Decoction to Drain the Lung	葶苈大枣泻肺汤
Tong Mai Si Ni Tang	Unblock the Pulse Decoction for Frigid Extremities	通脉四逆汤
Tong Qiao Huo Xue Tang	Unblock the Orifices and Invigorate the Blood Decoction	通窍活血汤
Tong Xie Yao Fang	Important Formula for Painful Diarrhea	痛泻要方
Tou Nong San	Discharge Pus Powder	透脓散
Tuo Li Xiao Du Yin	Drain the Interior and Detoxify Decoction	托里消毒饮
Wan Dai Tang	End Discharge Decoction	完带汤
Wei Jing Tang	Reed Decoction	苇茎汤

Pinyin Names	Translational Names	Chinese Names
Wei Ling Tang	Calm the Stomach and Poria Decoction	胃苓汤
Wei Rui Tang	Polygonatum Odoratum Decoction	葳蕤汤
Wen Dan Tang	Warm the Gallbladder Decoction	温胆汤
Wen Jing Tang	Warm the Menses Decoction	温经汤
Wen Pi Tang	Warm the Spleen Decoction	温脾汤
Wen Qing Yin	Warming and Clearing Decoction	温清饮
Wu Hu Zhui Feng San	Five-Tiger Powder to Pursue Wind	五虎追风散
Wu Ji San	Five-Accumulation Powder	五积散
Wu Ji Wan	Wu Ji Pill	戊己丸
Wu Lin San	Five-Ingredient Powder for Painful Urinary Dysfunction	五淋散
Wu Ling San	Five-Ingredient Powder with Poria	五苓散
Wu Mei Wan	Mume Pills	乌梅丸
Wu Mo Yin Zi	Five Milled-Herbs Decoction	五磨饮子
Wu Pi Yin	Five-Peel Decoction	五皮饮
Wu Ren Wan	Five-Seed Pills	五仁丸
Wu Wei Xiao Du Yin	Five-Ingredient Decoction to Eliminate Toxins	五味消毒饮
Wu Yao Shun Qi San	Lindera Powder to Smooth the Flow of Qi	乌药顺气散
Wu Zhu Yu Tang	Evodia Decoction	吴茱萸汤
Xi Gan Ming Mu San	Wash the Liver and Brighten the Eyes Powder	洗肝明目散
Xi Jiao Di Huang Tang	Rhinoceros Horn and Rehmannia Decoction	犀角地黄汤
Xian Fang Huo Ming Yin	Sublime Formula for Sustaining Life	仙方活命饮
Xiang Lian Wan	Aucklandia and Coptis Pills	香连丸
Xiang Ru San	Elsholtzia Powder	香薷散
Xiang Ru Yin	Elsholtzia Decoction	香薷饮
Xiang Sha Liu Jun Zi Tang	Six-Gentlemen Decoction with Aucklandia and Amomum	香砂六君子汤
Xiang Sha Ping Wei San	Cyperus and Amomum Powder to Calm the Stomach	香砂平胃散
Xiang Sha Yang Wei Tang	Nourish the Stomach Decoction with Aucklandia and Amomum	香砂养胃汤
Xiang Sha Zhi Zhu Wan	Aucklandia, Amomum, Immature Bitter Orange, and Atractylodes Macrocephala Pills	香砂枳术丸
Xiang Sheng Po Di San	Loud Sound Resembling Broken Bamboo Powder	响声破笛散
Xiang Su Cong Chi Tang	Cyperus, Perilla Leaf, Scallion, and Prepared Soybean Decoction	香苏葱豉汤
Xiang Su San	Cyperus and Perilla Leaf Powder	香苏散
Xiao Ban Xia Jia Fu Ling Tang	Minor Pinellia and Poria Decoction	小半夏加茯苓汤
Xiao Chai Hu Tang	Minor Bupleurum Decoction	小柴胡汤
Xiao Cheng Qi Tang	Minor Order the Qi Decoction	小承气汤
Xiao Er Hui Chun Dan	Return of Spring Special Pill (Pediatric)	小儿回春丹
Xiao Feng San	Eliminate Wind Powder	消风散
Xiao Huo Luo Dan	Minor Invigorate the Collaterals Special Pill	小活络丹
Xiao Ji Yin Zi	Cephalanoplos Decoction	小蓟饮子
Xiao Jian Zhong Tang	Minor Construct the Middle Decoction	小建中汤
Xiao Luo Wan	Reduce Scrofula Pill	消瘰丸
Xiao Qing Long Jia Shi Gao Tang	Minor Bluegreen Dragon Decoction plus Gypsum	小青龙加石膏汤
Xiao Qing Long Tang	Minor Bluegreen Dragon Decoction	小青龙汤
Xiao Xian Xiong Tang	Minor Sinking into the Chest Decoction	小陷胸汤
Xiao Xu Ming Tang	Minor Prolong-Life Decoction	小续命汤
Xiao Yao San	Rambling Powder	逍遥散
Xie Bai San	Drain the White Powder	泻白散
Xie Huang San	Drain the Yellow Powder	泻黄散
Xie Qing Wan	Drain the Green Pill	泻青丸
Xie Xin Tang	Drain the Epigastrium Decoction	泻心汤
Xin Jia Huang Long Tang	Newly-Augmented Yellow Dragon Decoction	新加黄龙汤
Xin Jia Xiang Ru Yin	Newly-Augmented Elsholtzia Decoction	新加香薷饮
Xin Yi Qing Fei Yin	Magnolia Decoction to Clear the Lung	辛夷清肺饮
Xin Yi San	Magnolia Flower Powder	辛夷散

Pinyin Names	Translational Names	Chinese Names
Xin Zhi Ju Pi Zhu Ru Tang	Newly-Formulated Tangerine Peel and Bamboo Shaving Decoction	新制橘皮竹茹汤
Xing Su San	Apricot Kernel and Perilla Leaf Powder	杏苏散
Xing Su Yin	Apricot and Perilla Decoction	杏苏饮
Xing Su Yin (Pediatric)	Apricot and Perilla Decoction (Pediatrics)	杏苏饮(幼科)
Xiong Gui Jiao Ai Tang	Cnidium, Tangkuei, Gelatin and Artemisia Decoction	芎归胶艾汤
Xiong Gui Tiao Xue Yin	Cnidium and Tangkuei Decoction to Regulate Blood	芎归调血饮
Xu Ming Tang	Prolong Life Decoction	续命汤
Xuan Fu Dai Zhe Shi Tang	Inula and Hematite Decoction	旋覆代赭石汤
Xue Fu Zhu Yu Tang	Drive Out Stasis in the Mansion of Blood Decoction	血府逐瘀汤
Yan Hu Suo San	Corydalis Powder	延胡索散
Yan Tang Tan Tu Fang	Salt Decoction to Induce Vomiting	盐汤探吐方
Yang He Tang	Yang-Heartening Decoction	阳和汤
Yang Xin Tang	Nourish the Heart Decoction	养心汤
Yang Yin Qing Fei Tang	Nourish the Yin and Clear the Lung Decoction	养阴清肺汤
Yi Gan San	Restrain the Liver Powder	抑肝散
Yi Gong San	Extraordinary Merit Powder	异功散
Yi Guan Jian	Linking Decoction	一贯煎
Yi Huang Tang	Benefit the Yellow [Discharge] Decoction	易黄汤
Yi Qi Cong Ming Tang	Augment the Qi and Increase Acuity Decoction	益气聪明汤
Yi Yi Fu Zi Bai Jiang San	Coicis, Prepared Aconite, and Patrinia Powder	薏苡附子败酱散
Yi Yi Ren Tang	Coicis Decoction	薏苡仁汤
Yi Yuan San	Benefit the Basal Powder	益元散
Yi Zi Tang	Yi Word Decoction	乙字汤
Yin Chen Hao Tang	Artemisia Scoparia Decoction	茵陈蒿汤
Yin Chen Si Ni Tang	Artemisia Scoparia Decoction for Frigid Extremities	茵陈四逆汤
Yin Chen Wu Ling San	Artemisia Scoparia and Five-Ingredient Powder with Poria	茵陈五苓散
Yin Hua Jie Du Tang	Honeysuckle Decoction to Relieve Toxicity	银花解毒汤
Yin Qiao San	Honeysuckle and Forsythia Powder	银翘散
Yin Qiao Tang	Honeysuckle and Forsythia Decoction	银翘汤
You Gui Wan	Restore the Right [Kidney] Pill	右归丸
You Gui Yin	Restore the Right [Kidney] Decoction	右归饮
Yu Nü Jian	Jade Woman Decoction	玉女煎
Yu Ping Feng San	Jade Windscreen Powder	玉屏风散
Yu Quan Wan	Jade Spring Pills	玉泉丸
Yu Ye Tang	Jade Fluid Decoction	玉液汤
Yu Zhen San	True Jade Powder	玉真散
Yue Bi Jia Zhu Tang	Maidservant from Yue Decoction plus Atractylodes	越婢加术汤
Yue Bi Tang	Maidservant from Yue Decoction	越婢汤
Yue Hua Wan	Moonlight Pills	月华丸
Yue Ju Wan	Escape Restraint Pill	越鞠丸
Zai Zao San	Renewal Powder	再造散
Zeng Ye Cheng Qi Tang	Increase the Fluids and Order the Qi Decoction	增液承气汤
Zeng Ye Tang	Increase the Fluids Decoction	增液汤
Zhe Chong Yin	Break the Conflict Decoction	折冲饮
Zhen Gan Xi Feng Tang	Sedate the Liver and Extinguish Wind Decoction	镇肝熄风汤
Zhen Ling Dan	Rouse the Spirits Special Pill	震灵丹
Zhen Ren Huo Ming Yin	True Man Decoction to Revitalize Life	真人活命饮
Zhen Ren Yang Zang Tang	True Man Decoction for Nourishing the Organs	真人养脏汤
Zhen Wu Tang	True Warrior Decoction	真武汤
Zhen Zhu Mu Wan	Mother of Pearl Pills	珍珠母丸
Zheng Gu Zi Jin Dan	Purple and Gold Pill for Righteous Bones	正骨紫金丹
Zhi Bai Di Huang Wan	Anemarrhena, Phellodendron, and Rehmannia Pills	知柏地黄丸
Zhi Gan Cao Tang	Honey-Fried Licorice Decoction	炙甘草汤
Zhi Jing San	Stop Spasms Powder	止痉散

Pinyin Names	Translational Names	Chinese Names
Zhi Shi Dao Zhi Wan	Immature Bitter Orange Pill to Guide Out Stagnation	枳实导滞丸
Zhi Shi Shao Yao San	Immature Bitter Orange and Peony Powder	枳实芍药散
Zhi Shi Xiao Pi Wan	Immature Bitter Orange Pill to Reduce Focal Distention	枳实消痞丸
Zhi Shi Xie Bai Gui Zhi Tang	Immature Bitter Orange, Chinese Chive, and Cinnamon Twig Decoction	枳实薤白桂枝汤
Zhi Sou San	Stop Coughing Powder	止嗽散
Zhi Suo Er Chen Tang	Two-Cured Decoction with Aurantium and Cardamon	枳缩二陈汤
Zhi Zhu Wan	Immature Bitter Orange and Atractylodes Macrocephala Pills	枳术丸
Zhi Zhuo Gu Ben Wan	Treat the Turbidity and Guard the Root Pills	治浊固本丸
Zhi Zi Bai Pi Tang	Gardenia and Phellodendron Decoction	栀子柏皮汤
Zhi Zi Chi Tang	Gardenia and Soja Decoction	栀子豉汤
Zhou Che Wan	Vessel and Vehicle Pill	舟车丸
Zhu Ling Tang	Polyporus Decoction	猪苓汤
Zhu Ru Wen Dan Tang	Bamboo Decoction to Warm the Gallbladder	竹茹温胆汤
Zhu Sha An Shen Wan	Cinnabar Pills to Tranquilize the Spirit	朱砂安神丸
Zhu Ye Shi Gao Tang	Lophatherum and Gypsum Decoction	竹叶石膏汤
Zi Cao Gen Mu Li Tang	Lithospermum and Oyster Shell Decoction	紫草根牡蛎汤
Zi Shen Ming Mu Tang	Nourish the Kidney to Bright the Eyes Decoction	滋肾明目汤
Zi Shen Tong Er Tang	Nourish the Kidney to Unblock the Ears Decoction	滋肾通耳汤
Zi Sheng Wan	Nourish Life Pill	资生丸
Zi Wan Tang	Aster Decoction	紫苑汤
Zi Yin Di Huang Wan	Rehmannia Pills to Nourish Yin	滋阴地黄丸
Zi Yin Jiang Huo Tang	Nourish Yin and Descend the Fire Decoction	滋阴降火汤
Zuo Gui Wan	Restore the Left [Kidney] Pill	左归丸
Zuo Jin Wan	Left Metal Pill	左金丸

Appendix 6 — Herbs Offering Beneficial Effects to Support Pregnancy

Certain herbs have been shown to offer beneficial effects during pregnancy. However, these herbs should be used only under supervision of a qualified healthcare professional, and only when benefits of using the herbs outweigh the risks.

Herbs	Restless Fetus	Nausea / Vomiting	Low Back Pain	Uterine Bleeding	Others
Ai Ye (Folium Artemisiae Argyi)				x	
Bai Shao (Radix Paeoniae Alba)	x				
Bai Zhu (Rhizoma Atractylodis Macrocephalae)	x			x	In cases of deficiencies
Ban Xia (Rhizoma Pinelliae)		x			
Bian Dou (Semen Lablab Album)		x			
Dang Gui (Radicis Angelicae Sinensis)	x		x	x	Breech presentation
Di Fu Zi (Fructus Kochiae)					Urinary tract infection
Dong Kui Zi (Semen Malvae)					Edema, dysuria
Du Zhong (Cortex Eucommiae)	x		x	x	
E Jiao (Colla Corii Asini)				x	
Fu Long Gan (Terra Flava Usta)		x			
Huang Qin (Radix Scutellariae)	x				
Huo Xiang (Herba Agastache)		x			
Ku Shen Gen (Radix Sophorae Flavescentis)					Dysuria
Sang Piao Xiao (Ootheca Mantidis)					Frequent urination
Sha Ren (Fructus Amomi)	x	x		x	In cases of deficiencies
Shu Di Huang (Radix Rehmanniae Preparata)	x				
Tu Si Zi (Semen Cuscutae)				x	
Xu Duan (Radix Dipsaci)	x			x	In cases of deficiencies
Yi Tang (Saccharum Granorum)	x				
Ze Xie (Rhizoma Alismatis)					Edema
Zhu Ru (Caulis Bambusae in Taenia)		x			
Zi Su Ye (Folium Perillae)	x	x			
Zong Lu Pi (Fibra Stipulae Trachycarpi)	x			x	

Appendix 7 — Cautions / Contraindications for Use of Herbs During Pregnancy

Certain herbs have a recognized potential to endanger or cause harm to a fetus during pregnancy, thus possibly causing birth defects or miscarriage. As a general rule, herbs with potent effects to regulate qi, move blood, or drain downwards should be avoided during pregnancy. These herbs are classified as **contraindicated** or for **use with caution** in treatment of pregnant women. Please note that these are not comprehensive lists—additional information is listed in each herb monograph.

Herbs	Caution	Contraindication
Ba Dou (Fructus Crotonis)		X
Bai Fu Zi (Rhizoma Typhonii)		X
Bai Guo (Semen Ginkgo)	X	
Bai Ji Li (Fructus Tribuli)		X
Ban Mao (Mylabris)		X
Ban Xia (Rhizoma Pinelliae)	X	
Bie Jia (Carapax Trionycis)		X
Bing Lang (Semen Arecae)	X	
Bing Pian (Borneolum Syntheticum)		X
Bu Gu Zhi (Fructus Psoraleae)	X	
Cang Er Zi (Fructus Xanthii)	X	
Cao Wu (Radix Aconiti Kusnezoffii)		X
Cha Chi Huang (Herba Stellariae Aquaticae)	X	
Chan Su (Venenum Bufonis)		X
Chuan Niu Xi (Radix Cyathulae)		X
Chuan Wu (Radix Aconiti Preparata)		X
Chuan Xin Lian (Herba Andrographis)	X	
Da Fu Pi (Pericarpium Arecae)	X	
Da Huang (Radix et Rhizoma Rhei)		X
Da Ji (Herba seu Radix Cirsii Japonici)	X	
Dai Zhe Shi (Haematitum)	X	
Dan Zhu Ye (Herba Lophatheri)	X	
Dang Gui (Radicis Angelicae Sinensis)	X	
Di Bie Chong (Eupolyphaga)		X
Di Long (Pheretima)	X	
Ding Jing Cao (Herba Linderniae)		X
E Zhu (Rhizoma Curcumae)		X
Fei Zi (Semen Torreyae)		X
Fu Zi (Radix Aconiti Lateralis Praeparata)		X
Gan Jiang (Rhizoma Zingiberis)	X	
Gan Qi (Resina Toxicodendri)		X
Gan Sui (Radix Euphorbiae Kansui)		X
Gou Qi Zi (Fructus Lycii)	X	
Guan Mu Tong (Caulis Aristolochiae Manshuriensis)		X
Guan Zhong (Rhizoma Dryopteridis)	X	
Gui Ban (Plastrum Testudinis)		X

Herbs	Caution	Contraindication
Hai Ma (Hippocampus)	x	
He Huan Pi (Cortex Albiziae)	x	
Hong Hua (Flos Carthami)		x
Hou Po (Cortex Magnoliae Officinalis)	x	
Hu Jiao (Fructus Piper)	x	
Hu Lu Ba (Semen Trigonellae)	x	
Hu Yao Huang (Herba Leucas Mollissimae)		x
Hu Zhang (Rhizoma Polygoni Cuspidati)		x
Hua Jiao (Pericarpium Zanthoxyli)	x	
Hua Rui Shi (Ophicalcitum)	x	
Huai Niu Xi (Radix Achyranthis Bidentatae)		x
Ji Xue Cao (Herba Centellae)	x	
Ji Xue Teng (Caulis Spatholobi)		x
Jiang Huang (Rhizoma Curcumae Longae)		x
Jiu Ceng Ta (Herba Ocimi Basilici)		x
Jue Ming Zi (Semen Cassiae)	x	
Lei Gong Teng (Radix Tripterygii Wilfordii)		x
Li Lu (Radix et Rhizoma Veratri)		x
Liu Huang (Sulfur)		x
Liu Ji Nu (Herba Artemisiae Anomalae)		x
Lu Cha (Folium Camellia Sinensis)	x	
Lu Hui (Aloe)		x
Lu Lu Tong (Fructus Liquidambaris)		x
Ma Bian Cao (Herba Verbenae)	x	
Ma Chi Xian (Herba Portulacae)	x	
Ma Huang (Herba Ephedrae)	x	
Ma Qian Zi (Semen Strychni)		x
Mang Xiao (Natrii Sulfas)		x
Meng Chong (Tabanus)		x
Mu Bie Zi (Semen Momordicae)		x
Niao Bu Su (Ramus Kalopanax Pictus)	x	
Niu Huang (Calculus Bovis)	x	
Pao Zai Cao (Herba Physalis Angulatae)		x
Pu Huang (Pollen Typhae)		x
Pu Yin (Radix Wikstroemia Indica)		x
Qi Ye Lian (Radix Schefflerae)	x	
Qian Niu Zi (Semen Pharbitidis)		x
Qing Fen (Calomelas)		x
Quan Xie (Scorpio)		x
Rou Gui (Cortex Cinnamomi)		x
Ru Xiang (Gummi Olibanum)		x
San Leng (Rhizoma Sparganii)		x
San Qi (Radix Notoginseng)	x	

Herbs	Caution	Contraindication
Shang Lu (Radix Phytolaccae)		x
She Gan (Rhizoma Belamcandae)		x
She Xiang (Moschus)		x
Shen Qu (Massa Fermentata)	x	
Shu Wei Huang (Herba Rostellulariae)		x
Shui Zhi (Hirudo)		x
Su Mu (Lignum Sappan)		x
Suan Zao Ren (Semen Zizyphi Spinosae)	x	
Tan Xiang (Lignum Santali Albi)	x	
Tao Ren (Semen Persicae)		x
Tian Hua Fen (Radix Trichosanthis)		x
Tian Xian Teng (Herba Aristolochiae)		x
Ting Li Zi (Semen Descurainiae seu Lepidii)		x
Wang Bu Liu Xing (Semen Vaccariae)		x
Wu Gong (Scolopendra)		x
Wu Ling Zhi (Excrementum Trogopteri seu Pteromi)		x
Xi Jiao (Cornu Rhinoceri)	x	
Xiang Yuan (Fructus Citri)	x	
Xiao Hui Xiang (Fructus Foeniculi)	x	
Xin Yi Hua (Flos Magnoliae)	x	
Xiong Huang (Realgar)		x
Xue Jie (Sanguis Draconis)		x
Ya Dan Zi (Fructus Bruceae)		x
Yi Mu Cao (Herba Leonuri)	x	
Yi Yi Ren (Semen Coicis)		x
Yu Jin (Radix Curcumae)	x	
Yuan Hua (Flos Genkwa)		x
Yuan Zhi (Radix Polygalae)	x	
Zao Jiao (Fructus Gleditsiae)		x
Zao Jiao Ci (Spina Gleditsiae)		x
Zao Xiu (Rhizoma Paridis)	x	
Zhang Nao (Camphora)		x
Zhi Ke (Fructus Aurantii)	x	
Zhi Shi (Fructus Aurantii Immaturus)	x	
Zhu Fan Hua Tou (Rhizoma Mirabilidis)	x	
Zhu Ye (Herba Phyllostachys)	x	

Appendix 8 — Dosing Guidelines

The dosages listed in this text refer to the daily dose for an adult of average height and weight, when using dehydrated herbs. However, the actual prescribed dosage will vary significantly, based not only on the characteristics of the illness and overall condition of the patient, but also on his or her size and age. Generally speaking, single herbs used individually require higher dosages, while herbs used as part of an herbal formula are chosen in smaller amounts. Treatment of an acute condition necessitates higher dosages, and treatment of a mild condition, smaller dosages. One must also consider the constitution of the patient. Those who are basically healthy and strong may tolerate larger doses, while weak and/or deficiency patients will need a smaller dose.

Recommended ingestion levels must be adjusted to reflect variations in age and body weight. The principle behind the *Age-to-Dose Guideline* is based on assessment of the maturity of the internal organs and their capacity to metabolize, utilize and eliminate herbs. This highly-detailed chart is especially useful for infants and younger children. The recommendations are taken from *Zhong Cao Yao* (Chinese Herbal Medicine), published by the Nanjing College of Traditional Chinese Medicine.

The principle behind the *Weight-to-Dose Guideline* is based on the effective concentration of the herbal medicine once it is distributed throughout different areas of the body. This dosing strategy is especially useful for patients whose body weight falls outside of the normal range. All calculations are based on Clark's Rule in '*Pharmaceutical Calculations*,' written by Mitchell Stoklosa and Howard Ansel.

These charts provide herbal practitioners a handy reference for dosing those patients who fall outside the definition of an "average adult." It is important to remember, however, that the charts serve only as guidelines—not as absolute rules. One must always remember to treat each patient as a unique individual, not as a statistic on a chart!

Age-to-Dose Dosing Guideline

Age	Recommended Daily Dosage
0 – 1 month	1/18 – 1/14 of adult dose
1 – 6 month	1/14 – 1/7 of adult dose
6 – 12 month	1/7 – 1/5 of adult dose
1 – 2 years	1/5 – 1/4 of adult dose
2 – 4 years	1/4 – 1/3 of adult dose
4 – 6 years	1/3 – 2/5 of adult dose
6 – 9 years	2/5 – 1/2 of adult dose
9 – 14 years	1/2 – 2/3 of adult dose
14 – 18 years	2/3 – full adult dose
18 – 60 years	**adult dose**
60 years and over	3/4 or less of adult dose

Weight-to-Dose Dosing Guideline

Weight	Recommended Daily Dosage
30 – 40 lbs	20% – 27% of adult dose
40 – 50 lbs	27% – 33% of adult dose
50 – 60 lbs	33% – 40% of adult dose
60 – 70 lbs	40% – 47% of adult dose
70 – 80 lbs	47% – 53% of adult dose
80 – 100 lbs	53% – 67% of adult dose
100 – 120 lbs	67% – 80% of adult dose
120 – 150 lbs	80% – 100% of adult dose
150 lbs	**adult dose**
150 – 200 lbs	100% – 133% of adult dose
200 – 250 lbs	133% – 167% of adult dose
250 – 300 lbs	167% – 200% of adult dose

Appendix 9 — Weights and Measures: Chinese, British and Metric Systems

CHINESE SYSTEM

1. Measure of Weight

1 *jin* (斤) = 16 *liang*
1 *liang* (两) = 10 *qian*
1 *qian* (钱) = 10 *fen*
1 *fen* (分) = 10 *li* (厘)

2. Measure of Volume

The standard unit is *sheng* (升) for measurement of volume. Historically, each *sheng* is approximately 1000 ml. Other units of measure, such as bowls and spoonfuls, are not discussed as they are quite vague and there are great differences in these standards in different regions.

BRITISH SYSTEM

1. Measure of Weight (Apothecary)

20 grains = 1 scruple
3 scruples (60 grains) = 1 drachm or dram
8 drachms (480 grains) = 1 ounce
12 ounces (5760 grains) = 1 pound

2. Measure of Weight (Avoirdupois)

437½ or 437.5 grains = 1 ounce
16 ounces (7000 grains) = 1 pound

3. Measure of Volume (Apothecary)

60 minims = 1 fluidrachm or fluidram
8 fluidrachms (480 minims) = 1 fluidounce
16 fluidounces = 1 pint
2 pints (32 fluidounces) = 1 quart
4 quarts (8 pints) = 1 gallon

METRIC SYSTEM

Multiples and Submultiples		Prefix	Symbol
1,000,000,000,000	(10^{12})	*tera-*	T
1,000,000,000	(10^{9})	*giga-*	G
1,000,000	(10^{6})	*mega-*	M
1,000	(10^{3})	*kilo-*	k
100	(10^{2})	*hecto-*	h
10	(10)	*deka-*	da
0.1	(10^{-1})	*deci-*	d
0.01	(10^{-2})	*centi-*	c
0.001	(10^{-3})	*milli-*	m
0.000,001	(10^{-6})	*micro-*	μ or mc
0.000,000,001	(10^{-9})	*nano-*	n
0.000,000,000,001	(10^{-12})	*pico-*	p
0.000,000,000,000,001	(10^{-15})	*femto-*	f
0.000,000,000,000,000,001	(10^{-18})	*atto-*	a

1. Measure of Weight

1 kilogram (kg) = 1000.000 grams
1 hektogram (hg) = 100.000 grams
1 dekagram (dag) = 10.000 grams
1 gram (g or gm) = 1.000 gram
1 decigram (dg) = 0.100 gram
1 centigram (cg) = 0.010 gram
1 milligram (mg) = 0.001 gram
1 microgram (μg or mcg) = 0.000,001 gram

1 gram (g or gm) = 0.001 kilogram
= 0.010 hektogram
= 0.100 dekagram
= 10 decigrams
= 100 centigrams
= 1000 milligrams
= 1,000,000 micrograms

2. Measure of Volume

1 kiloliter (kL) = 1000.000 liters
1 hektoliter (hL) = 100.000 liters
1 dekaliter (daL) = 10.000 liters
1 liter (L) = 1.000 liter
1 deciliter (dL) = 0.100 liter
1 centiliter (cL) = 0.010 liter
1 milliliter (mL) = 0.001 liter
1 microliter (μL) = 0.000,001 liter

1 liter = 0.001 kiloliter
= 0.010 hektoliter
= 0.100 dekaliter
= 10 deciliters
= 100 centiliters
= 1000 milliliters
= 1,000,000 microliters

CONVERSIONS

Weight Conversion (Chinese Units : Metric : Avoirdupois)

Chinese Units	Grams	Ounces
1 *jin*	500	17.87
1 *liang*	31.25	1.116875
1 *qian*	3.125	0.111688
1 *fen*	0.3125	0.011169
1 *li*	0.03125	0.001117

Volume Conversion (Chinese Units : Metric : Apothecary)

Chinese Units	Liter	Fluid Ounces
1 *sheng*	1	33.815

Appendix 10 — Convention on International Trade in Endangered Species (CITES)

Trade in herbs and animals listed in Appendix I of Convention on International Trade in Endangered Species (CITES) is strictly prohibited. The discussion of these substances in this text is included only to offer 1) the accurate history of its critically important usage in traditional herbal medicine, and 2) models for appropriate usage of effective substitute substances and alternatives. The information should not be interpreted as condoning illegal use of these endangered species.

Endangered Species	Status	Alternatives
Hu Gu (Os Tigris)	Appendix I	***Zhu Gu*** (Os Porcus)
Xi Jiao (Cornu Rhinoceri)	Appendix I	***Shui Niu Jiao*** (Cornu Bubali)
Xiong Dan (Fel Ursi)	Appendix I	***Niu Dan*** (Fel Bovis)

Bibliography of Historical Texts

Pinyin Names (Translated Names)	Chinese Names
Bai Rai Shin Shu (A New Study of Dermatomycosis and Dermatitis) by Tsursure Katakura	
Bai Yi Xuan Fang (Selected Formulas)	百一选方
Bao Ying Cuo Yao (Synopsis of Caring for Infants) by Xue Kai in 1555	保婴撮要
Bei Ji Qian Jin Yao Fang (Thousands of Golden Prescriptions for Emergencies)	备急千金要方
Ben Cao Bei Yao (Essentials of the Materia Medica) by Wang Ang in 1751	本草备要
Ben Cao Cong Xin (Thoroughly Revised Materia Medica) by Wu Yi-Luo in 1751	本草从新
Ben Cao Fa Hui (Elaboration of the Materia Medica) by Xu Yan-Chun in Ming Dynasty	本草发挥
Ben Cao Gang Mu (Materia Medica) by Li Shi-Zhen in 1578	本草纲目
Ben Cao Gang Mu Shi Yi (Omissions from the Grand Materia Medica) by Zhao Xue-Min in 1765	本草纲目拾遗
Ben Cao Hui Yan (Treasury of Words on the Materia Medica) by Ni Zhu-Mo in 1624	本草汇言
Ben Cao Jing Ji Zhu (Collection of Commentaries on the Classic of the Materia Medica) by Tao Hong-Jing in 480-498 B.C.	本草经集注
Ben Cao Meng Quan (Hidden Aspects of the Materia Medica) by Chen Jia-Mo in 1565	本草蒙荃
Ben Cao Pin Hui Jing Yao (Essentials of Materia Medica) by Liu Wen-Tai in 1505	本草品汇精要
Ben Cao Qiu Zheng (Verification of Materia Medica) by Huang Gong-Xiu in 1769	本草求正
Ben Cao Shi Yi (Omissions from the [Classic of the] Materia Medica) by Chen Cang-Qi in 741 A.D.	本草拾遗
Ben Cao Yan Yi (Extension of the Materia Medica) by Kou Zong-Shi in 1116	本草衍义
Ben Cao Yan Yi Bu Yi (Supplement to the Extension of the Materia Medica) by Zhu Zhen-Heng in 1347	本草衍义补遗
Ben Cao Yuan Shi (Origins of the Materia Medica) by Li Zhong-Li in Ming Dynasty	本草原始
Ben Cao Zai Xin (Renewed Materia Medica)	本草再新
Ben Cao Zheng (Rectification of the Materia Medica)	本草正
Ben Cao Zheng Yi (Truth and False Information of Materia Medica) by Zhang Shan-Lei in 1920	本草正义
Ben Jing (Divine Husbandman's Classic of the Materia Medica) in the second century	本经
Ben Jing Feng Yuan (Journey to the Origin of the Classic of Materia Medica) by Zhang Lu in 1670	本经逢原
Bian Zheng Lun (Records of Differential Diagnosis)	辨证论
Bo Ai Xin Jian (Manual of Universal Lover from the Heart)	博爱心鉴
Bu Yao Xiu Zhen Xiao Er Fang Lun (Supplement to the Pocket-Sized Discussion of Formulas for Children)	补要袖诊小儿方论
Chang Yong Zhong Cao Yao Shou Ce (Handbook of Commonly Used Traditional Chinese Herbs) by Guangzhou People's Liberation Army Medical Brigade	常用中草药手册
Cheng Fang Bian Du (Convenient Reader of Established Formulas) by Zhang Bing-Cheng in 1904	成方便读
Cheng Fang Qie Yong (Practical Formulas) by Wu Yi-Luo in 1761	成方切用
Chong Ding Tong Su Shang Han Lun (Revised Popular Guide to the Discussion of Cold-Induced Disorders) by Yu Gen-Chu in Qing Dynasty	重订通俗伤寒论
Chong Lou Yu Yao (Jade Key to Many Towers) by Zheng Mei-Run in 1838	重楼玉钥
Ci Shi Nan Zhi (Hard-Won Knowledge) by Wang Hao-Gu in 1308	此事难知
Dan Xi Xin Fa (Teachings of [Zhu] Dan-Xi) by Zhu Zhen-Heng in 1481	丹溪心法
Dan Xi Xin Fa Fu Yu (Additions to the Teachings for [Zhu] Dan-Xi) by Fang Guang-Lei in 1536	丹溪心法附余
De Pei Ben Cao (Materia Medica of Combinations)	得配本草
Dong Tian Ao Zhi (Profound Purpose from the Heavenly Abode) by Chen Shi-Duo in 1694	洞天奥旨
Dong Yi Bao Jian (Precious Mirror of Oriental Medicine) by Xu Sun in 1611	东医宝鉴
Dou Zhen Shi Yi Xin Fa (Teachings of Generations of Physicians about Pox) by Wan Quan in 1568	痘疹世医心法
Fang Ji Xue (Traditional Chinese Medical Formulas) by Shanghai College of Traditional Chinese Medicine in 1975	方剂学
Fu Ke Chan Lun Fang (Discussion of Formulas for Obstetrics and Gynecology)	妇科常论方
Fu Qing Zhu Nu Ke (Women's Diseases According to Fu Qing-Zhu) by Fu Shan in 1827	傅青主女科
Fu Ren Liang Fang (Fine Formulas for Women) by Chen Zi-Ming in 1237	妇人良方
Fu Shou Jing Fang (Exquisite Formulas for Fostering Longevity) by Wu Min in 1530	扶寿精防
Gu Jin Yi Jian (Medical Mirror of the Past and Present) by Gong Xin-Zuan in Ming Dynasty	古今医鉴
Gu Jin Yi Tong Da Quan (Comprehensive Collection of Medicine Past and Present) by Xu Chun-Fu in 1556	古今医通大全
Guang Wen Yi Lun (Discussion of Widespread Warm Epidemics) by Dai Tian-Zhang in 1722	广温疫论

Pinyin Names (Translated Names)	**Chinese Names**
Guangxi Zhong Yao Zhi (Guangxi Journal of Chinese Herbal Medicines)	广西中药志
Guizhou Min Jian Yao Wu (Folk Medicina from Guizhou)	贵州民间药物
Hai Yao Ben Cao (Materia Medica of Herbs from [Across the] Seas) by Li Xun in 907-960 A.D.	海药本草
Han Shi Yi Tong (Comprehensive Medicine According to Master Han) by Han Mao in 1522	韩氏医通
Huang Di Su Wen Xuan Ming Lun Fang (Formulas from the Discussion Illuminating the Yellow Emperor's Basic Questions) by Liu Yuan-Su in 1172	黄帝素问宣明论方
Huo Luan Lun (Discussion of Sudden Turmoil Disorders) by Wan Shi-Xiong in 1862	霍乱论
Ji Sheng Fang (Formulas to Aid the Living) by Yan Yong-He in 1253	济生方
Jia You Ben Cao (Materia Medica of the Jia You Era) by Zhang Yu-Xi and Su Song in 1057-1060	嘉佑本草
Jiang Su Zhi Wu Zhi (Jiangsu Journal of Botany)	江苏植物志
Jiao Zhu Fu Ren Liang Fang (Revised Fine Formulas for Women) by Bi Li-Zhai in 16th Century	校注妇人良方
Jin Gui Yao Lue (Essentials from the Golden Cabinet) by Zhang Zhong-Jing in Eastern Han	金匮要略
Jing Shi Zheng Lei Bei Ji Ben Cao (Differentiation and Application of Materia Medica) by Tang Shen-Wei in 1082	经史证类备急本草
Jing Xiu Tang Yao Shuo (Herbal Teachings from the Respectfully Decorated Hall) by Qian Shu-Tian	敬修堂药说
Jing Yue Quan Shu (Collected Treatises of [Zhang] Jing Yue) by Zhang Jie-Bing (Zhang Jing-Yue) in 1624	景岳全书
Jiu Huang Ben Cao (Materia Medica to Rescue Emergencies)	救荒本草
Kai Bao Ben Cao (Materia Medica of the Kai Bao Era) by Ma Zhi in 973-974 A.D.	开宝本草
Lan Shi Mi Cang (Secrets from the Orchid Chamber) by Li Ao in 1336	兰室秘藏
Lei Bian Zhu Shi Ji Yan Yi Fang (Effective Medical Formulas Arranged by Category by Doctor Zhu) by Zhu Zuo in 1266	类编朱氏集验医方
Lei Gong Pao Zhi Lun (Grandfather Lei's Discussions of Herb Preparation) by Lei Xiao in 470 A.D.	雷公炮制抡
Lei Zheng Huo Ren Shu (Book to Safeguard Life Arranged According to Pattern) by Zhu Gong in 1108	类证活人书
Liang Fang Yi Ye (Small Collection of Fine Formulas) by Xie Yuan-Qing in 1842	良方集腋
Lin Zheng Zhi Nan Yi An (Case Histories from the Compass of Clinical Patterns) by Ye Tian-Shi in 1746	临证指南医案
Ling Nan Cai Yao Lu (Records of Picking Herbs in Guangdong)	岭南采药录
Liu Zhou Yi Hua (Medical Dialogues from Liuzhou)	柳州医话
Lu Chan Yan Ben Cao (Materia Medica from Steep Mountainsides)	履巉岩本草
Ming Yi Za Zhu (Miscellaneous Records of Famous Physicians) by Tao Hong-Jing in 500 A.D.	名医杂著
Ming Yi Zhi Zhang (Displays of Enlightened Physicians) by Huang Fu-Zhong in 16th Century	名医指掌
Nanning Shi Yao Wu Zhi (Nanning City Medicines)	南宁市药物志
Nei Jing Shi Yi Fang Lun (Enumeration of Formulas Omitted from the Inner Classic) by Luo Long-Ji in Song Dynasty	内经拾遗方论
Nei Ke Zhai Yao (Summary of Internal Medicine) by Wen Sheng in Mid-19th Century	内科摘要
Nei Wai Shang Bian Huo Lun (Clarifying Doubts about Injury from Internal and External Causes) by Li Ao in 1247	内外伤辨惑论
Pi Wei Lun (Discussion of the Spleen and Stomach) by Li Ao in 1249	脾胃论
Pin Hui Jing Yao (Essentials of (Herbal) Distinctions)	品汇精要
Pu Ji Ben Shi Fang (Formulas of Universal Benefit from My Practice) by Xu Shu-Wei in 1132	普济本事方
Pu Ji Fang (Formulas of Universal Benefit)	普济方
Qi Xiao Hai Shang Xian Fang Mi Ben (Secret Text of Extraordinary Effective Beneficial Formulas from Across the Seas)	奇效海上仙方秘本
Qian Jin Yao Fang (Thousand Ducat Prescriptions) by Sun Si-Miao in 581-685 A.D.	千金要方
Qian Jin Yi Fang (Supplement to the Thousand Ducat Formulas) by Sun Si-Miao in 682 A.D.	千金翼方
Qing Cao Shi Jie (The World of Herbs) by Zhong Ding-Chuan in 1992	青草世界
Qing Cao Yao Han Shou Jiao Cai (Textbook of Botanical Medicine) by Zhong Ding-Chuan in 1992	青草药函授教材
Quan Guo Zhong Cheng Yao Chu Fang Ji (National Collection of Chinese Herbal Prepared Medicines) in 1949	全国中成药处方剂
Ren Zhai Zhi Zhi (Straight Directions of Benevolent Aid) by Yang Tu-Ying in 1264	仁斋直指
Ri Hua Zi Ben Cao (Materia Medica of Ri Hua-Zi) by Ri Hua-Zi in 713 A.D.	日华子本草
Ri Yong Ben Cao (Household Materia Medica) by Wu Rui in 1330	日用本草
Ru Men Shi Qin (Confucians' Duties to their Parents) by Zhang Cong-Zheng in 1228	儒门事亲

Pinyin Names (Translated Names)	Chinese Names
San Yin Ji Yi Bing Zheng Fang Lun (Discussion of Illnesses, Patterns, and Formulas Related to the Unification of the Three Etiologies) by Chen Yan in 1174	三因即一病证方论
Shang Hai Shi Zhong Cheng Yao Zhi Ji Gui Fan (Shanghai Municipal Standards for the Manufacturing of Chinese Prepared Medicines) in 1970	上海市中成药制剂规范
Shang Han Biao Ben Xin Fa Lei Cui (Collection of Methods Related to the Manifestation and Root of Cold-Induced Disorders)	伤寒标本心法类萃
Shang Han Liu Shu (Six Texts on Cold-Induced Disorders) by Tao Hua in 1445	伤寒六书
Shang Han Lun (Discussion of Cold-Induced Disorders) by Zhang Zhong-Jing in Eastern Han	伤寒论
Shang Han Lun Ming Li Lun (Clarification of the Theory of Cold Induced Disorders) by Cheng Wu-Ji in 1156	伤寒论明指论
Shang Han Zhi Ge Fang Lun (Direct Investigations of Formulas for Cold-Induced Disorders) by Liu Yuan-Su in Jin Dynasty	伤寒直格方论
She Sheng Mi Pou (Secrets Investigations Into Obtaining Health) by Hong Ji in 1638	摄生秘剖
She Sheng Zhong Miao Fang (Marvelous Formulas for the Health of Multitudes) by Zhang Shi-Che in 1550	摄生众妙方
Shen Nong Ben Cao Jing (Divine Husbandman's Classic of the Materia Medica) in the second century	神农本草经
Shen Nong Ben Cao Jing Shu (Revised Divine Husbandman's Classic of the Materia Medica) by Miao Xi-Yong in 1625	神农本草经书
Shen Shi Yao Han (Scrutiny of the Priceless Jade Case) by Fu Ren-Yu in 1644	审视瑶函
Shen Shi Zun Sheng Shu (Master Shen's Book for Revering Life) by Shen Jin-Ao in 1773	沈氏尊生书
Shi Bing Lun (Discussion of Seasonal Diseases) by Lei Feng in 1882	时病论
Shi Fang Ge Kuo (Collected Songs about Contemporary Formulas) by Chen Nian-Zi in 1801	时方歌括
Shi Liao Ben Cao (Materia Medica of Diet Therapy) by Meng Shan in the seventh Century	食疗本草
Shi Wu Ben Cao (Food As Materia Medica) by Lu He-Ming in 701-704 A.D.	食物本草
Shi Yao Shen Shu (Miraculous Book of Ten Remedies) by Ge Qian-Sun in 1348	十药神书
Shi Yi De Xiao Fang (Effective Formulas from Generations of Physicians) by Wei Yi-Lin in 1345	世医得效方
Shi Yong Tian Ran Yao Wu (Practical Natural Medicine) by Zheng Bing-Chuan in 1997	实用天然药物
Shou Shi Bao Yuan (Achieving Longevity by Guarding the Source) by Gong Ting-Xian in Early 17th Century	寿世保元
Shu Ben Cao (Materia Medica of Sichuan) by Han Bao-Sheng in 935-960 A.D.	蜀本草
Sichuan Zhong Yao Zhi (Sichuan Journal of Chinese Herbal Medicines)	四川中药志
Su Wen Bing Ji Qi Yi Bao Ming Ji (Collection of Writings on the Mechanism of Illness, Suitability of Qi, and the Safeguarding of Life as Discussed in the Basic Questions) by Zhang Yuan-Su in 1186	素问病机气宜保命集
Tai Ping Hui Min He Ji Ju Fang (Imperial Grace Formulary of the Tai Ping Era) by Imperial Medical Department in 1078-85	太平惠民和济局方
Tai Wan Min Jian Yao (Folk Medicine of Taiwan) by Gao Mu-Chun in 1985	台湾民间药
Tai Wan Zhi Wu Yao Cai Zhi (Medicinal Plants of Taiwan)	台湾植物药材志
Tang Ben Cao (Tang Materia Medica) by Su Jing in 659 A.D.	唐本草
Tang Ye Ben Cao (Materia Medica for Decoctions) by Wang Hao-Gu in 1306	汤液本草
Ti Ren Hui Bian (Compilation of Materials of Benevolence for the Body) by Peng Yong-Guang in 1549	体仁汇编
Tong Su Shang Han Lun (Plain Version of Discussion of Cold-Induced Disorder)	通俗伤寒论
Tu Jing Ben Cao (Illustrated Classic of the Materia Medica) by Su Song in 1061	图经本草
Wai Dan Ben Cao (Materia Medica for External Elixirs)	外丹本草
Wai Ke Zheng Zhi Quan Sheng Ji (Complete Collection of Patterns and Treatments in External Medicine) by Wang Wei-De in 1740	外科症治全生集
Wai Ke Zheng Zhi Zhun Sheng (Standards of Patterns and Treatments in External Medicine) by Wang Ken-Tang in Ming Dynasty	外科症治准绳
Wai Ke Zheng Zong (True Lineage of External Medicine) by Chen Shi-Gong in 1617	外科正宗
Wai Tai Mi Yao (Arcane Essentials from the Imperial Library) by Wang Tao in 752 A.D.	外台秘要
Wan Bing Hui Chun (Restoration of Health from the Myriad Diseases) by Gong Ting-Xian in 1587	万病回春
Wei Sheng Bao Jian (Precious Mirror of Health) by Luo Tian-Yi in Yuan Dynasty	卫生宝鉴
Wei Yao Tiao Bian (Cataloged Diffentiation of Erroneous Medicines)	伪药条辩

Pinyin Names (Translated Names)	**Chinese Names**
Wen Bing Tiao Bian (Systematic Differentiation of Warm Diseases) by Wu Ju-tong in 1798	温病条辨
Wen Re Jing Wei (Warp and Woof of Warm-Febrile Diseases) by Wang Meng-Ying in 1852	温热经纬
Wen Yi Lun (Discussion of Epidemic Warm Diseases) by Wu You-Xing in 1642	温疫论
Wu Pu Ben Cao (Wu Pu's Materia Medica)	吴普本草
Xi Yuan Ji Lu Jiao Yi (Correction and Explanation of the Wrongly Accused)	洗冤集录校译
Xian Dai Shi Yong Zhong Yao (Modern Practical Chinese Medicines)	现代实用中药
Xian Xing Zhai Yi Xue Guang Bi Ji (Wide-Ranging Medical Notes from the First-Awakened Studio) by Miao Xi-Yong in 1613	先醒斋医学广笔记
Xiao Er Yao Zheng Zhi Jue (Craft of Medicinal Treatment for Childhood Disease Patterns) by Qian Yi in 1119	小儿药症直决
Xin Xiu Ben Cao (Newly Revised Materia Medica) by Su Jing in 657-659 A.D.	新修本草
Xu Ming Yi Lei An (Continuation of Famous Physicians' Cases Organized by Categories) by Wei Zhi-Xiu in 1770	续名医类案
Yan Fang Xin Bian (New Compilation of Time-Tested Formulas) by Bao Xiang-Ao in 1846	验方新编
Yang Ke Xin De Ji (Collection of Personal Expertises Concerning Skin Lesions) by Gao Bing-Jun in 1805	疡科心得集
Yang Shi Jia Zang Fang (Collected Formulas of the Yang Family) by Yang Tan in 1178	杨氏家藏方
Yao Cai Xue (Study of Medicinal Substances)	药材学
Yao Pu (Medicinal Recipes) by Hou Ning-Ji	药谱
Yao Xing Ben Cao (Materia Medica of Medicinal Properties) by Zhen Quan in 600 A.D.	药性本草
Ye Shi Nu Ke (Ye's Women's Diseases)	叶氏女科
Yi Bian (Ordinary Medicine) by Wang San-Cai in 1587	医便
Yi Fang Ji Jie (Analytical Collection of Medical Formulas) by Wang Ang in 1682	医方集解
Yi Fang Kao (Investigation of Medical Formulas) by Wu Kun in 1584	医方考
Yi Fang Xin Jie (New Explanations of Medical Formulas) by Ma You-Du in 1980	医方新解
Yi Ji (Levels of Medicine)	医级
Yi Ji Bao Jian (Precious Mirror for Advancement of Medicine) by Dong Xi-Yuan in 1777	医籍宝鉴
Yi Lin Gai Cuo (Corrections of Errors Among Physicians) by Wang Qing-Ren in 1830	医林改错
Yi Lue Liu Shu (Six Texts on the Essentials of Medicine)	医略六书
Yi Men Fa Lu (Precepts for Physicians) by Yu Chang in 1658	医门法律
Yi Xue Fa Ming (Medical Innovations) by Li Ao in Jin Dynasty	医学发明
Yi Xue Qi Yuan (Origins of the Medicine) by Zhang Yuan-Su in Yuan Dynasty	医学启原
Yi Xue Ru Men (Introduction to Medicine) by Li Ting in 1575	医学入门
Yi Xue Xin Wu (Medical Revelations) by Cheng Guo-Peng in 1732	医学心悟
Yi Xue Zheng Zhuan (True Lineage of Medicine) by Yu Tian-Min in 1515	医学正传
Yi Xue Zhong Zhong Can Xi Lu (Records of Heart-Felt Experiences in Medicine With Reference to the West) by Zhang Xi-Chun in 1918-34	医学衷中参西录
Yi Yuan (Bases of Medicine) by Shi Shou-Tang in 1861	医原
Yi Zhen Yi De (Achievements Regarding Epidemic Rashes) by Yu Shi-Yu in 1794	疫疹一得
Yi Zong Jin Jian (Golden Mirror of the Medical Tradition) by Wu Qian in 1742	医宗金鉴
Yin Pian Xin Can (New References of Prepared Medicines)	饮片新参
Yin Shan Zheng Yao (Correct Guide to Eating and Drinking)	饮膳正要
Yong Lei Qian Fang (Everlasting Categorization of Seal Formulas)	永类钤方
Yuan Ji Qi Wei (Explanation of the Subtitles of the Original Mechanism) by Ni Wei-De in 1370	原机启微
Yuan Nan Yang (Asada's Prescriptions) by Sohaku Asada	
Za Bing Yuan Liu Xi Zhu (Wondrous Lantern for Peering into Origin and Development of Miscellaneous Diseases) by Shen Jin-Ao in 1773	杂病源流犀烛
Za Bing Zheng Zhi Xin Yi (New Significance of Patterns and Treatment in Miscellaneous Diseases)	杂病证治新义
Zhang Shi Yi Tong (Comprehensive Medicine According to Master Zhang) by Zhang Lu-Xuan in 1695	张氏医通
Zhen Nan Ben Cao (Materia Medica of South Yunnan) by Lan Mao in Qing Dynasty	滇南本草
Zhen Zhu Nang (Pouch of Pearls) by Zhang Yuan-Su in 1186	珍珠囊
Zeng Bu Nei Jing Shi Yi (Supplement to the Formulas Omitted from the Inner Classic)	增补内经拾遗
Zheng He Sheng Ji Zong Lu (Comprehensive Recording of Sage-Like Benefit from the Zheng He Era) by Sheng Fu in 1122	政和圣济总录

Pinyin Names (Translated Names)	Chinese Names
Zheng Lei Ben Cao (Materia Medica Arranged According to Pattern) by Tang Shen-Wei in 1082	证类本草
Zheng Shi Jia Chuan Nu Ke Wan Jin Fang (Zheng's Family Formulas for Women's Disorders)	郑氏家传女科万金方
Zheng Ti Lei Yao (Catalogued Essentials for Correcting the Body) by Bi Li-Zhai (Ji) in 1529	正体类要
Zheng Yin Mai Zhi (Pattern, Cause, Pulse, and Treatment) by Qin Jing-Ming in 1702	证因脉治
Zheng Zhi Zhun Sheng (Standards of Patterns and Treatments) by Wang Ken-Tang in 1602	症治准绳
Zhi Wu Ming Shi Tu Kao (Illustrated Guide for Nomenclature and Identification of Botanical Products)	植物名实图考
Zhong Guo Guo Yao Gu You Cheng Fang Xuan Ji (A Selection of Traditional Prescriptions of Chinese Medicine) by Chinese Herbal Medicine Committee of the Ministry of the Interior in 1967	中国国药故有成方选集
Zhong Guo Yao Dian (Dictionary of Chinese Medicine) in 1977	中国药典
Zhong Guo Yao Yong Zhi Wu Zi (Chinese Journal of Medicinal Botanicals)	中国药用植物志
Zhong Guo Zhi Wu Zi (Chinese Journal of Botany)	中国植物志
Zhong Xi Yi Jie He Zhi Liao Ji Fu Zheng (Combined Chinese and Western Medical Treatment of the Acute Abdomen) by Nankai Hospital of Tianjin in 1973	中西医结合治疗急腹症
Zhong Yao Zhi (Journal of Traditional Chinese Herbal Medicines)	中药志
Zhong Yao Zhi Ji Shou Ce (Handbook of Traditional Chinese Medicinal Preparations)	中药制剂手册
Zhong Yi Fu Ke Zhi Liao Xue (Traditional Chinese Medical Treatment of Women's Disorders) by Chengdu College of Traditional Chinese Medicine in 1970	中医妇科治疗学
Zhong Yi Nei Ke Xue (Traditional Chinese Internal Medicine) by Shanghai College of Traditional Chinese Medicine in 1970	中医内科学
Zhong Yi Shang Ke Xue (Traditional Chinese Traumatology) in 1949	中医伤科学
Zhong Yi Yan Ke Xue (Traditional Chinese Opthalmology) by Chengdu College of Traditional Chinese Medicine in 1970	中医眼科学
Zhong Zang Jing (Treasury Classic)	中藏经
Zhou Hou Bei Ji Fang (Emergency Formulas to Keep Up One's Sleeve) by Ge Hong in 341 A.D.	肘后备急方
Zhou Hou Fang (Formulas to Keep Up One's Sleeve)	肘后方

Bibliography of Contemporary References

Pinyin Names (Translated Names)	**Chinese Names**
Ai Zheng (Cancer)	癌症
An Hui Yi Xue (Anhui Medicine)	安徽医学
An Hui Zhong Yi Xue Yuan Xue Bao (Journal of Anhui University School of Medicine)	安徽中医学院学报
An Yi Xue Bao (Anyi Medical Journal)	安医学报
Bai Qiu En Yi Ke Da Xue Xue Bao (Journal of Baiqiuen University of Medicine)	白求恩医科大学学报
Bei Jing Yi Ke Da Xue Xue Bao (Journal of Beijing University of Medicine)	北京医科大学学报
Bei Jing Yi Xue (Beijing Medicine)	北京医学
Bei Jing Yi Xue Yuan Xue Bao (Journal of Beijing School of Medicine)	北京医学院学报
Bei Jing Zhong Yi (Beijing Chinese Medicine)	北京中医
Bei Jing Zhong Yi Xue Yuan Xue Bao (Journal of Beijing University School of Medicine)	北京中医学院学报
Bei Jing Zhong Yi Yao Da Xue Xue Bao (Journal of Beijing University of Medicine and Medicinals)	北京中医药大学学报
Bei Jing Zhong Yi Za Zhi (Beijing Journal of Chinese Medicine)	北京中医杂志
Ben Cao Cong Xin (Revised Herbal Materia Medica)	本草从新
Chang Chun Zhong Yi Xue Yuan Xue Bao (Journal of Changchun University of Chinese Medicine)	长春中医学院学报
Chang Yong Zhong Yao Cheng Fen Yu Yao Li Shou Ce (A Handbook of the Composition and Pharmacology of Common Chinese Drugs)	常用中药成分与药理手册
Chang Yong Zhong Yao De Ying Yong (Application of Commonly-Used Chinese Herbs)	常用中药的应用
Chang Yong Zhong Yao Xian Dai Yan Jiu Yu Lin Chuang (Recent Study & Clinical Application of Common Traditional Chinese Medicine)	常用中药现代研究与临床
Chen Tzu Yen Chiu (Acupuncture Research)	针灸研究
Cheng Du Zhong Yi Xue Yuan Xue Bao (Journal of Chengdu University of Traditional Chinese Medicine)	成都中医学院学报
Chi Jiao Yi Sheng Za Zhi (Journal of Barefoot Doctors)	赤脚医生杂志
Chong Qing Yi Yao (Chongching Medicine and Herbology)	重庆医药
Chuan Dong Zhong Yi Za Zhi (Chuandong Journal of Chinese Medicine)	川东中医杂志
Da Zhong Yi Xue (Public Medicine)	大众医学
Dang Dai Ming Yi Lin Zhen Jing Hua Zhong Liu Juan Ji (Essential Clinical Experience of Famous Modern Doctors- Cancer Volume)	当代明医临证精华-肿瘤卷辑
Di Er Jun Yi Da Xue Xue Bao (Journal of Second Military University of Medicine)	第二军医大学学报
Di Yi Jun Yi Da Xue Xue Bao (Journal of First Military University of Medicine)	第一军医大学学报
Dong Bei Zhi Wu Zhi (Northeast Journal of Herbal Medicine)	东北植物志
Dong Jing Yi Shi Xin Zhi (Tokyo Journal of Medicine)	东京医师新知
Dong Wu Xue Za Zhi (Journal of Zoology)	动物学杂志
Fang She Yi Xue (Journal of Radiology)	放射医学
Fu Chan Ke Bing Shi Yong Fang (Practical Formulas for OB/GYN Disorders)	妇产科病实用方
Fu Chan Ke Qing Bao Zi Liao (Journal of gynecology)	妇产科情报资料
Fu Jian Jun Qu Wei Sheng Bu (Health Department of Fujian Military)	福建军区卫生部
Fu Jian Sheng Yi Yao Yan Jiu Suo (Fujian Province Institute of Medicine and Herbal Research)	福建生医药研究所
Fu Jian Yi Xue Yuan Xue Bao (Journal of Fujian University of Medicine)	福建医学院学报
Fu Jian Yi Yao Za Zhi (Fujian Journal of Medicine and Herbology)	福建医药杂志
Fu Jian Yi Za Zhi (Fujian Journal of Chinese Medicine)	福建医杂志
Fu Jian Zhong Yi Yao (Fujian Chinese Medicine and Herbology)	福建中医药
Fu Ke Jing Sui (Essence of Ob/Gyn)	妇科精髓
Fu Ke Lin Chuang Jing Hua (Clinical Pearl of Ob/Gyn)	妇科临床精华
Fu Zhou Yi Yao (Fuzhou Medicine and Medicinals)	福州医药
Gan Su Zhong Yi Xue Yuan Xue Bao (Journal of Gansu University of Chinese Medicine)	甘肃中医学院学报
Guang Dong Yi Xue (Guangdong Medicine)	广东医学
Guang Dong Yi Yao Za Zhi (Guangdong Journal of Medicine and Herbology)	广东医药杂志
Guang Dong Zhong Yi (Guangdong Chinese Medicine)	广东中医
Guang Xi Chi Jiao Yi Sheng (Guangxi Barefoot Doctor)	广西赤脚医生
Guang Xi Wei Sheng (Guangxi Province Public Health)	广西卫生
Guang Xi Yi Xue (Guangxi Medicine)	广西医学

Pinyin Names (Translated Names)	Chinese Names
Guang Xi Yi Xue Yuan Xue Bao (Journal of Guangxi University of Medicine)	广西医学院学报
Guang Xi Zhi Wu (Guangxi Plants)	广西植物
Guang Xi Zhong Yi Yao (Guangxi Chinese Medicine and Herbology)	广西中医药
Guang Zhou Yi Yao (Guangzhou Medicine and Medicinals)	广州医药
Guang Zhou Zhong Yi Xue Yuan Xue Bao (Journal of Guangzhou University of Chinese Medicine)	广州中医学院学报
Gui Yang Yi Xue Yuan Xue Bao (Journal of Guiyang Medical University)	贵阳医学院学报
Gui Zhou Yao Xun (Guizhou Journal of Herbology)	贵州药讯
Gui Zhou Yi Yao (Medicine and Medicinals from Guizhou)	贵州医药
Guo Wai Yao Xue Zhi Wu Yao Fen Ce (Foreign Study of Medicine: Herbology)	国外药学植物药分册
Guo Wai Yi Xue (Foreign Medicine)	国外医学
Guo Wai Yi Xue Can Kao Za Zhi (Foreign Journal of Medicine)	国外医学参考杂志
Guo Wai Yi Xue Can Kao Zi Liao (Foreign Reference of Medicine)	国外医学参考资料
Guo Wai Yi Xue Zhong Yi Zhong Yao Fen Ce (Monograph of Chinese Herbology from Foreign Medicine)	国外医学中医中药分册
Guo Wai Yi Yao Zhi Wu Yao Fen Ce (Monograph of Foreign Botanical Medicine)	国外医药植物药分册
Ha Er Bing Yi Ke Da Xue (Haerbing University of Medicine)	哈尔滨医科大学
Ha Er Bing Yi Ke Da Xue Xue Bao (Journal of Haerbing University of Medicine)	哈尔滨医科大学学报
Ha Er Bing Zhong Yi (Haerbing Chinese Medicine)	哈尔滨中医
Ha Yi Da Xue Bao (Journal of Ha Medical University)	哈医大学报
Hai Jun Yi Xue (Navy Medicine)	海军医学
Hai Yang Yao Wu Za Zhi (Journal of Herbs from the Sea)	海洋药物杂志
Hai Yao Ben Cao (Sea of Herbal Pharmacopia)	海药本草
Han Fang Yi Xue (Kampo Medicine)	汉方医学
He Bei Xin Yi Yao (Hebei New Medicine and Herbology)	河北新医药
He Bei Yi Yao (Hebei Medicine and Herbology)	河北医药
He Bei Zhong Yi (Hebei Chinese Medicine)	河北中医
He Bei Zhong Yi Za Zhi (Hebei Journal of Chinese Medicine)	河北中医杂志
He Han Yi Yao Xue Hui Zhi (Hehan Journal of Medicine and Herbology)	和汉医药学会志
He Nan Yi Ke Da Xue Xue Bao (Journal of Henan University School of Medicine)	河南医科大学学报
He Nan Yi Xue Yuan Xue Bao (Journal of Henan University of Medicine)	河南医学院学报
He Nan Yi Yao (Henan Medicine and Herbology)	河南医药
He Nan Zhong Yi (Henan Chinese Medicine)	河南中医
He Nan Zhong Yi Xue Yuan Xue Bao (Journal of University of Henan School of Medicine)	河南中医学院学报
Hei Long Jiang Zhong Yi Yao (Heilongjiang Chinese Medicine and Herbology)	黑龙江中医药
Hu Bei Wei Sheng (Hubei Health)	湖北卫生
Hu Bei Yi Sheng (Hubei Doctor)	湖北医生
Hu Bei Yi Xue Yuan Xue Bao (Journal of Hubei College of Medicine)	湖北医学院学报
Hu Bei Zhong Yi Xue Yuan Xue Bao (Journal of Hubei University of Medicine)	湖北中医学院学报
Hu Bei Zhong Yi Za Zhi (Hubei Journal of Chinese Medicine)	湖北中医杂志
Hu Nan Sheng Jie He Bing Yan Jiu Yuan (Hunan Treatment and Research Center of Tuberculosis)	湖南省结核病研究院
Hu Nan Wei Sheng Fang Yi Tong Xun (Hunan Journal of Preventative Health)	湖南卫生防疫通讯
Hu Nan Yi Cao Gong Ye Yan Jiu (Hunan Research and Industry of Medicine and Medicinals)	湖南医草工业研究
Hu Nan Yi Ke Da Xue Xue Bao (Journal of Hunan University School of Medicine)	湖南医科大学学报
Hu Nan Yi Xue (Hunan Medicine)	湖南医学
Hu Nan Yi Xue Yuan Xue Bao (Medical Journal of Hunan University of Medicine)	湖南医学院学报
Hu Nan Yi Yao Za Zhi (Hunan Journal of Medicine and Herbology)	湖南医药杂志
Hu Nan Zhong Yi (Hunan Journal of Traditional Chinese Medicine)	湖南中医
Hu Nan Zhong Yi Xue Yuan Xue Bao (Journal of Hunan University of Traditional Chinese Medicine)	湖南中医学院学报
Hu Nan Zhong Yi Za Zhi (Hunan Journal of Chinese Medicine)	湖南中医杂志
Hua Xi Kou Qiang Yi Xue Za Zhi (Huaxi Journal of Stomatology)	华西口腔医学杂志
Hua Xi Yao Xue Za Zhi (Huaxi Herbal Journal)	华西药学杂志
Hua Xi Yi Xue Za Zhi (Huaxi Medical Journal)	华西医学杂志
Hua Xue Xue Bao (Journal of Chemistry)	化学学报

Pinyin Names (Translated Names)	**Chinese Names**
Huo Xue Hua Yu Yan Jiu (Research on Blood-Activating and Stasis-Eliminating Herbs)	活血化瘀研究
Ji Lin Wei Sheng (Jilin Public Health)	吉林卫生
Ji Lin Yi Sheng (Jilin Doctor)	吉林医生
Ji Lin Yi Xue (Jilin Medicine)	吉林医学
Ji Lin Yi Xue Yuan Xue Bao (Journal of Jilin University of Medicine)	吉林医学院学报
Ji Lin Zhong Yi Yao (Jilin Chinese Medicine and Herbology)	吉林中医药
Jiang Su Xin Yi Xue Yuan (New Jiangsu University of Medicine)	江苏新医学院
Jiang Su Yi Ke Da Xue Xue Bao (Journal of Jiangsu Universidy of Medicine)	江苏医科大学学报
Jiang Su Yi Xue (Jiangsu Medical Journal)	江苏医学
Jiang Su Yi Yao (Jiangsu Journal of Medicine and Herbology)	江苏医药
Jiang Su Zhong Yi (Jiangsu Chinese Medicine)	江苏中医
Jiang Su Zhong Yi Yao (Jiangsu Medicine and Herbology)	江苏中医药
Jiang Su Zhong Yi Za Zhi (Jiangsu Journal of Chinese Medicine)	江苏中医杂志
Jiang Xi Xin Yi Yao (Jiangxi New Medicine and Herbology)	江西新医药
Jiang Xi Yi Xue Yuan Xue Bao (Medical Journal of Jiangxi University of Medicine)	江西医学院学报
Jiang Xi Yi Yao (Jiangxi Medicine and Herbology)	江西医药
Jiang Xi Yi Yao Za Zhi (Jiangxi Journal of Medicine and Herbology)	江西医药杂志
Jiang Xi Zhong Yi Yao (Jiangxi Chinese Medicine and Herbology)	江西中医药
Jing Xian Dai 25 Wei Zhong Yi Ming Jia Fu Ke Jing Yan (Experiences of 25 Modern Ob/Gyn Experts)	近现代二十五位中医名家妇科经验
Jin Yi Ke Ji (Jinyi Science and Technology)	锦医科技
Jin Zhou Yi Xue Yuan Xue Bao (Journal of Jinzhou University of Medicine)	锦州医学院学报
Jing Fang Yan Jiu (Research of Experienced Formulas)	经方研究
Jun Shi Yi Xue Jian Xun (Military Medicine Notes)	军事医学简讯
Kang Sheng Su (Antibiotic)	抗生素
Ke Ji Tong Bao (Newspaper of Science and Technology)	科技通报
Ke Ji Tong Xun (Journal of Science and Technology)	科技通讯
Ke Ji Zi Liao (Scientific Techniques and Knowledge)	科技资料
Ke Xue Chu Ban She (Scientific Press)	科学出版社
Ke Xue Tong Bao (Journal of Science)	科学通报
Ke Yan Tong Xun (Journal of Science and Research)	科研通讯
Lan Zhou Yi Xue Yuan Xue Bao (Journal of Lanzhou University of Medicine)	兰州医学院学报
Lao Nian Xue Za Zhi (Journal of Geriatrics)	老年学杂志
Liao Ning Yi Xue (Liaoning Medicine)	辽宁医学
Liao Ning Yi Xue Za Zhi (Liaoning Journal of Medicine)	辽宁医学杂志
Liao Ning Yi Yao (Liaoning Medicine and Herbology)	辽宁医药
Liao Ning Zhong Ji Yi Kan (Liaoning Journal of Medium Medicine)	辽宁中级医刊
Liao Ning Zhong Yi (Liaoning Chinese Medicine)	辽宁中医
Liao Ning Zhong Yi Za Zhi (Liaoning Journal of Chinese Medicine)	辽宁中医杂志
Lin Chuang Gan Dan Bing Za Zhi (Clinical Journal of Hepatic and Gallbladder Diseases)	临床肝胆病杂志
Lin Chuang Pi Fu Ke Za Zhi (Journal of Clinical Dermatology)	临床皮肤科杂志
Lin Chuang Shou Ce You Du Zhong Yao Shi Yong (Clinical Handbook on Applications of Toxic Chinese Herbs)	临床手册有毒中药实用
Lin Chuang Yi Shi Zhen Liao Ji Qiao (Clinical Treatment & Techniques)	临床医师诊疗技巧
Lin Chuang Zhong Yao Xue (Clinical Chinese Pharmacology)	临床中药学
Liu Feng Wu Fu Ke Jing Yen (Experience of OB/GYN Master Liu Feng Wu)	刘奉五妇科经验
Lu Zhou Yi Xue Yuan Xue Bao (Journal of Luzhou Institution of Medicine)	泸州医学院学报
Mei Rong Mei Fa Zhong Yi Gu Fang (Ancient Chinese Formulas for Beautiful Face and Hair)	美容美发中医古方
Mei Rong Yu Wu Guan Bing Wai Zhi Du Te Xin Liao Fa (New Treatments for Cosmetology and the Five Senses)	美容与五官病外之独特新疗法
Min Guo Yi Xue Za Zhi (Medical Journal of People's Repblic of China)	民国医学杂志
Ming Yi Bie Lun (Theories of Famous Doctors)	名医别论
Nan Jing Yi Xue Yuan Xue Bao (Journal of Nanjing University of Medicine)	南京医学院学报

Pinyin Names (Translated Names)	Chinese Names
Nan Jing Zhong Yi Xue Yuan Xue Bao (Journal of Nanjing University of Traditional Chinese Medicine)	南京中医学院学报
Nan Jing Zhong Yi Yao Da Xue Xue Bao (Journal of Nanjing University of Traditional Chinese Medicine and Medicinals)	南京中医药大学学报
Nei Ke (Internal Medicine)	内科
Nei Meng Gu Zhong Yi Yao (Traditional Chinese Medicine and Medicinals of Inner Magnolia)	内蒙古中医药
Pi Fu Bing Fang Zhi Yan Jiu Tong Xun (Research Journal on Prevention and Treatment of Dermatological Disorders)	皮肤病防治研究通讯
Qing Dao Yi Xue Yuan Bao Dao (Medical Journal of Qingdao Institution)	青岛医学院报道
Qing Dao Yi Xue Yuan Xue Bao (Journal of Qingdao Institution of Medicine)	青岛医学院学报
Qing Hai Yi Yao Za Zhi (Qinghai Journal of Medicine and Herbology)	青海医药杂志
Quan Guo Zhong Yi Er Ke Xue (National Chinese Pediatrics)	全国中医儿科学
Ren Min Jun Yi (Military Reserve Medicine)	人民军医
Ren Min Wei Sheng Chu Ban She (Journal of People's Public Health)	人民卫生出版社
Ri Ben Yao Li Xue Za Zhi (Japanese Journal of Herbology)	日本药理学杂志
Ri Ben Yao Wu Xue Za Zhi (Japan Journal of Pharmacology)	日本药物学杂志
Shan Dong Ke Xue Ji Shu Chu Ban She (Shandong Science Publication)	山东科学技术出版社
Shan Dong Yi Kan (Shandong Medical Journal)	山东医刊
Shan Dong Yi Ke Da Xue Xue Bao (Journal of Shandong University of Medicine)	山东医科大学学报
Shan Dong Yi Xue Yuan Xue Bao (Journal of Shandong University School of Medicine)	山东医学院学报
Shan Dong Yi Yao (Shandong Medicine and Herbology)	山东医药
Shan Dong Yi Yao Gong Ye (Shandong Pharmaceutical Industry)	山东医药工业
Shan Dong Zhong Yi Xue Yuan Xue Bao (Journal of Shandong University School of Chinese Medicine)	山东中医学院学报
Shan Dong Zhong Yi Za Zhi (Shandong Journal of Chinese Medicine)	山东中医杂志
Shan Xi Xin Yi Yao (New Medicine and Herbology of Shanxi)	陕西新医药
Shan Xi Xin Zhong Yi (New Shanxi Chinese Medicine)	陕西新中医
Shan Xi Yi Kan (Shanxi Journal of Medicine)	陕西医刊
Shan Xi Yi Xue Za Zhi (Shanxi Journal of Medicine)	陕西医学杂志
Shan Xi Yi Yao (Shanxi Medicine and Herbology)	陕西医药
Shan Xi Yi Yao Za Zhi (Shanxi Journal of Medicine and Herbology)	陕西医药杂志
Shan Xi Zhong Yi (Shanxi Chinese Medicine)	陕西中医
Shan Xi Zhong Yi Xue Yuan Xue Bao (Journal of Shanxi University School of Chinese Medicine)	陕西中医学院学报
Shan Xi Zhong Yi Za Zhi (Shanxi Journal Chinese Medicine)	陕西中医杂志
Shang Hai Chi Jiao Yi Sheng Za Zhi (Shanghai Journal of Barefoot Doctors)	上海赤脚医生杂志
Shang Hai Di Er Yi Ke Da Xue Xue Bao (Journal of Second Shanghai University College of Medicine)	上海第二医科大学学报
Shang Hai Di Yi Xue Yuan Xue Bao (Journal of First Shanghai Medical College)	上海第一学院学报
Shang Hai Ke Xue Ji Shu Chu Ban She (Shanghi Science and Technology Publishing Company)	上海科学技术出版社
Shang Hai Ren Min Chu Ban She (People's Press of Shanghai)	上海人民出版社
Shang Hai Yao Wu Shi Yan (Shanghai Research of Medicine)	上海药物实验
Shang Hai Yi Ke Da Xue Xue Bao (Journal of Shanghai University of Medicine)	上海医科大学学报
Shang Hai Yi Xue (Shanghai Medicine)	上海医学
Shang Hai Yi Yao Za Zhi (Shanghai Journal of Medicine and Herbology)	上海医药杂志
Shang Hai Zhong Yi Xue Yuan Xue Bao (Journal of Shanghai University of Chinese Medicine)	上海中医学院学报
Shang Hai Zhong Yi Yao Za Zhi (Shanghai Journal of Chinese Medicine and Herbology)	上海中医药杂志
Shen De Yan Jiu (Research of Kidney)	肾的研究
Shen Jing Jing Shen Ji Bing Za Zhi (Journal of Psychiatric Disorders)	神经精神疾病杂志
Shen Nong Ben Cao Jing (Shen Nong Materia Medica)	神农本草经
Shen Yang Yao Xue Yuan Xue Bao (Journal of Shenyang College of Pharmacy)	沈阳药学院学报
Shen Yang Yi Xue Yuan Xue Bao (Journal of Shenyang University of Medicine)	沈阳医学院学报
Sheng Li Xue Bao (Physiology News)	生理学报
Sheng Wu Hua Xue Yu Sheng Wu Wu Li Xue Bao (Journal of Biochemistry and Biophysiology)	生物化学与生物物理学报
Sheng Yao Xue Za Zhi (Journal of Raw Herbology)	生药学杂志

Pinyin Names (Translated Names)	Chinese Names
Shi Yong Kou Qiang Yi Xue Za Zhi (Journal of Medical Stomatology)	实用口腔医学杂志
Shi Yong Nei Ke Za Zhi (Practical Journal of Internal Medicine)	实用内科杂志
Shi Yong Yi Xue Za Zhi (Practical Journal of Medicine)	实用医学杂志
Shi Yong Zhong Liu Xue Za Zhi (Practical Journal of Cancer)	实用肿瘤学杂志
Shi Yong Zhong Xi Yi Jie He Fu Ke Xue (Practical Integrated Medicine: OB/GYN)	实用中西医结合妇科学
Shi Yong Zhong Xi Yi Jie He Za Zhi (Practical Journal Integrated Chinese and Western Medicines)	实用中西医结合杂志
Shi Yong Zhong Xi Yi Jie He Zhen Duan Zhi Liao Xue (Practical Diagnostic and Therapeutics of Integrated Traditional Chinese and Western Medicine)	实用中西医结合诊断治疗学
Shi Yong Zhong Yi Mei Rong Jian Shen 3000 Fang (3000 Practical TCM Cosmetology Formulas) 3000	实用中医美容健身3000方
Shi Yong Zhong Yi Nei Ke Za Zhi (Journal of Practical Chinese Internal Medicine)	实用中医内科杂志
Shi Yong Zhong Yi Za Zhi (Journal of Practical Chinese Medicine)	实用中医杂志
Shi Zhen Guo Yao Yan Jiu (Research of Shizhen Herbs)	时珍国药研究
Shou Pi Guo Jia Ji Ming Lao Zhong Yi Xiao Yan Mi Fang Jing Xuan (Experienced Secret Formulas from Nationally Infamous TCM Doctors)	首批国家级名老中医效验秘方精选
Si Chuan Sheng Zhong Liu Fang Zhi Zi Liao Xuan Bian (Sichuan Journal of Cancer Prevention and Treatment)	四川省肿瘤防治资料选编
Si Chuan Yi Xue (Sichuan Medicine)	四川医学
Si Chuan Yi Xue Yuan Xue Bao (Journal of Sichuan School of Medicine)	四川医学院学报
Si Chuan Zhong Cao Yao Tong Xun (Sichuan Journal of Chinese Herbology)	四川中草药通讯
Si Chuan Zhong Yi (Sichuan Chinese Medicine)	四川中医
Su Zhou Yi Xue Yuan Xue Bao (Journal of Suzhou University of Medicine)	苏州医学院学报
Tai Wan Yi Xue Hui Za Zhi (Journal of Taiwan Medical Association)	台湾医学会杂志
Tai Wan Zhi Wu Yao Cao (Manual of Vegetable Drugs in Taiwan)	台湾植物药草
Te Chan Ke Xue Shi Yan (Research of Special Scientific Projects)	特产科学实验
Tian Jing Yi Xue Za Zhi (Journal of Tianjing Medicine and Herbology)	天津医学杂志
Tian Jing Yi Yao (Tianjing Medicine and Herbology)	天津医药
Tian Jing Yi Yao Tong Xun (Publication of Tianjing Medicine and Herbology)	天津医药通讯
Tian Jing Yi Yao Za Zhi (Journal of Tianjing Medicine and Herbology)	天津中医药杂志
Tian Jing Zhong Yi (Tianjing Chinese Medicine)	天津中医
Tie Dao Yi Xue (Tiedao Medicine)	铁道医学
Tong Ji Yi Ke Da Xue Xue Bao (Journal of Tongji University of Medicine)	同济医科大学学报
Wu Han Xin Yi Yao (Wuhan New Medicine and Herbology)	武汉新医药
Wu Han Xin Zhong Yi (Wuhan New Chinese Medicine)	武汉新中医
Wu Han Yi Xue Yuan Xue Bao (Journal of Wuhan University School of Medicine)	武汉医学院学报
Wu Han Yi Xue Za Zhi (Wuhan Journal of Medicine)	武汉医学杂志
Wu Shi Er Bing Fang (Fivety-two Disease Patterns & Formulas)	五十二病方
Xi An Yi Ke Da Xue Xue Bao (Journal of Xian University School of Medicine)	西安医科大学学报
Xi An Yi Xue Yuan Xue Bao (Journal of Xian University School of Medicine)	西安医学院学报
Xi Bei Yi Yao Za Zhi (Northwest Journal of Herbal Medicine)	西北医药杂志
Xi Xue Xue Bao (Academic Journal of Medicine)	西学学报
Xi Yao Yan Jiu Tong Xun (Research Journal of Medicine and Herbology)	西药研究通讯
Xian Dai Ben Cao Gang Mu (Contemporary Materia Medica)	现代本草纲目
Xian Dai Shi Yong Yao Xue (Practical Applications of Modern Herbal Medicine)	现代实用药学
Xian Dai Zhong Yao Yao Li Xue (Contemporary Pharmacology of Chinese Herbs)	现代中药药理学
Xiang Cun Yi Xue (Suburban Medicine)	乡村医学
Xiang Gang Zhong Yi Yao Nian Jian (Chinese Medicine and Medicinals of Hong Kong)	香港中医药年鉴
Xin Hua Ben Cao Gang Mu (New Chinese Materia Medica)	新华本草纲目
Xin Jiang Zhong Yi Yao (Xinjiang Chinese Medicine and Herbology)	新疆中医药
Xin Yao Yu Lin Chuang (New Medicine and the Clinical Application)	新药与临床
Xin Yi Xue (New Medicine)	新医学
Xin Yi Yao Tong Xun (Journal of New Medicine and Herbology)	新医药通讯
Xin Yi Yao Xue Za Zhi (New Journal of Medicine and Herbology)	新医药学杂志
Xin Zhang Xue Guan Ji Bing (Cardiovascular Diseases)	心脏血管疾病

Pinyin Names (Translated Names)	Chinese Names
Xin Zhong Yao Xue (New Chinese Herbal Medicine)	新中药学
Xin Zhong Yi (New Chinese Medicine)	新中医
Yao Jian Gong Zuo Tong Xun (Journal of Herbal Preparations)	药检工作通讯
Yao Li Shi Yan Fang Fa Xue (Research Methodology of Herbal Medicine)	药理实验方法学
Yao Li Xue (Pharmacology)	药理学
Yao Wu Fen Xi Za Zhi (Journal of Herbal Analysis)	药物分析杂志
Yao Xue Qing Bao Tong Xun (Journal of Herbal Information)	药学情报通讯
Yao Xue Tong Bao (Report of Herbology)	药学通报
Yao Xue Xue Bao (Journal of Herbology)	药学学报
Yao Xue Za Zhi (Journal of Medicinals)	药学杂志
Yao Yong Zhi Wu Da Ci Dian (Encyclopedia of Medicinal Herbs)	药用植物大辞典
Yi Fang Xin Jie (New Explanation for Medical Formulas)	医方新解
Yi Xue Ji Shu Zi Liao (Resource of Medical Techniques)	医学技术资料
Yi Xue Qing Kuang Jiao Liu (Medical Information Exchange)	医学情况交流
Yi Xue Wei Sheng Tong Xun (Journal of Medicine and Sanitation)	医学卫生通讯
Yi Xue Xue Bao (Report of Medicine)	医学学报
Yi Xue Yan Jiu Tong Xun (Report of Medical Studies)	医学研究通讯
Yi Xue Zhong Yang Za Zhi (Central Journal of Medicine)	医学中央杂志
Yi Yao Gong Ye (Pharmaceutical Industry)	医药工业
Yi Yao Ke Ji Za Zhi (Journal of Medical Technology)	医药科技杂志
Yi Yao Wei Sheng (Medicine, Medicinals, and Sanitation)	医药卫生
Yi Yao Xue (Study of Medicine and Medicinals)	医药学
Yi Yao Yan Jiu Tong Xun (Research Journal of Medicine and Medicinals)	医药研究通讯
Yi Yao Za Zhi (Journal of Medicine and Herbology)	医药杂志
Ying Yang Xue Bao (Report of Nutrition)	营养学报
Yu Bei Yi Xue Zhuan Ke Xue Xiao (Yubei University of Medicine)	预备医学专科科学校
Yun Nan Yi Xue Za Zhi (Yunan Journal of Medicine)	云南医学杂志
Yun Nan Yi Yao (Yunan Medicine and Herbology)	云南医药
Yun Nan Zhong Yao Zhi (Yunan Journal of Chinese Herbal Medicine)	云南中药志
Yun Nan Zhong Yi (Yunnan Journal of Traditional Chinese Medicine)	云南中医
Yun Nan Zhong Yi Xue Yuan Xue Bao (Journal of Yunnan University School of Medicine)	云南中医学院学报
Yun Nan Zhong Yi Za Zhi (Yunan Journal of Chinese Medicine)	云南中医杂志
Zhe Jiang Min Jian Chang Yong Cao Yao (Commonly Used Herbs in Zhejiang)	浙江民间常用草药
Zhe Jiang Wei Sheng Shi Yan Yuan (Zhejiang Department of Health Research)	浙江卫生实验院
Zhe Jiang Yao Xue (Zhejiang Journal of Chinese Herbology)	浙江药学
Zhe Jiang Yi Ke Da Xue Xue Bao (Journal of Zhejiang Province School of Medicine)	浙江医科大学学报
Zhe Jiang Yi Xue (Zhejiang Journal of Medicine)	浙江医学
Zhe Jiang Zhong Yi Xue Yuan Xue Bao (Journal of Zhejiang University of Chinese Medicine)	浙江中医学院学报
Zhe Jiang Zhong Yi Yao (Zhejiang Chinese Medicine and Herbology)	浙江中医药
Zhe Jiang Zhong Yi Za Zhi (Zhejiang Journal of Chinese Medicine)	浙江中医杂志
Zhi Wu Yao You Xiao Cheng Fen Shou Ce (Manual of Plant Medicinals and Their Active Constituents)	植物药有效成份手册
Zhi Wu Zi Yuan Yu Huan Jing (Source and Environment of Plants)	植物资源与环境
Zhong Cao Tong Xun (Journal of Chinese Herbs)	中草通讯
Zhong Cao Yao (Chinese Herbal Medicine)	中草药
Zhong Cao Yao Cheng Fen Hua Xue (Composition and Chemistry of Chinese Herbs)	中草药成分化学
Zhong Cao Yao Fang Ji De Ying Yong (Applications of Chinese Herbal Formulas)	中草药方剂的应用
Zhong Cao Yao Tong Xun (Journal of Chinese Herbal Medicine)	中草药通讯
Zhong Cao Yao Xue (Study of Chinese Herbal Medicine)	中草药学
Zhong Cao Yao Yao Li Xue (Herbology of Chinese Medicinals)	中草药药理学
Zhong Cheng Yao (Study of Chinese Patent Medicine)	中成药
Zhong Cheng Yao Yan Jiu (Research of Chinese Patent Medicine)	中成药研究
Zhong Guo Bing Li Sheng Li Za Zhi (Chinese Journal of Pathology and Biology)	中国病理生理杂志
Zhong Guo Fang Lao (Chinese Prevention of Tuberculosis)	中国防劳
Zhong Guo Fang Lao Za Zhi (Chinese Journal on Prevention of Tuberculosis)	中国防劳杂志

Pinyin Names (Translated Names)	Chinese Names
Zhong Guo Gang Chang Bing Za Zhi (Chinese Journal of Proctology)	中国肛肠病杂志
Zhong Guo Gang Chang Za Zhi (Chinese Journal of Anus and Intestines)	中国肛肠杂志
Zhong Guo Kang Fu Yi Xue Za Zhi (Chinese Journal of Rehabilitation)	中国康复医学杂志
Zhong Guo Mian Yi Xue Za Zhi (Chinese Journal of Immunology)	中国免疫学杂志
Zhong Guo Nong Cun Yi Xue (Chinese Agricultural Medicine)	中国农村医学
Zhong Guo Shen Jing Jing Shen Ke Za Zhi (Chinese Journal of Psychiatric Disorders)	中国神经精神科杂志
Zhong Guo Sheng Li Ke Xue Hui, Di Er Ci Hui (Chinese Convention on Biophysiology, 2nd Annual Convention)	中国生理科学会第二次会
Zhong Guo Shi Yong Nei Ke Za Zhi (Chinese Journal of Practical Internal Medicine)	中国实用内科杂志
Zhong Guo Shou Yi Za Zhi (Chinese Journal of Husbandry)	中国兽医杂志
Zhong Guo Xiang Cun Xin Xi (Suburb Doctors of China)	中国乡村信息
Zhong Guo Yao Chai Xue (Chinese Herbal Botany)	中国药柴学
Zhong Guo Yao Ci Dian (Journal of Chinese Medicinal Plants)	中国药辞典
Zhong Guo Yao Ke Da Xue Xue Bao (Journal of University of Chinese Herbology)	中国药科大学学报
Zhong Guo Yao Li Tong Xun (Journal of Chinese Herbal Studies)	中国药理通讯
Zhong Guo Yao Li Xue Bao (Chinese Herbal Pharmacology Journal)	中国药理学报
Zhong Guo Yao Li Xue Tong Bao (Journal of Chinese Herbal Pharmacology)	中国药理学通报
Zhong Guo Yao Li Xue Yu Du Li Xue Za Zhi (Journal of Herbology and Toxicology)	中国药理学与毒理学杂志
Zhong Guo Yao Xue Da Ci Dian (Grand Dictionary of Chinese Herbal Medicine)	中国药学大辞典
Zhong Guo Yi Ke Da Xue Xue Bao (Journal of University of Chinese Medicine)	中国医科大学学报
Zhong Guo Yi Xue Ke Xue Xue Bao (Journal of Chinese Medical Science University)	中国医学科学学报
Zhong Guo Yi Yao Bao (Chinese Journal of Medicine and Medicinals)	中国医药报
Zhong Guo Yi Yao Ke Xue Yuan Lun Wen Zhai Yao (Abstract from Chinese University of Medicine and Science)	中国医药科学院论文摘要
Zhong Guo Yi Yao Xue Bao (Chinese Journal of Medicine and Herbology)	中国医药学报
Zhong Guo Yi Yuan Yao Xue Za Zhi (Chinese Hospital Journal of Herbology)	中国医院药学杂志
Zhong Guo Zhong Xi Yi Jie He Za Zhi (Chinese Journal of Integrative Chinese and Western Medicine)	中国中西医结合杂志
Zhong Guo Zhong Yao Za Zhi (People's Republic of China Journal of Chinese Herbology)	中国中药杂志
Zhong Hua Bing Li Xue Za Zhi (Chinese Journal of Pathology)	中华病理学杂志
Zhong Hua Er Bi Hou Ke Za Zhi (Chinese Journal of ENT)	中华耳鼻喉科杂志
Zhong Hua Er Ke Za Zhi (Chinese Journal of Pediatrics)	中华儿科杂志
Zhong Hua Fu Chan Ke Za Zhi (Chinese Journal of OB/GYN)	中华妇产科杂志
Zhong Hua Ji Sheng Chong Chuan Ran Bing Za Zhi (Chinese Journal of Infectious Parasitic Diseases)	中华寄生虫传染病杂志
Zhong Hua Jie He Bing Ke Za Zhi (Chinese Journal of Tuberculosis)	中华结核病科杂志
Zhong Hua Kou Qiang Ke Za Zhi (Chinese Journal of Stomatology)	中华口腔科杂志
Zhong Hua Mi Niao Wai Ke (Chinese Journal of Urology and External Medicine)	中华泌尿外科
Zhong Hua Nei Ke Xue Za Zhi (Journal of Chinese Internal Medicine)	中华内科学杂志
Zhong Hua Nei Ke Za Zhi (Chinese Journal of Internal Medicine)	中华内科杂志
Zhong Hua Pi Fu Ke Xue Za Zhi (Chinese Journal of Dermatology)	中华皮肤科学杂志
Zhong Hua Ren Min Gong He Guo Yao Dian (Chinese Herbal Pharmacopoeia by People's Republic of China)	中华人民共和国药典
Zhong Hua Shen Jing Jing Shen Ke Za Zhi (Chinese Journal of Neurology and Psychiatry)	中华神经精神科杂志
Zhong Hua Wai Ke Za Zhi (Chinese Journal of External Medicine)	中华外科杂志
Zhong Hua Xin Xue Guan Bing Za Zhi (Chinese Journal of Cardiology)	中华心血管病杂志
Zhong Hua Xin Yi Xue Bao (Chinese Journal of New Medicine)	中华新医学报
Zhong Hua Xue Yi Xue Za Zhi (Chinese Journal on Study of Hematology)	中华血液学杂志
Zhong Hua Xue Yi Za Zhi (Chinese Journal of Hematology)	中华血液杂志
Zhong Hua Yan Ke Za Zhi (Chinese Journal of Ophthalmology)	中华眼科杂志
Zhong Hua Yi Liao Za Zhi (Journal of Chinese Therapies)	中华医疗杂志
Zhong Hua Yi Xue Za Zhi (Chinese Journal of Medicine)	中华医学杂志
Zhong Hua Yi Yao Xue Bao (Chinese Journal of Medicinal and Herbology)	中华医药学报
Zhong Hua Yu Fang Yi Xue Za Zhi (Chinese Journal of Preventative Medicine)	中华预防医学杂志

Pinyin Names (Translated Names)	**Chinese Names**
Zhong Hua Zhong Liu Za Zhi (Chinese Journal of Cancer)	中华肿瘤杂志
Zhong Ji Yi Kan (Medium Medical Journal)	中级医刊
Zhong Liu Bian Bing Zhuan Fang Zhi Liao (Differential Diagnosis and Treatment for Cancer)	肿瘤辨病专方治疗
Zhong Liu Yu Fang Yan Jiu (Tumor Prevention and Research)	肿瘤预防研究
Zhong Liu Yu Zhi Tong Xun (Journal of Prevention and Treatment of Cancer)	肿瘤预治通讯
Zhong Xi Yi Jie He Fang Zhi Yan Jiu Xue Guan Zhi Liao (Research on Prevention and Treatment of Cardiovascular Disorders Using Integrated Chinese and Western Medicines)	中西医结合防治研究血管治疗
Zhong Xi Yi Jie He Yan Jiu Zi Liao (Research Information on Ingration of Chinese and Western Medicine)	中西医结合研究资料
Zhong Xi Yi Jie He Za Zhi (Journal of Integrated Chinese and Western Medicine)	中西医结合杂志
Zhong Xi Yi Yao Za Zhi (Journal of Chinese and Western Medicine)	中西医药杂志
Zhong Yao Bu Liang Fan Ying Yu Zhi Liao (Adverse Reactions and Treatment of Chinese Herbal Medicine)	中药不良反应与治疗
Zhong Yao Cai (Study of Chinese Herbal Material)	中药材
Zhong Yao Cai Ke Ji (Science and Technology of Chinese Herbal Material)	中药材科技
Zhong Yao Ci Hai (Encyclopedia of Chinese Herbs)	中药辞海
Zhong Yao Da Ci Dian (Dictionary of Chinese Herbs)	中药大辞典
Zhong Yao Du Li Xue (Toxicology of Chinese Herbs)	中药毒理学
Zhong Yao Lin Zheng Ying Yong (Clinical Applications of Chinese Herbs)	中药淋症应用
Zhong Yao Tong Bao (Journal of Chinese Herbology)	中药通报
Zhong Yao Xian Dai Yan Jiu Yu Ying Yong (Modern Study of Traditional Chinese Medicine)	中药现代研究与应用
Zhong Yao Xue (Chinese Herbology)	中药学
Zhong Yao Yan Jiu (Research of Chinese Herbology)	中药研究
Zhong Yao Yao Li Du Li Yu Lin Chuang (Pharmacology, Toxicology and Clinical Applications of Chinese Herbs)	中药药理毒理与临床
Zhong Yao Yao Li Xue (Study of Chinese Herbology)	中药药理学
Zhong Yao Yao Li Yu Du Li Za Zhi (Journal of Pharmacology and Toxicology of Chinese Herbs)	中药药理与毒理杂志
Zhong Yao Yao Li Yu Lin Chuang (Pharmacology and Clinical Applications of Chinese Herbs)	中药药理与临床
Zhong Yao Yao Li Yu Ying Yong (Pharmacology and Applications of Chinese Herbs)	中药药理与应用
Zhong Yao Yu Jian Mei (Chinese Herbs and Beauty)	中药与健美
Zhong Yao Zhi (Chinese Herbology Journal)	中药志
Zhong Yi Er Ke Za Zhi (Chinese Medical Journal of Pediatrics)	中医儿科杂志
Zhong Yi Fang Ji De Yao Li Yu Ying Yong (Pharmacology and Applications of Chinese Herbal Formulas)	中医方剂的药理与应用
Zhong Yi Fang Ji Xian Dai Yan Jiu (Modern Study of Medical Formulae in Traditional Chinese Medicine)	中医方剂现代研究
Zhong Yi Fu Ke Xue (TCM OB/GYN)	中医妇科学
Zhong Yi Han Shou Tong Xun (Reports of Chinese Medicine)	中医函授通讯
Zhong Yi Yan Jiu Yuan (Research Hospital of Chinese Medicine)	中医研究院
Zhong Yi Yao Li (Pharmacology of Chinese Herbs)	中医药理
Zhong Yi Yao Xin Xi (Information on Chinese Medicine and Herbology)	中医药信息
Zhong Yi Yao Xue Bao (Report of Chinese Medicine and Herbology)	中医药学报
Zhong Yi Yao Yan Jiu (Research of Chinese Medicine and Herbology)	中医药研究
Zhong Yi Yao Yan Jiu Can Kao (Research and Discussion of Chinese Medicine and Herbology)	中医药研究参考
Zhong Yi Yao Yan Jiu Zi Liao (Research and Resource of Chinese Medicine and Herbology)	中医药研究资料
Zhong Yi Za Zhi (Journal of Chinese Medicine)	中医杂志
Zhong Yuan Yi Kan (Resource Journal of Chinese Medicine)	中原医刊

Glossary

The first column consists of the terms used in the body of the text. Subsequent columns provide correlation to the Chinese characters, pinyin transliteration, previous translation by Wiseman and Feng, and finally, a definition of the term.

When a Chinese term is important to the understanding of a theoretical or clinical concept, or when it is a term familiar to many students and practitioners of Chinese Herbal Medicine, that term is given in pinyin in the text, with an accompanying translation, if needed. However, for lesser-known terms, English translations have been used in the body of the text, with the glossary provided to assist interested individuals in making connections with the Chinese.

The authors have carefully considered the translation of each term and have offered the clearest and most practical translation they could discover, based on consideration both of the Chinese terminology and nuances of standard American English usage. In some cases, this differs slightly from translations offered by Wiseman and Feng, which we have included here for purposes of assisting researchers already familiar with their work. These small differences in no way diminish our respect for and appreciation of the diligence with which our esteemed colleagues have worked to provide thorough, extensive and effective bridges in understanding via their work.

Terminology	Chinese	Pinyin	Wiseman & Feng	Definition
5 a.m. diarrhea	五更泄	*Wu Geng Xie*	fifth-watch diarrhea	Characterized by early morning (approximately 5 a.m.) diarrhea, this is often caused by Kidney deficiency.
accumulation	积聚	*Ji Ju*	accumulation and gathering	An inclusive term describing the accumulation of *ji* (yin substances) and *ju* (yang substances), that may occur in any organ. Clinical presentation differs, depending on the area(s) and organ(s) affected.
ah shi point	阿是穴	*Ah Shi Xue*	a-shi point	A type of acupuncture point having no fixed location or name, but corresponding to an underlying disorder. Stimulating an *ah shi* point elicits tenderness and pain.
Ba Gang Bian Zheng (Eight Principle Differentiation)	八纲辨证	*Ba Gang Bian Zheng*	eight-principle pattern identification	A system of differential diagnosis based on patterns of imbalance or disharmony of the eight factors of exterior and interior location, cold and hot attributes, deficiency and excess states, and yin and yang qualities.
ben tun (running piglet)	奔豚	*Ben Tun*	running piglet	A sensation of qi rushing upwards from the lower abdomen to the chest, epigastrium and throat. There will generally be concurrent pain, discomfort, alternation of heat and cold, and palpitations.
beng lou (flooding and spotting)	崩漏	*Beng Lou*	flooding and spotting	A condition that includes massive uterine bleeding at irregular intervals and incessant dripping of blood from the uterus.
bi zheng (closed disorder)	闭证	*Bi Zheng*	block pattern	Characterized by clenched jaws, tight fists, unconsciousness, warm body and cold extremities, this generally occurs in wind stroke or febrile disorders, with heat attacking *ying* (nutritive) and *xue* (blood) levels.
bi zheng (painful obstruction syndrome)	痹证	*Bi Zheng*	impediment pattern	A pain condition characterized by stagnation and obstruction that may affect any tissue and/or organ.

Terminology	Chinese	Pinyin	Wiseman & Feng	Definition
blood	血	*Xue*	blood	The red viscous fluid in the body that comprises nutrients, body fluids and Kidney *jing* (essence).
blood deficiency	血虚	*Xue Xu*	blood vacuity	Pale, lusterless face, pale lips, dizziness, vertigo, palpitations, insomnia, coldness and numbness of the extremities, and a thready, weak pulse illustrate this condition, caused by loss of blood, excessive thinking and worrying, the presence of parasites, or injury to the internal organs.
blood dessication	血枯	*Xue Ku*	blood desiccation	Following profuse loss of blood, a condition characterized by dizziness, feeling of weightlessness of the extremities, and amenorrhea.
blood stagnation/stasis	血瘀	*Xue Yu*	blood stasis	A condition characterized by obstructed blood flow, leading to dark purplish skin color, dried or scaly skin, pain at a fixed location, pain that intensifies with pressure, fullness and distention of the lower abdomen, amenorrhea, black tarry stools, and a dark purple tongue with black spots. Blood stagnation/stasis may be caused by external injuries, menstrual irregularities, qi stagnation and cold stagnation. Blood stagnation refers to mild to moderate obstruction of blood circulation. Blood stasis refers to moderate to severe obstruction of blood circulation, possibly with clotting.
body fluids	津液	*Jin Ye*	fluids	An all-inclusive term that describes all the fluids in the body, including tears, saliva, sweat, blood and fluids that lubricate the joints.
breast abscess	乳痈	*Ru Yong*	mammary welling-abscess	A hard breast abscess accompanied by distention and pain, chills and fever, and obstructed flow of breast milk, this is generally caused by Liver qi stagnation, Stomach fire, and stasis of breast milk.
chang feng (intestinal wind)	肠风	*Chang Feng*	intestinal wind	A condition caused by wind attacking the intestines, leading to the presence of bright red blood in the stools.
chi position	尺	*Chi*	cubit	The third (most proximal) position on the wrist for pulse diagnosis, it represents Kidney yang (right hand) and Kidney yin (left hand).
chong (thoroughfare) channel	冲脉	*Chong Mai*	thoroughfare vessel	One of the eight extraordinary vessels, it controls the twelve channels. Also known as the "Sea of Blood," as it has functions related to blood and gynecology.
clumping	结	*Jie*	bind	This describes the formation of a solid mass or masses from one or more substances, such as phlegm, heat or cold.
cold	寒	*Han*	cold	Cold is a yin pathogenic factor that attacks both the outside and inside of the body and is characterized by contraction and stagnation. Clinical presentation of cold includes chills, shivering, aversion to cold, cold extremities, pale face and lips, the presence of undigested food in the stools, and clear urine.

Terminology	Chinese	Pinyin	Wiseman & Feng	Definition
collapse	厥	*Jue*	reversal	A condition of sudden collapse and loss of consciousness, that generally can be reversed. The causes of collapse include cold, heat, phlegm and dietary injury, among others.
controlling sequence	相克	*Xiang Ke*	restraining	A concept of *wu xing* (five element) theory that describes the orderly sequence in which one element controls the growth of another.
cun position	寸	*Cun*	cun	The first (most distal) position on the wrist for pulse diagnosis, it represents the Lung (right hand) and the Heart (left hand).
dai (girdle) channel	带脉	*Dai Mai*	girdling vessel	Another of the eight extraordinary vessels, this one serves to bind all of the channels together, and influences lower extremity function.
damp	湿	*Shi*	damp	Damp is a pathogenic factor that occurs mainly in the late summer or in places with high humidity. Dampness is characterized by heaviness and turbidity, which may lead to such symptoms as feeling heaviness in the head and extremities, general fatigue, and fullness in the chest and epigastrium. Dampness is also characterized by increased viscosity of substances and stagnation, such as in cases of abscesses, oozing ulcers, leukorrhea with foul discharge, and arthritis.
de qi (arrival of qi)	的气	*De Qi*	obtaining qi	Qi sensation (numbness, pressure, swelling, warmth or other) that follows insertion and manipulation of acupuncture needles.
debilitation	劳	*Lao*	taxation	Generalized weakness resulting from persistent mental and physical wear and tear on the body.
deficiency	虚	*Xu*	vacuity	Deficiency refers to a state of insufficiency (such as deficiency of qi, blood, yin or yang), or decreased ability of the organ to carry out its normal physiological functions (Spleen deficiency, Kidney deficiency, and so on). Deficiency occurs due to congenital deficiency, lack of nourishment, or long-term illness.
dian kuang (mania and withdrawal)	癫狂	*Dian Kuang*	mania and withdrawal	An inclusive term for various types of mental illness. *Dian* (withdrawal) represents yin disorders: the individual is quiet and socially inactive. *Kuang* (mania) represents yang disorders: the individual is irritable, restless, and physically active.
drooling phlegm	痰涎	*Tan Xian*	phlegm-drool	Characterized by profuse dripping of saliva in children, this is generally caused by wind-heat attacking the Spleen, resulting in its inability to properly process water.
drum-like abdominal distention	鼓胀	*Gu Zhang*	drum distention	Characterized by severe fullness and distention, resulting in the abdomen resembling a drum, this may be caused by emotional constraint, inappropriate diet, excessive use of alcohol, or intestinal parasites.

Terminology	Chinese	Pinyin	Wiseman & Feng	Definition
dryness	乾	*Gan*	dry	Dryness is a pathogenic factor that invades the body in late autumn when there is a lack of moisture in the environment. Dryness consumes yin and body fluids, and may lead to clinical presentations such as dry and chapped skin, dryness of the mouth and throat, thirst, dry cough with little sputum, and so on.
du (governing) channel	督脉	*Du Mai*	governing vessel	Confluence of all yang vessels, one of the eight extraordinary vessels, also known as the "Sea of Yang Qi." It influences brain and spinal column functioning.
dysentery	痢疾	*Li Ji*	dysentery	A disorder characterized by abdominal pain, increased frequency but decreased volume of bowel movements, tenesmus, and the presence of undigested food, mucus, and blood in the stool.
earth	土	*Tu*	earth	Another of the five elements, earth corresponds to ripeness and late summer, to sweet flavors, transformation, and centeredness. The corresponding organ is the Spleen.
epidemic toxin	疫毒	*Yi Du*	epidemic toxin	An epidemic pathogenic factor that attacks and affects the entire community, regardless of individual health and constitution.
epilepsy	痫证	*Xian Zheng*	epilepsy pattern	Characterized by altered consciousness and muscle convulsions, this disorder occurs frequently in children because they have not yet gained fully-developed defenses against external pathogens. Factors commonly causing seizure include wind, heat, phlegm and inappropriate diet.
excess	实	*Shi*	repletion	Excess refers to the state of surplus or overload that creates a pathologic condition in the body, such as when there is excess heat, formation or accumulation of phlegm, or blood stagnation, among others. Excess conditions occur in the case of invasion of exogenous pathogenic factors or in disharmony of the internal organs.
exterior	表	*Biao*	exterior	The outside of the body, such as the skin, mouth, nose and nostrils. Pathogenic factors are often said to attack the exterior prior to invading the interior. The clinical presentation of an exterior syndrome includes headache, muscle aches and pain, nasal congestion, coughing and so on.
exterior and interior	表里	*Biao Li*	exterior and interior	A term used to indicate differentiation between the exterior and interior parts of the body.
febrile diseases	热病	*Re Bing*	heat disease	A term that describes all externally-contracted diseases characterized by heat.
fire	火	*Huo*	fire	Fire is one of the five elements, associated with upward movement of energy, the sparkling flaring of fire, and summer. The corresponding organ is the Heart. In disease terminology, fire is a yang pathogenic factor representing a severe form of heat.

Terminology	Chinese	Pinyin	Wiseman & Feng	Definition
five elements	五行	*Wu Xing*	five phases	A theory which evaluates all things according to elements of water, wood, fire, earth and metal. The theory is also used to explain anatomy, physiology, and pathology of the human body, as well as treatment strategies.
floating edema	浮肿	*Fu Zhong*	puffy swelling	A symptom characterized by fluid accumulation in superficial parts of the body, this is generally caused by Lung, Spleen or Kidney deficiency, and the consequent inability to properly regulate water metabolism pathways.
focal distention	痞满	*Pi Man*	glomus fullness	Fullness, distention and oppression in the chest and abdomen, caused by food retention, phlegm stagnation, and/or damp-heat accumulation.
fright and palpitations	惊悸	*Jing Ji*	fright palpitations	A condition of emotional instability and increased sensitivity to stimulus caused by Heart qi deficiency.
frightened wind	惊风	*Jing Feng*	fright wind	Literally "frightened wind," this describes seizures and convulsions in children. It is most common in children under the age of five, with incidence gradually decreasing with increased age. Clinical presentation includes high fever, red eyes, convulsion, opisthotonos, clenched jaws, tight fists, eyes rolled up, and urinary and bowel incontinence.
fu (hollow organ)	腑	*Fu*	bowel	The hollow organs of the body are the Small Intestine, Large Intestine, Gallbladder, Stomach and Urinary Bladder.
Gallbladder	胆	*Dan*	gallbladder	Paired with the Liver, the Gallbladder stores bile and excretes it to the intestines to facilitate digestion.
gan ji (infantile malnutrition)	疳疾	*Gan Ji*	gan disease	A disorder characterized by the inability of the Spleen and Stomach to properly transform and transport food. Generally occurring in children under five years of age, *gan ji* is characterized by sallow facial appearance, weight loss, thin hair, poor appetite, abdominal distention, and irregular bowel movements.
gao lin (cloudy dysuria)	膏淋	*Gao Lin*	unctuous strangury	A urinary tract disorder in which the urine has a milky or cloudy appearance, and may be slightly pink (an indication of bleeding). This is caused by damp-heat attacking the Urinary Bladder, leading to the bladder's inability to clear turbid substances.
generating sequence	相生	*Xiang Sheng*	engendering	A concept of *wu xing* (five element) theory that describes the orderly sequence in which one element promotes the generation of another.
gu (food) *qi*	谷气	*Gu Qi*		Qi that is derived from the ingestion and absorption of food.
guan position	关	*Guan*	bar	The second (middle) position on the wrist for pulse diagnosis represents the Spleen (right hand) and the Liver (left hand).

Terminology	Chinese	Pinyin	Wiseman & Feng	Definition
half-body perspiration	半身汗	*Ban Shen Han*		Half-body perspiration refers to sweating only on half of the body, such as the left or right side, or upper or lower half. This condition occurs because of obstruction of the channels and collaterals caused by wind-phlegm or wind-damp. It may also be caused by disharmony of qi and blood, or of *ying* (nutritive) and *wei* (defense) levels.
he (uniting) point	合穴	*He Xue*	uniting point	Known as "uniting" or "sea" points, these represent the flow of qi where it is vast and deep, near the elbows or knees.
he xi feng (crane's knee wind)	鹤膝风	*He Xi Feng*	crane's-knee wind	A condition in which the knees are swollen and enlarged, but the muscles above and below the knees are atrophied.
Heart	心	*Xin*	heart	The Heart functions to control the blood channels and house the *shen* (spirit). It connects to the Small Intestine and opens to the tongue, and is associated with the fire element.
heat	热	*Re*	heat	Heat is a yang pathogenic factor that attacks both external and internal aspects of the body; it is characterized by the tendency to disperse outwards and to consume yin and fluids. Clinical presentations of heat include a wide variety of signs and symptoms, such as fever, inflammation, infection, bleeding, and others.
heat in the blood	血热	*Xue Re*	blood heat	A condition characterized by nosebleeds, coughing of blood, and late-afternoon fever, because of heat affecting the *xue* (blood) level.
hernial disorder	疝气	*Shan Qi*	mounting qi	Historically, this TCM term covers a wide variety of disorders related to both internal and external genitalia, in men and women. More recently, it refers specifically to disorders of the male external genitalia (testicles and scrotum).
hui (influential) point	会穴	*Hui Xue*	meeting point	Referred to as "meeting" or "influential" points, these eight points individually represent either *zang*, *fu*, qi, blood, tendons, channels, bones or marrow.
hun (ethereal soul)	魂	*Hun*	ethereal soul	Similar to the Western interpretation of "soul" or "spirit," the *hun* functions to maintain mental and psychological health and well-being. It has been said that the Liver stores blood, and blood contains *hun*. Therefore, disorders of the *hun* are often secondary to the inability of the Liver to store blood; or, secondary to deficiency of Liver blood.
insulting sequence	相侮	*Xiang Wu*	rebellion	A concept of *wu xing* (five element) theory that describes the situation in which an element normally controlled by another reverses the sequence and suppresses or reduces what is normally the controlling element.

Terminology	Chinese	Pinyin	Wiseman & Feng	Definition
interior	里	*Li*	interior	Internal aspects of the body, such as organs, bone marrow, and the *qi* (energy) and *xue* (blood) levels. Pathogenic factors may affect the interior of the body directly or indirectly (via the exterior). Clinical presentation of interior conditions varies significantly, depending on the area and/or organs affected.
intestinal abscess	肠痈	*Chang Yong*	intestinal welling-abscess	Intestinal abscesses generally arise from inappropriate diet or emotional disturbances (excessive anger or worry), and are characterized by abdominal pain.
irritability	烦	*Fan*	vexation	A state of impatience, anger, annoyance, and increased sensitivity to stimulus.
jin (thin body fluid)	津	*Jin*	liquid	An inclusive term that describes body fluids of lesser density, such as tears, saliva and sweat.
jing (essence)	精	*Jing*	essence	The basic substance that makes up the human body and sustains the vital functions of the internal organs. Derived prenatally from one's parents, and postnatally from food, essence is stored in the Kidney.
jing (river) point	经穴	*Jing Xue*	river point	Commonly referred to as either "traversing" or "river" points, these suggest that the flow of qi at the forearms or lower legs has attained a large volume.
jing (well) point	井穴	*Jing Xue*	well point	"Well" points represent the beginning of qi circulation within channels, at the most distal parts of the body, where qi flow is still small and shallow.
jueyin	厥阴	*Jue Yin*	reverting yin	The last of six stages in the paradigm of yin and yang. This describes the degree of pathology of disease according to the *Shang Han Lun* (Cold-Induced Disorders) text. It also identifies the level attributed to the Liver and Pericardium channels that travel throughout the body.
Kidney	肾	*Shen*	kidney	The Kidney controls growth, maturation, reproduction and aging. It produces marrow that forms the brain and spinal cord, and it promotes production of bones and blood. Furthermore, it dominates body fluids and receives qi from air via the Lung. Associated with the water element, the Kidney connects with the Urinary Bladder, opens to the ears, and houses the faculty of *zhi* (will power).
lao lin (fatigue dysuria)	劳淋	*Lao Lin*	taxation strangury	A urinary tract disorder involving increased frequency of urination, especially with physical stress and exertion. Accompanying symptoms include fatigue, lower back and knee soreness and pain, with dribbling urine, but no pain during urination. This is caused when prolonged exertion leads to Spleen and Kidney exhaustion and inability to control the normal flow of water and urination.
Large Intestine	大肠	*Da Chang*	large intestine	Connected to the Small Intestine, the Large Intestine absorbs nutrients and water from food.

Terminology	Chinese	Pinyin	Wiseman & Feng	Definition
leg *qi*	脚气	*Jiao Qi*	leg qi	A disorder of the leg(s) characterized by numbness, soreness, pain, weakness, possible swelling and cramps, and possible atrophy of leg muscles. Accompanying symptoms may include nausea, vomiting, dyspnea, incoherent speech, and palpitations. Generally caused by wind, damp, and toxins attacking the legs, it overlaps in symptomology with beriberi.
lin zheng (dysuria syndrome)	淋证	*Lin Zheng*	strangury pattern	Dysuria syndrome refers to a condition of frequent and painful urination, abdominal pain, and/or pain radiating to the lower back.
Liu Jing Bian Zheng (Six Stages Differentiation)	六经辨证	*Liu Jing Bian Zheng*	six-channel pattern identification	A system of differential diagnosis based on identifying patterns of disharmony by relationship to the energetic stages *taiyang, yangming, shaoyang, taiyin, shaoyin,* and *jueyin.*
Liver	肝	*Gan*	liver	The Liver stores blood, maintains proper flow of qi, and controls tendons. It connects to the Gallbladder, opens to the eyes, and is associated with the wood element.
loss of qi with hemorrhage	气随血脱	*Qi Sui Xue Tuo*	qi deserting with the blood	A dangerous dynamic in which qi is lost because it flows out with the blood in severe bleeding.
lower *jiao*	下焦	*Xia Jiao*	lower burner	The lower *jiao* represents the hypogastrium, and includes the functions of the Kidney and the Urinary Bladder.
Lung	肺	*Fei*	lung	The Lung controls breathing and the flow of air, regulates water passages, and dominates the skin and hair. It connects with the Large Intestine, opens to the nose, and is associated with the metal element.
lung abscess	肺痈	*Fei Yong*	pulmonary welling-abscess	A disorder characterized by cough, chest fullness, fever and chills, rapid pulse, dry throat without thirst, foul-smelling sputum, and profuse discharge of sputum. It is generally caused by wind-heat attacking the Lung.
luo (connecting) point	络穴	*Luo Xue*	network point	Known as "connecting" or "vessel" points, these assist communication between the yang external and yin internal channels. Fifteen points in all represent each of the twelve channels and one on each of the front, back and side of the trunk.
malaria	疟疾	*Nue Ji*	malaria	An infectious disorder characterized by alternation of chills, fever and perspiration. This disorder occurs most frequently in summer and fall, and is diagnosed as wind, cold, summer-damp, and damp attacking the *ying* (nutritive) and *wei* (defense) levels.
mammary aggregation	乳癖	*Ru Pi*	mammary aggregation	A breast nodule of variable size, slightly mobile, not painful, not of cold or hot origin, does not cause a change in local skin color, nor erupt or cause ulceration. These form primarily because of Liver qi stagnation.

Terminology	Chinese	Pinyin	Wiseman & Feng	Definition
mammary 'rock'	乳岩	*Ru Yan*	mammary rock	Single or multiple breast nodules similar in size to jujubes, that do not cause pain, itching, redness or heat sensations, and may continue to grow in size. Most common in women past middle age, this is caused by emotional constraint and obstructed flow of Liver and Spleen qi.
metal	金	*Jin*	metal	One of the five elements, metal has inward or contracting movement, represents autumn and harvest, and is associated with the Lung.
middle *jiao*	中焦	*Zhong Jiao*	middle burner	The middle *jiao* represents the epigastrium, and includes the functions of the Spleen and Stomach.
ming men (life gate)	命门	*Ming Men*	life gate	This is key to the overall vitality of the individual. A strong *ming men* (life gate) often indicates that an individual is in great health and will age slowly. A weak *ming men* is often evident in persons who look older than their actual age, and suffer from numerous age-related illnesses.
mu (collecting) point	募穴	*Mu Xue*	alarm point	Commonly referred to as "alarm" or "collection" points, these twelve points individually represent where the qi of a specific internal organ passes on the chest and abdomen.
mumps	痄腮	*Zha Sai*	mumps	An acute infectious disorder commonly seen in children. Clinical presentation includes swelling and pain of the parotid glands, chills and fever, difficulty chewing, and discomfort of the entire body. Most common in winter and spring, it may occur in any season, and is caused by wind-heat (entering the body through the mouth and nose) that becomes blocked in the *shaoyang* channels.
night perspiration	盗汗	*Dao Han*	night sweating	Night perspiration refers to sweating that occurs during sleep, and stops when one awakes. It is an indication of yin deficiency.
over-acting sequence	相乘	*Xiang Cheng*	overwhelming	A concept of *wu xing* (five element) theory that describes a situation in which a controlling element suppresses or reduces the controlled element instead of controlling its growth or activity.
Pericardium	心包	*Xin Bao*	pericardium	The Pericardium is the external covering of the Heart. It functions as the protective barrier of the Heart against pathological factors, and connects with the *San Jiao*.
persistent, indeterminate hunger	嘈杂	*Cao Za*	clamoring stomach	An uncomfortable sensation that mimics pain yet is not painful, that mimics hunger yet the person is not hungry. This condition is usually caused by fire, phlegm accumulation, qi stagnation, or food retention.
perspiration of the palms and soles	手足心汗	*Shou Zhu Xin Han*	sweating in the (heart of the) palms and soles	Profuse perspiration of the hands and feet is an indication of yin deficiency with heat. It is often caused by excessive thinking and worrying that leads to injuries of the Heart and Spleen.

Terminology	Chinese	Pinyin	Wiseman & Feng	Definition
phlegm	痰	*Tan*	phlegm	Phlegm is a by-product formed from water and damp stagnation. The presence of phlegm may obstruct healthy flow and cause illness throughout the body, damaging the Lung, Heart, Stomach, peripheral channels and collaterals, throat and skin.
plum pit syndrome	梅核气	*Mei He Qi*	plum-pit qi	Globus hystericus – the feeling of having a foreign substance obstructing the throat which cannot be expectorated nor swallowed.
po (corporeal soul)	魄	*Po*	corporeal soul	A term that refers to basic human instinct and reaction, such as the ability to smell, taste, see, distinguish between cold and hot, and the ability of the newborn to nurse and feed. The main function of *po*, which resides in the Lung, is to maintain physical awareness in order to react and adapt to the external environment.
post-decoct	后下	*Hou Xia*	add at end	A specific instruction when preparing a decoction, to add specific herbs near the end of the cooking process and then continue cooking the herbs for approximately 5 to 10 additional minutes.
pre-decoct	先煎	*Xian Jian*	predecoct	Instruction to cook a certain herb or herbs first (usually for 30 minutes, but this varies) before adding the rest of the herbs to cook a decoction.
profuse sweating	大汗	*Da Han*	great sweating	Profuse perspiration often leads to depletion of body fluids. It may occur because of excessive heat or yang collapse.
qi	气	*Qi*	qi	Qi represents the vital energy needed for proper functioning and existence of the organs and the body.
qi (energy) level	气分	*Qi Fen*	qi aspect	*Qi* (energy) level refers to the second of four levels of febrile infections. Heat attacking the qi level may affect such organs as the Stomach, Lung, Intestines, Gallbladder and Spleen. Clinical presentations will vary depending on the organ(s) affected.
qi and blood deficiency	气血两虚	*Qi Xue Liang Xu*	dual vacuity of qi and blood	Insufficiency of both qi and blood, which influences basic organ functions more strongly than insufficiency of either one alone.
qi and blood stagnation	气滞血瘀	*Qi Zhi Xue Yu*	qi stagnation and blood stasis	Obstructed flow of both qi and blood.
qi collapse	气陷	*Qi Xian*	qi fall	Severe insufficiency of qi results in collapse of vital functions.
qi deficiency	气虚	*Qi Xu*	qi vacuity	A condition in which insufficient quantity of qi affects body or organ functions.
qi deficiency bleeding	气虚失血	*Qi Xu Shi Xue*	qi vacuity bleeding	Bleeding caused by insufficiency of qi, and its consequent inability to properly guide the flow of blood.

Terminology	Chinese	Pinyin	Wiseman & Feng	Definition
qi lin (qi dysuria)	气淋	*Qi Lin*	qi strangury	A urinary tract disorder characterized by obstructed urinary flow, lower abdominal distention and pain, and green-blue tongue color. It is caused by Liver stagnation leading to obstructed flow of qi and urine.
qi stagnation	气滞	*Qi Zhi*	qi stagnation	Obstructed qi flow in internal organs or peripheral channels and collaterals, caused by a variety of factors, including inappropriate diet, emotional disturbance, environmental factors, or external injuries.
Qi Xue Jin Ye Bian Zheng (Qi, Blood, and Body Fluid Differentiation)	气血津液辨证	*Qi Xue Jin Ye Bian Zheng*	qi, blood and fluids pattern identification	A system of differential diagnosis based on patterns of disharmony of qi, blood, and body fluids.
re bi (heat painful obstruction)	热痹	*Re Bi*	heat impediment	One type of *bi zheng* (painful obstruction syndrome) characterized by local redness, swelling, burning sensations and pain. The development of heat is often caused by prolonged obstruction of the channels and collaterals by wind, cold or damp.
re lin (heat dysuria)	热淋	*Re Lin*	heat strangury	A urinary tract disorder characterized by frequent urination, painful and burning sensations upon urination, yellow urine, muscle cramps and pain in the lower abdomen, and a bitter taste in the mouth. This condition is caused by damp-heat attacking the lower *jiao*.
rebellious qi	气逆	*Qi Ni*	qi counterflow	Rebellious qi is the flow of qi opposite of its normal or appropriate direction, such as the flow of Lung qi upwards, that leads to coughing.
ren (conception) channel	任脉	*Ren Mai*	conception vessel	The confluence of all yin vessels, one of the eight extraordinary vessels. Also known as the "Sea of Yin Qi," it relates to urogenital, gynecological and obstetrical functions.
restless fetus	胎动不安	*Tai Dong Bu An*	stirring fetus	Constant downward movement of the fetus, abdominal pain, sore back, and perhaps bleeding, are generally caused by qi deficiency, blood deficiency, Kidney deficiency, heat in the blood, or external injuries.
rock-like breast abscess	乳石痈	*Ru Shi Yong*	rock-like mammary welling-abscess	A rock-hard breast abscess.
San Jiao	三焦	*San Jiao*	triple burner	The *San Jiao* is not an anatomical organ, but a generalization of different sections of the body compartment. The *San Jiao* is divided into upper, middle and lower sectors.
San Jiao Bian Zheng (Triple Burner Differentiation)	三焦辨证	*San Jiao Bian Zheng*	triple burner pattern identification	A system of differential diagnosis based on locating patterns of disharmony in the upper *jiao*, middle *jiao*, or lower *jiao*.
seven emotions	七情	*Qi Qing*	seven affects	Joy, anger, melancholy, meditation, grief, fear and fright. An excess of any of the seven emotions may create illness.

Terminology	Chinese	Pinyin	Wiseman & Feng	Definition
shang han (cold damage)	伤寒	*Shang Han*	cold damage	A collective term for disorders caused by cold externally-contracted pathogens, diagnosed and treated via *Liu Jing Bian Zheng* (Six Stages Differentiation).
Shang Han Lun (Discussion of Cold-Induced Disorders)	伤寒论	*Shang Han Lun*	On Cold Damage	A text written by Zhang Zhong-Jing in Eastern Han (see bibliography) that focused on diagnosis and treatment of cold-induced disorders. The basic principles of diagnosis and treatment are based on *Liu Jing Bian Zheng* (Six Stages Differentiation).
shaoyang	少阳	*Shao Yang*	lesser yang	Third of six stages in the paradigm of yin and yang. This term identifies the degree of pathology of disease according to the *Shang Han Lun* (Cold-Induced Disorders) text. It also describes the level attributed to the Gallbladder and *San Jiao* channels that travel throughout the body.
shaoyin	少阴	*Shao Yin*	lesser yin	The fifth of six stages in the paradigm of yin and yang. This term describes the degree of pathology of disease according to the *Shang Han Lun* (Cold-Induced Disorders) text. It also identifies the level attributed to the Heart and Kidney channels that travel throughout the body.
shen (spirit)	神	*Shen*	spirit	A term that refers to the entire presentation of the human being, including energy levels, the state of consciousness, and ability to think and reason. Because it is housed in the Heart, disorders affecting the Heart may also lead to disturbance of the *shen*.
shi lin (stone dysuria)	石淋	*Shi Lin*	stone strangury	A urinary tract disorder characterized by lower abdominal tightness and pain, the presence of sandy particles (and possibly blood) in the urine, difficult and painful urination, or sudden termination of the stream of urine. This is caused by damp-heat attacking the lower *jiao*, drying fluids, and leading to the formation of stones.
shi-re lin (damp-heat dysuria)	湿热淋	*Shi Re Lin*	damp-heat strangury	A urinary tract disorder characterized by frequent urination, painful and burning sensations upon urination, yellow urine, muscle cramps and pain in the lower abdomen, and a bitter taste in the mouth, all caused by damp-heat attacking the lower *jiao*. Other symptoms of damp-heat may include nausea, vomiting, constipation, a yellow, greasy tongue coat, and slippery, rapid pulse.
shivering perspiration	战津液汗	*Zhan Han*	shivering	Shivering perspiration is a phenomenon that occurs when the body fights against pathogenic factors. The prognosis is good if the patient has a normal temperature after perspiring. The prognosis is poor if the patient becomes fidgety and irritable after perspiring.
shu (stream) point	输穴	*Shu Xue*	stream point	Commonly referred to as "stream" or "transporting" points, these are usually located near the wrists or ankles and suggest that the flow of qi is now of sufficient quantity to carry out these functions.

Terminology	Chinese	Pinyin	Wiseman & Feng	Definition
shu (transport) point	俞穴	*Shu Xue*	transport point	Known as "associated points of the back," or "transporting" points, these are twelve points on the upper and lower back where the qi of the internal organs passes. Each represents an organ.
Small Intestine	小肠	*Xiao Chang*	small intestine	Connecting to the Stomach and Large Intestine, the Small Intestine absorbs nutrients from food.
sores	疮疡	*Chuang Yang*	sore	An inclusive term for skin lesions, boils, ulcers, carbuncles and furuncles.
Spleen	脾	*Pi*	spleen	The Spleen governs the transportation and transformation of food, controls blood, and dominates muscle. It connects with the Stomach, opens to the mouth, and represents the earth element.
spontaneous sweating	自汗	*Zi Han*	spontaneous sweating	Spontaneous perspiration, especially after only mild physical activities, is an indication of *wei* (defensive) *qi* deficiency.
summer heat	暑	*Shu*	summerheat	Summer heat is a yang pathogenic factor that occurs only in the summer, and is comprised of both heat and damp characteristics, including upward direction and dispersion. Clinical presentations of summer heat include excessive perspiration, thirst, shortness of breath, fatigue, elevated body temperature, heavy sensations in the extremities, poor appetite, and a feeling of congestion in the chest.
sweaty head	头汗	*Tou Han*	sweating head	Head perspiration generally arises from heat affecting the upper and middle *jiaos*, possibly accompanied by irritability, thirst, a yellow tongue coating, and a rapid pulse.
taiyang	太阳	*Tai Yang*	greater yang	First of six stages in the paradigm of yin and yang, identifying the degree of pathology of disease according to the *Shang Han Lun* (Cold-Induced Disorders) text. It also names the level attributed to the Small Intestine and Urinary Bladder channels that travel throughout the body.
taiyin	太阴	*Tai Yin*	greater yin	The fourth of six stages in the paradigm of yin and yang. This term describes the degree of pathology of disease according to the *Shang Han Lun* (Cold-Induced Disorders) text. It also identifies the level attributed to the Spleen and Lung channels that travel throughout the body.
tan yin (phlegm retention)	痰饮	*Tan Yin*	phlegm-rheum	Phlegm retention caused by accumulation of water and dampness, this may occur at various organs and tissues in the body, leading to different illnesses and clinical presentations.
tong bi (extremely painful obstruction)	痛痹	*Tong Bi*	painful impediment	One type of *bi zheng* (painful obstruction syndrome) characterized by cold. Similar to cold that is stationary and constricting, *tong bi* is distinguished by severe pain at a fixed location. This type of pain intensifies with exposure to cold, and is relieved by exposure to warmth.

Terminology	Chinese	Pinyin	Wiseman & Feng	Definition
toxin	毒	*Du*	toxin	A toxin is any substance that is potentially harmful to the body. 'Toxin' also describes a pathogenic factor that may cause illness either on the exterior or in the interior of the body. Clinical manifestations of toxicity include pus, abscesses, sores, ulcerations, swelling and inflammation.
tuo zheng (abandoned syndrome)	脱证	*Tuo Zheng*	desertion pattern	Characterized by profuse sweating, cold extremities, open mouth and closed eyes, and urinary incontinence, this condition occurs when there is severe exhaustion of yin, yang, qi and blood.
upper *jiao*	上焦	*Shang Jiao*	upper burner	The upper *jiao* represents the chest, and includes functions of the Heart and the Lung.
Urinary Bladder	膀胱	*Pang Guang*	bladder	The Urinary Bladder stores and excretes urine.
uroschesis	癃闭	*Long Bi*	dribbling urinary block	A disorder in which there is little or no urination, brought about by any of the following: heat in the Urinary Bladder, Kidney yang deficiency, qi deficiency, qi stagnation, or body fluid deficiencies.
wan bi (stubborn painful obstruction)	顽痹	*Wan Bi*	insensitive impediment	One type of *bi zheng* (painful obstruction syndrome) that generally occurs after chronic or repetitive injuries to the same areas, causing stiffness, numbness, and lack of mobility.
water	水	*Shui*	water	Water is one of the five elements, associated with winter, with the Kidney, downward movement, and the ability to store or accumulate.
water and fluid stagnation	水液停滞	*Shui Ye Ting Zhi*		Obstructed flow of water and thick fluids in the body.
wei (atrophy) syndrome	痿证	*Wei Zheng*	wilting pattern	A condition involving decreasing muscle mass and physical strength of the extremities, especially the legs; generally caused by the concurrent presence of excess and deficiency factors.
wei (defense) level	卫分	*Wei Fen*	defense aspect	The first of four levels affected by febrile infections. Heat attacking the *wei* (defense) level is characterized by disorders of the Lung, with such symptoms as fever, headache, dry mouth, thirst, cough, and sore throat, and a red tongue, and superficial, rapid pulse.
wei (defensive) *qi*	卫气	*Wei Qi*	defense qi	A type of yang qi responsible for warming the exterior, nourishing the skin and muscles, circulating under the skin to prevent invasion by external pathogenic factors, and controlling the skin pores and perspiration. It is generated by the Spleen and Stomach from the essence of food, controlled by the Lung, and resides in the upper *jiao*.
wei bi (atrophic painful obstruction)	痿痹	*Wei Bi*	wilting impediment	One type of *bi zheng* (painful obstruction syndrome) caused by deficiency of the Liver and Kidney, with such presentations as atrophy, weakness and pain of the muscles and bones.

Terminology	Chinese	Pinyin	Wiseman & Feng	Definition
Wei Qi Ying Xue Bian Zheng (Defensive, Qi, Nutritive, Blood Differentiation)	卫气营血辨证	*Wei Qi Ying Xue Bian Zheng*	four aspect pattern identification	A system of differential diagnosis based on patterns of disharmony found in the *wei* (defense) level, *qi* (energy) level, *ying* (nutritive) level or *xue* (blood) level.
wen bing (warm diseases)	温病	*Wen Bing*	warm disease	Acute illnesses caused by externally contracted heat factors: diagnosed and treated based on *Wei Qi Ying Xue Bian Zheng* (Defensive, Qi, Nutritive, Blood Differentiation) and *San Jiao Bian Zheng* (Triple Burner Differentiation).
wheezing and dyspnea	哮喘	*Xiao Chuan*	wheezing and panting	A disorder characterized by wheezing, dyspnea and hurried respiration.
wind	风	*Feng*	wind	Wind is a pathogenic factor that attacks the body through the pores. Wind is a yang pathogenic factor characterized by upward, outward dispersion. Clinical presentation of exterior wind includes headache, nasal obstruction, sore throat, aversion to wind and sweating.
wind rash	风疹	*Feng Zhen*	wind papules	An infectious skin disorder commonly seen during winter and spring in children under five years of age. Generally caused by wind-heat attack, it is characterized by itching, rashes and wheals of various sizes.
wood	木	*Mu*	wood	One of the five elements, wood represents the expansive energy of Spring, moving outward in all directions, and is associated with the Liver.
wu shu (five transport) points	五输穴	*Wu Shu Xue*	five transport points	Located below the knees and elbows, these points represent the growth of qi from small to large volume. Their name suggests images of the flow of water. It starts with only a small quantity in a *jing* (well), gushes out into a *ying* (spring), flows from shallow to deep as a *shu* (stream), traverses like a *jing* (river) through the continent, and finally unites with the *he* (sea).
wu xin re (five-center heat)	五心热	*Wu Xin Re*	vexing heat in the five hearts	A condition characterized by yin-deficiency heat in which there is a warm sensation at the center of the palms, the soles and the chest.
xi (cleft) point	郄穴	*Xi Xue*	cleft point	"Accumulating" or "cleft" points represent the holes or crevices where circulating qi accumulates. There are a total of sixteen such points, one for each of the twelve regular channels, as well as the *yangqiao, yinqiao, yangwei* and *yinwei* channels.
xiao ke (wasting and thirsting) syndrome	消渴	*Xiao Ke*	dispersion-thirst	A pathological condition characterized by increased intake of water and food, increased frequency of urination, and decreased body weight.
xing bi (mobile painful obstruction)	行痹	*Xing Bi*	moving impediment	One type of *bi zheng* (painful obstruction syndrome) caused by wind attacking the body. Similar to wind that is light and mobile, xing bi is characterized by pain in the upper body, specifically pain that travels from one area to another.

Terminology	Chinese	Pinyin	Wiseman & Feng	Definition
xiong bi (painful obstruction of the chest)	胸痹	*Xiong Bi*	chest impediment	Characterized by feelings of chest congestion, pain and discomfort, this condition is usually caused by factors such as cold excess, yang deficiency, or phlegm stagnation.
xue (blood) level	血分	*Xue Fen*	blood aspect	*Xue* (blood) level refers to the fourth level of febrile infections. Heat attacking the *xue* level is characterized by disorders of the Heart and Liver, with such symptoms as high fever, anger, mania, various types of bleeding, delirium, convulsions and clenched jaws.
xue bi (blood painful obstruction)	血痹	*Xue Bi*	blood impediment	One type of *bi zheng* (painful obstruction syndrome) that is related to blood. Dull pain may be caused by blood deficiency and the inability to nourish the tendons and bones. Sharp pain is often related to blood stagnation blocking the channels and collaterals.
xue lin (bloody dysuria)	血淋	*Xue Lin*	blood strangury	A urinary tract disorder characterized by the presence of blood or blood clots in the urine, and burning sensations and pain during urination. Accompanying symptoms may include fatigue, back pain, a pale red tongue, and a thready, rapid pulse. This condition is caused by damp-heat attacking the lower *jiao*, leading to bleeding and obstructed flow of qi and urine.
yang	阳	*Yang*	yang	Yang is the complement to and opposite of yin. Anatomically, it represents the upper, posterior and exterior parts of the body. Physiologically, it represents body functioning, such as the energy level, rate of metabolism, and state of awareness. Pathologically, it represents disharmony or imbalance of body organs.
yangming	阳明	*Yang Ming*	yang brightness	Second of the six stages in the paradigm of yin and yang, this term describes the degree of pathology of disease according to the *Shang Han Lun* (Cold-Induced Disorders) text. It also identifies the level given the Stomach and Large Intestine channels that travel throughout the body.
yangqiao (movement) channel	阳跷脉	*Yang Qiao Mai*	yang springing vessel	Another of the eight extraordinary vessels, this one pairs with *yinqiao* to maintain proper sleep cycles and control movement and balance.
yangwei (linking) channel	阳维脉	*Yang Wei Mai*	yang linking vessel	Of the eight extraordinary vessels, this one dominates the exterior in cooperation with *yinwei*, to balance yin and yang in the four extremities.
ye (thick body fluid)	液	*Ye*	humor	An inclusive term that describes body fluids of higher density, such as the fluid that lubricates the joints and moistens the bone marrow.
yi (intellect)	意	*Yi*	intellect	The ability to think, study, memorize, focus, understand, and all other cognitive activities. It resides in the Spleen. Therefore, excessive use of *yi* may consume the Spleen, and deficiency of the Spleen may interfere with the optimal performance of *yi*.

Terminology	Chinese	Pinyin	Wiseman & Feng	Definition
yin	阴	*Yin*	yin	Yin is the complement to and opposite of yang. Anatomically, it represents the lower, anterior and interior parts of the body. Physiologically, it represents the substances of the body, such as blood, sweat, saliva and body fluids. Pathologically, it represents the disharmony or imbalance of body organs.
yin (invisible phlegm)	饮	*Yin*	rheum	*Yin* (invisible phlegm) is the by-product formed from stagnation of water and dampness. *Yin* is the less viscous form of *tan* (phlegm).
ying (nutritive) level	营分	*Ying Fen*	construction aspect	The *ying* (nutritive) level refers to the third of four levels of febrile infections. Heat attacking the *ying* level is characterized by disorders of the Heart, with such symptoms as fever, thirst, irritability, delirium, red tongue and thready, rapid pulse.
ying (spring) point	荥穴	*Ying Xue*	spring point	"Gushing" or "spring" points are located in distal parts of the body; their name suggests that qi has begun to flow in larger quantity.
yinqiao (movement) channel	阴跷脉	*Yin Qiao Mai*	yin springing vessel	Another of the eight extraordinary vessels; see *yangqiao*.
yinwei (linking) channel	阴维脉	*Yin Wei Mai*	yin linking vessel	Another of the eight extraordinary vessels: in cooperation with *yangwei*, this one dominates the interior; to balance yin and yang in the four extremities.
yuan (source) point	原穴	*Yuan Xue*	source point	Known as "source" points, these are locations to which the qi of the organs flows and is retained. There are twelve such points, each representing a channel and an organ.
yuan (source) *qi*	原气	*Yuan Qi*	source qi	The most basic and most important qi in the body, *yuan* (source) *qi* is derived pre-natally from the *jing* (essence) of one's parents, and post-natally from the essence of food. It is distributed throughout the body to maintain health and well-being.
zang (solid organ)	脏	*Zang*	viscus	Solid organs of the body, including the Heart, Lung, Spleen, Liver and Kidney.
zang fu	脏腑	*Zang Fu*	bowels and viscera	The general term for the five *zang* (solid) and six *fu* (hollow) organs.
Zang Fu Bian Zheng (Organ Pattern Differentiation)	脏腑辨证	*Zang Fu Bian Zheng*	organ pattern identification	A system of differential diagnosis based on patterns of disharmony of *zang* (solid) organs and *fu* (hollow) organs.
zang zao (dry organ) disorder	脏燥	*Zang Zao*	visceral agitation	In middle-aged to geriatric women, this disorder is characterized by symptomology such as emotional instability, mental confusion, crying, episodes of extreme sadness or happiness, and increased sensitivity to stimulus.

Terminology	Chinese	Pinyin	Wiseman & Feng	Definition
zheng (upright) *qi*	正气	*Zheng Qi*	right qi	A term that summarizes the positive strength generated by healthy functioning of the organs. In comparison to the pathogenic factors, *zheng* (upright) *qi* also represents one's immunity.
zhi (will-power)	志	*Zhi*	mind	A term that encompasses will-power and memory. Stored by the Kidney, *zhi* controls drive, determination, motivation, memory and will-power.
zhong (central) *qi*	中气	*Zhong Qi*	center qi	The qi of the middle *jiao* represents the healthy functioning of the Spleen and Stomach to transport and transform food and nutrients.
zhong feng (wind stroke)	中风	*Zhong Feng*	wind stroke	An acute disorder of semi- or un-consciousness, deviation of the eyes or mouth, hemiparalysis, and difficulty with speech. The cause of the illness is predominantly wind, but this may be accompanied by blood deficiency, phlegm, fire, or other pathogens.
zhou bi (generalized painful obstruction)	周痹	*Zhou Bi*	generalized impediment	One type of *bi zheng* (painful obstruction syndrome) characterized by generalized pain that also affects the bones and joints.
zhuo bi (fixed painful obstruction)	着痹	*Zhuo Bi*	fixed impediment	One type of *bi zheng* (painful obstruction syndrome) that often occurs when damp affects specific, fixed areas. Similar to dampness that is heavy and sinking, *zhuo bi* is characterized by pain and swelling in the lower extremities.
zong (essential) *qi*	宗气	*Zong Qi*	ancestral qi	Zong (essential) *qi* is derived from air taken in by the Lung, and nutrients absorbed by the Spleen and Stomach. It functions to maintain proper ventilation of the Lung and circulation of the Heart.

About the Authors and Contributors

Authors:

John K. Chen, PhD, PharmD, OMD, LAc

Dr. John Chen actively participates in education, research and the frontiers of contemporary application of herbal medicine. In addition to developing professional continuing education seminars and serving as a senior lecturer through the widely-respected Lotus Institute of Integrative Medicine, Dr. Chen speaks at seminars and conferences for universities and local, state, national and international educational and professional organizations. A professor at Yo San University of Traditional Chinese Medicine, Emperor's College of Traditional Oriental Medicine, and the University of Southern California School of Pharmacy, Dr. Chen is also a member of the Herbal Medicine Committee for the American Association of Oriental Medicine (AAOM) and an herbal consultant for the California State Oriental Medicine Association (CSOMA). A recognized authority on Chinese herbal medicine and western (allopathic) pharmacology, Dr. Chen has written extensively on Oriental medicine and alternative complementary/integrative medicine for professional publications, journals and texts, drawing on his wealth of specialty post-graduate training and experience in mainland China in herbology as applied in internal medicine, and on his doctoral degrees from the University of Southern California (USC) School of Pharmacy and South Baylo University of Oriental Medicine. An editorial board member for the peer-reviewed journal of the American Academy of Medical Acupuncture (AAMA), *Medical Acupuncture*, John Chen was also a board member of the 1999 *Los Angeles Times* Festival Honorary Committee and speaker on Herbal Medicine for the City of Los Angeles First Annual Festival of Health. Appearing in the Discovery Channel 1999 six-hour documentary on alternative and complementary medicine, Dr. Chen served as the expert resource on Traditional Chinese Medicine. He also was guest speaker on herb-drug interactions in 1998 for the annual USC Bergen Brunswig convention, during which he addressed over 400 pharmacists and medical doctors. Dr. Chen maintains his consulting practice in Southern California.

Tina T. Chen, MS, LAc

Tina Chen is an active and respected educator in Oriental medicine and Chinese herbal medicine. In addition to lecturing on TCM Gynecology and Cosmetology across North America through the widely-respected Lotus Institute of Integrative Medicine, Ms. Chen is active on the faculty of South Baylo University of Oriental Medicine and has been an active contributor to professional journals and publications. She has served as Southern California Chair of the Education Committee for the California State Oriental Medical Association (CSOMA), and as an examiner for the California State License Exam for acupuncturists, and from 1996-2001 maintained private practice of acupuncture and herbal medicine through Chen's Clinic in La Puente, California. Her teaching and consulting is grounded in extensive post-graduate training in herbal medicine, TCM gynecology and cosmetology in numerous hospitals in mainland China. This included concentrated training sponsored by the World Health Organization (WHO) in Guang-An-Men Hospital of Traditional Chinese Medicine, Beijing, in the People's Republic of China, specializing in internal medicine, acupuncture and gynecology; also intensive clinical training in internal medicine and gynecology at First Tien-Jin Hospital, People's Republic of China; and at An-Hui Hospital, People's Republic of China, advanced training in internal medicine. Tina Chen's expertise in translation includes serving as translation specialist for the International Association of Integrating East-West Medicine from 1996-2000, the 1996 Third Annual International Acupuncture and Massage Conference sponsored by the Acupuncture and Massage Institute of America, and the California State Association of Oriental Medicine (CSOMA) in 1990. Licensed by the Acupuncture Board in California, Tina Chen also holds certification from the World Health Organization in internal medicine and gynecology. A graduate of South Baylo University of Oriental Medicine, she also earned a B.A. from the University of California at Irvine School of Humanities, in East Asian Language and Literature. She maintains a consulting practice in Southern California.

About the Authors and Contributors

Laraine Crampton, MPW, MLA, MATCM, LAc

Active on the faculty of Yo San University of Traditional Chinese Medicine since 1995, Laraine Crampton practices Traditional Chinese Medicine (TCM) through her private practice in Santa Monica, California. From July 1999 through late 2000, she was the charter Traditional Chinese Medicine Specialist in practice and patient education lecturer for B'shert Integrative Oncology Services (BIOS), the integrative medicine center of California Hematology Oncology Medical Group in Los Angeles. For the Torrance Memorial Medical Center in Torrance, California, Ms. Crampton served as a speaker and consultant on Traditional Chinese Medicine in integrative medicine settings through the Advantage public education program in 2000 and 2001. She received her graduate degree in TCM from Yo San University, and holds board licenses in Acupuncture and Herbology through the State of California Acupuncture Board and the National Certification Commission for Acupuncture and Oriental Medicine. Ms. Crampton has long been active as a writer and editor. Her previous publication experience includes having served as consultant, researcher, writer and editor for Affinity Communications in Los Angeles, contributing editor for Pacific Rim Business Journal, editor for the University of Southern California's Student Health Center publications, and ghostwriter for medical doctors publishing in journals such as the *Annals of Plastic Surgery*. Former Adjunct Professor in writing and Business Communications at the University of Southern California, Ms. Crampton also reported for the Los Angeles *Weekly* and National Public Radio's *Living on Earth*, as well as co-producing, co-writing and editing KCRW's award-winning *Arts/L.A.*, and serving as a founding producer for the respected daily public affairs broadcast *Which Way, L.A.?*

Editors

Vanessa G. Au, LAc, DC

Dr. Au received her Doctorate of Chiropractic from Los Angeles College of Chiropractic in 1998, and Master of Science in Acupuncture and Oriental Medicine from South Baylo University in 1999. She maintains a private practice in Acupuncture and Chiropractic in San Jose, California.

Colleen Burke, DOM, LAc, Dipl Ac & CH

Dr. Burke has written and/or contributed to articles on Chinese herbal medicine in a variety of publications. Specializing in environmental illness, immune dysfunction, arthritis, women's health, and the mind-body connection, Dr. Burke maintains a private practice in Santa Fe, New Mexico.

Christian DellaCorte, PhD

Dr. Christian DellaCorte is neurochemist with an interest in the pharmacological basis of Chinese herbs. She graduated from the University of Southern California (USC) and received training in herbology from Emperor's College in California. She currently teaches cellular and biomedical physiology and participates in research in the BioEngineering Department at the California Institute of Technology, Pasadena, California.

Joerg Fritschi, MD

Dr. Fritschi graduated from the University of Basel School of Medicine in 1981. He also received extensive training in traditional Chinese medicine, studying acupuncture at the Donghzhimen World Health Organization Collaborating College in Beijing, the People's Republic of China, Chinese herbology at Five Branches Institute in Santa Cruz, CA, USA, and Scalp Acupuncture (with Prof. Ming Qing Zhu) in La Jolla, CA, and Shanghai, PRC. He has served as a board member of the Swiss Society of TCM (Herbology), vice-president of the Swiss Society of Internal Medicine, expert member at the Swissmedic Study Group for the Regulation of Asian Herbs, and board member of the Swiss Society of Internal Medicine. Dr. Fritschi has an integrative medical practice in Pfeffingen, Switzerland.

About the Authors and Contributors

Steve Given, LAc, Dipl Ac
Steve Given holds a master's degree in traditional Oriental medicine from Emperor's College of Traditional Oriental Medicine. He is administrator and a faculty member of the Bastyr Center for Natural Health and a faculty member at Bastyr University. He is a site visitor for the Accreditation Commission for Acupuncture and Oriental Medicine, and Secretary of the Council of Colleges of Acupuncture and Oriental Medicine. Prior to his appointment at Bastyr, Given was Director of Clinical Education and a faculty member in western sciences at Yo San University of Traditional Chinese Medicine and specialized in addiction education and treatment. Steve Given resides in Seattle, Washington.

Glenn Grossman, MS, LAc, Dipl Ac & CH
Mr. Grossman has a bachelor's degree with honors and a master's degree from Samra University of Oriental Medicine. After graduation, Mr. Grossman did extensive training in TCM at Anhui College of Traditional Chinese Medicine and the China Beijing Acupuncture Institute. He is currently affiliated with the American Association of Oriental Medicine (AAOM) and Michigan Association of Acupuncture and Oriental Medicine (MAAOM). Mr. Grossman has a private practice in Okemos, Michigan, where he also teaches Herbology for Healthcare Professionals through the nursing program at Lansing Community College.

Lily Huang, LAc
Ms. Huang graduated from the University of California, Los Angeles with magna cum laude honors. She graduates from South Baylo University of Oriental Medicine in 2003, and is a licensed acupuncturist candidate living in Los Angeles.

Steven M. Jarsky LAc, Dipl Ac & CH
Steven Jarsky, Los Angeles-based acupuncturist and herbalist, specializes in internal medicine. Licensed in acupuncture and Chinese herbology by the state of California, board certified through the National Certification Commission of Acupuncture and Oriental Medicine (NCCAOM), he has been working as a Chinese herbalist since 1995, and graduated from Yo San University of Traditional Chinese Medicine with highest honors in a Master's degree in TCM.

Jing-Lih Lily Ko, LAc
Ms. Ko is a PhD candidate in the Acupuncture and Oriental Medicine Program of Yuing University in Compton, California. She is currently in private practice in Temple City, California.

Anita Chen Marshall, Pharm.D., MS, Dipl Ac, LAc
Dr. Anita Chen Marshall practices acupuncture and herbal medicine at the Sequoia Healing Center in Alameda, California. She holds a BS in Pharmacy from the University of Washington and a Pharm. D. from the University of the Pacific, and a Masters degree in Oriental Medicine from the Academy of Chinese Culture and Health Science. Dr. Marshall has more than 20 years of experience in all areas of pharmacy, including serving as Director of Pharmacy at a hospital. Nationally certified in both acupuncture and herbology, she is devoted to using her training and experience in helping to build the bridge between Eastern and Western medicine.

Cathy McNease, Dipl CH
Cathy McNease holds a Diplomat in Chinese Herbology from the National Certification Commission of Acupuncture and Oriental Medicine (NCCAOM), a B.S. in Biology and Psychology from Western Michigan University and two Master Herbalist certificates from Emerson College of Herbology in Canada and East-West Course in Herbology. She has co-authored two books, *Tao of Nutrition* and *101 Vegetarian Delights*. Currently on the faculty at Santa Barbara College of Oriental Medicine, Ms. McNease is chairperson of the herbal department and Director of the Herbal Clinic. She is also on the faculties of Emperor's College of

About the Authors and Contributors

Traditional Oriental Medicine and Yo San University of Traditional Chinese Medicine. In addition to her teaching and professional activities, Cathy McNease maintains a Chinese herbal pharmacy business, *Best Blends Herbs.*

Lawrence Miller, LAc, Dipl Ac & CH
Lawrence Miller specializes in cancer recovery and detoxification, as well as orthopedic pain management in his practice in Santa Monica, California. A graduate of Yo San University of TCM, Miller is also a Qualified Medical Evaluator and acupuncture detoxification specialist.

William R. Morris, DOM, LAc
Dr. Morris is Dean of Clinical Education at Emperor's College of Traditional Oriental Medicine and serves as a board member for the American Association of Oriental Medicine (AAOM). He has developed expertise in a subspecialty in pulse diagnosis since 1980, beginning with Nan Jing methods and subsequent work in the Ting family lineage of John H.F. Shen. A published author and teacher, Dr. Morris is also an editorial consultant for Elsevier Science on texts related to Chinese Medicine. His private practice is in Santa Monica, California.

Minh Thanh Nguyen, LAc
Ms. Nguyen graduated summa cum laude from the University of California, Riverside in 1994, and received her Master of Arts in English Literature from Cornell University in 1998. She studied naturopathic medicine at Bastyr University in 2001-2002, and is currently studying acupuncture and Oriental medicine at South Baylo University of Oriental Medicine in Los Angeles.

Daoshing Ni, DOM, PhD, LAc, Dipl CH
Co-founder and president of Yo San University of Traditional Chinese Medicine, Dr. Ni is well known and respected for his specialty in reproductive and gynecological medicine, and is a member of the American Society for Reproductive Medicine, the Pacific Coast Fertility Society, and the National Academy of Acupuncture and Oriental Medicine. He has served as an examiner for the California Acupuncture Committee and in development of the Chinese Herbology Exam for the National Certification Commission of Acupuncture and Oriental Medicine (NCCAOM). He pursued post-doctoral training in Beijing and Nanjing, and taught at Emperor's College and Samra University before becoming president of Yo San University. Author of numerous articles, books and videos on TCM, qigong, endometriosis and infertility, Dr. Ni maintains a full-time practice in Santa Monica, California.

Ray Rubio, LAc
Ray Rubio co-founded the Traditional Healing Arts Center in Los Angeles, and is on the staff of the Toluca Lake Health Center, a busy out-patient medical clinic. He serves on the academic and clinical faculties of Emperor's College of Traditional Oriental Medicine in Santa Monica.

Index

Words in **bold** indicate **primary herb** and **chapter names**.
Page numbers in **bold** indicate entries in the **Appendices**.
Page numbers in *italics* indicate entries in the *Glossary*.

Index

Index

Index

Index

Index

Index

Index

Index

Index

INDEX In

Index

Index

Index

Index

Index

Index

INDEX
In

Index

Index

Index

Index

Index

Index

Index

Index

Index

Index

Index

Index

Index

Index

Index

Index

INDEX
In

Index

Index

Index

Index

Index

Index

Index

Index

Index

Index

Index

Index

Index

Index

Index

Index

Index

Index

Index

Index

Index

Index

Index

Index

Index

Index

INDEX

In

Index

Index

Index

Index

Index

Index

Index

Index

Index

Index

Index

Index

Index

INDEX In

Index

Index

Index

Index

Index

Notes